BEHRMAN'S **Neonatal-perinatal medicine**

BEHRMAN'S Neonatal-perinatal medicine

DISEASES OF THE FETUS AND INFANT

EDITED BY

AVROY A. FANAROFF
M.B., F.R.C.P. (Edinburgh), D.C.H.

Professor of Pediatrics, Case Western Reserve University School of Medicine, University Hospitals (Rainbow Babies and Childrens Hospital), Cleveland, Ohio

RICHARD J. MARTIN
M.B., F.R.A.C.P., F.R.C.P. (Canada)

Assistant Professor of Pediatrics, Case Western Reserve University School of Medicine, University Hospitals (Rainbow Babies and Childrens Hospital), Cleveland, Ohio

ASSOCIATE EDITOR

IRWIN R. MERKATZ, M.D.

Professor and Chairman, Department of Obstetrics and Gynecology, Albert Einstein College of Medicine, New York, New York

THIRD EDITION

with **642** illustrations

The C. V. Mosby Company

ST. LOUIS • TORONTO • LONDON   1983

MOSBY

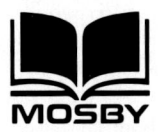

A TRADITION OF PUBLISHING EXCELLENCE

Editor: Karen Berger
Assistant editor: Theresa Van Schaik
Manuscript editors: Marjorie L. Sanson, Susan K. Hume
Book design: Jeanne Bush
Production: Carol O'Leary, Judy England, Jeanne A. Gulledge

THIRD EDITION

Copyright © 1983 by The C.V. Mosby Company

All rights reserved. No part of this publication may be reproduced, stored in a retrieval system, or transmitted, in any form or by any means, electronic, mechanical, photocopying, recording, or otherwise, without prior written permission from the publisher.

Previous editions copyrighted 1973, 1977

Printed in the United States of America

The C.V. Mosby Company
11830 Westline Industrial Drive, St. Louis, Missouri 63141

Library of Congress Cataloging in Publication Data

Main entry under title:

Behrman's Neonatal-perinatal medicine.

  Rev. ed. of: Neonatal-perinatal medicine /
edited by Richard E. Behrman. 2nd ed. 1977.
  Includes bibliographies and index.
  1. Infants (Newborn)—Diseases. 2. Fetus—
Diseases. I. Behrman, Richard E., 1931-
II. Fanaroff, Avroy A. III. Martin, Richard J.
IV. Neonatal-perinatal medicine. [DNLM: 1. Fetal
diseases. 2. Infant, Newborn, Diseases. WS
420 N439]
RJ254.B453   1983   618.92′01   82-6371
ISBN 0-8016-0580-6   AACR2

TS/CB/B 9 8 7 6 5 4 3 2 1   01/C/009

Contributors

GARY M. AMUNDSON, M.D.
Assistant Professor, Alberta Children's Hospital, University of Calgary, Department of Pediatrics, Calgary, Alberta, Canada

THOMAS L. ANDERSON, M.D.
Assistant Professor of Pediatrics, Department of Pediatrics, University of South Alabama College of Medicine, Mobile, Alabama

JACOB V. ARANDA, M.D., Ph.D.
Associate Professor, Pediatrics, Pharmacology and Therapeutics; Director of Developmental Pharmacology and Perinatal Research Unit, McGill University, Montreal Children's Hospital, Montreal, Quebec, Canada

TOM P. BARDEN, M.D.
Professor and Chairman, Department of Obstetrics and Gynecology, University of Cincinnati, Cincinnati, Ohio

RICHARD E. BEHRMAN, M.D.
Professor, Department of Pediatrics, and Dean, Case Western Reserve University School of Medicine, Cleveland, Ohio

KURT BENIRSCHKE, M.D.
Professor of Pathology and Reproductive Medicine, Pathology Department and Reproductive Medicine Department, University of California, San Diego; Director of Research, San Diego Zoo, La Jolla, California

JAY BERNSTEIN, M.D.
Director, Department of Anatomic Pathology, William Beaumont Hospital, Royal Oak, Michigan

THOMAS A. BLUMENFELD, M.D.
Director of Medical Affairs and Associate Professor of Clinical Pathology, Presbyterian Hospital, Columbia University College of Physicians and Surgeons, New York, New York

JEFFREY L. BLUMER, Ph.D., M.D.
Assistant Professor, Departments of Pediatrics and Pharmacology, Case Western Reserve University School of Medicine, Cleveland, Ohio

ALFRED W. BRANN, Jr., M.D.
Professor, Departments of Pediatrics and Gynecology/Obstetrics, Emory University, Atlanta, Georgia

PATRICK J. BRYAN, M.B., F.R.C.R.
Associate Professor of Radiology, Case Western Reserve University, Cleveland, Ohio

LUIS A. CABAL, M.D.
Assistant Professor of Pediatrics, University of Southern California School of Medicine; Director of Newborn Intensive Care Unit, Los Angeles, California

DEBORAH L. CALLANAN, M.D.
Pediatric Intensive Care Fellow and Resident, Baylor College of Medicine, Houston, Texas

ROBERT K. DANISH, M.D.
Assistant Professor of Pediatrics, Case Western Reserve University School of Medicine; Pediatric Endocrinologist, Cleveland Metropolitan General Hospital, Cleveland, Ohio

HAROLD M. DICK, M.D.
Clinical Professor of Orthopaedic Surgery, Department of Orthopaedics, Columbia University College of Physicians and Surgeons; Chief of Pediatric Orthopaedic Surgery, Babies Hospital, Columbia-Presbyterian Medical Center, New York, New York

LEROY J. DIERKER, M.D.
Assistant Professor, Department of Obstetrics and Gynecology, Cleveland Metropolitan General Hospital, Case Western Reserve University, Cleveland, Ohio

JOHN M. DRISCOLL, Jr., M.D.
Associate Professor of Clinical Pediatrics; Director of Neonatal ICU, Premature and Normal Nurseries, Department of Pediatrics, Columbia University College of Physicians and Surgeons, New York, New York

METHOD A. DUCHON, M.D.
Assistant Professor, Department of Reproductive Biology, Case Western Reserve University, Cleveland, Ohio

CHESTER M. EDELMANN, Jr., M.D.
Professor of Pediatrics and Associate Dean for Clinical Affairs, Albert Einstein College of Medicine; Attending Pediatrician, Bronx Municipal Hospital Center, Montefiore Hospital Medical Center, and Hospital of the Albert Einstein College of Medicine, Bronx, New York

NANCY B. ESTERLY, M.D.
Head, Division of Dermatology, Department of Pediatrics, The Children's Memorial Hospital; Professor of Pediatrics and Dermatology, Northwestern University Medical School, Chicago, Illinois

AVROY A. FANAROFF, M.B., F.R.C.P. (Edinburgh), D.C.H.
Professor of Pediatrics, Case Western Reserve University School of Medicine, University Hospitals (Rainbow Babies and Childrens Hospital), Cleveland, Ohio

PHILIP M. FARRELL, M.D., Ph.D.
Professor, Department of Pediatrics, University of Wisconsin Center for Health Sciences, Madison, Wisconsin

RALPH D. FEIGIN, M.D.
J.S. Abercrombie Professor and Chairman, Department of Pediatrics, Baylor College of Medicine; Physician-in-Chief, Texas Children's Hospital; Physician-in-Chief, Pediatric Service, Harris County Hospital District; Chief, Pediatric Service, The Methodist Hospital, Houston, Texas

BARRY D. FLETCHER, M.D., C.M.
Professor of Radiology, Case Western Reserve University; Director, Division of Pediatric Radiology, Rainbow Babies and Childrens Hospital, University Hospitals, Cleveland, Ohio

WILLIAM W. FOX, M.D.
Associate Professor of Pediatrics, University of Pennsylvania School of Medicine, Philadelphia, Pennsylvania

ROGER K. FREEMAN, M.D.
Medical Director, Women's Hospital, Memorial Hospital Medical Center of Long Beach; Professor, Obstetrics and Gynecology, University of California at Irvine, Orange, California

LAWRENCE M. GARTNER, M.D.
Professor and Chairman, Department of Pediatrics, Pritzker School of Medicine, University of Chicago; Director, Wyler Children's Hospital, Chicago, Illinois

†LOWELL A. GLASGOW, M.D.
Professor and Chairman, Department of Pediatrics, University of Utah School of Medicine; Medical Director, Primary Children's Medical Center, Salt Lake City, Utah

MORTON F. GOLDBERG, M.D.
Professor and Head, Department of Ophthalmology, University of Illinois, Chicago, Illinois

ELIZABETH M. GORDON, M.D.
Assistant Clinical Professor of Pediatrics, Case Western Reserve University School of Medicine, Cleveland, Ohio

JUDITH GIBBS, M.D., C.M.
Director of Neonatology, Allentown Hospital, Allentown, Pennsylvania

STANLEY N. GRAVEN, M.D.
Professor, Department of Child Health; Director of International Health, University of Missouri School of Medicine, Columbia, Missouri

SAMUEL GROSS, M.D.
Professor of Pediatrics, University of Florida, College of Medicine, Gainesville, Florida

MICHAEL T. GYVES, M.D.
Assistant Professor, Department of Reproductive Biology, Case Western Reserve University, Cleveland, Ohio

MAUREEN HACK, M.B., Ch.B.
Associate Professor, Department of Pediatrics; Director of High Risk Follow-up Program, Case Western Reserve University, Cleveland, Ohio

BARBARA F. HALES, Ph.D.
Assistant Professor, Department of Pharmacology and Therapeutics, McGill University, Montreal, Quebec, Canada

WILLIAM C. HEIRD, M.D.
Associate Professor of Pediatrics, Columbia University College of Physicians and Surgeons, New York, New York

ROGER H. HERTZ, M.D.
Associate professor, Department of Obstetrics and Gynecology, Cleveland Metropolitan General Hospital, Case Western Reserve University, Cleveland, Ohio

†Deceased.

JOAN E. HODGMAN, M.D.

Professor of Pediatrics, University of Southern California School of Medicine; Director, Newborn Division, Los Angeles County, University of Southern California Medical Center, Los Angeles, California

L. STANLEY JAMES, M.D.

Professor of Pediatrics and Obstetrics and Gynecology; Director, Division of Perinatology, Department of Pediatrics, Columbia University College of Physicians and Surgeons, New York, New York

SHELBY E. JARRELL, M.D.

Assistant Professor of Clinical Obstetrics and Gynecology, Medical College of Virginia, Richmond, Virginia

MAJIDA N. JASSANI, M.D.

Assistant Professor of Obstetrics and Gynecology and Radiology, Case Western Reserve University, Cleveland, Ohio

JOHN KATTWINKEL, M.D.

Director, Newborn Services, and Associate Professor of Pediatrics, University of Virginia Medical Center, Charlottesville, Virginia

JOHN H. KENNELL, M.D.

Professor of Pediatrics, Case Western Reserve University, Rainbow Babies and Childrens Hospital, Cleveland, Ohio

KATHERINE C. KING, M.D.

Associate Professor of Pediatrics, Case Western Reserve University; Director, Neonatal Intensive Care Unit and Newborn Service, and Co-director, Perinatal Clinical Research Center, Cleveland Metropolitan General Hospital, Cleveland, Ohio

MARSHALL H. KLAUS, M.D.

Professor and Chairman, Department of Pediatrics and Human Development, Michigan State University, East Lansing, Michigan

ROBERT M. KLIEGMAN, M.D.

Assistant Professor of Pediatrics, Case Western Reserve University, Rainbow Babies and Childrens Hospital and Cleveland Metropolitan General Hospital, Cleveland, Ohio

THADDEUS W. KURCZYNSKI, M.D. Ph.D.

Director, Genetics Center; Associate Professor of Pediatrics and Neuroscience, Department of Pediatrics, Medical College of Ohio, Toledo, Ohio

ROBERT E. LASKY, Ph.D.

Assistant Professor of Clinical Pediatrics, Department of Pediatrics, University of Texas Health Sciences Center at Dallas, Dallas, Texas

KWANG-SUN LEE, M.D.

Associate Professor of Pediatrics and Director of Newborn Services, Pritzker School of Medicine, University of Chicago, Chicago, Illinois

MARTIN H. LEES, M.D., F.R.C.P.

Professor of Pediatrics and Perinatology, Department of Pediatrics, Oregon Health Sciences University, Portland, Oregon

LAWRENCE D. LILIEN, M.D.

Attending Neonatologist, Cook County Children's Hospital; Assistant Professor of Pediatrics, Abraham Lincoln School of Medicine, University of Illinois College of Medicine, Chicago, Illinois

HENRY H. MANGURTEN, M.D.

Director, Section of Neonatology, Lutheran General Hospital, Park Ridge; Associate Professor of Clinical Pediatrics, Abraham Lincoln School of Medicine, University of Illinois College of Medicine, Chicago, Illinois

RICHARD J. MARTIN, M.B., F.R.A.C.P., F.R.C.P. (Canada)

Assistant Professor of Pediatrics, Case Western Reserve University School of Medicine, University Hospitals (Rainbow Babies and Childrens Hospital), Cleveland, Ohio

JOHN S. McDONALD, M.D.

Professor and Chairman, Department of Anesthesiology, Ohio State University College of Medicine, Columbus, Ohio

MICHAEL T. MENNUTI, M.D.

Associate Professor of Obstetrics and Gynecology, Human Genetics, and Pediatrics, Department of Obstetrics and Gynecology, University of Pennsylvania School of Medicine, Philadelphia, Pennsylvania

IRWIN R. MERKATZ, M.D.

Professor and Chairman, Department of Obstetrics and Gynecology, Albert Einstein College of Medicine, New York, New York

CHARLES H. MITCHELL, M.D.

Pediatric Gastroenterologist, Madigan Army Medical Center, Fort Lewis, Washington

RACHEL MORECKI, M.D.

Professor, Department of Pathology, Albert Einstein College of Medicine, Bronx, New York

AKIRA MORISHIMA, M.D., Ph.D.

Associate Professor and Director, Division of Pediatric Endocrinology, Department of Pediatrics, Columbia University College of Physicians and Surgeons, New York, New York

JEFFREY P. MORRAY, M.D.
Assistant Professor of Anesthesiology, University of Washington School of Medicine, Seattle, Washington

MARTIN A. NASH, M.D.
Associate Professor and Clinical Pediatrics, Columbia University College of Physicians and Surgeons; Director of Pediatric Nephrology, Babies Hospital, Columbia-Presbyterian Medical Center, New York, New York

MICHAEL R. NEUMAN, Ph.D., M.D.
Associate Professor of Biomedical Engineering in Reproductive Biology, Department of Reproductive Biology and Perinatal Clinical Research Center, Case Western Reserve University, Cleveland, Ohio

JOHN F. NICHOLSON, M.D.
Associate Professor of Pediatrics and Pathology, Columbia University College of Physicians and Surgeons; Director of Children's Diabetic Clinic; Director of Clinical Chemistry Service; Associate Attending Physician in Pediatrics, Columbia-Presbyterian Hospital and Medical Center, New York, New York

EMI OKAMOTO, M.D.
Assistant Professor of Pediatrics, Columbia University College of Physicians and Surgeons, New York, New York

JAMES C. OVERALL, Jr., M.D.
Professor of Pediatrics and Pathology; Chief, Pediatric Infectious Diseases; Director, Diagnostic Virology Laboratory, University of Utah School of Medicine, Salt Lake City, Utah

ROBERT H. PERELMAN, M.D.
Assistant Professor, Department of Pediatrics, University of Wisconsin Center for Health Sciences, Madison, Wisconsin

PAUL H. PERLSTEIN, M.D.
Professor of Pediatrics, Obstetrics and Gynecology, University of Cincinnati College of Medicine and Cincinnati Children's Hospital Medical Center, Cincinnati, Ohio

ROSITA S. PILDES, M.D.
Chairman, Division of Neonatology, Cook County Children's Hospital; Professor of Pediatrics, Abraham Lincoln School of Medicine, University of Illinois College of Medicine, Chicago, Illinois

ROY M. PITKIN, M.D.
Professor and Chairman, Department of Obstetrics and Gynecology, University of Iowa, College of Medicine, Iowa City, Iowa

WILLIAM B. PITTARD III, M.D.
Assistant Professor of Pediatrics, Case Western Reserve University School of Medicine, Cleveland, Ohio

RICHARD A. POLIN, M.D.
Associate Professor of Pediatrics, University of Pennsylvania, Philadelphia, Pennsylvania

STEPHEN H. POLMAR, Ph.D., M.D.
Professor of Pediatrics, Washington University School of Medicine; Director, Division of Allergy and Immunology, St. Louis Children's Hospital, St. Louis, Missouri

JOHN T. QUEENAN, M.D.
Professor and Chairman, Department of Obstetrics and Gynecology, Georgetown University School of Medicine, Washington, D.C.

JOHN E. READ, M.D.
Clinical Associate Professor, Department of Ophthalmology, University of Illinois, Chicago, Illinois

TOVE S. ROSEN, M.D.
Assistant Professor of Pediatrics, Columbia University College of Physicians and Surgeons, New York, New York

THOMAS V. SANTULLI, M.D.
Professor of Surgery, Columbia University College of Physicians and Surgeons; Attending Surgeon, Columbia-Presbyterian Medical Center, New York, New York

JAMES F. SCHWARTZ, M.D.
Professor, Departments of Pediatrics and Neurology, Emory University, Atlanta, Georgia

THOMAS H. SHAFFER, Ph.D.
Associate Professor of Physiology, Temple University School of Medicine, Philadelphia, Pennsylvania

SUSAN B. SHURIN, M.D.
Assistant Professor of Pediatrics, Case Western Reserve University School of Medicine, Cleveland, Ohio

BIJAN SIASSI, M.D.
Associate Professor of Pediatrics, University of Southern California, School of Medicine, Los Angeles, California

FRANK R. SINATRA, M.D.
Assistant Professor of Pediatrics and Director of Pediatric Gastroenterology Program, University of Southern California School of Medicine, Childrens Hospital of Los Angeles, Los Angeles, California

JOHN C. SINCLAIR, M.D.
Professor, Departments of Pediatrics and Clinical Epidemiology and Biostatistics, McMaster University, Hamilton, Ontario, Canada

MARY ELLEN L. SKALINA, M.D.

Staff Neonatologist, Cooper Medical Centre; Assistant Clinical Professor, University of Medicine and Dentistry, Rutgers Medical School, Camden, New Jersey

LAWRENCE M. SOLOMON, M.D.

Professor and Head, Department of Dermatology, University of Illinois, Chicago, Illinois

RICARDO U. SORENSEN, M.D.

Associate Professor of Pediatrics, Case Western Reserve University, Cleveland, Ohio

ADRIAN SPITZER, M.D.

Professor of Pediatrics and Director of Division of Nephrology, Department of Pediatrics, Albert Einstein College of Medicine; Attending Pediatrician, The Hospital of the Albert Einstein College of Medicine and Montefiore Hospital Medical Center, Bronx, New York

JEAN J. STEICHEN, M.D.

Associate Professor of Pediatrics, Obstetrics and Gynecology, Department of Newborn Pediatrics, University of Cincinnati College of Medicine, Cincinnati, Ohio

CECILLE O. SUNDERLAND, M.D.

Professor of Pediatrics, Oregon Health Sciences University, Portland, Oregon

PHILIP SUNSHINE, M.D.

Professor of Pediatrics, Stanford University Medical Center, Palo Alto, California

REGINALD C. TSANG, M.B.B.S.

Professor of Pediatrics, Obstetrics and Gynecology, Department of Newborn Pediatrics, University of Cincinnati College of Medicine, Cincinnati, Ohio

DAVID TUDEHOPE, M.B.B.S. (Monash), M.R.A.C.P., F.R.A.C.P.

Director of Neonatology, Mater Mothers Hospital, South Brisbane, Queensland, Australia

JON E. TYSON, M.D.

Assistant Professor of Pediatrics and Obstetrics and Gynecology, Department of Pediatrics, University of Texas Health Science Center at Dallas, Dallas, Texas

BARRY S. YULISH, M.D.

Assistant Professor of Radiology, Division of Pediatric Radiology, Case Western Reserve University School of Medicine, Rainbow Babies and Childrens Hospital, University Hospitals, Cleveland, Ohio

FREDERICK P. ZUSPAN, M.D.

Professor and Chairman, Department of Obstetrics and Gynecology, The Ohio State University, Columbus, Ohio

27 Postnatally acquired infections, 650
Ralph D. Feigin
Deborah L. Callanan

28 Viral and protozoal perinatal infections, 692
Lowell A. Glasgow
James C. Overall, Jr.

29 The blood and hematopoietic system, 708
Samuel Gross
Susan B. Shurin
Elizabeth M. Gordon

30 Jaundice and liver disease, 753

PART ONE Unconjugated hyperbilirubinemia, 754
Lawrence M. Gartner
Kwang-Sun Lee

PART TWO Conjugated hyperbilirubinemia, 771
Rachel Morecki
Lawrence M. Gartner
Kwang-Sun Lee

31 The kidney and urinary tract, 785
Adrian Spitzer
Jay Bernstein
Chester M. Edelmann, Jr.

32 Inborn errors of metabolism, 815
John F. Nicholson

33 Metabolic and endocrine disorders, 845

PART ONE Carbohydrate metabolism in the fetus and neonate, 845
Rosita S. Pildes
Lawrence D. Lilien

PART TWO Disorders of calcium and magnesium metabolism, 870
Reginald C. Tsang
Jean J. Steichen

PART THREE Thyroid disorders, 883
Akira Morishima

PART FOUR Abnormalities of sexual differentiation, 900
Robert K. Danish

PART FIVE Infants of addicted mothers, 933
Tove S. Rosen

34 The skin, 939
Nancy B. Esterly
Lawrence M. Solomon

35 The eye, 967
John E. Read
Morton F. Goldberg

36 Orthopedic problems, 1004
Harold M. Dick

37 Genetic disease and chromosomal abnormalities, 1013
Richard A. Polin
Michael T. Mennuti

38 Congenital malformations, 1035
Thaddeus W. Kurczynski

39 Diagnostic radiology, 1064
Barry D. Fletcher
Barry S. Yulish
Gary M. Amundson

Appendix A Blood specimen collection in the newborn, 1089
Thomas A. Blumenfeld

B Therapeutic agents, 1092
Jeffrey L. Blumer
Thomas A. Blumenfeld

C Tables of normal values, 1098
Thomas A. Blumenfeld

To
Roslyn and **Patricia**

Preface

The goal of this third edition of *Neonatal-Perinatal Medicine* is to present a comprehensive description of the disorders that affect the fetus and neonatal infant. The emphasis remains on the pathophysiology, clinical and laboratory manifestations, and prevention and treatment of diseases that have their onset in utero or during the neonatal period. We hope that this text will provide obstetricians, pediatricians, family physicians, and nurses with a basis for understanding and managing a broad spectrum of clinical problems, as well as provide them with an overall perspective about a field in which there continues to be a rapid acceleration of knowledge and technology.

Recognizing the increasing problems related to administration of neonatal intensive care units, as well as the critical educational roles of tertiary centers, we have addressed these issues in this edition. Furthermore, pharmacologic principles related to the fetus and newborn have been introduced, and expanded knowledge concerning the sensorimotor development of preterm infants has been included. Many new authors have been solicited in an attempt to update, revise, and more graphically present all sections.

We gratefully acknowledge the sterling efforts of our many contributors, Karen Berger, Terry Van Schaik, and Marjorie Sanson at Mosby, as well as Connie McSweeney and Ellen Rome, without whose valuable assistance this book could not have been completed.

Avroy A. Fanaroff
Richard J. Martin
Richard E. Behrman

Contents

1 The field of neonatal-perinatal medicine, 1
   Richard E. Behrman

2 Organization of nursery services, 4
   PART ONE The organization of perinatal health services, 4
   Stanley N. Graven
   Avroy A. Fanaroff
   PART TWO Perinatal outreach education, 11
   John Kattwinkel
   PART THREE Stress and the performance of the intensive care unit staff, 15
   Jon E. Tyson
   Robert E. Lasky

3 Diabetes in pregnancy, 22
   Method A. Duchon
   Michael T. Gyves
   Irwin R. Merkatz

4 Preeclampsia-eclampsia (pregnancy-induced hypertension), 27
   Frederick P. Zuspan

5 Erythroblastosis fetalis, 34
   John T. Queenan

6 Polyhydramnios and oligohydramnios, 44
   John T. Queenan

7 Intrauterine growth retardation: determinants of aberrant fetal growth, 49
   Robert M. Kliegman
   Katherine C. King

8 Antenatal ultrasound, 81
   Patrick J. Bryan
   Majida N. Jassani

9 Estimation of the placental function and reserve, 95
   PART ONE Fetal heart rate monitoring, 95
   Roger K. Freeman
   PART TWO Antepartum fetal assessment, 107
   Leroy J. Dierker
   Roger H. Hertz
   PART THREE Intrapartum fetal assessment, 112
   Roger H. Hertz
   Shelby E. Jarrell

10 Neonatal clinical cardiopulmonary monitoring, 119
   Luis A. Cabal
   Bijan Siassi
   Joan E. Hodgman

11 Obstetric management of prematurity, 133
   PART ONE Estimation of fetal maturity, 133
   Roy M. Pitkin
   PART TWO Premature labor, 139
   Tom P. Barden

12 Developmental pharmacology, 150
   Jacob V. Aranda
   Barbara F. Hales
   Judith Gibbs

13 Anesthesia for labor and delivery, 174
   John S. McDonald

Contents

14 Emergencies in the delivery room, 179
  L. Stanley James

15 Birth weight, gestational age, and neonatal risk, 196
  John C. Sinclair
  David I. Tudehope

16 Placental pathology, 206
  Kurt Benirschke

17 Birth injuries, 216
  Henry H. Mangurten

18 Care of the mother, father, and infant, 240
  Marshall H. Klaus
  John H. Kennell

19 Routine and special care, 254
  PART ONE Physical examination, 254
  John M. Driscoll, Jr.
  PART TWO Physical environment, 259
  Paul H. Perlstein
  PART THREE Biomedical engineering aspects of neonatal monitoring, 277
  Michael R. Neuman
  PART FOUR Care of the newborn, 289
  John M. Driscoll, Jr.

20 Nutrition, body fluids, and acid-base homeostasis, 302
  PART ONE Nutritional requirements of the low birth weight infant, 302
  William C. Heird
  Emi Okamoto
  Thomas L. Anderson
  PART TWO Methods of nutrient delivery for the low birth weight infant, 308
  William C. Heird
  Thomas L. Anderson
  PART THREE Provision of water and electrolytes, 314
  Martin A. Nash
  PART FOUR Disturbances of acid-base equilibrium, 320
  William C. Heird

21 The sensorimotor development of the preterm infant, 328
  Maureen Hack

22 Central nervous system disturbances, 347
  Alfred W. Brann, Jr.
  James F. Schwartz

23 The respiratory system, 404
  PART ONE The developmental biology of the lung, 404
  Philip M. Farrell
  Robert H. Perelman
  PART TWO Assessment of pulmonary function, 419
  William W. Fox
  Thomas H. Shaffer
  PART THREE The respiratory distress syndrome and its management, 427
  Richard J. Martin
  Avroy A. Fanaroff
  Mary Ellen L. Skalina
  PART FOUR Other pulmonary problems, 443
  Avroy A. Fanaroff
  Richard J. Martin
  PART FIVE Chronic pulmonary diseases of the neonate, 467
  William W. Fox
  Jeffrey P. Morray
  Richard J. Martin

24 The gastrointestinal system, 477
  PART ONE Development, 477
  Philip Sunshine
  Frank R. Sinatra
  Charles H. Mitchell
  Thomas V. Santulli
  PART TWO Gastrointestinal emergencies, 483
  Philip Sunshine
  Frank R. Sinatra
  Charles H. Mitchell
  Thomas V. Santulli
  PART THREE Gastrointestinal disorders, 490
  Philip Sunshine
  Frank R. Sinatra
  Charles H. Mitchell
  Thomas V. Santulli

25 The cardiovascular system, 536
  Martin H. Lees
  Cecille O. Sunderland

26 Immunology, 632
  Stephen H. Polmar
  Ricardo U. Sorenson
  William B. Pittard III

BEHRMAN'S Neonatal-perinatal medicine

CHAPTER 1 The field of neonatal-perinatal medicine

The term *perinatal* is used to designate the period from the twelfth week of gestation through the twenty-eighth day after birth. The *neonatal period* is defined as the first 4 weeks of life and is the period of the greatest mortality in childhood, with the highest risk occurring during the first 24 hours of life. The continuing high mortality and morbidity during this period are closely related to the fact that it is part of a continuum of fetal growth and development. Factors acting during gestation and delivery, as well as during the postnatal period, have a major impact on the health of both the fetus and neonate. Social, economic, and cultural influences are superimposed on genetic, metabolic, and physiologic intrauterine and extrauterine environmental effects.

The high incidence of disease during the perinatal period and the excessive neonatal and perinatal death rates make it important to identify as early as possible those fetuses and infants who are at greatest risk. Of equal importance is the need to lower the morbidity, especially for handicapping conditions such as mental retardation, resulting from untoward prenatal and neonatal factors. Our development as a species ultimately depends on the quality of the babies who are produced and their potential talents. There is increasing evidence that early recognition of the high-risk pregnancy and high-risk infant and appropriate antenatal and intrapartum management along with special neonatal intensive care will reduce the incidence of handicapping conditions and will reduce both the perinatal and neonatal death rates (p. 5).

Despite changes in population growth, little change has occurred in the incidence of infants of low birth weight (defined as infants weighing less than 2,500 gm) in the United States. It has remained at a mean rate of about 8% of total births with a range of 6% to 16+% for decades. The lower figure is usually approached by middle to upper income communities, and the higher figure is approached in urban ghettos and deprived rural communities. The latter figure is probably underestimated, since a number of babies born to the poor may not be included in the statistics. Of the 250,000 low birth weight babies born each year, in the United States, 40,000 to 45,000 die within the first month of life, and about as many term fetuses die each year in utero. This represents a substantial improvement in survival over past decades in all weight classes, but especially for infants weighing from 1,000 to 2,000 gm. Improvement in survival has also occurred in infants under 1,000 gm.

A number of infants will live a long life but remain significantly afflicted with disease or disability. The infants of very low birth weight are particularly vulnerable. Those who die are a source of anguish and grief to their parents and relatives for a varying but relatively brief period, whereas those who survive with disabilities and disease may be a continuing source of pain, anguish, and loss of resources for their parents and society, in addition to the personal suffering they may endure. They may also impose a very real biologic burden on future generations. Tragically, there are at least three times as many of these unfortunate infants in the black portion of the population in the United States. It has been estimated that about 60,000 of the 250,000 low birth weight babies born each year may be at high risk for serious lifetime disability. In addition to the human tragedy, the fiscal impact of this problem on our society is estimated to be in the billions of dollars each year. The major problems of cerebral palsy, mental retardation, sensory and cognitive disabilities, and a diminished ability to successfully adapt socially, psychologically, and physically to an increasingly complex environment are some of the results observed in children and adults who were low birth weight infants.

Table 1-1. Fetal organ blood flows (percent of the cardiac output ± SD)

	Brain	Heart	Lungs	Kidneys	Adrenal glands	Placenta
Control	15.7 ± 2.8	2.7 ± 0.9	10.7 ± 6.4	2.7 ± 1.0	0.4 ± 0.1	47.5 ± 4.9
Fetal distress	30.6 ± 11.3	4.9 ± 1.5	3.2 ± 2.4	1.9 ± 1.4	0.8 ± 0.5	29.2 ± 9.4
Statistical significance	$p < 0.01$	$p < 0.02$	$p < 0.05$	NS*	$p < 0.05$	$p < 0.005$

Adapted from Behrman, R. E., and others: Am. J. Obstet. Gynecol. **108:**956, 1970.
*NS, Not significant. Mean values ± 1 SD are presented.

In addition to these population and societal dimensions of the field of neonatal-perinatal medicine, it is becoming increasingly evident that important antecedents of many adult diseases, such as coronary artery disease, chronic renal and liver disease, obesity, and other human maladies, may be present in early development, at which stage there is real opportunity for prevention. Further improvement in longevity and decreased morbidity are likely to result from increased understanding of the origins of adult diseases in fetal life and infancy and the prevention and early management of these diseases.

More immediate clinical by-products are likely to result from the continuing expansion of our understanding of and ability to measure fetal physiologic and biochemical homeostasis. As our appreciation of the mechanics controlling the protective circulatory adjustments of the fetus to the stress of hypoxia continues to increase along with our understanding of fetal pharmacology, we are likely to develop new means not only to detect but also to medically treat the fetus before and during labor. In 1960 our ability to detect *fetal asphyxia* consisted of clinical auscultation of the fetal heart rate during labor and observation of the amniotic fluid for meconium staining when the membranes ruptured. We now know the sequence of events in the fetus that occurs in response to maternal hypotension, or hypoxia. The heart rate and blood pressure initially increase; then with the rapid onset of fetal bradycardia and hypotension the fetus develops a mixed metabolic and "placental" respiratory acidosis. The cardiac output and umbilical blood flow decrease sharply. A greater portion of the oxygenated umbilical vein blood is shunted past the liver into the inferior vena cava and returned to the heart. The cardiac output to the brain, heart, and adrenals is preferentially maintained so that tissue perfusion of these organs does not decrease significantly (Table 1-1). In contrast, the fetal lungs and cortex of the kidneys have a decreased perfusion. The oxygen consumption of the fetus decreases by over 50%. When this sequence of events becomes far enough advanced in the Rhesus monkey, baboon, and probably in the human, the problem is detectable by continuous monitoring of the fetal heart rate and uterine pressure curves; characteristic high-risk patterns such as those for cord occlusion or placental insufficiency can be identified (p. 101). Nevertheless, the treatments for fetal asphyxia currently available are limited to surgical intervention, oxygen, or position changes. Monitoring of fetal transcutaneous oxygen and carbon dioxide tensions provides us with more sensitive tools to detect early fetal hypoxia, and improved understanding of the hormonal and neural regulation of the patterns of fetal pathophysiologic response may broaden our pharmacologic approach to treatment before birth. Our ability to diagnose and/or treat some diseases before birth, such as erythroblastosis, respiratory distress syndrome (hyaline membrane disease), and a large number of genetic defects, has changed dramatically in recent years.

Research on the pregnant sheep and nonhuman primate is likely to continue to produce important models for the human but the focus of investigation has changed from systems and organs to the cellular level of development. We have progressed from simple determinations of whether a substance crosses the placenta, and the characterization of placental permeability by the molecular weights of the solutes transferred and the anatomic description of the placenta, to an appreciation of the interactions of the lipid membrane transport systems of the placenta, the kinetics of maternal uterine and fetal umbilical blood flows, and the protein binding of solutes and gases in these two circulations. This has laid the groundwork for developing a real pharmacology for the uterus, placenta, and fetus, which may be critical to our understanding the control of labor and thus, eventually, to our ability to decrease the incidence of low birth weight or premature infants. Prenatal diagnosis and biochemical and ultrasonic fetal monitoring may be the first steps to future treatments that may include hybridization of cells in the early blastocyst or embryo to correct inborn errors of metabolism, the stimulation of embryogenesis of organs, and the acceleration of organ maturation. The latter has already proved to be effective in the prevention of respiratory distress syndrome by treating mothers of selected third trimester fetuses with betamethasone (Chapter 23).

Finally, advances in the field of neonatal-perinatal medicine have focused attention on a number of ethical and legal issues. There is mounting concern about life and death decision making in neonatal intensive care units. New and complex physician-patient-family–nursing staff–societal relationships exist in these units, and this development has had an enormous impact on the process of making medical decisions. Regionalization has brought these issues into a sharper and more demanding focus. Criteria have to be formulated for making certain decisions that previously were made on a chance basis of access to the health system, which was strongly influenced by the economic position of a family. For example, should a 750-gm infant with a poor prognosis for intact survival be accepted in a regional neonatal intensive care unit when it means one cannot accept a 2,000-gm infant who is at high risk but has a good prognosis if he or she survives, just because the referring physician in the case of the 750-gm infant calls first or because the infant is born in the same hospital where the intensive care unit is located? The nature of the evolving customs or prelegal restraints differ in some important respects from those impinging on the traditional physician-patient relationship outside neonatal intensive care centers. Participation in discussions antecedent to decision making involves a diversity of people, the discussions are more explicitly informative, and the demands on the physician's ability to perceive what is meant from what is said are more exacting. Ironically, but not surprisingly, as the technology of care increases in these units, the difficult choices for the physician are not the technical medical decisions, but matters of judgment that require evaluating, analyzing, and interpreting the complex human interests and concerns of the relatives, their friends and advisors, and the staff, and the various consequences for the people involved. These have always been the most challenging and demanding decisions for physicians that cannot be delegated to others. The new elements are the frequency and complexity of these judgments in regional neonatal intensive care centers.

Whatever decision-making process is used to improve the quality of care provided to the individual patient, certain principles are important, but often not easy to apply. The fundamental responsibility of all who are concerned is to do no harm or, at least, no harm without a reasonable expectation of a compensating benefit for the patient. A corollary principle is that there must be continuous objective, critical scientific evaluation of the care being currently provided and of proposed innovations. Activities should not be initiated or continued that on balance do harm to the well-being of a newborn infant. The definition of "well-being" is the major problem, since the varying ethical values, religious commitments, and life experiences of all those who care for and about the infant, as well as legal restraints, must be taken into consideration. In general, the elements of well-being include a life prolonged beyond infancy, without excruciating pain, and with the potential of participating in human experience to a minimal degree.

Awareness of the above diverse considerations has contributed to the impetus for further clinical specialization within pediatrics, and obstetrics and gynecology, resulting in the formation of a field of clinical medicine for the fetus and neonatal infant: neonatal-perinatal medicine. This field has already expanded to encompass the developing embryo before as well as after organ formation and older infants whose immaturity or disease process makes them best cared for in neonatal intensive care centers.

Richard E. Behrman

BIBLIOGRAPHY

Behrman, R.E., and others: Distribution of the circulation in the normal and asphyxiated fetal perinate, Am. J. Obstet. Gynecol. **108:**956, 1970.

Hodgen, G.D.: Antenatal diagnosis and treatment of fetal skeletal malformations, J.A.M.A. **246:**1079, 1981.

Janis, A.R., and others: Critical issues in newborn intensive care: a conference report and policy proposal, Pediatrics **55:**756, 1975.

Report and recommendations research on the fetus, The National Commission for the Protection of Human Subjects of Biomedical and Behavioral Research, Department of Health, Education, and Welfare Pub. No. (OS) 76-127, 1975.

CHAPTER 2 # Organization of nursery services

PART ONE
The organization of perinatal health services

The successful delivery of high-quality care to perinatal patients requires not only excellence from physicians, nurses, and other health professionals as individuals, but also community involvement and a mechanism or system of organization that permits them to function as cohesive and well-coordinated teams.

Regionalization implies the development, within a geographic area, of a coordinated cooperative system of maternal and perinatal health care in which, by mutual agreements between hospitals and physicians and based upon population needs, the degree of complexity of maternal and perinatal care each hospital is capable of providing is identified so as to accomplish the following objectives: quality care to all pregnant women and newborns, maximal utilization of highly trained perinatal personnel and intensive care facilities, and assurance of reasonable cost effectiveness.*

BACKGROUND AND HISTORICAL PERSPECTIVE

Before 1940, perinatal care services were delivered in the United States, Canada, and Europe without any particular organization or structure. Most of the care was provided by an individual physician or midwife. In many areas the majority of the deliveries occurred in the home. A number of maternity hospitals developed in the larger urban areas, usually serving as teaching hospitals. These maternity hospitals often had home delivery services and neighborhood clinics serving a geographic area.

During the 1940s and early 1950s a number of cities developed centers for the care of premature infants. Most of these centers were located in urban areas. In Illinois, premature centers were located to serve the rural areas as well. In the late 1940s and 1950s many of the European countries, particularly in Scandinavia and the Netherlands, developed systems of care for the perinatal patient based on the development of primary prenatal care clinics staffed largely by midwives with district and regional hospitals for the care of mothers with complications. During the 1950s a number of states developed maternal mortality committees. These committees developed data that were used as a basis for activities directed at preventing maternal mortality.

From 1964 to 1968, studies were undertaken in Massachusetts, Wisconsin, and Arizona to analyze causes of neonatal mortality and morbidity. In Massachusetts the studies led to the development of standards and regulations for maternity units. Their implementation resulted in a decrease in the number of maternity units in Massachusetts from 102 in 1967 to 65 in 1975. In Wisconsin the studies led to the development of a statewide education-consultation program and regional newborn intensive care centers. These units subsequently evolved into regional perinatal centers. In 1967, as a result of a study of premature mortality, Arizona developed a statewide transport program for premature and other high-risk neonates. Three additional factors that promoted the movement toward the development of regional care plans were the study and report of the Joint Committee of the Society of Obstetricians and Gynaecologists of Canada and the Canadian Paediatric Society, entitled

*From Ryan, G.M.: Toward improving the outcome of pregnancy, Report of the Committee on Perinatal Health (AAFP, AAP, ACOG, AMA), 1976, Obstet. Gynecol. 46:375, 1975. Reprinted with permission from The American College of Obstetricians and Gynecologists.

"Regional Services in Reproductive Medicine"; the adoption of a statement on regionalization of perinatal care by the American Medical Association; and the report of the joint Committee on Perinatal Health of the American Medical Association, the American College of Obstetricians and Gynecologists, the American Academy of Family Physicians, and the American Academy of Pediatrics, entitled "Toward Improving the Outcome of Pregnancy." These reports, along with the data from Wisconsin, Massachusetts, and Arizona, have stimulated activities in most states toward development of regional organizations for perinatal care services. Additional impetus has been derived from the establishment of regional perinatal centers in the United States by the Robert Wood Johnson Foundation.

NEED FOR AN ORGANIZED PERINATAL CARE SYSTEM

There are marked disparities in the perinatal mortality for various nations. These disparities are particularly striking among various European nations, the United States, and Canada. There are also marked differences between states or districts within a country and between areas within the same district or state. Marked differences in perinatal mortality exist between census tracts within the same urban area. Those nations with well-organized systems for perinatal care have better perinatal mortality and morbidity statistics.

Often high fetal and neonatal mortality is attributed to socioeconomic conditions, educational deficiencies, and related social factors. In some areas, however, high perinatal mortality may exist simultaneously with very low mortality for older age groups, suggesting that the lack of adequate health care services for the pregnant woman and neonate is a major factor responsible for the high perinatal mortality.

In the studies from Massachusetts and Wisconsin, 30% to 65% of the fetal and neonatal mortalities were judged preventable. Of the preventable deaths, approximately half were judged preventable within the resources of the community hospital and its staff; the other half required the resources of a specialized regional center with team-derived resources. Studies of infants following neonatal intensive care have shown a marked reduction in the frequency of permanent neurologic sequelae. Thus the development of neonatal intensive care results not only in reduction in mortality but also in a reduction in serious morbidity. Maternal intensive care units and high-risk obstetric programs decrease fetal mortality and also reduce the frequency of neonatal problems requiring intensive care. The decrease in the number of deaths and improvement in the outcome for the survivors of both maternal and neonatal intensive care have justified the cost investment in these programs.

PRINCIPLES OF ORGANIZATION

There are general principles that form the basis for the development of regional health care services for perinatal patients. These principles derive from an understanding of the care needs of the mother, fetus, and family during pregnancy, and of the mother, newborn, and family following birth.

Accountability for population

Regionalization denotes a geographic area or population with definable care needs. The regional center and the network of related institutions are accountable for the overall perinatal health care for the region. The data on mortality and morbidity, frequency of problems, and quality of care are assessed for the entire population in the area. The availability and quality of care in any given institution become the responsibility of all the institutions, including the perinatal center.

One standard of quality

Regionalization is based on the premise that there should be a single standard of quality perinatal care. Any mother or infant should have equal access to all the components of a functioning perinatal system (see Table 2-1).

Differing care capabilities of institutions

Institutions operating within a region will differ in their capability for providing perinatal care. These differences reflect number of patients, educational background and experience of medical and nursing staff, and availability of equipment and facilities. Each institution is expected to deliver high-quality care up to the level of its capability. When care requirements exceed its capability, the patient is referred to the closest facility that has the capability.

The majority (60% to 80%) of problems associated with increased risk for the mother, fetus, or newborn are detectable sufficiently in advance of the crises to permit either the appropriate care resources to be made available locally or transfer of the patient to where appropriate resources are available. Even under ideal circumstances certain patients will have to move from one facility to another during the course of care. Thus institutions within a region must be effectively linked to permit ease of patient movement.

Minimal patient movement

The organization of the regional care network should be designed to make it possible for patients to receive care appropriate to their needs as close to their homes as possible. Only those patients with care needs exceeding that of their community facility should need to be referred to another institution. Through outreach education (see Chapter 2, part two) and consultation programs, efforts should be made to continually develop and expand the care capabilities of each institution to minimize the number of patients who must be dislocated while receiving care.

Optimum use of facilities and personnel

The concept of regionalization is designed to permit optimal use of both facilities and personnel. With the use of a regional perinatal center it is possible to have sufficient numbers of high-risk mothers and neonates concentrated in a single location to economically justify the staffing and equipment necessary to meet their care needs. In addition, personnel who have frequent opportunities to use their skills are able to maintain and enhance these skills. Institutions with small patient loads can avoid the expense of developing staff and equipment for services that are infrequently used.

Differing care needs for different groups

Groups within a population have differing care needs by virtue of socioeconomic conditions, education, ethnic background, personal health care practices, age, and other factors. The organization of facilities and personnel involved in perinatal care must reflect these varying needs.

Perinatal care: a team service

The health care needs of the perinatal patient require a close working relationship between the various disciplines involved to prevent fragmentation and gaps in care.

ORGANIZATION

Those countries with better perinatal mortality and morbidity statistics have carefully organized and universally available primary care for a mother during pregnancy and an estalished mechanism for referral of mothers and infants from primary care institutions to district or center hospitals when the needs of the patient indicate. They have placed less emphasis on tertiary care or intensive care because of the relatively low demand for such services. By contrast, the perinatal health services of the United States and Canada place great emphasis on the specialized hospital services for the perinatal patient, but the primary care services available to the mother during her pregnancy are disorganized and inconsistent. The number of perinatal patients requiring intensive in-hospital care is inversely related to the quality and availability of primary services, as well as to the general health status of the mothers before pregnancy.

An organized system for providing care to the maternity patient and her neonate consists of six types of units or facilities: physicians' offices and clinics, level I or community hospital facilities, level II hospital facilities, level III hospital facilities, regional perinatal centers, and specialized units such as children's hospitals and cardiac centers.

Physicians' offices and clinics

The basic or primary care units for care during pregnancy as well as for care of the mother and infant following delivery are physicians' offices and general clinics. These units need to have the capability for obtaining a complete health history, careful physical assessment of the mother or infant, systematic risk assessment (using one of the available risk scoring systems), and laboratory resources for determination of hematocrit or hemoglobin concentration and urinalysis.

Level I facilities

Level I (community hospital) facilities are those designed primarily for the care of the maternal and neonatal patients who have no complications. These units exist primarily because of geographic or cultural situations that limit access to units with greater care capabilities. Since even uncomplicated maternal and neonatal patients have a potential for unexpected complications, level I units must have the resources to provide competent emergency services when the need arises. The necessary services for a level I facility are shown in Table 2-1 and include a normal newborn nursery (Chapter 9, part four).

Level II facilities

Level II facilities are those hospitals which have larger maternity and newborn services. These hospitals will be located in urban and suburban areas serving larger communities. In addition to providing a full range of maternal and newborn services for perinatal patients who have no complications, they will provide services for some of the obstetric and neonatal patients who have complications. The range of obstetric and neonatal complications that fall within the capabilities of a given institution will depend on the resources available. The services available in level II units are presented in Table 2-1 and include both a normal newborn nursery and a transitional care nursery (Chapter 9, part four).

Level III facilities

In addition to the resources and capabilities of a level II unit, level III facilities are able to provide for a full range of maternal complications and newborn intensive care. The neonatal intensive care unit needs to have a full range of services for the neonate, with the possible exception of an occasional infant with congenital heart disease or other complex congenital anomaly who requires a specialized unit. The services offered by level

Table 2-1. Services provided by perinatal facilities

Services	Level I	Level II	Level III
Complete prenatal care for maternity patient with no complications or with minor complications	X	X	X
Complete prenatal care for maternity patients with most complications		X	X
A special diagnostic and management clinic for high-risk prenatal patients			X
Risk identification scoring system	X	X	X
Management of uncomplicated labor and delivery of normal term fetus	X	X	X
Prompt management of unexpected complications occurring during labor and delivery, including anesthesia, cesarean section, and blood administration	X	X	X
Management of complicated labor and delivery		X	X
Intrapartum intensive care			X
In-house anesthesia service		X	X
Electronic fetal monitoring	±	X	X
Physically separated facilities for obstetrics	X	X	X
Capability for resuscitation of depressed neonate at every delivery	X	X	X
Care for the healthy newborn	X	X	X
Stabilization and risk assessment of all neonates	X	X	X
Intravenous fluid administration to neonates	X	X	X
Management of most neonates who have complications up to short-term assisted ventilation		X	X
Continuous neonatal monitoring capability		X	X
Blood gases available on 24-hour basis		X	X
Neonatal intensive care including assisted ventilation and hyperalimentation			X
Neonatal surgical capability			X
Availability of pediatric subspecialists in cardiology, genetics, and hematology			X
Care of mothers with no postpartum complications	X	X	X
Management of unexpected postpartum complications including hemorrhage and sepsis	X	X	X
Management of most postpartum complications		X	X
Data collection on performance and outcome	X	X	X
Laboratory services for electrolytes, bilirubin, blood glucose, calcium on 24-hour basis	X	X	X
X-ray services with portable film capability on 24-hour basis	X	X	X
Laboratory services to assess fetal well-being and maturity		X	X
Diagnostic x-ray and ultrasound facilities		X	X
Nutritional consultation		X	X
Social service		X	X
Respiratory therapy consultation		X	X
Sterilization and family planning services	X	X	X
Follow-up developmental assessment clinic			X

III facilities are listed in Table 2-1 and include a neonatal intensive care nursery (Chapter 9, part four).

Regional perinatal center

A regional perinatal center is a level III facility that also has responsibility for coordination and management of special services, including transportation, that are needed for the region. In areas where there is only one level III facility, it is expected to function as the regional perinatal center. In areas where there is more than one unit with level III capabilities, one of the units would serve as the regional perinatal center. The regional perinatal center must offer outpatient and inpatient consultation and diagnostic services for level I and level II facilities within the region, including ultrasonography, laboratory analysis of amniotic fluid, gestational assessment, genetic studies, and other studies of fetal health. It also should provide specialized nursing services and consultation in nutrition, social services, respiratory therapy, and laboratory and radiology services. The center is responsible for carrying on an active outreach education program for the institutions, health professionals, and public within the region (see Chapter 2, part two).

A regional perinatal center has unique personnel needs. It should be directed by a full-time physician with extensive training and experience in perinatal medicine as well as in administration. There also should be a director of obstetric services and a director of neonatal services. The director of obstetric services should be a full-time physician with training and experience in fetal-maternal medicine, including maternal intensive care. The director of neonatal services should be a full-time neonatologist with training and experience in neonatal care, including newborn intensive care. The perinatal nursing services should be directed by a clinical nurse specialist with advanced experience in maternal and neonatal nursing and experience in administration. The center also may require a full-time director of the outreach education program to coordinate the active participation from physicians in obstetrics and newborn care, nurses in obstetrics and newborn care, nutritionists, social workers, and other specialized personnel. The obstetric and newborn care units, including the newborn intensive care unit, should have clinical nurse specialists in obstetrics and neonatal care, respectively, responsible for organizing the nursing programs and coordinating the patient care needs.

Frequency of risk problems

It is important to estimate the number of pregnant women who may need specialized obstetric and neonatal services within the area of a given regional perinatal center. The percentage of pregnancies at increased risk may vary from 10% for general populations, such as an entire state or country, to over 90% in some urban hospitals. In an Ontario perinatal study 32% of pregnancies had some increased risk factor that resulted in 60% of the neonatal problems. In the Nova Scotia Fetal Risk Project 11% of 9,483 patients accounted for 50% of the stillbirths and 75% of the neonatal deaths.

The number of neonatal care beds and neonatal intensive care days needed for a given population is most influenced by the frequency of premature birth and low birth weight. There are great differences in these frequencies between countries and between populations within a country. Low birth weight infants comprise less than 5% of the births in the Scandinavian countries and 6% to 9% of infants in some states in the United States; in some institutions the frequency may run as high as 15% to 20%.

Swyer calculated a need for neonatal intensive care beds at 0.7 beds per 1,000 live births on the basis of a 7% low birth weight rate. Transitional or intermediate bed and convalescent bed needs were approximately 4 per 1,000 live births. The Wisconsin Perinatal Care Program predicted a need for 12 intensive care beds for 6,000 live births (7% low birth weight rate).

Other services in a regional care system

An effective public health nursing system and availability of public health services are essential ingredients for effective perinatal care. Home visits during pregnancy and after birth provide a dimension of care not met by physician's offices or community hospitals. Finally, a perinatal center and hospital network must develop close working relationships with regional blood banks and with state or regional laboratories that provide special services to meet the unique needs of the perinatal patient.

EFFECTS OF REGIONAL ORGANIZATION OF PERINATAL SERVICES

The development of newborn intensive care units and transport systems has been associated with marked reduction in neonatal mortality (Fig. 2-1) as well as reduction in the frequency of neurologic sequelae. In Quebec the perinatal mortality survey demonstrated reduced mortality in hospitals using referral to a neonatal intensive care unit. In Toronto the neonatal mortality was reduced nearly 50% over a 10-year period with the development of a neonatal intensive care unit. Similar reductions in mortality have been demonstrated in Halifax, Nova Scotia, and Madison, Wisconsin. The development of statewide regional perinatal programs in Wisconsin, Massachusetts, and Arizona has likewise produced marked statewide reductions in perinatal mortali-

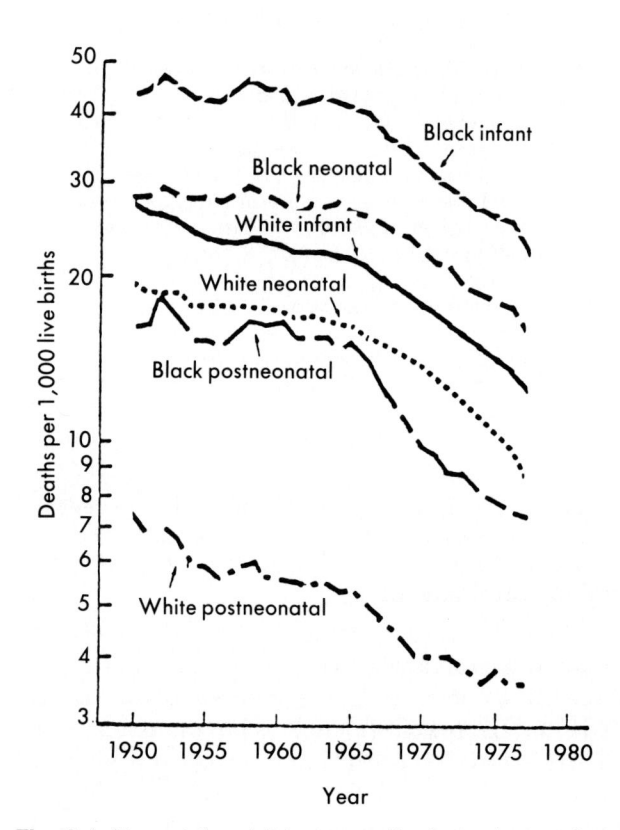

Fig. 2-1. Neonatal and infant mortality in the United States since 1950. (From National Center for Health Statistics. Computed by the Division of Analysis from data compiled by the Division of Vital Statistics.)

ty attributed to the statewide teaching program as well as to the development of regional centers. Following the development of a statewide infant transport program for regional neonatal intensive care units in Arizona there was a decrease in the state neonatal mortality from 17.3 to 11.5 deaths per thousand live births over a 5-year period. Infant mortality decreased and care practices improved within 2 years of the development of a statewide perinatal care program in Iowa.

PROBLEMS OF REGIONALIZATION

One of the most common disorders of regionalization is centralization in place of regionalization. This is the end product of a regional center that operates with no outreach education program or other mechanisms for continuing the development and improvement of services in the other hospitals of the region. With such a system the central hospital continues to receive the referrals of high-risk mothers or high-risk neonates but makes no effort to help the referring hospital develop programs for preventing the problems. This may be particularly true in university medical centers where outreach education and service are not considered a regular academic or hospital activity. Recently this problem appears to have diminished, particularly with "reverse transports," in which neonates no longer requiring tertiary level care are transported back to their community hospitals.

A second common disorder of regionalization is unnecessary duplication of units. This includes the unnecessary duplication of both level I and level II units within rural or urban areas and competing level III units, particularly in the smaller urban areas. The duplication results in difficulties in recruiting and maintaining the necessary personnel for such care units as well as in increased cost per patient for such care. Such duplication invariably is a result of competing institutions and competing medical staffs who view maternal intensive care and neonatal intensive care units as important to their business, income, or institutional image.

Many regional centers are staffed with inadequate or inappropriately trained personnel. One of the most common problems is the staffing of maternal and infant intensive care nurseries with inexperienced house staff as the primary responsible physicians, particularly during night hours and weekends. Such units often have only a single neonatologist or fetal-maternal obstetrician available, thus placing a great reliance on house staff. In such circumstances house staff also may become involved in answering requests for consultations from outlying hospitals and in other activities for which they are inadequately prepared. An equally serious problem of medical supervision is seen in those intensive care units which operate with no full-time in-hospital staff. The coverage and time commitment available from busy general pediatric practitioners does not permit the attention necessary for intensive care or the development of expertise. Inadequate or inappropriate staffing is also often manifested in the use of licensed practical nurses by hospitals in place of experienced professional nurses in the care of high-risk mothers and high-risk neonates. This is usually done as a cost-saving measure with inadequate understanding of the value of experienced professional nurses in the delivery of high-risk perinatal care. There is likewise a reluctance to use clinical nurse specialists and nurse clinicians because of the cost and lack of understanding of their role in patient care.

A number of regional networks have no integrated system for transportation. This results in many patients, particularly high-risk infants, being transported in poorly equipped vehicles with poorly trained or inexperienced staff. Such regions have consistently increased mortality and morbidity as a direct result of problems associated with transport.

Finally, in most regions there are some institutions and physicians that consistently fail to appropriately use the resources of a regional center when the care of the patient clearly indicates such a need. The hospitals that make least use of the center may be located closest to the center. Fear of loss of patients, physician ego, and failure to recognize problems promptly are the major inhibitors to appropriate use of perinatal center resources.

MEASUREMENTS OF EFFECTIVENESS OF CARE ORGANIZATION

When the effectiveness of any care system as well as of its individual components is measured, it is essential to analyze data for the entire region. There are many examples of dramatic changes in mortality or morbidity statistics for a given hospital in the course of a single year, not as a result of improvement of care, but as a result of movement of patients with particular problems to another institution. If the geographic boundaries of a region are well designed, there will be limited patient movement from region to region. This permits consistent year-to-year evaluation of the care within the region.

Maternal mortality has declined to the point that it is no longer a satisfactory index of quality care. Fetal and neonatal mortality is still a reasonable indicator of perinatal care. In their evaluation within a region, the data must link the hospital in which the death is recorded with the institution and community in which the birth occurred or the care was initiated. Fetal and neonatal mortalities should also be divided by weight groups. The weight groups should be in 500-gm increments or less, beginning with 500 gm. If possible, the gestational age distribution and cause of death for the fetal or neonatal deaths should be established. Such practices make it possible to identify those areas or institutions within a region in which there are major problems with care. Infant mortality (those deaths occurring between 28 days and 1 year after birth) is an indicator of socioeconomic conditions and living standards as well as the availability and quality of health care.

When maternal, fetal, or neonatal mortality or morbidity rates are used, certain other information is necessary to permit useful interpretation. For maternal mortalities it is essential to separate those maternal deaths during or as a result of pregnancy associated with other maternal disease, such as severe cardiac disease or malignancy, from those deaths associated primarily with the pregnancy. This requires individual analysis of each death and assignment to preventable or nonpreventable categories. For evaluation of neonatal programs and regionalization, the frequency of 1-minute Apgar scores of 3 or under and 5-minute Apgar scores of 5 and under should be recorded. Also helpful in assessing effectiveness of care are the frequency of sepsis, traumatic delivery, respiratory distress syndrome, and neurologic problems, the number of intensive care days, and the number of patient transfers from community institutions to institutions of greater care capability.

All high-risk mothers and neonates should have systematic follow-up. Those infants at high risk for developmental, neurologic, or learning problems should be followed into school age with careful neurologic and educational testing. The incidence of child abuse and failure to thrive may also reflect parenting disorders having antecedents in the perinatal period.

FINANCIAL CONSIDERATIONS

The facilities within a regional network, including a regional perinatal center, are financially dependent on patient revenue or public support or both for the care of neonatal patients. With carefully coordinated use of resources and facilities the cost of care delivery can be contained. It is essential that the health insurance programs provide adequate coverage for obstetric and neonatal conditions and that charges reflect the cost of delivering the services. Medical assistance and other forms of payment as well as direct support of state and county hospitals must be adequate for the care needs. There must be adequate nursing staff, physician coverage, equipment, and supplies to achieve an acceptable quality of care. The reimbursement schemes should provide for patient transfer between institutions without multiplication of deductibles or major financial hardship to the patient. The cost of emergency transport of high-risk maternal and newborn patients should be covered. The financial incentives should promote the use of the resources appropriate to the patient care needs.

IMPLICATIONS FOR EDUCATION

In the organization of most perinatal regions the educational needs of health care professionals must be carefully integrated with the needs of the patient and family. It is essential that the patient's needs for privacy, care, professional attention, and time for personal interactions among infant, family, and other important caretakers be recognized by those participating in patient care: nurses, medical students, house staff, and so forth. However, quality care is, in large part, dependent on undergraduate and graduate education programs that are an integral part of the responsibilities of a regional perinatal center. Senior staff physicians and nurses must accept direct responsibility for patient care and major management decisions while at the same time fulfilling their educational responsibilities toward those in training or in practice in the community.

Stanley N. Graven
Avroy A. Fanaroff

BIBLIOGRAPHY

American Medical Association, House of Delegates: Report J, Atlantic City, N.J., 1971, The Association.

Aubry, R.H., and Nesbitt, R.E.L., Jr.: High risk obstetrics. 1. Perinatal outcome in relation to a broadened approach to obstetrical care for patients at special risk, Am. J. Obstet. Gynecol. **105**:241, 1969.

Bacola, E., and others: Perinatal and environmental factors in late neurogenic sequelae. 1. Infants having birth weights under 1500 grams, Am. J. Dis. Child. **112**:359, 1966.

Callon, H.F.: Regionalizing perinatal care in Wisconsin, Nurs. Clin. North Am. **10**:263, 1975.

Callon, H.F.: Unpublished data.

Committee on Perinatal Welfare: Report on perinatal and infant mortality in Massachusetts, 1967 and 1968, Boston, 1971, Massachusetts Medical Society.

Drillien, C.M.: Growth and development in a group of children of very low birth weight, Arch. Dis. Child. **33**:10, 1958.

Drillien, C.M.: The long term prospects for babies of low birth weight, Hosp. Med. **1**:937, 1967.

Erickson, S.: Infant I.C.U.'s save lives but too many units may add cost and hamper growth, Mod. Hosp. **15**:80, 1970.

Goodwin, J.W., Dunne, J.T., and Thomas, B.W.: Antepartum identification of the fetus at risk, Can. Med. Assoc. J. **101**:458, 1969.

Grassy, R.G., and Zachman, R.D.: The growth and development of low birth weight infants receiving neonatal intensive care, Clin. Pediatr. **15**:549, 1976.

Graven, S.N., and Callon, H.F.: Perinatal care in Wisconsin, 1964-1974 (unpublished report), 1976.

Graven, S.N., Howe, G., and Callon, H.F.: Perinatal health care studies and program results in Wisconsin, 1964-1970. In Stetson, J.B., and Swyer, P.R., editors: Neonatal intensive care, St. Louis, 1975, Warren H. Green, Inc.

Hackel, A.: Interregional transport of high risk infants, Columbus, Ohio, 1974, Sixty-sixth Ross Conference on Pediatric Research.

Hobel, C.J., and others: Prenatal and intrapartum high risk screening, Am. J. Obstet. Gynecol. **117:**1, 1973.
Indyk, L.: Evaluation of equipment in transport systems, Columbus, Ohio, 1974, Sixty-sixth Ross Conference on Pediatric Research.
Knobloch, H., and others: Neuropsychiatric sequelae of prematurity: a longitudinal study, J.A.M.A. **161:**581, 1956.
Leonard, T.: History of the Wisconsin maternal mortality study and survey committee, Wis. Med. J. **69:**75, 1970.
Lubchenco, L.O., and others: Evaluation of premature infants of low birth weights at ten years of age, Am. J. Dis. Child. **106:**101, 1963.
Merkatz, I.R., and Fanaroff, A.A.: The regional perinatal network. In Caplan, R.M., and Sweeney, W.J., editors: Advances in obstetrics and gynecology, Baltimore, 1978, The Williams & Wilkins Co.
Meyer, H.B.P.: Regional perinatal care in Arizona, Columbus, Ohio, 1974, Sixty-sixth Ross Conference on Pediatric Research.
Ontario Perinatal Mortality Study Committee: Second report of the perinatal mortality study in ten university teaching hospitals in Ontario, Canada, 1967, Ontario Department of Health.
Pettigrew, A.H.: The role of the state department of health in regionalized perinatal care, Columbus, Ohio, 1974, Sixty-sixth Ross Conference on Pediatric Research.
Pomerance, J.J., and others: Cost of living for infants weighing 1,000 grams or less at birth, Pediatrics **61:**908, 1978.
Rawlings, G., and others: Changing prognosis for infants of very low birth weight, Lancet **1:**516, 1971.
Robertson, A.M., and Crichton, J.U.: Neurological sequelae in children with neonatal respiratory distress: infants with low birth weights, Am. J. Dis. Child. **117:**271, 1969.
Ryan, G.M.: Toward improving the outcome of pregnancy: recommendations for the regional development of perinatal health services, Obstet. Gynecol. **46:**375, 1975.
Ryan, G.M., and Fogerty, S.: Regionalization of perinatal health services (unpublished report), 1976.
Schneider, J.H., and Graven, S.N.: Regionalized obstetric/gynecology care in Wisconsin perinatal centers, Contemp. Ob/Gyn **3:**35, 1974.
Scott K.E.: Report of the Committee on Maternal and Perinatal Health of the Province of Nova Scotia, Nova Scotia Med. Bull. **49:**81, 1970.
Segal, E.S., editor: Transport of high risk newborn infants, Toronto, 1972, The Foetus and Newborn Committee of the Canadian Paediatric Society.
Silverman, W.A.: Dunham's premature infants, New York, 1961, Harper & Row, Publishers.
Stewart, A.L., Reynolds, E.O.R., and Lipscomb, A.P.: Outcome for infants of a very low birthweight: survey of world literature, Lancet **1:**1038, 1981.
Swyer, P.R.: The regional organization of special care of the neonate, Pediatr. Clin. North Am. **17:**761, 1970.
Swyer, P.R., and Goodwin, J.W., editors: Regional services in reproductive medicine, Toronto, 1973, The Joint Committee of the Society of Obstetricians and Gynaecologists of Canada and the Canadian Paediatric Society.
Toward improving the outcome of pregnancy (report of Committee on Perinatal Health of the American Medical Association, American College of Obstetrics and Gynecologists, American Academy of Pediatrics, and American Academy of Family Physicians), New York, 1975, National Foundation–March of Dimes.
Vapaavuori, E.K., and Raiha, N.C.R.: Intensive care of small premature infants: indications and results of treatment, Acta Paediatr. Scand. **59:**353, 1970.
World Health Organization Technical Report, Series No. 457, p. 7, as reported by Swyer, P.R.: Pediatr. Clin. North Am. **17:**761, 1970.

PART TWO

Perinatal outreach education

RATIONALE

The basic tenet of regionalized perinatal care is that all fetuses and newborn infants should receive optimum care consistent with their degree of illness or risk and regardless of their place of residence. Since over 80% of pregnancies are managed outside of regional perinatal centers, the main responsibility for early identification of the high risk patient resides with community-based practitioners. These individuals must assume responsibility for providing optimum resuscitation and stabilization for the 20% to 40% of high-risk newborns not identified before delivery. In rural areas the number of babies requiring such stabilizing care is even higher because of the inadvisability of transporting a woman in advanced labor over long distances. Thus, if perinatal statistics are to improve, the community-based perinatal professionals should be the main target population for teaching optimum perinatal principles and techniques. It is with sound basis, therefore, that the regional perinatal concept assigns outreach education as one of the major responsibilities of each regional perinatal center.

CLASSIC APPROACHES

Most of the traditional programs of continuing education have been based on the regional center's perception of the community hospital's needs. The most familiar of these is the 1- to 3-day lecture series organized for referring physicians and held at the regional center. Content often covers those subject areas which are appealing to the program director or which are particularly current in the medical literature. Usually the mistaken assumption is that the audience has a significant and uniform background fund of knowledge on which the speakers can build fairly complex concepts. There is frequently little attempt made to evaluate the practitioners' needs and then to design a program around those needs.

A fairly recent form of continuing education has been the "mini-residency," in which practicing physicians and/or community hospital nurses visit the regional center for several days or even weeks to function as short-term staff members. Although this format gives the practitioner more "hands-on" experience than does the lecture approach, generally the patients cared for have more complex problems and the equipment used is more sophisticated than will be dealt with or needed in the participant's local environment.

Most regional centers have developed a traveling outreach program in which a neonatologist, perinatologist, and perinatal nurse spend several hours in each of their referring hospitals giving lectures, critiquing the hospital's perinatal facilities, and reviewing the course of patients recently referred to the regional center. This format is often more successful than the others because it makes a significant attempt to tailor the educational experience to the unique needs of the community hospital. Disadvantages are that it is a relatively brief educational experience, it tends to attract the least busy individuals who often need the teaching the least, it is viewed with skepticism by many busy practitioners, and it is relatively time consuming for regional center personnel.

In general, each of these classic approaches is structured after the traditional teaching model of medical education (e.g., classroom lectures, apprentice training, education of each professional group separately). However, modern perinatal medicine does not function in a classic format of a single physician treating a single patient. The obstetrician relies on consultation from the pediatrician, the practicing physician cannot prescribe rational therapy for the infant without the expertise of the nurse at the bedside, and the perinatal patient with complex problems requires an intricate interdigitation of respiratory therapist, laboratory technician, social worker, nutritionist, and perinatal nurses and physicians to receive quality care. Community hospital perinatal medicine may rely on a smaller team size, but the same interdigitation of medical, nursing, and support disciplines is essential. Thus, although many of the classic teaching methods may be quite useful, they are not likely to have a significant effect on altering care practices unless they are incorporated as part of a comprehensive program that is team oriented and uses local resources.

PRINCIPLES OF OUTREACH EDUCATION
Community base

It is important that program participants be able to relate what they learn to their available resources for new knowledge to be translated into altered care practices. Also, because of the nature of community hospital staffing patterns and private practice demands, it is virtually impossible for more than several individuals to leave their jobs at one time. Therefore, for a program to be effective in changing patient care and to reach the most individuals, it should require a minimum of off-the-job travel time. The community hospital/office-based program is ideal for this purpose.

Multidisciplinary orientation

The most successful perinatal educational program will be aimed at the same multidisciplinary team that is involved with taking care of the patient in the clinical setting. Thus pediatricians, obstetricians, perinatal nurses, and supporting professionals, such as respiratory therapists, must be exposed to the same concepts simultaneously. A program aimed at just nurses or just physicians will generally not have a reflection in clinical practice without the endorsement of the other team members. Likewise, for maximum acceptability and practicality of subject matter, it is just as important that the program be developed and introduced to the community by the same type of multidisciplinary group. The minimum components of a regional center outreach education team include a perinatal physician and nurse. Optimally, all the disciplines just mentioned should be represented on this team.

Local participation in teaching process

It is extremely beneficial to have some of the program's activities coordinated by local personnel. This is particularly valuable if the program is anticipated to last several weeks or months or, preferably, to be a continuous experience. In most regional systems, geography and staffing limitations prohibit frequent interaction between center and community personnel. Also, in general, new concepts and skills will be more readily accepted and adapted to local care practices if first introduced by local community professionals. Therefore the most efficient and useful program will use selected local physicians and/or nurses as teachers and coordinators.

Content matched to patient care goals

Program content should be selected to match the complexity of care anticipated. If, for example, it is hospital practice and consistent with the state's regional plan for babies requiring respirator therapy or exchange transfusion to be referred to another center, then these subjects should be deleted from the program for that specific hospital. There are certain basic topics, such as resuscitation of the newborn, that are appropriate for all perinatal professionals; however, the overall content should be flexible to meet specific community patient care goals. In some regions these goals will have already been determined through the regionalization planning process. In others a process of identification of goals and resources must precede the educational program. An outline of the content for perinatal outreach education follows.

A. Fetal evaluation
  1. High-risk pregnancies
  2. Fetal maturity and well-being
      a. Skill: amniocentesis*
  3. Fetal monitoring
      a. Skill: fetal monitoring techniques
B. Immediate newborn assessment
  1. Resuscitation
      a. Skill: Apgar scoring

*Optional unit or skill. Included only for those community hospitals with the appropriate facilities and patient care goals.

        b. Skill: bag and mask ventilation
        c. Skill: endotracheal intubation
        d. Skill: cardiac massage
        e. Skill: medication administration
    2. Gestational age and size assessment
        a. Skill: physical/neurologic examination
C. Newborn care concepts and procedures
    1. Temperature control
        a. Skill: operation of radiant warmers
        b. Skill: operation of incubators
    2. Oxygen therapy
        a. Skill: measurement of oxygen concentration
        b. Skill: mixing, heating, and humidifying oxygen and compressed air
    3. Respiratory distress and apnea
        a. Skill: arterial sampling/transcutaneous monitoring
        b. Skill: continuous positive airway pressure*
    4. Umbilical catheters
        a. Skill: umbilical catheterization
    5. Blood pressure
        a. Skill: blood pressure measurement
    6. Hypoglycemia
        a. Skill: blood glucose screening
    7. IV therapy
        a. Skill: starting peripheral IVs
    8. Feeding
        a. Skill: tube feedings*
    9. Hyperbilirubinemia
        a. Skill: exchange transfusion*
    10. Infections
    11. Preparation for transport
    12. Continuing care for infants at risk

COMPONENTS OF A COMPREHENSIVE PROGRAM

The following items should be included in any comprehensive outreach education program. Each step builds on the accomplishments of the preceding one and anticipates the existence of the subsequent step. Therefore a regional center should have organized an entire plan (including provisions for funding, personnel, and software) before the potential participants are approached.

Initial contact

Unless a close rapport has already been developed between the community hospital and regional center, the proposed program often will be viewed with skepticism at this stage. Physicians will be concerned about regulation of care practices, nurses will anticipate unrealistic demands on staff time, and administrators will predict that the program will impose an unneeded expense on the hospital budget. Therefore community leaders from all three groups (medicine, nursing, and hospital administration) should be contacted simultaneously to prevent misconceptions from developing.

Commitment

Some general commitment to participate should be secured from the hospital and signed by the individuals just noted. At this time the commitment should be no more than an agreement between the community hospital and regional center to devote the staff time and funds (if any) to the program. Issues, such as referral contracts or patient care agreements, should be avoided or at least postponed until after the educational program. By that time a much closer working relationship will have developed, and all parties will be aware of the resources required for delivery of various intensities of care.

Inventory process

Before any education is provided it is important to define goals and identify resources. It is pointless to teach procedures or concepts that will never be used, either because the appropriate type of patient will not be managed locally or because the necessary equipment will not be available in the local hospital. Therefore local practitioners should be encouraged to define their patient care goals and hospital personnel should be asked to define the facilities, staffing, and equipment available for patient care before any educational intervention. There should then be an attempt to compare the goals and resources so that the facilities can be expanded to accommodate the stated goals. In some cases the practitioners may elect to change their goals rather than acquire the recommended resources. As much as possible this process of goal setting and resource identification should take place at the local level with regional center personnel acting as advisors rather than prescribers.

Regional center workshop

At this point it is beneficial to have selected nurses and physicians visit the regional center to learn the new concepts and skills that will be introduced to the entire local staff during the upcoming program. This type of workshop differs from the classic mini-residency in that the participants should learn through structured sessions oriented toward community hospital medicine rather than through focus on care practices appropriate for a tertiary care center.

Cognitive program

Educational content areas for the program will vary depending on the patient care goals of each community hospital (see preceding outline). However, several areas (e.g., resuscitation of the newborn) are basic for any hospital with a delivery service. Several different formats have been developed (e.g., self-instructional books, mediated programs, programed texts, organized lecture series), and many are available commercially. Comparative studies indicating preference for one type of program over another have not been performed.

Skills acquisition

Many of the new concepts introduced in the cognitive program require the performance of newly acquired skills before they can be translated into altered care practices. Teaching of new skills often requires hands-on practice sessions in addition to a written or mediated lesson. Models such as manikins, sections of human umbilical cords, or anesthetized cats can provide subjects for the practice of certain complex skills, such as umbilical catheterization or endotracheal intubation.

Continuation (review/update)

All hospitals should have a comprehensive basic educational program available for orientation of new staff. The local professionals who have visited the regional center should be responsible for maintaining this availability. The regional center should periodically update the basic program, as well as provide a mechanism for teaching new concepts and skills to the individuals who have previously completed the basic program. One format that has been suggested for a periodic update is the transport-referral conference, in which physicians and nurses from the regional center and community hospitals meet to discuss the management of previously referred antenatal and neonatal patients. These conferences are particularly valuable after the community participants have been exposed to the basic program but may prove overly controversial and threatening if sufficient background knowledge has not been acquired.

EVALUATION

The type of evaluation process used should depend on three factors: the purpose of the evaluation, the size of the population being evaluated, and the extent of evaluation resources. Measures can be made of ultimate outcomes (such as changes in perinatal mortality and morbidity) or of intermediate outcomes (such as changes in patient care practices or referral patterns). Ultimate outcomes require longer analysis periods and larger populations and are therefore affected by more variables than are intermediate outcomes. On the other hand, if intermediate outcomes are used as a measure of effectiveness, one must make the assumption that a change in intermediate outcome will lead to a corresponding change in ultimate outcome. (For example, one must assume that, if arterial oxygen tensions are measured more frequently, there will be a reduced incidence of retrolental fibroplasia.) In general, ultimate outcomes are of particular value for analyzing the effects of multifactorial programs on large populations (such as the statewide effects of a perinatal regionalization program), whereas intermediate outcomes are more valuable for measuring specific changes in a small population (such as the effects of an educational program on the perinatal care delivered by a specific hospital).

Baseline preprogram measurements

There are two purposes in obtaining baseline measurements. First, it is helpful to determine which communities are in greatest need of an educational program. Second, to measure the effects of a program, preintervention data must be collected for comparison with data obtained after program activities.

The perinatal mortality data are probably the simplest and most accessible data for determining which communities are in greatest need of an educational program. However, as just mentioned, mortality data are not reliable for small populations, and therefore one should be extremely cautious about interpreting mortality data collected from individual hospitals, particularly if the birth rate is low. Therefore, for the purposes of determining educational need, only perinatal mortality trends occurring over several years should be examined. Estimates of educational need may also be derived from an analysis of patient status at the time of referral or by preprogram administration of one of the instruments listed in Table 2-2.

Measures of program effectiveness

For an educational program to be truly effective, it must be used by the community professionals and result in improved knowledge; the hospital facilities required for delivery of optimum care must improve; the care delivered to patients must change; and, ultimately, the number of babies dying or damaged must decrease (Table 2-2). Only two of these measures (changes in cogni-

Table 2-2. Measure of program effectiveness

Evaluation measure	instrument
Program use	Completion rates Evaluation forms
Changes in cognitive knowledge	Preprogram vs. postprogram test scores
Changes in facilities	Preprogram vs. postprogram inventory survey
Changes in care practices	Chart review Patient status at transport Referral patterns
Changes in patient outcome	Mortality Morbidity

tive knowledge and facilities) require that prospective, preprogram measurements be made. The others (e.g., changes in patient records or referral patterns) are best analyzed retrospectively to avoid having the evaluation process directly affect the outcome.

Program use is easily assessed by comparing the number of program participants to the total number of available personnel in each professional group. Most programs also include an evaluation form asking for the participants' assessment of the programs' format and appropriateness.

Cognitive knowledge change is classically measured by a written test administered before and after the program. However, good test questions are difficult to prepare and require extensive validity analysis before one can be confident of the results. Tests can also be threatening to the community hospital participants, particularly if administered on a pass/fail basis. If possible, answers should be returned to the participants so that the test becomes part of the learning process. A particularly valuable form of testing is the patient management problem of the branching tree or algorithm format. However, again, it is difficult to prepare such problems without ambiguity, and considerable validation testing of large populations is advisable.

Changes in hospital facilities can be measured by a simple postprogram repetition of the self-inventory process suggested for analysis of the hospital's baseline resources.

Changes in care practices are the most important of the intermediate outcomes to measure. Unfortunately, they also require the most time-consuming and expensive evaluation techniques. Also, they generally will be among the slowest to show change as the result of an education effort. It is not unusual for perinatal professionals to know intellectually the appropriate clinical action but then not practice it in the field. For example, although a physician may answer a test question correctly regarding the increased incidence of hypoglycemia in infants large for gestational age, considerable time may pass before a change in hospital policy will result in all babies large for gestational age receiving a blood glucose screen. A hospital chart review or analysis of patient status at the time of transport can be used to document various care practices. Translation of learned knowledge into altered care practices can be facilitated by returning the analysis results to the participants (see section on continuation [review/update]).

Change in patient outcome cannot be measured reliably on a short-term basis and therefore is of limited value for assessing the results of a specific educational intervention. A reflection in mortality statistics will require many thousands of births to occur, and true morbidity cannot be tested reliably in neonates. However, with appropriate resources, large populations, and sufficient follow-up time these ultimate outcomes provide the most convincing evidence of true change.

John Kattwinkel

BIBLIOGRAPHY

American Academy of Pediatrics: Standards and recommendations for hospital care of newborn infants, ed. 6., Evanston, Ill., 1978, American Academy of Pediatrics.

Clarke, T.A., Levy, L., and Mannino, F.: Use of the placenta as a teaching model, Pediatrics **62:**234, 1978.

Hein, H.A.: Regionalization of perinatal care in rural areas based on the Iowa experience, Semin. Perinat. **1:**241, 1977.

Jennings, P.B., Alden, E.R., and Brenz, R.W.: A teaching model for pediatric intubation utilizing ketamine-sedated kittens, Pediatrics **53:**283, 1974.

Kattwinkel, J., and others: Improved perinatal knowledge and care in the community hospital through a program of self-instruction, Pediatrics **64:**451, 1979.

March of Dimes Proceedings of the Conference on Outreach Programs: Their integral parts and processes, White Plains, N.Y., 1978 and 1980, The March of Dimes Birth Defects Foundation.

Oh, W., and others: Role of an educational program in the regionalization of perinatal health care, Semin. Perinatol. **1:**279, 1977.

Ryan, G.M.: Toward improving the outcome of pregnancy. Recommendations for the regional development of perinatal health services, Obstet. Gynecol. **46:**375, 1975.

Task Force on Pediatric Education: The future of pediatric education, Evanston, Ill., 1978, American Academy of Pediatrics.

Wirtschafter, D.D., and others: Continuing medical education: an assessment of impact upon neonatal care in community hospitals, Annu. Conf. Res. Med. Educ. **18:**252, 1979.

PART THREE

Stress and the performance of the intensive care unit staff

The ability of nurses and physicians to function effectively has a major bearing on the outcome of high-risk newborns. Near optimum performance is required of nursery staff to prevent death or handicap among the sickest of infants. The awareness of this fact is but one stress experienced by nursery personnel. This section considers the sources of stress in the intensive care unit, the reaction of nursery staff to stress, the effect of stress on personnel performance, and the management of stress in the intensive care unit.

SOURCES OF STRESS IN THE INTENSIVE CARE UNIT

Few work environments combine the multiple stresses common in intensive care units. These stresses result from a variety of sources, including fatigue, crowding, repetitive disturbing stimuli, complex tasks, role conflict, ethical uncertainties, and frequent exposure to death.

Traditional duty schedules result in considerable sleep loss for physicians. Nurses often experience chronic fatigue from an excessive work load, extra duty, or shift changes. Laube and Stehle surveyed 359 nurses from 30 randomly selected neonatal units. An occupancy rate exceeding 100% was reported for 26% of these units. In 48% of units, nurses work 6 to 8 consecutive days; in 70%, some nurses work double shifts. Circadian rhythms do not adjust well to shift changes scheduled more often than once monthly, and disturbed sleep patterns have been noted for nurses working night shifts.

Turner and co-workers have shown that the background noise in intensive care units is quite high relative to that recommended for hospitals. Unpleasant and unpredictable noise, such as monitor alarms, is known to increase errors, lower efficiency, and stress frustration (Chapter 19, part two).

Staff conflict and role confusion result from the variation in skills among staff members and the need to provide prompt expert care to seriously ill newborns. Traditional concepts of the physician-nurse hierarchy have been challenged as nurses have become skilled in tasks previously considered the responsibility of physicians (e.g., starting intravenous infusions, performing arterial punctures, identifying cases of pneumothorax, conducting resuscitation). Role confusion and conflict may have a major effect on staff performance. These problems can be minimized but not avoided by an emphasis on the team approach.

Ethical problems are also an unavoidable source of major stress in the intensive care unit. The attitudes of staff members toward ethical problems differ according to physician age, religious background, marital status, and specialty. In a study of medical intensive care units, Younger and co-workers found that, as a group, nurses were similar to physicians in their attitudes toward ethical issues. However, a significant minority of physicians and nurses were unhappy with group decisions involving ethical problems. Nurses were more dissatisfied than physicians with the method of reaching ethical decisions and the communication between staff and family members. Lippincott has emphasized that discordant values within groups are particularly stressful to intensive care unit personnel.

The strong feelings about death common to physicians in general may be even more intense among those who work in neonatal units. Neonatal staff members are generally highly conscientious persons who seem especially vulnerable to feelings of guilt. Todres and associates found that pediatricians reported more distress associated with patient death than did anesthesiologists.

The stresses in neonatal units are, of course, somewhat different from those in units for older patients. Neonatal staff do not have to deal with patients who may question or resist treatment or with whom they can easily identify. However, nursery staff face stresses peculiar to neonatal units: the frequency of congenital malformations, the occurrence of iatrogenic diseases of the newborn (e.g., birth trauma, retrolental fibroplasia, and kernicterus), and the disruption of parent-infant attachment. Neonatal staff are also burdened by the extent to which their errors may affect the development and longevity of their patients.

REACTION OF INTENSIVE CARE UNIT STAFF TO STRESS

The reaction of physicians to stress in neonatal units has received little study. However, Todres and co-workers interviewed house officers in Boston about their experience in a pediatric intensive care unit. Of those interviewed during the last week of their rotation, 41% reported discontent concerning staff relationships; 36% reported excessive fatigue; 36% reported depression related to death of patients; and 25% had feelings of incompetence. Frader reported similar feelings among pediatric residents interviewed about their rotation in a pediatric intensive care unit in Philadelphia.

More information has been gathered about nurses. Of those surveyed by Laube and Stehle, 29% reported that the most stressful problem they face is neonatal death; 17% cited a heavy work load; and 12% reported conflict with other medical personnel. These same problems were included in those considered most stressful by 87 nurses surveyed by Jacobson. The nurses in the Jacobson study also cited feelings of incompetence as a cause of stress; even experienced nurses mentioned these feelings. Lancaster and Korones asked neonatal nurses to grade both the frequency and the severity of various kinds of stresses. These nurses cited the admission of out-born infants at times of high census as a frequent and severe stress. Ethical concerns, although commonly experienced, were generally regarded as only moderately stressful. Other moderately disturbing sources of stress included a generally heavy work load, a maldistribution of nurses among the three 8-hour work periods, inadequate nursing time for emotional support of parents, and difficulties associated with working with house officers, including the frequent perception that house officers ignore the early signs of deterioration reported to them by nurses.

Gentry and co-workers have compared nurses working in intensive care unit and non–intensive care unit settings by their responses to a detailed questionnaire and a battery of psychologic tests. More depression, hostility, anxiety, and dissatisfaction occurred among intensive care unit nurses. No differences in self-esteem, guilt feelings, and general personality patterns were observed between the two groups. The authors related the difficulties of the intensive care unit nurses to situational stress associated with crowding, communication problems with physicians, and an excessive workload.

Since nurses and physicians working in the same unit have not been previously compared, we surveyed the feelings of our own house officers and neonatal nurses. A questionnaire was completed by 14 of 15 nurses who regularly work in our intensive care unit and by all 36 house officers who had previous rotations through the neonatal unit and who were working in our center when the survey was completed. Eleven sources of stress were rated from 0 (absolutely nonstressful) to 10 (unbearably stressful), considering both the frequency and the intensity of stress they produce. The mean score of all items was significantly higher for physicians ($x = 5.8$; SD = 2.2) than for nurses ($x = 4.8$; SD = 2.4) ($p < 0.01$). However, there was generally good agreement between physicians and nurses when the sources of stress were ranked from highest to lowest mean score ($r = 0.56$). A difference of more than three places in the rank order assigned by physicians and by nurses was observed for only two of the 11 sources of stress. The physical environment of our nursery (crowding, noise, heat, odors, etc.) was ranked first by nurses and sixth by physicians. Feelings associated with brain damage in surviving infants was ranked third by physicians and tenth by nurses.

The overall importance of each of the various sources of stress in our nursery was evaluated by averaging the mean score of physicians with that of nurses. In descending order, the three sources with the highest average scores (6.1 to 6.2) were support service deficiencies, fatigue, and concern that an unreasonable work load would compromise patient care. Intermediate scores (4.9 to 5.9) were calculated for physical environment, staff conflict, parental reactions (anger, grief, guilt, etc.) feelings associated with brain damage among surviving infants, and feelings associated with prolonged care of infants likely to die. The lowest average scores (4.1 to 4.9) were recorded for feelings associated with death, ethical qualms about intensive care for very immature, chronically ill, or brain-damaged infants, and concern that one's level of expertise (relative to that expected) would compromise patient care. The low scores for these items were unexpected and may relate to the use of denial as a defense mechanism among nursery staff.

The perceived effect of stress on personnel performance, well-being, and social relationships was also evaluated. Most house officers and nurses felt that stress had only a mild effect on their performance and well-being. House staff reported significantly more stress-related effects than did nurses, particularly for the effect of stress on their social relationships. Twenty-five percent of the house officers (9 of 36) attributed major difficulties involving family members or close friends to stress during their rotation in the nursery.

In contrast to the minimal health and social difficulties noted by our nurses, Laube and Stehle found that 35% of neonatal intensive care unit nurses reported stress-related illnesses, including headaches, gastrointestinal disturbances, and hypertension. Oskins found that a significant proportion (15%) of intensive care nurses scored in the high-risk range on the Rahe Life Change Event Scale, a scale alleged to relate level of stress to risk of illness. Considerable attention has been paid to the association of stress and illness in nonmedical professions, for example, the high incidence of hypertension, diabetes, and ulcer disease among air traffic controllers. Whether stressful occupations (irrespective of the personality and life-style of persons who choose these occupations) increase the likelihood of serious illness has not been determined.

There is limited information about the methods by which neonatal staff cope with various stresses. According to Lippincott, physicians are notable for their poor stress management and their use of denial. Denial, rationalization, and preoccupation with technology and pathophysiology are often used by physicians to shield themselves from the awareness of stress. Oskins has studied the coping methods and defense mechanisms reported by 79 nurses working in adult units in five hospitals. In dealing with stressful situations, these nurses noted a variety of coping behaviors. The three most common behaviors involved direct efforts to eliminate the source of stress. For the most stressful situations they also reported palliative and sometimes detrimental responses that most commonly included anxiety, anger, and the use of humor. Laube and Stehle, in their study of neonatal nurses, noted that the two most common coping responses involved "talking it out" and direct efforts to reduce the stress. About half of the nurses' responses involved indirect methods of coping (exercise, hobbies, eating, smoking, etc.).

EFFECT OF STRESS ON PERSONNEL PERFORMANCE

Although an optimum level of stress may improve performance, stress of the kind and degree present in neonatal units is more likely to impair performance. Psychologists have shown deleterious effects of crowding, noise, and role conflict in nonmedical settings; the effect of work load, work schedule, and sleep loss has been extensively investigated in military, aerospace, and industrial personnel. Performance deteriorates at night. This deterioration occurs among those who regularly work at night as well as among those who rotate from the day to the night shift. Maximum adaptation to night work cannot be expected from nurses who change shifts every few weeks. The decline in mental and motor abilities at night is aggravated by extended periods of duty and sleep loss. A survey in England, Wales, and Scotland indicated that 49% of obstetric house staff and 40% of pediatric house staff believed that their work was always or often impaired by their long periods of duty. Friedman and co-workers reported that house staff errors in the interpretation of electrocardiograms increase following nights on call. Stanley and Alberman noted an increased neonatal mortality at night in London hospitals in association with diminished staffing during the same hours.

We have compared the quality and outcome of newborn care during the day with that at night in a 22-bed neonatal unit at McMaster University, Hamilton, Ontario. At the same time the study was conducted, nursing staff routinely worked 12-hour shifts in teams of 8 to 11 nurses. Often one less nurse worked at night than during the day. Nurses changed shifts every 2 weeks and worked 7 days and 7 nights during each 4-week period. Three residents and two to four fellows worked in the unit each weekday. At night and on weekends one resident and one fellow remained in the hospital on duty for a continuous period of 28 to 32 hours. Thus, as in other neonatal units, the number and supervision of staff declined at night as levels of fatigue increased.

We found that during the night (2101 to 0900 hours) intravenous infusions infiltrated more often, and the tidal volume of ventilators was regulated less often (p <0.01) than during the day (0901 to 2100 hours). Blood pH values less than 7.20 (excluding values within 12 hours of admission) were recorded more often and in more patients at night (p <0.05). In addition, significantly more deaths occurred at night whether or not the infants who died within 12 hours of admission were excluded (p <0.05). When weekdays were compared to weekends, pH values less than 7.20 tended to occur more often on weekends. However, neither acidosis nor death occurred significantly more often on weekends. The fewest deaths occurred in the middle of the week in the periods beginning at 0901 on Tuesday, Wednesday, and Thursday. A progressive increase in deaths occurred on Friday, Saturday, Sunday, and Monday.

In a second study we related the time of admission to the subsequent development of infants admitted to the neonatal unit at Parkland Memorial Hospital, Dallas, Texas. With the support of the Robert Wood Johnson Foundation we have performed follow-up evaluations for infants who weigh less than 1500 gm at birth and infants who require ventilatory therapy. The Bayley Scales of Infant Development have been used to assess all infants at 92 weeks after conception (1 year corrected age). Data for the first 50 patients have been analyzed. Those infants admitted on weekdays have had a significantly greater mental score ($\bar{x} = 89$) than have those admitted on the weekends ($\bar{x} = 71$; p <0.05). Sizable differences in mental and motor scores (5 to 10 points) have been observed between those admitted during the day and those admitted at night. However, with only 50 patients the differences were not statistically significant. Of all infants, those admitted during the day on weekdays have had the highest mental score ($x = 96$) and motor score ($x = 99$).

The increased frequency of acidosis and death among newborns at night may result from endogenous diurnal rhythms unrelated to care and environment. However, such rhythms have not been identified in the first weeks after birth. A change in the quality of care seems a more likely explanation for the deterioration of infants at night as well as the impaired subsequent development of those admitted during times of reduced staffing.

This explanation is supported by a study we performed using time-lapse photography to assess the effect of time-related and clinical variables on bedside care in the McMaster neonatal unit. The activities of physicians and random samples of nurses assigned to the four-bed study area were photographed. To allow staff to adjust to the presence of the camera, photographs taken during the first weeks were discarded. As shown for the residents in Fig. 2-2, physicians were observed providing bedside care significantly less often at night than during the day. Total resident and fellow time devoted to bedside care was also significantly less on weekends. Much of this difference was due to a reduced number of house officers at night and on weekends. Physician time devoted to bedside care increased abruptly for patients with the greatest care needs as measured by our infant care score, which was calculated each day for each infant. The scores were determined independently by a senior nurse and based on a detailed list of observations and treatment methods used in our unit.

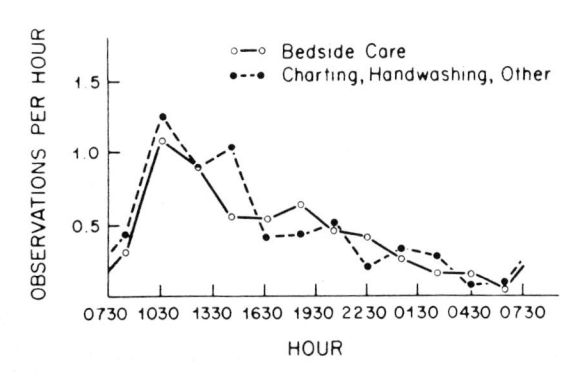

Fig. 2-2. Activities of neonatal residents during an average 24-hour period at McMaster University Medical Centre.

In contrast to that observed for physicians, bedside nursing time was unaffected by time-related variables (day vs. night, weekday vs. weekend, consecutive days or nights of work, or various nursing rotations). Regression analysis showed a linear twofold to threefold increase in bedside nursing with increasing infant care score.

The importance of individual differences among nursery personnel is suggested by multivariate analysis, which indicated that differences between individual nurses accounted for as much of the total variation of bedside care (30%) as did differences between infants in their care needs. The differences between nurses were not explained by traditional biographic information—age, marital status, rank in nursing school, nursing degree, and duration of intensive care unit nursing experience.

The influence of the infant on his care is suggested by the observation that 7% of the total variation in bedside care resulted from differences between infants unrelated to care scores. Several infants acknowledged as nursing favorites consistently received more bedside care than expected from their infant care scores; one ventilator-dependent infant with end-stage bronchopulmonary dysplasia consistently received less than expected. This study suggests that the deterioration of infants at night is likely to relate to a marked reduction in physician time devoted to bedside care during hours of diminished mental and motor skills as a result of fatigue. Our observations also suggest that many as yet undefined factors affect the individual or group performance of nursery personnel. However, it is likely that the care needs of patients (assessed in this study by infant care score) can be used to define appropriate staff numbers for units with differing or changing patient populations.

METHODS TO MANAGE STRESS IN THE INTENSIVE CARE UNIT

The deleterious effects of stress on the morale and performance of staff can be minimized by attention to the following areas.

Physical environment, staff number, and staff schedules

For many units an improvement in working conditions is the single change most likely to prevent undue stress. When asked to suggest one improvement for their intensive care unit, 43% of nurses surveyed by Laube and Stehle indicated the need for either more space or more staff. An increase in staff number as well as a reduction in crowding, disorganization, or stressful stimuli may be required to reduce the rapid nursing turnover in many neonatal units. The extra responsibility and stress associated with intensive care would seem to justify fewer hours and more pay. The cost of changes that increase retention of experienced nurses is likely to be offset by a reduction in the cost of iatrogenic disease and, as shown by Consolvo, the cost of training new staff.

Physician staffing practices should be reconsidered. The education of house officers and the welfare of high-risk infants may be best served by fewer duty hours for house officers in neonatal units, more equitable staffing at night, and/or increased responsibilities for properly trained nurses.

Professional growth and satisfaction of neonatal staff

Much of intensive care nursing involves highly repetitive activities. An active and ongoing in-service education program is essential to maintain the interest and increase the sophistication of nursing staff. Rotations to less stressful areas of the perinatal services are enjoyed by some but not all nurses. Nurses should be encouraged to attend conferences and workshops in other centers. Experienced nurses should be given new responsibilities stimulating to their development and the development of their unit (e.g., performance of procedures, participation in the transport program, the follow-up clinic, or the in-service, outreach, or parent education programs). Lateral promotions should be feasible for experienced nurses who prefer bedside care to administration.

In university hospitals the house staff teaching program should be carefully designed to meet specified educational goals at each level of training. House staff enthusiasm and effectiveness are likely to be increased by the feeling that education is an important goal of those responsible for the unit. If time permits, house officers should be encouraged to participate in teaching conferences and in the review of literature related to the management of difficult problems.

Although formal conferences may be quite educational, the greatest opportunity for professional growth for both house officers and nurses occurs at the bedside. Neonatal nurses surveyed by Laube and Stehle noted that their most satisfying experiences involved seeing infants improve and working with parents. Supervision, encouragement, and evaluation from the attending physician are crucial to the continuing improvement of staff performance and professional satisfaction.

Staff interaction

As emphasized by Marshall and Kasman, any effective program to manage stress in the intensive care unit will include continuous attention to staff interaction. Increased interpersonnel conflict is often the first result of the unusual stresses experienced by intensive care unit staff members. Such conflict should be appreciated before an increase in incident reports, staff illness, resignations, or other more obvious stress-related problems occur.

Some sources of staff conflict can be prevented by measures that are not only inexpensive but actually cost saving. These measures include well-defined nursery policies, clear communication of treatment plans, adequate training of new nursery staff, and recognition of skilled performance. Conflict between house officers and nurses should be minimized by emphasis on the team approach to patient care. Ethical dilemmas are more tolerable if the issues are clearly identified and discussed with the understanding that their resolution is ultimately the responsibility of the attending physician and often the parents.

Regularly scheduled meetings are widely recommended as a forum to improve communication and interaction among neonatal staff. Dubovsky and co-workers have performed the most careful study to document the value of such meetings. Changes in personnel performance were evaluated in a coronary care unit following the initiation of staff meetings attended by a consulting psychiatrist. A similar unit without these meetings was also studied. More favorable changes in charting, time spent in direct patient care, and patient mortality were observed in the unit with a psychiatric consultant.

Attempts to establish regular group discussions between physicians and neonatal nurses have not been universally successful. Attendance is often limited by clinical demands and scheduling problems, especially if the meetings are not perceived as particularly helpful. Both Frader and Rosini found a significant proportion of house officers were unenthusiastic about these meetings. The effectiveness of these discussions depends in part on whether there is sufficient leadership to maintain a healthy interaction between staff members and to improve problem areas once they are clearly identified. Even with expert leadership, difficult transition periods can be expected during the course of these meetings. However, such meetings can be used to identify problems in the operation of the unit, to resolve unnecessary misunderstanding or misinterpretation, to increase the appreciation of individual staff members for the opinions and concerns of others, and to communicate that anxiety, guilt, and uncertainty are common and acceptable feelings among neonatal staff. Neonatal units unable to establish these meetings successfully should consider a liaison with specialists skilled in leading group discussions.

Staff meetings should not supersede private discussions needed to promptly resolve strong personnel conflict. Very stressful events (e.g., iatrogenic disease, ethical dilemmas, and neonatal deaths) often require immediate discussion between senior staff members and those experiencing the most distress. In some instances a series of discussions is helpful, especially for those coping with death or ethical dilemmas for the first time. Following the death of infants, meetings between the parents and close staff members are often therapeutic for all involved. The strong relationships developed with families of seriously ill infants can be enriching and fulfilling to nursery staff, despite the frequent occurrence of death in neonatal units.

Investigation

Considerable research is needed to answer a variety of questions vital to the effective function of nursery personnel: What stresses most disrupt staff performance? What are practical ways to minimize serious stress and facilitate effective coping strategies? How can individual staff members having the most difficulty be identified and helped? What is the relationship of staff number to quality of care? What work schedule is most effective for neonatal personnel? What factors contribute most to personnel satisfaction, and how can they be used to maximize retention of experienced staff?

In summary, multiple sources of stress in neonatal units affect nursery personnel and compromise the outcome of seriously ill infants. However, excessive stress is preventable. With effective stress management, the operation of neonatal units can be modified to support the best possible performance of nursery staff and an optimum outcome for high-risk infants.

Jon E. Tyson
Robert E. Lasky

BIBLIOGRAPHY
Sources of stress in the intensive care unit

Cherniss, C., Egnatios, E.S., and Wacker, S.: Job stress and career development in new public professionals, Prof. Psych. **7**:428, 1976.

Cohen, H.H.: Working efficiency as a function of noise level, work pace, and time at work, Diss. Abst. Int. **33**:(8B):3975, 1973.

Jacobson, S.P.: Stressful situations for neonatal intensive care nurses, Am. J. Matern. Child Nursing, May/June, 1978.

Laube, J., and Stehle, J.: Profile of the neonatal intensive care nurse: personal characteristics, self-perceived stresses, and coping. Part I (submitted for publication).

Parasuraman, S.: Sources and outcomes of organizational stresses: a multidimensional study of the antecedents and attitudinal and behavioral indices of job stress, Diss. Abst. Int. **38**(9A):5584, 1978.

Todres, I.D., and others: Pediatrician attitudes affecting decision making in defective newborns, Pediatrics **60**:197, 1977.

Turner, A., King, C., and Craddock, J.: Measuring and reducing noise, Hospitals **49**:85, 1975.

White, L.P.: The self-image of physicians and the care of dying patients, Ann. N.Y. Acad. Sci. **164**:822, 1969.

Younger, S., Jackson, D.L., and Allen, M.: Staff attitudes towards the care of the critically ill in the medical intensive care units, Crit. Care Med. **7**:35, 1979.

Reactions of intensive care unit staff to stress

Frader, J.: Difficulties in providing intensive care, Pediatrics **64:**10, 1979.

Gentry, W.D., Foster, S.B., and Froehling, S.: Psychologic responses to situational stress in intensive and nonintensive nursing, Heart Lung **1:**793, 1972.

Jacobson, S.: Stressful situations for neonatal intensive care nurses, Am. J. Matern. Child Nurs. **3:**144, 1978.

Lancaster, J., and Korones, S.: Stress factors for nurses in iatrogenic problems in neonatal intensive care, The 69th Ross Conference on Pediatric Research, 1975.

Lippincott, R.C.: Psychological stress factors in decision making, Heart Lung **8:**1095, 1979.

Oskins, S.L.: Identification of situational stresses and coping methods by intensive care nurses, Heart Lung **8:**933, 1979.

Rahe, R.: Life change measurement as a predictor of illness, Proc. Roy. Soc. Med. **61:**1124, 1968.

Rahe, R., and others: Social stress and illness onset, J. Psychosom. Res. **8:**35, 1964.

Rose, R., Jenkins, C.D., and Hurst, M.W.: Health change in air traffic controllers: a prospective study. I. Background and description, Psychosomatics **40:**142, 1978.

Todres, I.D., Howell, M.C., and Shannon, D.C.: Physicians' reactions to training in a pediatric intensive care unit, Pediatrics **53:**375, 1974.

Effect of stress on personnel performance

Alluisi, E.: Sustained performance, work rest scheduling, and diurnal rhythms in man, Acta Psychol. **27:**436, 1967.

Ax, A., and others: Quantitative effects of sleep deprivation, J. Exp. Psychol. **66:**439, 1963.

Conroy, R.T.W.L., and Mills, J.N.: Human circadian rhythms, London, 1975, J. & A. Churchill, Ltd.

Finkleman, J.M., and Glass, D.C.: Reappraisal of the relationship between noise and performance by means of a subsidiary task measure, J. Appl. Psychol. **54:**211, 1970.

Friedman, R.C., Bigger, J.T., and Kornfield, D.S.: The intern and sleep loss, N. Engl. J. Med. **285:**201, 1971.

Glass, D.C., Singer, J.E., and Friedman, L.N.: Psychic cost of adaptation to an environmental stressor, J. Pers. Soc. Psychol. **12:**200, 1969.

Mills, J.N.: Development of circadian rhythms in infancy. In Davis, J.A., and Dobbing, J., editors: Scientific foundations of pediatrics, London, 1974, Heinemann Medical Books, Ltd.

Stanley, F.J., and Alberman, E.D.: Infants of very low birthweight. I. Perinatal factors affecting survival, Dev. Med. Child. Neurol. **20:**300, 1978.

Tyson, J., and others: Diurnal variation in the quality and outcome of newborn intensive care, J. Pediatr. **95:**277, 1979.

Tyson, J., and others: Analysis of newborn intensive care by time-lapse photography, Crit. Care Med. **9:**780, 1981.

Wilkinson, R.T.: After effect of sleep deprivation, J. Exp. Psychol. **66:**439, 1963.

Wilkinson, R.T., Tyler, P.D., and Varey, C.A.: Duty hours of young hospital doctors: effects on the quality of work, J. Occup. Psychol. **48:**219, 1975.

Williams, W.L., Lubin, A., and Goodnow, J.: Impaired performance with acute sleep loss, Psychol. Monogr. **73:**1, 1959.

Methods to manage stress in the intensive care unit

Bilodeau, C.B.: The nurse and her reactions to critical care nursing, Heart Lung **2:**358, 1973.

Cassem, N.H., and Hackett, T.P.: Stress on the nurse and therapist in the intensive care unit and the coronary care unit, Heart Lung **4:**252, 1975.

Consolvo, C.: Nurse turnover in the newborn intensive care unit, J. Obstet. Gynecol. Neonatol. Nurs. **8:**201, 1979.

Drotar, D.: Consultation in the intensive care nursery, Int. J. Psychiatr. Med. **7:**69, 1976.

Dubovsky, S., and others: Impact on nursing care and mortality: psychiatrists on the coronary care unit, Psychosomatics **18:**18, 1977.

Frader, J.E.: Difficulties in providing intensive care, Pediatrics **64:**10, 1979.

Hay, D., and Oken, D.: The psychological stresses of intensive care nursing, Psychosom. Med. **34:**109, 1972.

Marshall, R.E., and Kasman, C.: Burnout in the neonatal intensive care unit, Pediatrics **65:**1161, 1980.

Rosini, L.A., and others: Group meetings in a pediatric intensive care unit, Pediatrics **53:**371, 1974.

CHAPTER 3 Diabetes in pregnancy

The challenges offered to the obstetric-neonatal team by the occurrence of diabetes in pregnancy have served to stimulate many of the recent advances in perinatal medicine. Maternal metabolic disturbances and those resulting in both fetus and neonate fully test the integrated medical, nursing, nutritional, and supportive skills of a perinatal unit undertaking care of high-risk patients. Despite acknowledged challenges to both maternal and infant well-being, with no other condition has it been more readily demonstrated that comprehensive perinatal care can be effective in normalizing pregnancy outcome. Although many problems remain unsolved, the elucidation of the basic pathophysiology affecting the maternal-fetal relationship has led to better clinical results for both the diabetic woman and her offspring.

The scope of the problem of diabetes in pregnancy can be appreciated by a 1973 Health Interview Survey, which reported 443,000 women of childbearing age with diabetes mellitus in the United States. The prevalence of overt diabetes complicating pregnancy has been estimated to approximate 0.5% of all gestations in the United States; an additional 3% of women demonstrate transient biochemical abnormalities that are unmasked only during their pregnancies. Without appropriate care those women who are diabetic prior to pregnancy evidence a perinatal mortality 10 times that of a normal population, whereas those with diabetes only during gestation still have a twofold to threefold increase in rate of loss. The latter group requires special identification so that appropriate preventive efforts be initiated to ensure careful supervision of the developing fetus.

The overt or juvenile-onset diabetic woman presents more of a management than a diagnostic challenge. Under ideal circumstances, in her early reproductive years she will have been referred to an experienced center for contraceptive services, prepregnancy counseling, and advice with respect to later pregnancy supervision. However, a woman with a more subtle form of carbohydrate intolerance presents an additional problem of detection. Too often her diagnosis may be unsuspected or missed, and an unanticipated fetal death ensues. In the past, much of the pregnancy-focused diabetic testing was inappropriately performed in the early puerperium, at a point when it is now understood that insulin antagonism is no longer operative. Furthermore, traditional glucose testing during pregnancy had usually been confined only to selected high-risk categories. Women with histories of stillbirth, macrosomic infants, or first-degree family members affected with diabetes were the ones most commonly suspected of having latent diabetes mellitus. Studies have now shown that such clinical risk factors are by themselves insensitive indicators for patients with gestational diabetes. Therefore, routine diabetic screening is currently advocated for all pregnant women. Although not yet universally practiced, this approach appears to offer particular benefit in identifying those women at increased risk for carbohydrate-related perinatal loss, macrosomia, and birth injury. For example, Merkatz and associates in Cleveland have been offering a 2-hour capillary screening test following a 75-gm oral glucose load to all pregnant women throughout the community. Results indicate that, with modest inconvenience and cost, a significantly improved identification of gestational diabetes occurs. It is further suggested that, with minimal obstetric and nutritional interventions, the excess perinatal mortality and morbidity for these women can be effectively eliminated.

Unfortunately there are as yet no universally accepted criteria for a diagnosis of glucose intolerance during pregnancy. A 1979 Workshop on Gestational Diabetes (sponsored by the American Diabetes Association) examined various potential alternatives and could only define

Table 3-1. O'Sullivan-Mahan criteria for diabetes in pregnancy*

FBS	105 mg/dl
1 hour	190 mg/dl
2 hour	165 mg/dl
3 hour	145 mg/dl

*Based on overnight fast with 100-gm oral glucose load. Values are for plasma glucose with two abnormal values needed for diagnosis.

gestational diabetes as "glucose intolerance with its recognition of onset during pregnancy." It has been recommended that, at least for the present, the original published blood glucose values of O'Sullivan and Mahan be the ones employed to establish the diagnosis (Table 3-1). Although it may eventually be proved that these values do not pertain to pregnant women of all ages, weights, and stages of gestation, they remain as yet the most extensively studied.

The White classification groups pregnant diabetic women according to age of onset and duration of their disease as well as to the presence or absence of vascular complications. Although generally helpful as a prognostic guide to care, the system has its greatest potential value in comparing outcome results of clinical series reported by various institutions. The classification should not be used by itself to set guidelines for the timing of a particular patient's delivery, since irrespective of the White class that decision is now more appropriately based on a concept of individualized patient management. Following is a breakdown of the White classification of diabetes.

Class A: Gestational diabetes
Class B: Age of onset over 20 or duration of disease under 10 years with no vascular disease
Class C: Age of onset between 10 and 20 or duration of disease between 10 and 20 years with no vascular disease
Class D: Age of onset under 10, disease longer than 20 years, or retinopathy
Class E: Calcification of pelvic vessels
Class F: Nephropathy
Class R: Proliferative retinopathy

Pedersen and Pedersen originally identified co-risk factors known as "prognostically bad signs during pregnancy" that could be shown to adversely affect the outcome of the diabetic pregnancy. They demonstrated in all White categories that a fetus remains at increased risk if the mother experiences pyelonephritis, ketoacidosis, toxemia, or neglect of care. The obstetrician must be vigilant in identifying such factors promptly and in taking aggressive therapeutic steps to ameliorate or prevent their deleterious effects.

Changes in carbohydrate metabolism are characteristic of the normal pregnant state. Early in gestation, improved glucose utilization is typical for all, so for the diabetic woman an episode of hypoglycemia may sometimes provide the first clue that conception has occurred. This physiologic alteration usually begins in the first trimester and lasts for about 8 to 12 weeks. In the second half of pregnancy there occurs a decrease in the ability of endogenous insulin to translocate glucose into cells. The diabetic woman evidences a progressive increase in her insulin requirement. Rising levels of maternal progesterone, estrogen, and human chorionic somatomammotropin (HCS) all appear to play a role in this "insulin resistance" of pregnancy, but HCS has been primarily implicated. After delivery of the placenta the typical insulin refractoriness is abruptly lost, and the diabetic patient then becomes exquisitely sensitive to exogenous therapy. Thus normal and diabetic women alike are subjected to a series of metabolic alterations throughout both gestation and the puerperium.

INTRAPARTUM COMPLICATIONS
Unstable metabolic condition

Recent physiologic studies conducted in the controlled environment of the metabolic unit have provided 24-hour profiles of blood insulin levels, glucose concentrations, amino acids, and other metabolic parameters throughout normal and diabetic pregnancies. In particular, the fasting blood glucose level has been clearly shown to be lower during pregnancy than in the nonpregnant state. Furthermore, there is a marked constancy of blood glucose levels throughout the day, with plasma levels rarely exceeding 100 mg/dl except during the first hour following meals. In diabetic pregnancies, on the other hand, there appears a much greater flux in the concentrations of all fuels between fed and fasted states. With respect to glucose there is a tendency toward hyperglycemia after breakfast and nocturnal hypoglycemia. Thus the extremely stable metabolic milieu for the fetus that appears to characterize normal pregnancy is lost in the pregnancy complicated by diabetes. These observations now provide the clinician with a rational basis of blood glucose regulation during both the gestational and overt diabetic pregnancy.

It is prudent in both of these pathological situations that the maternal metabolic condition be stabilized by all available means to reapproximate the normal physiology of pregnancy. For the insulin-dependent patient dietary management, insulin therapy, and maternal activity are integrated to maintain euglycemia throughout the day. For most gestational diabetic patients dietary therapy alone suffices in achieving this objective. Although achieving normal blood glucose levels is important, the purpose of the diet is first to ensure an adequate maternal weight gain during pregnancy. Caloric intake is not restricted, since every attempt is made to meet both the calorie and protein requirements of normal gestation. Most patients consume a 2,200 to 2,400-calorie diet to satisfy both their own and the fetal energy demands. With obesity or adolescence, more rather than fewer calories are often needed to prevent the potentially deleterious effects of ketonemia. A nutritionist experienced with pregnant diabetic patients thus becomes an essential member of the health care team. Diets are constructed and modified in accordance with individual needs and preferences. Attention is focused on the total caloric intake as well as its individual components at various times during the day. To avoid marked fluctuations in the blood glucose level, an even distribution of calories and carbohydrates is suggested among meals and snacks. At least 20% of the diet should comprise protein totaling up to 115 gm. Carbohydrates usually provide 45% or more of the total calories, but monosaccharides are to be avoided, except for those available in natural sources.

If, after the establishment of an appropriate diet, blood glucose levels are not normalized throughout the day, insulin therapy is instituted. The data currently indicate that about 15% of gestational diabetic women need insulin treatment comparable to that for the overt diabetic. Combinations of intermediate and short-acting insulins divided between morning and evening doses appear to be most effective; approximately two thirds of the insulin is administered before breakfast and the remainder prior to the evening meal. Especially for patients unaccustomed to such insulin regimens, a period of adjustment and training in the hospital is often useful at midpregnancy. Corresponding to the times of peak insulin effect, four blood glucose determinations are obtained daily. Adjustments in one or more of the four insulin components can then be made in order to approximate the desired constant euglycemia.

It is, of course, difficult to simulate normal activity under such hospital conditions, so insulin requirements may be overestimated. Therefore, once a general strategy of dietary and insulin therapies has been established, continued ambulatory management is preferred. More exquisite metabolic control can be obtained when activity or frank exercise is used as a third therapeutic modality. As shown by Jovanovic and others, this ambulatory management has now become markedly facilitated through the availability of home glucose-monitoring techniques. The pregnant diabetic woman is currently able to closely supervise her own glucose profiles and to periodically adjust her diet, insulin, or activity accordingly. As pregnancy advances and the phenomenon of insulin antagonism becomes more influential, periodic modifications in the regimen are mandated. Blood glucose values in the range of 60 to 80 mg/dl fasting and less than 120 mg/dl post prandial reflect optimum maternal-fetal homeostasis. It should be underscored that oral hypoglycemic agents are not to be employed during pregnancy because of their potentially teratogenic effects in the first trimester and because of their capacity to induce profound and prolonged hypoglycemia in the neonate.

Fetal hyperinsulinism

Insulin has been implicated as the primary growth hormone for intrauterine development. For example, when fetal insulin is absent, marked intrauterine growth retardation occurs. On the other hand, when fetal hyperinsulinism is present as the result of maternal and fetal hyperglycemia, marked anabolic actions of insulin become manifest. There ensues an accelerated protein synthesis together with a deposition of excessive glycogen and fat stores. The typical macrosomic, plethoric infant of the diabetic mother results. This is the infant most at risk for the neonatal complications of hypoglycemia, hypocalcemia, hyperviscosity, and hyperbilirubinemia (Chapter 33, part one). Evidence from in vitro studies and from clinical observations among gestational diabetic women has recently been used to modify the original Pedersen hypothesis so that it now recognizes elevated maternal levels of amino acids and free fatty acids along with hyperglycemia as factors in promoting the development of fetal macrosomia. A surfeit of all metabolic fuels presented to the fetus in the presence of fetal hyperinsulinism is now understood to represent the basic pathologic mechanism in the diabetic pregnancy. Nevertheless, clinical efforts can as yet only be focused primarily on the control of maternal plasma glucose concentrations.

Maternal ketoacidosis

An episode of *maternal ketoacidosis* with its accompanying metabolic derangements represents the greatest threat to the life and well-being of the pregnant diabetic woman and her fetus. The mortality for the unborn baby resulting from such an episode may be as high as 50% or greater. With such a high degree of risk it must be concluded that only by early and aggressive management or, better still, through prevention will the contribution of diabetic ketoacidosis to overall perinatal mortality be significantly reduced. Each diabetic patient must be instructed to report early signs of infection and any suggestion of loss of metabolic control. A healthy dialogue must be established between physician and patient to ensure adherence to therapeutic regimens, and the entire obstetric team must be receptive to the patient's own concerns and observations. Maternal fasting and dehydration act in concert to augment the production of ketone bodies and to decrease their rate of eventual excretion. Superimposed on the normal accelerated physiologic ketosis of pregnancy, disturbances in oral intake coupled with nausea and vomiting serve to set the stage for a ketoacidotic episode. This risk is heightened particularly during protracted nausea and vomiting in late gestation. Patients may unwisely choose to eliminate an insulin dose. If there is a delay in diagnosis or continued disturbances in oral intake, serious decompensation of the diabetes may result. Therefore, when any potentially dangerous signs or evidence of serious alterations in metabolic regulation appear, the patient should be hospitalized and appropriately evaluated.

With overt ketoacidosis the maternal status, the insulin therapy, and fluid and electrolyte balance are best followed with a flow sheet. The fetal condition is appraised with external cardiotachometry. Maternal acidosis is often reflected in uterine hyperactivity together with a loss of fetal heart rate variability and/or the appearance of late decelerations. These changes usually resolve when maternal and fetal homeostasis has been restored. Intravenous insulin by bolus or continuous infusion is a primary component of therapy. The other principal need is for adequate replacement of body fluids, particularly to restore the depleted intravascular compartment. Therapy proceeds along physiologic lines to achieve metabolic stability. An initial use of isotonic (0.9%) saline solution is favored with a subsequent employment of more dilute fluids. Serum electrolytes, pH, and bicarbonate levels are followed closely. There is a reluctance to employ bicarbonate therapy in correcting maternal acidosis because of experimental data suggesting that it may paradoxically accentuate acidosis in the fetus. As metabolic equilibrium is restored, the diet and usual insulin regimen are resumed while antibiotics and other specific therapies are instituted to correct any underlying pathologic condition.

Stillbirth

Whether or not ketoacidosis, toxemia, polyhydramnios, or other serious complications develop during the course of a diabetic pregnancy, the risk of a sudden stillbirth at or near term cannot be totally discounted. For this reason, as the pregnancy advances, careful confirmation of fetal well-being is mandatory. The insulin-dependent patient may still have to be admitted to the hospital for a period of fetal surveillance prior to delivery. With more severe diabetes or with documentation of inadequate metabolic control, admission as early as 34 weeks' gestation may be prudent. When the maternal condition has been stable and there are no ominous signs, admission may be delayed until much closer to term. The gestational diabetic patient whose blood glucose profile remains normal with dietary regulation alone and who develops no other complication is typically followed on an ambulatory basis until labor begins spontaneously or until the duration of pregnancy becomes prolonged. If the pregnancy is to be carried much beyond 40 weeks, hospitalization should then be considered and the same intensive fetal surveillance provided as that for the insulin-dependent woman. Daily maternal plasma or 24-hour urinary estriol determinations reflect the size of the fetoplacental mass and provide a reassuring parameter of continued fetal well-being. Stress or nonstress cardiotachometry (p. 108) provides evidence of placental respiratory reserve and the status of fetal autonomic function. It has been sufficiently substantiated that this conservative approach is preferable to one which formerly recommended routine preterm delivery for all diabetic women.

Premature births

In the past, programatic attempts to prevent intrauterine deaths resulted instead in many iatrogenic premature births with an attendant high rate of neonatal loss and long-term serious hazard. Contemporary control of maternal diabetes and the available tools permitting adequate fetal supervision now facilitate the prevention of such prematurity. In particular, through amniocentesis and the analysis of amniotic fluid, the degree to which fetal pulmonary development has progressed may be ascertained prior to birth (p. 134). An induction of labor or scheduled cesarean section is postponed unless indices of surfactant synthesis are available and indicative of functional pulmonary maturity. When blood biochemical control has been present during late gestation, the usual lecithin/sphingomyelin ratio appears dependable for the diabetic pregnancy. However, in the absence of maternal physiologic stability, false positive test results occur more frequently, and an additional determination of amniotic fluid phosphatidylglycerol has been recommended prior to delivery.

Induction of labor is best initiated early in the morning when the entire perinatal team can be alerted and adequately prepared for delivery. From most reports it appears that, with modern management, as many as half of pregnant diabetics can now have safe vaginal deliveries.

Congenital anomalies

By correcting the metabolic abnormalities of diabetes in pregnancy and by individualizing the timing of delivery, we can minimize the incidence of stillbirths and neonatal deaths. Congenital anomalies, however, continue to be a significant problem for the offspring of diabetic women. Infants with major anomalies are born to diabetic women two to three times more often than they are to women in the general obstetric population. These anomalies most commonly arise during the first 7 weeks of embryonic life, which is before most women come under the care of their obstetricians and also before metabolic control is normalized. Thus there remains an irreducible minimum of perinatal mortality and morbidity that is secondary to fetal anomalies. Poor control in early pregnancy as evidenced by elevated maternal hemoglobin A_{1c} is associated with an increased risk of major structural malformations. There is some evidence that the establishment of euglycemia prior to conception and through the first trimester will reduce the incidence of congenital anomalies to approximate that of the general obstetric population. Thus further reductions in perinatal mortality and morbidity beyond the "irreducible minimum" may in time be feasible.

POSTPARTUM CARE

Post partum, the diabetic woman must continue under close supervision. Because of her potential sensitivity to exogenous therapy, long-acting insulins are usually withheld for the first 24 hours or more, and usually as little as half the prepregnancy dosage is the starting point for resumption of therapy. A prompt return to oral feedings following cesarean delivery aids in the restoration of normal control.

Lactation

It has been observed for years that lactation may be poor with maternal diabetes, and the problem remains unsolved today. Considerable support by the nursing staff and encouragement by all professionals are essential in aiding the well-motivated woman to establish adequate milk production. Good nutrition and continued attention to metabolic control help to overcome initial obstacles to successful breast-feeding.

Family planning

Finally, comprehensive perinatal care for the diabetic patient must also provide appropriate family planning advice and services. The postpartum period is a time when patients are eager for contraceptive counseling and most receptive to educational efforts. In general, barrier methods entail the least medical risk along with satisfactory levels of effectiveness for the motivated diabetic woman. Studies have also shown that the IUD may be employed without undue risk of infection. Oral contraceptive treatment entails potential problems with diabetic regulation and long-term cardiovascular complications. Nevertheless, with careful supervision this contraceptive modality may also be considered.

Method A. Duchon
Michael T. Gyves
Irwin R. Merkatz

BIBLIOGRAPHY

Goodlin, R.C.: Maternal-fetal acidosis. In Care of the fetus, New York, 1979, Masson Publishing USA, Inc.

Gyves, M.T., and others: A modern approach to management of pregnant diabetics: a two year analysis of outcomes, Am. J. Obstet. Gynecol. **128:**606, 1977.

Hill, E.: Effect of insulin on fetal growth. In Merkatz, I.R., and Adam, P.A.J., editors: The diabetic pregnancy: a perinatal perspective, New York, 1979, Grune & Stratton, Inc.

Jovanovic, J., and others: Feasibility of maintaining normal glucose profiles in insulin-dependent pregnant diabetic women, Am. J. Med. **68:**105, 1980.

Linzey, E.M.: Controlling diabetes wiht continuous insulin infusion, Contemp. Ob/Gyn, **12:**43, 1978.

Merkatz, I.R., and others: A pilot community based screening program for gestational diabetes, Diabetes Care **3:**453, 1980.

Merkatz, R.B., Budd, K., and Merkatz, I.R.: Psychological and social implications of scientific care for pregnant diabetic women. In Merkatz, I.R., and Adam, P.A.J. editors: Diabetes in pregnancy, Semin. Perinatol. (2):373, 1978.

Miller, E., and others: Elevated maternal hemoglobin A_{1c} in early pregnancy and major congenital anomalies in infants of diabetic mothers, N. Engl. J. Med. **304:**1331, 1981.

O'Sullivan, J.B., and Mahan, C.M.: Criteria for the oral glucose tolerance test in pregnancy, Diabetes **13:**278, 1964.

Pedersen, J., Molsted-Pedersen, L., and Anderson, B.: Assessors of fetal perinatal mortality in diabetic pregnancy, Diabetes **23:**302, 1974.

Rodman, H.M., and others: The diabetic pregnancy as a model for modern perinatal care. In New, M.I., and Fiser, R.H., Jr., editors: Diabetes and other endocrine disorders during pregnancy and in the newborn, Progress in Clinical and Biological Research, vol. 10, New York, 1976, Alan R. Liss, Inc.

Summary and Recommendations, Report of the Workshop Chairmen: Symposium on Gestational Diabetes, Diabetes Care **3:**499, 1980.

White, P.: Pregnancy complicating diabetes, Am. J. Med. **7:**609, 1949.

CHAPTER 4 Preeclampsia-eclampsia (pregnancy-induced hypertension)

Preeclampsia-eclampsia, toxemia, or *pregnancy-induced hypertension* is a disease peculiar to pregnancy and is found only in humans. It occurs clinically after the twenty-fourth week of pregnancy and is characterized by the sequential appearance of edema, hypertension, and proteinuria. Its onset is often subtle, and its etiology remains obscure. The pathophysiology of toxemia is well documented and affects both mother and fetus, indicating that therapy should be directed at both.

DIAGNOSIS

The term toxemia of pregnancy or, more appropriately, pregnancy-induced hypertension may resemble several specific categorical diagnoses if the patient is seen for the first time in the third trimester of pregnancy:
1. True preeclampsia (glomeruloendotheliosis)
2. Chronic hypertension
3. Renal disease
4. Transient hypertension

The differentiation of these diagnoses is often difficult and can be accomplished by a retrospective evaluation of each case or a renal biopsy during the first 5 postpartum days. In the Chicago Lying-In Hospital study 75% of primigravida patients with a clinical diagnosis of preeclampsia had biopsy-confirmed lesions of glomeruloendotheliosis. However, various combinations of these diagnoses may occur in the same patient (e.g., true preeclampsia, true preeclampsia and renal disease).

Mild preeclampsia is defined as the development of one or more of the following conditions after the twenty-fourth week of pregnancy:
1. Edema of the face or hands
2. A systolic blood pressure of at least 140 mm Hg or a rise of 30 mm or more above the usual level
3. A diastolic pressure of 90 mm Hg or more or a rise of 15 mm above the usual level
4. Proteinuria

In general, the following chronologic sequence occurs: edema, an increase in blood pressure, and the appearance of proteinuria. Edema is almost always present; without fluid retention, the diagnosis of pregnancy-induced hypertension should be questioned. Variations in the blood pressure obtained by the same observer may be caused by the vasospasm present in the disease, different environment, position of the pregnant patient, anxiety, activity, and time of day. The highest reading of the blood pressure is the most significant and indicates the cardiovascular reactivity of the patient. Proteinuria should be present in a clean-catch urine specimen on 2 or more successive days. If proteinuria is present in a significant amount (2+), this most likely indicates the renal lesion of glomeruloendotheliosis.

The normal decrease in peripheral resistance and blood pressure in the middle trimester of pregnancy must be considered. A 90/50 blood pressure reading may be observed during the middle trimester; thus an increment of 30 mm systolic or 15 mm diastolic would result in a blood pressure of less than 140/90. If such a patient has edema, the possibility of preeclampsia must be considered. The absolute values in blood pressure may not be as important as a change from baseline pressures. A recently observed phenomenon (roll test) is the increase in blood pressure when the position of a patient is changed. An increase of 20mm Hg or more diastolic blood pressure from when the patient is on her side after stabilization to when she is rolled on her back (positive) correlates with an increased risk of subsequently developing preeclampsia. This test should be done on *all* primigravida patients on each visit (preferably no longer than 2 weeks apart) starting at 24 weeks of gestation. If the roll test remains negative, it is unusual for the patient to develop preeclampsia.

Severe preeclampsia is diagnosed if one of the following signs or symptoms is present:
1. Systolic blood pressure of 160 mm Hg or a diastolic pressure of at least 110 mm Hg on two occasions, 6 hours apart, with the patient resting in bed
2. Proteinuria of 5 gm or more in 24 hours, which for practical purposes is a 4+ urinary protein level
3. Oliguria of less than 400 ml in 24 hours
4. Cerebral or visual disturbances
5. Pulmonary edema or cyanosis

The connotations for both mother and fetus are significant in severe preeclampsia.

Chronic hypertension is diagnosed by comparison of blood pressure values in a woman during pregnancy and in a nonpregnant state. In addition, pregnancy may unmask latent hypertension. A strong family history of hypertension is also helpful information. The long-term follow-up of patients who manifest hypertension during pregnancy is a means of retrospectively diagnosing whether the patient had preeclampsia or whether she had chronic vascular or renal disease. Preeclampsia does not cause hypertension in subsequent pregnancies or later in life.

ETIOLOGY

The cause or causes of this disease are still unknown. However, certain factors must be included in any etiologic theory of preeclampsia (toxemia). Preeclampsia is primarily a disease of the primigravida. Predisposing influences include multiple pregnancy, hydatidiform mole, and hydramnios. Preeclampsia is seen more often in certain regions of the world, particularly in the southeastern region of the United States. The condition occurs more frequently among indigent than private patients, and it is more prevalent as term approaches. It disappears once the uterus is empty. A renal lesion (glomeruloendotheliosis) is usually present and disappears after pregnancy. Some disruption of pregnancy homeostasis triggers events that eventually lead to preeclampsia.

EPIDEMIOLOGY

The incidence of preeclampsia throughout the United States is estimated to be 5% to 7% of all pregnancies. The geographic location, number of indigent patients, whether the hospital is a general hospital or a referral hospital, method of reporting, and other factors affect this incidence. Therefore reliable statistics on the incidence for large segments of the United States are not available. The problem is compounded further by erroneous diagnoses often made in this disease syndrome, and the recording of statistics is customarily an inpatient hospital procedure rather than an outpatient responsibility. In their international survey of eclampsia, Doll and Hanington cite the incidence in different countries as varying between 1.2 and 2.6 per 1,000 deliveries.

PATHOGENESIS

The normal homeostatic relationship during pregnancy (Fig. 4-1) becomes disrupted in acute pregnancy-induced hypertension. During uncomplicated pregnancies the placenta produces an increased amount of progesterone, which contributes to a minor sodium loss, since progesterone is a mild diuretic. This sodium loss results in contraction of the blood volume in the vascular compartment, which in turn activates the stretch receptor afferent arteriole and the juxtaglomerular apparatus to produce renin. Renin activates α_2-globulin in the blood, which is converted to angiotensin I and, by another enzyme, to angiotensin II. The angiotensin, in turn, acts on the zona glomerulosa of the adrenal gland to produce an increased amount of aldosterone as a compensatory mechanism. This increases the reabsorption of sodium from the renal tubule and subsequently reexpands the water in the vascular compartment, thus decreasing the stimulus on the stretch receptors, which decreases renin production.

In toxemia of pregnancy this homeostatic mechanism is altered by the pathophysiology seen in preeclampsia, including (1) a disease of arterioles, (2) a compromised metabolic function, (3) an increased central nervous system (CNS) irritability, (4) a decrease in renal function, (5) increased catabolism, and (6) altered (decreased) vascular volume. The scheme in Fig. 4-2 represents the development of the altered homeostasis in preeclampsia. The increased steroids and binding hormones contribute to the sodium retention and weight gain seen in normal pregnancy. There is also an increased aldosterone secretion rate in normal pregnancy, which is associated with an increased retention of fluid. The unaffected pregnant patient can easily handle this excess salt load. The beginning of preeclampsia may be aortic-renal compression. Renin activation triggers events that, along with sodium retention in vessel walls, contribute to the altered cardiovascular reactivity. The preeclamptic patient hyperresponds to pressor infusions such as epinephrine, norepinephrine, and angiotensin. Relative uterine ischemia develops and there is intravascular fibrin deposition, which may contribute to the development of the "toxemic lesion" (glomeruloendotheliosis); this may decrease the glomerular filtration rate and result in increased proteinuria. Glomeruloendotheliosis consists of a reversible swelling of the endothelial cytoplasm without involving other structures. The severe preeclamptic patient may also become oliguric.

Vasospasm and altered cardiovascular reactivity are

Preeclampsia-eclampsia (pregnancy-induced hypertension) 29

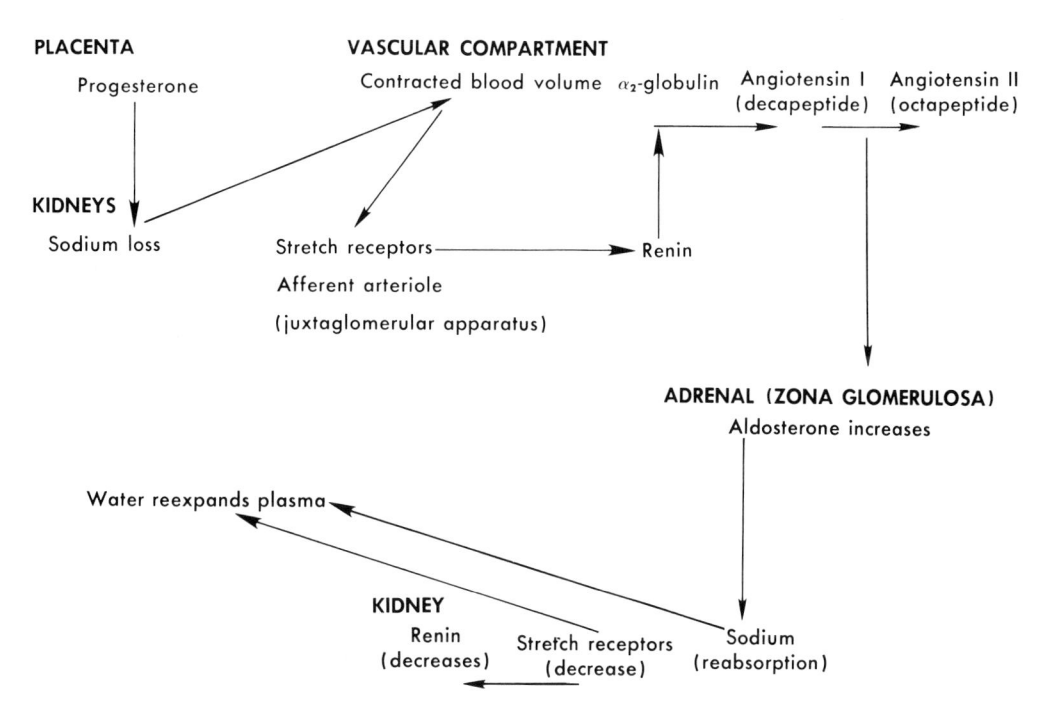

Fig. 4-1. Homeostatic relationships in normal pregnancy.

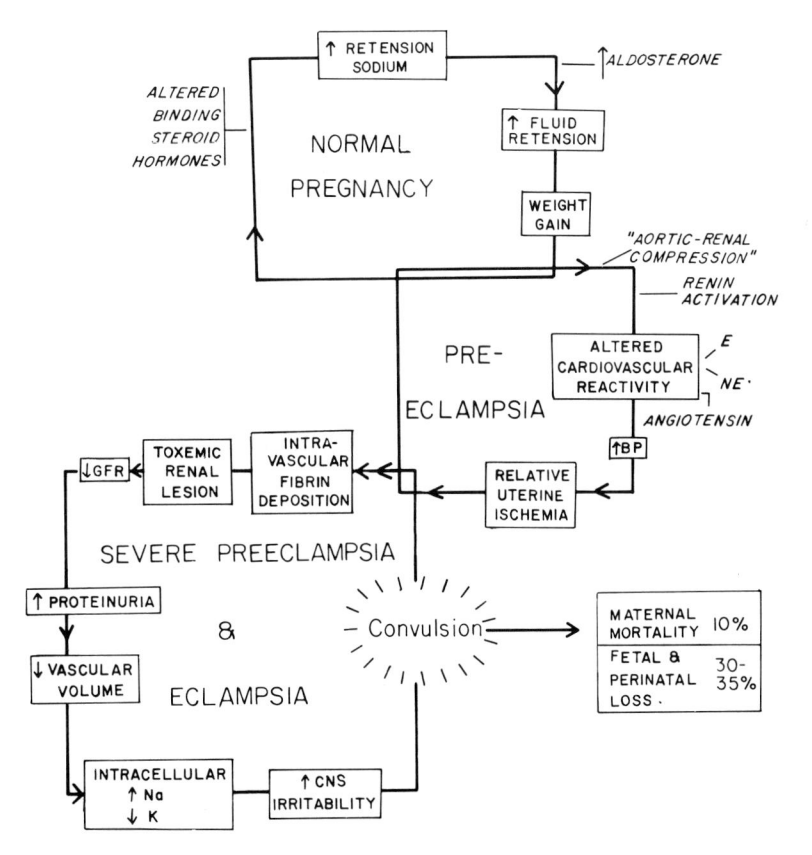

Fig. 4-2. Pathogenesis of preeclampsia. (From Zuspan, F.P.: J. Reprod. Med. **2**:116, 1969.)

hallmarks of acute pregnancy-induced hypertension. Pressor substances may contribute to this hyperreactivity. The vasospasm of the arterioles decreases blood flow to vital organs, especially the uterus, compromising placental function and placing the fetus in a precarious position for survival. It is not unusual to observe intrauterine growth retardation due to poorer placental nutrition. In all probability this altered uterine blood flow and decreased placental nutrition contribute to the large number of stillbirths that occur in the severe forms of preeclampsia.

Sodium is retained in patients with preeclampsia. There is an increase in the sodium space and in the total exchangeable sodium. Severe disease is associated with an increase in intracellular sodium concentration and decreased intracellular potassium concentration. These changes in sodium balance may explain both the increased cardiovascular reactivity and the increase in CNS irritability. The latter is easily demonstrated by testing for hyperactive reflexes. As preeclampsia worsens, the CNS irritability increases. Signs of CNS irritability, such as apprehension and anxiety, often precede a convulsion and are difficult to evaluate.

Hemoconcentration also occurs as the preeclamptic condition worsens. Fluid and electrolytes may shift to the third space and contract the blood volume. The serum electrolytes usually are normal. The blood volume of the relatively severe preeclamptic patient may approach that of a nonpregnant patient; a deficit of 1,000 ml or more is not unusual. The hematocrit value is high from hemoconcentration when the ill preeclamptic-eclamptic patient is initially seen. Subsequently, therapy and mobilization of fluid from the extracellular compartment, as diuresis occurs, lead to a decreased hematocrit value and can be viewed as a positive response to therapy. A positive nitrogen balance is usually seen in the unaffected pregnant patient; however, in the eclamptic patient there is a negative antepartum nitrogen balance and a positive postpartum nitrogen balance.

CLINICAL MANIFESTATIONS

It is often difficult to distinguish between abnormal fluid retention in the pregnant patient and early signs of preeclampsia. Once the disease is fully manifested, no form of therapy will reverse the process until delivery takes place. Intrauterine growth retardation is not present in most cases of preeclampsia but has been observed in cases of severe preeclampsia and eclampsia where the disease was present for some time.

Laboratory studies in all but the severe cases are usually within normal limits except that the hematocrit reading may show hemoconcentration. As the disease progresses, more abnormal findings may appear, as indicated in Table 4-1.

The most severe maternal and fetal complications obviously result in death. Maternal mortality varies from 0% to 13%, whereas perinatal mortality ranges from 10% to 37%. During the past four decades maternal mortality associated with preeclampsia-eclampsia has gradually decreased to less than 10% in the United States. Perinatal mortality, however, continues to remain excessive. The incidence of maternal and fetal mortality is in direct proportion to the severity of the toxemia. There is an increased frequency of prematurity and neonatal deaths in pregnancies complicated by severe toxemia. Mild and severe preeclampsia results in a perinatal mortality of 8% to 9%, whereas eclampsia may result in a perinatal loss of 24%. The overall perinatal mortality per 1,000 total births is increased two to three times over the expected perinatal mortality in unaffected patients. Perinatal mortality is partially dependent on the stage of gestation when severe preeclampsia occurs.

Abruptio placentae occurs more frequently in patients who have acute hypertension during pregnancy and is more common in patients who have preeclampsia. Madry's review of 39 cases of *hypofibrinogenemia* revealed that 54% were associated with abruptio placentae and 23% with preeclampsia-eclampsia. Hypofibrinogenemia is not clinically diagnosed until the fibrinogen level is 100 mg or less. The patient with severe toxemia

Table 4-1. Increased positive laboratory findings with level of hypertension

Condition	Hematocrit	Electrolytes	Serum creatinine (mg/dl)	Liver enzymes	Fibrinogen and split enzymes	Proteinuria	Estriol
Normal	↓	Normal	0.4-0.6	Normal	Normal	0	Normal
Mild preeclampsia	↓	Normal	0.4-0.6	Normal	Normal	Trace	Normal
Severe preeclampsia	↑	Normal	0.6-0.8	Normal	Normal	2+	Normal
Eclampsia	↑↑	Normal	Above 0.8	Elevated	Occasional ↓ fibrinogen and ↑ split products	4+	May be decreased

of pregnancy should be followed with serial fibrinogen and other coagulation determinations.

The severe preeclamptic patient occasionally may exhibit clinical signs of hemolysis as manifested by jaundice and dark-colored urine, which should be considered a bad omen. It is not known whether this represents hepatocellular damage or red blood cell destruction from other causes. These patients may have abnormal liver enzyme function and a decrease in fibrinogen. Periportal necrosis of the liver is a common autopsy finding in eclampsia.

Cerebral hemorrhage is the most common cause of death in toxemia of pregnancy. Convulsions may occur secondary to hemorrhage or to electrolyte imbalance and create added risks of aspiration, pneumonia, and trauma. Temporary loss of vision lasting for as long as 7 days has been observed. Hemorrhage occasionally occurs in the eyegrounds of a patient and should warn the clinician of an impending vascular accident. These patients require vigorous antihypertensive therapy.

Intrauterine growth retardation may be associated with preeclampsia-eclampsia if the disease is present for a protracted time period (p. 57).

PREVENTION

To prevent toxemia of pregnancy, one would have to eliminate many of the ills of society, including poor nutrition with low protein intake, overcrowding, limited antenatal care, and poor education on reproduction. Therefore the health care team's main effort in prevention must be in the identification and optimum management of those patients in whom the risk of pregnancy-induced hypertension is known to be greatest. All primigravidas should be considered at high risk. Prevention should include (1) a nutritious diet high in protein (1 gm protein/kg/day), (2) bed rest at noon for 90 minutes, (3) recognition of patient responsibility for pregnancy, and (4) frequent prenatal visits to the physician (every 2 weeks).

The characteristics of patients at risk are:
1. Primigravida
2. Poor
3. Lower level of education
4. Poor protein intake
5. Teenage primigravidas
6. Diabetes, renal disease, chronic hypertension, twins, and hydramnios

Patients with the above profile should be seen more frequently (every 2 weeks), since intensive perinatal care is essential to prevent development of severe forms of toxemia. The roll test should be used regularly, and if it remains negative, it gives reassurance that impending preeclampsia is *not* present. Fig. 4-3 illustrates that eclampsia is frequently a disease of teenage primigravidas. When identified early in pregnancy and seen at frequent intervals, these patients can be managed with a regimen that will prevent severe forms of preeclampsia. Hospitalization is mandatory once a patient progresses beyond the clinical stage of abnormal fluid retention. The incidence of severe preeclampsia-eclampsia can be significantly decreased by early recognition of toxemia and by its aggressive hospital management. Outpatient diuretic and antihypertensive therapies have no place in the management of preeclampsia.

TREATMENT

All therapy for preeclampsia-eclampsia is empiric, since the basic etiologic mechanism is unknown. Early hospitalization and proper care will almost completely eliminate the severe manifestations of preeclampsia and decrease maternal and fetal mortality and morbidity. Longterm prophylactic use of diuretics in pregnancy does not alter the incidence of preeclampsia, hypertension, prematurity, congenital anomalies, or perinatal mortality.

Once a patient is hospitalized and receiving therapy, convulsions should rarely occur. If reflexes are hyperactive, an intravenous infusion of magnesium sulfate is given. The concern in the preeclamptic patient is primarily for the fetus, since maternal mortality is rare. The time of delivery should be determined by a mature lecithin/sphingomyelin (L/S) ratio (p. 135) and other clinical factors.

The *mild preeclamptic patient* should be placed in the

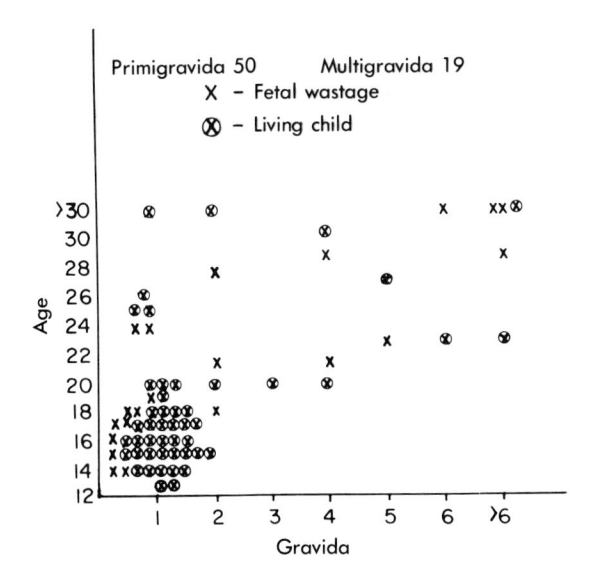

Fig. 4-3. Sixty-nine eclamptic patients show the disease to be one indigenous to the teenage primigravida. If a multigravida develops eclampsia, fetal prognosis is worse. (From Zuspan, F.P.: Clin. Obstet. Gynecol. **9**:964, 1966.)

hospital at complete bed rest but given bathroom privileges; she should be positioned on her side. She should be restricted to a sodium intake of less than 2 gm per day, given a protein intake of 70 gm or more per day, and given mild sedatives, such as phenobarbital (30 mg four times a day). Diuresis should be achieved within 18 to 36 hours by this regimen. If there is a mild blood pressure rise, it usually returns to normal. Diuretics are usually not needed if diuresis occurs within 48 to 72 hours after admittance to the hospital. The disease usually improves symptomatically, and often in 3 to 5 days the patient may be discharged from the hospital *under careful outpatient care*. However, if the gestation period is 38 weeks or more, the patient should be considered for induction of labor following control of the preeclampsia.

The patient with *severe preeclampsia* should be hospitalized and placed on her side at bed rest with bathroom privileges. She is weighed daily; intake and output are recorded; baseline laboratory studies are done, which include a 24-hour urine specimen, collected for protein and estriol determinations. An amniocentesis should be performed to evaluate fetal maturity. A 2-gm sodium diet containing 70 gm of protein is given, and the patient is given mild sedatives, such as phenobarbital (30 mg four times a day). The blood pressure is observed every 4 hours. Diuresis can be expected to occur within 24 to 48 hours, and the patient's condition should improve. If the patient has preeclampsia, her weight loss while she is on this regimen should exceed 2 kg in 3 days.

Unfortunately, some patients do not improve, and their condition deteriorates in spite of hospital management. Delivery must be considered in these patients. If the mother's condition and therapeutic control permit, induction of labor should be delayed until fetal pulmonary maturity is documented in the amniotic fluid. If the patient is beyond 34 weeks' gestation or the pulmonary maturity is adequate, the fetus should be delivered. The fetus of a severely preeclamptic-clamptic patient usually has few problems with respiratory distress syndrome. The toxemic patient may have a vaginal delivery by oxytocin induction regardless of the condition of the cervix; delivery should occur in less than 18 hours or a cesarean section is done. Abdominal delivery may be indicated for maternal reasons or for fetal distress or because of insufficient progress of labor with oxytocin induction.

The reflexes may be hyperactive in the severe preeclamptic patient, and this may be an indication for magnesium sulfate therapy. The magnesium sulfate is administered by infusion pump or by an intravenous infusion: 10 to 20 gm of magnesium sulfate is added to 1,000 ml of 5% dextrose and water. The rate of administration is approximately 1 gm per hour after a slowly administered loading dose of 4 gm. If magnesium sulfate is administered, the reflexes are monitored at frequent intervals; urinary output should be in excess of 100 ml every 4 hours. Once clinical improvement ensues, the magnesium sulfate is gradually decreased and often may be discontinued. Diuretics or hypotensive agents should not be used routinely in severe preeclampsia or eclampsia. Antihypertensive therapy should be given to prevent a cerebrovascular accident; diastolic pressure above 100 mm Hg should be an indication for hypotensive therapy. If a hypotensive agent is used, however, the diastolic pressure should not be reduced below 85 to 90. Hydralazine hydrochloride (Apresoline) by bolus injection, later followed by infusion pump administration, has been used successfully in controlling hypertension. Methyldopa (Aldomet) may also be given; this medication takes longer to act, however. Diazoxide is not indicated in these acute problems in pregnancy, since hypotension often develops after therapy, which is especially hazardous to the fetus.

The uterus should be emptied within a short period of time. When labor is induced, the severely preeclamptic patient delivers the fetus readily because of the characteristically increased uterine activity in the toxemic patient. Oxytocin is given by infusion pump in small doses, such as 2 to 4 milliunits, and increased to achieve the desired uterine activity. Uterine pressures and fetal heart rate (FHR) should be monitored electronically during labor. Cesarean section is reserved for obstetric indications, not for preeclampsia-eclampsia itself, unless the fetus is less than 1,500 gm; then cesarean section can be considered.

Once a patient with pregnancy-induced hypertension develops a convulsion and eclampsia is diagnosed, the survival statistics for both mother and fetus decrease dramatically. The following treatment regimen has resulted in zero maternal mortality and 10% fetal mortality if the fetus was alive when the eclamptic patient was seen. The basic therapy is with magnesium sulfate. No diuretics are used, and antihypertensive therapy (hydralazine) is used if the diastolic blood pressure exceeds 100 mm Hg.

Self-injury to the oral passages can be prevented during a convulsion by use of padded tongue blades. They should be available at the bedside in labor and delivery rooms. A plastic airway is inserted following the convulsion, and oxygen is administered. Adequate suctioning of the oral passages and the Trendelenburg position are necessary to prevent aspiration. The stomach contents should be aspirated by a nasogastric tube, preferably after adequate control with magnesium sulfate has been achieved. If this is done, an antacid should be instilled before removal of the tube. The antacid will increase the pH of the gastric contents and help prevent aspiration complications. Magnesium sulfate, 4 to 6 gm, is given *slowly* and intravenously over a period of 5 minutes to control the convulsion. A Foley catheter is inserted, and urinary output is recorded hourly; the specific gravity and albumin of the urine are determined every 6 to 8 hours and in pooled 24-hour specimens. If the patient is not convulsing, the initial loading dose of magnesium sulfate is 2 to 4 gm given intravenously, followed by 1 gm per hour. Infusion pump administration is preferable. If additional magnesium sulfate is needed because of hyperactive patellar reflexes, it can be injected into the intravenous tubing. Therapeutic amounts of magnesium also act as a mild sedative. Calcium gluconate should be kept at the bedside and 1 gm administered intravenously for magnesium overdosage (rare). Patellar reflexes should always be present but hypoactive when optimum magnesium sulfate therapy has been achieved. The urinary output should exceed 25 to 30 ml per hour if magnesium sulfate is being administered. If urinary excretion decreases below this level, the magnesium sulfate dosage should be decreased or stopped; if diuresis occurs, the dosage should be increased.

Because magnesium sulfate is a potentially dangerous drug, maternal reflexes, respiratory rate, blood pressure, heart rate, and urinary output must be monitored during its administration. The clinical manifestations of increasing levels of magnesium sulfate are a disappearance of knee jerks, a decrease in respiration, and cardiac arrest. Furthermore, it is synergistic when used with curarelike drugs. Although it is not a hypotensive drug, an initial transient decline in blood pressure may be observed, and it often decreases variability on a fetal heart pattern tracing. When administered for appropriate indications, in the optimum dose with adequate monitoring, the benefits of magnesium sulfate for the toxemic mother and her fetus outweigh the fetal and neonatal risks. The magnesium level in the newborn is the same as in the mother; thus, if a cord blood magnesium level is not measured, a maternal value is equally good. The magnesium is usually excreted by the newborn in the first 4 to 6 hours of life. Intensive observation of the newborn is indicated for signs of neuromuscular depression (Chapter 33, part two).

The mild forms of preeclampsia are not associated with an increased fetal or maternal loss; however, the severe forms of preeclampsia-eclampsia are associated with an increase in fetal loss and in maternal mortality. If the cause of hypertension during pregnancy is not diagnosed, a renal biopsy may be indicated during the postpartum period. The long-term prognosis of both mother and fetus needs critical evaluation. Adequate studies on infants born of toxemic mothers have not been done. Follow-up studies on the long-term prognosis for the mother have shown that eclampsia does not contribute to residual cardiovascular disease.

Frederick P. Zuspan

BIBLIOGRAPHY

Brewer, T.H.: Role of malnutrition, hepatic dysfunction, and gastrointestinal bacteria in the pathogenesis of acute toxemia of pregnancy, Am. J. Obstet. Gynecol. 84:1253, 1962.

Bryans, C.I., Jr., Southerland, W.L., and Zuspan, F.P.: Eclampsia; a longterm follow-up study, Obstet. Gynecol. 21:701, 1963.

Chesley, L.C.: Toxemia of pregnancy in relation to chronic hypertension, West. J. Surg. 64:284, 1956.

Claireaux, E.A.: Perinatal mortality in toxemia of pregnancy, Pathol. Microbiol. (Basel) 24:607, 1961.

Cobo, E.: Uterine hypercontractility in toxemia of pregnancy, Am. J. Obstet. Gynecol. 90:505, 1964.

Corkill, T.F.: Experience of toxemia control in Australia and New Zealand, Pathol. Microbiol. (Basel) 24:428, 1961.

Doll, R., and Hanington, E.: International survey of eclampsia and preeclampsia, 1958-1959: epidemiologic aspects, Pathol. Microbiol. (Basel) 24:531, 1961.

Gant, N.F., Worley, R., and Chand, S.: A clinically useful, simple method for the early identification of gravidas destined to develop preeclampsia, Presented at the Twenty-First Annual Meeting of the Society for Gynecologic Investigations, Los Angeles, March 27-29, 1974.

Hendricks, C.H.: Patterns of fetal and placental growth: second half of normal pregnancy, Obstet. Gynecol. 24:357, 1964.

Madry, J.T.: Blood coagulation defects during pregnancy, Obstet. Gynecol. 20:235, 1962.

Plentl, A.A., and Gray, M.J.: Total body water, sodium space, and total exchangeable sodium in normal and toxemic pregnant women, Am. J. Obstet. Gynecol. 78:472, 1959.

Pritchard, J.A.: Changes in the blood volume during pregnancy and delivery, Anesthesiology 26:393, 1965.

Pritchard, J.A.: Personal communication, 1976.

Pritchard, J.A., and Stone, S.R.: Clinical and laboratory observations on eclampsia, Am. J. Obstet. Gynecol. 99:754, 1967.

Raab, W., and others: Vascular reactivity and electrolytes in normal and toxemic pregnancy, J. Clin. Endocrinol. 16:1196, 1956.

Spargo, B., McCartney, C.P., and Winemiller, R.: Glomerular capillary endotheliosis in toxemia of pregnancy, Arch. Pathol. 68:593, 1959.

Talledo, O.E., Chesley, L.C., and Zuspan, F.P.: Renin-angiotensin system in normal and toxemic pregnancies. III. Differential sensitivity to angiotensin II and norepinephrine in toxemia of pregnancy, Am. J. Obstet. Gynecol. 100:218, 1968.

Talledo, O.E., and Zuspan, F.P.: Spontaneous uterine contractility in eclampsia, Clin. Obstet. Gynecol. 9:910, 1966.

Vande Wiele, R.L., and others: The secretory rate of progesterone and aldosterone in normal and abnormal late pregnancy. In First International Congress of Endocrinology, Copenhagen, 1960.

Zuspan, F.P.: Toxemia of pregnancy (foreword), Clin. Obstet. Gynecol. 9:857, 1966.

Zuspan, F.P.: Treatment of severe preeclampsia and eclampsia, Clin. Obstet. Gynecol. 9:954, 1966.

Zuspan, F.P.: Problems encountered in the treatment of pregnancy-induced hypertension, Am. J. Obstet. Gynecol. 131:591, 1978.

Zuspan, F.P., and Bell, J.D.: Variable salt-loading during pregnancy with preeclampsia, Obstet. Gynecol. 18:530, 1961.

Zuspan, F.P., Nelson, G.H., and Ahlquist, R.P.: Epinephrine infusions in normal and toxemic pregnancy. I. Nonesterified fatty acids and cardiovascular alterations, Am. J. Obstet. Gynecol. 90:88, 1964.

Zuspan, F.P., and Talledo, O.E.: Factors affecting delivery in eclampsia: condition of the cervix and uterine activity, Am. J. Obstet. Gynecol. 100:672, 1968.

Zuspan, F.P., and Ward, M.C.: Improved fetal salvage in eclampsia, Obstet. Gynecol. 26:893, 1965.

CHAPTER 5 Erythroblastosis fetalis

ERYTHROBLASTOSIS FETALIS

Erythroblastosis fetalis is a condition of the fetus and newborn caused by the transplacental passage of maternal IgG antibodies, which react with antigens on the fetal red blood cells (RBCs). In most instances the mother becomes immunized by the antigen on the fetal erythrocytes from a previous pregnancy, abortion, or blood transfusion. During a subsequent pregnancy the destruction of the fetal RBCs by maternal antibodies causes a severe hemolytic anemia that may result in congestive heart failure and fetal death. Severely affected neonates show the characteristic stigmata of hydrops fetalis: edema, hepatosplenomegaly, cardiomegaly, and extramedullary erythropoiesis. Rh immunization generally progresses in severity with successive pregnancies. See Chapter 29 for a discussion of this disorder.

History

Accounts of erythroblastosis fetalis date as far back as 400 BC, when Hippocrates described a syndrome similar to hydrops fetalis. Although many descriptive reports appeared subsequently, the etiology of the condition was not discovered until 1939, when Levine and Stetson described an atypical agglutinin in the blood of a woman who had a transfusion reaction when transfused with apparently compatible blood following the birth of a stillborn, macerated fetus. They postulated that the maternal immunization was the result of a fetal antigen inherited from the father and lacking in the mother.

Epidemiology

Before the advent of passive immunization with Rh immune globulin, erythroblastosis fetalis occurred in approximately 1% of pregnancies. Increasing use of Rh immune globulin, beginning in 1968, has markedly decreased the frequency of this condition. However, there are many individuals still in their childbearing years who are already immunized. In addition, a significant number of newly immunized pregnancies occur each year due to three causes: immunizations occurring during pregnancy, failure to administer the Rh immune globulin after delivery, and failure to administer a dose of Rh immune globulin sufficient to cover a large antigenic stimulus. Before effective treatment of this condition, 20% of the affected infants were stillborn and another 50% died in the neonatal period or suffered permanent brain damage. Today the practices of early identification of the patient at risk, serial antibody titers, amniotic fluid analysis for bilirubin, fetal maturity studies, preterm delivery, neonatal exchange transfusions, and occasionally intrauterine transfusions have contributed to a lowered perinatal mortality of 8% to 9%.

Diagnosis

Erythroblastosis fetalis encompasses a broad clinical spectrum. It can vary from mild disease that the newborn can overcome without therapy, to moderate disease requiring postnatal exchange transfusions, to severe fetal disease necessitating intrauterine transfusions. A careful history should include data on previous pregnancies and possible blood transfusions. ABO and Rh blood types should be determined in all patients, and antibody screening should be done on the initial antepartum visit regardless of the blood type of the individual. Antibody titers should be repeated at 24, 28, 32, 36, and 40 weeks' gestation in all Rh-negative patients. Even patients given Rh immune globulin in previous pregnancies should have routine antibody screening. Although erythroblastosis fetalis is usually more severe in pregnancies following the initial immunization, as many as 20% of fetuses in the first Rh-immunized pregnancy are severely affected, and the perinatal mortality in this group is significant.

The incidence of immunization in the first full-term pregnancy in the absence of a history of exposure to Rh-positive blood is 1% to 2% at the time of delivery.

IgM (saline-reacting) antibodies may be detected in early immunizations. These are generally transient. IgG (albumin-reacting) antibodies are detected when the IgM antibodies appear or shortly thereafter. Although the IgM antibodies disappear, the IgG antibodies do not. When a patient is immunized to the Rh antigen, she is immunized for life. The titer may decrease to a level where it is barely detectable, but further exposure to the Rh antigen generally invokes an anamnestic response with a substantial rise in the antibody titer.

In the *first immunized pregnancy* serial antibody determinations showing a rise in antibody titer indicate that the fetus is Rh positive. Serial antibody titers in this instance will usually reflect the condition of the fetus. Each laboratory should establish the "critical level" below which intrauterine death due to erythroblastosis fetalis has not occurred. For the optimum management of the Rh-negative patient, it is necessary to know when the anti-Rh$_O$(D) antibody first appeared. Once antibodies have been detected, titers should be repeated frequently until the "critical titer" is reached. At this point amniotic fluid analysis is required to assess the severity of the condition.

In *subsequent immunized pregnancies* the antibody titer may be of value only for indicating when other diagnostic procedures should be employed. If the antibody titer is low, a significant rise may indicate an Rh-positive fetus. If the antibody titer is high initially, the titer may rise, fall, or remain unchanged irrespective of the antigenic properties of the fetal RBCs. Therefore, in patients who have been previously immunized, serial antibody titers are not a reliable method of evaluating the status of the fetus. In these instances the amniotic fluid must be evaluated to assess the fetal condition. The time of the initial amniocentesis depends primarily on the patient's obstetric history and antibody titer. In general, the first amniocentesis should be performed at about 28 weeks' gestation unless a poor obstetric history or an antibody titer indicates that it should be performed earlier. Rarely is amniocentesis required before 23 weeks' gestation, since experience has shown that fetuses requiring an intrauterine transfusion earlier than 24 weeks' gestation are rarely salvaged. Once amniocentesis is initiated, it should be repeated at regular intervals until delivery.

Clinical manifestations

In 1956 Bevis reported a correlation between increased amniotic fluid blood pigments and the severity of erythroblastosis fetalis. There are several methods of analyzing amniotic fluid, all of which are based on the amount of indirect bilirubin pigment present; they provide an excellent index of the fetal condition. The various methods of analyzing the amniotic fluid have the same objectives: (1) to prevent intrauterine death of the affected fetus and (2) to prevent premature delivery of the unaffected or the mildly affected fetus. Most methods use a spectrophotometric scan of amniotic fluid to quantitate the amount of bilirubin pigments present. The pattern of these pigments is compared with the normal amniotic fluid pattern one would expect in an unaffected fetus at that stage of gestation. Based on the bilirubin values, the trend of these values, and studies of fetal maturity, a decision as to the appropriate time for delivery or the need for an intrauterine transfusion can be made. In general, rising bilirubin levels indicate a poor prognosis, whereas decreasing bilirubin levels indicate a good prognosis.

Most affected infants should be delivered before term. Mildly affected fetuses should be allowed to remain in utero until 38 weeks. More severely affected infants should be delivered as soon as fetal maturity is established or at that point at which the risk of infant death from prematurity is less than the expected mortality (5% per procedure by an experienced team) from intrauterine transfusions. In the very severely affected fetus

Table 5-1. Management of erythroblastosis fetalis

Status	Management
No antibodies	No disease
	Repeat antibody determinations at 24 weeks and every 4 weeks thereafter.
First immunized pregnancy	Antibodies less than critical value indicate a good prognosis
	Follow every 2 to 3 weeks with Rh titer to detect significant rise and avoid amniocentesis
	Antibodies at critical level or greater
	Amniocentesis after 25 to 26 weeks' gestation: low values indicate repeat amniocenteses every 2 to 3 weeks; high values indicate repeat amniocenteses every 1 to 2 weeks to establish trend
Subsequent immunized pregnancy	Amniocentesis indicated after 24 weeks' gestation: low values indicate repeat amniocenteses every 2 to 3 weeks; high values indicate repeat amniocenteses every 1 to 2 weeks to establish trend

requiring intrauterine transfusions, amniotic fluid frequently is not a reliable means of assessing the condition of the fetus after the first transfusion. The amniotic fluid may be contaminated with blood or meconium. In these instances, once an intrauterine transfusion has been performed, it is continued at regular intervals of 10 to 20 days until delivery. In addition to the analysis of amniotic fluid, some indication of fetal well-being can be obtained by observing fetal heart size, progressive absorption of blood, and absence of fetal ascites with ultrasound scanning. The oxytocin challenge tests (OCTs) and maternal estriol values (pp. 108 and 110) may also be helpful. Although high maternal estriol levels indicate the adequacy of metabolic pathways, dependent on a well-functioning fetoplacental unit, the values themselves are not good indices of the severity of erythroblastosis fetalis.

Management

See Table 5-1.

Amniocentesis should always be preceded by placental localization with ultrasound to decrease the chance of placental injury. Fig. 5-1 is a transverse ultrasound section of a patient with a large anterior placenta. The transabdominal approach is always used. Fig. 5-2 shows how ultrasound scanning can be used to find a placenta-free window for amniocentesis. The needle is usually directed toward the area of the fetal small parts (Fig. 5-3). However, occasionally the placenta overlies this area, and an amniocentesis in the area posterior to the fetal neck is indicated. Rarely, an amniocentesis may be done by displacing the fetal head upward, holding the head with one hand, and inserting the needle with the other. Objections to this technique are that it is cumbersome and manipulative and that the amniocentesis is done in the area of the maternal bladder. The needle puncture site is also closer to the cervix, and leakage of amniotic fluid may be more likely.

If a bloody specimen of amniotic fluid is obtained, a Kleihauer-Betke smear should be done to determine if the blood is fetal. In 90% of instances the blood is maternal. There have been no reported cases of severe maternal hemorrhage due to amniocentesis. If fetal blood is obtained and the fetus is viable, then the fetal heart rate (FHR) should be monitored for several hours to detect potential serious fetal hemorrhage.

A *spectrophotometric scan* is made of the amniotic fluid from 350 to 750 mμ. The optical density or absorbance is plotted against the wavelength. To determine the magnitude of the deviation from normal, a line is projected from 375 to 525 mμ delineating the approximate absorbance of amniotic fluid in the absence of bilirubin pigment. The deviation from normal is determined by calculating the increased absorbance due to indirect bilirubin pigments at 450 mμ. Fig. 5-4 is a spectrophotometric scan of a patient with severe erythroblastosis fetalis. The deviation in optical density at 450 mμ is 0.37. This value is used to evaluate the condition of the fetus.

Liley constructed a graph that he divided into three prognostic zones (Fig. 5-5). Zone 1, the low zone, indicates a nonaffected or mildly affected fetus. The upper zone, zone 3, indicates a severely affected fetus. In the middle zone, serial bilirubin values are used to assess the condition of the fetus. Those showing a decreasing trend of amniotic fluid bilirubin value usually have mild erythroblastosis fetalis. Those with increasing values have more severe disease.

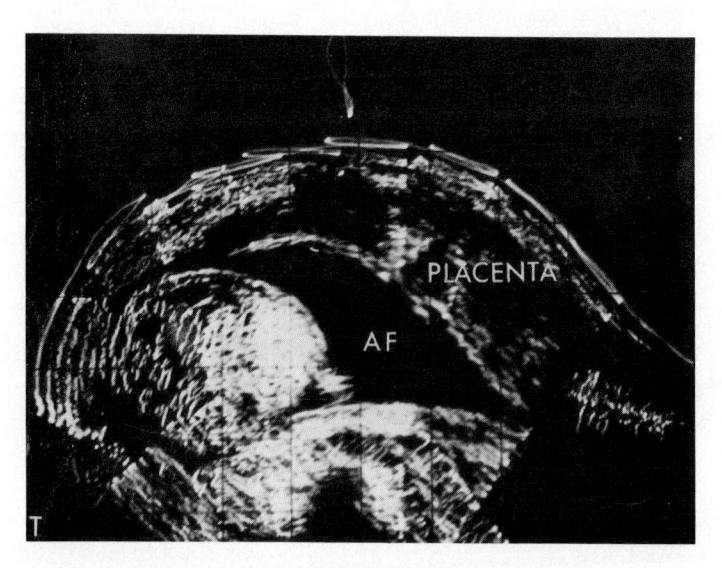

Fig. 5-1. Transverse ultrasound section of a patient with a large anterior placenta. Note the pocket of amniotic fluid *(AF)* and the fetal thorax on the patient's right side.

Queenan and Goestchel noted, on serial determinations, a decreasing value of ΔOD at 450 mμ with moderately affected, mildly affected, and unaffected fetuses. An increasing or horizontal trend occurred when the pregnancy terminated in intrauterine or neonatal death. A graph of their data is shown in Fig. 5-6. If the initial amniotic fluid bilirubin value is below the area of overlap, the fetus will almost certainly survive, but serial amniocenteses are still necessary to find the rare case in which the trend begins to rise later in gestation. Generally, two to four amniotic fluid samples are needed in these patients. If the initial value is above the area of overlap, the fetus is in danger of intrauterine or neonatal death. A repeat value in 1 week is indicated to verify the value and to determine the trend. If the value is constant or rising, the risk of an intrauterine transfusion must be weighed against the risk of the loss of the fetus due to complications of prematurity if delivered. If the risk to

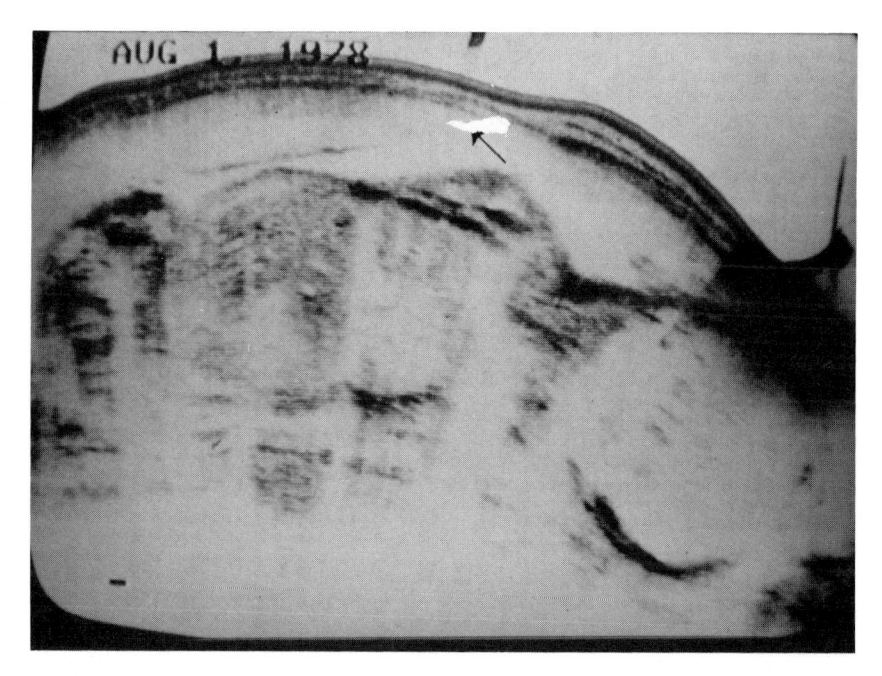

Fig. 5-2. Longitudinal ultrasound scan of patient with an anterior placenta. The arrow points to the lower edge of the placenta.

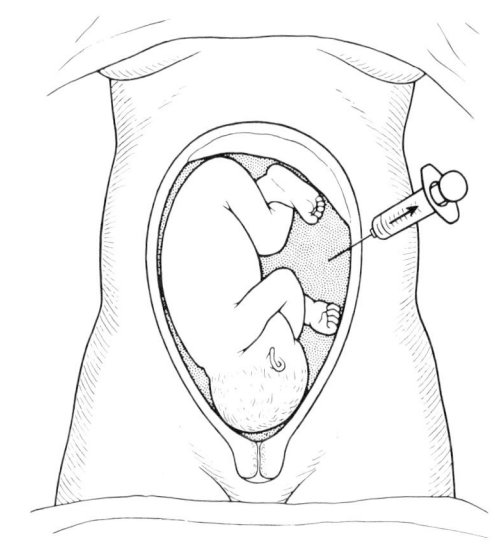

Fig. 5-3. Amniocentesis in the area of the fetal small parts. (From Queenan, J.T.: Clin. Obstet. Gynecol. **9:**491, 1966.)

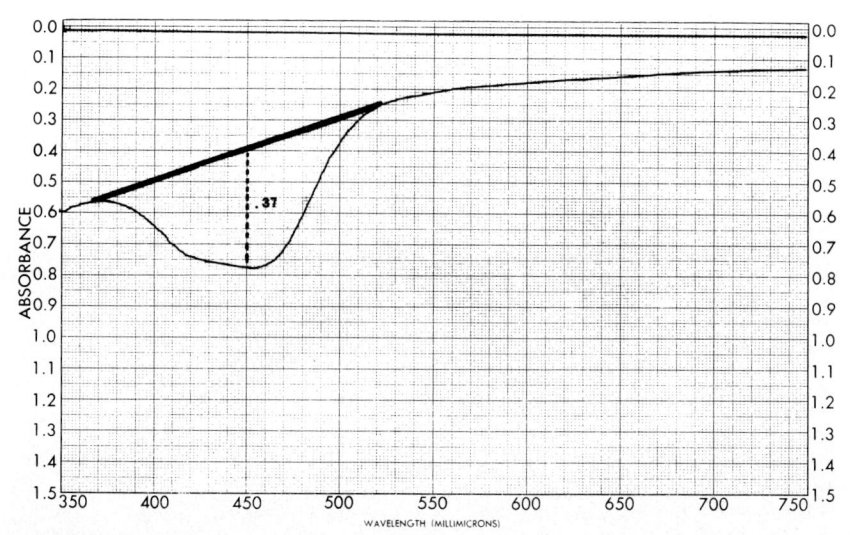

38 Behrman's neonatal-perinatal medicine: diseases of the fetus and infant

Fig. 5-4. Spectrophotometric scan demonstrating a typical "bilirubin hump" in a patient with severe erythroblastosis fetalis. The deviation in optical density at 450 mμ is 0.37. (From Queenan, J.T.: Clin. Obstet. Gynecol. **9**:491, 1966.)

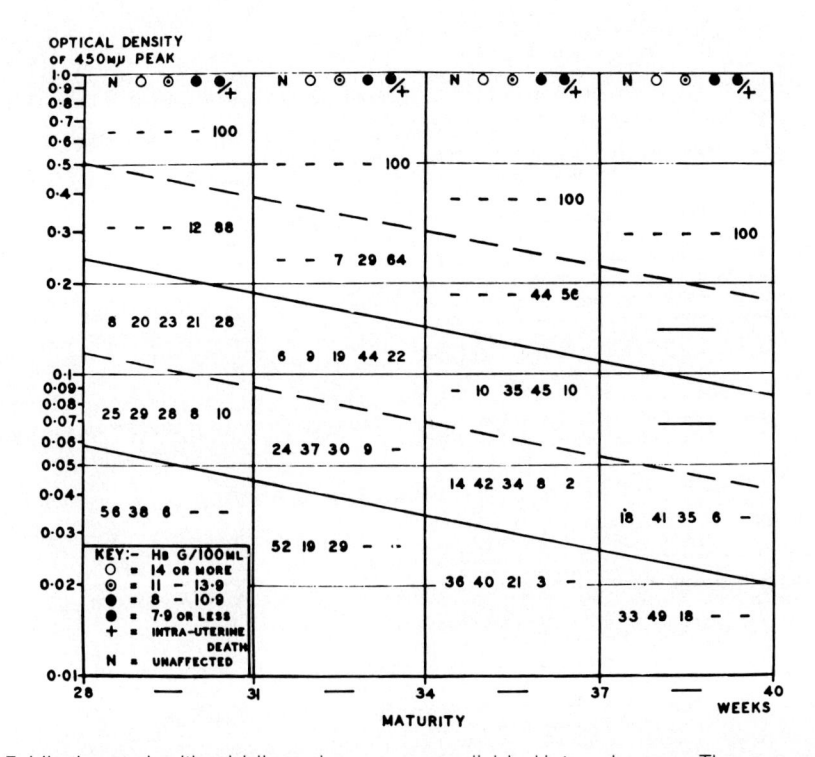

Fig. 5-5. Liley's graph with middle and upper zones divided into subzones. The percentage probability of various grades of affliction for the single amniotic fluid specimen is presented. (From Liley, A.W.: Am. J. Obstet. Gynecol. **82**:1359, 1961.)

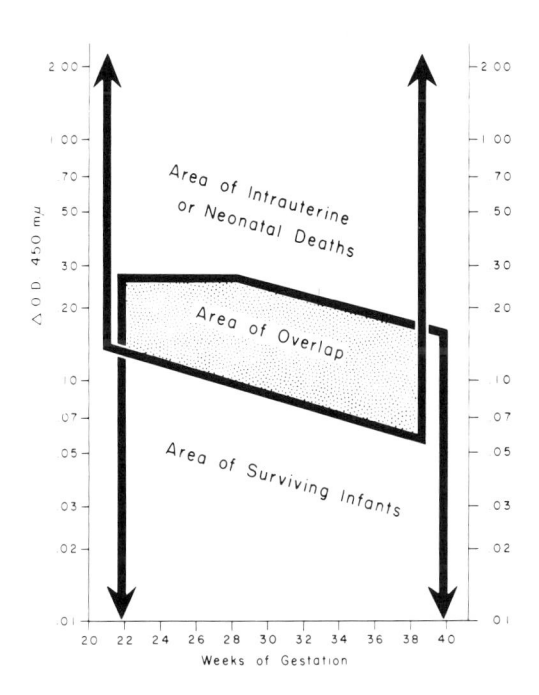

Fig. 5-6. Graphic representation of the distribution of amniotic fluid values from surviving infants and those with intrauterine and neonatal death. (From Queenan, J.T.: Modern management of the Rh problems, New York, 1967, Hoeber.)

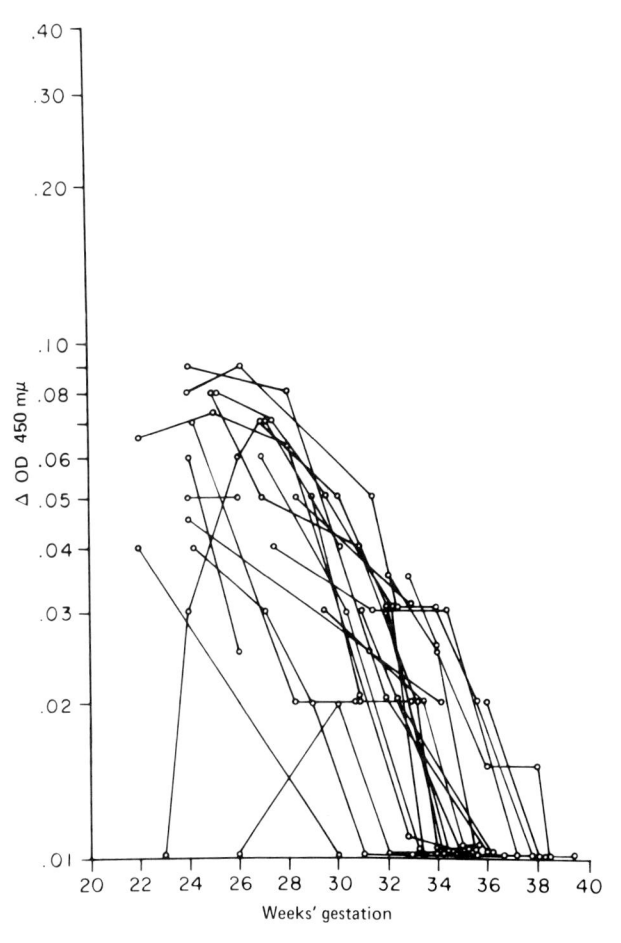

Fig. 5-7. Amniotic fluid bilirubin values from Rh-negative, immunized patients delivering Rh-negative (unaffected) infants. Values are recorded as change in absorbance at 450 mµ (Δ OD). Serial values are connected by lines; note the downward trend. (Reprinted with permission from Queenan, J.T., editor: Modern management of the Rh problem, ed. 2, New York, 1977, Harper & Row, Publishers.)

the fetus of delivery is greater than that of an intrauterine transfusion, then a transfusion is indicated unless the fetus is severely hydropic, as determined by ultrasonography. Generally, the earliest an intrauterine transfusion is performed is 24 weeks' gestation. If the fetus is truly at risk of dying earlier in pregnancy, intrauterine transfusions will not salvage the fetus. The latest that an intrauterine transfusion is initiated is 32 weeks' gestation. To be successful, the fetus must be well enough to survive long enough to absorb the intraperitoneal blood. When a fetus reaches 33 to 34 weeks' gestation, intensive neonatal management is far superior to intrauterine transfusion.

If the initial amniotic fluid bilirubin value is in the area of overlap, a single value is of little prognostic help, and repeat studies are necessary to establish a trend. Repeat amniocenteses indicating a decreasing trend denote a favorable prognosis. An exception to this generalization is seen in the case of polyhydramnios, which can dilute the bilirubin value and give a falsely low result. If the trend is horizontal or rising, the fetus is in jeopardy. Again, if the risk of intrauterine transfusion is less than the risk of perinatal death due to complications of prematurity, then an intrauterine transfusion should be performed.

Further study of amniotic fluid in the Rh-immunized pregnancies was undertaken. Particular attention was paid to the trend of amniotic fluid ΔOD at 450 mµ values. Fig. 5-7 shows the trend of amniotic fluid bilirubin values in patients delivering Rh-negative (unaffected) babies. The trend is distinctly downward. When patients delivering mildly affected babies (cord blood hemoglobin 14 gm/dl or greater) were studied, the amniotic fluid bilirubin trends were almost identical. When patients delivering moderately affected babies (cord blood hemoglobin 10 to 14 gm/dl) were studied, the values were similar and the trend was almost always downward. Patients whose fetuses died in utero were studied. The trend was almost always horizontal or rising, as shown in Fig. 5-8. These findings led to the establishment of the method of determining fetal condition by the amniotic fluid bilirubin trend.

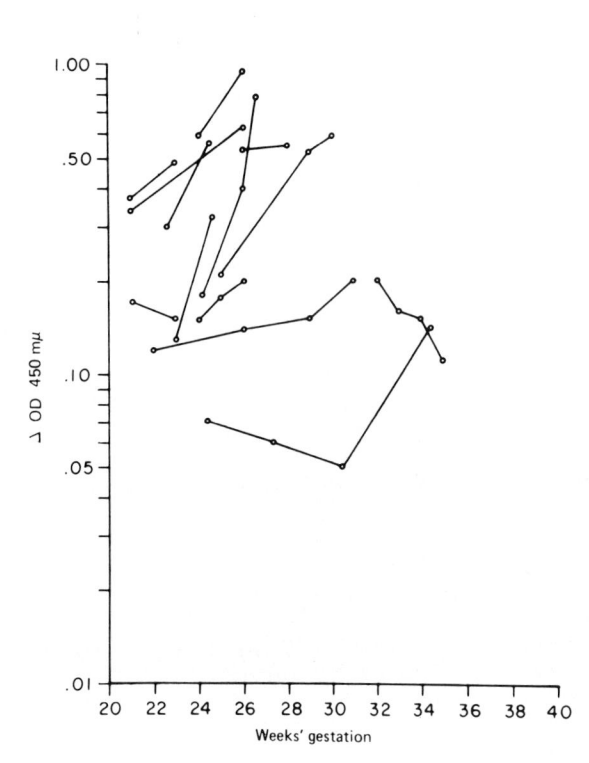

Fig. 5-8. Amniotic fluid bilirubin values from Rh-negative immunized patients whose fetuses died in utero. Serial values are connected by lines; note the upward trend. (Reprinted with permission from Queenan, J.T., editor: Modern management of the Rh problem, ed. 2, New York, 1977, Harper & Row, Publishers.) 1977.

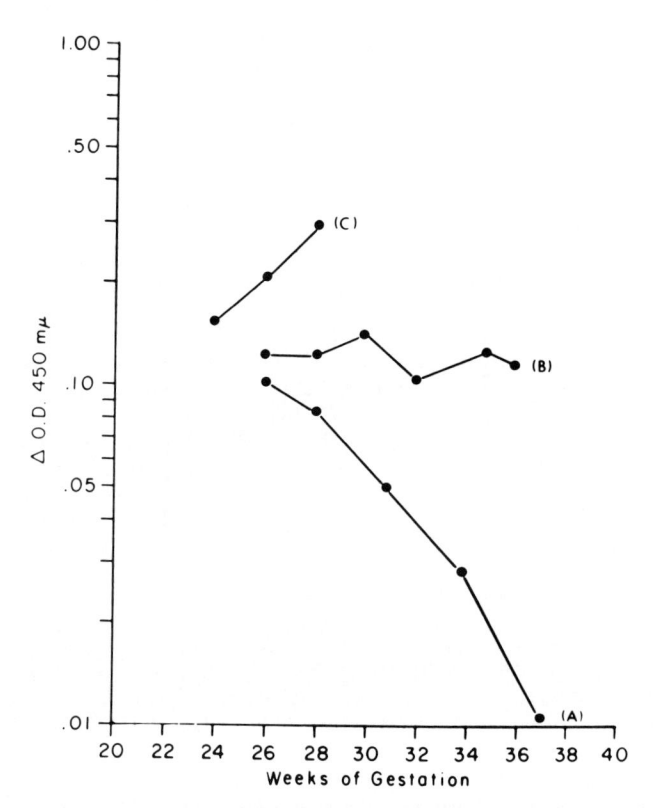

Fig. 5-9. Examples of various amniotic fluid bilirubin trend patterns. A, Decreasing trend, favorable outcome; B, horizontal or rising trend after 32 weeks indicates delivery; C, rising trend prior to 32 weeks may indicate intrauterine transfusion.

Clinical application

This method is based on the principle that the amniotic fluid bilirubin trend is extremely reliable in predicting the outcome of pregnancy in the Rh-immunized patient. The following protocol is suggested:
1. Do the initial amniocentesis at 28 to 29 weeks' gestation unless the patient's obstetric history or antibody titer indicates it should be done earlier.
2. Repeat amniocenteses at 1- to 3-week intervals, depending on the level of the ΔOD at 450 mμ.
3. Study serial ΔOD values to determine the trend (see Fig. 5-9). If the trend is falling, the fetus is safe until scheduled delivery at 38 weeks' gestation. If the trend is rising or horizontal, do an intrauterine transfusion between 25 and 32 weeks. If the trend is rising or horizontal after 32 weeks, perform preterm delivery.
4. Do amniotic fluid maturity studies in conjunction with ΔOD measurements to determine the optimum time to deliver.

When amniotic fluid bilirubin levels indicate that the fetus is affected with erythroblastosis fetalis, the clinician has a number of options to evaluate the fetal condition further. Amniography, once very important for detecting scalp edema and determining the amount of fetal swallowing, is rarely used today because ultrasound scanning has largely displaced this modality. Fetal scalp edema, as shown on the amniogram in Fig. 5-10, and decreased fetal activity are poor prognostic signs.

The major fetal surveillance in erythroblastosis fetalis is done by ultrasound scanning. The heart size may be noted to increase when the fetus is apparently developing congestive heart failure. Additionally, fetal ascites suggests that the fetus may die in utero. Fig. 5-11 shows an ultrasound scan in cross section of a fetus without ascites. Fig. 5-12 shows an ultrasound scan of another fetus at the level of the umbilical vein with ascites present. Whereas amniotic fluid analysis will identify the fetus that is affected and will potentially die in utero, further information may be gained by ultrasound scanning.

Fetal activity, both perceived and observed, is very important in determining when a fetus may die in utero. In the setting of a severely compromised fetus, a marked decrease in perceived fetal activity should warn the clinician that a fetal death could occur. Additionally, the

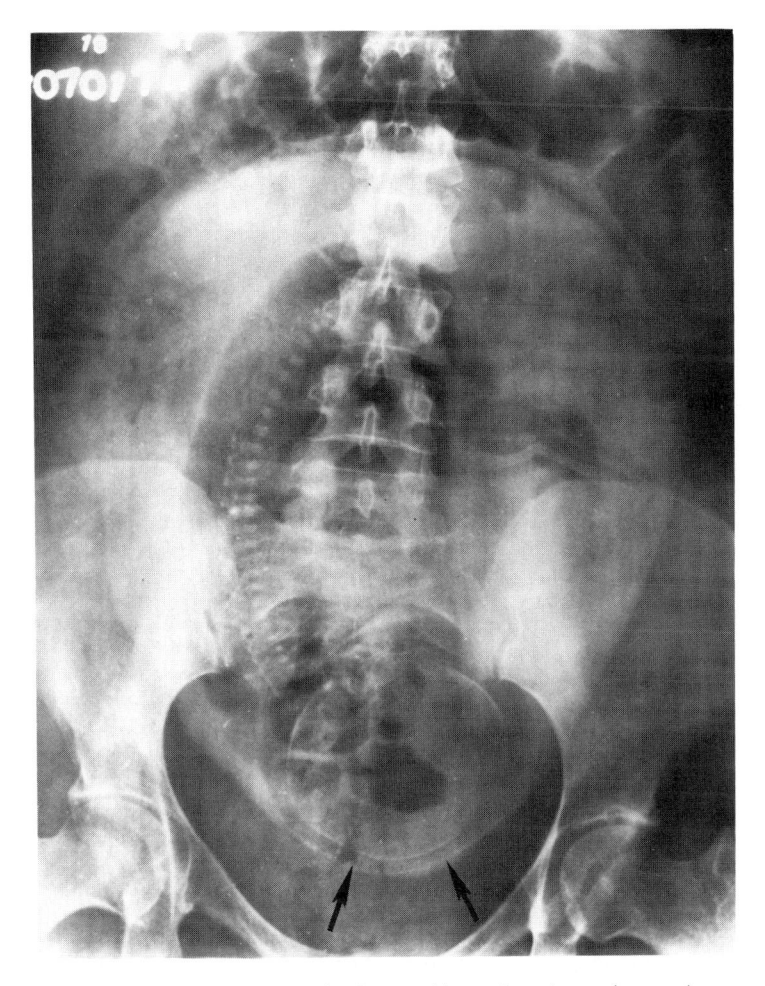

Fig. 5-10. Amniogram of a fetus with scalp edema *(arrows)*.

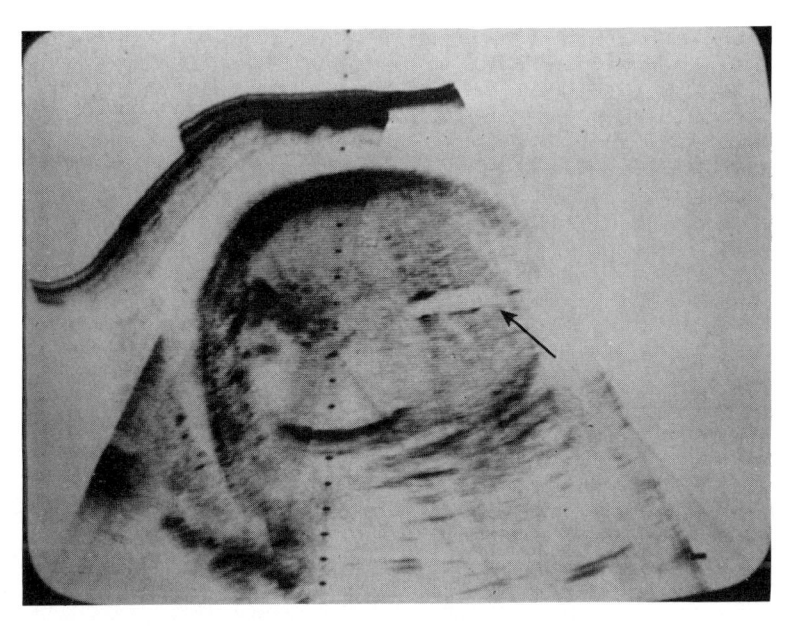

Fig. 5-11. Ultrasound cross section of the fetal abdomen in a normal pregnancy. The arrow points to the umbilical vein.

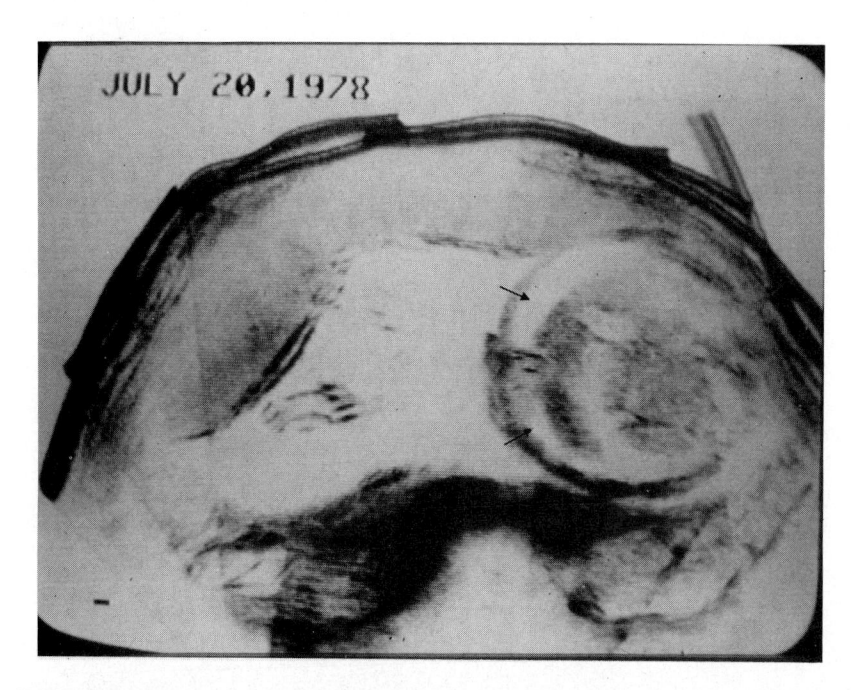

Fig. 5-12. Ultrasound scan of a fetus with moderate ascites *(arrows)*. Note that the placenta has a homogenous edematous appearance.

decreased activity of a mildly hydropic fetus appears to be a bad prognostic sign.

When the decision to deliver the fetus has been made, the method of delivery must be chosen. If the fetal presentation and the condition of the cervix are favorable and continuous FHR monitoring is available throughout labor, an induction of labor is indicated. With an unfavorable fetal presentation, long uneffaced cervix, or a premature infant, cesarean section is indicated to prevent exposing the already compromised fetus to the risk of labor.

ABO incompatibility

Halbrecht was the first to describe ABO erythroblastosis in 1954. These infants may develop early severe jaundice but rarely show signs of fetal hemolysis. The mother's and infant's major blood groups are incompatible; the mother's is usually group O and the infant's group A or B. Coombs' test may be negative in ABO hemolytic disease. When a positive Coombs test does occur, it is different from that seen in Rh hemolytic disease; a small weak agglutination appears after 3 to 8 minutes, rather than the complete agglutination that comes in less than 1 minute with Rh erythroblastosis fetalis. The antenatal prediction of ABO erythroblastosis is not possible with any degree of certainty. Since anti-A and anti-B occur naturally, they may be present in maternal serum without clinical disease in the infant. ABO erythroblastosis fetalis is about three times as common as Rh erythroblastosis fetalis. Since there is no risk of intrauterine death with ABO incompatibility, amniocentesis is not indicated and intrauterine transfusion is never required. There are no indications for preterm delivery of these infants. A history of previous ABO incompatibility can alert the obstetrician and pediatrician of an impending problem. Routine umbilical cord blood Coombs' tests at delivery and careful observation of the neonate are generally adequate to detect ABO disease. Because of the recent trend toward early discharge, the physician should be particularly careful to rule out the possibility of ABO incompatibility. Treatment of the newborn with this condition is the same in other types of erythroblastosis fetalis (Chapter 29).

Other antibodies

Theoretically, any blood group antigen present on the fetal RBCs and not present on maternal erythrocytes could cause erythroblastosis fetalis. The incidence of antibodies to other blood group antigens in an obstetric population is in the range of 1% to 2%. Some Rh(D)-negative women will be immunized to other antigens, and it is therefore important to identify the antibody present rather than to assume that an Rh-negative woman is immunized to $Rh_O(D)$. As many as half the obstetric patients with other antibodies will be Rh positive; therefore it is important to screen Rh-positive and Rh-negative patients to detect the possibility of erythroblastosis fetalis. Anti-(C), anti-(E), anti-Fy^a, and anti-Kell have been shown to cause erythroblastosis severe enough to require exchange transfusion. Rh-positive women can be immunized to "c" or "e" if they have received a transfusion of O Rh-negative *cde* blood.

Prevention

The long-term solution to management is passive immunization through the administration of adequate amounts of Rh immune globulin. Maternal immunization usually occurs at delivery, and the administration to the patient of $Rh_O(D)$-immune globulin binds Rh-positive antigenic sites on transfused fetal RBCs. Spontaneous abortions carry a 3% to 4% risk of immunization, whereas induced abortions have a slightly higher risk. The first full-term pregnancy has approximately a 1% to 2% risk of immunization up to the time of delivery. Subsequent term pregnancies carry a 10% risk of immunization. Ectopic pregnancies can also result in immunization. An antibody excess is required to protect the patient from Rh immunization. In general, a dose of 300 μg of $Rh_O(D)$-immune globulin is in excess of the dose necessary for the prevention of maternal immunization. However, more than this dose of immunoglobulin should be given for suspected large transplacental hemorrhage. It is mandatory that all unimmunized, Rh-negative women delivering Rh-positive infants receive Rh immune globulin. Unimmunized, Rh-negative patients with either spontaneous or induced abortions as well as ectopic pregnancies should also receive prophylaxis.

Recently, considerations have been given to antepartum administration of $Rh_O(D)$-immune globulin. When an Rh-negative patient undergoes genetic amniocentesis, she runs the risk of Rh immunization if the needle interrupts the integrity of the fetoplacental circulation. The phenomenon of immunization as a consequence of amniocentesis has been definitely demonstrated by numerous investigators. The ability of $Rh_O(D)$-immune globulin to protect against immunologic response to transplacental hemorrhage seems like an excellent possibility. If this is administered for a genetic amniocentesis from 16 to 18 weeks' gestation, the administration of $Rh_O(D)$-immune globulin should be repeated again at 28 to 32 weeks, thus maintaining an effective antibody level to prevent enhancement.

The antepartum administration of $Rh_O(D)$-immune globulin between 28 and 32 weeks' gestation has been suggested to decrease the likelihood of becoming immunized by transplacental hemorrhage. Although this is a relatively expensive program to embark on when the incidence of immunization is low and the Rh type of the fetus is unknown, it is likely that it would be helpful in preventing Rh immunization. If such a program is done in the United States, it is imperative that the clinician remember to give $Rh_O(D)$-immune globulin post partum if the baby is Rh positive.

John T. Queenan

BIBLIOGRAPHY

Bevis, D.C.A.: Bood pigments in haemolytic disease of the newborn, J. Obstet. Gynaecol. Br. Emp. **63**:68, 1956.

Freda, V.J.: The Rh problem in obstetrics and a new concept of its management using amniocentesis and spectrophotometric scanning of amniotic fluid, Am. J. Obstet. Gynecol. **92**:341, 1965.

Goplerud, C.P., and others: The first Rh-isoimmunized pregnancy, Am. J. Obstet. Gynecol. **115**:632, 1973.

Halbrecht, I.: Role of hemagglutinins anti-A and anti-B in pathogenesis of jaundice of the newborn (icterus praecox neonatorum), Am. J. Dis. Child. **68**:248, 1954.

Levine, P., and Stetson, R.E.: Unusual causes of intragroup agglutination, J.A.M.A. **113**:126, 1939.

Liley, A.W.: Liquor amnii analysis in management of pregnancy complicated by rhesus sensitization, Am. J. Obstet. Gynecol. **82**:1359, 1961.

Queenan, J.T.: Amniocentesis and transamniotic fetal transfusion for Rh disease, Clin. Obstet. Gynecol. **9**:491, 1966.

Queenan, J.T.: Role of spontaneous abortion in Rh immunization, Am. J. Obstet. Gynecol. **110**:128, 1971.

Queenan, J.T.: Modern management of the Rh problems, ed. 2, New York, 1977, Harper & Row, Publishers.

Queenan, J.T.: Management of high-risk pregnancy, Oradell, N.J., 1980, Medical Economics Co.

Queenan, J.T., and Goetschel, E.: Amniotic fluid analysis for erythroblastosis fetalis, Obstet. Gynecol. **32**:120, 1968.

Queenan, J.T., and others: Role of induced abortion in Rh immunization, Lancet **1**:815, 1971.

Queenan, J.T., and others: Irregular antibodies in the obstetric patient, Obstet. Gynecol. **34**:767, 1969.

CHAPTER 6 Polyhydramnios and oligohydramnios

POLYHYDRAMNIOS

Polyhydramnios is a pathologic accumulation of excess amniotic fluid; an amniotic fluid volume exceeding 2,000 ml in the third trimester constitutes polyhydramnios. The amniotic fluid volume increases gradually during normal pregnancy, although the turnover of amniotic fluid is rapid. Fetal urine and tracheobronchial tree secretions contribute to the net increase in the amniotic fluid volume; fetal swallowing tends to reduce volume. In addition, water and solute are exchanged between the mother and the amniotic fluid across the placental membranes. In a normal patient this volume increases less than 10 ml per day until the thirty-fourth week of gestation, after which it slowly diminishes (Fig. 6-1). The volumes vary widely in normal pregnancies, a volume of 500 to 2,000 ml at term is normal. Various maternal and fetal conditions may disturb the dynamic equilibrium of the amniotic fluid volume. Esophageal atresia, which prevents normal swallowing, is usually associated with polyhydramnios, whereas fetal renal agenesis may be associated with oligohydramnios. Occasionally the volume increases without a recognizable maternal or fetal cause.

Clinical manifestations

The diagnosis of polyhydramnios is often first suggested by the patient's symptoms. She may complain of pressure, rapidly increasing size of the abdomen, or of a protuberant abdomen. Later she may complain of pain, contractions, dyspnea, or orthopnea. Physical signs include a rapidly enlarging uterus reflected in a disproportionate increase in fundal height, abdominal girth, weight gain, and abdominal striae. The fetal head can usually be ballotted, but the fetal extremities are difficult to outline. The fetal heart is difficult to hear; it is usually detectable with the Doppler ultrasound sensor, but the signal may be lost intermittently because of the mobility of the fetus in the abnormally large volume of amniotic fluid. The presentation may vary from examination to examination, and there is an increased frequency of breech and oblique lie with a single fetus.

The acute form of polyhydramnios is rare, occurring in 1 out of every 50 instances of polyhydramnios. The fluid accumulates rapidly, and the uterus is tense and tender. It is usually diagnosed by 23 to 25 weeks' gestation.

Chronic polyhydramnios, the most common form, is a problem of the third trimester. Occasionally the diagnosis is not made until the patient has a dysfunctional labor or until an abnormally large amount of amniotic fluid is noted during delivery. Most commonly the diagnosis is made by abdominal examination during the third trimester or by ultrasound scan. Prolonged pregnancy is rare except in association with anencephaly. The reported incidence of chronic polyhydramnios varies from 1 in 150 deliveries to 1 in 400 deliveries.

Laboratory evaluation

Ultrasound is very useful in confirming the diagnosis of polyhydramnios. The increased amniotic fluid is evident as a large sonolucent echo-free area on the ultrasound scan (Fig. 6-2). Associated conditions, such as multiple gestations and congenital malformations, also may be appreciated. A roentgenogram can detect polyhydramnios but exposes the patient and the fetus to unnecessary radiation. Amniography, which entails the same radiation exposure as a roentgenogram, may rarely be indicated to detect certain congenital malformations. Measurement of polyhydramnios with a dye dilution technique (para-aminohippuric acid) is safe but of little practical value, since ultrasound scanning gives a good estimate of amniotic fluid volume.

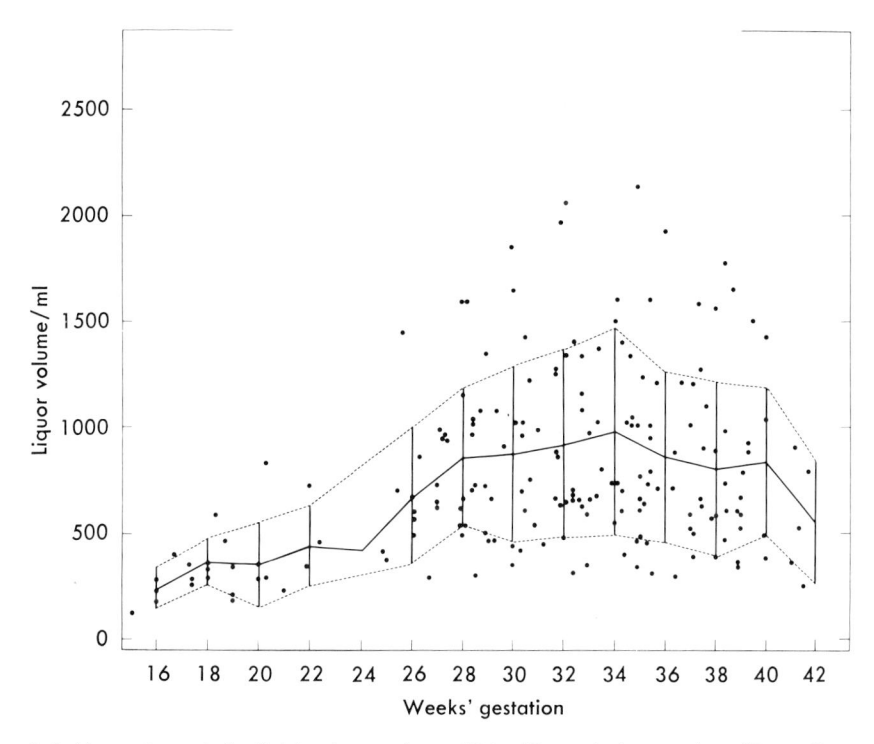

Fig. 6-1. Normal amniotic fluid volumes from 16 to 42 weeks' gestation. (From Queenan, J.T., and others: Am. J. Obstet. Gynecol. **114:**34, 1972.)

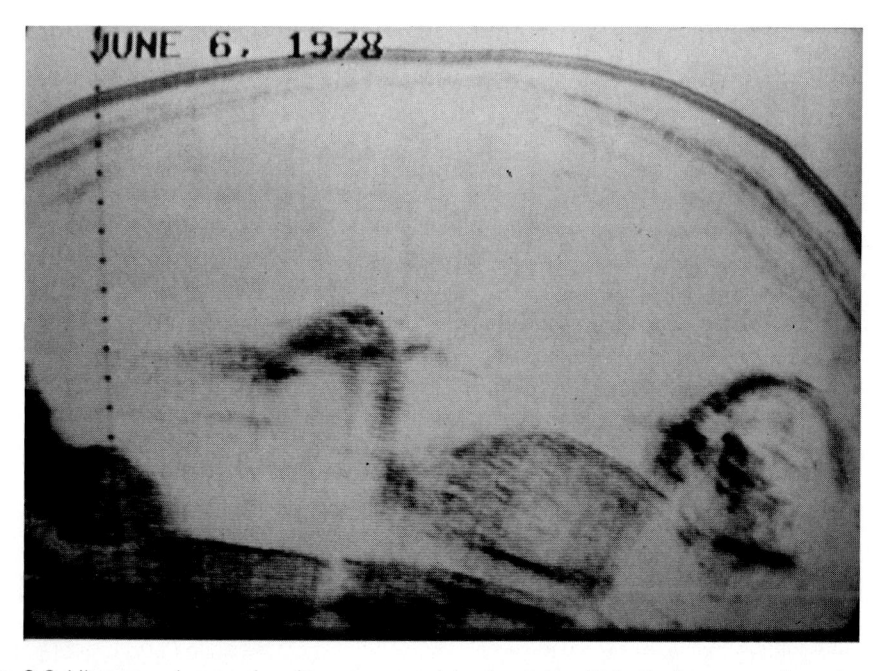

Fig. 6-2. Ultrasound scan showing severe polyhydramnios. Note the large sonolucent area.

Associated conditions

In a study reported in 1970, 358 instances of polyhydramnios were found in 86,000 deliveries, a frequency of 0.41%. The associated conditions were diabetes mellitus (25%), congenital malformations (20%), erythroblastosis fetalis (11%), and multiple gestations (8%). Thirty-four percent had no apparent prenatal or postnatal cause. Acute polyhydramnios occurred in 2%. Polyhydramnios appeared to be more prevalent with severe diabetes than with mild disease. When polyhydramnios is associated with erythroblastosis fetalis, there is usually hydrops fetalis. Multiple gestations, especially monochorionic twins, are more common than expected in pregnancies associated with polyhydramnios. There is also an increased incidence of postpartum hemorrhage due to overdistention of the uterus. The most frequently reported congenital anomaly is anencephaly; approximately 50% of pregnancies associated with anencephaly are found to have polyhydramnios. Hydrocephalus and both duodenal and esophageal atresia are also frequently associated with this condition. Ultrasound examination frequently can localize the site of gastrointestinal obstruction in the fetus. Neuromuscular disorders associated with impaired swallowing and reduced fetal activity frequently are complicated by polyhydramnios. Fig. 6-3 shows the interval between diagnosis and delivery according to diagnosis. The average birth weights are displayed on the vertical axis (see Chapter 37).

Treatment

If diabetes or erythroblastosis fetalis is the cause of polyhydramnios, appropriate therapy for these disorders should be undertaken. If twins are diagnosed, limitation of activity is indicated. Some major gastrointestinal anomalies can be corrected with prompt surgery during the neonatal period; but if gross multiple anomalies are found, interruption of the pregnancy may be indicated.

Chronic polyhydramnios without underlying disease should be managed with bed rest, restricted activity, and a high-protein diet. An abdominal binder can sometimes relieve symptoms. Diuretics are not indicated. Rarely, amniocentesis is required to relieve maternal symptoms; fluid should be removed slowly to avoid causing premature labor or premature separation of the placenta. In contrast, acute recurrent polyhydramnios may require multiple amnioceneteses. In one patient approximately 20,000 ml of amniotic fluid was removed during the third trimester, and the fetus developed to viability.

Prognosis

The overall prognosis for the fetus of a pregnancy complicated by polyhydramnios is poor. The incidence of stillborn infants is 10% to 20%. The perinatal mortality is 35% to 40%. The perinatal mortality is significantly higher with acute polyhydramnios. The prognosis for the infant depends on the associated conditions that are

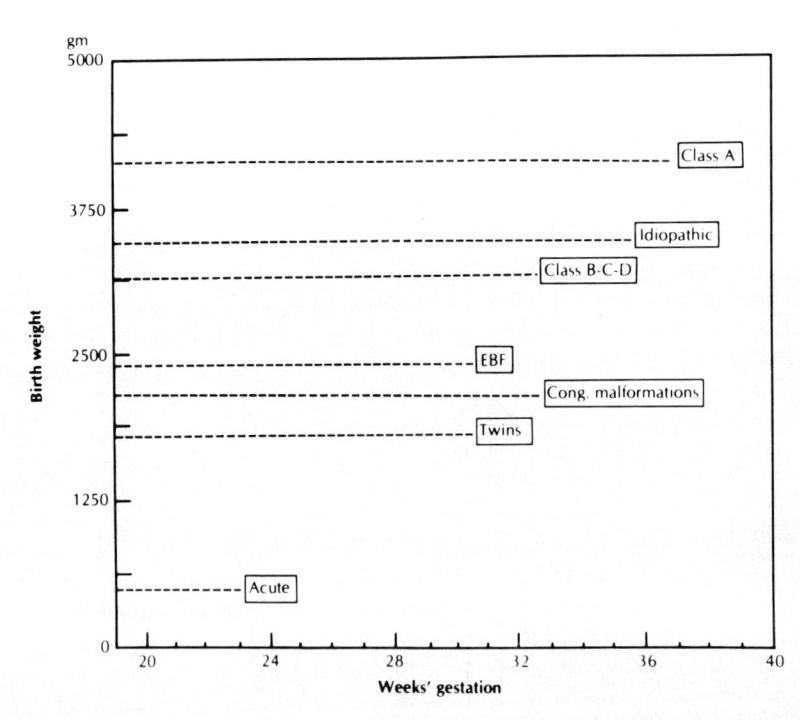

Fig. 6-3. Interval between diagnosis and delivery according to causes of polyhydramnios. (From Queenan, J.T., and Gadow, E.C.: Am. J. Obstet. Gynecol. **108:**349, 1970.)

present. In 1970 Queenan reported a perinatal mortality in class A diabetic patients of 8%, whereas when class B, C, and D diabetes were associated with polyhydramnios, the perinatal mortality was 17.5%. The perinatal mortality in twin gestations associated with polyhydramnios was 45% in this study. Polyhydramnios associated with erythroblastosis fetalis portends a poor outcome for two reasons. Polyhydramnios is often associated with the development of hydrops fetalis, and second, the excess fluid can dilute the amniotic fluid bilirubin values and mask the severity of the disease. The perinatal mortality of patients with erythroblastosis fetalis and polyhydramnios in Queenan's series was 73%. In patients with polyhydramnios and congenital abnormalities the perinatal mortality reached 87%.

OLIGOHYDRAMNIOS

Oligohydramnios refers to diminished amounts of amniotic fluid. The occurrence of a very small amniotic fluid volume, a few ounces or less, is recorded less frequently than polyhydramnios. This can be attributed to the fact that generally the associated condition has caused no maternal distress and, if after rupture of the membranes during labor there is little fluid, it is often erroneously assumed that the rupture had occurred earlier and the fluid escaped. During the later stages of pregnancy the fetal urine is a major source of amniotic fluid, which is maintained in continuous equilibrium by being swallowed and reabsorbed by the fetus. A marked deficit of fetal urine production or excretion can lead to oligohydramnios. The clinical importance of significant decreases in amniotic fluid volume lies mainly in the increased incidence of fetal abnormality. Severe oligohydramnios is most often associated with major renal malformations, including renal aplasia with dysplastic kidneys as well as obstructive lesions of the lower urinary tract.

There has also been an association of small amniotic fluid volumes with fetal growth retardation attributed in initial reports to excessive fetal swallowing due to fetal hunger. Liley, however, demonstrated that fetuses small for gestational age actually swallow at a low rate. Wallenberg documented ultrasonographically a decreased urine production and concluded that, in fetuses small for gestational age, the kidneys play a more important role in the regulation of amniotic fluid volume than in normally nourished fetuses. The underlying mechanism of the oligohydramnios in growth-retarded infants thus is not known.

The diagnosis of oligohydramnios is usually subjective, since precise values of amniotic fluid determinations are rarely available. Furthermore, because conditions associated with oligohydramnios other than premature rupture of membranes and prolonged leakage of amniotic fluid cause little or no distress to the mother, antenatal recognition may be difficult. More precise quantitation of amniotic fluid volume may be accomplished ultrasonographically, or the pathologist may confirm the diagnosis by documenting the presence of amnion nodosum (Chapter 16). These gray-yellow amniotic nodules consist histologically of clumps of vernix, desquamated fetal epidermal cells, and appendages of the skin on the amnion. The amniotic epithelium under the nodules may be completely intact. Amnion nodosum is thought to arise as a

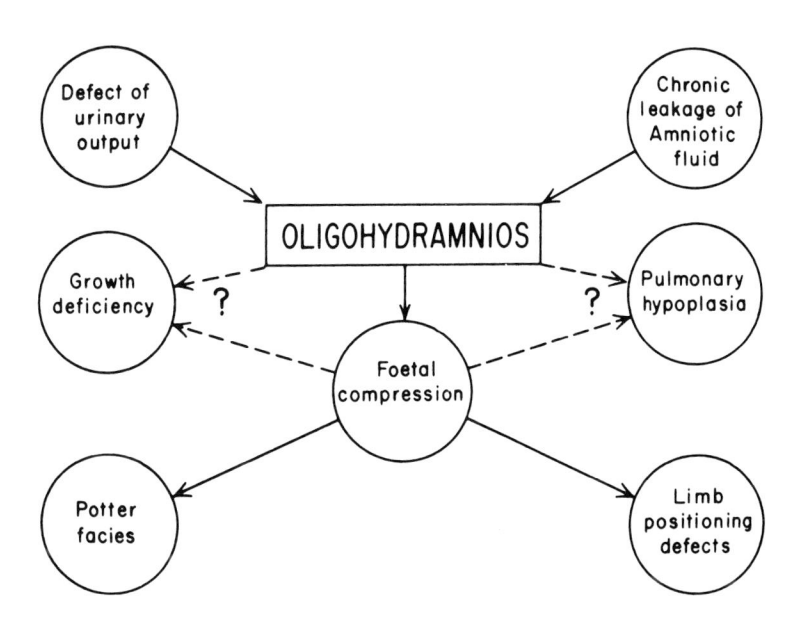

Fig. 6-4. Major nonrenal malformations caused by oligohydramnios. (From Thomas, I.T., and Smith, D.W.: J. Pediatr. 84:811, 1974.)

result of close contact between fetal skin and amnion resulting from oligohydramnios. Whereas amnion nodosum may imply oligohydramnios, oligohydramnios, especially when secondary to amniorrhea, does not necessarily imply amnion nodosum. Furthermore, although the oligohydramnios syndrome frequently accompanies renal agenesis, the features of the oligohydramnios syndrome may be absent if a defect in fetal swallowing coexists. The defects in fetal swallowing could compensate for fetal anuria, preventing oligohydramnios and its effects. The oligohydramnios tetrad of anomalies consists of facial anomalies, limb positioning defects, pulmonary hypoplasia, and fetal growth deficiency; when accompanied by bilateral renal agenesis, it is typically referred to as Potter's syndrome (Chapter 31). The characteristic facial appearance includes a flattened nose, recession of the chin, and a prominent fold that runs downward and outward from the inner canthus of the eye. The ears are often low set, aberrantly folded, and usually flattened to the side of the head. There are limb defects such as spadelike hands and talipes equinovarus. Additionally, these infants are usually growth deficient if delivered after 34 weeks, the lungs are hypoplastic, and there is most commonly a urinary tract defect such that urine production or flow is grossly deficient or absent. It has been assumed that the oligohydramnios which accompanies most cases of renal agenesis is the cause of the major nonrenal malformations, including pulmonary hypoplasia and the facial features (Fig. 6-4).

That oligohydramnios may cause fetal compression and so explain the facial appearance and limb defects is supported by the production of similar anomalies in rat fetuses subjected to amniocentesis. Fetuses unable to excrete urine into the amniotic space, but for unusual reasons having adequate amniotic fluid present, have none of these secondary features of Potter's syndrome. Furthermore, all the nonrenal features of Potter's syndrome can be present as a consequence of oligohydramnios secondary to chronic leakage of amniotic fluid in fetuses who have no problems of urine production. For any infant who has a low Apgar score or severe respiratory distress together with features of the oligohydramnios tetrad a prompt suprapubic tap and detailed evaluation of the genitourinary tract should be undertaken.

John T. Queenan

BIBLIOGRAPHY
Polyhydramnios

Jacoby, H.E., and Charles, D.: Clinical conditions associated with hydramnios, Am. J. Obstet. Gynecol. **94**:910, 1966.

Kramer, E.E.: Hydramnios, oligohydramnios and fetal malformations, Clin. Obstet. Gynecol. **9**:508, 1966.

Kucera, M.: Rate and type of congenital anomalies among offspring of diabetic women, J. Reprod. Med. **7**:61, 1971.

Pitkin, R.M.: Acute polyhydramnios recurrent in successive pregnancies, Obstet. Gynecol. **48**:425, 1976.

Prindle, R.A., and others: Maternal hydramnios and congenital anomalies of the central nervous system, N. Engl. J. Med. **252**:555, 1955.

Queenan, J.T.: Recurrent acute polyhydramnios, Am. J. Obstet. Gynecol. **106**:625, 1970.

Queenan, J.T., and Gadow, E.C.: Polyhydramnios: chronic vs. acute, Am. J. Obstet. Gynecol. **108**:349, 1970.

Queenan, J.T., and others: Amniotic fluid volume in normal pregnancies, Am. J. Obstet. Gynecol. **114**:34, 1972.

Oligohydramnios

Brown, D.R., Doshi, N., and Taylor, P.M.: Oligohydramnios and fatal pulmonary hypoplasia without amnion nodosum, J. Reprod. Med. **20**:293, 1978.

Liley, A.W.: Disorders of amniotic fluid. In Assali, N.S., editor: Pathophysiology of gestation, New York, 1972, Academic Press, Inc.

Thomas, I.T., and Smith, D.W.: Oligohydramnios, cause of the nonrenal features of Potter's syndrome, including pulmonary hypoplasia, J. Pediatr. **84**:811, 1974.

Wallenberg, H.C.S, and Wladimiroff, J.W.: The amniotic fluid. II. Polyhydramnios and oligohydramnios, J. Perinatol. Med. **6**:233, 1977.

CHAPTER 7 Intrauterine growth retardation: determinants of aberrant fetal growth

Fetal development is characterized by sequential patterns of tissue and organ growth and maturation that are determined by the maternal environment, uteroplacental function, and the inherent genetic growth potential of the fetus. When circumstances are optimal, none of these factors has a rate-limiting effect on fetal growth and development. Thus the healthy fetus should achieve complete functional maturity and somatic growth, with the anticipation of an uncomplicated intrapartum course, and thus a smooth neonatal cardiopulmonary and metabolic adaptation to extrauterine life.

However, fetal growth and development do not always occur under optimum intrauterine conditions. Those neonates subjected to aberrant maternal, placental, or fetal circumstances that restrain growth are a high-risk group and are categorized as small for gestational age (SGA). The cumulative effects of both adverse environmental conditions and aberrant fetal growth (intrauterine growth retardation, IUGR) threaten continued intrauterine survival, and labor, delivery, and neonatal adaptation become increasingly hazardous. Similarly, postneonatal growth and development may be impaired as a result of intrauterine growth retardation and the subsequent problems encountered during the neonatal period. This chapter discusses normal and aberrant fetal growth and its sequelae.

Following is a list of synonyms for SGA*:
1. Small for dates
2. Small for gestational age
3. Light for dates
4. Chronic fetal distress
5. Hypotrophic fetus
6. Intrauterine growth retardation
7. Intrauterine malnutrition
8. Dysmature
9. Clifford syndrome
10. Postdates
11. Postmaturity
12. Failure to thrive in utero
13. Fetal deprivation syndrome
14. Pseudoprematurity

FETAL GROWTH AND BODY COMPOSITION

Through anthropomorphic measurements that include fetal weight, length (crown-heel), and head circumference, fetal growth standards have been determined for different reference populations from various locations. Although the range of birth weight at each gestational age in these populations may vary (Table 7-1), the overall pattern of fetal growth (Fig. 7-1) is representative for each of these groups. Both early and late fetal growth appear to be linear beginning at approximately 20 weeks' gestation and lasting until 38 weeks; thereafter the rate of weight gain begins to decline. Reasonably equivalent data have been recorded when fetal dimensions are examined by ultrasound (see further). Included in Fig. 7-1 are growth curves corrected for parity, race, and fetal sex, factors to be discussed in later sections. Fig. 7-2 demonstrates a similar linear relationship between fetal weight and gestational age. Near-term fetal weight gain appears to decelerate; following birth it again assumes the intrauterine rate. Fetal weight gain (grams per day) is constant during the second trimester, then accelerates during the majority of the third trimester, but declines near term. During the neonatal period the rate of gain accelerates again. This relative slowing of growth as the

---

*From Brandt, Ingeborg: Growth dynamics of low birth weight infants with emphasis on the perinatal period. In Falkner, F., and Tanner, J.M., editors: Human growth, vol. 2: Postnatal growth, New York, 1978, Plenum Press.

Table 7-1. Birth weights from six sources

Nearest week of gestation	Mean birth weight (gm) ± 1 SD					
	Denver	Baltimore	Montreal	Portland	Chapel Hill	12 US cities (cluster method)
28	1,150 ± 259	1,050 ± 310	1,113 ± 150	1,172 ± 344	1,150 ± 272	1,165 ± 109
29	1,270 ± 294	1,200 ± 350	1,228 ± 165	1,322 ± 339	1,310 ± 299	1,295 ± 94
30	1,395 ± 341	1,380 ± 370	1,373 ± 175	1,529 ± 474	1,460 ± 340	1,440 ± 115
31	1,540 ± 375	1,560 ± 400	1,540 ± 200	1,757 ± 495	1,630 ± 340	1,601 ± 117
32	1,715 ± 416	1,750 ± 410	1,727 ± 225	1,881 ± 437	1,810 ± 381	1,760 ± 128
33	1,920 ± 505	1,950 ± 420	1,900 ± 250	2,158 ± 511	2,010 ± 367	1,955 ± 138
34	2,200 ± 539	2,170 ± 430	2,113 ± 280	2,340 ± 552	2,220 ± 395	2,160 ± 202
35	2,485 ± 526	2,390 ± 440	2,347 ± 315	2,518 ± 468	2,430 ± 408	2,387 ± 208
36	2,710 ± 519	2,610 ± 440	2,589 ± 350	2,749 ± 490	2,650 ± 408	2,621 ± 274
37	2,900 ± 451	2,830 ± 440	2,868 ± 385	2,989 ± 466	2,870 ± 395	2,878 ± 288
38	3,030 ± 451	3,050 ± 450	3,133 ± 400	3,185 ± 450	3,030 ± 395	3,119 ± 302
39	3,140 ± 403	3,210 ± 450	3,360 ± 430	3,333 ± 444	3,170 ± 408	3,210 ± 434
40	3,230 ± 396	3,280 ± 450	3,480 ± 460	3,462 ± 456	3,280 ± 422	3,351 ± 448
41	3,290 ± 396	3,350 ± 450	3,567 ± 475	3,569 ± 468	3,360 ± 435	3,444 ± 456
42	3,300 ± 423	3,400 ± 460	3,513 ± 480	3,637 ± 482	3,410 ± 449	3,486 ± 463
43		3,410 ± 490	3,416 ± 465	3,660 ± 502	3,420 ± 463	3,473 ± 502

From Naeye, R., and Dixon, J.: Pediatr. Res. **12**:987, 1978. With permission.

normal fetus approaches term is thought to be caused by some restraint of fetal growth. These restraining factors may be related to uterine size or placental function (see further). During the neonatal period growth resumes and approaches the in utero rate once this restraint has been eliminated.

Although weight gain per day is maximum prior to term, when growth is expressed as percent increment per day it is greatest during embryonic and early fetal development (Fig. 7-2). However, the nature of fetal growth is different during early and later fetal life. During the embryonic and early fetal growth period, tissues and organs increase in cell number rather than cell size (the hyperplastic phase of cell growth, when total DNA content increases in new tissues). Later phases of growth include a period when cell size also increases (protein and RNA content), along with continued enhancement of cell number (mixed hyperplastic and hypertrophic phase). In muscle and brain this phase of growth may continue through adolescence and the second year of life, respectively. The final stage of growth is a purely hypertrophic phase, when only cell size increases.

The contribution of each tissue to body weight changes during fetal and postnatal development is depicted in Table 7-2. Muscle represents only 25% of fetal and neonatal body weight; once full adult maturity has been achieved, it accounts for 40% of the body's mass. Fetal muscle growth, as well as all protein synthesis in the fetus, depends on active transport of amino acids across the placenta. Once provided with these precursors, fetal protein synthesis is autonomous and results in the net synthesis of proteins that have amino acid patterns equivalent to those in the adult. Although the building blocks may be the same, developmentally the fetal muscle has a lower fibrillar protein content, whereas the sarcoplasmic protein concentration remains unchanged as maturation proceeds. Aside from those immunoglobulins which cross the placenta, all protein present in the fetus has been synthesized de novo within fetal tissue.

Paralleling the patterns of fetal growth, the macromolecular composition of the body also undergoes sequential patterns of change. One general trend includes a decrease of total body and extracellular water content as the fetus and infant mature (Fig. 7-3; Table 7-3). Simultaneously, there is an increment of body protein and fat content (Fig. 7-4). Whereas the increase of tissue protein is gradual during development, the increment of fetal body fat is delayed until the third trimester. Once initiated, the deposition of subcutaneous and deep body adipose tissue accelerates more rapidly than the rate of protein accumulation.

Coinciding with the changes of the extracellular fluid space, the sodium and chloride concentration in the fetus declines while the expansion of the intracellular fluid space results in an increase of potassium concentration. The decline of the total body sodium is less than that for chloride, since sodium is also a component of fetal bone. Calcium, phosphorus, and magnesium are nevertheless the major minerals in bone. By term the total body calcium/phosphorus ratio is 1.7:1.8 with 98% of calcium, 80% of phosphorus, and 60% of magnesium deposited within the bone. To summarize, the composition and rate of new tissue deposited during each period of gestation varies (Fig. 7-4). As development proceeds toward

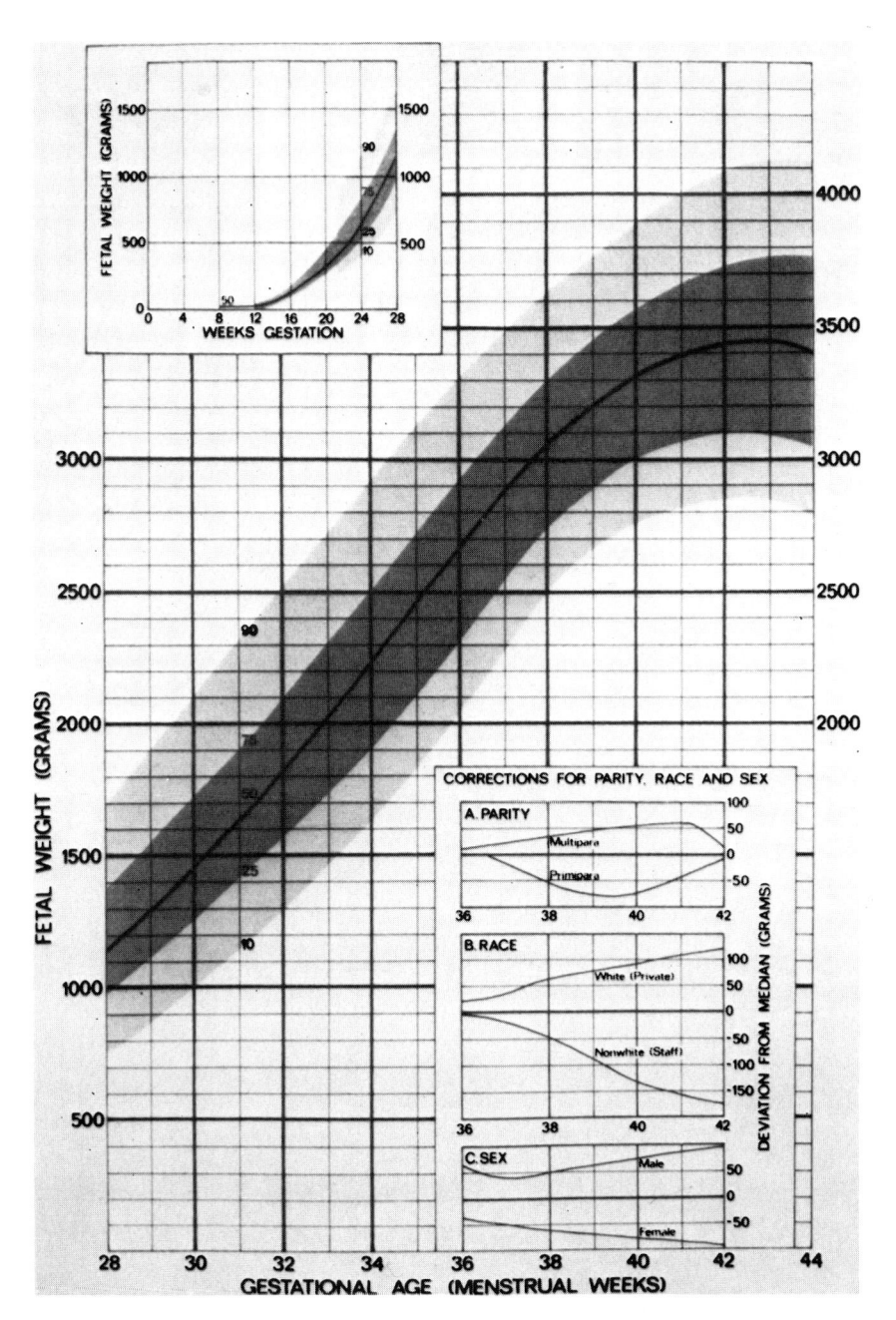

Fig. 7-1. Fetal weight with correction for parity, race (socioeconomic), and sex derived from 31,202 prostaglandin abortions and "spontaneous" deliveries. (From Brenner, W., and others: Am. J. Obstet. Gynecol. **126**:555, 1976.)

Fig. 7-2. Smoothed curves for fetal and postnatal growth in grams and grams gained per day and expressed as percent increment of body weight. (From Usher, R., and McLean, F. In Davis, J., and Dobbing, J., editors: Scientific foundations of pediatrics, Philadelphia, 1974, W.B. Saunders Co.)

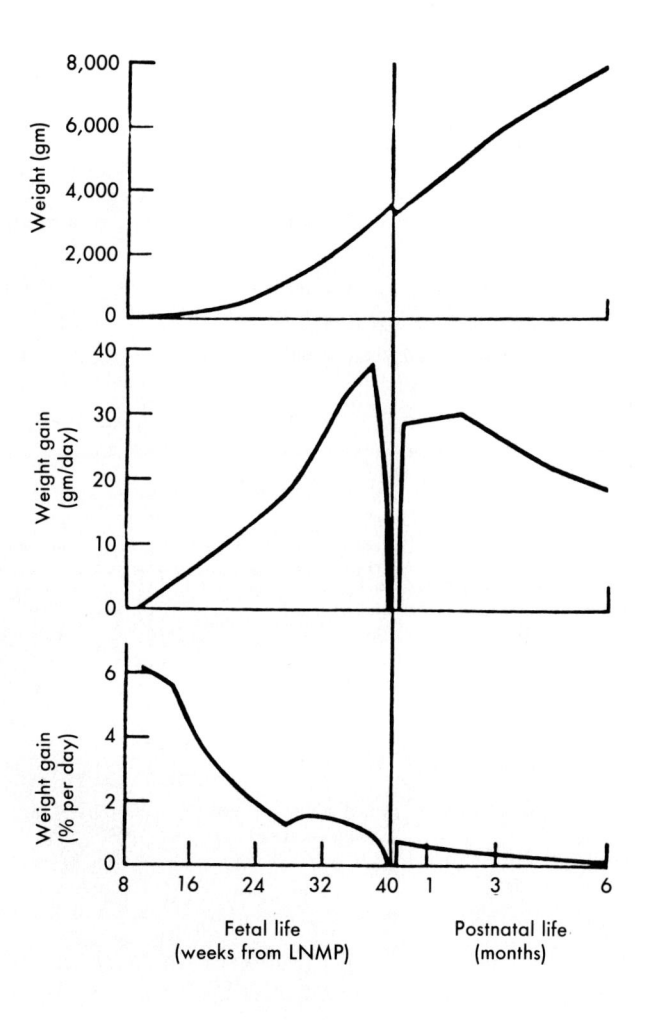

Fig. 7-3. Developmental alterations of fluid space distribution. (From Uttley, W., and Habel, A.: Clin. Endocrinol. Metabol. **5:**3, 1976.)

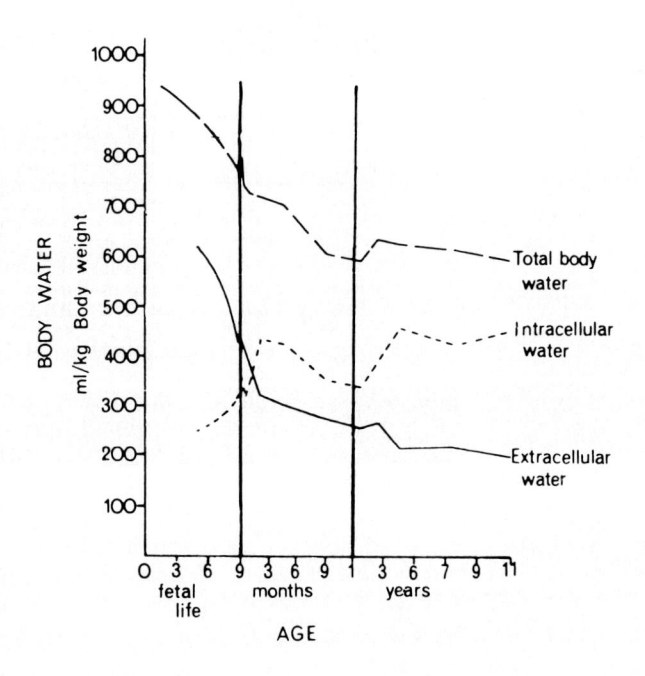

Table 7-2. Contribution of organs to body mass during development

Tissue	Fetus 20-24 weeks %	Full-term baby %	Adult %
Skeletal muscle	25	25	43
Skin	13	15	7
Skeleton	22	18	18
Heart	0.6	0.5	0.4
Liver	4	5	2
Kidneys	0.7	1	0.5
Brain	13	13	2

From Widdowson, E. In Assali, N., editor: Biology of gestation, vol. 2, New York, 1968, Academic Press, Inc. With permission.

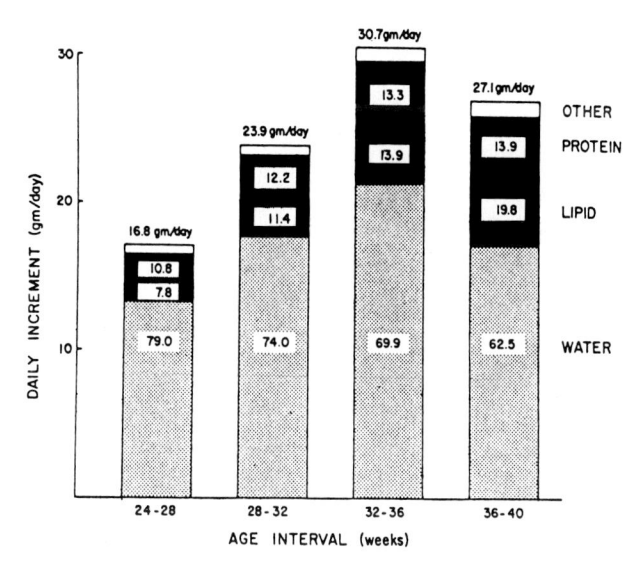

Fig. 7-4. Composition of fetal weight gain. (From Ziegler, E., and others: Growth **40**:329, 1976.)

Table 7-3. Body composition of the reference fetus

Gestational age (weeks)	Body weight (gm)	Per 100 gm body weight					Per 100 gm fat-free weight						
		Water (gm)	Protein (gm)	Lipid (gm)	Other (gm)	Water (gm)	Protein (gm)	Ca (mg)	P (mg)	Mg (mg)	Na (mEq)	K (mEq)	Cl (mEq)
24	690	88.6	8.8	0.1	2.5	88.6	8.8	621	387	17.8	9.9	4.0	7.0
25	770	87.8	9.0	0.7	2.5	88.4	9.1	615	385	17.6	9.8	4.0	7.0
26	880	86.8	9.2	1.5	2.5	88.1	9.4	611	384	17.5	9.7	4.1	7.0
27	1010	85.7	9.4	2.4	2.5	87.8	9.7	609	383	17.4	9.5	4.1	6.9
28	1160	84.6	9.6	3.3	2.4	87.5	10.0	610	385	17.4	9.4	4.2	6.9
29	1318	83.6	9.9	4.1	2.4	87.2	10.3	613	387	17.4	9.3	4.2	6.8
30	1480	82.6	10.1	4.9	2.4	86.8	10.6	619	392	17.4	9.2	4.3	6.8
31	1650	81.7	10.3	5.6	2.4	86.5	10.9	628	398	17.6	9.1	4.3	6.7
32	1830	80.7	10.6	6.3	2.4	86.1	11.3	640	406	17.8	9.1	4.3	6.6
33	2020	79.8	10.8	6.9	2.5	85.8	11.6	656	416	18.0	9.0	4.4	6.5
34	2230	79.0	11.0	7.5	2.5	85.4	11.9	675	428	18.3	8.9	4.4	6.4
35	2450	78.1	11.2	8.1	2.6	85.0	12.2	699	443	18.6	8.9	4.5	6.3
36	2690	77.3	11.4	8.7	2.6	84.6	12.5	726	460	19.0	8.8	4.5	6.1
37	2940	76.4	11.6	9.3	2.7	84.3	12.8	758	479	19.5	8.8	4.5	6.0
38	3160	75.6	11.8	9.9	2.7	83.9	13.1	795	501	20.0	8.8	4.5	5.9
39	3330	74.8	11.9	10.5	2.8	83.6	13.3	836	525	20.5	8.7	4.6	5.8
40	3450	74.0	12.0	11.2	2.8	83.3	13.5	882	551	21.1	8.7	4.6	5.7

From Ziegler, E., and others: Growth **40**: 329, 1976. With permission.

term gestation, water represents a smaller component of each gram of fetal weight while lipid and protein contribute a greater percentage to the mean increment of daily weight gain.

FETAL METABOLISM

Although the fetus is described as the perfect parasite, maternal and fetal nutritional deprivations can adversely affect fetal growth. The fetus depends on maternal nutrient intake and maternal endogenous substrate stores as precursors for fetal tissue synthesis and fuel for fetal oxidative metabolism. The oxygen consumed by the fetus in turn provides energy to support essential fetal "work," such as maintenance of transmembrane potentials and replacement of tissue components that are continuously being renewed. In addition, fetal oxygen consumption is required for net synthesis of complex macromolecules such as DNA, RNA, protein, and lipid. Each gram of protein synthesized requires the expenditure of 7.5 Cal, whereas a gram of triglycerides requires 11.6 Cal. Since 4.85 Cal use 1 L of oxygen, net tissue synthesis represents a substantial proportion of fetal oxygen consumption, which is approximately 4 to 6 ml/kg/minute. The energy cost of neonatal growth among premature infants constitutes the energy stored in tissue plus that expended for the synthesis of that tissue. Total energy cost per gram of new tissue is approximately 5.7 Cal, whereas that remaining in structural or depot macromolecules represents 4.0 Cal. Therefore 1.7 Cal are used to produce 1 gm of new tissue. A similar relationship should occur in the third-trimester fetus, since energy requirements for growth should not change following birth.

Maternal metabolic adjustments during pregnancy are characterized by fuel and hormonal alterations that attempt to secure a continuous provision of substrates for use by the fetus. During periods of alimentation, sufficient substrates are presented to the uteroplacental circulation while maternal fuel stores are simultaneously enriched. When fasting occurs during pregnancy, fuel mobilization is accelerated, as is evident by the rapid rise of maternal free fatty acids and ketone bodies. This accelerated mobilization of maternal adipose tissue stores is facilitated by a rapid decline of insulin levels and an enhanced secretion of human placental somatomammotropin. This latter placental hormone has lipolytic activity and may also diminish maternal glucose oxidation directly. In addition, maternal glucose utilization is attenuated because free fatty acids and ketones replace glucose as a fuel in maternal tissues, whereas hypoinsulinemia reduces glucose uptake in the insulin-dependent tissue of the mother. Thus fetal glucose provision may be continued. In addition, alternate substrates such as ketones cross the placenta, attempting to maintain fetal growth and development. Ketones may be oxidized or

Table 7-4. Oxidizable substrates in the ovine fetus*

Substrate	Total oxygen consumption accounted for (%)
Glucose	50
Amino acids	25
Lactate	20
Acetate	5 to 10
Free fatty acids	Not significant
Fructose	Not significant
Glycerol	Not significant
Keto acids	Not significant

From Milley, J., and Simmons, M.: Clin. Perinatol. **6**:365, 1979. With permission.
*Sheep placenta is impermeable to FFA and ketones, in contrast to that of other mammals, which may use these substrates.

serve as precursors for fetal lipid or protein synthesis. This accelerated mobilization of fuels can ensure fetal growth during short periods of maternal fasting; however, prolonged periods of starvation will adversely affect fetal outcome (see further).

The substrates used to maintain fetal oxygen consumption have been most accurately determined in the ovine fetus (Table 7-4). Glucose accounts for approximatey 50% of fetal energy production in sheep when the mother is maintained in a high nutritional plane. Amino acids, in addition to functioning as precursors for fetal protein synthesis, serve as an oxidizable fuel; they may contribute to 25% of ovine fetal oxygen uptake. Taken together, lactate and acetate may supply an additional 25%. Data from human pregnancies suggest that glucose oxidation may contribute a greater proportion of fetal energy production than that in the ovine fetus.

Similarly, fetal respiratory quotient has been estimated to be close to 1.0 in other mammalian species, which suggests that carbohydrate oxidation is the predominant source for fetal oxidative metabolism. As discussed previously, fasting during human pregnancy may result in an alteration of substrates presented to the fetus when maternal and subsequently fetal ketone bodies increase in concentration. Ketones may then serve as fuels for energy production and also as precursors for amino acids, proteins, and lipids. Although free fatty acids, especially the essential fatty acids, must cross the placenta, their role in fetal energy production is limited, since they probably are deposited in structural or depot tissues (Fig. 7-5).

In addition to the provision of substrates for fetal oxygen consumption and growth, tissue growth also depends on an appropriate fetal endocrine milieu. Among the hormones, insulin has been implicated as the "growth hormone" of the fetus. Since insulin does not cross the placenta, this growth-enhancing hormone must

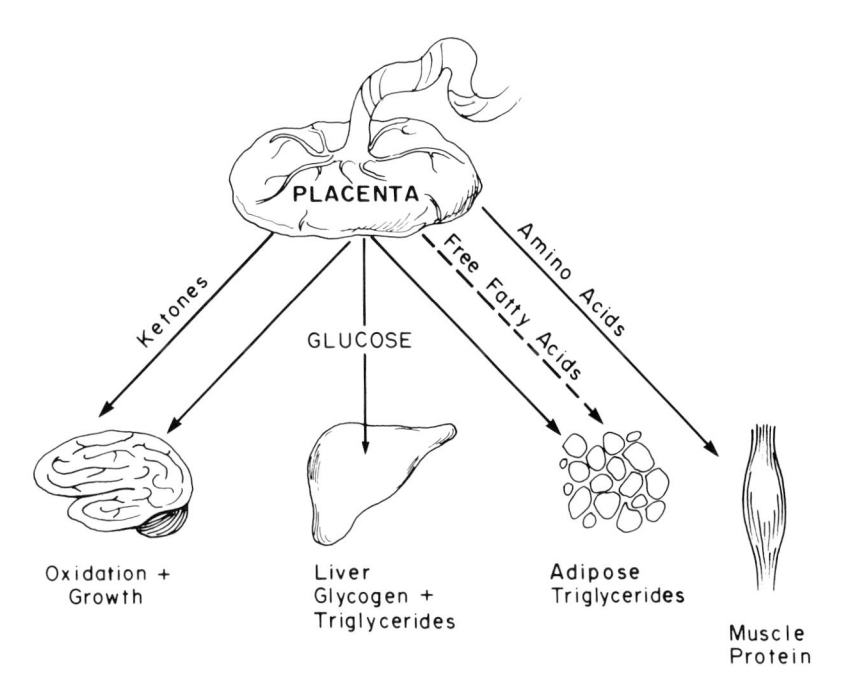

Fig. 7-5. Placental nutrient support and disposition of substrates. (Modified from Adam, P.A.J.: Metabolism in pregnant woman and fetus. In Falkner, F., and Tanner, J.: Human growth, vol. 1, New York, 1978, Plenum Press.)

be of fetal origin. Insulin promotes fetal deposition of adipose and glycogen stores while potentially stimulating amino acid uptake and protein synthesis in muscle. In the absence of fetal insulin production, as in conditions such as pancreatic aplasia, transient neonatal diabetes mellitus, or congenital absence of the islets of Langerhans, fetal growth is impaired. Also, when the peripheral action of insulin is attenuated by diminished receptor or postreceptor events, as in leprechaunism, fetal growth may be impaired. On the other hand, those neonates experiencing prolonged periods of hyperinsulinism in utero, such as infants of diabetic mothers or infants with Beckwith's syndrome or nesidioblastosis, demonstrate enhanced adipose and muscle tissue mass resulting in excessive birth weight (Chapters 24 and 33, part one).

Growth hormone is another hormone that can influence fetal growth. Although its role is not as important as that of insulin, its effect has been inferred from infants born with anencephaly, since these neonates are frequently SGA. However, this alteration of fetal growth may depend more on cerebral cortical signals or other neuroendocrine hormones such as prolactin, since anencephaly is not purely a growth hormone deficiency state. The birth weight of a panhypopituitary fetus is not different from that of a normal fetus, suggesting that other growth regulatory factors may contribute to the low birth weight of the anencephalic fetus. However, the final common pathway of growth hormone action is mediated by the generation of insulin-like growth regulatory factors, the somatomedins. The concentration of these substances in cord blood correlates with fetal weight. SGA infants may have diminished somatomedin values, whereas neonates with a deficiency of somatomedin generation are born with diminished birth length (Larson's dwarf). Additional growth hormone–dependent "growth factors" include multiplication-stimulating action factor and insulin growth factors 1 and 2. Other growth hormone–independent factors, such as fibroblast growth factor, nerve growth factor, and epidermal growth factor, have been investigated only in cell culture.

The role of other hormones, notably corticosteroids and thyroid hormone, has not been well defined for fetal growth. With thyroid hormone deficiency, for example, in the human athyrotic cretin, birth weight is not altered. These hormones, however, probably have a more significant role as regulatory signals for the initiation of maturation and differentiation in fetal tissues.

MATERNAL CONTRIBUTIONS TO ABERRANT FETAL GROWTH
Physical environment

Certain otherwise normal mothers are prone to repeated delivery of SGA infants. Many of these women themselves were born SGA, raising the possibility of nongenetic horizontal transmission of a physical regulator of fetal growth. A proportion of these women also remain small throughout life and are identifiable by low prepregnancy weight and stature. These women may

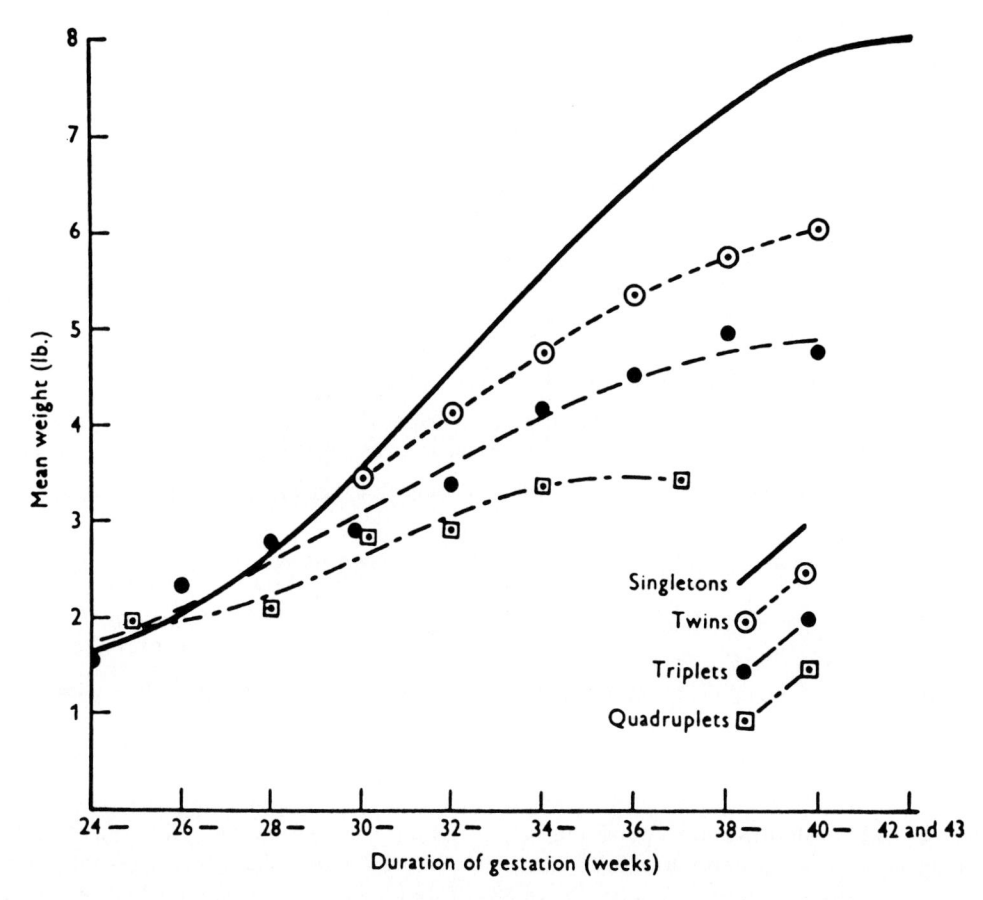

Fig. 7-6. Birth weight–gestational age relationships in multiple gestation denoting origin of aberrant fetal growth. (From McKeown, T., and Record, R.: J. Endocrinol. **8**:386, 1952.)

exert a restraint on fetal growth by some unknown regulator, possibly related to their own stature or uterine capacity. This may be analogous to the breeding experiments between Shetland ponies and Shire horses. The offspring resulting from breeding a male Shire to a female Shetland is similar in birth weight to a Shetland pony, whereas that born to a cross between a male Shetland and a female Shire approaches the birth weight of a Shire. The smaller Shetland female apparently exerts a growth restraint on the genetic potential derived from the larger Shire male. Similar constraints may be exerted during multiple gestations, since fetal growth declines when the number of fetuses increases. The onset of growth retardation in multiple gestations is also related to the number of fetuses, since growth restraint begins sooner with triplets than twins (Fig. 7-6). In multiple gestations the uterine constraint appears to occur when combined fetal size approaches 3 kg. Placental implantation site, vascular anastomoses, and nutritional factors may also interfere with growth in these pregnancies. The uterine capacity itself may also place a constraint on optimum fetal growth.

Maternal nutrition

Prepregnancy weight and pregnancy weight gain are two important independent variables that affect fetal growth. Underweight mothers and those affected with malnutrition deliver infants with diminished birth weight. Weight gain during pregnancy in nonobese patients correlates significantly with fetal birth weight. The effect of prepregnancy weight in obese women is independent of pregnancy weight gain and offsets the frequently observed poor weight gain of these overweight women. SGA infants are unusual for obese women, which may be related to large maternal nutrient stores.

The effects of maternal nutritional status on fetal growth are minimal during the first trimester of pregnancy. This is related to the large surfeit of nutrients presented to the relatively small, undemanding embryo and early fetus. As fetal growth accelerates, the requirements for fetal growth increase and may not be sufficiently provided by an inadequate maternal diet. In an otherwise healthy population of Dutch women experiencing a short period of famine during the Hunger Winter of 1944-

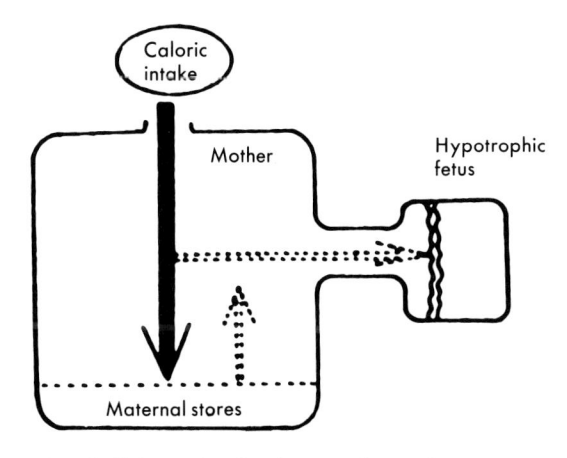

Fig. 7-7. "Selfish mother" enhances her substrate stores at the expense of fetal nutritional deficiency. Possible causes include (1) excessive maternal insulin release, (2) deficient insulin resistance, and (3) deficient destruction of insulin. (From Frydman, R., and others: Fifth European Congress of Perinatal Medicine Proceedings, vol. 203, 1976.)

1945, fetal growth was most severely affected when deprivation occurred in the third trimester. Substrate deficiency during this period resulted in an overall reduction of birth weight of 300 gm. Maternal weight gain and placental weight were even more drastically reduced, demonstrating preferential use of nutrients for the fetus. Similar observations occurred during a more severe and prolonged famine in Leningrad, where birth weight was reduced by 500 gm at term.

Attempts at improving the low birth weight outcome in high-risk populations (characterized by having poor nutritional histories) have demonstrated a positive effect of nutritional supplementation. Additional calories, rather than protein supplementation, correlate best with enhanced fetal weight. Caloric supplements greater than 20,000 calories per pregnancy reduced the number of low birth weight infants; each 10,000 calories supplemented above the standard diet improved fetal weight by an average of 29 gm. Protein supplementation may even have adverse neurodevelopmental effects on the fetus. Aside from periods of famine and geographic areas where malnutrition is endemic, other conditions associated with poor maternal nutrition and suboptimum fetal growth are included in the following list.* Adolescent women, in particular, are at risk because of their own growth requirements in addition to those of the fetus.

1. Adolescents, especially those who are not married
2. Women with low prepregnancy weights
3. Women with inadequate weight gain during pregnancy
4. Women with low income or for whom food purchase is an economic problem
5. Women with a history of frequent conceptions
6. Women with a history of infants having low birth weight
7. Women with diseases that influence nutritional status—diabetes, tuberculosis, anemia, drug addiction, alcoholism, or mental depression
8. Women known to be dietary faddists or with frank pica

Certain maternal metabolic aberrations are associated with suboptimum fetal growth. Mothers who demonstrate excessively low fasting blood glucose values and those who fail to elevate their blood glucose sufficiently following an oral glucose tolerance test are at risk to deliver an SGA infant. A "selfish mother" hypothesis has been proposed to explain the poor growth of these infants (Fig. 7-7). Rather than providing for their fetus, these mothers store glucose and fatty acids in their own depot tissues, thus limiting placental transfer. Maternal hyperinsulinism and enhanced insulin action may mediate these events, which may diminish the provision of substrates available for fetal growth.

Chronic disease

Of all disease mechanisms that interfere with fetal growth, those resulting in uterine ischemia and/or hypoxia have the most marked effect. Chronic maternal hypertension due to either primary renal parenchymal disease, such as nephritis, or those extrinsic to parenchymal disorders, such as essential hypertension, significantly alters fetal growth and well-being. This effect is related to the duration of hypertension and to the absolute elevation of the diastolic pressure and is most severe in the presence of end-organ disorders, such as retinopathy.

Pregnancy-induced hypertension is of paramount importance to perinatologists in relation to its effect on fetal growth and well-being (see Chapter 4). This disease, which may affect uteroplacental perfusion and fetal growth long before clinical signs of edema, proteinuria, and hypertension develop, reduces uterine blood flow as determined by ^{24}Na and dehydroisoandrosterone clearance studies. Preeclampsia is characterized by an unusual sensitivity of maternal blood vessels to vasoactive compounds, resulting in enhanced and pathologic vasoconstriction. In pregnancies complicated by eclampsia, fetal growth deviates from the expected norm from 32 weeks onward (Fig. 7-8). Vascular insufficiency resulting from advanced maternal diabetes mellitus, especially in the presence of end-organ disease in the kidney or retina, also produces intrauterine growth retardation despite

---
*From Robertson, W. In Quilligan, E., and Kretchmar, N., editors: Fetal and maternal medicine, New York, 1980, John Wiley & Sons, Inc.

the presence of maternal hyperglycemia (Chapter 3).

Another major category associated with diminished fetal weight gain is that resulting from maternal hypoxemia. Severe cyanotic congenital heart disease, such as tetralogy of Fallot or Eisenmenger's complex, is the best example of this mechanism, whereas sickle cell anemia is representative of diseases that can produce local uterine hypoxia and ischemia. Nutritional anemias are not usually associated with aberrant fetal growth. In sickle cell anemia the abnormal cells may interfere with local uterine perfusion during episodes of sickling, and growth retardation is observed.

A common and nonpathologic factor related to maternal hypoxia is the diminished environmental oxygen saturation that is present at high altitudes. Infants born in the mountains of Peru demonstrate lower birth weights than do Peruvian infants born at sea level. Placental mass has hypertrophied in these newborns in an attempt to compensate for the lower circulating maternal oxygen concentration. Interestingly, these neonates are not born with polycythemia as a response to fetal hypoxia, as proposed in other SGA infants.

Drugs

The effects of maternal drug administration on the fetus are usually considered primarily in terms of teratogenicity. However, a continuum of fetal compromise may be present, since many malformation syndromes are associated with diminished birth weight, whereas other agents may interfere only with fetal growth. Drugs associated with intrauterine growth retardation are included in the following list:

1. Amphetamines
2. Antimetabolites (aminopterin, busulfan, methotrexate, etc.)
3. Bromides
4. Cigarettes (carbon monoxide, nicotine)
5. Ethanol
6. Heroin
7. Hydantoin
8. Methadone
9. Phencyclidine
10. Polychlorinated biphenyls (PCB)
11. Propranolol
12. Steroids (prednisone)
13. Trimethadione (Tridione)
14. Warfarin

Many of the commonly abused drugs have been implicated as agents producing fetal growth retardation by reducing maternal appetite and by being associated with lower socioeconomic groups. However, at least for heroin, methadone, and ethanol, a direct cellular toxic effect acting directly on cell replication and growth appears to be involved. This is most evident in the fetal alcohol syndrome in that the prenatal onset of growth retardation persists during postnatal periods despite adequate food intake. A placental transfer block for specific amino acids has been observed, resulting in the fetal alcohol syndrome.

Cigarette smoking during pregnancy reduces eventual

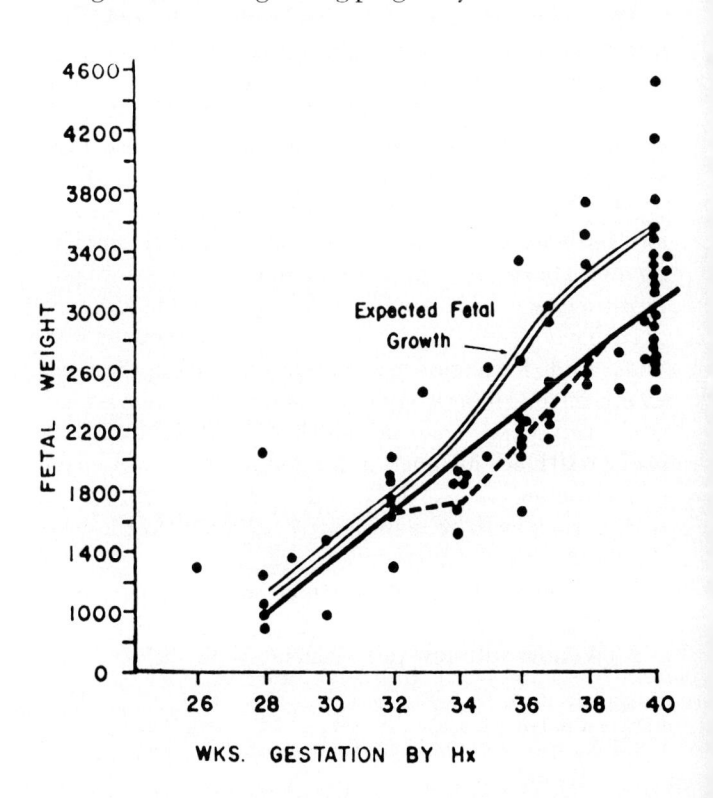

Fig. 7-8. Fetal weight following eclampsia. Broken line demonstrates mean weight alteration. (From Zuspan, F.: Clin. Obstet. Gynecol. **9:**954, 1966.)

fetal birth weight and is related directly to the amount of cigarettes consumed. Birth weight at term is reduced an average of 170 gm if more than 10 cigarettes are consumed per day; consumption of more than 15 per day may reduce weight by 300 gm. The mechanism of fetal growth retardation is uncertain, but nicotine and subsequent catecholamine release may produce uterine vasoconstriction and fetal hypoxia, whereas carbon monoxide and cyanide may cause a more direct effect. Following binding to hemoglobin, carbon monoxide and cyanide may diminish oxygen unloading from the mother to the fetus and from the fetus to its tissues.

Drugs such as propranolol and corticosteroids probably have a direct effect on the fetus, although the confounding influences of the chronic maternal illness for which these agents are prescribed may also contribute to intrauterine growth retardation.

Socioeconomic status

Poor environmental conditions related to lower socioeconomic status have been associated with infant malnutrition of both prenatal and postnatal onset. With improvement of these conditions, birth weight is enhanced. This was extensively studied following the improvements in living conditions that occurred in postwar Japan. The improvement of birth weight during this era occurred only in infants born during the latter part of the third trimester, as nutritional or environmental effects seem greatest during this period of fetal growth.

Many of the maternal factors, such as drug abuse, poor nutritional habits, and cigarette smoking, are interrelated and are covariables associated with poor socioeconomic status. Factors such as adverse environmental living conditions and chronic maternal illness are more prevalent among reproductive-age women of lower socioeconomic status. Adolescent and single-parent families and those who seek little prenatal advice are also more common variables among women in this bracket. Many investigations have demonstrated that these groups of women are at risk for intrauterine growth retardation. Newer evidence has been proposed which suggests that if chronic maternal illness and certain behavioral characteristics are eliminated, the remaining women of lower socioeconomic status do not have a higher incidence of SGA infants. The specific behavioral characteristics more common among poor women include the following:

1. Unmarried status
2. Age less than 17 or greater than 35
3. Low prepregnancy weight
4. Poor pregnancy weight gain
5. Drug abuse
6. Cigarette smoking
7. Failure to seek antenatal care

These behavioral variables may be related to an attitude difference among these women, who choose a different life-style and constitute a subgroup, and not specifically representing the entire population; thus they may be based on choice and not necessarily environment.

PLACENTAL DETERMINANTS

Optimum fetal growth depends on efficient placental function as both nutrient supply line and organ of gaseous exchange. Placental functional integrity requires additional energy production, since placental oxidative metabolism may equal that of the fetus. This large energy requirement is essential to maintain its growth-promoting roles, which include the active transport of amino acids, synthesis of protein and steroid hormones, and support of placental maturation and growth. Placental growth parallels that of the fetus; however, toward term there is a greater decline in the rate of placental weight gain than that in the fetus. During this decline of placental weight the fetus also exhibits a decrement in its rate of weight change, suggesting that placental function, as well as its weight, has declined, leading to reduced fetal growth (see preceding material). However, despite the change in placental weight, the placenta continues to mature. Placental villous surface area continues to increase with advancing gestational age (Fig. 7-9) while

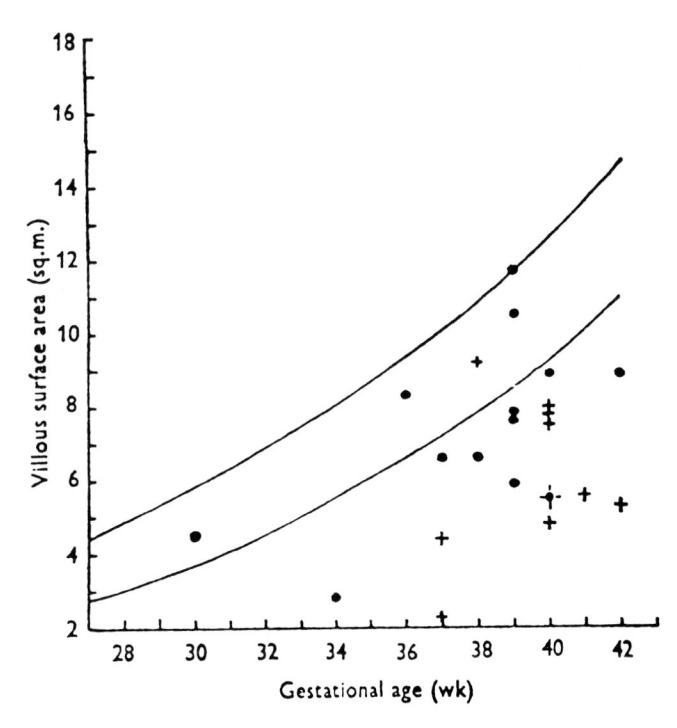

Fig. 7-9. Area of chorionic surface area in normal and abnormal pregnancies. ●, Maternal hypertension; +, normotensive, IUGR. (From Aherne, W., and Dunnill, M.: J. Pathol. Bacteriol. **91:**132, 1966.)

Fig. 7-10. Urea permeability per gram of the ovine placenta. ●, Singletons; ○, twins. (From Kulhanek, J., and others: Am. J. Physiol. **226:**1257, 1974.)

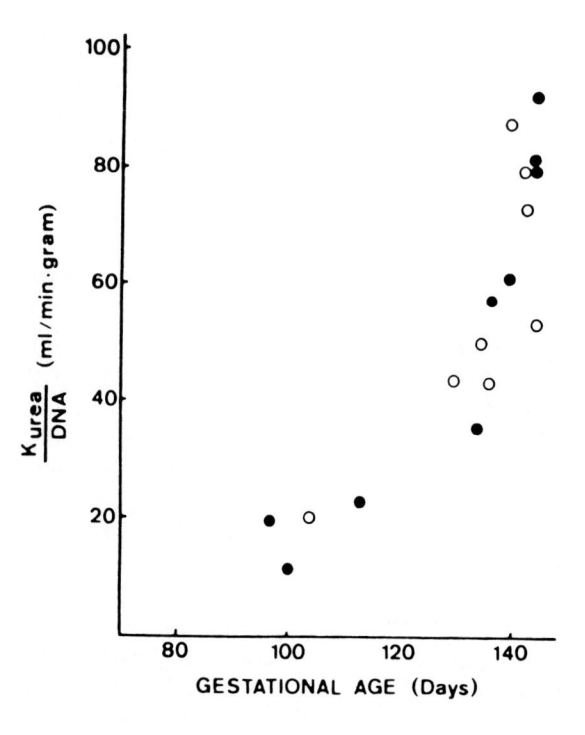

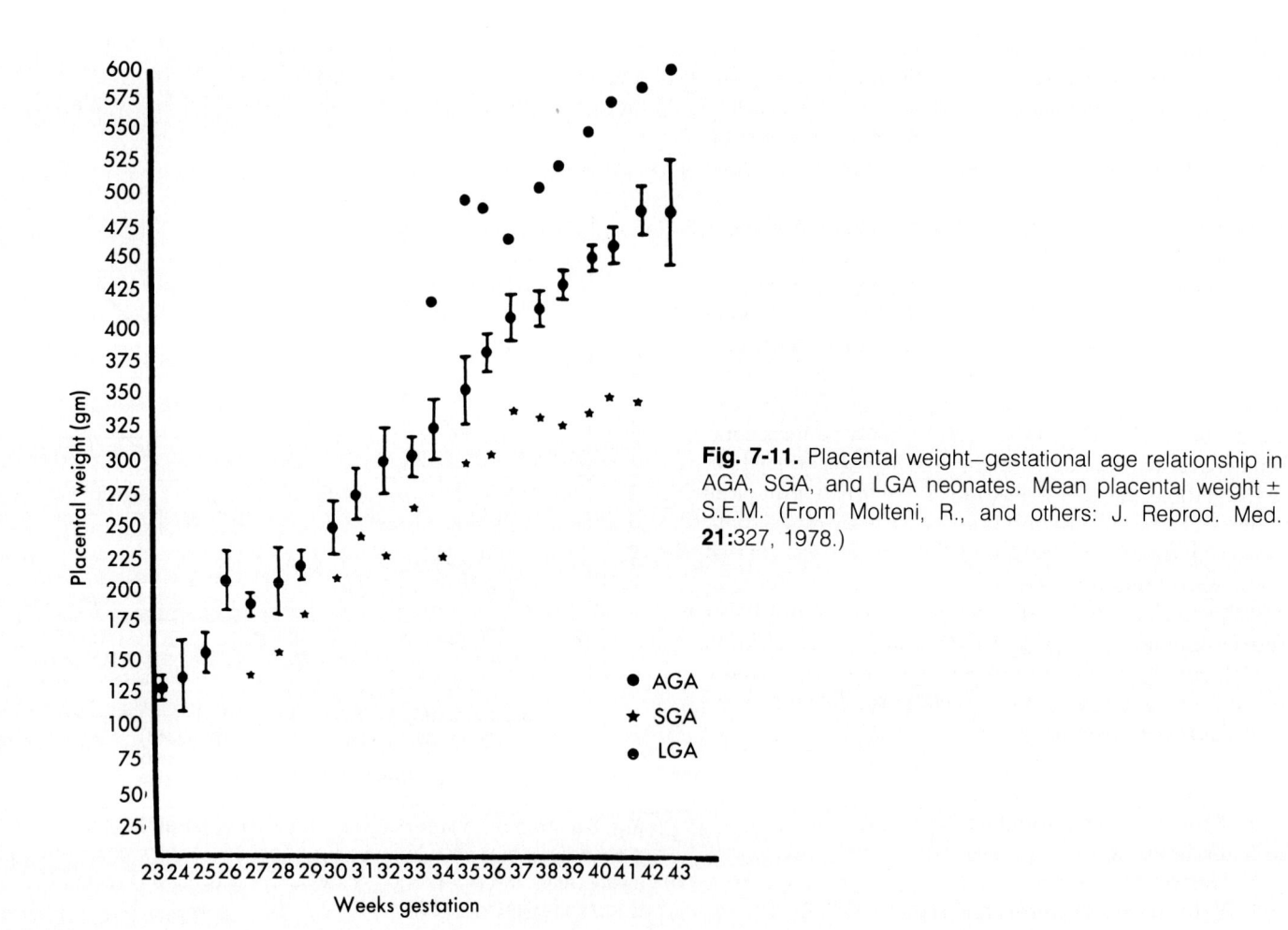

Fig. 7-11. Placental weight–gestational age relationship in AGA, SGA, and LGA neonates. Mean placental weight ± S.E.M. (From Molteni, R., and others: J. Reprod. Med. **21:**327, 1978.)

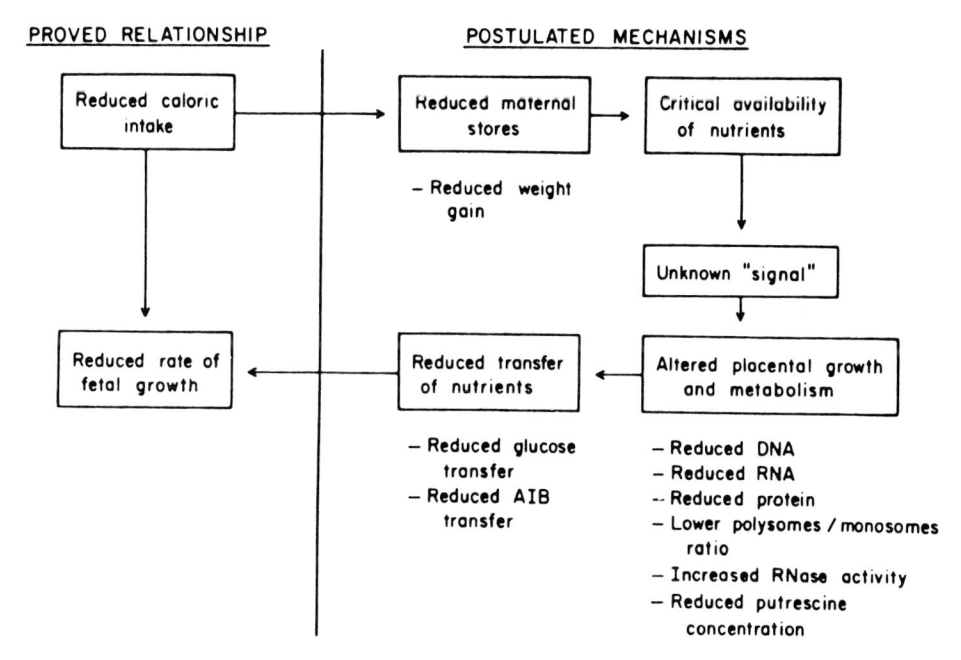

```
PROVED RELATIONSHIP          |  POSTULATED MECHANISMS

[Reduced caloric intake] ──→ [Reduced maternal stores] ──→ [Critical availability of nutrients]
                                  – Reduced weight gain                    │
       │                                                                    ▼
       │                                                          [Unknown "signal"]
       │                                                                    │
       ▼                                                                    ▼
[Reduced rate of fetal growth] ←── [Reduced transfer of nutrients] ←── [Altered placental growth and metabolism]
                                    – Reduced glucose transfer      – Reduced DNA
                                    – Reduced AIB transfer          – Reduced RNA
                                                                    – Reduced protein
                                                                    – Lower polysomes / monosomes ratio
                                                                    – Increased RNase activity
                                                                    – Reduced putrescine concentration
```

Fig. 7-12. Effect of maternal undernutrition on fetal growth. (From Russo, P., and others. In Young, D., and Hicks, J., editors: The neonate, New York, 1976, John Wiley & Sons, Inc.)

simultaneously, the syncytial trophoblast layer continues to thin out and vascularization of the terminal villi continues to improve. Functionally, urea clearance is enhanced toward term in the ovine placenta (Fig. 7-10), suggesting that permeability and diffusing distance improve as the placenta approaches term. Birth weight has been correlated to placental weight (Fig. 7-11) and villous surface area (Fig. 7-9), suggesting that macroscopic and microscopic events are related to optimum placental function.

When placental insufficiency occurs, there may be a functional failure of the placenta as a respiratory or nutritive organ or both. Placental insufficiency associated with maternal nutritional deficiency has more than one effect on fetal growth. In addition to diminished fetal substrate provision, placental metabolism will be altered directly, as proposed in Fig. 7-12. Diminished placental growth will adversely affect total nutrient transfer, whereas reduced placental production of chorionic somatomammotropin will attenuate maternal mobilization of fuels to her fetus. Reduced placental energy production and protein synthesis will limit active transport of amino acids and facilitative transport of glucose.

When placental insufficiency complicates maternal vascular disease such as preeclampsia, there is also diminished placental weight and volume. In addition, there is a decline in villous surface area (Fig. 7-9) and a relative increase of nonexchanging tissue. At the same time, these placentas demonstrate thickening of the capillary basement membrane. Unfortunately, such detailed microscopic analyses of villous surface area are not available at most medical centers; therefore we are often left with only gross macroscopic and screening microscopic examination of the placenta in SGA infants.

Following is a list of common findings in placental disorders associated with diminished birth weight.

1. Twins (implantation site)
2. Twins (vascular anastomoses)
3. Chorioangioma
4. Villitis (TORCH)
5. Villitis (unknown etiology)
6. Avascular villi
7. Ischemic villous necrosis
8. Multiple infarcts
9. Syncytial knots
10. Chronic separation (abruptio)
11. Diffuse fibrinosis
12. Hydatidiform change
13. Abnormal insertion
14. Single umbilical artery
15. Fetal vessel thrombosis
16. Circumvallate placenta

Multiple gestations may produce significant placental disorders, both in suboptimum sites of implantation or, more often, related to abnormal vascular anastomoses in diamnionic monochorionic twinning (Fig. 7-13). As a result of arteriovenous interconnections, one twin serves as the donor and develops intrauterine growth retarda-

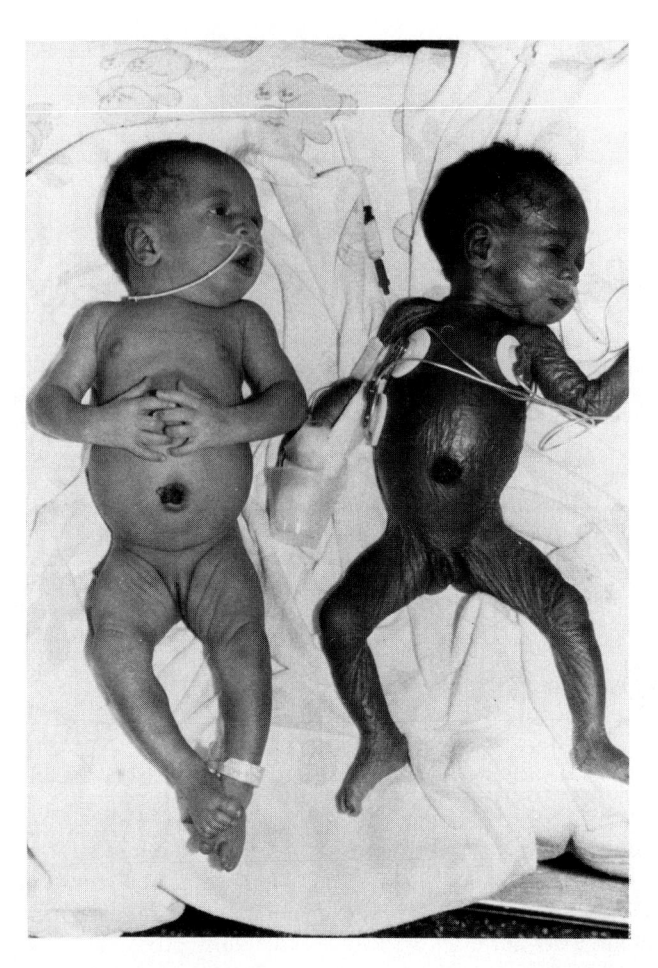

Fig. 7-13. Diamnionic monochorionic twins, 36 weeks gestational age, with birth weights of 1.3 and 2.0 kg.

tion, losing its nutrient supplies, while the other is the recipient and has satisfactory growth. These anastomoses may be detectable on careful gross examination of the placenta. Other detectable potential causes related to aberrant fetal growth include chorioangiomas, large retroplacental infarcts and hemorrhages, abnormal cord insertion patterns, and (questionably) single umbilical artery. The remaining pathologic findings may be detected with microscopic examination of appropriately selected sections of the placenta.

FETAL DETERMINANTS

Optimum fetal growth depends on adequate provision of substrates, their effective placental transfer, and the inherited regulatory factors within the fetal genotype. In addition to substrates, oxygen must be transferred and an appropriate hormonal milieu must be present. There must also be sufficient room within the uterus. In the absence of adverse environmental effects, the inherent growth potential of the fetus may be achieved.

Genetic determinants of fetal growth are inherited from both parents, and population norms must be established to detect aberrant fetal growth. For example, the average birth weight of Cheyenne Indians is 3,800 gm at term, whereas that for the New Guinea Luni tribe is 2,400 gm. Such genetic potentials are the major determinants of early fetal growth, since nutritional and environmental problems should not affect the fetus until the requirements for tissue growth increase during the third trimester.

Approximately 20% of birth weight variability in a given population is determined by the fetal genotype; maternal hereditary and environmental factors contribute an additional 65%; the remaining contributing factors are unknown. Birth order affects fetal size: infants born to primiparous women weigh less than subsequent siblings (Fig. 7-1). The second and each additional child weigh an average of 180 gm more than the firstborn. Male sex of the fetus is associated with enhanced birth weight, beginning to become predominant after 32 weeks' gestation (Fig. 7-1). At term males weigh approximately 150 gm more than female infants. A male twin, in addition to affecting its own somatic growth, can also enhance the growth of its female co-twin. Androgenic hormonal stimulation of fetal growth may contribute to these observed differences. There is also a theory stating that maternal-fetal antigenic differences are responsible for this effect. These antigenic differences result in enhanced placental trophoblastic invasion of the decidua, improving placental and subsequent fetal growth. As a corollary, interference with maternal immunologic function may inhibit this antigenic growth advantage and explain in part the diminished birth weights following maternal immunosuppressive therapy.

Alternately, chromosomes may carry growth-determining genes, as genetic material on the Y chromosome may enhance the growth of the male fetus. Similarly, chromosomal deletions or imbalances result in diminished fetal growth. For example, Turner's syndrome (XO) is associated with diminished birth weight. The converse is not true, since additional X chromosomes beyond the norm are associated with reduced fetal growth. For each additional X chromosome (in excess of XX), birth weight may be reduced 300 gm. Similarly, autosomal trisomies such as Down's syndrome are also associated with abnormal fetal growth. Chromosomal aberrations often result in diminished fetal growth by interfering with cell division. An intrinsic defect in cultured fibroblasts from trisomy 21 patients has been observed in tissue culture. In addition, placental function may be altered. Single-gene defects may also reduce fetal growth. The inborn errors most notably associated with diminished fetal weight are included in the following outline. Many syndromes with either autosomal recessive, dominant, polygenetic, or unknown inheritance are also associated with poor fetal growth and occasionally may produce marked intrauterine growth retardation.

Infectious agents are commonly sought as being responsible for early onset of intrauterine growth retardation. Of these, cytomegalovirus and rubella virus are the most important identifiable agents associated with marked fetal growth retardation. Following maternal viremia, both agents invade the placenta, producing varying degrees of villitis, and then subsequently gain access to fetal tissues. The effects of placentitis itself on fetal growth are unknown, but once congenital fetal infection has occurred, these viral agents have direct adverse effects on fetal development. Intracellular rubella virus inhibits cellular mitotic activity in addition to producing chromosomal breaks and subsequently cytolysis. In addition, this virus produces an obliterative angiopathy that further compromises cell viability. Cytomegalovirus also causes cytolysis, resulting in areas of focal tissue necrosis. These viral agents therefore reduce cell number and subsequent birth weight by simultaneously inhibiting cell division and producing cell death.

Following are examples of factors affecting fetal growth.

A. Chromosome disorders associated with intrauterine growth retardation
   1. Trisomies 8, 13, 18, 21
   2. Short-arm deletion 4
   3. Long-arm deletion 13
   4. Long-arm deletion 21
   5. Triploidy
   6. XO
   7. XXY, XXXY, XXXXY
   8. XXXXX
B. Metabolic disorders associated with diminished birth weight
   1. Agenesis of pancreas
   2. Congenital absence of islets of Langerhans
   3. Congenital lipodystrophy
   4. Galactosemia (?)
   5. Generalized gangliosidosis type I
   6. Hypophosphatasia
   7. I cell disease
   8. Leprechaunism
   9. Maternal PKU
   10. Maternal renal insufficiency
   11. Maternal Gaucher's disease
   12. Menke's syndrome
   13. Transient neonatal diabetes mellitus
C. Syndromes associated with diminished birth weight
   1. Aarskog's syndrome
   2. Anencephaly
   3. Bloom's syndrome
   4. Cornelia de Lange syndrome
   5. Dubowitz syndrome
   6. Dwarfism (achondrogenesis, achondroplasia, etc.)
   7. Ellis–van Creveld syndrome
   8. Familial dysautonomia
   9. Fanconi pancytopenia
   10. Meckel-Gruber syndrome
   11. Microcephaly
   12. Möbius syndrome
   13. Osteogenesis imperfecta
   14. Potter's syndrome
   15. Prader-Willi syndrome
   16. Progeria
   17. Prune belly syndrome
   18. Radial aplasia; thrombocytopenia
   19. Robert's syndrome
   20. Russell-Silver dwarf
   21. Seckel's syndrome
   22. Smith-Lemli-Opitz syndrome
   23. VATER and VACTERL syndromes
   24. William's syndrome
D. Congenital infections associated with intrauterine growth retardation
   1. Rubella
   2. Cytomegalovirus
   3. Toxoplasmosis
   4. Malaria
   5. Syphilis
   6. Varicella (?)
   7. Others (?)

THE SGA INFANT
Definition

Since the introduction of gestational age assessment and further subdivision of each neonatal age period into large, appropriate, and small for gestational age categories, it has become increasing apparent that the low birth weight infant (< 2,500 gm) is not always premature (< 37 weeks). On a worldwide basis, between 30% and 40% of these infants are born at term gestation and are therefore undergrown, or SGA. As discussed previously, population norms need to be determined for each specific genetic group, especially those characterized by unusual inherited patterns of fetal growth. In general, these population norms established in various North American and European cities describe the usual fetal growth pattern for industrial societies and may be used as the reference norms for similar ethnic groups (Fig. 7-1; Table 7-1). Each curve defines either standard deviations or percentile units that include the normal variability or distribution of birth weights at each gestational age. By definition, infants less than two standard deviations or those less than the third percentile (tenth for Denver curves due to the lower birth weight at higher altitudes) will be classified as SGA. Therefore, between 2.5% and 10% of each population are SGA. The use of population means, however, is at times misleading. Within a sibship, fetal birth weight is less variable and more consistent than that for an entire population. Compared with family members, 80% of infants with congenital rubella infection were classified as SGA, whereas only 40% were SGA using population standards. Fetal growth assessment must therefore be considered in the context of both prior reproductive history and clinical examination of the newborn (see further).

Aberrant fetal growth patterns

Fetal growth retardation may have its origins early or late during fetal development. Infants who demonstrate reduced fetal growth early in gestation constitute approximately 30% of all SGA infants. They are symmetrically growth retarded, since head circumference, weight, and length are proportionately affected to equivalent degrees. These fetuses and infants continue to grow, albeit with reduced net effect (Fig. 7-14, A). Besides inherent genetic growth constraint, other factors may produce diminished growth potential in these neonates. Congenital viral infections usually have their worst effect if infection occurs during the first trimester, when they have a significant effect on cell replication and subsequently birth weight. Similarly, abnormal genetic factors such as single gene deletions and chromosomal disorders also reduce the intrauterine growth rate at an early stage of development. Characteristics and examples of intrauterine growth retardation are listed on p. 66.

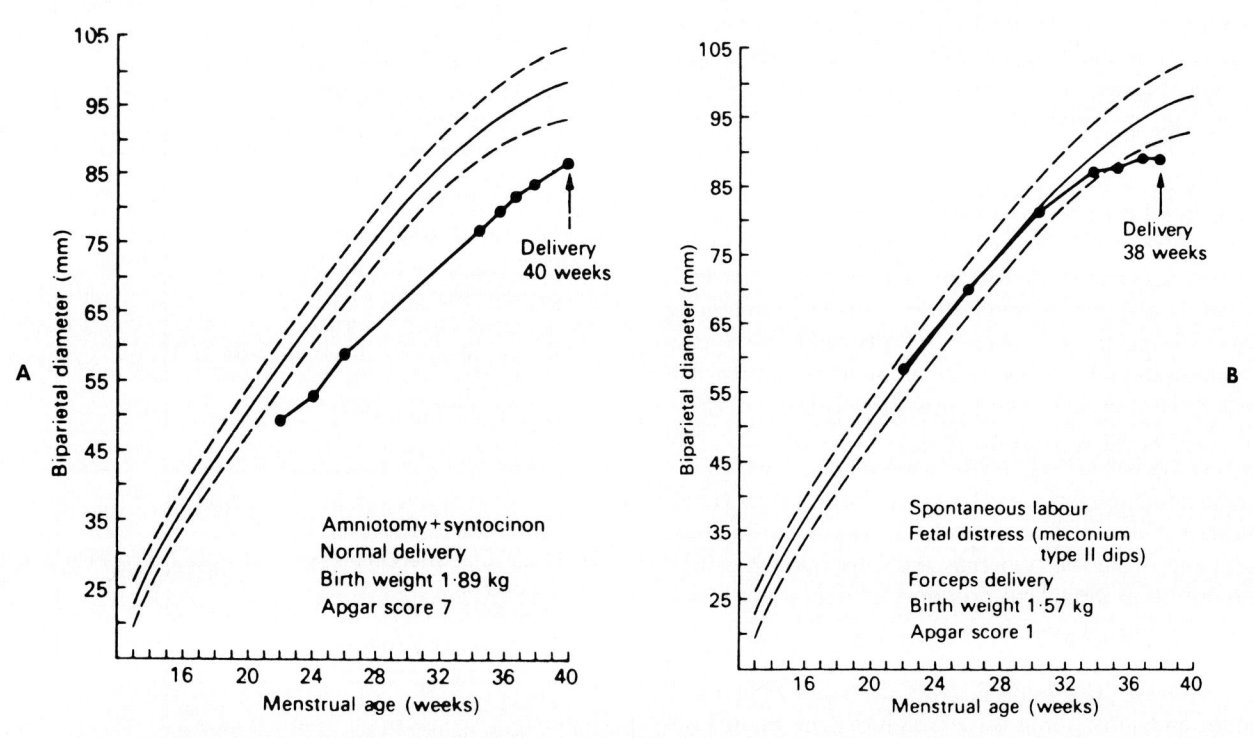

Fig. 7-14. Low profile **(A)** and late flattening **(B)** patterns of IUGR. (From Campbell, S. In Beard, R., and Nathanielsz, P., editors: Fetal physiology and medicine, Philadelphia, 1976, W.B. Saunders Co.)

Intrauterine growth retardation: determinants of aberrant fetal growth

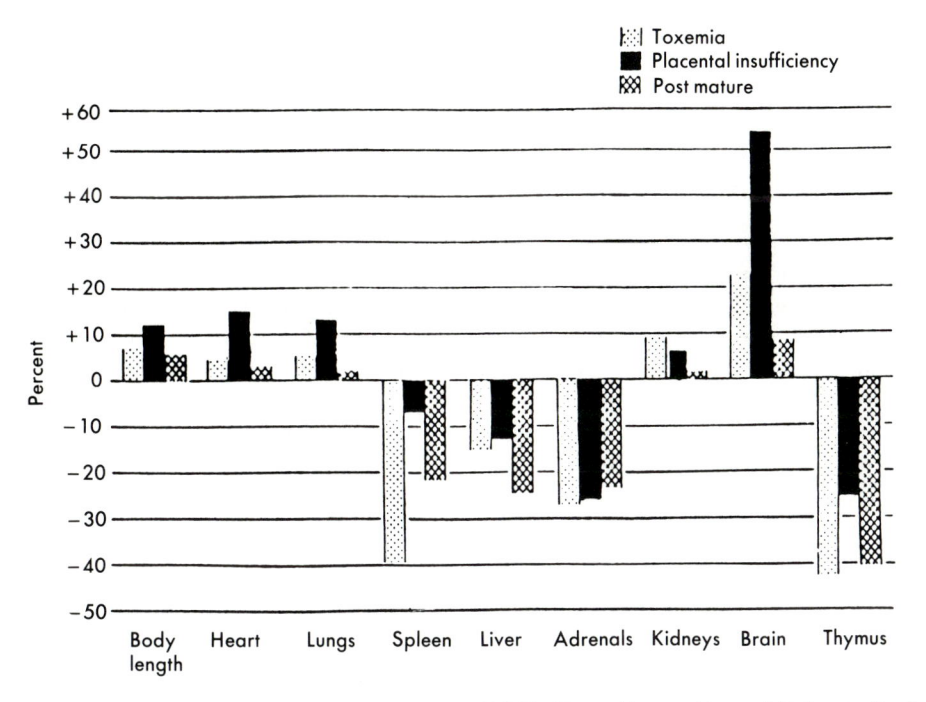

Fig. 7-15. Deviation of organ weights following IUGR. (From Naeye, R., and Kelly, J.: Pediatr. Clin. North Am. **13:**849, 1966.)

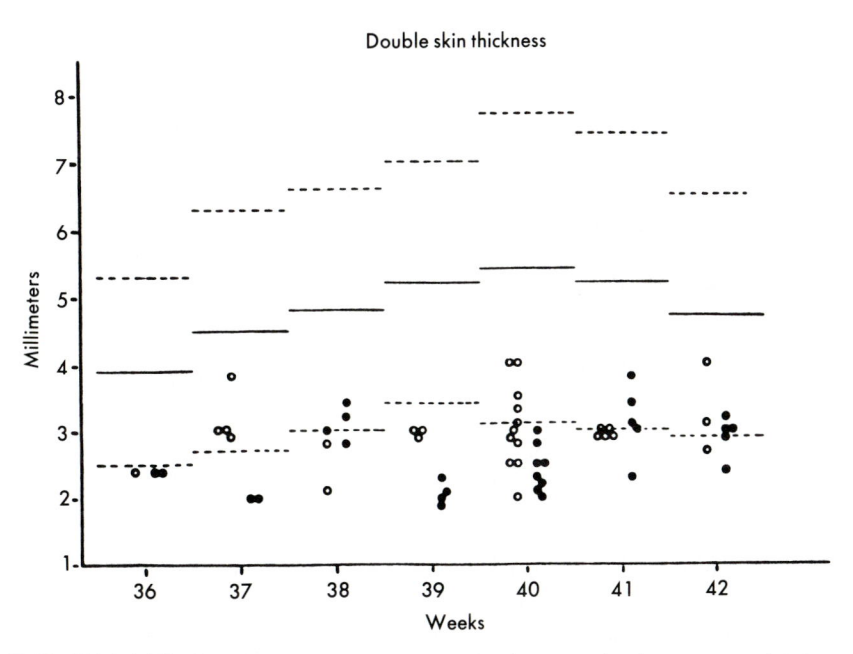

Fig. 7-16. Skinfold thickness is a major determinant of neonatal subcutaneous fat deposits. Fetal malnutrition with (●) and without (○) severe clinical signs of wasting. (From Usher, R.: Pediatr. Clin. North Am. **17:**169, 1970.)

Characteristics

Early onset	Late onset
Symmetrical	Asymmetrical
Constitutional	Environmental
Low-profile BPD	Late flattening BPD
↓ Growth potential	Growth arrest

Examples

Genetic	Preeclampsia
TORCH	Chronic hypertension
Chromosomal	Diabetes classes D to F
Syndromes	Nutrition

Growth retardation of a later onset is usually associated with impaired uteroplacental function or nutritional deficiency during the third trimester (Fig. 7-14, B). Nutrient supplies and uteroplacental perfusion are in excess of their requirements during early fetal development and should not interfere with fetal growth until the growth rate exceeds the provision of substrates and/or oxygen. During the last trimester the fetal growth rate and net tissue accretion increase markedly; if the uteroplacental supply line is compromised, intrauterine growth retardation will develop. The anthropomorphic findings among these infants demonstrate a relative sparing of head growth, whereas body weight and somatic organ growth are more seriously altered. Spleen, liver, adrenal, thymus, and adipose tissue growth is affected to the greatest extent in these late-onset SGA newborns (Figs. 7-15 and 7-16). The relative sparing of fetal head (brain) growth may be due to preferential perfusion of the brain with well-oxygenated blood containing adequate substrates following redistribution of the cardiac output during periods of fetal distress.

ANTENATAL CARE
Diagnosis

Antenatal diagnosis of intrauterine growth retardation has proved an extremely difficult task. Usually these infants deliver at or beyond term without prior antenatal detection. At the very best, when looked for with careful maternal physical examination, accurate dating, and risk assessment analysis, only 50% of these infants may be detected before birth. Antenatal detection is an essential component of care for these infants, since they require intensive obstetric and neonatal management to reduce their excessive perinatal morbidity and mortality. This poor outcome is associated with unexplained antepartum fetal demise, intrapartum fetal death, neonatal asphyxia, and other major neonatal adaptive problems. Antenatal detection and intensive perinatal care of mother, fetus, and, later, the neonate are imperative components that result in improved outcome for these infants.

Currently, careful measurement and recording of the fundal height at each antenatal visit is the best clinical screening aid for the diagnosis of intrauterine growth retardation. When dates are confirmed by onset of quickening, audible heart tones, and accurate menstrual history, size-dates discrepancy (i.e., fundal height smaller than or lagging behind gestational age) is suggestive of intrauterine growth retardation. Historical findings that may be components of a risk assessment score for intrauterine growth retardation include a past history of an SGA infant, vaginal bleeding, multiple gestation, low prepregnancy weight, and poor pregnancy weight gain. Chronic maternal illness and preeclampsia are also high-risk situations indicating possible intrauterine growth retardation.

Laboratory tests potentially helpful in detecting intrauterine growth retardation include analysis of serum human placental lactogen concentration and serum or urinary estriol (E_3) determinations (see Chapter 9). Both are placental hormones secreted into the maternal circulation and in part related to placental mass, gestational age, and birth weight. However, these are not consistently helpful. Urinary estriol determinations are probably more important for serial monitoring of placental function and fetal well-being. Other determinants of fetal well-being and growth include maternal plasma assays of oxytocinase, diamine oxidase, alkaline phosphatase, and alpha-fetoprotein. The former three enzymes are of placental origin; however, their usefulness in detecting fetal well-being and growth has declined in recent years. In contrast, alpha-fetoprotein is of fetal origin, and elevated levels have been associated with intrauterine growth retardation.

On the basis of maternal risk assessment and size-date discrepancy, fetal body measurement by ultrasonography is the best available method for the estimation of fetal weight and the diagnosis of intrauterine growth retardation (see also Chapter 8). In addition to small size, the SGA fetus may have a smaller placenta; reduced fetal urine production may also result in less amniotic fluid. These individual components result in a diminished total uterine volume. The determination of this volume is tedious but useful in diagnosing intrauterine growth retardation. Classically, serial biparietal diameters (BPD) before 32 weeks' gestation, analyzed according to their absolute numerical values and to rate of change, have been established as a reliable means to determine fetal weight, maturity, and aberrant growth patterns (Figs. 7-14, 7-17, and 7-18). However, in asymmetrical growth retardation, fetal head growth is spared relative to the degree of wasting of extracerebral tissues. Serial BPD determinations may not detect such affected infants. Newer parameters such as truncometry may be employed by measuring the abdominal circumference at the level of the umbilical vein (Fig. 7-19). This permits more accurate determination of the asymmetrically

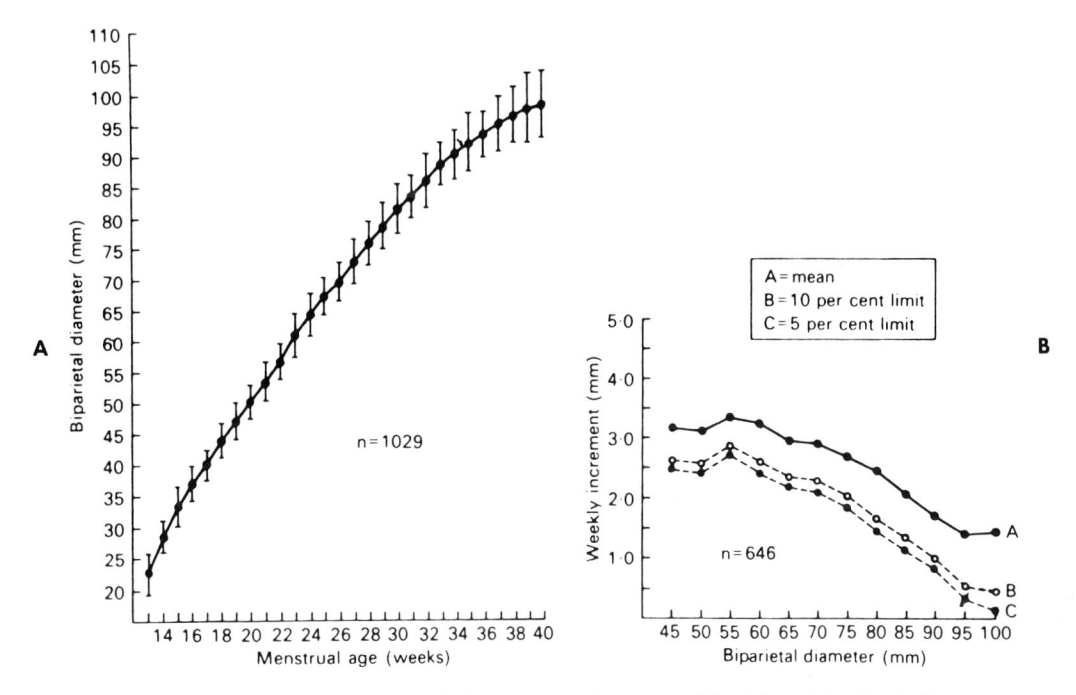

Fig. 7-17. Absolute measurement **(A)** and rate of change **(B)** of fetal biparietal diameter. (From Campbell, S.: Size at birth, Amsterdam, 1974, Elsevier Scientific Publications.)

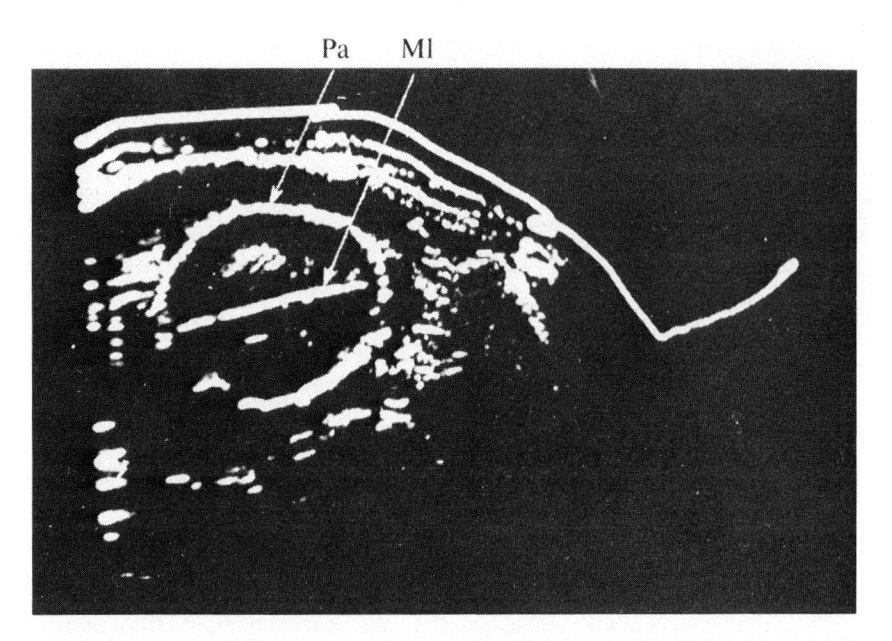

Fig. 7-18. Sonogram demonstrating determination of the BPD. *Pa,* Parietal bone; *Ml,* midline echo. (From Campbell, S. In Beard, R., and Nathanielsz, P., editors: Fetal physiology and medicine, Philadelphia, 1976, W.B. Saunders Co.)

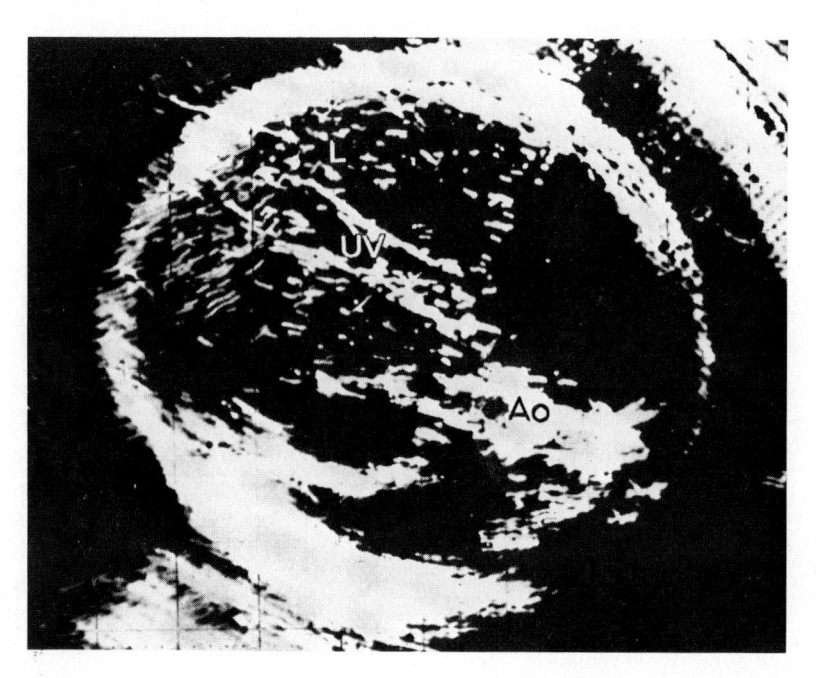

Fig. 7-19. Truncometry at the level of fetal liver *(L)*, umbilical vein, *(UV)*, and aorta *(Ao)*. (From Campbell, S.: Size at birth, Amsterdam, 1974, Elsevier Scientific Publications.)

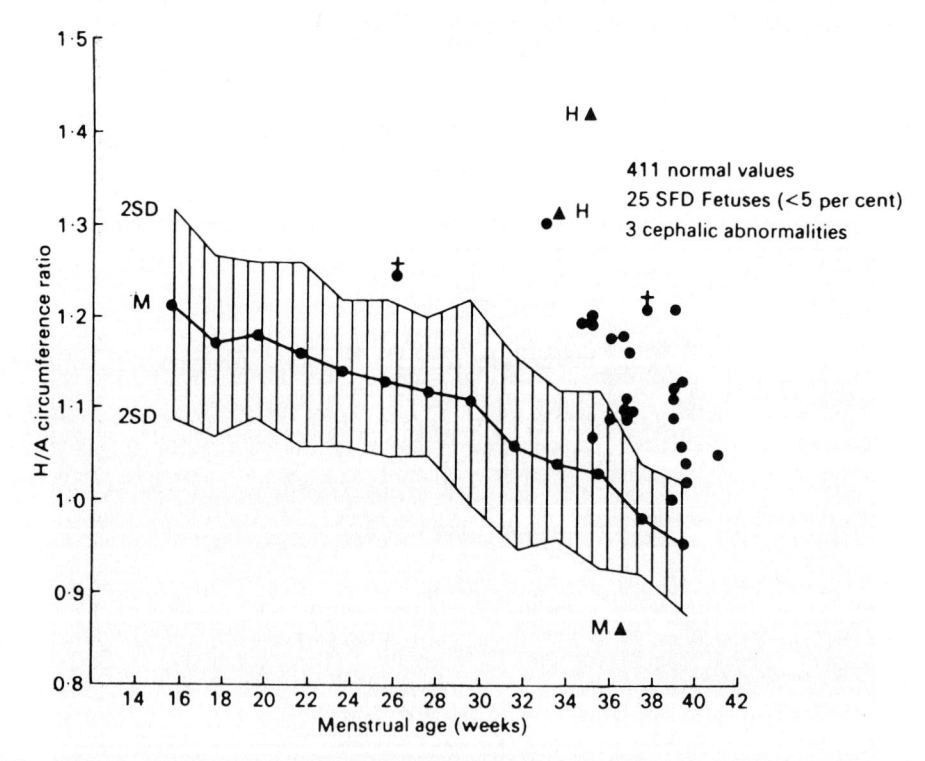

Fig. 7-20. Assessment of aberrant fetal growth by the head-abdomen circumference ratio. *H,* Hydrocephalus; *M,* microcephalus; +, fetal demise. (From Campbell, S. In Beard, R., and Nathanielsz, P., editors: Fetal physiology and medicine, Philadelphia, 1976, W.B. Saunders Co.)

growth-retarded fetus. More recently, combining these data and investigating the ratio between fetal head and abdominal circumference has added even greater accuracy to the determination of intrauterine growth retardation (Fig. 7-20).

Antenatal management

Once the diagnosis of intrauterine growth retardation is suspected and strengthened by ultrasonography, it is essential to institute appropriate maternal-fetal care and closely monitor the well-being of the fetus. Maternal activity should be limited and bed rest initiated with the mother assuming a left lateral recumbent position to ensure optimum uterine blood flow. Chronic illness should be strictly managed to prevent further deterioration of the fetal environment; nutritional intake should be optimal. Serial ultrasonography will help define the pattern of growth retardation and the degree of growth arrest. An integral part of ultrasonography is to search carefully for evidence of congenital malformations, since these anomalies are common among the early onset, low-profile group of SGA infants.

Assessment of fetal well-being should be instituted once the diagnosis is entertained and the fetus has approached a gestational age compatible with extrauterine survival. An inexpensive screening procedure is for the mother to record a log of fetal activity, since this is a reasonable sign of well-being. A specific time period should be monitored, such as after a meal, and fetal activity recorded each day. In addition to this maternal record, a systematic approach to fetal evaluation should be performed routinely and frequently. Classically, the oxytocin challenge test (OCT) has been used to predict the potential for fetal demise or an acute intrapartum death in a marginally oxygenated, compromised fetus. This test requires the intravenous administration of oxytocin, which must result in three uterine contractions within 10 minutes. If no late (type II) fetal heart rate decelerations occur with these three contractions, the OCT is read as negative (see Chapter 9). These late decelerations denote relative uteroplacental insufficiency and suggest that the oxygenation of the fetus may be impaired. A positive OCT (three late decelerations with three contractions) also suggests that, in addition to uteroplacental insufficiency, the fetus may be unable to tolerate the contractions that occur during labor. This is not a universal observation, since as many as 50% of these infants may be able to withstand spontaneous or oxytocin-induced labor, without the recurrence of late decelerations or the development of fetal acidosis (see further). Any decelerations less than that of a positive OCT should be considered suspicious and be repeated (along with technically unsatisfactory tracings) within the next 24 to 48 hours.

Because there are technical and time difficulties related to the OCT and because there are contraindications for its use, such as a previous classic cesarean section, placenta previa, and concern about inducing premature labor, non-stress testing (NST) has been employed. This test examines fetal well-being by determining the acceleration of the fetal heart rate following spontaneous fetal movement. A healthy fetus (nonhypoxic) will respond to its own body movements with a mean acceleration of 15 beats per minute above baseline heart rate. In addition, the frequency of fetal movements should be ascertained; at the same time, examination of beat-to-beat and long-term variability can offer additional useful information. The NST can also supplement the OCT, since fetuses with a positive OCT but a reactive NST and normal beat-to-beat variability are more likely to tolerate labor without untoward problems. Under stable maternal conditions and signs of fetal well-being (negative OCT and/or reactive NST) these tests may be repeated weekly.

An additional aid in assessing fetal well-being is the use of urinary or plasma estriol levels (p. 110). A single determination is not helpful, since estriol levels are usually depressed in intrauterine growth retardation; therefore serial determinations are more important. Low, but persistently rising, estriol levels are reassuring. A decline of greater than 35% over the mean of the prior 3 days is an ominous finding and is evidence of potential fetal distress. Plasma unconjugated estriol determinations have been replacing urinary estriol determinations because they obviate the inconveniences of the latter, which are also seriously affected by maternal renal function.

With continued careful fetal surveillance and a stable maternal-fetal environment a course of nonintervention is indicated. If the OCT turns positive and estriol levels decline, the fetus should be delivered regardless of the functional state of fetal lung maturity, since fetal viability may be in jeopardy. If the OCT is positive while estriol levels remain stable or rise, or if the OCT is negative but the estriol levels abruptly decline, an amniocentesis should be performed to determine fetal pulmonary maturity. If there is evidence of adequate maturation, delivery should be planned as soon as possible. If fetal maturation is not complete, repeated assessment of fetal well-being should be intensified to detect further deterioration of the fetus.

The mode of delivery is not necessarily dictated by the abnormalities recorded by biochemical or electrophysiologic surveillance of the fetus. Many patients can tolerate labor following a positive OCT, with oxygen administration and a left lateral recumbent position. However, it would be judicious to avoid labor in those situations complicated by a nonreactive NST, a flat baseline, and a positive OCT. Similarly, SGA premature infants, in particular those with a breech presentation, and those whose mothers have a completely unfavorable cervix should be delivered by the abdominal route. Particular attention should be given to the asymmetrically (late flattening) growth-retarded fetus, who tolerates labor poorly and readily develops signs of fetal distress, compared with both the symetrically undergrown and the normal fetus. Whether labor is induced or spontaneous, continuous intrapartum fetal heart rate monitoring combined with appropriate use of fetal scalp pH determinations must be employed (p. 115). If late decelerations become evident, scalp blood pH must be evaluated and, if fetal acidosis has developed, delivery should be expedited.

During labor, uterine contractions may further compromise marginal placental perfusion and fetal gas exchange. The myocardium of these fetuses may have diminished glycogen stores, a key energy source partially responsible for the fetal ability to withstand asphyxia. Because there is a high incidence of intrapartum birth asphyxia, it is essential that the delivery be coordinated with the neonatal team, who should be prepared to resuscitate a depressed or asphyxiated newborn. In addition, combined obstetric-pediatric management is indicated if meconium is present in the amniotic fluid. This event often follows periods of fetal hypoxia and stress, occurring with greatest frequency in the SGA term or postterm neonate. Obstetric management should include oropharyngeal suctioning immediately following delivery of the head. Immediately following the birth the neonatal team should further clear the oropharynx and then the trachea of additional meconium (see also Chapter 33, part four).

One problem that often comes up in managing these pregnancies is what to do when the fetus stops growing. Unfortunately, under stable maternal conditions and if the fetus demonstrates no other detectable signs of compromise, the best alternative is to leave the fetus in utero, ensure bed rest (preferably in-hospital), provide good nutrition, and continue fetal surveillance. The question of whether to deliver these fetuses should be tempered by the accuracy of the diagnosis and the ability to efficiently manage all potential neonatal problems, including appropriate alimentation.

APPROACH TO THE SGA INFANT

Following birth the SGA infant may develop significant neonatal problems (Table 7-5). In the delivery room it is essential to ensure optimum neonatal cardiopulmonary physiologic adaptation while ensuring minimal heat loss in a warm environment. Once stabilization has been established, a careful physical examination should be performed.

When infants with obvious anomalies and syndromes and those born to mothers with severe illness or malnutrition are excluded, there still remains a heterogenous population of SGA infants. These infants have a characteristic physical appearance; the heads look relatively large for their undergrown trunks and extremities, which seem wasted. The abdomen is scaphoid, misleading one to suspect a diaphragmatic hernia. The extremities have a paucity of subcutaneous tissue and fat, best exemplified by a reduced skinfold thickness (Fig. 7-16). In addition, the skin appears to hang, is rough, dry, and parchment-like, and desquamates quite easily. Fingernails may be long, and the hands and feet of these infants tend to look too large for the rest of the body. The facial appearance suggests to many observers the look of a "wise old person," especially in reference to that of premature infants (Fig. 7-21). Cranial sutures may be widened or overriding; the anterior fontanel is larger than expected, representing diminished membranous bone formation. Similarly, epiphyseal ossification at the knee (chondral bone) is also retarded. When meconium is passed in utero, there is often yellow-green staining of the nails, skin, and umbilical cord, which may also appear thinner than usual.

Gestational age assessment of the SGA infant may

Table 7-5. Perinatal adaptive problems

Problem	Pathogenesis	Prevention
Perinatal asphyxia	↓ Placental reserve (insufficiency)	Antepartum, intrapartum FHR monitoring
	↓ Cardiac glycogen stores	
Meconium aspiration	Hypoxic/stress phenomenon	Oral-pharyngeal-tracheal suction
Fasting hypoglycemia	↓ Hepatic glycogen	Early alimentation
	↓ Gluconeogenesis	
Alimented hyperglycemia	"Starvation diabetes"	Avoid excessive carbohydrate loads
Polycythemia-hyperviscosity	Fetal hypoxia, ↑ erythropoietin	Neonatal partial exchange transfusion
	Placental transfusion	
Temperature instability	↓ Adipose tissue	Ensure neutral thermal environment
	↑ Heat loss	
Pulmonary hemorrhage (rare)	Hypothermia/↓ O_2/DIC	Avoid cold stress/hypoxia
Immunodeficiency	"Malnutrition" effect	Unknown

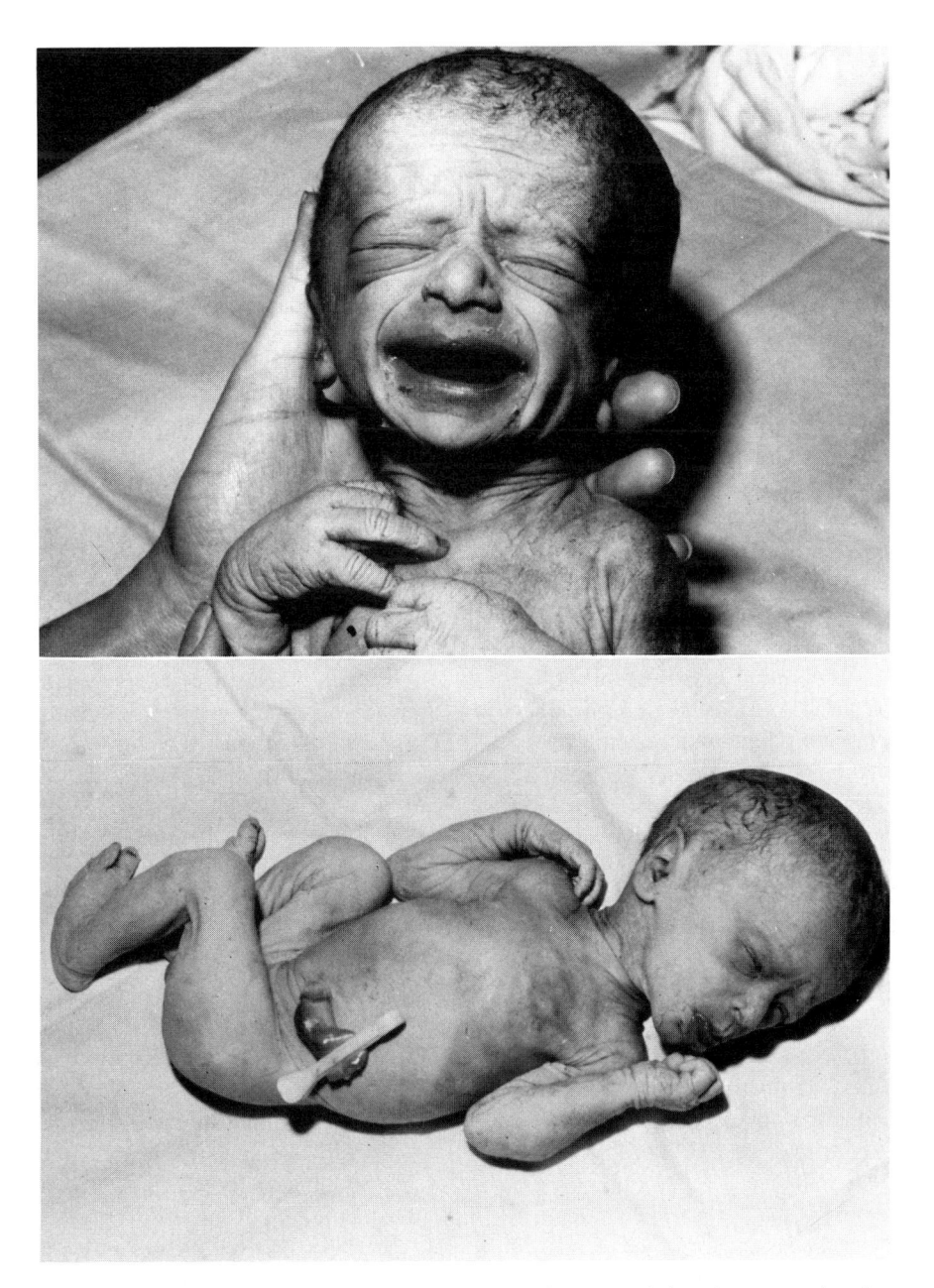

Fig. 7-21. Term SGA infant, demonstrating wizened facies and dry, desquamating, hanging skin. Birth weight, 1,500 gm.

result in misleading data when based on physical criteria alone. Vernix caseosa is frequently reduced or absent, resulting from diminished skin perfusion during periods of fetal distress or from depressed synthesis of estriol, which enhances vernix production. In the absence of this protective covering the skin is continuously exposed to amniotic fluid and will begin to desquamate following birth. Sole creases are determined, in part, by exposure to amniotic fluid and therefore will appear more mature. Breast tissue formation also depends on peripheral blood flow and estriol levels and will become markedly reduced in SGA infants. In addition, the female external genitalia will appear less mature, due to the absence of the perineal adipose tissue covering the labia. Ear cartilage, as noted in bone ossification, may also be diminished.

Neurologic examination for gestational age assessment is on safer grounds than that for the physical criteria. Intrauterine growth retarded infants functionally achieve appropriate for gestational age neurologic maturity despite a hostile in utero environment. Peripheral nerve conduction velocity and visual or auditory evoked responses correlate well with gestational age in normal neonates and are not impaired following intrauterine growth retardation. These aspects of neurologic maturity are not sensitive to deprivation, and occasionally maturity may even become accelerated (see further). Since intrauterine growth retardation does not grossly affect neurologic maturity, this assessment will be more appropriate in the determination of gestational age than will the physical score. Determinants of active or passive tone and posture should be reliable in SGA infants, assuming that those infants with significant central nervous system and metabolic disorders are excluded.

Specific organ maturity occurs despite diminished somatic growth. Cerebral cortical convolutions, renal glomeruli, and alveolar maturation all relate to gestational age and are not retarded with intrauterine growth retardation. As a result of stress in utero these infants may occasionally accelerate the maturity of specific organ systems, such as the lung, thus explaining the paucity of respiratory distress syndrome in SGA preterm neonates.

When examined in closer detail, SGA infants do demonstrate specific behavioral characteristics which suggest that, despite the presence of electrical neurologic maturity, functional central nervous system maturity may be impaired. In the absence of significant central nervous system disease these neonates demonstrate abnormal sleep cycles, diminished muscle tone, reflexes, activity, and excitability. This hypoexcitability suggests an adverse effect on polysynaptic reflex propagation and implies that central nervous system functional maturity does not necessarily proceed independently of the intrauterine events which result in intrauterine growth retardation.

Once stabilized and assigned a gestational age, the SGA neonate should be examined in more detail to direct the diagnostic work in a rational manner, as detailed in the following outline.

A. History and physical examination
B. Accurate growth parameters
C. Findings
    1. Dysmorphic features
        a. Chromosomes
        b. Syndrome
        c. Drugs
    2. Blueberry-muffin rash, petechiae, hepatosplenomegaly, ocular pathology
        a. Rubella
        b. CMV
        c. Other
    3. Neither
        a. Constitutional
        b. Genetic
        c. Nutritional
        d. Toxins
        e. Placenta-twins
        f. Unknown

Dysmorphic features, "funny looking faces," abnormal hands, feet, and palmar creases, in addition to gross anomalies, suggest congenital malformation syndromes, chromosomal defects, or teratogens. Ocular disorders such as chorioretinitis, cataracts, glaucoma, cloudy cornea, in addition to hepatosplenomegaly, jaundice, and a blueberry-muffin rash, should suggest a congenital infection (p. 698). The remaining infants constitute a heterogenous group that represents the majority of SGA neonates. Multiple gestations are the most recognizable etiology in this category. TORCH infections resulting in SGA infants are unusual in the absence of other clinical signs of congenital infection; however, a screening determination on cord blood for IgM values may be indicated. Radiographic examination of long bones and skull (or ultrasonography of the head) may be diagnostically useful. Careful data related to the present and past reproductive history of the mother, in addition to ongoing neonatal management and close observation, are indicated in the remaining large number of SGA neonates whose underlying diagnoses may never be determined.

NEONATAL PROBLEMS (Table 7-5)
Asphyxia

Perinatal asphyxia and its sequelae constitute the most significant problem of SGA infants. As discussed, uterine contractions may add an additional hypoxic stress on the marginally functioning placenta. The ensuing fetal hypoxia, acidosis, and cerebral depression may result in fetal demise or neonatal asphyxia. With repeated episodes of fetal asphyxia or persistent hypoxemia, myocardial glycogen reserves are depleted, further limiting the fetal cardiopulmonary adaptation to hypoxia. If inadequate resuscitation occurs at birth and Apgar scores are low, both intrapartum and neonatal asphyxia place the infant in double jeopardy for a continuum of central nervous system insult. The sequelae of perinatal asphyxia include multiple organ system dysfunction potentially characterized by ischemic-hypoxic encephalopathy, ischemic congestive heart failure, persistent fetal circulation, gastrointestinal perforation, and acute tubular necrosis. Concomitant with these sequelae there may be metabolic derangements such as hypoglycemia (see further). Hypocalcemia is due in part to excessive phosphate release from damaged cells, acidosis, and its correction with sodium bicarbonate and diminished calcium intake. Meconium aspiration syndrome, if managed inappropriately in the delivery room, may complicate the clinical picture and further embarrass respiratory function and oxygenation with the development of pneumonitis and pneumothorax.

Neonatal metabolism

Fasting hypoglycemia develops in SGA infants more than any other neonatal subgroup or category. The propensity for hypoglycemia is greatest during the first 3 days of life; however, some of these infants develop ketotic hypoglycemia months later. Key to the occurrence of hypoglycemia is the diminished hepatic glycogen stores (Fig. 7-22). Glycogenolysis constitutes the predominant source of glucose for the neonate during the immediate hours after birth. Later in the day, when glycogen stores become depleted, fasting glucose production results from the incorporation of lactate and gluconeogenic amino acid precursors into glucose. SGA infants demonstrate an inability to increase blood glucose concentration following oral or intravenous administration of the key gluconeogenic amino acid, alanine. Hypoglycemic SGA infants have elevated alanine and lactate levels, suggesting that substrate availability is not rate limiting for gluconeogenesis. Nonhypoglycemic SGA infants do demonstrate equivalent rates of gluconeogenesis from alanine compared with nonhypoglycemic AGA neonates.

Immediately following birth, fasting SGA infants may develop lower plasma free fatty acid levels than normally growing infants. In addition, once fed, SGA infants have a deficient utilization of intravenous triglycerides. Following the intravenous administration of triglyceride emulsion, SGA infants develop high free fatty acid and triglyceride levels, but ketone body formation is attenuated. This suggests that the utilization and oxidation of free fatty acids and triglycerides are diminished in SGA neonates. Free fatty acid oxidation is important because it spares peripheral tissue use of glucose while the hepatic oxidation of free fatty acids may contribute the reducing equivalents and energy required for hepatic gluconeogenesis. Deficient provision and/or oxidation of fatty acids may, in part, be responsible for the development of

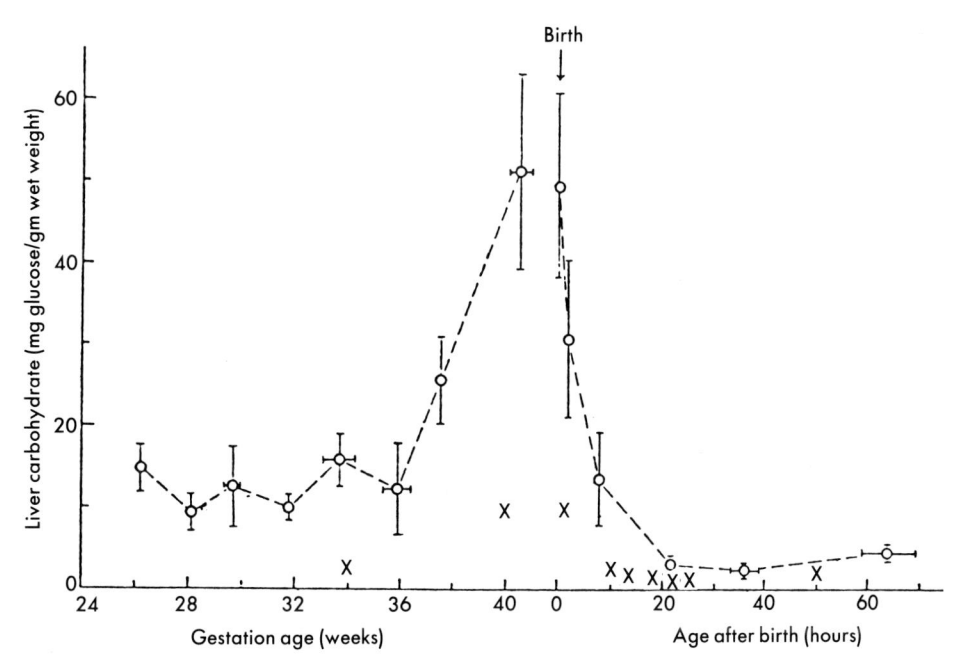

Fig. 7-22. Fetal and neonatal hepatic glycogen content *(X)* in IUGR patients. (From Shelly, H., and Neligan, G.: Br. Med. Bull. **22:**34, 1966.)

fasting hypoglycemia in these infants (Fig. 7-23).

Endocrine alterations have also been implicated in the pathogenesis of hypoglycemia in SGA infants. Catecholamine release is deficient in these neonates during periods of hypoglycemia. Although basal glucagon levels may be elevated, exogenous administration of glucagon fails to enhance glycemia. These data suggest an abnormality of counterregulatory hormonal mechanisms during periods of neonatal hypoglycemia in SGA infants.

With improved standards of care and attempts at early feeding or intravenous alimentation, fasting hypoglycemia in the SGA neonate is a rare event. Prior to the onset of alimentation, careful monitoring with Dextrostix for determination of blood glucose values will detect infants with asymptomatic hypoglycemia. If whole blood glucose concentrations decline to less than 30 mg/dl during the first 3 days in term infants or 20 mg/dl in preterm infants and no untoward symptoms have occurred, glucose infusion initially at 4 to 8 mg/kg/minute should be commenced. Following this initial rate the infusion should be titrated until blood glucose values achieve normal levels. If the hypoglycemia is symptomatic, particularly when seizure activity intervenes, an intravenous minibolus of D10W at 200 mg/kg should be given, followed by an infusion as just described. Infants at greatest risk for the development of hypoglycemia are those who have been asphyxiated and those who appear most undergrown according to the ponderal index (Fig. 7-24). Similarly, breast-fed twins who are not supplemented with a carbohydrate source are at risk, particularly the smaller co-twin, and should be monitored carefully.

Temperature regulation

Following the birth of an infant complicated by uteroplacental insufficiency, the neonate's initial body temperature may actually be elevated. When placental function fails, its heat-eliminating capacity also becomes deficient, resulting in fetal hyperthermia. On exposure to the cold environment of the delivery room, SGA infants can increase their heat production (oxygen consumption) appropriately, since brown adipose tissue stores are not necessarily depleted during intrauterine growth retardation. However, their core temperature drops if the cold stress continues, implying that heat loss has exceeded heat production. Heat loss in these infants is due in part to the large body surface area exposed to cold and the deficiency of an insulating layer of subcutaneous adipose tissue stores. The SGA infant therefore has a narrower neutral thermal environment than full-term infants but a broader one than that in premature neonates. In SGA infants hypoglycemia and/or hypoxia interferes with heat production and may contribute to the thermal instability of these infants. In all infants, particularly the SGA infant, a neutral thermal environment should be sought

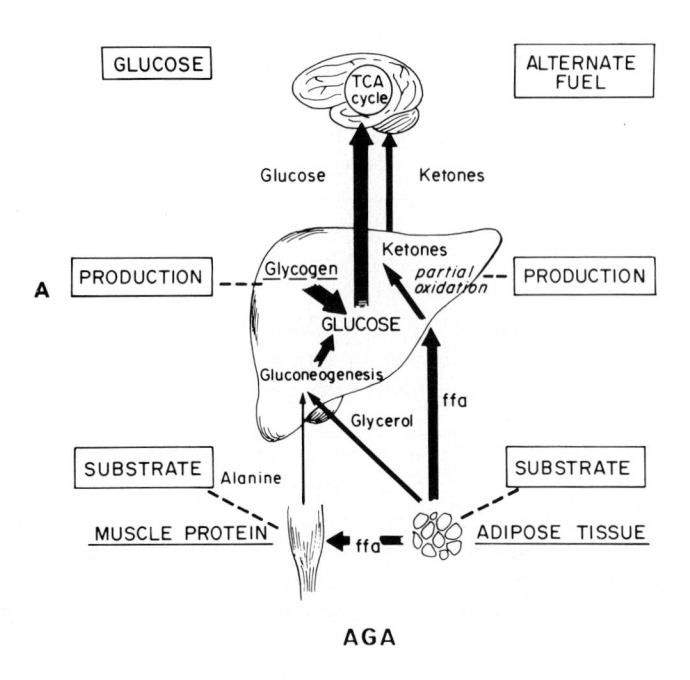

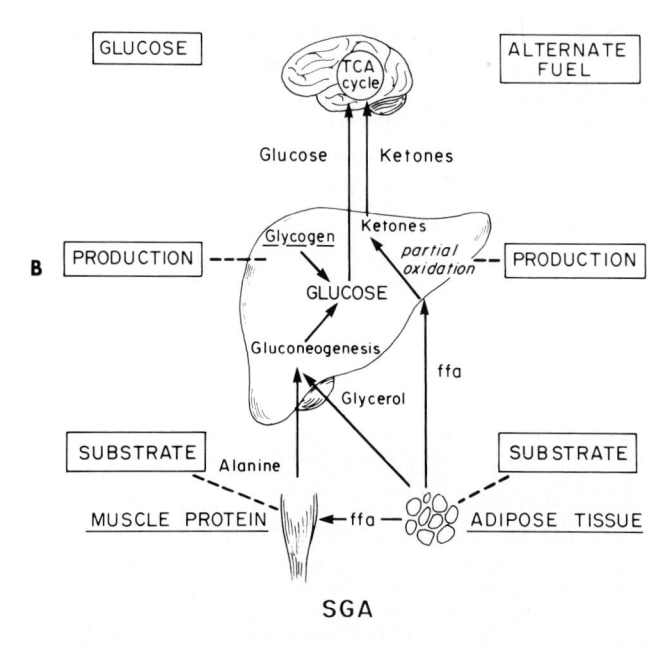

Fig. 7-23. Postnatal glucose and fatty acid metabolic relationships in AGA **(A)** and SGA **(B)** neonates. Arrows depict magnitude of flux. SGA infants demonstrate both diminished glycogen stores and gluconeogenesis. In addition, they may have attenuated fatty acid oxidation. (Modified from Adam, P.A.J.: Metabolism in pregnant woman and fetus. In Falkner, F., and Tanner, J.: Human growth, vol. 1, New York, 1978, Plenum Press.)

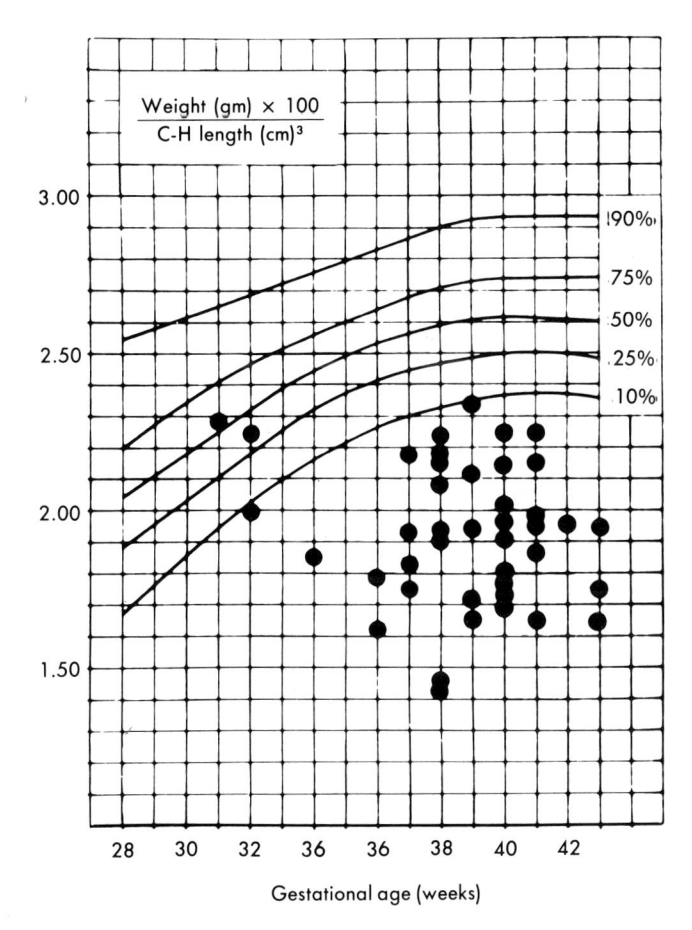

Fig. 7-24. Relationship between ponderal index and neonatal hypoglycemia in IUGR. ●, Hypoglycemic infants. (From Jarai, I., and others: Early Hum. Dev. **1:**25, 1977.)

to prevent excessive heat loss and to promote appropriate postnatal weight gain.

When nursed in a neutral thermal environment, SGA infants demonstrate the usual decline of the respiratory quotient following birth, representing a shift toward free fatty acid oxidation. During the first 12 hours after birth, basal oxygen consumption may be diminished in SGA neonates. Similar observations have been recorded in utero among spontaneously SGA fetal lambs, suggesting in both situations that there is a deficiency of potentially oxidizable substrates. Supporting this hypothesis is the marked increment of oxygen consumption that occurs in well-alimented SGA infants. This latter observation is also analogous to the rise of energy production following the nutritional rehabilitation of infants with marasmus-kwashiorkor. The increment of oxygen consumption following fetal or infantile malnutrition represents the energy cost of growth. SGA infants have a significantly smaller postnatal weight loss because they are maturationally capable of achieving an adequate caloric intake earlier than premature neonates. Due to this enhanced caloric intake, SGA infants have a higher oxygen consumption than less mature neonates. There is, however, a group of SGA neonates who do not demonstrate an elevation of oxygen consumption following appropriate caloric intake. These infants have had low-profile intrauterine growth and may be considered examples of "primordial fetal growth retardation." Their growth is set and fixed at a slower rate while their eventual growth potential is reduced. The diminished body cell number in congenitally infected infants and those with chromosomal disorders exemplifies these primordial growth-retarded neonates.

Hyperviscosity-polycythemia syndrome

The plasma volume of SGA infants immediately following birth averages 52 ml/kg, as opposed to 43 ml/kg in appropriately grown infants. Once equilibrated at 12 hours of life, the plasma volume becomes equivalent in the two groups. In addition to an enhanced plasma space, the circulating red blood cell mass is expanded. Fetal hypoxia and subsequent erythropoietin synthesis may induce excessive red blood cell production. Alternately, a placental-fetal transfusion during labor or periods of fetal asphyxia may result in a shift of placental blood to the fetus. Be that as it may, the elevation of the hematocrit potentially increases blood viscosity, which interferes with vital tissue perfusion. The altered viscosity adversely affects neonatal hemodynamics and results in an abnormal cardiopulmonary and metabolic postnatal adaptation, producing hypoxia and hypoglycemia. In the event polycythemia is present (central hematocrit > 65%) with such symptoms, appropriate therapy should be directed at correcting hypoxia and hypoglycemia while a partial exchange transfusion to reduce blood viscosity and improve tissue perfusion should be considered (Chapter 29).

Other problems

Recent evidence has demonstrated that the immunologic function of SGA infants may be depressed as it is in older infants with the postnatal onset of malnutrition. Neonates with congenital rubella syndrome have functional deficiencies of both T and B lymphocytes. This may, however, be related to continued intracellular viral infection. Other SGA infants may also manifest varying degrees of immunologic dysfunction that persists into childhood. Deficiencies have been demonstrated in lymphocyte number and function, which include decreased spontaneous mitogenesis and reduced response to phytohemagglutinin. Similarly, these infants tend to develop lower immunoglobulin levels during infancy and demonstrate an attenuated antibody response to oral polio vaccine.

Additional problems and their management are noted in Table 7-5.

FOLLOW-UP

Excluding the severely affected SGA infants with serious congenital malformations and viral infections, the remaining neonates should benefit from optimum antenatal detection, exquisite management of pregnancy, and avoidance of hypoxic fetal distress. In addition, with ideal neonatal intensive care the morbidity and mortality of SGA infants should be reduced to a minimum, and postnatal developmental handicaps should be diminished. Unfortunately, in the best medical centers only 50% of these infants are recognized before delivery. These latter infants will continue to contribute to the excessive fetal and neonatal morbidity and mortality associated with intrauterine growth retardation. Neonatal mortality is greater than that of full-term but less than that in premature neonates, whereas the incidence of fetal demise remains higher than in both other groups. Besides the etiologic events that lead to the development of intrauterine growth retardation, these infants have additional multisystem problems that further compromise survival and future growth or development. Among these fetuses the perinatal mortality is 10 times that of appropriately grown infants. Intrauterine fetal demise is greatest among the most severely undergrown infants. Both antepartum and intrapartum events contribute to fetal mortality. Lethal congenital malformations and birth asphyxia are the two leading causes of death among SGA neonates.

Developmental outcome

When infants with congenital infections and severe malformations are excluded, there remains a heterogenous group of undergrown neonates. Intellectual and neurologic function in these remaining infants depends on the presence or absence of adverse perinatal events, in addition to the specific etiology resulting in intrauterine growth retardation. Cerebral morbidity will be adversely affected by the hypoxic-ischemic encephalopathy subsequent to birth asphyxia and the postnatal problems of hypoxia and hypoglycemia. Therefore the prognosis must consider all the adverse perinatal circumstances in addition to intrauterine growth retardation. When these perinatal problems are minimal or are avoided, the SGA neonate may still demonstrate cerebral developmental handicaps, especially in the presence of relative head growth retardation (microcephaly). If term, appropriately grown neonates are used as a standard, term SGA infants demonstrate developmental problems when they are examined at follow-up at 2 years, 5 years, and older. Even when compared with premature neonates, term SGA infants continue to have developmental disadvantages. Follow-up of these term SGA infants reveals little differences in intelligence quotient or neurologic sequelae; however, their school performance is poor, partly because of behavioral and learning disorders. SGA infants contributed a disproportionately high incidence to those Swedish children with psy-

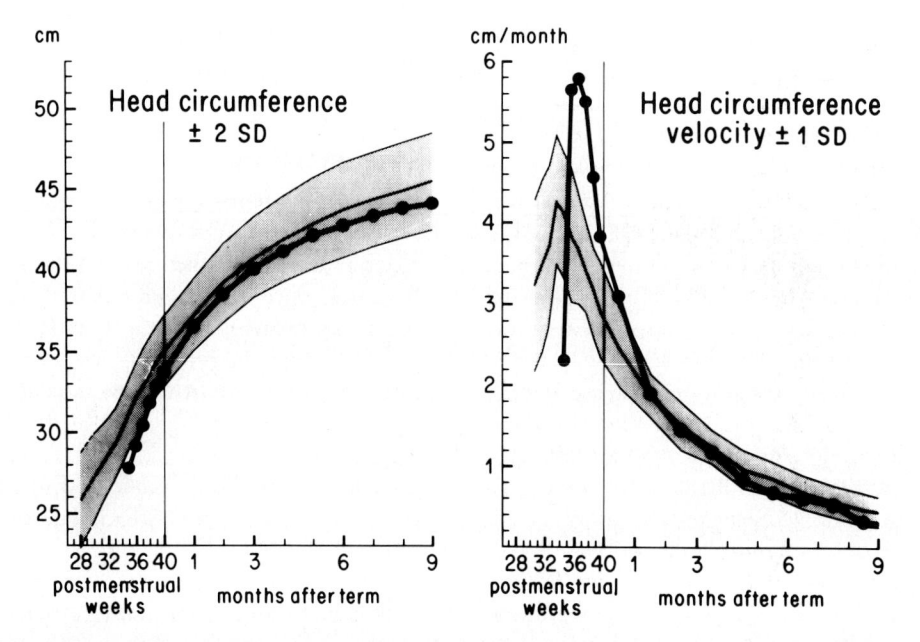

Fig. 7-25. Postnatal catch-up growth following IUGR. (From Brandt, I.: Growth dynamics of low birth weight infants with emphasis on the perinatal period. In Falkner, F., and Tanner, J., editors: Human growth, vol. 2, Postnatal growth, New York, 1978, Plenum Press.)

chomotor retardation and cerebral palsy in the early 1970s. Preterm SGA infants may have an even greater percentage of abnormal neurodevelopmental outcome than term SGA neonates. Those early onset SGA infants demonstrating decreased BPD growth before 26 weeks' gestation have diminished developmental quotients in infancy. However, some follow-up observations on both term and preterm SGA neonates are very favorable, as these neonates compared well to their appropriately grown counterparts. SGA infants are a heterogenous group, and the different populations investigated may vary in the severity of neurodevelopmental handicap; similarly, antenatal detection and perinatal management vary among high-risk centers. It would therefore appear that these latter favorable reports may represent the outcome following optimum obstetric management and neonatal care.

Another major determining influence on neonatal neurodevelopmental outcome in SGA infants is the family's socioeconomic status. Parent educational background, place of rearing, and environmental conditions all have a strong effect on outcome. SGA infants born to families of higher socioeconomic status demonstrated little developmental differences on follow-up, whereas those born to poorer families have significant developmental handicaps. The same environmental influences have related to the developmental outcome following severe malnutrition in infancy, suggesting that adequate environmental stimulation is essential for the ideal outcome of SGA infants.

Growth

Postnatal growth following intrauterine growth retardation depends in part on the cause of the growth retardation, the postnatal nutritional intake, and the social environment. Although birth weight correlates best to

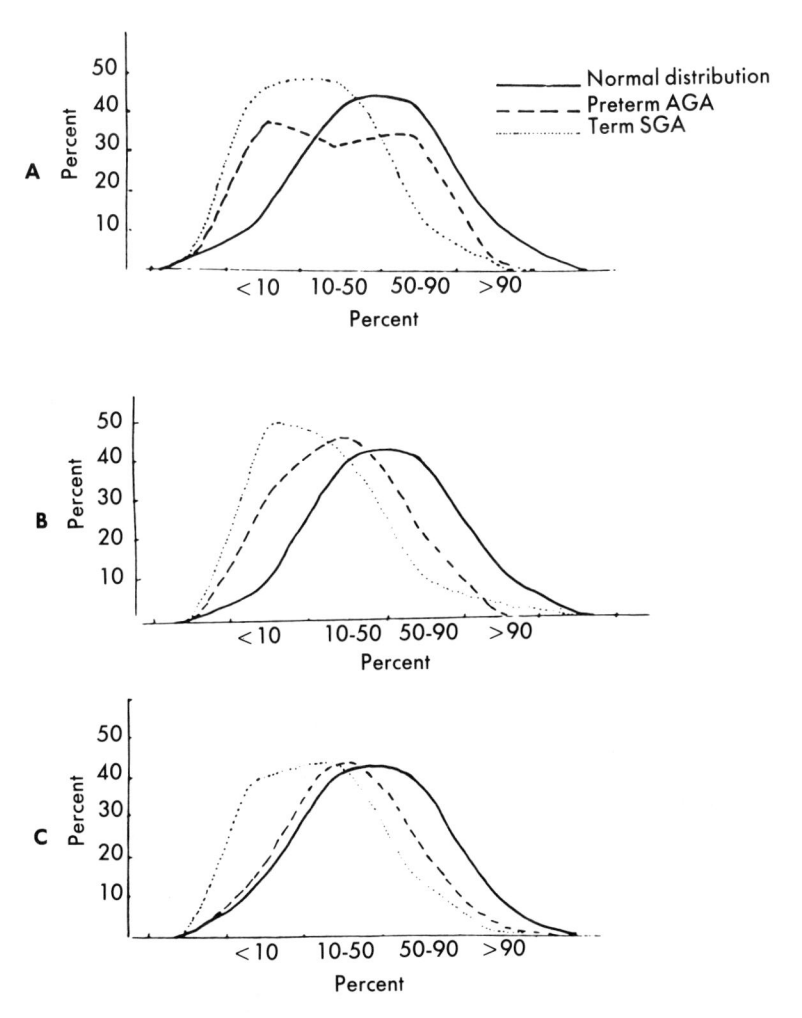

Fig. 7-26. Eventual physical growth of SGA term, AGA premature, and term neonates at 4 years of age. **A,** Height; **B,** weight; **C,** head circumference. (From Lubchenco, L.: The high-risk infant, Philadelphia, 1976, W.B. Saunders Co.)

maternal weight, postnatal growth is related to both maternal and paternal growth characteristics. SGA neonates who have primordial growth retardation related to congenital viral, chromosomal, or constitutional syndromes will remain small throughout life. Those infants whose intrauterine growth was inhibited late in gestation due to uterine constraint, placental insufficiency, or nutritional deficits will have catch-up growth after birth and approach their inherited growth potential when provided with an optimum environment. These latter infants have an accelerated growth phase once adequate postnatal caloric intake has been established, suggesting release of an in utero constraining factor following birth (Fig. 7-25). This postpartum acceleration of growth must occur within the first 6 months of life, placing the infant on a new percentile growth tract (Fig. 7-25). Despite the catch-up period, many of these infants remain significantly smaller than appropriately grown neonates (Fig. 7-26), especially those who had the onset of growth retardation before 34 weeks.

The goal of future management plans for the improvement of the growth and developmental outcome of SGA neonates must have its origins close to the onset of intrauterine growth retardation. Once growth retardation has developed, early identification and careful avoidance of undue hypoxic stress and nutritional deficits should enhance the survival and quality of these high-risk neonates.

Robert M. Kliegman
Katherine C. King

BIBLIOGRAPHY
General

Cheek, D.: Fetal and postnatal cellular growth, New York, 1975, John Wiley & Sons, Inc.

Ciba Foundation Symposium 27: Size at birth, Amsterdam, 1974, Elsevier.

Creasy, R., and Resnick, R.: Intrauterine fetal growth retardation. In Milunsky, A., Friedman, E., and Gluck, L., editors: Advances in perinatal medicine, vol. 1, New York, 1981, Plenum Press.

Falkner, F., and Tanner, J.: Human Growth, vols. 1 and 2, New York, 1978, Plenum Press.

Miller, H., and Merritt, T.: Fetal growth in humans, Chicago, 1979, Year Book Medical Publishers, Inc.

Roberts, D., and Thomson, A.: The biology of human fetal growth, New York, 1976, Taylor & Francis, Ltd.

Usher, R., and McLean, F.: Normal fetal growth and the significance of fetal growth retardation. In Davis, J., and Dobbin, J., editors: Scientific foundations of pediatrics, Philadelphia, 1974, W.B. Saunders Co.

Fetal growth

Brenner, W., Edelman, D., and Hendricks, C.: A standard of fetal growth for the United States of America, Am. J. Obstet. Gynecol. **126**:555, 1976.

Lubchenco, L., and others: Intrauterine growth as estimated from liveborn birth weight data at 24 to 42 weeks of gestation, Pediatrics **32**:793, 1963.

Naeye, R., and Dixon, J.: Distortions in fetal growth standards, Pediatr. Res. **12**:987, 1978.

Robinson, J.: Growth of the fetus, Br. Med. Bull. **35**:137, 1979.

Vorherr, H.: Factors influencing fetal growth, Am. J. Obstet. Gynecol. **142**:577, 1982.

Ziegler, E., and others: Body composition of the reference fetus, Growth **40**:329, 1976.

Fetal metabolism

Adam, P.A.J., and Felig, P.: Carbohydrate, fat, and amino acid metabolism in the pregnant woman and fetus. In Falkner, F., and Tanner, J., editors: Human growth, vol. 1, New York, 1978, Plenum Press.

Battaglia, F., and Meschia, G.: Principal substrates of fetal metabolism, Physiol. Rev. **58**:499, 1978.

Brooke, O., Alvear, J., and Arnold, M.: Energy retention, energy expenditure, and growth in healthy immature infants, Pediatr. Res. **13**:215, 1979.

Milley, J., and Simmons, M.: Metabolic requirements for fetal growth, Clin. Perinatol. **6**:365, 1979.

Fetal endocrinology

Brinsmead, M., and Liggins, G.: Somatomedins and other growth factors in fetal growth. In Scarpelli, E., and Cosmi, E., editors: Reviews in perinatal medicine, vol. 3, New York, 1979, Raven Press.

Hill, D.: Insulin and fetal growth. In Diabetes and other endocrine disorders during pregnancy and in the newborn, New York, 1976, Alan R. Liss, Inc.

Liggins, G.: The drive to fetal growth. In Beard, R., and Nathanielsz, P., editors: Fetal physiology and medicine, Philadelphia, 1976, W.B. Saunders Co.

Maternal factors

Bakketerg, L., Hoffman, H., and Harley, E.: The tendency to repeat gestational age and birth weight in successive births, Am. J. Obstet. Gynecol. **135**:1086, 1979.

Johnstone, F., and Inglis, L.: Familial trends in low birth weight, Br. Med. J. **3**:659, 1974.

Ounsted, M., and Ounsted, C.: Maternal regulation of intra-uterine growth, Nature **220**:995, 1966.

Ounsted, M., and Ounsted, C.: Rate of intrauterine growth, Nature **220**:559, 1966.

Nutrition

Hytten, F.: Nutrition in pregnancy, Postgrad. Med. J. **55**:295, 1979.

Metcoff, J.: Asociation of fetal growth with maternal nutrition. In Falkner, F., and Tanner, J., editors: Human growth, vol. 1, New York, 1978, Plenum Press.

Miller, H., and Hassanein, K.: Fetal malnutrition in white newborn infants: maternal factors, Pediatrics **52**:504, 1973.

Naeye, R., Blanc, W., and Paul, C.: Effects of maternal nutrition on the human fetus, Pediatrics **52**:494, 1973.

Niswander, K., and others: Weight gain during pregnancy and prepregnancy weight, Obstet. Gynecol. **33**:482, 1969.

Philipps, C., and Johnson, N.: The impact of quality of diet and other factors on birth weight of infants, Am. J. Clin. Nutr. **30**:215, 1977.

Stein, Z., Susser, M., and Rush, D.: Prenatal nutrition and birth weight: experiments and quasi-experiments in the past decade, J. Reprod. Med. **21**:287, 1978.

Maternal disease and socioeconomic status

Clarren, S., and Smith, D.: The fetal alcohol syndrome, N. Engl. J. Med. **298**:1063, 1978.

Gruenwald, P., and others: Influence of environmental factors on fetal growth in man, Lancet **1**:1026, 1967.

Lichty, J., and others: Studies of babies born at high altitude, Am. J. Dis. Child. 93:666, 1957.
Long, P., Abell, D., and Beischer, N.: Fetal growth retardation and pre-eclampsia, Br. J. Obstet. Gynecol. 87:13, 1980.
Meyer, M.: How does maternal smoking affect birth weight and maternal weight gain? Am. J. Obstet. Gynecol. 131:888, 1978.
Miller, H., Nassanein, K., and Hensleigh, P.: Effects of behavioral and medical variables on fetal growth retardation, Am. J. Obstet. Gynecol. 127:643, 1977.
Miller, H., Hassanein, K., and Hensleigh, P.: Maternal factors in the incidence of low birth weight infants among black and white mothers, Pediatr. Res. 12:1016, 1978.
Naeye, R., and others: Fetal complications of maternal heroin addiction: abnormal growth, infections and episodes of stress, J. Pediatr. 83:1055, 1973.
Rantakallio, P.: The effect of maternal smoking on birth weight and the subsequent health of the child, Early Hum. Devel. 2:371, 1978.
Raye, J., Dubin, J., and Blechner, J.: Fetal growth retardation following maternal morphine administration: nutritional or drug effect? Biol. Neonate 32:222, 1977.
Redmond, G.: Effect of drugs on intrauterine growth, Clin. Perinatol. 6:5, 1979.
Resnik, R.: Maternal disease associated with abnormal fetal growth, J. Reprod. Med. 21:315, 1978.
Zuspan, F.: Treatment of severe preeclampsia and eclampsia, Clin. Obstet. Gynecol. 9:954, 1966.
Zuspan, F.: Problems encountered in the treatment of pregnancy-induced hypertension, Am. J. Obstet. Gynecol. 131:591, 1978.

Placental factors

Aherne, W., and Dunnill, M.: Quantitative aspects of placental structure, J. Pathol. Bacteriol. 91:123, 1966.
Altshuler, G., Russell, P., and Ermocilla, R.: The placental pathology of small for gestational age infants, Am. J. Obstet. Gynecol. 121:351, 1975.
Molteni, R., Stys, S., and Battaglia, F.: Relationship of fetal and placental weight in human beings: fetal/placental weight ratios at various gestational ages and birth weight distributions, J. Reprod. Med. 21:327, 1978.
Rosso, P., and others: Effects of maternal undernutrition on placental metabolism and function. In Young, D., and Hicks, J., editors: The neonate, New York, 1976, John Wiley & Sons, Inc.
Saintonge, J., and Rosso, P.: Placental blood flow and transfer of nutrient analogs in large, average, and small guinea pig littermates, Pediatr. Res. 15:152, 1981.
Stuart, M., and others: Decreased prostacyclin production: a characteristic of chronic placental insufficiency syndromes, Lancet 1:1126, 1981.

Fetal factors

Jones, O.: Genetic factors in the determination of fetal size, J. Reprod. Med. 21:305, 1978.
Knox, G.: Influence of infection on fetal growth and development, J. Reprod. Med. 21:352, 1978.
Ounsted, C., and Ounsted, M.: Effect of Y chromosome on fetal growth rate, Lancet 2:857, 1970.
Reisman, L.: Chromosome abnormalities and intrauterine growth retardation, Pediatr. Clin. North Am. 17:101, 1970.
Smith, D.: Recognizable patterns of human malformation, ed. 3, Philadelphia, 1982, W.B. Saunders Co.

Antenatal diagnosis

Belezan, J., and others: Diagnosis of intrauterine growth retardation by a simple clinical method: measurement of uterine height. Am. J. Obstet. Gynecol. 131:643, 1978.

Campbell, S.: Fetal growth. In Beard R., and Nathanielsz, P., editors: Fetal physiology and medicine, Philadelphia, 1976, W.B. Saunders Co.
Crane, J., and others: Abnormal fetal growth patterns, Obstet. Gynecol. 54:597, 1979.
Darkoku, N., and others: The relative significance of human placental lactogen in the diagnosis of retarded fetal growth, Am. J. Obstet. Gynecol. 135:516, 1979.
Galbraith, R., and others: The clinical prediction of intrauterine growth retardation, Am. J. Obstet. Gynecol. 133:281, 1979.
Ghari, P., Berkowitz, R., and Hobbins, J.: Prediction of intrauterine growth retardation by determination of fetal intrauterine volume, Am. J. Obstet. Gynecol. 127:255, 1977.
Low, J., and Galbraith, R.: Pregnancy characteristics of intrauterine growth retardation, Obstet. Gynecol. 44:122, 1974.
Persson, P., and others: Fetal biparietal diameter and maternal plasma concentrations of placental lactogen, chorionic gonadotrophin, estriol, and alpha-fetoprotein in normal and pathological pregnancies, Br. J. Obstet. Gynecol. 87:25, 1980.
Wladimiroff, J., Bkoemsma, C., and Wallenburg, H.: Ultrasonic assessment of fetal head and body sizes in relation to normal and retarded fetal growth, Am. J. Obstet. Gynecol. 131:857, 1978.

Antenatal management

Bashore, R., and Westlake, T.: Plasma unconjugated estriol values in high risk pregnancy, Am. J. Obstet. Gynecol. 128:371, 1977.
Boegelsmann, U.: The uses of estriol as a monitoring tool, Clin. Obstet. Gynecol. 6:223, 1979.
Evertson, L., and others: Antepartum fetal heart rate testing, Am. J. Obstet. Gynecol. 133:29, 1979.
Huddleston, J., and others: Oxytocin challenge test for antepartum fetal assessment, Am. J. Obstet. Gynecol. 135:609, 1979.
Lin, C., and others: Oxytocin challenge test and intrauterine growth retardation, Am. J. Obstet. Gynecol. 140:282, 1981.
Long, P., Abell, D., and Beischer, N.: Fetal growth and placental function assessed by urinary estriol excretion before the onset of pre-eclampsia, Am. J. Obstet. Gynecol. 135:344, 1979.
Luther, E., and others: The effect of maternal glucose infusion on breathing movements in human fetuses with intrauterine growth retardation, Am. J. Obstet. Gynecol. 142:600, 1982.
Rosen, M., and others: Monitoring fetal movement, Clin. Obstet. Gynecol. 6:325, 1979.
Spellacy, W., and others: Oxytocin challenge test results compared with simultaneously studied serum human lactogen and free estriol levels in high risk pregnant women, Am. J. Obstet. Gynecol. 135:917, 1979.

The SGA infant

Bhatia, V., Katiyar, G., and Agarwal, K.P.: Effect of intrauterine nutritional deprivation on the neuromotor behaviour of the newborn, Acta Pediatr. Scand. 68:561, 1979.
Bhatia, V., and others: Sleep cycle studies in babies of undernourished mothers, Arch. Dis. Child. 55:134, 1980.
Gruenwald, P.: Chronic fetal distress and placental insufficiency, Biol. Neonatol. 5:215, 1963.
Jones, M., and Battaglia, F.: Intrauterine growth retardation, Am. J. Obstet. Gynecol. 127:540, 1977.
Naeye, R., and Kelly, J.: Judgement of fetal age, Pediatr. Clin. North Am. 13:849, 1966.
Schulte, F., Hinz, G., and Schrempf, G.: Maternal toxemia, fetal malnutrition and bioelectric brain activity of the newborn, Neuropediatr. 2:439, 1971.
Schulte, F., Schrempf, G., and Hinze, G.: Maternal toxemia, fetal malnutrition, and motor behaviours of the newborn, Pediatrics. 48:871, 1971.

Turner, G.: Recognition of intrauterine growth retardation by considering comparative birth weights, Lancet **2**:1123, 1971.

Usher, R.: Clinical and therapeutic aspects of fetal malnutrition, Pediatr. Clin. North Am. **17**:169, 1970.

Metabolism

Andrew, G., Chan, G., and Schiff, D.: Lipid metabolism in the neonate, J. Pediatr. **92**:995, 1978.

Frazer, T., and others: Direct measurement of gluconeogenesis from [2, 3^{13}C$_2$] alanine in the human neonate, Am. J. Phys. E., vol. 615, 1981.

Harris, R.: Plasma nonesterified fatty acid and blood glucose levels in healthy and hypoxemic infants, J. Pediatr. **84**:578, 1974.

Haymond, M., Karl, I., and Pagliara, A.: Increased gluconeogenic substrates in the small for gestational age infant, N. Engl. J. Med. **291**:322, 1974.

Jarai, I., and others: Body size and neonatal hypoglycemia in intrauterine growth retardation, Early Hum. Devel. **1**:25, 1977.

LeDune, M.: Response to glucagon in small for dates hypoglycemic and nonhypoglycemic newborn infants, Arch. Dis. Child. **47**:754, 1972.

Mestyan, J., Schultz, K., and Horvath, M.: Comparative glycemic responses to alanine in normal term and small for gestational age infants, J. Pediatr. **85**:286, 1974.

Sable, K.: Metabolic adaptation in small for gestational age newborn infants, Göteburg, Sweden, 1978, University of Göteburg.

Shelly, H., and Neligan, G.: Neonatal hypoglycemia, Br. Med. Bull. **22**:34, 1966.

Stern, L., Sourkes, T., and Raiha, N.: The role of the adrenal medulla in the hypoglycemia of fetal malnutrition, Biol. Neonatal. **11**:129, 1967.

Williams, P., and others: Effect of oral alanine on blood glucose, plasma glucagon, and insulin concentration in small for gestational age infants, N. Engl. J. Med. **292**:612, 1975.

Other neonatal problems

Bard, H.: Neonatal problems of infants with intrauterine growth retardation, J. Reprod. Med. **21**:359, 1978.

Bhakoo, O., and Scopes, J.: Minimal rates of oxygen consumption in small for dates babies during the first week of life, Arch. Dis. Child. **49**:583, 1974.

Chandra, R.: Fetal malnutrition and postnatal immunocompetence, Am. J. Dis. Child. **128**:456, 1975.

Chandra, R.: Serum thymic hormone activity and cell-mediated immunity in healthy neonates, preterm infants, and small-for-gestational-age infants, Pediatrics **67**:407, 1981.

Ferguson, S.: Prolonged impairment of cellular immunity in children with intrauterine growth retardation, J. Pediatr. **93**:52, 1978.

Sinclair, J.: Heat production and thermoregulation in the small for date infant, Pediatr. Clin. North Am. **17**:147, 1970.

Spiers, P.: Does growth retardation predispose the fetus to congenital malformation? Lancet **1**:312, 1982.

Follow-up

Brandt, I.: Growth dynamics of low birth weight infants with emphasis on the perinatal period. In Falkner, F., and Tanner, J., editors: Human growth, New York, 1978, Plenum Press.

Chamberlain, R., and Simpson, R.: Cross-sectional studies of physical growth in twins, postmature, and small for dates children, Acta Pediatr. Scand. **66**:457, 1977.

Fancourt, R., and others: Follow-up study of small for dates babies, Br. Med. J. **1**:1435, 1976.

Fitzhardinge, P., and Steven, E.: The small-for-date infant. I. Later growth patterns, Pediatrics **49**:671, 1972.

Fitzhardinge, P., and Steven, E.: The small-for-date infant. II. Neurological and intellectual sequelae, Pediatrics **50**:50, 1972.

Francis-Williams, J., and Davies, P.: Very low birthweight and later intelligence, Dev. Med. Child. Neurol. **16**:709, 1974.

Harvey, D., and others: Abilities of children who were small for gestational age babies, Pediatrics **69**:296, 1982.

Lipper, E., and others: Determinants of neurobehavioral outcome in low birth weight infants, Pediatrics **67**:502, 1981.

Low, J., and others: Intrauterine growth retardation: a preliminary report of long-term morbidity, Am. J. Obstet. Gynecol. **130**:534, 1978.

Low, J., and others: Intrauterine growth retardation: a study of long-term morbidity, Am. J. Obstet. Gynecol. **142**:620, 1982.

Lubchenco, L.: The high-risk infant, Philadelphia, 1976, W.B. Saunders Co.

Neligan, G., and others: Born too soon or born too small, London, 1976, Spastics International Medical Publications.

Sable, K., Olegard, R., and Victorin, L.: Remaining sequelae with modern perinatal care, Pediatrics **57**:652, 1976.

Vohr, B., and others: The preterm small for gestational age infant: a two-year follow-up study, Am. J. Obstet. Gynecol. **133**:426, 1979.

CHAPTER 8 Antenatal ultrasound

The use of ultrasound in evaluation of the pregnant uterus was first described by Donald in 1958. Since then ultrasound has replaced all other imaging modalities, including radiography and radionuclide scanning, in the evaluation of the uterus and fetus. The development of gray-scale instrumentation in the mid-1970s provided greatly improved visualization of fetal anatomic structures. More recently the use of high-resolution real-time scanners has made possible the routine evaluation of fetal anatomy in great detail.

In addition to its accuracy, ultrasound has the major advantage of safety. In contrast to x rays, ultrasound is nonionizing. Although very high-intensity sound is known to produce definite biologic effects, such as heat production, cavitation, shearing stresses, changes in cell membrane permeability, and chromosomal damage, the intensity at which these effects occur is many times greater than that used in diagnostic ultrasound. Average intensities in most commercial ultrasound instruments are less than 10 mW/cm^2; no biologic ill effect has been confirmed at these low intensities.

PRINCIPLES OF ULTRASONOGRAPHY

Ultrasound is defined as sound above the human hearing range, i.e., 20,000 cycles per second (cps). In obstetric ultrasonography the frequency used is usually in the region of 2 to 5 million cps (2 to 5 MHz). Ultrasound is a form of mechanical energy produced by applying a voltage across a crystal that has what is known as a piezoelectric property, which can convert the electrical energy of the applied voltage to mechanical energy in the form of ultrasound. The ultrasound beam is propagated through tissue mainly as a longitudinal waveform. The velocity of sound varies in different tissues, with the average velocity being about 1,540 m/second. Different tissues also have varying densities. The product of the density of the tissue and the velocity of sound in the tissue is referred to as its acoustic impedance. When sound encounters an interface between two tissues of different acoustic impedances, it behaves very much like light in that a portion of the sound is reflected at the interface. If the interface is large in relation to the wavelength of the sound beam, e.g., the surface of an organ, it acts as a specular reflector, and the angle of reflection is equal to the angle of incidence. Reflected echoes will return to the transducer only if the angle of incidence is within a few degrees of perpendicular to that interface. Ultrasound is also scattered by interfaces that are small in relation to the wavelength of the beam, such as the microarchitecture of tissues. Sound is then scattered in every direction, and the resultant echoes are very much weaker than those from specular reflectors. These weak, scattered echoes give the characteristic tissue texture echoes seen in a gray-scale display.

Since the velocity of sound in a given tissue is constant, the wavelength is inversely proportional to the frequency. The lower the frequency, i.e., the longer the wavelength, the greater distance the sound beam will penetrate because it will interact with fewer interfaces within tissue. Conversely, high-frequency sound with very short wavelengths has much less penetration, but because of the short wavelengths, the resolution improves as frequency increases. The frequency actually employed for any given application is a trade-off between the desirability of getting high resolution with increased frequency and the necessity to penetrate to a sufficient depth, which may require a lower frequency. In practice, the highest frequency that will provide adequate penetration should always be used, and this will vary in obstetric applications, usually between 3 and 5 MHz. The higher frequency can be used in thin patients and in the evaluation of early pregnancy, whereas obese people will require a lower frequency, perhaps even as low as 2 MHz, to provide adequate penetration.

Two basic types of ultrasonic equipment are used in obstetric ultrasonography. The traditional static B-scanner is still widely used and has the advantage of providing a complete cross section of the uterus and its contents on a single scan. This can be particularly useful in showing the exact position of the fetus and placenta in the uterus. The other main type of ultrasonic instrument used in obstetrics is the real-time scanner, which provides a dynamic image of the fetus at a frame rate of 15 to 30 frames per second. With a real-time scanner it is possible to continuously scan the fetus without interruption and also to observe fetal movements. One can obtain much more detailed information in a very short time with real-time scanning and, in our opinion, it should always be the primary method used in evaluating the pregnant uterus and fetus. Two general designs of real-time scanners are available. One is a so-called sector scanner, which produces a diverging scanning field, narrower near the surface and becoming wider with depth. Such a sector scanner can use a single oscillating crystal, multiple rotating crystals, or, in a somewhat more sophisticated design, a phased array of crystals can be electronically steered to produce the beam pattern. The other main type of real-time scanner is the linear array, which produces a rectangular scan. In general, the linear array scan produces better resolution in the near field and the sector scanner is superior for deep structures. Overall, the linear array scanners are probably preferable for obstetric examinations from the second trimester onward, whereas sector scanners are superior in early pregnancy and for gynecologic examinations.

For examination of the uterus, the bladder should be moderately distended with urine. This is particularly crucial in early pregnancy because the distended bladder displaces bowel out of the pelvis and provides an acoustic window to the posteriorly situated uterus. In later pregnancy, bladder distension is also desirable but not quite as crucial. It is important, however, that the bladder is not overdistended, since this can compress the lower uterine segment and cause a false impression of a low-lying placenta.

DIAGNOSIS OF EARLY PREGNANCY AND ESTIMATION OF GESTATIONAL AGE

Pregnancy can be diagnosed sonographically as early as 5 weeks after the last menstrual period. A gestational sac is seen within the uterus. The actual embryo can be seen at 6 to 7 weeks, and cardiac movement can be documented by real-time scanning (Fig. 8-1).

A blighted ovum will be seen as an empty gestational sac, which is inappropriately small for the duration of amenorrhea. The gestational sac may be distorted and

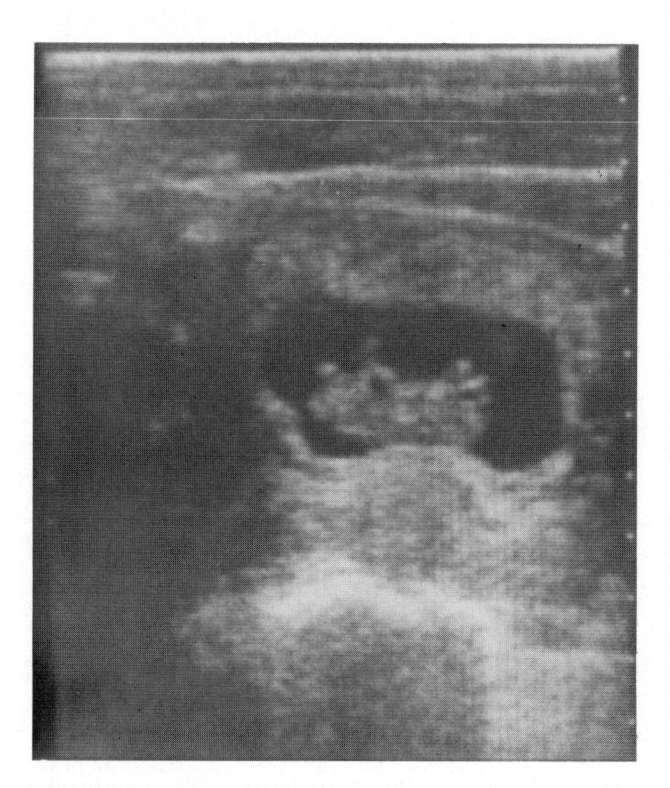

Fig. 8-1. First trimester pregnancy. The embryo is seen within the gestational sac. The crown-rump length can be measured on this image for estimation of gestational age.

collapsed and may also be situated unusually low in the uterine cavity. The diagnosis of blighted ovum can be confirmed by repeating the study after 7 to 10 days and documenting no interval growth or appearance of an embryo.

The most accurate method of estimating gestational age is by measuring the crown-rump length in the first trimester. This has an accuracy of ±3 days. Measurement of gestational sac diameter also can be used for estimating gestational age during the first trimester, although it is not as accurate as the crown-rump length, since its shape can be quite variable.

Cephalometry

From the beginning of the second trimester onward, the most widely used method of estimating gestational age is the biparietal diameter (BPD). Campbell described a technique for obtaining accurate BPDs using static B-scanners in 1968, and his method became universally adopted. Since the advent of high-resolution real-time scanners, it has become possible to obtain reliable and reproducible BPDs quickly and easily. Details of intracranial anatomy should be seen routinely from the second trimester onward (Figs. 8-2 and 8-3). The midbrain and cerebral peduncles can almost always be iden-

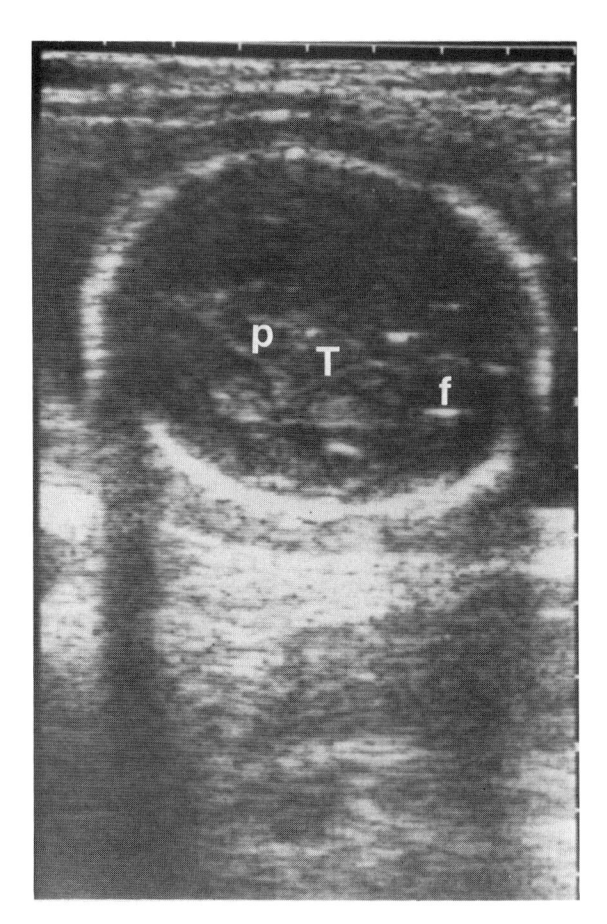

Fig. 8-2. Normal intracranial structures. *p,* Cerebral peduncles; *T,* thalamus; *f,* frontal horn of lateral ventricle.

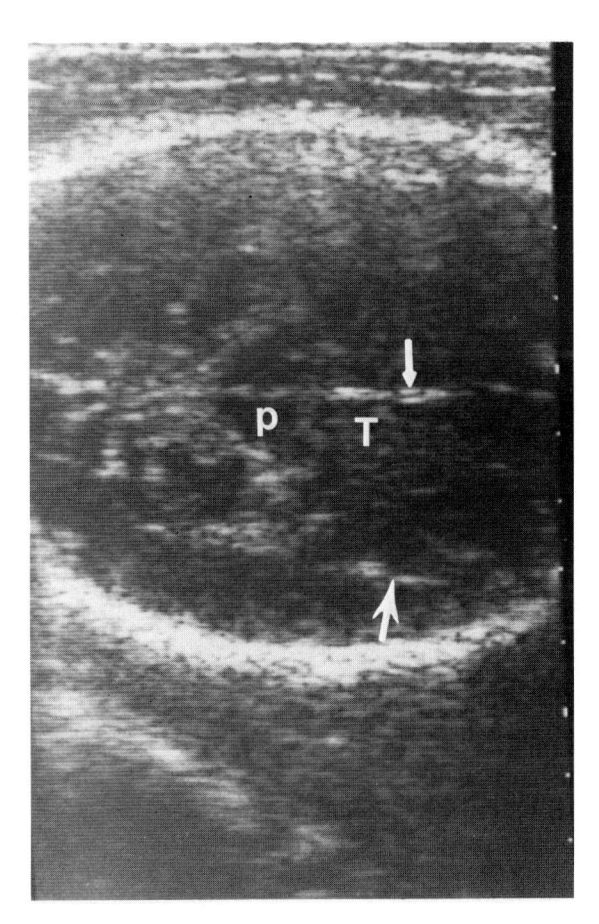

Fig. 8-3. Normal anatomy. Small arrow shows third ventricle; large arrow shows sylvian fissure. *p,* Cerebral peduncle; *T,* thalamus.

tified as relatively echo-free structures, and the basilar artery can be seen pulsating on the anterior aspect of the midbrain. The thalami can be seen also as relatively hypoechoic structures on either side of the third ventricle, but the third ventricle itself is sometimes not seen as a discrete structure due to its small size. The pulsations of the internal carotid arteries can be seen in the region of the circle of Willis, and branches of the middle cerebral artery can be seen producing pulsations in the sylvian fissures, which appear as linear echogenic structures parallel to the skull vault and approximately two thirds of the distance from the midline to the periphery. A strong midline echo is routinely seen; it represents the interhemispheric fissure and falx at more superior levels and the septum pellucidum and third ventricle at more caudal levels. The lateral ventricles can be seen routinely from the beginning of the second trimester onward. In the second trimester the lateral ventricles are relatively large compared with the size of the brain and may extend as far as two thirds of the way from the midline to the periphery at 15 weeks' gestation. As pregnancy progresses toward term, the brain grows at a relatively faster rate than the lateral ventricles, and at term the ratio should be less than 35%. The measurement done from the midline echo to the lateral margin of the lateral ventricle does not represent the true size of the lateral ventricle but also includes a portion of the corpus callosum medially. The medial wall of the normal lateral ventricle is frequently not seen, since it is not perpendicular to the sound beam. When the ventricle becomes dilated, the medial wall frequently does become perpendicular to the beam, and the true size of the lateral ventricle can then be measured. It should never exceed 13 mm. The normal choroid plexus is seen as a strongly echogenic structure within the lateral ventricle. In the presence of hydrocephalus, the ventricle can be seen to contain predominantly clear fluid and, as mentioned previously, both walls of the ventricle can be seen when it is dilated. The occipital horn is frequently the first portion of the ventricle to dilate.

To consistently obtain BPDs in a reproducible fashion and at the maximum levels, the structures around the region of the thalamus should be included in the plane of measurement. The cross section of the head will then be

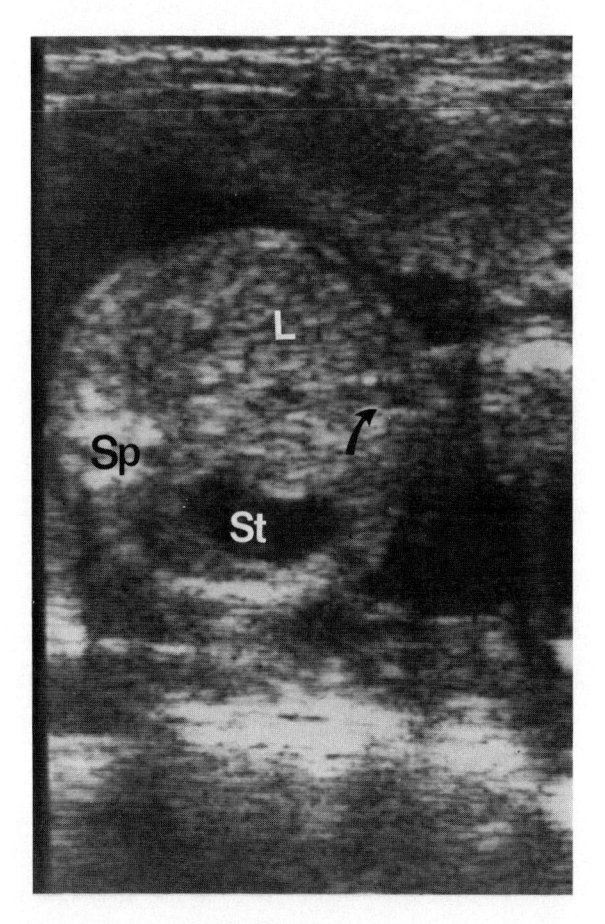

Fig. 8-4. Cross section of abdomen at level of umbilical vein (arrow). *L*, Liver; *St*, stomach; *Sp*, spine.

ovoid when it is scanned in the axial plane. If the head is measured at the level of the interhemispheric fissure, the diameter will usually not be maximal and the measurement derived may underestimate the gestational age by several weeks. The accuracy of BPD estimations is ±10 days up to about 34 weeks, and thereafter, due to a falling off in the rate of growth, the accuracy diminishes to ±3 weeks.

Other methods of estimating gestational age

In addition to the BPD, the fetal abdominal diameter should be measured. This is conventionally done at the level of the liver, and the umbilical vein is used as a reproducible landmark to indicate the appropriate level (Fig. 8-4). Either average fetal body diameter (average of anteroposterior and lateral diameters) or abdominal circumference can be used. We have found that using the average diameter is simpler and just as useful as measuring the circumference. In the presence of intrauterine growth retardation, head growth tends to be preserved at the expense of body growth, and the abdominal diameter will lag behind the BPD (Chapter 7). They should normally be within 5 mm of each other, with the head being larger up to about 34 weeks and the body becoming larger thereafter.

The length of the fetal femur can easily be measured, particularly using real-time scanning, and this also proves to be a reliable indicator of gestational age. It is particularly useful if an adequate BPD measurement cannot be obtained due to fetal position. Some workers use estimates of total intrauterine volume both to estimate gestational age and to assess the presence of intrauterine growth retardation. Accurate measurements of total intrauterine volume are difficult to obtain and have a wide normal variation. We have not found them to be sufficiently useful to warrant the time it takes to perform such estimates on a routine basis.

PLACENTAL LOCALIZATION

The arrival of B-mode ultrasonography quickly replaced all other modalities in evaluating and localizing the placenta. Apart from being noninvasive, it is by far the most accurate method because it directly images the placenta and shows its precise position as well as any abnormalities that may be present. Up to about 30 weeks the placenta appears as a homogenous echogenic structure that is parallel to the uterine wall. After 30 weeks, changes appear in the placenta that are normal accompaniments of placental maturity. These include echogenic ringlike structures, which probably represent fibrosis, and also calcifications of the basal plate and of the placenta itself. Placental calcification increases as term is approached and is usually not very prominent until after 34 weeks. It has been reported to occur at an earlier stage in the presence of intrauterine growth retardation.

The major importance of accurate placental localization is to detect placenta previa. Placenta previa may be clinically suspected whenever there is vaginal bleeding during pregnancy or when the fetus is other than in a cephalic presentation, i.e. breech, transverse, or unstable lie. Whenever a patient has vaginal bleeding, one must look for evidence of abruptio placentae (retroplacental hematoma) in addition to ruling out placenta previa. Abruptio may be seen as an area of separation of the placenta from the uterine wall, which may contain either echo-free or echogenic blood. Sometimes the blood is not contained in a hematoma but tracks along the uterine wall in an extraamniotic plane and may be seen distant from the placenta. It may also escape entirely from the uterus, and ultrasound then will show no evidence of hematoma.

A placenta that appears to be low lying in early or middle pregnancy frequently migrates away from the lower uterine segment as pregnancy progresses. Such placental migration was first described by King in 1973 and may be due to differential growth of the lower uterine segment relative to the upper. King also hypothesized a process of dynamic placentation in which the placenta continuously separates and reattaches itself a small portion at a time. Some such process appears likely, since the proportion of the uterine wall covered by the placenta progressively diminishes during the course of pregnancy. Because of this phenomenon of placental migration, one must never make the diagnosis of placenta previa or low-lying placenta early in pregnancy. Whenever the placenta is seen in a low position at this stage, a repeat study should be done after 34 weeks to reassess its position. In about 80% of cases it is found to have assumed a normal position on the repeat study. The diagnosis of placenta previa should be made only when it is seen to reach or cross the internal os after 34 weeks. A final diagnosis of low-lying placenta that reaches within a few centimeters of the internal os likewise should not be made until the last few weeks of pregnancy. Apparent change in placental position is occasionally seen immediately after the patient alters her position, e.g., after lying on her side to relieve the inferior vena caval compression syndrome. The placenta then appears to have changed from a lateral to an anterior or posterior position or vice versa. It can also appear to change its distance from the internal os. This is thought to be due to uterine rotation around its long axis.

Whenever multiple pregnancy is found, an attempt should be made to identify an equal number of placentae. However, the separate placentae frequently cannot be identified even in the presence of fraternal twins, since the placentae tend to merge into each other. In that case the separating amniotic membranes will almost always be clearly seen.

Amniocentesis

Amniocentesis should always be done under ultrasonic guidance. The exact position of the fetus can be determined, and thus the possibility of injury by the amniocentesis needle can be avoided. In particular, one should choose a site away from the fetal head and thorax. A suitable pool of amniotic fluid can usually be found around the lower extremities. One should also try to avoid traversing the placenta with the needle, but this is sometimes not possible when the placenta is located anteriorly.

DIAGNOSIS OF FETAL ANOMALIES

Ultrasonography now offers the opportunity to evaluate selected high-risk pregnancies for the presence of fetal malformations that are amenable to corrective measures as well as those that are incompatible with life. Although radiography has been applied with some success in detection of fetal malformations involving osseous structures, invasive amniography has heretofore usually been required for the diagnosis of soft tissue or gastrointestinal abnormalities. Ultrasonography has now virtually replaced x rays for the diagnosis of fetal anomalies, since, in addition to its being safe and noninvasive, it also provides vastly superior detail of fetal anatomy. During a 3-year period, Jassani and associates observed major fetal malformations in 1% of 6,050 cases that underwent antenatal ultrasonographic evaluation. Statistics from this study follow:

Number of patients examined	6,050
Structurally abnormal fetuses	60
Multiple abnormalities	10
Organ systems involved	
Central nervous	29
Gastrointestinal	9
Genitourinary	13
Skeletal	2
Cardiopulmonary	5
Other	14

This incidence is probably higher than that to be expected in the general population, since the series included high-risk patients referred from a population of about 5 million. Hobbins and co-workers found an approximately equal incidence of fetal anomalies in a series of 2,548 scans on high-risk patients. The major fetal anomalies can be diagnosed as early as 15 to 16 weeks of gestational age. Indications for antenatal ultrasound follow.

A. Dating pregnancy
   1. No accurate dates
   2. Uterine size/dates discrepancy
      a. Suspected growth retardation
      b. Suspected large for dates; rule out:
         (1) Multiple gestation
         (2) Polyhydramnios
         (3) Macrosomia
         (4) Uterine abnormality, e.g., fibroid
         (5) Molar pregnancy
B. Fetal/placental localization
   1. Confirm pregnancy
   2. Suspected missed abortion
   3. Suspected ectopic pregnancy
   4. Suspected placenta previa
   5. Prior to amniocentesis
   6. Prior to fetal transfusion/surgery
C. Survey of fetal anatomy; rule out congenital malformation, especially with:
   1. History of previous malformation
   2. Elderly mother
   3. Diabetic pregnancy
   4. Polyhydramnios/oligohydramnios
   5. Abnormal presentation
   6. Exposure to teratogens
   7. Elevated serum alpha-fetoprotein levels

Normal fetal anatomy

In addition to the normal intracranial structures previously described, many other fetal organs can be routinely seen (Figs. 8-4 and 8-5). Structures that should always be identified include the heart, liver, kidneys, stomach, umbilical vein, urinary bladder, spine, and extremities. Organs that are usually seen but can sometimes be obscured by an unfavorable fetal position include the gallbladder, individual cardiac chambers, aorta, vena cava, and external genitalia (Figs. 8-6 and 8-7).

Genitourinary abnormalities

The kidneys can be identified as early as 14 weeks' gestation as two circular structures situated on either side of the fetal spine (Fig. 8-5). The bladder can be seen as early as 14 or 15 weeks' gestation. If serious renal malfunction such as severe obstruction or renal agenesis is present, the absence of fetal urine production causes severe oligohydramnios. Thus, whenever oligohydramnios is encountered on an ultrasound examination, particular attention should be paid to the fetal urinary tract. The fetal bladder should always be visualized after about 15 weeks, and if it is not seen at the first attempt, the patient should be rescanned at 30-minute intervals in case the failure to see it on the first attempt is due to recent voiding. Unfortunately, the lack of surrounding amniotic fluid makes it much more difficult to see details of fetal anatomy. Nevertheless, if the bladder and kidneys cannot be seen in the presence of oligohydramnios, this is strongly suggestive of renal agenesis. The fetal adrenals are relatively much larger than they are in later life, and sometimes the adrenals can be seen and misinterpreted as kidneys in cases of renal agenesis.

Hydronephrosis may be unilateral due to pelviureteric junction obstruction or bilateral due to lower urinary tract obstruction, such as posterior urethral valves. In mild cases only a dilated pelvis will be seen, and the renal parenchymal thickness will be normal. However, if the degree of hydronephrosis is severe, a markedly dilated pelvis and calyces can be seen with thinning of the renal parenchyma (Fig. 8-8). Minimal dilatation of the renal pelvis can sometimes be seen in normal kidneys, and the presence of minimal dilatation does not necessarily indicate obstruction.

Multicystic renal dysplasia is the most common cause of an abdominal mass in the newborn and is readily diagnosable in the fetus. It appears as a multicystic mass in the renal fossa alongside the spine with cysts of varying sizes that lack any apparent organization (Fig. 8-9). This is in contrast to the findings in severe hydronephrosis, where there is an orderly arrangement of a large renal pelvis surrounded by smaller calyces (Fig. 8-8). (See Chapter 31.)

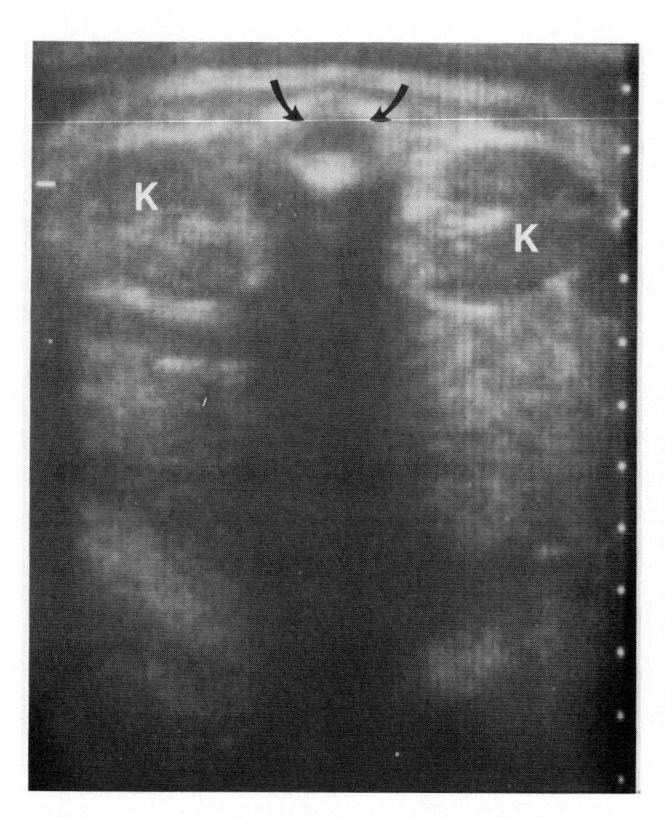

Fig. 8-5. Normal fetal kidneys *(K)* and spinal canal *(arrows).*

In posterior urethral valves a distended bladder will usually be seen in addition to hydronephrosis, which is most often bilateral but may be unilateral.

Gastrointestinal malformations

Obstruction at various levels of the gastrointestinal tract can be easily diagnosed by ultrasound. Obstruction of the proximal alimentary canal interferes with the normal process of amniotic fluid turnover, which involves swallowing and absorption of the amniotic fluid by the fetus. Thus, in bowel obstruction, polyhydramnios is an invariable finding (Chapter 6).

In esophageal atresia, absence of the stomach and bowel loops in association with polyhydramnios should alert the examiner to the diagnosis. In duodenal atresia, the presence of a distended stomach and duodenum provides a so-called double-bubble sign and make the diagnosis almost certain. Similarly, ileal atresia can be diagnosed by the presence of multiple dilated loops of bowel (Fig. 8-10). The same pattern can be seen in meconium ileus and anal atresia.

Abdominal wall defects are among the more common abnormalities detected in the neonate with an approximate incidence of 1 in 2,500 births. The presence of the abdominal viscera in the base of the umbilical cord is an

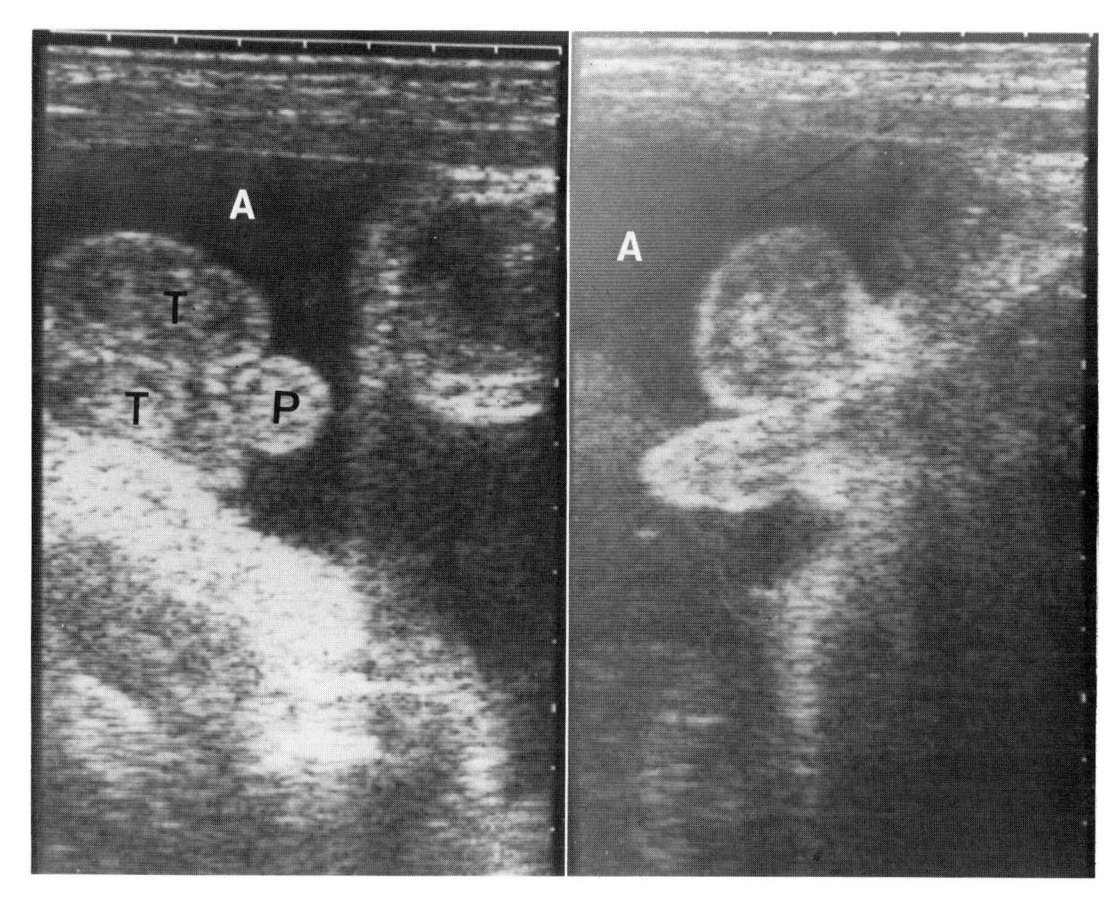

Fig. 8-6. Two scans showing external genitalia of a male fetus. *T*, Testis; *P*, penis; *A*, amniotic fluid.

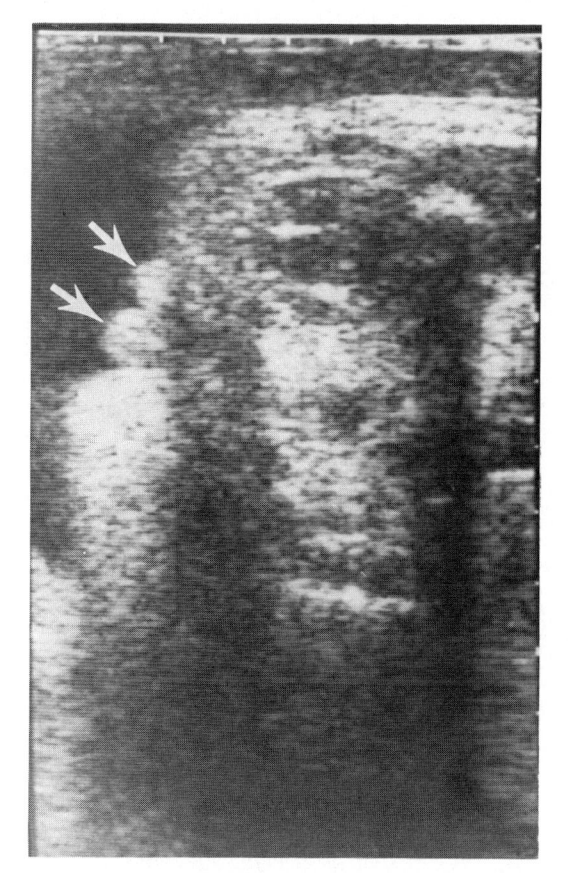

Fig. 8-7. Labia majora *(arrows)* of a female fetus.

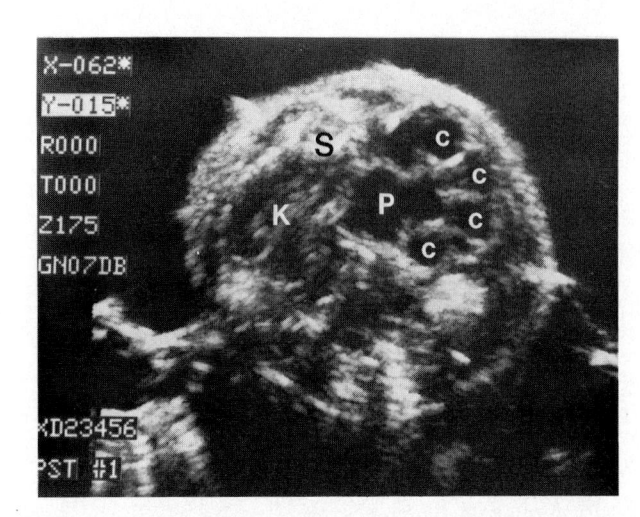

Fig. 8-8. Unilateral hydronephrosis in a newborn. Note the orderly arrangement of dilated pelvis (P) and calyces (c). The contralateral kidney (K) appears normal. S, Spine.

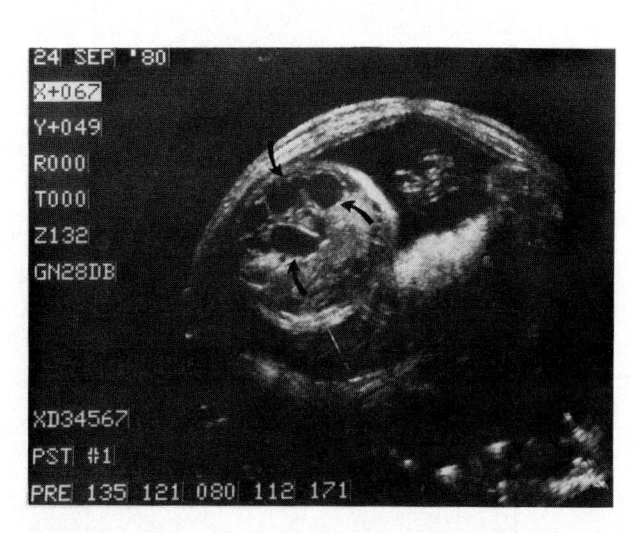

Fig. 8-9. Multicystic dysplastic kidney (arrows). The cysts appear as echo-free structures of varying sizes without apparent organization.

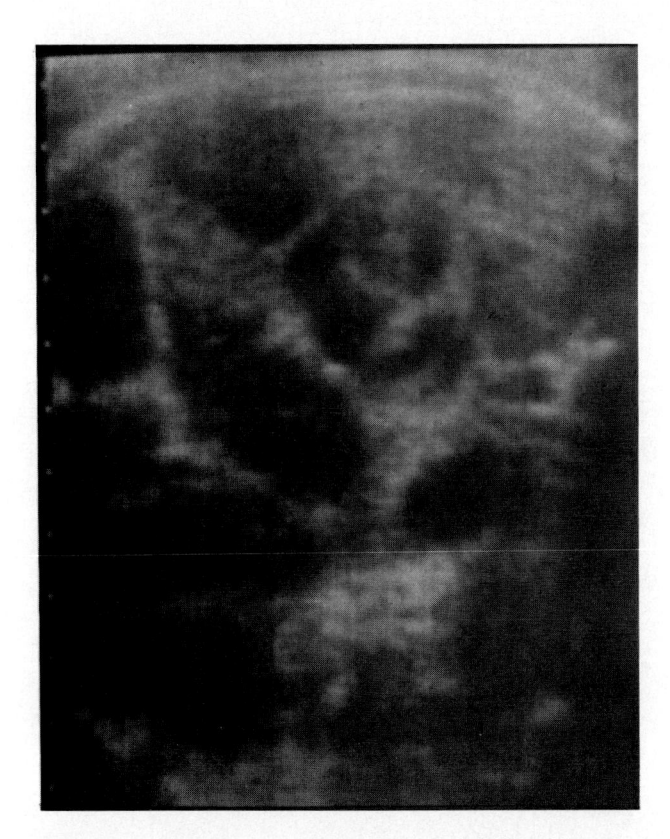

Fig. 8-10. Ileal atresia. Multiple dilated fluid-filled loops of bowel are seen in the fetal abdomen.

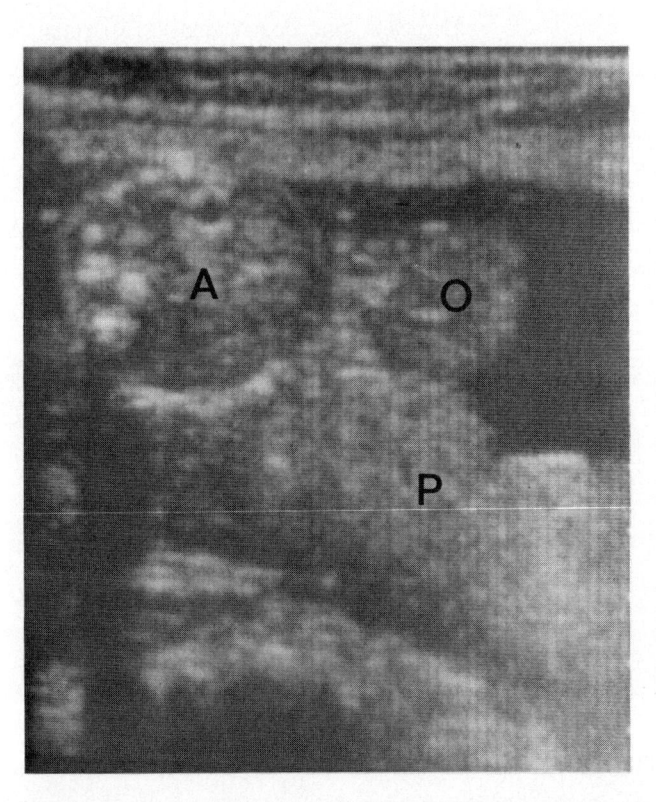

Fig. 8-11. An omphalocele (O) is seen adjacent to the fetal abdomen (A). P, Placenta.

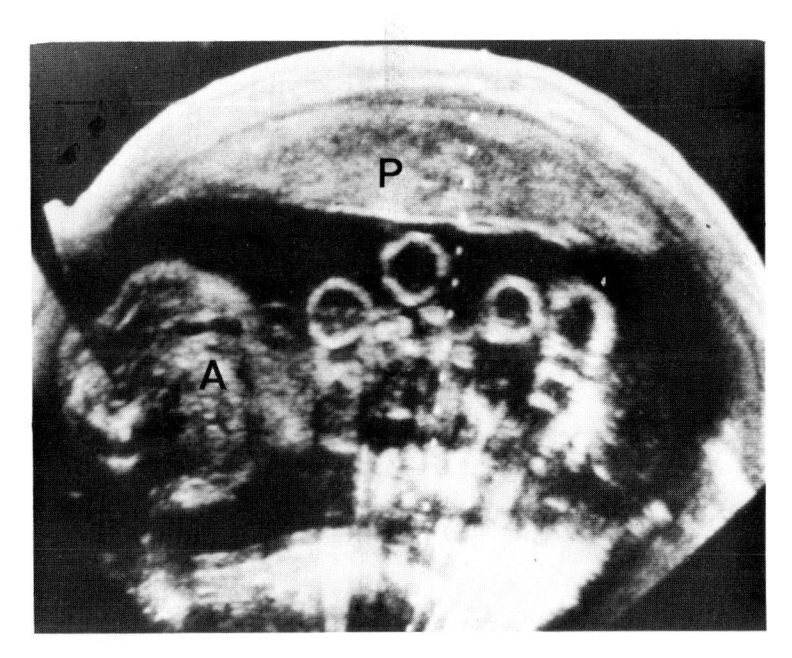

Fig. 8-12. Gastroschisis. Multiple loops of bowel are seen floating freely in the amniotic fluid. The fetal abdomen *(A)* is relatively small, and there is polyhydramnios. *P,* Placenta.

ultrasonic characteristic of omphalocele (Fig. 8-11), whereas in gastroschisis free bowel loops and liver are seen floating in the amniotic cavity and the defect is usually lateral to the cord insertion (See Chapter 24.)

Central nervous system

As described previously, the lateral ventricle can be visualized from 15 weeks' gestation. Hydrocephalus can be diagnosed as early as 17 weeks by dilatation of the lateral ventricle (Fig. 8-13). The dilatation, in general, occurs before any change in the BPD.

Meningoencephaloceles can be identified as a defect in the calvaria with projection of a membrane containing cerebrospinal fluid or brain tissue outside the skull (Fig. 8-14).

Spina bifida

The spine can be examined by ultrasound in both longitudinal and transverse planes. Longitudinally the spine appears as two parallel lines, and in transverse sections the spinal canal is seen as a circular structure (Fig. 8-5). In the presence of spina bifida, increased separation of the two lines will be noted longitudinally, and a V-shaped or U-shaped defect will be seen in the transverse section (Figs. 8-15 and 8-16). With meningomyelocele a membrane can be seen bulging from the spine.

Anencephaly

Absence of the normal cranium can be detected by approximately 14 to 15 weeks' gestation (Fig. 8-17). There is usually associated polyhydramnios.

Microcephaly

Microcephaly can be diagnosed by ultrasound as early as 19 weeks' gestation by the presence of a small head relative to the size of the body. We have had one case in which we made the diagnosis at approximately 21 weeks' gestation after repeating the examination three times. We noted that the abdominal diameter was larger than the head, which in itself is abnormal at that stage of gestation. In addition, we noted a decrease in the rate of the growth of the BPD in the 3-week period during which we repeated the study. Postmortem examination of the fetus confirmed the diagnosis.

Skeletal system

A variety of congenital malformations of the fetal limbs can be detected by ultrasound after 16 weeks' gestation. Both upper and lower extremities can be measured by real-time ultrasonography from 16 weeks' gestation, and the length can be ascertained and compared with O'Brien and associates' data.

We have diagnosed several cases of dwarfism and one case of osteogenesis imperfecta.

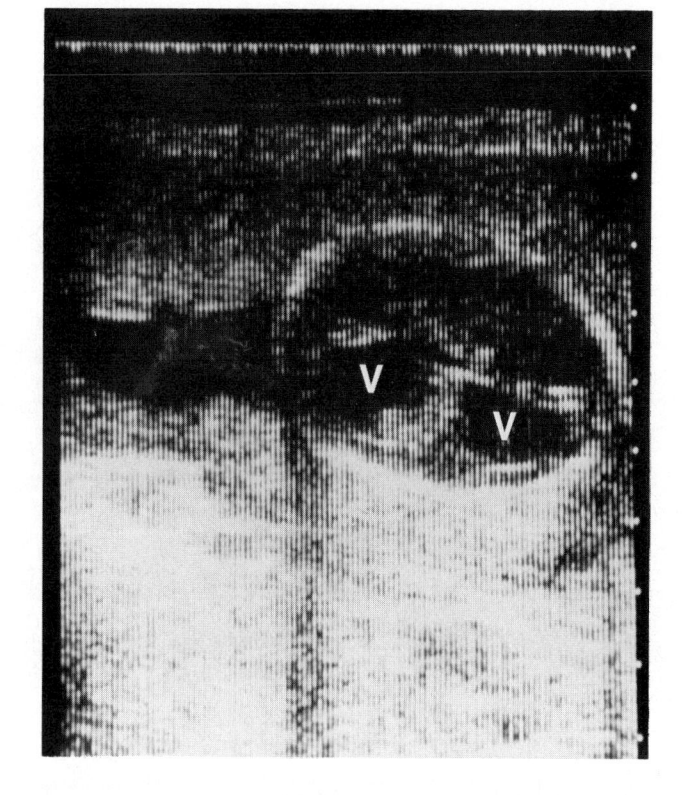

90 Behrman's neonatal-perinatal medicine: diseases of the fetus and infant

Fig. 8-13. Hydrocephalus. The occipital and frontal horns of the lateral ventricles *(V)* are seen to be dilated, and there is thinning of the cerebral mantle.

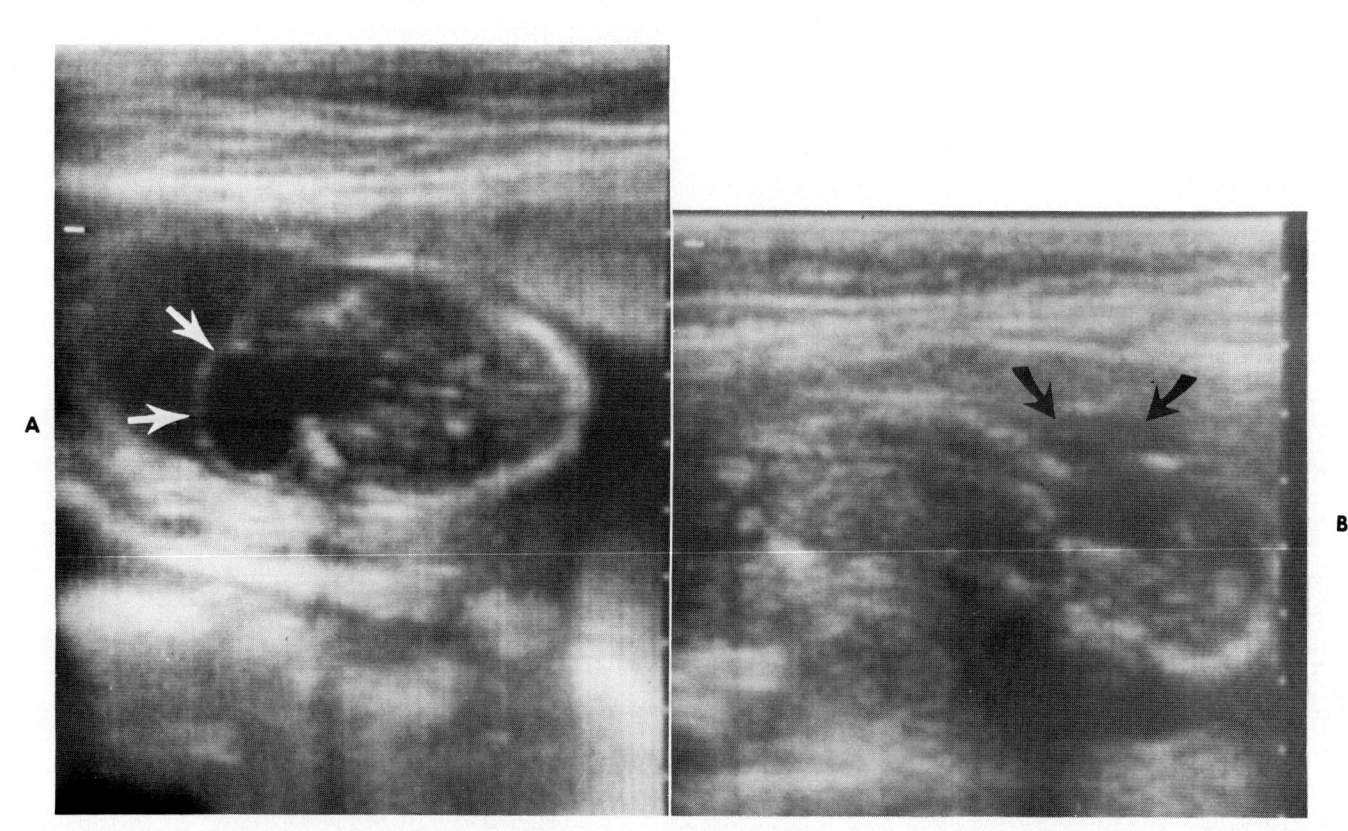

Fig. 8-14. Occipital meningocele. A transverse axial scan (**A**) shows the defect in the calvaria with the membrane *(arrows)* projecting out into the amniotic fluid. A longitudinal scan (**B**) shows the meningocele *(arrows)* at the base of the occiput.

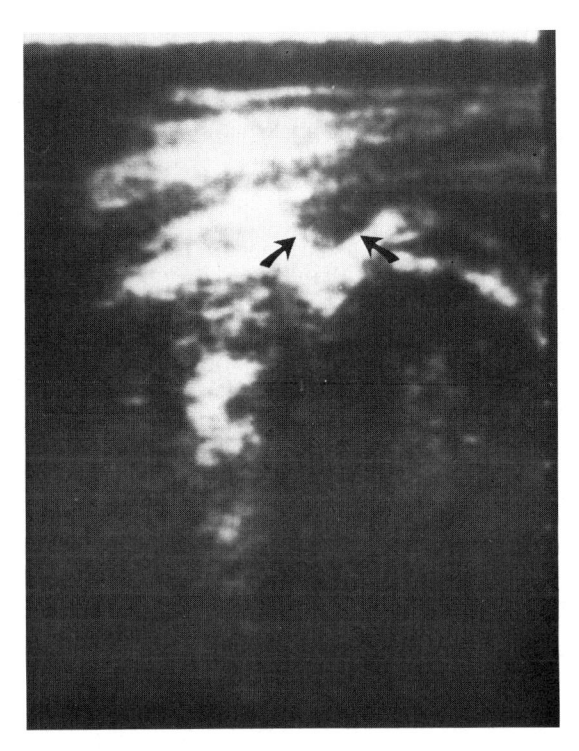

Fig. 8-15. Spina bifida. A V-shaped defect is seen on this transverse scan *(arrows)*.

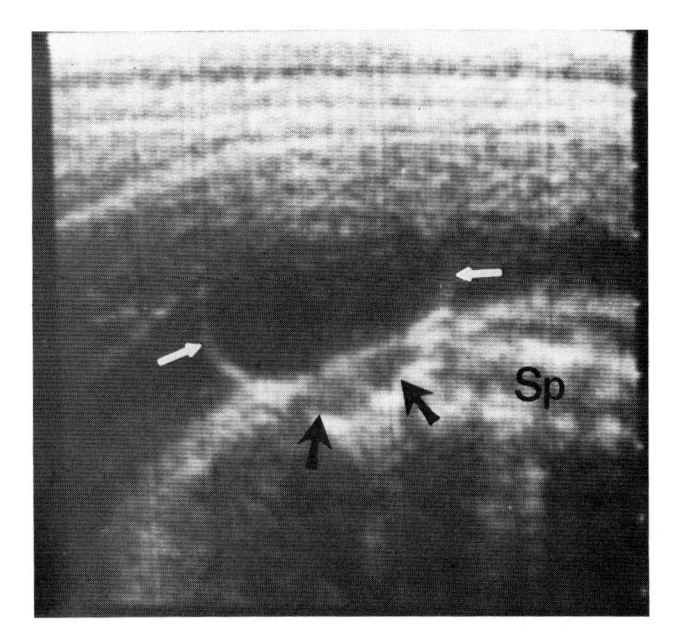

Fig. 8-16. Longitudinal scan of fetus showing spina bifida with meningocele *(small arrows)*. The normal spine *(Sp)* superior to the defect is seen as parallel lines. The posterior line is interrupted at the level of the spina bifida *(large arrows)*.

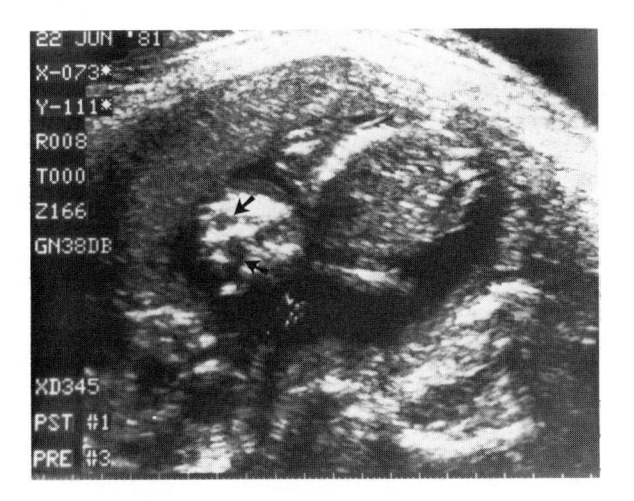

Fig. 8-17. Anencephaly. The fetal body and facial bones are seen, but there is no cranial vault. Arrows point to the orbits.

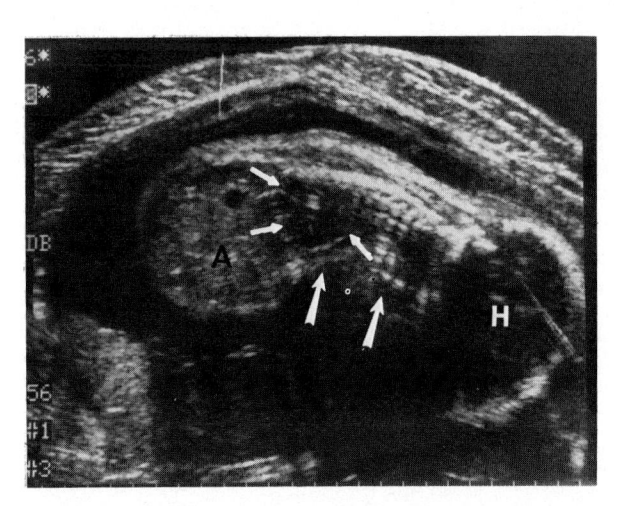

Fig. 8-18. Small thorax in a thanatophoric dwarf, secondary to hypoplasia of the lungs. Note the small diameter of the thorax relative to the abdomen *(A)*. Large arrows show the thorax; small arrows show the fetal heart. *H,* Head.

Abnormalities of the chest, such as hydrothorax, microthorax due to hypoplastic lungs (Fig. 8-18), diaphragmatic hernia, and major cardiac abnormalities, can be diagnosed by ultrasound.

Diagnosis of fetal death

Absence of the visible fetal heartbeat by real-time imaging is the most reliable method of diagnosing intrauterine fetal death. Other signs include absence of fetal limb movement and collapse of the bones of the calvaria. The latter occurs about a week after fetal demise and was a valuable sign before the availability of good real-time equipment.

USE OF ULTRASOUND IN HIGH-RISK PREGNANCY

Intrauterine growth retardation is associated with a significantly increased rate of perinatal mortality and long-term morbidity (Chapter 7). Improved perinatal outcome is contingent on accurate early identification. Confirmation of the diagnosis of intrauterine growth retardation (IUGR) by hormonal studies is inadequate. Campbell assessed the value of urinary estrogen in 85 small for dates infants and found that only 53% had abnormal estrogens; a similar finding was reported by Martin and associates. Therefore considerable attention has been focused recently on the use of ultrasonography in the diagnosis of growth retardation.

Campbell and Dewhurst used serial BPD measurements to predict intrauterine growth retardation. They studied a series of 140 pregnancies complicated by intrauterine growth retardation and found that in 82% the BPD growth was below normal. They reported two different patterns of abnormal BPD growth. In the first pattern there is normal growth until the third trimester, with flattening of the growth rate thereafter. In the second pattern the BPD shows steady but abnormally low growth rate, usually very early in pregnancy, and this is the so-called low-profile growth. However, other investigators using BPD measurements alone could predict growth retardation in only 50% of cases.

Another method used for detection of growth retardation is the head/body ratio. This is of value because in growth retardation the brain is relatively spared and the body diameter or circumference will lag behind the head, reflecting reduced growth of the fetal liver. Normally the average fetal body diameter measured at the level of the umbilical vein should be within 5 mm of the BPD, and in late pregnancy it is usually greater than the BPD. A body diameter in excess of 5 mm less than the BPD indicates probable growth retardation.

Hobbins used total intrauterine volume measurements for diagnosis of growth retardation and found that when the volume was more than 1.5 standard deviations below the mean for the gestational age most of the fetuses were growth retarded. However, other investigators could not confirm those findings. Other methods of diagnosing growth retardation include using combined head/body ratio, placental appearance, and amniotic fluid volume. Many authorities agree that there is no single placental abnormality that is common to small for gestational age (SGA) fetuses. However, there are certain lesions that occur with high frequency in the placentae of such neonates, including infarction, villous vascularity, fibrosis, and a nonspecific villous inflammation. With advances in ultrasound techniques it is possible to study the placental structure in detail prior to delivery. Calcification and fibrous maturity rings are found in most placentae near term. However, excessive calcification prior to 36 weeks' gestation indicates possible fetal compromise. Amniotic fluid volume also tends to be reduced in IUGR. Once identification of possible growth retardation has been made, hospitalization is imperative.

Ultrasound is of particular value in following the growth of twin gestations. In early pregnancy the BPDs of twins are always identical. In later stages of pregnancy the abdominal circumference or abdominal diameter is more helpful in diagnosis of growth retardation in twin gestations than is the BPD. Because of increased pressure, the BPD may be altered due to variations in the shape of the baby's head, such as dolichocephaly.

Rh incompatibility

Hobbins described the sequence of events in Rh disease observed on ultrasonography (Chapter 5). The first sign of fetal compromise is excessive accumulation of amniotic fluid, followed by increase in the placental thickness to more than 5 cm. The next change is in the fetal liver with development of hepatomegaly. Usually the abdominal diameter or the abdominal circumference is larger than normal in relation to the head. The last sign is the appearance of fetal ascites (Fig. 8-19). Ultrasound is valuable not only in localizing for amniocentesis but also to follow the progress of the fetus in conjunction with the ΔOD. Once the decision is made for intrauterine transfusion, the procedure nowadays is usually performed under direct real-time ultrasound guidance, with the needle tip being monitored into the fetal abdomen. Its presence in the peritoneal cavity is then confirmed by injecting a small amount of contrast material and obtaining a radiograph (Fig. 8-20). The success of the procedure is confirmed by seeing the transfused blood in the peritoneal cavity.

Diabetes

The ultrasound findings in diabetes vary according to the class. From classes A to C the general picture is that

Antenatal ultrasound 93

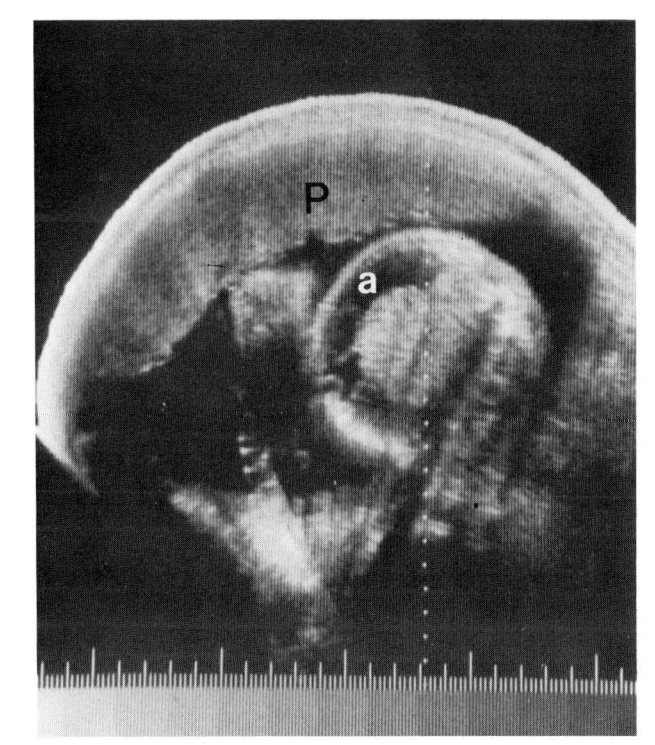

Fig. 8-19. Rh incompatibility with fetal ascites *(a)*. The placenta *(P)* is thickened.

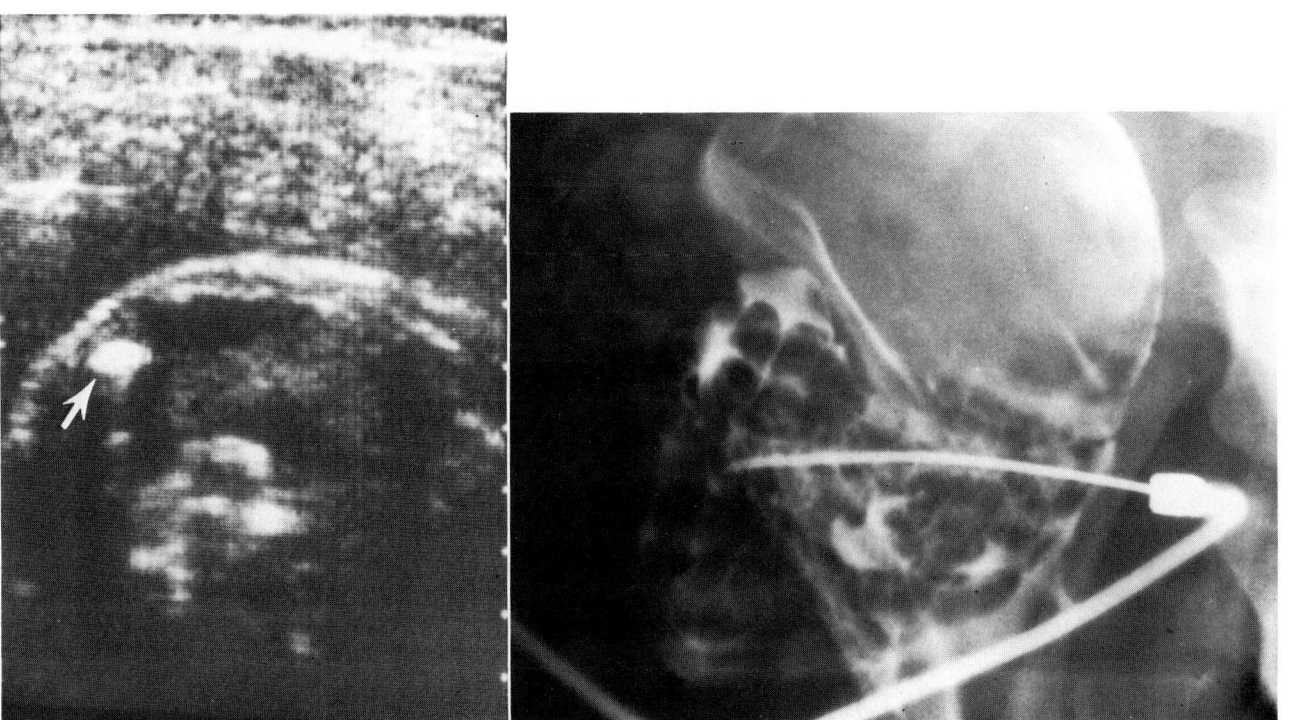

Fig. 8-20. Intrauterine transfusion for Rh incompatibility. **A,** The needle produces a strong echo *(arrow)* in the fetal abdomen. **B,** Radiograph obtained after injection of a small amount of contrast through the needle shows loops of bowel and liver outlined by the contrast. This confirms the intraperitoneal location of the needle tip.

of an abdominal diameter that is large relative to that of the head, increase in amniotic fluid volume, and a placenta that is thicker than normal. The degree of macrosomia of the fetus can be followed by the rate of growth of the fetal head and by the head/abdomen ratio. In classes D to F diabetes there is an increased incidence of growth retardation due to vascular involvement, and the patient should be followed for possible intrauterine growth retardation (Chapter 3).

CONCLUSION

With recent improvements in technology, ultrasound has become the most important modality for evaluating the pregnant uterus and the fetus. The growth and well-being of the fetus can be evaluated and several major fetal anomalies diagnosed antenatally. This may be crucial because it alerts the pediatricians and pediatric surgeons to the need for immediate corrective therapy or surgery after birth.

Patrick J. Bryan
Majida N. Jassani

BIBLIOGRAPHY

Adam A.H., and Robinson, H.P.: An evaluation of real-time scanning in the first trimester of pregnancy. In Bennett, M.J., and Campbell, S., editors: Real-time ultrasound in obstetrics, Boston, 1980, Blackwell Scientific Publications.

Azimi, F., Bryan, P.J., and Marangola, J.P.: Ultrasonography in obstetrics and gynecology: historical notes, basic principles, safety considerations, and clinical applications, CRC Critical Reviews in Clinical Radiology and Nuclear Medicine, 1976.

Bennett, M.J.: Real-time ultrasound in the second and third trimesters of pregnancy. In Bennett, M.J., and Campbell, S., editors: Real-time ultrasound in obstetrics, Boston, 1980, Blackwell Scientific Publications.

Bryan, P.J., and Champlin, F.M.: Apparent placental migration caused by uterine rotation. In White, D., and Brown, R.E., editors: Ultrasound in medicine, vol. 3A, New York, 1977, Plenum Publishing Corp.

Campbell, S.: An improved method of fetal cephalometry by ultrasound, J. Obstet. Gynaecol. Br. Commonw. **75:**568, 1968.

Campbell, S., and Little, D.J.: Clinical potential of real-time ultrasound. In Bennett, M.J., and Campbell, S., editors: Real-time ultrasound in obstetrics, Boston, 1980, Blackwell Scientific Publications.

Campbell, S., and Dewhurst, C.J.: Diagnosis of small-for-dates fetus by serial ultrasonic cephalometry, Lancet **2:**1002, 1971.

Campbell, S.: The prediction of fetal maturity by ultrasonic measurement of the biparietal diameter, J. Obstet. Gynaecol. Br. Commonw. **76:**603, 1969.

Deter, R.L., and others: The use of ultrasound in the assessment of normal fetal growth: a review, J. Clin. Ultrasound **9:**481, 1981.

DeVore, G.R., and Hobbins, J.C.: Fetal growth and development: the diagnosis of intrauterine growth retardation. In Hobbins, J.C., editor: Diagnostic ultrasound in obstetrics, New York, 1979, Churchill Livingstone.

Donald, I.: Sonar: a new diagnostic echo-sounding technique in obstetrics and gynaecology, Proc. R. Soc. Med. **55:**637, 1962.

Donald I., and Brown, T.G.: Demonstration of tissue interfaces within the body of ultrasonic echo sounding, Br. J. Radiol. **34:**539, 1961.

Donald, I., MacVicar, J., and Brown, T.G.: Investigation of abdominal masses by pulsed ultrasound, Lancet **1:**1188, 1958.

Fadel, H.E., and Martin, S.: Realtime sonographic diagnosis of fetal dysplastic kidney, Int. J. Gynaecol. Obstet. **18:**140, 1980.

Grannum, P., and others: Assessment of fetal kidney size in normal gestation by comparison of ratio of kidney circumference to abdominal circumferences, Am. J. Obstet. Gynecol. **136:**249, 1980.

Grannum, P. Berkowitz, R.L., and Hobbins, J.C.: The ultrasonic changes in the maturing placenta and their relation to fetal pulmonic maturity, Am. J. Obstet. Gynecol. **133:**915, 1979.

Grossman, M., and others: Pitfalls in ultrasonic determination of total intrauterine volume, J. Clin. Ultrasound **10:**17, 1982.

Hadlock, F.P., Deter, R.L., and Park, S.K.: Real-time sonography: ventricular and vascular anatomy of the fetal brain in utero, Am. J. Roentgenol. **136:**133, 1981.

Hobbins, J.C., and Venus, I.: Congenital anomalies. In Hobbins, J.C., editor: Diagnostic ultrasound in obstetrics, New York, 1979, Churchill Livingstone.

Hobbins, J.C., and others: Ultrasound in the diagnosis of congenital anomalies, Am. J. Obstet. Gynecol. **134:**331, 1979.

Hobbins, J.C.: Use of ultrasound in complicated pregnancies. In Berkowitz, R.L., editor: Clinics in perinatology, vol. 7, Philadelphia, 1980, W.B. Saunders Co.

Jassani, M.N., and others: Twin pregnancy with discordancy for Down's syndrome, Obstet. Gynecol. **55**(3):45S, 1980.

Jassani, M.N., and others: A perinatal approach to the diagnosis and management of gastrointestinal malformations, Obstet. Gynecol. **59**(1):33, 1982.

Johnson, M.L., and others: Evaluation of fetal intracranial anatomy by static and real-time ultrasound, J. Clin. Ultrasound **8:**311, 1980.

Keirse, M., Meerman, D., and Meerman, R.H.: Antenatal diagnosis of Potter syndrome, Obstet. Gynecol. **52**(1):64S, 1978.

King, D.L.: Placental migration demonstrated by ultrasonography, Radiology **109:**167, 1973.

Kossoff, G., and Garrett, W.J.: Intracranial detail in fetal echograms, Invest. Radiol. **7:**159, 1972.

Martin, J.D., and others: Urinary oestrogen excretion in women with intra-uterine fetal growth retardation, Aust. N.Z.J. Obstet. Gynaec. **12:**102, 1972.

McGahan, J.P., and others: Sonographic spectrum of retroplacental hemorrhage, Radiology **142:**481, 1982.

Meire, H.B.: Diagnosis of renal agenesis using ultrasonography, Br. J. Radiol. **53:**381, 1980.

O'Brien, G.D., Queenan, J.T., and Campbell, S.: Assessment of gestational age in the second trimester by real-time ultrasound measurement of the femur length, Am. J. Obstet. Gynecol. **139:**540, 1981.

Platt, L.D., and Manning, F.A.: Real-time ultrasound in special procedures. In Hobbins J.C., editor: Diagnostic ultrasound in obstetrics, New York, 1979, Churchill Livingstone.

Queenan, J.T., and Kubarych, S.F.: Detecting and managing polyhydramnios, Contemp. Ob/Gyn **16:**113, 1980.

Spirt, B.A., Cohen, W.N., and Weinstein, H.M.: The incidence of placental calcification in normal pregnancies, Radiolgy **142:**707, 1982.

CHAPTER 9 # Estimation of the placental function and reserve

PART ONE
Fetal heart rate monitoring

Electronic fetal heart rate (FHR) monitoring during labor has been practiced commonly in the United States for almost 10 years. The principle involves continuous instantaneous beat-to-beat FHR recording on one channel of a two-channel recorder with simultaneous recording of uterine activity on the other channel. The original and still most effective method involves a direct fetal scalp electrode application after membranes have ruptured to provide a fetal ECG complex for counting the heart rate. The uterine activity is measured directly by a transvaginal uterine catheter hooked to a strain gauge. External techniques for heart rate monitoring are less accurate but allow recording when membranes are intact or the fetal presenting part is not accessible. The methods include phonocardiography, Doppler ultrasound technique, and abdominal fetal electrocardiography. The Doppler technique is the only indirect external method that currently works adequately for labor monitoring. Uterine activity is measured by a tocodynamometer from the mother's abdominal wall when external uterine activity recording is desired. This gives only qualitative information about the frequency and duration of contractions and does not provide quantitative data on the amplitude of contractions.

This section is designed to acquaint pediatricians and neonatologists with an overview of this technique in order to familiarize them with principles and terminology involved in the interpretation of FHR data that may be important in their evaluation of the neonate.

BASELINE FETAL HEART RATE

The average FHR between periodic changes is referred to as the baseline FHR. Generally one needs to observe a tracing for 20 minutes or more to establish the true baseline FHR, especially if there are frequent periodic changes occurring. The baseline heart rate normal range is usually considered to be between 120 and 160 beats per minute (Fig. 9-1). However, when the baseline heart rate is outside this so-called range, one must consider the possibilities for the causes of this deviation, since often it does not represent any intrinsic fetal problem. When the baseline FHR rises, it is referred to as tachycardia, either relative or absolute. When the baseline FHR is low, it is referred to as bradycardia, either absolute or relative. Later, when we talk about periodic changes, we refer to accelerations and decelerations. It is important to use this terminology.

Fetal tachycardia is most commonly caused by maternal fever and is a normal fetal response to hyperthermia (Fig. 9-2). Sometimes fetal tachycardia will be seen even before the mother becomes febrile, as in chorioamnionitis. Certain drugs will also cause the FHR to rise. These include parasympatholytic agents such as atropine, sympathomimetic agents such as ritodrine, and other drugs that may decrease uterine blood flow, producing fetal hypoxia and secondary tachycardia. Rarely one sees a patient who is pregnant and has hyperthyroidism; in a small percentage of these patients there will be fetal tachycardia, perhaps due to the presence of LATS, which crosses the placenta, whereas T_4 and T_3 do not cross sufficiently to produce fetal tachycardia.

The most significant cause of fetal tachycardia is fetal hypoxia. The mechanism probably represents β-adrenergic activity stimulated by the hypoxemia itself. It is usually seen following a hypoxic episode and often is part of the recovery process (Fig. 9-3). Sometimes, however, tachycardia will be seen during a more gradual onset of fetal hypoxemia and may even precede the development of late deceleration. For the clinician, a rising baseline FHR may signify developing or recovering hypoxemia in the fetus as well as maternal fever, drug effects, or hyperthyroidism in the mother. It is therefore a nonspecific

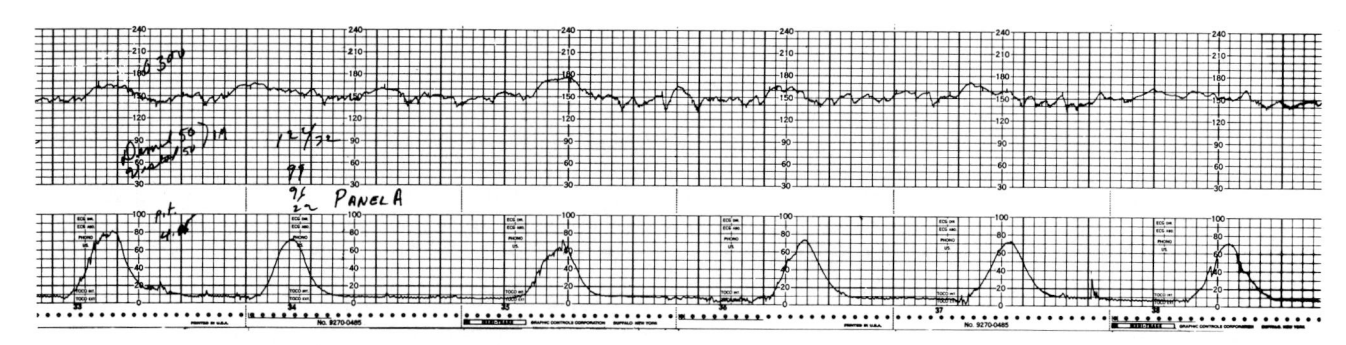

96 Behrman's neonatal-perinatal medicine: diseases of the fetus and infant

Fig. 9-1. Normal FHR pattern. (From Freeman, R., and Garite, T.: Fetal heart rate monitoring, Baltimore. Copyright 1981, The Williams & Wilkins Company. Reproduced by permission.)

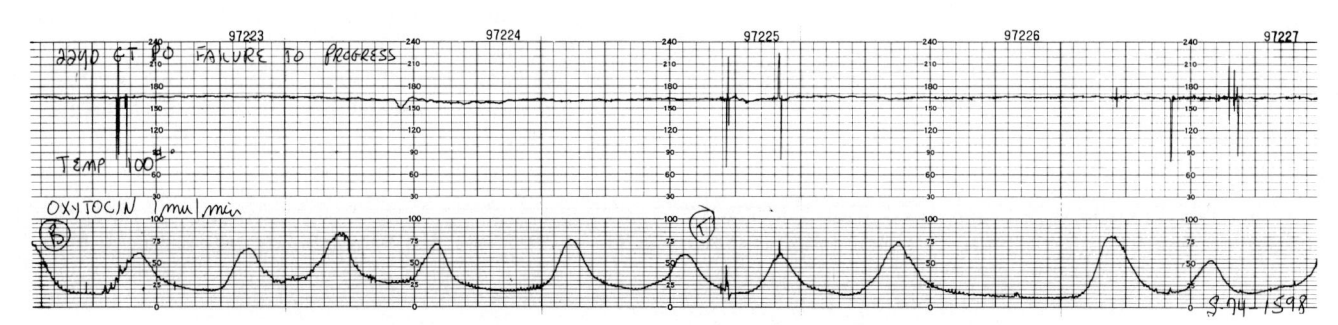

Fig. 9-2. Fetal tachycardia; fetal heart rate 165 beats per minute. This tachycardia is associated with maternal fever (note temperature). Also note the associated loss of variability. The absence of associated decelerations and presence of an explanation (fever) makes hypoxia an unlikely cause. (From Freeman, R., and Garite, T.: Fetal heart rate monitoring, Baltimore. Copyright 1981, The Williams & Wilkins Company. Reproduced by permission.)

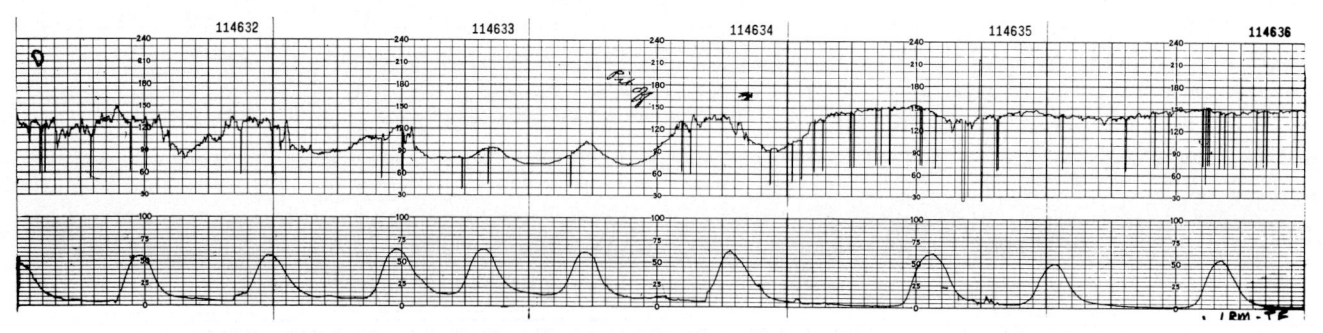

Fig. 9-3. Late deceleration associated with uterine hyperstimulation with oxytocin. Note compensatory relative fetal tachycardia developing as recovery occurs. (From Freeman, R., and Garite, T.: Fetal heart rate monitoring, Baltimore. Copyright 1981, The Williams & Wilkins Company. Reproduced by permission.)

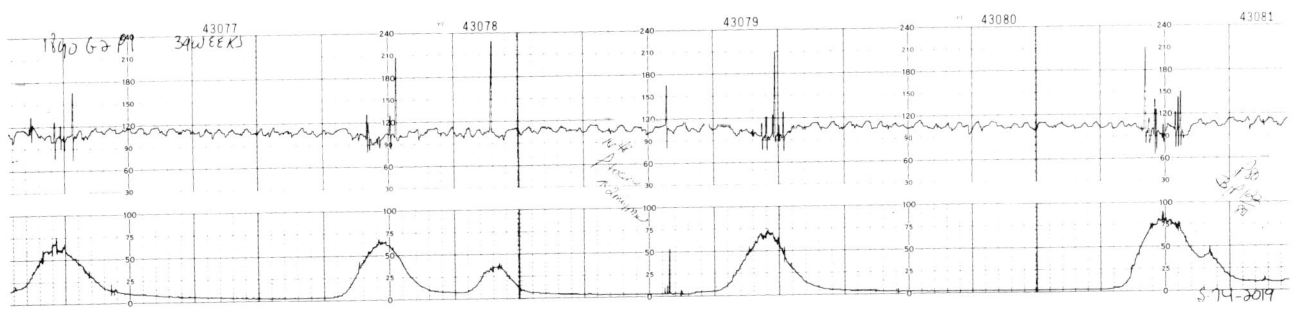

Fig. 9-4. Fetal bradycardia. The heart rate is 110. There is normal variability present by direct (internal scalp electrode) monitoring. Four hours later, the patient delivered a 3,025-gm baby with Apgar scores of 9 at 1 minute and 10 at 5 minutes. Mother and baby did well. (From Freeman, R., and Garite, T.: Fetal heart rate monitoring, Baltimore. Copyright 1981, The Williams & Wilkins Company. Reproduced by permission.)

change that should be interpreted along with other clinical information available as well as other aspects of the FHR tracing.

Very rarely a fetus may be noted to have an FHR in the range of 220 to 300 beats per minute. This probably represents supraventricular tachycardia that may be either paroxysmal or constant. Such fetuses are at great risk for death in utero. Although maternal digitalization may be helpful for the fetus, we have not had great success with this approach. Death appears to be due to fetal heart failure, since the fetuses are hydropic. It is therefore recommended to deliver such fetuses if there is evidence of lung maturity; if not, we follow them with serial sonograms, looking for fetal ascites, placental thickening, and fetal edema. If the fetus begins to become hydropic, it would seem best to deliver even in the absence of confirmed fetal lung maturity.

Fetal bradycardia was originally thought to be a sign of fetal hypoxemia. However, except in preterminal situations where the FHR has previously been higher and there is no FHR variability, fetal bradycardia with good FHR variability is not a sign of fetal hypoxemia (Fig. 9-4). Many times a baseline FHR of 100 to 120 beats per minute may be just the normal heart rate.

The other characteristic of the baseline FHR is its variability. Recently most authorities have paid more attention to the FHR variability than was originally the case. FHR variability has two characteristics. The short-term FHR variability represents the actual beat-to-beat interval differences and can be appreciated only with direct fetal scalp ECG as a signal source because external Doppler methods are using an ultrasonic signal source that is not precise enough to allow this measurement to be made accurately. Long-term variability is defined as the fetal heart rate change that has a cyclicity of 3 to 6 per minute and is made up of FHR change that includes series of FHR changes in a positive or negative direction. There has been no satisfactory method developed to quantitate either the short- or the long-term variability in a clinically useful way, so we are forced to rely on our visual inspection of tracings for this interpretation (Figs. 9-5 and 9-6).

It is well known that when good long- and short-term variability are present, it is very unlikely that a fetus is suffering from significant hypoxemia at the time the recording is made. Conversely, I have never seen a fetus die that did not first lose its FHR variability. Unfortunately, there are many causes for loss of FHR variability that are not related to fetal asphyxia, and the loss of variability becomes a rather nonspecific warning sign. Clearly, in the face of periodic FHR changes suggesting fetal hypoxia (late deceleration or severe variable deceleration), the absence of FHR variability greatly increases the likelihood of poor outcome as indicated by Apgar score and/or fetal metabolic acidosis.

Causes for the loss of FHR variability include:
1. Narcotic drugs
2. Local anesthetics
3. Sedatives
4. Parasympatholytic drugs
5. β-Adrenergic blocking agents
6. Fetal sleep states
7. Fetal heart block
8. Fetal tachycardia from any cause
9. Fetal hypoxia

Recently it has become known that mild fetal hypoxia may be characterized by exaggerated FHR variability. The mechanism probably represents initial fetal chemoreceptor stimulation by hypoxemia, resulting in a reflex fetal adrenergic response causing fetal hypertension and fetal baroreceptor stimulation, resulting in a reflex vagal output. The end result is an increase in both parasympathetic and sympathetic tone and a general increase in FHR variability. Clinically these increases in FHR variability should only be a warning to keep a close eye on the tracing because at worst it signifies only transient

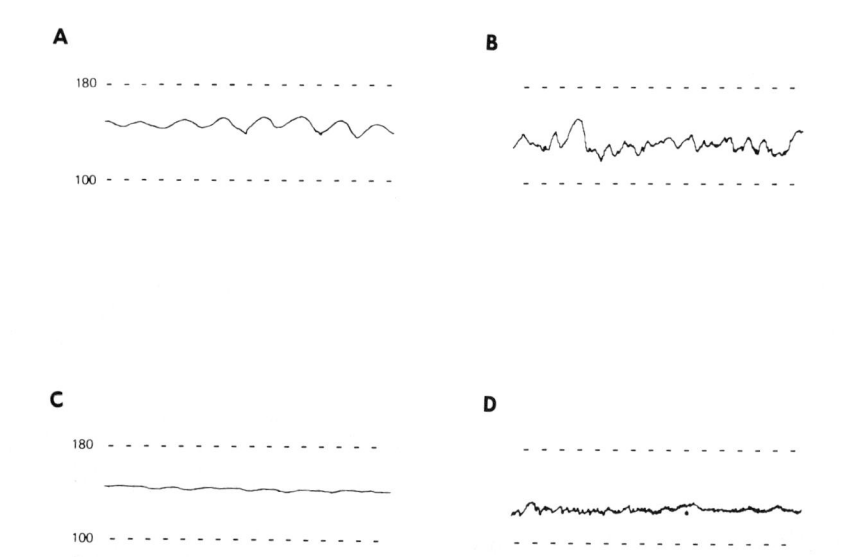

Fig. 9-5. Components of FHR variability for fetal ECG-derived FHR. **A,** Long-term without short-term variability. **B,** Long-term and short-term variability. **C,** No long-term and no short-term variability. **D,** Short-term without long-term variability. (From Zanani B., and others: Am. J. Obstet. Gynecol. **136**:43, 1980.)

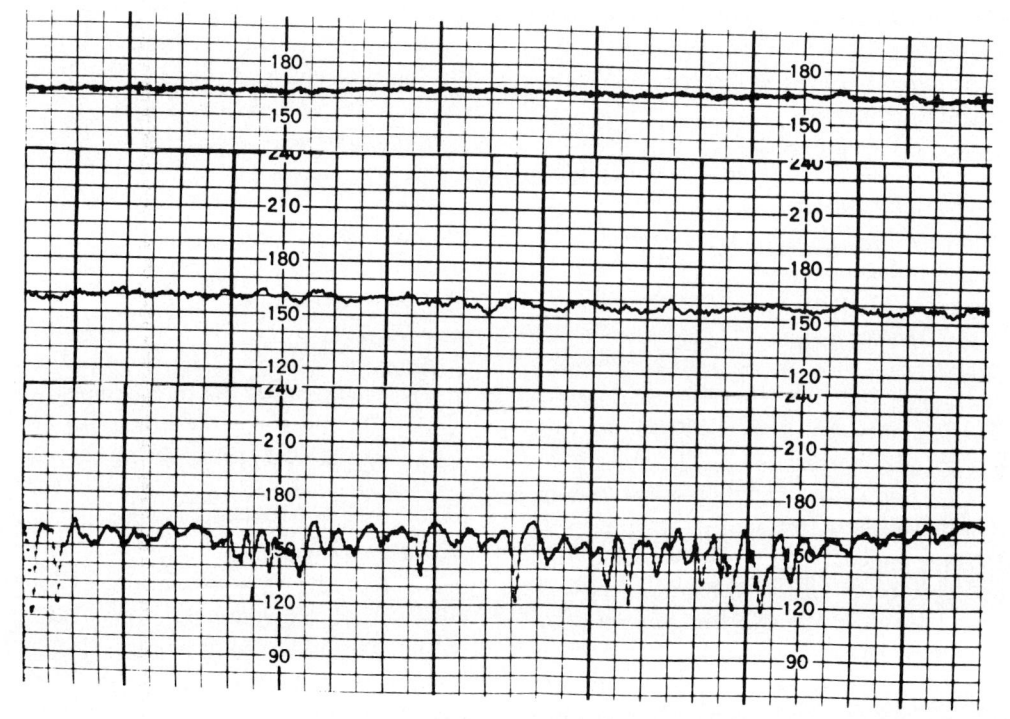

Fig. 9-6. Reduced FHR variability (top), average FHR variability (middle), and increased FHR variability (bottom).

mild hypoxemia. If the hypoxemia worsens or is longer standing, one would then expect to see the development of late deceleration and eventually the loss of variability and metabolic acidosis as the fetus becomes more hypoxic.

PERIODIC FHR CHANGES

Periodic FHR changes include accelerations and decelerations. They are usually related to some event such as a uterine contraction, an episode of fetal movement, external stimulation, or a form of compromise such as maternal hypotension or sudden hypoxemia.

Accelerations are frequently present during the antepartum period and are usually associated with measurable fetal movements (Fig. 9-7). Recent studies with real-time ultrasound reveal that, when fetal movements are not appreciated by the mother or the monitoring device at the time of FHR acceleration, fetal movements are almost always present even though not detectable by the usual methods. Hence the term *reactivity* (which has been used to refer to FHR acceleration in association with fetal movement) can probably be applied to any significant FHR acceleration, whether or not fetal movement is demonstrable. The magnitude of these accelerations, with respect to both amplitude and duration, has been shown to increase with advancing gestational age. The frequency of these episodes also increases with gestational age. Some require a duration of 15 seconds and an amplitude of 15 beats per minute in order to classify an episode of FHR acceleration as fetal reactivity. It would appear, however, that lesser magnitudes of acceleration may suffice at very early gestational ages. Usually these episodes of acceleration are present in groups over periods of 20 to 30 minutes, and then the fetal reactivity may cease or markedly decrease for similar periods of time. These cycles make it necessary to observe the FHR for sufficient time (30 to 60 minutes) to be sure that a fetus is indeed nonreactive. After labor has begun, fetal reactivity may continue or it may disappear without having ominous connotations. The accelerations associated with fetal movement have been referred to by some as nonuniform accelerations to distinguish them from those uniform appearing accelerations which are commonly associated with uterine contractions during labor.

The significance of fetal reactivity (acceleration with fetal movement) has been related to an association with fetal well-being prior to labor and forms the basis for the nonstress test. Indeed, the presence of fetal reactivity is extremely reassuring in demonstrating that the fetus is in good condition at the time of the recording, but it is not a good measure of the uteroplacental reserve. The absence of FHR accelerations (nonreactivity) may indicate that the fetus is indeed in jeopardy, or it may be related to drug therapy or often to fetal sleep states. The loss of fetal reactivity is the end point of the NST, and it should indicate the need for a stress test to determine the significance of this finding.

Accelerations appearing with uterine contractions (Fig. 9-8) are seen in 30% to 40% of patients at some time during labor. Accelerations with contractions have not been associated with fetal compromise as evidenced by fetal metabolic acidosis or low Apgar scores. Renou has shown that these accelerations are blocked by propranolol. Recently it has been suggested that these "uniform" accelerations associated with contractions may be caused by low-grade umbilical cord compression. The evidence for this is that, often as labor continues, these accelerations begin to dip in the center and may actually evolve into variable decelerations (Fig. 9-9). Accelerations are also seen more often in association with breech presentation where presumed umbilical cord entanglement is more common than with cephalic presentations. Recent studies have shown that with selective umbilical venous occlusion there is transient fetal hypotension resulting from the decreased venous return. There is then an FHR acceleration in response to the fetal hypotension. Since

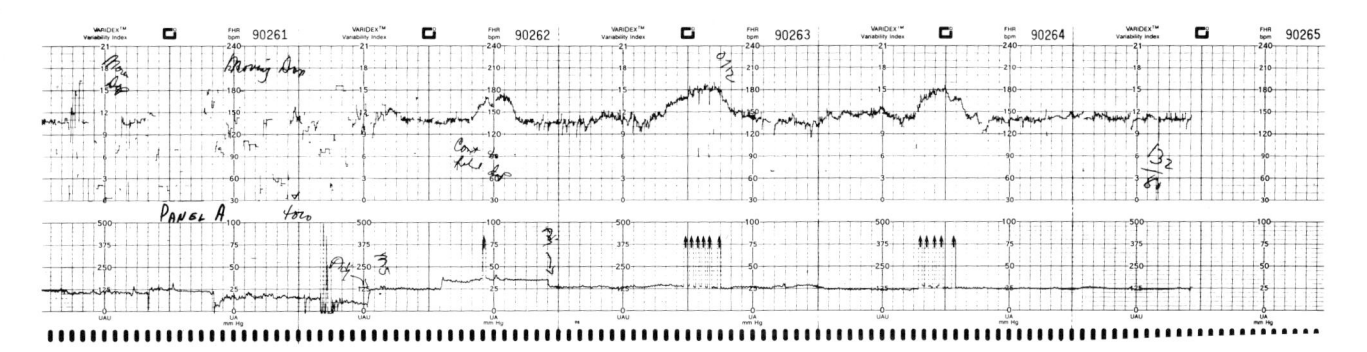

Fig. 9-7. Acceleration occurring with fetal movement, which is noted by arrows on contraction channel. (From Freeman, R., and Garite, T.: Fetal heart rate monitoring, Baltimore. Copyright 1981, The Williams & Wilkins Company. Reproduced by permission.)

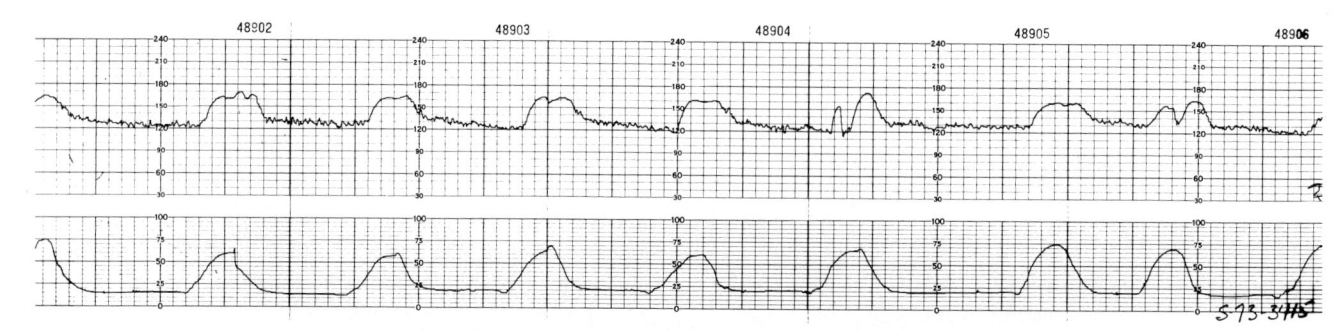

Fig. 9-8. Accelerations of the fetal heart rate are seen with each contraction. Baseline heart rate and variability are normal. Such a pattern is reassuring. (From Freeman, R., and Garite, T.: Fetal heart rate monitoring, Baltimore. Copyright 1981, The Williams & Wilkins Company. Reproduced by permission.)

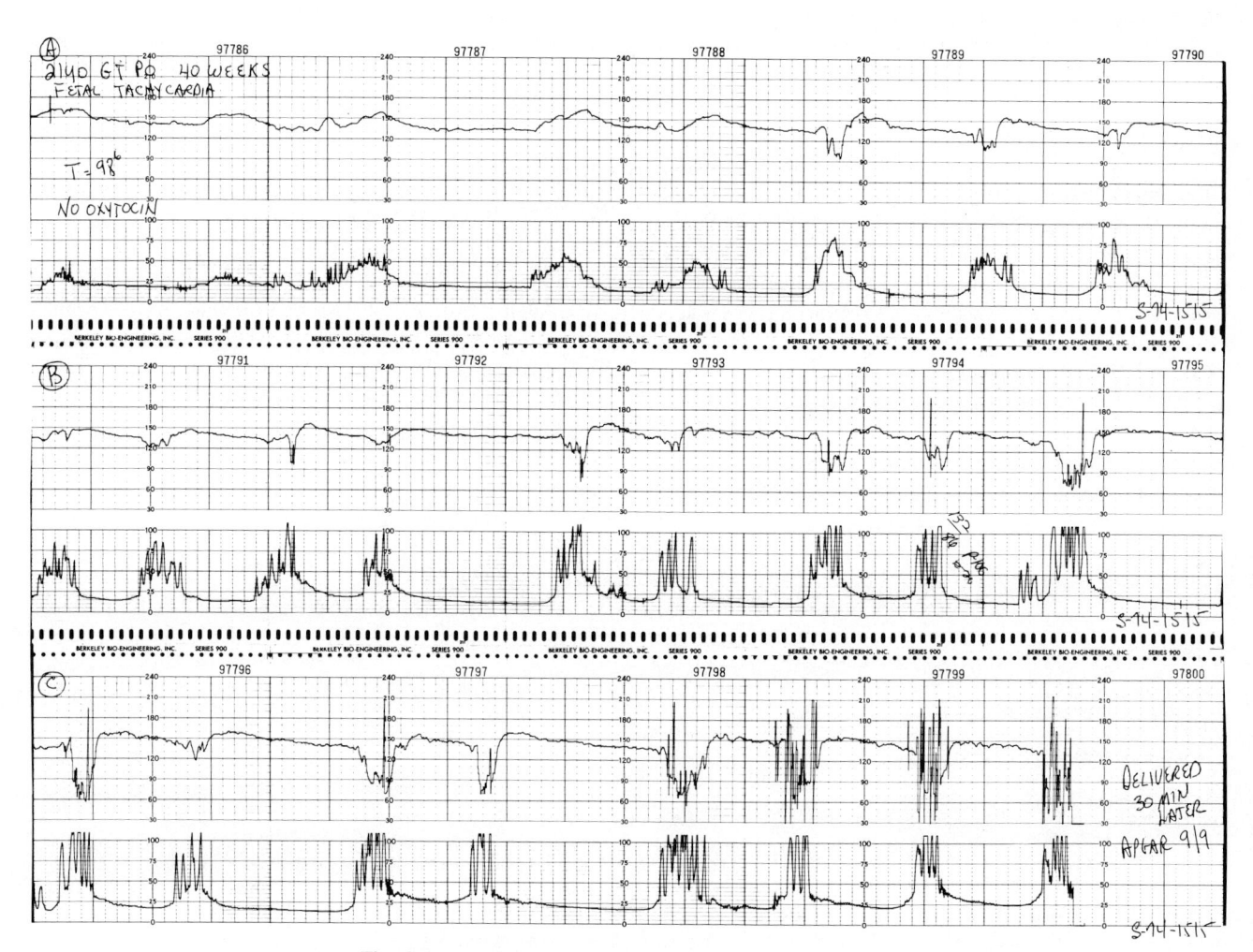

Fig. 9-9. Acceleration leading to variable deceleration.

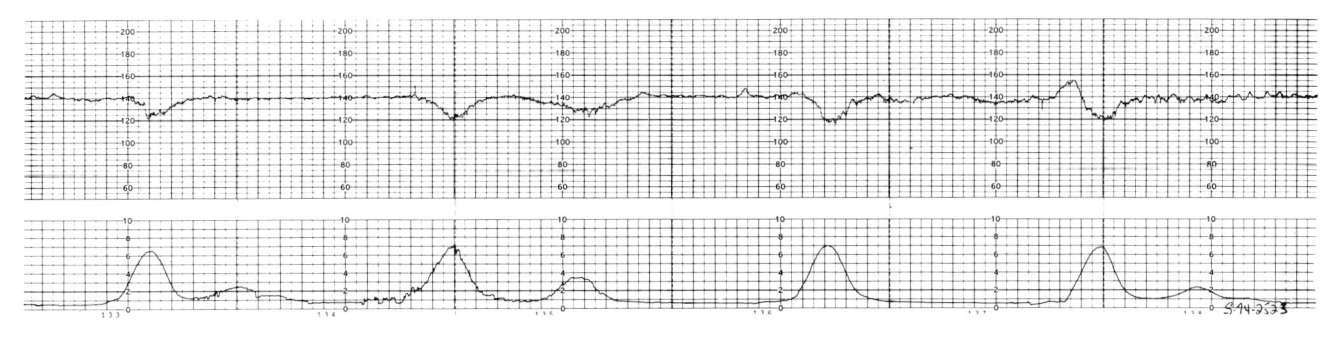

Fig. 9-10. Early decelerations are seen with each contraction on this panel. They are uniform, mirror the contractions, and decelerate only 10 to 20 beats per minute. (From Freeman, R., and Garite, T.: Fetal heart rate monitoring, Baltimore. Copyright 1981, The Williams & Wilkins Company. Reproduced by permission.)

the umbilical vein has a lower internal pressure than the umbilical artery, it would stand to reason that mild cord compression may result in selective venous occlusion and the appearance of acceleration. Whether the underlying cause for all accelerations with contractions is umbilical venous compression certainly cannot be proved, but the explanation is plausible, and there is some experimental animal work to support the explanation. This also opens the possibility that nonuniform acceleration seen with fetal movement (reactivity) during the antepartum period may sometimes be related to mild umbilical cord compression associated with fetal movement. Clinically the important aspect of acceleration is that it is in all instances a healthy fetal response, never representing fetal compromise, and, whether indicating mild umbilical cord compression or not, it is reassuring to the clinician.

FHR deceleration patterns have best been described by Hon. They consist of three basic responses to uterine contractions. Early deceleration is ascribed to fetal head compression, variable deceleration is ascribed to umbilical cord occlusion, and late deceleration has been felt to be caused by uteroplacental insufficiency. These three patterns have now been well studied, and the underlying physiologic mechanisms are reasonably well understood.

Early deceleration is characterized as a uniform pattern with gradual onset and gradual offset, resembling a mirror image of the uterine contraction (Fig. 9-10). It tends to be uniform in shape from one contraction to the next and tends to parallel the amplitude of the contraction, with higher amplitude contractions eliciting deeper decelerations and lower amplitude contractions eliciting more shallow decelerations. The deceleration begins early in the contraction, peaks simultaneously with the nadir of the contraction, and returns to baseline during the decline of the contraction so that the FHR is back to baseline by the time uterine activity is back to baseline. The baseline FHR is usually in the normal range, and the FHR variability is most often normal. The FHR deceleration is quite shallow, and seldom does it drop below 120 beats per minute.

Clinically, early deceleration is usually seen between about 4 and 7 cm dilatation. Hon has shown that this corresponds to the time that the edge of the cervix is crossing the anterior fontanel, and he has reproduced this in neonates by exerting pressure with doughnut pessaries from 4 to 7 cm over the fetal vertex. Since the anterior fontanel is the area most vulnerable to external pressure that may affect cerebrovascular hemodynamics, this clinical observation fits well with the physiologic studies of Quilligan, showing that the mechanism for early deceleration appears to be central vagal stimulation caused by altered cerebral blood flow. The vagus then causes the heart rate to slow in direct proportion to the pressure being exerted on the anterior fontanel, resulting in the uniform pattern previously described. Both animal and human studies have shown that this pattern is blocked or markedly altered by the administration of atropine, thus confirming the vagal reflex nature of the early deceleration pattern.

Clinically the importance of this pattern relates to its similarity in appearance to late deceleration. Early deceleration is associated with normal fetal pH, normal Apgar scores, and no other evidence of fetal compromise. To the clinician it is a reassuring FHR pattern and should not indicate any form of intervention.

Variable deceleration is the most common FHR deceleration pattern seen during labor (Fig. 9-11). It is observed at some time in over 50% of labors, it is more commonly seen after rupture of membranes, and it is especially common during the second stage of labor.

The pattern of variable deceleration is characterized by a rapid and profound descent of the FHR to levels that are usually well below 120, often 60, beats per minute. The duration, shape, and timing of the pattern are non-

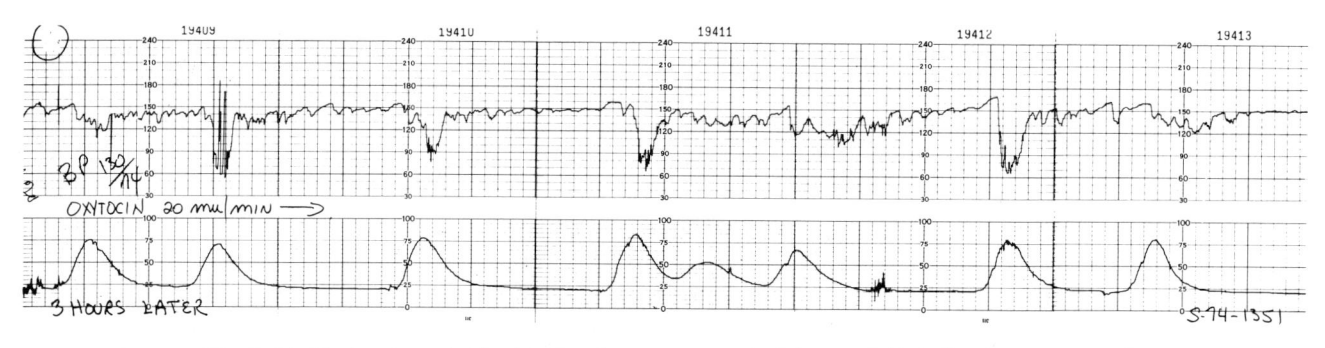

Fig. 9-11. Moderate variable decelerations are seen in this panel. Baseline heart rate and variability are normal. (From Freeman, R., and Garite, T.: Fetal heart rate monitoring, Baltimore. Copyright 1981, The Williams & Wilkins Company. Reproduced by permission.)

uniform, hence the name *variable deceleration*. It is often associated with acceleration preceding the development of this pattern, and after the variable deceleration again another acceleration, referred to by some as "shoulders."

The mechanism of variable deceleration is believed to be umbilical cord compression, with the acceleration portion described previously representing umbilical venous occlusion and the variable deceleration itself being due to additional compression of the umbilical arteries. Physiologically, it is believed that, when the umbilical arteries are occluded, there is a sudden and rapid fetal hypertension resulting from the cutoff of the low-resistance placental circuit. This brings forth a baroreceptor response, resulting in a vagal FHR deceleration. Indeed, it has been shown that atropine will alter this response, and Barcroft showed many years ago that sectioning the vagal nerve in exteriorized fetal goats caused a delay in the deceleration resulting from umbilical cord occlusion. It would therefore appear that the FHR deceleration associated with umbilical cord compression is vagally mediated, but if the occlusion is prolonged and severe, the deceleration is of a hypoxic nature, probably due to fetal myocardial depression.

During variable deceleration there may be a rapid decline in the fetal Po_2, a rapid rise in the fetal Pco_2, and a concomitant fall in the fetal pH. This transient fetal hypoxemia and respiratory acidosis are reversed as soon as the umbilical artery is released and circulation is restored to the intact placenta, where gas exchange and equilibration are rapid. However, if cord compression is prolonged or severe or if there is reduced placental function due to some other cause, such as abruptio placentae or maternal hypertensive vascular disease, the hypoxemia and respiratory acidosis may not be rapidly corrected, and the fetus may become significantly hypoxic with resultant fetal anaerobic metabolic production of lactic acid. This will, of course, be manifested by an accumulating base deficit and a corresponding metabolic acidosis. When this occurs, there will also usually be a rise in the baseline FHR, a reduction in the FHR variability, and a slow return of the variable deceleration to the baseline, representing the above-described myocardial depression seen in the hypoxic phase of severe variable deceleration.

The clinical implications of these acid-base and FHR changes are related to the role of fetal scalp blood sampling and the interpretation of the FHR changes with respect to fetal compromise. Since most all variable decelerations are associated with fetal respiratory acidosis, it becomes important to determine either the Pco_2 or the base deficit when variable deceleration is present, especially if the timing of the fetal scalp sample is during the deceleration. Clearly, it is best to sample between contractions in such instances. We have not found scalp sampling to be of great help in the management of variable deceleration because the pattern is quite unpredictable from one contraction to the next, and a normal pH 5 minutes previously may not be beneficial when the pattern suddenly deteriorates. For this reason we manage severe variable deceleration patterns strictly on the basis of the FHR change.

For clinical purposes we have set the following criteria as describing variable decelerations that may be regarded as reassuring and, other than attempts at position change, do not demand any intervention:

1. The variable deceleration should not be below 80 beats per minute for more than 45 seconds.
2. The baseline FHR should not be rising.
3. The baseline FHR variability should not be decreasing.
4. The return to baseline should be abrupt.

With these guidelines in mind, one should then look at the clinical situation to determine appropriate intervention if the situation warrants it. For example, often during the second stage of labor variable decelerations get progressively more prolonged and may actually exceed 60 or 70 seconds (Fig. 9-12). This is because, with the

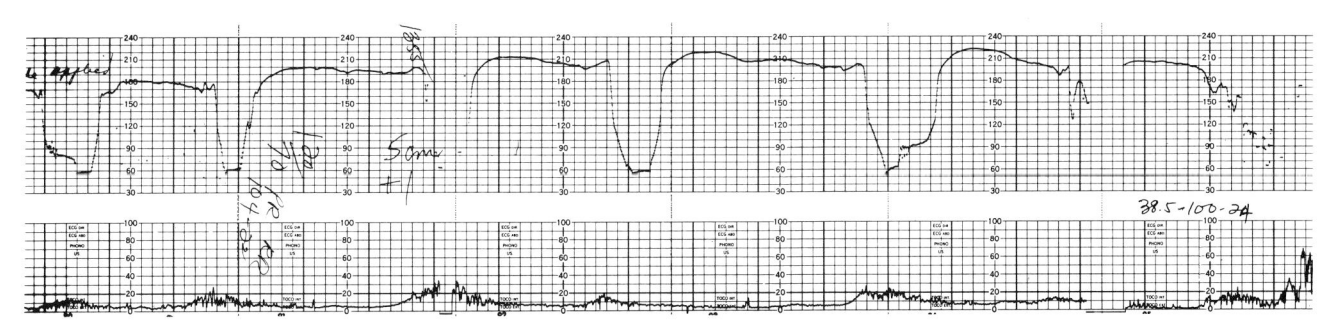

Fig. 9-12. Severe ominous variable decelerations are seen with rising baseline heart rate to 210 beat per minute and virtually absent variability. A premature baby was delivered by cesarean section with Apgar scores of 1 at 1 minute and 2 at 5 minutes. (From Freeman, R., and Garite, T.: Fetal heart rate monitoring, Baltimore. Copyright 1981, The Williams & Wilkins Company. Reproduced by permission.)

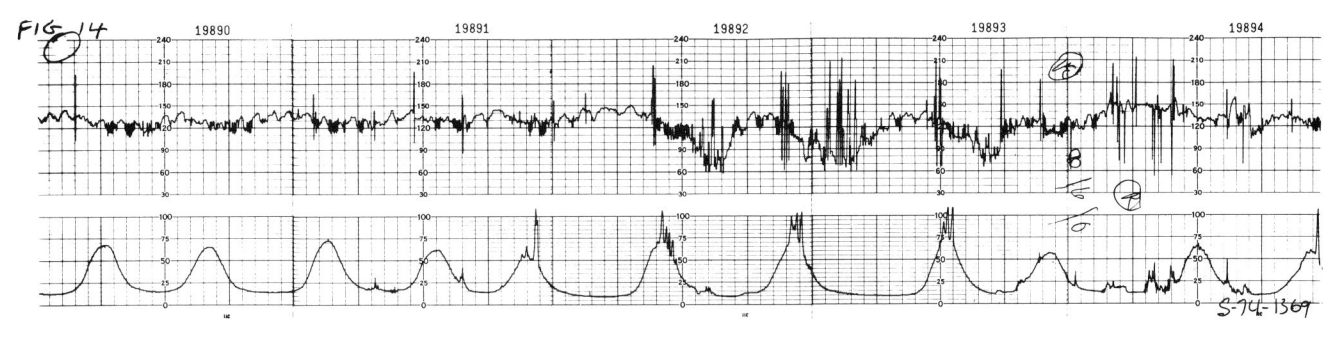

Fig. 9-13. Late deceleration with good variability. (From Freeman, R., and Garite, T.: Fetal heart rate monitoring, Baltimore. Copyright 1981, The Williams & Wilkins Company. Reproduced by permission.)

descent of the presenting part during the second stage, there is more compression of an entrapped cord, such as when it is around the fetal neck. At this point the baseline rate and variability may allow one to avoid intervention by midforceps delivery or cesarean section because these factors reflect the current condition of the fetus and its response to the cord occlusion. Also, one anticipates that, since the second stage of labor has been reached, the likelihood of a long period of continued prolonged variable decelerations is low. On the other hand, if variable decelerations are lasting 60 seconds and are not correctable with maternal position change in a patient early in the first stage of labor, the likelihood of achieving a vaginal delivery without significant fetal compromise would seem less, and a lower threshold for intervention may be justified.

Late deceleration must be regarded as nonreassuring under all circumstances. The pattern is characterized by its uniformity in shape and timing. Late deceleration usually begins at or soon after the peak of the uterine contraction. The onset is gradual, the nadir of the deceleration follows the nadir of the contraction, and the return to baseline is also gradual and follows the return of the contraction to the baseline (Fig. 9-13). The pattern tends to be related to the amplitude of the contraction, with larger amplitude contractions eliciting larger amplitude decelerations. Most often the deceleration does not go below 120 beats per minute, but it may. With persistence of late deceleration, it is common to see a rise in the baseline FHR and a decrease in the baseline FHR variability.

The physiologic mechanism of late deceleration has two components as described by Martin. With mild fetal hypoxemia there is chemoreceptor stimulation that results in an adrenergic fetal hypertensive response. This hypertension then causes a baroreceptor vagal reflex resulting in late deceleration. The delay in the deceleration is due to the lag in time for fetal hypoxemia to develop, since the uterine contraction decreases uterine blood flow. Most fetuses tolerate the contraction-induced decreased uterine blood flow without developing late deceleration, but, if the oxygen-transferring capacity of

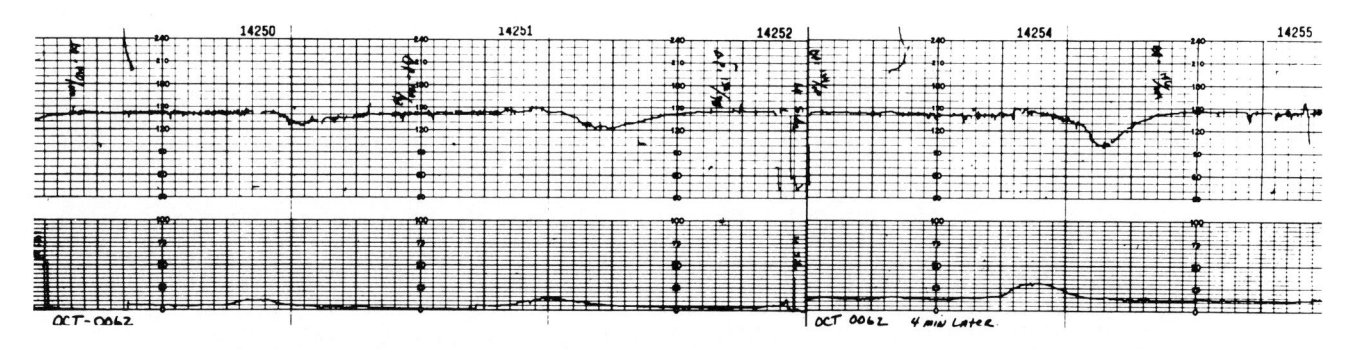

Fig. 9-14. Late deceleration with absent variability. (From Freeman, R., and Garite, T.: Fetal heart rate monitoring, Baltimore. Copyright 1981, The Williams & Wilkins Company. Reproduced by permission.)

the placenta is reduced, the fetus will develop a progressive oxygen debt with each episode of contraction-induced transient decrease in oxygen transfer. This late deceleration due to mild hypoxemia in the fetus is of reflex origin, as described, but when hypoxia becomes more severe, the fetus produces lactic acid as a result of the anaerobic metabolism of glucose, resulting in fetal metabolic acidosis, and it appears that at this point the late deceleration is no longer a simple vagal reflex but is caused by fetal myocardial depression (Fig. 9-14).

With fetal metabolic acidosis and myocardial depression, a reduction in FHR variability is seen and subsequently low Apgar scores. On the contrary, when persistent late deceleration is present with good variability, fetal metabolic acidosis is not usually present, and the neonates are usually not depressed at birth.

Clinically, the indicated course of management for late deceleration follows:
1. Turn mother on her side to maximize uterine blood flow.
2. Turn off any oxytocics to decrease uterine activity.
3. Administer oxygen with a tight face mask to raise the mother's Po_2 and increase the gradient of oxygen between the mother and fetus.
4. Correct any maternal hypotension, preferably by raising the legs, infusing IV fluids to restore volume, and changing position to take uterine pressure off the vena cava and aortoiliac vessels. Only as a last resort are pressor agents indicated, and ephedrine is currently the agent of choice.

Late deceleration appears to be a relatively early warning sign of fetal hypoxia and, when variability remains good, there may be a role for serial fetal scalp blood sampling for pH with the avoidance of operative intervention, as long as the pH is normal (above 7.25) and there is not a downward trend. This approach requires sampling at least every 30 minutes as long as the pattern persists. Most authorities would not recommend fetal scalp blood sampling when the variability of the FHR is reduced or there is significant tachycardia not due to maternal fever or drugs. In this situation expeditious operative intervention is indicated. Clearly, depending on the logistics of the obstetric service, to follow the serial scalp sampling routine just described, one must act rapidly after deciding to intervene, and, if this is not the case, to opt for intervention without scalp sampling even when good variability is present.

OTHER OMINOUS PATTERNS

Prolonged decelerations may occur de novo. They are usually believed to be due to sudden profound and prolonged umbilical cord compression and in such cases may be quite ominous. When there is no obvious cause, one must assume this mechanism and, if the deceleration lasts several minutes and recovers, it may be reasonable to watch it very closely. If the pattern recurs, we advise immediate intervention. Many prolonged decelerations, however, are due to identifiable causes such as:
1. Tetanic uterine contraction (Fig. 9-15)
2. Paracervical block
3. Hypotension following conduction anesthesia
4. Direct stimulation from a vaginal examination or when applying a fetal scalp electrode
5. Prolapsed cord (Fig. 9-16)

If the prolonged deceleration occurs with one of the above, the management is dictated by the cause, with intervention for delivery only being indicated with the prolasped cord, whereas the other causes are usually self-limited and would not warrant delivery.

Occasionally a flat FHR with complete absence of variability and no periodic changes is seen (Fig. 9-17). This pattern cannot be interpreted, and one must realize that this could be a profoundly hypoxic fetus with a fixed heart rate that no longer responds to any stimulus. However, in our experience most of these fetuses have normal pH and some will behave normally postnatally. Others will show signs of brain damage that probably occurred at some previous time, and the pH is now nor-

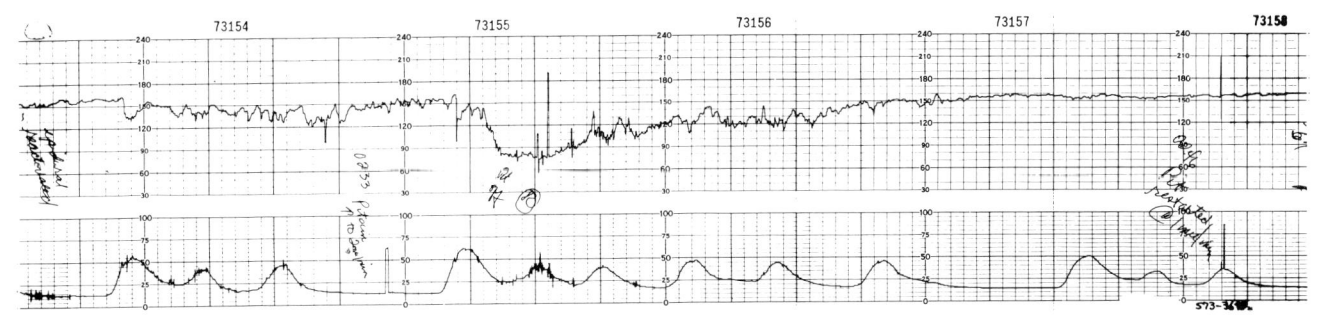

Fig. 9-15. Here a prolonged deceleration is seen associated with excessive uterine activity secondary to oxytocin hyperstimulation. Again, a rebound tachycardia with decreased variability follows the prolonged deceleration. Pitocin was stopped and restarted at a lower rate, and the heart rate subsequently returned to normal. (From Freeman, R., and Garite, T.: Fetal heart rate monitoring, Baltimore. Copyright 1981, The Williams & Wilkins Company. Reproduced by permission.)

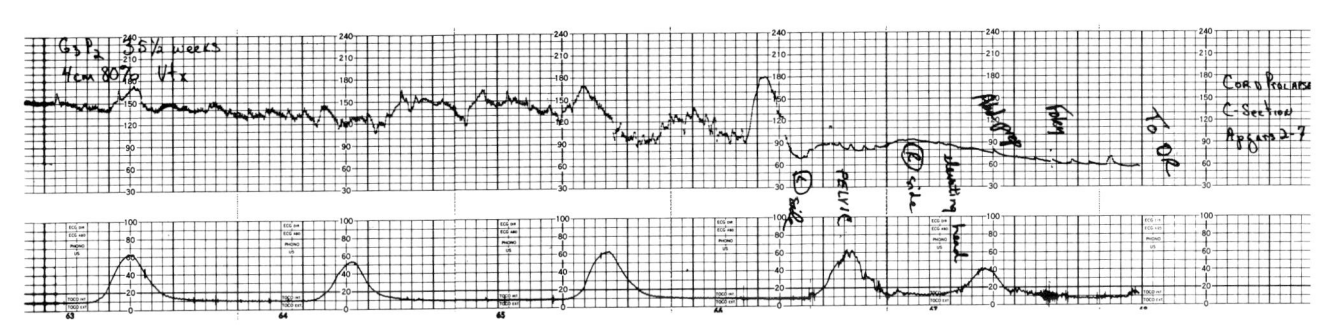

Fig. 9-16. A sudden prolonged deceleration is seen in this patient in the early active phase of labor. Immediate pelvic examination revealed cord prolapse, and cesarean section was performed. (From Freeman, R., and Garite, T.: Fetal heart rate monitoring, Baltimore. Copyright 1981, The Williams & Wilkins Company. Reproduced by permission.)

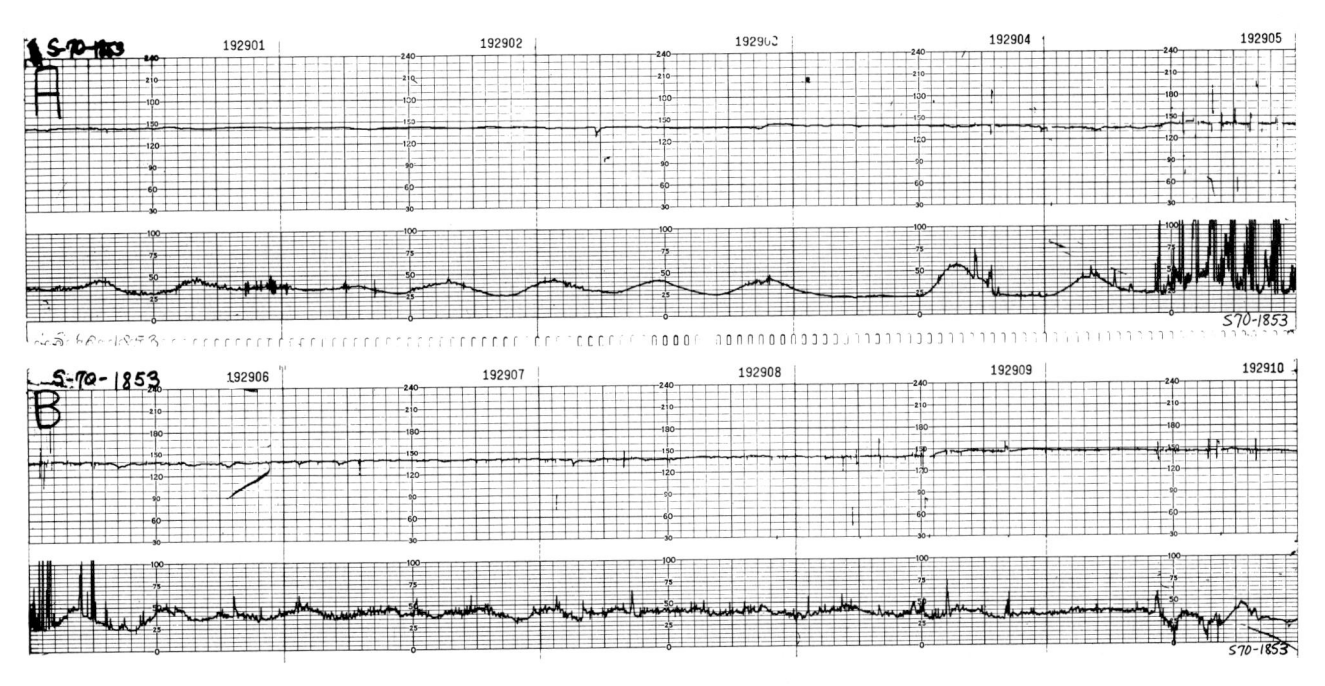

Fig. 9-17. Complete absence of FHR variability without any decelerations. (From Freeman, R., and Garite, T.: Fetal heart rate monitoring, Baltimore. Copyright 1981, The Williams & Wilkins Company. Reproduced by permission.)

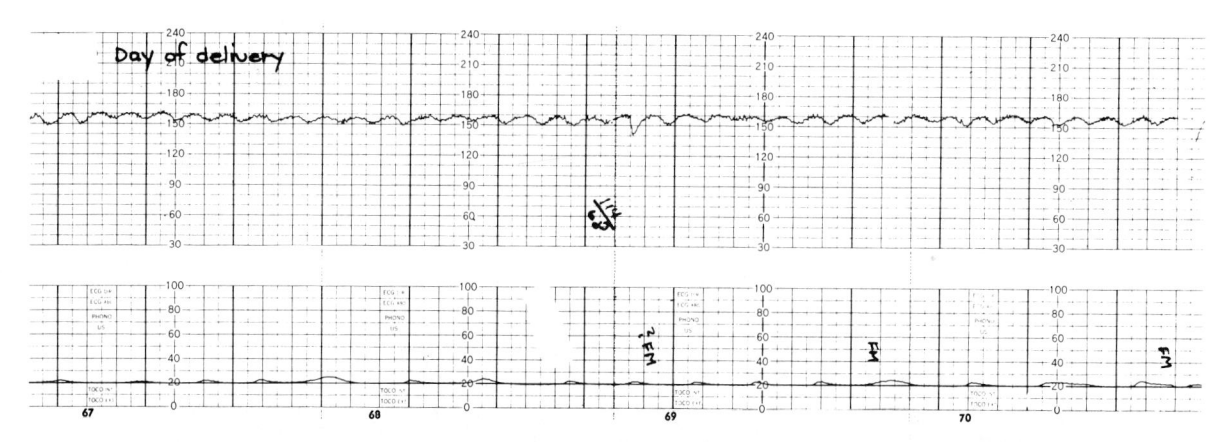

Fig. 9-18. Sinusoidal FHR pattern in patient with fetal hydrops from Rh sensitization. (From Freeman, R., and Garite, T.: Fetal heart rate monitoring, Baltimore. Copyright 1981, The Williams & Wilkins Company. Reproduced by permission.)

mal. The flat heart rate may also be due to a cardiac or CNS anomaly where fetal oxygenation is normal. This pattern of absent variability without periodic changes with a normal pH does not demand intervention. If the pH is low, we recommend expeditious delivery, recognizing that CNS damage may have already occurred.

Sinusoidal FHR patterns are very rare. They are characterized by no short-term variability and a uniform oscillation resembling a sine wave (Fig. 9-18). Many patterns have been mistaken for this rare finding because the observers did not look for absent short-term variability. In addition, if there is normal heart rate preceding and/or following the pattern in question, we do not consider this an ominous sinusoidal pattern. Classically this pattern was first described in association with severe fetal anemia in hydropic Rh-sensitized fetuses. More recently it has also been seen with fetal anemia caused by fetomaternal transfusion and with intrapartum hypoxia. All these conditions are obviously ominous. However, recently the pattern has been seen following the administration of alphaprodine analgesia by the intravenous route, lasting about 20 minutes and not being associated with poor fetal outcome. One Rh-sensitized patient had a sinusoidal pattern that persisted in the neonate despite adequate oxygenation but disappeared following exchange transfusion. The actual mechanism of this pattern remains obscure.

THE BENEFIT OF FETAL MONITORING

Recently there has been a great deal of discussion about the risks and benefits of electronic FHR monitoring (EFM). Critics have said that the method does not improve outcome but does increase the cesarean section rate. As one looks critically at this new technology it becomes apparent that there have been insufficient prospective randomized studies to answer this question. However, there are adequate numbers in retrospective studies that clearly point to the benefit of EFM with respect to intrapartum fetal death, neonatal death, and low Apgar score. Clearly there does appear to be an increase in the cesarean section rate that has been temporally related to the increased use of EFM. It appears, however, that the contribution of EFM to this increased cesarean section rate is small, and most of the increase is related to other factors, such as performing a section for most breech presentations, giving up difficult midforceps operations, and intervening on premature babies with malpresentations or fetal distress who would not have been considered salvageable previously.

The NIH consensus report of 1979 suggested that the low-risk patient may not need EFM if guaranteed auscultatory surveillance is available every 15 minutes during the first stage of labor and every 5 minutes during the second stage. Most hospitals try to provide this level of coverage, but too often other duties do not allow the labor room nurse to guarantee this type of surveillance. At Memorial Hospital we monitor all patients electronically during labor and have only had one fetal death in 15,000 deliveries that was not considered hopeless because of extreme prematurity. In that one case, clear EFM evidence of fetal distress was present but was not recognized.

In conclusion, EFM appears to be a useful tool if properly applied and interpreted in a setting where appropriate timely intervention is available. With experience, most labor nurses and obstetricians can avoid the unexpected compromised fetus, and it would appear that neonatologists and pediatricians caring for infants today have a better chance with many of them because of what this technology has allowed obstetricians to do for the fetus.

Roger K. Freeman

BIBLIOGRAPHY

Antenatal diagnosis, U.S. Department of Health, Education, and Welfare, Public Health Service, National Institute of Health Publication No. 79-1973, April, 1979.

Barcroft, J.: Researches on prenatal life, Oxford, England, 1946, Blackwell Scientific Publications, Inc.

Baskett, T.F., and Koh, K.S: Sinusoidal fetal heart pattern: a sign of fetal hypoxia, Obstet. Gynecol. **44**:379, 1974.

Bottoms, S., Rosen, M., and Sokol, J.: The increase in the cesarean birth rate, N. Engl. J. Med. **302**:559, 1980.

Druzen, M., and others: A possible mechanism for the increase in FHR variability following hypoxemia. Presented at the twenty-sixth annual meeting of the Society for Gynecological Investigation, San Diego, Calif., March 23, 1979.

Elliott, J.P., and others: The significance of fetal and neonatal sinusoidal heart rate pattern: further clinical observations in Rh incompatibility, Am. J. Obstet. Gynecol. **138**:227, 1980.

Gray, J.H., and others: Sinusoidal fetal heart rate pattern associated with alphaprodine administration, Obstet. Gynecol. **52**:678, 1978.

Hon, E.H., Bradfield, A.H., and Hess, O.W.: The electronic evaluation of the fetal heart rate. V. The vagal factor in fetal bradycardia, Am. J. Obstet. Gynecol. **82**:291, 1961.

Hon, E.H., and Quilligan, E.J.: Classification of fetal heart rate. II. A revised working classification, Conn. Med. **33**:779, 1967.

James, L.S., and others: Umbilical vein occlusion and transient acceleration of the fetal heart rate: experimental observations in subhuman primates, Am. J. Obstet. Gynecol. **126**:276, 1976.

Klein, A., Holzman, I., and Austin, E.: Fetal tachycardia prior to the development of hydrops. Attempted pharmacologic cardioversion: case report, Am. J. Obstet. Gynecol. **134**:347, 1979.

Lee, C.V., Di Loreto, P.C., and O'Lane, J.M.: A study of fetal heart rate acceleration patterns, Obstet. Gynecol. **45**:142, 1975.

Martin, C.B., and others: Mechanisms of late deceleration in the fetal heart rate: a study of autonomic blocking agents in fetal lambs, Eur. J. Obstet. Gynecol. Reprod. Biol. **9**:361, 1979.

Modanlou, H., and others: Sinusoidal fetal heart rate pattern and severe fetal anemia, Obstet. Gynecol. **49**:537, 1977.

Neutra, R., Greenland, S., and Friedman, E.: The effect of fetal monitoring on Cesarean-section rate, Obstet. Gynecol. **55**:2, 197, 1980.

Paul, W.M., Quilligan, E.J., and MacLachlan, T.: Cardiovascular phenomena associated with fetal head compression, Am. J. Obstet. Gynecol. **90**:824, 1964.

Paul, R.H., and others: Clinical fetal monitoring. VII. the evaluation and significance of intrapartum baseline FHR variability, Am. J. Obstet. Gynecol. **123**:206, 1975.

Platt, L., and others: Antepartum detection of fetal A-V dissociation utilizing real time B-mode ultrasound, Obstet. Gynecol. **53**:595, 1979.

Renou, P., Warwick, N., and Wood, C.: Autonomic control of fetal heart rate, Am. J. Obstet. Gynecol. **105**:949, 1969.

Schifferli, P., and Caldeyro-Barcia, R.: Effects of atropine and beta adrenergic drugs on the heart rate of the human fetus. In Boreus, L., editor: Fetal pharmacology, New York, 1973, Raven Press.

PART TWO

Antepartum fetal assessment

The obstetrician is the only primary physician with the responsibility of caring for two patients, the mother and the fetus. Major life-affecting decisions that preclude direct communication with or examination of one of these patients (the fetus) are necessary, and situations exist where the interest of one patient may have to be compromised in the interests of the other. For example, in severe preeclampsia the fetus may have to be delivered prematurely, with its attendant risks, to halt the progression of maternal illness and associated complications. Similarly, with rupture of membranes early in the third trimester or in a premature breech, the mother may be exposed to the risks of infection on one hand or to operative intervention on the other to minimize risks to the neonate.

In the past, traditional methods of fetal evaluation were limited to auscultation of the fetal heart rate, clinical observation of fetal size and growth, and crude estimation of fetal activity based on maternal perception of fetal movement. Only recently has additional information regarding fetal health been obtained. It is the purpose of this section to discuss newer methods of physiologic and biochemical fetal assessment and to relate how this information is used in clinical patient care. Sonographic assessment of fetal growth and development is considered in Chapters 7 and 8.

ELECTROPHYSIOLOGIC MONITORING

An increasing awareness that measurable intrapartum events were related to perinatal outcome, together with Benson's observation that intermittent auscultation of the fetal heart rate (FHR) *during* labor did not significantly improve neonatal outcome, was the stimulus for Hon and others to advance and develop the technology of continuous electrophysiologic monitoring of fetal heart rate and intrauterine pressure. Pose and Hammacher were the first to suggest that the stress of labor could be simulated by administering oxytocin to the mother. The induced contractions decrease placental blood flow and result in a transient (relative) hypoxic stress to the fetus. Their hypothesis was that the healthy fetus would tolerate contraction-induced transient hypoxia without a change in heart rate, whereas the compromised fetus would demonstrate periodic heart rate changes. The evaluation of FHR response to induced uterine contractions became known as the oxytocin challenge test (OCT) or contraction stress test. This is of value in predicting fetal compromise (or distress) as measured by fetal death in utero, meconium staining of the amniotic fluid, or other signs of fetal distress during labor.

At approximately the same time that he was evaluating the OCT as a clinical tool, Hammacher suggested that an evaluation of FHR variability, even in a steady, nonstressed state, could be used to predict fetal health. Hammacher, Rochard, Lee, and others demonstrated an association between the "silent" (flat) FHR pattern and fetal distress on one hand and normal FHR patterns and normal fetuses on the other. The presence of FHR accelerations in association with fetal movements is considered further evidence of a healthy fetus. The emergence of nonstress testing (NST) has thus rekindled interest in one of the oldest methods of fetal assessment—the mother's perception of fetal movement. Additionally, fetal chest wall movement patterns (fetal breathing) and fetal cardiac time intervals have been suggested as predictors of fetal health.

FETAL MOVEMENT AND THE "MOVEMENTS ALARM SIGNAL"

Quickening is usually perceived by the mother between the sixteenth and twentieth week of gestation. The frequency and intensity of perceived fetal movements increase, peaking between 28 and 38 weeks of gestation and then gradually declining until delivery. Although perceived decreases in the frequency of fetal movement in the latter part of the third trimester may be related to the increasing length of fetal quiet periods, behavior that may be the fetal analogue of quiet sleep in the neonate, *absence* of fetal movement has long been noted to be a sign of potential fetal distress. Sadovsky and co-workers instructed pregnant women to count the number of fetal movements for two 30-minute periods during the day. Based on these periods of maternal observation the number of fetal movements was extrapolated over a 12-hour period. The authors noted that, when there were fewer than four fetal movements per 12-hour period, there was a significant association with fetal death in utero. They described less than four extrapolated movements within 12 hours as a "movements alarm signal," a situation requiring immediate, intensive evaluation. Similar findings and conclusions were reached by Pearson and associates. The obvious advantages of maternal perception of movement and the movements alarm signal as predictors of fetal health are that it is applicable to virtually the entire population, it is inexpensive, and it can be performed anywhere. The disadvantage is that the test is subjective, and the mother may not perceive or count movements accurately. Not infrequently, absence of fetal movement for a prolonged period will be reported, only to have movements appear during the first few minutes of a formalized NST. Nonetheless, this is a simple, reliable technique for outpatient monitoring of fetal health.

NONSTRESS (UNSTRESSED) FETAL MONITORING

Nonstress fetal monitoring involves external monitoring of the FHR using electronic instrumentation (e.g., transabdominal fetal electrocardiogram, phonocardiogram, or sonocardiogram for detection of fetal cardiac activity).

Fetal movements and uterine activity are documented using a tocodynamometer (an external strain gauge) as well as the notation of fetal movements by the patient or an observer.

The nonstress test (NST) is interpreted as reactive (normal), nonreactive (abnormal), or suspicious. The presence of at least two FHR accelerations of at least 15 beats per minute above the baseline FHR in association with fetal movements over a 20-minute period is the criterion for a *reactive* NST. The criterion of a *nonreactive* NST is the absence of FHR accelerations in the presence of fetal movements. When no fetal movements occur and normal baseline FHR variability is seen, the test falls into the suspicious category. Reactive NSTs are felt to indicate fetal health and to represent an intact functional central nervous system.

Variations of the NST have been described by Miller and co-workers and include sound stimulation. Generated acoustic impulse is the stimulus, and associated FHR accelerations are the response. The ability to demonstrate an intact stimulus-response reaction is considered to indicate a healthy fetus, whereas the absence of a response to a sufficient stimulus is a worrisome sign. Stimulus-response testing has been suggested as being potentially more efficient than a standard NST, since a sufficient stimulus should "awaken" the fetus from a quiet period during which there would be a relatively lower, less variable FHR baseline and few, if any, fetal movements. Further evaluation of responses and habituation by the fetus is necessary.

OXYTOCIN CHALLENGE TEST

The oxytocin challenge test (OCT) is an attempt to produce an intermittent, hopefully standardized stress to the fetus. The stress consists of three contractions of moderate intensity lasting 40 to 60 seconds during a 10-minute interval. FHR and uterine contractions are monitored externally. An OCT is considered positive (abnormal) when there are repetitive, uniform decelerations of the FHR following the peak of the intrauterine pressure (late decelerations), a pattern which has been shown to result from fetal hypoxia (Po_2 of <20 mm Hg).

Indications for fetal physiologic testing include conditions associated with *chronic* placental insufficiency such as hypertensive cardiovascular disorders, diabetes mellitus, collagen vascular disease, or chronic renal disease. Additional indications include patients with a previous stillbirth of undetermined etiology, decreased maternal perception of fetal movement, and situations in which clinical and/or laboratory data suggest abnormal patterns of growth.

Positive OCTs occur in 3% to 10% of cases and are felt to reflect uteroplacental insufficiency. The correlation between positive OCTs and presumptive signs of fetal distress, such as meconium or FHR decelerations during labor, depressed Apgar scores (≤6) at birth, or fetal death in utero, is far from perfect. The OCT has a false positive rate exceeding 50% in some studies. False positive results may arise for a variety of reasons, including the Poseiro effect, i.e., distal aortic compression by the contracting uterus resulting in decreased distal aortic pressure and decreased placental blood flow, or supine hypotension as a result of maternal vena caval compression. Any of these conditions may result in a hypoxia-induced late deceleration of maternal rather than fetal origin, which would not be present if the mother's position were changed. Another potential cause of false positive OCT results arises from the lack of true standardization of the stress, i.e., the resting (baseline) intrauterine pressure as well as the intensity and duration of the contractions, three factors that affect the quantity of blood flow, and thus oxygenation, in the intervillous space. Thus the "standard" stress of three contractions during a 10-minute period varies with respect to its effect from patient to patient. On the other hand, the false negative rate of the OCT is quite low. Less than 1% of negative OCTs are associated with fetal death in utero within 1 week of its performance. It is important to emphasize that this test, or for that matter any other test, is not infallible in predicting fetal survival. This is because pregnancy is a dynamic, rather than a static, state, and these tests are predictors of chronic rather than acute conditions. Although the association of a negative OCT and fetal survival is very high, a negative (normal) OCT does not preclude signs of fetal distress during labor (such as meconium, late decelerations, and bradycardia).

The OCT remains an inconvenient method of evaluating fetal condition because its performance requires approximately 2 hours, systemic infusion of oxytocin, and an attendant to monitor that infusion, restricting the number of tests that can be performed with limited personnel. In addition, several clinical conditions preclude the induction of uterine contractions, such as placenta previa, premature rupture of fetal membranes, and previous classic cesarean section. The NST can be performed safely on all patients. Rochard has observed the NST to be of value in erythroblastosis, a condition in which the OCT appears to be of limited value.

Reactive NSTs correlate well with negative OCTs and with in utero fetal survival (usually for at least 1 week), *provided* that the clinical course remains stable. A false negative rate of less than 1% with respect to fetal survival is noted. The rate of nonreactive NSTs and the false positive rate are similar to those seen with the OCT. Thus less than 10% of NSTs are positive even when performed in high-risk populations. Approximately 50% of those fetuses exhibiting a nonreactive FHR pattern will be clinically normal.

A variant of the nonreactive NST pattern that is considered abnormal is the *sinusoidal* pattern, seen primarily in fetuses with severe erythroblastosis fetalis. Rochard found a perinatal mortality of approximately 50% in patients with erythroblastosis secondary to Rh sensitization who had a sinusoidal FHR pattern on NST evaluation.

False positive NSTs may be related to fetal sleep, decreased beat-to-beat variability due to maternal medication (e.g., phenobarbital), and unrecognized vena caval compression.

FETAL BREATHING

Human fetal breathing movements may be observed by using several techniques. The original description of fetal breathing movements was based on visual observation of rhythmic fetal chest wall movements that were transmitted through the uterus to the maternal anterior abdominal wall. Ahlfeld documented these movements using primitive mechanical strain gauges, which have been replaced by more sophisticated electromagnetic or piezoelectric transducers (tocodynamometers). Although breathing movements may be recorded with external tocodynamometers, this technique remains difficult and, at times, incomplete. More commonly used techniques involve Doppler ultrasound, which is used to detect changes in thoracic venous blood flow occurring as a consequence of fetal chest wall activity. However, the most commonly used technique today is direct observation of fetal chest wall movements using real-time ultrasound scanners. This technique allows for long-term direct visual observation and video recording of chest wall movements.

Observation of fetal respiratory patterns in animal models suggests that these respiratory movements are a sensitive indicator of fetal health. Animal fetuses that failed to recover from experimental surgical procedures lacked normal respiratory movement patterns observed in apparently healthy surviving fetuses and frequently demonstrated a "gasping" respiratory pattern. The absence of respiratory movements often preceded any other overt evidence of fetal distress. Encouraged by these findings in their animal models, Boddy and co-workers evaluated fetal breathing movements in high-risk human pregnancies, noting an association of apnea and gasping patterns within 72 hours of death in fetuses who were subsequently stillborn. Several investigators have since noted a strong association between normal fetal breathing patterns and a normal outcome. Using these techniques, clinicians usually define abnormality as the absence of fetal chest wall movement during a variable period of observation. As with other tests of fetal well-being, a normal study correlates well with normal fetal outcome. One limitation of this technique, however, is that fetal breathing movements may be absent from 2 to 4 hours in apparently healthy, normal fetuses. Abnormal results should therefore be interpreted cautiously and in conjunction with other methods of fetal evaluation.

ANTENATAL BIOCHEMICAL FETAL ASSESSMENT

For almost half a century physicians have been searching for a specific chemical predictor of fetal health. In some perinatal centers, use of various biochemical tests is proliferating, whereas others are questioning whether even the most accepted analyses, such as estriol, are cost effective in the management of high-risk pregnancies.

Amniotic fluid

During the early middle trimester the direct measurement of amniotic fluid constituents for the presence or absence of specific enzymes or chromosomal studies may be helpful in determining the presence or absence of congenital disease. Later in pregnancy the concentration of various substances can be measured in an attempt to identify infants with growth abnormalities or infants that are in distress. Amniotic fluid pH, PO_2, lactate, ketone bodies, osmolarity, glucose, insulin, BUN, and amino acids have been evaluated, as have most steroid hormones (e.g., estriol and estetrol). Currently none of these tests has significant clinical value. The measurement of the lecithin/sphingomyelin (L/S) ratio, as well as the measurement of specific phospholipids such as phosphatidyl glycerol, has been used to predict accurately the risk of respiratory distress syndrome (see Chapter 23). In addition, the relationship between these amniotic fluid constituents and both fetal size and estimated fetal gestational age is useful in discriminating accelerated versus delayed fetal maturity as well as small for gestational age (SGA) infants versus large for gestational age (LGA) infants.

In cases of erythroblastosis fetalis a change in optical density (ΔOD) at 450 mμ is the primary determinant in ongoing management and is used to determine whether intrauterine transfusion is necessary or when premature delivery becomes indicated (see Chapter 5). Occasionally amniocentesis will be used to determine whether meconium is present, since the demonstration of meconium in amniotic fluid requires focused intensive care. Depending on the circumstances, this might mean hospitalization with careful electronic monitoring, daily estriol analysis (see further), or delivery.

Placental proteins and enzymes

In the past, activities of enzymes such as placental alkaline phosphatase and cystine amniopeptidase have been suggested as predictors of placental function. Currently, however, they have no value in clinical management. Human placental lactogen (HPL), now renamed human chorionic somatomammotropin (HCS), a placental protein similar in structure to human growth hormone, is secreted into the maternal circulation where it exerts an anti-insulin (diabetogenic) effect. HPL has been extensively studied because of the many important metabolic effects that this protein hormone has on maternal metabolism. Spellacy and associates have reported that HPL values of less then 4 μg/ml (the "fetal danger zone") are associated with significantly increased risk of fetal death in utero. HPL is a high–molecular weight protein and is not excreted by the maternal kidneys. Maternal levels of HPL are therefore independent of renal function. It has been suggested that HPL may be particularly valuable in cases of toxemia or renal disease, conditions that can alter significantly the reliability of estriol levels as indicators of fetal well-being. Unfortunately, the problem with HPL, as with other biochemical tests of fetal well-being, is that normal values are sometimes associated with chronic fetal distress and abnormally low values may be quite consistent with normal fetuses. The number of false negative and false positive results makes individual interpretations difficult. HPL has not been shown to be more accurate than estriol in the prediction of fetal distress, and therefore its value remains in doubt.

Fetoplacental steroid hormones

The placenta synthesizes or participates in the synthesis of a large number of steriod hormones, including progesterone, esterone, estradiol, and estriol. Progesterone can be entirely synthesized within the placenta without maternal or fetal precursors. Since up to 20% of the daily placental production of progesterone may be recovered in maternal urine as the metabolite pregnanediol, early investigators attempted to use pregnanediol excretion as an index of placental function but abandoned it because of lack of sensitivity and specificity. Estradiol produced by the placenta and estetrol produced by the fetus have occasionally been used as tests of fetal well-being. However, from a clinical perspective, except in erythroblastosis fetalis, the most important estrogen is estriol.

Estriol production depends on both fetal and placental function; its excretion is related to maternal renal function. Today it is the most widely used biochemical estimator of fetoplacental function, and, except in rare cases, 90% of all pregnancy estrogen is estriol. The primary exceptions to this rule are cases complicated by anencephaly, placental sulfatase deficiency, and fetal adrenal hypoplasia. Abnormalities in maternal urinary excretion of estriol may arise from altered renal function, usually associated with a rise in serum estriol levels, inflammatory bowel disease, or drugs (e.g., ampicillin) that can affect estriol levels by altering the intestinal bacterial metabolism and subsequent reabsorption of the conjugated estriol into the enterohepatic circulation. Additionally, certain corticosteroids may suppress fetal adrenal function and thus lower both maternal serum and urinary estriol levels. Other drugs (e.g., mandelamine) can affect the assay for estriol.

The usefulness of estriol as a measure of fetoplacental function arises from the fact that critical enzymatic steps in its synthesis occur in both the fetus and the placenta with the rate-limiting enzymatic step occurring in the fetal adrenal glands. For normal amounts of estriol to be secreted, there must be a functional fetal hypothalamic-pituitary-adrenal axis, a functioning fetal liver, a functioning fetal placenta, and functioning maternal liver, gastrointestinal tract, and kidneys.

A functioning fetal hypothalamic-pituitary-adrenal axis is required to stimulate fetal adrenal activity, which results in the synthesis of estriol precursors from substrates supplied by the mother. The fetal adrenal glands excrete dehydroepiandrosterone (DHEA) and some 16-hydroxy-dehydroepiandrosterone (16-OH-DHEA) as sulfates. In passage through the fetal liver, additional DHEA is converted to 16-OH-DHEA. Desulfatation and aromatization take place in the placenta. The product of 16-OH-DHEA metabolism in the placenta is estriol, and the synthetic product of DHEA in the placenta is estradiol.

Estriol passes into the maternal circulation and is carried to the maternal liver, where it is conjugated either at the 3- or 16-carbon with either sulfate or glucuronic acid. From the liver, conjugates are excreted into the gastrointestinal tract, where further metabolism by intestinal bacteria occurs with subsequent reabsorption into the enterohepatic circulation. Although the estriol-3-sulfate-16-glucuronide predominates in maternal plasma, in maternal urine estriol-16-glucuronide represents most of the estrogen measured in 24-hour urine collections. The amount and form of estriol conjugates present in blood and urine relate to how those conjugates are cleared by the kidneys; only conjugated estrogens are excreted in maternal urine. Under normal circumstances 90% of all estriol in the maternal compartment will be in the conjugated form and thus available for excretion in the urine.

Smith first introduced the use of estriol into obstetric practice in 1927. Over the past 15 years, many factors affecting fluctuations in estriol excretion have been identified. Although mean estriol levels correlate with fetal size, the normal range of estriol levels is so wide that macrosomia and intrauterine growth retardation can seldom be diagnosed solely on the basis of an estriol level. Rarely, an unusually high level of estriol will lead to the recognition of multiple gestation. Finally, because significant diurnal variations in *urinary* estriol excretion have been noted when analyzing successive 6-hour collections, the 24-hour urine collection remains most suitable. Diurnal variations in plasma estriol are less evident. It appears that unconjugated serum estriol decreases in the late morning, and total plasma estriol decreases during the late afternoon and evening. Diurnal variations in plasma estriol levels in the range of 15% are overshadowed by much larger day-to-day fluctuations. It seems prudent to collect all plasma specimens at approximately the same time each day. Although the literature evaluating the efficacy of various serum estriol assays remains confusing, it is suggested that the free or unconjugated estriol may be more reliable than urinary estriol collections. Goebelsmann reported that free serum estriol showed less variability and was more accurate in predicting clinically significant changes than either total serum estriol or 24-hour urinary estriol in diabetic patients. Long-term trends in either urinary or serum estriols should be similar.

The only worthwhile data available relating decreased estriol excretion and fetal distress are based on the management of diabetic pregnancies. Data presented by Katagiri and co-workers suggest that a significant drop in urinary estriol levels is defined as a drop of 35% from the mean value of the *preceding 3* days. A significant drop in plasma estriol requires a drop in excess of 40% of the mean value of the previous 3 days. Whether this information applies to nondiabetic pregnancies is still speculative. Deviations from the mean of the 3 previous days are required because the daily fluctuations in the estriol levels are so large. Since daily estriol levels are required and acute changes may be missed, the cost effectiveness of this method of monitoring fetal health is controversial.

The dehydroepiandrosterone-sulfate (DHEA-S) loading test has been proposed by Gant and associates as a dynamic test of placental function. In this test the infusion of DHEA-S to the mother results in an acute, measurable increase in placental estrogen synthesis. This is currently an investigational test that may be useful in testing placental reserve, particularly in pregnancies complicated by intrauterine growth retardation. This test may also be used to identify pregnancies associated with placental sulfatase deficiency. Additional clinical experience with this test is indicated prior to its widespread use.

CLINICAL APPLICATIONS OF ANTEPARTUM MONITORING

Clinicians have been relying on electrophysiologic rather than biochemical testing because of increased experience with electrophysiologic monitoring, the expense of biochemical testing, and the less frequent (weekly) patient testing. Nonstressed fetal monitoring is the primary test used in antepartum fetal assessment because of the reliability, lack of risk, and minimal personnel involvement. The NST is performed in high-risk patients once or twice a week, depending on the stability of the clinical situation. When a clearly abnormal or very suspicious NST is encountered, an oxytocin challenge test is performed. If the OCT is normal, NST is resumed once or twice a week. When the OCT is suspicious or hyperstimulation is encountered, the test is repeated in 24 hours, and daily estriol collections are initiated. When the OCT is abnormal and questions regarding lung maturity exist, an amniocentesis is performed. When the amniocentesis reveals meconium and when a positive L/S ratio is confirmed, delivery is undertaken. When amniotic fluid studies reveal an immature L/S ratio, observation is considered if daily estriol levels have been normal. If estriol levels are low or falling, delivery is initiated. If estriol levels are stable and continue to remain normal, serial estriol collections are evaluated, and the patient is stabilized on bed rest in a lateral recumbent position to maximize placental perfusion. Expectant therapy is continued with daily NSTs until serial normal NSTs are documented or abnormal biochemical changes are documented.

Leroy J. Dierker
Roger H. Hertz

BIBLIOGRAPHY

Ahlfeld, F.: Uber bisher noch nicht beschreibene intrauterine bewegungen des kindes, Verh Dtsch. Ges. Gynaekol. **2**:203, 1888.

Benson, R.C., and others: Fetal heart rate as a predictor of fetal distress, Obstet. Gynecol. **32**:259, 1968

Bieniarz, J., and others: Aortocaval compression by the uterus in late human pregnancy, Am. J. Obstet. Gynecol. **100**:203, 1968.

Boddy, K., and Dawes, G.S.: Fetal breathing, Br. Med. Bull. **31**:3, 1975.

Dawes, G.S., and others: Respiratory movements and rapid eye movement sleep in the foetal lamb, J. Physiol. **22**:119, 1972.

Distler, W., Gabbe, S.G., and Goebelsmann, U.: Estriol in pregnancy. V. Unconjugated and total plasma estriol in the management of pregnant diabetic patients, Am. J. Obstet. Gynecol. **130**:424, 1978.

Gant, N.F., and others: The metabolic clearance rate of dehydroisoandrosterone sulfate. IV. Acute effects of induced hypertension, hypotension, and naturesis in normal and hypertensive pregnancies, Am. J. Obstet. Gynecol. **124**:143, 1976.

Hammacher, K.: The clinical significance of cardiotocography. In Huntingford, P.S., Huter, E.A., and Saling, E., editors: Perinatal medicine, New York, 1969, Academic Press, Inc.

Hon, E.H.: Detection of fetal distress. In Wood, C., editor: Fifth World Congress of Gynecology and Obstetrics, London, 1967, Butterworths.

Katagiri, H., and others: Estriol in pregnancy. IV. Normal concentrations, diurnal and/or episodic variations and day-to-day changes of unconjugated and total estriol in late pregnancy plasma, Am. J. Obstet. Gynecol. **124**:272, 1976.

Kubli, F.W., and others: Observations on heart rate and pH in the human fetus during labor, Am. J. Obstet. Gynecol. **104**:1190, 1969.

Lee, C.Y., DiLoreto, P.C., and Logrand, B.: Fetal activity acceleration determination for the evaluation of fetal reserve, Ob./Gyn. **48**:19, 1976.

Pearson, J., and Weaver, J.: Fetal activity and fetal well-being: an evaluation, Br. Med. J. **1**:1305, 1976.

Pose, S.V., and others: Test of fetal tolerance to induced uterine contractions for the diagnosis of chronic distress. In Perinatal factors affecting human development, Washington, D.C., 1969, World Health Organization Scientific Publication no. 185.

Preyer, W.F.: Specielle physiologie des embryos: Uetersuchungenuber die lebenserscheiunungen vor der gebart, Leipzig, 1885, Grieben.

Queen, J.T.: Modern management of the Rh problem, New York, 1977, Harper & Row, Publishers.

Read, T.A., and Miller, F.C.: Fetal heart rate acceleration in response to acoustic stimulation as a measure of fetal well-being, Am. J. Obstet. Gynecol. **129**:512, 1977.

Rochard, F., and others: Non-stressed fetal heart rate monitoring in the antepartum period, Am. J. Obstet. Gynecol. **126**:699, 1976.

Sadovsky, E., and Polishuk, W.: Fetal movements in utero: Nature, assessment, prognostic Value, timing of Delivery, Ob./Gyn. **50**:49, 1977.

Smith, O.W., Smith, G.V., and Joslin, E.P.: Prolan and estrin in the serum and urine of diabetic and nondiabetic women with special reference to late pregnancy toxemia, Am. J. Obstet. Gynecol. **33**:365, 1937.

Spellacy, W.N., and others: Value of human chorionic somatommammotropin in managing high-risk pregnancies, Am. J. Obstet. Gynecol. **109**:588, 1971.

PART THREE

Intrapartum fetal assessment

ELECTROPHYSIOLOGIC MONITORING

Although labor is tolerated safely by a large majority of fetuses, for some it is a perilous time. Analysis of continuous fetal heart rate/intrauterine pressure tracings and intermittent microbiochemical analysis of fetal scalp blood samples are the cornerstones of intrapartum fetal assessment. Newer techniques, including the evaluation of various components of fetal cardiac time intervals (e.g., pre-ejection period, ventricular ejection time), the fetal electroencephalogram, continuous pH and PO_2 evaluation, as well as computer-assisted evaluation and integration of multiple techniques of fetal monitoring, are receiving attention in laboratory and clinical research

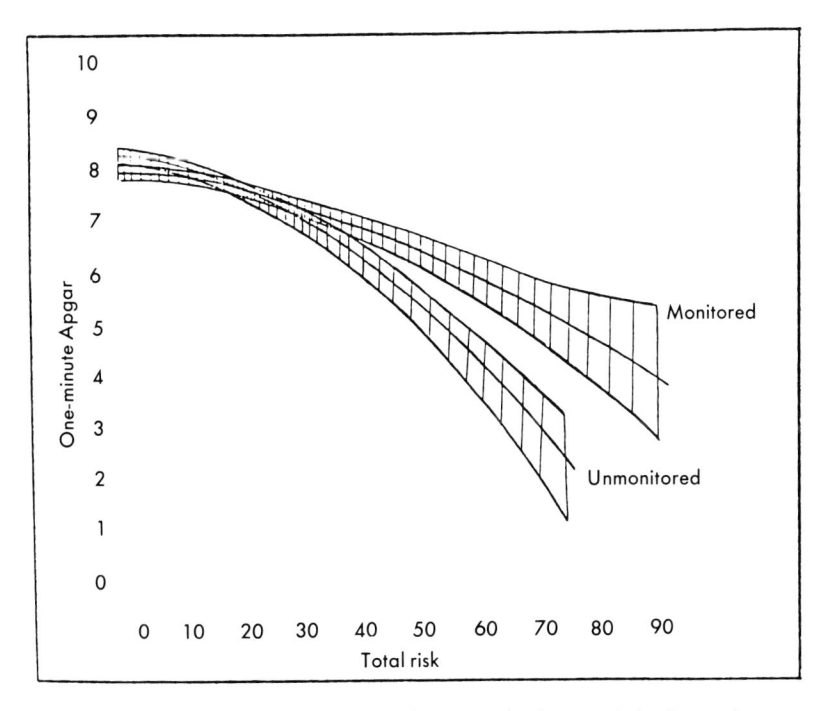

Fig. 9-19. Relationship between electronic fetal monitoring and 1-minute Apgar scores. Note more depressed babies among fetuses who were not monitored. (From Sokol, R., and others: Antenatal diagnosis: report of a consensus development conference sponsored by NICHD, March 1979, NIH Pub. no. 79-1973, April 1979.)

settings. While the efficacy of these newer methods of fetal assessment are under study, the clinician must rely on bedside analysis of fetal heart rate/intrauterine pressure and intermittent fetal scalp blood analysis data.

For the fetal metabolic milieu to remain normal, *nutrient flow* (O_2, glucose, etc.) in both the maternal and fetal compartments must remain sufficient to meet fetal metabolic requirements. Significant changes in nutrient flow in either compartment will result in a metabolic abnormality that, when severe, will lead to depression, asphyxia, or death. Physiologically the flow component (e.g., maternal placental blood flow or fetal umbilical blood flow) is the more vulnerable component of nutrient flow to and from the fetus. The relatively steady-state flow dynamics prior to labor are altered by increasing baseline uterine pressures, increasing strength and length of uterine contractions (uterine systole), and decreasing contraction-free intervals (uterine diastole) as labor progresses. Thus, as normal labor progresses, a combination of lengthening intermittent interruptions of steady-state flow and the decreasing interval for metabolic recovery (longer, more frequent contractions) results in a gradually decreasing pH, even in normal labors.

Who should be monitored during labor

During normal labor diminished placental blood flow, as a consequence of uterine contractions and elevated uterine tone, may represent a physiologic stress; thus any fetus entering labor already in an "at risk" status should be considered a candidate for electrophysiologic fetal monitoring. Sokol and Rosen, using a modified Hobel antepartum/intrapartum risk assessment scale, confirmed that the higher the risk, the lower the 1-minute Apgar score (Fig. 9-19). They examined the 1- and 5-minute Apgar scores in over 3,000 consecutive deliveries, of which 1,212 (39.4%) were monitored and 1,964 (60.6%) were not monitored. High-risk patients had higher Apgar scores if they were monitored, and they concluded that monitoring neither increased maternal risks nor worsened the neonatal outcome in patients at low risk. Analysis of their data indicated that patients entering labor with diabetes mellitus, cardiovascular or renal disease, or severe medical-obstetric complications such as collagen disease, third trimester bleeding, premature rupture of the membranes, nonvertex presentations, and low birth weight fetus (preterm and/or growth-retarded fetuses) benefited the most (Table 9-1).

The presence of meconium has traditionally been considered a presumptive sign of fetal distress. Although the majority of these fetuses tolerate labor and have a normal Apgar score at delivery, 15% to 20% will have a metabolic acidosis (pH less than 7.25) at the time of delivery. The presence of meconium at the onset of labor, even when not associated with fetal heart rate (FHR) abnormalities

Table 9-1. The risk of low Apgar score and reduction in excess risk with monitoring by weight and gestational duration

	Low apgar score in unmonitored group (%)	Reduction in excess risk (%)
Weight (gm)		
500-1,000	94.6	191.3
1,001-2,000	63.0	139.0
2,001-2,500	26.4	66.7
2,501-4,000	10.5	0.0
>4,000	16.6	6.8
Weeks gestation (OB)		
21-31	81.0	230.2
32-37	20.8	16.0
38-42	11.2	0.0
>42 (post dates)	25.0	65.0
Definite preterm	59.9	178.2
Definite IUGR	24.3	21.1
Definite LGA	20.6	38.7

Table 9-2. Variations in normal baseline intrauterine pressure

	Baseline pressure	Peak pressure
Early first stage (latent phase)	<5 mm Hg	25-40 mm Hg
Late first stage (active phase)	8-12 mm Hg	30-50 mm Hg
Second stage	10-20 mm Hg	>80 mm Hg

during labor, appears to increase the risk of immediate neonatal depression. The incidence of depression and asphyxia are significantly increased in those cases complicated by both meconium and FHR abnormalities. It is therefore preferable to monitor closely fetuses presenting with meconium-stained amniotic fluid prior to labor as well as those fetuses who pass fresh meconium during labor.

Patients who develop abnormal patterns of uterine contraction, including tachysystole, polysystole (with or without an elevated baseline pressure), and tetanic contractions, should be monitored closely and, since the use of oxytocin may result in decreased placental blood flow resulting from baseline intrauterine pressure abnormalities as well as contraction pattern abnormalities, patients whose labor has been induced or augmented with oxytocin are candidates for increased fetal surveillance.

Monitoring techniques

Routine modern fetal surveillance includes evaluation of the intrauterine pressure and the corresponding FHR responses and evaluation of the metabolic status based on micro–blood gas analysis of fetal blood taken directly from the presenting part.

With internal monitoring the pressure tracing is obtained from intrauterine pressure transmitted to a pressure transducer via a fluid-filled catheter. With appropriate catheter placement a quantitative pressure is obtained. In addition, the time of onset and the end of the contraction are more accurately recorded, and the baseline intrauterine pressure between contractions can be measured. Disadvantages of internal pressure monitoring are that the membranes must be ruptured and skilled personnel must insert the catheter. In addition, there is a small risk for morbidity (e.g., uterine or placental perforation, umbilical prolapse, and infection).

Uterine activity can be evaluated from the baseline pressure and the uterine contraction pattern. Baseline uterine pressure is defined as the intrauterine pressure present between contractions that can be obtained only by the internal monitoring technique after appropriate zeroing of the intrauterine pressure system. Zeroing is accomplished by opening the pressure transducer to atmosphere, placing it at the level of the midportion of the uterine cavity (assuming that this is the approximate position of the catheter tip within the uterus), and then adjusting the pen reading to zero. Normal baseline pressure varies with the stage of labor (Table 9-2). *Elevations in baseline* may occur in conditions such as abruptio placentae, occiput posterior position, and cephalopelvic disproportion and as a consequence of the use of oxytocin. The physiologic significance of elevated baseline intrauterine pressure stems from its interference with uteroplacental nutrient flow. Thus, when the pressure is elevated, the fetus cannot recover from uterine contractions readily, resulting in a significant metabolic abnormality.

The second aspect of intrauterine pressure analysis concerns evaluation of the contraction pattern. Normal contractions are bell shaped and last 30 to 60 seconds. The length of the contraction as well as the peak intrauterine pressure during the contraction varies with the stage of labor (Table 9-2). Abnormal contractions are significant because, once intrauterine pressure exceeds spiral arteriolar pressure, the flow of oxygenated blood into the intervillous space ceases. A period of increasing hypoxia then develops until intrauterine pressure falls below that required to allow resumption of blood flow through the placental bed.

Six abnormal contraction patterns have been described by Stookey (Fig. 9-20):
1. Skewed contractions: prolongation of the relaxation phase of the uterine contraction
2. Polysystole: a contraction containing more than one peak in the uterine pressure tracing
3. Paired contractions: a normal contraction with return

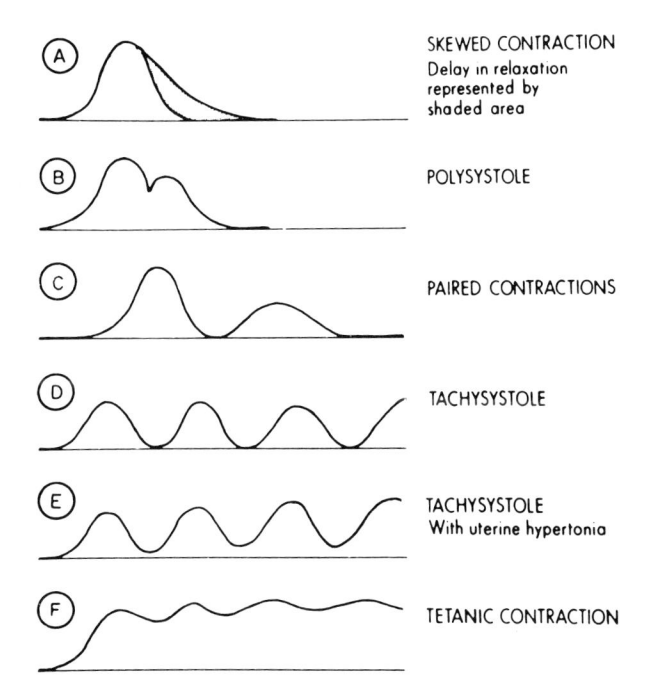

Fig. 9-20. Contraction pattern abnormalities during induction of labor. Resting potential represented by horizontal line. (From Stookey, R., Sokol, R., and Rosen, M.: Obstet. Gynecol. **45**:359, 1973.)

- A — SKEWED CONTRACTION: Delay in relaxation represented by shaded area
- B — POLYSYSTOLE
- C — PAIRED CONTRACTIONS
- D — TACHYSYSTOLE
- E — TACHYSYSTOLE With uterine hypertonia
- F — TETANIC CONTRACTION

to a normal baseline followed closely by a second normal contraction (though usually of a lower magnitude)
4. Tachysystole: normal contractions occurring more frequently than every 2 minutes
5. Tachysystole with uterine hypotonia: an abnormally high baseline pressure between the contractions
6. Tetanic contractions: a sustained contraction with one or more peaks that does not return to baseline for approximately 5 minutes

These contraction pattern abnormalities may result in a decrease in nutrient flow to the intervillous space. With skewed contractions, polysystole, and tetanic contractions, uterine systole is prolonged. Uterine diastole is shortened with paired contractions and tachysystole. In each of these cases the ratio of the duration of uterine systole to diastole is significantly increased, resulting in decreased placental perfusion and fetal hypoxia. When fetal hypoxia is uncorrected, major metabolic and physiologic alterations, including FHR abnormalities and acidosis, occur (see Chapter 9, part one).

Abnormal contraction patterns may occur with either spontaneous or stimulated labor and are often associated with other labor abnormalities. Thus the initiation of oxytocin stimulation or continued augmentation in the face of abnormal labor progress must be undertaken with caution and should be monitored using internal pressure monitoring techniques to acquire absolute rather than relative baseline and peak intrauterine pressure data.

INTRAPARTUM ASSESSMENT OF FETAL pH

Over 90% of all fetuses will be vigorous at birth when the FHR/IUP tracing is normal. On the other hand, even when FHR/IUP patterns are suggestive of fetal distress, most fetuses will still have normal Apgar scores at birth. Thus knowledge of whether abnormal heart rate patterns or prolonged labor is causing significant metabolic alterations in the fetus will facilitate optimum timing of delivery by the most appropriate route. Indeed, extensive clinical experience has shown that appropriate use of FHR/IUP and fetal pH monitoring will significantly reduce perinatal morbidity and mortality. The purpose of this section is to define normal and abnormal acid-base relationships and to discuss the rationale and the technique of fetal blood sampling.

FETAL pH

With the development of microbiochemical techniques and with the introduction of clinical fetal blood sampling by Saling, intrapartum biochemical monitoring became a practical reality. A fetal acid-base profile can be determined from as little as 100 λ (0.1 ml) of fetal blood. It was found that under normal conditions the pH of fetal blood is chronically lower than that of maternal blood. The lower fetal pH (mean of 7.34 in the fetus versus 7.44 in the mother) is primarily the result of the higher concentration of Pco_2 in the fetal circulation (Pco_2 of 44.2 mm Hg in the fetus versus 32.2 mm Hg in the mother). Fetal bicarbonate ion concentration is only slightly higher than the mother's (23.1 versus 21.1). Therefore, by adult standards, the fetus may be viewed as having a partially compensated respiratory acidosis.

Fetal pH is maintained by the rapid diffusion of CO_2 and by the equilibration of HCO_3^- across the placenta. The exact mechanism involved in the transfer of HCO_3^- across the placenta remains controversial.

Carbon dioxide and water are the by-products of aerobic metabolism in the fetus. In the presence of an adequate oxygen-nutrient supply and adequate maternal, placental, and umbilical blood flow, normal fetomaternal gradients are maintained and the fetal pH remains normal and stable. Whenever there is a reduction in nutrient flow, whether in the maternal or the fetal compartment, resulting in a significant reduction in oxygen delivery, the fetus becomes hypoxic and a metabolic acidosis develops. When the fetus becomes hypoxic, a shift from aerobic to the much less efficient anaerobic metabolism occurs. This leads to an accumulation of lactic acid with depletion of buffer-base stores (HCO_3^-) and the development of a metabolic acidosis. When there is a reduction of umbilical blood flow (secondary to cord entanglement), there is interference in both oxygen delivery and CO_2 excretion. Thus the concentration of both lactic acid and CO_2 may arise in the fetus, resulting in a combined metabolic and "respiratory" acidosis. Thus, from the theoretical standpoint, the determination of fetal pH appears to be a measure of the significance of fetal hypoxia, whereas determination of fetal bicarbonate ion concentration appears to be a measure of the fetus's ability to withstand further metabolic insult.

Subscribing to the concept that the final common metabolic pathway in fetal distress is acidosis, Saling developed the technique of fetal micro-blood sampling and established normative values for fetal pH, Pco_2, and HCO_3^- that have withstood the test of time. Based on his large prospective series, fetal scalp pH values above 7.25 were considered normal, pH values between 7.20 and 7.25 were considered to be "preacidotic," and pH values of less than 7.20 were considered to be acidotic. In his original series of 850 patients, Saling found that 85% of infants described as vigorous, lively, or only mildly depressed had a pH equal to or greater than 7.20, whereas 80% of the infants whose last pH was less than 7.20 were significantly depressed with Apgar scores of 6 or less. The development of the clinical technique of micro-blood sampling was particularly significant in light of the relationship between neonatal acidosis, Apgar score, and asphyxia demonstrated by James and co-workers.

Bowe critically examined the reliability of scalp sampling in the prediction of neonatal depression. They confirmed Saling's observations, finding an excellent correlation between the pH value of 7.22 or less and an Apgar score of 6 or less ($p < 0.001$). MacDonald showed that all of his severely depressed infants (Apgar scores < 4) had pH's of 7.20 or less. De la Rama found that only 8% of 178 infants with scalp pH's greater than 7.25 required extensive resuscitation (with most of these being associated with difficult operative deliveries after the last biochemical study had been performed), whereas 59% of their patients with a pH of less than 7.20 required extensive resuscitation.

A comparison of biochemical with FHR/IUP monitoring clearly shows that fetal scalp blood sampling is the more specific method for predicting fetal distress at birth. Edington and associates monitored 806 patients by continuous FHR tracings and obtained fetal blood samples in 158 of these patients. In this study only 30% of the fetuses with suspicious or abnormal FHR tracings were actually acidotic. Thomas, in his retrospective study covering a 34-month period, showed that with late decelerations the incidence of fetal distress (pH less than 7.25 or a 1-minute Apgar score of less than 6) was less than 50%. Tejani and co-workers reported on a series of 216 patients monitored with both continuous FHR tracings and scalp pH and confirmed previous reports that, with a normal baseline FHR and no periodic changes, there was a less than 10% chance of fetal acidosis. In that study the incidence of acidosis varied from 23% to 47% depending on the type, depth, and frequency of FHR decelerations. Tejani went one step further and correlated FHR patterns and fetal scalp pH with neonatal outcome. In the absence of FHR changes, they found that 92% of the neonates had Apgar scores of 7 or more. Late decelerations were associated with an Apgar score of less than 7 in 37% of the cases. By comparison, if the last pH was equal to or greater than 7.25, 88% of the infants had Apgar scores of 7 or more, whereas if the last pH was less than 7.20, 80% of the infants were depressed with Apgar scores of 6 or less.

Measurement of the bicarbonate ion concentration (or the negative base excess) reflects the fetuses' residual buffer-base capacity. This measurement is useful in predicting the metabolic severity of the fetal distress and will give an indication of how difficult and how long therapeutic intervention will be required during the neonatal period. Other blood gas parameters (e.g., Po_2) change too rapidly to be of value in predicting fetal outcome and should not be used to diagnose fetal distress at this time.

TECHNIQUE OF FETAL BLOOD SAMPLING

The technique for obtaining the small amount of fetal blood required for biochemical analysis is relatively simple, with a reported complication rate of less than 1%. To perform fetal blood sampling, the chorioamnionic membrane must be ruptured, the cervix adequately dilated, and the presenting part known and low enough in the birth canal so as to be relatively immobile. If the presenting part is not fixed, an assistant must stabilize it by applying sufficient fundal pressure. Appropriate positioning of the mother is extremely important and may be best accomplished in the delivery room. Fetal blood sampling can be done with the patient either in the lithotomy position with a slight lateral tilt to prevent supine hypotension or, when the presenting part is on the perineum, in the lateral (Sims) position.

After prepping and draping of the perineum has been done, the endoscope should be placed against the fetal presenting part. The sample site, preferably not over a suture or fontanel, must be cleaned and dried. Blood, mucus, meconium, or any amniotic debris should be removed. The sample site should be isolated from further contamination by maintaining *gentle* pressure on the endoscope. Excessive pressure may reduce local blood flow or dislodge the presenting part and therefore should be avoided. A thin layer of silicone gel may be applied to the presenting part to enhance beading of the blood droplet. Using a microscalpel, a 1- to 2-mm deep puncture is made in the skin. Blood collection is facilitated when the puncture is performed at the beginning of a contraction. As the blood droplet forms, a heparinized capillary tube is inserted into the endoscope; it should make contact with the blood droplet but should not touch the fetal scalp. This will minimize contamination and/or obstruction of blood flow by foreign material. A single pH determination requires approximately 100 λ (0.1 ml) of blood. If blood flow is adequate, a second tube should be collected for comparison. These tubes are handed to an assistant, who seals one end, inserts a small metal mixing rod, and seals the second end to prevent diffusion of respiratory gases. The mixing rod is moved within the tube using a magnet to facilitate heparinization of the sample. The fetal blood sample is placed on crushed ice and carried to the laboratory for biochemical study. Meanwhile, the operator maintains pressure on the sample site for several minutes. Whenever possible, the sample site is then visualized through a contraction to be sure that hemostasis has been achieved. Additional pressure is applied whenever necessary.

Results of fetal blood sampling

When fetal blood sampling has been undertaken and the fetal pH is greater than 7.25 with a base deficit (base excess) within normal limits, the obstetrician can be reassured that labor may be allowed to continue. If the abnormality that prompted the fetal blood sampling disappears, no further sampling is required. However, if the abnormality persists, fetal sampling should be repeated on an hourly basis when the abnormality is mild, and sooner if the visual data are ominous or worse.

When the pH is between 7.20 and 7.25, the fetus is said to be preacidotic and fetal sampling should be repeated every 15 to 30 minutes, depending on the indications and the bicarbonate ion concentration, until a trend is established. When the pH is less than 7.20, the obstetrician should consider either repeating the fetal blood sampling immediately to establish a trend or moving toward delivery if the FHR abnormality is severe (severe baseline bradycardia, severe variable decelerations with a slow return to baseline). When the pH is *less than* 7.10 and this result is consistent with other clinical data, immediate delivery by the most expeditious route should be considered. A skilled neonatologist should be summoned, and the delivery of a severely asphyxiated infant should be anticipated.

Three very important precautions must be observed if fetal blood sampling is to be used most effectively:

1. Prolonged attempts to collect fetal blood should be avoided when there is qualitative evidence of severe peripheral fetal vasoconstriction or fetal hypotension, i.e., there is no blanching when endoscopic pressure is applied and little or no blood flow when the presenting part is incised. When this circumstance is encountered in patients with significant FHR abnormalities, immediate delivery should be considered and delivery of a very depressed infant should be anticipated.
2. The clinician should try to avoid acting on the basis of a single pH determination. To minimize technical errors, whenever the clinical situation permits, additional fetal blood sampling to confirm or establish a trend should be obtained.
3. Maternal acidosis as the cause for fetal blood gas abnormality must be ruled out. This can be done easily by obtaining a maternal venous sample drawn without the use of a tourniquet. Fetal hypoxic acidosis can be distinguished from maternal acidosis by comparing metabolic components of the acid-base status in the mother to that of the fetus. This can best be done by measuring the actual pH and Pco_2 of both maternal and fetal blood and then using the Siggard-Anderson nomogram to determine the base deficit of both samples at a hemoglobin concentration of 5 gm/dl. This corresponds to the base deficit and at the tissue level. If the value obtained after subtracting the fetal base deficit value from the maternal base deficit value is greater than 0, the acidosis is maternal in origin. If a value of less than 0 is obtained, the acidosis is of fetal origin. This relationship is valid *only* when the base deficit values are calculated at a hemoglobin value of 5 gm/dl.

A second means of distinguishing maternal from fetal acidosis is by comparing the pH of maternal and fetal blood after both are equilibrated at a Pco_2 of 40 mm Hg. Equilibrating both samples at the same CO_2 tension removes the respiratory component of the pH. A difference between the two values of less than 0.05 pH units virtually rules out fetal hypoxia as a cause of the acidosis. Bowe feels that excluding maternal acidosis as the cause for abnormal fetal pH will virtually eliminate the 10% false positive rate reported by some authors.

Complications

The complication rate for fetal blood sampling is less than 1%. Although uncommon, complications from sampling include persistent bleeding from the puncture site, blade breakage, and infection. Significant bleeding rarely occurs without some underlying coagulation defect. When bleeding does occur, it can almost always be controlled with additional pressure at the puncture site. A small suture may be required in an extremely rare case. Breakage of the blade may result from improper seating of the blade in the scalpel or through excessive force. Occasionally a defective blade may be the cause. Should this occur, the broken blade can usually be removed with a long clamp. Rarely, removal must await delivery and roentgenologic localization. When blade breakage occurs, the fetus must be closely observed for evidence of persistent bleeding.

Local infection, including scalp abscess, may occur following scalp sampling. Infection is usually well localized and responds to local therapy and antibiotics. Careful observation in the nursery and prompt intervention will minimize the effects of this complication.

Contraindications to fetal blood sampling are few and include the following:
1. A presenting part that is not easily accessible or clearly defined
2. A mother who is a known carrier of hemophilia with a male fetus
3. A mother with a bleeding disorder that might be transmitted to the fetus (especially idiopathic thrombocytopenic purpura)
4. A genital infection (e.g., herpes, CMV, gonorrhea, or β-hemolytic streptococci)

FUTURE OUTLOOK

Continuous transcutaneous fetal scalp pH monitoring is under evaluation as a research procedure. A pH electrode has been incorporated into the spiral scalp FHR electrode, providing the clinician with both a continuous FHR tracing and a transcutaneous pH evaluation every 15 seconds. This arrangement may overcome many of the technical difficulties and inconveniences encountered in intermittent fetal blood sampling. If the tissue pH electrode provides data that are comparable with data from intermittent fetal blood sampling, it will represent a significant advance in intrapartum fetal assessment. Further improvement in fetal assessment may result from computer-assisted trend analysis of continuously acquired FHR/IUP/pH data.

Continuous transcutaneous oxygen (TcPo$_2$) monitoring offers a noninvasive technique for recording changes in oxygenation (Chapter 23). Although this technique has been used successfully in the intensive care unit, there have been limited reports of fetal surveillance during labor. Löfgren has reported that when the electrode is applied properly, the technique is useful for documenting fetal oxygenation. Thus, together with the other criteria already outlined, TcPo$_2$ broadens the data base concerning fetal hypoxemia, permitting a more rational therapeutic approach to fetal asphyxia.

CONCLUSION

Fetal blood gas sampling is a relatively simple procedure, has a low complication rate, and is a reliable predictor of neonatal depression. Fetal blood gas analysis allows the obstetrician to determine more accurately the fetal condition and measure its metabolic reserve. Fetal blood sampling allows specific identification of fetuses not tolerating the stress of labor based on the screening technique of FHR/IUP monitoring. Thus it allows the clinician to distinguish between FHR/IUP tracings that represent "benign" stresses and those which represent "malignant" stresses. Therefore concerned clinicians who wish to avoid unnecessary operative interventions must use fetal blood gas determinations to supplement data acquired from electrophysiologic monitoring.

Roger H. Hertz
Shelby E. Jarrell

BIBLIOGRAPHY

Balfour, H., and others: Complications of fetal blood sampling, Am. J. Obstet. Gynecol. **107:**288, 1970.

Bowe, E.T.: Reliability of fetal blood sampling, Am. J. Obstet. Gynecol. **107:**279, 1970.

Bretscher, J., and Saling, E.: pH values in the human fetus during labor, Am. J. Obstet. Gynecol. **97:**906, 1967.

Chan, W., Paul, R., and Toews, J.: Intrapartum fetal monitoring, Obstet. Gynecol. **41:**7, 1973.

Chang, A., and Wood, C.: Fetal-acid-base balance, Am. J. Obstet. Gynecol. **125:**61, 1976.

Davenport, H.W.: The ABC's of acid-base chemistry, Chicago, 1974, University of Chicago Press.

DeGruyter, W.: J. Perinat. Med. vol. 1, 1973.

DeLaRama, X., and Merkatz, I.: Evaluation of fetal scalp pH with a proposed new clinical assessment of the neonate, Am. J. Obstet. Gynecol. **107:**94, 1970.

Edington, P.T., and Beard, R.W.: Influence on clinical obstetrics of routine intrapartum fetal monitoring, Br. Med. J. **3:**341, 1975.

Fetal blood sampling, American College of Obstetricians and Gynecologists Technical Bulletin No. 42, 1976.

Hon, E.: Biochemical studies of the fetus, Obstet. Gynecol. **33:**219, 1967.

James, L.S., and others: The acid-base status of human infants in relation to birth asphyxia and the onset of respiration, J. Pediatr. **52:**379, 1958.

Lee, W., and Baggish, M.: The effect of unselected intrapartum fetal monitoring, Obstet. Gynecol. **47:**516, 1976.

Löfgren, O.: Continuous transcutaneous oxygen monitoring in fetal surveillance during labor, Am. J. Obstet. Gynecol. **141:**729, 1981.

Low, J.A.: Acid-base, lactate and pyruvate characteristics of the normal obstetric patient and fetus during the intrapartum period, Am. J. Obstet. Gynecol. **120:**762, 1974.

Low, J.A., and others: The acid-base and biochemical characteristics of intrapartum fetal asphyxia, Am. J. Obstet. Gynecol. **121:**446, 1975.

MacDonald, J.: Evaluation of fetal blood pH as a reflection of fetal well being, Am. J. Obstet. Gynecol. **97:**912, 1967.

Mondanlou, H., and others: Complications of fetal blood sampling during labor, Clin. Pediatr. **12:**603, 1973.

Paul, R.: Clinical fetal monitoring, Am. J. Obstet. Gynecol. **115:**573, 1972.

Saling, E.: Foetal and neonatal hypoxia, London, 1966, Edward Arnold Publishers, Ltd.

Saling, E., and Schneider, D.: Biochemical supervision of the fetus during labor, J. Obstet. Gynecol. Brit. Commonwealth **74:**799, 1967.

Schenker, L.: Clinical experiences with fetal heart rate monitoring of one thousand patients in labor, Am. J. Obstet. Gynecol. **115:**1111, 1973.

Tejani, N., Mann, L., and Bhakthavathsalan, A.: Correlation of fetal heart rate patterns and fetal pH with neonatal outcome, Obstet. Gynecol. **48:**460, 1976.

Tejani, N., and others: Correlation of fetal heart rate—uterine contraction patterns with fetal scalp blood pH, Obstet. Gynecol. **46:**392, 1975.

Thomas, G.: The aetiology, characteristics and diagnostic relevance of late deceleration patterns in routine obstetric practice, Br. J. Obstet. Gynecol. **82:**121, 1975.

CHAPTER 10

Neonatal clinical cardiopulmonary monitoring

A computer does not substitute for judgment any more than a pencil substitutes for literacy.

Robert S. McNamara

Monitoring of biophysical and biochemical parameters is an integral part of neonatal intensive care (Chapter 19, part three). When monitoring a patient it is important to determine what parameters need to be followed and to understand the characteristics of what is being measured. Knowledge of principles and techniques by which instruments operate should be shared by all members of the team responsible for patient care. Furthermore, review of monitoring records is a valuable teaching tool and objective method of quality control of care.

NEONATAL HEART RATE MONITORING

The clinical evaluation of neonatal heart rate (NHR) has been based on stethoscopic auscultation or electrocardiographic tracings. These techniques average the counted heart beats and, in addition to the loss of large amounts of data, detect only marked tachycardia or bradycardia, not transient changes. This is illustrated in Fig. 10-1, which shows the comparison of instantaneous and average heart rate counting techniques and illustrates the increased detail of the instantaneous heart rate, which is obtained using a cardiotachometer that displays beat-to-beat heart rate after each cardiac cycle. The bioengineering aspects of neonatal heart rate monitoring are further discussed in Chapter 19.

Normal heart rate

The baseline NHR is related to gestational age, postnatal age, race, and state of sleep or wakefulness. Variations in this baseline level reflect differences in the degree of neurocirculatory control exerted at specific times and in different sleep states. Heart rate can be properly interpreted only when sleep state is taken into account, since variability is markedly increased during active as compared with quiet sleep. From the first minute of life the NHR appears to be a good indicator of how the infant has tolerated the stress of labor and delivery and reflects the adequacy of adaptation to extrauterine life. Following delivery of a vigorous infant the NHR will change rapidly, with a higher baseline observed at this time than during labor. The mean NHR of healthy term infants is 175 beats per minute at 1 minute; within 2 minutes the NHR rises to a mean of 189 beats per minute and then declines, falling by 20 beats at 5 minutes and by 40 beats at 20 minutes. The NHR of healthy preterm infants follows a similar pattern after birth but shows a significantly lower peak and a slower rate of decline.

The baseline NHR as a function of postnatal age during the first week of life is shown in Fig. 10-2 for healthy and sick preterm infants. After the first week of life the heart rate reaches a maximum of 148 and 132 for preterm and term infants between 4 and 8 weeks of age. Thereafter it rapidly decreases during the remainder of the first six months. In small for gestational age infants, changes in NHR follow a similar pattern to that of appropriately grown neonates.

Baseline changes

The interpretation of NHR recordings requires a classification of changes in heart rate levels. Four alterations of the baseline heart rate have been described according to the direction and duration of the changes. *Tachycardia* or *bradycardia* is defined as baseline levels above or below the normal limits for the patient's age and maturity. More transient rises or falls from baseline levels are often referred to as *accelerations* or *decelerations*. Continuous beat-to-beat NHR recordings show rapid alterations in the NHR associated with changes in respiratory rate and pattern of respiration, with procedures, as a response to medications, and as a manifestation of various clinical entities. Following is an outline of entities or procedures that may elicit such alterations. Neonatal cardiac arrhythmias are discussed in Chapter 25.

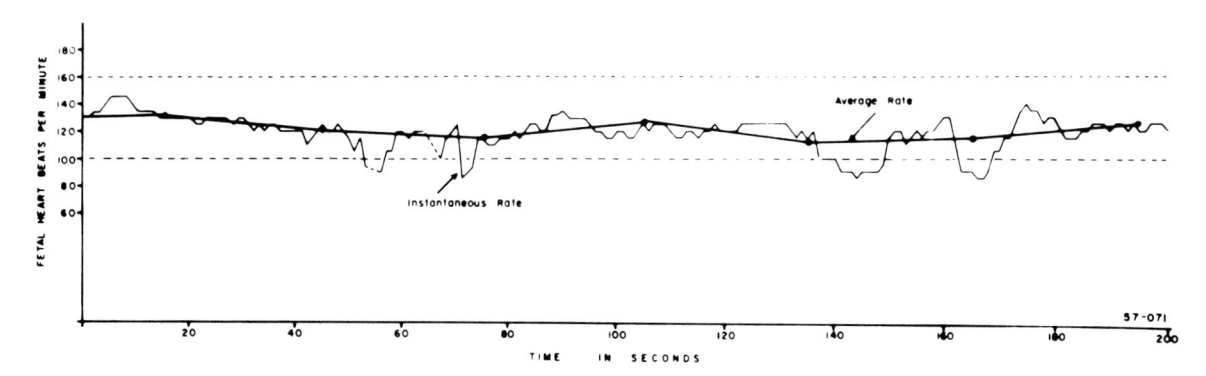

Fig. 10-1. Comparison of instantaneous and average heart rates. (From Hon, E., Cabal, L., and Zanini, B.: An introduction to neonatal heart rate monitoring, North Haven, Conn., 1975, W. Mack Publishing Co.)

Fig. 10-2. Mean (± SEM) heart rate levels as a function of postnatal age in healthy preterm infants (*n* = 38) and sick preterm infants with severe RDS (*n* = 19).

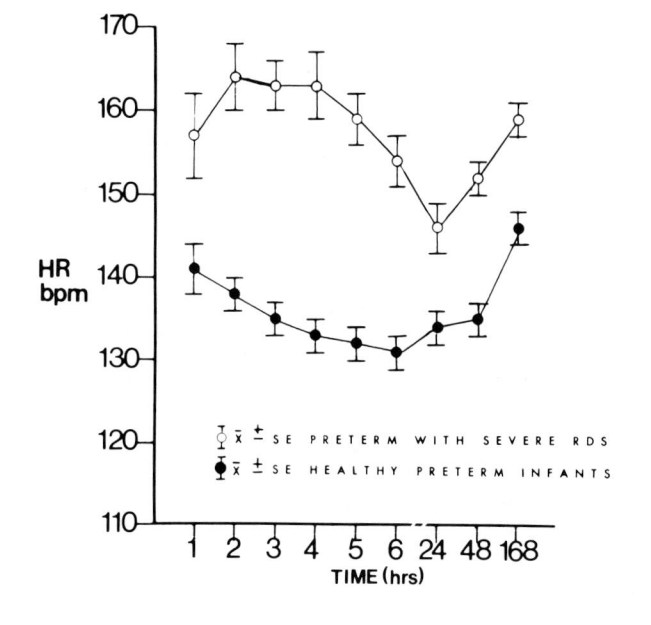

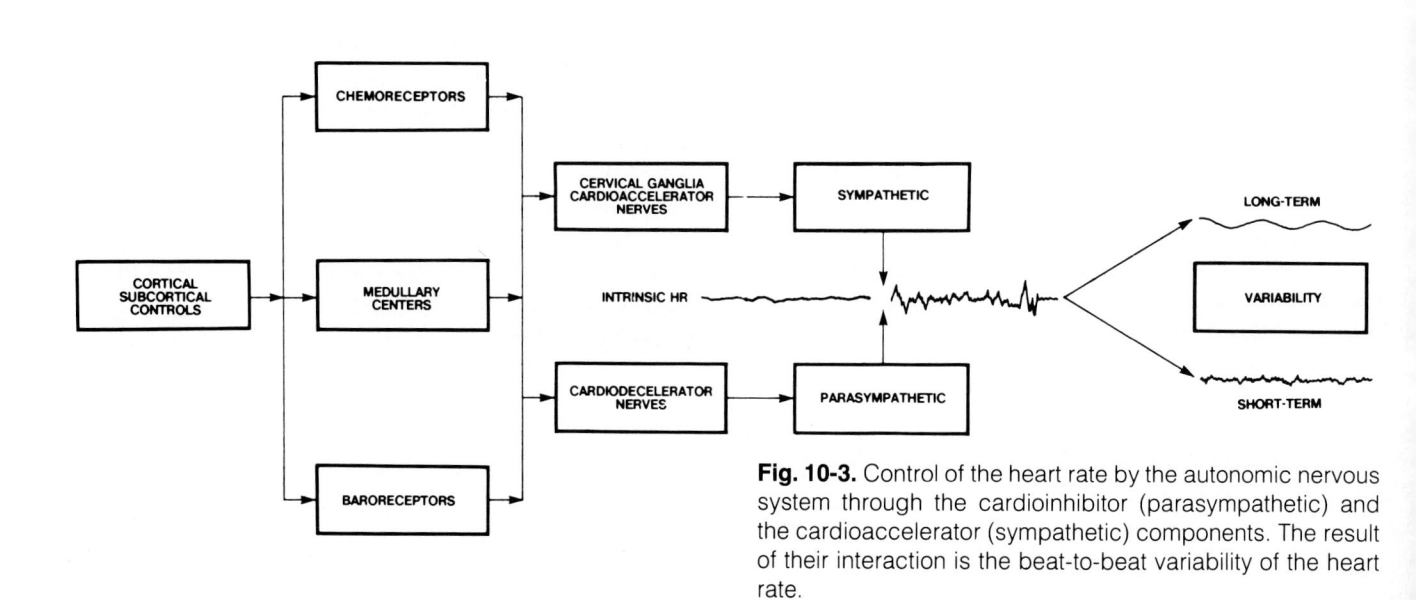

Fig. 10-3. Control of the heart rate by the autonomic nervous system through the cardioinhibitor (parasympathetic) and the cardioaccelerator (sympathetic) components. The result of their interaction is the beat-to-beat variability of the heart rate.

A. Causes of neonatal tachycardia
   1. Physiologic reactions
      a. Somatic activity (prolonged)
      b. Post delivery
   2. Maneuvers and procedures
      a. Hyperventilation
      b. Heat stress
      c. Cold stress
      d. Painful stimuli
   3. Drugs
      a. Isoproterenol
      b. Tolazoline
      c. Atropine
      d. Pancuronium bromide
      e. Epinephrine
      f. Aminophylline
      g. Glucagon (IV)
   4. Pathologic conditions
      a. Hypoxia
      b. Shock
      c. Hypercapnia
      d. Fever
      e. Anemia
      f. Sepsis
      g. Patent ductus arteriosus
      h. Congestive heart failure
      i. Cardiac arrhythmias
      j. Postasphyxic states
      k. Metabolic disorders
      l. Hyperammonemia
      m. Hyperthyroidism
      n. Pheochromocytoma
B. Causes of neonatal bradycardia
   1. Physiologic reactions
      a. Swallowing
      b. Micturition
      c. Defecation
      d. Vomiting
      e. Head compression
      f. Carotid compression
      g. Ocular compression
   2. Maneuvers and procedures
      a. Pharyngeal stimulation
      b. Tracheal stimulation
      c. Gavage feedings
      d. Airway suction
      e. Abdominal compression
      f. Visceral manipulation during surgery
      g. Excessive transpulmonary pressure
   3. Drugs
      a. Propranolol
      b. Digitalis
      c. Atropine (during hypoxia)
      d. Local anesthetics
      e. Calcium infusions
   4. Pathologic conditions
      a. Hypoxia
      b. Acidosis (severe)
      c. Hypothermia (severe)
      d. Shock (late)
      e. Apnea
      f. Congestive heart failure
      g. Pneumothorax-pneumopericardium
      h. Airway obstruction
      i. Hyperkalemia
      j. Cardiac arrhythmias
      k. Pulmonary hemorrhage
      l. Hydrocephalus
      m. Intracranial bleeding
      n. Convulsions
      o. Diaphragmatic hernia
      p. Hypothyroidism
      q. Bile pigments

Heart rate variability

In normal subjects, heart rate is determined by the intrinsic rhythm of the sinoatrial node pacemaker modified by the interaction of the different physiologic control systems. Fig. 10-3 illustrates the heart rate control by the autonomic nervous system through the cardioinhibitor (parasympathetic) and the cardioaccelerator (sympathetic) components. Sympathetic control is via the cardioaccelerator nerves and parasympathetic primarily via the vagus nerve. The sympathetic and parasympathetic systems are physiologic antagonists in their controlling action over the sinoatrial node and, because of their changing tone and different time constants, the result of their interaction is the beat-to-beat variability of heart rate, reflecting the reactivity of each system at a specific time.

Heart rate variability has been shown to have at least two components: (1) long-term variability (LTV), defined as the difference between the minimum and maximum oscillations of heart rate within a time period, and (2) short-term variability (STV), obtained from the mean of successive R-R interval length differences. LTV is thought to result from the dynamic balance between the sympathetic and parasympathetic divisions of the autonomic nervous system, whereas STV is generated by the oscillations of vagal tone controlling the heart rate. Variability is an integral part of the neonatal heart rate, and its absence may reflect damage, obtundation, or immaturity of the autonomic nervous system control over the heart. Furthermore, since the mechanisms of heart rate control include the reflex interaction with other higher centers and peripheral receptors, the quantification of variability thereby provides a technique for evaluating pathophysiologic and pharmacologic fetal and neonatal responses. Most of the studies dealing with NHR vari-

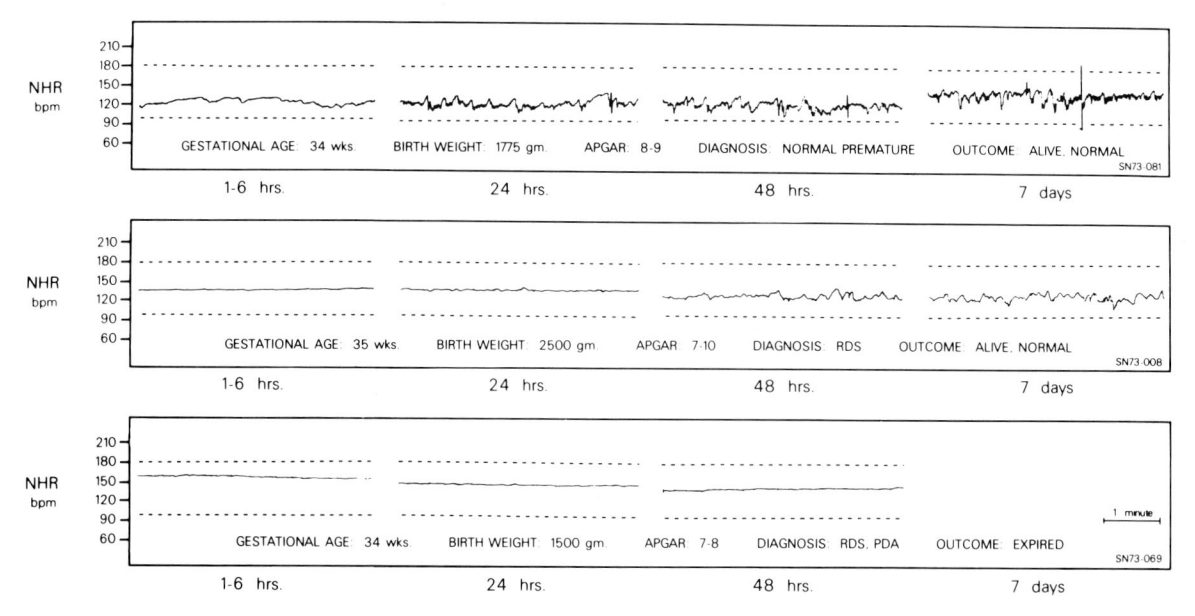

Fig. 10-4. Recordings illustrating the baseline NHR variability of three infants with different clinical conditions at varying ages of life.

ability have been performed in healthy term infants, and only a few are available in preterm infants.

Recent studies have provided quantitative data of NHR variability. They show that in healthy preterm infants the baseline heart rate is stable during the first 48 hours of life and increases by 7 days. There is an inverse relationship between neonatal heart rate variability and baseline heart rate levels. Interpretation of heart rate variability can be done only when the heart rate levels in beats per minute or as R-R intervals are taken into account. NHR variability, corrected for heart rate levels, increases with advancing postnatal age in healthy infants, suggesting maturation and stabilization of the autonomic nervous system control.

Our studies, as well as those of others, have demonstrated that heart rate variability corrected for heart rate levels is remarkably decreased in preterm infants with respiratory distress syndrome (RDS). The decrease in heart rate variability is proportional to the increasing severity of the RDS. The lack of variability is reversible in infants who recover from RDS and persists in infants dying from this disorder (Fig. 10-4). In infants recovering from RDS the return of variability heralds a good prognosis. Decreased heart rate variability found in infants with RDS may reflect suppression of the cardioregulatory centers.

RESPIRATION

Respiration can be monitored by direct and indirect methods (Table 10-1). Direct methods sense the air exchange between the infants airway and an outside source. Indirect methods detect body motion or measure physical property changes of the body caused by breathing. Some of the direct methods not only sense a change occurring with breathing but also may add information regarding the effectiveness of respiration, i.e., the volume exchanged or the degree to which CO_2 is removed from the lungs. Table 10-2 summarizes the advantages and disadvantages of the various methods used for respiratory monitoring; the bioengineering aspects of the commonly employed techniques are discussed in Chapter 19, part three.

Patterns of breathing

The description of the various patterns of breathing is based on the relationship between the rate and depth of breathing, either from one respiratory cycle to another or over longer periods of time. The patterns of breathing found in newborn infants are regular breathing, irregular breathing, periodic breathing, paradoxical (disorganized) breathing, oscillatory breathing, sighs, gasping, Cheyne-Stokes and Biot-like breathing, and apnea (Fig. 10-5).

Regular breathing is the pattern during which breath-to-breath intervals are nearly equal and individual breaths are of similar depth. This pattern is commonly found in mature infants during quiet (non-REM) sleep. Irregular breathing is characterized by marked variability of the depth and timing of respiration; it is commonly found in preterm infants and is usually present—even in mature infants—during active (REM) sleep (Chapter 23, part four). Short, repeated cessations of air exchange for 3 seconds or longer, occurring at regular intervals, are

Table 10-1. Techniques for monitoring respiration

System	Elements	Operation
Thermistor	Thermistor in face mask, nasal prongs, or under nose	Resistance of thermistor changes as it is warmed or cooled by inhaled air
Pneumotachograph	Fine mesh screen placed across patient's airway	Detects air flow by measurement of pressure drop across screen
Spirometer	Reservoir connected to patient's airway	Measures volume of air breathed by patient
Phonopneumograph	Microphone under nose or on skin over upper airway	Detects air flow by sensing inspiratory and expiratory breath sounds
Capnograph	Infrared light connected to patient's airway	Detects CO_2 (% or PCO_2) change during inspiration and expiration by sensing changes in infrared light absorption
Impedance pneumograph	A 10- to 100-kHz electric current of approx. 50 μA is passed through 2 chest electrodes placed across thorax	Change in chest air and blood volume with each breath causes impedance that generates voltage change
Body plethysmograph	Infant placed in airtight box with face exposed to the outside; box is connected with strain gauge or with pneumotachometer	Volume of air displaced with each breath is sensed by pneumotachometer or pressure transducer
Radar/Doppler	Radiotransmitter/receiver of signals directed to infant's chest	Detects changes in signals reflected from infant during breathing motion
Mercury-in-rubber strain gauge	Encircles abdomen and/or thorax	Senses pressure changes generated by expansion and contraction with breathing movements
Air-filled tubing pneumograph	Two small, hollow, corrugated rubber tubes strapped around chest and/or thorax and connected to an air tambour	Air tambour senses air displacement caused by thoracoabdominal motion during breathing
Capacitance pneumograph	Patient lies between 2 conductive plates that form a capacitor	Detects changes in capacitance between plates caused by breathing movements
Photoelectric pneumograph	Photoelectric cell emitting particular wavelengths of light to chest tissue	Detects breathing-induced alterations in absorption of light by blood in underlying tissue
Air mattress	Tubing connected to heated thermistor	Breathing movements displace air in coiled air-filled tubing: displaced air cools heated thermistor
Capacitive mattress	Two capacitors in mattress interspaced with fine wire mesh	Vertical components of breathing movements induce changes in capacitance, which are interpreted as breathing
Pressure transducer mattress	Pressure transducer in mattress or pad	Respiratory movements alter pressure on mattress, and these pressure changes are interpreted as breathing
Magnet mattress/pad	Magnet placed on patient's abdomen or chest and coiled wire placed in the mattress or pad	Magnet movements during breathing induce voltage changes in coiled wire which are amplified and interpreted as breathing
Airway pressure	A tap between endotracheal tube and ventilator circuits is connected to pressure transducer	Detects pressure changes occurring with patient's spontaneous respiration and with cycling of ventilator
Central venous and esophageal pressures	A central venous and a water-filled esophageal catheter or balloon placed at lower third of esophagus and connected to strain gauges	Detect changes in pleural pressures caused during inspiration, expiration, and cycling of ventilator

Table 10-2. Advantages and disadvantages of respiratory monitoring methods

	Impedance	Thermistor	Capnograph	Phonopneumograph	Mattress	Magnets
Disadvantages						
Easily damaged, deteriorated, or lost		X			X	X
Sensitive to noise, humidity, air currents, or magnetic materials		X	X	X		X
Sensitive to cardiovascular artifacts	X		X			
Sensitive to vibration					X	X
Sensitive to body movements	X				X	X
Others	Skin trauma; possibility of electrical shock	May increase airway resistance; difficult to clean	Changes with circulation		Displacement of infant or sensor	Radiopaque
Advantages						
Easy setup				X	X	X
Easy to operate	X	X	X	X	X	X
No electrical contact with baby			X	X	X	X
No direct contact with baby			X		X	
Others	Uses ECG electrodes; reflects chest volume changes			Identifies inspiratory and expiratory phases	Radiolucent	

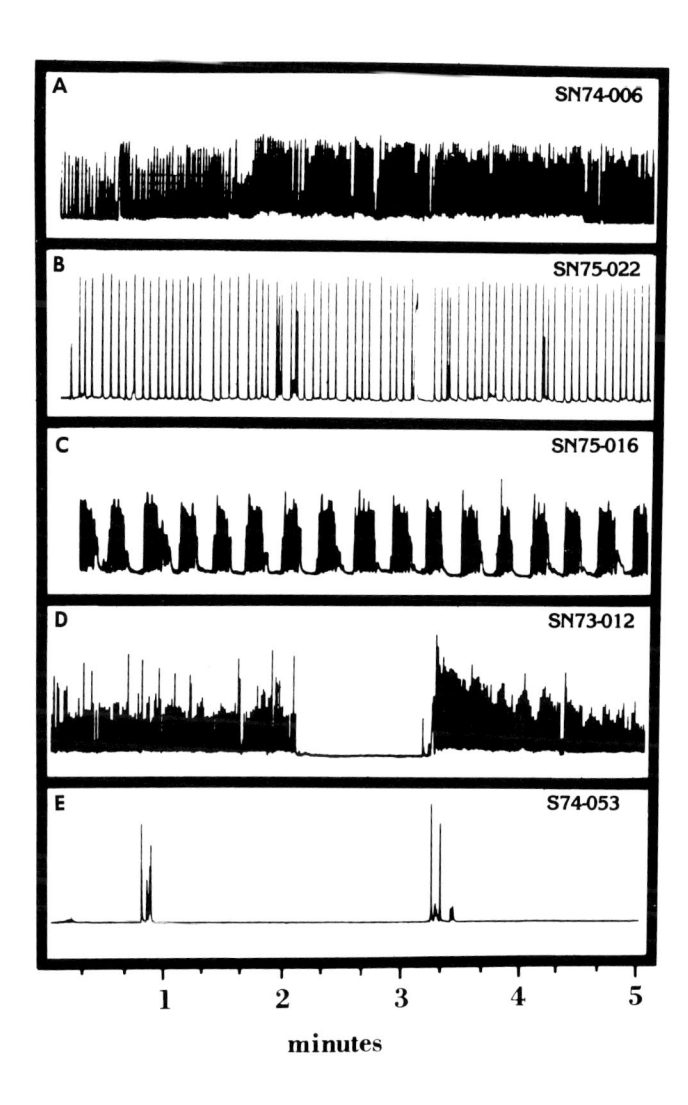

Neonatal clinical cardiopulmonary monitoring **125**

Fig. 10-5. Various patterns of breathing found in newborn infants. **A,** Fast and regular; **B,** slow and regular; **C,** periodic; **D,** apnea; **E,** terminal gasping.

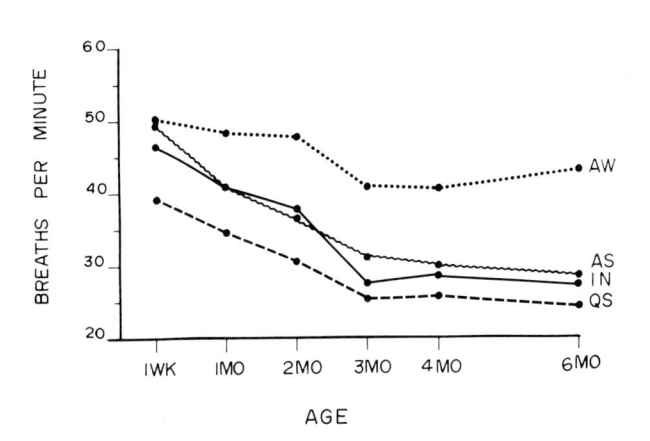

Fig. 10-6. Average median respiratory rate obtained from eight healthy term infants at various ages while awake *(AW)* and in active *(AS)*, quiet *(QS)*, and indeterminate *(IN)* sleep states. (From Hoppenbraouwers, T., Hodgman, J., and Harper, R.: Pediatr. Res. **12:**120, 1978.)

defined as periodic breathing. The breathing pattern of preterm infants is typically periodic and irregular; as gestation advances, the pattern becomes less periodic and more regular. The rate of respiration decreases markedly in all sleep states from the first week to the third month of life (Fig. 10-6).

There is no agreement in the literature on the duration of nonbreathing periods that either can be defined as apnea or classified as pathologic (Chapter 23, part four). For sleep studies, apnea of greater than 2 seconds has been considered significant; however, the clinical definition of significant apnea ranges between greater than 10 seconds up to 60 seconds. Apnea has been considered more significant when it is associated with heart rate decelerations and/or evidence of impaired oxygenation.

ARTERIAL BLOOD PRESSURE

Close attention to the technical details of measurement and cautious interpretation of the pressure values are essential in monitoring arterial blood pressure in the newborn infant. It should also be borne in mind that the so-called normal blood pressure values reported for small premature infants might have been influenced by the abnormal transitional circulation that may have occurred during the immediate neonatal period. Finally, the temptation to equate low arterial blood pressure with hypovolemia should be vigorously avoided, and the arterial blood pressure should be interpreted in the context of the clinical condition of the infant.

The pressure pulse is generated in the arterial system as a result of cardiac ejection. The maximum pressure reached in the arterial system during cardiac ejection is the systolic pressure. During the diastolic phase of the cardiac cycle the arterial pressure falls progressively, reaching the minimum pressure, or the diastolic pressure. Mean blood pressure is determined by integration of pulse contour during the interval of the cardiac cycle. The pulse pressure is the difference between systolic and diastolic pressure. A very crude estimate of the mean blood pressure may be obtained by adding one third of the pulse pressure to the diastolic pressure.

Mean blood pressure is equal to the cardiac output times the total peripheral resistance. The systolic pressure depends on the stroke volume, cardiac contractility, and arterial distensibility; the diastolic pressure depends on the level of systolic pressure, peripheral resistance, heart rate, and arterial elastic recoil.

Methods of measurement

With the exception of the intraarterial pressure measurement, all other methods use a blood pressure cuff that interrupts blood flow on inflation; the pressure may be detected at or beyond the cuff during deflation. The width of the pressure cuff should be 25% greater than the diameter of the arm or leg where blood pressure is being measured. Several methods for determining blood pressure are in use. The biophysical aspects of various techniques for pressure measurement are discussed in Chapter 19.

1. *Auscultation*. This is based on detection of Korotkoff sounds during cuff deflation. The systolic pressure corresponds to the point at which the initial Korotkoff sounds are heard. Muffling of the sound is the best index of the diastolic pressure.
2. *Palpation*. This technique is not particularly useful in the neonatal period, since the pulse may be difficult to feel in either the arm or the leg beyond the cuff.
3. *Flush technique*. This method consists of placing a suitable cuff around the forearm or the calf, raising and squeezing the limb while quickly inflating the cuff, and on deflation detecting the earliest appearance of cutaneous flush. The level of the pressure is obtained when the flush first appears in the blanched area. This pressure reading is more likely to be a mean pressure.
4. *Oscillometry*. Pressure changes are transmitted through the arterial wall to the pressure cuff, and the oscillations are detected by a sensitive pressure indicator.
5. *Doppler ultrasound technique*. A Doppler ultrasound transducer detects arterial wall oscillations that produce the major components of Korotkoff sounds. The frequency analysis of these oscillations accurately indicates the systolic pressure and to a lesser degree of accuracy the diastolic pressure.
6. *Direct measurement of arterial blood pressure*. A saline-filled catheter connected to the arterial line is attached to a strain gauge pressure transducer. The strain gauge is zeroed to the midaxillary line while the infant is lying supine in a horizontal position. In this manner it is possible to record the arterial pressure and the pressure wave.

Analysis of aortic pulse wave

An undamped aortic pressure pulse recorded through an umbilical arterial catheter can be analyzed for pulse wave characteristics providing potentially useful information. The pulse contour in the aorta shows a rapid upstroke during systole, interrupted by the anachrotic notch and a slower rise to peak pressure. The end of systole with the sudden closure of the aortic valve is indicated by the dicrotic notch. During diastole, as the blood flows out of the aorta into the peripheral vessels, initially the diastolic pressure decreases more rapidly and then more slowly (Fig. 10-7).

In the absence of aortic stenosis the rate of aortic systolic pressure rise gives a rough indication of the state of contractility of the left ventricle. In the presence of valvular aortic stenosis the upstroke of the aortic pressure is decreased. The rate of aortic diastolic pressure decay gives an indication of systemic vascular resistance. A rapid aortic diastolic pressure drop may be present in infants with left-to-right shunt through the ductus arteriosus.

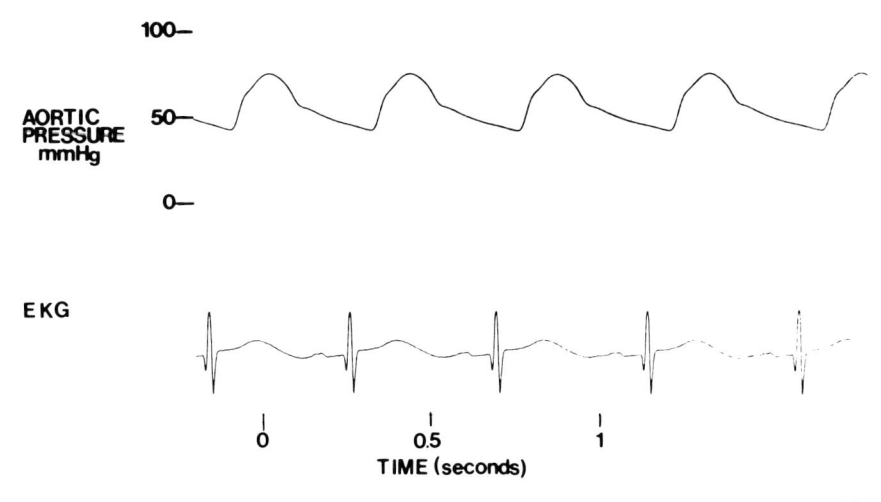

Fig. 10-7. Aortic pressure pulse. Note rapid upstroke during early systole interrupted by an anacrotic shoulder. The end of systole is heralded by a dicrotic notch followed by the diastolic phase.

Pitfalls in the measurement and interpretation of arterial blood pressure

The indirect methods of arterial blood pressure measurement should be considered an approximation of the true arterial pressure in the neonate. Most indirect techniques are reasonably reliable in determining the systolic pressure, whereas the diastolic pressure is measured less accurately. The indirect methods of pressure measurements are less reliable in neonates in shock. The Doppler ultrasound technique is generally considered to give the most reliable noninvasive pressure measurements.

Direct arterial pressure recording provides the most accurate measure of the arterial pressure, provided that (1) the catheter and the connecting tube systems are leak free, (2) clots and air bubbles are excluded, (3) the lumen of the indwelling catheter and needle is large enough, (4) the connecting tube is nondistensible, and (5) the transducer is defect free, properly calibrated, and zeroed accurately. If a small-lumen indwelling catheter (lumen of small caliber or decreased by fibrin deposition) is used or when an air bubble is present in the pressure system, a damped pressure is recorded. Under these circumstances the systolic pressure will be decreased, and the diastolic pressure will be altered (increased, decreased, or unchanged). Therefore the mean pressure will be either unaltered or decreased, and the pulse wave will be diminished with disappearance of the dicrotic notch. Furthermore, intraarterial pressure obtained from small distal arteries (radial, temporal, or dorsalis pedis) will be diminished or even disappear in circulatory shock and in other conditions with peripheral vasoconstriction.

Arterial blood pressure of neonates is best correlated with body weight (Fig. 10-8) (see also Chapter 25 and Appendix B). In general, a neonatal diastolic pressure lower than 25 mm Hg and a mean pressure less than 30 mm Hg should cause concern. Conversely, a diastolic pressure greater than 50 mm Hg in preterm and 60 mm Hg in term infants, or a mean pressure greater than 60 mm Hg in preterm and 70 mm Hg in term infants, should be considered beyond normal range. The underlying causes of alteration in arterial pressure should be investigated with awareness of the pathophysiology. Following is an outline of some of the disease states that can alter arterial blood pressure. Furthermore, some of the commonly accepted clinical manipulations may have profound transient effect on the arterial pressure.

A. Systolic and diastolic hypertension
   1. Renal hypertension
      a. Renal parenchymal disease: acute renal failure, hydronephrosis, polycystic kidneys
      b. Renovascular hypertension
   2. Neurogenic hypertension
      a. Increased intracranial pressure: intracranial hemorrhage, hydrocephalus, meningitis, hyperammonemia
   3. Endocrine hypertension
      a. Hyperthyroidism
      b. Pheochromocytoma
      c. Congenital adrenal hyperplasia
   4. Coarctation of the aorta
   5. After cardiac surgery
      a. Patent ductus arteriosus ligation
      b. Ligation of arteriovenous fistula
      c. Miscellaneous
   6. Idiopathic (essential hypertension?)
   7. Drugs: phenylephrine, epinephrine, dopamine, pancuronium
B. Systolic hypertension
   1. Patent ductus arteriosus
   2. Anemia

3. Fever
4. Aortic regurgitation
5. Arteriovenous fistula
6. Thyrotoxicosis
7. Drugs: isoproterenol
C. Systolic and diastolic hypotension
 1. Cardiogenic shock
  a. Myocardial dysfunction: asphyxia, hypoglycemia, hypocalcemia
  b. Severe cardiac arrhythmias, heart block, tachyarrhythmia
  c. Mechanical restrictions of cardiac function or venous return: tension pneumothorax, diaphragmatic hernia, cardiac tamponade
  d. Congenital cardiac defects: hypoplastic left side of heart, coarctation of the aorta, critical aortic stenosis, patent ductus with left ventricular failure, arteriovenous fistula, critical pulmonary stenosis, cor triatriatum
 2. Hypovolemic shock
  a. Antepartum blood loss: placenta previa, abruptio placentae, fetomaternal and twin-to-twin transfusions, birth injuries
  b. Postpartum blood loss: vitamin K deficiency, disseminated intravascular coagulation, iatrogenic causes
  c. Fluid and electrolyte loss: heat stress, GI abnormalities, iatrogenic causes
 3. Neurogenic shock
  a. Massive intracranial hemorrhage
  b. Severe hypoxic damage
 4. Septic shock
  a. Gram positive: group B *Streptococcus, Staphylococcus, Listeria* infections
  b. Gram negative: *E. coli, Pseudomonas, Klebsiella, Proteus* infections
 5. Drug toxicity: digitalis, barbiturates, phenothiazines, diuretics, vasodilators
D. Diastolic hypotension
 1. Patent ductus arteriosus
 2. Bradycardia
 3. Early sepsis
 4. Arteriovenous fistula
 5. Vasodilators

CENTRAL VENOUS PRESSURE (CVP)

The value of central venous or right atrial pressure measurement in the critically ill child and adult is well established. It has been useful mainly as an aid for fluid replacement, in postoperative management of patients undergoing cardiac surgery, and in the management of shock. There is less agreement about the value of CVP monitoring during infancy; however, it is now generally agreed that similar factors affecting CVP in older children and adults are operative during infancy. In general,

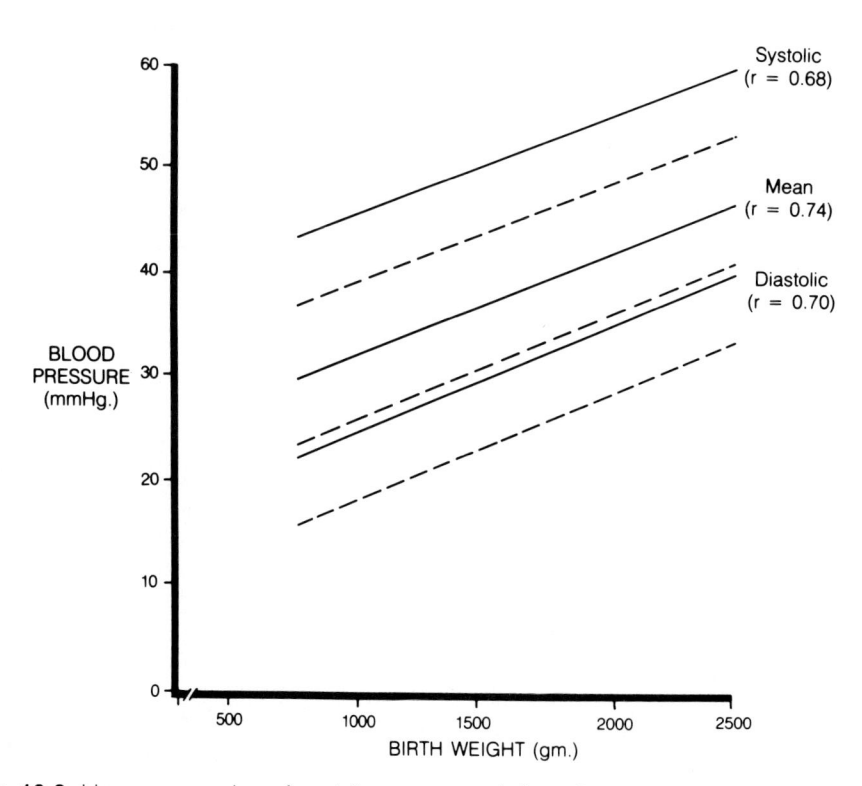

Fig. 10-8. Linear regression of systolic, mean, and diastolic blood pressure versus birth weights during the first 24 hours of life in 59 premature infants (*n* = 120). The dotted lines represent lowest systolic, diastolic, and mean pressure at 90% confidence level.

right atrial pressure is affected by the pumping effectiveness of the right ventricle, the systemic venous return, and the pressure surrounding the heart. Acute left ventricular failure is not usually associated with right-sided heart failure. Accordingly, premature infants with patent ductus arteriosus and left ventricular failure often have normal right atrial pressure, except during terminal stages when combined ventricular failure with cardiogenic shock supervenes. In contrast, in severe right ventricular failure, such as in hypoplastic left ventricle, CVP is almost invariably increased. Changes in venous return as a determinant of right atrial pressure are the basis for the use of CVP to determine adequacy of fluid replacement. Large intravascular volume expansion is required to affect the CVP in patients with normal cardiopulmonary systems. Neonates with borderline right ventricular failure, however, may show significant changes in CVP after moderate intravascular volume expansion. The changes in pressure surrounding the heart have the most dramatic effect on the right atrial pressure. Thus development of tension pneumothorax or cardiac tamponade is associated with immediate rise in CVP in newborn infants.

Method of measurement

Since central venous or right atrial pressures fluctuate within a few millimeters of mercury, an accurately calibrated and zeroed strain gauge transducer should be employed for their measurement. The catheter tip should be located in the right atrium, inferior vena cava, or superior vena cava close to the right atrium. Special care should be taken when measuring CVP through the umbilical vein, since a catheter blindly introduced can be located at any of the following sites: umbilical vein, portal vein, ductus venosus, interior vena cava, right atrium, superior vena cava, or left atrium. The location of the tip of the catheter can be determined from the length inserted, pressure wave analysis, and oxygen saturation measurements and should be confirmed by a chest radiograph. The transducer should be zeroed to the midaxillary line while the infant is resting in a supine horizontal position.

Pressure wave analysis (Table 10-3)

Central venous and atrial pressures are influenced by cardiac action and respiration. Two major pressure waves are generated as the result of cardiac action: the a wave is generated by atrial contraction, whereas the v wave is produced by atrial filling against a closed atrioventricular valve. During spontaneous respiration the negative intrathoracic pressure generated during inspiration is transmitted to the central veins and atria and is inscribed as a negative pressure wave, whereas during intermittent positive pressure respiration a positive pressure wave is transmitted during mechanical inspiration. The pressure waves are minimal or absent in peripheral veins, portal vein, and ductus venosus and are prominent in central veins and the atria. Normally the right atrial a wave is higher than v wave, whereas in the left atrium both a and v waves are prominent (Fig. 10-9).

Although slightly higher normal values for central venous and atrial pressures have been reported in later childhood and adulthood, during the early neonatal period the central venous and atrial pressures are not correlated with birth weights. Infants with atrioventricular valve insufficiency have prominent v waves in the corresponding atrial tracings. Prominent a waves are seen with nodal beats, and giant a waves are seen in atrial tracings due to superimposition of atrial and ventricular contractions.

Risk of central venous pressure monitoring

The benefit of central venous pressure monitoring should be weighed against the risks of prolonged right atrial or central venous catheterization. Indwelling central venous or right atrial catheterization carries an increased risk for thromboembolism, infection, and vascular perforation. This could be minimized by shortening the duration of catheterization and adhering strictly to aseptic catheter maintenance techniques. The central

Table 10-3. Venous pressure: site, characteristics, and normal range

Site	Pressure level	Venous waves	Changes with respiration	Average range	
Portal system	High	Absent	Slight ↑ with inspiration	Mean pressure 6.5 (2.5 to 10.5) mm Hg	
Right atrium	Low	Present; $a > v$ wave	Prominent ↓ with inspiration	a Wave Inspiratory wave Mean pressure	4.9 (+2 to +8) mm Hg −3.2 (0 to −8) mm Hg 1.4 (−3 to +4) mm Hg
Left atrium	Low	$v \geq a$ wave	Prominent ↓ with inspiration	a Wave v Wave Mean pressure	6.5 (+3 to +10) mm Hg 8.5 (+5 to +12) mm Hg 3.5 (+1 to +6) mm Hg

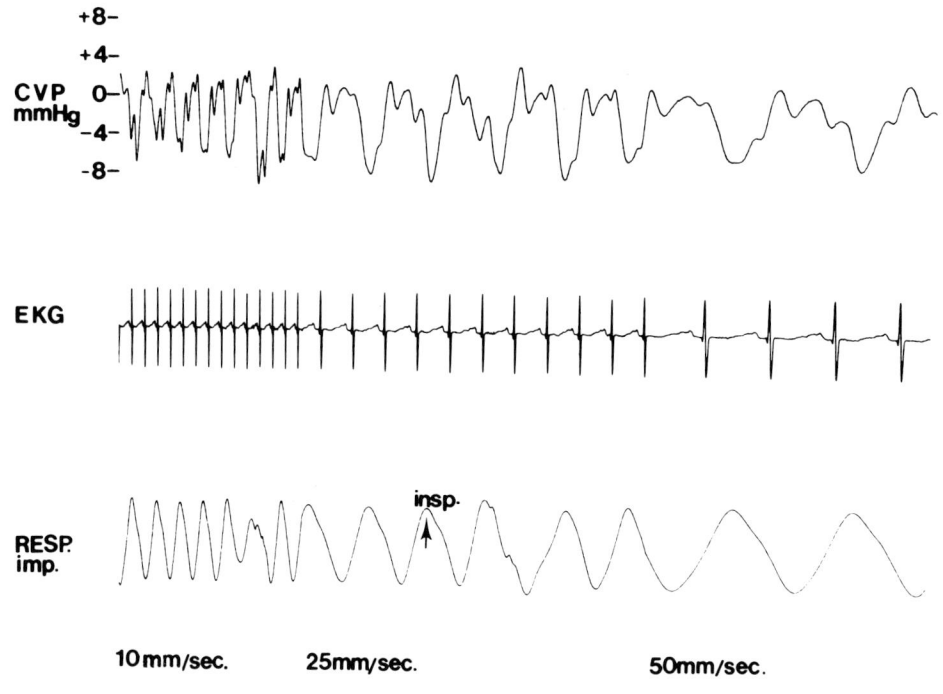

Fig. 10-9. Right atrial pressure measurement in a premature infant with RDS. Note a, v, and inspiratory waves.

venous line should be closed off to the patient to prevent the possibility of air embolism during the negative pressure created by the infant's inspiratory efforts.

PULMONARY ARTERY PRESSURE

The most crucial change that occurs during the transition from a fetal to a neonatal circulation is the sharp decrease in pulmonary vascular resistance and pressure below systemic levels. Except occasionally during the first hour of life, pulmonary artery pressure in healthy newborn infants remains lower than systemic arterial pressure and should be below 50% of systemic pressure by 24 hours of life. If pulmonary vascular resistance remains higher than systemic vascular resistance after birth, right-to-left shunt may persist across fetal channels, leading to neonatal cyanosis. The persistence of pulmonary hypertension (or persistence of the fetal circulation) may be primary or occur in a number of entities involving diseases or abnormalities of the heart and lungs. Some of the factors that affect pulmonary artery pressure follow.

Increased
1. Hypoxemia
2. Acidosis
3. Polycythemia
4. Primary increase in pulmonary artery smooth muscle
5. Chronic intrauterine stress
6. Fetal systemic hypertension
7. Perinatal asphyxia
8. Decreased cross-sectional area of pulmonary vascular bed: diaphragmatic hernia, pulmonary hypoplasia, lobar emphysema
9. Congenital cardiac defect with left-to-right shunts: ventricular septal defect, patent ductus arteriosus, transposition of great vessels
10. Left-sided heart failure: myocardial dysfunction, congenital cardiac defects
11. Obstruction to pulmonary venous return: diaphragmatic hernia, tension pneumothorax, congenital lobar emphysema, total anomalous pulmonary venous return, cor triatriatum
12. Pulmonary parenchymal disease: meconium aspiration, respiratory distress syndrome, pneumonia
13. Mechanical ventilation with high mean airway pressure
14. Pulmonary edema
15. Drugs: Norepinephrine, dopamine (high doses), epinephrine

Decreased
1. Hyperoxia
2. Decrease in pulmonary arterial smooth muscle
3. Drugs: isoproterenol, chlorpromazine, tolazoline, acetylcholine

Persistent pulmonary hypertension can be evaluated indirectly by echocardiographically determining the ratio of right ventricular preejection period/right ventricular ejection time (Chapter 25). Although clinically use-

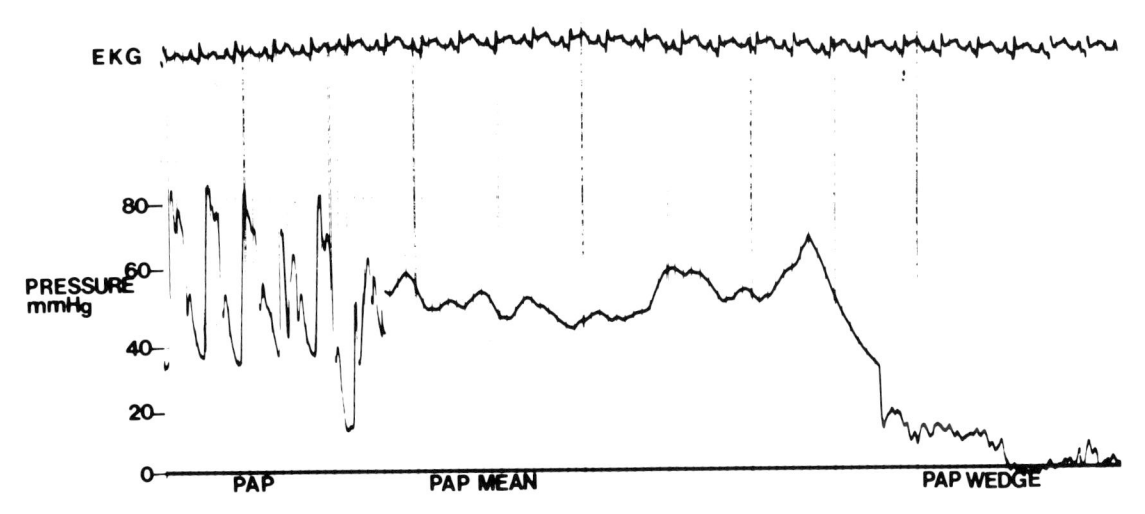

Fig. 10-10. Pulmonary arterial pressure *(PAP)* in a 3-day-old, full-term infant with meconium aspiration and persistent pulmonary hypertension. Note elevated pulmonary artery pressure and normal wedge pressure. In this case pulmonary artery pressure was monitored through a no. 5F Swan-Ganz balloon catheter; the wedge pressure was obtained after inflation of the balloon to occlude the right pulmonary artery.

ful, these measurements are not direct measurements of pulmonary hypertension. Continuous direct monitoring of pulmonary artery pressure through an indwelling catheter has become an accepted practice in critically sick adults. Recent experience with indwelling pulmonary artery catheters in critically ill neonates suggests potential usefulness of such a technique in selected cases.

Methods of measurement

Pulmonary artery catheters can be inserted percutaneously through umbilical or femoral veins and by cutdown technique through external jugular or femoral veins. Usually a no. 5F catheter (with or without ballooned tip) is manipulated under fluoroscopic control through the right ventricle and is left with its tip in the right or the left pulmonary arteries. Although balloon flotation catheters are placed routinely without fluoroscopy in older children and adults, we feel it is safer to place the catheter under direct vision in newborn infants. The pulmonary arterial pressure is measured using a strain gauge transducer, similar to the technique of direct arterial pressure monitoring (Fig. 10-10).

Risks of direct pulmonary arterial pressure monitoring

Perforation of the pulmonary artery, pulmonary embolism, infection, and massive pulmonary hemorrhage have been reported in adult patients with prolonged indwelling pulmonary arterial catheters. In view of the limited experience in the neonate, the risks of such procedures are not well evaluated. It is reasonable, however, to assume that the dangers are similar to those of prolonged central venous catheterization. To minimize such risks, we restrict direct pulmonary arterial pressure monitoring to critically ill full-term infants and limit the duration to less than 72 hours. Further experience with this technique will define the relative risk/benefit ratio of this procedure.

Luis A. Cabal
Bijan Siassi
Joan E. Hodgman

BIBLIOGRAPHY
Heart rate

Cabal, L.A., and others: Factors affecting heart rate variability in preterm infants, Pediatrics **65:**50, 1980.

Kero, P.: Heart rate variation in infants with respiratory distress syndrome, Acta Paediatr. Scand. Suppl. **250:**3, 1974.

Rudolph, A.J., and others: Cardiodynamic studies in the newborn. III. Heart rate patterns in infants with idiopathic respiratory distress syndrome, Pediatrics **36:**551, 1965.

Urbach, J.R., and others: Instantaneous heart rate patterns in newborn infants, Am. J. Obstet. Gynecol. **93:**965, 1965.

Valimaki, I.: Heart-rate variation in full-term newborn infants, Am. J. Obstet. Gynecol. **110:**343, 1971.

Valimaki, I., and Tarlo, P.A.: Heart rate patterns in newborn infants, Am. J. Obstet. Gynecol. **110:**343, 1971.

Respiration

Cherniack, N., and Longobardo, G.: Cheyne-Stokes breathing: an instability in physiological control, N. Engl. J. Med. **288:**952, 1973.

Hoppenbrouwers, T., and others: Polygraphic studies of normal infants during the first six months of life. II. Respiratory rate and variability as a function of state, Pediatr. Res. **12:**120, 1978.

Parmelee, A.H., Stern, E., and Harris, M.A.: Maturation of respiration in premature and young infants, Neuropaediatrie **3:**294, 1972.

Arterial blood pressure

Barr, P.A., Bailey, P.E., and Summers, J.: Relation between arterial blood pressure and blood volume and effect of infused albumin in sick preterm infants, Pediatrics **60:**282, 1977.

Brown, E.G., and others: Blood volume and blood pressure in infants with respiratory distress, J. Pediatr. **87:**1133, 1975.

Cabal, L.A., and Hodgman, M.: Neonatal monitoring: arterial and venous pressure. In Gregory, G., and Thibeault, D., editors: Neonatal pulmonary care, Menlo Park, Calif., 1979, Addison-Wesley Publishing Co., Inc.

Central venous and pulmonary artery pressure

Guyton, A.C., and Jones, C.E.: Central venous pressure: physiologic significance and clinical implications, Am. Heart J. **86:**431, 1973.

Peckham, G.C., Fox, W.W., and Blesa, M.: Continuous pulmonary artery pressure monitoring in persistent pulmonary hypertension of the newborn, Pediatr. Res. **11:**397, 1977.

Riemenschneider, T.A., and others: Disturbances of the transitional circulation: spectrum of pulmonary hypertension and myocardial dysfunction, J. Pediatr. **89:**622, 1976.

Siassi, B., and others: Central venous pressure in preterm infants, Biol. Neonate **37:**285, 1980.

Swan, H.J.C., and Ganz, W.: Use of balloon flotation catheters in critically ill patients, Surg. Clin. North Am. **55:**520, 1975.

CHAPTER 11 Obstetric management of prematurity

PART ONE
Estimation of fetal maturity

Termination of pregnancy by induction of labor or cesarean section late in gestation is an important therapeutic decision in obstetrics; often it represents the only effective means of treatment. It may be *indicated* for maternal or fetal well-being or both in a number of conditions, such as hypertensive disorders, Rh isoimmunization, and diabetes mellitus. It is also sometimes used *electively*, as in induction of labor for patient or physician convenience or scheduled repeat cesarean section. Selection of the proper time for termination of pregnancy requires, among other things, an ability to estimate gestational duration and the degree of maturity of the fetus. The extent to which estimated fetal maturity influences the timing of pregnancy termination varies with the reason for which the termination is being done. It frequently is the most important determinant.

Conventionally, pregnancy is dated from the last menstruation, and the mean interval from the onset of the last menstrual period (LMP) to the estimated date of confinement (EDC) is 280 days or 40 weeks. *Duration of pregnancy* refers to the number of *completed* weeks since the onset of the last menstruation, with the assumption that ovulation (and thus conception) occurred approximately 14 days after the LMP. *Gestational age* is a term applied to the fetus or newborn regarding the duration of pregnancy. Gestational age calculated from the maternal history may be corroborated by physical and neurologic examination of the newborn (Chapter 19, part one). *Fetal maturity* refers to the state of developmental maturation of the fetus or newborn in relation to its ability to adapt to extrauterine life. As a general term it applies to the totality of physiologic processes involved. Variation exists with respect to both overall maturity from fetus to fetus at a given gestational age and maturation of specific functional processes in the same fetus. In general, fetal maturity is regarded as occurring at a gestational age of 37 weeks.

CLINICAL MANIFESTATIONS

Several clinical characteristics are useful in estimating duration of pregnancy and, indirectly, fetal maturity. The *menstrual history* may yield unreliable estimates for a variety of reasons. The preovulatory interval may have been unexpectedly long (as in the patient who conceives immediately after a period of taking ovulatory suppressive drugs), or conception may have followed an unrecognized early spontaneous abortion without intervening menstruation. Both circumstances would result in overestimation of pregnancy duration. At the other extreme, bleeding in early pregnancy might masquerade as a menstrual period, leading to an underestimate of gestational length. Finally, the use of menstrual history depends on subjective data, that is the recollection of an isolated event occurring some time previously. Thus, whereas the menstrual history is reasonably precise for population groups, it may give unreliable results in individual patients.

Quickening, the time a pregnant woman first perceives fetal movement, normally occurs at 18 to 20 weeks' gestation. However, quickening is also highly subjective, and patients rarely recall it with precision.

By far the most reliable clinical index is the *uterine size* estimated on physical examination in the *first trimester*. As pregnancy progresses, however, the accuracy of this method decreases progressively. By the third trimester it becomes quite unreliable because of normal variation in fetal and placental size and amniotic fluid volume. Even if the correlation between fetal size and gestational age were close—which it is not—estimates of fetal size by abdominal palpation exhibit a tendency to overestimation of the small fetus and underestimation of the large fetus.

A reliable clinical sign is the time the *fetal heart* is heard with a stethoscope, which normally occurs at 20 weeks. Unfortunately, this index is rarely available because either patients are not seen frequently at this interval or careful auscultation is not done. When applicable, however, such information gives a reasonably reliable estimation of pregnancy duration.

RADIOGRAPHY AND ULTRASOUND

See also Chapters 8 and 39.

The most commonly used radiographic procedure in estimating fetal maturity involves the appearance of *epiphyseal centers* about the knee, the distal femoral and proximal tibial epiphyses. The distal femoral epiphysis may appear as early as 32 weeks and is nearly always present at 40 weeks, whereas the proximal tibial epiphysis may appear as early as 36 weeks and is present in 50% to 75% of fetuses at 40 weeks. Thus the *absence* of the distal femoral epiphysis indicates prematurity (but its presence does not confirm maturity), and the *presence* of the proximal tibial epiphysis connotes maturity (but its absence does not mean prematurity). Accordingly, the presence of a distal femoral epiphysis and the absence of a proximal tibial epiphysis leave the question of maturity in doubt. Unfortunately, this is the commonest finding on abdominal x-ray film in late pregnancy. Moreover, the time of epiphyseal appearance seems to relate more closely to size than to maturity, and differences with sex and race occur. For all of these reasons and the desire to minimize radiation exposure, radiographic methods of estimating fetal maturity have fallen into disfavor.

A substantially more useful index of fetal maturity is *ultrasonic cephalometry*, which permits reasonably precise measurement of fetal head diameters (p. 82). Biparietal diameter (BPD) growth is essentially linear up to 29 or 30 weeks, but after this point it both slows and becomes more variable. The question of whether the fetal BPD relates more closely to fetal size or to maturity is not entirely settled. A close correlation with birth weight ($r = 0.82$) has been found. However, others have described a better correlation with maturity than with size, even in pathologic conditions such as maternal diabetes associated with abnormal fetal growth. The BPD probably reflects both age and size.

AMNIOTIC FLUID ANALYSIS

A large number of amniotic fluid constituents have been proposed for use in estimating fetal maturity. These may be considered conveniently on the basis of whether they reflect the property of surface tension lowering or "surfactant" activity in the lung.

Surfactant tests

The theoretical basis of measuring indices of surfactant activity in amniotic fluid for estimation of fetal maturity rests on the role of these substances in the pathophysiology of respiratory distress syndrome (RDS) (Chapter 23, part three). The airway is normally lined with substances that lower surface tension so that alveoli do not collapse completely with expiration but are stabilized in expiration, retaining an appropriate functional residual capacity. In the absence of these substances, complete collapse follows expiration, and each subsequent inspiration requires high intrathoracic negative pressure. Thus an extraordinary amount of work is necessary for each breath; the capacity to maintain this effort is soon exceeded, and the result is progressive atelectasis, hypoxia, and ultimately the outpouring of the proteinaceous material recognized histologically as hyaline membrane.

The principal pulmonary surfactant is a specialized phospholipid, dipalmitoyl lecithin or phosphatidyl choline, synthesized by the type II alveolar cell (Chapter 23, part one). The earlier an infant is born, the more likely it will be to exhibit the effects of pulmonary surfactant deficiency. The use of amniotic fluid surfactant tests assumes that surfactant activity levels in amniotic fluid reflect those in the fetal lung, although extrapulmonary sources of amniotic fluid phospholipids have been described. Thus the tests permit conclusions about the state of maturation of the fetal lung.

The determination of the amniotic fluid concentration of lecithin relative to that of sphingomyelin (a phospholipid lacking surfactant properties), originally described by Gluck, is the most widely used amniotic fluid surfactant test. Lecithin and sphingomyelin are present in similar concentrations (thus the L/S ratio is 1) until the middle of the third trimester. At this point, the level of lecithin begins to increase, whereas that of sphingomyelin remains relatively constant. By 35 weeks, on the average, the L/S ratio approximates 2, indicating a concentration of lecithin at least twice that of sphingomyelin. The analytic method for determination of the L/S ratio involves lipid extraction and concentration, cold acetone precipitation (which separates surfactant from nonsurfactant lecithin), thin-layer chromatographic separation of lecithin and sphingomyelin, and densitometric determination of their relative concentrations. The technique involved is of moderate complexity although well within the capability of a good laboratory; meticulous attention to detail is required.

Lecithin and sphingomyelin are present in similar concentrations until the middle of the third trimester. Thus the L/S ratio is normally 1 or less until 30 to 32 weeks' gestation, reaches 2 at approximately 35 weeks, and continues to increase to and beyond term (Fig. 11-1). These observations are based on average values in normal pregnancy; under certain circumstances the course may be

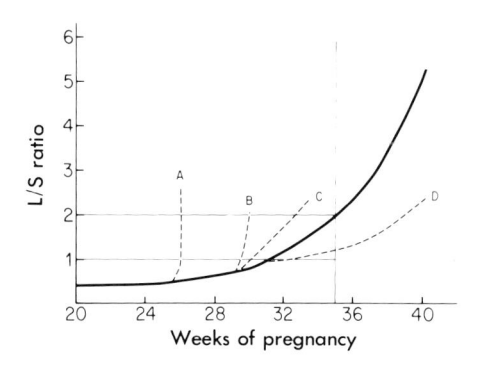

Fig. 11-1. Patterns of lecithin/sphingomyelin (L/S) ratio during the last half of pregnancy. Heavy dark line indicates the average normal pattern. *A, B,* and *C* indicate various types of accelerated patterns; *D* indicates a retarded pattern (see text). (Based on data from Gluck, L., and others: Am. J. Obstet. Gynecol. **120:**142, 1974.)

either accelerated or retarded. Rapid maturation early in pregnancy may occur with catastrophic intrauterine events, such as severe (but nonfatal) premature separation of the placenta (Fig. 11-1, *A*). Rapid maturation (for example, over 24 or 48 hours) may follow premature spontaneous rupture of the fetal membranes (Fig. 11-1, *B*). A more gradual acceleration of maturity apparently accompanies maternal narcotic addiction and hypertensive and renal-vascular diseases (Fig. 11-1, *C*). All of these conditions are thought to involve some type of fetal stress, and it is hypothesized that glucocorticoid output by the fetus in response to stress prematurely activates the enzyme systems involved in surfactant production. In contrast, delay in pulmonary maturation seems to occur in hydrops fetalis and some cases of maternal diabetes without vascular disease (Fig. 11-1, *D*).

The L/S ratio indicating a low risk for developing RDS varies somewhat from laboratory to laboratory, probably as a result of modifications of the analytical methodology. The likelihood of RDS approaches zero with L/S ratios of 2 or more. With L/S ratios less than 2, the reported incidence of RDS ranges from 40% to 80%; the lower the ratio the greater the risk.

Several artifacts may influence the L/S ratio. Maternal and fetal serum has an L/S ratio of approximately 1.4, and addition of quantities as low as 2.5 ml can lower a "mature" amniotic fluid value into the "immature" range. Blood may raise an immature ratio slightly but never enough to give a false positive value. Thus blood contamination probably will not alter the significance of a mature ratio but renders an immature one suspect. Meconium contamination of amniotic fluid may make L/S determinations unreliable, but the nature of the effect is uncertain; both elevation and depression of the results have been reported. Storage conditions may also affect the L/S ratio; values are lowered within 24 hours at room temperature and within 3 days in a refrigerator, but frozen specimens yield valid results after indefinite storage. Centrifugation of the amniotic fluid also may influence the L/S ratio by removing more lecithin than sphingomyelin, thereby lowering the ratio. If centrifugation is necessary to remove particulate matter, it should be limited to low speeds.

The incidence of "false negative" L/S ratios in which an immature value is associated with an infant who does not exhibit respiratory distress is at least 20% to 25%. False positive values in which RDS occurs in spite of a mature L/S ratio are much less frequent and seem to be principally related to acute perinatal complications and maternal diabetes. Hypoxia and acidosis immediately before or after birth or hypothermia in the neonatal period predisposes to RDS presumably by causing constriction of pulmonary blood vessels and suboptimal surfactant production. Thus an infant experiencing these complications, particularly before 35 weeks, might develop RDS even though the amniotic fluid L/S ratio measured before labor indicated pulmonary maturity. Maternal diabetes mellitus adversely affects the reliability of the association between the L/S ratio and RDS. Milder forms of maternal diabetes are sometimes associated with delayed lung maturation, but severe diabetes with vascular disease may accelerate lung maturity. Maternal diabetes rarely may be responsible for false positive results in which RDS may occur with a mature L/S ratio (Chapter 3).

An alternative to the widely used L/S ratio is the *rapid surfactant, bubble stability,* or *shake test.* It involves the shaking of amniotic fluid (undiluted and in various saline dilutions) with an equivalent volume of 95% ethanol. The test is read as positive if a complete ring of bubbles persists at the meniscus (Fig. 11-2). The greatest advantage of this semiquantitative test is its simplicity. It is a bedside test, although scrupulous attention is needed in making certain that all detergent is removed from the tubes before their use. Positive tests in dilutions of 1:2 or greater correlate well with the absence of RDS and with high lecithin concentrations and L/S ratios; this indicates the validity of the method as an index of pulmonary maturity. There is a relatively high incidence of false negative results, however, and a negative test should be further evaluated by the L/S ratio before use in clinical management.

The relative frequency of indeterminate L/S ratios (1.5 to 2.0) has stimulated further investigation of the amniotic fluid phospholipids in search for more accurate, early identification of biochemical maturation (Table 11-1). Although an L/S ratio of 1.5 to 2.0 identifies a group of infants with a significant risk for developing RDS, many of them are sufficiently mature to be delivered without delay. It has been suggested that the "lung profile" consisting of four measurements, the L/S ratio, and the percentages of disaturated lecithin, phosphatidyl inositol,

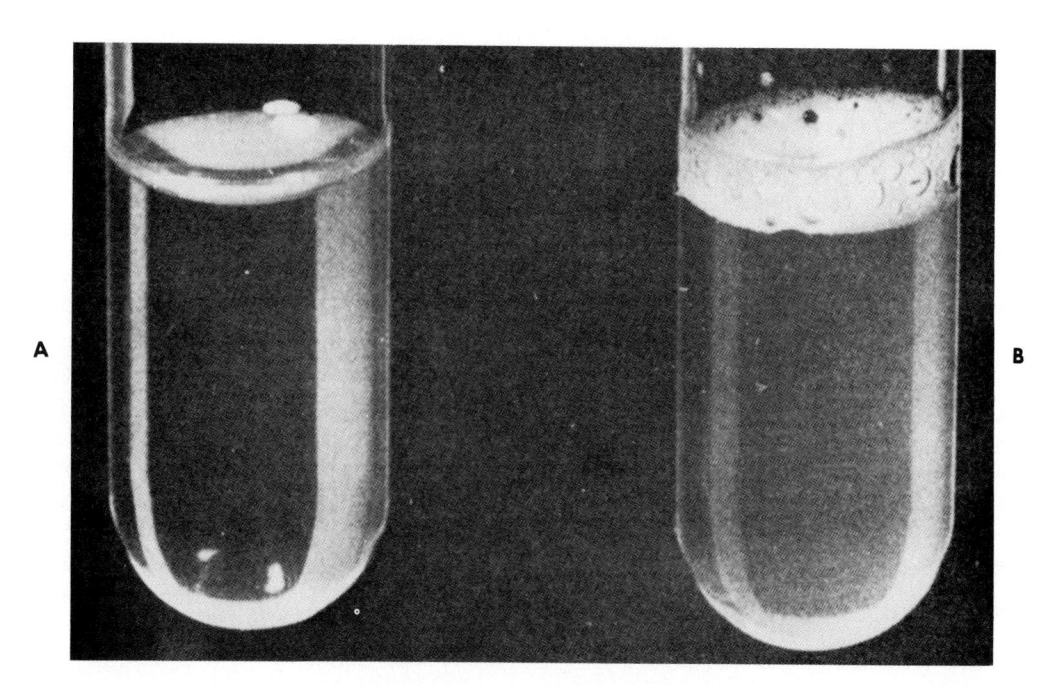

Fig. 11-2. Negative **(A)** and positive **(B)** tubes in the amniotic fluid rapid surfactant or shake test. (From Shepherd, B., and Spellacy, W.N.: Obstet. Gynecol. **43:**558, 1974.)

Table 11-1. Assessment of fetal pulmonary maturity

Test	Advantages	Disadvantages
L/S ratio	Few false positives, not altered by changes in amniotic fluid volume	Many false negatives, special laboratory equipment required
Lung profile	Reduces false negative L/S ratios	Requires more time and equipment than L/S ratio
Lecithin	Few false positives	Altered by changes in amniotic fluid volume, time consuming
Microviscosimeter	Few false positives, fast, easily performed	Requires expensive equipment
"Shake test"	Few false positives, fast, easily performed	Many false negatives
Optical density	Few false positives, fast, easily performed	Many false negatives

From Gabbe, S.G.: Recent advances in the assessment of fetal maturity, J. Reprod. Med., **23:**228, 1979.

and phosphatidyl glycerol would provide a more accurate indication of biochemical maturation. All components can be measured with relatively little modification of the standard technique. Two-dimensional thin-layer chromatography replaces one-dimensional chromatography. The measurement of phosphatidyl glycerol, a phospholipid that appears at about 36 weeks gestation and increases to term, greatly enhances the information derived from amniocentesis. It is possibly the most reliable indicator of pulmonary maturation, even in diabetic pregnancy. A unique advantage is that phosphatidyl glycerol is found only in pulmonary surfactant, so that contamination of amniotic fluid with blood, meconium, or vaginal secretions does not confuse the interpretation.

Another approach to the assay of surfactant concentration is the measurement of the viscosity of amniotic fluid. This technique of fluorescent polarization (microviscometry) is based on the fact that surface tension and viscosity are related physical characteristics and both are affected by surfactant concentration. Clinical experience with this technique is still very limited. It appears to be rapid, simple to perform, and accurate although the cost of instrumentation is significant.

The relationship between the optical density of fresh amniotic fluid at 650 nm and the traditional L/S ratio has also been evaluated. Optical density is thought to evaluate the turbidity changes in amniotic fluid, which are dependent on the total amniotic fluid phospholipid concentration. Although a wavelength of 400 nm was initially used, interference by pigments of meconium, bilirubin, and hemolyzed blood led to the subsequent use of 650 nm. False-negative results ranged from 6% to 8% in initial studies but have subsequently exceeded 30%.

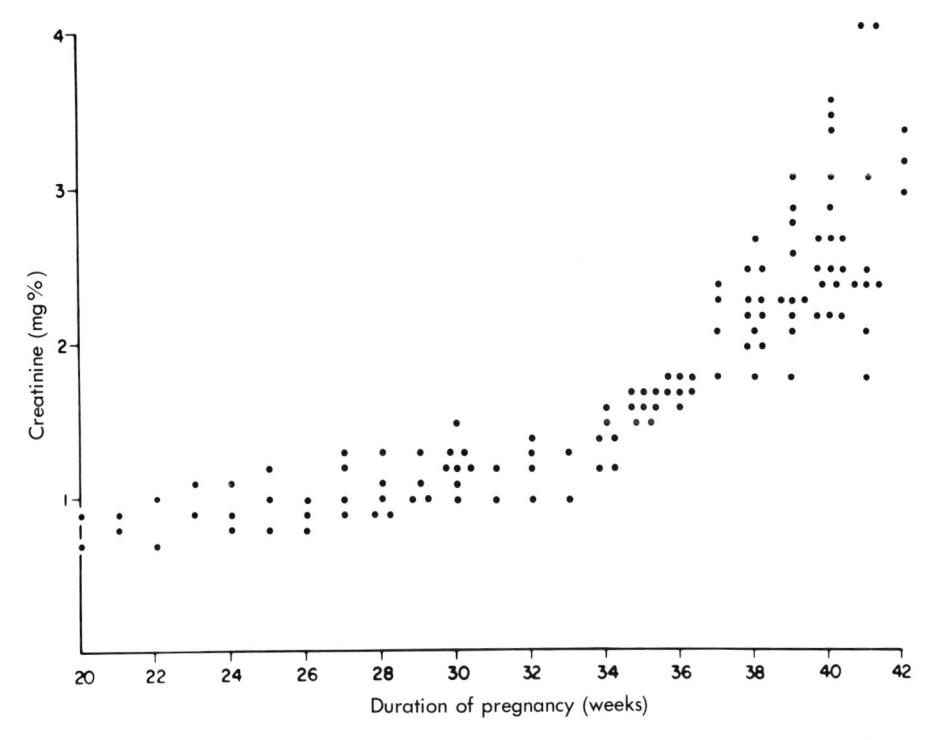

Fig. 11-3. Creatinine concentration in (untreated) amniotic fluid during the last half of pregnancy. (From Pitkin, R.M., and Zwirek, S.J.: Am. J. Obstet. Gynecol. **98:**1135, 1967.)

Amniotic fluid optical density at 650 nm requires further evaluation but may prove to be a valuable screening test when a positive result is obtained.

Nonsurfactant tests

The concentration of *creatinine* in amniotic fluid is a useful index of gestational age. Amniotic fluid creatinine is derived from the fetus. During the first half of pregnancy, levels are similar in maternal plasma, fetal plasma, and amniotic fluid. After approximately the midpoint of gestation, a time coincident with the onset of fetal urination, amniotic fluid creatinine values increase progressively, reaching levels over twice those found in plasma by 37 weeks (Fig. 11-3). That the mechanism of transfer in late gestation involves fetal urine is confirmed by a parallel pattern of urine production and creatinine concentration over the last 8 weeks of pregnancy. Increasing fetal urinary creatinine excretion probably reflects maturing renal function rather than growth of fetal muscle mass. A "mature" creatinine level does not ensure the absence of RDS.

The standard alkaline picrate method for measuring creatinine in body fluids is applicable to amniotic fluid. When this method is used on untreated fluid, maturity is indicated by a level of 2 mg/dl or more. Pretreatment with Lloyd's reagent (aluminum silicate) or tungstate to remove nonspecific chromogens may lower this value by as much as 0.5 mg/dl. In at least 95% of instances in which the level is above 1.5 to 2 mg/dl (depending on methodology), the fetus will be at least 37 weeks' gestational age by physical findings and neonatal behavior. Alternatively, 10% to 20% of values below 2 mg/dl are associated with mature fetuses. Thus the test is somewhat more reliable as a predictor of maturity than as a predictor of prematurity. Blood contamination, at least up to 4% or 5%, has minimal effect on the validity of the test.

Elevated maternal blood creatinine levels are reflected in the amniotic fluid; studies in patients in whom the maternal serum value exceeds 1 mg/dl must be interpreted cautiously. In such instances the amniotic fluid–maternal serum ratio may be a useful clinical guide. Most studies have noted creatinine to be equally reliable in normal and complicated pregnancies if the maternal serum value is normal. Rh sensitization is a possible exception; there may be a slight lowering of the amniotic fluid creatinine level with this condition. In contrast, levels may be higher with preeclampsia or hypertensive disorders. Maternal diuretic treatment may raise the amniotic fluid creatinine level as a reflection of an increased maternal plasma concentration associated with a decline in plasma volume. Variations in amniotic fluid volumes seem to have little influence on the validity of creatinine concentration. False negative results may occur more frequently with polyhydramnios, but mature values are reliable in that condition. False positive results in oligohydramnios do not usually represent a cause for concern, because of the relatively low chance of successful amniocentesis with oligohydramnios.

In addition to its use in estimating gestational age, creatinine may have value in evaluating fetal status. A failure of progressive increases or a paradoxical decline with advancing gestation has been noted with severe Rh sensitization and diabetes mellitus.

Amniotic fluid *cytology*, the other major nonsurfactant test of fetal maturity, depends on the presence of epithelial cells, principally from the fetal skin, in amniotic fluid. Thus the test measures maturity of the fetal skin and is more reliable in predicting maturity than in predicting prematurity. For genetic uses of amniocentesis see Chapter 37.

SUMMARY

The accurate estimation of gestational age is important to obstetric management. Menstrual history and uterine size evaluated by an experienced examiner in early pregnancy are particularly helpful in the estimation. Serial ultrasound measurement of the fetal BPD initiated before the third trimester can be used to approximate gestational age with a degree of reliability generally sufficient for clinical use. With respect to amniotic fluid indices of gestational age or fetal maturity or both, virtually all have low false positive rates but appreciable false negative rates. Thus they are valid tests of maturity but are less reliable in indicating immaturity. Tests measuring surfactant activity are particularly valuable because they reflect lung maturity; the major immediate problem facing the premature newborn is respiratory function. The most widely used surfactant test is the L/S ratio. Simpler methods such as the shake test are reliable as indicators of maturity, but negative results should be checked with a more precise method. Nonsurfactant indices of value in estimating gestational age are amniotic fluid creatinine and cytology. In general, the use of multiple tests is more reliable than any single test.

Roy M. Pitkin

BIBLIOGRAPHY

Abramovich, D.R., Keeping, J.D., and Thom, H.: The origin of amniotic fluid lecithin, Br. J. Obstet. Gynaecol. **82**:204, 1975.

Bergnaud, W.P., Jr., and others: Amniotic fluid creatinine for prediction of fetal maturity, Obstet. Gynecol. **34**:7, 1969.

Bishop, E.H., and Corson, S.: Estimation of fetal maturity by cytologic examination of amniotic fluid, Am. J. Obstet. Gynecol. **102**:654, 1968.

Brosens, I., and Gordon, H.: The estimation of maturity by cytologic examination of the liquor amnii, J. Obstet. Gynaecol. Br. Commonw. **73**:88, 1966.

Buhi, W.C., and Spellacy, W.N.: Effects of blood and meconium on the determination of the amniotic fluid lecithin/sphingomyelin ratio, Am. J. Obstet. Gynecol. **121**:321, 1975.

Campbell, S., and Newman, G.B.: Growth of the fetal biparietal diameter during normal pregnancy, J. Obstet. Gynaecol. Br. Commonw. **78**:513, 1971.

Cassady, G., and others: Amniotic fluid creatinine in pregnancies complicated by diabetes, Am. J. Obstet. Gynecol. **122**:13, 1975.

Chan, W.H., Willis, J., and Woods, J.: The value of the Nile blue sulphate stain in the cytology of the liquor amnii, J. Obstet. Gynaecol. Br. Commonw. **76**:193, 1969.

Christie, A., and others: The estimation of fetal maturity by roentgen studies of osseous development, Am. J. Obstet. Gynecol. **60**:133, 1950.

Clements, J.A., and others: Assessment of the risk of the respiratory distress syndrome by a rapid test for surfactant in amniotic fluid, N. Engl. J. Med. **286**:1077, 1972.

Cohen, W.N.: The prenatal determination of fetal maturity by B-scan ultrasound, Radiology **103**:171, 1972.

Condorelli, S., Cosmi, E.v., and Scarpelli, E.M.: Extrapulmonary source of amniotic fluid phospholipids, Am. J. Obstet. Gynecol. **118**:842, 1974.

Dancis, J.: Predictors of fetal maturation. In Antenatal diagnosis, NIH Report, 1979.

Donald, I.R., and others: Clinical experience with the amniotic fluid lecithin/sphingomyelin ratio, Am. J. Obstet. Gynecol. **115**:547, 1973.

Droegmueller, W., and others: Amniotic fluid examination as an aid in the assessment of gestational age, Am. J. Obstet. Gynecol. **104**:424, 1969.

Duenhoelter, J.H., and Pritchard, J.A.: Human fetal respiration, II. Fate of intra-amniotic hypaque and ^{51}Cr labelled red cells, Obstet. Gynecol. **43**:878, 1974.

Frantz, T., and others: Phospholipids in amniotic fluid. II. Lecithin fatty acid patterns related to gestation, maternal disease and fetal outcome, Acta Obstet. Gynecol. Scand. **54**:33, 1975.

Gabbe, S.G.: Recent advances in the assessment of fetal maturity, J. Reprod. Med. **23**:228, 1979.

Gabert, H.A., Bryson, M.J., and Stenchever, M.A.: The effect of cesarean section on respiratory distress in the presence of a mature lecithin sphingomyelin ratio, Am. J. Obstet. Gynecol. **116**:366, 1973.

Gauthier, C., Dosjardins, P., and McLean, F.: Fetal maturity: amniotic fluid analysis correlated with neonatal assessment, Am. J. Obstet. Gynecol. **112**:334, 1970.

Gibbons, J.M., Huntley, T.E., and Corral, A.G.: Effect of maternal blood contamination of amniotic fluid analysis, Obstet. Gynecol. **44**:657, 1974.

Gluck, L., and Kulovich, M.V.: Lecithin-sphingomyelin ratios in amniotic fluid in normal and abnormal pregnancy, Am. J. Obstet. Gynecol. **115**:539, 1973.

Gluck, L., and others: Diagnosis of the respiratory distress syndrome by amniocentesis, Am. J. Obstet. Gynecol. **109**:440, 1971.

Gluck, L., and others: Interpretation and significance of the lecithin-sphingomyelin ratio in amniotic fluid, Am. J. Obstet. Gynecol. **120**:142, 1974.

Harrison, R.F.: Amniotic fluid creatinine levels in the normotensive and pre-eclamptic patient, J. Obstet. Gynaecol. Br. Commonw. **80**:544, 1973.

Hinkley, D., O'Neill, L., and Cassady, G.: Amniotic fluid creatinine in the Rh-sensitized pregnancy, Am. J. Obstet. Gynecol. **117**:544, 1973.

Keniston, R.C., and others: A prospective evaluation of the lecithin/sphingomyelin ratio and the rapid surfactant test in relation to fetal pulmonary maturity, Am. J. Obstet. Gynecol. **121**:324, 1975.

Kulkarni, B.D., and others: Determination of lecithin-sphingomyelin ratio in amniotic fluid, Obstet. Gynecol. **40**:173, 1792.

Lemons, J.A., and Jaffe, R.B.: Amniotic fluid lecithin/sphingomyelin ratio in the diagnosis of hyaline membrane disease, Am. J. Obstet. Gynecol. **115**:223, 1973.

Lind, T., Billewicz, W.Z., and Cheyne, G.A.: Composition of amniotic fluid and maternal blood through pregnancy, J. Obstet. Gynaecol. Br. Commonw. 78:505, 1971.

Lindback, T., and Frantz, T.: Effect of centrifugation of amniotic fluid phospholipid recovery, Acta Obstet. Gynecol. Scand. 54:101, 1975.

Lindback, T., Skjaeraasen, J., and Carcedo, L.: Amniotic fluid phospholipid determination by bubble stability test and quantitative lipid analysis, Acta Obstet. Gynecol. Scand. 53:359, 1974.

McAllister, C.J., Stull, C.G., and Courey, N.G.: Amniotic fluid levels of uric acid and creatinine in toxemic patients, possible relation to diuretic use, Am. J. Obstet. Gynecol. 115:560, 1973.

Morgan, T.E.: Pulmonary surfactant, N. Engl. J. Med. 284:1185, 1971.

Morrison, J.C., and others: Nile blue staining of cells in amniotic fluid for fetal maturity. I. A reappraisal, Obstet. Gynecol. 44:355, 1974.

Murata, Y., and Martin, C.B., Jr.: Growth of the biparietal diameter of the fetal head in diabetic pregnancy, Am. J. Obstet. Gynecol. 115:252, 1972.

Nelson, G.H.: Risk of respiratory distress syndrome as determined by amniotic fluid lecithin concentration, Am. J. Obstet. Gynecol. 121:753, 1975.

Nelson, G.H.: Determination of amniotic fluid total phospholipid phosphorus as a test for fetal lung maturity, Am. J. Obstet. Gynecol. 115:933, 1973.

Olson, E.B., Jr., and others: The use of amniotic fluid bubble stability, L/S ratio, and creatinine concentration in the assessment of fetal maturity, Am. J. Obstet. Gynecol. 122:755, 1975.

Pitkin, R.M.: Prenatal estimation of fetal maturity, Int. J. Gynaecol. Obstet. 7:199, 1969.

Pitkin, R.M.: Amniotic fluid creatinine in estimating fetal maturity, Contemp. Ob/Gyn 4:13, 1974.

Pitkin, R.M., and Reynolds, W.A.: Creatinine flux between mother, fetus, and amniotic fluid, Am. J. Physiol. 228:231, 1975.

Pitkin, R.M., and Zwirek, S.J.: Amniotic fluid creatinine, Am. J. Obstet. Gynecol. 98:1135, 1967.

Roopnarinesingh, S., and Morris, D.: Amniotic fluid urea and creatinine in normal pregnancy and preeclampsia, J. Obstet. Gynaecol. Br. Commonw. 78:29, 1971.

Roux, J.F., Nakamura, J., and Brown, E.G.: Further observation on determination of gestational age by amniotic fluid analysis, Am. J. Obstet. Gynecol. 116:633, 1973.

Sabbagha, R.E., and others: Sonar BPD and fetal age: definition of relationship, Obstet. Gynecol. 43:7, 1974.

Schirar, A., and others: Amniotic fluid phospholipids and fatty acids in normal pregnancies, Am. J. Obstet. Gynecol. 121:633, 1975.

Shepherd, B., and Spellacy, W.N.: Critical analysis of the amniotic fluid shake test, Obstet. Gynecol. 43:558, 1974.

Weiss, R.R., and others: Amniotic fluid uric acid and creatinine as measures of fetal maturity. Obstet. Gynecol. 44:208, 1974.

PART TWO

Premature labor

EFFECTS OF PREMATURITY

Premature birth, defined as either low birth weight or as birth prior to term gestation, remains the major contributing factor to neonatal morbidity and mortality. The National Center for Health Statistics reported that of the 3,333,279 live births in the United States during 1978, 7.1% weighed 501 to 2,500 gm and 8.9% occurred at less than 37 weeks' gestation. Although there is convincing evidence that recent advances of medical care serve to increase the chance of survival and decrease the likelihood of serious sequelae in survivors, premature birth is still associated with over 70% of neonatal deaths and infants with permanent neurologic damage. United States natality statistics from 1968 through 1978 revealed that the incidence of low birth weight was relatively static at approximately 7.5%; however, during the same period the neonatal death rate steadily declined from approximately 16 to 10 per 1,000 live births. The improving neonatal survival rate, presumably due to advances in obstetric and newborn care, improved standards of living, and reduced birth rates, served to emphasize the growing influence of premature birth in morbidity and mortality statistics.

MECHANISMS OF LABOR

In seeking an optimum clinical approach to the management of premature labor, one logically must consider the mechanisms of onset of labor. Current evidence suggests that humans and nonhuman primates, in contrast to other mammalian species, do not have major alterations of maternal hypothalamohypophyseal function or placental hormone production prior to the onset of labor. Liggins and associates proposed that labor onset is probably associated with changes in target tissue sensitivity to placental steroids rather than by major alterations of their production rates. In contrast, Csapo proposed that decreasing production of progesterone by the placenta in late pregnancy serves to remove a local block of myometrial activity beneath the implantation site, which then permits the onset of labor. The Csapo hypothesis was supported by the report of Kumar and associates, who found higher concentrations of progesterone in myometrial samples from beneath the placental site than elsewhere in the uterus. Although the administration of progesterone during pregnancy delays the onset of labor in many animal species, Brenner and Hendricks found no evidence that medroxyprogesterone, taken orally during late human pregnancy, had any influence on the onset of labor. However, in a series of patients at risk for premature labor, Johnson and associates reported that prophylactic administration of 17-α-hydroxyprogesterone caproate was highly effective in preventing premature labor when compared with placebo treatment. The inhibitory effect of progesterone on myometrial activity was also suggested by observations of Bengtsson in which injections of medroxyprogesterone into the anterior wall of the uterus successfully inhibited labor in 9 of 10 patients in clinical premature labor. Also, Scommegna and associates observed that human labor was partially inhibited by intravenous infusion of pregnenolone, the immediate precursor of placental progesterone. Thus the weight of available evidence suggests that progesterone serves to promote relaxation of the uterus. This action of progesterone may be accomplished through its role in the production of prostaglandins.

The oxytocic properties of prostaglandins, plus their appearance in amniotic fluid and maternal blood with the onset of labor, strongly suggest a physiologic role in the mechanism of labor onset. Arachidonic acid, the immediate precursor of prostaglandins, is stored in fetal membranes and uterine decidua in its esterified, inactive form as glycerophospholipids. Progesterone serves to stabilize lysosomal phospholipase A_2, an enzyme located in fetal membranes and uterine decidua, which converts glycerophospholipids to arachidonic acid. The withdrawal of progesterone or the introduction of a physical stress, as with hyperosmolar conditions or even distension of the uterus, serves to labilize lysosomes and causes release of phospholipase A_2 and the subsequent production of prostaglandins. The physiologic role of prostaglandins in human parturition was suggested when Karim observed their appearance in amniotic fluid and maternal blood at the onset of labor. Kloeck and Jung reported that stretch of in vitro myometrial strips stimulated the release of prostaglandins. The increase of uterine activity often apparent after manipulation of fetal membranes, following rupture of membranes, with amnionitis, or after uterine manipulation during abdominal surgery probably is mediated through the production of prostaglandins.

The role of oxytocin in the mechanism of human labor now appears to be rather minor. This contrasts with the earlier belief that maternal hypophyseal release of oxytocin is the primary mechanism of labor onset in humans, a theory that was enforced by the report by Ferguson in 1941 that the uterine contractility usually observed after stimulation of the rabbit cervix did not occur after transection of the spinal cord or destruction of the pituitary. He suggested that cervical stimulation produces a cord reflex that triggers release of oxytocin from the pituitary. More recently, Fuchs reported that infusion of ethanol in rabbits inhibited uterine activity, presumably by blocking release of oxytocin from the maternal pituitary. Subsequent studies, to be described later, revealed that intravenous infusion of ethanol in humans would inhibit term or preterm labor. However, the virtual absence of oxytocin in maternal blood until late labor, as detected by the sensitive radioimmunoassay technique, rather strongly suggests that maternal oxytocin release is not a major component of the labor onset mechanism in humans. In contrast, fetal oxytocin release may be a very important component of the mechanism. Chard and associates found significantly higher levels of oxytocin in umbilical cord blood than in maternal blood at delivery. Also, it is now known that oxytocin levels are higher in umbilical artery than in umbilical vein blood, which rather strongly implies a fetal source of oxytocin. Myometrial sensitivity to oxytocin is enhanced by the increasing production of estrogens during late human pregnancy. Also, pregnancies complicated by placental sulfatase deficiency have extremely low estrogen production and usually fail to develop labor until post term. In contrast, Raja and associates found higher levels of plasma estradiol in patients who subsequently developed spontaneous premature labor than others who delivered at term.

Hippocrates was probably the earliest to suggest that the fetus initiates labor when intrauterine conditions are no longer satisfactory. In addition to fetal oxytocin release, this may be accomplished through fetal adrenal gland production of estrogen and cortisol. The importance of fetal cortisol production in the mechanism of human labor onset is suggested from the frequent association of prolonged pregnancy and fetal anencephaly where there is marked hypoplasia of adrenal glands. Anderson and associates observed that adrenal glands were heavier in a series of premature infants dying soon after birth when there was no recognizable cause of premature labor than in another series of infants of similar weights where an obvious obstetric complication had been associated with premature birth. From studies in sheep it was found that destruction of the fetal pituitary or bilateral fetal adrenalectomy was usually followed by prolongation of pregnancy, whereas infusion of glucocorticoids to fetal lambs was followed by premature delivery. In contrast, bilateral fetal adrenalectomy in rhesus monkeys failed to influence the timing of labor onset. There have been many conflicting observations of cortisol levels in human umbilical cord blood after spontaneous versus oxytocin-induced labor, or following vaginal delivery versus delivery by cesarean section. Thus the exact role of fetal adrenal function in the mechanism of labor onset has not been clearly established for human pregnancy.

Alterations of uterine blood flow may influence any of the various uterine, placental, or fetal systems known to participate in the mechanism of labor onset. In general, reduced uterine blood flow is associated with increased uterine activity, whereas increased blood flow promotes uterine relaxation. Brotanek and associates found evidence of decreased blood flow with oxytocin stimulation of uterine activity, and increased blood flow when the uterus was relaxed. A relative reduction of uterine blood flow may be the common factor that frequently triggers premature labor in patients with toxemia, chronic hypertensive disease, multiple pregnancy, hyponutritive states, and heavy smoking habits. Uterine blood flow may also be altered by endogenous catecholamines, but the response is not entirely predictable, since the myometrial reaction to blood flow changes may be contrary to the response mediated through adrenergic receptors.

For example, in rhesus monkeys maternal stress or administration of catecholamines may produce fetal distress due to reduced uterine blood flow but often without influencing uterine activity.

PATHOGENESIS OF PREMATURE LABOR

Despite our rapidly expanding knowledge of the mechanisms of labor onset, the pathogenesis of premature labor in most patients is obscure. However, many clinical and social factors are known to relate to the incidence of premature birth. Iatrogenic reasons for premature delivery may be purposeful in response to clinical evidence of deterioration of fetal or maternal condition or accident, as results from miscalculation of gestational age prior to elective delivery. The latter should be virtually eliminated by appropriate use of ultrasonic evaluation of gestational age and tests of fetal pulmonary maturation (pp. 82 and 134). There is an obvious relationship between low socioeconomic status and higher incidence of premature delivery, which in turn may relate to risk factors such as poor nutrition, pregnancy in very young patients, frequent genitourinary infections, greater stress of living, and inadequate prenatal care. Although the frequency of premature births among blacks is more than twice that of whites, the rates are essentially the same among black and white cohorts of comparable economic status. A previous premature delivery is known to increase the risk of premature labor in the current pregnancy to approximately 20%, compared with about 5% in other patients. Other risk factors of premature labor include first or second trimester uterine bleeding, incompetent cervix, placenta previa, abruptio placentae, multiple pregnancy, hydramnios, fetal anomalies, uterine anomalies, severe toxemia, asymptomatic bacteriuria, acute pyelonephritis, and smoking during pregnancy. The relationship of urogenital bacterial infection to premature labor and delivery is relatively obscure. Although mycoplasma colonization is more prevalent among patients who deliver before term, the same organism is found more often in patients with multiple sexual partners or more sexual activity. Goodlin and associates reported that the incidence of sexual orgasm in pregnancy was higher in patients who subsequently delivered prematurely than in those who delivered at term. This finding may relate to the oxytocic role of prostaglandins which are now considered partially responsible for orgasm.

Risk factors of premature labor are of particular clinical importance when they are recognized in early pregnancy and are amenable to some form of treatment. For example, the recognition and treatment of asymptomatic bacteriuria or incompetent cervix should reduce the risk of subsequent premature labor. Patients with multiple pregnancy, uterine malformation, or a history of previous premature births should be placed under very careful surveillance and encouraged to avoid smoking and coitus, to maintain good nutrition, and to spend a considerable portion of their pregnancy resting in bed.

CLINICAL EVALUATION AND MANAGEMENT

The diagnosis of premature labor is based on a clinical evaluation of uterine activity and cervical changes that are consistent with labor, plus evidence of preterm gestation. The determination of gestation has been greatly facilitated by the use of ultrasonic techniques and by tests for amniotic fluid maturity indices. The use of ultrasonography to determine fetal growth patterns during pregnancy has greatly facilitated the recognition of pregnancies complicated by growth retardation. Obviously, if fetal distress were manifested by premature labor as well as by severe fetal growth retardation, any attempt to stop such a labor would be quite inappropriate. However, a fetus with mild growth retardation could potentially benefit from further intrauterine development (p. 69). Several other clinical factors are considered relative or absolute contraindications to specific treatment for inhibition of labor. For example, the presence of intrauterine infection, a major premature separation of the placenta, fetal death, a fetal malformation incompatible with survival, and severe toxemia are absolute contraindications to inhibition of labor. The management of patients in premature labor with ruptured membranes remains controversial. Delay of delivery presents an increasing risk of intrauterine infection, but it also permits time for advancement of fetal maturity by either endogenous mechanisms or by administration of corticosteroids. However, there is concern that corticosteroids may potentially either enhance the risk of intrauterine infection and possibly produce long-term aftereffects in the infant. Also, several reports have described a reduction in the incidence of respiratory distress syndrome among infants exposed to a tocolytic agent without concomitant corticosteroid therapy. Thus with further observations it may be possible to conclude that treatment with a tocolytic agent alone is as effective as the combination of a tocolytic agent and a corticosteroid in reducing the incidence of respiratory distress syndrome. The management of premature labor in a pregnancy complicated by possible placental insufficiency, as with diabetes mellitus or hypertensive disease, should be based upon a judgement of the method which offers the least of potential risks to mother and fetus.

The management of premature labor is complicated by the inherent difficulty of recognizing early labor versus "false labor." By delaying active management until there is definite progress of labor, one may miss the opportunity to successfully inhibit premature labor. Although it is not entirely clear to what extent "doing something" influences the treatment of premature labor, placebo-controlled trials of specific tocolytic agents have reported that from 38% to 71% of labors are successfully delayed by placebo treatment. Bed rest, specifically in the lateral decubitus position in which uterine blood flow is maximal, is a very important adjunct to more specific forms of treatment of premature labor. When we exclude the patients in whom premature labor ceases with bed rest alone and also those in whom inhibition of labor is either contraindicated or likely to fail due to advanced labor, there remain those who are candidates for treatment with tocolytic agents.

DRUG THERAPY FOR PREMATURE LABOR

Historically the most popular agents used to inhibit premature labor were many varieties of sedatives, tranquilizers, hormonal substances, vasodilators, and neuromuscular agents. Although sedative and analgesic drugs enjoyed a reputation as uterine relaxants, quantitative studies of some have indicated that they cause an increase of uterine activity. Although most clinical experience has failed to demonstrate any effect of progesterone on established labor, Bengtsson reported temporary inhibition of labor when it was injected directly into the uterine wall. However, the intramyometrial injection of a drug has obvious clinical shortcomings. Various biologic formulations prepared from mammalian ovaries have been reputed to relax the uterus, but none has been subjected to controlled studies that might establish efficacy and safety for clinical use. Vasorelaxing agents such as amyl nitrite and epinephrine will temporarily relax the uterus, but they are not suitable for prolonged inhibition of premature labor because of their excessive cardiovascular effects. Likewise, the uterine relaxation produced by inhalation anesthetic agents such as ethyl ether or fluothane cannot be sustained for effective management of premature labor. European investigators have reported that calcium antagonists serve to enhance the tocolytic effects of β-mimetic agents.

Aminophylline

Aminophylline, a dimethylxanthine derivative used for its bronchial relaxant effect, also causes relaxation of the uterus. It acts by blocking the action of intracellular phosphodiesterase, which normally serves to degrade cyclic adenosine monophosphate (cAMP). The resulting accumulation of cAMP in the myometrial cell promotes movement of calcium to intracellular storage sites or across the cell membrane, which in turn results in relaxation of the cell. Coutinho and Vieira Lopes reported that intravenous injection of 240 to 480 mg of aminophylline briefly relaxed the uterus of nonpregnant women. Liu and associates reported delay of premature labor by 24 hours or more in 80% of a series of patients treated with aminophylline (250 mg intravenously over 15 minutes) followed by an intravenous infusion of approximately 50 mg per hour for up to 48 hours and then 100 mg orally every 8 hours. Lipshitz, in a series of oxytocin-induced term labor patients, reported that intravenous injection of 250 mg of aminophylline over 5 minutes produced a modest decrease of uterine activity with a marked maternal tachycardia. He concluded that aminophylline, compared with the β-sympathomimetic drugs, has an unfavorable cardiovascular/tocolytic ratio. Thus further studies of aminophylline are needed to establish its potential value in treatment of premature labor.

Diazoxide

Diazoxide is a benzothiadiazine structurally related to chlorothiazide but without its diuretic properties. It was introduced as an antihypertensive agent but was also found to relax smooth muscle, suppress insulin, and elevate glucose. Several reports have indicated that diazoxide will inhibit labor but that it has a rather narrow margin of safety from effective uterine relaxation to excessive vasodilatation with maternal hypotension. However, Wilson and associates reported that diazoxide, and not the β-adrenergic agents (ritodrine, isoproterenol, and metaproterenol), inhibited prostaglandin $F_{2\alpha}$–induced uterine activity. Considering the importance of prostaglandins in the pathophysiology of human labor, diazoxide may deserve further evaluation in the treatment of premature labor. For now, diazoxide has not been evaluated by controlled trials and is not approved for the treatment of premature labor.

Magnesium sulfate

Magnesium sulfate (p. 32), commonly used for its neurostabilization effects in management of toxemia of pregnancy, is a potentially useful tocolytic agent. Its effect on uterine activity may be mediated by a direct effect on myometrial cells, as well as indirectly through improved uterine blood flow. Several investigators have reported that intravenous infusion of magnesium sulfate inhibits spontaneous and oxytocin-induced labor in humans. Steer and Petrie, in a partially randomized trial, found magnesium sulfate more effective than intravenous ethanol or dextrose solution for control of premature labor. Magnesium sulfate was administered intravenously as a 4-gm loading dose and then as an infusion of 2 gm per hour until uterine contractions stopped. Delivery was delayed for at least 24 hours in 24 of 31 patients (77%) treated with magnesium sulfate and 14 of 31 patients (45%) treated with ethanol. Although suggestive of potential clinical value, this study lacked the proper design to fully establish efficacy or safety of magnesium sulfate as a tocolytic agent. At present, magnesium sulfate is not approved for treatment of premature labor.

Antiprostaglandins

Indomethacin and other nonsteroidal antiinflammatory drugs inhibit myometrial activity by blocking endogenous production of prostaglandins. Studies in rats and primates revealed that administration of aspirin, indomethacin, and naproxen during pregnancy was followed by a significant delay in the onset of labor. Lewis and Schulman reported that human labor was delayed in onset and somewhat longer in a series of patients who had taken large doses of aspirin during pregnancy in treatment of arthritis. Zuckerman and associates reported successful inhibition of premature labor in 40 of 50 patients treated with indomethacin (100 mg by rectal suppository followed by 25 mg by mouth every 6 hours for 5 days). This report, in 1974, stimulated widespread clinical use of indomethacin in the U.S. However, the popularity of indomethacin in treatment of premature labor soon waned as additional studies in animals revealed that such antiprostaglandin compounds may promote closure of the fetal ductus arteriosus and fetal death (Chapter 25). Subsequently, however, indomethacin was used to successfully treat newborns with patent ductus arteriosus, preventing the need for surgical closure. Other potentially serious side effects of antiprostaglandin agents are thrombocytopenia, peptic ulceration, and allergic reactions. In a placebo-controlled, double-blind trial, Niebyl and associates reported that treatment with indomethacin delayed delivery at least 24 hours in 14 of 15 patients (93%) treated with indomethacin, in contrast to 6 of 15 patients (40%) receiving a placebo treatment. These investigators found no evidence of premature closure of the ductus arteriosus, pulmonary hypertension, or bleeding problems among the infants exposed to indomethacin in utero. Despite these encouraging results, antiprostaglandin drugs have not been subjected to adequate controlled trials to warrant their approval for treatment of premature labor. They remain experimental and should not be used clinically for their tocolytic effects.

Ethanol

Ethanol, administered by intravenous infusion, has been one of the most popular methods for treatment of premature labor in the United States. In 1966 Fuchs reported that intravenous infusion of ethanol in rabbits inhibits pituitary release of oxytocin. More recently Gibbens and Chard, using a radioimmunoassay technique, reported a reduction in the frequency of spurt release of oxytocin during intravenous infusion of ethanol administered to women in spontaneous labor. In 1967 Fuchs and associates reported on the first clinical studies of intravenous ethanol for treatment of premature labor in which 35 of 52 patients (67%) were successfully delayed for 3 days or more. Later Zlatnik and Fuchs reported on a placebo-controlled trial of ethanol therapy of premature labor in which 17 of 21 patients (81%) treated with intravenous ethanol and only 8 of 21 patients (38%) treated with intravenous dextrose solution were delayed for 72 hours or more. The dosage schedule for intravenous ethanol recommended by Fuchs and associates consists of 7.5 ml of a 9.5% ethanol solution per kilogram of body weight per hour for 2 hours as a loading dose, and then 1.5 ml per kilogram of body weight per hour for 10 hours or more. This dosage schedule produces maternal blood ethanol concentrations of 178 ± 42 mg/dl at the end of the loading dose and approximately 150 ± 45 mg/dl during the maintenance dose. Legal intoxication exists when blood ethanol concentrations are 150 mg/dl. The most common maternal side effects of intravenous infusion of ethanol are inebriation, nausea, vomiting, headache, and restlessness; however, occasional patients develop severe acidosis, respiratory depression, and aspiration, which in one case led to death. There are relatively few fetal side effects of maternal treatment with intravenous ethanol despite rapid equilibration of fetal and maternal blood concentrations. Zerroudakis and associates reported that infants born within 12 hours after administration of ethanol had significantly lower 1-minute Apgar scores and a significantly higher incidence of respiratory distress syndrome. Occasional infants have marked central nervous system depression with lethargy, poor tone, and apnea, whereas others manifest signs of withdrawal. Ethanol has not been approved for treatment of premature labor by the United States Food and Drug Administration. The clinical popularity of ethanol for treatment of premature labor has dramatically declined during recent years because of the clinical emergence of other more effective tocolytic agents with fewer side effects.

β-Mimetic drugs

β-Mimetic drugs are compounds structurally related to epinephrine and isoproterenol that inhibit uterine contractions through their action on β-adrenergic receptors of myometrial cells. Their action on myometrial cells results consecutively in the intracellular formation of cAMP, activation of protein kinases, movement of calcium to sequestration sites, and cellular relaxation. Lands and associates described evidence of two populations of β-adrenergic receptors, the $β_1$-receptors located predominantly in the heart, smooth muscle of the small intestine, and adipose tissue, and the $β_2$-receptors located in the smooth muscle of the uterus, bronchi, and arterioles. Stimulation of $β_1$-receptors produces an increase of heart rate, relaxation of the small intestine, and lipolysis; stimulation of $β_2$-receptors produces relaxation of the uterus and bronchi, vasodilatation, and muscle glycogenolysis. An ideal drug for treatment of premature labor would stimulate only the $β_2$-receptors of the uterus, but unfortunately all the existing β-mimetic drugs act to some degree on both $β_1$- and $β_2$-receptors. Thus the usual side effects of these drugs, in the dosage needed to inhibit uterine contractions, include elevation of heart rate, lowering of blood pressure, and elevation of blood glucose levels.

Through mid-1980 the only β-mimetic drugs generally available in the United States and suitable for parenteral administration were isoproterenol (Isuprel), isoxsuprine (Vasodilan), and terbutaline (Bricanyl, Brethine). None of these agents had been classified as suitable for treatment of premature labor by the FDA. Isoproterenol and terbutaline were approved for treatment of bronchospasm, and isoxsuprine was classified as possibly effective for relief of cerebral and peripheral vascular insufficiency. The unfavorable balance of cardiovascular to tocolytic effects of isoproterenol prevented its use in treatment of premature labor. However, because of the unavailability of an FDA-approved drug, both isoxsuprine and terbutaline became popular for management of premature labor. Another β-mimetic drug, ritodrine (Yutopar), which had previously been available for clinical use in 23 other countries, was approved for treatment of premature labor by the United States FDA in June 1980. Thus ritodrine became the only β-mimetic drug, and the only drug of any class, to be approved in the United States for treatment of premature labor. Although ritodrine quickly became the dominant β-mimetic drug for treatment of premature labor, isoxsuprine and terbutaline will also be discussed for a historical perspective.

Isoxsuprine

Isoxsuprine hydrochloride was found to have a favorable balance of tocolytic to cardiovascular activity in a series of animal studies reported by Lish and associates in 1960. A year later Bishop and Woutersz reported that, of 156 patients in premature labor who were treated with isoxsuprine, 117 (75%) were delayed from delivery for more than 24 hours, and 33 (21%) were delayed for more than 7 days. In 1969 Das reported that, among 50 patients presenting in premature labor, delivery was delayed for 7 days or more in 36 of those treated with isoxsuprine and bed rest, compared with none treated by bed rest alone. More recently Csapo and Herczeg reported on a placebo-controlled trial of isoxsuprine in a series of 36 patients in premature labor with an average gestation of 31 weeks. Among the 17 patients treated with the placebo the average delay of delivery was 13.6 days, and 5 (29%) delivered infants weighing over 2,500 gm. In contrast, of the 19 patients treated with isoxsuprine the average delay of delivery was 46.3 days, and 16 (84%) delivered infants weighing more than 2,500 gm.

The usual dosage regimen for isoxsuprine consists of an intravenous infusion of 250 to 500 mg per minute, which, if successful, is continued for 8 to 12 hours. When successful, the infusion is followed by oral administration of 5 to 10 mg every 3 to 6 hours, continued until term gestation. The intravenous infusion of isoxsuprine is repeated if labor recurs.

The usual side effects of isoxsuprine administered by intravenous infusion include maternal tachycardia, tremor, nervousness, restlessness, palpitations, and mild hypotension. However, occasional patients develop marked hypotension with reduced uterine blood flow and fetal distress. From the widespread clinical experience with isoxsuprine, obvious effects on the fetus or newborn have been very rare; but from retrospective observations Brazy and Pupkin reported more common neonatal hypocalcemia, hypoglycemia, ileus, hypotension, and neonatal death among infants exposed to isoxsuprine within 48 hours of birth, compared with infants of similar birth weight who did not receive the drug. Approximately 50% of infants in each group developed respiratory distress syndrome. In contrast, Kero and associates reported that respiratory distress syndrome developed in only 2 of 26 (7.7%) premature infants with an average birth weight of 1,720 gm and average gestation of 31.6 weeks after unsuccessful treatment of premature labor with isoxsuprine. Similar results have been reported with other tocolytic agents, including ritodrine, but there have been no properly controlled prospective studies to confirm this apparent beneficial side effect.

Terbutaline

Terbutaline sulfate was initially described in 1970 by Persson and Olsson as a selective $β_2$-receptor stimulator with effects mainly on the β-receptors of the bronchi, peripheral vessels, and uterus. Clinical studies conducted in Sweden concluded that terbutaline was an effective inhibitor of nonpregnant and pregnant uterine activity with few cardiovascular or other side effects. In 1976 Ingemarsson reported on a double-blind, placebo-controlled study of terbutaline in a series of 30 patients in premature labor. The average gestation of patients entering the study was approximately 35 weeks. Terbutaline was administered by intravenous infusion, starting with a dosage of 10 μg per minute and increasing by 5 μg per minute every 10 minutes until contractions ceased, or to a maximum dosage of 25 μg per minute. After 1 hour the dosage was reduced by 5 μg per minute every 30 minutes to reach the lowest effective dose, which was then continued for 8 hours. Next, with continued absolute bed rest, terbutaline was administered by a subcutaneous injection of 250 μg every 6 hours for 3 days and then by oral administration of 5 mg every 8 hours, continued until the end of the thirty-sixth week of gestation. Maternal and fetal side effects were minimal and considered of no clinical consequence. Among the 30 patients, 12 of 15 (80%) who received terbutaline and only 3 of 15 (20%) who received the placebo reached 37 weeks' gestation. From a noncontrolled study of terbutaline treatment of premature labor, Wallace and associates reported that, although 47 of 50 patients were initially arrested, there were 11 (22%) treatment failures, 21 (42%) required more than one intravenous infusion, and gestation was prolonged beyond 36 weeks in only 24 (48%). In this study terbutaline was administered by intravenous infusion of 10 to 80 µg per minute, only until contractions were controlled. Then patients were permitted to ambulate and were given terbutaline (250 µg subcutaneously every 4 hours for 24 hours and then 2.5 mg orally every 4 hours). From the results of these two reports one may surmise that bed rest is a very important component of the successful treatment of premature labor.

The usual side effects of terbutaline are quite similar to those of the other β-mimetic drugs, with maternal tachycardia, slight elevation of fetal heart rate, increased pulse pressure with a modest rise of systolic and fall of diastolic blood pressure, elevation of maternal and fetal blood glucose levels, palpitations, nervousness, and tremor. Occasional patients treated with terbutaline have developed acute pulmonary edema. Although this serious adverse effect apparently occurs more often with terbutaline than with other tocolytic drugs, it has also been encountered with ritodrine, fenoterol, and magnesium sulfate. In almost all instances maternal pulmonary edema developed when patients had received combined therapy of the tocolytic drug and a glucocorticoid, such as betamethasone, hydrocortisone, or dexamethasone, used to enhance fetal pulmonary maturation in anticipation of possible premature delivery. Specific risk factors for the development of pulmonary edema include multiple pregnancy, fluid overload, hypokalemia, anemia, and preexisting cardiac disease.

Ritodrine

Ritodrine hydrochloride was developed specifically for obstetric applications because of its favorable balance of uterine relaxant to cardiovascular properties. In 1971 Wesselius-de Casparis and associates from seven hospitals in four European countries reported on a double-blind placebo-controlled study of ritodrine treatment of premature labor in 63 patients with an average gestation of 31.5 weeks at the beginning of treatment. The treatment consisted of an intravenous infusion of ritodrine (200 µg per minute) or a placebo for 24 to 48 hours, followed by a course of oral ritodrine or placebo tablets for the next 5 to 7 days. Bed rest was maintained for the first 4 days and followed by gradual ambulation. Side effects during ritodrine therapy were limited to a moderate increase of maternal heart rate and a slight rise in systolic blood pressure. Delivery was delayed at least 7 days in 80% of the ritodrine group and in 48% of the placebo group. Among the 51 patients with intact membranes the mean gain per case was 28.2 days in the ritodrine group and 17.4 days in the placebo group.

Subsequent studies of ritodrine conducted in Europe and in the United States confirmed its effectiveness in relaxing uterine contractions of preterm and term labor. Brettes and associates reported evidence that ritodrine produced an increase of uterine blood flow in patients with hypertension but no change in those who were normotensive. Miller and associates reported that 4 of 25 toxemic patients had an apparent increase in frequency of premature ventricular contractions during and immediately after the intravenous infusion of ritodrine. From fetal scalp blood sampling they reported that the mean fetal serum glucose level rose from 87.2 to 122.8 mg/dl during the administration of ritodrine. Spellacy and associates reported that, in a series of patients treated with ritodrine for inhibition of premature labor, the maternal blood glucose level rose from approximately 80 to 150 mg/dl, with a simultaneous rise of plasma insulin from about 20 to 100 µ units/ml. Kauppila and associates reported that ritodrine was more potent than isoxsuprine in causing increased levels of cAMP, glucose, insulin, and triglycerides. They also noted that both drugs caused a significant fall in serum iron and potassium levels during intravenous infusions lasting 6 hours or more. Placental blood flow responses to ritodrine were studied by Suonio and associates using a radionucleotide accumulation method. Following maternal intramuscular injection of 10 mg of ritodrine, placental perfusion increased 19% in normotensive patients, 24% in preeclamptic patients, and 45% in patients with chronic hypertension. Ragni and associates, using a phonocardiographic technique to measure cardiac intervals and plethysmography to record peripheral blood flow, concluded that the intravenous infusion of ritodrine (400 µg per minute) caused a significant increase of both cardiac output and peripheral blood flow. Thus it has become apparent that ritodrine, as well as other β-mimetic drugs, should not be used in patients with serious cardiac disease and should be used very cautiously in patients with hypertensive disease, hyperthyroidism, anemia, diabetes mellitus, or multiple pregnancy.

Ritodrine was compared with ethanol in treatment of premature labor in a randomized controlled study among three medical centers in the United States; it was reported on by Lauersen and associates in 1977. The average gestation of patients entering the study was 31 weeks. There were 67 patients who received ethanol and 68 treated with ritodrine. Delivery was delayed 72 hours or more in 61 (90%) of the ritodrine group and in 48 (73%) of the ethanol group. The average delay to delivery was 44 days in the ritodrine group and 27.6 days in the ethanol group. The side effects of treatment with the two drugs were judged as roughly equivalent. Thus from the data presented one must conclude that ritodrine is more effective than ethanol for treatment of premature labor.

Creasy and associates reported on a trial of continuing treatment with oral ritodrine versus oral placebo in 55 patients who initially had premature labor inhibited by treatment with intramuscular ritodrine. The number of relapses of premature labor requiring repeat intramuscular treatment was 1.11 in the ritodrine group versus 2.71 in the placebo group. Also, the mean interval between beginning oral treatment and the first relapse or delivery was 5.8 days in the oral placebo group and 25.9 days among those receiving oral ritodrine. Thus the effectiveness of oral ritodrine therapy is strongly supported by these results.

The approval of ritodrine hydrochloride for treatment of premature labor by the FDA in 1980 was preceded by the collaborative studies of 13 investigators at 11 university centers in the United States that were conducted from 1972 to 1977. The data were derived from treatment of 366 women in premature labor who received parenteral ritodrine (223), intravenous ethanol (77) or an intravenous placebo (66). With the ethanol and placebo treatment designated as the controls and by considering only the highest risk subgroup of patients who had labor onset prior to 33 weeks of gestation, the mean time gained in utero for infants of mothers treated with ritodrine was 40.9 days and 24.4 days for the controls. In the same subgroup the incidence of newborn respiratory distress was 13% in the ritodrine group and 29% in the controls, whereas the incidence of neonatal death was 8% in the ritodrine group and 24% in the control group. All these differences between the ritodrine and control groups were statistically significant.

The dosage schedule for treatment of premature labor with ritodrine consists of an initial intravenous infusion of 50 to 100 μg per minute, which is increased by 50 μg per minute increments every 10 minutes until contractions stop, unacceptable side effects develop, or the maximum dose of 350 μg per minute is reached. The patient remains in bed in the lateral decubitus position. Uterine activity, maternal heart rate, maternal blood pressure, and fetal heart rate are monitored frequently during the infusion. If unacceptable side effects develop, the dosage is reduced to a tolerable level. The infusion is stopped if labor persists for more than 30 minutes at the maximum dose. If contractions are successfully inhibited, the infusion is maintained for 12 to 24 hours. Oral therapy at a dosage of 10 mg is started 30 minutes before the infusion is stopped, and is continued at 10 mg every 2 hours for the next 24 hours (maximum dose 120 mg/day). The oral dose is continued as 10 to 20 mg every 4 to 6 hours until term, or earlier if so dictated by obstetric judgment.

Ambulation is resumed gradually after 48 hours. If premature labor recurs and there are no new obstetric or medical contraindications, ritodrine may again be administered by intravenous infusion.

Other β-mimetic drugs

Other β-mimetic drugs that have been evaluated in treatment of premature labor include salbutamol, orciprenaline and fenoterol. From several comparative studies we may conclude that fenoterol, orciprenaline, and isoxsuprine are less β_2-receptor specific than are ritodrine and terbutaline. From South Africa, Lipshitz and associates reported on their comparisons of fenoterol, ritodrine, salbutamol, and hexoprenaline. By comparing the uterine and cardiovascular responses of these drugs, they concluded that hexoprenaline was the most β_2-receptor selective.

CONCLUSIONS

The search for the best possible drug therapy for premature labor is far from over despite the current enthusiasm over the availability of ritodrine. The evaluation of drug therapy of premature labor is complicated by the inherent difficulty of diagnosing true versus false labor, the clinical variables that influence the onset of premature labor, the beneficial effect of bed rest alone, and the variety of ways that success or failure may be judged. However, there is now considerable evidence that 75% to 80% of patients in premature labor may be prevented from delivering for at least 48 hours by treatment with a variety of drugs. Although the safety of glucocorticoids administered for their effect on fetal pulmonary maturation has not yet been completely established, the tocolytic agents currently available are usually able to delay delivery long enough for the desired effect. Even if glucocorticoids are not used, any delay of premature delivery is potentially beneficial to the fetus. In the future a more complete understanding of the pathogenesis of premature labor and the role of the fetus in its initiation will undoubtedly permit our more intelligent use of tocolytic agents.

Tom P. Barden

BIBLIOGRAPHY

Ahlquist, R.P.: A study of the adrenotropic receptors, Am. J. Physiol. **153**:586, 1948.

Akerland, M., Andersson, K.E., and Ingemarsson, I.: Effects of terbutaline on myometrial activity, uterine blood flow, and lower abdominal pain in women with primary dysmenorrhea, Br. J. Obstet. Gynaecol. **83**:673, 1976.

Anderson, A.B.M., and others: Fetal adrenal weight and the course of premature delivery in human pregnancy, J. Obstet. Gynaecol. Br. Commonwealth **78**:481, 1971.

Andersson, K.E., Ingemarsson, I., and Persson, C.G.A.: Effects of terbutaline on human uterine motility at term, Acta Obstet. Gynecol. Scand. **54**:165, 1975.

Baillie, P., Meehan, F.P., and Tyack, A.J.: Treatment of premature labor with orciprenaline, Br. Med. J. 4:154, 1970.

Barden, T.P.: Effect of ritodrine on human uterine motility and cardiovascular responses in term labor and the early postpartum state, Am. J. Obstet. Gynecol. 112:645, 1972.

Barden, T.P., Peter, J.B., and Merkatz, I.R.: Ritodrine hydrochloride: a betamimetic agent for use in preterm labor. I. Pharmacology, clinical history, administration, side effects, and safety, Obstet. Gynecol. 56:1, 1980.

Bengtsson, L.P.: Experiments on the suppressive effect of a synthetic gestagen on the activity of the pregnant human uterus, Acta Obstet. Gynecol. Scand. 41:124, 1962.

Bieniarz, J., Motew, M., and Scommegna, A.: Uterine and cardiovascular effects of ritodrine in premature labor, Obstet. Gynecol. 40:65, 1972.

Bishop, E.H., and Woutersz, T.B.: Isoxsuprine, a myometrial relaxant: a preliminary report, Obstet. Gynecol. 17:442, 1961.

Blackard, W.G., and Aprill, C.N.: Mechanism of action of diazoxide, J. Lab. Clin. Med. 69:960, 1967.

Boog, G., Ben Brahim, M., and Gaudar, R.: Beta-mimetic drugs and possible prevention of respiratory distress syndrome, Br. J. Obstet. Gynaecol. 82:285, 1975.

Brazy, J.E., and Pupkin, M.J.: Effects of maternal isoxsuprine administration on preterm infants, J. Pediatr. 94:444, 1979.

Brenner, W.E., and Hendricks, C.H.: Effect of medroxyprogesterone acetate upon the duration and characteristics of human gestation and labor, Am. J. Obstet. Gynecol. 82:1094, 1961.

Brettes, M.P., Renaud, R., and Grander, R.: A double-blind investigation into the effects of ritodrine on uterine blood flow during the third trimester of pregnancy, Am. J. Obstet. Gynecol. 124:164, 1976.

Brotanek, V., Hendricks, C.H., and Yoshida, T.: Importance of changes in uterine blood flow in initiation of labor, Am. J. Obstet. Gynecol. 105:535, 1969.

Carsten, M.E.: Hormonal regulation of myometrial calcium transport, Gynecol. Invest. 5:269, 1974.

Castren, O., Gummerus, M., and Saarikoski, S.: Treatment of imminent premature labor, Acta Obstet. Gynecol. Scand. 54:95, 1975.

Cawson, M.J., and others: Cortisol, cortisone, and 11-deoxy-cortisol levels in human umbilical and maternal plasma in relation to the onset of labour, J. Obstet. Gynaecol. Br. Commonwealth 81:737, 1974.

Characteristics of births, United States 1973-1975, Series 21, No. 30, National Center for Health Statistics, Vital and Health Statistics, U.S. Department of Health, Education, and Welfare.

Chard, T., and others: Release of oxytocin and vasopressin by the human foetus during labour, Nature 234:352, 1971.

Coutinho, E.M., and Vieria Lopes, A.C.: Inhibition of uterine motility by aminophylline, Am. J. Obstet Gynecol. 110:726, 1971.

Creasy, R.K., Gummer, A., and Liggins, G.C.: System for predicting spontaneous preterm birth, Obstet. Gynecol. 55:692, 1980.

Creasy, R.K., and others: Oral ritodrine in treatment of preterm labor, Am. J. Obstet. Gynecol. 137:212, 1980.

Csapo, A.I.: Progesterone "block," Am. J. Anat. 98:273, 1956.

Csapo, A.I.: Defense mechanism of pregnancy. In Ciba Foundation Study Groups: Progesterone and the defense mechanism of pregnancy, Boston, 1961, Little, Brown & Co.

Csapo, A.I.: The prospects of PG's in postconceptional therapy, Prostaglandins 3:245, 1973.

Csapo, A.I., and Csapo, E.E.: The prostaglandin step: a bottleneck in the activation of uterus, Life Sci. 14:719, 1974.

Csapo, A.I., and Herczeg, J.: Arrest of premature labor by isoxsuprine, Am. J. Obstet. Gynecol. 129:482, 1977.

Csapo, A.I., and others: Volume and activity of the pregnant human uterus, Am. J. Obstet. Gynecol. 85:819, 1963.

Csapo, A.I., and others: Effect of massive progestational hormone treatment on the parturient human uterus, Fertil. Steril. 17:621, 1966.

Csapo, A.I., and others: Delay of spontaneous labor by naproxin in the rat model, Prostaglandins 3:827, 1973.

Dandavino, A., and others: Circulatory effects of magnesium sulfate in normotensive and renal hypertensive pregnant sheep, Am. J. Obstet. Gynecol. 127:769, 1977.

D'Angelo, L., and Sokol, R.J.: Prematurity: recognizing patients at risk, Prenatal Care 10(2):16, 1978.

Das, R.K.: Isoxsuprine in premature labor, J. Obstet. Gynaecol. India 19:566, 1969.

Daywood, M.Y., and others: Fetal contribution to oxytocin in human labor, Obstet. Gynecol. 52:205, 1978.

Daywood, M.Y., and others: Oxytocin in human pregnancy and parturition, Obstet. Gynecol. 51:138, 1978.

Drost, M., and Holm, L.W.: Prolonged gestation in ewes after foetal adrenalectomy, J. Endocrinol. 40:293, 1968.

Elliot, H.R., and Abdulla, U.: Pulmonary edema associated with ritodrine infusion and betamethasone administration in premature labor, Br. Med. J. 2:799, 1978.

Elliott, J.P., and others: Pulmonary edema associated with magnesium sulfate and betamethasone administration, Am. J. Obstet. Gynecol. 134:717, 1979.

Ferguson, J.K.W.: A study of the motility of the intact uterus at term, Surg. Gynecol. Obstet. 73:359, 1941.

Fuschs, A.R.: The inhibitory effect of ethanol on the release of oxytocin during parturition in the rabbit, J. Endocrinol. 35:125, 1966.

Fuchs, F., and others: Effect of alcohol on threatened premature labor, Am. J. Obstet. Gynecol. 99:627, 1967.

Fuchs, A.R., and others: Effect of ethanol on the activity of the non-pregnant human uterus and its reactivity to neurohypophyseal hormones, Am. J. Obstet. Gynecol. 101:1968.

Gibbons, G.L.D., and Chard, T.: Observations on maternal oxytocin release during human labor and the effect of intravenous alcohol administration, Am. J. Obstet. Gynecol. 126:243, 1976.

Goodlin, R.C., Keller, D.W., and Raffin, M.: Orgasm during late pregnancy, Obstet. Gynecol. 38:916, 1971.

Gustavii, B.: Release of lysosomal acid phosphatase into the cytoplasm of decidual cells before the onset of labor in humans, Br. J. Obstet. Gynaecol. 82:177, 1975.

Harbert, G.M., Cornell, G.W., and Thornton, W.N., Jr.: Effect of toxemia therapy on uterine dynamics, Am. J. Obstet. Gynecol. 105:94, 1969.

Heymann, M.A., Rudolph, A.M., and Silverman, N.H.: Closure of the ductus arteriosus in premature infants by inhibition of prostaglandin synthesis, N. Engl. J. Med. 295:530, 1976.

Ingemarsson, I.: Effect of terbutaline on premature labor: a double-blind placebo-controlled study, Am. J. Obstet. Gynecol. 125:520, 1976.

Jacobs, M.M., Knight, A.B., and Arias, F.: Maternal pulmonary edema resulting from beta mimetic and glucocorticoid therapy, Obstet. Gynecol. 56:56, 1980.

Johnson, J.W.C., and others: Efficacy of 17a-hydroxyprogesterone caproate in the prevention of premature labor, N. Engl. J. Med. 293:675, 1975.

Karim, S.M.M.: Identification of prostaglandins in human amniotic fluid, J. Obstet. Gynaecol. Br. Commonwealth 73:903, 1966.

Karim, S.M.M.: Appearance of prostaglandin F_2 in human blood during labour, Br. Med. J. 4:618, 1968.

Karim, S.M.M., and Devlin, J.: Prostaglandin content of amniotic fluid during pregnancy and labor, J. Obstet. Gynaecol. Br. Commonwealth 74:230, 1967.

Kauppila, A., and others: Effects of ritodrine and isoxsuprine with and without dexamethasone during late pregnancy, Obstet. Gynecol. 51:288, 1978.

Kero, P., Hirvonen, T., and Valimaki, I.: Prenatal and postnatal isoxsuprine and respiratory distress syndrome, Lancet 2:198, 1973.

Kloeck, F.K., and Jung, H.: In vitro release of prostaglandins from the human myometrium under the influence of stretching, Am. J. Obstet. Gynecol. 115:1066, 1973.

Korda, A.R., Lyneham, R.C., and Jones, W.R.: The treatment of premature labour with intravenously administered salbutamol, Med. J. Aust. 1:744, 1974.

Kumar, D., Goodno, J.A., and Barnes, A.C.: Isolation of progesterone from human pregnant myometrium, Nature 195:1204, 1962.

Kumar, D., Zourlas, P.A., and Barnes, A.C.: In vitro and in vivo effects of magnesium sulfate on human uterine contractility, Am. J. Obstet. Gynecol. 86:1036, 1963.

Landesman, R., and others: The inhibitory effect of diazoxide in normal term labor, Am. J. Obstet. Gynecol. 103:430, 1969.

Landesman, R., and others: The relaxant action of ritodrine, a sympathomimetic amine, on the uterus during term labor, Am. J. Obstet. Gynecol. 110:111, 1971.

Lands, A.M., and others: Differentiation of regular systems activated by sympathomimetic amines, Nature 214:597, 1967.

Lauersen, N.H., and others: Inhibition of premature labor: a multicenter comparison of ritodrine and ethanol, Am. J. Obstet. Gynecol. 127:837, 1977.

Lewis, R.B., and Schulman, J.D.: Influence of acetylsalicylic acid, and inhibitor of prostaglandin synthesis, on duration of human gestation and labor, Lancet 2:1159, 1973.

Liggins, G.C.: Premature delivery of foetal lambs infused with glucocorticoids, J. Endocrinol. 45:515, 1969.

Liggins, G.C., and Howie, M.B.: A controlled trial of antepartum glucocorticoid treatment for prevention of the respiratory distress syndrome in premature infants, Pediatrics 50:515, 1972.

Liggins, G.C., Kennedy, P.C., and Holm, L.W.: Failure of initiation of parturition after electrocoagulation of the pituitary of the fetal lamb, Am. J. Obstet. Gynecol. 98:1080, 1967.

Liggins, G.C., and Vaughn, G.S.: Intravenous infusion of salbutamol in the management of premature labour, J. Obstet. Gynaecol. Br. Commonwealth 80:29, 1973.

Liggins, G.C., and others: Control of parturition in man, Biol. Reprod. 16:39, 1977.

Lipshitz, J.: Uterine and cardiovascular effects of aminophylline, Am. J. Obstet. Gynecol. 131:716, 1978.

Lipshitz, J., Baillie, P., and Davey, D.A.: A comparison of the uterine beta$_2$-adrenoreceptor selectivity of fenoterol, hexoprenaline, ritodrine and salbutamol, S. Afr. Med. J. 50:1969, 1976.

Lish, P.M., Hillyard, I.W., and Dungan, K.W.: The uterine relaxant properties of isoxsuprine, J. Pharmacol. Exp. Ther. 129:438, 1960.

Liu, D.T.Y., Measday, B., and Melville, H.A.H.: Premature labour parameters for comparison employing methylxanthine therapy, Aust. N.Z. J. Obstet. Gynaecol. 15:145, 1975.

Manniello, R.L., and Farrell, P.M.: Analysis of United States neonatal mortality statistics from 1968 to 1974, with specific reference to changing trends in major causalities, Am. J. Obstet. Gynecol. 129:667, 1977.

Mayer, P.S., and Wingate, M.B.: Obstetric factors in cerebral palsy, Obstet. Gynecol. 51:399, 1978.

Merkatz, I.R., Peter, J.B., and Barden, T.P.: Ritodrine hydrochloride: a betamimetic agent used in preterm labor, II. Evidence of efficacy, Obstet. Gynecol. 56:7, 1980.

Milewich, L., and others: Initiation of parturition. VIII. Metabolism of progesterone by fetal membranes of early and late human gestation, Obstet. Gynecol. 50:45, 1977.

Miller, F.C., and others: Effects of ritodrine hydrochloride on uterine activity and the cardiovascular system in toxemic patients, Obstet. Gynecol. 47:50, 1976.

Monthly Vital Statistics Report, U.S. Department of Health and Human Services, 29(suppl. 1):1, 1980.

Mosler, K.H.: The treatment of threatened premature labor by tocolytics, Ca^{++}antagonists and anti-inflammatory drugs, Arzneim. Forsch. 25:263, 1975.

Mueller-Heubach, E., Myers, R.E., and Adamsons, K.: Effects of adrenalectomy on pregnancy length in the rhesus monkey, Am. J. Obstet. Gynecol. 112:221, 1972.

Niebyl, J.R., and others: The inhibition of premature labor with indomethacin, Am. J. Obstet. Gynecol. 136:1014, 1980.

Nochimson, D.J., and others: The effects of ritodrine hydrochloride on uterine activity and the cardiovascular system, Am. J. Obstet. Gynecol. 118:523, 1974.

Novy, M.J., Cook, M.J., and Manaugh, L.: Indomethacin block of normal onset of parturition in primates, Am. J. Obstet. Gynecol. 118:412, 1974.

Persson, H., and Olsson, T.: Some pharmacological properties of terbutaline 1-(3,5-dihydroxyphenyl)-2-(T-butylamino)-ethanol: a new sympathomimetic β-receptor-stimulating agent, Acta Med. Scand. 512 (suppl.):11, 1970.

Petrie, R.H., and others: The effect of drugs on uterine activity, Obstet. Gynecol. 48:431, 1976.

Ragni, N., and others: Poly-plethysmographic study on the effects of ritodrine on the cardiovascular system of patients in labour, Br. J. Obstet. Gynaecol. 86:866, 1979.

Raja, R.L., Anderson, A.B.M., and Turnbull, A.C.: Endocrine changes in premature labor, Br. Med. J. 4:67, 1974.

Rayburn, W.F., and Wilson, E.A.: Coital activity and premature delivery, Am. J. Obstet. Gynecol. 137:972, 1980.

Renard, M., and Gauder, R.: The use of ritodrine in the treatment of premature labour, J. Obstet. Gynaecol. Br. Commonwealth 81:182, 1974.

Riffel, H.D., and others: Effects of meperidine and promethazine during labor, Obstet. Gynecol. 42:738, 1973.

Robinson, G.A., Butcher, R.W., and Sutherland, E.W.: Cyclic AMP, Am. Rev. Biochem. 37:149, 1968.

Schwarz, B.E., and others: Initiation of human parturition. IV. Demonstration of phsopholipase A$_2$ in the lysosomes of human fetal membranes, Am. J. Obstet. Gynecol. 125:1089, 1976.

Scommegna, A., and others: Effect of pregnenolone sulfate on uterine contractility, Am. J. Obstet. Gynecol. 108:1023, 1970.

Sokol, R.J., and others: Risk, antepartum care, and outcome: impact of a maternity and infant care project, Obstet. Gynecol. 56:150, 1980.

Spellacy, W.N., and others: The acute effects of ritodrine infusion on maternal metabolism: measurements of levels of glucose, insulin, glucagon, triglycerides, cholesterol, placental lactogen, and chorionic gonadotropin, Am. J. Obstet. Gynecol. 131:637, 1978.

Stander, R.W., and others: Fetal cardiac effects of maternal isoxsuprine infusion, Am. J. Obstet. Gynecol. 89:792, 1964.

Steer, C.M., and Petrie, R.H.: A comparison of magnesium sulfate and alcohol for prevention of premature labor, Am. J. Obstet. Gynecol. 129:1, 1977.

Stubblefield, P.G.: Pulmonary edema occurring after therapy with dexamethasone and terbutaline for premature labor: a case report, Am. J. Obstet. Gynecol. 132:341, 1978.

Suonio, S., Oikkonen, H., and Lahtinen, T.: Maternal circulatory response to a single dose of ritodrine hydrochloride during orthostasis in normal and hypertensive late pregnancy, Am. J. Obstet. Gynecol. 130:745, 1978.

Sutherland, E.W., and Rall, T.W.: Relation of adenosine 3'5'-phosphate and phosphorylase to the actions of catecholamines and other hormones, Pharmacol. Rev. 12:265, 1960.

Vane, J.R.: Inhibition of prostaglandin synthesis as a mechanism of action for aspirin-like drugs, Nature 231:232, 1971.

Wagner, L., Wagner, G., and Guerrero, J.: Effect of alcohol on premature newborn infants, Am. J. Obstet. Gynecol. 108:308, 1970.

Wallace, R.L., and others: Inhibition of premature labor by terbutaline, Obstet. Gynecol. 51:387, 1978.

Wesselius-deCasparis, A., and others: Results of double-blind, multicentre study with ritodrine in premature labour, Br. Med. J. 3:144, 1971.

Wilson, K.H., and others: Effects of diazoxide and beta adrenergic drugs on spontaneous and induced uterine activity in the pregnant baboon, Am. J. Obstet. Gynecol. 118:499, 1974.

Zervoudakis, I.A., and others: Infants of mothers treated with ethanol for premature labor, Am. J. Obstet. Gynecol. 137:713, 1980.

Zlatnik, F.J., and Fuchs, F.: A controlled study of ethanol in threatened premature labor, Am. J. Obstet. Gynecol. 112:610, 1972.

Zuckerman, H., Reiss, U., and Rubinstein, I.: Inhibition of human premature labor by indomethacin, Obstet. Gynecol. 44:787, 1974.

Zuspan, F.P., coordinator: Progestational therapy during pregnancy: an invitational symposium, J. Reprod. Med. 3:225, 1969.

Zuspan, F.P., Cibils, L.A., and Pose, S.V.: Myometrial and cardiovascular responses to alterations in plasma epinephrine and norepinephrine, Am. J. Obstet. Gynecol. 84:841, 1962.

Zuspan, F.P., and others: Premature labor: its management and therapy, J. Reprod. Med. 9:93, 1972.

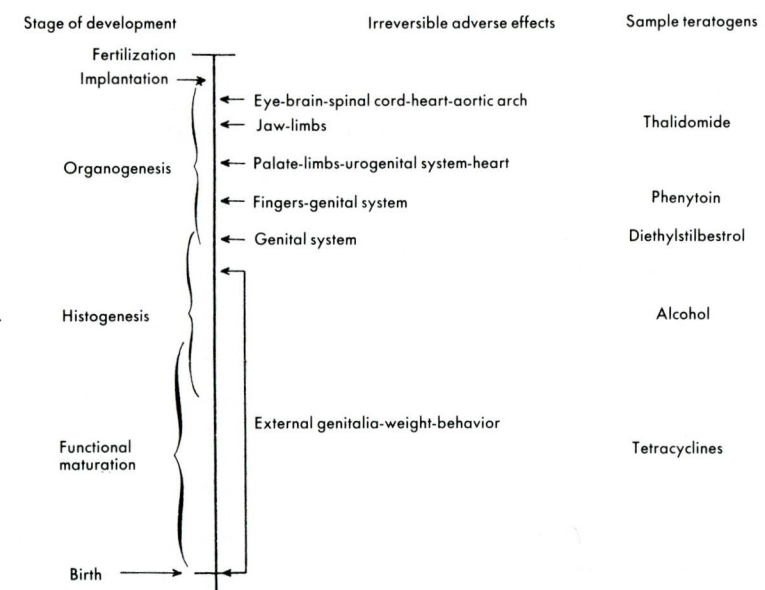

Fig. 12-2. Critical periods in human embryogenesis.

Stage of development	Irreversible adverse effects	Sample teratogens
Fertilization		
Implantation	Eye-brain-spinal cord-heart-aortic arch	
	Jaw-limbs	Thalidomide
Organogenesis	Palate-limbs-urogenital system-heart	
	Fingers-genital system	Phenytoin
	Genital system	Diethylstilbestrol
Histogenesis		Alcohol
	External genitalia-weight-behavior	
Functional maturation		Tetracyclines
Birth		

spermatozoa and consequently alter the developmental process of fertilized eggs.

Although many methodologic problems face the researcher investigating the relationship between paternal drug ingestion and perinatal outcome in humans, it is likely over the next few years that we will become aware of a larger number of paternally mediated teratogenic effects.

Effect of drugs on the fetus

The adverse effects of in utero exposure to drugs can vary from reversible effects such as transient changes in clotting time or fetal breathing movements to irreversible effects such as fetal death, intrauterine growth retardation, structural malformations, or mental retardation. The specific drug, the dosage, the route of administration, the timing of treatment, and the genotype of the mother or the fetus all may be critical determinants of the effect of a drug on the fetus. The disease being treated may be an important consideration. The factors that may combine to influence the outcome of drug administration include diet and coadministration of drugs. It is at best difficult to control these parameters in humans, and thus the incontrovertible establishment of a drug as a teratogen in humans requires the combination of extreme situations such as those just outlined for thalidomide. Consequently it has been necessary to rely heavily on animal studies to assess the teratogenic potential of drugs.

The *timing* of drug exposure is frequently a critical determinant of the effect of the drug on the fetus (Fig. 12-2). The first week after fertilization is the "period of the zygote" (cleavage and gastrulation); during this time the most common adverse effect of drugs is termination of pregnancy, which may occur even before the woman knows she is pregnant. Exposure of the preimplantation embryo to embryotoxic drugs may also retard its development, perhaps by decreasing cell number in the blastocyst. The second to the eighth weeks of gestation are the "period of the embryo." It is mainly during this period of organogenesis that drugs produce dramatic and catastrophic structural malformations. Other adverse effects during this phase may include fetal wastage, transplacental carcinogenesis (e.g., diethylstilbestrol), and intrauterine growth retardation. From the third to ninth months of gestation, the "period of the fetus," differentiation of the central nervous system and reproductive system continues. Drugs given during this time have been implicated as behavioral teratogens. In this period, drugs may cause disproportionate growth retardation (infants whose head growth has been spared, after 30 or more weeks) or may alter the external genitalia.

Consideration of irreversible adverse effects of drugs on development usually stops with birth. However, it is well known that sensory and other higher nervous system functions are not fully developed until well after birth. Thus birth is not really a termination point but only another milestone in development. Little is known about the long-term or delayed adverse effects of drugs administered to the mother during labor and delivery or directly to the neonate. Antitumor agents such as cyclophosphamide can have long-term effects on the histogenesis of the cerebellum, on growth and development, and on reproductive function when administered postnatally.

The effects of individual drugs on the fetus are highly

Table 12-2. Drugs associated with congenital malformations in humans

Drugs	Fetal growth	Growth retardation	Mental retardation	Central nervous system	Cardiovascular	Musculoskeletal	Urogenital	Eye and ear	Thyroid
Antimicrobials									
Tetracycline						X			
Streptomycin								X	
Quinine?								X	
Antineoplastics									
Methotrexate	X	X		X	X				
Busulfan, chlorambucil, cyclophosphamide				X	X	X	X		
CNS drugs									
Diazepam					X				
Phenothiazines	X								
Lithium?					X				
Narcotic analgesics									
Morphine, methadone, heroin	X	X							
Anticonvulsants									
Phenytoin		X	X		X			X	
Barbiturates			X		X	X			
Trimethadione			X		X	X		X	
Steroid hormones									
Androgens							X		
Diethylstilbestrol							X		
Estrogens/progestins				X			X		
Iodine, propylthiouracil									X
Warfarin		X			X	X			
Propranolol		X							
Alcohol	X	X		X	X	X	X		
Tobacco smoking	X	X			X	X			

Developmental pharmacology

respect to teratogenic potential. Thalidomide was withdrawn from the market because of its marked effect on the fetus. However, glutethimide (with the same dioxopiperidine ring as thalidomide) is not teratogenic. It is obvious that more information on how drugs induce malformations is needed before knowledge of their molecular structure or pharmacologic action will permit prediction of teratogenicity. The decision as to whether to give a drug during pregnancy is difficult. Some of the information available on the potential adverse effects of pharmacologic classes of drugs often administered during pregnancy is summarized in Table 12-2.

Table 12-3 summarizes the results of studies on the teratogenicity of various commonly used therapeutic agents.

Self-administered nontherapeutic agents

Chronic alcohol intake during pregnancy is associated with a readily identifiable fetal alcohol syndrome (Chapter 33, part five) and has been cited as the most frequently documented cause of mental deficiency in the Western world. Prenatal and postnatal growth retardation, mental deficiency, persistent microcephaly, and minor anomalies of the face, eyes, heart, joints, and genitalia have been identified. The Collaborative Perinatal study reported a mortality of 17% and mental retardation in 44% of infants of alcoholic mothers.

There may be a dose-response relationship between the severity of fetal alcohol syndrome and the alcohol consumption by the mother. Among babies born to mothers who drank 1.5 oz or more of absolute alcohol daily, 63% demonstrated neurologic impairment, 16% were born prematurely, and 28% were small for gestational age; 32% of the infants born to heavy drinkers had congenital malformations, and 16% had major malformations. The mechanisms whereby alcohol produces teratogenic effects on the fetus are unknown.

There now seems to be no question that maternal smoking substantially reduces birth weight of offspring (p. 59). There is a significant dose-response relationship, and early cessation of smoking can result in birth weights similar to those among offspring of nonsmoking mothers. The largest studies also document a 30% to 35% increase in mortality due to abruptio placentae, placenta previa, prematurity, and respiratory disease. Some studies also report an increased incidence of spontaneous abortion in smoking mothers.

There are conflicting data concerning an association between smoking during pregnancy, congenital heart defects, and cleft palate and lip in the infant. Others report no association between maternal smoking and congenital malformations. In addition to potential morphologic effects of cigarette smoking, there may be important functional consequences for the fetus, such as

dependent on the specific drug involved. There are no infallible means for predicting which drug will be "selectively toxic" to the fetus. Within some groups of drugs each individual drug can cause the same type of malformation. The anticonvulsants exemplify a family of drugs in which the core structure necessary for activity as an anticonvulsant appears also to fulfill the requirements for inducing characteristic malformations. In other instances, such as the sedative-hypnotics, individual drugs with common therapeutic effects differ markedly with

Table 12-3. Teratogenicity of physician- or self-administered therapeutic agents

Specific agents	Studies reported	Results and recommendations
Antineoplastic agents (antimetabolites, alkylating agents, antitumor antibiotics, etc.)		As a group these are the most potent teratogens known. It is difficult to delineate one agent because of frequent combined uses in addition to irradiation.
Antimetabolites (purine analogs, pyrimidine analogs, folic acid antagonists)	Nicholson; Milunsky	Most potent teratogens of this group; associated with skeletal defects.
Alkylating agents (busulfan, chlorambucil, cyclophosphamide, nitrogen mustard)	Schardein; Diamond; Shottran; Greenberg; Garrett	Some reports have described drug-related defects, but cases with no drug-related defects have also been reported. Avoid use during first trimester; less critical after this time but may still result in IUGR.
Antimicrobials		
Sulfonamides	Schardein; Richards	Conflicting reports on teratogenicity; should be avoided in third trimester because of risk of kernicterus
Tetracyclines	Colhan	Result in staining of dentition; should be avoided in second and third trimesters and early childhood. Permanent teeth unaffected.
Penicillins Cephalosporins Chloramphenicol Aminoglycosides	Nelson	Appear to be safe when administered at any phase of pregnancy.
Streptomycin; dihydrostreptomycin Antituberculars	Scheinhorn; Warkany (1979)	Auditory nerve defects and ocular nerve damage in infants following prenatal exposure.
Isoniazid (INH)	Monnet	Five children with severe encephalopathies after prenatal exposure; recommend prophylactic administration of vitamin B_6 to pregnant women receiving INH.
Ethionamide; ethambutol; rifampin	Schardein	No clear relationship with abnormal fetal development.
Antiparasitics	Schardein	Quinidine—deafness; others—no definite teratogenicity.
Anticonvulsants	Smith	Women requiring anticonvulsant therapy should be counseled prior to becoming pregnant as to the nature and magnitude of risk to the fetus; overall risk of having a malformed child is about 1 in 10.
Hydantoins Phenytoin	Hanson	Typical *fetal hydantoin syndrome* with mild to moderate growth and mental deficiencies, limb anomalies, and dysmorphic facies (low nasal bridge, short nose, mild ocular hypertelorism).
Barbiturates; deoxybarbiturates Primidone; phenobarbital; secobarbital; amobarbital	Bethenod; Heinonen	Postnatal effects similar to those in fetal hydantoin syndrome; associated cardiovascular malformations.
Oxazoladinediones Trimethadione	Goldman	Fetal trimethadione syndrome with developmental delay, speech difficulty, V-shaped eyebrows, epicanthus, low-set ears, palatal anomaly, and irregular teeth.
Psychotropic agents		The teratogenicity of most psychotropics is not established; caution is necessary in administering them during pregnancy; all minor tranquilizers should be avoided during pregnancy.
Thalidomide	Schardein	Tremendously teratogenic to humans when administered in the first to eighth weeks of pregnancy; limb reduction anomalies reported.
Meprobamate Benzodiazepines Diazepam; chlordiazepoxide	Safra; Saxen; Heinonen; Milkovich (1974)	Greatly conflicting results; increased incidence of cleft lip, with or without cleft; ingestion before parturition may cause hypotonia, apnea, and hypothermia.

Table 12-3. Teratogenicity of physician- or self-administered therapeutic agents—cont'd

Specific agents	Studies reported	Results and recommendations
Psychotropic agents—cont'd		
Phenothiazines	Heinonen; Rumeau-Rouquette	In general, associated with slight increase in incidence of malformations.
Chlorpromazine	Sobel	Increased incidence of spontaneous abortion when administered in first 4 months of pregnancy.
Prochlorperazine	Hill	Cardiovascular deformities and complications of extrapyramidal activity.
Lithium	Nora	Cardiovascular anomalies and congenital heart disease; infants of women who begin labor with high plasma levels may develop respiratory distress and cyanosis lasting for up to 10 days post partum.
Tricyclic antidepressants	Schardein	Possible increased incidence of malformation.
Monoamine oxidase inhibitors	Samojlik	Little data available for humans; only phenelzine is reported as embryotoxic in rats.
Antinauseants; antihistamines	Heinonen; Shapiro; Smithells; Paterson	No evidence of association to malformation in humans; chlorcyclizine and meclizine are teratogenic in lab animals but not in humans.
Nonnarcotic analgesics, antiinflammatory, antipyretic agents	Eriksson	Little evidence to associate these with malformations (see specific exceptions following). As a group, considering wide usage, they are not considered to be teratogenic in humans.
Salicylates	Turner; Shapiro	Conflicting results regarding perinatal mortality and birth weight; great concern exists regarding effects on platelet function that could cause hemorrhagic complications in a traumatic birth. Possible intrauterine closure of PDA, pulmonary hypertension.
p-Aminophenols Acetaminophen	Schardein	May be related to development of cataracts, but a causal relationship has not been confirmed.
Narcotic analgesics	Rothstein	Appear to be nonteratogenic to humans; withdrawal symptoms may occur in infants of narcotic-addicted women.
Hormones and hormone antagonists		
Androgens	Forsberg	Increased risk of masculinization or pseudohermaphroditism in humans.
Antiandrogens Cyproterone acetate	Forsberg	Associated with abnormal sexual development in male laboratory animals; effects in humans unknown.
Progestins Ethisterone; norethindrone	Wilkins	Associated with equivocal or frankly masculinized external genitalia of varying degrees related to the treatment period during pregnancy.
Estrogens Diethylstilbestrol	Ulfelder; Herbst; Barnes; Henderson	Associated with high risk of vaginal adenocarcinoma in young women exposed in utero; also benign alterations in genital tract of exposed females; in exposed males there was increased incidence of genitourinary tract disturbances but no increase in cancer incidence.
Antiestrogens Clomiphene	Oakley	Multiple pregnancy.
Oral contraceptive agents	Levy; Yasuda; Nora; Orti-Perez; Rothman	Conflicting reports of results; some uncorroborated evidence of increased incidence of limb reduction malformations and great vessel malformations; it seems reasonable to conclude that there are no large risks of malformation facing offspring born after oral contraceptive use.
Corticosteroids (natural and synthetic mineralocorticoids and glucocorticoids)	Schardein	All are teratogens in animals and have possibly been associated with cleft palate, limb anomalies, and heart defects in humans.
Antithyroid agents (iodides and propylthiouracil)		May produce neonatal goiter and tracheal obstruction; also may be associated with hypospadias, aortic atresia, and developmental retardation.
Hypoglycemic drugs (tolbutamide; chlorpropamide)	Landauer (1972)	Generally, hypoglycemic drugs have little if any teratogenic potential in humans; possible increased incidence of caudal dysplasia (agenesis of sacrum and coccyx).
Insulin	Schardein	Teratogenic to mice and rabbits but *not* in humans.

Continued.

Table 12-3. Teratogenicity of physician- or self-administered therapeutic agents—cont'd

Specific agents	Studies reported	Results and recommendations
Vitamins and iron		Used almost universally by pregnant women with only rare reports of associated malformations (see following).
Vitamin A	Schardein; Bernhardt; Pilotti	Hypervitaminosis appears to be teratogenic in animals, and 2 cases of related urinary malformations have been reported in humans.
Vitamin D		Supravalvular aortic stenosis.
Iron-containing drugs	Nelson; McBride	Association with congenital malformations has been reported but remains unconfirmed by other studies.
Diuretics		In general, not associated with congenital malformations.
Benzothiadiazides	Rodriguez; Torilla	Thrombocytopenia, altered carbohydrate metabolism, and hyperbilirubinemia have been reported in infants exposed late in gestation.
Cardiovascular drugs (antiarrhythmics; digitalis glycosides; antihypertensives)		Very few reports relate these to malformations in humans.
Propranolol	Pruyn; Oakes	Associated with decreased uterine blood flow and intrauterine growth retardation; bradycardia and hypoglycemia in the newborn.
Anticoagulants		
Warfarin	Schardein; Warkany (1976)	Of this group only warfarin has shown teratogenicity in humans. Exposure during the first trimester has been related to chondrodysplasia punctata and nasal hypoplasia associated with roentgenographic stippling of the epiphyses (Conradi syndrome). Exposure in the third trimester is known to cause fetal or placental hemorrhage; thus it is recommended that patients requiring anticoagulant therapy be treated with an agent that will not cross the placenta.
Cough and cold medicines		
Bronchodilators; centrally acting antitussive agents; decongestants; expectorants	Schardein	Of these, only the iodide expectorants have been associated with adverse effects (fetal hypothyroidism and goiter).
Sympathomimetic amines (phenylephrine; phenylpropanolamine; ephedrine; dextroamphetamine)	Heinonen	Have been associated with facial malformations, inguinal hernia, and clubfoot; it is difficult to determine if these malformations were caused by these agents or by the viral infection being treated.

decreased fetal breathing movements and increased fetal heart rate. Several studies have reported a significant relationship between maternal smoking during pregnancy and low achievement, increased hyperactivity, and "minimal cerebral dysfunction" in the offspring.

Exactly which ingredient(s) in cigarette smoke causes the effects and whether it is a direct effect on the fetus or is mediated via the mother are unknown. There does not seem to be a significant beneficial effect on birth weight or perinatal mortality from reduction in nicotine and tar content or filtering of cigarettes. Prevention of the harmful effects of tobacco on the fetus can apparently only come from the cessation of smoking.

Although caffeine has been found to be teratogenic in high doses in animal experiments, these reports suggest little teratogenic danger to humans. Administration of caffeine does alter ovine fetal respiratory activity, and the presence of caffeine in most cord plasma samples suggests that it alters human fetal respiratory activity or even neonatal breathing patterns.

Smoking and consumption of alcohol and caffeine are highly correlated. The potential interaction of these influences plus other drug and environmental factors should be considered systematically in future studies.

Environmental chemicals

There are many chemicals in the environment. Fortunately, few of these chemicals have shown teratogenic potential in animals or humans. In Ireland the prevalence of anencephaly and spina bifida has been related to heavy dietary consumption of blighted potatoes, although this has not been confirmed. Intrauterine methylmercury poisoning (Minamata disease) was characterized by severe neurologic symptoms and convulsions.

It has been suggested that the abuse of gasoline by

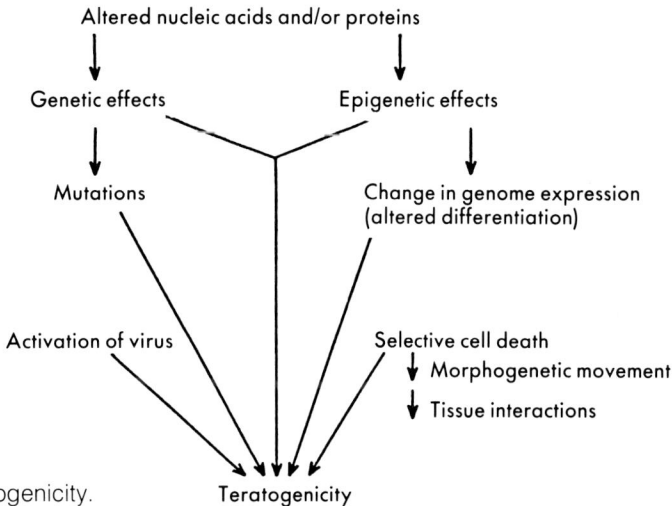

Fig. 12-3. Potential mechanisms of drug-induced teratogenicity.

inhalation could cause congenital malformations characterized by profound retardation, initial hypotonia progressing to hypertonia, scaphocephaly, a prominent occiput, poor postnatal head growth, and additional minor abnormalities. Polycyclic aromatic hydrocarbons and halogenated aromatic hydrocarbons (insecticides) are embryotoxic in animals; future studies may demonstrate that these environmental chemicals are also fetotoxic in humans.

In summary, it is interesting to consider the specificity of the adverse effects of various drug groups. Exposure to hormones, antimicrobials, and many CNS drugs during gestation produces fetal effects involving only one or two organ systems. In contrast, the antineoplastics, anticonvulsants, alcohol, and cigarette smoke have adverse effects on the fetus encompassing a variety of diverse organ systems.

Factors modifying the fetal response to drugs
Genetic background

In addition to the drug itself, the dosage, timing during gestation, and genetic background of the individual fetus and/or mother may play an important role in determining susceptibility to the teratogenic effects of a drug.

Recent experiments in mice differing at one allele demonstrated the importance of both the maternal and fetal genotype in determining the outcome of exposure to a toxic drug. Fraser and co-workers have demonstrated genetic (strain) differences in the susceptibility of inbred mice to development of a cortisone-induced cleft palate. Thus congenital malformations may be under multifactorial control.

Drug-drug interactions

Individuals taking drugs rarely consume a single drug; rather, various combinations are used. Animal experiments have provided examples of instances where the administration of one drug can modify the teratogenicity of another. For example, treatment of rats with phenobarbital increased the teratogenicity of the antitumor drug cyclophosphamide. It is thought that phenobarbital pretreatment induced maternal hepatic cytochrome P_{450}, increasing the activation of cyclophosphamide to mutagenic and/or teratogenic metabolites.

Mechanisms of drug toxicity in the fetus

A wide variety of mechanisms has been postulated for the adverse effects of drugs on the fetus. These include mutations, altered differentiation, inhibition of the biosynthesis of structural proteins (e.g., collagen), inhibition of tissue interactions, and altered morphogenetic movements due to selective cell death (Fig. 12-3).

We now know that many chemical carcinogens (or mutagens) are "precarcinogens" (or "premutagens") and must be metabolically activated to reactive electrophilic metabolites or "ultimate carcinogens" to initiate the cell damage leading to cancer. Experiments with limb bud and whole embryo culture techniques suggest that at least one teratogen, cyclophosphamide, also requires activation to its "ultimate teratogen." There is also some evidence that thalidomide, phenytoin, chlorcyclizine, and diethylstilbestrol require metabolic activation to be teratogenic. The mechanisms whereby such active metabolites produce their effects are thought to involve reactions with DNA (causing base substitution or frame shift mutations), with proteins (blocking crucial steps in cell metabolism), or with structural lipids (promoting lipid peroxidation). We know that many active metabolites, because of their instability, react with any available cell nucleophile. Thus, in fact, a combination of the above mechanisms may be involved.

Such reactive electrophilic metabolites can be detoxified by conjugation with nucleophiles like glutathione, catalyzed by the glutathione S transferases. Animal experiments have revealed the presence of enzymes during development that may result in other deactivation processes, including hydration, glucuronidation, acetylation, or sulfation.

Determination of adverse drug effects in the fetus

Human studies of the effects of drugs during pregnancy are almost all retrospective. Amniocentesis and ultrasound can be used to screen for some birth defects, but pregnancy is already well advanced by the time these can be used. Epidemiologic studies can, after the fact, correlate a drug with a defect and thus prevent exposure of future fetuses. However, to delineate the effects of drugs taken either alone or in combination on unidentified multiple factors in development is difficult in humans, even in large epidemiologic studies. Exposure to drugs associated with malformations can be prevented or minimized in women of childbearing age.

Fortunately, animal models are now available to study the effects of these drugs. Such studies permit the definition of dosage of the drug, its timing during gestation, environment, and genotype and allow controls matched for weight and xenobiotic exposure. The definition of genotype and environment that these studies allow has increased understanding of the mechanisms of drug-induced toxicity in teratogenicity. Rodents (specifically, mice and rats) are frequently chosen as animal models because they are easy to breed, inexpensive, and have short gestational periods. Although animal models are generally useful in identifying teratogens, certain limitations must be kept in mind. Thalidomide is an unfortunate example of a human teratogen that is not teratogenic in rodents. Aspirin (acetylsalicylic acid) is an example of a drug that is not a human teratogen but is teratogenic in rodents.

Further study of the mechanisms of drug-induced teratogenicity may permit the development of antiteratogens to prevent the fetotoxic effects of drugs essential for the mother during pregnancy. A variety of such compounds (e.g., nicotinamide, ascorbate, cysteine, and vitamins) has been studied in laboratory experiments.

New, quick, and inexpensive screening tests for teratogens need to be developed. Preferably such tests should include routes of metabolism of the drug similar to those in humans. Perhaps organ culture techniques (limb bud, palate) will be developed to test teratogens in vitro. Such systems could have drug-metabolizing enzymes incorporated (in liposomes or intact liver parenchymal cells) to activate any preteratogen such as thalidomide or cyclophosphamide. Other studies have suggested that the inhibition of attachment of tumor cells in vitro may be useful in the prediction of drug teratogenicity in vivo.

DRUG USE, DISPOSITION, AND METABOLISM IN THE NEWBORN

At birth a full-term infant in North America receives at least three types of drugs: an ophthalmic antimicrobial agent (e.g., silver nitrate), vitamin K, and triple dye for the cord. Low birth weight and sick infants in a neonatal intensive care unit additionally receive an increasing number of drugs (Table 12-4), with the constant introduction of old drugs with new indications (e.g., caffeine and theophylline for apnea, indomethacin for closure of the ductus arteriosus) and new drugs (e.g., bumetanide) in the neonatal therapeutic armamentarium. Thus the overall xenobiotic exposure of the fetus and newborn exceeds current estimates, particularly when environmental agents (e.g., lead, methylmercury, volatile hydrocarbons) and drugs of habits (e.g., caffeine, alcohol) are taken into consideration. Since many of these agents are pharmacologically active, their effects may be significant if sufficient amounts reach the fetus or newborn. Besides the usual oral or parenteral routes, unintentional portals of drug entry include the transplacental route, inadvertent direct fetal injection, pulmonary, skin, or conjunctival entry, or via breast milk. Lack of awareness or underestimation of the degree of drug entry through these routes and of altered drug disposition and metabolism in the perinatal period have led to well-recognized therapeutic misadventures in neonatology. Possible prevention of drug toxicity and a rational and safe use of drugs require a thorough understanding of the various pharmacologic profiles of each drug used in the neonate.

Fig. 12-4 illustrates many of the interrelationships of the absorption, distribution, binding, biotransformation, and excretion of a drug and its concentration at the locus of action. To produce its characteristic effect, a drug must be present in appropriate concentrations at its sites of action or the receptor sites. The concentration of drug at the receptor site depends not only on the amount of drug administered but also on the aforementioned interrelationships (Fig. 12-4). Those factors which have been evaluated in the newborn infant differ substantially relative to the adult and even to the young infant beyond the neonatal period.

Absorption of drugs in the newborn

Drug absorption is the passage of a drug from its site of administration into the circulation. In the sick neonate there exists a preferential utilization of the intravenous route because of ease of delivery, accuracy of dosage, possible poor peripheral perfusion, and poor gastrointestinal function. In neonates who can tolerate gastric feedings the oral route of drug administration is the most convenient and probably the safest. Absorption of a drug or substance through the gastrointestinal system may be

Table 12-4. Comparative plasma half-lives (in hours) of antimicrobial drugs excreted by the kidneys in newborns and adults

Drug	Birth weight (gm)	Newborn <7 days	Newborn >7 days	Adults*	Approximate relative prolongation <7 days	Approximate relative prolongation >7 days	Reference
Aminoglycosides							
Neomycin	Term	5.6	3-4	8	—	—	Axline (1964)
Streptomycin		7	—	2.5	2.5	—	Axline (1964); Sereni (1968)
Kanamycin	<2,000	7.7	5.2	3-4	2	1.4	Howard (1975)
	>2,000	5.3	3.8		1.5	—	
Gentamicin	<2,000	All infants	All infants	2	6	—	McCracken (1971)
	>2,000	5	3.2		2.5	1.6	
Tobramycin	<2,000	8.5	5.1	2	4	2.5	Kaplan (1973);
	>2,000	6	4		3	2	McCracken (1976)
Amikacin	<2,000	6.6	5.5	2	3	2.5	McCracken (1976);
	>2,000	5.8	4.9		2.5	2.4	Bodey (1974)
Cephalosporins							
Cephalothin	Term	1.5-2	—	0.5-0.8	2	—	Grossman (1965)
Cefazolin	Term	4.5-3	3	1.5	3	2	Nakasawa (1970)
Penicillins							
Penicillin G	<2,000	4.9	2.6	0.5	9	5	McCracken (1975);
	>2,000	2.6	2.1		5	4	Braude (1976)
Ampicillin	<2,000	6.4	2.2	1.5	4	1.4	McCracken (1977);
	>2,000	4.9	2.3		3	1.5	Eickoff (1965)
Carbenicillin	<2,000	5.7	3.6	1.5	6	4	Morehead (1972)
	>2,000	4.2	2.1		4	2	
Methicillin	<2,000	2.8	1.8	0.5	6	4	McCracken (1977);
	>2,000	2.2	1.1		4	2	Howard (1975)
Oxacillin	Premature	3	1.5	0.5	6	3	Axline (1967)
Tetracycline		15-18 (1 day)†	6-8 (1 mo-11 yr)†	6.9	2	—	Sereni (1965)
Sulfisoxazole		12.4	7.8	5	2	1.3	Krauer (1975)

*Adult data derived from Weinstein, L.: Chemotherapy of microbial disease: antimicrobial therapy. In Goodman, L., and Gilman, A., editors: The pharmacological basis of therapeutics, ed. 5, New York, 1975, Macmillan Publishing Co., Inc.
†Age at study.

Fig. 12-4. Interrelationships of absorption, distribution, biotransformation, and excretion of a drug and its concentration at the receptor site.

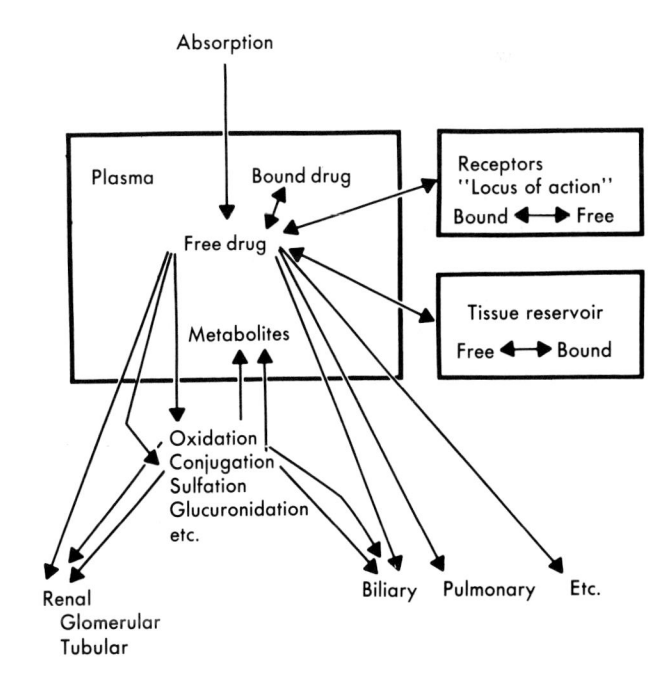

comprehensively defined as the net movement of a drug from the gastrointestinal lumen into the systemic circulation draining this organ. This process entails the movement of drugs across the gastrointestinal epithelium, which behaves as a semipermeable lipid membrane and constitutes the main barrier to absorption. The various processes operating to induce transepithelial membrane movement of drug molecules include (1) simple diffusion through lipid membranes or through aqueous pores of the membrane, (2) filtration through aqueous channels or membrane pores, and (3) carrier-mediated transport such as active transport or facilitated diffusion and vesicular transport such as pinocytosis. Of these, the most important is the process of simple diffusion, since most drugs administered orally are absorbed via this route. This is evident from the direct proportionality between the concentration of the drug in the intestine and the amount of drug absorbed over a wide range of concentrations. Moreover, one drug does not compete with another for transfer, indicating that the process of absorption is a simple, nonsaturatable one.

The rate and extent of drug absorption are partly determined by the physical and chemical characteristics of the drug. Polarity, nonlipid solubility, and large molecular size tend to decrease absorption. In contrast, nonpolarity, lipid solubility, and small molecular size increase absorption. The degree of ionization, determined by the pK_a of the drug and the pH of the solution in which it exists, is an important determinant in drug absorption. The gastrointestinal epithelium is more permeable to the nonionized form, since this portion is usually lipid soluble and favors absorption. The degree of drug ionization will change as the pH increases from the stomach through the distal portion of the gut. The slow gastric emptying time in the newborn may retard drug absorption and could be rate limiting. This is because the major absorption occurs in the proximal bowel, which has the greatest absorptive surface area. On the other hand, a slow transit time or slow intestinal motility may facilitate the absorption of some drugs.

These physiologic processes do, however, undergo substantial changes during the neonatal period. Gastric acid production is generally low at birth, and the gastric pH is usually 6 to 8, decreasing within a few hours to pH values of 3 to 1. Acid secretion is low in the first 10 days of life; it tends to rise thereafter and approaches adult values around 6 to 8 months. Intestinal motility is slow in the newborn, and transit time from the stomach to the cecum is generally prolonged relative to that in the adult. The gastric emptying time after milk feeding is considerably prolonged in the neonate and approaches adult values at ages 6 to 8 months. The precise influence of milk feeding on neonatal drug absorption has not been studied.

Drug absorption requires an intact splanchnic vascular circulation. In sick neonates, especially those with hypotension, perfusion of the gut may decrease to maintain adequate perfusion of vital organs, resulting in decreased drug absorption.

Current evidence indicates that the amount of absorption of most drugs is independent of age, although the rate of absorption of certain drugs shows a nonlinear correlation with age. Heimann studied the enteral absorption of various drugs (i.e., sulfonamides, phenobarbital, digoxin, methyldigoxin, D[−]xylose and L[−]arabinose) and found reduced absorption rates in neonates relative to older children. There is very little specific information concerning other drugs; however, available information indicates that gastrointestinal absorption of drugs is relatively slow in the newborn and undergoes maturational changes similar to those found in drug distribution, metabolism, and disposition. Although the neonatal drug absorptive deficit may influence the achievement of a desired pharmacologic effect, it is very likely that its significance is minor relative to the age-related alterations in drug distribution, metabolism, and disposition.

Protein binding of drugs in the newborn

The unbound drug in the plasma is considered to be the pharmacologically active fraction of the drug. For some drugs, including theophylline, phenytoin, phenobarbital, penicillin, and salicylates, the binding to plasma protein in the newborn is decreased compared to that in the nonpregnant adult. This suggests that a more intense pharmacologic response may be obtained in the newborn than in the adult for the same total drug concentration. The developmental changes in protein-drug binding and the postnatal age at which adultlike binding is achieved have not been defined with confidence. Some drugs, like phenytoin, may exhibit adultlike binding before the infant reaches 3 months.

The reasons underlying this deficient plasma protein binding of drugs at birth have not been definitely established. Possible explanations include decreased plasma albumin concentrations, possible qualitative differences in neonatal plasma proteins, and competitive binding by many endogenous substrates, such as hormones. Hyperbilirubinemia may accentuate this competition by displacing a drug, such as phenytoin, from its albumin-binding site. This contrasts to the well-known bilirubin drug-protein binding interaction, where drugs such as sulfonamides may displace bilirubin from its binding site.

Deficient plasma protein binding is not usually considered in calculating neonatal drug dosages. This factor must be considered in the application of adult therapeutic plasma concentrations to the neonatal patient. Moreover, decreased protein binding will influence calculations of apparent volumes of distribution based on plasma concentrations of total drug. In terms of therapeutic monitoring, drug concentrations obtained from saliva reflect the concentrations of the unbound fraction in plasma.

Drug metabolism and disposition in the newborn

Many drugs administered to the newborn infant need to undergo metabolism for efficient elimination from the body (Fig. 12-4). In the past decade, spurred by the chloramphenicol gray baby syndrome and the increased awareness of altered drug disposition in the newborn, the pharmacokinetic disposition and metabolism of some drugs have been studied in the neonate, and available data permit the following generalizations:
1. The rates of drug biotransformation and overall elimination are slow.
2. The rate of drug elimination from the body exhibits marked interpatient variability.
3. The maturational changes in drug metabolism and disposition as a function of postnatal age are extremely variable and depend on the substrate (or drug) being used.
4. Neonatal drug biotransformation and elimination are vulnerable to pathophysiologic states.
5. Neonates may exhibit activation of alternate biotransformation pathways.

The observation that drug elimination is slower in the neonate relative to adults is well recognized, although the magnitude and duration of this deficit as a function of specific drugs have not been adequately appreciated. Tables 12-4 and 12-5 shows the approximate prolongation of the plasma half-lives of certain drugs in the newborn relative to adults. Drugs that are closely related structurally, such as caffeine and theophylline, may even vary significantly. Thus application of dose rates for theophylline to caffeine in the treatment of neonatal apnea led to marked accumulation of caffeine in the blood. One apparent exception to this observed functional deficit is carbamazepine. Transplacentally acquired carbamazepine was eliminated in four of five infants in the immediate postnatal period as rapidly as in adults. In contrast,

Table 12-5. Comparative plasma half-lives of miscellaneous drugs in newborns and adults*

Drug	Plasma half-life (hours) Newborn	Plasma half-life (hours) Adult	Approximate prolongation†	References (first authors)
Analgesics-antipyretics				
Acetaminophen	2.2-5.0(3.5)	1.6-2.8(2.2)	1.5-2	Levy (1975)
Aminopyrine	30-40	2-4	11	Reinecke (1970)
Phenylbutazone	21-34	12-30	1-1.5	Gladtke (1968)
Indomethacin	(7.5-51)	2-11(6)	4	‡
Meperidine	22	3-4	5-6	Caldwell (1976)
Anesthetics				
Bupivacaine	25	1.3	19	Caldwell (1976)
Mepivacaine	8.7	3.2	2.5-3	Moore (1978)
Antiepileptics				
Phenytoin				
Premature	(75)	—	3	Loughnan (1977)
Term	21	11-29	—	Rane (1974)
Carbamazepine	8-28	21-36	—	Rane (1975)
Phenobarbital	82-199	24-140	1.5-2	Boreus (1978) Harvey (1980)
Other drugs				
Amobarbitol	17-60	12-27	2	Kramer (1973)
Caffeine	40-231 (100)	(6)	17	Aranda (1979)
Theophylline	14-57 (30)	(6)	5	Aranda (1976)
Tolbutamide	10-40 (30)	4.4-9 (7)	4	Nitowesky (1966)
Chloramphenicol	14-24	2.5	5-9	Hodgman (1961) Weiss (1960)
Salicylates	4.5-11.5	2.7	1.3-4.5	Levy (1975)
Digoxin				
Premature	90	31-40	2.5-1.3	Wettrell (1977)
Term	52	—	1.3	Wettrell (1977)

*Values are expressed as ranges or individual values. Numbers in parentheses indicate mean.
†Approximate prolongation calculated from the mean values if available.
‡Derived from several authors as compiled from Aranda, J.V., and others: Therapeutic Drug Monitoring **2**:39, 1980.

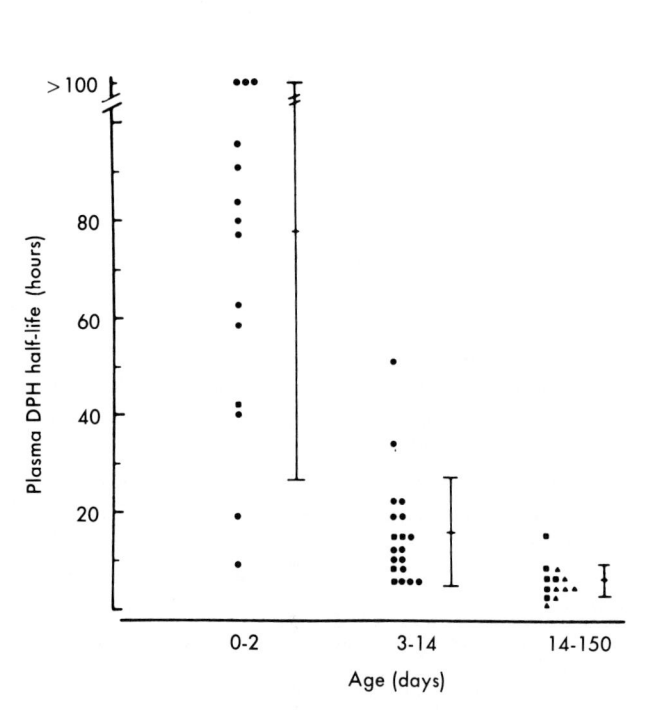

Fig. 12-5. Plasma phenytoin *(DPH)* half-lives measured in infants grouped according to postnatal age. Each infant received the drug via transplacental transfer (●) or as an initial therapeutic dose (■). Half-lives derived from steady-state plasma phenytoin as shown (▲). Bars indicate mean and standard deviations. Data were obtained from several published studies. (Reproduced, with permission, from Neims, A.H., and others: Annu. Rev. Pharmacol. Toxicol. **16**:427, 1976. © 1976 by Annual Reviews Inc.)

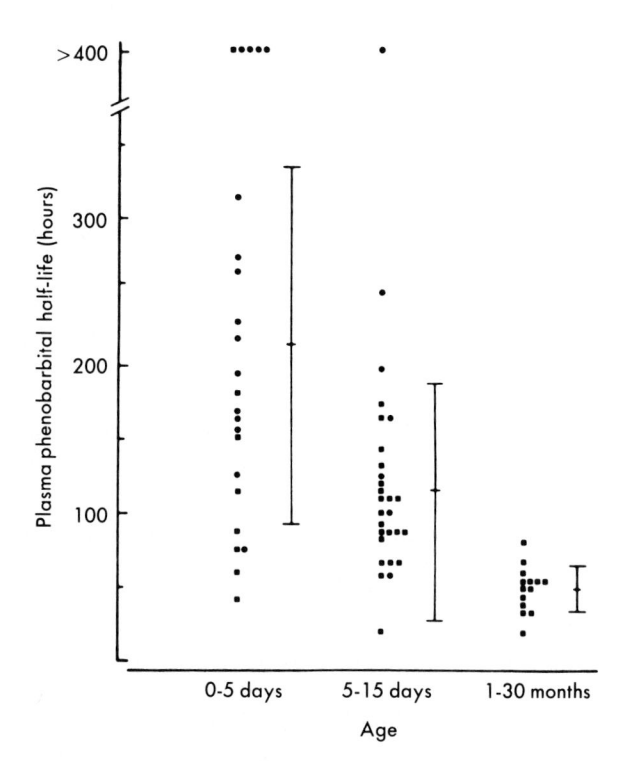

Fig. 12-6. Plasma half-lives of phenobarbital administered transplacentally (●) or postnatally (■) in infants, plotted as a function of postnatal age. Data were obtained from several published sources; means and standard deviation are shown. (Reproduced, with permission, from Neims, A.H., and others: Annu. Rev. Pharmacol. Toxicol. **16**:427, 1976. © 1976 by Annual Reviews Inc.)

some drugs, such as indomethacin, caffeine, and theophylline, are eliminated much more slowly.

One possible basis for this difference in oxidative biotransformation and elimination capability relates to the existence of multiple forms of cytochrome P_{450}, each with its own distinctive substrate specificity. The cytochrome P_{450} monooxygenases are hemoproteins localized at the smooth endoplasmic reticulum of the liver microsomes that catalyze many oxidative drug biotransformation processes by the liver. Data on the comparative measurements of the hemoprotein cytochrome P_{450} in the human fetal, neonatal, and adult liver do not, however, fully explain the observed deficiency in drug biotransformation and elimination. Drugs that undergo conjugation may exhibit characteristics similar to those of drugs requiring oxidative biotransformation for elimination. Glucuronidation is virtually absent in midgestational human fetal liver, and this deficit persists at birth, whereas sulfation is active in the neonate. Acetylation and other synthetic or conjugative reactions, such as those with glutathione, are likely to be somewhat deficient at birth.

The time after birth at which adult rates of elimination are achieved and the rates at which these maturational changes occur vary with the drug used. Rapid increases in rate of elimination during the first week postnatally have been observed with phenytoin and phenobarbital (Figs. 12-5 and 12-6). Large interindividual variability in plasma half-lives was observed at birth but rapidly diminished with increasing postnatal age. This means that some neonates receiving a standard recommended dose may exhibit subtherapeutic drug concentrations in the plasma, whereas others may exceed the upper limit of the presumed therapeutic range. In neonates given phenobarbital for seizures, repeated doses of 5 mg/kg/day yielded mean plasma concentrations of about 40 mg/L during the first week, whereas a lower dosage (2.5 to 5 mg/kg/day) yielded plasma concentrations below 15 mg/L by the second and third weeks. The rapidity at which these developmental changes occur would warrant monitoring of plasma concentrations, since dose rates for many drugs usually held constant during the neonatal period may result in poor or exaggerated clinical responses that may be partly attributed to plasma drug

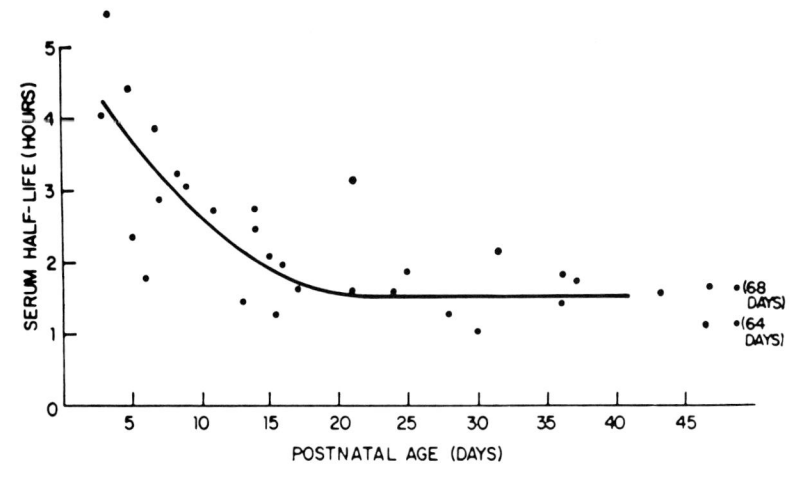

Fig. 12-7. Postnatal changes in the serum half-life of ampicillin. (From Axline, S.G., and others: Pediatrics **39**:97, 1967. Copyright American Academy of Pediatrics 1967.)

concentrations below or above the presumed therapeutic range. Adjustment of dosage based on plasma concentrations of the drug and accounting for a rapid postnatal increase in drug clearance may result in maintenance of plasma concentrations of phenobarbital within the suggested therapeutic range (15 to 25 mg/L). In contrast, caffeine exhibits negligible maturational changes in the neonatal period. Adult rates of elimination are achieved at about 3 to 4 months and may be exceeded thereafter.

The need to eliminate xenobiotic compounds from the body in the face of decreased oxidative and conjugative pathways in the fetus and neonate may lead to activation and/or use of available biotransformation pathways. For example, premature neonates given theophylline may produce caffeine via methylation pathways, which are active as early as the first trimester, as shown in human hepatic organ culture studies. Since minimum oxidative function is present at this stage of gestation, the relative increase in activity of the methylase pathway leads to the production of caffeine as one of the major metabolites of theophylline in the human fetus and newborn. Both caffeine and theophylline exhibit similar pharmacologic activity but of variable specific potency; therefore interpretation of clinical effect must account for both methylxanthines.

Disease states (e.g., congestive heart failure, liver disease) are well recognized in adults as factors that alter drug elimination. The presence of pathophysiologic states (e.g., hypoxia, asphyxia) in neonates can further diminish a deficient drug elimination capability, thus allowing the accumulation of drug in the plasma. For example, neonates with seizures who experienced perinatal asphyxia may have higher steady-state plasma concentrations of phenobarbital than those without asphyxia.

The dynamicity and variability in neonatal drug disposition and metabolism make generalization of dosage schedules and application of data obtained from one drug to another extremely difficult if not dangerous. Available data further reinforce the need for acquisition of specific pharmacologic data for each drug used in the neonatal period.

Renal excretion of drugs

The kidneys are the most important organs for drug elimination in the newborn, since the most commonly used drugs, such as antimicrobial agents, are excreted via these organs. Renal elimination of these drugs reflects and is dependent on neonatal renal function characterized by low glomerular filtration rate, glomerular preponderance, nephron heterogenicity, low effective renal blood flow, and low tubular function compared to that in the adult (Chapter 31). Neonatal glomerular filtration rate is about 30% of the adult value and is greatly influenced by gestational age at birth. The most rapid changes occur during the first week of life, and these events are reflected by the plasma disappearance rates of aminoglycosides, which are eliminated mainly by glomerular filtration. These changes have been considered in the dosage regimen recommended by McCracken for these drugs and other antibiotics.

Effective renal blood flow may influence the rate at which drugs are presented to and eliminated by the kidneys. Effective renal blood flow as measured by para-aminohippurate (PAH) clearance is substantially lower in infants relative to adult values, even when PAH extraction values are correlated (i.e., PAH extraction is 60% in infants compared with greater than 92% in adults). Recent data suggest a low effective renal blood flow during the first 2 days of life (34 to 99 ml/minute/1.73 m^2), which increases to 54 to 166 ml/minute/1.73 m^2 by 14 to

21 days and further increases to adult values of about 600 ml/minute/1.73 m² by age 1 to 2 years.

The pharmacokinetic behavior of drugs eliminated via the neonatal kidneys exhibits characteristics similar to those underlying hepatic biotransformation. For instance, the half-life of many antimicrobials such as ampicillin (Fig. 12-7) shows marked interindividual variability at birth, which narrows somewhat with advancing age. The plasma half-life also shortens progressively after birth, achieving adult rates of elimination within 1 month postnatally. The drug-dependent variability in the elimination process may reflect, in part, the major renal mechanism of drug excretion. Those drugs which undergo substantial elimination via glomerular filtration (e.g., aminoglycosides) may be excreted more rapidly than those requiring substantial tubular excretion (e.g., penicillins). These differences may reflect neonatal glomerular preponderance.

As with hepatic metabolism, renal excretion of certain drugs may be as efficient as in adults. For example, colistin, an antibiotic, is eliminated by neonates at rates similar to those in adults. However, as a rule, drug excretion via the neonatal kidneys is deficient relative to that in the adult. Pathophysiologic insults further compromise the inherent deficiency in drug elimination, thus complicating individual drug dosage regimens. Moreover, very small infants who receive the greatest number of drugs in the neonatal population exhibit the worst functional deficiency in drug elimination. This could result in overdosage, as in the case of digoxin. Neonates weighing less than 1,000 gm achieved steady-state plasma concentrations of digoxin three times higher than their full-term counterparts. Hypoxemia further decreases the slow glomerular and tubular function in the neonates, thus leading to slower renal excretion of drugs, as has been shown with amikacin. A linear relationship between oxygen tension and hepatic oxidation has been reported, so drugs that require hepatic biotransformation or renal excretion may be excreted much more slowly in the phase of hypoxemia. Determinations of plasma concentration of drugs, coupled with appropriate caution and clinical awareness, will help in optimum and safe drug therapy in the neonate.

PHARMACOKINETIC CONSIDERATIONS, DOSAGE GUIDELINES, AND THERAPEUTIC MONITORING IN NEONATAL DRUG THERAPY

Knowledge of the kinetic profile of a drug allows manipulation of the dosage to achieve and maintain a given plasma concentration. Many drugs administered in the newborn period exhibit a plasma disappearance curve (Fig. 12-8). In this example the log of the plasma concentration decreases linearly as a function of time with a brief but fast distributive (α) phase and a slower elimination (β) phase. This exemplifies a two-compartment model and first-order kinetics, that is, a certain fraction (not amount) of the drug remaining in the body is eliminated with time, and after the distribution phase, the plasma concentration reflects or is proportional to the concentration of drug in other portions of the body. This model is applicable to a wide variety of drugs used in the neonatal period, although some drugs (e.g., gentamicin,

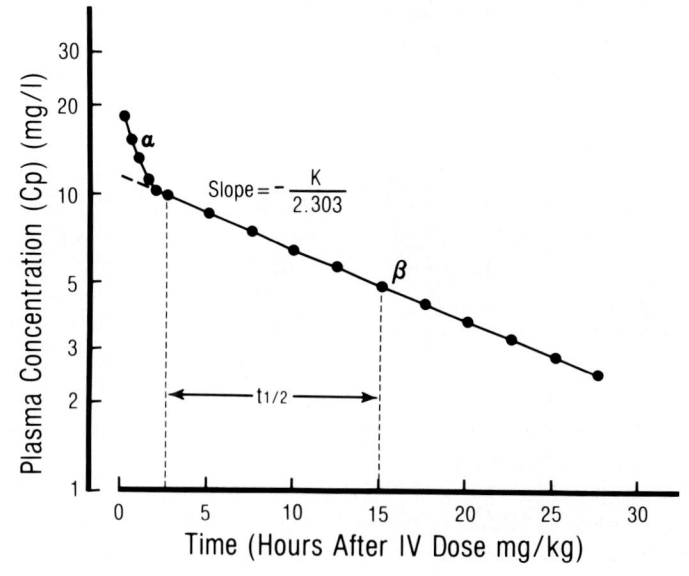

Fig. 12-8. Representative plasma disappearance curve of a drug given intravenously, plotted semilogarithmically as a function of time. A fast distribution phase (α) is followed by a slower elimination phase (β).

about 0.005 mg/kg/day. Nonetheless, there are no known harmful effects to the infant from the ingestion of human milk contaminated to this degree.

Many other pesticides have been found in human milk, and this reflects the current commercial use in the region or country. *Dieldrin*, for instance, which was banned in the United States after 1974, is decreasing in concentration in breast milk.

Industrial by-products

The extremely toxic dioxin *TCDD* (2,3,7,8-tetrachlorodibenzo-*p*-dioxin) caused environmental contamination in Seveso, Italy, in 1976. Children who were directly exposed developed chloracne; further effects remain to be determined. This toxin has been found in human milk.

There has been great public interest in the *polychlorinated biphenyls* (PCBs). This class of compounds has had 50 years of industrial usage, primarily in the manufacture of electrical apparatus (transformers, capacitors), although such usage seems to be declining. Because of contamination of rivers and lakes by industrial effluent, PCBs are widely distributed in fresh-water fish and in those animals which eat them. Like organic pesticides, PCBs remain in body fat stores and are excreted with the fat of breast milk. An epidemic of poisoning by PCBs (Yusho disease) occurred in 1968 in Japan, when a commercial rice oil product was inadvertently contaminated with PCBs. Fetuses exposed in utero suffered growth retardation both antenatally and postnatally. Several infants whose only exposure was via human milk developed weakness and apathy. It is of great concern that milk levels of PCBs in North America appear to be increasing. In Canada in 1979, the average PCB level in human milk was 12 ng/gm, whereas women who are exposed occupationally to PCBs or who consume game fish from contaminated waters may have much higher levels in milk.

The *polybrominated biphenyls (PBBs)* were brought to attention by an incident in Michigan in 1973 and 1974, in which several hundred pounds of PBBs, normally used as fire retardants in the plastics industry, accidently contaminated cattle feed; widespread intoxication of farm animals resulted. PBBs have the usual propensity to lodge in fat tissue and to persist in the body. To date, no ill effects have been noted in infants exposed to PBBs through their mother's milk. In Michigan, breast milk PBB surveillance has provided an accurate picture of the contamination of the general population. This method of epidemiologic analysis for fat-soluble poisons has much to recommend it, since the collection of milk samples is far easier than the collection of adipose tissue specimens. Breast milk PBB levels in the contaminated areas of Michigan averaged 0.07 parts per million.

Conclusion

Like the helpless fetus in utero, the nursing infant is exposed to nearly everything entering the body of its mother. The dangers, especially over the long term, are quite unclear. Environmental pollutants are almost impossible to avoid, and elimination of nontherapeutic (recreational) compounds involves changing life-styles. Drug administration is the easiest to control, yet often a difficult choice must be made between maternal therapy and potential infant harm. The following are some simple guides to be observed:

1. A lactating woman should not receive a drug that one would be reluctant to give directly to her infant at that particular postnatal or gestational age.
2. Drug secretion into milk is so variable that one should not attempt to *treat* an infant by administering the drug to the lactating mother.
3. Milk that is donated to milk banks must be free from contamination.
4. When maternal drug administration is necessary, one may attempt to minimize the dosage to the infant by withholding nursing at the time of maximum secretion of the drug into milk.
5. Signs and symptoms in a nursing child should be correlated with drug ingestion by the mother. In investigation it is perhaps most useful to measure levels of the drug and its metabolites in the infant's body fluids, rather than at isolated times in maternal blood or milk.

Jacob V. Aranda
Barbara F. Hales
Judith Gibbs

BIBLIOGRAPHY
Drugs and the fetus

Anon: Occupational disease among operating room personnel: a rational study, Anesthesiology **41**:321, 1974.

Barnes, A.B., and others: Fertility and outcome of pregnancy in women exposed in utero to diethylstilbestrol, N. Engl. J. Med. **302**:609, 1980.

Bernhardt, I.B. and Dorsey, D.J.: Hypervitaminosis A and congenital renal anomalies in a human infant, Obstet. Gynecol. **43**:750, 1974.

Bethenod, M., and Frederich, A.: Les enfants des antiepileptiques, Pediatrie **30**:227, 1975.

Bleyer, W.A., and others: Studies on the detection of adverse drug reactions in the newborn. I. Fetal exposure to maternal medication, J.A.M.A. **213**:2046, 1970.

Bongiovanni, A.M., and McPadden, A.J.: Steroids during pregnancy and possible fetal consequences, Fertil. Steril. **11**:181, 1960.

Braun, A.G., Emerson, D.J., and Nichinson, B.B.: Teratogenic drugs inhibit tumour cell attachment to lectin-coated surfaces, Nature **282**:507, 1979.

Butler, N.R., and Goldstein, H.: Smoking in pregnancy and subsequent child development, Br. Med. J. **4**:573, 1973.

Chung, L.W.K., and others: Perinatal toxicology: the question of delayed and residual effects. In Sellers, E.M., editorial: Pharmacology of psychoactive drugs, Toronto, 1975, Alcohol and Addiction Foundation.

Clarren, S.K., and Smith, D.W.: The fetal alcohol syndrome, N. Engl. J. Med. **298**:1063, 1978.

Cohlan, S.Q.: Tetracycline staining of teeth, Teratology **15**:127, 1977.

partum, ensuring that lactation is already well established, and to use the lowest dosage possible. The infants should be followed with some care, since there have been reports of gynecomastia and changes in vaginal epithelium. A study of late effects in exposed infants is urgently needed.

Other drugs

Cimetidine, a histamine-H_2-receptor antagonist, has been reported in breast milk in concentrations three to twelve times greater than in maternal blood; this drug may be actively transported into milk. Until there is more information concerning its effects in infants, cimetidine should not be used during lactation. *Theobromine* from chocolate has been found in milk at a level of 80% of maternal serum. *Theophylline* ingestion by the mother has been associated with infant irritability. Extracts of *ergot* have been responsible for toxic reactions in nursing infants and should be avoided. The use of *isotopes* for diagnosis or therapy should be avoided during lactation. An acceptable level of an isotope in milk is not known. It has been suggested that women not nurse for 10 days after exposure to ^{131}I, for 3 days after ^{99m}Tc exposure, and for 2 weeks following ^{67}Ga exposure.

"Nontherapeutic" agents in human milk
Caffeine

One hour after the ingestion of an average cup of coffee, a peak milk caffeine level of about 1.5 μg/ml is obtained. Caffeine levels in milk are about half the corresponding maternal blood level. Although the daily amount of caffeine consumed by a nursing infant might be small, the long half-life of caffeine could cause symptoms such as wakefulness or jitteriness.

Ingredients of cigarettes

The *nicotine* content of breast milk from women smoking one pack per day has been found to be about 100 to 500 parts per billion. No symptoms have been ascribed to this degree of contamination. *Thiocyanate*, which is elevated in the blood of smoking women, does not appear in elevated amounts in their milk.

Ethanol

Ethanol, a small molecule, diffuses freely into milk and achieves levels equivalent to those in blood. The metabolite acetaldehyde does not appear in milk. Excessive ethanol intake by the mother may depress the infant's central nervous system.

Narcotics

Heroin, methadone, morphine, and other opiate derivatives have been found in milk and may be responsible for both addiction and withdrawal symptoms in the nursing infant. Opiates used briefly appear to have little clinical effect. It has been suggested that women receiving methadone maintenance doses take their daily dose after the last breast-feeding in the evening, since milk methadone levels are found to peak about 4 hours after administration of the drug by mouth.

Environmental pollutants in human milk
Lead

Lead has been found in both bovine and human milk, as well as in commercial infant formulas. The lead content of human milk has remained rather constant over the past four decades, in contrast to levels of some other pollutants. One study found the lead level in human milk in the United States to be about 0.03 μg/ml. There are no reports of signs and symptoms of lead toxicity from this source.

Mercury

Metallic or inorganic mercury poisoning in adults has usually been in association with occupational exposure. There are no reports of metallic mercury poisoning from human milk. Organic mercury, more specifically *methylmercury*, has been used industrially in fungicides, in pulp and paper factories, and in chlor-alkali plants. In the late 1950s Minamata Bay in Japan was contaminated with industrial wastes containing methylmercury; the compound found its way into humans through contaminated fish. There was a high incidence of neurologic abnormalities in children born in this area, probably related to in utero exposure to the chemical rather than to exposure during lactation. Methylmercury was found in human milk in a concentration about 5% of that in blood; the half-life for disappearance of mercury from milk was estimated to be about 70 days.

Several epidemics in Iraq in the last 15 years were traceable to the contamination of grains with methylmercury fungicides. A number of nursing infants ingested enough methylmercury in milk to achieve blood levels above the toxic limit.

Pesticides

Organic pesticides are concentrated in body fat, and milk production, with its export of large quantities of lipid, is a very efficient way for the female to rid her body of these poisons. The nursing human infant thus becomes the highest animal in the "food chain." *DDT* was first identified in breast milk in 1951, and milk levels have been falling slowly since its use was restricted in North America in the early 1970s. Current levels of DDT in human milk vary geographically and are related to agricultural use of the compound. In Canada in 1979, average milk DDT was 44 ng/gm of human milk. A 5-kg infant ingesting 1 kg of breast milk each day would thus take in about 0.009 mg/kg/day. The FAO/WHO recommendations for maximum allowable intake by an adult is

of the drug's potential for displacement of bilirubin from serum albumin.

Compounds in human milk
Anticoagulants

Heparin does not enter breast milk. Oral anticoagulants of the *inandione* group as well as *bishydroxycoumarin* and ethyl *biscoumacetate* are found in milk and have been associated with infant coagulopathies. *Warfarin* must be considered the drug of choice, since by virtue of its acidity as well as its high degree of protein binding it is undetectable in human milk.

Antiinflammatory and analgesic drugs

Acetylsalicylic acid (ASA) appears to be without danger when used occasionally. Older infants have been found to receive about 0.2% to 0.3% of a single dose of ASA administered to the mother. Although detailed studies do not exist, *acetaminophen* seems to be safe.

Antimicrobial drugs

Fortunately, most antimicrobial agents in human milk appear safe for the nursing infant. Drugs of the *penicillin* group may change the infant's intestinal flora and cause diarrhea and thrush; in theory they could also incite hypersensitivity. The *cephalosporins* appear to be secreted in insignificant amounts in milk. The passage of the various *sulfonamide* derivatives is influenced by their differing degrees of ionization and protein binding; all of them have the potential to displace bilirubin from albumin. Ingestion of *salicylazosulfapyridine* leads to the appearance of the metabolite sulfapyridine in milk; it has been estimated that the infant of a mother chronically using this drug will receive about 0.3% of the maternal dose per day. *Erythromycin* is present in milk in higher concentration than in maternal plasma, suggesting that the infant could receive a significant dose. The *tetracyclines* in milk have the theoretical potential to cause dental staining. Most authors recommend that *chloramphenicol* not be taken by lactating women, even though the drug levels in milk do not lead to a dose as large as those associated with the "gray baby" syndrome. The *aminoglycosides* are poorly absorbed from the infant's gastrointestinal tract. *Isoniazid* and *PAS* have not been associated with ill effects to the nursing infant. *Metronidazole* remains contraindicated until it has been proved definitely noncarcinogenic to humans.

Drugs affecting the cardiovascular system

The amount of *digoxin* present in milk depends on the maternal dose; infants whose mothers received 0.25 mg per day did not ingest enough digoxin in milk to have detectable blood levels. *Diuretics* in general seem to be harmless, although if a nursing woman were to become dehydrated because of diuretic use, lactation would be greatly depressed. The effects of diuretics on milk composition are unclear. *Spironolactone* and its less active metabolite are secreted in milk, and an estimated 0.2% of the mother's daily dose is received by the infant. *Chlorthalidone* appears in small amounts in milk but could potentially accumulate in the young infant. *Propranolol* seems to be safe. *Quinidine* is secreted in milk to a concentration about 60% that of maternal blood, but no ill effects have been observed.

Drugs affecting the central nervous system

Diazepam is converted in the body to an active metabolite, desmethyldiazepam, and both are excreted in milk. Both these compounds have a prolonged half-life in infants, and chronic use of diazepam by nursing women has been associated with lethargy and weight loss in their babies. The *barbiturates* appear in milk in concentrations that depend on their different degrees of ionization and lipid solubility. In anticonvulsant doses they seem to be safe. *Chlordiazepoxide* in breast milk has been linked to depression in the nursing infant. *Meprobamate* should probably be avoided, since the drug achieves milk concentrations several times greater than the maternal plasma levels.

Lithium is definitely contraindicated during lactation, since it has been found to cause significant cardiovascular and CNS signs in the infant. The *phenothiazines* and *tricyclic antidepressants* have been found in breast milk but appear to be safe in modest doses. The *amphetamines* also appear in milk and may cause jitteriness.

Phenytoin is found in milk in concentrations about one-fifth those of maternal blood. *Primidone* and *ethosuximide* both achieve milk levels near that of maternal blood, although significant symptoms in the infants have not been noted.

Drugs affecting the endocrine system

Drugs of the *thiouracil* family, *methimazole*, *carbimazole*, and *iodides*, are contraindicated during breast-feeding; they achieve a high milk concentration and can suppress the infant's thyroid. On the other hand, *thyroxin* and other thyroid hormone preparations seem to be safe; endogenous thyroid hormone naturally secreted in breast milk may mask congenital cretinism during breast-feeding. The long-term effects of exogenous *glucocorticoids* and their derivatives in milk are not known. Women receiving *prednisone* and *prednisolone* excrete very small amounts of these compounds in milk.

A common dilemma is the use of *oral contraceptives* during lactation. Little is known about the effects of long exposure to small doses of these compounds in milk. Contraceptives with a high concentration of estrogen and progestin will depress lactation, especially if they are begun soon after parturition. If their use is imperative, it would seem wise to start treatment about 4 weeks post

diazepam, digoxin) fit a multicompartmental model; others (e.g., ethanol) exhibit saturation kinetics, i.e., a certain amount (not fraction) of the drug is eliminated per unit time. In the newborn, where the elimination (or β) phase is extremely prolonged relative to the distribution (α) phase, the relative contribution of the distributive phase to overall elimination and to dosage computations may not be significant. Thus the entire body may behave kinetically as though it were a single compartment.

The administration of a loading dose (mg/kg) to achieve quickly a given plasma drug concentration depends on the rapidity with which the onset of drug action is required. For many drugs used in neonates loading doses would generally be greater, relative to older children or adult subjects. The prolonged half-life warrants a substantially lower maintenance dosage given at longer intervals to prevent toxicity or overdosage. The rapid postnatal changes in drug elimination require adjustment of maintenance dosage rates (mg/kg/day) with advancing postnatal age; this adjustment may also be a function of the drug being used. Monitoring of drug concentrations is extremely useful if the desired pharmacologic effect is not attained or if adverse reactions occur. Moreover, therapeutic drug monitoring seems prudent, especially for drugs with a narrow therapeutic index used during a period in which there is rapid change in drug elimination.

DRUGS AND LACTATION

Until recently, investigations of drugs and other compounds in breast milk were hampered by the very small numbers of lactating women studied and the insensitivity of drug assay methods. Much of the earlier literature concerns isolated case reports and a small selection of drugs. Several recent papers review these data. At the present time a higher incidence of breast-feeding provides a larger number of situations in which lactating women are exposed to various medications, and we can expect to see an increasing number of useful studies of these drugs in milk.

In addition to pharmaceuticals, environmental pollutants and nontherapeutic or "social" chemicals find their way into human milk. Public awareness of these problems is high, and the physician is often called on for counseling.

Passage of exogenous compounds from maternal blood to milk

The presence and concentration of compounds in human milk depend on molecular weight, degree of ionization, protein binding in blood, lipid solubility, and specific uptake by mammary tissue. Drugs that are not absorbed after oral ingestion will obviously not appear in milk.

Small compounds with molecular weight of less than about 200 appear freely in milk and are presumed to have passed through pores in the mammary alveolar cell. Large compounds such as insulin or heparin do not pass into milk. Intermediate-size compounds must penetrate the lipoprotein cell membrane by diffusion or active transport.

In general, drugs that are not ionized at blood pH will traverse the alveolar cell membrane with greater ease than will highly ionized compounds. Since milk pH is about 7 or slightly less, milk will act as a trap for weak bases.

Drugs pass the cell membrane only in their free form; thus highly protein-bound drugs are less available for passage. Drugs or other chemicals that are very lipid soluble readily cross the alveolar cell, and, since milk contains a considerable amount of lipid, these compounds are also trapped in milk.

Finally, certain compounds are actively taken up by mammary tissue and are found in milk in concentrations substantially higher than in blood.

Modifications of passage of compounds into milk

Drugs may be metabolized by the maternal body to active or inactive metabolites. These derivatives may then be secreted into milk less readily than is the parent compound. The timing of maternal ingestion of a drug in relation to the time of milk synthesis may influence the concentration of the drug in any particular milk feeding.

In animals, changes in mammary gland blood flow control the amount of drug presented to sites of uptake. Mammary tissue itself can metabolize certain compounds. Drugs already secreted into milk may be secreted back into the alveolar cell and thence into blood. Last, the stage of lactation plays a role; drugs may be secreted more easily in the colostral phase.

Delivery of compounds to, and disposition by, the infant

The total volume of milk consumed in a known period of time determines the dosage to the infant. Since daily volume intake of breast milk is exceedingly variable and impractical to routinely measure, one could assume a *high average* daily milk consumption to be about 1 L.

To produce an effect, the drug in the milk must either act locally in the gut or be absorbed. It is possible that the proteins of milk will bind certain drugs and thereby impede absorption; it is also possible that the bowel of a very young infant may permit absorption of normally excluded large molecules.

The infant's disposition of the drug in milk will change with postnatal age; in addition, one must always be aware

Diamond, I., Anderson, M.M., and McCreadie, S.R.: Transplacental transmission of busulfan (Myleran) in a mother with leukemia: production of fetal malformation and cytomegaly, Pediatrics 25:85, 1960.

Doering, P.L., and Stewart, R.B.: The extent and character of drug consumption during pregnancy, J.A.M.A. 239:843, 1978.

Dunn, H.G., and others: Maternal cigarette smoking during pregnancy and the child's subsequent development. II. Neurological and intellectual maturation to the age of 6½ years, Can. J. Public Health 68:43, 1977.

Ellenhorn, M.J.: The FDA and the prevention of drug embryopathy, J. New Drugs 4:12, 1964.

Ericson, A., Kallen, B., and Westerholm, P.: Cigarette smoking as an etiologic factor in cleft lip and palate, Am. J. Obstet. Gynecol. 135:348, 1979.

Eriksson, M., Catz, C.S., and Yaffe, S.J.: Drugs and pregnancy, Clin. Obstet. Gynecol. 16:199, 1973.

Fantel, A.G., and others: Teratogenic bioactivation of cyclophosphamide in utero, Life Sciences 25:67, 1979.

Fedrick, J., Alberman, E., and Goldstein, H.: Possible teratogenic effect of cigarette smoking, Nature 231:529, 1971.

Forsberg, J.G., and Jacobsohn, D.: The reproductive tract of males delivered by rats given cyproterone acetate from days 7 to 21 of pregnancy, J. Endocrinol. 44:461, 1969.

Fraser, F.C.: The multifactorial/threshold concept—uses and misuses, Teratology 14:267, 1976.

Garrett, M.J.: Teratogenic effects of combination chemotherapy, Ann. Intern. Med. 80:667, 1974.

Goldman, A.S., and Yaffe, S.J.: Fetal trimethadione syndrome, Teratology 17:103, 1978.

Greenberg, L.H., and Tanaka, K.R.: Congenital anomalies probably induced by cyclophosphamide, J.A.M.A. 188:423, 1964.

Hales, B.F.: Modification of the mutagenicity and teratogenicity of cyclophosphamide in rats with inducers of the cytochromes P-450, Teratology 24:1, 1981.

Hales, B.F., and Jaine, R.: Characteristics of the activation of cyclophosphamide to a mutagen by rat liver, Biochem. Pharmacol. 29:256, 1980.

Hales, B.F., and Neims, A.H.: Developmental aspects of glutathione S-transferase B (ligandin) in rat liver, Biochem. J. 160:231, 1976.

Hanson, J.W.: Fetal hydantoin syndrome, Teratology 13:185, 1976.

Hanson, J.W., and others: Risks to the offspring of women treated with hydantoin anticonvulsants, with emphasis on the fetal hydantoin syndrome, J. Pediatr. 89:662, 1976.

Hanson, J.W., Streissguth, A.P., and Smith, D.W.: The effects of moderate alcohol consumption during pregnancy on fetal growth and morphogenesis, J. Pediatr. 92:457, 1978.

Harada, M.: Congenital Minamata disease: intrauterine methylmercury poisoning, Teratology 18:285, 1978.

Heinonen, O.P., Slone, D., and Shapiro, S.: Birth defects and drugs in pregnancy, Littleton, Mass., 1977, Publishing Sciences Group, Inc.

Henderson, B.E., and others: Urogenital tract abnormalities in some of women treated with diethylstilbestrol, Pediatrics 58:505, 1976.

Herbst, A.L., and others: Prenatal exposure to stilbestrol: a prospective comparison of exposed female offspring with unexposed controls, N. Engl. J. Med. 292:334, 1975.

Hill, R.M., Desmond, M.M., and Kay, J.L.: Extrapyramidal dysfunction in an infant of a schizophrenic mother, J. Pediatr. 69:589, 1966.

Hunter, A.G.W., Thompson, D., and Evans, J.A.: Is there a fetal gasoline syndrome? Teratology 20:75, 1979.

Joffe, J.M.: Influence of drug exposure of the father on perinatal outcome, Clin. Perinatol. 6:21, 1979.

Jones, K.L., and others: Pattern of malformation in offspring of chronic alcoholic mothers, Lancet 1:7815, 1973.

Kline, J., and others: Smoking: a risk factor for spontaneous abortion, N. Engl. J. Med. 297:793, 1977.

Lamba, P.A., and Sood, N.N.: Congenital microphthalmus and colobomata in maternal vitamin A deficiency, J. Pediatr. Ophthalmol. 5:115, 1968.

Lambert, G.H., and Nebert, D.W.: Genetically mediated induction of drug-metabolizing enzymes associated with congenital defects in the mouse, Teratology 16:147, 1977.

Landauer, W.: Is insulin a teratogen? Teratology 5:129, 1972.

Landauer, W.: Antiteratogens as analytical tools. In Persaud, T.V.N., editor: Teratogenic mechanisms: advances in the study of birth defects, Baltimore, 1979, University Park Press.

Landesman-Dwyer, S., and Emanuel, I.: Smoking during pregnancy, Teratology 19:119, 1979.

Lenz, W.: Kindliche Missbildungen nach Medikamenteinnahme während der graviditat? Dtsch. Med. Wochenschr. 86:2555, 1961.

Levy, E.P., Cohen, A., and Fraser, F.C.: Hormone treatment during pregnancy and congenital heart defects, Lancet 1:611, 1973.

Manning, F.A., and Feyerabend, C.: Cigarette smoking and fetal breathing movements, Br. J. Obstet. Gynaecol. 83:262, 1976.

Manson, J.M., and Simons, R.: In vitro metabolism of cyclophosphamide in limb bud culture, Teratology 19:149, 1979.

Maren, T.H.: Teratology and carbonic anhydrase inhibition, Arch. Ophthalmol. 85:1, 1971.

Martz, F., Failinger, C., III, and Blake, D.A.: Phenytoin teratogenesis: correlation between embryopathic effect and covalent binding of putative arene oxide metabolite in gestational tissue, J. Pharmacol. Exp. Ther. 203:231, 1977.

McBride, W.G.: Thalidomide and congenital abnormalities, Lancet 2:1358, 1961.

McBride, W.G.: The teratogenic action of drugs, Med. J. Aust. 2:689, 1963.

Metzler, M., and McLachlan, J.A.: Oxidative metabolites of diethylstilbestrol in the fetal, neonatal, and adult mouse, Biochem. Pharmacol. 27:1087, 1978.

Milkovich, L., and van den Berg, B.J.: Effects of prenatal meprobamate and chlordiazepoxide hydrochloride on human embryonic and fetal development, N. Engl. J. Med. 291:1268, 1974.

Milkovich, L., and van den Berg, B.J.: An evaluation of the teratogenicity of certain antinauseant drugs, Am. J. Obstet. Gynecol. 125:244, 1976.

Milunsky, A., Graef, J.W., and Gaynor, M.F.: Methotrexate-induced congenital malformations, J. Pediatr. 72:790, 1968.

Monnet, P., Kalb, J.C., and Pujol, M.: Doit on craindre un influence teratogene eventuelle de l'isoniazide? Rev. Tuberc. (Paris) 31:845, 1967.

Mulvihill, J.J.: Caffeine as teratogen and mutagen, Teratology 8:69, 1973.

Naeye, R.L.: Relationship of cigarette smoking to congenital anomalies and perinatal death, Am. J. Pathol. 90:289, 1978.

Nelson, M.M., and Forfar, J.O.: Associations between drugs administered during pregnancy and congenital abnormalities of the fetus, Br. Med. J. 1:523, 1971.

Newcombe, R.G.: Cigarette smoking in pregnancy (letter), Br. Med. J. 2:755, 1976.

Nicholson, H.O.: Cytotoxic drugs in pregnancy, J. Obstet. Gynaec. Brit. Cowlt. 75:307, 1968.

Nishimura, H., and Nakai, K.: Congenital malformations in offspring of mice treated with caffeine, Proc. Soc. Exp. Biol. Med. 104:140, 1960.

Nora, J.J., and Nora, A.H.: Birth defects and oral contraceptives, Lancet 1:941, 1973.

Nora, J.J., and others: Maternal exposure to potential teratogens, J.A.M.A. 202:1065, 1967.

Nora, J.J., Nora, A.H., and Toews, W.H.: Lithium, Ebstein's anomaly, and other congenital heart defects, Lancet 2:594, 1974.

Oakes, G.K., and others: Effect of propranolol infusion in the umbilical and uterine circulations of pregnant sheep, Am. J. Obstet. Gynecol. 126:1038, 1976.

Oakley, G.P., and Flynt, J.W.: Increased prevalence of Down's syndrome (mongolism) among the offspring of women treated with ovulation-inducing agents, Teratology 5:264, 1972.

Ortiz-Perez, H.E., and others: Abnormalities among offspring of oral and non-oral contraceptive users, Am. J. Obstet. Gynecol. 134:512, 1979.

Paterson, D.C.: Congenital deformities associated with Bendectin, Can. Med. Assoc. J. 116:1348, 1977.

Peer, L.A., Bernhard, W.G., and Gordon, H.W.: Vitamin deficiency as a cause for birth deformities, Acad. Med. N.J. Bull. 10:140, 1964.

Phelan, J.P.: Diminished fetal reactivity with smoking, Am. J. Obstet. Gynecol. 136:230, 1980.

Piercy, W.N., and others: Alteration of ovine fetal respiratory-like activity by diazepam, caffeine and doxapram, Am. J. Obstet. Gynecol. 127:43, 1977.

Pilotti, G., and Scorta, A.: Hypervitaminosis A during pregnancy and neonatal malformations of the urinary apparatus, Minerva Ginecol. 17:1103, 1965.

Poland, A., and Glover, E.: 2,3,7,8-Tetrachlorodibenzo-p-dioxin: segregation of toxicity with the Ah locus, Mol. Pharmacol. 17:86, 1980.

Posner, H.S., and others: Experimental alteration of the metabolism of chlorcyclizine and the incidence of cleft palate in rats, J. Pharmacol. Exp. Ther. 155:494, 1967.

Pruyn, S.C., Phelan, J.P., and Buchanan, G.C.: Long-term propranolol therapy in pregnancy: maternal and fetal outcome, Am. J. Obstet. Gynecol. 135:485, 1979.

Renwick, J.H.: Spina bifida, anencephaly, and potato blight, Lancet 2:967, 1972.

Rhead, W.J.: Smoking and SIDS (letter), Pediatrics 59:791, 1977.

Richards, I.D.G.: A retrospective inquiry into possible teratogenic effects of drugs in pregnancy. In Klingberg, M.A., Abramovici, A., and Chemke, J., editors: Drugs and fetal development, New York, 1972, Plenum Press.

Rodriguez, S.O., Leikin, S.L., and Hiller, M.C.: Neonatal thrombocytopenia associated with ante-partum administration of thiazide drugs, N. Engl. J. Med. 270:881, 1964.

Rothman, K.J., and Louik, C.: Oral contraceptives and birth defects, N. Engl. J. Med. 299:522, 1978.

Rothstein, P., and Gould, J.B.: Born with a habit: infants of drug-addicted mothers, Pediatr. Clin. North Am. 21:307, 1974.

Rumeau-Rouquette, C., Goujard, J., and Huel, G.: Possible teratogenic effect of phenothiazines in human beings, Teratology 15:57, 1977.

Safra, M.J., and Oakley, G.P.: Association between cleft lip with or without cleft palate and prenatal exposure to diazepam, Lancet II:478, 1975.

Samojlik, E.: Effect of monoamine oxidase inhibition on fertility, fetuses, and reproductive organs of rats. I. Effect of monoamine oxidase inhibition on fertility, fetuses and sexual cycle, Endokrynol. Pol. 16:69, 1965.

Sarma, V.: Maternal vitamin deficiency and fetal microcephaly and anophthalmia, Obstet. Gynecol. 13:299, 1959.

Saxen, I., and Saxen, L.: Association between maternal intake of diazepam and oral clefts, Lancet II:498, 1975.

Schardein, J.L.: Drugs as teratogens, Cleveland, Ohio, 1976, CRC Press, Inc.

Scheinhorn, D.J., and Angelillo, V.A.: Antituberculous therapy during pregnancy, West. J. Med. 127:195, 1977.

Scott, J.R.: Fetal growth retardation associated with maternal administration of immunosuppressive drugs, Am. J. Obstet. Gynecol. 128:668, 1977.

Shapiro, S., and others: Antenatal exposure to doxylamine succinate and dicyclomine hydrochloride (Bendectin) in relation to congenital malformations, perinatal mortality rate, birth weight and intelligence quotient score, Am. J. Obstet. Gynecol. 128:480, 1977.

Shapiro, S., and others: Perinatal mortality and birth weight in relation to aspirin taken during pregnancy, Lancet 1:1375, 1976.

Short, R.D., and Gibson, J.E.: Development of cyclophosphamide activation and its implications in perinatal toxicity to mice, Toxicol. Appl. Pharmacol. 19:103, 1971.

Shottan, D., and Monie, I.W.: Possible teratogenic effect of chlorambucil on a human fetus, J.A.M.A. 186:180, 1963.

Sieber, S.M., and Adamson, R.H.: Toxicity of antineoplastic agents in man: chromosomal aberrations, antifertility effects, congenital malformations, and carcinogenic potential, Adv. Cancer Res. 22:57, 1975.

Smith, D.J., and Joffe, J.M.: Increased neonatal mortality in offspring of male rats treated with methadone or morphine before mating, Nature 253:202, 1975.

Smith, D.W.: Teratogenicity of anticonvulsive medications, Am. J. Dis. Child. 131:1337, 1977.

Smithells, R.W., and Sheppard, S.: Teratogenicity testing in humans: a method demonstrating safety of Bendectin, Teratology 17:31, 1978.

Sobel, D.E.: Fetal damage due to ECT, insulin coma, chlorpromazine, or reserpine, Arch. Gen. Psychiatry 2:606, 1960.

Soyka, L.F., Peterson, J.M., and Joffe, J.M.: Lethal and sublethal effects on the progeny of male rats treated with methadone, Toxicol. Appl. Pharmacol. 45:797, 1978.

Spiers, P.S., and others: Human potato consumption and neural-tube malformation, Teratology 10:125, 1974.

Terrila, L., and Vartieinen, E.: The effects and side-effects of diuretics in the prophylaxis and toxaemia of pregnancy, Acta Obstet. Gynecol. Scand. 50:351, 1971.

Turner, G., and Collins, E.: Fetal effects of regular salicylate ingestion in pregnancy, Lancet 2:338, 1975.

Ulfelder, H.: DES-Transplacental teratogen—and possibly also carcinogen, Teratology 13:101, 1976.

Underwood, P.B., and others: Parental smoking empirically related to pregnancy outcome, Obstet. Gynecol. 29:1, 1967.

Van Waes, A., and Van de Veldi, E.: Safety evaluation of haloperidol in the treatment of hyperemesis gravidarum, J. Clin. Pharmacol. 9:224, 1969.

Warkany, J.: Warfarin embryopathy, Teratology 14:205, 1976.

Warkany, J.: Antituberculosis drugs, Teratology 20:133, 1979.

Wilkins, L.: Masculinization of female fetus due to use of orally given progestins, J.A.M.A. 172:1028, 1960.

Wilson, J.G.: Teratogenic effects of environmental chemicals, Fed. Proc. 36:1698, 1977.

Yasuda, M., and Miller, J.R.: Prenatal exposure to oral contraceptives and transposition of the great vessels in man, Teratology 12:239, 1975.

Drug use, disposition, and metabolism in the newborn

Agunod, M., and others: Correlative study of hydrochoric acid, pepsin, and intrinsic secretion in newborns and infants, Am. J. Dig. Dis. 14:400, 1969.

Aranda, J.V., and Turmen, T.: Methylxanthines in apnea of prematurity, Clin. Perinatol. 6:87, 1979.

Aranda, J.V., and others: Pharmacokinetic aspects of theophylline in premature newborns, N. Engl. J. Med. 295:413, 1976.

Aranda, J.V., and others: Pharmacokinetic profile of caffeine in the premature newborn with apnea, J. Pediatr. 94:665, 1979.

Axline, S.G., and Simon, J.G.: Clinical pharmacology of antimicrobials in premature infants. I. Kanamycin, streptomycin and neomycin, Antimicrob. Agents Chemother. 135:141, 1964.

Axline, S.G., Yaffe, S.J., and Simon, H.J.: Clinical pharmacology of antimicrobials in premature infants. II. Ampicillin, methicillin, oxacillin, neomycin, and colistin, Pediatrics 39:97, 1967.

Bada, H.S., Khanna, N.N., Somani, S.M., et al.: Interconversion of theophylline and caffeine in newborn infants, J. Pediatr. 94:993, 1979.

Bodey, G., Valdiviero, M., Feld, R., et al.: Pharmacology of amikacin in humans, Antimicrob. Agents Chemother. 5:508, 1974.

Boreus, L.O., Jalling, B., and Walling, A.: Plasma concentrations of phenobarbital in mother and child after combined prenatal and postnatal administration for prophylaxis of hyperbilirubinemia, J. Pediatr. 93:695, 1978.

Bory, C., and others: Metabolism of theophylline to caffeine in the premature newborn infant, J. Pediatr. 94:988, 1979.

Braude, A.I.: Antimicrobial drug therapy. In Smith, L.H., Jr., editor: Major problems in internal medicine, vol. 8, Philadelphia, 1976, W.B. Saunders Co.

Caldwell, J., and others: Pharmacokinetics of bupivacaine administered epidurally during childbirth, Br. J. Clin. Pharmacol. 3:956P, 1976.

Caldwell, J., and others: Maternal and neonatal disposition of pethidine in childbirth—a study using quantitating gas chromatography mass spectrometry, Life Sci. 22:589, 1978.

Cumming, J.F., and Manngering, G.J.: Effect of phenobarbital administration on the oxygen requirement for hexobarbital metabolism in the isolated perfused rat liver and in the intact rat, Biochem. Pharmacol. 19:973, 1970.

Dauber, I.M., and others: Renal failure following perinatal anoxia, J. Pediatr. 88:851, 1976.

Ehrnebo, M., and others: Age differences in drug binding by plasma proteins: studies on human fetuses, neonates, and adults, Eur. J. Clin. Pharmacol. 3:189, 1971.

Eickhoff, T.C., Kislak, J.W., and Finland, M.: Sodium ampicillin—absorption and secretion of intramuscular and intravenous doses in normal young men, Am. J. Med. Sci. 249:163, 1965.

Faucett, D.W.: Surface specialization of absorbing cells, J. Histochem. Cytochem. 13:75, 1965.

Gladtke, E.: Pharmacokinetic studies on phenylbutazone in children, Farmaco. (Sci.) 23:897, 1968.

Grossman, M., and Tichnor, W.: Serum levels of ampicillin, cephalothin, cloxacillin, and nafcillin in the newborn infant, Antimicrob. Agents Chemother. 5:214, 1965.

Guignard, J.P., and others: Glomerular filtration rate in the first three weeks of life, J. Pediatr. 87:268, 1975.

Guignard, J.P., and others: Renal function in respiratory distress syndrome, J. Pediatr. 88:845, 1976.

Harvey, S.C.: Hypnotics and sedatives. In Gilman, A.G., Goodman, L.S., Gilman, A. (eds.): The pharmacological basis of therapeutics, New York, MacMillan Publishing Co., Inc., p. 339.

Heimann, G.: Enteral absorption and bioavailability in children in relation to age, Eur. J. Clin. Pharmacol. 18:43, 1980.

Hodgman, J.E., and Burns, L.E.: Safe and effective chloramphenicol dosages for premature infants, Am. J. Dis. Child. 101:140, 1961.

Howard, J.B., and McCracken, G.H.: Pharmacologic evaluation of amikacin in neonates, Antimicrob. Agents Chemother. 8:86, 1975.

Howard, J.B., and McCracken, G.H.: Reappraisal of kanamycin usage in neonates, J. Pediatr. 86:949, 1975.

Jalling, B.: Plasma concentrations of phenobarbital in treatment of seizures in newborns, Acta Paediatr. Scand. 64:514, 1975.

Kaplan, J.M., and others: Clinical pharmacology of tobramycin in newborns, Am. J. Dis. Child. 125:656, 1973.

Krauer, B.: The development of diurnal variation in drug kinetics in the human infant. In Morselli, P.L., Garattini, S., and F. Sereni, editors: Basic and therapeutic aspects of perinatal pharmacology, New York, 1975, Raven Press.

Krauer, B., and others: Elimination kinetics of amobarbital in mothers and their newborn infants, Clin. Pharmacol. Ther. 14:442, 1973.

Levy, G., and others: Pharmacokinetics of acetaminophen in the human neonate: formation of acetaminophen glucuronide and sulfate in relation to plasma bilirubin concentration and D. glucaric acid excretion Pediatrics 55:818, 1975.

Loughnan, P.M., and others: Pharmacokinetic observations of phenytoin disposition in the newborn and young infant, Arch. Dis. Child. 52:302, 1977.

McCracken, G.H., West, N.R., and Horton, L.F.: Urinary excretion of gentamicin in the neonatal period, J. Infect. Dis. 123:257, 1971.

McCracken, G.H., Jr., and others: Clinical pharmacology of penicillin in newborn infants, J. Pediatr. 82:692, 1973.

McCracken, G.H., Jr., and Nelson, J.D.: Commentary: an appraisal of tobramycin usage in pediatrics, J. Pediatr. 88:314, 1976.

McCracken, G.H., Jr., and Nelson, J.D.: Antimicrobial therapy for newborns, Monogr. Neonatol. New York, 1977, Grune & Stratton, Inc.

Mirhig, N., Reeves, M.D., and Roberts, R.J.: Effects of hypoxia on amikacin pharmacokinetics, (Abstr.) Pediatr. Res. 10:192A, 1976.

Moore, R.G., and others: The pharmacokinetics and metabolism of the anilide local anesthetics in neonates. III. Mepivacaine. Eur. J. Clin. Pharmacol. 14:203, 1978.

Morehead, C.D., and others: Pharmacokinetics of carbenicillin in neonates of normal and low birth weights, Antimicrob. Agents Chemother. 2:267, 1972.

Morselli, P.L., and Ronel, V.: Placental transfer of pethidine and norpethedine and their pharmacokinetics in the newborn, Eur. J. Clin. Pharmacol. 18:25, 1980.

Morselli, P.L., and others: Diazepam elimination in premature and full term infants and children, J. Perinat. Med. 1:133, 1973.

Nakazawa, S., and others: Studies on cefazolin in the pediatric field, Chemotherapy 18:659, 1970.

Neims, A.H., and others: Developmental aspects of the hepatic cytochrome P450 monooxygenase system, Annu. Rev. Pharmacol. Toxicol. 16:427, 1976.

Nitowsky, H.M., Matz, L., and Berzofsky, J.A.: Studies on oxidative drug metabolism in the full term newborn infant, J. Pediatr. 69:1139, 1966.

Odell, G.B.: The dissociation of bilirubin from albumin and its clinical implications, J. Pediatr. 55:268, 1959.

Painter, M.J., and others: Phenobarbital and diphenylhydantoin levels in neonates with seizures, J. Pediatr. 92:315, 1978.

Pinsky, W.W., and others: Serum digoxin levels in premature infants, Pediatr. Res. 10:196A, 1976.

Rane, A., Bertillson, L., and Palmer, L.: Disposition of placentally transferred carbamazepine in the newborn, Eur. J. Clin. Pharmacol. 8:283, 1975.

Rane, A., and others: Plasma protein binding of diphenylhydantoin in normal and hyperbilirubinemic infants, J. Pediatr. 78:877, 1971.

Rane, A., and others: Plasma disappearance of transplacentally transferred diphenylhydantoin in the newborn studied by mass fragmentography, Clin. Pharmacol. Ther. 15:39, 1974.

Reineche, C., and others: Die Wirkung von phenylbutazon and phenobarbital auf die amidopyrin-elimination, die bilirubin-gisamtkonzentration im serum und einige Blutgerin-nungsfatoren bie neugeborenen kinderm, Pharmacol. Clin. 2:167, 1970.

Schanker, L.S., and others: Absorption of drug from the rat small intestine, J. Pharmacol. Exp. Ther. 123:81, 1958.

Schedl, H.D., and Clifton, J.A.: Small intestinal absorption of steroids, Gastroenterol. 41:491, 1961.

Seigel, S.R., and Oh, W.: Renal function as a marker of human fetal maturation, Acta Paediatr. Scand. 65:481, 1976.

Sereni, F., and Principi, N.: Developmental pharmacology, Annu. Rev. Pharmacol. Toxicol. 8:453, 1968.

Sereni, F., and others: Tissue distribution and urinary excretion of a tetracycline derivative in newborn and older infants, J. Pediatr. 67:299, 1965.

Sertel, H., and Scopes, J.: Rates of creatinine clearance in babies less than one week of age, Arch. Dis. Child. 48:717, 1973.

Sjoqvist, F., and others: Plasma disappearance of nortriptyline in a newborn infant following placental transfer from an intoxicated mother: evidence for drug metabolism, J. Pediatr. 80:495, 1972.

Weinstein, L.: Chemotherapy of microbial diseases: antimicrobial therapy. In Goodman, L., and Gilman, A., editors: Pharmacologic basis of therapeutics, ed. 5, New York, 1975, Macmillan Publishing Co., Inc.

Weiss, C.F., Glazko, A.J., and Weston, J.K.: Chloramphenicol in the newborn infant: a physiologic explanation of its toxicity when given in excessive doses, N. Engl. J. Med. 262:787, 1960.

Welbrandt, W., and Rosenberg, T.: The concept of carrier transport and its corollaries in pharmacology, Pharmacol. Rev. 13:109, 1961.

Wettrel, G., and Anderson, K.W.: Clinical pharmacokinetics of digoxin in infants, Clin. Pharmacokinet. 2:17, 1977.

Drugs and lactation

Ananth, J.: Side effects in neonates from psychotropic agents excreted through breast-feeding, Am. J. Psychiatry 135:801, 1978.

Anderson, P.O.: Drugs and breast-feeding, Semin. Perinatol. 3:271, 1979.

Bagnell, P.C., and Ellenberger, H.A.: Obstructive jaundice due to a chlorinated hydrocarbon in breast milk, Can. Med. Assoc. J. 117:1047, 1977.

Berlin, C.M., and Yaffe, S.J.: Disposition of salicylazosulfapyridine (Azulfidine) and metabolites in human breast milk, Dev. Pharmacol. Ther. 1:31, 1980.

Binkiewica, A., Robinson, M.J., and Senior, B.: Pseudo-Cushing syndrome caused by alcohol in breast milk, J. Pediatr. 93:965, 1978.

Brilliant, L.B., and others: Breast-milk monitoring to measure Michigan's contamination with polybrominated biphenyls, Lancet 2:643, 1978.

Chan, V., Tse, T.F., and Wong, V.: Transfer of digoxin across the placenta and into breast milk, Br. J. Obstet. Gynaecol. 85:605, 1978.

DeSwiet, M., and Lewis, P.J.: Excretion of anticoagulants in human milk, N. Engl. J. Med. 297:1471, 1977.

Dickey, R.P.: Drugs affecting lactation, Semin. Perinatol. 3:279, 1979.

Dickinson, R.G., and others: Transmission of valproic acid (Depakene) across the placenta: half-life of the drug in mother and baby, J. Pediatr. 94:832, 1979.

Eeg-Olofsson, O., and others: Convulsions in a breast-fed infant after maternal indomethacin, Lancet 2:215, 1978.

Erickson, S.H., and Oppenheim, G.L.: Aspirin in breast milk, J. Fam. Prac. 8:189, 1979.

Erickson, S.H., Smith, G.H., and Heidrich, F.: Tricyclics and breast feeding, Am. J. Psychiatry 136:1483, 1979.

Erkkola, R., and others: Excretion of methylergometrine (methylergonovine) into the human breast milk, Int. J. Clin. Pharmacol. 16:579, 1978.

Finely, J.P., and others: Digoxin excretion in human milk, J. Pediatr. 94:339, 1979.

Fumita, M., and Takabatake, E.: Mercury levels in human maternal and neonatal blood, hair and milk, Bull. Environ. Contam. Toxicol. 18:205, 1977.

Gelenberg, A.J.: Amoxapine, a new antidepressant, appears in human milk, J. Nerv. Ment. Dis. 167:635, 1979.

Ghodse, A.H., Reed, J.L., and Mack, J.W.: The effect of maternal narcotic addiction on the newborn infant, Psychol. Med. 7:667, 1977.

Giacoia, G.P., and Catz, C.S.: Drugs and pollutants in breast milk, Clin. Perinatol. 6:181, 1979.

Hill, L.M., and Malkasian, G.D.: The use of quinidine sulfate throughout pregnancy, Obstet. Gynecol. 54:366, 1979.

Jonsson, V., and others: Chlorohydrocarbon pesticide residues in human milk in Greater St. Louis, Missouri, 1977, Am. J. Clin. Nutr. 30:1106, 1977.

Kaneko, S., Sato, T., and Suzuki, K.: The levels of anticonvulsants in breast milk, Br. J. Clin. Pharmacol. 7:624, 1979.

Karim, A.: Spironolactone: disposition, metabolism, pharmacodynamics, and bioavailability, Drug Metab. Rev. 8:151, 1978.

Karpow, S., Gotz, V., and Lauper, R.D.: Cimetidine, J.A.M.A. 239:402, 1978.

Koup, J.R., Rose, J.Q., and Cohen, M.E.: Ethosuximide pharmacokinetics in a pregnant patient and new newborn, Epilepsia 19:535, 1978.

Kuwabara, K., and others: Levels of polychlorinated biphenyls in blood of breast-fed children whose mothers are non-occupationally exposed to PCB's, Bull. Environ. Contam. Toxicol. 21:458, 1979.

Lawrence, R.A.: Breast-feeding: a guide for the medical profession, St. Louis, 1980, The C.V. Mosby Co.

Levy, M., Granit, L., and Lanfer, N.: Excretion of drugs in human milk, N. Engl. J. Med. 297:789, 1977.

Loughnan, P.M.: Digoxin excreted in human breast milk, J. Pediatr. 22:1010, 1979.

Mandelli, M., Tognoni, G., and Garattini, S.: Clinical pharmacokinetics of diazepam, Clin. Pharmacokinet. 3:72, 1978.

Meberg, A., and others: Smoking during pregnancy: effects on the fetus and on thiocyanate levels in mother and baby, Acta Paediatr. Scand. 68:547, 1979.

Mes, J., and Davids, D.J.: Presence of polychlorinated biphenyl and organochlorine pesticide residues and the absence of polychlorinated terphenyls in Canadian human milk samples, Bull. Environ. Contam. Toxicol. 21:381, 1979.

Mischler, T.W., and others: Cephradine and epicillin in body fluids of lactating and pregnant women, J. Reprod. Med. 21:130, 1978.

Mulley, B.A., and others: Placental transfer of chlorthalidone and its elimination in maternal milk, Eur. J. Clin. Pharmacol. 13:329, 1978.

Niebyl, J.R., and others: Carbamazepine levels in pregnancy and lactation, Obstet. Gynecol. 53:139, 1979.

Nilsson, S., Nygren, K., and Johansson, E.D.B.: d-Norgestrel concentrations in maternal plasma, milk, and child plasma during administration of oral contraceptives to nursing women, Am. J. Gynecol. Obstet. 129:178, 1977.

Nilsson, S., Nygren, K., and Johansson, E.D.B.: Transfer of estradiol to human milk, Am. J. Obstet. Gynecol. 132:653, 1978.

Olszyna-Marzys, A.E.: Contaminants in human milk, Acta Paediatr. Scand. 67:571, 1978.

Orme, M.L., and others: May mothers given warfarin breast-feed their infants? Br. Med. J. 1:1564, 1977.

Pagliaro, L.A., and Levin, R.H., editors: Problems in pediatric drug therapy, Hamilton, Ill., 1979, Drug Intelligence Publications.

Phelps, D.L., and Karim, A.: Spironolactone: relationship between concentrations of dethioacetylated metabolite in human serum and milk, J. Pharm. Sci. 66:1203, 1977.

Pynnonen, S., and others: Carbamazepine: placental transport, tissue concentrations in fetus and newborn, and level in milk, Acta Pharmacol. Toxicol. 41:244, 1977.

Resman, B.H., Blumenthal, H.P., and Jusko, W.J.: Breast milk distribution of theobromine from chocolate, J. Pediatr. 91:477, 1977.

Somogyi, A., and Gugler, R.: Cimetidine excretion into breast milk, Br. J. Clin. Pharmacol. 7:627, 1979.

Sovner, R., and Orsulak, P.J.: Excretion of imipramine and desipramine in human breast milk, Am. J. Psychiatry 136:451, 1979.

Tyrala, E.E., and Dodson, W.E.: Caffeine secretion into breast milk, Arch. Dis. Child. **54:**787, 1979.

Update: drugs in breast milk, Med. Lett. Drugs Ther. **21:**21, 1979.

Vuori, E., and others: The occurrence and origin of DDT in human milk, Acta Paediatr. Scand. **66:**761, 1977.

Wiles, D.H., Orr, M.W., and Kolakowska, T.: Chlorpromazine levels in plasma and milk of nursing mothers, Br. J. Clin. Pharmacol. **5:**272, 1978.

Yoshida, S., and Nakamura, A.: Residual status after parturition of methylsulfone metabolites of polychlorinated biphenyls in the breast milk of a former employee in a capacitor factory, Bull. Environ. Contam. Toxicol. **21:**111, 1979.

Yoshioka, H., and others: Transfer of cefazolin into human milk, J. Pediatr. **94:**151, 1979.

CHAPTER 13 Anesthesia for labor and delivery

A reduction in perinatal mortality and morbidity is in part dependent on the quality of obstetric anesthesia and analgesia. These procedures require close, continuing cooperation between obstetrician, anesthesiologist, and neonatalogist. Various methods of pain relief that do not interfere with the first and second stages of labor will be covered in this chapter.

ANALGESIA FOR NORMAL LABOR AND DELIVERY

The first stage of labor begins with the onset of progressive dilatation and effacement of the cervix. For the most part, patients need minimal analgesia in the early first stage of labor. Poorly prepared, anxious patients may benefit from the use of a mild tranquilizing agent to offset anxiety; much of this anxiety can be prevented if the changes of pregnancy and the various facets of labor have been carefully explained to the patient in a detailed fashion. In general, systemic drugs used in the first stage of labor should be injected intravenously in small increments to minimize total drug exposure and to more effectively adjust the dose to counteract discomfort as cervical dilatation progresses. The most frequently used analgesic drugs are meperidine hydrochloride (Demerol) and alphaprodine (Nisentil); hydroxyzine hydrochloride (Atarax and Vistaril) or promethazine hydrochloride (Phenergan) is often administered as a tranquilizer. Meperidine has attained its prominence in obstetric analgesia by virtue of its relatively short duration of effect in the mother and relatively low CNS penetration in the fetus and neonate when compared with morphine. Nonetheless, neonatal depression can occur and appears to be related to the amount of unmetabolized meperidine that has been transferred from mother to fetus rather than to the presence of the active metabolite normeperidine, as had been previously suspected. Potential neonatal depression correlates best with the injection-delivery interval. Intervals of less than 1 hour are associated with essentially no ill effects. Neonatal depression occurs most often when meperidine is administered 2 to 3 hours before delivery. Alphaprodine is structurally similar to meperidine with a shorter duration of effect, although fewer pharmacologic data are available for this drug than for meperidine. Single-agent opiate therapy can provide good analgesia with the possibility of essentially complete pharmacologic reversibility (Chapter 14).

The paracervical block is also a very effective first-stage analgesic method, but it may have untoward effects on the fetus in high-risk pregnancies. Therefore it should be used sparingly in such patients. The segmental lumbar epidural block is another very useful technique that provides excellent first-stage analgesia combined with the possibility of later second-stage pain relief. It also minimizes the complications that formerly were associated with the larger volume sympathetic block. An alternative approach is the use of the lumbar epidural block for the first stage and the caudal epidural block for the second stage of labor. This difficult technique allows the physician to insert the epidural catheters when the patient is not so uncomfortable and to administer less medication subsequently, when the patient's discomfort demands pain relief.

Second-stage pain relief can also be managed with a low spinal block, often erroneously referred to as a "saddle block." A low spinal block consists of an initial injection of a small amount of either tetracaine hydrochloride (0.4 mg in a hyperbaric solution) or lidocaine (Xylocaine) (25 mg of a 5% solution), followed by positioning the patient to achieve an effect at a T10 upper level. In addition, inhalation analgesia with nitrous oxide–oxygen (50% concentration) or subanesthetic concentrations of halothane, enflurane, or isoflurane can be used to manage an otherwise extremely uncomfortable or uncooperative patient in the acute delivery phase. Psychoprophylaxis also may be effective in relieving the discomfort of the second stage; it takes a competent staff dedicated to the technique and a suitably motivated patient. Ideally, the combination of psychoprophylaxis for early labor and the lumbar epidural or the lumbar epidural/caudal epidural technique for added relief and comfort later is an optimum combination for management of the patient and protection of the fetus.

The premature infant is at an increased risk of central nervous system depression from obstetric anesthesia and analgesia. Therefore narcotic analgesics for discomfort in the first stage of labor should be severely restricted. Relief of pain during the first stage of labor can be effected by use of selective regional analgesia, while maternal and fetal homeostasis is maintained. Segmental lumbar epidural analgesia is recommended with a minimal amount of longer-lasting local anesthetic (bupivacaine hydrochloride [Marcaine], 8 ml of 0.25% solution) to reduce maternal and fetal drug accumulation. The technique of lumbar epidural analgesia for first-stage labor and caudal epidural analgesia for second-stage labor may also be used. The use of a paracervical block in labors with a premature fetus should be limited because of the hazard of inadvertently elevated fetal anesthetic drug levels due to fetal injection.

There are several alternative forms of analgesia for the second stage of labor in the case of premature labor. A subarachnoid block may be restricted to the sacral area by manipulating the patient's position and using a hyperbaric solution. A bilateral pudendal block or local infiltration may also be used for restricted perineal analgesia.

Psychoprophylaxis may be an important adjunct to the management of premature labor because of high maternal motivation. The combination of psychoprophylaxis for the early first stage of labor followed by segmental lumbar epidural analgesia alone or with the segmental caudal epidural analgesia may be optimal in premature labor.

ANESTHESIA FOR SPECIAL CIRCUMSTANCES
Diabetes and postmaturity

See pp. 23 to 25.

Maternal diabetes and fetal postmaturity present similar serious problems in regard to providing anesthesia in the face of a reduced uteroplacental reserve. The anesthesiologist should participate in the management of the patient from the beginning of hospitalization. Maternal hypotension, which may further reduce maternofetal placental exchange and thus precipitate an episode of intrapartum asphyxia, must be prevented. It is also advisable to prevent or minimize systemic depressants that easily cross the placenta and increase the hazard of birth asphyxia and later neonatal depression. The fetuses of diabetic mothers may be excessively large, thus causing problems in the mechanics of the first stage of labor. Therefore analgesia should not depress first-stage uterine contractility but should provide optimum conditions for an atraumatic application of forceps for facilitated vaginal delivery when forceps extraction is contemplated. Regional segmental lumbar epidural analgesia for the first and second stages or the use of caudal epidural analgesia in the second stage is effective. A subarachnoid block may also be used in the second stage with special attention being focused on preventing maternal hypotension caused by excessive spread of the block.

Toxemia

See p. 27.

Toxemic and chronic hypertensive patients merit special consideration, since the use of regional blockade in these patients may result in serious sequelae for both mother and fetus. Management of toxemic and chronic hypertensive patients must include a careful evaluation by the anesthesiologist. Special attention should be given to fluid balance, electrolyte stability, and urinary output. If the patient appears to have mild preeclampsia, preference should be given to a segmental epidural block with small increments of anesthetic. This technique is preferred in preeclampsia, not only because there is minimal effect on blood pressure after adequate fluid replacement, but also because it can be instituted with minimal agitation to the patient. Second-stage analgesia may be attained by either a saddle, restricted caudal, or pudendal block.

In severe toxemia, physiologic changes are exaggerated, and regional blockade, in the face of a restricted intravascular volume, may result in a considerable depression of blood pressure. Profound reductions in maternal systemic pressure may occur when standard epidural or low subarachnoid blocks are given, for example, a large-volume (usually 12 to 15 ml) deposition of local anesthetic in the epidural space. However, the restricted segmental lumbar epidural block has been safely used in patients with toxemia when careful attention is paid to management of intravascular blood volume and the use of small doses of local anesthetics (not greater than 5 ml of drug with restriction of the analgesic block to the T10 to L2 levels). All patients are kept on their sides to offset the effect of the vena cava syndrome. For the second stage of labor modified caudal analgesia, again with only S2 to S5 block, or a true saddle block may also be the anesthetic technique of choice. Alternatively, if the patient has severe preeclampsia with evidence of moderately reduced fetal reserve, an analgesic technique that minimizes swings in maternal arterial pressure may be preferred, for example, first-stage systemic medication or second-stage inhalation analgesia or pudendal block.

Vacuum extraction

Vacuum extraction may be useful when the fetal position is not easily ascertainable or there is need to avoid using a space-occupying instrument in tight pelvic conditions. It has been associated with reports of fetal damage such as scalp lacerations, cephalohematomas, and intracranial hemorrhage.

Analgesic requirements for vacuum extraction are not demanding. Some relief of discomfort and adequate vaginal relaxation during the introduction of the examiner's hand and manipulation of the extraction cup are all that is necessary. If one has a cooperative patient with a sufficiently relaxed vagina, this may be performed without analgesia or anesthetic. When the parturient is not cooperative and the obstetrician has difficulty in actual placement of the cervical cup, a saddle block may be performed to provide adequate vaginal analgesia and relaxation. This denervates only sacral fibers and is compatible with continued uterine contractions and good Valsalva maneuvers when required for descent and rotation of the fetal head. Lumbar epidural, caudal epidural, and pudendal analgesia also suffice to reduce pelvic diaphragmatic muscle tension and may be used successfully to aid in ease of application.

Midforceps deliveries

Recent critical appraisal of fetal and maternal trauma subsequent to midforceps deliveries has stringently curbed the use of this procedure. In midforceps maneuvers the operator is faced with the use of an additional space-occupying instrument in a restricted pelvic area. Therefore both profound vaginal tract and perineal analgesia and muscular relaxation are indicated before starting the procedure. Since timing and certain specific requirements for rotation may be necessary, the obstetrician should determine these factors and, with the anesthesiologist, decide on the most suitable technique and agent for each patient. During the induction of anesthesia, the patient should not be stimulated by application of the forceps or attempted rotation until the anesthesiologist is ready to proceed. Vigorous suprafundic pressure should be avoided during the expulsion phase.

Regional anesthesia is the preferred method, since it provides complete analgesia and relaxation without significant maternal or fetal depression. Lumbar epidural or combined lumbar epidural and caudal analgesia or subarachnoid block will provide sensory analgesia and motor relaxation adequate for these procedures by obtunding thoracic segments T10 to T12 and L1 and sacral segments S2, S3, and S4. Pudendal block is not adequate for midforceps rotational maneuvers and even when combined with light inhalation analgesia usually will not provide sufficient relaxation to protect the mother and fetus during these maneuvers. An inhalation analgesia/anesthesia combination with a potent uterine relaxant may be used and produces good results in expert hands, but it is rarely required, since uterine relaxation is an unusual requirement for obstetric midforceps operative procedures.

Low forceps deliveries

Elective or prophylactic forceps deliveries require minimal analgesia restricted to the perineum and lower portion of the vagina. In addition, relaxation is not always necessary; a cooperative patient may often aid the descent and delivery with moderate Valsalva maneuvers. The duration of perineal analgesia needed is very short, since no manipulation is required and the time of traction is minimal. Local analgesia by infiltration and supplemental N_2O/O_2 inhalation analgesia or pudendal block may be all that is required in a cooperative patient. Saddle block, low caudal epidural, and lumbar epidural analgesia also may be used in low forceps delivery with good results.

Breech presentations

Breech presentations (frank, complete, incomplete, and footling) may occur in 3% to 5% of all mothers in labor. The perinatal mortality in breech delivery is significantly greater than that associated with vertex delivery. In many centers all breech presentations, except frank breech, are considered best managed by cesarean section. Frank breech presentation may provide a wedge to the cervix of sufficient diameter to produce cervical dilatation and simultaneously protect the fetal umbilical cord from prolapse during dilatation, descent, and rotation. In the frank breech subjected to vaginal delivery the obstetrician and anesthesiologist should be prepared for the necessity of immediate inhalation anesthesia and profound uterine relaxation.

The primary life-threatening situation to the fetus is entrapment of the fetal head after delivery of the smaller diameter pelvic girdle and shoulders. This is a special threat in a premature infant whose head size is proportionately greater than the shoulder or pelvic girdle size. The midpelvis may also present a secondary threat to delivery of the fetal head; the cervix cannot be relaxed and dilated with a suitable uterine relaxant, since its lower portion is primarily connective tissue. Normally, it takes 1 hour for each 2 cm of cervical dilatation; this process cannot be accelerated even when there is profound myometrial relaxation caused by profound inhalation anesthesia. Persistent forceful attempts at dilatation will only produce maternal trauma, possible rupture of the lower uterine segment, and fetal injury. In contrast, many cases of breech delivery involve only increased tone of the lower uterine segment, which traps the fetal head, and of the levator ani and coccygeus muscles, which hinders manipulation. The use of the inhalation anesthetic technique for emergency vaginal delivery may be the indicated treatment under these circumstances. The two phases of general anesthesia for emergency vaginal delivery include the preparatory phase, which may be performed during prepping and draping of the patient for delivery, and phase II for induction.

A. Preparatory
 1. Antacid, 30 ml
 2. Denitrogenation
 3. Glycopyrrolate, 0.2 mg IV
 4. d-Tubocurarine chloride, 3 mg IV
B. Induction
 1. Thiopental sodium, 2.5 mg/kg IV
 2. Cricoid pressure
 3. Succinylcholine chloride, 80 mg IV
 4. Avoid positive pressure
 5. Endotracheal intubation
 6. Halothane, 2%-3%

A pudendal block may be used during the descent of the breech to the introitus. When descent is adequate, as shown by delivery of the umbilicus to the perineum, induction is started. This gives the anesthesiologist adequate time to place an endotracheal tube and begin administration of halothane 2% with oxygen 50% while the obstetrician is delivering the lower extremities followed by the upper extremities and thorax of the fetus. By this time, both lower uterine segment and pelvic relaxation should be adequate for manipulation of the fetal head by either Piper forceps or the Mauriceau maneuver. In situations where halothane is administered and where the anesthesiologist increases alveolar ventilation to effect rapid myometrial relaxation, endotracheal intubation and blood pressure monitoring to safeguard against possible hypotension are essential. It cannot be stressed too emphatically that, if an anesthesiologist is called only at the time an obstetrician encounters difficulty with entrapment of the fetal head, it will be practically impossible for him to safely and effectively anesthetize the mother and provide optimum conditions for an atraumatic delivery.

Twins and version-extraction

Internal podalic version and extraction is principally of historic significance. It has been associated with uterine rupture, cervical and perineal laceration, hemorrhage, and puerperal sepsis. A very high incidence of maternal death has been associated with the procedure. Nevertheless, under optimum conditions of uterine relaxation and full cervical dilatation, internal podalic version and extraction may be useful in management of a second twin with fetal distress immediately after extraction of the first twin. Maternal and fetal safety depends on an experienced obstetrician working with a competent obstetric anesthesiologist. Unless conditions are optimal, cesarean section delivery is the procedure of choice.

Success with version and extraction depends on adequate uterine relaxation. Before version and extraction, the patient is prepared for general anesthesia in the routine fashion. In emergency circumstances some of the steps may be abbreviated, such as elimination of the curare and reduction of the preoxygenation period to 15 seconds of hyperventilation. Once the endotracheal tube is inserted, halothane and oxygen are administered in an appropriate concentration and duration to rapidly achieve the uterine relaxation necessary for complete version and extraction without postpartum excess residual atony. This requires close communication and interaction of the obstetrician and anesthesiologist during delivery. If at any time the obstetrician believes that manipulation is too difficult, a cesarean section should be performed.

Cesarean section

Ideally, general anesthesia for cesarean section should permit the mother to be unconscious, analgesic, and to experience no unpleasant recall of the procedure, without jeopardizing the fetus and neonate. The N_2O relaxant technique for cesarean section has gained substantial popularity in the United States because it is not explosive, it reduces the use of more potent inhalation anesthetics that cause myometrial and neonatal depression, and it involves a minimum risk of maternal hypotension. Thiobarbiturates, muscle relaxants, N_2O, and O_2 are commonly used during the interval between induction and delivery. The analgesic effect of N_2O is often less than optimal until after delivery. This approach is unlikely to produce hypotension; it should, in skilled hands, produce ideal fetal and neonatal conditions even in cases of known maternal, fetal, or uteroplacental compromise. The technique consists of:

1. Antacid, 30 ml
2. Glycopyrrolate, 0.2 mg IV
3. d-Tubocurarine, 3 mg
4. Thiopental sodium, 2.5 mg/kg IV
5. No positive airway pressure
6. Cricoid pressure
7. Succinylcholine, 80 mg IV for intubation
8. N_2O/O_2, 50% mixture

The antacid regimen before induction is intended to elevate the gastric pH. The d-tubocurarine prevents fasciculations from succinylcholine chloride and subsequent increased intragastric pressure that may release gastric air and acid fluid into the esophagus. Misdirected positive pressure in the esophagus could worsen this problem. Cricoid pressure against the vertebral body of the upper cervical spine effectively closes the esophagus and reduces the incidence of gastric fluid escape into the upper airway. For maternal amnesia and fetal protection, 2.5 mg/kg of thiopental sodium is optimal. If there is fetal distress, an increased maternal ventilation with O_2 is indicated in spite of the possibility of greater maternal recall.

A maternal FIO_2 of 0.5 is adequate for the inhalation technique of cesarean section; there is no significant improvement in fetal oxygenation when maternal PaO_2 values rise above 300 mm Hg.

John S. McDonald

BIBLIOGRAPHY

Baraka, A.: Correlation between maternal and foetal pO_2 and pCO_2 during cesarean sections, Br. J. Anaesth. **42:**434, 1970.

Belfrage, P., and others: Neonatal depression after obstetrical analgesia with pethidine: the role of the injection-delivery time interval and of the plasma concentrations of pethidine and norpethidine, Acta Obstet. Gynecol. Scand. **60:**43, 1981.

Bonica, J.J.: Principles and practices of obstetric analgesia and anesthesia, Philadelphia, 1967, F.A. Davis Co.

Caldeyro-Barcia, R., and others. In Cassels, D.E., editor: The heart and circulation in the newborn and infant, New York, 1966, Grune & Stratton, Inc., pp. 7-36.

Fanning, G., and Golgan, F.: The efficacy of cricoid pressure in preventing regurgitation of gastric contents, Anesthesiology **32:**553, 1970.

Finster, M., and others: Plasma thiopental concentrations in the newborn following delivery under thiopental nitrous oxide anesthesia, Am. J. Obstet. Gynecol. **95:**621, 1966.

Freeman, R.K., and others: Fetal cardiac response to paracervical block anesthesia, Am. J. Obstet. Gynecol. **113:**583, 1972.

Hellman, L.M., and Pritchard, J.A., editors: Williams obstetrics, ed. 14, New York, 1971, Appleton-Century-Crofts.

Joyce, T.H., III, editor: Clinical symposium on obstetric anesthesia and analgesia, Clin. Perinatol., vol. 9, 1982.

Kivalo, I., Timonen, S., and Castren, O.: The influence of anesthesia and the induction delivery interval on the newborn delivered by cesarean section, Ann. Chir. Gynaecol. Fenn. **60:**71, 1971.

Kosaka, Y., Takahashi, T., and Mark, L.: Intravenous thiobarbiturate anesthesia for cesarean section, Anesthesiology **31:**489, 1969.

Kuhnert, B.R., and others: Meperidine and normeperidine levels following meperidine administration during labor. II. Fetus and neonate, Am. J. Obstet. Gynecol. **133:**909, 1979.

Miller, R., and Walter, W.: Inhibition of succinylcholine induced increased intragastric pressure by nondepolarizing muscle relaxants and lidocaine, Anesthesiology **34:**185, 1971.

Rorke, M.J., Davey, D.A., and DuToit, H.J.: Foetal oxygenation during cesarean section, Anaesthesiology **23:**585, 1968.

Sjostedt, J.E.: The vacuum extractor and forceps in obstetrics: a clinical study, Acta Obstet. Gynecol. Scand. **48** (Suppl. 10), 1967.

Taylor, G., and Pryse-Davies, J.: The prophylactic use of antacids in the prevention of the acid-pulmonary-aspiration syndrome (Mendelson's syndrome), Lancet **1:**288, 1966.

Westholm, H., Magno, R., and Berg, A.: Experiences with paracervical block: a double blind study with bupivacaine, Acta Obstet. Gynecol. Scand. **49:**335, 1970.

CHAPTER 14

Emergencies in the delivery room

Emergencies in the delivery room encompass two main areas: resuscitation of the asphyxiated or depressed newborn infant and the diagnosis of certain congenital anomalies that may require immediate treatment.

ONSET OF BREATHING AND PHYSIOLOGIC CHANGES AT BIRTH

To understand the principles of resuscitation, the normal cardiopulmonary events that take place with the onset of respiration must be understood. The healthy newborn infant makes respiratory efforts within a few seconds of birth, and after the first few breaths the lungs are almost completely expanded. As the chest emerges from the birth canal, there is an elastic recoil that can draw in between 7 and 42 ml of air to replace fluid squeezed out during the final stages of delivery. This explains the cough that occasionally precedes the first inspiratory effort. Glossopharyngeal muscular movement (frog breathing) may force down an additional 5 to 10 ml. The first inspiration is usually followed by a cry as the infant expires against a partially closed glottis, creating a positive intrathoracic pressure of up to 40 cm H_2O. Within a few minutes, functional residual capacity reaches about three fourths of final aeration.

Although the intrathoracic pressures recorded during the first breaths are high, often initial lung expansion appears to require little effort. The work for initial lung expansion is undeniably greater than that for quiet breathing, but it is not greater than that required many times a day during vigorous crying.

The first breath is caused by the integrated activity of several stimuli; the most important are hypoxia and acidosis (asphyxia), cord occlusion, and thermal changes. During the final stages of labor and delivery there is a reduction in exchange of oxygen and carbon dioxide between fetus and mother leading to a moderate degree of asphyxia at birth. The average value for oxygen saturation in the arterial blood at birth is 22%, and in nearly one fourth of all neonates it is less than 10%. The relatively low oxygen levels are accompanied by varying degrees of hypercapnia and acidosis, the average carbon dioxide pressure (P_{CO_2}) being 58 mm Hg and the average pH 7.28; lower pH and higher P_{CO_2} are associated with lower oxygen levels. The respiratory drive during asphyxia depends on the presence of carotid and aortic chemoreceptors, which are known to be functional in the newborn. Cord occlusion is associated with a prompt rise in blood pressure and stimulation of both the aortic baroreceptors and the sympathetic nervous system. Finally, thermal stimuli immediately after birth are intense. Calculations based on the rate of fall of skin temperature in the first minutes of extrauterine life indicate that at room temperature the newborn human infant loses about 600 calories per minute. It is difficult to prevent this initial heat loss even if the infant is immediately placed under a radiant heater. If this initial stimulus is completely prevented, apnea may follow.

With the onset of respiration and lung expansion, pulmonary vascular resistance falls. This is caused largely by the direct effect of oxygen and carbon dioxide on the blood vessels; resistance decreases as oxygen tension (P_{O_2}) rises and P_{CO_2} falls. Lung expansion alone contributes to lowering of the pulmonary vascular resistance. There then follows a gradual transition from the fetal to the adult type of circulation; the foramen ovale and ductus arteriosus remain open for varying lengths of time (Chapter 25).

Pressure in the left atrium falls in the first few hours of life to levels below those in the normal adult; by 24 hours it may be less than 1 mm Hg above that in the right atrium. This small pressure difference probably accounts for right-to-left shunt through the foramen ovale for 24 hours or longer, particularly with episodes of crying. Pulmonary arterial pressure remains relatively high for several hours. As the pulmonary vascular resistance falls, the direction of blood flow through the ductus arteriosus reverses. In the first hours of extrauterine life the flow is bidirectional, but the shunt eventually becomes entirely left-to-right and by 15 hours of age is functionally insignificant.

The ductus arteriosus constricts in response to an increase in arterial oxygen tension (PaO_2). Sympathomimetic amines and prostaglandin also cause it to constrict. Hypoxemia can cause a constricted ductus to reopen and at the same time may reestablish the fetal pattern of circulation by increasing the pulmonary vascular resistance. This response of the ductus arteriosus to oxygen or hypoxia is thus opposite to that of the pulmonary arterioles, enabling the right ventricle to contribute a variable fraction of its output to placental perfusion during fetal life. The different reactivity of these vessels during hypoxia, although an asset to the fetus, becomes a liability for the newborn infant. Hypoxic episodes in early neonatal life can lead to a rise in pulmonary vascular resistance and opening of the ductus arteriosus, increasing any residual right-to-left shunt.

Failure to breathe at birth

Depression of the fetal central nervous system is the basic cause for failure to breathe at birth. This may be caused by asphyxia, by analgesic or anesthetic agents administered to the mother, and/or by trauma.

Fetal asphyxia may be caused by maternal factors, including compression of the inferior vena cava and aorta by the heavy gravid uterus, particularly if the mother is supine; strong uterine contractions that occlude arterioles leading to the intervillous space impeding blood flow; hypotension caused by regional anesthesia, hyperventilation, or pharmacologic agents administered to the mother for hypertension; systemic vascular disease, including toxemia of pregnancy; and anemia or methemoglobinemia.

Fetal factors that may lead to asphyxia include mechanical occlusion of the umbilical cord or fetal hypotension as a result of depressant drugs that have crossed the placenta. Abnormalities of the placenta itself may impair its diffusion capacity (p. 206), for example, its small size, underdevelopment, aging, edema, infarcts, partial or complete separation, or inflammatory changes.

Neonatal factors also may lead to asphyxia. Most common is depression of the respiratory center from hypnotic, analgesic, or anesthetic agents administered to the mother. The second most common neonatal cause is immaturity of the lung (Chapter 23); this may relate to abnormalities in enzyme systems responsible for the release of surfactant to alveolar lining cells, to the vasculature, or to the lung parenchyma itself. The end result is difficulty in lung expansion and establishment of a normal pulmonary circulation. A third category is mechanical airway obstruction from aspiration of meconium and intrauterine pneumonia (pp. 443 and 446). Finally, various congenital anomalies may prevent or impede lung expansion; these include choanal atresia, a laryngeal web, hypoplastic lungs (usually associated with diaphragmatic hernias or large abdominal masses), hydrothorax or ascites, certain cardiac anomalies, and congenital myasthenia gravis.

The effect of trauma is more difficult to evaluate and to separate from the effect of asphyxia. It undoubtedly plays a role, particularly in precipitous labors or in difficult forceps deliveries.

Fetal respiratory responses—normal and abnormal

The normal mammalian fetus makes respiratory movements in utero from time to time. These are relatively rapid (80 to 120 per minute) and are noted during the latter half of gestation. It is unlikely that the rapid breathing movements result in a tidal flow of amniotic fluid.

There is a considerable quantity of fluid in the fetal lung before delivery. This fluid appears to be an ultrafiltrate of plasma; it is more acidic and has a higher chloride content than plasma or amniotic fluid. With the onset of extrauterine respiration, reabsorption of this fluid is quite rapid. Its low protein concentration, together with the fall in pulmonary artery pressure occurring when the lung expands, facilitates this process. The difference in composition of tracheal fluid compared with amniotic fluid is strong evidence against aspiration of amniotic fluid occurring as a normal phenomenon.

Cardiovascular, respiratory, and biochemical changes occurring during asphyxia under controlled conditions are predictable. Information on this subject has been obtained experimentally in a variety of newborn mammals. During the initial phase of asphyxia of the unanesthetized newborn primate, respiratory efforts increase in depth and frequency for up to 3 minutes. This period, which is called primary hyperpnea, is followed by primary apnea lasting for approximately 1 minute. Rhythmic gasping then begins and is maintained at a fairly constant rate of 8 to 10 gasps per minute for several minutes. The gasps finally become weaker and slower. Their cessation marks the beginning of secondary apnea.

There is some variation in the period of gasping (time to the last gasp) during the course of complete asphyxiation in different species, depending on the initial acid-base state, drugs given to the mother, environmental temperature, and degree of maturity of the species at

Emergencies in the delivery room   **181**

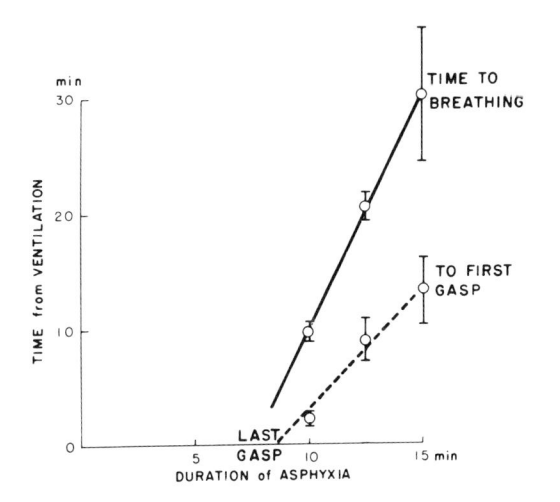

Fig. 14-1. Time from ventilation to first gasp and to rhythmic breathing in newborn monkeys asphyxiated for 10, 12.5, and 15 minutes at 30° C. Mean time from onset of asphyxia until last gasp was 8.42 ± 0.24 (SE) min. (From Adamsons, K., and others: J. Pediatr. **65:**807, 1964.)

birth. At a given environmental temperature the principal determinant of duration of gasping in the nonanesthetized animal is the initial arterial pH. Narcotics and systemic anesthetic agents administered to the mother can abolish the period of primary hyperpnea and prolong primary apnea; large doses can suppress all respiratory efforts. Gasping is always prolonged at lower body temperatures.

During primary apnea a variety of stimuli such as pain, cold, and analeptics can initiate gasping. Once the stage of secondary apnea has been reached, these stimuli are without effect. Gasping can, however, be reinitiated by artificial ventilation or correction of acidosis by administration of base. There is a linear relationship between the duration of asphyxia and recovery of respiratory function after resuscitation. In newborn monkeys, for each minute after the last gasp that artificial ventilation is delayed, there is a further delay of 2 minutes before rhythmic breathing is established (Fig. 14-1). The longer artificial ventilation is delayed during secondary apnea, the longer it will take to resuscitate the infant.

One of the most potent stimuli to gasping in utero is occlusion of the umbilical cord. This has been observed experimentally in both the fetal lamb and monkey. After 2 to 3 minutes of cord occlusion, when the fetus has become partially asphyxiated, deep gasping efforts commence. These respiratory efforts continue for 10 to 20 minutes following release of the cord occlusion. The presence of meconium and squamous cells in the lung periphery of mature infants dying after chronic intrauterine asphyxia indicates that aspiration may occur in the older fetus.

Preparation for resuscitation

The delivery room should be prepared for adequate and prompt treatment of severe asphyxia at birth, whether it is expected or not. All members of the delivery room team should be trained in methods of resuscitation, since both mother and baby may be in difficulty at the same time.

Every piece of apparatus necessary for emergency resuscitation should be carefully checked as present and functioning before each delivery. There should be suction apparatus, a plastic oropharyngeal airway, a laryngoscope equipped with a pencil handle and a blade, and a plastic endotracheal tube. Oxygen should be available. In addition, the container for receiving the infant should be warm, and some form of radiant heat should be available to help in maintaining body temperature.

Although thermal stimuli may be important in the initiation and establishment of breathing by increasing the state of activity of the reticular system, prolonged exposure of the naked infant to room temperature leads to progressive metabolic acidosis, particularly in the depressed infant or in the infant with impaired pulmonary function. If depression of the newborn is caused by excessive maternal medication, a fall in body temperature will prolong the effect of most analgesic and anesthetic drugs. The mean blood glucose level is also decreased at lower body temperatures.

If electronic monitoring of the fetal heart rate (FHR) (p. 95) is not available, the FHR should be determined between every contraction during the final stages of labor. A rate below 100 or above 160 per minute between contractions or the passage of meconium is an urgent warning sign of fetal distress. If these signs develop, the staff should be alerted for an emergency and the baby delivered as soon as possible. Analysis of capillary samples from the fetal scalp for pH and capillary or transcutaneous blood gases will provide a more precise evaluation of fetal condition (Chapter 9).

EVALUATION AT BIRTH—APGAR SCORE

Immediately after delivery the baby should be restrained with the head slightly dependent while the cord is clamped and cut. The infant should then be placed supine on a table, the head kept low with a slight lateral tilt. A nurse or assistant should listen to the heartbeat immediately, indicating the rate by finger movement. If help is not available, the rate may be detected from pulsation of the umbilical cord. A strong beat with a rate of over 100 per minute indicates that there is no immediate emergency. A slow rate indicates severe depression, calling for resuscitative measures. While the nurse is listening to the heart, the physician should aspirate secretions from the mouth, the pharynx, and the nose with a catheter. This suction should be brief. From

Table 14-1. Apgar score

Sign	0	1	2
Heart rate	Absent	Slow (below 100)	Over 100
Respiratory effort	Absent	Slow, irregular	Good, crying
Muscle tone	Flaccid	Some flexion of extremities	Active motion
Reflex irritability	No response	Grimace	Vigorous cry
Color	Pale	Cyanotic	Completely pink

birth to completion of suctioning should take about 1 minute. Lightly slapping the soles or rubbing the infant often aids in initiating a deep breath and crying.

During the course of these initial procedures the infant should be carefully observed for any evidence of central nervous system (CNS) depression or inability to breathe. Particular attention should be paid to the first few breaths and the evenness and ease of respiration. A congenital laryngeal web or bilateral choanal atresia (p. 460) can cause complete airway obstruction; both require immediate treatment. A diaphragmatic hernia with abdominal viscera in the chest, abdominal distention from ascites (p. 532), congenital cystic lung disease, or intrauterine pneumonia may all cause initial respiratory difficulty and may even prevent lung expansion.

The Apgar score was introduced to quantitate the initial evaluation of the infant. It focuses on five vital signs: heart rate, respiratory effort, muscle tone, reflex irritability, and color, all judged 60 seconds after complete delivery of the infant (Table 14-1). This particular time interval was chosen because it coincides with maximum depression. A score of 0 is given for each of the following: no heart beat, no respiratory effort, no muscle tone, no reflex response to a slap on the soles of the feet, and a blue or pale color. A score of 1 is given for a slow heart beat (less than 100), slow or irregular respiratory effort, some flexion of the extremities, a grimace to a slap on the soles of the feet, and a pink body with blue extremities. Finally, a score of 2 is given for a heart rate over 100, good respiratory effort accompanied by crying, fully flexed limbs, a vigorous cry in response to a slap on the feet, and a completely pink coloration.

The majority of infants are vigorous, with a score of 7 to 10, and cry or cough within seconds of delivery. No resuscitative procedures are necessary for these babies. Mildly to moderately depressed infants form the largest group requiring some form of resuscitation at birth. These babies score 4 to 6. They are pale or blue at 1 minute after birth, do not have sustained respirations, and may be nearly flaccid. However, their heart rate and reflex irritability are good. The most severely depressed infants score 0 to 3. They are pale or cyanotic, apneic, hypotonic, have a reduced or absent reflex response, and their heart rates are slow or inaudible; artificial ventilation should be started immediately in these infants.

Order of disappearance of signs

The foregoing five signs disappear in a predictable fashion during asphyxiation of the newborn. In vigorous infants who cry lustily as soon as they are born, heart rate, reflex response, and tone are all present to the full extent; the signs to which the observer has to pay attention are color and respiration. Mildly depressed babies are cyanotic (1 for color), but heart rate and reflex response are usually normal; attention has to be focused primarily on tone and respiration. In severely depressed infants who are pale (0 for color), apneic (0 for respiration), and usually flaccid (0 for tone), attention has to be paid primarily to heart rate and reflex response.

All the signs but reflex response can be seen—respiration from chest movement, tone from flexed or moving extremities, and heart rate from movement of the index finger of the nurse who listens to the heart with a stethoscope. A normal reflex cry is present in all vigorous infants. This sign need be elicited only in those infants scoring 6 or less and forms part of the resuscitation procedure during the first minute of life.

The heart rate is usually slow (under 100) or fast (over 160). In the high score group the heart rate is fast probably in response to catecholamine release due to elevated PCO_2 and the cold stimulus at birth. In those scoring 6 or less who are not breathing, it is slow either as a result of baroreceptive reflex or from myocardial depression. Initially the physician may have some difficulty in evaluating the five signs at once. A mental note of the total clinical picture should be made when 1 minute has elapsed; then a value for each of the clinical signs can be assigned.

Value of scoring
Clinical picture at a glance

The scoring system serves many useful purposes. It teaches the delivery room personnel to observe more than one sign at a time and ensures that the infant will be observed closely during the first minute of life.

Need for resuscitation

Scoring also serves as a guide as to the need for resuscitation; having made a rapid evaluation the physician can decide whether the infant should be resuscitated rather than waiting hopefully to see whether the infant will respond spontaneously.

Serial score—index of recovery

A physician or nurse can readily evaluate the infant at 1, 2, 5, and 10 minutes using the scoring system as a semiquantitative shorthand method to describe the recovery rate of an infant whose condition may change rapidly from moment to moment. This is extremely valuable on a busy obstetric service where there may not be time for detailed notation of the changing clinical state.

Defining infants at high risk

A further advantage of the scoring system is to identify the infants at high risk with regard to both mortality and morbidity. The mortality in low score infants is nearly 15 times that in the high score group, and respiratory distress syndrome (RDS) occurs significantly more frequently in low score than high score infants.

Time to assign the score

A simple alarm timer should be firmly fixed on the delivery room wall and set for 60 seconds. When the head and feet of the infant are visible, the timer is started, and when the alarm sounds at 60 seconds, the score is assigned.

Person to score

The person delivering the infant should not be the one to assign the score. He or she is usually emotionally involved with the outcome of the delivery and with the family and may not make an objective evaluation. It is ideal to have a specially trained observer regularly present (physician or nurse), but this situation is seldom possible. If a pediatrically oriented person is not routinely present for all deliveries, the anesthesiologist should assign the score, and the infant should be placed in a bassinet near the head of the delivery table.

Five-minute score

The 5-minute score is more predictive of survival or neurologic abnormality at 1 year of age than the 1-minute score. This is not surprising, since the longer asphyxia exists, the more likely death or permanent damage will occur. Furthermore, if the first observation is made as late as 5 minutes, a number of asphyxiated infants will remain untreated, with subsequent higher mortality and morbidity.

Limitations

While the Apgar score is useful, it is no substitute for a careful physical examination or for serial observations over the first few hours of life. Although it is of value in estimating the probability of survival and morbidity in groups of infants, it will not predict neonatal survival of individual infants or their long-term prognoses.

TREATMENT OF MODERATELY DEPRESSED INFANTS

If initial resuscitative measures have produced no response by 1½ minutes after delivery, the progressing asphyxia usually leads to diminished muscular tone and a fall in the heart rate. A small plastic oropharyngeal airway should then be inserted into the mouth and oxygen applied under pressure of 16 to 20 cm H_2O for 1 or 2 seconds. Although this pressure is insufficient to expand the alveoli, some oxygen will reach the respiratory bronchioles. The rise in intrabronchial pressure stimulates pulmonary stretch receptors. This stimulus, added to that of the chemoreceptors, initiates a gasp in about 85% of the cases.

If there is no respiratory effort and the heart rate continues to fall, with the infant becoming completely flaccid, the larynx should be visualized with the laryngoscope and the infant intubated. This is not a difficult procedure, but skill should be obtained by practice on stillborn infants.

Intubation is best accomplished with the infant lying supine on a flat surface. A folded towel under the head and slight extension of the neck will place him in a position resembling a sniffing posture. The head should be steadied with the right hand and kept in line with the body. The laryngoscope is held in the left hand, and the blade is introduced at the right corner of the mouth and advanced between tongue and palate for about 2 cm. As it is advanced, the blade is swung to the midline. This moves the tongue to the left of the blade. The operator looks along the blade for the rim of the epiglottis. The laryngoscope is gently advanced into the space between the base of the tongue and the epiglottis. Slight elevation of the tip of the blade will expose the glottis as a vertical dark slit bordered posteriorly by pink arytenoid cartilages.

If foreign material such as small blood clots, meconium-stained mucus, or vernix obstructs the larynx, quick brief suction is indicated. When the glottis is seen to be patent, a curved endotracheal tube is introduced at the right corner of the mouth and inserted through the cords until the flange of the tube rests at the glottis. Care must be taken not to intubate the esophagus. The laryngoscope is then withdrawn. Rarely, the glottis is obstructed by a laryngeal web. If the web is partial or thin, it may be perforated, or the opening may be enlarged with an endotracheal tube. The presence of a thick membrane requires immediate tracheostomy.

If stimuli from these procedures have not initiated a spontaneous gasp, positive pressure should be applied to the endotracheal tube. Brief puffs of air blown through the tube with enough force to cause the lower chest to rise gently will usually start spontaneous respiration. If the stomach rises, however, the esophagus has been intubated instead of the trachea, and the position of the tube must be corrected. Pressures between 25 and 35 cm H_2O are necessary to expand normal alveoli initially and can be applied safely for 1 or 2 seconds. Experience in applying such pressures should be gained by puffing into a spring manometer. Oxygen-enriched gas may be delivered to the infant by placing a tube carrying oxygen in the operator's mouth. The endotracheal tube should, however, be fitted with appropriate-sized adapters that can be connected to a rubber bag of oxygen or oxygen-enriched gas mixture or to one of the mechanical devices for applying positive pressure.

Artificial expansion of the lungs can initiate a spontaneous gasp. With the first or second application of positive pressure the infant usually makes an effort to breathe. The endotracheal tube may be withdrawn after the infant has established sustained spontaneous ventilation.

TREATMENT OF SEVERELY DEPRESSED INFANTS

No time should be lost in establishing ventilation. The glottis should be inspected immediately with the laryngoscope. If meconium or thick meconium-stained mucus has been aspirated into the trachea, it must be suctioned out at once before inflation of the lungs. It is usually possible to accomplish this within 1 minute after delivery. These severely depressed infants may require 3 to 8 minutes of artificial ventilation before a spontaneous gasp is taken. The endotracheal tube can be removed as soon as quiet and sustained respiration is established.

PROCEDURE FOR INFANT RESUSCITATION

During resuscitation, heat loss should be prevented or minimized by placing the infant under a radiant heat lamp. Three people should be available for optimum emergency resuscitation—one for establishing an airway and ventilating the infant, one for cardiac massage and monitoring the heart rate, and one for umbilical catheterization and the administration of alkali. When possible the procedure should be carried out under sterile conditions, including sterile gowns and gloves. All equipment, including laryngoscope, endotracheal tubes, and stethoscope, should be sterile. The resuscitation area should be covered with a sterile sheet previously warmed from an overhead heat lamp.

Attention must first be directed to establishing pulmonary ventilation in resuscitating the severely asphyxiated newborn. The steps should be as follows: establishment and maintenance of a clear airway, expansion of the lungs and continuation of ventilation with up to 100% oxygen at a rate of 30 to 40 inflations per minute. Ventilation should be interrupted every six or seven breaths and alternated with periods of cardiac massage as needed to maintain a rate of 120 beats per minute. Both ventilation and cardiac massage may be carried out by one person; if two people are involved, it is important that they coordinate their actions so that cardiac massage and artificial ventilation are not given simultaneously. This can result in a pneumomediastinum or a pneumothorax, since ventilation will be done against a compressed and distorted tracheobronchial tree. While these measures are being initiated, another physician should insert a catheter into the umbilical vein.

Aspiration syndrome

The importance of suctioning meconium from the trachea and bronchi deserves special emphasis. Meconium is passed following an asphyxial episode in utero. If the asphyxial episode is accompanied by prolonged gasping, meconium will be drawn deeply into the lungs. The fetus may recover from this episode with regard to his acid-base state and CNS responsiveness but may be born with his lungs full of meconium (p. 443). Such infants initially may be responsive and vigorously attempt to breathe. It is essential that the larynx be observed in all infants who have passed meconium during labor or who have meconium-stained amniotic fluid as soon as they are born, irrespective of their initial responsiveness. If there is thick meconium at the back of the pharynx, it should be suctioned out under direct vision and the larynx intubated with an endotracheal tube. Suction then should be applied directly to this tube, which is gradually withdrawn while suction is applied. In our unit we use mouth-to-tube suction. Not infrequently, a large piece of meconium, too thick to pass up the endotracheal tube, is observed clinging to the tip of the tube. If this occurs, the trachea should be reintubated immediately and the procedure repeated until only watery mucus is obtained. The fluid normally produced by the fetal lung continues to form and washes out meconium from the deeper radicals of the lung. If this procedure is followed in all cases of meconium aspiration, many subsequent complications can be avoided.

There are four conditions in which lung expansion is impossible in spite of proper intubation: massive aspiration of meconium that cannot be removed by suctioning, intrauterine pneumonia with organization of exudate, large bilateral diaphragmatic hernias with hypoplastic lungs, and congenital adenomatous cysts of the lung. Infants with the first two conditions are usually severely depressed at birth. However, those with hypoplastic lungs may be vigorous initially and score as high as 7 at 1 minute of age, making strenuous but ineffective respiratory efforts. At present there is no available treatment for this condition. Congenital adenomatous cysts of the lung are usually associated with hydrops fetalis, and the condition is usually fatal.

Cardiac massage

Blood pressure and heart rate fall during prolonged asphyxia. If the blood pressure is very low at the beginning of resuscitation, positive pressure ventilation is unlikely to be successful unless cardiac massage is employed. Cardiac massage should not be initiated until after the lungs have been well expanded by two or three inflations. If the heartbeat cannot be heard or if a slow heartbeat has not increased in rate, cardiac massage should be commenced. External manual compression of the heart between the chest wall and vertebral column forces blood into the aorta. Relaxation of pressure allows the heart to fill with venous blood.

The technique consists of intermittent compression of the middle and lower third of the sternum 100 to 200 times per minute with the index and middle fingers. Initially massage is interrupted every 5 seconds to permit two or three inflations of the lung; subsequently, if the heart is responding, six or seven breaths should be alternated with massage. Cardiopulmonary resuscitation is most successful when there has been no clinical evidence of fetal distress and when a normal FHR has been heard between contractions up to the moment of birth.

Administration of alkali

The rationale for rapid correction of an acid pH from asphyxia is based in part on experiments in newborn monkeys. The maintenance of a normal pH during asphyxia by rapid intravenous infushions of alkali together with glucose prolongs gasping and delays cardiovascular collapse. Resuscitation is also facilitated if alkali and glucose are infused at the same time as artificial ventilation is started; oxygen consumption is greater, and the time for establishing spontaneous breathing is shorter. In addition, there is a significant decrease in combined cardiac output in fetal lambs in the face of hypoxemia plus acidosis. Pulmonary vascular resistance has been shown to vary directly with hydrogen ion concentration; a sudden rise in arterial pH improves pulmonary blood flow and PaO_2. Mortality from RDS was reduced with early administration of intravenous glucose and sodium bicarbonate, and the early treatment of neonatal acidosis in low birth weight infants was found to be associated with a reduced morbidity. Furthermore, the synthesis of lecithin is markedly reduced in the presence of acidosis. It has been proposed that the beneficial effects of pH correction are derived from a prolongation and acceleration of anaerobic glycolysis, a restitution of the oxygen-carrying capacity of hemoglobin, the increased response of cardiovascular muscle to sympathomimetic amines, and a fall in pulmonary vascular resistance.

The most severely asphyxiated infants—those with an arterial pH below 7.0—will have a base deficit of 26 mEq/L or greater in addition to a marked elevation in PCO_2. By means of artificial ventilation alone, the base deficit can be reduced by approximately 10 mEq/L in a matter of 5 to 10 minutes, provided that good alveolar ventilation is achieved and the infant does not remain in circulatory collapse. This change occurs as a result of a significant bicarbonate shift at PCO_2's greater than 70 mm Hg, which should be taken into consideration in calculations for the initial base administration to prevent overcorrection. It is advisable initially to attempt to correct half the residual metabolic component of the mixed acidosis. Thus a 3-kg infant would receive 8 mEq of base:

$$\frac{\text{Base deficit (26-10)}}{2} \times \frac{\text{Body weight (3 kg)}}{\text{ECV (3)}}$$

This working formula is only an approximation and assumes the extracellular volume (ECV) to be one third of the body weight (p. 320).

Sodium bicarbonate rather than tris(hydroxymethyl)aminomethane (THAM) is recommended because the latter solution is able to enter the cell and occasionally cause depression of the respiratory center and arrest of breathing. Sodium bicarbonate, as it is obtained from the commercial ampule, contains nearly 1 mEq/ml (44.7 mEq in 50 ml, 0.9M solution.) This solution has an osmolality of 1,400 and a pH of 7.8. It should be diluted in equal parts with distilled water to reduce its osmolality to 700 and infused at a rate not greater than 2 to 3 ml/minute. If the heart rate is slow and irregular, the infusion should be accompanied by intermittent cardiac massage. The alkali may be infused into either the umbilical vein or artery.

Subsequent alkali administration

The infant's response to alkali administration will vary according to the degree of asphyxia, the effectiveness of ventilation, and the responsiveness of the cardiovascular system. It is important, therefore, to have a measurement of his acid-base state as soon as the initial dose of sodium bicarbonate has been given. This can usually be made by 15 minutes of age. The required amount of sodium bicarbonate for subsequent correction to a pH of 7.3 may then be calculated.

Controversy and risk

Considerable concern has arisen following the demonstration of a significant association between intracranial hemorrhage, hypernatremia, and alkali administration in a retrospective study. In a controlled prospective trial the finding of intracranial hemorrhage in 4 of 26 infants who received alkali by rapid intravenous infusion has raised further doubts about this therapy. However, another retrospective study has failed to confirm the association between alkali therapy and intracranial hemorrhage, and in our experience the incidence of intracranial hemorrhage was actually higher in those infants who did not receive alkali. Examination of the effect of alkali administration in the presence of elevated $PaCO_2$ revealed that a further rise in $PaCO_2$ was transient, and bicarbonate appeared to be effective as a base for correcting acidosis.

From experimental work there seems little doubt that infusion of hypertonic solutions containing sodium can cause intracranial hemorrhage and may also cause hypocalcemia. When bicarbonate is administered in a "closed" system, the PCO_2 may rise and pH actually fall. Rapid infusion of bicarbonate to newborn puppies with mechanically fixed hypoventilation resulted in a rise in both $PaCO_2$ and osmolality.

Administration of alkali therefore is not without risk, which will outweigh the benefits if it is given in too high a concentration, in too great a quantity, and in the presence of severely impaired ventilation. There seems to be little doubt that the adverse effects of alkali have resulted from injudicious use, particularly in the presence of impaired CO_2 elimination. Sodium bicarbonate will be ineffective in correcting acidosis if a prompt increase in CO_2 excretion cannot be ensured.

In summary, the beneficial effects of alkali would appear to outweigh the risks in the immediate resuscitation of the newborn, provided that the lungs can be expanded promptly and pulmonary ventilation established.

Technique for catheterization of umbilical vein

A standard umbilical catheter, if advanced to a distance of 7 to 10 cm from the skin surface of the umbilical vein, will lie just beyond the ductus venosus in the inferior vena cava in a mature, term weight infant. If the catheter is even slightly curved, it may be deflected into one of the radicals in the portal system. Any tendency for the catheter to bounce back as it is advanced should suggest that it is not passing through the ductus venosus. Rapid verification of the correct site can be obtained if the catheter has been previously attached to a strain gauge and a recording polygraph. The moment the ductus venosus is passed, the venous pulsations (A, C, and V waves) can be readily seen, unless there is cardiac arrest. This means of verification of catheter position is more rapid and suitable for delivery room treatment than the use of an image-intensified roentgenogram (p. 129).

Technique for catheterization of umbilical artery

Only fine catheters should be used (3½ or 5, French). They should be nonrigid and pliable with a hole in the softly rounded tip. They should also be radiopaque for radiologic localization. The lumen of the artery should be carefully identified after cutting of the cord close to the abdominal wall with sharp scissors. Fine, curved, non- toothed forceps should be gently placed in the pinpoint clot that usually marks the vessel opening. Pressure on the forceps is then gradually released to allow the natural spring to open the vessel gradually. This procedure is repeated four or five times, the forceps gradually being advanced to a depth of ¼ to ½ inch. The catheter then may be introduced and will usually pass readily down to the region of the iliac artery. Occasionally, some obstruction is met ½ inch from the skin, but this rarely causes any difficulty. If resistance is felt at the entrance into the internal iliac artery, only moderate pressure should be applied. If the catheter will not advance, 0.5 ml of 0.5% procaine hydrochloride (Novocain) may be slowly infused. This may be sufficient to release any spasm and permit further advancement of the catheter. If this maneuver is unsuccessful and resistance persists, the second umbilical artery should be catheterized. If damage to the vessels is to be avoided, resistance in the region of the internal iliac artery should not be responded to aggressively; efforts to catheterize should be discontinued if unsuccessful after three attempts.

Once the venous or arterial catheter is in place, a lateral film should be taken to verify position. In the PA view the catheter cannot be distinguished from the maze of wires attached to the thermistors (Fig. 14-2). A catheter introduced into the umbilical vein may reach a variety of positions. If advanced far enough, it will pass directly through the ductus venosus and foramen ovale into the left atrium. It may also pass into the right or left branches of the portal vein, the superior or inferior mesenteric veins, or even the splenic vein. Lodged in these areas, catheters can occlude blood flow and serve to localize any solutions infused. The ideal position for the umbilical vein catheter is just beyond the ductus venosus in the inferior vena cava.

A catheter introduced into the umbilical artery will usually pass into the aorta from the internal iliac artery. Occasionally it will pass down the femoral artery or into the gluteal artery. The two latter sites are unsuitable for sampling and pressure measurements or for the infusion of alkali. Either of two positions in the aorta is recommended for the catheter placement—in the lower abdomen below the renal arteries and inferior mesenteric artery or just above the diaphragm. If left in the internal iliac or the region of the aortic bifurcation, the chances of arterial spasm are increased.

The status of the circulation is obviously of great importance when hypertonic or strongly alkaline solutions are administered. From a clinical point of view, blood flow can be fairly reasonably assessed from blood pressure, and, if low, cardiac massage is indicated during injection. If the umbilical vein is used for infusion, the catheter should be just beyond the ductus venosus, and the alkali administered into the inferior vena cava.

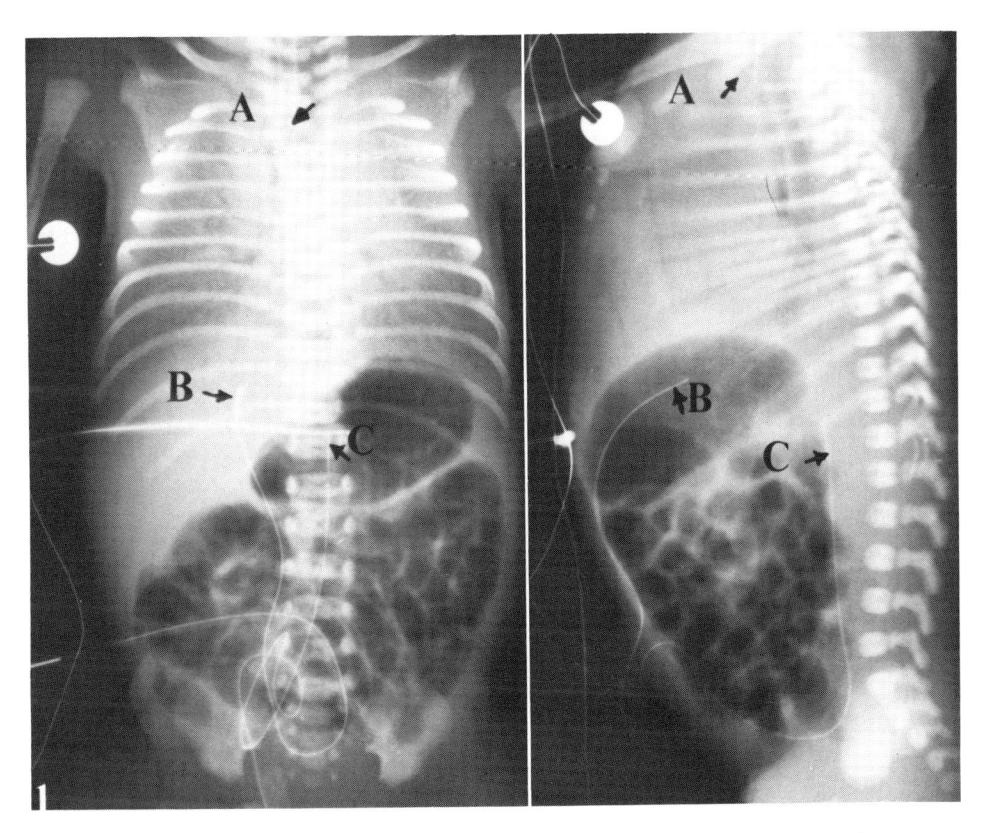

Fig. 14-2. AP x-ray film of infant with thermistors and an umbilical catheter in place; note that maze of wires prevents identification of catheter position in this veiw. The lateral view clearly identifies that catheter has been inserted into an umbilical vein and is lying in the portal system of the liver. *A*, Endotracheal tube; *B*, umbilical venous catheter at the juncture of the umbilical vein, ductus venosus, and portal vein; *C*, umbilical artery catheter passed up the aorta to T12. (Courtesy Walter E. Berdon, Babies Hospital: Infant with RDS. Note granular lungs, air bronchogram, and air-filled esophagus.)

Complications from umbilical catheterization

Although catheterization of the umbilical vein and artery are relatively simple maneuvers and allow easy infusion of fluids or blood sampling, the procedures are not without hazard. Complications relate to trauma during insertion, the duration of catheterization, the size of the catheters used, the state of the circulation when solutions are being infused, and the pH or tonicity of the solutions infused. Although the incidence of complications is relatively low, the procedure is not recommended as the usual route for fluid or drug therapy and should be used only in very ill infants or those at high risk when monitoring is essential for diagnosis and therapeutic management.

False lumen and perforation. If the lumen of the constricted artery is not localized accurately, it is possible to create a false lumen in the wall of the vessel. This may be erroneously interpreted as spasm when obstruction is met in the region of the internal iliac artery. If the catheter being inserted is rigid, the vessels may be perforated at this point, the catheter passing into the abdominal cavity. If undue force is exerted, even with a soft catheter, it may track extraperitoneally and result in retroperitoneal hemorrhage.

Blanching of the limb or alteration in pulse. This complication occurs in approximately 5% of infants. It is directly related to the relative size of the catheter in the aorta. It also has been seen when a cold solution is rapidly infused into the aorta. The signs will usually disappear after removal of the catheter. If the limb blanches, the catheter should be removed promptly. We do not advocate warming the contralateral limb as the initial procedure to cause vasodilatation of the affected limb because of the higher risk with such delay.

Accidental hemorrhage. This is associated with inexperience. The incidence is negligible when physicians and nursing personnel are accustomed to the use of stopcocks and connections and are experienced in the placement of catheters.

Infection. The incidence of infection is related to the

sterility conditions at the time of catheter placement and to maintenance procedures and the experience of the personnel.

Serious complications at necropsy. The incidence of serious complications at necropsy ranges from 1.5% to 7% and appears as a significant cause of death in less than 2% of cases. The lesions include embolization, thrombosis of hepatic vein, liver necrosis, aortic thrombi, and infarcts. Aortic thrombi are common, and their occurrence usually increases the longer the duration of the catheterization. A serious complication is thrombosis of the renal arteries and renal shutdown leading to death. A recent increase in the incidence of neonatal hypertension may be related in whole or part to renal vascular complications of umbilical arterial catheters. In newborn monkeys where the aorta is relatively small, occlusion of the inferior mesenteric arteries by the catheter with infarction of the bowel has been observed; the presenting sign was bloody stool.

Hemorrhagic necrosis of the liver has been observed in asphyxiated newborn human infants and newborn monkeys treated with strong alkalis (sodium bicarbonate or THAM). In relating liver necrosis to catheterization and the infusion of hypertonic solutions, it should be recalled that this complication also occurs following severe asphyxia alone. The incidence of intracranial hemorrhage also may be associated with hyperosmolar infusions causing hypernatremia, hypervolemia, or hypertension.

DEPRESSION FROM DRUGS VERSUS ASPHYXIA

An infant depressed primarily as a result of maternal analgesics or anesthetics can usually be distinguished by clinical signs from one depressed from asphyxia. The infant depressed from medication will not have passed meconium before birth; his skin may be cyanotic rather than pale, since he has not received an asphyxial stimulus to cause peripheral vasoconstriction; his heart rate may be slow but the pulse strong and full; the cord will be filled with blood, since his cardiovascular system has not been depressed by asphyxia; and he will usually not be completely hypotonic. In contrast, the infant depressed primarily as a result of asphyxia may be meconium stained and pale as a result of intense peripheral vasoconstriction; the heart rate will be slow and the sounds soft, distant, and occasionally irregular; the umbilical cord will be limp and contain little blood.

The Apgar score does not distinguish between depression from these two causes. Differentiation is useful, since the medicated infant will frequently respond quite promptly to simple resuscitative procedures—stimulation and positive pressure ventilation applied with a mask. Intubation and artificial inflation of the lungs are rarely necessary. Recognition of the infant depressed by medication is also important if drug antagonists are to be administered. On the other hand, the severely asphyxiated infant may require not only intubation, artificial ventilation, and cardiac massage, but also correction of a severe metabolic acidosis by infusion of alkali.

Use of analeptics, drug antagonists, and cardiovascular stimulants

Analeptics and drug antagonists should never be administered before the lungs have been expanded and the infant oxygenated by artificial ventilation. Analeptics, such as nikethamide, are not indicated in resuscitation of the newborn. Although they may shorten primary apnea, they are ineffective in secondary apnea and may cause hypotension and convulsions even if given in the recommended dosage. The morphine antagonist naloxone may be of value (Appendix B).

However, with the decreasing use of meperidine (Demerol) in obstetrics, the occasions when naloxone would be beneficial are quite infrequent. We recommend its use only when the infant remains depressed after effective lung expansion and oxygenation. Furthermore, the possibility that naloxone could interfere with the normal process of adaptation through its antagonism of endorphins should also be considered.

In general, the use of a wide variety of cardiovascular stimulants that are administered in cardiopulmonary resuscitation, particularly in adults and older children, are not recommended for resuscitation at birth. Unlike that in the adult and older child, neonatal cardiac arrest occurs very late in the course of asphyxiation. Consequently the severely asphyxiated infant who does not respond to cardiac massage and effective lung expansion is likely to have already suffered damage to the brain and other vital organs.

Toxicity from local anesthetics

Rarely, local anesthetics may be injected accidentally into the fetus during an attempted caudal anesthesia or paracervical block. The infant may be profoundly depressed at birth. However, as soon as he is oxygenated during the course of resuscitation and the responsiveness of the CNS is partially restored, generalized convulsions may occur. The presenting part of the infant should be carefully examined for a needle puncture if accidental injection is suspected and the convulsion treated promptly with IV phenobarbital, 10 to 15 mg/kg. It may be necessary to repeat the barbiturate and maintain the infant on a ventilator. As soon as possible a 2- to 3-volume exchange transfusion should be performed.

Delayed depression from maternally administered analgesia and anesthesia

Drugs that cross the placenta enter the fetus through the umbilical vein and the ductus venosus. A significant but variable portion of the umbilical vein flow also passes to the inferior vena cava through the liver and hepatic veins and not through the ductus venosus. This places the liver in a strategic position for uptake of drugs, particularly those with a high fat solubility. From the liver they can be released slowly over a period of hours. Thus infants delivered soon after the mother has been given a drug may initially appear vigorous but develop a marked CNS depression 2 to 4 hours later. Therefore, when relatively large doses of sedatives or narcotics have been given to the mother and the infant breathes well at birth, he should nevertheless be carefully observed for delayed secondary depression. This may be so severe as to require an exchange transfusion.

Drug-addicted newborn infant

See Chapter 33, part five.

Signs of drug withdrawal are not usually seen for 12 to 24 hours after birth. However, if the mother has not taken a dose of narcotic recently, both mother and infant may be in a state of withdrawal at the time of delivery.

ACUTE HEMORRHAGE

Acute blood loss may occur under several circumstances: placenta previa, as a complication of fetal blood sampling, in multiple pregnancy, with cord occlusion, or at cesarean section (Chapter 29). If the blood loss has occurred during the final stages of delivery, the infant will appear pale, but the onset of respiration will not be inhibited. If it has occurred at a longer interval before delivery and the fetus has become hypotensive, severe asphyxia will be superimposed, and the infant will be depressed and unresponsive at birth. The mechanism of blood loss in placenta previa is obvious. Its occurrence as a complication of fetal blood sampling is described below. However, in the other three conditions hemorrhage may not be immediately apparent or suspected. In multiple pregnancy one fetus may bleed into another, or there may be partial placental separation with hemorrhage at the time of delivery of the first infant (p. 206). Mild cord occlusion sufficient to constrict the vein but not arteries is occasionally seen; under these circumstances the fetus literally bleeds into the placenta. Such blood loss is usually not severe, being limited by the capacity of the placental vascular bed. Blood loss at cesarean section also occurs into the placenta. When the infant is removed from the uterus, he is usually held up by the feet while the cord is clamped. In a few seconds a considerable volume of blood can flow into the placenta from the arteries, and venous blood can be prevented from returning from the placenta to the infant as a result of the hydrostatic pressure caused by the infant's being held in the air. The venous blood loss by this mechanism is usually not severe. Nevertheless, unless special precautions are taken to prevent this occurrence, such as placing the infant on the mother's abdomen and milking the umbilical cord once or twice toward the infant before clamping the cord, the hematocrit value of the infant at 3 hours of age will be 6% to 12% lower than that in healthy infants delivered vaginally. Blood "loss" or redistribution into the placenta does not occur in infants delivered normally, since they are usually held at the level of their mother's perineum, and the uterus, having expelled the infant, is firmly clamped on the placenta.

The hemoglobin and hematocrit values should be measured in all circumstances where blood loss may have occurred if there is any abnormality such as low Apgar score, slow, delayed, or difficult breathing, pallor, or cyanosis. If there is pallor and peripheral vasoconstriction, a hematocrit reading from the peripheral capillaries will not be reliable, and a sample should be taken from the umbilical vein as soon as is practical after delivery. If blood loss has occurred acutely at delivery, it will not be reflected in the hematocrit value of central circulating blood during the first minutes of life. Therefore measurement should be repeated at 3 hours, the time usually necessary for readjustment of blood volume and circulating red blood cells after birth. In normal infants the mean hematocrit value usually increases from 48% to 52% during this time (Chapter 29). If the hematocrit value is below 40% at birth or if there is a significant fall in the first 3 hours of life accompanied by pallor and respiratory distress, the infant should be given a transfusion of blood.

PNEUMOTHORAX AND PNEUMOMEDIASTINUM

Pneumothorax and pneumomediastinum usually occur spontaneously and in association with aspiration syndromes. Occasionally they may be a result of incorrect or injudicious resuscitative procedures. If mild they will not be recognized clinically and may only be discovered accidentally when a roentgenogram is taken of the infant for another reason.

Pneumomediastinum should be suspected if heart sounds become distant or suddenly cannot be heard in an infant who otherwise appears normal. It should also be suspected if the anteroposterior diameter is increased. No treatment is necessary. The infant should be observed carefully after a chest roentgenogram has been taken, since this complication may progress to pneumothorax.

A tension pneumothorax is a serious complication that requires immediate treatment (p. 448). It presents as respiratory distress that becomes progressively more severe. The respirations are often rapid rather than labored. The heart will be shifted away from the affected side, which will move little and may appear hyperinflated. The infant usually appears pale rather than cyanotic. Since a diaphragmatic hernia may present similarly, particularly when the stomach and small bowel become filled with air, it is important first to pass a catheter into the stomach and attempt to suck out any air (Chapter 24). If symptoms are not relieved by this procedure, transillumination of the chest should be performed and, if positive in an infant with severe respiratory distress, a needle may need to be inserted into the thoracic cavity in the midaxillary line at about the level of the sixth rib and the air pressure released. Following this, a tube should be inserted surgically and connected to underwater drainage. If the pneumothorax is not under tension, it is usually possible to obtain a roentgenogram of the chest to confirm the clinical diagnosis and aid in deciding on the management, which may require oxygen administration, placement of a chest tube, or a combination of these therapies.

SEVERE ERYTHROBLASTOSIS

In severe cases of erythroblastosis with hydrops (Chapter 29) certain emergency procedures in the delivery room may be indicated. These all focus on promptly establishing good cardiopulmonary function and ensuring that the oxygen-carrying capacity of the blood is satisfactory. If the infant is born by vagina, a blood sample should be obtained from the cord or from a peripheral venous site for Coombs' test, for determination of hemoglobin or hematocrit value, and for crossmatching with compatible blood. It is also possible to obtain a sample of capillary blood from the presenting part before delivery. If delivery is by cesarean section, O negative blood compatible with the mother's should be available before delivery. The red blood cells should be partially packed. The blood should be in readiness on the resuscitation table together with umbilical catheters, a laryngoscope, an endotracheal tube, and a 20-gauge needle.

As soon as the infant is delivered he should be intubated, the lungs expanded, and positive pressure ventilation initiated. This is necessary because these infants are prone to develop pulmonary edema, since lung capillary permeability is increased and serum proteins are usually low. If there is marked abdominal distention from ascites or a recent intrauterine infusion of blood, a 20-gauge needle may need to be inserted in the lateral flank to remove fluid and relieve pressure on the diaphragm. Although fluid is usually present in the thoracic cavity of such infants, we do not recommend removal as a blind emergency procedure. Positive pressure ventilation should be continued until the infant is stabilized in the neonatal intensive care unit and can be closely observed for the development of pulmonary edema.

During the initial resuscitation, blood should be withdrawn from a clamped segment of the cord for measurement of the central hematocrit value and from the umbilical artery for a pH measurement. These results should be available to the physician within 5 to 6 minutes of delivery. If the infant is severely anemic, both umbilical vein and artery should be quickly catheterized and the blood administered through the vein, approximately 20 ml/kg, while an equal quantity is slowly withdrawn from the artery if there are signs of congestive cardiac failure. The speed of infusion and withdrawal should be about 10 ml/minute to prevent any sudden change in hemodynamics. If a hematocrit reading has been obtained from fetal capillary blood during labor, catheterization and administration of blood can proceed while the infant is being intubated and ventilated. Freshly drawn heparinized blood is desirable but is rarely available in the delivery room. This will have a pH in the range of 7.3. CPD blood that has a pH of about 7.25 is an adequate substitute for heparinized blood. If only citrated blood is available, the pH will be 6.9 or less. This pH should be corrected with sodium bicarbonate. Citrated blood also has a high potassium content.

During these procedures every effort should be made to prevent heat loss by having a warm container ready for the infant, with an overhead radiant heat source turned on well in advance of delivery. Prompt oxygenation and restoration of the oxygen-carrying capacity of the blood are essential if these infants are to be given an optimum chance to survive.

IMMATURE INFANT

Immature infants require the application of all the principles of resuscitation just described. Because of their relatively large surface area, particular attention should be paid to preventing heat loss by drying the infant promptly and ensuring that the resuscitation area is warmed with a radiant heater and is as draft free as possible. This is sometimes difficult in modern air-conditioned delivery rooms. The small size of the infant and the delicacy of immature tissues demand greater manual dexterity and gentleness if intubation is to be performed rapidly and without trauma. Intubation, if necessary, is facilitated by the physician placing the fifth finger of the left hand, which holds the laryngoscope, over the larynx. Gentle pressure on the larynx as the blade is tilted will bring the glottis into view.

COMPLICATIONS OF FETAL BLOOD SAMPLING

Two major complications following fetal blood sampling have been observed. The first is abscess formation in the area of the sampling incision, and the second is hemorrhage from the incision itself. These complications have occurred in about 1% of cases (p. 117).

Abscess formation has been seen where the incision was made in an area that had been previously traumatized, with the subsequent formation of a cephalhematoma, or where the tissue had become traumatized during delivery, from the application of either forceps or a vacuum extractor at the incision site. There also is an increased risk of infection following sampling in the breech presentation, since healing of incisions in the sacral region is poor. Although there is no way to be certain that bacteria are introduced at the time of sampling, the fact that abscesses do occur underscores the importance of careful aseptic techniques in the fetal blood sampling procedure.

Hemorrhage may occur if the incision is made over a small artery. It will usually stop when firm pressure is applied, but occasionally the incision may have to be sutured. This is a potentially lethal complication. It is important that the incision area be observed directly for two or three contractions after a blood sample has been taken to ensure that hemostasis is present. Clotting studies have been abnormal in a number of infants who have bled from the scalp sampling site. Most of the infants reported to have bled following fetal scalp sampling have suffered from chronic intrauterine asphyxiation, and this is sometimes associated with depletion or deficiency in certain clotting factors, particularly the labile factors V and VII. It is therefore important that neonates who bleed readily from sampling incisions have a screening coagulation study (Chapter 29). Postnatal bleeding from a sampling incision may be the first manifestation of a severe neonatal coagulation disorder.

If the scalp appears pale when visualized through the amnioscope and does not blanch when compressed by the instrument, severe peripheral vasoconstriction and hypotension are likely. Under these circumstances it may be difficult to obtain blood when an incision is made. If blood does not flow readily from the first incision, the temptation is to make multiple incisions. However, after delivery and alleviation of asphyxia, the peripheral circulation will improve; the infant then may bleed from several sites and sustain substantial blood loss.

Maternal intrapartum or postpartum infection has been seen more frequently in mothers of infants who develop complications from fetal blood sampling. Therefore infants whose mothers develop infections should be observed very closely for infection and hemorrhage at the site of a sampling incision.

IMMEDIATE COMPLICATIONS OF ASPHYXIA

Major signs of dysfunction of the central nervous system in the full-term infant following intrauterine asphyxia include abnormal respiratory pattern, stereotyped movements, fixed posturing, poor suck and feeding, reduced oculovestibular response, abnormal pupillary response, and fullness of the anterior fontanel. The sign that appears to be the most indicative of the degree of insult to the nervous system is the loss of tone. Loss of tone in the infant is the last of the components of the Apgar score to return following recovery from asphyxia.

For this reason it appears to be one of the best and earliest clinical indicators of the severity of the intrauterine insult. If the tone returns to normal within 1 or 2 hours, the infant has a good chance of surviving with an intact nervous system. However, if the infant remains significantly hypotonic during the first 4 to 5 days of life, there is an increased chance that the child will not survive the neonatal period, or if the child survives, there will be severe cerebral damage. If hypotonia is replaced with marked hypertonia and increased activity during the first 24 hours, chances of survival increase greatly, but there is an increased incidence of cerebral damage (Chapter 22).

Pathologic features

In the full-term infant pathologic features depend on the length and severity of the intrauterine asphyxial episode, the care of the patient in the neonatal period, and the length of survival of the patient. Patients who die in the first few hours after birth may show no gross or microscopic changes. Those patients dying after the first 24 hours of age frequently have brain swelling and cerebral necrosis. Full-term infants who survive the intrauterine asphyxial episode and the neonatal period have been described as having two primary neuropathologic conditions: ulegyria and status marmoratus of the basal ganglia. The principal focus of damage is in the cortical mantle and not in the paraventricular region of brain, as in the premature infant.

There has been much discussion regarding the issue of whether brain swelling occurs prior to or subsequent to cerebral necrosis. It is likely that the initial swelling is intracellular, occurring first at the depths of the sulci. The extent and pattern of ulegyria obviously depend on the degree and location of the cerebral ischemia and subsequent cerebral necrosis. The presence of gross brain swelling is simply the end result of the increasing focal areas of cerebral swelling and ischemia, leading not only to the generalized brain swelling but also to generalized cerebral necrosis. If the infant survives, the existing areas of cerebral necrosis, through the reparative process of brain gliosis, are converted into areas of ulegyria.

In the preterm infant the most common brain lesion at autopsy is subependymal hemorrhage/intraventricular hemorrhage (SEH/IVH) (p. 367). Most observations regarding SEH/IVH, prior to the advent of computerized tomography, have come from autopsy studies which indicate that the incidence of SEH/IVH in the neonate varies from 25% to 75%, with a higher incidence of hemorrhage occurring in the more immature infant.

Clinical signs that are statistically related to SEH/IVH are the following:
1. Fall in hematocrit level

2. Failure of rise in hematocrit level when transfusion of packed red cells is given
3. Tight anterior fontanel
4. Decrease in spontaneous activity
5. Decrease in tone
6. Abnormal eye signs
7. Seizures

The quantity of blood appears to be prognostically significant with regard to survival.

Two areas of concern regarding the outcome of neonates who survive SEH/IVH are progressive posthemorrhagic hydrocephalus and long-term neurobehavioral abnormalities. Contrary to previous belief, progressive hydrocephalus is not always an invariable outcome in patients with documented significant hydrocephalus. There is spontaneous resolution of hydrocephalus in a significant number of patients without any therapy whatsoever.

Effect of hypoxia on other organ systems

Other organs, which can be dispensed with functionally by the fetus, are likely to be more severely compromised than is the brain. Blood flow to the gut, kidneys, and lungs is decreased with redistribution to the myocardium and CNS during asphyxia (p. 2). The blood flow to the adrenals is also maintained during asphyxia in experimental models, but the role of the adrenals and their hormone products has been incompletely studied. Thus, if there is evidence of brain damage in an asphyxiated infant, there is almost always evidence of more profound damage to other organs. The degree of damage and the extent of the interaction between compromised gut, lungs, and kidneys will depend on a large number of factors, including gestational age.

The effect of intrauterine asphyxia on the lungs is reflected in the development of RDS in immature infants and in persistence of the fetal circulation and meconium aspiration in the more mature infants. There is a significant relationship both to the development of RDS and its severity with intrapartum and neonatal asphyxia. The reduction in blood flow to the lungs of the fetus leads to damage to the cells lining the tracheobronchial tree, resulting in loss of function and in the severest cases cellular destruction. In the liver, despite preferred perfusion, processes that cause compromise of oxygen delivery from the placenta can result in anything from extremes of necrosis to subtle hepatic functional changes related to problems of hypoglycemia and hyperbilirubinemia. The importance of the alteration in hepatic enzyme function that occurs with perinatal asphyxia and hypoxia is incompletely defined yet may play a critical role in the handling of maternal drugs and endogenous metabolic products. The gut is a target organ for profound cellular damage in the presence of any compromise to blood flow or oxygenation. There is evidence to suggest that hypoxia plays a leading role in preparing the neonatal gut for necrotizing enterocolitis.

Particularly wide variation in renal function is incurred during and following perinatal hypoxia. As yet there has been no systematic investigation of the neonatal kidney's ability to maintain homeostatic adjustments of water and electrolytes and thus body composition in the face of perinatal asphyxia. Active research in fetal and neonatal animals has begun to elucidate the mechanisms by which hypoxia may cause alterations in renal function or varying degrees and patterns of renal failure. The derangements in function related to hypoxia and acidosis have been shown to depend not only on the duration and degree of insult, but also on the actions of vasopressin, angiotensin and catecholamines. High concentrations of these hormones are found in fetal plasma during and subsequent to asphyxial insult.

There is evidence that decreased activity of the converting enzyme during asphyxia leads to some of the pathophysiologic consequences of asphyxia. Inhibition of this enzyme's activity with hypoxia could be a primary event in mediating the changes in blood flow patterns in the asphyxiated newborn, as well as the interactions between this system and adrenergic vasoactive compounds. There is also evidence linking the blood coagulation system with the potent edematogenic agent bradykinin and vasoactive compounds that might well underlie some of the pathophysiologic changes in the various organs affected by hypoxia. The agents responsible for the modulation of blood flow in the fetus and newborn during hypoxia have complex interactions. Further research in this area should yield important new knowledge.

DIAGNOSIS OF CONGENITAL ANOMALIES
Incidence

The incidence of congenital defects has been estimated to be between 1% and 7% of all live births (p. 200). This incidence will depend on the kind of conditions that are included, but probably 2% to 3% of all live-born infants show one or more significant congenital malformations that may require medical attention soon after birth. Disorders of the skeleton are the commonest of these malformations and comprise approximately one third of all defects. Most of these can be seen or felt and can be verified by roentgenography. However, a number of defects are not immediately apparent on visual examination. About 20% of deaths in the third trimester of gestation and about 15% in the neonatal period may be attributed to gross congenital malformations. Prompt diagnosis of the anomalies as soon as the patient is born may enable life-saving medical and surgical treatment to be instituted.

Polyhydramnios

See Chapter 6.

A congenital anomaly should be suspected if the mother has either polyhydramnios or oligohydramnios. Congenital anomalies associated with hydramnios follow:
A. Anencephaly
B. Hydrocephaly
C. Microcephaly
D. Spina bifida
E. Mongolism
F. Volvulus
   1. With atretic upper jejunum
   2. With congenital bands of upper jejunum
   3. With common mesentery and herniation of liver
G. Tracheoesophageal fistula with atretic esophagus
H. Imperforate anus
I. Cleft palate
J. Congenital heart disease
K. Pyloric stenosis
L. Genitourinary disease
M. Deformed extremities
N. Agenesis of ears (Oligohydramnios is frequently associated with renal agensis or other anomalies of the genitourinary tract. See further.)
O. Neuromuscular disorders

Choanal atresia and laryngeal stenosis

During the initial appraisal of the newborn particular attention should be paid to the evenness and ease of respiration. If respiratory difficulty is present and persists after pharyngeal suctioning, choanal atresia or laryngeal stenosis should be suspected. Although rare, these anomalies are emergencies. Choanal atresia is a bony or membranous obstruction between the nose and pharynx (p. 463). Clinically, although the airway from the mouth to the larynx is patent, this anomaly may result in complete respiratory obstruction, since infants are obligatory nose breathers. Respiratory difficulty at birth may require intubation and artificial ventilation. However, this anomaly usually presents as respiratory distress or apnea after the onset of breathing at 5 to 10 minutes of age. Once breathing is established, choanal atresia is diagnosed by occluding the mouth and the right or left nostril. It may also be diagnosed by inserting a catheter first into one nostril and then into the other, then ventromedially along the floor of the nose. The catheter should pass with ease for 3 to 4 cm. A temporary airway should be promptly provided. This is best achieved by inserting a small plastic infant airway between the tongue and the palate. Once ventilation is established, the infant will then breathe through his mouth while awake. During sleep, however, he will attempt to revert to his obligatory nose breathing. If laryngeal stenosis is present, it will be recognized immediately when the glottis is visualized with the laryngoscope. Immediate tracheostomy is imperative. Under these emergency conditions this is most easily done through the cricothyroid membrane.

Diaphragmatic hernia and congenital adenomatous lung cysts

A diaphragmatic hernia with abdominal viscera (p. 488) in the chest or congenital cysts of the lungs (p. 455) may cause immediate respiratory difficulty. The lungs may be hypoplastic if the diaphragmatic hernia is large and bilateral. These two congenital anomalies are likely to be diagnosed during the course of resuscitation. Following intubation for respiratory difficulty, strong resistance is felt when an attempt is made to expand the lungs by positive pressure. Two other conditions must be considered in the differential diagnosis of this type of respiratory obstruction: massive aspiration of meconium that cannot be removed by suctioning and intrauterine pneumonia with organization of exudate. Infants with hypoplastic lungs or congenital adenomatous cysts of the lungs may be vigorous initially and score as high as 7 at 1 minute of age, making strenuous but ineffective respiratory efforts. In contrast, infants with meconium aspiration or intrauterine pneumonia are usually severely depressed at birth. Congenital adenomatous cysts of the lungs may be associated with hydrops.

A small or unilateral diaphragmatic hernia may not be apparent initially. However, with deep respiratory efforts additional gut may be drawn into the thorax from the abdomen and prevent lung expansion on one side. This is usually manifested in the first 10 to 15 minutes of life as respiratory difficulty and may be verified by observing asymmetry of chest movements and diminution or absence of air sounds on the affected side. In some circumstances the diaphragmatic hernia is not apparent for the first 30 to 60 minutes of life or even later. Manifestation of the anomaly in these instances appears to be dependent on the infant's swallowing air and the gradual distention of gut in the thorax by this swallowed air.

Tracheoesophageal fistula

Atresia of the esophagus with tracheoesophageal fistula should be looked for in every baby (p. 496). As soon as good ventilation is established, a catheter should be introduced into the mouth on either the left or right side of the tongue and advanced down into the esophagus and stomach. The outline of the tip of the catheter is usually seen in the left half of the abdomen as it is gently advanced. If not, the examiner's hand is placed over the upper quadrant, and a puff of air is blown into the catheter. A bubble is immediately felt. It may also be detected by listening over the stomach with a stethoscope. If the catheter does not enter the stomach, the esophagus probably ends in a blind pouch. The longer this anomaly remains undiagnosed the greater is the risk of aspiration pneumonia. In rare instances a fistula occurs with a patent esophagus. This condition is difficult to diagnose. The anomaly should be suspected if the infant coughs during feeding. It may be verified using a barium swallow and cineradiography.

Anomalies of the upper gastrointestinal tract

If complete intestinal obstruction is above the midjejunum, the stomach may contain a large volume of fluid (Chapter 24). The average volume of fluid found in healthy infants delivered by the vaginal route is 5.7 ml (range, 1 to 20 ml); for those delivered in breech position, 4.3 ml; and for those delivered by cesarean section, 7.2 ml (range, 0 to 50 ml). The smallest amount of fluid that has been associated with a high gastrointestinal obstruction is 38 ml. A catheter should be passed into the newborn's stomach and the contents removed. If more than 15 ml of fluid are present in the stomach, a roentgenogram of the abdomen should be obtained during the first 3 hours of life to detect the presence of gas. The absence of gas below the pylorus may indicate obstruction and necessitate early exploration. Under normal circumstances the upper intestine is filled with air within 3 hours. When obstruction is present, the roentgenogram has an even, flat, opaque appearance. A small amount of contrast air is seen only in the stomach and duodenum. Duodenal or jejunal atresia, malrotation of the gut, or an annular pancreas may be the cause.

High gastrointestinal obstructions should be suspected if the mother has polyhydramnios. Normally there is a constant equilibrium of amniotic fluid between the mother and baby. Swallowing of fluid by the fetus and subsequent absorption from his intestinal tract into the circulation is one of the principal modes by which fluid returns to the placenta and finally to the mother. Any anomaly of the gastrointestinal tract that interferes with this process may cause amniotic fluid to accumulate and produce polyhydramnios. CNS anomalies that interfere with swallowing may also produce polyhydramnios. In these cases as much as 170 ml of fluid has been aspirated from the baby's stomach.

Perforation of the stomach by a catheter may occur in the newborn period, but this is rare (Chapter 24) provided that the catheter used for gastric aspiration is soft and flexible.

Anal atresia

A catheter should be used to rule out anal atresia (p. 508). With the infant's thighs flexed, the catheter should be introduced through the anal opening as far as it can be easily passed. If it passes for 3 cm, obstruction is unlikely.

Skeletal anomalies

Anomalies of the skeleton are usually readily verified visually or by palpation. The association between chromosomal abnormalities and congenital defects particularly relates to the skeletal system. The anterior fontanel is normally open and should be palpated for size and tension. Bulging is diagnostic of increased intracranial pressure and may indicate hydrocephalus and intracranial hemorrhage. The posterior fontanel is normally closed and is frequently difficult to outline because of scalp edema and molding of the sutures. A small or closed anterior fontanel occurs in craniosynostosis (p. 382) and is not infrequently accompanied by microcephaly or an abnormally shaped head. Soft spots in the skull (craniotabes), usually located in the parietal areas, are present in about one third of all newborns. Rarely, a cranial bone may be absent, indicating osteogenesis imperfecta. The sacral region should be examined for pigmentation and abnormal hair, which is commonly associated with occult spina bifida.

Cleft palate

The mouth should be carefully examined for the presence of a cleft palate. This may occur even if the upper lip is normal. A small-sized laryngoscope with a premature blade is an ideal instrument with which to visualize both the hard and soft palate. The extent of the defects may vary from a small round hole to a large triangular opening with the base at the site of the uvula. Although treatment for this anomaly is not an emergency, feeding problems and an increased risk of aspiration may be anticipated.

Anomalies of the genitourinary system

Malformations of the external ear are associated with renal anomalies. If the ears are low set or the configuration is deformed, the infant should be closely observed for the passage of urine. The abdomen should be carefully palpated, both for the verification of normal position of the liver and spleen and for the presence of abnormal masses. In the first few minutes of life, before the infant has swallowed sufficient gas to distend the gut and while the tone of the abdominal wall is somewhat reduced, the kidneys may be readily felt for verification of their normal position, size, and shape. Congenital obstruction of the bladder outlet or urethra will usually be associated with a distended bladder readily palpable as a firm, central, dome-shaped structure in the lower abdomen. Finally the umbilical, inguinal, and femoral regions should be examined for hernias. The presence of both testes in the scrotum should be determined and the possibility of hypospadias should be evaluated.

PROGNOSIS

The outcome of a difficult and complex resuscitation is not always a happy one. With the introduction of new life-saving techniques that include more effective and efficient artificial ventilation, cardiac massage, and correction of pH, we now have the means of salvaging infants with brain damage who would otherwise have died. The decision not to resuscitate a severely brain-damaged infant is extremely difficult. The answer to this dilemma undoubtedly lies in the development of better means of diagnosing congenital anomalies, assessing the fetal condition before the onset of labor, measuring the capacity of the placenta to support the infant during labor, and evaluating the fetus as labor progresses. These measures will provide the obstetrician with more information from which he can make the best judgment to deliver the infant in optimum condition. When these advances in preventive medicine are achieved and introduced into obstetric practice, the birth of severely asphyxiated infants requiring a complex resuscitation should become a rare occurrence.

L. Stanley James

BIBLIOGRAPHY

Adamsons, K., Gandy, G., and James, L.S.: The influence of thermal factors upon oxygen consumption of the newborn infant, J. Pediatr **66:**495, 1965.

Adamsons, K., and others: The treatment of acidosis with alkali and glucose during asphyxia in fetal rhesus monkeys, J. Physiol. (London). **169:**679, 1963.

Adamsons, K., and others: Resuscitation by positive pressure ventilation and tris-hydroxymethyl-aminomethane of rhesus monkeys asphyxiated at birth, J. Pediatr. **65:**807, 1964.

Apgar, V., and James, L.S.: Further observations on the newborn scoring system, AM. J. Dis. Child. **104:**419, 1962.

Apgar, V., and others: Evaluation of the newborn infant—second report, J.A.M.A. **168:**1985, 1958.

Baker, D.H., Berdon, W.E., and James, L.S.: Proper localization of umbilical, arterial and venous catheters by lateral roentgenograms, Pediatrics **43:**34, 1969.

Banker, B.Q., and Larroche, J.: Periventricular leucomalacia of infancy, Arch. Neurol. **7:**386, 1962.

Bland, R.D., Clark, T.I., and Harden, L.B.: Rapid infusion of sodium bicarbonate and albumin into high-risk premature infants soon after birth: a controlled, prospective trial, Am. J. Obstet. Gynecol. **124:**263, 1976.

Cockburn, F., and others: The effect of pentobarbital anesthesia on resuscitation and brain damage in fetal rhesus monkeys asphyxiated on delivery, J. Pediatr. **75:**281, 1969.

Cohn, H.E., and others: Cardiovascular responses to hypoxemia and acidemia in fetal lambs, Am. J. Obstet. Gynecol. **120:**817, 1974.

Cole, V.A., and others: Pathogenesis of intraventricular haemorrhage in newborn infants, Arch. Dis. Child. **49:**772, 1974.

Corbet, A.J., and others: Controlled trial of bicarbonate therapy in high-risk premature newborn infants, J. Pediatr. **91:**771, 1977.

Daniel, S.S., and James, L.S.: Abnormal renal function in the newborn, J. Pediatr. **38:**856, 1976.

Daniel, S.S., and others: Analeptics and resuscitation of asphyxiated monkeys, Br. Med. J. **2:**562, 1966.

Finberg, L., Luttrell, C., and Redd, H.: Pathogenesis of lesions in the nervous system in hypernatremic states. II. Experimental studies of gross anatomic changes and alterations of chemical composition of the tissues, Pediatrics **33:**46, 1959.

Gandy, G.M., and others: Thermal environment and acid-base homeostasis in human infants during the first few hours of life, J. Clin. Invest. **43:**751, 1964.

Goldstein, G.W.: Pathogenesis of brain edema and hemorrhage: role of the brain capillary, Pediatrics **96:**357, 1979.

Hagberg, B., and others: Incidence of cerebral palsy according to cause, Acta Paediatr. Scand. **64:**187, 1975.

Haglund, U., and others: The intestinal mucosal lesions in shock, (2 parts), Eur. Surg. Res. **8:**435, 448, 1976.

Harding, R., and others: Cardiovascular changes in new-born lambs during apnoea induced by stimulation of the laryngeal receptors with water, J. Physiol. (Lond.) **256:**35P, 1975.

Hobel, C.J., and others: Early versus late treatment of neonatal acidosis in low birth weight infants: relation to respiratory distress syndrome, J. Pediatr. **81:**1178, 1972.

James L.S.: Acidosis of the newborn and its relation to birth asphyxia, Acta Paediat. (Upps) **49**(suppl. 122):17, 1960.

James L.S.: Physiology of respiration in newborn infants and in the respiratory distress syndrome, Pediatrics **24:**1969, 1969.

James, L.S., and Adamsons, K.: Respiratory physiology of the fetus and newborn infant, N. Engl. J. Med. **271:**1403, 1964.

Leuenberger, P.J., and others: Decrease in angiotensin I conversion by acute hypoxia in dogs, Proc. Soc. Exp. Biol. Med. **158:**586, 1978.

Merritt, T.A., and Farrell, P.M.: Diminished pulmonary lecithin synthesis in acidosis: experimental findings related to RDS, J. Pediatr. **57:**32, 1976.

Moya, F., and others: Hydramnios and congenital anomalies, J.A.M.A. **173:**1552, 1960.

Moya, F., and others: Cardiac massage in the newborn infant through the intact chest, Am. J. Obstet. Gynecol. **84:**798, 1962.

Ostrea, E.M., Jr., and Odell, G.B.: The influence of bicarbonate administration on blood pH in a "closed system": clinical implications, J. Pediatr. **80:**671, 1972.

Rudolph, A.M., and Yuan, D.: Response of the pulmonary vasculature to hypoxia and H^+ ion concentration changes, J. Clin. Invest. **43:**399, 1966.

Russell, G., and Cotton, E.K.: Effects of sodium bicarbonate by rapid injection and of oxygen in high concentration in respiratory distress syndrome of the newborn, Pediatrics **41:**1063, 1968.

Simmons, M.A., and others: Hypernatremia and intracranial hemorrhage in neonates, N. Engl. J. Med. **291:**6, 1974.

Stalcup, S.A., and others: Inhibition of converting enzyme activity by acute hypoxia in dogs, J. Appl. Physiol. **46:**227, 1979.

Steichen, J.J., Kleinman, L.I.: Effect of HCO_3 therapy on acid-base homeostasis in newborn dogs with and without ventilatory restriction, Pediatr. Res. **11:**543, 1977.

Thorne, I.: Cerebral symptoms in the newborn, Acta Paediatr. Scand. (suppl.) 915, 1969.

Usher, R.: Reduction of mortality from respiratory distress syndrome of prematurity with early administration of intravenous glucose and sodium bicarbonate, Pediatrics **32:**966, 1963.

CHAPTER 15 Birth weight, gestational age, and neonatal risk

Neonatal risk, particularly that due to adaptive disorders, is largely a function of the birth weight and gestational age of the newborn. Birth weight is easily measured with an accuracy of ±10 gm in most hospitals and is routinely taken in the delivery room or on admission to the newborn nursery. Gestational age, calculated from the maternal menstrual history, can usually be determined but is sometimes unknown or uncertain. However, gestational age may be estimated by studies of the fetus, amniotic fluid, and newborn. (Methods for prenatal and postnatal estimate of gestational age are reviewed on p. 257.) Thus it is possible to classify babies soon after birth according to *size* (birth weight classes), *age* (gestational age classes), and *size for age* (birth weight for gestational age classes). Many neonatal risks occur much more commonly within some classes of babies than within others. The classification of newborns by weight and gestational age is inherently useful for many descriptive, correlative, and evaluative purposes. Most important for the clinician, the association of neonatal risk (both general and specific) with birth weight and gestational age enables the clinical tasks of *prediction* (prognosis) and *diagnosis* to be performed more skillfully.

CLASSIFICATION OF NEONATES
Classification of babies by birth weight

The Expert Committee on Maternal and Child Health of the World Health Organization has recommended that babies be classified in birth weight groups at 500-gm intervals. A strong argument can be made for the use of narrower class intervals (such as 250 gm), especially below a birth weight of 1,500 gm. The most commonly employed convention is a simple binary classification that distinguishes babies of birth weight of 2,500 gm or less ("low birth weight") from the remaining births. The incidence of low birth weight is generally highest in those countries where the mean birth weight is lowest; it varies from about 5% to 25% of live births. The incidence of low birth weight in the United States Collaborative Perinatal Study was 7.1% for whites and 13.4% for blacks.

Classification of babies by gestational age

Gestational age, calculated from the maternal menstrual history, is expressed in completed weeks (so that 40 weeks = 280 to 286 days). When babies are grouped in gestational age classes, three groups and definitions are suggested: preterm (less than 259 days, that is, less than 37 weeks), term (259 to 293 days, 37 to 41 weeks), and postterm (294 days or more, 42 weeks or more). In contrast to the striking difference between countries with respect to birth weight and its distribution, cross-population differences in length of gestation are quite minor. The incidence of preterm delivery in the United States Collaborative Perinatal Study was 7.1% for whites and 17.9% for blacks. These numbers have not changed significantly in the last decade.

Classification of babies by birth weight for gestational age

By relating the birth weight (or other external dimensions) to the gestational age of the newborn, we assess the *rate* of intrauterine growth. Standards for intrauterine growth have been constructed for several different populations. The difficulties inherent in the construction of an intrauterine growth standard are in some respects similar to those encountered in the construction of the postnatal growth standard but in other respects are unique. A problem common to establishing both prena-

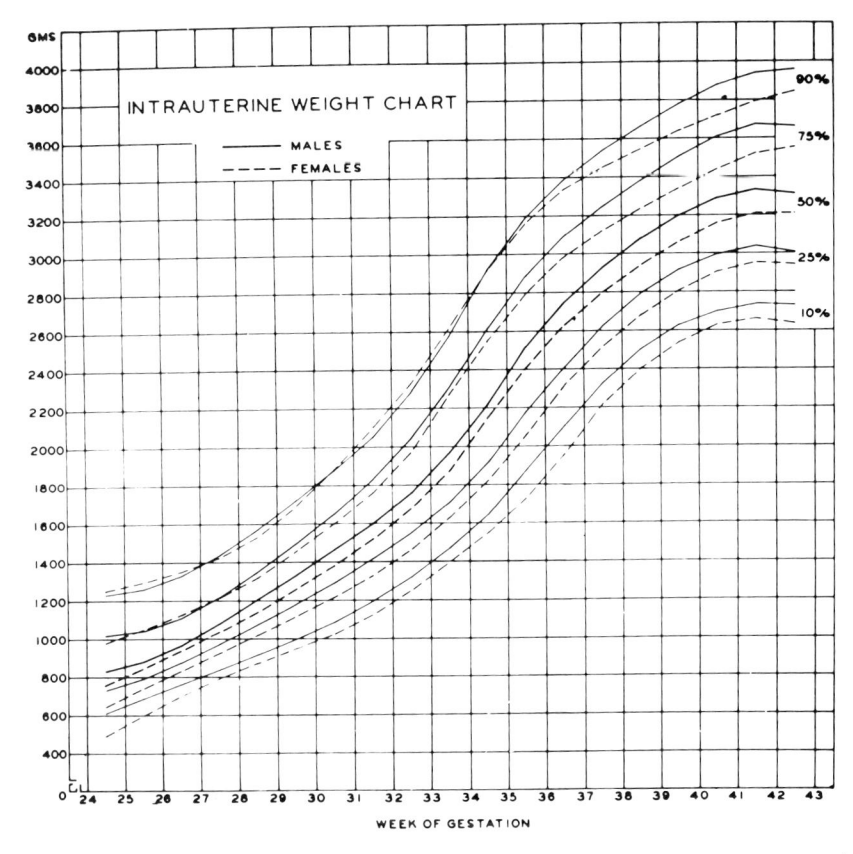

Fig. 15-1. Percentile distribution of birth weight for gestational age. (From Lubchenco, L.O., and others: Pediatrics **32:**794, 1963.)

tal and postnatal growth standards is that of defining a "normal" population. When an intrauterine growth standard is constructed, multiple births and babies with major congenital malformations are usually excluded. (Often other possibly deviant groups are excluded as well, such as infants of diabetic or toxemic mothers.) For prenatal as for postnatal growth, there is a sex-related difference in growth rate, so that sex-specific standards for intrauterine growth are necessary. A difficulty unique to the measurement of fetal size and growth rate is that the normal population is inaccessible for direct, serial measurement. This problem is being partly overcome by the application of new techniques, such as ultrasound (p. 81). In general, however, measurement of fetal size is limited to measurement of size at birth. The assumption is made that those babies born at a given gestational age are representative of those of the same age who are still in the uterus. Tanner argues that this assumption may be weak when the length of pregnancy is particularly deviant (for example, when gestational age is less than 32 weeks).

A widely used American intrauterine growth standard is given in Fig. 15-1. For each gestational age in the range from 24 to 42 weeks, the tenth, twenty-fifth, fifti-

Table 15-1. Variation in fetal growth: weights for boys at 40 weeks' gestational age

Author	Country	Median (gm)	Tenth percentile (gm)
Bjerkedahl and others (1973)	Norway	3,650	3,080
Sterky and others (1970)	Sweden	3,630*	3,040
Thomson and others (1968)	UK	3,560	2,980
1958 British Perinatal Mortality Survey	UK	3,460	2,920
Lubchenco and others (1963)	USA	3,290	2,700
Freeman and others (1970)	USA	3,210	2,680

*Mean value.

eth, seventy-fifth and ninetieth percentiles of newborn weight have been calculated. The percentile points have been joined by graphic smoothing. Similar charts are available relating newborn length and head circumference to gestational age. However, considerable difference exists between various population standards for intrauterine growth (Table 15-1); Norwegian and Swedish babies are about 350 gm heavier at term than the Denver babies described by Lubchenco (p. 49).

The size-for-age relationship displayed in Fig. 15-1 defines three classes of newborn infants: birth weight in the tenth to ninetieth percentiles (appropriate for gestational age, AGA), birth weight above the ninetieth percentile (large for gestational age, LGA), and birth weight below the tenth percentile (small for gestational age, SGA). There is a lack of agreement as to the class limits of size for age that should be applied when designating babies as appropriate, large, or small for gestational age. This uncertainty arises because (1) there are considerable differences between populations in the rate of fetal growth and (2) nonuniform practices have been used to express within-population variation (standard deviation [SD] or percentile distribution) and to define cutoff points for limiting the normal range (for example, third, fifth, or tenth percentile, −2 SD).

Given the large differences between various standards for fetal growth (Table 15-1), what standard should be used in evaluating the growth of an individual baby? There are two alternatives: either to use the fetal growth standard constructed on the population from which the baby was drawn and to adjust the standard, when possible, for demographic factors known to be associated with systematic deviations in growth rate; or to use a universal "ideal" standard, constructed on a population known to be healthy and of lowest risk (for example, the Norwegian or Swedish standards). Systematic differences in fetal growth have been described in association with maternal size, birth order, sibling weight, social class, maternal smoking habit, and other factors. The impact of each factor on fetal growth has been quantitated (p. 55). Methods have been devised for the adjustment (upward and downward) of the population intrauterine growth standard for maternal size, birth order, and sibling weight. These practices may provide more accurate and potentially useful assessments of deviant fetal growth. For example, within-family standards for birth weight identify more babies with rubella embryopathy as having had fetal growth retardation than do the conventional population birth weight standards. In general, it remains to be determined how much of the variation in birth weight between various subgroups is due to extrafetal (environmental) factors rather than to genetic differences in growth potential. Much more work needs to be done before we are in a position to confidently evaluate a baby's fetal growth in relation to his genetic growth potential.

NEONATAL MORTALITY

Neonatal mortality (number of deaths before 28 days of age per 1,000 live births) is highly dependent on birth weight. Fig. 15-2 shows the relationship between neonatal mortality and birth weight in data reported separately from New York, Baltimore, Denver, and Portland (Ore.). As birth weight increases from 500 to 3,000 gm, there is a fairly strict logarithmic decrease in neonatal mortality. Neonatal mortality is lowest in babies weighing between 3 and 4 kg at birth and then rises among babies of very high birth weight.

Neonatal mortality is also highly dependent on gestational age (Fig. 15-3). For every increase of 2 weeks in

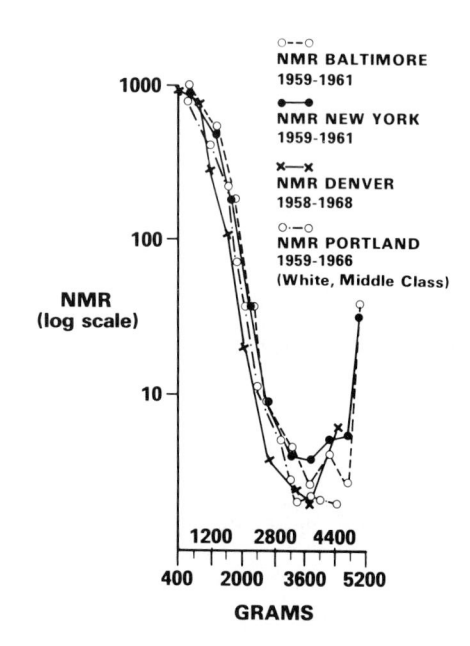

Fig. 15-2. Neonatal mortality (number of neonatal deaths under 28 days per 1,000 live births) by birth weight. The Denver data are limited to live-born infants delivered at the University of Colorado Medical Center.

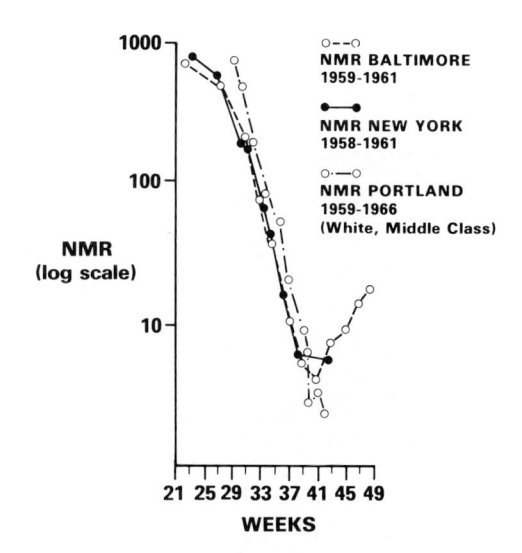

Fig. 15-3. Neonatal mortality (number of neonatal deaths under 28 days per 1,000 live births) by gestational age.

gestational age, from 25 to 37 weeks, neonatal mortality decreases by approximately half. The lowest neonatal mortality occurs in babies of 37 to 41 weeks' gestational age. From Figs. 15-2 and 15-3 it can be seen that there is no sharp break in the decline in mortality at either 2,500 gm or 37 weeks' gestational age. Therefore these values, although widely used demographically in the classification of babies by birth weight and gestational age, do not have unique biologic meaning. Recent data on the outcome of very low birth weight infants is seen in Table 15-2.

Since most neonatal mortality occurs within the first hours and days after birth, the outlook improves rapidly with increasing postnatal survival. Kitchen and Gaudry have shown how increasing postnatal age improves the potential for survival of babies in their nursery weighing 1,500 gm or less, particularly among those with respiratory distress syndrome (RDS) (hyaline membrane disease) (Fig. 15-4). It should be noted, however, that recent advances in perinatal care have resulted in an extension of the mortality period beyond the first days of life and even into the postnatal period.

Neonatal morbidity follows the same pattern as neonatal mortality, with babies in the highest mortality zones also showing the highest morbidity. Such data are useful in identifying those babies in need of special care, in determining the required capacity, equipment, and staffing of special care units, and in evaluating cost-benefit and other measures of the impact of perinatal service programs.

SPECIFIC NEONATAL RISKS BY BIRTH WEIGHT AND GESTATIONAL AGE

The incidence of certain neonatal risks varies greatly according to birth weight, gestational age, and birth weight for gestational age. Small babies, whether born prematurely or SGA, are poorly insulated against heat loss and are therefore at risk of hypothermia when placed in an environment providing thermal comfort for larger, better insulated babies. Conversely, babies who are very large, regardless of gestational age, have a higher incidence of birth injuries, such as cervical and brachial plexus injury, phrenic nerve damage with paralysis of the diaphragm, fractured clavicle, cephalhematoma, and ecchymosis of the head and face. Preterm babies are predisposed to a large number of special neonatal risks. These include RDS, recurrent apnea, infection, hypoglycemia, hypocalcemia, hyperbilirubinemia, necrotizing enterocolitis, and intraventricular hemorrhage (IVH). Babies who are born post term are at special risk for perinatal asphyxia, meconium aspiration, and pneumothorax. SGA babies also have increased risk of perinatal

Table 15-2. Survival to discharge of very low birth weight infants born to Hamilton-Wentworth residents, 1964-1969 versus 1973-1977

	1964-1969		1973-1977	
Birth weight	Livebirths (number)	Survival (number [%])	Livebirths (number)	Survival (number [%])
500-999 gm	160	17 (11)	98	22 (22)
1,000-1,499 gm	213	133 (62)	167	129 (77)
Totals	373	150 (40)	265	151 (57)

From Horwood, S.P., and others: Pediatrics **69**:613, 1982. Copyright American Academy of Pediatrics 1982.

Fig. 15-4. Nomogram for prediction of survival of infants weighing 1,000 to 1,500 gm with respiratory distress syndrome. (From Kitchen, W.H., and Gaudry, E.: Aust. Pediatr. J. **10**:282, 1974.)

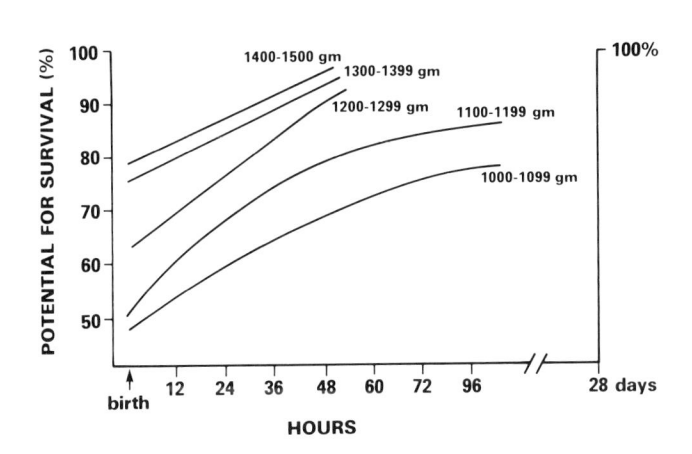

asphyxia and its sequelae; in addition, they show an increased incidence of symptomatic hypoglycemia, polycythemia, congenital malformation, chronic intrauterine infection, and massive pulmonary hemorrhage. Babies born to diabetic mothers are often LGA. The infant of the diabetic mother (Chapter 33, part one) is especially prone to RDS, hypoglycemia, hypocalcemia, and hyperbilirubinemia.

Several important factors may affect the reported incidence of neonatal risks. These include the nature of the clinical service, the diagnostic criteria applied, and the increasing impact of preventive antenatal and intrapartum care in reducing the incidence of neonatal disorders. The experience of a referral unit dealing with selected high-risk pregnancies or sick babies will differ greatly from a unit dealing with a less selected population. Both diagnostic criteria and surveillance methods differ between centers, as applied to the clinical recognition of neonatal conditions such as RDS, patent ductus arteriosus (PDA), major and minor congenital malformations, and necrotizing enterocolitis. Incidence figures based on mortality approximate the true incidence for highly fatal conditions such as massive pulmonary hemorrhage or massive IVH. However, reporting of mortality figures will variably underestimate the true incidence of conditions such as RDS, whose case fatality rate is highly responsive to the quality of neonatal care. Improved antenatal and intrapartum care can substantially reduce the incidence of neonatal morbidity due to birth asphyxia, RDS, hypoglycemia, and other disorders.

Congenital malformations

Estimates of the incidence of congenital malformations in all live births vary widely, ranging from 1% to 7% (Chapter 38). McIntosh and associates show that less than half of malformations diagnosed during infancy are suspected or noted at birth. The incidence of malformations is higher in infants of low birth weight than in all live births; this increase is due to a higher malformation rate both in preterm births and in full-term small for dates (SFD) infants. Van den Berg and Yerushalmy computed the incidence of nontrivial and severe malformations among 367 infants of birth weights of 1,600 to 2,500 gm divided into gestational quartiles (Table 15-3). Infants whose intrauterine growth rates were slowest were found to have a striking increase in incidence of malformations.

The overall incidence of congenital heart disease is at least 7.7 per 1,000 live births (Chapter 25). The incidence of ventricular septal defect is much higher in infants of birth weight less than 2,500 gm or gestational age less than 34 weeks, or both, than among infants larger or gestationally older at birth. However, spontaneous closure of the defect occurs with the same incidence among low birth weight infants as among full-size babies

Table 15-3. Incidence of congenital malformations by gestation quartiles in infants of birth weights of 1,600 to 2,500 gm

Gestation quartiles (weeks)	Type of malformation	
	Severe (%)	Nontrivial (%)
33-35	3	12
35-37	3	6
37-39	3	12
39-41	16	22

with ventricular septal defect. Except for PDA (see further), there is little information on the incidence of other specific cardiac lesions by birth weight and gestational age classes. Babies with transposition of the great vessels have a mean birth weight that is higher than that of babies with other cyanotic cardiac lesions, but the difference is not large enough to be of reliable clinical value. Babies with chromosomal anomalies (such as trisomy 21 or trisomy 18) and babies with congenital rubella infection have a very high incidence of congenital heart disease and tend to be SGA. Babies with surgical lesions, such as meconium ileus and other causes of intestinal obstruction, and those with gastroschisis and omphalocele are often born prematurely, especially if hydramnios is present, and are sometimes SGA.

Patent ductus arteriosus

Persistent patency of the ductus arteriosus beyond the third day of life has been noted frequently in low birth weight infants, particularly in those with pulmonary disorders (p. 438 and Chapter 25). Siassi and associates studied 100 consecutively born preterm infants surviving at least to the third day and weighing 2,000 gm or less at birth and another 50 consecutively born babies with birth weights of 2,001 to 2,500 gm. In these groups they found an overall incidence of clinically diagnosed PDA of 21%. The incidence of PDA was related inversely to increasing gestational age and birth weight (Fig. 15-5). In common with other investigators, they found a high degree of association between PDA and respiratory distress syndrome. Spontaneous closure of the ductus occurred in 79% of affected infants that survived the neonatal period.

Respiratory distress syndrome

RDS remains the most important cause of morbidity and mortality among anatomically normal infants during the first few days of life. The occurrence of RDS has been tabulated on the basis of both its clinical diagnosis and its pathologic diagnosis in those who die. The incidence of the clinical disorder is highest in babies of shortest gestation and falls progressively with increasing gestational

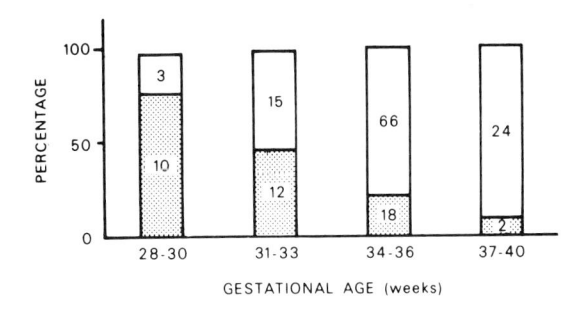

Fig. 15-5. Incidence of persistent patency of patent ductus arteriosus (PDA) in relation to gestational age and birth weight. Numbers within bars indicate number of infants with and without PDA. (From Siassi, B., and others: Pediatrics **57:**348, 1976.)

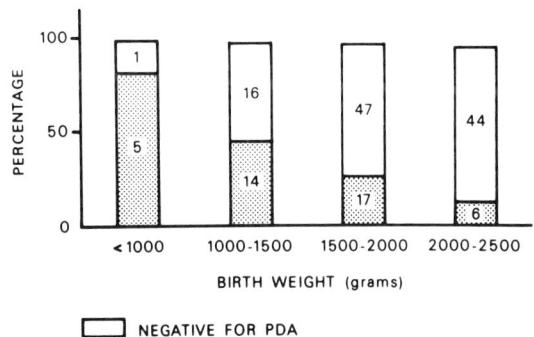

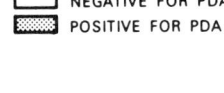

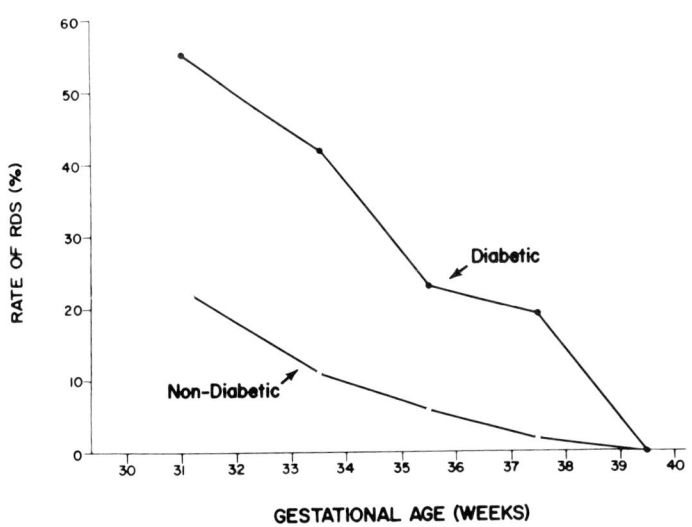

Fig. 15-6. Incidence of RDS related to gestational age in diabetic and nondiabetic pregnancy. (From Robert, M.F., and others: N. Engl. J. Med. **294:**357, 1976. Reprinted by permission of the New England Journal of Medicine.)

age. The disorder is very rare in babies born within 2 weeks of term. Preterm infants who have experienced chronic fetal stress and are retarded in body growth have a lower than expected incidence of RDS; conversely, infants of diabetic mothers (who are often LGA) have a much increased risk (Fig. 15-6).

The antenatal prediction of risk of RDS is crucially important in the weighing of neonatal versus fetal risk in those clinical situations where elective early delivery is considered. In the past, prediction of RDS risk was based mainly on gestational age. This practice has now been superseded by the assessment of fetal lung maturity from the amniotic fluid lecithin/sphingomyelin (L/S) ratio (p. 134) (Fig. 15-7). The increased accuracy of this approach, together with the possibility of enhancing fetal lung maturity with corticosteroids in fetuses at risk, makes it likely that a sizable reduction in incidence of RDS can be achieved.

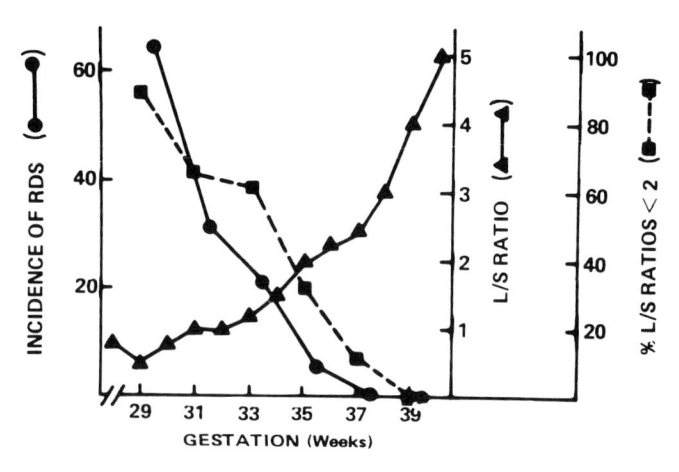

Fig. 15-7. Relationship between incidence of RDS, ratio of lecithin/sphingomyelin (L/S) in amniotic fluid, and gestational age. (From Farrell, P.M., and Avery, M.E.: Am. Rev. Resp. Dis. **111**:657, 1975.)

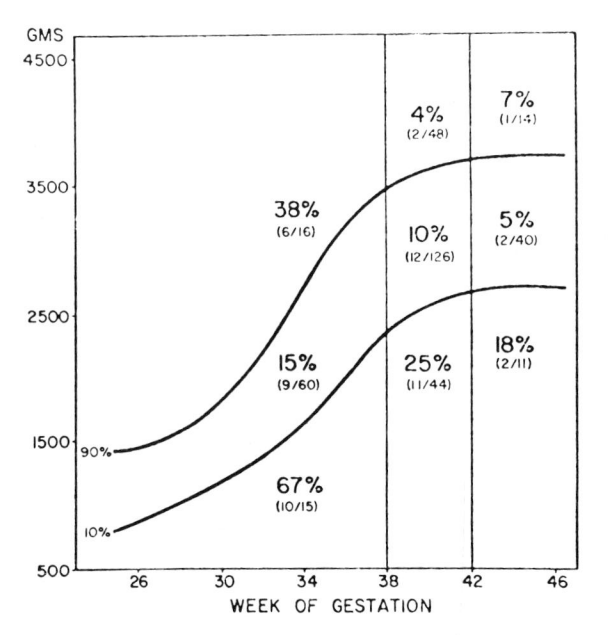

Fig. 15-8. Incidence of hypoglycemia by birth weight and gestational age. (Glucose levels <30 mg/100 ml before first feeding at about 3 to 6 hours of age.) The tenth and ninetieth percentiles of birth weight for gestational age are shown. (From Lubchenco, L.O., and Bard, H.: Pediatrics **47**:832, 1971.)

Disturbances in glucose homeostasis

The recognition by Cornblath and associates that babies who develop symptomatic neonatal *hypoglycemia* tend to be SGA provided much early impetus to the study of neonatal risks in relation to birth weight and gestational age. In the case of hypoglycemia it was soon learned that babies could have low blood glucose concentrations with no apparent symptoms ("asymptomatic hypoglycemia"). Therefore there has been considerable uncertainty as to the diagnostic criteria to be applied. Cornblath and Schwartz surveyed a nursery population and found that the lower end of the normal range (2 SD below the mean) for blood glucose during the first few days of life was 30 mg/100 ml for full-size babies and 20 mg/100 ml for low birth weight babies. However, these values may be unphysiologically low for the newborn, and a lower limit of 40 mg/100 ml, regardless of birth weight, has been proposed. Pildes and associates found that 5.7% of low birth weight infants showed two consecutive blood glucose concentrations below 20 mg/100 ml; all such babies were symptomatic, and symptoms disappeared during glucose administration. Lubchenco and Bard measured the blood glucose concentration before the first feeding at 3 to 6 hours of age in babies classified into 9 birth weight/gestational age groups (Fig. 15-8). A particularly high incidence of hypoglycemia was reported for SGA term infants (25%) and for SGA preterm infants (67%). Lugo and Cassady also found that SGA infants have a high incidence of hypoglycemia (12% in their series) compared with their gestational age peers (6%) and birth weight peers (8%). The infant of the diabetic mother (both gestational diabetic and insulin dependent) has a high incidence of neonatal hypoglycemia that is usually transient and asymptomatic. Such infants are usually LGA and are often preterm. See also Chapter 33, part one.

Hyperglycemia is a common problem in extremely premature infants receiving intravenous glucose infusion and occasionally in SGA infants (Chapter 33, part one). Dweck and Cassady showed that 43 of 50 infants of birth weights less than 1,100 gm developed hyperglycemia (blood glucose >125 mg/100 ml) while receiving an IV glucose infusion of 6 mg/kg/minute. Babies with the uncommon syndrome of transient neonatal diabetes are generally SGA.

Recurrent apnea

Apnea is usually defined as cessation of breathing for more than 15-20 seconds or cessation of breathing prolonged enough to produce cyanosis and/or bradycardia (p. 456). Buckfield used this definition when surveying 6,078 live-born infants grouped according to Yerushalmy's classification (Table 15-4). There was a very high incidence of recurrent apnea in babies under 1,500 gm. Buckfield's study includes babies with apnea that was symptomatic of a disease process. Other studies have shown babies under 32 weeks gestational age to be at an even higher risk.

Necrotizing enterocolitis

Necrotizing enterocolitis, formerly an uncommonly diagnosed illness, is now being recognized with alarming

Table 15-4. Incidence of recurrent apnea

Birth weight (gm)	Gestational age (weeks)	Total babies (number)	Babies with apnea (number)	Incidence (percent)
<1,500	All	63	34	54.0
1,500-2,500	<37	144	14	9.8
1,500-2,500	>37	113	0	0
>2,500	<37	90	8	3.3
>2,500	>37	5,115	8	0.2

Table 15-5. Incidence of necrotizing enterocolitis, McMaster University Medical Centre Neonatal Unit, 1973 to 1975

Birth weight class (gm)	Inborn	Outborn
<1,500	6/76 (8%)	15/140 (11%)
1,500-2,499	5/152 (3%)	10/145 (7%)
≥2,500	2/441 (0.5%)	6/151 (4%)

Data from Yu, V.Y.H., Tudehope, D.I., and Gill, G.J.: Med. J. Aust. **1**(19):685, 1977.

frequency in neonatal intensive care units (p. 512). The incidence of the condition varies greatly between centers and is highest in babies of lowest birth weight. Table 15-5 gives the incidence of the condition in the special care Neonatal Unit at McMaster University Medical Centre. The criteria for diagnosis included the clinical syndrome of abdominal distention, delayed gastric emptying, and blood in stool, and, in addition, either definite intramural gas on abdominal roentgenogram or pathologic confirmation of the diagnosis. The highest incidence was seen among babies below 1,500 gm birth weight. An incidence as high as 27% has been reported among babies of birth weights of less than 1,200 gm cared for in a referral center receiving mostly babies born elsewhere.

USES OF THE CLASSIFICATION OF BABIES BY BIRTH WEIGHT AND GESTATIONAL AGE
Description

The birth weight/gestational age classification allows the association of a variety of antecedents or outcomes with the distribution of gestational age, birth weight, or weight for age. The preceding section contains many examples of the descriptive value of the classification in relation to neonatal outcomes.

Prediction (prognosis)

The *prediction of general risk* of neonatal mortality or morbidity by birth weight and gestational age classes allows the identification of *groups* of neonates at increased risk at birth who would benefit most from admission to a special care nursery and aids in the formulation of nursery policies for the care of the high-risk infant (such as admission to a special care unit or screening for hypoglycemia). On the other hand, the clinician or parent who wishes to know, in absolute terms, the prognosis of an *individual baby* is very unlikely to obtain a valid answer from a table of neonatal mortality by birth weight and gestational age classes. The three most important reasons for this are (1) the individual baby and his environment may not be typical of the population on which the table was constructed; (2) no existing table can reflect the continuing trend favoring better outcome of the high-risk infant; (3) most tables reflect prognosis at birth and cannot be applied to older infants without adjustment for improving prognosis with increasing postnatal age.

Characteristic associations of specific neonatal risks with gestational age and birth weight allow the clinician, in *predicting specific risk* (such as RDS or neonatal hypoglycemia), to anticipate their occurrence and employ appropriate techniques for prevention and treatment. For example, babies under 32 weeks' gestational age, because of their high incidence of recurrent apnea, are expectantly monitored for apneic spells. Babies under 2,000 gm birth weight, because of their poor insulation and risk of hypothermia, are expectantly placed in incubators. Babies who are SGA, because of their increased risk of symptomatic hypoglycemia, have their blood glucose concentrations monitored. As the science of neonatal pediatrics advances, there is decreasing reason to base prediction of specific neonatal outcomes solely on gestational age class or birth weight class. For example, although the incidence of RDS is correlated (inversely) with both gestational age and with birth weight the measurement of the L/S ratio in amniotic fluid (p. 134) greatly improves the predictive accuracy in pregnancies at high risk.

Diagnosis

Consideration of the baby's birth weight and gestational age often can help in weighing diagnostic possibilities. For example, consider the baby with the symptom complex of tachypnea, grunting, chest retractions, and cyanosis. If the baby is preterm, RDS is a more likely possibility than meconium aspiration; if the baby is term or postterm, the reverse is true. However, the clinician should be cautioned against overplaying this approach to diagnosis. It is the individual baby's condition that must be diagnosed. *Preoccupation with probabilities based on birth weight and gestational age should not be allowed to intrude into the more relevant process of an objective diagnostic evaluation of the individual baby.*

Correlation

Birth weight and its distribution are readily measured and recorded variables that have been used in a variety of correlative studies, not only in perinatology but also in epidemiology and demography. For example, birth weight has been found to be highly correlated with selected independent variables at a community level and may prove more useful and effective than infant mortality statistics for many purposes for which death data are now used.

Evaluation

Neonatal outcome is highly correlated with birth weight and gestational age. To evaluate outcome, whether in the context of clinical research, audit of a neonatal unit's performance over time, or comparison between different units, it is crucial to take into account the impact of the distribution of birth weight and gestational age in affecting the observed outcome. Techniques exist ("prognostic stratification") for minimizing the difficulties in evaluation that arise because of differences (for example, between treatment groups, between years, or between regions) in the distribution of birth weight, gestational age, or any other characteristic that is highly correlated with outcome.

John C. Sinclair
David I. Tudehope

BIBLIOGRAPHY
Classification by birth weight

Niswander, K.R., and Gordon, M.: Collaborative perinatal study: the women and their pregnancies, Philadelphia, 1972, W.B. Saunders Co.

Public health aspects of low birth weight, Third Report of the Expert Committee on Maternal and Child Health, World Health Organization Technical Report Series no. 217, 1961.

Rosa, F.W., and Turshen, M.: Fetal nutrition, Bull. W. H. O. **43**:785, 1970.

Classification by gestational age

Niswander, K.R., and Gordon, M.: Collaborative perinatal study: the women and their pregnancies, Philadelphia, 1972, W.B. Saunders Co.

Working party to discuss nomenclature based on gestational age and birth weight, Arch. Dis. Child. **45**:730, 1970.

World Health Organization Technical Report Series no. 25, 1950.

Classification by birth weight for gestational age

Babson, S.G., Behrman, R.E., and Lessel, R.: Fetal growth: liveborn birth weights for gestational age of white middle class infants, Pediatrics **45**:937, 1970.

Bjerkedahl, T., Bakketeig, L., and Lehmann, E.H.: Percentiles of birth weights of single live births at different gestation periods, Acta Paediatr. Scand. **62**:449, 1973.

Butler, N.R., and Alberman, E.D.: Perinatal problems, Second Report of the 1958 British Perinatal Mortality Survey, Edinburgh, 1969, E. and S. Livingstone Ltd.

Butler, N.R., and Bonham, D.G.: Perinatal mortality, First Report of the 1958 British Perinatal Mortality Survey, Edinburgh, 1963, E. and S. Livingstone Ltd.

Freeman, M.G., Graves, W.L., and Thomson, R.L.: Indigent Negro and Caucasian birth weight gestational age tables, Pediatrics **46**:9, 1970.

Lubchenco, L.O., Hansman, C., and Boyd, E.: Intrauterine growth in length and head circumference as estimated from live births at gestational ages from 26 to 42 weeks, Pediatrics **37**:403, 1966.

Lubchenco, L.O., and others: Intrauterine growth as estimated from liveborn birth weight data at 24 to 42 weeks of gestation, Pediatrics **32**:793, 1963.

Sterky, G.: Swedish standard curves for intrauterine growth, Pediatrics **46**:7, 1970.

Tanner, J.M.: Standards for birth weight or intrauterine growth, Pediatrics **46**:1, 1970.

Tanner, J.M., Lejarraga, H., and Turner, G.: Within family standards for birth weight, Lancet **2**:193, 1972.

Tanner, J.M., and Thomson, A.M.: Standards for birth weight at gestation periods of 32 to 42 weeks allowing for maternal height and weight, Arch. Dis. Child. **45**:566, 1970.

Thomson, A.M., Billewicz, W.Z., and Hytten, F.E.: The assessment of foetal growth, J. Obstet. Gynecol. Br. Commw. **75**:903, 1968.

Usher, R., and McLean, F.: Intrauterine growth of liveborn Caucasian infants at sea level: standards obtained from measurements in 7 dimensions of infants born between 25 and 44 weeks of gestation, J. Pediatr. **74**:901, 1969.

Neonatal mortality by birth weight and gestational age

Battaglia, F.C.: Intrauterine growth retardation, Am. J. Obstet. Gynecol. **106**:1103, 1970.

Battaglia, F.C., Frazier, T.M., and Hellegers, A.E.: Birth weight, gestational age and pregnancy outcome with special reference to the high birth weight, low gestational age infant, Pediatrics **37**:417, 1966.

Behrman, R.E., Babson, G.S., and Lessel, R.: Fetal and neonatal mortality in white middle class infants, Am. J. Dis. Child. **121**:486, 1971.

Erhardt, C.L., and others: Influences of weight and gestation on perinatal and neonatal mortality by ethnic group, Am. J. Public Health **54**:1841, 1964.

Hack, M., and others: Changing trends of neonatal and postneonatal deaths in very low birth weight infants, Am. J. Obstet. Gynecol. **137**:797, 1980.

Horwood, S.P., and others: Mortality and morbidity of 500 to 1499 gram birth weight infants liveborn to residents of a defined geographic region before and after neonatal intensive care, Pediatrics **69**:613, 1982.

Kitchen, W.H., and Guadry, E.: Prediction of survival of very low birth weight infants, Aust. Paediatr. J. **10**:281, 1974.

Lubchenco, L.O., Searls, D.T., and Brazie, J.V.: Neonatal mortality rate: relationship to birth weight and gestational age, J. Pediatr. **81**:814, 1972.

Yerushalmy, J.: The classification of newborn infants by birth weight and gestational age, J. Pediatr. **71**:164, 1967.

Yerushalmy, J.: The low birth weight baby, Hosp. Pract. **3**:62, 1968.

Congenital malformations

McIntosh, R., and others: The incidence of congenital malformations, Pediatrics 14:505, 1954.

Mehrizi, A., and Drash, A.: Birth weight of infants with cyanotic and acyanotic congenital malformations of the heart, J. Pediatr. 59:715, 1961.

Mitchell, S.C., Berendes, H.W., and Clark, W.M.: The normal closure of the ventricular septum, Am. Heart J. 73:334, 1967.

Mitchell, S.C., Korones, S.B., and Berendes, H.W.: Congenital heart disease in 56,109 births, Circulation 43:323, 1971.

Van den Berg, B.J., and Yerushalmy, J.: The relationship of the rate of intrauterine growth of infants of low birth weight to mortality, morbidity, and congenital anomalies, J. Pediatr. 69:531, 1966.

Warkany, J.: Congenital malformations, Chicago, 1971, Year Book Medical Publishers, Inc.

Patent ductus arteriosus

Kitterman, J.A., and others: Patent ductus arteriosus in premature infants, N. Engl. J. Med. 287:473, 1972.

Siassi, B., and others: Incidence and clinical features of patent ductus arteriosus in low birth weight infants, Pediatrics 57:347, 1976.

Respiratory distress syndrome

Dunn, P.M.: The respiratory distress syndrome of the newborn: immaturity versus prematurity, Arch. Dis. Child. 40:62, 1965.

Farrell, P.M., and Avery, M.E.: Hyaline membrane disease, Am. Rev. Resp. Dis. 111:657, 1975.

Fedrick, J., and Butler, N.R.: Certain causes of neonatal death. 1. Hyaline membranes, Biol. Neonate 15:229, 1970.

Miller, H.C., and Fatiakul, P.: Birth weight, gestational age and sex as determining factors in the incidence of respiratory distress syndrome of prematurely born infants, J. Pediatr. 72:628, 1968.

Robert, M.F., and others: Association between maternal diabetes and the respiratory distress syndrome in the newborn, N. Engl. J. Med. 294:359, 1976.

Roberton, N.R.C., and Tizard, J.P.M.: Prognosis for infants with idiopathic respiratory distress syndrome, Br. Med. J. 3:271, 1975.

Usher, R.H., Allen, A.C., and McLean, F.H.: Risk of respiratory distress syndrome related to gestational age, route of delivery, and maternal diabetes, Am. J. Obstet. Gynecol. 111:826, 1971.

Disturbances in glucose homeostasis

Cornblath, M., Odell, G.B., and Levin, E.Y.: Symptomatic neonatal hypoglycemia associated with toxemia of pregnancy, J. Peidatr. 55:545, 1959.

Cornblath, M., and Schwartz, R.: Disorders of carbohydrate metabolism in infancy, Philadelphia, 1966, W.B. Saunders Co.

Dweck, H.S., and Cassady, G.: Glucose intolerance in infants of very low birth weight. 1. Incidence of hypoglycemia in infants of birth weights 1,100 grams or less, Pediatrics 53:189, 1974.

Lubchenco, L.O., and Bard, H.: Incidence of hypoglycemia in newborn infants classified by birth weight and gestational age, Pediatrics 47:831, 1971.

Lugo, G., and Cassady, G.: Intrauterine growth retardation, Am. J. Obstet. Gynecol. 109:615, 1971.

Pagliara, A.S., and others: Hypoglycemia in infancy and childhood (part I), J. Pediatr. 82:365, 1973.

Pildes, R., and others: The incidence of neonatal hypoglycemia—a completed survey, J. Pediatr. 70:76, 1967.

Robert, M.F., and others: Association between maternal diabetes and the respiratory distress syndrome in the newborn, N. Engl. J. Med. 294:357, 1976.

Schiff, D., Colle, E., and Stern, L.: Metabolic and growth patterns of transient neonatal diabetes, N. Engl. J. Med. 287:119, 1972.

Other conditions

Book, L.S., and others: Necrotizing enterocolitis in low birth weight infants fed an elemental formula, J. Pediatr. 87:602, 1975.

Buckfield, P.M.: Neonatal at risk factors, N. Z. Med. J. 75:266, 1972.

Fedrick, J., and Butler, N.R.: Certain causes of neonatal death. II. Massive pulmonary hemorrhage, Biol. Neonate 18:253, 1971.

Fedrick, J., and Butler, N.R.: Certain causes of neonatal death. IV. Massive pulmonary hemorrhage, Biol. Neonate 18:253, 1971.

Haracke, T.M., and others: Perinatal cerebral intraventricular hemorrhage, J. Pediatr. 80:37, 1972.

Yu, V.Y.H., Tudehope, D.I., and Gill, G.J.: Neonatal necrotizing enterocolitis: clinical aspects, Med. J. Austr. 1:685, 1977.

Uses of the classification of babies by birth weight and gestational age

Feinstein, A.R.: Clinical biostatics. XIV. The purposes of prognostic stratification (part I), Clin. Pharmacol. Ther. 13:285, 1972.

Hack, M., Fanaroff, A.A., and Merkatz, I.R.: The low birth weight infant—evaluation of a changing outlook, N. Engl. J. Med. 301:1162, 1979.

Lewis, R., Charles, M., and Patwary, K.M.: Relationships between birth weight and selected social, environmental and medical care factors, Am. J. Public Health 63:973, 1973.

CHAPTER 16 # Placental pathology

Neonatal diagnosis and therapy are greatly enhanced by the availability of the placenta. This organ may reflect many of the intrauterine events that affect the infant's health, and a quick but knowledgeable examination of this organ before it is discarded can save valuable hours of differential diagnosis and laboratory work. The neonatologist should know what the normal placenta looks like so that the pathologic specimen can be recognized immediately.

EXAMINATION

The placenta is examined in the fresh state, before fixation or freezing. Its cord and membranes are positioned to assume approximately the shape they occupied in utero before a systematic examination is begun. The external surface of the membranes, the chorion laeve, is examined for presence of old or fresh blood; the point of rupture of the membranes is noted; and the membranes are trimmed off the edge of the placenta proper. Next, the cord is studied. Its normal position is near the center of the organ; less commonly it inserts at the margin or even on the membranes. If the latter occurred, then the blood vessels that ramify from this velamentous cord must be examined for tears, thrombi, or calcification. The cord is cut and the number of vessels counted on a fresh-cut surface. Next, the fetal surface of the placenta is inspected carefully. Is it shiny, opacified, or discolored? Are there possible needle punctures from amniocentesis, and can nodules of amnion nodosum be identified? Similarly, the surface of the umbilical cord should be inspected for the presence of nodules that may signify *Candida* infection, and its color is noted. Thereafter the placenta should be weighed and the maternal surface inspected after removing the loosely attached jellylike clots that form after delivery. In my experience, a majority of *retroplacental hematomas* are overlooked clinically, and this is the time when they may be recognized. The old retroplacental blood appears brown and has a dry, granular appearance. Often a hue of yellow or green from blood breakdown pigments is present, and the villous tissue beneath may be firmer and infarcted. Calcification is noted as fine yellow stippling and has no known pathologic significance, even when excessive; it connotes maturity of the organ. Finally, the placenta is sectioned into strips with a long, sharp knife. The color is noted, and abnormalities such as infarcts, thrombi, and choriangiomas are both palpated and visualized. Unusual congestion suggests the possibility of maternal glucose intolerance; unusual pallor connotes fetal anemia. At this point sections are taken for fixation and future histologic analysis because some lesions, such as inflammatory ones, often cannot be suspected by macroscopic examination.

MEMBRANES

The inner surface is composed of the amnion. It can easily be stripped off the chorion; such disruption occurs often at the time of delivery, so inspection of the sac may be confusing. The amnion contains no blood vessels, and its integrity depends on nutrition from the underlying chorion and its adjacent tissue. Between amnion and chorion lies the yolk sac whose minute (0.3 cm) yellow remnants must not be considered a pathologic lesion. The chorionic sac is covered on the outside by remains of villi, trophoblast enmeshed in fibrin, and decidua capsularis. The latter often shows extensive degeneration and is yellow and friable. The membranes may tear with greater or lesser ease at examination, but this feature has not been correlated with any specific pathologic lesion and is not indicative of inflammation or time of rupture of membranes in the course of delivery.

The point of rupture of the membranes identifies

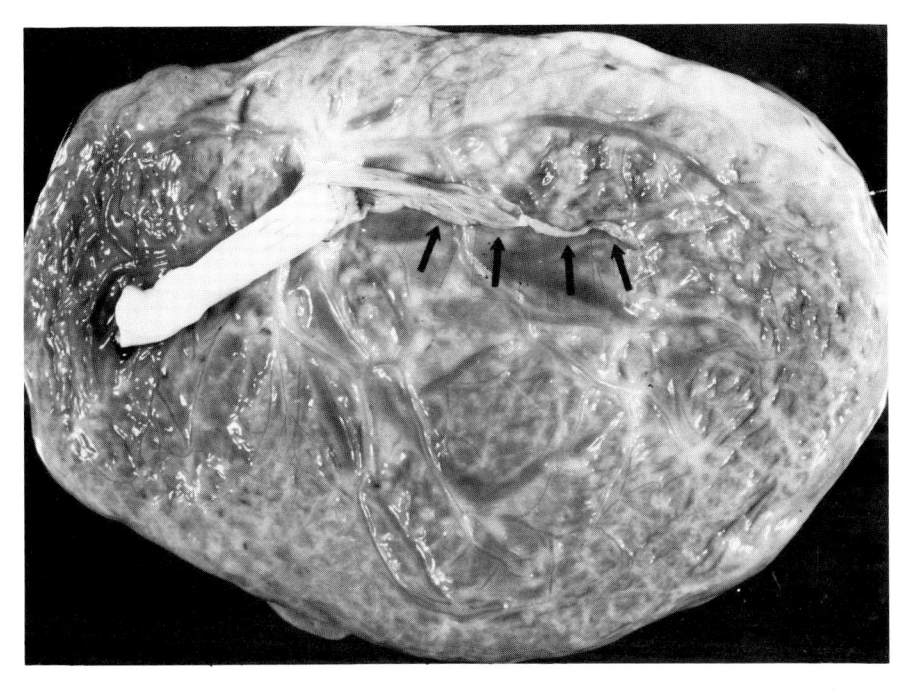

Fig. 16-1. Placenta from a term infant with amputation of terminal phalanx, several toes, and deep constriction of muscles in the calf. There were clubbed feet and only 60 ml of dark amniotic fluid. Remains of amnion are extending into thin band at arrows.

approximately the position of the placenta within the uterus. Thus, when a margin of membranes exists all around a vaginally delivered placenta, the examination rules out placenta previa. On rare occasion one can determine from the shape of the membranous sac, particularly when it is distended under water as Torpin advocates, that a uterine anomaly, such as a bicornuate uterus, was present. The presence of succenturiate lobes on the membrane also may indicate an anomaly of implantation, but for the neonatologist it is more important to ascertain whether the fetal vessels that supply this extra lobe have become disrupted by the tear in the membranes, leading to fetal anemia.

A final but significant deduction that may be made from observations of the rupture of the membranes is the rare event of extramembranous gestation. In such patients the hole within the membranes is too small for the passage of the fetus; only the cord emanates through the opening. The fetus had its growth within the endometrial cavity, having escaped earlier through a tear in the membranes, which then collapsed. Fetal growth retardation, pulmonary hypoplasia, misshapen extremities, circumvallate placentation, and amniorrhea are all sequelae of this abnormal event.

The amnion alone may tear before delivery during the first 3 months of development. Remnants of amnion are frequently found, particularly around the cord (Fig. 16-1), as bands or sheets with stringlike extensions. *Amniotic bands* may strangulate the cord, leading to abortion; they may entangle the extremities, leading to amputations, severe constrictions, or other deformities (Chapter 36); they may adhere to the skull of anencephalics; and their presence may be correlated with other anomalies. Since the fetus resides within the chorionic sac, outside the (destroyed) amnion, the chorionic surface and its vessels are opacified and thickened. The etiology of amnion ruptures is obscure.

Oligohydramnios secondary to deficient fetal urine production or prolonged amniorrhea is associated with *amnion nodosum*. Pulmonary hypoplasia is the common cause of neonatal respiratory distress of infants with this placental abnormality (p. 47). Amnion nodosum represents the deposition of impacted granules of vernix on the degenerating amnion. Usually the amnion epithelium undergoes necrosis first, and then the vernix is deposited. It is most readily recognized on the placental surface but also can be seen on the free membranes. The surface sheen of the amnion is usually lost, the membranes are slightly opacified, and yellow-brown granules of irregular size are found. They must be differentiated from the normal nodules of squamous metaplasia (Fig. 16-2). The latter are present in most mature placentas and are distributed primarily around the insertion of the cord. They are rarely found in the periphery of the placenta and never on the membranes.

Discoloration of the fetal surface occurs frequently.

Fresh meconium may be wiped off. After a short time the pigmented material is taken in by a large number of resident macrophages within the amnion, and then after some 3 hours or more it is passed onto the chorionic macrophages. Thus a very rough guide exists from examining the placenta as to how long meconium was present in the sac. Bilirubin stains the cord and membranes green-yellow, whereas yellow-brown colors are imparted by hemosiderin and hematoidin from marginal or retromembranous hemorrhages as well as from fetal hemorrhages into the amniotic sac.

Inflammation is the only other important process to be observed in the membranes. Polymorphonuclear leukocytes migrate into the amniotic cavity exclusively in

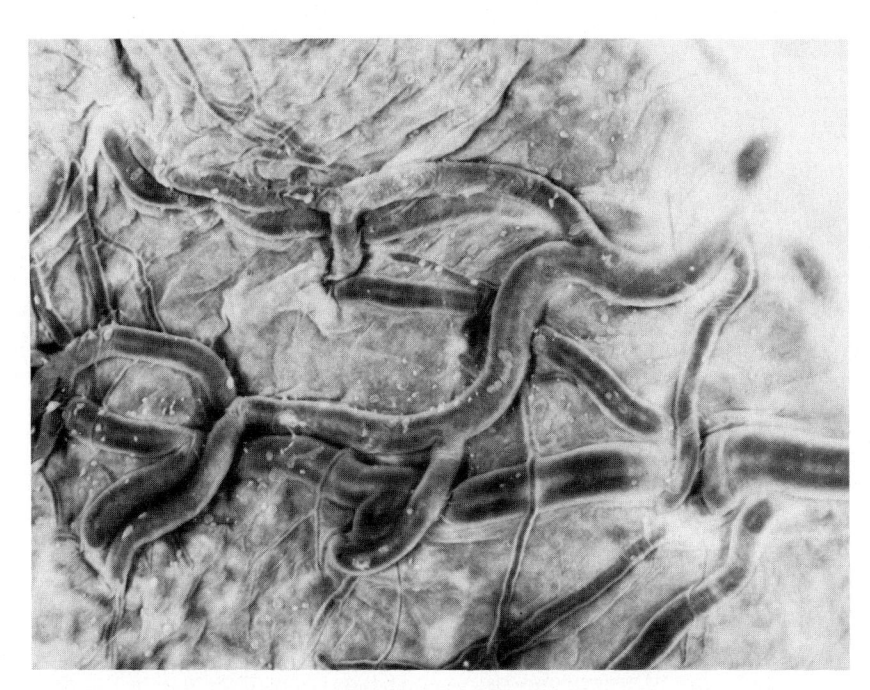

Fig. 16-2. Plaques of squamous metaplasia on the amnion of a normal placenta are prominent over fetal vessels near the insertion of umbilical cord. This must not be confused with amnion nodosum secondary to oligohydramnios (see text).

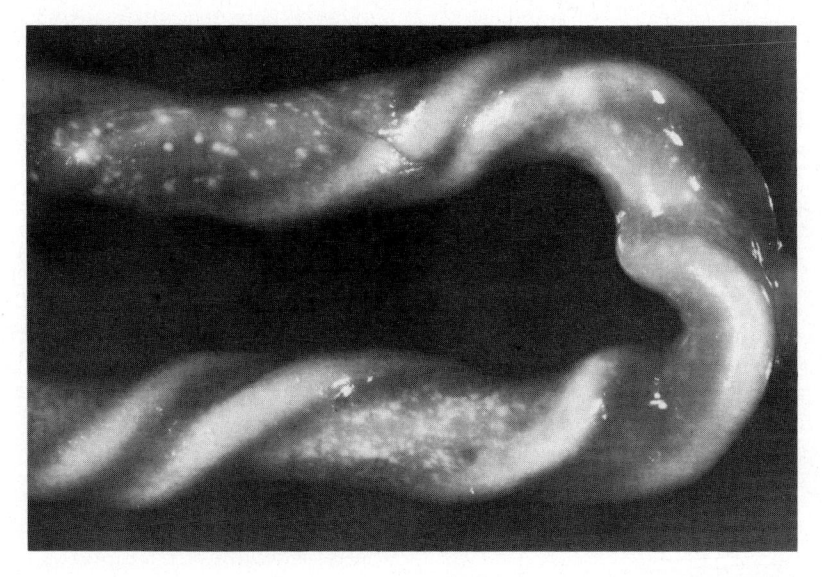

Fig. 16-3. Typical small granules of candidiasis on surface of a discolored umbilical cord.

response to infection of the amniotic fluid. The older concept that chorioamnionitis also represents a response to hypoxia or changes in pH can no longer be accepted. Polymorphonuclear leukocytes come from the decidual (maternal) vessels in the free membranes, from the intervillous space (maternal) on the placental surface, and from the cord and its vascular ramifications (fetal). In general, the most severe infiltration usually exists around the point of rupture of the membranes; it is inferred from this and other correlations that it is usually related to an ascending, transcervical infection. Organisms may be found in large numbers at times, while at other times they cannot be identified at all. A significant degree of inflammation can be identified grossly because it renders the surface of the placenta opaque. In particular, the normally blue fetal vessels appear whitish, and the luster of the surface is gone. At times the surface is malodorous. To assess the nature and degree of this inflammation more accurately, one must prepare histologic sections. Touch preparations and smears prepared from a clean placental surface or after removal of the amnion may also identify the polymorphonuclear leukocytes. A late sequel of severe inflammation is mural thrombosis of surface vessels, which then appear to have yellow-white streaks. Lymphocytic infiltration of the membranes is most uncommon, but a plasmacellular response is, on occasion, seen with virus infections or with syphilis.

Infection with *Candida albicans* is a special form of amniotic sac infection that is readily recognized by placental examination. It is more common than hitherto recognized and may be accompanied by a diffuse or pustular rash in the neonate. Aside from the chorioamnionitis, the surface of the cord has a characteristic appearance (Fig. 16-3). Small whitish nodules appear distributed irregularly on a brownish discolored Wharton's jelly. These nodules are composed of inflammatory exudate and fungi. While the hyphae of *C. albicans* are nearly always present, infections with *C. parapsilosis* (lacking hyphae), a fungus with wide distribution, are now recognized.

UMBILICAL CORD

Normally the cord measures between 50 and 60 cm, but extremes occur in association with abnormal fetal development. Thus unusually *short cords* exist in some chromosomal anomalies and with omphalocele; they occasionally tear on delivery, with fetal blood loss. Excessively *long cords* are prone to knot or entangle around fetal parts; thrombosis and fetal death may be sequelae. Nothing is known of the factors that regulate the length of the cord except that, in rats, removal of amniotic fluid leads to short cords and various fetal positional anomalies.

Angiomas occur on occasion within the cord, usually at its placental insertion, and present a grave prognosis (Fig. 16-4). They may partially calcify or thrombose and probably represent a variation of the more common *chorangioma* of the placental tissue (p. 211).

The most common anomaly of the cord is a *single umbilical artery* (Fig. 16-5). In the Collaborative Perinatal Study, single umbilical artery occurred in 0.9% of deliveries; it is slightly more frequent in white than in black infants and in multiple pregnancies (my own obser-

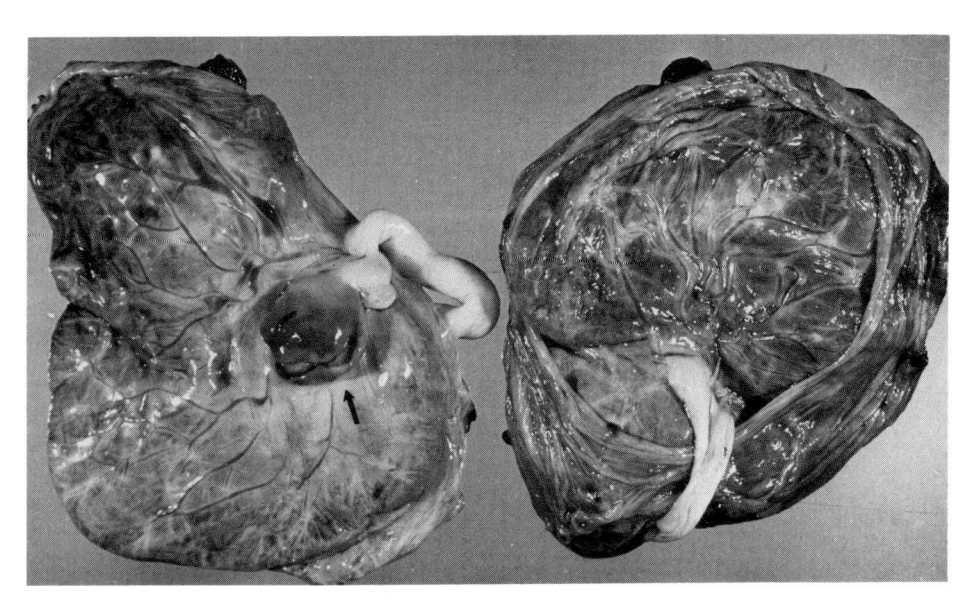

Fig. 16-4. Placentas of premature dizygotic twins. The arrow at left points to an angioma at the insertion of the umbilical cord. This infant had no congenital anomalies but died in the neonatal period.

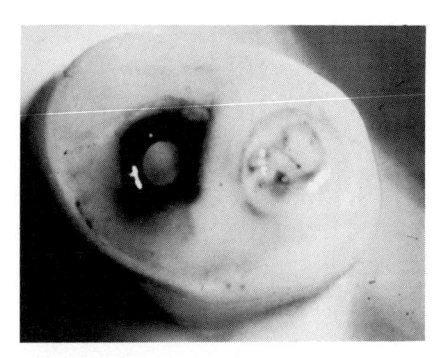

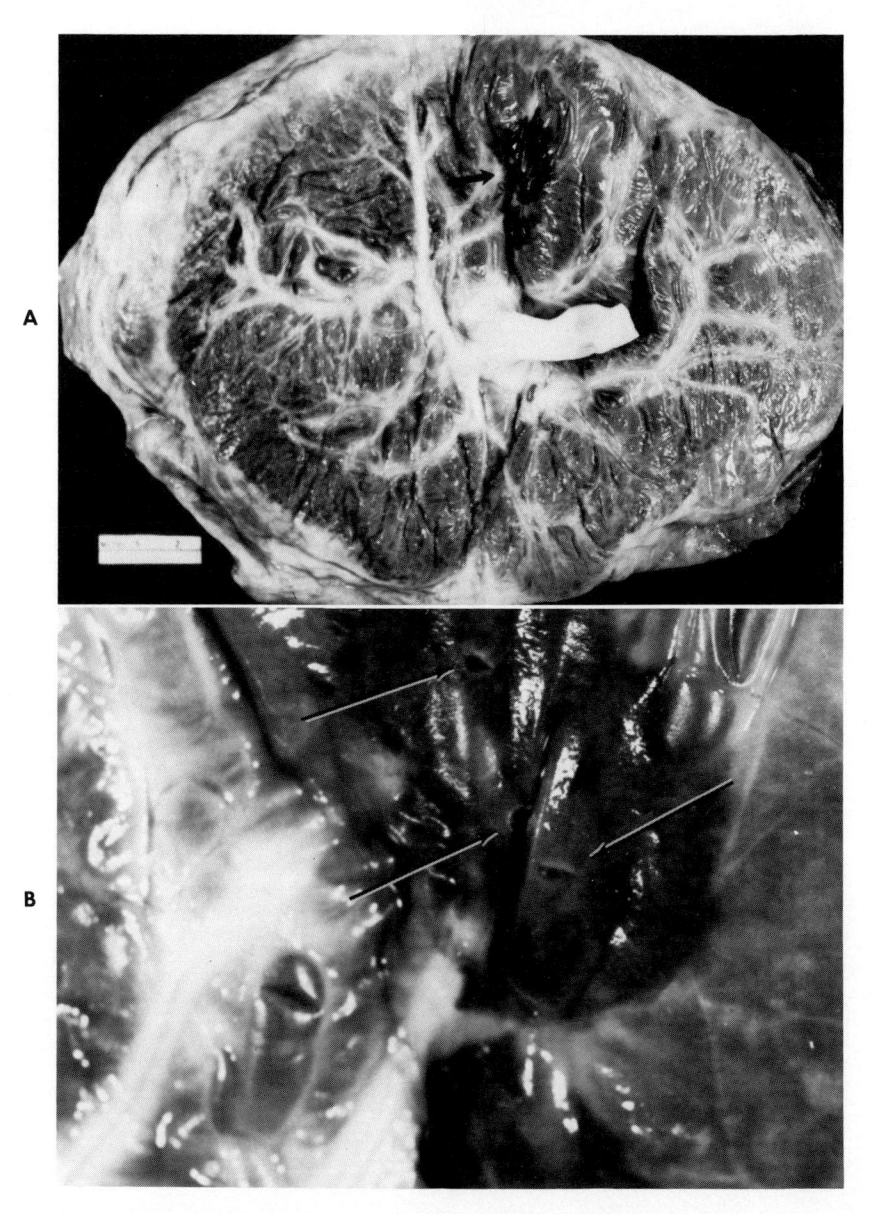

Fig. 16-5. Single umbilical artery of newborn with renal agenesis and velamentous insertion of cord.

Fig. 16-6. A, Placenta of 38 weeks' gestation following cesarean section performed because the fourth amniocentesis, performed to ascertain the lecithin/sphingomyelin ratio in a patient with class B diabetes, led to recognition of fetal bleeding. Infant survived following neonatal transfusion. A small area of subamnionic hemorrhage is seen at arrow. **B,** Higher magnification of hemorrhagic area from **A.** At arrows are three distinct puncture sites of fetal vessels from which fetal bleeding occurred.

vations indicate a frequency of 3.5%; Soma and associates found 6.2%). Single umbilical artery is an indicator of possible hidden anomalies. The Collaborative Perinatal Study indicated that 14% of infants with this anomaly die perinatally and that 53% of these infants have congenital abnormalities; among the survivors, anomalies are identified in only 4%, and when followed to age 4 years there is a significant increase of inguinal hernias. When single umbilical artery is diagnosed, the pediatrician should be notified so that there may be a detailed search for congenital anomalies. Urogenital anomalies are not more common than other types of maldevelopment. Sections of the cord frequently reveal remnants of an atrophying second artery; the frequency of anomalies is the same as with complete single umbilical artery.

Single umbilical artery often occurs with *velamentous cords*. Normally the cord comes from near the center of the placenta, but in about 7% of placentas it inserts marginally—the battledore placenta. In velamentous cords (1.6% of singletons, 5% of twins) the vessels ramify over the membranes from the marginal cord insertion toward the placenta. If they pass over the internal os of the uterus, then the possibility of rupture of such "vasa previa" has to be considered, an event more common in multiple pregnancy. In addition to acute exsanguination during labor when such vasa previa rupture, the membranous vessels predispose to thrombosis and are more readily compressed by the fetal head during labor. Thrombosis can be widespread in such vessels and is, on occasion, associated with signs of disseminated intravascular coagulation in the neonate (Chapter 29). Calcification also may occur in such vessels. The etiology of velamentous insertion is in dispute. However, there is ultrasonographic evidence that it results from a wandering away of the placenta in the course of development from its original site of implantation.

With the increased use of amniocentesis as a diagnostic tool (p. 134), placentas may be observed with holes in the surface, at times in fetal vessels, from which the fetus may exsanguinate. Often the amnion and chorion are discolored because of hemosiderin deposition subsequent to bleeding. Even with ultrasonic verification of placental site, the placenta cannot always be avoided by the needle. At times the tip of the needle has injured the placental fetal surface vessels on the opposite side of the uterus (Fig. 16-6). The defects in the fetal vessels may be very small, but they are very distinctive and may be recognized by careful inspection of the surface. Occasional spontaneous fetus-to-mother hemorrhage has no recognizable placental lesion (Chapter 29).

THE PLACENTA PROPER

The weight of this portion of the placenta alone, membranes and cord trimmed off, is of limited use in assessing fetal/placental ratio. It is usually between 5 or 6:1, but major deviations from this ratio occur with normal neonates. The fetal surface may suggest several diagnoses. The opacity referred to previously allows one to suspect infection. An unusually blue surface, mottled with less than normal patches of subchorial fibrin, suggests maternal diabetes. There may be associated placental congestion, thickness, and an unusual spongy consistency. Conversely, unusual pallor, particularly on cut sections, is indicative of fetal anemia, since the color of this organ is imparted primarily by its content of fetal blood. Thus it is very pale in erythroblastosis, α-thalassemia, and in the donor of the transfusion syndrome. When erythroblastosis is not the obvious cause of marked placental anemia, a careful study is warranted. Fetal blood should be obtained for electrophoresis, and placental tissue samples should be taken to rule out such conditions as syphilis, viral infections, and storage diseases.

The surface also displays *cysts* on occasion (Fig. 16-7). They are usually in a subchorial position, have a mucinous content, and may be blood tinged. These cysts arise in placental septa and are formed by the secretory activity of the so called X cells, trophoblastic derivatives without known function. The presence of cysts in septa or under the surface, in general, connotes maturity, as does the presence of fine, yellow calcium stippling on the maternal surface. On very rare occasions a surface cyst exists that represents a twin pregnancy with a minute fetus papyraceus inside.

Inspection of the surface also may identify the *circumvallate placenta*. This is produced when chronic circumferential hemorrhages detach the membranes from the edge. It may recur in successive pregnancies and is responsible for some premature terminations. A direct correlation with low birth weight infants has not been substantiated. Other abnormal outlines of the placenta, such as elongate, bilobed, or succenturiate lobed, may reflect some abnormality of implantation or uterine shape, but they have no known influence on fetal growth.

Chorangiomas occur perhaps once in 1,000 placentas. Some bulge on the fetal surface and weigh up to 600 gm, whereas others are small and multiple, detectable only on sectioning or palpation. They are fleshy, congested, and often septated masses of sinusoids or capillaries and have a tendency to infarct. They are fetal vascular anomalies—hamartomas—and are associated with a higher incidence of fetal angiomas and other anomalies. Chorangiomas are always benign, but their presence often leads to prematurity, abruptio placentae, hydramnios, and other complications. Because they represent a peripheral mass of high resistance or arteriovenous fistulas, the fetal heart may be hypertrophied or the fetus may be in heart failure. They also may bleed during pregnancy, resulting in fetomaternal blood loss.

The maternal surface should be freed from its loosely

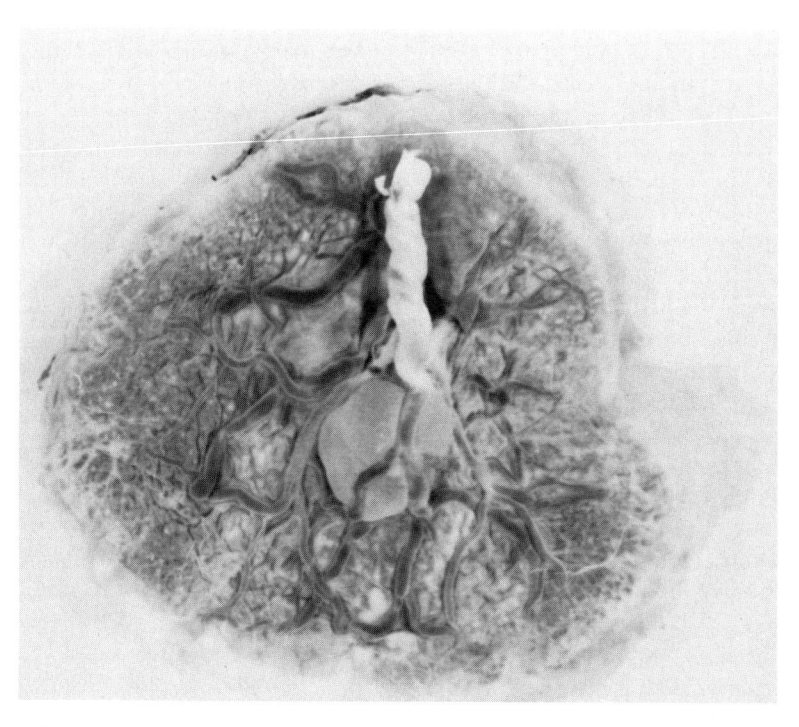

Fig. 16-7. Fetal surface of a mature placenta displaying a subchorionic cyst without pathologic significance.

attached postpartum clot and the lighter color from oxygen exposure not mistaken for pathologic events. The only important lesion identified on examination of the maternal surface is *abruptio placentae*. In its classic form abruptio placentae is a retroplacental hemorrhage associated with abdominal pain and often stillbirth and is followed by many maternal problems. In such patients there is a large, somewhat firm retroplacental blood clot compressing the placenta; it may cause subjacent villous infarction. More often, *retroplacental hematomas* are found on examination of the placenta of patients who do not have classic symptoms or have no clinical syndrome. Their recognition is important in the assessment of growth retardation. Blood undergoes hemolysis relatively rapidly in vivo. Consequently, retroplacental hematomas discolor within a day or more. They become dry, flaky, brown-yellow, and then green. Sometimes they are very large and, because the blood interposes between the supplying maternal vessels and the intervillous space, the placental tissue is often infarcted and necrotic.

Infarcts are the result of deficient intervillous perfusion and are most often secondary to decidual vascular occlusion or interposing hemorrhage. They are at first red but firmer than the adjacent normal tissue. Later they lose fetal blood color and become yellow and then white, firm, and contracted. They never "organize" but only shrink with time. They are readily felt on palpation, and the estimation of their total mass reflects in some measure the total transfer membrane available. The maternal vascular lesions that are the cause of the retroplacental hemorrhages or infarcts are often not identifiable by placental examination. They are destroyed in the infarctive process or are more proximal in the uterine bed. Curettage (placental bed biopsy) discloses thrombosis or the atherosis of preeclampsia and other complex vascular changes. Maternal vascular lesions may exist in the absence of clinical symptoms and signs of toxemia. Sectioning of infarcts or intervillous thrombi is usually useless for diagnostic purposes. Their quantitation and the documentation of vascular changes are relevant to the diagnosis of fetal growth retardation (p. 59).

Few additional lesions are recognized when the fresh placenta is sectioned with a long knife. It is probably more important to save a complete cross section in an appropriate fixative (Bouin's solution; formalin) so that the structures can be studied if the infant has an abnormal course. This practice is of particular importance in growth-retarded newborns, when the placenta has unusual color or consistency.

Chronic villitis is a condition of varied etiology that has no precise macroscopic counterpart. Villi are infiltrated with lymphocytes, macrophages, and particularly with plasma cells (Fig. 16-8). It may be confined to only a few terminal villi or be scattered throughout the villous tissue. At times it is associated either with small hemor-

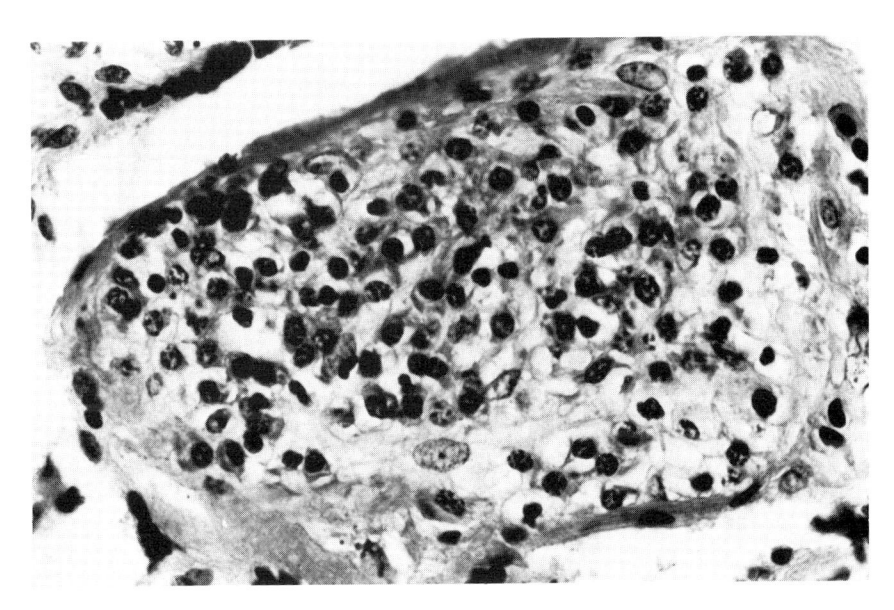

Fig. 16-8. Chronic villitis in the placenta of a premature infant with cytomegalovirus hepatitis and nephritis. This unusually dense infiltrate is composed largely of plasma cells and lymphocytes. Some are degenerating; fetal vessels are occluded, and thus the placenta is pale. Inclusion bodies, fibrosis, and hemosiderin were present in other villi. The infant survived with defects. The placenta was examined only because of maternal "porphyria." (From Benirschke, K., and others: Virchows Arch. [Cell Pathol.] **16:**121, 1974.) (H & E, ×650.)

rhages and hemosiderin or with fetal vascular thrombosis, while at other times it leads to dissolution or fibrosis of many villi. Up to 3% of placentas are affected. Known causes include the TORCH complex, syphilis, and Chagas' disease. Cytomegalovirus is the most common etiologic agent. A microscopic evaluation of the placenta is indicated in evaluating small for dates infants to diagnose chronic villitis (p. 59). It is important to recognize that the severity of fetal disease is not necessarily reflected in the extent of villitis. In the placenta, scarring of villi after previous villitis may lead to an underestimation of the extent of disease. Finally, massive and at times recurrent destructive villitis has been observed with fetal death or intrauterine growth retardation in patients in whom no etiologic agent has been identified. The impact and pathogenesis of this varied lesion are not yet fully understood, but it must be considered in the differential diagnosis of the small for dates infant.

Listeriosis (Chapter 27) may require rapid diagnosis and therapy. The placenta acquires typical features in this transplacental infection. Aside from funisitis and chorioamnionitis, the fetal septicemic process leads to placental villous abscesses that have been interpreted as granulomas. In contrast to the more common chronic villitis, in listeriosis the villi contain polymorphonuclear exudate in which the gram-positive rods are readily seen. Occasional macroscopic nodules are found, representing a more chronic state of infection.

Some storage diseases (Chapter 32) can be diagnosed by the histology of their placental lesions. GM_1-gangliosidosis causes a recognizable trophoblastic vacuolization. Powell and colleagues have recently studied five stillborn infants in whose pale placentas masses of stored products produced diffuse vacuolization. In at least one patient, I cell disease could be identified as the causative defect. This suggests that placental study should become an integral part of all newborn examinations and perinatal autopsies. It also should be recognized that a tissue culture from the placenta can be established that represents the fetal genome. This technique is even possible with macerated stillbirths. The ideal tissue to sample sterilely is the chorionic membrane, after the amnion has been stripped off the surface. Villous tissue also can be established in culture but grows less rapidly.

In *trisomies* (Chapter 39) no specific placental anomalies exist, but small, malformed placentas and single umbilical artery are more common.

MULTIPLE PREGNANCY

Examination *and* recording of the appearance of the placenta should be done for all multiple births. *Monozygosity* can be firmly established by inspection of the membranes in the majority of identical twins. Also, the markedly increased perinatal mortality in twin pregnancies can be understood only by placental examination of the twins; such study may have therapeutic implications.

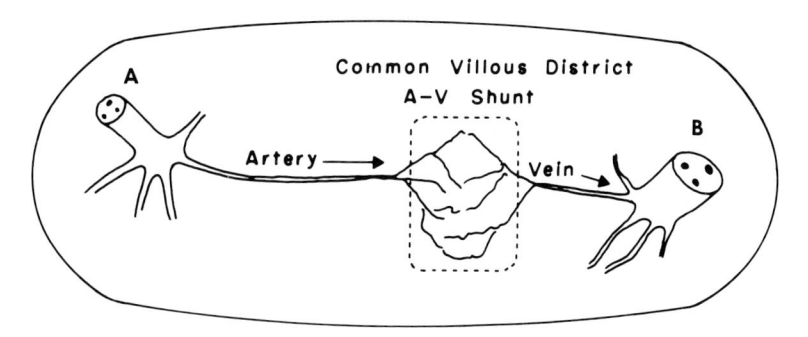

Fig. 16-9. Diagrammatic relationship of arteriovenous shunt in the transfusion syndrome of monochorial, monozygotic twins. The donor A delivers blood to a cotyledon, which in turn is drained through a vein into twin B. The latter (recipient) becomes plethoric and hypertrophied. The twins may differ by 10 gm of hemoglobin and over 1,000 gm and still be "identical." (From Benirschke, K., and Driscoll, S.G.: The pathology of the human placenta, New York, 1967, Springer-Verlag New York, Inc.)

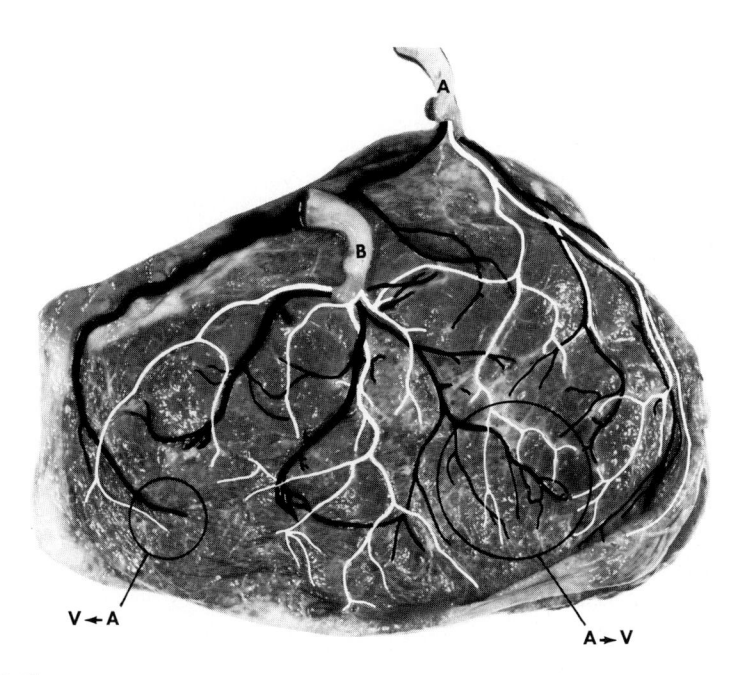

Fig. 16-10. These premature twins (26 weeks) delivered with severe hydramnios and had the prenatal transfusion syndrome. The diamnionic membranes of this placenta have been stripped; a single chorion remains. The placental area of the donor (A) is much smaller than that of the recipient (B). Several arteriovenous shunts from A to B are present in the central right portion, whereas only one arteriovenous shunt (lower left) compensates partly for this transfusion.

It should begin with identification of the cords of each infant, A and B. This is best accomplished at the time of delivery, with appropriate ties around the cut ends. The sacs are reconstructed and the dividing membranes examined. They may be composed of two amnions or of two amnions plus two chorions. Rarely, no dividing membrane exists (monoamnionic), in which case the monozygotic twins suffer a 50% mortality from entangling of the cords. Monochorionic placentation (two amnions only) is diagnostic of identical twins, and almost invariably the placenta is a single mass. Dichorionic, diamnionic placentation is usually the mode of fraternal twin placentation. Nevertheless, one third of monozygotic (like-sex) twins also have this membrane relationship, and their zygosity can be ascertained only by blood grouping, conveniently and harmlessly from umbilical cord blood, or more detailed immunologic study.

Twins have a higher incidence of velamentous cords, ruptured vasa previa, single umbilical artery, and other anomalies. A study of their vascular relationships is most important. Anastomoses exist, for all intents and purposes, only in monochorionic placentas. They are studied most easily after careful stripping of the amnion and with the placental tissue kept intact. In monochorionic placentas the fetal vasculature is almost invariably joined, sometimes in a very complex manner. Artery-to-artery communications cross *over* placental veins and, when anastomoses are present, blood can readily be stroked from one side into the other fetal vascular bed. Such vessels have the least significance. Vein-to-vein communications are less common and similarly recognized. Artery-to-artery plus vein-to-vein anastomoses form the basis for the development of an *acardiac fetus*. Single umbilical artery is nearly always present, and the normal twin may have cardiac hypertrophy and other problems. A monozygotic twin, differing in karyotype through postmeiotic chromosomal nondisjunction (the so-called heterokaryotic twin) also may be a lymphocyte mosaic because the blood passes through such anastomoses and establishes clones.

More important are arteriovenous shunts in the twin placenta that take the course diagrammatically shown in Fig. 16-9. In essence, these twins share one cotyledon. An artery from one delivers blood that is drained through the vein of the other. The latter becomes plethoric, large, and often has accompanying hydramnios, whereas oligohydramnios, anemia, and smaller size characterize the donor in this transfusion syndrome (p. 62 and Chapter 29). It is now well recognized in neonatology, but the recognition of the causal placental shunt is rarely accomplished. Injection with milk may facilitate identification of the causal placental shunt. Several types of anastomoses may coexist in the same placenta, whose sum flow determines the disparity of fetal development and blood content. The complexity of the vascular relationship may be appreciated from Fig. 16-10.

Recognition of the placental abnormalities in multiple birth placentas is important not only for immediate therapy of newborns; their record is also needed for the future care of the child. For instance, it is now recognized that congenital anomalies are more common in monozygotic twins than in fraternal sets. Moreover, one of the monozygotic twins may be abnormal (discordant), and this has a bearing for future genetic counseling.

Kurt Benirschke

BIBLIOGRAPHY

Altshuler, G., and Russell, P.: The human placental villitides: a review of chronic intrauterine infection, Curr. Top. Pathol. **60**:63, 1975.

Altshuler, G., Russell, P., and Ermocilla, R.: The placental pathology of small-for-gestational age infants, Am. J. Obstet. Gynecol. **121**:351, 1975.

Altshuler, G., Tsang, R.C., and Ermocilla, R.: Single umbilical artery: correlation of clinical status and umbilical cord histology, Am. J. Dis. Child. **129**:697, 1975.

Benirschke, K.: Diseases of the placenta. In Gluck, L., editor: Modern perinatal medicine, Chicago, 1974, Year Book Medical Publishers, Inc.

Benirschke, K.: Placental causes of maldevelopment. In Berry, C.L., and Poswillo, D.E., editors: Teratology, trends and application, New York, 1975, Springer-Verlag New York, Inc.

Benirschke, K., and Driscoll, S.G.: The pathology of the human placenta, New York, 1967, Springer-Verlag New York, Inc.

Benirschke, K., Mendoza, G.R., and Bazeley, P.L.: Placental and fetal manifestations of cytomegalovirus infection, Virchows Arch. (Cell Pathol.) **16**:121, 1974.

The Collaborative Perinatal Study of the National Institute of Neurological Diseases and Stroke; the women and their pregnancies, DHEW Publ. No. (NIH) 73-379, Washington, D.C., 1972, Department of Health, Education, and Welfare.

Froehlich, L.A., and Fujikura, T.: Follow-up of infants with single umbilical artery, Pediatrics **52**:6, 1973.

Gruenwald, P.: Pathology of the deprived fetus and its supply line. In Size at birth (Ciba Foundation Symposium 27), Amsterdam, 1974, Elsevier Publishing Co., p. 3.

Kellogg, S.G., Davis, C., and Benirschke, K.: *Candida parapsilosis*: previously unknown cause of fetal infection; a report of two cases, J. Reprod. Med. **12**:159, 1974.

King, D.L.: Placental migration demonstrated by ultrasonography: a hypothesis of dynamic placentation, Radiology **109**:167, 1973.

Lowden, J.A., and others: Prenatal diagnosis of GM_1-gangliosidosis, N. Engl. J. Med. **288**:225, 1973.

Poswillo, D.: Fetal posture and causal mechanisms of deformity of palate, jaws and limbs, J. Dent. Res. **45**:584, 1966.

Powell, H.C., and others: Foamy changes of placental cells in fetal storage disorders, Virchows Arch. (Pathol. Anat.) **369**:191, 1976.

Schirar, A., and others: Congenital mycosis (*Candida albicans*), Biol. Neonate **24**:273, 1974.

Sieracki, J.C., and others: Chorangiomas, Obstet. Gynecol. **46**:155, 1975.

Shanklin, D.R.: The influence of placental lesions on the newborn infant, Pediatr. Clin. North Am. **15**:25, 1970.

Soma, H., and others: Fetal abnormalities associated with twin placentation, Teratology **12**:211, 1975.

Torpin, R.: The human placenta: its shape, form, origin and development, Springfield, Ill., 1969, Charles C Thomas, Publisher.

CHAPTER 17 **Birth injuries**

Birth injuries are those sustained during the birth process (including labor and delivery). They may be avoidable, or they may be unavoidable and occur despite skilled and competent obstetric care, as in an especially hard or prolonged labor or with an abnormal presentation. Fetal injuries related to amniocentesis (Chapter 37) and intrauterine transfusions (p. 37) and neonatal injuries following resuscitation procedures (p. 183) are not considered birth injuries. However, injuries related to the use of intrapartum monitoring of fetal heart rate (FHR) and collection of fetal scalp blood for acid-base assessment will be discussed here. Factors predisposing the infant to birth injury include macrosomia, prematurity, cephalopelvic disproportion, dystocia, prolonged labor, and abnormal presentation.

The incidence of birth injuries is 2 to 7 per 1,000 live births. In an autopsy study Valdes-Dapena and Arey found birth injuries in 2% of all infants studied and in 11% of those weighing over 2,500 gm. Birth injuries rank eighth in overall importance as a cause of neonatal mortality; in the group weighing over 2,500 gm, they rank fourth. These figures represent a decreased incidence in recent years. This has been attributed to refinements in obstetric techniques, the increased choice of cesarean section over difficult vaginal deliveries, and elimination (or decreased use) of difficult forceps, vacuum extractors, and version and extraction.

Despite this decrease, birth injuries still represent an important problem to the clinician. They are frequently readily apparent to the parents, provoking anxiety and providing the clinician with the opportunity to provide important counseling and supportive service. Many of the injuries are mild and self-limited; observation is often the best treatment. However, some injuries may be latent or initially subtle, only to develop manifestations suddenly, with rapid progression.

INJURIES TO SOFT TISSUES
Erythema and abrasions

Erythema and abrasions frequently occur when there has been dystocia during labor secondary to cephalopelvic disproportion or when forceps have been used during delivery. Injuries secondary to dystocia occur over the presenting part; forceps injury occurs at the site of application of the instrument. The latter injury frequently has a linear configuration across both sides of the face outlining the position of the forceps. The affected areas should be kept clean to minimize the risk of secondary infection. These lesions usually resolve spontaneously within several days with no specific therapy.

Petechiae

Occasionally, petechiae are present over the head, neck, upper chest, and lower back at birth following a difficult delivery; they are more frequently observed after breech deliveries.

Etiology. Petechiae are probably caused by a sudden increase in intrathoracic and venous pressures during passage of the chest through the birth canal. An infant born with the cord tightly wound around the neck may have petechiae only above the neck.

Differential diagnosis. Petechiae may be a manifestation of an underlying hemorrhagic disorder. The birth history, early appearance of the petechiae, and absence of bleeding from other sites help to differentiate petechiae secondary to increased tissue pressure or trauma from petechiae caused by hemorrhagic disease of the newborn (Chapter 29). The localized distribution of the petechiae, the absence of subsequent crops of new lesions, and a normal platelet count exclude neonatal thrombocytopenia. The platelet count may also be low secondary to infections or disseminated intravascular coagulation. The former may be clinically distinguished from traumatic

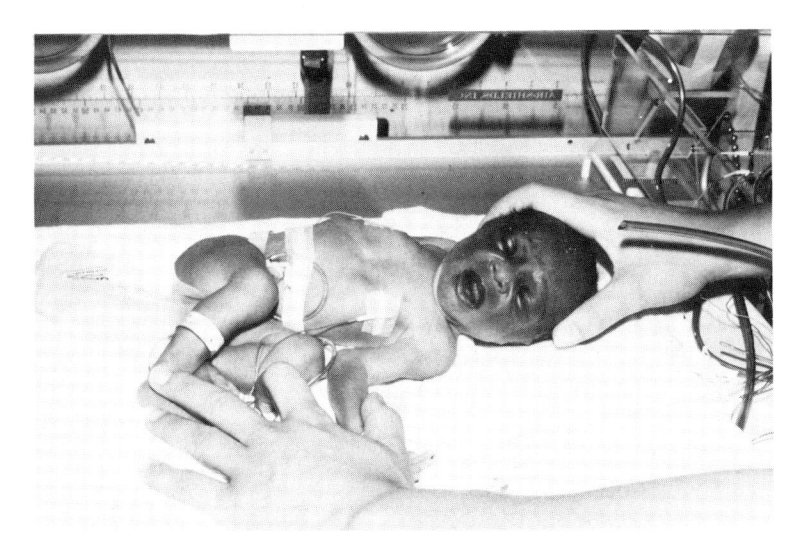

Fig. 17-1. Marked bruising of the entire face of a 1,490-gm female born vaginally after face presentation. Less severe ecchymoses were present on the extremities. Despite use of phototherapy from the first day, icterus was noted on the third day, and exchange transfusions were required on the fifth and sixth days.

petechiae by the presence of other signs and symptoms. The latter is usually associated with excessive and persistent bleeding from a variety of sites. Petechiae are usually distributed over the entire body when associated with systemic disease.

Treatment. If the petechiae are caused by trauma, neither steroids nor heparin should be used. No specific treatment is necessary.

Prognosis. Traumatic petechiae usually fade within 2 or 3 days.

Ecchymoses

Ecchymoses may occur after traumatic or breech deliveries. The incidence is increased in premature infants, especially after a rapid labor and poorly controlled delivery. When extensive, ecchymoses may reflect blood loss severe enough to cause anemia and, rarely, shock. The reabsorption of blood from an ecchymotic area may result in significant hyperbilirubinemia (Fig. 17-1).

Treatment. No local therapy is necessary. The rise in serum bilirubin that follows severe bruising may be decreased by the use of phototherapy (Chapter 30). Ecchymoses rarely result in significant anemia.

Prognosis. The ecchymoses usually resolve spontaneously within 1 week.

Subcutaneous fat necrosis

Subcutaneous fat necrosis is characterized by well-circumscribed indurated lesions of the skin and underlying tissue.

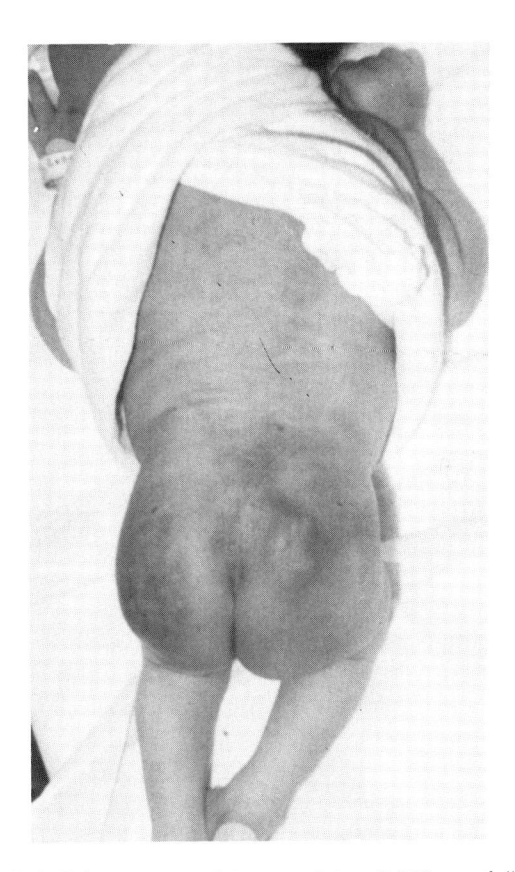

Fig. 17-2. Subcutaneous fat necrosis in a 2,900-gm, full-term infant delivered vaginally; pregnancy, labor, and delivery were completely uncomplicated. Note nodular raised lesion over the right buttock that is surrounded by erythema (darkened area). (Courtesy Dr. Rajam Ramamurthy, Cook County Hospital, Chicago.)

Etiology. Obstetric trauma is the most likely cause of subcutaneous fat necrosis. Many of the affected infants are large and have been delivered by forceps or after a prolonged, difficult labor involving vigorous fetal manipulation. The distribution of the lesions is usually related to the site of trauma. Other etiologic factors that have been implicated include hypoxia, local ischemia, and excessive cooling.

Pathology. Initially, histopathologic studies reveal endothelial swelling and perivascular inflammation in the subcutaneous tissues. This is followed by necrosis of fat and a dense granulomatous inflammatory infiltrate containing foreign body–type giant cells with needle-shaped crystals resembling cholesterol.

Clinical manifestations. Necrotic areas usually appear between 6 and 10 days of age but may be noted as early as the second day or as late as the sixth week. They occur on the cheeks, neck, back, shoulders, arms, buttocks, thighs, and feet, with relative sparing of the chest and abdomen. The lesions vary in size from 1 to 10 cm; rarely they may be more extensive. They are irregularly shaped, hard, plaquelike, and nonpitting (Fig. 17-2). The overlying skin may be colorless, red, or purple. The affected areas may be slightly elevated above the adjacent skin; small lesions may be easily movable in all directions. There is no local tenderness or increase in skin temperature.

Differential diagnosis. This includes lipogranulomatosis and sclerema neonatorum, which present a grave prognosis, and nodular nonsuppurative panniculitis, which is usually associated with fever, hepatosplenomegaly, and tender skin nodules.

Treatment. These lesions require only observation. Surgical excision is not indicated.

Prognosis. The lesions slowly soften after 6 to 8 weeks and completely regress within several months. Occasionally minimal residual atrophy, with or without small calcified areas, is observed.

Lacerations

Accidental lacerations may be inflicted with a scalpel during cesarean section. They usually occur on the scalp, buttocks, and thighs but may occur on any part of the body. If the wound is superficial, the edges may be held in apposition with butterfly adhesive strips. Deeper, more freely bleeding wounds should be sutured with the finest material available, preferably 7-0 nylon. Rarely the amount of blood loss and depth of wound require suturing in the delivery room. After repair, the wound should be left uncovered unless it is in an area of potential soiling such as the perineal area; in such locations the wound should be sprayed with protective plastic. Healing is usually rapid, and the sutures may be removed after 5 days.

INJURIES TO THE HEAD
Skull
Caput succedaneum

Caput succedaneum, a frequently observed lesion, is characterized by a vaguely demarcated area of edema over that portion of the scalp which was the presenting part during a vertex delivery.

Etiology. Serum or blood or both accumulate above the periosteum in the presenting part during labor. This extravasation results from the higher pressure of the uterus or vaginal wall on those areas of the fetal head which border the caput. Thus in a left occiput–transverse presentation the caput succedaneum occurs over the upper and posterior aspect of the right parietal bone; in a right-sided presentation it occurs over the corresponding area of the left parietal bone.

Clinical manifestations. The soft swelling is usually a few millimeters thick and may be associated with overlying petechiae, purpura, or ecchymoses. Because of its location external to the periosteum, a caput succedaneum may extend across the midline of the skull and across suture lines. After especially difficult labors an extensive caput may obscure various sutures and fontanels.

Differential diagnosis. Occasionally a caput succedaneum may be difficult to distinguish from a cephalhematoma, particularly when the latter occurs bilaterally. Careful palpation usually indicates whether the bleeding is external to the periosteum (a caput) or beneath the periosteum (a cephalhematoma).

Treatment. Usually no specific treatment is indicated. Rarely a hemorrhagic caput may result in shock and require blood transfusion.

Prognosis. A caput succedaneum usually resolves within several days.

Cephalhematoma

Cephalhematoma is an infrequently seen subperiosteal collection of blood overlying a cranial bone. The incidence is 0.4% to 2.5% of live births; the frequency is higher in male infants and in infants born to primiparous mothers.

Etiology. A cephalhematoma is caused during labor or delivery by a rupture of blood vessels that traverse from skull to periosteum. Repeated buffeting of the fetal skull against the maternal pelvis during a prolonged or difficult labor and mechanical trauma caused by use of forceps in delivery have been implicated.

Clinical manifestations. The bleeding is sharply limited by periosteal attachments to the surface of one cranial bone; there is no extension across suture lines. The bleeding usually occurs over one or both parietal bones. Less commonly it involves the occipital bones and, very rarely, the frontal bones. The overlying scalp is not discolored. Because subperiosteal bleeding is slow, the

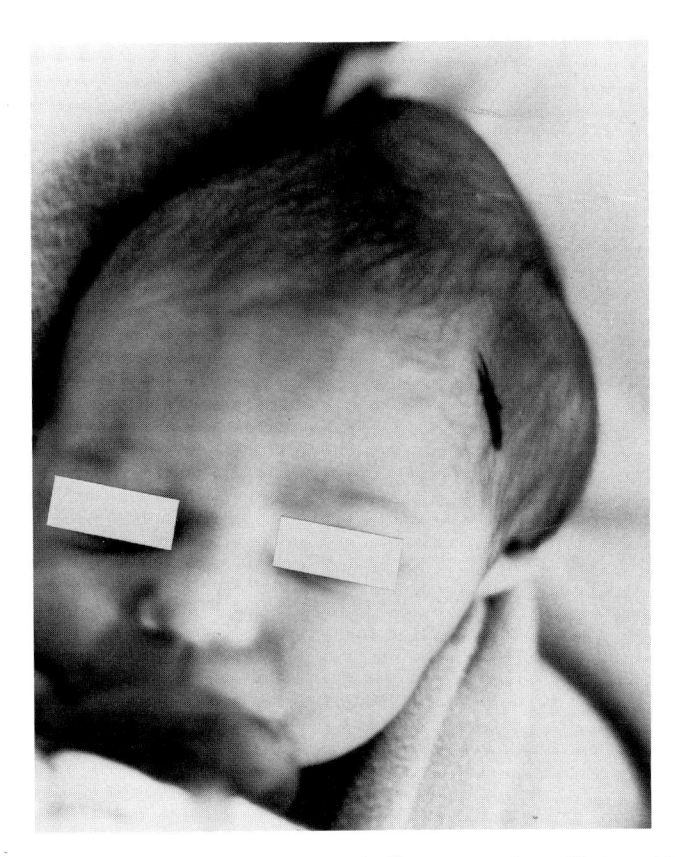

Fig. 17-3. Massive, persistently enlarging cephalhematoma in a 13-day-old female, who had been delivered by midforceps after occiput-posterior presentation. Surgical drainage revealed 300 ml of yellowish material that cultured *Escherichia coli.*

swelling may not be apparent for several hours or days after birth. The swelling is often larger on the second or third day, when sharply demarcated boundaries are palpable. The cephalhematoma may feel fluctuant and is often bordered by a slightly elevated ridge of organizing tissue that gives the false sensation of a central bony depression. In 1952 Kendall and Woloshin noted an underlying skull fracture in 25% of cephalhematomas; a recent study by Zelson and associates indicated an incidence of 5.4%. These fractures are almost always linear and nondepressed.

Roentgenographic manifestations. These vary with the age of the cephalhematoma. During the first 2 weeks bloody fluid results in a shadow of water density. At the end of the second week bone begins to form under the elevated pericranium at the margins of the hematoma; the entire lesion is progressively overlaid with a complete shell of bone.

Differential diagnosis. A cephalhematoma may be differentiated from caput succedaneum by (1) its sharp periosteal limitations to one bone, (2) the absence of overlying discoloration, (3) the later initial appearance of the swelling, and (4) the longer time period before resolution. Cranial meningocele is differentiated from cephal-

hematoma by pulsations, increase in pressure during crying, and the demonstration of a bony defect by roentgenogram. An occipital cephalhematoma may be confused initially with an occipital meningocele and with cranium bifidum because all occupy the midline position.

Treatment. Therapy is not indicated for the uncomplicated cephalhematoma. Rarely a massive cephalhematoma may result in blood loss severe enough to require transfusion. Significant hyperbilirubinemia may also result, necessitating phototherapy or other treatment of jaundice (Chapter 30).

The most common associated complications are skull fracture and intracranial hemorrhage. Linear fractures do not require specific therapy, but roentgenograms should be taken at 4 to 6 weeks to ensure closure and to exclude formation of leptomeningeal cysts; depressed fractures require immediate neurosurgical consultation. Specific treatment for blood loss or hyperbilirubinemia or both may be indicated if there has been an intracranial hemorrhage. Incision or aspiration of a cephalhematoma is contraindicated because of the risk of introducing infection. Rarely bacterial infections of cephalhematomas occur, usually in association with septicemia and

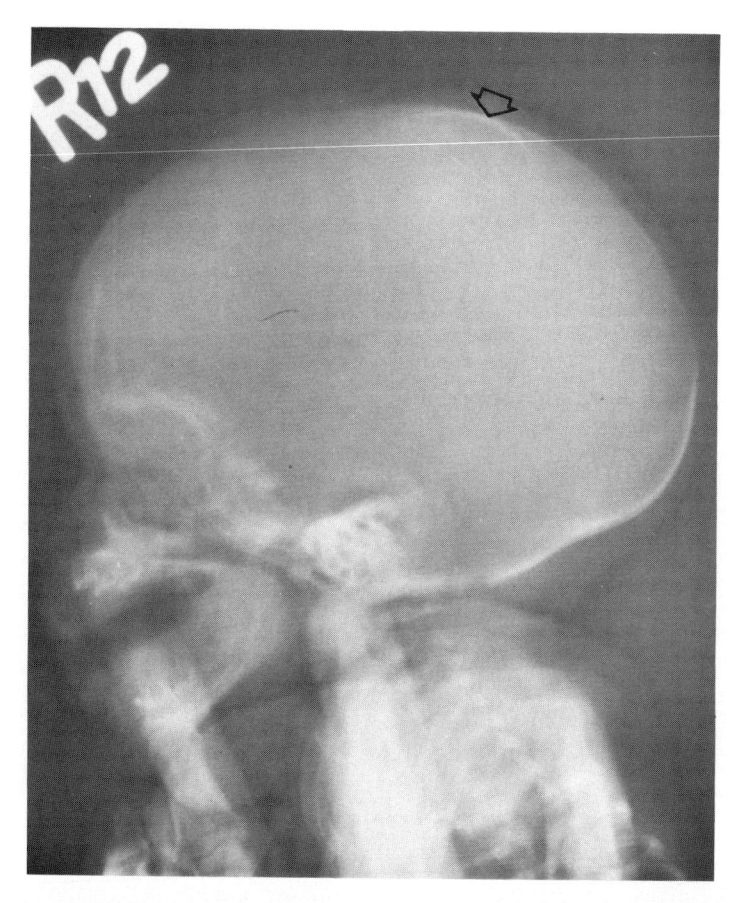

Fig. 17-4. Calcified cephalhematoma in left parietal region of a 5-week-old female. Infant weighed 1,410 gm at birth and was delivered rapidly because of prolapsed cord. Hard left parietal swelling was detected at 5 weeks by nurses while feeding the infant.

meningitis. Focal infection should be suspected when there is a sudden enlargement of a static cephalhematoma during the course of a systemic infection, a relapse of meningitis or sepsis after treatment with antibiotics, or the development of local signs of infection over the cephalhematoma (Fig. 17-3). Diagnostic aspiration may be indicated. If a local infection is present, surgical drainage and specific antibiotic therapy should be instituted.

Prognosis. Most cephalhematomas are resorbed within 2 weeks to 3 months, depending on their size; the majority are resorbed by 6 weeks. In a few patients, calcium is deposited (Fig. 17-4), causing a bony swelling that may persist for several months and, rarely, up to 1½ years.

Roentgenographic findings persist after disappearance of clinical signs. The outer table remains thickened as a flat irregular hyperostosis for several months. There may be a persistent (for years) widening of the space between the new shell of bone and the inner table; the space originally occupied by hematoma usually develops into normal diploic bone, but cystlike defects may persist at the sites of the hematoma for months or years. Rarely a neonatal cephalhematoma may persist into adult life as a symptomless mass, the *cephalhematoma deformans of Schüller*.

Skull fractures

Fracture of the neonatal skull is uncommon, since the bones of the skull are less mineralized at birth and thus more compressible. In addition, the separation of the bones by membranous sutures usually permits enough alteration in the contour of the head to allow its passage through the birth canal without injury.

Etiology. Skull fractures usually follow a forceps delivery or a prolonged, difficult labor with repeated forceful contact of the fetal skull against the maternal symphysis pubis, sacral promontory, or ischial spine. Most of the fractures are linear. Depressed fractures almost always result from forceps application. Occipital bone fractures usually occur in breech deliveries as a consequence of traction on the hyperextended spine of the infant when the head is fixed in the maternal pelvis.

Clinical manifestations. Linear fractures over the convexity of the skull are frequently accompanied by soft

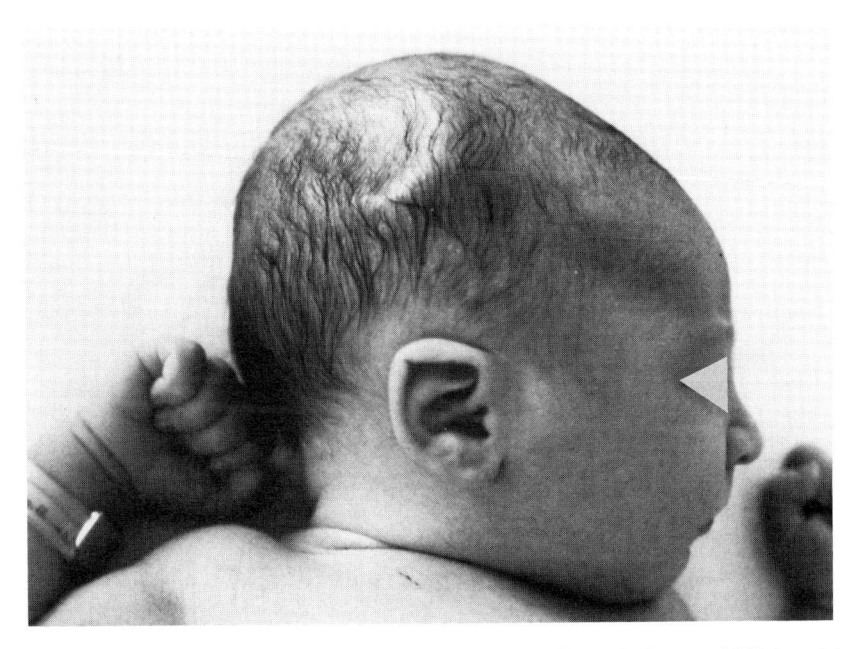

Fig. 17-5. Depressed skull fracture in a full-term male delivered after rapid (1 hour) labor. The infant was delivered by occiput-anterior presentation after rotation from occiput-posterior position.

tissue changes and cephalhematoma. Usually the infant's behavior is normal unless there is an associated concussion or hemorrhage into the subdural or subarachnoid space. Fractures at the base of the skull with separation of the basal and squamous portions of the occipital bone almost always result in severe hemorrhage caused by disruption of the underlying venous sinuses. The infant may develop shock, neurologic abnormalities, and drainage of bloody cerebrospinal fluid from the ears or nose.

Depressed fractures are visible and palpable indentations in the smooth contour of the skull, similar to dents in a Ping-Pong ball (Fig. 17-5). The infant may be entirely asymptomatic unless there is associated intracranial injury.

Roentgenographic manifestations. The diagnosis of a simple linear or fissure fracture is seldom made without roentgenograms, where they appear as lines and strips of decreased density. Depressed fractures appear as lines of increased density. On some views they are manifested by an inward buckling of bone with or without an actual break in continuity. Either type of fracture may be seen on only one view.

Differential diagnosis. Occasionally the fragments of a linear fracture may be widely separated and simulate an open suture. Conversely, parietal foramina, the interparietal fontanel, mendosal sutures, and innominate synchondroses may be mistaken for fractures. In addition, normal vascular grooves, "ripple lines" that represent soft tissue folds of the scalp, and lacunar skull may be mistaken for fractures.

Treatment. Uncomplicated linear fractures over the convexity of the skull usually do not require treatment. Fractures at the base of the skull often necessitate blood replacement for severe hemorrhage and shock, in addition to other supportive measures. If cerebrospinal fluid rhinorrhea or otorrhea is present, antimicrobial coverage is indicated to prevent secondary infection of the meninges.

Small (less than 2 cm) "Ping-Pong" fractures may be observed without surgical treatment. Loeser and associates recently reported three infants with depressed skull fractures in whom spontaneous elevation of the fractures occurred within 1 day to 3½ months of age. Follow-up at 1 to 2½ years revealed normal neurologic development in all three.

Several nonsurgical methods have been described for elevation of depressed skull fractures in certain infants:

1. A thumb is placed on opposite margins of the depression and gentle, firm pressure exerted toward the middle. After several minutes of continuous pressure the area of depression gradually disappears.
2. A hand breast pump is applied to the depressed area. Petroleum jelly placed on the pump edges ensures a tighter seal, and gentle suction for several minutes results in elevation of the depressed bone.
3. A vacuum extractor is placed over the depression, and a negative pressure of approximately 0.2 to 0.5 kg/cm^2 is maintained for approximately 4 minutes.

Since these methods are technically easier and less traumatic, they may be preferable to surgical intervention in an asymptomatic infant with an isolated lesion.

Comminuted or large fractures associated with neurologic signs or symptoms should be treated by immediate surgical elevation of the indented segment to prevent underlying cortical injury from pressure. Other indications for surgical elevation include manifestations of cerebrospinal fluid beneath the galea and failure to elevate the fracture by nonsurgical manipulation.

Prognosis. Simple linear fractures usually heal within several months without sequelae. Rarely a leptomeningeal cyst may develop from an associated dural tear, and meninges or part of the brain may protrude through the fracture. The fracture line may widen rapidly within weeks, or a large defect in the skull may be noted many months later. If detected early, the cyst may be excised successfully and brain atrophy prevented. It is therefore advisable to repeat skull roentgenograms within 2 to 3 months to detect early widening of the fracture line.

Basal fractures carry a grave prognosis. When separation of the basal and squamous portions of the occipital bone occurs, the outcome is almost always fatal; surviving infants have an extremely high incidence of neurologic sequelae.

The prognosis for a depressed fracture is usually good when treatment is early and adequate. When therapy is delayed, especially with a large depression, death may occur from pressure on vital areas of the brain. Since the natural history of depressed skull fractures in neonates has not been clearly elucidated, the outcome is uncertain for infants with smaller lesions that have been treated either by simple observation or by surgery after significant delays. Despite the apparently normal outcome in the three infants reported by Loeser and associates, one cannot completely exclude the possibility of subtle neurologic sequelae developing years later.

Intracranial hemorrhage

See Chapter 22.

Face

Facial nerve palsy

Facial nerve palsy in the neonate may follow birth injury or rarely may result from agenesis of the facial nerve nucleus. The latter condition is occasionally hereditary but is usually sporadic.

Etiology. Traumatic facial nerve palsy most commonly follows compression of the peripheral portion of the nerve, either near the stylomastoid foramen through which it emerges or where the nerve traverses the ramus of the mandible. The nerve may be compressed by forceps, especially when the fetal head has been grasped obliquely. The condition also occurs after spontaneous deliveries following prolonged pressure by the maternal sacral promontory. Less commonly injury is sustained in utero, often in association with a mandibular deformity, by the persistent position of the fetal foot against the superior ramus of the mandible. An extremely rare cause is the pressure of a uterine tumor on the nerve.

A traumatic facial nerve palsy may follow a contralateral injury to the central nervous system (CNS), such as a temporal bone fracture or hemorrhage or tissue destruction or both to structures within the posterior fossa. This central nerve injury is less frequent than a peripheral nerve injury.

Clinical manifestations. Paralysis is usually apparent on the first or second day but may be present at birth. It usually does not increase in severity unless there is considerable edema over the area of nerve trauma. The type and distribution of paralysis are different for central facial paralysis compared with peripheral paralysis.

Central paralysis is a spastic paralysis limited to the lower half or two thirds of the contralateral side of the face. The paralyzed side is smooth and full and often appears swollen. The nasolabial fold is obliterated, and the corner of the mouth droops. When the infant cries, the mouth is drawn to the normal side, the wrinkles are deeper on the normal side, and movement of the forehead and eyelid is unaffected. Usually there are other manifestations of intracranial injury, most commonly a sixth nerve palsy.

Peripheral paralysis is flaccid and, when complete, involves the entire side of the face. When the infant is at rest, the only sign may be a persistently open eye on the affected side caused by paralysis of the orbicular muscle of the eye. With crying the findings are the same as those in a central facial nerve injury, with the addition of a smooth forehead on the involved side. Since the tongue is not involved, feeding is not affected.

A small branch of the nerve may be injured with involvement of only one group of facial muscles. Paralysis is then limited to the forehead, eyelid, or mouth. Peripheral paralysis secondary to nerve injury distal to the geniculate ganglion may be accompanied by a hematotympanum on the same side.

Differential diagnosis. Central and peripheral facial nerve palsies must be distinguished from *nuclear agenesis* (Möbius' syndrome). The latter frequently results in bilateral facial nerve palsy; the face is expressionless and immobile, suggesting muscle fibrosis. Other cranial nerve palsies and deformities of the ear, palate, tongue, mandible, and other bones may be associated with *Möbius' syndrome*. Congenital absence or hypoplasia of the depressor muscle of the angle of the mouth may also simulate congenital facial palsy and has been associated with an increased incidence of other congenital anomalies.

Treatment. No specific therapy is indicated for most facial palsies. If the paralysis is peripheral and complete, initial treatment should be directed at protecting the cornea with an eye pad and 1% methylcellulose drops instilled every 4 hours. The functional state of the nerve should be followed closely. If there is no evidence of improvement within 7 to 10 days, electrodiagnostic tests should be performed to determine whether there is neuropraxia or degeneration with interruption of the anatomic continuity of the nerve. If the latter condition is present, surgical intervention should be considered. The best surgical results are obtained with decompression or neuroplasty or both. The ideal time for surgery is not known. Occasionally facial tone may be improved after anastomosis of the facial nerve to the hypoglossal or accessory nerves. Adrenocorticotropic hormone (ACTH) is not indicated.

Prognosis. The majority of facial palsies resolve spontaneously within several days; total recovery may require several weeks or months. Electrodiagnostic testing is beneficial in predicting recovery; repeatedly normal nerve excitability indicates a good prognosis, but decreased or absent excitability early in the course suggests a poor outlook. The subsequent appearance of muscle fibrillation potentials indicates nerve degeneration. The prognosis in surgically treated infants worsens with increasing age at treatment.

Fractures and dislocations of facial bones

Facial bone fractures may occur during passage through the birth canal, during forceps application and delivery, and during obstetric manipulation (most commonly the Mauriceau maneuver for delivery of the fetal head in a breech presentation). The latter may result in mandibular fractures and mandibular joint damage but is rarely severe enough to cause separation of the symphysis of the mandible. Fracture of the nose may result in early respiratory distress and feeding difficulties. The most frequent nasal injury is dislocation of the cartilaginous part of the septum from the vomerine groove and columella. This may result from intrauterine factors (such as a uterine tumor or persistent pressure on the nose by fetal small parts) or during delivery from pressure on the nose by the symphysis pubis, sacral promontory, or perineum. The presence of nasal septal dislocation may be differentiated from the more common normal variant of misshapen nose by a simple compression test, in which the tip of the nose is compressed (Fig. 17-6). In the presence of septal dislocation the nostrils collapse and the deviated septum becomes more apparent; in the normal nose no nasal deviation occurs with compression.

Treatment. Early reduction and immobilization are advised for fracture of the mandible because rapid, firm union may occur as early as 10 to 14 days. Fractures of the maxilla, lacrimal bones, and nose unite even faster, with fixation in 7 to 10 days. Therefore nasal fractures

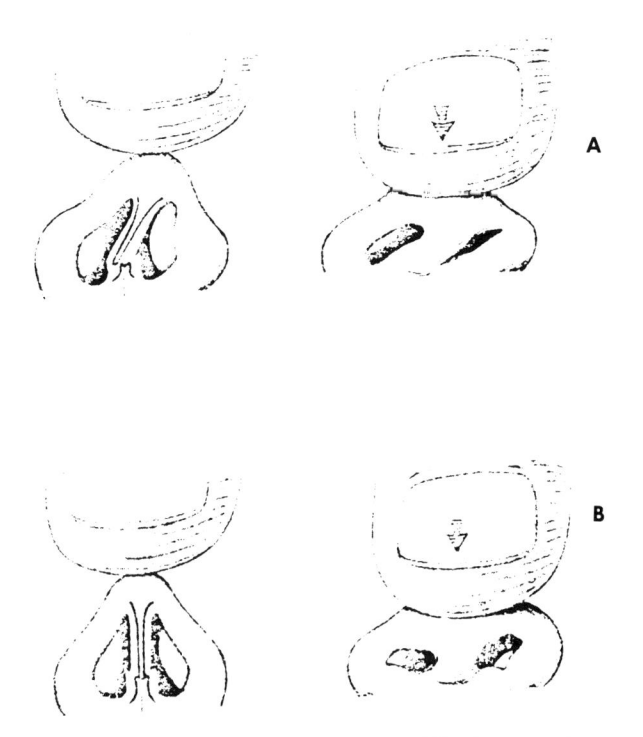

Fig. 17-6. Result of finger compression **(A)** when nasal septum is dislocated. Normal septal relationship **(B)** results in no nasal deviation with pressure. (From Daily, W., and Davis, W.E.: Missouri Med. **74:**381, 1977.)

should be treated even sooner. Since nasal trauma frequently requires extensive surgery, the pediatrician should request immediate consultation with a physician with expertise in nasal surgery. While waiting, the pediatrician should provide an oral airway to relieve respiratory distress. Often the surgeon can grasp the traumatized nose and elevate and remold it manually, resulting in relief of respiratory distress. Fractures of the septal cartilage may also be reduced by simple manual remolding, but most are associated with hematomas that should be promptly incised and drained. The surgeon can visualize the deformity with an infant nasal speculum, place a septal elevator in the nose, and guide the septal cartilage into the vomerine groove; an audible and palpable click indicates return of the septum into position.

Prognosis. If the fracture is reduced and fixated within a few days, rapid healing without complication is the usual course. If treatment is inadequate, missed, or delayed, subsequent developmental deformities are common. Ankylosis of the mandible in the second year of life is thought to result from birth trauma to the temporomandibular joint. Recently a young child was described with unilateral mandibular hypoplasia, which was thought to be a result of fibrous ankylosis secondary to perinatal trauma to the condylar cartilage of the ipsilateral temporomandibular joint. Other deformities may not become apparent until adolescence or young adulthood.

Eyes

See also Chapter 35.

Mechanical trauma to various regions of the neonatal eye usually occurs during abnormal presentation, in dystocia from cephalopelvic disproportion, or as a result of inappropriate forceps placement in normal deliveries. Most of the injuries are self-limited, mild, and require no specific treatment.

Eyelids

Edema, suffusion, and ecchymoses of the eyelids are common, especially after face and brow presentations or forceps deliveries. Severely swollen lids should be forced open by an ophthalmologist for examination of the eyeball; retractors may be necessary. These findings usually resolve within a week without treatment, although an infant was recently reported with totally everted upper eyelids that required suturing for 4 days before remaining in the normal position. It is felt by some that these injuries represent a possible cause of congenital ptosis.

Lagophthalmos, the inability to close an eye, is an occasional finding thought to result from facial nerve injury by forceps pressure. It usually is unilateral. The exposed cornea should be protected by an eye pad and methylcellulose drops instilled every 4 hours. The condition usually resolves within a week.

Orbit

Orbital hemorrhage and fracture may follow direct pressure by the apex of one forceps blade, most commonly in high forceps extractions. In most instances immediate death occurs. Surviving infants demonstrate traumatic eyelid changes, disturbances of extraocular muscle movements, and exophthalmos. The presence of the latter two findings warrants immediate ophthalmologic consultation. Subsequent management may also require neurosurgical and plastic surgery consultations.

Sympathetic nervous system

Horner's syndrome, resulting from cervical sympathetic nerve trauma, frequently accompanies lower brachial plexus injury (p. 226). The syndrome consists of miosis, partial ptosis, slight enophthalmos, and anhidrosis of the homolateral side of the face. Although small, the pupil reacts to light. The presence of neurologic signs indicating brachial plexus injury helps to distinguish this syndrome from intracranial hemorrhage as a cause of anisocoria. Pigmentation of the homolateral iris is frequently delayed to several months of age; occasionally pigmentation never occurs. Resolution of other signs of the syndrome depends on whether the injury to the nerve is transient or permanent.

Subconjunctival hemorrhage

Subconjunctival hemorrhage, characterized by bright red patches on the bulbar conjunctiva, is a relatively common finding in the neonate. It may be found after a difficult delivery but often is noted after easy, completely uncomplicated deliveries. If the baby is otherwise well, treatment consists of reassuring the parents. The blood is usually absorbed within 1 to 2 weeks. As the blood pigments break down and are absorbed, the color changes from bright red to orange and yellow.

External ocular muscles

Injury involving the external ocular muscles may result from direct trauma to the cranial nerve (in the form of compression or surrounding hemorrhages) or from hemorrhage into the muscle sheath, with subsequent fibrosis. The sixth nerve (abducens) is the most frequently injured cranial nerve because of its long intracranial course; the result is paralysis of the lateral rectus muscle. This injury may follow a tentorial laceration with extravasation of a small amount of blood around the intracranial portion of the nerve. The involvement may be mild and transient; internal strabismus noted at birth may resolve gradually within 1 to 2 months. The seventh nerve may be injured simultaneously with the sixth nerve by compression with forceps. Improvement in lateral gaze of the affected eye may appear within 1 to 2 months. Alternate patching of either eye in the severely affected infant maintains visual acuity until, with time, maximum improvement has occurred. At 6 months the degree of nerve regeneration may be evaluated. Some infants subsequently require surgical repair of their strabismus.

Fourth nerve (trochlear) palsy is uncommon. It may follow small brainstem hemorrhages with nuclear damage. The affected muscle is the superior oblique, which mainly turns the eye inferiorly and medially. This is difficult to identify in the newborn. Surgical correction may be necessary at a later time.

Third nerve (oculomotor) palsy, when complete, causes paralysis of the inferior oblique and medial, superior, and inferior rectus muscles. This results in ptosis, a dilated fixed pupil, and outward and downward deviation of the eye, with inability to adduct or elevate up and in or up and out or to depress down and out. This palsy may also occur in partial form, with or without pupillary involvement. Partial palsies may recover function spontaneously within several months, whereas complete palsies usually require surgical intervention.

Optic nerve

The optic nerve may be directly injured by a fracture in the region of the optic canal or from a shearing force on the nerve, with resultant hemorrhage into the nerve sheath. The latter injury is seldom recognized because of the more apparent and severe changes in the sensorium.

Occasionally a fracture through the optic foramen results in formation of callus, which slowly compresses the nerve. A difficult forceps delivery is a frequent preceding event. If optic nerve injury is not diagnosed within several hours with prompt surgical intervention, irreversible damage is likely. The result is optic atrophy and blindness. This is characterized by a blue-white optic disc, in contrast to the grayish disc of the normal newborn. In primary optic atrophy (for example, that caused by birth trauma), the disc margin is well defined, and fine vessels are rarely present in the disc tissue. In secondary atrophy the disc margin is blurred; there is a central gray area and evidence of intraocular disease.

Cornea

A diffuse or streaky haziness of the cornea is relatively common. This is usually caused by edema related to the birth process but may also follow use of a silver nitrate solution more concentrated than 1%. The haziness usually disappears in 7 to 10 days. When it persists, a rupture of Descemet's membrane has probably occurred; usually this results from malpositioning of forceps at delivery. The consequence of a ruptured Descemet's membrane is a leukoma or diffuse white opacity of the cornea. This results from interstitial damage of the substantia propria by fluids entering through the tear in the membrane. These leukomas are often permanent and are accompanied by a high incidence of amblyopia and strabismus (Chapter 35).

Intraocular hemorrhage

Trauma at birth may result in retinal hemorrhage, hyphema, or vitreous hemorrhage. Retinal hemorrhage is the most common, with a reported incidence of 2.6% to 50% of all births. The extreme variability in incidence is probably related to the infant's age when first examined; the incidence is higher with earlier observations. The cause is most likely compression of the fetal head, resulting in venous congestion. The fetal head has been shown to be compressed two to four times more forcefully than other fetal parts during the second stage of labor. Retinal hemorrhage is more common in primiparous deliveries and after forceps or vacuum extraction; it is rare after cesarean section. It may occur in normal deliveries. The most common lesion is the flame-shaped or streak hemorrhage found mainly near the disc and sparing the macula and extreme periphery; it usually disappears within 1 to 3 days (occasionally 5 days) with no residual effects. Rarely hemorrhages may take up to 21 days to resolve. Retinal hemorrhages may reduce the resolving power of the macula, either bilaterally to produce nystagmus or unilaterally to produce amblyopia, which may not always respond to prolonged covering of the fixing eye with improvement of the amblyopic eye.

Hyphemas and vitreous hemorrhages usually result from misplaced forceps and are often associated with ruptures of Descemet's membrane. Recently an infant was reported in whom a hyphema developed in one eye following spontaneous delivery. The hyphema usually is clear of gross blood within 5 days; during this time the infant should be handled gently and fed frequently to minimize crying and agitation. If blood persists or secondary hemorrhage occurs, systemic administration of acetazolamide (Diamox) and surgical removal of blood may be necessary.

Vitreous hemorrhage is manifested by large vitreous floaters, blood pigment seen with the slit lamp, and an absent red reflex. The prognosis is guarded; if resolution does not occur in 6 to 12 months, surgical correction should be considered.

Ears

The proximity of ears to the site of application of forceps make them susceptible to injury at birth. Most of the injuries are mild and self-limited, but serious injuries may occur because of slipping or misplacement of forceps.

Abrasions and ecchymoses

Abrasions must be cleansed gently to minimize the risk of secondary infection. Ecchymoses, if extensive and involving other areas of the body, may result in hyperbilirubinemia.

Hematomas

Hematomas of the external ear, if not treated promptly, liquefy slowly, followed by early organization and development of cauliflower ear. Wide incision and evacuation of the hematoma may be indicated.

Lacerations

Lacerations of the auricle may be repaired by the pediatrician if they are superficial and involve only skin. After thorough cleansing and draping, the wound edges are sutured with interrupted 6-0 or 7-0 nylon sutures, with exact edge-to-edge approximation. If the laceration involves cartilage, surgical consultation should be obtained because of the tendency for postoperative perichondritis, which is refractory to treatment and leads to subsequent deformities. A sterile field and more meticulous presurgical preparation are essential. A contour pressure dressing is applied postoperatively.

Vocal cord paralysis

Unilateral or bilateral paralysis of the vocal cords is uncommon in the neonate.

Etiology. Unilateral paralysis may be a consequence of excessive traction on the head during a breech delivery or lateral traction with forceps in a cephalic presentation. The recurrent laryngeal branch of the vagus nerve in the neck is injured. The left side is more commonly involved because of this nerve's lower origin and longer course in the neck. Bilateral paralysis may be caused by peripheral trauma involving both recurrent laryngeal nerves, but more commonly it is caused by a CNS insult, such as hypoxia or hemorrhage involving the brainstem.

Clinical manifestations. An infant with a unilateral paralysis may be completely asymptomatic when resting quietly, but crying is usually accompanied by hoarseness and mild inspiratory stridor. Bilateral paralysis results in more severe respiratory symptoms. At birth the infant may have difficulty in establishing and maintaining spontaneous respiration; later dyspnea, retractions, stridor, cyanosis, or aphonia may develop.

Differential diagnosis. Unilateral paralysis of the vocal cords must be distinguished from congenital laryngeal malformations that produce neonatal stridor (p. 193). A history of difficult delivery, especially involving excessive traction on the fetus, may suggest laryngeal paralysis; the diagnosis can be confirmed only by direct laryngoscopic examination. Bilateral paralysis also must be distinguished from a number of causes of respiratory distress in the neonate (p. 460); stridor should suggest the larynx as the site of disturbance. Direct laryngoscopy is necessary to establish the diagnosis.

Treatment. Infants with unilateral paralysis should be closely observed until there is evidence of improvement. Gentle handling and frequent small feedings will aid in keeping the infant quiet and minimizing the risk of aspiration. Bilateral paralysis necessitates immediate tracheal intubation to establish an airway. Tracheostomy is required subsequently in most patients. Laryngoscopic examinations then should be performed at intervals to look for evidence of return of vocal cord function; early extubation may be attempted if there is complete return within a short period of time.

Prognosis. The infant with unilateral paralysis usually improves rapidly without treatment, and complete resolution occurs within 4 to 6 weeks. The prognosis of bilateral paralysis is more variable. If untreated, the infant may develop a funnel deformity in the lower sternal area; this may appear as early as the fifteenth day of life. After tracheostomy a decrease in the severity of the deformity may occur within several weeks. Some of the affected infants subsequently regain normally shaped chests; others may have residual fixed depressions, occasionally severe enough to require surgical correction. The recovery of vocal cord function varies in time and degree. Some infants may show partial recovery within a few months, with several years elapsing before complete movement of the cords is restored. Other infants who have been followed for years show no improvement. Bilateral paralysis of central origin may improve completely if it is caused by cerebral edema or hemorrhage that rapidly resolves.

INJURIES TO THE NECK AND SHOULDER GIRDLE
Fracture of the clavicle

The clavicle is the most commonly fractured bone during labor and delivery. Most clavicular fractures are of the greenstick type, but occasionally the fracture is complete.

Etiology. The major causes of clavicular fractures are difficult delivery of the shoulders in vertex presentations and extended arms in breech deliveries. Usually there has been vigorous, forceful manipulation of the arm and shoulder.

Clinical manifestations. Usually a greenstick fracture is not associated with any signs or symptoms but is first detected after the appearance of an obvious callus at 7 to 10 days of life. Complete fractures and some greenstick fractures may be apparent shortly after birth; there is decreased or absent movement of the arm on the affected side. Deformity and, occasionally, discoloration may be visible over the fracture site with obliteration of the adjacent supraclavicular depression as a result of sternocleidomastoid muscle spasm. Passive movement of the arm elicits cries of pain from the infant. Palpation reveals tenderness, crepitus, and irregularity along the clavicle. The Moro reflex on the involved side is characteristically absent. Roentgenograms confirm the diagnosis of fracture.

Differential diagnosis. A similar clinical picture of impaired movement of an arm with absent Moro reflex may follow fracture of the humerus or brachial palsy. The former is confirmed by roentgenograms; the latter is accompanied by additional clinical findings.

Treatment. Therapy is directed toward minimizing the infant's pain. The affected arm and shoulder should be immobilized with the arm abducted above 60 degrees and the elbow flexed above 90 degrees. A callus forms, and pain usually subsides by 7 to 10 days, when immobilization may be discontinued.

Prognosis. Prognosis is excellent, with growth resulting in restoration of normal bone contour after several months.

Brachial palsy

Brachial palsy is a paralysis involving the muscles of the upper extremity that follows mechanical trauma to the spinal roots of the fifth cervical through the first thoracic nerves, the brachial plexus, during birth. Three main forms occur, depending on the site of injury: (1) Duchenne-Erb, or upper arm, paralysis, which results from injury of the fifth and sixth cervical roots and is by far the most common; (2) Klumpke's, or lower arm, paralysis, which results from injury of the eighth cervical and first thoracic roots and is extremely rare; and (3) paralysis of the entire arm, which occurs slightly more often than the Klumpke type.

Etiology. Most cases of brachial palsy follow a prolonged and difficult labor culminating in a traumatic delivery. The affected infant is frequently large, relaxed, and asphyxiated and thereby vulnerable to excessive separation of bony segments, overstretching, and injury to soft tissues. Injury of the fifth and sixth cervical roots may follow a breech presentation with the arms extended over the head; excessive traction on the shoulder in the delivery of the head may result in stretching of the plexus. The same injury may follow lateral traction of the head and neck away from one of the shoulders while attempting to deliver the shoulders in a vertex presentation. More vigorous traction of the same nature will result in paralysis of the entire arm. The mechanism for isolated lower arm paralysis is uncertain; it is thought to result from stretching of lower plexus nerves under and against the coracoid process of the scapula during forceful elevation and abduction of the arm. Excessive traction on the trunk during a breech delivery may result in avulsion of the lower roots from the cervical cord. In most patients the nerve sheath is torn and the nerve fibers are compressed by the resultant hemorrhage and edema. Less commonly the nerves are completely ruptured and the ends severed, or the roots are avulsed from the spinal cord with injury to the spinal gray matter.

Clinical manifestations. The infant with upper arm paralysis holds his affected arm in a characteristic position, reflecting involvement of the shoulder abductors and external rotators, forearm flexors and supinators, and wrist extensors. The arm is adducted and internally rotated, with extension at the elbow, pronation of the forearm, and flexion of the wrist. When the arm is passively abducted, it falls limply to the side of the body. The Moro, biceps, and radial reflexes are absent on the affected side. There may be some sensory deficit on the radial aspect of the arm, but this is difficult to evaluate in the neonatal infant. The grasp reflex is intact. Any signs of respiratory distress may indicate an accompanying homolateral phrenic nerve root injury (p. 228).

Lower arm paralysis involves the intrinsic muscles of the hand and the long flexors of the wrist and fingers. The hand is paralyzed, and voluntary movements of the wrist cannot be made. The grasp reflex is absent; the deep tendon reflexes are intact. Sensory impairment may be demonstrated along the ulnar side of the forearm and hand. Frequently, dependent edema and cyanosis of the hand and trophic changes in the fingernails develop. After some time there may be flattening and atrophy of the intrinsic hand muscles. Usually a homolateral *Horner's syndrome* (ptosis, miosis, and enophthalmos) is also present because of injury involving the cervical sympathetic fibers of the first thoracic root. Often this is associated with delayed pigmentation of the iris, sometimes of more than 1 year's duration.

When the entire arm is paralyzed, it is usually completely motionless, flaccid, and powerless, hanging limply to the side. All reflexes are absent. The sensory deficit may extend almost up to the shoulder.

Differential diagnosis. The presence of a flail arm in a neonate may be caused by cerebral injury or by a number of injuries about the shoulder. The former is usually associated with other manifestations of CNS injury. A careful roentgenographic study of the shoulder (including lower cervical spine, clavicle, and upper humerus) should be made to exclude tearing of the joint capsule, fracture of the clavicle, and fracture, dislocation, or upper epiphyseal detachment of the humerus.

Treatment. The basic principle of treatment is prevention of contractures while awaiting recovery of the brachial plexus. This is accomplished by partial immobilization during the first 1 to 2 weeks, appropriate positioning, and an exercise program. Active physical therapy should be avoided initially because of a painful traumatic neuritis that usually affects the brachial plexus. By 7 to 10 days of age gentle range of motion exercises may be started.

In upper arm paralysis the arm should be abducted 90 degrees with external rotation at the shoulder, 90 degrees flexion at the elbow, full supination of the forearm, and slight extension at the wrist so that the palm of the hand is turned toward the face. This may be done with cautious use of a splint or brace during the first 1 to 2 weeks, until the traumatic neuritis has resolved. Current authorities warn against the potential risk of abduction contractures occurring following prolonged or persistent splinting. In fact, many question whether splinting results in any beneficial effects other than decreasing the pain that would accompany movement of the affected limb. Accordingly, splinting should only be administered intermittently throughout the day; a useful routine is to immobilize the affected limb while the infant is asleep, between feedings, followed by removal of the splint during the feeding. After the first 1 to 2 weeks gentle massage and passive range of motion exercises are indicated to prevent development of contractures. If the infant is otherwise stable, the parents may be easily instructed in the exercise procedures, thereby permitting discharge of the infant. The infant must be followed closely and active and passive corrective exercises continued until normal scapulohumeral rhythm has been reestablished. Patients who demonstrate persistent lack of abduction and external rotation may benefit from a teres major tendon transfer to the rotator cuff. Most authorities recommend delaying this procedure until the child is approximately 3 or 4 years of age to permit a valid preoperative muscle assessment.

In lower arm paralysis the forearm and wrist should be splinted in a neutral position, and padding should be placed in the fist. Passive range of motion exercises of the wrist, hand, and fingers should be gently performed.

When the entire arm is paralyzed, the same treatment principles should be followed: immobilization in a neutral position, padding of the fist, massage, and range of motion exercises.

Routine neurosurgical exploration and repair of the injury are not indicated. Mild injuries are self-limited, and severe injuries usually involve avulsion of the roots from the cord, making suture of the nerves impossible. Dissection of the plexus is so difficult that more damage may be inflicted, resulting in formation of additional scar tissue and symptoms years after the operation. Matson has explored the brachial plexus and performed neurolysis on infants who showed no improvement after 3 to 6 months and in whom there was palpable thickening in the supraclavicular fossa or swelling or ecchymosis over the plexus during the acute phase of injury. Although the results have been generally discouraging, several infants have shown a greater degree of improvement following surgery than would have been expected to occur spontaneously.

Prognosis. If the nerve roots are intact, return of function may appear within several days as the local hemorrhage and edema resolve. The rate of recovery varies with the degree of injury. In some infants recovery is complete within a few weeks. The majority of appropriately treated infants will recover completely within 3 to 6 months. An occasional infant with severe injury may show continued improvement over a period of up to 2 years. Even where recovery of function appears complete, close examination will usually reveal peculiar posturing of the arm in abduction at the shoulder, tightness in internal rotation, difficulty in forearm supination, and minimal winging of the scapula.

Lower arm paralysis is associated with a relatively poor prognosis; a claw deformity may develop. Paralysis of the entire arm may show recovery of some function eventually.

Electrodiagnosis is helpful in distinguishing a neuropraxis lesion from a root avulsion. An infant with a severe lesion of the former type may be predicted to have partial, and possibly total, return of function, whereas an infant with an avulsion injury may be predicted to have permanent paralysis. In avulsion injuries and untreated stretch injuries, residual contractures and bony deformities develop. The former may be treated with gentle stretching in the infant and by tenotomies in the older patient. Bony deformities may be treated by osteotomies or tendon transfers. These procedures produce no increase in muscle power but may make motion of the arm less awkward.

Phrenic nerve paralysis

See also pp. 374 and 460.

Phrenic nerve paralysis results in diaphragmatic paralysis and rarely occurs as an isolated injury in the neonatal infant. The majority of injuries are unilateral and are associated with a homolateral upper brachial plexus palsy.

Etiology. The most common cause is a difficult breech delivery. Lateral hyperextension of the neck results in overstretching or avulsion of the third, fourth, and fifth cervical roots, which supply the phrenic nerve.

Clinical manifestations. The first sign may be recurrent episodes of cyanosis, usually accompanied by irregular and labored respirations. The respiratory excursions of the involved side of the diaphragm are largely ineffectual, and the breathing is therefore almost completely thoracic so that no bulging of the abdomen occurs with inspiration (Fig. 17-7, A and B). The thrust of the diaphragm, which often may be felt just under the costal margin on the normal side, is absent on the affected side. Dullness and diminished breath sounds are found over the affected side. In a severe injury tachypnea, weak cry, and apneic spells may occur.

Roentgenographic manifestations. Roentgenograms taken during the first few days may show only slight elevation of the affected diaphragm, occasionally so subtle that it may be considered normal. Repeated films will show the more apparent elevation of the diaphragm, with displacement of the heart and mediastinum to the opposite side (Fig. 17-7, C). Frequently areas of atelectasis appear bilaterally. Early diagnosis can be confirmed only by fluoroscopy, which reveals an abnormal elevation of the affected hemidiaphragm and seesaw movements of the two hemidiaphragms with respiration (elevation of the affected side and descent of the normal side during inspiration); opposite movements occur during expiration. Fluoroscopy reveals a shift of the mediastinum toward the normal side during inspiration. In questionable cases diagnosis can be further enhanced by transvenous electrical stimulation of the phrenic nerve.

Differential diagnosis. Careful physical examination should allow differentiation between CNS, cardiac, and pulmonary causes of neonatal respiratory distress. The diagnosis can be confirmed by fluoroscopy and/or electrical stimulation of the phrenic nerve.

Treatment. Most infants require only nonspecific medical treatment. The infant should be positioned on the involved side, and oxygen should be administered for cyanosis and/or hypoxemia. Intravenous fluids may be necessary the first few days. If the infant begins to show improvement, progressive oral or gavage feedings may be started. Antibiotics are indicated if pneumonia occurs.

Infants with more severe respiratory distress, particularly those with bilateral phrenic nerve palsy, may require assisted ventilation shortly after delivery. Other modes of therapy that have been successfully used include continuous positive airway pressure by nasal can-

Birth injuries 229

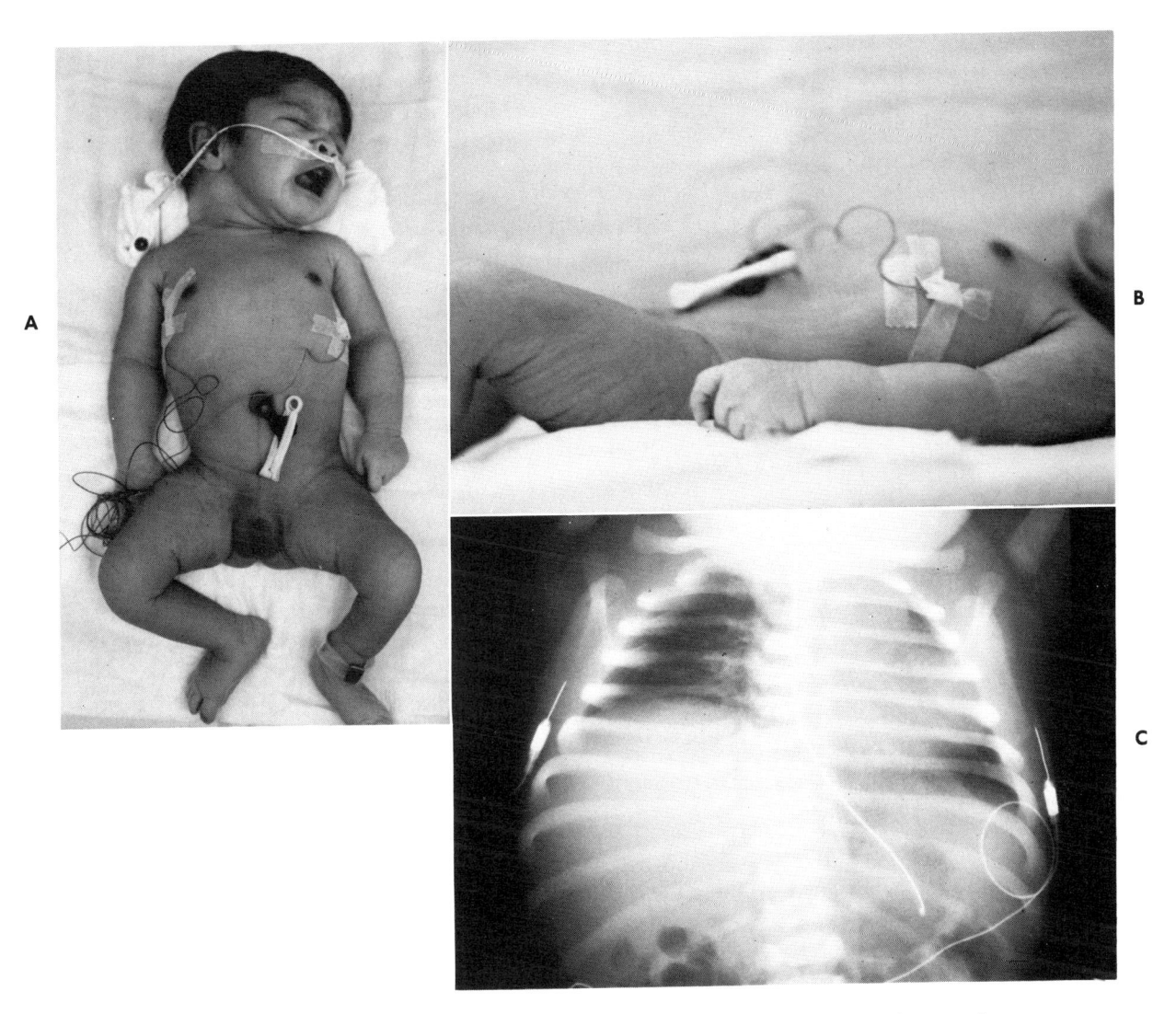

Fig. 17-7, A. Nine-hour-old 3,190-gm, female born after difficult total breech extraction; during delivery cervix clamped down on head, necessitating extensive tugging and pulling on both arms. Note markedly hyperexpanded chest and classic appearance of both upper extremities in Erb's palsy positions. **B,** Lateral view of same infant, demonstrating increased AP diameter of chest as well as close-up of left upper extremity adducted at shoulder, extended at elbow, and pronated and flexed at wrist. **C,** Significant elevation of right hemidiaphragm to T5 level in same infant, compatible with paralysis of the right hemidiaphragm. Note significant shifting of the heart and mediastinum to the left.

nula and continuous negative pressure via a negative-pressure respirator. These forms of therapy may be used either primarily or secondarily to facilitate weaning the infant off the respirator. Electrical diaphragmatic pacing may also be used as an adjunct to assisted ventilation if the diaphragm shows significant contraction following electrical stimulation of the phrenic nerve.

Surgical intervention should be considered for the infant with severe or increasing respiratory distress despite medical management, or for the infant who, after 3 or 4 months, is only mildly symptomatic but has shown no roentgenographic evidence of recovery of function of the affected hemidiaphragm. Electrical stimulation of the phrenic nerve is helpful in deciding on the advisability of surgical treatment. The infant who demonstrates absence of diaphragmatic contraction following phrenic nerve stimulation has probably incurred nerve damage below the level of stimulation or diaphragmatic muscle atrophy and should be considered a candidate for surgery. The procedure of choice is either plication or excision of part of the paralyzed diaphragm. This results in a tightening of the diaphragm and brings the dome of the diaphragm down to a normal level, allowing the mediastinum to return to its normal position.

Prognosis. Most infants recover spontaneously. This may be complete by 6 weeks but usually takes several months. If avulsion of the cervical nerves has occurred, spontaneous recovery is not possible, and in the absence of surgery the infant is susceptible to pneumonia in the atelectatic lung. Many of these infants die before 3 months of age. Infants treated surgically do well, with no recurrence of pneumonia and no late pulmonary or chest wall complications. The repaired hemidiaphragm remains in a satisfactory position despite permanent paralysis of the phrenic nerve. The accuracy of prognosis may be improved by electrical phrenic nerve stimulation. If the stimulation results in adequate diaphragmatic contraction, nerve injury below the level of stimulation is unlikely and diaphragmatic muscle fibers are intact. If diaphragmatic contraction does not occur, nerve damage has probably occurred below the level of stimulation.

Injury to the sternocleidomastoid muscle

This injury is also designated muscular torticollis, congenital torticollis, or sternocleidomastoid fibroma. Its cause and pathology have been a matter of controversy.

Etiology. The birth trauma theory suggests that the muscle or fascial sheath is ruptured during a breech or difficult delivery involving hyperextension of the muscle. A hematoma develops and is subsequently invaded by fibrin and fibroblasts with progressive formation of scar tissue and shortening of the muscle. The intrauterine theory postulates abnormal pressure, position, or trauma to the muscle during intrauterine life. Another theory suggests a hereditary defect in the development of the muscle. Still others have noted pathologic findings resembling infectious myositis, suggesting an infection in utero or a muscle injured at delivery.

Clinical manifestations. A mass in the midportion of the sternocleidomastoid muscle may be evident at birth, although usually it is first noted 10 to 14 days after birth. It is 1 to 2 cm in diameter, hard, immobile, fusiform, and well circumscribed; there is no inflammation or overlying discoloration. The mass enlarges during the following 2 to 4 weeks and then gradually regresses and disappears by the age of 5 to 8 months.

A transient torticollis produced by contracture of the involved muscle appears soon after birth. The head tilts toward the involved side, and the chin is somewhat elevated and rotated toward the opposite shoulder. The head cannot be moved passively into normal position. If the deformity persists beyond 3 or 4 years, the skull becomes foreshortened. Flattening of the frontal bone and bulging of the occipital bone occur on the involved side, whereas the contralateral frontal bone bulges and the occiput is flattened. The ipsilateral eyebrow is slanted; the clavicle and shoulder become elevated compared with the opposite normal side, and the ipsilateral mastoid process becomes more prominent. If treatment is not instituted, a lower cervical–upper thoracic scoliosis subsequently develops. Rarely calcification develops in the affected muscles.

Differential diagnosis. Careful roentgenographic examination should be made of the cervical spine and shoulders to rule out Sprengel's deformity or Klippel-Feil syndrome, cervical myelodysplasia, and occipitalization of the atlas.

Treatment. Treatment should be instituted as early as possible. The involved muscle should be stretched to an overcorrected position by gentle, even, and persistent motion with the baby supine. The head is flexed forward and away from the affected side, and the chin is rotated toward the affected side. The mother can be instructed to repeat this maneuver several times a day. The infant should also be stimulated to turn the head spontaneously toward the affected side; the crib may be positioned so that he must turn to the desired position of overcorrection in looking for window light or at a mobile or favorite rattle; during sleep the baby should be placed on the side of the torticollis; in this position sandbags should be placed on each side of his body for fixation. An alternative approach recently described involves a helmet that is custom made for the infant. Rubber straps made of surgical drain tubing attached to the helmet are in turn fixed to the side rails of the crib at night, with appropriate adjustments made to force the infant to sleep on the prominent side of the head. This results in stretching of the shortened sternocleidomastoid muscle.

Conservative therapy should be continued for 6 months. If the deformity has not been fully corrected, surgery should be considered to prevent permanent skull and cervical spine deformities. Removal of the tumor is not necessary and will needlessly deform the outline of the neck. The procedure of choice is lengthening and division of the sternal portion of the muscle from the mastoid process at its origin; the neck outline is preserved. After surgery the head should be immobilized in an overcorrected position for several weeks, followed by an exercise program.

Prognosis. Most infants treated conservatively show complete recovery within 2 to 3 months. If surgery is necessary and if it is performed early, the facial asymmetry will disappear almost entirely.

INJURIES TO THE SPINE AND SPINAL CORD

See p. 373.

Birth injuries to the vertebral spine and spinal cord are rarely diagnosed. It is not certain whether the low incidence is real, reflecting improved obstetric techniques, or represents a tendency for postmortem examination to overlook spine and spinal cord lesions.

Etiology. These injuries almost always result from breech deliveries, especially difficult ones where version and extraction were used. Other predisposing factors include brow and face presentations, dystocia (especially shoulder), prematurity, primiparity, and precipitous delivery.

The injuries are usually caused by stretching of the cord and not by compression. The most common mechanism responsible is probably forceful longitudinal traction on the trunk while the head is still firmly engaged in the pelvis. When combined with flexion and torsion of the vertebral axis, this becomes a more significant problem. Occasionally a snap is felt by the obstetrician while exerting traction. Although cesarean section has been recommended as the optimum delivery for infants in breech presentation with a hyperextended head, several reports have appeared documenting vertebral or spinal cord injury following cesarean section. The patient reported on by Maekawa and co-workers demonstrated weak fetal movements during the third trimester, suggesting that injury was occurring prior to delivery. Difficulty in delivery of the shoulders in cephalic presentations may result in a similar mechanism of injury. The spinal cord is very delicate and inelastic. Its attachments are the cauda equina below and the roots of the brachial plexus and medulla above. Because the ligaments are elastic and the muscles delicate, the infant's vertebral column may be stretched quite easily. In addition, the dura is more elastic in the infant than in the adult. Consequently, strong longitudinal traction may be expected to cause elongation of the spinal column and to stretch the spinal cord and its membranes. The possible result is vertebral fracture or dislocation or both and cord transection. Most often, hemorrhage and edema produce a physiologic transection. The lower cervical and upper thoracic regions are most commonly involved, but occasionally the entire length of the spinal canal contains a heavy accumulation of blood.

Clinical manifestations. Affected infants may follow one of four clinical patterns. Those in the first group are either stillborn or in poor condition from birth, with respiratory depression, shock, and hypothermia. They deteriorate rapidly; death occurs within several hours, often before neurologic signs are obvious. These infants are usually victims of a high cervical or brainstem lesion.

The second group consists of infants who at birth may appear normal or show signs similar to group one; these infants die after several days. Cardiac function is usually relatively strong. Within hours or days the central type of respiratory depression, which is initially present, may be complicated by respiratory distress of pulmonary origin, usually pneumonia. The spinal lesion, usually in the upper or midcervical region, frequently is not recognized for several days, when flaccidity and immobility of the legs are noted. Occasionally urinary retention may be the first symptom. Paralysis of the abdominal wall is manifested by a relaxation of the abdominal wall and bulging at the flanks when the baby is held upright. The intercostal muscles may be affected if the lesion is high enough. Sensation is absent over the lower half of the body. Deep tendon reflexes and spontaneous reflex movements are absent. The infant is constipated. The brachial plexus is involved in about 20% of all cases. The spinal column is usually clinically and roentgenographically normal.

The third group, with lesions at C8 to T1 or lower, is composed of infants who survive for long periods, some for years. Paraplegia noted at birth may be transient. The lesion in the cord may be mild and reversible, or it may result in permanent neurologic sequelae with no return of function of the lower cord segments. The skin over the involved part of the body is dry and scaly, predisposing the infant to bed sores and ulcers. Muscle atrophy, severe contractures, and bony deformities follow. Bladder distention and constant dribbling persist, and recurring urinary tract infections and pneumonia are common. Within several weeks or months this clinical picture is replaced by a stage of reflex activity or paraplegia-in-flexion. This is characterized by return of tone and rigid flexion of the involved extremities, improvement in skin condition with healing of decubiti, and periodic mass reflex responses composed of tonic spasms of the extremities, spontaneous micturition, and profuse sweating over the involved part of the body.

Infants in the fourth group have subtle neurologic signs of spasticity thought to represent cerebral palsy. These patients have incurred partial spinal cord injuries and occasional cerebrovascular accidents.

Differential diagnosis. During the first few weeks of life, injuries to the spinal cord may be confused with amyotonia congenita or myelodysplasia associated with spina bifida occulta (p. 385). The former may be differentiated by the generalized distribution of the weakness and hypotonia and by the presence of normal sensation and sphincter control. The latter is usually associated with some cutaneous lesions over the sacral region such as dimples, angiomas, or abnormal tufts of hair; it is always associated with defects in the spinal lamina. Other conditions less commonly considered include transverse myelitis and spinal cord tumors, particularly in infants who demonstrate paralysis following an apparently normal labor and delivery. Cerebral hypotonia should be considered in infants who also demonstrate cranial nerve abnormalities, persistent primitive reflexes, and a dull facial appearance, contrasting with the bright, alert facies of the spinal cord trauma victim. However, the concomitant occurrence of cerebral damage in an infant with spinal cord injury may confound the diagnosis. A final consideration is the infant with bilateral brachial plexus palsy with associated motor and sensory loss, or Horner's syndrome; the demonstration of normal lower extremity function should rule out spinal cord injury.

Treatment. Therapy is supportive and usually unsatisfactory. The infant affected at birth requires basic resuscitative and supportive measures. Infants who survive present a therapeutic challenge that can be met only by the combined and interested efforts of the pediatrician, neurologist, neurosurgeon, urologist, psychiatrist, orthopedist, nurse, physical therapist, and occupational therapist.

While the infant is reasonably stable, cervical and thoracic spine roentgenograms should be obtained. In the rare occurrence of vertebral fracture or dislocation or both, immediate neurosurgical consultation is necessary for reduction of the deformity and relief of cord compression, followed by appropriate immobilization. Lumbar puncture in the acute period is of little practical value and may aggravate existing cord damage if the infant is excessively manipulated during the procedure. After several days, however, a persistent spinal fluid block may be demonstrated and may be an indication for exploratory laminectomy at the site of trauma. This possibility should be suspected in an infant with partial paraplegia and normal roentgenograms.

Prompt and meticulous attention must be given to skin, bladder, and bowel care. The position of paralyzed parts should be changed every 2 hours. Areas of anesthetic skin should be washed, dried, and gently massaged daily. Lamb's-wool covers are helpful in preventing pressure necrosis of skin. Benzoin tincture applications help protect the skin in pressure areas. A decubitus ulcer is treated by scrupulous cleansing and complete freedom from weight bearing and friction. An indwelling urethral catheter should be inserted within several hours after severe cord trauma at any level. In the smaller infant a no. 3 feeding tube may be used. Repeated instrumentation should be avoided. Cultures of urine should be obtained at least weekly and antibiotic therapy employed only in the presence of infection. After several weeks the infant reaches the stage of paraplegia-in-flexion, and urinary retention is usually replaced by regular episodes of spontaneous voiding. If this is accompanied by a decrease in bladder size to normal, the catheter is removed. In the infant in whom prompt return of bladder function does not occur, urologic assistance should be sought in catheter management and planning of further procedures (for example, suprapubic cystostomy and wet ureterostomies).

The first infection should be treated with the appropriate antibiotic for 2 weeks. After the neonatal period, this should be followed by suppressive therapy with sulfisoxazole (Gantrisin), 50 to 75 mg/kg/day for 3 to 6 months, assuming that cultures remain negative. Subsequent antibiotic therapy should be governed by the spectrum of sensitivity of cultured organisms.

Fecal retention is also a common problem, especially after total cord transection. Appropriate dietary balance should aid in keeping the stools soft. Early use of glycerin suppositories at regular intervals will encourage automatic defecation. Digital manipulation may be necessary to relieve fecal impactions.

Finally, physical rehabilitation should be instituted early in an attempt to minimize deformity. After several years orthopedic procedures may still be necessary to correct contractures and bony deformities.

Prognosis. The prognosis varies with the severity of the injury. Most severe injuries result in death shortly after birth. Infants with cord compression from vertebral fractures or dislocations or both may recover with reasonable return of function if prompt neurosurgical removal of the compression is performed. Infants with mild injuries or partial transections may recover with minimal sequelae. Infants who exhibit complete physiologic cord transection shortly after birth without vertebral fracture or dislocation have an extremely poor outlook for recovery of function. Many die in infancy of ascending urinary tract infection and sepsis. Long-term survivors have been reported to live into their third decade. These are extremely rare, and although the child may have normal intelligence and learn to walk with special appliances, he faces the late complications of pain, spasms, autonomic dysfunction, bony deformities, and genitourinary, psychiatric, and school problems.

INJURIES TO INTRAABDOMINAL ORGANS

Although birth trauma involving intraabdominal organs is uncommon, it frequently must be considered by the physician who manages neonatal infants because deterioration can be fulminant in an undetected lesion, and therapy can be very effective when a lesion is diagnosed early. Intraabdominal trauma should be suspected in any newborn infant with shock and abdominal distention or pallor, anemia, and irritability without evidence of external blood loss.

Rupture of the liver

The liver is the most commonly injured abdominal organ during the birth process. The autopsy incidence varies from 0.9% to 9.6%.

Etiology. Birth trauma is the most significant contributing factor. The condition usually occurs in large infants, infants with hepatomegaly (for example, erythroblastosis fetalis and infants of diabetic mothers), and breech deliveries. Manual pressure on the liver during delivery of the head in a breech presentation is probably a common mechanism of injury. Prematurity and postmaturity also have been felt to predispose the infant to this injury. Other contributing factors include asphyxia and coagulation disorders. Trauma to the liver more commonly results in subcapsular hematoma than actual laceration of the liver.

Clinical manifestations. The infant usually appears normal the first 1 to 3 days and rarely for as long as 7 days. Nonspecific signs related to loss of blood into the hematoma may appear early; these include poor feeding, listlessness, pallor, jaundice, tachypnea, and tachycardia. A mass may be palpable in the right upper quadrant. The hematocrit and hemoglobin values may be stable early in the course, but serial determinations will suggest blood loss. These manifestations are followed by sudden circulatory collapse, usually coincident with rupture of the hematoma through the capsule and extravasation of blood into the peritoneal cavity. The abdomen then may be distended, rigid, and dull to percussion, occasionally with a bluish discoloration of the overlying skin, which may extend over the scrotum. Abdominal roentgenograms may reveal uniform opacity of the abdomen, indicating free intraperitoneal fluid. Paracentesis confirms the presence of free blood in the peritoneal cavity.

Differential diagnosis. This lesion is one of several that can result in hemoperitoneum; others include trauma to the adrenals, kidneys, gastrointestinal tract, and spleen. Presence of a right upper quadrant mass suggests trauma to the liver, but absence of a mass does not rule it out. Abdominal roentgenograms, ultrasonography, and intravenous pyelography may assist in pinpointing the site of trauma, but ultimately a definite diagnosis can be made only by laparotomy.

Treatment. Immediate management consists of prompt transfusion with whole blood to restore the blood volume and of recognition and correction of any coagulation disorder. This should be followed by laparotomy with evacuation of the hematoma and repair of any laceration with sutures placed over a hemostatic agent. Any fragmented, devitalized liver tissue should be removed to prevent subsequent fatal secondary hemorrhage. Because of the successful treatment of two infants with blood transfusion only and because of hemostatic difficulty in one infant at surgery, it has been suggested that blood transfusion and the tamponade of intraabdominal pressure might be adequate therapy in some infants.

Prognosis. In unrecognized liver trauma with formation of a subcapsular hematoma, shock and death may result if the hematoma ruptures through the capsule, reducing the pressure tamponade and resulting in new bleeding from the liver. Recognition of the possibility of liver rupture in infants with a predisposing birth history, followed by early diagnosis and prompt therapy, should improve the prognosis. Early diagnosis and correction of any existing coagulation disorder will also improve the prognosis.

Rupture of the spleen

Rupture of the spleen in the newborn occurs much less often than rupture of the liver. However, recognition of this condition is equally important because of its similar potential for fulminant shock and death if the diagnosis is delayed.

Etiology. The condition is most common in large babies, babies delivered in breech position, and babies with erythroblastosis fetalis or congenital syphilis, in whom the spleen is enlarged and more friable and thereby susceptible to rupture either spontaneously or after minor trauma. An underlying clotting defect has also been implicated. Rupture of the spleen has occurred in normal-sized infants with uneventful deliveries and no underlying disease.

Clinical manifestations. Clinical signs indicating blood loss and hemoperitoneum are similar to those described for hepatic rupture. The hemoglobin and hematocrit values decrease, and abdominal paracentesis may reveal free blood. Several infants have been described in whom the blood was circumscribed within the leaves of the phrenicolineal ligament and therefore not clinically detectable. Occasionally a left upper quadrant mass may be palpable, and films of the abdomen may show medial displacement of the gastric air bubble.

Differential diagnosis. Rupture of the liver and trauma to the adrenals, kidneys, and gastrointestinal tract must be distinguished.

Treatment. Whole blood should be transfused promptly, and any coexisting clotting defect should be corrected. This should be followed by immediate exploratory laparotomy. In contrast to earlier recommendations in favor of splenectomy, the current philosophy is to attempt repair and preservation of the spleen to prevent the subsequent increased risk of infection. Matsuyama and associates reported on an infant in whom the almost transected spleen was successfully repaired surgically.

Prognosis. With early recognition and emergency surgery, survival should approach 100%.

Adrenal hemorrhage

Neonatal adrenal hemorrhage is more common than previously suspected; some autopsy studies have revealed a high incidence of subclinical hemorrhage. Massive hemorrhage is much less common, and the incidence is difficult to determine, since the diagnosis is often unsuspected and only considered retrospectively years later when calcified adrenals are unexpectedly found on roentgenograms or at autopsy.

Etiology. The most likely cause is birth trauma; the frequency is higher in infants with macrosomia, in infants

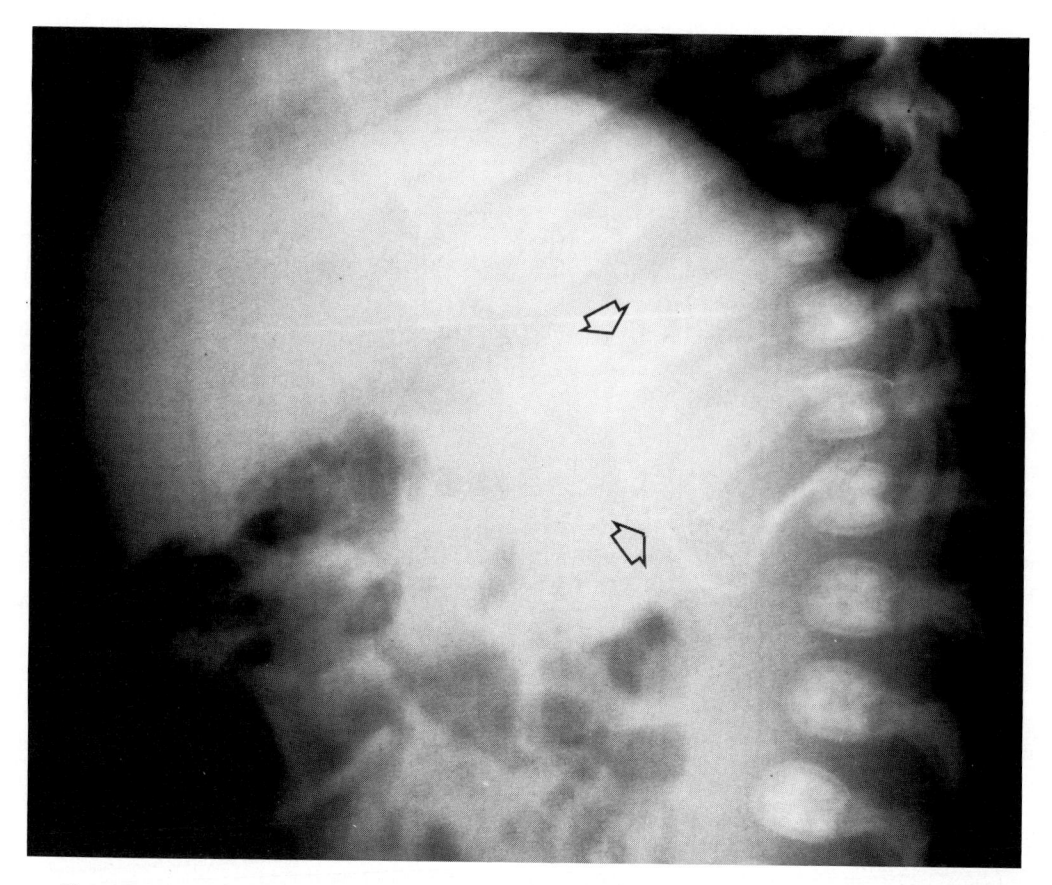

Fig. 17-8. Lateral abdominal roentgenogram of a 5,312-gm male delivered vaginally, with difficulty after shoulder dystocia. At 48 hours fever, icterus, and slow feeding were noted, and a mass was palpable above the left kidney. At 31 days there was dense, retracted calcification, assuming the configuration of the adrenal gland.

of diabetic mothers, in breech presentation, in infants with congenital syphilis, and when there is dystocia. Placental hemorrhage, anoxia, hemorrhagic disease of the newborn, prematurity, and, more recently, neuroblastoma have been implicated. Pathologic findings vary from unilateral minute areas of bleeding to massive bilateral hemorrhage. The increased size and vascularity of the adrenal gland at birth may predispose it to hemorrhage.

Clinical manifestations. Signs vary with the degree and extent of hemorrhage. The classic findings are fever, tachypnea out of proportion to the degree of fever, yellowish pallor, cyanosis of the lips and fingertips, a mass in either flank with overlying skin discoloration, and purpura. Findings suggesting adrenal insufficiency include poor feeding, vomiting, diarrhea, obstipation, dehydration, abdominal distention, irritability, hypoglycemia, uremia, skin rash, listlessness, coma, convulsions, and shock.

Roentgenographic manifestations. Initial roentgenographic manifestations may be limited to widening of the retroperitoneal space with forward displacement of stomach and duodenum or downward displacement of intestines or kidneys. In time, calcification may appear. Typically this is rimlike and has been observed as early as the twelfth day of life. After several weeks the calcification becomes denser and retracted and assumes the configuration of the adrenal gland (Fig. 17-8). The increased experience with ultrasound in the neonate provides another adjunctive method of diagnosis. Abdominal ultrasound performed during the first several days may reveal a solid lesion in the location of the adrenal hemorrhage; this is felt to represent either clot fragmentation or diffuse clotted blood throughout the adrenal gland. If adrenal hemorrhage is suspected, ultrasound should be repeated at 3- to 5-day intervals. If adrenal hemorrhage has occurred, the lesion will change from a solid to a cystic appearance, coincident with liquefaction, degeneration, and lysis of the clot.

Differential diagnosis. Adrenal hemorrhage must be distinguished from other causes of abdominal hemorrhage. In addition, when a mass is palpable, the differential diagnosis must include the multiple causes of flank masses in the newborn infant, such as genitourinary anomaly, Wilms' tumor, and neuroblastoma. If the infant is large or the delivery is traumatic or breech, an adrenal hemorrhage is most likely. Neuroblastoma may be distinguished by persistent demonstration of a solid lesion on serial ultrasound examinations, as well as by increased excretion of vanillylmandelic acid (VMA) and other urinary catecholamines in 85% to 90% of affected infants. Blood pressure measurements and roentgenograms may also help to evaluate this possibility.

Treatment. Significant blood loss should be replaced with whole blood transfusion. Suspicion of adrenal insufficiency may warrant use of intravenous fluids and steroids. The decision for surgical intervention is dictated by the location and degree of hemorrhage. If it appears to be retroperitoneal and limited by the perinephric fascia, some authors recommend blood replacement and careful observation in the hope of spontaneous control by tamponade; often this approach is successful and surgery is not necessary. If paracentesis reveals blood or if blood loss exceeds replacement, exploratory laparotomy is indicated. Surgery may involve evacuation of hematoma, vessel ligation, and adrenalectomy with or without nephrectomy. When the hemorrhagic process extends to the peritoneal cavity, peritoneal exploration and evacuation of clots are indicated.

Prognosis. Small hemorrhages are probably often asymptomatic and have no associated significant morbidity, judging from the unexpected discovery of calcified adrenals on abdominal films taken for other reasons later in infancy and childhood. If hemoperitoneum or adrenal insufficiency or both develop, the outlook depends on the speed with which diagnosis is made and appropriate therapy instituted. Surviving infants should be followed closely after discharge from the hospital. Adrenal function should be tested with ACTH stimulation at a later date to determine whether a normal response occurs in the urinary excretion of 17-hydroxycorticosterone.

INJURIES TO THE EXTREMITIES
Fracture of the humerus

After the clavicle, the humerus is the bone most often fractured during the birth process.

Etiology. The most common mechanisms responsible are difficult delivery of extended arms in breech presentations and of the shoulders in vertex presentations. Besides traction with simultaneous rotation of the arm, direct pressure on the humerus is also a factor. This may account for the occurrence of fracture of the humerus in spontaneous vertex deliveries. The fractures are usually in the diaphysis. They are often greenstick, although complete fracture with overriding of the fragments occasionally occurs.

Clinical manifestations. A greenstick fracture may be overlooked until a callus is noted. A complete fracture with marked displacement of fragments presents an obvious deformity that calls attention to the injury. Often the initial manifestation of the fracture is immobility of the affected arm. Palpation reveals tenderness, crepitation, and hypermobility of the fragments. The homolateral Moro response is absent. Roentgenograms confirm the diagnosis.

Differential diagnosis. This includes all the previously noted lesions that cause immobility of the arm. An associated brachial plexus injury occasionally occurs.

Treatment. The affected arm should be immobilized in adduction for 2 to 4 weeks. This may be accomplished by maintaining the arm in a hand-on-hip position with a triangular splint and a Velpeau bandage, by strapping the arm to the chest, or by application of a cast.

Prognosis. The prognosis is excellent. Healing is associated with marked callus formation. Moderate overriding and angulation disappear with time because of the excellent remodeling power of infants. Complete union of the fracture fragments usually occurs by 3 weeks. Fair alignment and shortening of less than 1 inch indicate satisfactory closed reduction. Long bone fractures in infants always result in epiphyseal stimulation; the closer the fracture to the epiphyseal cartilage, the greater the degree of subsequent overgrowth.

Fracture of the femur

Although a relatively uncommon injury, fracture of the femur is by far the most common fracture of the lower extremity in the newborn.

Etiology. This injury usually follows a breech delivery, when the leg is pulled down after the breech is already partially fixed in the pelvic inlet or when the infant is improperly held by one thigh during delivery of the shoulders and arms.

Clinical manifestations. Usually there is an obvious deformity of the thigh; as a rule the bone breaks transversely in the upper half or third, where it is relatively thin. Less commonly the injury may not be appreciated until several days post partum when swelling of the thigh is noted; this may be caused by hemorrhage into adjacent muscle. The infant refuses to move the affected leg or cries in pain during passive movement or palpation over the fracture site. Roentgenograms almost always show overriding of the fracture fragments.

Treatment. Optimum treatment is traction-suspension of both lower extremities, even if the fracture is unilateral. The legs are immobilized in a spica cast; and with Bryant's traction the infant is suspended by the legs from an overhead frame with the buttocks and lower back just raised off the crib. The legs are extended and the thighs flexed on the abdomen. The weight of the infant's body is enough to overcome the pull of the thigh muscles and thereby reduce the deformity. The infant is maintained in this position for 3 to 4 weeks until adequate callus has formed and new bone growth has started. During the treatment period, special attention should be given to careful feeding and protection of bandages and casts from soiling with urine and feces.

Prognosis. The prognosis is excellent; complete union and restoration without shortening are expected. Extensive calcification may develop in the areas of surrounding hemorrhage; this is resorbed subsequently.

Dislocations

Dislocations caused by birth trauma are rare. Often an apparent dislocation is actually a displaced fracture through an epiphyseal plate. Since the epiphyseal plate is radiolucent, a fracture occurring adjacent to an unmineralized epiphysis will give a radiographic picture simulating a dislocation of the neighboring joint. This type of injury has been termed pseudodislocation. Since the humeral and proximal femoral epiphyses are usually not visible on roentgenograms at birth, a pseudodislocation can occur at the shoulder, elbow, or hip.

Of the true dislocations, those involving the hip and knee are probably not caused by the trauma of the birth process. Most likely they are either intrauterine positional deformities or true congenital malformations. A true dislocation resulting from birth trauma is that involving the radial head. This has been associated with traumatic breech delivery. Examination reveals adduction and internal rotation of the affected arm, with pronation of the forearm; the Moro response is poor, and palpation reveals lateral and posterior displacement of the radial head. This is confirmed by roentgenograms. With supination and extension the radial head can be readily reduced. This should be done promptly, followed by immobilization of the infant in this position in a circular cast for 2 to 3 weeks. Early recognition and treatment should result in normal growth and function of the elbow.

Epiphyseal separations

Like dislocations, epiphyseal separations are rare. They occur mostly in primiparity, dystocic deliveries, and breech presentations, especially those requiring manual extraction or version and extraction; any delivery associated with vigorous pulling may predispose the infant to this injury. The upper femoral and humeral epiphyses are most commonly involved. Usually on the second day the soft tissue over the affected epiphysis develops a firm swelling with reddening, crepitus, and tenderness. Active motion is limited, and passive motion is painful. If the injury is in the upper femoral epiphysis, the infant assumes the frog position with external rotation of the leg.

Early roentgenograms will show only soft tissue swelling, with occasional superolateral displacement of the proximal femoral metaphysis. Since the neonatal femoral capital epiphysis is not ossified, this can be interpreted mistakenly as congenital hip dislocation. However, the presence of pain and tenderness would make the latter condition unlikely. Besides plain roentgenograms of the hips, an infant with a history and physical examination compatible with traumatic epiphysiolysis should also be studied by arthrography before attempting manipulation. Hip arthrography in such an infant would demonstrate a normal femoroacetabular relationship, in contrast to abnormal findings in septic arthritis and congenital hip dislocation. In addition, in the presence of traumatic epiphysiolysis, the femoral head and neck would not be continuous, in contrast to the findings of septic arthritis and congenital hip dislocation. Further differentiation between traumatic epiphysiolysis and septic arthritis can be provided by arthrocentesis; in the former the joint does not contain excess fluid, and what is obtained may be serosanguineous, whereas in the latter, purulent fluid is obtained. After 1 to 2 weeks extensive callus appears, confirming the nature of the injury; during the third week subperiosteal calcification appears.

If possible, treatment should be conservative. Closed reduction and immobilization are indicated within the first few days before rapidly forming fibrous callus prevents mobilization of the epiphysis. The hip is immobilized in the frog-leg position as in congenital dislocation. Poorly immobilized fragments may require temporary fixation with a Kirschner wire. Union usually occurs within 10 to 15 days. Untreated or poorly treated epiphyseal injuries may result in subsequent growth distortion and permanent deformities such as coxa vara. Mild injuries carry a good prognosis.

Other peripheral nerve injuries

In contrast to the brachial plexus and phrenic and facial nerves, other peripheral nerves are injured less often at birth, and usually in association with trauma to the extremity. Radial palsy has occurred following difficult forceps extractions, both from pressure of incorrectly applied forceps and in association with fracture of the arm. Occasionally the palsy occurs later when the radial nerve is enmeshed within the callus of the healing fracture. Frequently there is associated subcutaneous fat necrosis overlying the course of the radial nerve along the lateral aspects of the upper arm. The presence of isolated wrist-drop with weakness of the wrist, finger, and thumb extensors, skin changes overlying the course of the nerve, and absence of weakness above the elbow serve to distinguish this from brachial plexus injury. Palsies of the femoral and sciatic nerves have occurred after breech extractions; the sciatic palsy has followed extraction by the foot. Passive range of motion exercises are usually the only therapy required. Complete recovery usually occurs within several weeks or months.

TRAUMA TO THE GENITALIA

Soft tissue injuries involving the external genitalia are not uncommon, especially after breech deliveries and in large babies.

Scrotum and labia majora

Edema, ecchymoses, and hematomas can occur in the scrotum and labia majora, especially when these are the presenting parts in a breech presentation. Since the newborn male has a pendulous urethra that is vulnerable to compression or injury, it is possible for significant trauma to occur following a protracted labor in the breech position; the mechanism is felt to be compression of the urethra against a firm structure in the maternal bony pelvis. Cromie recently managed four male infants who developed marked temporary hydronephrosis following delivery in the breech position. The hydronephrosis resolved within 3 days. Because of laxity of the tissues, the degree of swelling and discoloration occasionally is extreme enough (Fig. 17-9) to evoke considerable concern among the medical and nursing staff, especially regarding deeper involvement (for example, periuretheral hemorrhage and edema), which might hinder normal micturition. However, generally this has not been a problem, and frequently these babies void shortly after arriving in the nursery. Spontaneous resolution of edema occurs within 24 to 48 hours and of discoloration within 4 to 5 days. Treatment is not necessary. Secondary ulceration, necrosis, or eschar formation is rare unless there is an associated underlying condition such as herpes simplex infection.

Deeper structures

Much less often birth trauma may involve the deeper structures of the genitalia. If the tunica vaginalis is injured and blood fills its cavity, a hematocele is formed. Absence of transillumination distinguishes this from a hydrocele. If the infant appears to be in pain, the scrotum may be elevated and cold packs applied. Spontaneous resolution is the usual course.

The testes may be injured, often in association with injury to the epididymis. Usually the involvement is bilateral. The testes may be enlarged, smoothly rounded, and insensitive. The infant may be irritable, with vomiting and poor feeding. Urologic consultation is indicated; occasionally exploration and evacuation of blood are necessary, especially with increasing size of the testes. Severe trauma may result in atrophy or failure of the testes to grow. The occasional finding in older children of a circumscribed fibrous area within the testicular tissue is thought to represent old birth trauma to the gland.

INJURIES RELATED TO INTRAPARTUM FETAL MONITORING

Continuous monitoring of the FHR and the intermittent sampling of fetal scalp blood for determination of acid-base status are often employed to monitor the fetus

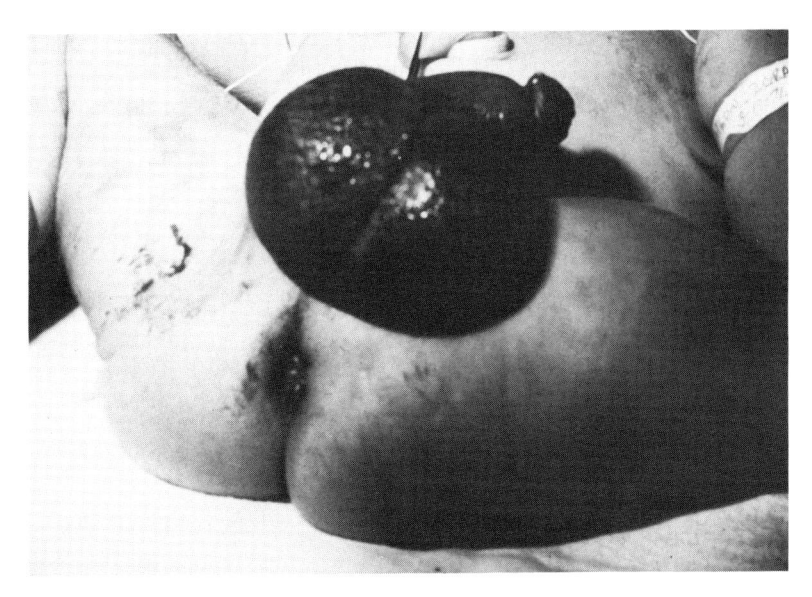

Fig. 17-9. Hematoma of scrotum and penis in a 3,895-gm male delivered vaginally after frank breech presentation. The infant voided at 22 hours and regularly thereafter. Swelling diminished appreciably within 5 hours and was gone by the third day. Discoloration was markedly diminished by the second day.

during labor. Thousands of patients have now been monitored by these methods (pp. 117 and 190). The relative infrequency of complications indicates that in experienced hands these procedures are generally safe. However, certain specific complications have occurred.

Injuries related to direct FHR monitoring

Direct monitoring of the FHR during labor depends on application of an electrode to the fetal scalp or other presenting part. Superficial abrasions, lacerations, and hematomas have occurred at the site of application of the electrode. These complications require no specific therapy beyond local treatment.

A number of investigators have reported abscesses of the scalp associated with application of scalp electrodes. These have, for the most part, been sterile and have required only local treatment. Systemic signs or symptoms require evaluation for possible septicemia.

More recently, Thomas and Blackwell reported a potentially more serious complication related to use of a spiral fetal scalp electrode. At delivery this electrode was noted to have penetrated the substance of an eyelid, with considerable secondary local edema and minimal scleral hematoma. The complication was believed to have resulted from movement of the fetus before application of the electrode. The electrode was removed, and the infant recovered without sequelae.

Injuries related to fetal scalp blood sampling

Fetal biochemical monitoring requires puncture of the presenting part, usually the scalp, with a 2-mm blade and the collection of blood under direct visualization in a heparinized tube. The major complications that have occurred are excessive bleeding and accidental breakage of the blades. The bleeding can be stopped by pressure but on occasion may require sutures. Several infants have required blood replacement. It is important to obtain a detailed family history of bleeding disorders before initiation of this procedure.

The second major complication has been breakage of the blade within the fetal scalp. Removal soon after delivery has been recommended to prevent secondary infection. This has been accomplished by use of a magnet attached to a small forceps that probes the puncture site and elicits a click as the blade is attracted to the magnet. On occasion radiographic localization followed by a small incision is necessary for withdrawal of the blade.

Henry H. Mangurten

BIBLIOGRAPHY
General
Altemus, L.A., and Ferguson, A.D.: The incidence of birth injuries, J. Natl. Med. Assoc. **58**:333, 1966.

Ehrenfest, H.: Birth injuries of the child, ed. 2, New York, 1931, Appleton-Century-Crofts.

Valdes-Dapena, M.A., and Arey, J.B.: The causes of neonatal mortality: an analysis of 501 autopsies on newborn infants, J. Pediatr. **77**:366, 1970.

Injuries to soft tissues
Davis, J.A., and Schiff, D., Bruising as a cause of neonatal jaundice, Lancet **1**:636, 1966.

Injuries to the head
Berger, S.S., and Stewart, R.E.: Mandibular hypoplasia secondary to perinatal trauma: report of case, J. Oral Surg. **35**:578, 1977.

Besio, R., and others: Neonatal retinal hemorrhages and influence of perinatal factors, Am. J. Ophthalmol. **87**:74, 1979.

Birrell, J.F.: The ear, nose, and throat diseases of children, London, 1960, Cassell & Co., Ltd.

Cavanagh, F.: Vocal palsies in children, J. Laryngol. Otolaryngol. **69**:399, 1955.

Chasler, C.N.: The newborn skull (the diagnosis of fracture), Am. J. Roentgenol. Radium Ther. Nucl. Med. **100**:92, 1967.

Daily, W., and Davis, W.E.: Nasal septal dislocation in the newborn, Missouri Med. **74**:381, 1977.

Ferguson, C.F.: Congenital abnormalities of the infant larynx, Otolaryngol. Clin. North Am. **3**:185, 1970.

Hepner, W.R., Jr.: Some observations on facial paresis in the newborn infant: etiology and incidence, Pediatrics **8**:494, 1951.

Jaworski, S., and Dudkiewicz, Z.: Mandibular fractures in the course of labor in a newborn infant, Pediatr. Pol. **48**:1501, 1973.

Jeppesen, F., and Windfeld, I.: Dislocation of the nasal septal cartilage in the newborn, Acta Obstet. Gynecol. Scand. **51**:5, 1972.

Kendall, N., and Woloshin, H.: Cephalhematoma associated with fracture of the skull, J. Pediatr. **41**:125, 1952.

Lee, Y., and Berg, R.B.: Cephalhematoma infected with *Bacteroides*, Am. J. Dis. Child. **121**:77, 1971.

Loeser, J.D., Kilburn, H.L., and Jolley, T.: Management of depressed skull fracture in the newborn, J. Neurosurg. **44**:62, 1976.

McHugh, H.E.: Facial paralysis in birth injury and skull fractures, Arch. Otolaryngol. **78**:443, 1963.

Pohjanpelto, P., Niemi, K., and Sarmela, T.: Anterior chamber haemorrhage in the newborn after spontaneous delivery: a case report, Acta Ophthalmol. **57**:443, 1979.

Rainin, E.A.: Eversion of upper lids secondary to birth trauma, Arch. Ophthalmol. **94**:330, 1976.

Raynor, R., and Parsa, M.: Nonsurgical elevation of depressed skull fracture in an infant, J. Pediatr. **72**:262, 1968.

Saunders, B.S., and others: Depressed skull fracture in the neonate: report of three cases, J. Neurosurg. **50**:512, 1979.

Schrager, G.O.: Elevation of depressed skull fracture with a breast pump, J. Pediatr. **77**:300, 1970.

Sezen, F.: Retinal haemorrhages in newborn infants, Br. J. Ophthalmol. **55**:248, 1971.

Silverman, S.H., and Leibow, S.G.: Dislocation of the triangular cartilage of the nasal septum, J. Pediatr. **87**:456, 1975.

Tan, K.L.: Elevation of congenital depressed fracture of the skull by the vacuum extractor, Acta Paediatr. Scand. **63**:562, 1974.

Zelson, C., Lee, S.J., and Pearl, M.: The incidence of skull fractures underlying cephalhematomas in newborn infants, J. Pediatr. **85**:371, 1974.

Injuries to the neck and shoulder girdle
Bennet, G.C., and Harrold, A.J.: Prognosis and early management of birth injuries to the brachial plexus, Br. Med. J. **1**:1520, 1976.

Bingham, J.A.W.: Two cases of unilateral paralysis of the diaphragm in the newborn treated surgically, Thorax **9**:248, 1954.

Bishop, H.C., and Koop, C.E.: Acquired eventration of the diaphragm in infancy, Pediatrics **22**:1088, 1958.

Claren, S.K., Smith, D.W., and Hanson, J.W.: Helmet treatment for plagiocephaly and congenital muscular torticollis, J. Pediatr. 94:43, 1979.

Eng, G.D.: Brachial plexus palsy in newborn infants, Pediatrics 43:18, 1971.

Harris, G.B.C.: Unilateral paralysis of the diaphragm in the newborn, Postgrad. Med. 50:51, 1971.

Hoffer, M.M., Wickenden, R., and Roper, B.: Brachial plexus birth palsies: results of tendon transfers to the rotator cuff, J. Bone Joint Surg. 60-A:691, 1978.

Matson, D.D.: Neurosurgery of infancy and childhood, ed. 2, Springfield, Ill., 1969, Charles C Thomas, Publisher.

Sanerkin, N.G., and Edwards, P.: Birth injury to the sternomastoid muscle, J. Bone Joint Surg. 48-B:441, 1966.

Vassalos, E., Prevedourakis, C., and Paraschopoulou-Prevedouraki, P.: Brachial plexus paralysis in the newborn, Am. J. Obstet. Gynecol. 101:554, 1968.

Weisman, L., Woodall, J., and Merenstein, G.: Constant negative pressure in the treatment of diaphragmatic paralysis secondary to birth injury, Birth Defects: Original Article Series XII:297, 1976.

Yasuda, R., and others: Bilateral phrenic nerve palsy in the newborn infant: a case report, J. Pediatr. 89:986, 1976.

Zajkowski, E.J., and Kravath, R.E.: Bilateral diaphragmatic paralysis in the newborn infant: treatment with nasal continuous positive airway pressure, Chest 75:392, 1979.

Injuries to the spine and spinal cord

Brans, Y.W., and Cassady, G.: Neonatal spinal cord injuries, Am. J. Obstet. Gynecol. 123:918, 1975.

Koch, B.M., and Eng, G.M.: Neonatal spinal cord injury, Arch. Phys. Med. Rehabil. 60:378, 1979.

Maekawa, K., Masaki, T., and Kokubun, Y.: Fetal spinal-cord injury secondary to hyperextension of the neck: no effect of caesarean section, Dev. Med. Child. Neurol. 18:229, 1976.

Towbin, A.: Latent spinal cord and brain stem injury in newborn infants, Dev. Med. Child. Neurol. 11:54, 1969.

Walter, C.E., and Tedeschi, L.G.: Spinal injury and neonatal death, Am. J. Obstet. Gynecol. 106:272, 1970.

Injuries to intraabdominal organs

Drucker, V., and Rodriguez, C.E.: Extensive bilateral calcification within adrenal hemorrhage, Radiology 64:258, 1955.

Eraklis, A.J.: Abdominal injury related to trauma of birth, Pediatrics 39:421, 1967.

Gross, M., Kottmeier, P.K., and Waterhouse, K.: Diagnosis and treatment of neonatal adrenal hemorrhage, J. Pediatr. Surg. 2:308, 1967.

Holder, T.M., and Leape, L.L.: The acute surgical abdomen in the neonate, N. Engl. J. Med. 278:605, 1968.

Leape, L.L., and Bordy, M.D.: Neonatal rupture of the spleen, Pediatrics 47:101, 1971.

Matsuyama, S., Suzuki, N., and Nagamachi, Y.: Rupture of the spleen in the newborn: treatment without splenectomy, J. Peidatr. Surg. 11:115, 1976.

Mineau, D.E., and Koehler, P.R.: Ultrasound diagnosis of neonatal adrenal hemorrhage, Am. J. Roentgenol. 132:443, 1979.

Monson, D.O., and Raffensperger, J.G.: Intraperitoneal hemorrhage secondary to liver laceration in a newborn, J. Pediatr. Surg. 2:464, 1967.

Injuries to the extremities

Haliburton, R.A., Barber, J.R., and Fraser, R.L.: Pseudodislocation: an unusual birth injury, Can. J. Surg. 10:455, 1967.

Labelle, P.: Orthopedic anxieties in the newborn, Appl. Ther. 8:226, 1966.

Mortens, J., and Christensen, P.: Traumatic separation of the upper femoral epiphysis as an obstetrical lesion, Acta Orthop. Scand. 34:239, 1964.

Schubert, J.J.: Dislocation of the radial head in the newborn infant, J. Bone Joint Surg. 47:1019, 1965.

Towbin, R., and Crawford, A.H.: Neonatal traumatic proximal femoral epiphysiolysis, Pediatrics 63:456, 1979.

Wilson, J.C., Jr.: Fractures and dislocations in childhood, Pediatr. Clin. North Am. 14:659, 1967.

Trauma to the genitalia

Cromie, W.J.: Genitourinary injuries in the neonate, Clin. Pediatr. 18:292, 1979.

Hodgman, J.E., Friedman, R.I., and Levan, N.E.: Neonatal dermatology, Pediatr. Clin. North Am. 18:713, 1971.

Injuries related to intrapartum fetal monitoring

Chan, W.H., Paul, R.H., and Toews, J.: Intrapartum fetal monitoring: maternal and fetal morbidity and perinatal mortality, Obstet. Gynecol. 41:7, 1973.

Cordero, L., and Hon, E.H.: Scalp abscess: a rare complication of fetal monitoring, J. Pediatr. 78:533, 1971.

Modanlou, H., and others: Complications of fetal blood sampling during labor, Clin. Pediatr. 12:603, 1973.

Paul, R.H., and Hon, E.H.: Clinical fetal monitoring; a survey of current usage, Obstet. Gynecol. 37:779, 1971.

Thomas, G., and Blackwell, R.J.: A hazard associated with the use of spiral fetal scalp electrodes, Am. J. Obstet. Gynecol. 121:1118, 1975.

CHAPTER 18　**Care of the mother, father, and infant**

Much of the joy and sorrow of life revolves around attachments or affectional relationships: making them, breaking them, preparing for them, and adjusting to their loss. The bond between a mother and father and their newborn infant is one of these very special ties. Perhaps the parents' attachment to a child is the strongest bond in the human species. The power of this attachment is so great that it enables the mother and father to make the unusual sacrifices necessary for the care of their infant.

An "attachment" can be defined as a unique relationship between two people that is specific and endures through time. Although it is difficult to define this lasting relationship operationally, we have taken as indicators of this attachment behaviors such as fondling, kissing, cuddling, and prolonged gazing, behaviors that serve both to maintain contact and show affection to the particular individual. Although this definition is useful in experimental observations, it is important to distinguish between attachment and attachment behaviors. Close attachment can persist during long separations of time and distance even though there may at times be no visible sign of its existence. A call for help even after 40 years may bring a mother to her child and evoke attachment behaviors equal in strength to those of the first year.

The impetus to study intensively the mother-to-infant bond occurred 15 to 20 years ago when staffs of intensive care nurseries observed that sometimes, after extraordinary efforts had been taken to save small premature infants, they would return to emergency rooms battered and partially destroyed by their parents, even though they had been sent home intact and thriving. More careful studies of this phenomenon have consistently shown that battering and failure to thrive without organic cause appear in a disproportionate number of infants who were premature or hospitalized for other reasons during the newborn period. (Failure to thrive without organic disease is a syndrome in which the infant does not grow, gain, or develop normally at home during the early months of life, and yet shows leaps in development and weight gain with routine hospital care.) Table 18-1 presents observations on the incidence of infant battering and failure to thrive without organic disease and their relationship to separation in the early days of life. The occurrence of these and other mothering disorders has provided a continuing stimulus to unravel the process of parental attachment.

Over the last 15 years, more and more mothers have been allowed to enter premature nurseries in the United States. It is apparent from the data and definition of deprivation that most normal deliveries in the United States are followed by several days of deprivation for the mother. A woman who delivers a premature infant suffers complete deprivation from the first day if she can see her infant only through a glass window for 8 weeks. Only mothers who deliver at home and room in with their infants from the moment of birth experience no deprivation.

This chapter describes recent studies of the process by which a parent becomes attached to his or her infant and suggests applications of these findings to the care of the parents of a normal infant, a premature infant, and a malformed infant. In an attempt to determine what triggers, fosters, or disturbs a mother's attachment to her infant, information has been gathered from clinical observations during medical care procedures, naturalistic observations of mothering, long-term, in-depth interviews of a small number of mothers primarily by psychoanalysts, structured interviews or observations, and results from closely controlled studies on the parents of full-term infants.

Table 18-1. The incidence of early neonatal separation in infants who have been battered or show failure to thrive without organic disease

	Authors	Number in study	Percentage separated
Failure to thrive	Ambuel and Harris (1963)	100	27
	Shaheen and others (1968)	44	36
	Evans and others (1972)	40	22.5
Battering	Elmer and Gregg (1967)	20	30
	Skinner and Castle (1969)	78	13
	Klein and Stern (1971)	51	23.5
	Oliver and others (1974)	38	21
	Fomuford, Sinkford, and Levy (1975)	36	41.5
	Lynch (1975)*	25	40

*Separation in 35 sibling controls (6%).

Events that are important to the formation of a mother's attachment to her infant include the following:
A. Prior to pregnancy
 1. Planning the pregnancy
B. During pregnancy
 1. Confirming the pregnancy
 2. Accepting the pregnancy
 3. Fetal movement
 4. Accepting the fetus as an individual
C. After birth
 1. Birth
 2. Seeing the baby
 3. Touching the baby
 4. Giving care to the baby

By observing and studying the human mother according to these periods, we can begin to fit together the interlocking pieces that lay the foundations of attachment.

PRIOR TO PREGNANCY

The child development literature suggests that children are socialized by the powerful process of imitation or modeling. Their behavior is influenced by how they themselves were mothered or what they observed. Long before a woman herself becomes a mother, she has obtained a repertoire of mothering behaviors through observation, play, and practice. She has already learned whether infants are picked up when they cry, how much they are carried, and whether they should be chubby or thin. It is an interesting phenomenon that these modes of conduct, absorbed when children are very young, become unquestioned imperatives for them throughout later life. Unless adults consciously and painstakingly reexamine these learned behaviors, they will probably unconsciously repeat them when they become parents.

PREGNANCY

Caplan considers pregnancy to be a development crisis involving two particular adaptive tasks.

Acceptance of pregnancy

During the first stage of pregnancy a woman must come to terms with the knowledge that she will be a mother. When she first realizes that she is pregnant, a mother will often have mixed feelings. A large number of considerations, ranging from a change in her familiar patterns to more serious matters such as economic and housing hardships or interpersonal difficulties, all influence her acceptance of the pregnancy. This initial stage, as outlined by Bibring, is the mother's identification of the growing fetus as an "integral part of herself."

Perception of the fetus as a separate individual

The second stage involves a growing awareness of the baby in the uterus as a separate individual. It usually starts with the remarkably powerful event of quickening, the sensation of fetal movement. It probably occurs earlier for some mothers who see their baby and its movements on the screen during ultrasonography. During this period the woman must begin to change her concept of the fetus from a being that is a part of herself to a living baby who will soon be a separate individual. Bibring believes that this realization prepares the woman for birth and physical separation from her child. In turn, this preparedness lays the foundation for a relationship with the child.

After quickening, a woman will usually begin to have fantasies about what the baby will be like, attributing some personality characteristics and developing feelings of attachment. At this time she may further accept her pregnancy and show significant changes in attitude toward the fetus. Objectively, there will usually be some outward evidence of the mother's preparation. She may purchase clothes or a crib, select a name, and rearrange her home to accommodate a baby.

The production of a normal child is a major goal of most women. Yet most pregnant women have hidden fears that the infant may be abnormal or reveal some of their own secret inner weaknesses. Brazelton has clarified the importance of these changes and turmoil that occur during pregnancy for the subsequent development of attachment to the new infant*:

The prenatal interviews with normal primiparas, in a psychoanalytic interview setting, uncovered anxiety which often seemed to be of pathological proportions. The unconscious material was so loaded and distorted, so near the surface, that before delivery one felt an ominous direction for making a pre-

*From Brazelton, T.B.: Effect of maternal expectations on early infant behavior, Early Child Devel. Care **2:**259, 1973.

diction about the woman's capacity to adjust to the role of mothering. And yet, when we saw her in action as a mother, this very anxiety and the distorted unconscious material could become a force for reorganization, for readjustment to her important new role. I began to feel that much of the prenatal anxiety and distortion of fantasy could be a healthy mechanism for bringing her out of the old homeostasis which she had achieved to a new level of adjustment. The alarm reaction we were tapping in on was serving as a kind of shock treatment for reorganization to her new role. . . . I now see the shakeup in pregnancy as readying the circuits for new attachments, as preparation for the many choices which they must be ready to make in a very short critical period, as a method of freeing her circuits for a kind of sensitivity to the infant and his individual requirements which might not have been easily or otherwise available from her earlier adjustment. Thus, this very emotional turmoil of pregnancy and that in the neonatal period can be seen as a positive force for the mother's adjustment and for the possibility of providing a more individualized environment for the infant.

Cohen, however, emphasizes that any stress, such as moving to a new geographic area, marital infidelity, death of a close friend or relative, previous abortions, or loss of previous children, that leaves the mother feeling unloved or unsupported or that precipitates concern for the health and survival of either her infant or herself may delay preparation for the infant and retard bond formation. After the first trimester, behaviors that are a reaction to stress and suggest rejection of pregnancy include a preoccupation with physical appearance or negative self-perception, excessive emotional withdrawal or mood swings, excessive physical complaints, absence of any response to quickening, or lack of any preparatory behavior during the last trimester.

It is difficult to understand the factors that determine the interactional and parenting behavior of an adult human who has lived for 20 to 30 years. A mother and father's behavior toward their infant is derived from a complex combination of their own genetic endowments, the infant's responses to them, a long history of interpersonal relationships with their own families and with each other, experiences with this or previous pregnancies, the absorption of the practices and values of their cultures, and, probably most important, the way in which each was raised by his or her own parents. The mothering and fathering behavior of each woman and man, the ability of each to tolerate stresses, and the needs each has for special attention differ greatly and depend on a mixture of these factors.

Fig. 18-1 is a schematic diagram of the major influences on parental behavior and the resulting disturbances that we hypothesize may arise from them. At the time the infant is conceived, some of these determinants, such as the mothering the father and mother received when they were infants, the practices of their culture,

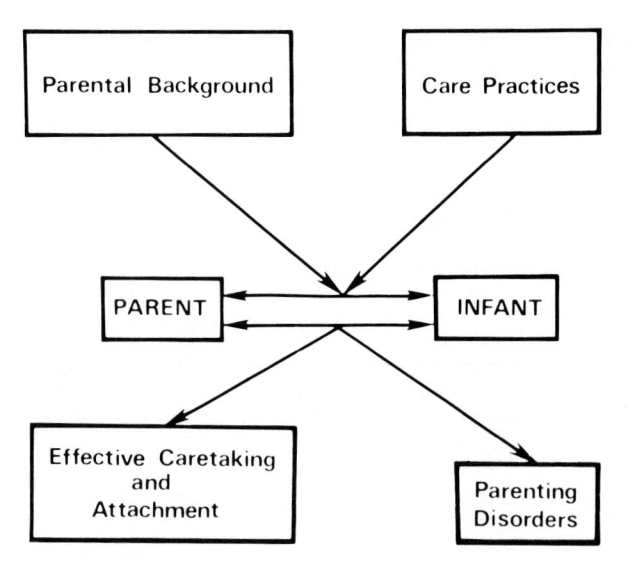

Fig. 18-1. Major influences on parent-infant attachment and the resulting outcomes.

their endowments, and their relationships with their own families, are contributed by the parents. We originally believed these determinants fixed and unchangeable. However, Harmon and Emde have argued that the influence of some of these may be changed during the crisis of birth. Other determinants relate to the hospital culture. For example, the attitudes, statements, and practices of the nurses and physicians in the hospital; whether there is separation from the infant in the first days of life; the infant's temperament; and whether he is healthy, sick, or malformed obviously also affect the relationship. Fig. 18-1 also shows a series of mothering disorders ranging from mild anxiety, such as persistent concerns about a baby after a minor problem that has been completely resolved in the nursery, to the most severe manifestation—the battered child syndrome. It is our hypothesis that some problems result in part from separation and other unusual circumstances which occur in the early newborn period as a consequence of present hospital care policies. Experiences during labor, parent-infant separation, and hospital practices during the first hours and days of life are the most easily manipulated variables in this scheme. Recent studies have partly clarified some of the steps in mother-infant attachment during this early period.

LABOR

Before childbirth moved from the home to the hospital, it was the practice in industrialized nations for family members to support the mother in labor, often with the assistance of a trained or untrained midwife. In all but one of 150 cultures studied by anthropologists, a family member or friend, usually a woman, remained with the mother during labor and delivery. Although more fathers, relatives, and friends have been allowed into labor and delivery rooms in the past 10 years, a significant number of mothers still labor and deliver in some hospitals without the presence of family members or close friends. There has been little systematic study of this issue since the Newtons reported that mothers who were quiet and relaxed and had better emotional relationships with their attendants during labor and delivery were more pleased at the first sight of their babies. A recent study in Guatemala was designed to investigate the effects of a supportive companion (Raphael termed such a person a *doula*) on the length of labor and mother-infant interaction after delivery, in an obstetric setting in which mothers routinely labor alone.

Initial assignment of mothers to the experimental (doula) or control group was random, but controls showed a higher rate ($p<0.001$) of subsequent perinatal problems (e.g., cesarean section, meconium staining). It was necessary to admit 103 control versus 33 experimental mothers to obtain 20 in each group with uncomplicated deliveries. In the final sample the length of time from admission to delivery was shorter in the experimental group (8.8 versus 19.3 hours; $p<0.001$). Significantly more mothers who had a doula present during labor remained awake after delivery and were more interactive with their infants during the time they were awake. These observations suggest there are major perinatal benefits of constant human support during labor.

AFTER BIRTH

Immediately after the birth parents enter a unique period during which events may have lasting effects on the family. This period, which lasts a short time, and during which the parents' attachment to their infant begins to blossom, we have named the *maternal sensitive period*. Because we believe this concept is crucial to the understanding of the bonding process, we will examine in detail the evidence supporting its existence. During this enigmatic period complex interactions between mother and infant help to lock them together. This must be distinguished from the sensitive time during which the infant establishes a stable, affectionate relationship with the mother, later in the first year. In this section we must emphasize that we are focusing on the process of attachment *from parent to infant*.

The clinical observations of Rose and Kennell suggested that affectional ties can be easily disturbed and may be permanently altered during the immediate postpartum period. Relatively mild illness in the newborn, such as slight elevations of bilirubin levels, slow feeding, additional oxygen for 1 to 2 hours, and the need for incubator care in the first 24 hours for mild respiratory distress,

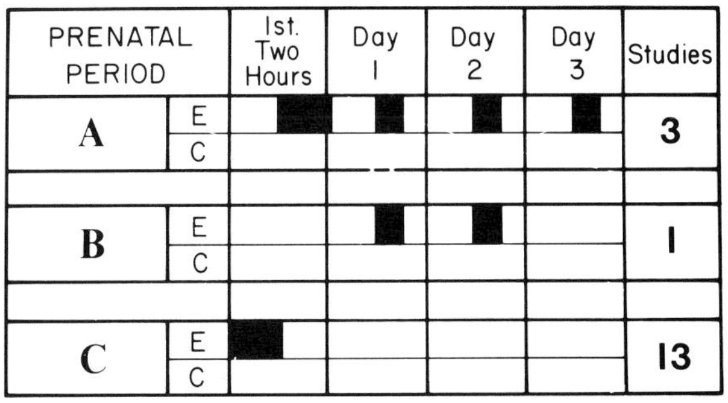

Fig. 18-2. Time patterns and number of three types of controlled studies in which one group of mothers has additional contact *(E)* with their infants compared with another group with routine contact *(C)*.

appear to affect the relationship between mother and infant. The mother's behavior is often disturbed during the first year or more of the infant's life, even though his problems are completely resolved prior to discharge and often within a few hours. That early events have long-lasting effects is one of our principles of attachment. Anxieties a mother has about her baby in the first few days after birth, even about a problem that is easily resolved, may affect her relationship with the child long afterward.

In the past 10 years, 17 separate studies have focused on whether additional time for close contact of the mother and infant in the first minutes, hours, and days of life alters the quality of the attachment.

Fig. 18-2 illustrates the timing of the contact in the 17 human studies. In three studies the extra time was added not only during the first 3 hours but also during the next 3 days of life. At 1 month the mothers in the group who had extra contact showed significantly more affectionate behavior toward their infants. They stood closer and watched over them more during the physical examination, soothed them more when they cried, engaged in more eye-to-eye contact and fondling during feeding, and were more reluctant to leave them with someone else. At 1 year the two groups of mothers were again significantly different, with extra-contact mothers spending more time assisting and soothing their infants during stressful office visits. At 2 years the linguistic behavior of the two groups was compared. Extra-contact mothers used longer sentences but fewer content words and imperatives than did the controls.

In 13 studies the additional mother-infant contact occurred only during the first hour of life. In 10 of these studies significant differences in the behavior of the mothers were noted. As an example DeChateau investigated the effects on maternal behavior of skin-to-skin contact and suckling during the first 30 minutes after delivery in 40 primiparous middle-class Swedish moth-

Table 18-2. Percentage of mothers breast-feeding at 2 or 3 months post partum after additional early mother-infant contact

	Number	Hospital routine	Early contact
Johnson (USA)	12	16	100
Sosa (Guatemala I)	60	92	74*
Sosa (Guatemala II)	60	58	70
Sosa (Social Security Hospital)	40	59	85
Sousa (Brazil)	200	27	47
De Chateau (Sweden)	40	26	58
Ali and Lowry (Jamaica)	100	27	57
Salariya and others (Canada)	108	50	60*
	30	20	60

*No significant difference.

ers. The mothers with early contact received only an additional 15 minutes of extra contact in the first 30 minutes of life. Following this both the control and experimental groups had a similar amount of time with their babies. When the infants were 3 months old, detailed observations at home revealed that early contact mothers spent significantly more time looking at their infants face to face and kissing them, whereas control mothers spent more time cleaning their babies. The infants of mothers with early contact cried significantly less and smiled significantly more than infants of control mothers. In 7 of 9 studies breast-feeding was significantly increased by permitting the mother additional time with her infant in the first hour (Table 18-2).

When additional time is given for close mother-infant contact following the first 8 hours post partum, there are also differences in later mothering behavior. In a study of 301 primiparous patients, O'Connor noted that increasing the time by 12 hours (6 hours on days 1 and 2) significantly decreased the number of mothering disorders with 10 such occurrences in the control group but only 2 in the group of mothers who received extra time with their infants. Siegel and associates in a group mainly of new and previous mothers did find differences in parenting at 4 and 12 months but no difference in mothering disorders (Table 18-3). A woman was defined as having a mothering disorder if her infant was battered, had nonorganic failure to thrive, was abandoned, or was given up for an unplanned adoption.

A number of questions come to mind. Is the time a mother spends with her newborn in the first hour as significant as a longer period together on the second or third day of life? Is the effect in the first hour due to the quiet, alert state of the infant or to the state of the mother? In the first hour after birth the newborn infant is in a heightened state of alertness and responsivity. Interestingly, no matter when increased amounts of contact between mother and infant are added in the first 3 postpartum days, there appears to be improved mothering behavior. At present it is not known why such striking alterations in caretaking have been noted when mother-infant contact is increased for such a short time in the first hours of life.

Those human studies which have attempted to unravel the components of this complex process have unfortunately been misinterpreted by some caretakers to suggest that the first hour is the critical and only time for attachment to occur. Recent observations by MacFarlane reveal that normal English women feel love for their baby or feel the baby is theirs over a prolonged period (41% during pregnancy, 34% at birth, 27% during the first week, and 8% after the first week).

The recent accumulation of information in a closely related field has greatly augmented our understanding of parent-to-infant attachment. Detailed studies of the amazing behavioral capacities of the normal neonate have shown that the infant sees, hears, and moves in rhythm to his mother's voice in the first minutes and hours of life, resulting in a beautiful linking of the reactions of the two and a synchronized "dance" between the mother and infant. The infant's appearance coupled with his broad array of sensory and motor abilities evokes responses from the mother and father and provides several channels of communication that are most helpful in the process of attachment and the initiation of a series of reciprocal interactions (Chapter 21).

Lang noted that, immediately after a home delivery, most mothers suckle their infants. The infants she observed did not suck but licked the area around the nipple. MacFarlane has shown that 6 days after birth the infant will have the ability to distinguish reliably by scent his own mother's breast pad from the breast pads of other women. The mother has an intense interest in looking at her newborn baby's open eyes. In the first 45 minutes of life the infant is awake and alert and will follow his mother for 180 degrees with his own eyes. The licking of the nipple will induce a marked increase in prolactin secretion in the mother, and at the same time oxytocin, to contract the uterus and decrease bleeding. With the mother's strong desire to touch and see her child, Nature has provided for the immediate and essential union of the two. The alert newborn rewards his mother for her efforts by following her with his eyes, thus maintaining their interaction and kindling the tired mother's fascination with her baby.

Lind and his associates in Stockholm have shown that a surprising increase in blood flow to the breast occurs when a mother hears the cries of her own infant. These intricate interactions have focused our attention on the

Table 18-3. Early and extended contact

Number of patients	Study and sample	Extra contact (EC)	Hospital routine (HR)	Results	Comments
28	Klaus and associates (1972); low-income U.S. mothers and infants, bottle feeding Kennell and associates (1974) Ringler and associates (1975)	1 hour with nude newborn within 3 hours of birth and 5 extra hours of contact daily for 3 days ($n = 14$) (mother gowned)	Glimpse of baby at birth; brief contact for identification at 6-12 hours, 20-30 minute contact every 4 hours for feeding ($n = 14$)	1. At 1 month EC mothers demonstrated more soothing, fondling, eye-to-eye contact during feeding. 2. At 1 year EC mothers soothed the infant more during physical examination. 3. At 2 years EC mothers used more questions, fewer imperatives, and more words/proposition.	Beginning evidence of early sensitive period for maternal bonding.
200	Sousa (1974)	Early and continuous contact; infant crib beside mother; Enthusiastic nurse encouraging nursing ($n = 100$)	Glimpse at birth; 12-24 hour separation, 30 minutes every 3 hours; infant in nursery ($n = 100$)	1. At 2 months EC = 77% lactating; HR = 27.4% lactating.	Many differences in care other than EC between HR and EC might explain results.
202	Siegel and associates (1980); low-income families	97 early and extended contact	105 routine care	1. At 4 and 12 months 2.5%-3.2% of variance explained by EC; 10%-22% of variance explained by background variables; no difference in child abuse (10 control, 7 EC)	
301	O'Connor and associates (1980); low-income U.S. mothers and infants	6 hours of extra contact daily for 2 days ($n = 143$)	20 minutes every 4 hours for feeding ($n = 158$)	During 17-month follow-up, more HR children (10) experienced abuse, neglect, abandonment, and nonorganic failure to thrive; 2 EC infants admitted for parenting failure.	Extra contact affected both later mothering and child health.
12	Johnson (1976); middle class	Initial breast-feeding 1 hour	Initial breast-feeding at 15 hours	At 2 months, 5/6 EC breast-feeding; 1/6 HR breast-feeding.	
60 68 40	Sosa and associates (1975) Roosevelt I Roosevelt II Social Security Poor Guatemalan mothers	45 mintues of skin-to-skin contact (1 hour of life)	Early separation Roosevelt: 12 hours Social Security: 24 hours	Duration of breast-feeding for EC longer at Social Security and Roosevelt I; EC greater weight gain 1 year at Social Security.	Roosevelt II EC and HR significant difference; socioeconomic index determined at home visit.
19	Kennell and associates (1975)	45 minutes of skin-to-skin contact (1 hour of life) ($n = 9$)	Glimpse at birth; 12-hour separation ($n = 10$)	At 12 hours EC mothers demonstrated more attachment behaviors.	Design inadequacy: study observations made when HR mothers first held infant.

Continued.

Table 18-3. Early and extended contact—cont'd

Number of patients	Study and sample	Extra contact (EC)	Hospital routine (HR)	Results	Comments
42	DeChateau and associates (1977, 1977); middle-class Swedish mothers and infants, breast-feeding	15 minute skin-to-skin contact and suckling within 20 minutes of birth; then treated according to HR	Nurses cared for baby for 30 minutes after birth; wrapped infant, then placed in crib next to mother for 1½ hours; mothers and babies then separated except for every 4-hour feeds for 3 days; on days 4-7 daytime rooming-in ($n = 20$)	1. At 26 hours EC mothers sitting up, holding, and cradling their infants more than HR mothers. 2. In hospital EC mothers carried their infants more on the left side and less in their hands away from their bodies. 3. At 3 months EC mothers kissed, looked en face more, and cleaned babies less during free play in the home. 4. At 3 months EC babies smiled and laughed more and cried less.	As little as 15 minutes early extra skin contact affected both maternal and infant behavior; more synchronous and positive mother-infant interaction apparently established.
60	Hales (1977); very low–income Guatemalan mothers and infants; breast-feeding	Early: 45 minutes of private skin-to-skin contact within minutes of birth ($n = 20$) Delayed: 45 minutes of private skin-to-skin contact at 12 hours ($n = 20$)	Glimpse of baby at birth; 12-hour separation, then daytime rooming-in for 2 days ($n = 20$)	At 36 hours early EC mothers showed more affectionate behaviors (smiling, kissing, en face, talking, fondling) and especially more en face than either delayed EC or HR; no difference in keeping babies close or caregiving.	Maternal behavior at 36 hours altered if mother and infant have early skin-to-skin contact.
100	Ali and Lowery (1981); poor Jamaican women	45 minutes early contact ($n = 50$)	Routine care ($n = 50$)	At 12 weeks EC had more gazing, standing near infant, and vocalizing; solely breast-feeding	

cascade of interlocking sensory patterns that quickly develop between mother and infant in the first hours of life.

There is suggestive evidence that many of these early interactions also take place between the father and his newborn child. Parke in particular has demonstrated that, when fathers are given the opportunity to be alone with their newborns, they spend almost exactly the same amount of time as mothers holding, touching, and looking at them.

In his work with a mother and her 3-month-old twins, Stern observed that the pattern of interaction between a mother and her child has a characteristic rhythm. Intricate interchanges occur within a period of a few seconds. And when these interactions are repeatedly out of phase, for example, if one partner looks away just as the other looks at him, many aspects of the relationship between the two individuals are disturbed. Our observations suggest that this dance of mother and infant, which may or may not be in rhythm, is first initiated in the immediate postpartum period. As Brazelton and his colleagues have stated, "This interdependency of rhythms seems to be at the root of their 'attachment' as well as communication." Thus it seems important that the family have privacy in the first hours of life, in which the new and older members may become attuned to each other.

On the basis of our observations and the reports of parents, we believe that every mother has a task to perform during the postpartum period. She must look and "take in" her real live baby and reconcile the fantasy of the infant she imagined with the one she actually delivered. Many cultures recognize this need by providing the mother with a doula, or "aunt," who mothers her and relieves her of other responsibilities so that she can devote herself completely to this task.

In an interesting and significant observation of fathers, Lind noted that paternal caregiving was markedly increased in the first 3 months of life when the father was

Table 18-3. Early and extended contact—cont'd

Number of patients	Study and sample	Extra contact (EC)	Hospital routine (HR)	Results	Comments
62	Carlsson and associates (1979); middle-class Swedish mothers and infants; breast-feeding	1 hour in bed with nude infant immediately after birth with suckling; then treated according to HR (n = 22) or allowed demand feeding, extra contact, nursing support (n = 20)	Infant placed in crib next to mother's bed for 4 hours; then every 4 hours contact for feeding (n = 20)	On second and fourth day EC mothers, regardless of later ward experience, showed more physical contact and physical affection (rubs, pets, rocks, touches, holds close in arms or lap) during breast-feeding than HR mothers; at 6 weeks no differences during feeding noted.	Early skin contact altered maternal behavior first 4 days.
48	Kontos (1978); middle-class Canadian mothers	1 hour of early contact 30-40 minutes after birth; skin-to-skin for first ½ hour, en face for second ½ hour (n = 24)	Holding wrapped infant 5-10 minutes after birth, then routine (n = 24)	Significantly greater attachment behaviors at 1 and 3 months with extra contact.	Observers were not always blinded.
100	Campbell and associates (1979); middle class	1 hour early contact (n = 50)	Routine care; mother and infant together 5 minutes (n = 50)	No differences in maternal-infant interaction at 3 days or 1 month.	Mothers in routine group had infant for 5 minutes in first hour.
30	Svejda and associates (1980); middle class	1 hour of early contact; 90 minutes at each feeding (n = 15)	Brief contact at delivery; 5 minutes in first hour; 30 minutes at every feeding (n = 15)	No significant differences in maternal behavior at 36 hours.	Mothers in routine group had their infant for 5 minutes in first hour.
30	Thomson and associates (1979); middle class Canadian women	Unwrapped infant on mother's chest; 15-30 minutes suckling (n = 15)	Brief contact at delivery (5 minutes); feedings every 4 hours (n = 15)	Significantly more mothers successfully nursing at 2 months.	Control male/female ratio 11/4, but experimental 6/9.

asked to undress the infant twice and establish eye-to-eye contact with him for 1 hour during the first 3 days of life.

It is our belief that other principles also govern the attachment process. Although solid evidence is scanty, the following additional rules appear to be important.

1. The process of attachment is structured so that the father and mother will become attached optimally to only one infant at a time. In 1958 Bowlby stated this principle for the attachment process in the other direction (infant to mother) and termed it *monotropy*.
2. During the early process of the mother's attachment to her infant it is necessary that the infant respond to the mother by some signal such as body or eye movements.
3. People who witness the birth process become strongly attached to the infant.
4. It is difficult and possibly mutually incompatible for some people to both become attached and detached at the same time, as in simultaneously attempting to go through the processes of attachment to one person while mourning the loss or threatened loss of the same or another person.
5. Early events have long-lasting effects. Anxieties in the first day about the well-being of a baby with a temporary disorder may result in long-lasting concerns that may adversely shape the development of the child.

PRACTICAL CONSIDERATIONS

In 1959 Bibring wrote, "What was once a crisis with carefully worked-out traditional customs of giving support to the woman passing through this crisis period has become at this time a crisis with no mechanisms within the society for helping the woman involved in this profound change of conflict-solutions and adjustive tasks." This deficiency accounts for the development of the many support systems in our society. The wide assortment of childbirth classes, which attempt to continue previous customs, are good examples. These groups help the mother through the delivery period as well as aiding her in later infant and child care. They also lessen the tensions, fears, and fantasies that occur during normal pregnancies. By joining a group of mothers with whom she can chat and share her feelings, a woman can alleviate many of the emotional upsets that occur during normal pregnancies. We therefore believe that these courses, particularly those in which mothers participate actively, have a valuable supportive role during pregnancy.

To minimize the number of unknowns for a mother while she is in the hospital, she and the father (or other supportive companion who will stay with her throughout labor and delivery) should visit the maternity unit to see where labor and delivery will take place. She should also learn about the anesthetic (if she is to receive one), delivery routines, and all the procedures and medication she will receive before, during, and after delivery. By reducing the possibility of surprise, such advance preparation will increase confidence during labor and delivery. For an adult, just as for a child entering the hospital for surgery, the more meticulously every step and event is detailed in advance, the less the subsequent anxiety. The less anxiety the mother experiences while delivering and becoming attached to her baby, the better will be her immediate relationship with him.

The mother must have continuing support and reassurance during her labor and delivery, whether from her husband, the father, her mother or other female family member or friend, a midwife, or a nurse. She also must be satisfied with the arrangements that have been made to maintain her home during her hospitalization.

In an effort to reduce the amount of tension on the mother, she should have a supportive companion with her and should labor and deliver in the same room, preventing the necessity of rushing to a delivery room in the last minutes of labor. Once the delivery is completed and the mother has had a quick glance at the infant, it is important for her to have a few seconds to regain her composure and, in a sense, catch her breath before she proceeds to the next task—taking on the infant. This breath-catching usually occurs during the period when the placenta is being delivered, while the mother is being cleansed and is having any necessary suturing. It has been our experience that it is best not to give a mother her baby until she indicates that she is ready. It should be her decision.

In many hospitals it is customary to put the baby on the mother's chest for 1 or 2 minutes shortly after delivery. This is helpful, but the short time period coupled with the lack of privacy and narrow table does not allow sufficient opportunity for the mother to touch and explore her baby. Even 5 or 10 minutes of contact, particularly without privacy, are probably not sufficient to optimize maternal attachment.

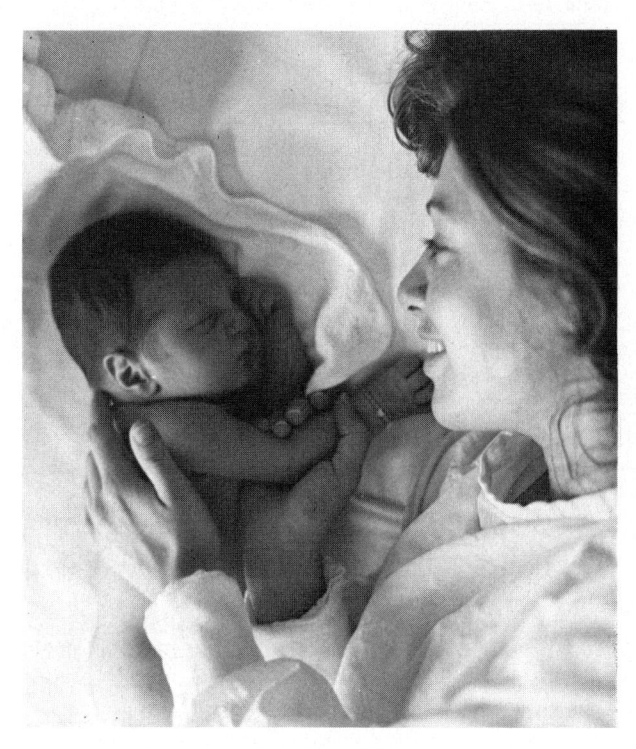

Fig. 18-3. A mother and her infant shortly after birth in a labor room. A heat panel (not shown) is above the infant and is maintaining the infant's temperature. (From Klaus, M.H., and Kennell, J.H.: Maternal-infant bonding, St. Louis, 1976, The C.V. Mosby Co.)

After delivery it is extremely valuable for the father, mother, and baby to have a period alone in either the delivery room or an adjacent room (i.e., a recovery room). Obviously this is only possible if the infant is normal and the mother is well. The mother should have and hold the infant with her on the bed. The infant should not be off in a bassinet where the face cannot be seen. She should be given the baby nude so that she can perform a complete inspection. We have found it valuable to encourage the mother to move over in her regular hospital bed, so that she only takes up about half of it, leaving the other half for her partially dressed or nude infant. A heat panel easily maintains or, if need be, increases the body temperature of the infant (Fig. 18-3). Several mothers have told us of the unforgettable experience of holding their nude baby against their own bare chest, so we recommend skin-to-skin contact. The father sits or stands at the side of the bed by the infant. This allows the parents and infant to become acquainted. Because the eyes are so important for both the parents and baby, we withhold the application of silver nitrate ($AgNO_3$) to the eyes until after this rendezvous.

We have found it valuable for the mother, father, and infant to be together for about 30 to 60 minutes. After 10 to 15 minutes the mother and baby often fall into a deep sleep. In Guatemalan hospitals, where drugs and anesthesia are used more sparingly, the majority of mothers were awake after 45 minutes of privacy with their infants. We must emphasize that this should be a private session. Affectional bonds are further consolidated in the succeeding 4 or 5 days through continued close association of baby and mother, particularly when she cares for him. Close contact with her husband and other children is also obviously important.

PREMATURE OR SICK NEONATES

We recommend the following procedures.

1. We have found it useful and safe when a premature baby weighing 1.5 to 2.5 kg is delivered and appears to be doing well without grunting and retractions for the mother to have the baby placed in her bed in the first hour of life with a heat panel above them. We do not recommend this approach unless the physician feels relaxed about the health of the infant.

2. A mother and her infant should be kept near each other in the same hospital, ideally on the same floor. When the long-term significance of early mother-infant contact is kept in mind, a modification of restrictions and territorial traditions can usually be arranged.

3. We have found it helpful, if the baby does have to be moved to a hospital with an intensive care unit, to give the mother a chance to see and touch her infant, even if he has respiratory distress and is in an oxygen hood. The house officer or the attending physician stops in the mother's room with the transport incubator and encourages her to touch and look at her baby at close hand. A comment about the baby's strength and healthy features may be long remembered and appreciated.

4. We encourage the father to follow the transport team to our hospital so he can see what is happening with his baby. He uses his own transportation so that he can stay in the premature unit for 3 to 4 hours. This extra time allows him to get to know the nurses and physicians in the unit, to find out how the infant is being treated, and to talk with the physicians in a relaxed fashion about what we expect will happen to the baby in the succeeding days. We allow him to come into the nursery and explain in detail everything that is going on with the infant, often offering him a cup of coffee. We ask him to help act as a link between us and his family by carrying information back to his wife, and we request that he come to our unit before he visits his wife so that he can let her know how the baby is doing. We suggest that he take a Polaroid photograph, even if the infant is on a respirator, so that he can describe the baby's care to his wife in detail.

5. Transportation of the mother from the community hospital before delivery to the maternity division of the medical center so she will be together with her baby after birth is occurring with increased frequency in many communities, as is transportation of the mother with the baby after delivery.

6. A mother should be permitted to enter the premature nursery as soon as she is able to maneuver easily. When she makes her first visit, it is important to anticipate that she may become faint or dizzy when she looks at her infant. We always have a stool nearby so that she can sit down, and a nurse stays at her side during most of the visit describing in detail the procedures being carried out, such as the monitoring of respiration and heart rate, the umbilical catheter, nasal CPAP, endotracheal tube, feeding through the various infusion lines, and the functioning of the incubator and ventilator.

7. We also encourage grandparents, brothers, sisters, and other relatives to view the infant through the glass window of the nursery so they will begin to know and to feel attached to the infant. We believe it is important to arrange for the grandparents and special close friends or relatives to enter the nursery and visit the baby, particularly when the baby is very ill or expected to die, so that they can provide firsthand support and understanding to the parents. We selectively allow siblings to enter the nursery when we believe it will truly relieve (and not aggravate) a child's confusion and anxiety.

8. It is necessary to find out what the mother believes is going to happen or what she has read about the problem. We try to move at her pace during any discussion to ensure that she understands.

9. In discussing the infant's condition by telephone with the mother, who is still in the referring hospital, we ask the father to stand nearby so that we can talk to them both at the same time and they can hear the same message. This group communication reduces misunderstandings and usually is helpful in assuring the mother that we are telling her the whole story.

10. If there is any chance that the infant will survive, we are optimistic with the parents from the beginning. There is no evidence that, if a favorable prediction proves to be incorrect and the baby expires, the parents will be harmed by early optimism. There is almost always time to prepare them before the baby actually dies. If the infant lives and the physician has been pessimistic, it is almost impossible for parents to become closely attached after they have figuratively dug a few shovelfuls of earth. We recognize that this recommendation is contrary to many old customs and places a heavy burden on the physician. It is our belief that, if the infant does expire, we must continue to work with the mother and father and help them with their mourning reactions.

11. Once the possibility that a baby has brain damage has been mentioned, the parents will not forget it. Therefore, unless we are convinced that the baby is dam-

aged, we do not mention the possibility of any brain damage or retardation to the parents.

12. It is important to emphasize that, if there is a clear objective finding such as a cardiac abnormality or a specific congenital malformation, we see no reason to hide it from the parents.

13. As soon as possible we describe to both the father and the mother the value of touching the infant in helping them get to know him, in reducing the number of apneic episodes (if this is a problem), and possibly increasing weight gain, thus hastening discharge from the unit.

14. It is important to remember that feelings of love for the baby are often elicited through eye-to-eye contact. Therefore, if an infant is under bilirubin lights, we turn them off and remove the eye patches so the mother and her infant can really see each other.

15. From our previous observations we have found that keeping a book in which to record parental phone calls and visits is useful in determining which mothers are likely to require additional help from a social worker or extra discussions about the health of their infant. If a mother visits the nursery less than three times in 2 weeks, the chance of her developing some sort of mothering disorder increases. Therefore, if the visiting pattern of the mother is less than that of most other mothers, she is given extra help in adapting to the hospitalization.

CONGENITAL MALFORMATIONS

The birth of an infant with a congenital malformation presents complex challenges to the physician who will care for the affected child and his family. Despite the relatively large number of infants with congenital anomalies, our understanding of how parents develop an attachment to a malformed child remains incomplete. Although previous investigators agree that the child's birth often precipitates major family stress, relatively few have described the process of family adaptation during the infant's first year of life. A major advance was Solnit and Stark's conceptualization of parental reactions. They emphasized that a significant aspect of adaptation is the necessity for parents to mourn the loss of the normal child they had expected. Other observers have noted the pathologic aspects of family reactions, including the chronic sorrow that envelops the family of a defective child. Less attention has been given to the more adaptive aspects of parental attachment to children with malformations.

Parental reactions to the birth of a child with a congenital malformation appear to follow a predictable course. For most parents initial shock, disbelief, and a period of intense emotional upset (including sadness, anger, and anxiety) are followed by a period of gradual adaptation that is marked by a lessening of intense anxiety and emotional reaction (Fig. 18-4). This adaptation is characterized by an increased satisfaction with and ability to care

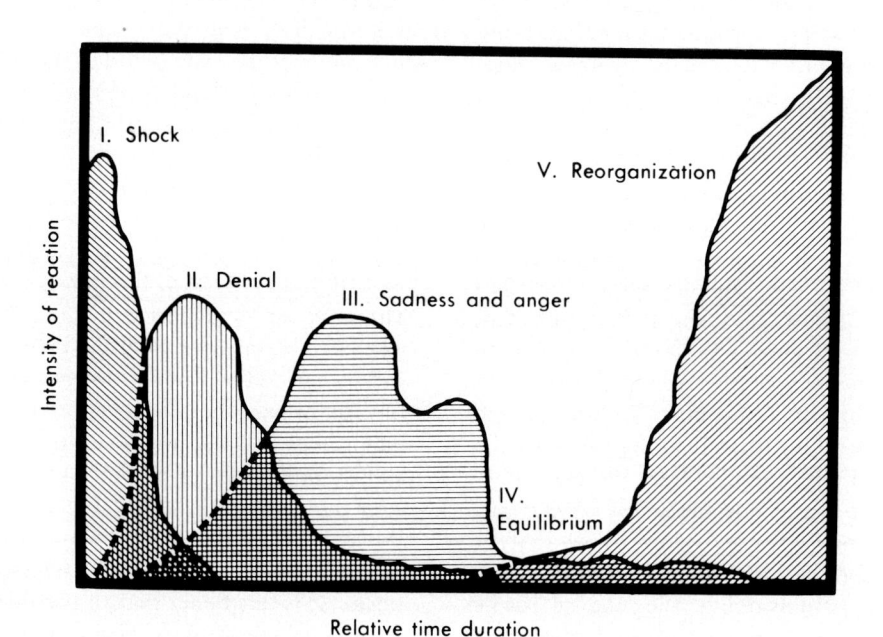

Fig. 18-4. Hypothetical model of a normal sequence of parental reactions to the birth of a malformed infant. (Adapted from Drotar, D., and others: Pediatrics **56**:710, 1975. Copyright American Academy of Pediatrics 1975.)

for the baby. These stages in parental reactions are similar to those reported in other crisis situations, such as terminally ill children. The shock, disbelief, and denial reported by many parents seem to be an understandable attempt to escape the traumatic news of the baby's malformation, so discrepant with usual parental expectations for a normal newborn.

Solnit and Stark have likened the crisis of the birth of a child with a malformation to the emotional crisis following the death of a child, in that the mother must mourn the loss of her expected, normal infant. In addition, she must become attached to her actual living, damaged child. However, the sequence of parental reactions to the birth of a baby with a malformation differs from that following the death of a child in yet another respect. The mourning or grief work appears not to take place in the usual manner because of the complex issues raised by continuation of the child's life and the demands of his physical care. The parents' sadness, which is important initially in their relationship with their child, diminishes in most instances once the parents take over the physical care. Most parents reach a point at which they are able to care adequately for their children and cope effectively with disrupting feelings of sadness and anger. The mother's initiation of the relationship with her child is a major step in the reduction of anxiety and emotional upset associated with the trauma of the birth. As with normal children, the parents' initial experience with their infant seems to release positive feelings which aid the mother-child relationship following the stresses associated with the news of the child's anomaly and, in many instances, the separation of mother and child in the hospital.

PRACTICAL SUGGESTIONS FOR PARENTS OF MALFORMED INFANTS

1. We have come to believe that it is better to leave the infant with the mother for the first 2 or 3 days, if medically feasible. If the child is rushed to the hospital where special surgery will eventually be done, the mother will not have enough opportunity to become attached to him. Even if the surgery is required immediately, as for bowel obstruction, it is best to bring the baby to the mother first, allowing her to touch and handle him and point out to her how normal he is in all other respects.

2. It is our impression that the parents' mental picture of the anomaly is often far more alarming than the actual problem. Any delay during which the parents suspect that there may be a problem greatly heightens their anxiety and causes their imaginations to run wild. Therefore we suggest that it is helpful to bring the baby to both parents when they are together as soon after delivery as possible.

3. We have arranged for the father to stay with the mother in her room on the maternity division on several occasions. We believe that this opportunity to support each other, to cry and curse and talk together, is highly beneficial. We use the process of early crisis intervention, meeting several times with the parents, whether the father lives in with the mother or not. During these discussions we ask the mother how she is doing, how she feels her husband is doing, and how he feels about the infant. We then reverse the questions and ask the father how he is doing and how he thinks his wife is progressing. The hope is that they will think not only about their own reactions but will begin to consider each other's as well.

4. We believe that parents should not be given tranquilizers. These tend to blunt their responses and slow their adaptation to the problem. A small dose of secobarbital (Seconal) at night, however, is often helpful.

5. It has been our clinical experience that parents who are initially adapting reasonably well often ask many questions and at times appear to be almost overinvolved in clinical care. In our unit we are pleased by this and more concerned about parents who ask few questions and who appear stunned and overwhelmed by the problem.

6. Many anomalies are very frustrating, not only to the parents but also to the physicians and nurses as well. There is a temptation for the physician to withdraw from the parents and their infant. The many questions asked by the parent who is trying to understand the problem are often very frustrating for the physician. The parent often appears to forget and asks the same questions over and over again.

7. Each parent may move through the process of shock, denial, anger, guilt, and adaptation at a different pace, so the two parents may not be synchronized with one another. If they are unable to talk with each other about the baby, there may be a marked disruption in their own relationship. We have found it best to move at the parents' pace. If we move too quickly, we run the risk of losing the parents along the way. It is beneficial *to ask* the parents how they view their infant: "Maybe you could tell me how you see the infant."

SUMMARY

Since the newborn baby is utterly dependent on his parents for his survival and optimum development, it is essential to understand the process of bonding as it develops from the first moments after the child is born. Although we have only a beginning understanding of this complex phenomenon, those responsible for the care of mothers and infants would be wise to reevaluate hospital procedures that interfere with early, sustained mother-infant contact, to consider measures that promote a mother's contact with her infant, and to help her appreciate the wide range of sensory and motor responses of her neonate.

Marshall H. Klaus
John H. Kennell

BIBLIOGRAPHY

Ambuel, J., and Harris, B.: Failure to thrive: a study of failure to grow in height or weight, Ohio Med. J. 59:997, 1963.

Barnett, C.R., and Grobstein, R.: Personal communication, 1974.

Barnett, C.R., and others: Neonatal separation: the maternal side of interactional deprivation, Pediatrics 45:197, 1970.

Bibring, C.: Some considerations of the psychological processes in pregnancy, Psychoanal. Study Child 14:113, 1959.

Bloom, R.: Definitional concepts of the crisis concept, J. Consult. Clin. Psychol. 27:42, 1963.

Bowlby, J.: Nature of a child's tie to his mother, Int. J. Psychoanal. 39:350, 1958.

Brazelton, T.B.: Effect of maternal expectations on early infant behavior, Early Child Devel. Care 2:259, 1973.

Brazelton, T.B., Koslowski, B., and Main, M. In Lewis, M., and Rosemblum, X., editors: The effect of the infant on its caregiver, New York, 1974, John Wiley & Sons, Inc.

Brazelton, T.B., Scholl, M., and Robey, J.: Visual responses in the newborn, Pediatrics 37:284, 1966.

Bronfenbrenner, U.: Early deprivation in mammals: a cross-species analysis. In Newton, G., and Levine, S., editors: Early experience and behavior, Springfield, Ill., 1968, Charles C Thomas, Publisher.

Budin, P.: The Nursling, London, 1907, Caxton Publishing Co.

Caplan, H.: Patterns of parenteral response to the crisis of premature birth, Psychiatry 23:365, 1960.

Cohen, R.L.: Some maladaptive syndromes of pregnancy and the puerperium, Obstet. Gynecol. 25:562, 1966.

Condon, W.S., and Sander, L.W.: Neonate movement is synchronized with adult speech: interactional participation and language acquisition, Science 183:99, 1974.

DeChateau, P., and Wiberg, B.: Long-term effect on mother-infant behaviour of extra contact during the first hour post partum. I. First observations at 36 hours, Acta Paediatr. Scand. 66:137, 1977.

DeChateau, P., and Wiberg, B.: Long-term effect on mother-infant behaviour of extra contact during the first hour post partum. II. Follow-up at three months, Acta Paediatr. Scand. 66:145, 1977.

Drotar, D., and others: The adaptation of parents to the birth of an infant with a congenital malformation: a hypothetical mode, Pediatrics 56:710, 1975.

Elmer, E., and Gregg, D.: Development characteristics of abused children, Pediatrics 40:596, 1967.

Emde, R.N., and Robinson, J.: The first two months: recent research in developmental psychobiology and the changing view of the newborn. In Noshpitz, J., and Call, J., editors: Basic handbook of child psychiatry, New York, Basic Books (in press).

Evans, S., Reinhart, J., and Succop, R.: A study of 45 children and their families, J. Am. Acad. Child Psychiatry 11:440, 1972.

Fanaroff, A.A., Kennell, J.H., and Klaus, M.H.: Follow-up of low birth-weight infants—the predictive value of maternal visiting patterns, Pediatrics 49:288:1972.

Friedman, S.B., and others: Behavioral observations on parents anticipating the death of a child, Pediatrics 32:610, 1963.

Geleerd, E.R.: Two kinds of denial: neurotic denial and denial in the service of the need to survive. In Schur, M., editor: Drives, affects and behavior, vol. 2, New York, 1965, International Universities Press.

Greenberg, M., Rosenberg, I., and Lind, J.: First mothers rooming-in with their newborns: its impact on the mother, Am. J. Orthopsych. 43:783, 1973.

Hare, E.H., and others: Spina bifida cystica and family stress, Br. Med. J. 2:757, 1966.

Hersher, L., Richmond, J., and Moore, A.: Maternal behavior in sheep and goats. In Rheingold, H., editor: Maternal behavior in mammals, New York, 1963, John Wiley & Sons, Inc.

Johns, N.: Family reactions to the birth of a child with a congenital abnormality, Med. J. Aust. 7:277, 1960.

Kennell, J., and Rolnick, A.: Discussing problems in newborn babies with their parents, Pediatrics 27:832, 1960.

Kennell, J.H., and others: Maternal behavior one year after early and extended post-partum contact, Dev. Med. Child Neurol. 16:172, 1974.

Klaus, M., and Fanaroff, A.: Care of the high-risk neonate, Philadelphia, 1973, W. B. Saunders Co.

Klaus, M.H., and Kennell, J.H.: Parent-infant bonding, ed. 2, St. Louis, 1981, The C. V. Mosby Co.

Klaus, M.H., and others: Human maternal behavior at the first contact with her young, Pediatrics 46:187, 1970.

Klaus, M.H., and others: Maternal attachment—importance of the first post-partum days, N. Engl. J. Med. 286:460, 1972.

Klein, M., and Stern, L.: Low birth weight and the battered child syndrome, Am. J. Dis. Child. 122:15, 1971

Klopfer, P.: Mother love! What turns it on? Am. Sci. 49:404, 1971.

Lang, R.: Birth book, Ben Lomond, Calif., 1972, Genesis Press.

Lang, R.: Personal communication, 1974.

Leifer, A., and others: Effects of mother-infant separation on maternal attachment behavior, Child Dev. 43:1203, 1972.

Lind, J., Vuorenkoski, V., and Wasz-Hoeckert, O.: The effect of cry stimulus on the temperature of the lactating breast primipara: a thermagraphic study. In Morris, N., editor: Psychosomatic medicine in obstetrics and gynaecology, Basel, Switzerland, 1973, S. Karger.

MacFarlane, J.A.: Olfaction in the development of social preferences in the human neonate. In The Parent-infant relationship, Ciba Foundation, Amsterdam, 1975, Elsevier.

MacFarlane, J.A., Smith, D.M., and Garrow, D.H.: The relationship between mother and neonate. In Kitzinger, S., and Davis, J.A., editors: The place of birth, New York, 1978, Oxford University Press.

McBryde, A.: Compulsory rooming-in in the ward and private newborn service at Duke Hospital, J.A.M.A. 45:625, 1951.

Meier, G.W.: Maternal behavior of feral- and laboratory-reared monkeys following the surgical delivery of their infants, Nature 206:492, 1965.

Michaels, J., and Shucman, H.: Observations on the psychodynamics of parents of retarded children, Am. J. Ment. Defic. 66:568, 1962.

National Association for Mental Health Working Party: The birth of an abnormal child: telling the parents, Lancet 2:1075, 1971.

Newton, N., and Newton, M.: Mother's reactions to their newborn babies, J.A.M.A. 181:206, 1962.

Oliver, J.E., and others: Severely ill-treated young children in North-East Wiltshire, Research Report no. 4, Oxford University Unit of Clinical Epidemiology.

Olshansky, S.: Chronic sorrow: a response to having a mentally defective child, Social Casework 43:190, 1962.

Parke, R.: Family interactions in the newborn period: some findings, some observations, and some unresolved issues. In Riegel, K., and Meacham, J.: Proceedings of the International Society for Study of Behavior Development, Oxford, 1974.

Raphael, D.: The tender gift: breastfeeding, Englewood Cliffs, N.J., 1973, Prentice-Hall, Inc.

Rappoport, L.: The state of crisis: some theoretical considerations. In Parad, H.J., editor: Crisis intervention, New York, 1965, Family Service Association.

Ringler, N.M., and others: Mother-to-child speech at two years: effects of early postnatal contacts, Behav. Pediatr. **86:**141, 1975.

Robson, K.: The role of eye-to-eye contact in maternal-infant attachment, J. Child Psychol. Psychiatry **8:**13, 1967.

Rose, J., Boggs, T., Jr., and Alderstein, A.: The evidence for a syndrome of "mothering disability" consequent to threats to the survival of neonates: a design for hypothesis testing including prevention in a prospective study, Am. J. Dis. Child. **100:**776, 1960.

Roskies, E.: Abnormality and normality: the mothering of thalidomide children, New York, 1972, Cornell University Press.

Rubin, R.: Maternal touch, Nurs. Outlook, p. 828, Nov. 1963.

Sackett, G.P., and Ruppenthal, G.G.: Some factors influencing the attraction of adult female macaque monkeys to neonates. In Lewis, M., and Rosenblatt, L., editors: The effect of the infant on its caregiver, New York, 1974, John Wiley & Sons, Inc.

Schneirla, T., Rosenblatt, J., and Tobach, E.: Maternal behavior in the cat. In Rheingold, J., editor: Maternal behavior in mammals, New York, 1963, John Wiley & Sons, Inc.

Shaheen, E., and others: Failure to thrive—a retrospective profile, Clin. Pediatr. **7:**225, 1968.

Siegel, E., and others: Hospital and home support during infancy: impact on maternal attachment, child abuse and neglect, and health care utilization, Pediatrics **66:**183, 1980.

Skinner, A., and Castle, R.: Seventy-eight battered children: a retrospective study, Report by the National Society for the Prevention of Cruelty to Children, 1969.

Solnit, A.J., and Stark, M.H.: Mourning and the birth of a defective child, Psychoanal. Study Child **16:**523, 1961.

Sosa, R., and others: The effect of a supportive companion on perinatal problems, length of labor, and mother-infant interaction, N. Engl. J. Med. **303:**597, 1980.

Sousa, P.L.R., and others: Attachment and lactation, Paper presented at Pediatria XIV: Nutrition, Toxicology and Pharmacology, Buenos Aires, Argentina, 1974.

Spitz, R.: The first year of life, New York, 1965, International Universities Press.

Stern, D.: A micro-analysis of mother-infant interaction, J. Am. Acad. Child. Psychiatry **10:**510, 1971.

Waterman, J.H.: Psychogenic factors in parental acceptance of feebleminded children, Dis. Nerv. Syst. **9:**184, 1948.

Winters, M.: The relationship of time of initial breastfeeding to success of breastfeeding, submitted thesis (nursing master's), University of Washington, 1973.

Yarrow, L.J.: Maternal deprivation: toward an empirical and conceptual re-evaluation, Psychol. Bull. **58:**459, 1961.

Zuk, G.H.: Religious factor and the role of guilt in parental acceptance of the retarded child, Am. J. Ment. Defic. **64:**145, 1950.

CHAPTER 19 # Routine and special care

PART ONE

Physical examination

The initial physical examination of the newborn should be done in the delivery room to detect significant anomalies, birth injuries, and cardiorespiratory disorders that may compromise a successful adaptation to extrauterine life. A more detailed examination should then take place in the nursery before advising the parents about their infant. The entire examination in the delivery room and nursery should be performed under a radiant heat source to prevent significant heat loss from the infant.

TRANSITION PERIOD

To detect disorders in adaptation soon after delivery, one must be aware of the normal features of the transitional stage. During labor there are a host of sensory inputs to the fetus, and at delivery a new set of stimuli influence fetal adaptation to the extrauterine environment. Both the intrapartum and the immediate neonatal events result in a sympathetic discharge that is reflected in changes in heart rate, color, respiration, motor activity, gastrointestinal function, and temperature of the infant.

During the late stages of labor the infant's heart rate normally fluctuates with a certain degree of variability around a baseline of 120 to 140. After delivery there is a rapid increase in the heart rate to the range of 160 to 180, lasting 10 to 15 minutes, with a gradual fall by 30 minutes to a baseline rate of between 100 and 120. During the *first* 15 minutes of life, respirations are irregular; peak respiratory rates range between 60 and 80 per minute. During this period rales are also present on auscultation; grunting, flaring, and retractions may also be noted, and there may be brief periods of apnea. Coincident with these changes in heart rate and respiratory rate, the infant is alert and his behavior is marked by spontaneous startle reactions, gustatory movements, tremors, crying, and movements of the head from side to side. This characteristic exploratory behavior is accompanied by a decrease in body temperature and a generalized increase in motor activity with increase in muscle tone.

In healthy infants who have not been subjected to adverse factors during labor there are characteristic changes accompanying the normal adaptation to extrauterine existence. The initial period of reactivity, previously described, is followed by a period of unresponsiveness and a second period of reactivity. The initial period of reactivity generally lasts 15 to 30 minutes. The gastrointestinal manifestations of this initial period of reactivity include the appearance of bowel sounds, the passage of meconium, and the production of saliva, all a result of parasympathetic discharges occurring during this period. The duration of this first period of reactivity, although varying between 15 and 30 minutes in healthy infants, is prolonged in term infants who have had an abnormal labor or delivery and in sick infants and normal premature infants.

Following this first period of reactivity the infant either sleeps or has a marked decrease in motor activity. The heart rate falls into the range of 100 to 120, and the infant becomes relatively unresponsive. This period of unresponsiveness, frequently accompanied by sleep, lasts from 60 to 100 minutes and is followed by a second period of reactivity, which lasts from 10 minutes to several hours. Periods of tachycardia and tachypnea, associated with changes in tone, color, and mucus production, are noted. Meconium is frequently passed during the second period of time (Fig. 19-1). Foreknowledge of the normal changes occurring during the transitional period

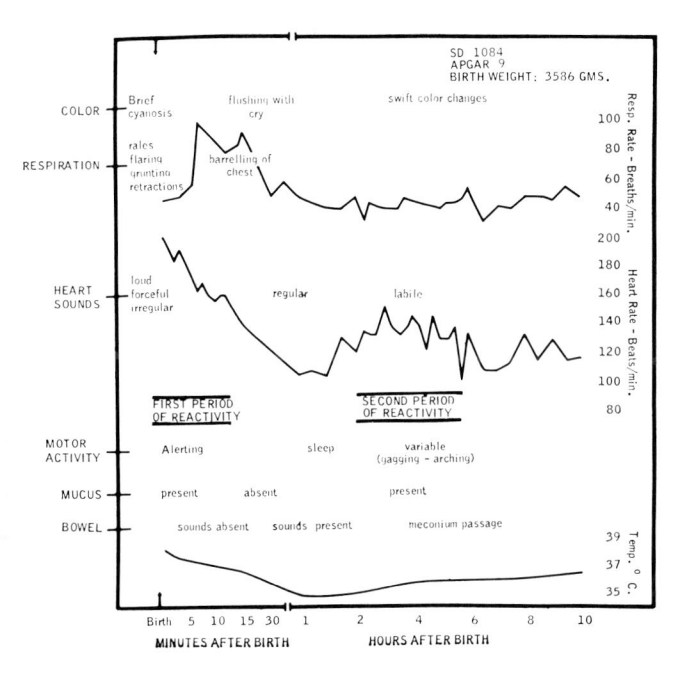

Fig. 19-1. Normal transition period. (From Desmond, M., Rudolph, A., and Phitakspharaiwan, P.: Pediatr. Clin. North Am. **13**:651, 1966.)

allows early recognition of the infant who is not making a normal extrauterine adaptation.

EXAMINATION IN THE DELIVERY ROOM

In the delivery room color is of immediate concern. Generalized cyanosis may indicate significant heart or lung disease or, rarely, the presence of methemoglobinemia. Differential cyanosis involving the lower extremities indicates persistence of a right-to-left shunt through the ductus, increased pulmonary vascular resistance, and, on occasion, a preductal coarctation (Chapter 25). Many normal infants have transient differential cyanosis that clears in the first minutes of life.

The pale infant either has been severely asphyxiated (asphyxia pallida) with the pallor caused by intense peripheral vasoconstriction or is severely anemic, secondary to acute blood loss from placenta previa, fetomaternal hemorrhage, or hemolysis from erythroblastosis fetalis (Chapters 5 and 29). An immediate decision regarding the cause is imperative if shock from acute blood loss is to be reversed by transfusion.

The meconium-stained infant should alert the examiner to the special risks of the acute or chronically asphyxiated infant (p. 184), who is often small for gestational age. Jaundice is seldom noted in the delivery room, even with severe erythroblastosis.

After determining the color of an infant, the examiner should evaluate the cardiopulmonary status. Initial inspection determines the respiratory rate. Tachypnea (a respiratory rate greater than 50 breaths per minute) should alert the examiner to possible pulmonary problems; bradypnea (less than 30 breaths per minute) or apnea or both should focus attention on the central nervous system and causes for central nervous system depression. Intercostal retractions, an audible grunt, and nasal flaring are additional signs of respiratory distress commonly present in the delivery room. Inspiratory or expiratory stridor should be noted and when present requires careful direct examination of the upper airway and magnification film of the airway if available.

Auscultation of the chest reveals the quality of breath sounds bilaterally, the presence or absence of rales, rhonchi, or expiratory wheezing, and the ease with which heart tones are heard. (Detailed examination of the cardiovascular system is covered in Chapter 25.) In the delivery room each infant's heart rate should be recorded as well as the quality of the heart tones; heart murmurs may be transient or may be indicative of significant heart disease. The absence, presence, and quality of peripheral pulses provide additional vital information.

The abdomen is inspected for protuberance, which may be secondary to abdominal masses, or concavity, which may be secondary to displacement of intestinal contents into the chest when there is a diaphragmatic hernia. Palpation and auscultation complete the initial examination of the abdomen. In the delivery room the relaxed muscle tone of the infant allows the best opportunity for abdominal examination; both kidneys should be palpated to exclude renal anomalies. The umbilical vessels should be counted to exclude the presence of a single umbilical artery, which correlates with an increased incidence of congenital anomalies.

The genitalia are examined to exclude the possibility of ambiguous genitalia before telling parents the sex of their infant (Chapter 33, part four).

The presence of significant choanal atresia should be excluded by manually occluding the mouth and each nostril and observing the infant for signs of respiratory distress or by passing a suction catheter through each naris into the stomach. The gastric contents should then be aspirated; the presence of more than 20 to 30 ml of gastric aspirate should raise the suspicion of upper intestinal obstruction. After the catheter has passed to a length that should be in the stomach, the instillation of 5 to 10 ml of air under direct gastric auscultation may be used to exclude the most common type of tracheoesophageal fistula. After exclusion of choanal atresia and upper intestinal anomalies, the same catheter can be used to establish the patency of the rectum.

The mental status and muscular tone of the infant should then be assessed. The neurologic examination is discussed in Chapter 22.

Before transfer of the infant from the delivery room,

significant anomalies should be sought (for example, clubfeet, cleft lip or palate, or meningomyelocele).

EXAMINATION IN THE NURSERY

See also Chapter 38.

The initial examination should be followed by a more detailed evaluation within the first 12 hours of life. Measurements of head and chest circumference and length and recordings of temperature and heart and respiratory rate should be included.

Jaundice is the most likely change in skin color to be noted on subsequent examination. In addition, cyanosis and pallor should be reevaluated. The infant should also be carefully examined for the presence of hemangiomas, pigmented or depigmented nevi, and mongolian spots.

The skull should be checked for overlapping sutures, the patency of sutures, caput succedaneum with its poorly defined margins, and cephalhematoma with its clearly demarcated margins. The eyes should be examined (Chapter 35). Approximately 40% of all infants will have conjunctival or retinal hemorrhages noted in the initial examination. The presence of a red reflex should be established, pupil size and reaction to light recorded, and the lens checked for the presence of cataracts. The size of the globes should be examined for possible microphthalmia.

The face should be examined for evidence of disorders that may present with distinctive facies (for example, trisomies and cretinism) (Chapter 38). The symmetry of the face should be evaluated to exclude possible facial nerve injuries following traumatic deliveries or in infants delivered by forceps.

Malformation of the ears may provide evidence of associated renal anomalies but more often is familial and only of cosmetic concern. The presence or absence of cartilage aids in establishing gestational age.

With the use of both a finger and a light with good direct visualization, both the soft and hard palates should be checked to exclude a cleft palate. High-arched palates as isolated findings are generally of no significance. Epithelial inclusion cysts are frequently noted along the gum margins and are benign entities requiring only parental reassurance. The tongue should be an appropriate size for its cavity; an inappropriately large tongue should raise the suspicion of a hemangioma or lymphangioma. The large tongue of cretinism is accompanied by other stigmata. The association of macroglossia with Beckwith's syndrome and Pompe's disease (type II glycogen storage disease) is well established. In infants with micrognathia a normal tongue may seem large. The well-known association of micrognathia, glossoptosis, and cleft palate (Pierre Robin syndrome) often presents initially as an upper airway obstruction and later becomes a cosmetic problem (Chapter 38).

The skinfolds of the neck should be checked for webbing or fistulous openings associated with either branchial clefts or thyroglossal duct cysts. During examination of the neck, each clavicle should be palpated for possible fracture. An asymmetric Moro reflex will often confirm a suspicious clinical finding noted on palpation.

The chest is examined for its musculature, bony structure, and location of nipples. By feeling for the pectoralis major in the axilla, one excludes absence of this muscle. Pectus excavatum or carinatum is of genuine concern to parents but only rarely is of clinical or cosmetic significance. The areolar size provides additional evidence on the gestational age of each infant.

The lungs and heart are again examined, but with particular attention to questionable findings previously noted at birth, especially transient heart murmurs or adventitial sounds. Radial, brachial, and femoral pulses should all be palpated and compared. Poor or diminished quality of pulses is an indication of inadequate cardiac output, whatever the cause. Absent femoral pulses are associated with coarctation of the aorta; bounding femoral pulses may be equally grave indicators of congenital heart disease. If pulses are suspect, a blood pressure taken either by flush or by the Doppler technique (p. 126) should be recorded in the upper and lower extremities.

The abdominal examination is also repeated to exclude the presence of a mass. Examination of the genitalia provides additional evidence for establishing gestational age. Males should be checked for hypospadias, to determine the location of the testes, and to exclude either inguinal hernias or hydrocele, the latter being far more common. Most female infants have a mucoid vaginal discharge in the first week of life that occasionally becomes sanguinous secondary to hormonal withdrawal. Either a large penis or clitoris should raise the question of adrenogenital syndrome, and there should be appropriate evaluation to exclude or confirm the diagnosis with its life-threatening sequelae (Chapter 33, part four).

The extremities of each infant are examined for the presence of structural anomalies, such as congenital dislocation of hip, clubfeet, and neurologic disorders.

At the end of the initial examination in the delivery room or transitional or normal nursery, the gestational age of each infant should be estimated. There are four methods employed to assess gestational age: physical criteria, neurologic examination, combined physical and neurologic examination, and examination of the lens. Table 19-1 lists the physical criteria used to establish gestational age. The characteristics progress in an orderly fashion during gestation. Close examination of sole creases, breast nodule diameter, scalp hair, cartilage in the earlobe, and testes and scrotum provides a rough guide to age that becomes more exact when using neurologic assessment.

Table 19-1. Estimation of gestational age

Evaluation		Approximate week of gestation when findings present								
		24	28	30	32	34	36	38	40	
Head circumference in cm ±2 SD			23-28.3	25-30.4	26.8-32.4	28.6-34	30.5-35.5	32-36.5	33-37	Based on 300 single live births —all Caucasian
Clinical	Sole creases	Anterior transverse crease only →					Occasional creases anterior two thirds →		Sole covered with creases →	
	Breast nodule diameter	Not palpable—absent →					2 mm	4 mm	7 mm	If small may represent fetal malnutrition
	Scalp hair	Fine and fuzzy Hard to distinguish individual strands →					Thick and silky Appear as individual strands →			
	Earlobe	Pliable—no cartilage →					Some cartilage	Stiffened by thick cartilage →		
	Testes and scrotum	Testes in lower canal Scrotum small—few rugae →					Intermediate	Testes pendulous, scrotum full, extensive rugae →		

From Behrman, R.E., Fisher, D., Paton, J.B., and Keller, J.: In utero disease and the newborn infant. In Schulman, I., editor: Advances in pediatrics, vol. 17, Chicago. Copyright © 1970 by Year Book Medical Publishers. Used by permission. (Adapted from Amiel-Tison, Brett, Koenigsbergh, and Usher.)

Although the physical criteria can be used to establish gestational age immediately following delivery, the neurologic criteria used to determine gestational age require the infant to be in an alert, rested state. In some infants this may not occur during the initial or subsequent examinations on the first day; in many infants accurate assessment of gestational age by neurologic criteria is not possible until the second or third day of life. Infants who are asphyxiated at the time of delivery, have a primary neurologic disorder, or are transiently depressed related to maternal medication characteristically underscore during neurologic examination. For this reason neurologic assessment should not be done until the infant is fully recovered. The assessment of gestational age using neurologic criteria was originally described by the French school and simplified by Amiel Tison. The examination involves assessment of posture, passive and active tone, reflexes, and righting reactions.

Using a system that combines the physical criteria and the neurologic assessment of gestational age, Dubowitz described and developed a combined scoring system. The scores from the physical and neurologic assessment are combined to give each infant a total score. The gestational age of the infant is calculated using the scores from the examination. The disadvantage of the Dubowitz scoring system is that it involves the assessment of 11 physical criteria and 10 neurologic findings. Although the physical criteria allow clear distinction of infants with varying gestational ages greater than 34 weeks, neurologic criteria are essential to differentiate infants between 26 and 34 weeks where the physical changes are less evident. Ballard and her colleagues abbreviated the Dubowitz scoring system to include six neurologic and seven physical criteria. These criteria are listed in Fig. 19-2. The accuracy and reliability of the abbreviated Ballard scoring system have been confirmed. The assessment can be performed in a significantly shorter period of time and thus facilitates accurate gestational age assessment, particularly of sick infants.

No matter what method of assessing gestational age is used, the infants should be examined in an optimum state of alertness and with strict adherence to the directions described by the original authors. Regardless of the method used, the assessment of gestational age using physical and neurologic criteria is accurate to ±2 weeks.

Hittner used the orderly disappearance of the anterior vascular capsule of the lens as a means of accurately assessing gestational age in premature infants between 26 and 34 weeks of gestation. She arbitrarily divided the disappearance of the anterior vascular capsule into four grades (Fig. 19-3). Examination requires observation with a direct ophthalmoscope following dilatation of the pupils. The examination should be done within the first

Neuromuscular Maturity

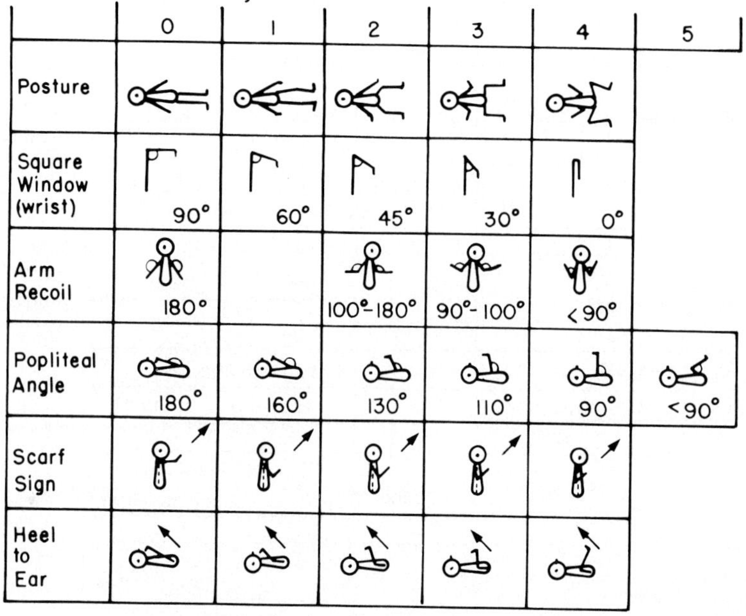

	0	1	2	3	4	5
Posture						
Square Window (wrist)	90°	60°	45°	30°	0°	
Arm Recoil	180°		100°–180°	90°–100°	<90°	
Popliteal Angle	180°	160°	130°	110°	90°	<90°
Scarf Sign						
Heel to Ear						

Apgars _____ 1 min _____ 5 min
Age at Exam _____ hrs
Race _____ Sex _____
B.D. _____
LMP _____
EDC _____
Gest. age by Dates _____ wks
Gest. age by Exam _____ wks
B.W. _____ gm. _____ %ile
Length _____ cm. _____ %ile
Head Circum. _____ cm. _____ %ile
Clin. Dist. None _____ Mild _____
            Mod. _____ Severe _____

PHYSICAL MATURITY

Skin	gelatinous red, transparent	smooth pink, visible veins	superficial peeling &/or rash few veins	cracking pale area rare veins	parchment deep cracking no vessels	leathery cracked wrinkled
Lanugo	none	abundant	thinning	bald areas	mostly bald	
Plantar Creases	no crease	faint red marks	anterior transverse crease only	creases ant. 2/3	creases cover entire sole	
Breast	barely percept.	flat areola no bud	stippled areola 1–2 mm bud	raised areola 3–4 mm bud	full areola 5–10 mm bud	
Ear	pinna flat, stays folded	sl. curved pinna; soft with slow recoil	well-curv. pinna; soft but ready recoil	formed & firm with instant recoil	thick cartilage ear stiff	
Genitals ♂	scrotum empty no rugae		testes descending, few rugae	testes down good rugae	testes pendulous deep rugae	
Genitals ♀	prominent clitoris & labia minora		majora & minora equally prominent	majora large minora small	clitoris & minora completely covered	

MATURITY RATING

Score	Wks
5	26
10	28
15	30
20	32
25	34
30	36
35	38
40	40
45	42
50	44

Fig. 19-2. Assessment of gestational age using the Ballard method. (From Ballard, J.L., Novak, K.Z., and Driver, M.: J. Pediatr. **95**:769, 1979.)

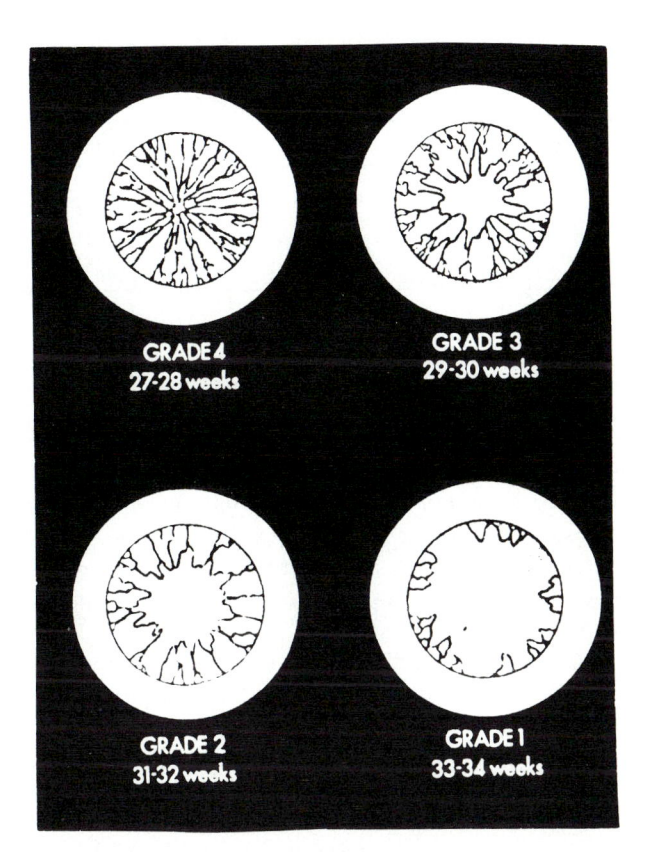

Fig. 19-3. Assessment of gestational age by examination of anterior vascular capsule of lens. (From Hittner, H.M., Hirsch, N.J., and Rudolph, A.J.: J. Pediatr. **91**:455, 1977.)

24 to 48 hours, since the vascular system changes rapidly within the first several days. Using this method the correlation between gestational age and the vascularity is highly significant.

After completion of the gestational assessment and physical examination, the parents of the new infant should be advised as to the infant's general health. Another examination should be carried out just before discharge from the nursery.

John M. Driscoll, Jr.

BIBLIOGRAPHY

Ballard, J.L., Novak, K.Z., and Driver, M.: A simplified score for assessment of fetal maturation of newly born infants, J. Pediatr. **95**:769, 1979.

Behrman, R.E., and others: In utero disease and the newborn infant, vol. 17, Advances in Pediatrics, Chicago, 1970, Year Book Medical Publishers, Inc.

Desmond, M., Rudolph, A., and Phitakspharaiwan, P.: The transitional care nursery, Pediatr. Clin. North Am. **13**:651, 1966.

Dubowitz, L., Dubowitz, V., and Goldberg, C.: Clinical assessment of gestational age in the newborn infant, J. Pediatr. **77**:1, 1970.

Hittner, H.M., Hirsch, N.J., and Rudolph, A.J.: Assessment of gestational age by examination of the anterior vascular capsule of the lens, J. Pediatr. **91**:455, 1977.

PART TWO

Physical environment

THE THERMAL ENVIRONMENT
Temperature and survival

Methods for protecting babies against heat loss developed in response to published evidence that such protection improved their survival (Table 19-2). In 1957 Silverman and Blanc reported that premature infants housed in incubators humidified to more than 80% had higher survival rates than babies housed in incubators humidified to less than 60%. The conclusion that these results could be related to thermal differences was reinforced in 1958, when Silverman reported that babies housed in humidified convectively heated incubators survived at a greater rate when the air temperature was controlled to 32° C as compared to 29° C. Premature sick infants largely contributed to the significant differences in mortality noted in these and subsequent studies. Whether thermal conditions affect the survival of full-term infants remains unknown.

In 1963 Agate and Silverman described an incubator warmed by a radiant heater controlled in servoresponse to the infant's skin temperature. The incubator control ensured that the infant had normal and stable body temperatures. Design of the incubator included an appreciation of the importance of radiant heat losses in simple convectively heated incubators (Fig. 19-4). The new incubator was used to compare survival rates of premature infants with similar skin temperatures but housed in two contrasting humidity settings. The results indicated that enhanced survival could not be credited to the nonthermal use of high humidity in an enclosed radiantly heated incubator. This report has been misinterpreted as providing proof that incubator environments do not have to be humidified; the results did not negate the earlier evidence that humidity may be important when warming infants in convectively heated incubators.

Subsequent studies demonstrated a thermal advantage for neonates housed in radiantly versus convectively heated incubators. Nonetheless, because of difficulties encountered in the fabrication of radiantly heated incubators, radiant heaters were replaced by convective heaters in the design of incubators for commercial distribution. Although elimination of the radiant heater did not compromise skin temperature stability, it did result in the production of an environment different from that produced in the radiantly heated incubator. In the radiantly heated enclosed incubator, the air temperature was stable, whereas in the convectively heated servocontrolled incubator air temperature can vary over short periods by 3° to 4° C and after severe disruptions by as much as 5° to 10° C (Fig. 19-5). These rapid excursions in

Table 19-2. Mortality of premature infants maintained in environments providing more or less protection against heat loss

	More		Less	
	Number	**Died (%)**	**Number**	**Died (%)**
Silverman and co-workers (1958)	91	16	91	32
Beutow and co-workers (1964)	89	42	69	54
Day and co-workers (1964)	60	23	65	37
Perlstein and co-workers (1976)	105	22	105	35
Totals	345	26	330	40

temperature have been correlated with apneic spells in some premature infants.

In 1976 Perlstein and associates reported improved survival of babies housed in computer-controlled incubators constrained to prevent wide thermal change in the environment. The stable thermal environment created by the computer-controlled system is similar to the environment created in the earlier radiantly heated enclosed incubators. In addition, while stabilizing the environmental temperature, the computer-controlled system uses logic that allows skin temperature to vary freely within the range of 35.5° and 37.0° C; the simpler radiantly heated systems assumed abnormality if the infant's skin temperature varied by more than ±0.2° C. Although documented to enhance survival, neither the radiantly heated nor computer-controlled incubator systems are commercially available. Of the commercially available incubator systems, none has been documented to improve infant survival when compared with other available systems.

Temperature and homeothermy

As a rule, babies are homeotherms who attempt to maintain their body temperatures within some narrow range. They respond to heat loss by generating more heat. The consequences of prolonged and maximum heat production include the conversion of life-sustaining substrates to acidic metabolic by-products (Fig. 19-6).

Infants are alerted to cold stress when thermal receptors in the skin are stimulated. The face is particularly sensitive, and even when the baby's body is warm, cooling of the face will cause a responsive rise in metabolic rate. Conversely, warming of the facial skin when the body is cold suppresses homeothermically induced hypermetabolism.

Measurement of body temperature alone is of limited value in assessing the probable metabolic state of an infant. An infant with a specific body temperature will become hypermetabolic if the environmental temperature drops sufficiently below the skin temperature to cause a rate of heat loss exceeding the rate of heat generated by the infant's basal metabolic activity. Even with a low body temperature, however, if the environmental temperature is rising or is close enough to the skin temperature to limit heat loss to a rate not exceeding the rate of basal heat production, a baby will not become hypermetabolic. High body temperatures also activate distress mechanisms that require an increase in metabolic work.

An infant can limit heat loss by changes in body posture that reduce the skin surface area exposed to the environment. This capability is compromised in premature, unconscious, sedated, and physically restrained babies. Infants also can reduce shunting of internal heat to body surfaces by vasoconstricting peripheral vessels. This mechanism can be defeated in shock and by some autonomic drugs (Fig. 19-6). An infant may generate heat by crying and becoming hyperactive when cold stressed to the point of jitteriness, although shivering does not appear to occur.

A cold-stressed baby primarily depends on mechanisms that cause chemical thermogenesis. When stimulated by cold, norepinephrine and thyroid hormones are released, inducing lipolysis in brown fat stores principally found in the interscapular, paraspinal, and perirenal areas. Although not all of the chemical pathways are known, triglycerides in the fat are broken down to fatty acids and glycerol. The former enter thermogenic metabolic paths that end in the common pool of metabolic acids. Glycolysis may be stimulated during severe stress when epinephrine, released from the adrenals, activates glycogen stores and may result in transient hyperglycemia. Hypoglycemia has also been reported by Cornblath in cold-stressed infants, possibly due to inhibition of glycolysis by lipolysis or to exhaustion of glycogen stores.

The absolute maximum or "summit" amount of heat production is affected by gestational and postnatal age and is demonstrably less during the first days of life. An infant not exposed to periodic cold stress may adapt to the protective environment and lose the ability to respond homeothermically when exposed to an unfamiliar cold stimulus.

Central nervous system damage, sedation, shock, hypoxia, and drugs may all reduce the metabolic response to

Routine and special care 261

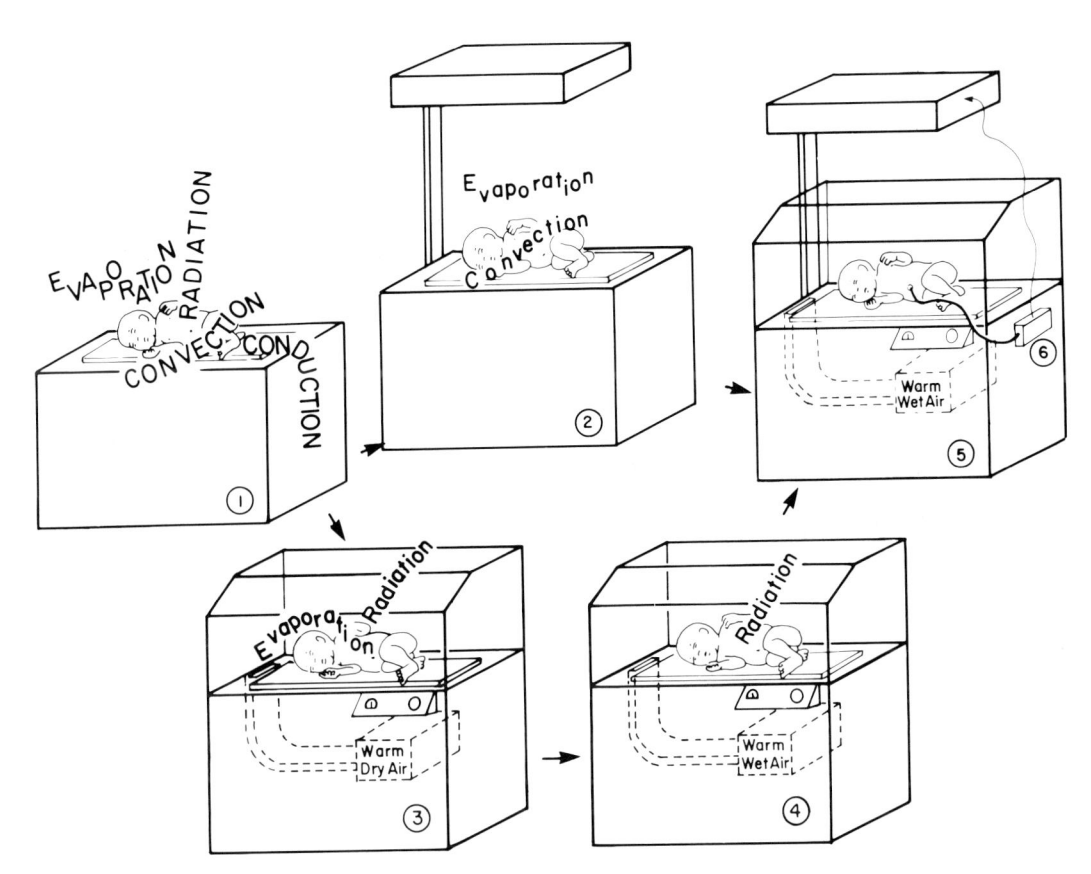

Fig. 19-4. Logic leading to development of skin servocontrolled radiantly heated convectively ventilated incubator. *1,* An unprotected baby loses body heat from skin surfaces by conduction, convection, evaporation, and radiation. *2,* A radiant heater eliminates radiant and conductive losses but not those caused by convection and evaporation. *3,* An unhumidified convectively heated incubator eliminates convective and conductive losses but not those caused by radiation and evaporation. *4,* Humidifying a convectively heated incubator eliminates all major heat losses except for the losses by radiation. *5,* Using a radiant heater to warm a convectively ventilated and humidified incubator should eliminate all sources of heat loss from the infant's skin. *6,* Normal infant temperature can be ensured by adding a controller to the incubator so that power is delivered to the radiant heater whenever the infant's skin temperature falls below a present value.

Fig. 19-5. Typical air temperatures in convectively heated incubator, servocontrolled to maintain infant's skin temperature at 36° C.

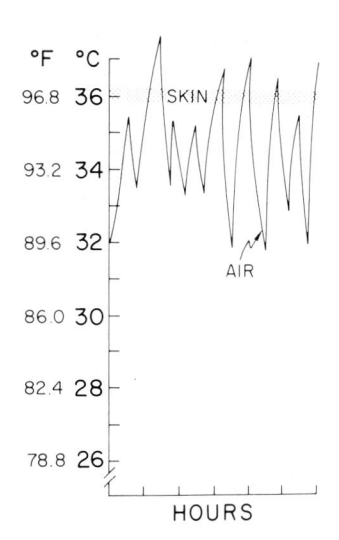

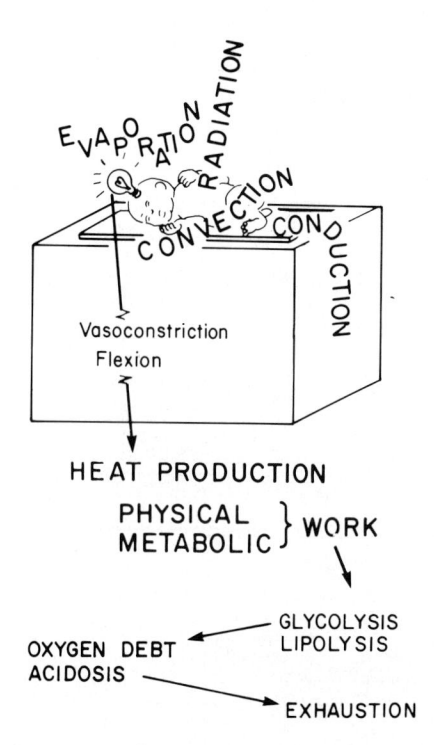

Fig. 19-6. Schematic of homeothermy in newborns. On sensing loss of body heat, the infant minimizes heat loss from the skin and increases metabolic rate. The increase in metabolism can produce acidosis and substrate depletion.

cold. This may represent a direct antimetabolic effect or be due to a blunting of the sensory mechanisms that alert the intact baby to the stress stimuli. After prolonged stress, depletion of hormonal and energy stores may reduce the ability to further respond.

The concept of an optimum thermal environment for newborn babies evolved during the 1960s. This idealized setting, called *neutral thermal environment,* is one in which a baby can maintain a normal body temperature while producing only the minimum amount of heat generated from basal life-sustaining metabolic processes. Maintenance of neutral thermal conditions is considered to be of greatest importance in the youngest, most immature infants, whose ability to generate additional heat in a heat-losing environment may be minimal. The ability to increase metabolic rate in these infants may be further hampered by impaired gas exchange in the lungs and/or restriction of caloric intake.

The physics of heat exchange

The temperature of an object is a measure of the balance between heat leaving and entering the object. Heat can only be lost from a substance that is warmer to one that is cooler. A baby will lose heat only when the surrounding environment is colder than the infant. The rate of heat loss is directly proportional to the magnitude of the difference between the infant's skin temperature and the temperature of the environment. This proportionality can be expressed mathematically by introducing a constant called the thermal transfer coefficient (h), the value of which depends upon the material of the substance transferring the heat:

Heat loss = h (Skin temperature − Environmental temperature) × (Surface area)

The exposed surface area of the infant is critical in the equation used to calculate heat loss. Thus a baby that is diapered or swaddled has less exposed surface than an unclothed infant.

The thermal transfer coefficient describes the rate at which heat leaves the body surface and is related to body shape, thickness of the boundary layer of air surrounding the body, and the characteristic way in which tissue absorbs or reflects radiant energy. Heat loss is also modified by the thermal conductance of an infant. The thermal conductance is computed using the difference between the baby's core and skin temperatures multiplied by a thermal coefficient describing the speed with which heat is transferred from the interior to the exterior of the body. This variable coefficient depends on body size, tissue composition and thickness, skin blood flow, and vascular shunting.

The differences between body shapes and sizes and tissue thickness result in babies having thermal conduction and transfer coefficients that are much higher than in adults. Because of this difference in coefficients, babies lose more heat than adults in identical heat-losing environments.

Definition of normal body temperature

Silverman and Agate in 1964 defined body temperature as a weighted value in which a colonic measurement contributed 60% and a skin measurement 40%. For practical purposes, however, it is traditional to rely on a single-site measurement. If an infant's internal temperature is within the range of 35.5° to 37.5° C, the infant's temperature can be considered normal. Since body temperature is a measure only of the balance between heat production and net heat loss, a normal body temperature should not be confused with a "normal" metabolic rate (Fig. 19-7).

Internal body temperature measurements

Although esophageal and tympanic membrane temperatures have been used in some physiologic studies, it is easier and traditional in a clinical setting to equate rectal temperature with the baby's internal body temperature.

In measuring the rectal temperatures of newborn

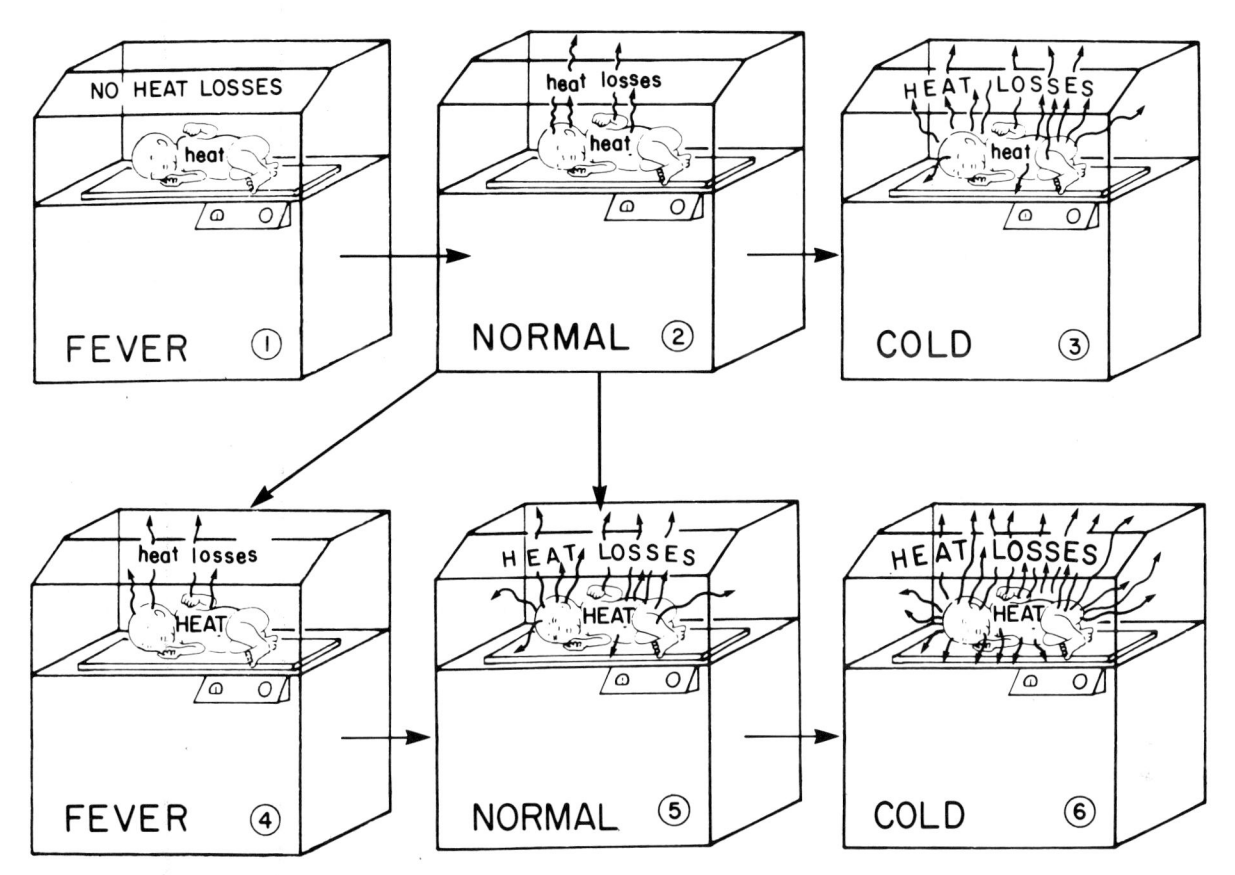

Fig. 19-7. *1,* Fever due to total elimination of heat losses from minimally metabolic baby. *2,* Normal temperature when heat losses are minimized and equal to heat produced by minimally metabolic baby (neutral thermal conditions). *3,* Hypothermia caused by large heat losses from baby who is temporarily poikilothermic. *4,* "Fever" when heat losses are less than heat produced by hypermetabolic baby. *5,* Normal temperature when heat losses are large but equal to heat produced by hypermetabolic infant. *6,* Hypothermia caused by very large heat losses that exceed the heat produced by a hypermetabolic infant.

Heat = greater than minimal heat production.
Fever = internal temperature of more than 37.5° C.
Normal = internal temperature of 35.5° to 37.5° C.
Cold = internal temperature less than 35.5° C.

babies, the depth of insertion of the thermometer is very important. Karlberg documented that the difference between rectal temperature measured by a thermistor inserted 1 cm and then 5 cm into the rectum can exceed 1.5° C. Serial readings should be taken at a common depth. Thermometers used for temperature transduction in babies ideally should be accurate to ±0.1° C and have a range that spans 33° to 40° C.

Over the years some concern has been expressed about the danger of perforation or other injury when using rigid thermometers or thermistors to transduce rectal temperatures. Measurement of axillary temperature has been suggested as a safer alternative. Although axillary temperatures have been found variably comparable to simultaneous measurements of rectal temperature, Torrance demonstrated that, if care is taken to place a thermometer firmly in the axilla with the infant's arm held against the body of the baby, accurate and comparable temperature readings can be obtained if a sufficient period of time is allowed for the transducer to reach its maximum reading.

Skin temperature measurements

Skin temperature is usually measured with thermocouples or thermistors attached to the skin. These three-dimensional temperature transducers sense the temperatures of their tops, sides, and bottoms. They are affected by the temperature of the transducing element and by the temperature of the wires used to connect the element to an electronic thermometer. They actually trans-

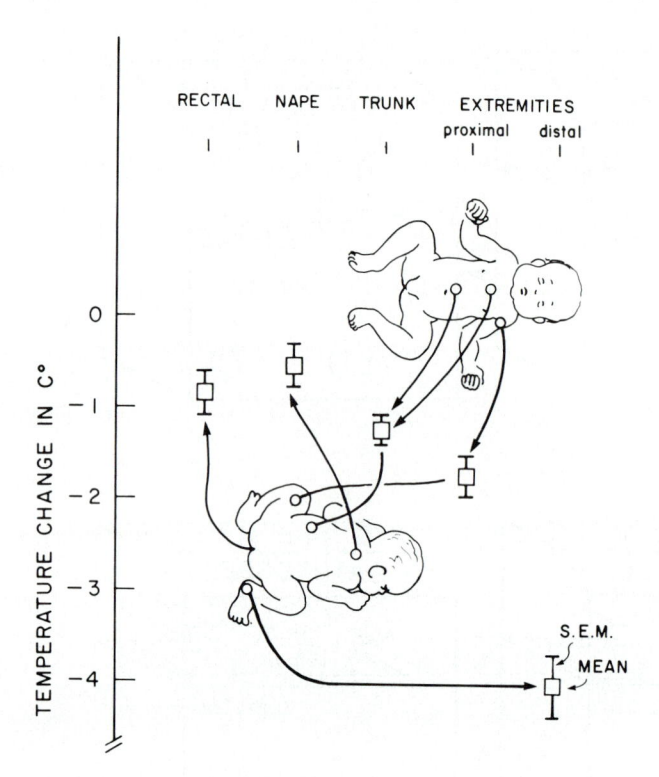

Fig. 19-8. Cooling of skin over different body surfaces after heat-losing exposure. Skin temperature changes measured in 16 infants of varying weights, gestations, and postnatal ages. Infants were exposed naked for 1 hour to room temperatures ranging between 23° and 29° C. (Adapted from Silverman, W.A., and others: Pediatrics **33**:984, 1964. Copyright American Academy of Pediatrics 1964.)

duce both skin temperature *and* environmental temperature. The relative contribution of each of these thermal sources to the final numerical readout of skin temperature is a function of the construction, insulation, location, and mode of attachment of the transducer. The attachment of a skin sensor also produces compression of underlying vessels, further causing a distortion of the true skin temperature value.

There is a very wide distribution of different temperatures over varying skin surface sites. These variations make interpretation of a single skin temperature difficult. It has been suggested that, when only a single skin temperature is to be sensed, the transducer be attached to the skin over the liver or between the umbilicus and the pubis. In a clinical setting, however, attachment sites sometimes need to be changed to prevent skin irritation. In addition, the rotation of babies into various positions requires attachment sites to be altered so that the infant's body does not cover the probe and cause a measurement of mattress instead of skin temperature.

In practice it is common to move single skin probes freely so that they are always on a skin surface exposed to the environment. In search of a "mean" surface temperature, the transducers are usually not attached over the least and most vasoreactive body regions. Bony prominences and the extremities, therefore, are the least favored attachment sites. It is also sensible to avoid placing probes on the skin overlying the metabolically reactive brown fat collections in the interscapular region (Fig. 19-8).

Environmental temperature measurements

The environment in which an object resides is defined as everything that surrounds the object. The components of the environment can be idealized by discussing the four simple mechanisms by which most heat is lost from the body: conduction, convection, radiation, and evaporation. This idealization is a useful way to emphasize the near independence of each of these mechanisms and the mistake in considering "air temperature" as a synonym for "environmental temperature." In fact, it has been suggested that an actual measurement of the true environmental temperature probably can only be idealized, and to avoid the implication of greater precision the word should probably be modified to an "operative" environment.

Conductive and convective heat losses

Conduction is a term that describes the transfer of heat between contacting solid objects of different temperatures. Convection can be thought of as a special subset of conduction referring to heat exchange between the dense material of a solid object to the solid but less dense material in the gaseous environment.

In ordinary circumstances, heat losses by conduction can be kept to a minimum by ensuring that an infant is lying on a warm mattress of very low conductivity, or if swaddled, that the infant is wrapped in prewarmed materials. If the mattress and swaddling materials are at the same temperature as the baby's skin, no heat loss or gain will occur by conduction. If, however, the baby is placed on a cold table or wrapped in a blanket at room temperature, these heat losses can become tremendous. Conversely, if placed close to a hot water bottle or heating pad that is warmer than the infant, the baby will gain heat at a rate directly proportional to the temperature difference between the conductive heat source and the baby's skin, and overheating may result.

Convective temperatures are usually equated with the simple measure of air temperature. Convective heat losses, however, are increased not only when the air cools but also with higher rates of air flow. The air temperature in an enclosed incubator must be thought of in terms of both its absolute value and the way this value is modified by an associated wind chill factor introduced by a circulating fan.

The measured air temperature should be that perceived by the infant. Thus, ideally the air temperature immediately adjacent to the infant's skin surface should be the temperature transduced. Measurement of air temperatures elsewhere in an incubator can introduce an error of up to 10° C, which is the span of temperature values that can coexist within an incubator chamber. Sometimes it is necessary to monitor multiple air temperatures influencing heat exchange over different body surfaces. When a baby is in a head hood flushed by air or oxygen, both incubator chamber and head hood temperature measurements are needed. Traditionally, convective losses were considered only as a heat transfer from the skin surfaces into the surrounding air, but consideration also must be given to heat exchanges that occur between the respiratory system and cooler gases delivered by respirators.

Radiant heat losses

Heat loss by radiation is heat loss at the speed of light. Objects can be characterized by their ability to absorb or emit energy in the infrared range of the electromagnetic spectrum. The degree to which infrared rays are absorbed or emitted is called the emissivity of an object and can range from near 0 for a perfectly reflecting substance such as shiny silver to the value of almost 1 for a substance that, like carbon black, absorbs and reemits all infrared energy received. Human skin is more like carbon than silver and for practical purposes is considered to have an emissivity of 1. Emissivity is related more to the tissue's moisture content, texture, and porosity than to its color.

Heat loss by radiation is heat loss from a warmer to a cooler object with which the warmer object is not in contact. Walls, windows, chairs, light bulbs, and other people are examples of surfaces with which babies exchange radiant heat. This route of heat exchange is essentially independent of all other routes. A baby can get cold in a room containing air warmer than the infant's skin if the walls and windows are sufficiently cold. A baby in the warm air of an incubator can get cold if the incubator walls are cold, and a baby in an incubator with cold air can get overheated if the walls are too hot.

Because of the radiant "greenhouse" effect, a baby in an incubator can get too hot even if the incubator walls are not subjected to any obvious heating. Because the acrylic plastic walls of most incubators are opaque to infrared waves, they behave like the glass in a greenhouse, through which visible short-wave light rays pass easily. On absorption of the short electromagnetic waves by the housed plants, the short waves are converted into heat energy and reemitted as long infrared rays that, upon reaching the glass inner surface, are absorbed and not transmitted. The glass is heated by the infrared energy, and this energy is reemitted toward the plants. In this way visible light can be used to generate heat, which is trapped in the greenhouse whose contents become warmer.

It is not uncommon to find babies in incubators near windows become cold in the evening when incubator wall radiate their heat to the night-chilled glass panes. The same infants can be found febrile in the morning when the bright sun streams through glass and plastic to warm the incubator occupant. Such environmental changes can occur without causing changes in incubator air temperature.

To define environmental temperature requires at least a measurement of surrounding wall temperatures with which the baby lives in radiant harmony. Since radiant exchanges are quantitatively related not only to absolute temperature gradients but also to the distance between the surfaces exchanging heat, to the angles subtended by electromagnetic rays traveling from one surface to the other, and to the emissivities of each of the radiant surfaces, no single measurement can provide any but a gross approximation of a baby's radiant world. When an infant is within the chamber of an enclosed incubator, however, the measurements are greatly simplified and the approximations more believable than those made when an infant is in an open crib.

Evaporative heat losses

With every milliliter of water that evaporates, approximately 0.58 Cal of body heat are lost. It is therefore theoretically possible to use insensible weight loss measurements to estimate the amount of heat that an infant has lost by this mechanism. Since insensible weight loss measurements are somewhat difficult to obtain, this form of monitoring is reserved for research purposes.

To understand heat loss by evaporation is to appreciate the distinction that exists between humidity and vapor pressure. The vapor pressure of water is the specific atmospheric pressure of water vapor at any given temperature at which water can exist in both its liquid and vaporous states. The partial pressure of water vapor is the actual pressure being exerted by water vapor at any given temperature. If the partial pressure equals the vapor pressure, the vapor is saturated. If the partial pressure is less than the vapor pressure, the vapor is unsaturated. Relative humidity is a percentage expression of this degree of saturation and is computed using the following relationship:

$$\text{Relative humidity (\%)} = 100 \times \frac{\text{Partial pressure of water vapor}}{\text{Vapor pressure at same temperature}}$$

Although relative humidity is easy to quantitate, it is not the relative humidity but the difference between the partial pressure of the water vapor in the boundary layers around the baby's body and the vapor pressure of water in the environment outside this boundary layer that actually sets up the driving force causing evaporative water losses. The vapor pressure rises with higher temperatures. As long as the baby's skin is warmer than the environment, evaporative losses can occur even when the humidity is 100%.

How to keep a baby warm

Prevention of heat loss is often best achieved by simple methods applied with the knowledge born from common sense. Since heat loss requires the presence of a thermal gradient, it is important to avoid exposing the baby to a cold environment by either warming the environment or covering the baby.

The delivery room

In utero a fetus is warmer than the mother. Born wet, warm, and naked into the usual environment of a delivery room, the newborn infant loses heat rapidly. Even if the oxygen consumption of a homeothermic infant increases to the maximum summit of 15 ml/kg/minute, the 0.075 Cal/kg/minute of heat produced is still two or three times less than the approximate rate of loss of 0.2 Cal/kg/minute. The variable consequences of this heat loss depend on many factors, including the general condition of the baby at birth. Gandy and associates in 1964 reported that poorly protected infants tend to have a metabolic acidosis mixed variably with a compensatory respiratory alkalosis. Based on various methods used to protect infants, it would appear that elimination of heat loss in a clinical setting can be effective but is seldom complete (Table 19-3).

In the delivery room a large proportion of heat loss is caused by evaporation. The skin should be dried with warm towels and evaporative losses severely limited using plastic bags or other swaddling materials to insulate the skin from the dry room air. Attention should be directed toward drying the head and face, since a brief clean-up with a dry towel in the delivery room may prevent the subsequent cold exposure that accompanies a prolonged cosmetic cleansing bath in the nursery. Even with the most careful drying of the newborn, it is almost impossible to completely dry the hair.

The resuscitation of a newborn should not be allowed to interfere with thermal protection. If, during resuscitation, access is needed to some body surface, then only that body surface and no other should be exposed. If the umbilicus is to be tied or cannulated, there is no need to unswaddle the infant's head, arms, chest, or legs. Closed cardiac chest massage can be performed without exposing the lower half of the body. Only one leg requires exposure when applying an identification band to an ankle, when taking an identifying footprint, or for that matter when starting an intravenous infusion in the extremity. It is reasonable to back up the protection of swaddling by using a radiant heater to add extra warmth to the area assigned for infant care in the delivery room. Radiant heaters in the delivery room can provide excellent protection that is almost equal to that provided by careful swaddling, and when used together the protection can be superb (Table 19-3).

The control over heat loss must not be loosened during the transfer of a baby from the delivery room to another care area. Even within the delivery room, the baby should remain swaddled when carried to a weighing scale or for display to the parents. Weighing scales should be placed under a radiant heater, and if the mother desires skin-to-skin contact with her baby, they should be "swaddled" together under warm blankets.

The nursery

If swaddling is to be discontinued either in the delivery room or nursery, then alternatives to swaddling must be considered. These alternatives can be reduced to three common choices:
1. Warm up the room.
2. Place the baby in a warm enclosed incubator.
3. Place the baby under an open radiant heater.

The warm room. Heating a room to the 36° to 37° C needed to keep some small and sick babies warm may distress personnel working in the nursery. These conditions also may be unfavorable for larger and healthier infants in the same area. For long-term care, heating and humidifying nurseries to appropriate temperatures is probably the least desirable method for limiting heat losses from infants, although in short-term situations such as in radiology departments, operating rooms, and treatment rooms this method of protection can be the most applicable and effective. Raising the room temperature to meet the needs of a small baby is an important responsibility of those who deliver infants at home. Ambulances used in transporting between institutions should always be warmed before initiating the transfer.

Convectively heated incubators. These are the most common devices available for creating a microclimate in which to care for an individual baby. They all provide a single- or double-layered plastic-walled chamber into which a baby is placed on an insulating mattress. The plastic walls of the chamber have portals in various places to provide hand access to the enclosed infant. All convectively heated incubators use fans to force filtered room air at various rates of flow over relatively large heaters and pans that can be optionally filled with water. The warmed and humidified air is directed into the plastic chamber at various locations in different incubators and is exhausted from the incubator chamber under differing influences. The heating of incubator air can be controlled

Table 19-3. Postnatal temperature fall within 30 minutes with various methods of limiting heat loss

Method	Source of data	30-Minute temperature (°C)*	30-Minute fall in temperature (°C)†
Infant placed in crib 30-40 cm under 60-W bulb covered with warm blanket; later dressed and put in incubator	Miller and Oliver	35.5 ± 0.16	2.6
Infant placed in preheated crib, covered loosely with warm blanket, and then bathed, dressed, and swaddled	Miller and Oliver	35.6 ± 0.14	2.5
Infant swaddled in warm, dry towel	Baum and Scopes	36.1 ± 0.59	2.0
Infant dried, placed in incubator (procedures through portholes)	Miller and Oliver	36.2 ± 0.15	1.9
Naked baby, 80 cm under 750-W radiant heater	Besch and associates	36.2 ± 0.10	1.9
Transparent swaddler without heat shield	Besch and associates	36.2 ± 0.11	1.9
Naked baby, 64 cm under 400-W radiant heater	Du and Oliver	36.4 ± 0.16	1.7
Silver swaddler	Baum and Scopes	36.6 ± 0.61	1.5
Transparent swaddler with head shield	Besch and associates	36.9 ± 0.09	1.2
Transparent swaddler with head shield and 750-W radiant heater at 80 cm	Besch and associates	37.3 ± 0.11	0.8

Adapted from Besch N.J., and others: N. Engl. J. Med. **284:**125, 1971.
*Mean ± SE.
†From fetal intrauterine temperature of 38.1° C.

variably by a thermostat referenced to the temperature within the chamber or the temperature under the incubator chamber base. The heating can also be controlled in a servo-loop that references the heater-on or heater-off decision to a narrow band of infant skin temperatures. Different brands of incubators use differing techniques and thermal limits to prevent excessive heating within the incubator chamber. Only a few studies of the differences between various convectively heated incubators have been published, but they all confirm that general statements assuming homeogeneity in their function are somewhat naive.

The differences become very clear when comparing how different incubators react when their control systems and environmental chambers are subjected to influences that potentially disrupt their integrity. As an example, Ahlgren demonstrated that, whereas incubators with solid acrylic plastic port doors cool rapidly when the doors are opened, incubators with flexible plastic sleeves as port covers can be entered with minimum change in incubator temperature. The first kind of incubator, however, probably provides the contained infant with more protection against radiant heat losses. In maintaining incubator air temperatures, positioning of the sensing thermistor may make it vulnerable to situations that might cause false temperature recordings. For example, the probe may be warmed by a covering of diapers and blankets lying in the incubator or artifactually cooled by a stream of cold oxygen from a resuscitation bag placed carelessly next to the infant.

In general, although incubator chambers can be cooled rapidly, they take a relatively long time to reach a stable thermal equilibrium during warming. Therefore, before placement of a baby within the chamber, the incubator should be prewarmed. A prewarmed incubator should always be ready and available in anticipation of the arrival of a sick infant. Prewarming an incubator so that the air is at 36° C will produce a thermal environment of about 35° C, which is sufficient to reduce heat loss from most infants. If oxygen is to be administered by head hood or respirator, the gas humidification chambers also should be prewarmed.

Since the initial care provided a sick baby ordinarily requires multiple entries into the incubator chamber, it is reasonable, especially when caring for very small babies, to provide the infant with some form of additional thermal protection. This protection can be provided by turning the incubator humidity control to a maximum setting, keeping the baby partially swaddled, or using a supplementary portable radiant heat source over the incubator top. The initial focus of thermal control should be the prevention of heat loss without excessive concern about optimizing the environment for long-term care.

There are various guidelines that can be used when adjusting incubator temperatures for infants of various sizes and ages. No available guidelines, however, negate the responsibility to measure and record the infant's core and skin temperatures along with incubator air temperatures periodically, if not continuously. Clear orders should specify the desired ranges for both incubator and baby temperatures, and the site of air temperature measurement should be that perceived by the baby. There are now many types of relatively inexpensive electronic thermometers commercially available for use in making these measurements. The incubator temperature should be increased and decreased in small stepwise degrees as frequently as needed to maintain the infant's temperature within the specified normal range. Because of the possible induction of apnea, rapid and large changes in temperature should be prevented, especially when the incubator houses a small, sick premature infant.

When thermostat control of the air temperature is not considered sufficiently exact, an incubator with skin servocontrol electronics can be used to control incubator air temperature more precisely. The skin probe need only be suspended in the airstream near the baby and the setpoint adjusted to the desired air temperature. As with any system, however, frequent adjustments may need to be made in the air temperature setpoint. Servocontrolling a convective heater to automatically maintain an infant's skin temperature at a specified level is best reserved for healthier, more mature infants. Since body warming is offset by environmental cooling in a skin servocontrolled incubator, an infant who becomes hypermetabolic because of sepsis or other cause may not become febrile, and the problem remains unrecognized. It is imperative, therefore, that careful records of skin and environmental temperatures be maintained to diagnose when an infant becomes infected. When using skin servocontrol, the thermistor probe must be firmly attached to the skin and carefully protected against artifacts that might interfere with the accurate transduction of the infant's true temperature. Since very little data exist to help in selecting a single appropriate skin temperature as a control point in a servocontrolled system, any value in the range between 35.5° and 37° C could probably be defended. Daily and co-workers observed more apneic spells when premature infants were controlled to skin temperatures of 36.5°, as opposed to 36° C.

During the ongoing monitoring of incubators in a busy intensive care nursery, Perlstein and associates found incubators out of predictable control more than 10% of the time because of unrecognized events that interfered with the equipment's proper functioning. Alarm systems can and have been designed to warn of such disruptions, but until these designs become generally available, only an understanding of incubator frailty, constant awareness, and unflagging attentiveness can reduce the response of incubated babies to unintended hazards. It

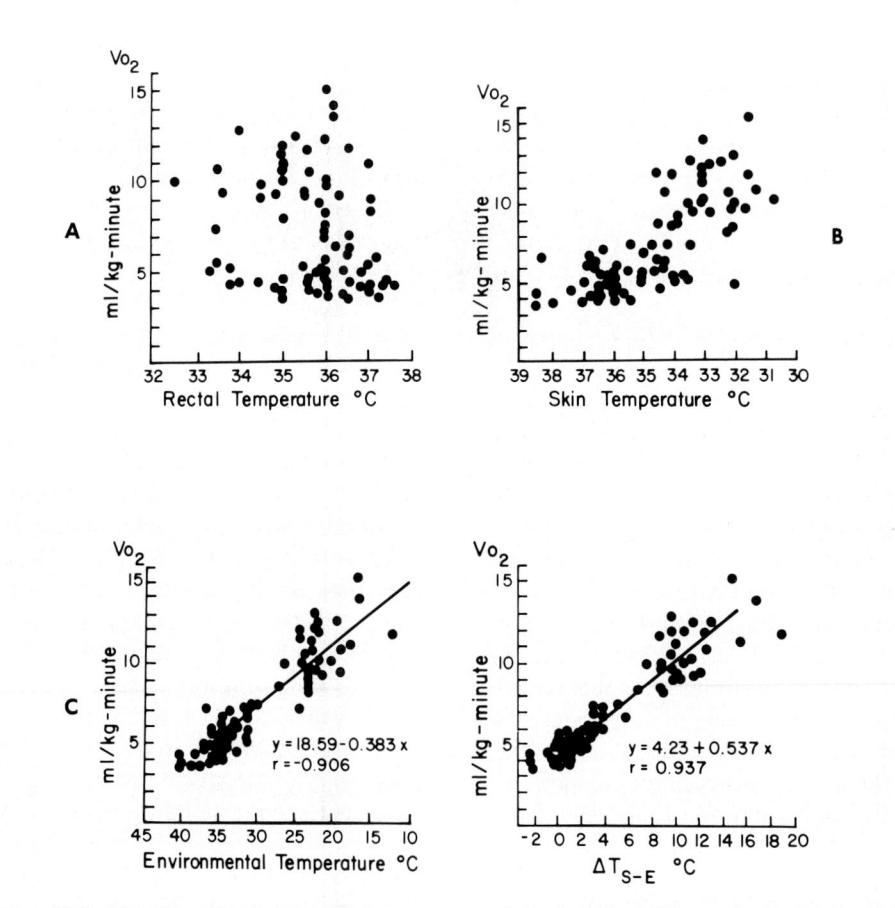

Fig. 19-9. Relationship between oxygen consumption and rectal temperature in various environments (**A**), skin temperature in various environments (**B**), and environmental temperature when incubator walls and air are within ±2° C of each other (**C**). (Adapted from Adamsons, K., Jr., Gandy, G.M., and James, L.S.: J. Pediatr. **66**:495, 1965.)

should also be obvious that enclosed incubators can be protective only when they are kept closed. If the limits of skill and requirements of care preclude keeping the incubator closed during care procedures, then the use of open radiantly heated beds should be considered.

Convective heating and thermoneutrality. The only way to certify that an infant with a normal body temperature is in a neutral thermal environment is to monitor the infant's metabolic rate continuously. This is usually done by measuring the baby's oxygen consumption, which requires techniques unsuited for ongoing clinical care. To estimate an infant's metabolic status, it also is possible to compare measurements of an infant's incubator temperature to the infant's skin temperature.

From the data of Adamsons it is probable that an infant is in a minimal metabolic state if the incubator environment is less than 2.5° C cooler than the infant's skin temperature (Fig. 19-9). Several difficulties are encountered when using this guideline. True environmental temperature is difficult to transduce and different from the air temperature in an incubator. A way around this problem has been provided by Hey, who determined that the incubator environmental temperature is approximately 1° C cooler than the incubator air temperature for every 7° C gradient that exists between incubator and nursery air temperatures. An incubator environment is therefore approximately 1° to 2° C cooler than the measured chamber air temperatures in the usual nursery environment.

Moreover, to believe that neutral thermal conditions always exist when the environment is no more than 2.5° C cooler than the infant's skin is to assume that an infant always has an oxygen consumption of less than 6 ml/kg/minute, and for each milliliter of oxygen used, 5 Cal of heat are produced. Basal oxygen consumption rates actually vary with an infant's gestational and postnatal ages, body size and shape, and weight (Fig. 19-10). It is difficult to certify, therefore, that any gradient is really appropriate when the assumptions ignore that basal metabolic rates vary with dynamic growth and development. A 2.5° C gradient would be excessively large, for example, for a newborn 1,500-gm infant with a basal

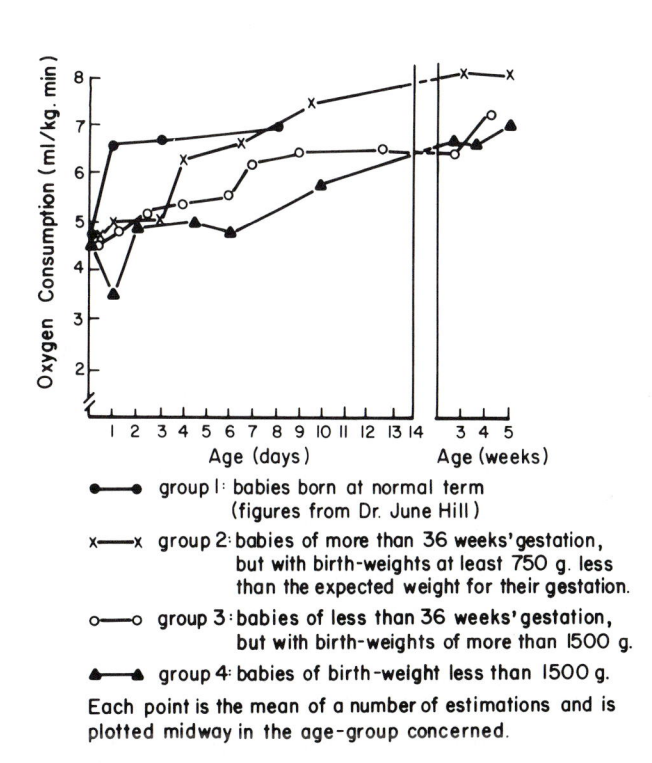

Fig. 19-10. Change in minimal oxygen consumption with age. (From Scopes, J.W.: Br. Med. Bull. **22:**88, 1966.)

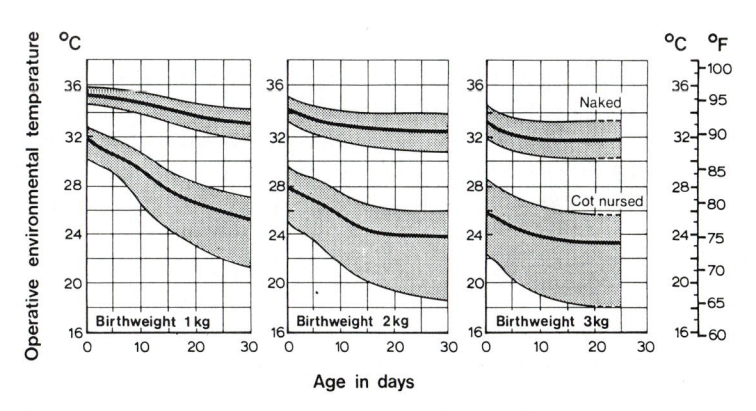

- group 1: babies born at normal term (figures from Dr. June Hill)
- group 2: babies of more than 36 weeks' gestation, but with birth-weights at least 750 g. less than the expected weight for their gestation.
- group 3: babies of less than 36 weeks' gestation, but with birth-weights of more than 1500 g.
- group 4: babies of birth-weight less than 1500 g.

Each point is the mean of a number of estimations and is plotted midway in the age-group concerned.

Fig. 19-11. Changes that usually occur with age in mean temperature to provide warmth for babies weighing 1-3 kg at birth, in draft-free, uniform temperature surroundings at 50% relative humidity. *Thick lines,* Usual "optimum" temperature; *shaded area,* range within which to maintain normal temperature without increasing heat production or evaporative water loss by more than 25%. The operative environmental temperature inside a single-walled incubator is *less* than the internal air temperature recorded by the thermometer; the effective environmental temperature provided by the incubator can, however, be estimated by subtracting 1° C from the air temperature for each 7° C by which incubator air temperature exceeds room temperature. (From Hey, E.N. In Gairdner and Hull: Recent advances in paediatrics, ed. 4, London, 1971, Churchill.)

oxygen consumption rate of 4.5 ml/kg/minute, and may be excessively constraining for the same infant 2 weeks later when the basal rate may have risen to 7 ml/kg/minute. Scopes has provided the most complete data for helping to resolve this problem of changing requirements with age and has reduced his observations to guidelines for incubator temperature settings, which should at least be close to the lower limit of the neutral thermal range expected for the specific infant (Fig. 19-11).

Open radiantly heated beds. The use of overhead radiant heaters to keep infants warm has become popular because they provide unimpeded access to infants receiving intensive care. Overhead radiant heaters are usually high-energy heat sources that require the use of skin servocontrol to ensure that babies do not become overheated when under their influence. The only exception to this requirement is when radiant heaters are used to protect infants for short periods immediately after birth. The heat loss from the wet body of a freshly delivered newborn is sufficiently great to balance even the heat provided by the 800-W potential in the largest radiant heaters. It is good that this balance exists, since the attachment of a skin servocontrol probe to the amniotic fluid–covered skin of a baby can be very difficult, and temperatures recorded may be unreliable.

Because of the known risk of causing hyperthermia when using a radiant heater, manufacturers have been adding increasing amounts of logic to the heater control designs. There is usually a provision to cause an alarm to sound if the skin probe becomes unattached. Failure to reactivate silenced alarms may expose infants under radiant heaters to a subsequent risk of hyperthermia; thus the safe use of a radiant heater requires an informed awareness of the specific way that the alarms operate in the heater employed. The proper attachment of a thermistor probe to the skin of an infant under a radiant heater remains undefined. Various authoritative opinions have been expressed that support techniques of attachment which both maximally and minimally shield the probe from the infrared energy emitted by the heater element. Since insulated probes do provide different information than exposed probes, a consistent technique is recommended during the care of any individual baby.

The radiantly heated open bed is unquestionably more convenient and allows superior access to the infant when compared with the enclosed convectively heated incubator. Data exist, however, to suggest some special problems to consider when using a radiant heat source. Babies under radiant heaters are known to have higher insensible losses of water than do infants housed in enclosed incubators (p. 314). Wu and Hodgman confirmed that infants in unhumidified enclosed incubators had age-dependent insensible losses ranging from means of 17.8 ml/kg/24 hours for infants weighing more than 1,500 gm to 37.4 ml/kg/24 hours for babies weighing less than 1,500 gm. In contrast, infants weighing more than 1,500 gm had insensible water losses (depending on the brand of heater) ranging between means of 32.4 and 51.6 ml/kg/24 hours when they were on open beds that were radiantly heated. Infants weighing less than 1,500 gm and under radiant heaters had insensible water losses that ranged between means of 55.2 and 88.9 ml/kg/24 hours. Although the metabolic implications of this increased evaporative loss are uncertain, at least the fluid and electrolyte management of babies under radiant heaters must be modified from that provided infants housed in enclosed incubators. Since the fluid and probably also electrolyte losses vary widely from infant to infant and from day to day, the specific replacement requirements can be determined only by carefully assessing the needs for each baby (p. 314). Some amelioration of this fluid loss problem is possible by using plastic sheets or bags to swaddle infants when they are under radiant heaters. It has also been suggested that the use of an acrylic plastic heat shield reduces insensible water loss under a radiant heater.

In some cases large evaporative losses from infants can be considered therapeutic. When dealing with an infant with decreased urinary output, the minimum amount of fluid required in administering drugs may exceed the usual fluid losses by insensible routes. Increasing these insensible losses by placing the infant under a radiant heater may diminish the danger of fluid overloading the baby. It is unclear whether the thermal cycling of an open radiant heater can induce apneic spells as has been observed when susceptible infants are housed in enclosed incubators.

The introduction of radiant heating has provided a valuable alternative way to keep babies warm. In some settings this is the only controllable way to protect babies against heat loss. The as yet unknown problems associated with this form of protection, however, exceed those associated with the use of enclosed convective incubators.

Radiant heating and thermoneutrality. Although it has been documented by several investigators that babies under radiant heaters can have minimum oxygen consumption, these demonstrations have all been made using head hoods for collecting and sampling the infant's expired air. A plastic head hood becomes warm under a radiant heater, and by heating a baby's face a warm head hood might suppress a hypermetabolic state. The available data therefore do not answer the important question about whether the radiant heating of babies who are not in head hoods would be sufficient to prevent the possible homeothermic stimulation from cold and dry air-conditioned convective currents in the open nursery. Nonetheless, the use of a plastic hood to cover the head of an infant under a radiant heater may provide a way to produce conditions consistent with thermoneutrality.

Helping a cold infant rewarm

Because of a reduced responsiveness to bacterial pyrogens, a baby may not become hypermetabolic and febrile when septic. Sepsis does, however, frequently suppress an infant's normal homeothermic reactions, and such an infant, although previously able to maintain a warm body temperature in a cool environment, may now get cold in the same environment. The probable mechanism is that the sepsis resulted in shock, which inhibited homeothermy, although it was the cold environment that made the infant hypothermic. Since rewarming some infants may induce apnea, an infant should be constantly observed and the environment carefully analyzed and controlled during the rewarming process.

Debates over the comparative virtues of rapid versus slow rewarming procedures notwithstanding, there is no convincing argument available to certify any method as being better than another. Tafari found no difference when comparing rapid and slow techniques of rewarming. The approach presented here has been developed partly from a logical use of known physical and physiologic principles and partly from numerous observations of infants of all weights and gestations during the rewarming process. The approach is pragmatic and absolutely dependent on multiple adjustments in environmental heating as indicated by the responses of the baby as the environmental and body temperatures increase.

As a first step in rewarming, produce a heat-gaining environment that eliminates any further significant heat losses from the baby. Warm the incubator air to 36° C and do not let the baby get colder. The existence of a heat-gaining environment can be certified only if the infant begins to get warmer, and simply warming the air temperature to a level that is higher than the baby's temperature is inadequate. It should be remembered that the actual environmental temperature in a convectively heated incubator is probably 1° to 2° C less than the measured air temperature. Evaporative losses should be minimized by raising the incubator humidity. Radiant losses should be minimized by protecting the incubator walls from excessive cooling or, as described by Hey, an inner incubator shield wall or heat shield can be inserted. If evaporative and radiant losses are minimized, the absolute air temperature becomes more meaningful, which is important, since it is the only really controllable heating factor in a convectively heated incubator.

A temperature-monitoring thermistor or thermometer should be suspended directly in the air over the infant's body to measure actual incubator air temperature. The 36° C air temperature should provide a sufficient heat-gaining gradient for any infant with a skin temperature below 35° C. The gradient should also be sufficiently narrow to prevent too rapid transfer of heat from the environment to the infant. The goal is to produce an environment in which the infant is rewarmed by the heat actually generated by the infant. Excessive external warming of an infant tends to cause vasodilatation of the skin vessels, which can result in the shunting and pooling of blood to a degree that produces sharp decreases in blood pressure. Continual monitoring of the rewarming infant's rectal temperature can be used to certify that heating of the skin temperature has not become excessive. The rate of warming should be such that the skin temperature never is more than 1° C warmer than the coexisting rectal temperature.

If in this initial environment the infant's temperature ceases to fall or slowly begins to rise, the settings should be maintained at that level and monitoring of all temperatures continued. If the temperature of the baby continues to fall, then raise the incubator temperature 1° to 37° C and carefully search for any previously undiscovered source of heat loss (Fig. 19-12). If within 15 minutes body temperature has not stabilized when the air temperature is 37° C, raise the air temperature to 38° C and, assuming that a heat sink still exists, look again for any further potential causes of heat loss. In these searches, incubator humidity should be measured and certified to be at a level of more than 70%. If, in spite of all these attempts, the baby continues to cool, call for someone else to evaluate the environment, since sometimes the obvious can be seen only by an outside observer.

Heating an incubator to an air temperature of more than 38° C is sometimes difficult because of overriding safety thermostats built into most incubators. If the source of heat loss escapes discovery when the air temperature is at 38° C, this failure does not provide reason to allow an infant to continue to cool. The baby can be swaddled, or a radiant heater can be suspended over the incubator and, with the probe attached to the plastic chamber, servocontrolled to raise the incubator wall temperature by slow 1° C increments to higher levels until heat losses are completely offset. If a baby becomes apneic during rewarming, the rate of warming should be slowed. On occasion, it may be necessary to completely halt the warming process for a period to allow the infant to adjust to the new conditions, even though the infant may still be hypothermic.

The baby who is too hot

It has been nearly 30 years since DuBois wrote "Fever is only a symptom, and we are not sure that it is an enemy. Perhaps it is a friend."

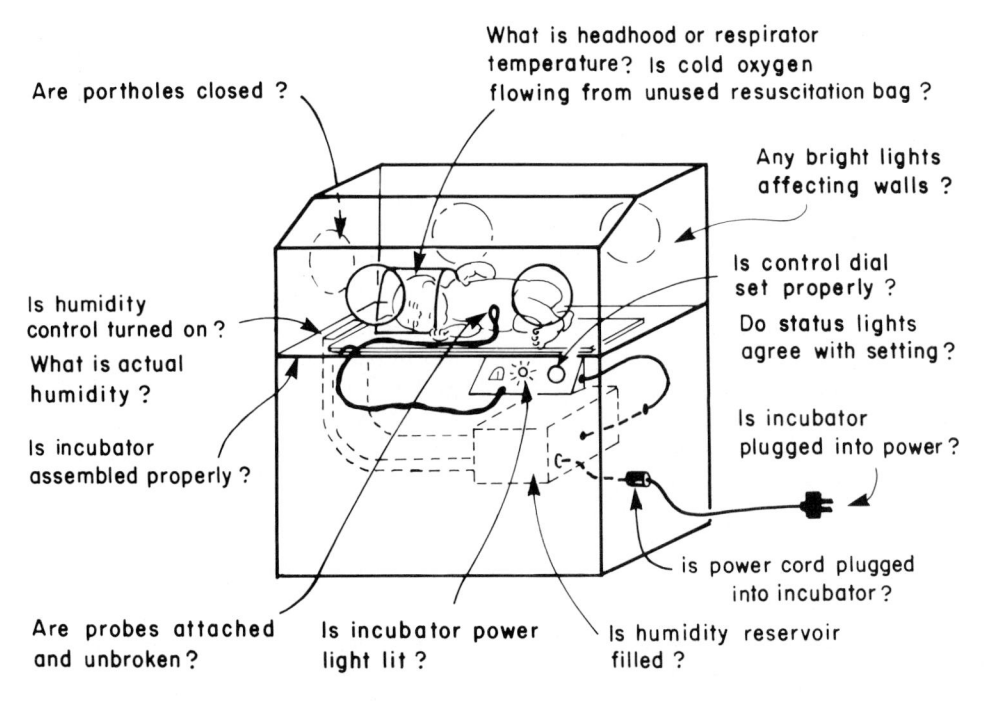

Fig. 19-12. "Troubleshoot" an incubator.

This fairly well summarizes what is known today about the febrile infant, although there is a new wave of scientific interest in the physiologic significance of fever. Most neonatal thermoregulatory studies have focused on the effects, prevention, and amelioration of hypothermia. Hyperthermia has been noted primarily as a sign of hypermetabolism when a baby is septic or otherwise stimulated. There is general agreement that it is probably beneficial to cool a baby who has become febrile because of exposure to an overheated environment. Whether it is good, however, to cool infants who are febrile because they are septic or otherwise stressed by internal conditions is less clear, although usually attempted.

An infant with a body temperature of more than 37.5° C may be considered abnormally warm. To determine whether the elevated temperature is due to an increase in heat production, as might occur if the baby were septic, or due to a decrease in heat loss, some simple presumptive clinical measures can be made.

A physiologically competent infant will respond to a hot environment by incorporating heat-losing mechanisms. The baby's skin vessels will dilate, the infant may appear to be flushed, and the hands and feet will be suffused and warm. Evaporative losses will increase and, although uncommonly observed in premature babies, active sweating may be noted in the full-term infant. If the heat stress is severe, the baby may begin to protest and complain, becoming hyperactive and irritable. The overheated skin of the infant will be warmer than the infant's core temperature.

An infant who is febrile because of an increase in endogenous heat production will reflect a state of stress. The baby will be vasoconstricted and, compared with the skin on the trunk, the extremities will appear pale and blue and feel cold. Unlike the gradients expected in overheated infants, the core temperature of the hypermetabolic infant will be warmer than the skin temperature.

Simultaneous measurements of rectal, abdominal skin, and foot temperatures will therefore often help to distinguish the infant who is febrile due to iatrogenic overheating from the infant hypermetabolic because of sepsis or stimulating drugs. In the afebrile and minimally metabolic baby the abdominal skin temperature usually will be no more than 1° to 2° C cooler than the infant's rectal temperature. The normal infant's foot temperature will be no more than 2° to 3° C colder than the abdominal skin temperature. In the febrile and hypermetabolic infant the rectal temperature will be warmer than the skin temperature and the foot temperature will be more than 3° C colder than the abdominal skin temperature. In the overheated infant the rectal temperature will be colder than the skin temperature and the foot temperature will be less than 3° C cooler than the abdominal skin temperature.

THE NONTHERMAL SENSORY ENVIRONMENT

Babies in incubators are exposed to continuous noise levels of between 50 and 86 decibels (dB) with frequent peaks that can reach levels of 90 to 100 and beyond. The addition of each new piece of life-support equipment can add 15 to 20 dB to the background noise. The American Academy of Pediatrics (AAP) Committee on Environmental Hazards has recommended that efforts be directed toward reducing the known high level of noise in nurseries. The industrial standard that allows the exposure of workers to 90 dB for an 8-hour day is probably too generous when establishing criteria for infants. Young animals suffer auditory damage at lower sound levels than do adults of their species. Drugs commonly used in the nursery, such as ethacrynic acid, furosemide, and the aminoglycosides streptomycin, kanamycin, neomycin, gentamicin, and tobramycin, are known from animal studies to potentiate noise-induced hearing loss.

Nurseries are too noisy, and the recommendation by the AAP Committee to reduce these noise levels to less than 70 dB is sensible. Noise can be reduced simply by asking personnel to care for the babies more quietly. As a first step to noise abatement, it is helpful to query whether all the beeping sounds from heart rate monitors are really helpful.

With rare exception the lighting in nurseries, the colors used to paint walls, the decorations, and windows with a view are examples of environmental factors designed to suit the observational and psychologic needs of adults who provide infants with care. There is little question that daylight-simulating illumination enhances the ability to observe color and other changes that occur in sick babies. It is, however, unclear whether the illumination is otherwise beneficial or harmful to the infants, although the near constant illumination of most special care nurseries is almost certainly perceived by the babies. The visual acuity and perception of infants are discussed in Chapter 21.

Along with the recent increase in the interest being paid to the social and educational development of babies, many programs are being introduced that use visual, auditory, tactile, and proprioceptive techniques to enhance the sensory stimulation of infants. There is nothing inherently wrong with the concept of socializing and educating newborns, but a critical stance must be maintained during the development of these programs. Babies respond to stimulation not only socially but also with a variety of autonomic responses, some of which may be detrimental to the sick neonate.

ENVIRONMENTAL POLLUTION

The questionable quality of the air we breathe is one of many environmental subjects generating debate in our society. It is rare to quantitatively analyze the composition of nursery or incubator air. The report by Waffarn in which 18 of 42 infant incubators were found to contain detectable concentrations of mercury vapor suggests that such quantitation may be appropriate.

Various combinations of metal pipes and plastic tubes are used to delivery gases to an incubator, into a head hood, or directly into a baby's lungs. Because of soldered and glued joints, protectively coated surfaces, and other sources of contamination, the air can contain oils, lead, cadmium, bismuth, mercury, and various other residues of organic and metallic salts. The gases also can contain bacteria and fungi. Many of these contaminants can be eliminated by appropriate filters, but the success of any filtering must be certified by laboratory testing.

As more studies are generated to evaluate the health impact of radiation, ultraviolet light, microwaves, radar, radioactivity, and other environmental components, it also is to be hoped that the specific susceptibility of babies to these potential hazards will be considered in research designs. The lack of existing awareness that radiation may be a hazard is suggested every time a baby's pelvis is included in a roentgenographic field when only a chest film is ordered (Chapter 39). It also is exemplified whenever a portable roentgenogram is taken in a nursery and the adults, concerned about their own exposure, run out of range of the x-ray unit or shield themselves with protective lead aprons while ignoring the exposure of the naked baby in the next incubator. At present insufficient data exist to express more than serious concern about potential environmental pollution in the nursery.

Paul H. Perlstein

BIBLIOGRAPHY
Thermoregulation
Subject reviews

Adamsons, K.: The role of thermal factors in fetal and neonatal life, Pediatr. Clin. North Am. 13:599, 1966.

Ahlgren, E.W.: Environmental control of the neonate receiving intensive care, Int. Anesthesiol. Clin. 12:173, 1974.

Bruck, K.: Heat production and temperature regulation. In Stave, U., editor: Perinatal physiology, New York, 1978, Plenum Publishing Corp.

Dawes, G.S.: Oxygen consumption and temperature regulation in the newborn. In foetal and neonatal physiology, 1968, Year Book Medical Publishers, Inc.

DeLue, N.A.: Climate and environmental concepts, Clin. Perinatol. 3:425, 1976.

Hey, E.N., and Katz, G.: The optimum thermal environment for naked babies, Arch. Dis. Child. 45:328, 1970.

Klaus, M., Fanaroff, A., and Martin, R.J.: The physical invironment. In Klaus, M.H., and Fanaroff, A.A., editors: Care of the high risk neonate, Philadelphia, 1979, W.B. Saunders Co.

Lutz, L., and Perlstein, P.H.: Temperature control in newborn babies, Nurs. Clin. North Am. 6:15, 1971.

Oliver, T.K.: Temperature regulation and heat production in the newborn, Pediatr. Clin. North Am. 12:765, 1965.

Scopes, J.W.: Thermoregulation in the newborn. In Avery, G.B., editor: Neonatology, Philadelphia, 1975, J.B. Lippincott Co..

Sinclair, J.C.: Metabolic rate and temperature control. In Smith, C.A., and Nelson, N.M., editors: The physiology of the newborn infant, Springfield, Ill. 1976, Charles C Thomas, Publisher.

Sinclair, J.C.: The effect of the thermal environment on neonatal mortality and morbidity. In Adamsons, K., and Fox, H.A., editors: Preventability of perinatal injury, New York, 1975, Alan R. Liss, Inc.

General

Adamsons, K., Jr., Gandy, G.M., and James, L.S.: The influence of thermal factors upon oxygen consumption of newborn human infant, J. Pediatr. **66**:495, 1965.

Agate, F.J., and Silverman, W.A.: The control of body temperature in the human premature infant by low energy infrared radiation, Anat. Rec. **136**:152, 1960.

Aherne, W., and Hull, D.: Brown adipose tissue and heat production in the newborn infant, J. Pathol. **91**:223, 1966.

Aynsley-Green, A., Roberton, N.R.C., and Rolfe, P.: Air temperature recordings in infant incubators, Arch. Dis. Child. **50**:215, 1975.

Babak, E.: Ueber die Warmeregulation der Neugeborenen, Pfleugers Arch. **89**:154, 1902.

Baum, J.D., and Scopes, J.W.: The silver swaddler: device for preventing hypothermia in the newborn, Lancet **1**:672, 1968.

Belgaumkar, T.K., and Scott, K.E.: Effects of low humidity on small premature infants in servocontrol incubators. I. Decrease in rectal temperatures, Biol. Neonate **26**:337, 1975.

Belgaumkar, T.K., and Scott, K.E.: Effects of low humidity on small premature infants in servocontrol incubators. II. Increased severity of apnea, Biol. Neonate **26**:348, 1975.

Bell, E.F., Weinstein, M.R., and Oh, W.: Heat balance in premature infants: comparative effects of convectively heated incubator and radiant warmers, with and without plastic heat shield, J. Pediatr. **96**:460, 1980.

Benedict, F.G., and Talbot, F.B.: The physiology of the newborn infant: character and amount of catabolism, Washington, D.C., Carnegie Institute, Publication no. 233, 1915.

Besch, N.J., and others: The transparent baby bag: a shield against heat loss, N. Engl. J. Med. **284**:121, 1971.

Blackfan, K.D., and Yaglou, C.P.: The premature infant, Am. J. Dis. Child. **46**:1175, 1933.

Bolton, D.R., Fox, A.M., and Kennaird, D.L.: Preliminary observations on the application of thermography to the study of brown adipose tissue in the human newborn, J. Physiol. (Lond.)**208**:23P, 1970.

Bruck, K.: Temperature regulation in the newborn infant, Biol. Neonate **3**:65, 1961.

Bruck, K.: Which environmental temperature does the premature infant prefer? Pediatrics **41**:1027, 1968.

Bruck, K., Parmalee, A.H., Jr., and Bruck, M.: Neutral temperature range and range of "thermal comfort" in premature infants, Biol. neonate **4**:32, 1962.

Budin, P.: The feeding and hygiene of premature and fullterm infants. In Dion, O., editor: The nursling, London, 1907, Caxton Publishing. (Translated by W.J. Maloney.)

Buetow, K.C., and Klein, S.W.: Effect of maintenance of "normal" skin temperature on survival of infants of low birth weight, Pediatrics **34**:163, 1964.

Clark, R.P., and others: Neonatal natural forced convection, J. Physiol. (Lond.) **284**:22, 1978.

Cornblath, J., and Schwartz, R.: Disorders of carbohydrate metabolism in infancy. In Major problems in clinical pediatrics, vol. 3, Philadelphia, 1966, W.B. Saunders Co.

Cree, J.E., Meyer, J., and Hailey, D.M.: Diazepam in labour: its metabolism and effect on the clinical condition and thermogenesis of the newborn, Br. Med. J. **3**:251, 1973.

Cross, K., Dawes, G.S., and Karlberg, P. In Oliver, T.K., Jr., editor: Neonatal respiratory adaptation, Public Health Service Publication no. 1432, Washington, D.C., 1966, p. 117.

Cross, K., Tizard, J.P.M., and Trythall, D.A.H.: The gaseous metabolism of the newborn infant, Acta Paediatr. Scand. **46**:265, 1957.

Cross, K., Tizard, J.P.M., and Trythall, D.A.H.: The gaseous metabolism of the newborn infant breathing 15 percent oxygen, Acta Paediatr. Scand. **47**:217, 1958.

Cross, K., and others: Lack of temperature control in infants with abnormalities of the central nervous system, Arch. Dis. Child. **46**:437, 1971.

Dahm, L.S., and James, L.S.: Newborn temperature and calculated heat loss in the delivery room, Pediatrics **49**:504, 1972.

Daily, W.J., Klaus, M., and Meyer, H.B.: Apnea in premature infants: monitoring, incidence, heart rate changes, and an effect of environmental temperature, Pediatrics **43**:510, 1969.

Dangman, B.C., and others: The variability of PO_2 in newborn infants in response to routine care, Pediatr. Res. **10**:422, 1976.

Daniel, S.S., and others: Hypothermia and the resuscitation of asphyxiated fetal rhesus monkeys, J. Pediatr. **68**:45, 1966.

Darnall, R.A., Jr., and Ariagno, R.L.: Minimal oxygen consumption in infants cared for under overhead radiant warmers compared with conventional incubators, J. Pediatr. **93**:283, 1978.

Darnall, R.A., Jr., and Ariagno, R.L.: Resting oxygen consumption of premature infants covered with a plastic thermal blanket, Pediatrics **63**:547, 1979.

Dawes, G.S.: Neonatal respiratory adaptation. In Proceedings of Interdisciplinary Conference on Neonatal Respiratory Adaptation, Public Health Service Pub. No. 1432, Washington, D.C., 1966, U.S. Government Printing Office.

Dawes, G.S., and Mott, J.C.: The increase in oxygen consumption of the lamb after birth, J. Physiol. **146**, 295, 1959.

Dawkins, M.J.R., and Scopes, J.W.: Non-shivering thermogenesis and brown adipose tissue in the human newborn infant, Nature **206**:201, 1965.

Day, R.: Regulation of body temperature during sleep, Am. J. Dis. Child. **61**:734, 1941.

Day, R.: Respiratory metabolism in infancy and childhood, Am. J. Dis. Child. **65**:376, 1943.

Day, R.L., and others: Body temperature and survival of premature infants, Pediatrics **34**:171, 1964.

Du, J.N.H., and Oliver, T.K., Jr.: The baby in the delivery room: a suitable microenvironment, J.A.M.A. **207**:1502, 1969.

Eckstein, A.: Ueber die Warmregulierung der Fruhgeborenen, Z. Kindelh. **42**:5, 1926.

Edwards, N.K.: Radiant warmers. In Iatrogenic problems in neonatal intensive care, Report of the 69th Ross Conference on Pediatric Research, 1976, p. 79.

Emergency Care Research Institute: Evaluation: infant radiant warmers, Health Devices **3**:4, 1973.

Fanaroff, A.A., and others: Insensible water loss in low birth weight infants, Pediatrics **50**:236, 1972.

Fenner, A., and List, M.: Observations of body temperature regulation in young, premature and full term newborns while being connected to a servocontrol temperature unit, Biol. Neonate **18**:300, 1971.

Fisher, D.A., and Oddie, T.H.: Neonatal thyroidal hyperactivity, Am. J. Dis. Child. **107**:574, 1964.

Fisher, D.A., and Odell, W.D.: Acute release of thyrotropin in the newborn, J. Clin. Invest. **48**:1670, 1969.

Foster, K.G., Hey, E.N., and Katz, G.: The response of the sweat glands of the newborn baby to thermal stimuli and to intradermal acetylcholine, J. Physiol. **203**:13, 1969.

Gandy, G.M., and others: Thermal environment and acid-base homeostasis on human infants during the first few hours of life, J. Clin. Invest. **43**:751, 1964.

Glass, L., Silverman, W.A., and Sinclair, J.C.: Effect of the thermal environment on cold resistance and growth of small infants after the first week of life, Pediatrics **41**:1033, 1968.

Glass, L., Silverman, W.A., and Sinclair, J.C.: Relationship of thermal environment and caloric intake to growth and resting metabolism in the late neonatal period, Biol. Neonate **14**:324, 1969.

Gold, A.J., and Zornitzer, A.: Effect of partial body cooling on man exercising in a hot environment, Aerospace Med. **39**;944, 1968.

Gordon, H.H.: Inclusions of studies, mostly of premature infants, Pediatrics **8**:163, 1951.

Grausz, J.P.: The effects of environmental temperature changes on the metabolic rate of newborn babies, Acta Paediatr. Scand. **57**:98, 1968.

Haroy, J.D.: Physiology of temperature regulation, Physiol. Rev. **41**:521, 1961.

Heim, T., Kellenmayer, M., and Dani, M.: Thermal conditions and the mobilization of lipids from brown and white adipose tissue in the human neonate, Acta Paediatr. Acad. Sci. Hung. **9**:109, 1968.

Hess, J.H.: Premature and congenitally diseased infants, Philadelphia, 1922, Lea & Febiger.

Hey, E.N.: The relation between environmental temperature and oxygen consumption in the newborn baby, J. Physiol. **200**:589, 1969.

Hey, E.N., and Katz, G.: Evaporative water loss in the newborn baby, J. Physiol. **200**:605, 1969.

Hey, E.N., and Katz, G: Temporary loss of a metabolic response to cold stress in infants of low birthweight, Arch. Dis. Child. **44**:323, 1969.

Hey, E.N., and Katz, G.: The optimum thermal environment for naked babies, Arch. Dis. Child. **45**:328, 1970.

Hey E.N., Katz, G., and O'Connell, B.: The total thermal insulation of the newborn baby, J. Physiol. (Lond.) **207**:683, 1970.

Hey, E.N., Kohlinsky, S., and O'Connell, B.: Heat losses from babies during exchange transfusion, Lancet **1**:335, 1969.

Hey, E.N., and Maurice, N.P.: Effect of humidity on production and loss of heat in the newborn baby, Arch. Dis. Child. **43**:166, 1968.

Hey, E.N., and Mount, L.E.: Temperature control in incubators, Lancet **2**:202, 1966.

Hey, E.N., and Mount, L.E.: Heat losses from babies in incubators, Arch. Dis. Child. **42**:57, 1967.

Hey, E.N., and O'Connell, B.: Oxygen consumption and heat balance in the cot-nursed baby, Arch. Dis. Child. **45**:335, 1970.

Hill, J.R.: Oxygen consumption of newborn and adult mammals: its dependence on oxygen tension in inspired air and on environmental temperature, J. Physiol. (Lond.) **149**:346, 1959.

Hill, J.R., and Rahimtulla, K.A.: Heat balance and the metabolic rate of newborn babies in relation to environmental temperature; and the effect of age and of weight on basal metabolic rate, J. Physiol. **180**:239, 1965.

Hull, D., and Segall, M.J.: The contribution of brown adipose tissue to heat production in the newborn rabbit, J. Physiol. (Lond.) **191**:449, 1965.

Indyk, L.: A dangerous situation encountered in the administration of oxygen to an infant in a baby warmer, Pediatrics **47**:503, 1971.

Jolly, H., Molyneux, P., and Newell, D.J.: A controlled study of the effect of temperature on premature babies, J. Pediatr. **60**:889, 1962.

Karlberg, P.: The significance of depth of insertion of the thermometer for recording rectal temperatures, Acta Paediatr. Scand. **38**:359, 1949.

Karlberg, P.: Determination of standard energy metabolism in normal infants, Acta Paediatr. Scand. (Suppl.) **41**:?, 1952.

Karlberg, P.: Proceedings of Interdisciplinary Conference on Neonatal Respiratory Adaptation, Public Health Service Publ. No. 1432, Washington, D.C., 1966, U.S. Government Printing Office.

Karlberg, P., Moore, R.E., and Oliver, T.K., Jr.: The thermogenic response of the newborn infant to noradrenalin, Acta Paediatr. Scand. **51**:284, 1962.

Levison, H., and Swyer, P.R.: Oxygen consumption and the thermal environment in newly born infants, Biol. Neonate **7**:305, 1964.

Lewis, H.E., and others: Aerodynamics of the human microenvironment, Lancet **50**:1273, 1969.

Mann, T.P., and Elliott, R.I.K.: Neonatal cold injury, Lancet **1**:229, 1957.

Marks, K.H., Friedman, Z., and Maisels, M.J.: A simple device for reducing insensible water loss in low birth weight infants, Pediatrics **60**:223, 1977.

Marks, K.H., and others: Intravenous alimentation and insensible water loss in low birth weight infants, Pediatrics **63**:54, 1979.

Mestyan, J., Jarai, I., and Fekete, M.: The total energy expenditure and its components in premature infants maintained under different nursing and environmental conditions, Pediatr. Res. **2**:161, 1968.

Mestyan, J., and others: Surface temperature versus deep body temperature and the metabolic response to cold of hypothermic premature infants, Biol. Neonate **7**:230, 1964.

Mestyan, J., and others: The significance of facial skin temperature in the chemical heat regulation of premature infants, Biol. Neonate **7**:243, 164.

Miller, D.L., and Oliver, T.K., Jr.: Body temperature in the immediate neonatal period: the effect of reducing thermal losses, Am. J. Obstet. Gynecol. **94**:964, 1966.

Miller, J.A., Jr., Miller, F.S., and Westin, B.: Hypothermia in treatment of asphyxia neonatorum, Biol. Neonate **6**:148, 1964.

Mordhorst, H.: Uber die chemische Warmeregulation fruhgeborener Sauglinge, Monatsschr. Kinderheilkd. **55**:174, 1932.

Motil, K.J., Blackburn, M.G., and Pleasure, J.R.: The effects of four different radiant warmer temperature set points used for rewarming neonates, J. Pediatr. **85**:546, 1974.

Mount, L.E.: The oxygen consumption of the newborn pig in relation to environmental temperature, J. Physiol. (Lond.) **142**:37p, 1958.

Nielsen, L., and others: Evaluation of the Porta-Warm mattress as a source of heat for neonatal transport, Pediatrics **58**:500, 1976.

Oh, W., and Karecki, H.: Phototherapy and insensible water loss in the newborn infant, Am. J. Dis. Child. **124**:230, 1972.

Oliver, T.K., Jr., and Karlberg, P.: Gaseous metabolism in newly born human infants—the effects of environmental temperature and 15 percent oxygen in the inspired air, Am. J. Dis. Child. **105**:427, 1963.

Perlstein, P.H.: Thermal control. In Iatrogenic problems in neonatal intensive care, Report of the 69th Ross Conference on Pediatric Research, 1976, p. 75.

Perlstein, P.H., Edwards, N.K., and Atherton, H.D.: Incubator control with computer assistance, Perinatol. Neonatal. **1**:16, 1977.

Perlstein, P.H., Edwards, N.K., and Sutherland, J.M.: Apnea in premature infants and incubator air temperature changes, N. Engl. J. Med. **282**:461, 1970.

Perlstein, P.H., Edwards, N.K., and Sutherland, J.M.: Age relationship to thermal patterns on the backs of cold stressed infants, Biol. Neonate **20**:127, 1972.

Perlstein, P.H., and others: Thermal patterns on the backs of cold stressed babies, Pediatr. Res. **4**:472, 1970.

Perlstein, P.H., and others: Adaptation to cold in the first three days of life, Pediatrics **54**:411, 1974.

Perlstein, P.H., and others: Computer-assisted newborn intensive care, Pediatrics **57**:494, 1976.

Pribylova, H., and Znamenacek, K.: The effect of body temperature on the level of carbohydrate metabolites and oxygen consumption in the newborn, Pediatrics **37**:743, 1966.

Schiff, D., Stern, L., and Leduc, J.: Chemical thermogenesis in newborn infants, Pediatrics **37:577, 1966.**

Scopes, J.W.: Metabolic rate and temperature control in the human body, Br. Med. Bull. **22**:88, 1966.

Scopes, J.W., and Ahmed, I.: Indirect assessment of oxygen requirements in newborn babies by monitoring deep rectal temperature, Arch. Dis. Child. **41**:25, 1966.

Scopes, J.W., and Ahmed, I.: Minimal rates of oxygen consumption in sick and premature newborn infants, Arch. Dis. Child. **41**:407, 1966.

Scopes, J.W., and Tizard, J.P.M.: The effect of intravenous noradrenaline on the oxygen consumption of newborn animals, J. Physiol. **165**:305, 1963.

Shvartz, E.: Effect of a cooling hood on physiological responses to work in a hot environment, J. Appl. Physiol. **29**:36, 1970.

Silverman, W.A.: Thermoregulation of the newly born, In Thompson, S.G., editor: Reports of Ross Conference on Pediatric Research, (Suppl. 2) Columbus, Ohio, 1964, Ross Laboratories.

Silverman, W.A.: Use and misuse of temperature and humidity in care of the newborn infant, Pedatrics **33:**276, 1964.

Silverman, W.A.: Incubator-baby side shows, Pediatrics **64:**127, 1979.

Silverman, W.A., and Agate, F.J.: Variations in cold resistance among small newborn infants, Biol. Neonate **6:**113, 1964.

Silverman, W.A., Agate, F.J., Jr., and Fertig, J.W.: A sequential trial of the nonthermal effect of atmospheric humidity on survival of newborn infants of low birth weight, Pediatrics **31:**719, 1963.

Silverman, W.A., and Blanc, W.A.: The effect of humidity on survival of newly born premature infants, Pediatrics **20:**477, 1957.

Silverman, W.A., Fertig, J.W., and Berger, A.P.: The influence of the thermal environment upon the survival of newly born premature infants, Pediatrics **22:**876, 1958.

Silverman, W.A., and Parke, P.C.: Keep him warm, Am. J. Nurs. **65:**81, 1965.

Silverman, W.A., Sinclair, J.C., and Agate, F.J.: The oxygen cost of minor changes in heat balance of small newborn infants, Acta Paediatr. Scand. **55:**294, 1966.

Silverman, W.A., and others: Warm nape of the newborn, Pediatrics **33:**984, 1964.

Sinclair, J.C., Scopes, J.W., and Silverman, W.A.: Metabolic reference standards for the neonate, Pediatrics **39:**724, 1967.

Sokal, M., and Sinclair, J.C.: Effect of temperature on growth of newborn rabbits, Biol. Neonate **28:**1, 1976.

Stephenson, J.M., Du, J.N., and Oliver, T.K., Jr.: The effect of cooling on blood gas tensions in newborn infants, J. Pediatr. **76:**848, 1970.

Stern, L., Lees, M.H., and Leduc, J.: Environmental temperature, oxygen consumption and catecholamine excretion in newborn infants, Pediatrics **36:**367, 1965.

Sulyok, E., Jequier, E., and Ryser, G.: Effect of relative humidity on thermal balance of the newborn infant, Biol. Neonate **21:**210, 1972.

Tafari, N., and Gentz, J.: Aspects on rewarming newborn infants with severe accidental hypothermia, Acta Paediatr. Scand. **63:**595, 1974.

Tahti, E., and others: Changes in skin temperature of the neonate at birth: a cine-thermographic study, Acta Paediatr. Scand. **61:**159, 1972.

Talbot, F.B., and others: The basal metabolism of prematurity. III. Metabolism finding in twenty-one premature infants, Am. J. Dis. Child. **26:**29, 1923.

Torrance, J.T.: Temperature readings of premature infants, Nurs. Res. **17:**312, 1968.

Turnell, R.: The influence of different environmental temperatures on pulmonary gas exchange and blood gas changes after birth, Acta Paediatr. Scand. **64:**57, 1975.

Walker, D., Walker, A., and Wood, C.: Temperature of the human fetus, Br. J. Obstet. Gynaecol. **76:**503, 1969.

Williams, R.A., and Chambers, A.B.: Effect of neck warming and cooling on thermal comfort, In Proceedings of the Second Conference of Portable Life Support Systems, N.A.S.A. **SP-302:**289, 1971.

Winslow, C.E.A., Herrington, L.P., and Gagge, A.P.: Physiological reactions of the human body to varying environmental temperatures, Am. J. Physiol. **120:**1, 1937.

Wolf, H., and Stave, U.: Free fatty acids and glycerol in plasma and tissue of normal, hypothermic, and hypotrophic newborn rabbits, Biol. Neonate **19:**132, 1971.

Wood, C., and Beard, R.W.: Temperature of the human fetus, Br. J. Obstet. Gynaecol. **71:**768, 1964.

Wu, P.Y.K., and Hodgman, J.E.: Changes in insensible water loss in infants with and without phototherapy, Clin. Res. **20:**284, 1972.

Wu, P.Y.K., and Hodgman, J.E.: Insensible water loss in preterm infants; changes with postnatal development and non-iodizing radiant energy, Pediatrics **54:**704, 1974.

Yeh, T.F., and others: Reduction of insensible water loss in premature infants under the radiant warmer, J. Pediatr. **94:**651, 1979.

Ylppo, A.: Zur Physiologie, Klinik und zur Schicksal der Fruhgeborenen, Z. Kinderh. **24:**1, 1919.

Young, I.M.: Vasomotor tone in the skin blood vessels of the newborn infant, Clin. Sci. **22:**325, 1962.

Nonthermal sensory environment

Bess, F.H., Peek, B.F., and Chapman, J.J.: Further observations on noise levels in infant incubators, Pediatrics **63:**100, 1979.

Blennow, G., Svenningsen, N.W., and Almquist, B.: Noise levels in infant incubators (adverse effects?), Pediatrics **53:**29, 1974.

Bower, T.G.R.: The object in the world of the infant, Sci. Am. **224:**30, 1971.

Dayal, V.S., Kokshanian, A., and Mitchell, D.P.: Combined effects of noise and kanamycin, Ann. Otol. Rhinol. Laryngol. **80:**897, 1971.

Dayton, G., and others: Developmental study of coordinated eye movements in the human infant. I. Visual acuity determined by electrooculography, Arch. Ophthalmol. **71:**865, 1964.

Doueck, E., and others: Effects of incubator noise on the cochlea of the newborn, Lancet **2:**1110, 1976.

Falk, S.A., and Farmer, J.C., Jr.: Incubator noise and possible deafness, Arch. Otolaryngol. **97:**385, 1973.

Falk, S.A., and Woods, N.F.: Hospital noise levels and potential health hazards, N. Engl. J. Med. **289:**774, 1973.

Falk, S.A., and others: Noise-induced inner ear damage in newborn and adult guinea pigs, Laryngoscope **84:**444, 1974.

Fantz, R.L.: Patterned vision in newborn infants, Science **140:**296, 1963.

Fitzgerald, H.E.: Autonomic pupillary reflex action during early infancy and its relation to social and non-social visual stimuli, J. Exp. Child. Psychol. **6:**470, 1968.

Gadeke, R., and others: The noise level in a children's hospital and the wake-up threshold in infants, Acta Paediatr. Scand. **58:**164, 1969.

Goren, C.C., Sarty, M., and Wu, P.Y.: Visual following and pattern discrimination of face-like stimuli by newborn infants, Pediatrics **56:**544, 1975.

Gorman, J.J., Cogan, D.G., and Gellis, S.S.: An apparatus for grading the visual acuity of infants on the basis of optokinetic nystagmus, Pediatrics **19:**1088, 1957.

Kiff, R., and Lepard, E.: Visual response of premature infants, Arch. Opthalmol. **75:**631, 1966.

Kirner, A., and others: Effects of waterbed flotation on premature infants: a pilot study, Pediatrics **56:**361, 1975.

Kramer, L., and Pierpont, M.: Rocking waterbed and auditory stimuli to enhance growth of preterm infants, J. Pediatr. **88:**297, 1976.

Long, J.G., Alistair, G.S., and Lucey, J.F.: Use of continuous TcPO$_2$ monitoring to avoid handling and pain as causes of hypoxemia, Pediatr. Res. **13:**499, 1979.

Long, J.G., Lucey, J.F., and Philip, A.G.S.: Noise and hypoxemia in the intensive care nursery, Pediatrics **65:**143, 1980.

Miller, R.W., and others: Noise pollution: neonatal aspects, Committee on Environmental Hazards, American Academy of Pediatrics, Pediatrics **54:**476, 1974.

Rosen, S.: Noise, hearing and cardiovascular function. In Welch, B., and Wesch, A.S., editors: Physiological effects of noise, New York, 1970, Plenum Press.

Scarr-Salapatek, S., and Williams, M.: The effects of early stimulation on low birth weight infants, Child. Dev. **44:**94, 1973.

Shenai, J.P.: Sound levels for neonates in transit, J. Pediatr. **90:**811, 1977.

Siqueland, E., and Lipsitt, L.: Learning ability and its enhancement. In Henkes, J., and Schein, R., editors: Learning disorders in children, Report of the 61st Ross Conference on Pediatric Research, Columbus, Ohio, 1971, Ross Laboratories.

Solkoff, N., and others: Effects of handling on the subsequent development of premature infants, J. Dev. Psych. **1**:765, 1969.

Vidyasagar, D., Joseph, M.E., and Hamilton, L.R.: Noise levels in the neonatal intensive care unit, J. Pediatr. **88**:115, 1976.

Welch, B.L., and Welch, A.S.: Physiological effects of noise, New York, 1970, Plenum Press.

Environmental pollution

Hamel, A.J., Deane, R.S., and Paquette, R.D.: Compressed air and oxygen supply lines as a source of contamination of respiratory therapy equipment, Items and Topics **22**:8, 1976.

Waffarn, F., and Hodgman, J.E.: Mercury vapor contamination of infant incubators: a potential hazard, Pediatrics **64**:640, 1979.

PART THREE
Biomedical engineering aspects of neonatal monitoring

See also Chapter 10.

Electronic instrumentation is assuming an ever-expanding role in neonatal intensive care. Although it is perhaps ambitious to expect neonatologists to have the expertise of engineers, a basic understanding of the principles involved in neonatal electronic instrumentation is important. By being aware of the various electronic techniques of physiologic measurement, the neonatologist not only can know the strengths and limitations of the instrumentation but also can avoid many errors that result from either incorrect application of the instrumentation or minor malfunctions. The manufacturers of neonatal electronic apparatus often have designed the apparatus as merely scaled-down versions of electronic monitoring devices for adults. The neonatologist, of course, is acutely aware that the neonate is certainly not a miniature adult but rather has unique characteristics and problems. Thus it is important that instrumentation for neonatal monitoring be specifically designed by engineers and physicians together to meet the special requirements of the neonate and not just be variations of adult monitors. The major requirements for neonatal monitoring equipment are as follows:

1. Safe for patients and personnel
2. Solid and resistant to wear
3. Small and space saving
4. Noninvasive and nonobstructive for patient care
5. Easy to use
6. Specific and sensitive

This section is devoted to cardiac, blood pressure, and respiration monitoring. Instrumentation for temperature and blood gas monitoring is in part four and in Chapter 23.

The basic arrangement of an electronic instrumentation system is shown in Fig. 19-13. For the physician the most important part is the interface between the instrumentation system and the patient. The sensor makes up the instrument side of this interface. It must detect accurately the physiologic variable being monitored but must not in itself provide constraints on the system that could change this variable. The portion of the instrumentation concerned with modifying and interpreting the signal from the sensor is known as the processor. It is in this block that most of the electronic manipulation of the data is carried out. The processor can be anything from a simple amplifier to a complex digital computer programmed to recognize and indicate normal and pathologic signs on the signal. The final block on the instrumentation system is again concerned with interface, but this time between the instrument and the clinical staff who uses it. This so-called display and recording section is concerned with indicating the variables being measured and providing a permanent record of them such as on a paper chart recorder or a magnetic tape recorder. This section should be designed to minimize communication errors between the machine and the clinical staff.

CARDIAC MONITORING

Cardiac monitoring, as considered here, is only the monitoring of the heart rhythm through the electrocardiogram and the monitoring of heart rate. The sensor function of a neonatal cardiac monitor is carried out by the skin biopotential electrodes. Their function is to con-

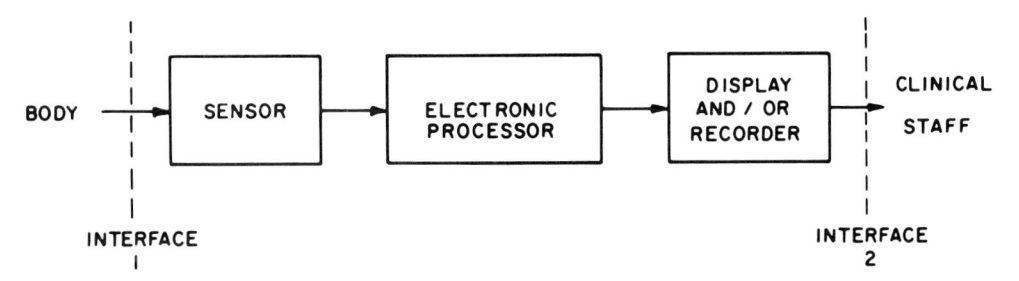

Fig. 19-13. Basic medical electronic instrumentation system. Interfaces *1* and *2* require special consideration for optimum clinical performance of the instrument.

vert the electrical signal in the body to one that can be handled by the remainder of the instrumentation system. The carriers of electrical charge in the body are the electrolyte ions, whereas in an electronic device electrical charge is transferred by electrons. Thus the biopotential electrodes must convert an ionic type of electrical signal to one that is electronic in nature. This means that an oxidation-reduction reaction must occur at the electrode surface. In this chemical reaction electrons are transferred from ions to the electrode or vice versa. At the surface of the electrode there must be available ions for the reaction, and once the reaction occurs, the products of the reaction must be removed. In addition, chemical differences between the electrode material and the ions in the body also can cause an accumulation or depletion of specific ionic species at the electrode surface. Thus it is fair to say that the concentration of ions near the surface of the electrode in general will be different from that in the body away from the electrode. This phenomenon is known as polarization, and it is responsible for many of the problems encountered with biopotential-measuring electrodes. For the best results it is therefore desirable to find electrodes that will minimize polarization. Unfortunately ideal nonpolarizable electrodes do not exist in practice; however, electrochemists have developed electrodes that come close to behaving as though they were nonpolarizable.

The silver–silver chloride electrode is one of these sensors which receives widespread application in cardiac monitoring. In its simplest form this electrode can be thought of as a silver surface which is coated with the salt silver chloride. This electrode is found to have high electrical stability and low polarization in chloride-containing electrolytic solutions. Since chloride is the principal anion of extracellular fluid in the body, it is reasonable to apply the silver–silver chloride electrode in biology.

Electrodes attached to the skin surface may not have appropriate ionic solutions coupling the extracellular fluid to their surface, and so it is necessary to provide such a coupling medium. This is the so-called electrolyte gel, which consists of an aqueous solution of ions in a gelatinous base to give it a high viscosity. Normally electrode gels are designed to have the same electrolyte content as that of the extracellular fluid; however, it is the belief of some neonatologists that the chloride content of the electrode gel causes excessive irritation of neonatal skin. For that reason new electrode gels for use with neonates that contain low or even no chloride are now available. When these gels, however, are used with silver–silver chloride electrodes, the advantages of the electrode stability are no longer present because of absence or reduced concentration of chloride ions in the gel. Thus, in instrumentation systems where silver–silver chloride electrodes are required for best performance, the use of these special electrode gels may compromise the overall operation of the system.

Polarization effects on biopotential electrodes also can be minimized by making certain that only an absolute minimum of electrical current flows across the electrode-body interface. Although theoretically a measurement can be made with zero current across this interface, in practice there always has to be some current. Nevertheless, by using processor electronic blocks that provide a very high electrical resistance between the electrode input connections (technically referred to as a processor with a high electrical input resistance or input impedance), one can minimize these polarization effects. Modern electronics has made it possible to routinely have input resistance on the order of 10^7 ohms (Ω) on medical electronic equipment. In many cases this is sufficiently high to make it possible to use pure silver or even stainless steel electrodes without severe polarization problems. In these cases low-chloride electrolyte gel can be used much more effectively. The processor must not inject current into the electrodes either. Thus another important feature of the processor is that this current (sometimes referred to as bias current) be very small.

Some special considerations should be made when dealing with neonatal skin electrodes. Because the neonate is much smaller than the adult, the radius of curvature and variations in the radius of curvature at different locations on the thorax will be much greater than they are for the adult. Thus, to effectively keep the neonatal skin electrodes in place and to maintain stable electrical operation, one must make some mechanical considerations as well as electrical ones. The electrodes must be small and flexible so that they conform to the skin surface. They must be attached in such a way that they are secure, but their method of attachment does not cause skin irritation. Finally, in addition to the electrolyte gel considerations previously described, one desires a gel material that will not rapidly dry out, requiring that the electrodes be frequently changed. Some of the problems related to the electrodes, their placement, or the adhesives are as follows:

1. Skin injury: erythema, vesiculation, ulceration, pigmentary changes
2. Infection
3. Pneumothorax (needle electrodes)
4. Poor contact (false alarms)
5. Size: interference with care

The remaining functions of the neonatal cardiac monitor are concerned with signal processing and display or recording (Fig 19-14). The first stage of signal processing is concerned with providing electrical isolation between the patient and the monitor. The isolation stage is necessary to prevent interaction between the cardiac monitor and any other electrical device that might come in

Routine and special care 279

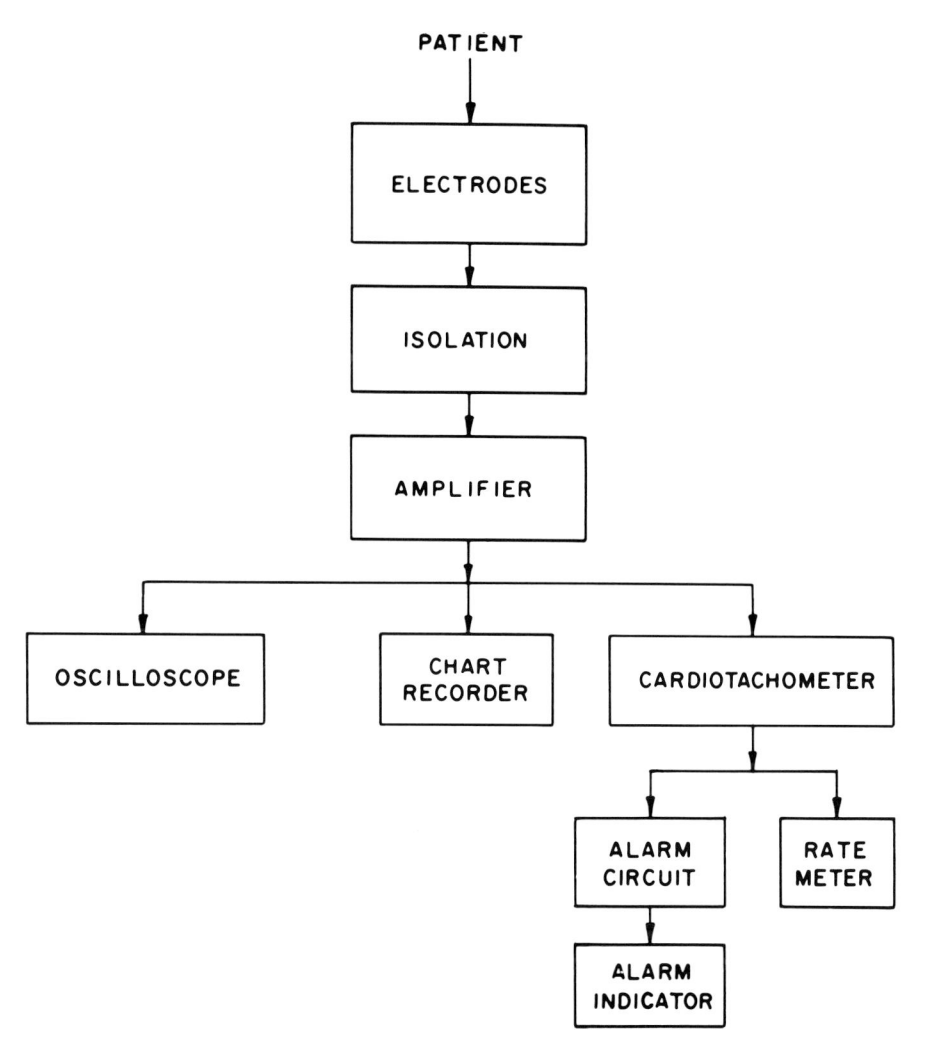

Fig. 19-14. Functional blocks of a typical neonatal cardiac monitor.

contact with the patient. Without isolation, electrical current from one device might flow through the patient to the other device, causing electrical shock.

The isolated electrocardiographic signal from the electrodes is now amplified to provide a strong enough signal to operate the remainder of the system. In the simplest cardiac monitors the display function is carried out by an oscilloscope that indicates the electrocardiogram as it is taken. Generally, a 6- to 10-second segment of the most recent electrocardiogram is shown on the oscilloscope. Another means of displaying the electrocardiogram is through the use of a chart recorder. Here a permanent record is made on a paper strip. Obviously this cannot be used for continuous monitoring because of the impractical lengths of the paper involved.

Most neonatal cardiac monitors determine heart rate. This is done by the functional blocks shown on the right side of Fig. 19-14. A cardiotachometer circuit determines the heart rate from the electrocardiogram in one of two ways. Instantaneous, or beat-to-beat, cardiotachometers measure the interval between each R wave, and a heart rate is calculated as though each and every RR interval of the electrocardiogram were the same. This process is updated at the completion of each RR interval, and the rate meter indicates heart rate as determined for the previously completed interval. Such a cardiotachometer is capable of determining the beat-to-beat variability in heart rate. In addition to the rate meter, some neonatal cardiac monitors have a chart recorder so that heart rate variability can be visualized as it is on a fetal monitor.

The other type of cardiotachometer determines an average heart rate. There are several ways in which this can be done, and the essence of each is that several RR intervals are averaged before a heart rate is determined. Thus the rate meter indicates the average heart rate as determined from several previous beats. This method cannot be used to determine beat-to-beat variability, since the averaging process eliminates some of that variability.

In addition to the oscilloscope and chart recorder, the clinician-machine interface is provided by the rate meter and the alarm system. Digital rate meters are becoming quite popular because they are easy to read. However, when they are used with beat-to-beat cardiotachometers, the new calculation of heart rate with each heart beat causes the meter to frequently change its indication. This can be confusing to the clinical staff and makes it difficult to read the indicator. Often this problem is avoided by having the digital meter display only averaged values of heart rate. An analog indicator such as a meter having a scale of heart rates and a pointer also is frequently used. A disadvantage of this system is that there can be errors introduced on reading the meter. The advantage of this type of indicator is the ease with which one can tell the relation of the present value to a predetermined limit.

The alarm system is used to indicate when the heart rate has fallen beneath or exceeded preset values. An alarm circuit compares the heart rate at the present time with the upper and lower limits, as determined by the operator; as long as the heart rate is between these limits, nothing happens. If this condition is not met, the alarm circuit activates the alarm indicator, which produces an audible and visible alarm.

A major concern in the application of neonatal electronic monitoring devices is the occurrence of false alarms. In some cases these occur so frequently that frustrated clinical staff members deactivate the alarm system altogether. False positive tachycardiac alarms are the result of artifactual signals that the cardiotachometer interprets as R waves. Thus the cardiotachometer registers extra erroneous "heart beats," resulting in a falsely elevated heart rate. An artifact of this type can be the result of electrode polarization and motion. If a layer of electrolyte ions builds up adjacent to the electrode surface, motion of the electrode with respect to this polarization layer in the electrolyte gel will result in a relocation of electrical charge, which manifests itself as a signal on the electrode. There are two ways to minimize this problem. One is to use a nonpolarizable electrode such as a silver–silver chloride electrode, and the second is to eliminate relative motion between the electrode and the electrolyte gel. Neither technique in itself can completely eliminate the problem. Thus it is best to attempt both. No matter what one does, the motion-induced polarization artifact cannot be entirely eliminated.

Another source of artifact that produces false positive tachycardiac alarms is interference from extraneous signals. These signals also have the possibility of fooling the cardiotachometer into interpreting them as R waves. Common sources of such signals are the electrical power lines, other pieces of electrical apparatus located near the patient and monitor, and other bioelectrical signals emanating from the patient. Power line interference often can be recognized on the oscilloscope or chart recorder of a cardiac monitor. A broad baseline on the electrocardiogram is the clue. Interference from other electrical devices is seen on the oscilloscope or the chart recorder as a sudden jump in the baseline. The best way to eliminate this source of artifact is to remove or repair the offending device whenever possible. When trying to locate an extraneous source of artifact of this type, one should first suspect electrical apparatus employing motors and/or heaters. The major biologic source of extraneous signals is the electromyogram. The influence of the electromyogram on the cardiotachometer can be minimized by choosing electrode positions that maximize the amplitude of the QRS complex of the electrocardiogram while minimizing the magnitude of any electromyogram derived from muscle groups underneath the electrodes.

Since the false positive tachycardic alarms result from the misrecognition of artifact, the problem can be minimized by developing more sophisticated cardiotachometers that can differentiate between true signal and artifact. Biomedical engineers have described various techniques for doing this ranging from electronic filters to computer recognition of the QRS complex. It is important for clinicians to be aware of any of these techniques which might be used in their monitors, since they could also result in the elimination of important data. For example, a cardiotachometer that is set to recognize only QRS complexes will miss ectopic ventricular beats because of their different wave shape. If a cardiotachometer uses extensive signal processing, it is desirable that the monitor incorporate a control to enable the clinician to turn off this processing if desired.

PRESSURE MONITORING

Physicists define pressure as the force exerted by a fluid on a surface of unit area; thus the measurement of pressure is really the measurement of a force. There are both direct and indirect methods to measure pressures. In the former the pressure sensor is in direct contact with the fluid being measured, whereas in the latter the fluid being measured is separated from the sensor.

The sensor function of pressure monitors is carried out by a pressure transducer. This device measures the force detected by a diaphragm in contact with the fluid being measured. The pressure in the fluid exerts a force on the diaphragm that deflects it, and this deflection is measured electrically to provide the signal for the processor portion of the instrument. Since pressure in the fluid being measured causes the diaphragm to deflect, some fluid must flow into the pressure transducer. It is thus possible to characterize a pressure transducer in terms of its compliance: the change in volume produced by a change in pressure divided by that change in pressure. It is noted that the definition of compliance of a pressure transducer is the same as that for the lungs, but, as is pointed out later, unlike the lungs, the pressure transducer should have a very low compliance.

Coupling the body to the sensor is an important problem in pressure-monitoring systems (interface 1, Fig. 19-13). In direct pressure measurement the fluid being measured must be coupled to the pressure transducer itself. This can be done through a fluid-filled tube or catheter. The fluid in the catheter should have properties similar to those of the fluid being measured. For example, physiologic saline solution can be used as the coupling medium in the catheter when one desires to make a direct measurement of blood pressure. As long as the distal end of the catheter is at the same level as the pressure transducer, Pascal's law tells us that the pressure at the transducer will be the same as the pressure at the distal tip of the catheter. This only applies to static (constant) pressures. If the pressure at the distal tip of the catheter is varying, fluid must flow along the catheter to the pressure transducer because of its nonzero compliance. The catheter offers resistance to this fluid flow, and this introduces distortion in the pressure measurement. The amount of fluid that must flow through the catheter is determined by the compliance of the pressure transducer, and so a pressure transducer with low compliance will require less fluid to flow; therefore catheter resistance effects will be minimized.

The compliance of the pressure transducer, the mass of the fluid, and the resistance of the catheter are responsible for another type of distortion that can occur in time-varying pressure measurements. This distortion is a result of mechanical resonance in the system and can produce additional undulations in the pressure waveform, as seen at the transducer, that were not present in the waveform at the distal tip of the catheter. This type of distortion can result in overshoot, which causes the instrument to read a peak pressure that is greater than the actual peak of the pressure waveform.

Additional artifact from the catheter can be seen as the result of movement. Even though a steady pressure is maintained at the distal tip of the catheter and the transducer is at the same height as the distal tip of the catheter, moving the catheter will produce transient pressure changes at the transducer. This type of motion-induced distortion is generally short lived but makes it difficult to make direct pressure measurements.

Thus, to measure neonatal arterial or venous blood pressure by the direct technique, a catheter must be placed in the appropriate umbilical vessel and advanced until it reaches the central circulation, i.e., the aorta or the inferior vena cava. A pressure transducer should be

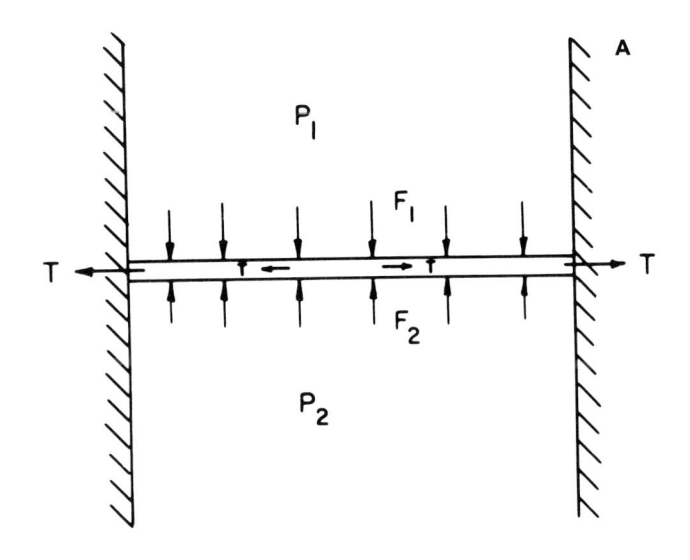

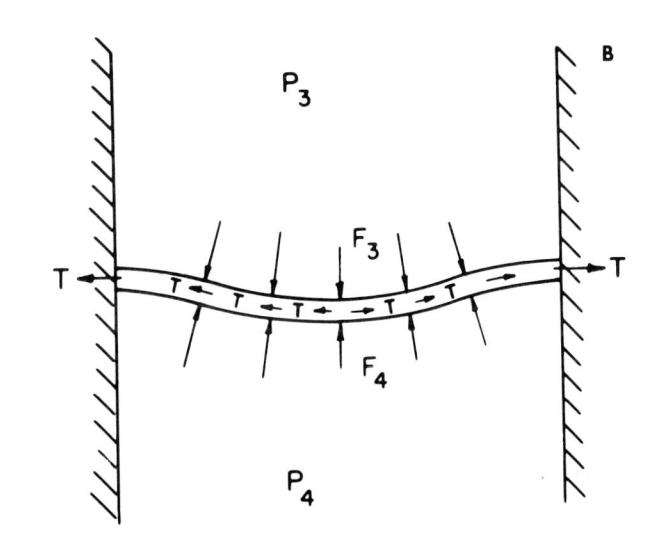

Fig. 19-15. Pressure difference across an elastic membrane under tension. **A,** Equal pressure on each side of the membrane. **B,** Pressure above the membrane is greater than that below the membrane.

attached to the proximal end of the catheter and positioned so that it is at the same height as the distal end of the catheter. In this way baseline errors are avoided. Even though these errors are not too damaging in the measurement of arterial blood pressure, they can be quite serious in the measurement of venous blood pressure. A 10-cm difference in height between the distal catheter and the pressure transducer results in an error of 7.7 mm Hg. The transducer and catheter also should be placed such that there is a minimum of motion so as to reduce artifact.

Pressure can be measured indirectly by tonometry. The basic principle is illustrated in Fig. 19-15. Depicted

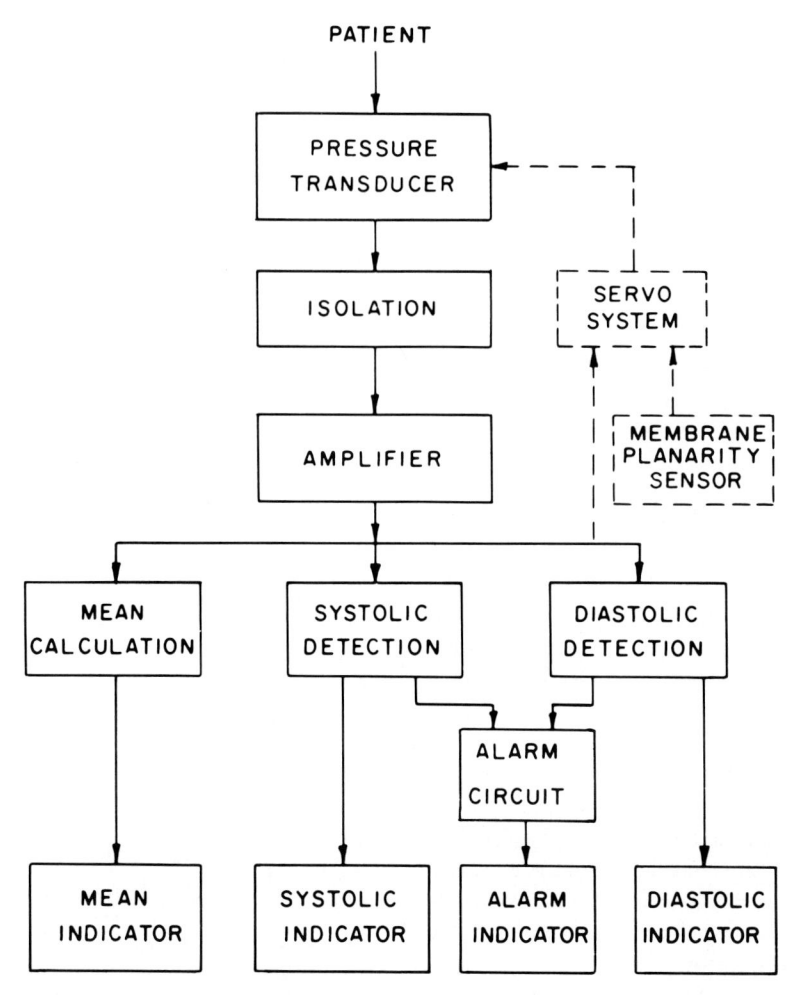

Fig. 19-16. Functional block diagram of a typical pressure monitor. The blocks indicated by dashed lines must be added when indirect tonometric monitoring is performed.

are two fluid-filled chambers separated by an elastic membrane of finite thickness and under tension (T). The pressure in the chamber above the membrane (P_1) and that in the chamber below the membrane (P_2) are equal. Since the areas of the membrane surface facing P_1 and P_2 are equal, the force exerted by the fluid on each side of the membrane must be the same, or in other words: $F_1 = F_2$. The membrane tends to assume the position in which it is stretched the least, i.e., where it is perpendicular to the sides of the container (Fig. 19-15, A).

In Fig. 19-15, B, where the pressure above the membrane is greater than the pressure beneath it, the force F_3 is greater than the force F_4. The membrane therefore will be stretched to the shape shown. The tension in the membrane (T) tends to flatten it out to a position where it is stretched the least. The membrane tension therefore exerts a force that aids F_4 and opposes F_3. This force is determined by the amount of curvature in the membrane and its tension. At equilibrium the sum of this force and F_4 will equal F_3. Since we do not know the membrane tension or curvature, it is not possible to determine pressure P_4 by measuring P_3. In the situation of Fig. 19-15, A, where the membrane is planar, it is possible to determine pressure P_2 by measuring pressure P_1. Thus, in general, one can measure the pressure on one side of an elastic membrane if one can determine the pressure on the other side and maintain the planarity of the membrane.

As seen in the preceding discussion, there are several possibilities for errors in pressure measurement by tonometry. Nevertheless there are some instances where it is the only safe method available. For example, several investigators have shown that transdural and transfontanel *monitoring of intracranial pressure* is efficacious. In the former case the dura and part of the pressure sensor serve as the membrane between the two compartments, whereas in the latter the effective membrane includes the scalp as well as the dura and pressure transducer.

The functional block diagram of a typical pressure-monitoring system is shown in Fig. 19-16, with the scheme for signal processing following the pressure transducer indicated. As is the case with the cardiac monitor, effective electrical isolation of the pressure transducer and thus the patient from the rest of the machine is essential for safe operation in all types of clinical environments. The isolated electrical pressure signal is then amplified, and special circuits are employed to determine the systolic and diastolic pressures from the pressure waveforms when arterial blood pressure is monitored. The instrument also contains some circuitry for calculating mean pressures. The monitor can consist of only these blocks when it is used for watching pressures that vary slowly such as venous blood pressure or cerebral spinal fluid pressure. Often monitors intended for this purpose have the pressure indicator connected directly to the amplifier, since the variations are so slow that it is not necessary to calculate a mean.

The alarm circuit in Fig. 19-16 is shown connected to the systolic and diastolic detectors for arterial blood pressure monitoring. This circuit compares systolic and diastolic pressures with preset limits, and, if either of the pressures is outside this predetermined range, an audible and visible alarm is activated. It is also possible to have the alarm circuit connected to the mean pressure channel.

In the indirect pressure-measurement system the signal processor must carry out additional functions. If the pressure below the membrane is to be measured, it is necessary to adjust the pressure above the membrane to produce membrane planarity. Thus a system must be included in the monitor that is capable of modifying the pressure above the membrane until membrane planarity is achieved. This sytem must sense the position of the membrane and adjust the pressure accordingly. Once the membrane is planar, the pressure above the membrane can be sensed, and the signal can be processed in the same way as the direct signal. The system for carrying out this function is known as a servo system, since it must adjust the pressure in the transducer to provide planarity of the membrane. The additional functional blocks in the instrumentation system are shown with dashed lines in Fig. 19-16.

As with the cardiac monitors, pressure monitors have several sources of error. Catheter artifact resulting in baseline and pressure transient errors already have been discussed. In addition, the catheter can become partially or fully obstructed, or an air bubble can form in the catheter. All these problems produce distortion of the pressure waveform. Leaks in the catheter system can result in abnormally low pressure readings or, when the leak is severe, can lead to rapid exsanguination of the patient when the catheter is placed in an artery. Thus it is extremely important that this problem be avoided. In the indirect method of measuring pressure additional errors can be introduced by the "membrane." The thickness of the membrane in Fig. 19-15 is relatively small compared with dimensions of the area over which pressure is measured, and the membrane itself was assumed to be homogenous. When the pressure is measured across a neonatal fontanel, the membrane is no longer thin with respect to the dimensions of the sensor, nor is it homogenous. Materials of varying elastic properties and tensions are found between the pressure transducer and the neonatal cerebral spinal fluid. One cannot even be certain that there is only cerebral spinal fluid in contact with the inner surface of the "membrane." The process of establishing planarity of the membrane most likely presses the central portion of the dura under the transducer against the cortex and perhaps might even cause minor distension of the cortex. In this case the cortex will exert a force against the membrane that is added to the force produced by the cerebral spinal fluid pressure (F_2 in Fig. 19-15). So for the pressure in the transducer to overcome this force, it is necessary that P_1 be greater than P_2; therefore the measurement is in error. In the indirect method one also has problems in maintaining stable contact between the pressure sensor and the body, as well as in making certain that this contact does not modify the membrane and its tension. Therefore, when indirect pressure-measurement techniques must be used, great care must be employed in their application, and the results must be viewed critically.

A discussion of neonatal pressure monitoring would not be complete without mentioning the measurement of neonatal blood pressure using a sphygmomanometer cuff and ultrasonic detection of the systolic and diastolic pressures. Even though this is not a method of continuous monitoring, it is the most frequently used technique for measuring neonatal blood pressure.

Conventional sphygmomanometry and auscultation cannot be used with neonates because of the difficulty in detecting Korotkoff's sounds. By adding an ultrasonic Doppler detection system to a conventional sphygmomanometer cuff, systolic and diastolic pressures can be determined. Ultrasound kinetoarteriography determines the systolic and diastolic pressures by sensing the movement of the wall of the brachial artery that is in the portion of the arm surrounded by the occluding cuff. An ultrasonic transducer is centrally placed under the cuff so that it is approximately over the brachial artery. A portion of the ultrasound beam illuminating the artery is reflected back to the transducer from the arterial wall. If the arterial wall moves with respect to the transducer under the cuff, the frequency of the reflected sound will be shifted in relation to the incident sound. This frequency change, known as a Doppler shift, is a basic physical property of propagating waves and is the same effect that causes the pitch of an automobile horn to sound higher than normal when the vehicle is approaching the listener and lower than normal as it speeds away. Thus, by electronically sensing the shift in frequency of the reflected ultrasound and converting this to an audible signal, it is possible to indicate arterial wall movements under the pneumatic cuff.

The arterial wall will move only when the pressure surrounding the artery and, roughly, the pressure in the cuff lie between the systolic and diastolic pressure. When the cuff pressure is greater than systolic pressure, the artery is collapsed, and blood cannot flow through it. As the cuff pressure drops beneath systolic arterial pressure, the blood pressure is able to force the artery open during systole, but the artery once again collapses when the blood pressure drops below the cuff pressure. Such arterial expansion and collapsing will cause two Doppler frequency shifts to occur during each cardiac cycle. The first is a result of the expanding of the artery during the rising phase of arterial pressure as it exceeds the cuff pressure. The second Doppler shift occurs as the arterial pressure falls below the cuff pressure and the artery collapses. When the cuff pressure is close to systolic blood pressure, the two Doppler shifts occur close together in time, and, when the cuff pressure is close to diastolic pressure, there is more time between the two Doppler shifts, since the artery is patent for a longer period.

Once the cuff pressure falls below the diastolic pressure, arterial pressure always will be higher than the cuff pressure; therefore there will be only slight changes in the arterial diameter, which result in only small Doppler shifts in the frequency of the reflected ultrasonic wave. Thus with ultrasonic kinetoarteriography it is possible to detect the systolic and diastolic pressures in a similar manner to the method of ausculation, but ultrasound rather than audible sound is used. The principal advantage of this method is the great ease with which blood pressures can be determined. Unlike auscultation, where Korotkoff's sounds are especially difficult to hear in premature neonates, ultrasound kinetoarteriography is relatively easy to perform. The ultrasonic sensors are unaffected by ambient noise; and because the ultrasonic signal is processed electronically and converted to audible sound, if the device is used in a noisy environment or the neonate is crying, one need only increase the sound level of the instrument to be able to conveniently detect systolic and diastolic pressures. Automated instruments are even available which automatically determine these points and indicate them on a scale.

The major disadvantage of this technique is that the ultrasonic system is sensitive not only to the motion of the arterial wall but also to any other structure that moves in the ultrasound beam. This includes the skin under the transducer and the ultrasound transducer itself. Thus for reliable results it is necessary for the subject to be relatively still. Even though this is not always possible, one can frequently obtain a useful signal, but a certain amount of caution is wise when making measurements on an active infant, and restraint of the limb during the measurement as well as a second check is a good idea for best results.

RESPIRATION MONITORING

The monitoring of respiratory gas exchange also can be done by direct and indirect methods. As is the case with pressure monitoring, the direct method is more invasive than the indirect methods; however, it also is more accurate. In the direct method airway flow is sensed by instrumentation that has direct access to the airway. If the therapy applied to the neonate already requires a direct connection to the airway such as an endotracheal cannula, direct instrumentation is no problem, but to make this connection for purposes of monitoring respiration usually is not justified.

The sensor in the airway must detect gas flow. There are many ways to do this, but one of the simplest is to place a low-mass temperature sensor that can be heated to above respiration gas temperature. The relatively cool gas being transported in the airway passes over this sensor and cools it; thus the temperature sensor is cooled on inspiration and on expiration. Its mass must be small so that it will quickly warm during zero-flow conditions such as those which occur at end inspiration or end expiration. A thermistor is a temperature sensor that can be made very small and has an electrical resistance which is related to its temperature. Its small size and high sensitivity and the fact that one can heat it using the same electrical signal that measures its resistance make it ideal for placement in the airway. It is also possible to place a thermistor over the neonatal nose and measure air passing through the nose. Placement of the thermistor in this case is somewhat difficult, and maintaining this placement also presents problems. In all applications of the thermistor for sensing airway gas transport the calibration is qualitative. One can tell that gas is being exchanged, but it is not possible to tell how much without having special temperature and moisture-content controls.

The indirect methods of measuring respiration involve detecting chest and abdominal wall movement, whole body movement, or changes in thoracic electrical impedence. Chest and abdominal wall movement can be sensed by several methods: by sensors attached to the neonate or by sensors not placed directly on the patient. A strain gauge—an electrical sensor that changes its electrical resistance when its dimensions are changed— can be taped on the neonate to detect dimensional changes in the chest and/or abdominal wall with breathing. It is important, when such a sensor is used, for it not to be stiff and not to alter the normal movement of that part of the body on which it is placed. A small permanent magnet (magnetometer) also can be taped on the anterior aspect of the chest or abdominal wall when the infant is supine. A magnetic field sensor such as an electrical coil then can be placed under the infant, and it produces an electrical signal that is related to the position of the magnet. In this way an electrical signal is produced which is related to chest or abdominal wall movement when the infant breathes.

A low-power beam of ultrasound or electromagnetic energy can be aimed at the neonate in the incubator. Some of this radiation will be reflected from the chest or abdominal walls, and the nature of this reflection will change with chest or abdominal wall position. Thus sensing this reflected signal enables one to qualitatively sense positional changes of the neonatal reflecting surface.

Neonatal body movements also can be detected by placing the patient on a special mattress that is sensitive to patient movement. When the infant moves, electrical signals are produced by the sensor, and these can be related to respiratory motion. The problem with this method and the external radiation method is that the sensors are also sensitive to nonrespiratory movements of the neonate, and it may be difficult to obtain an accurate respiration signal. Body movements during apneic periods may be interpreted erroneously as breaths.

One of the most frequently employed methods of sensing respiration is to measure changes in the transthoracic electrical impedence. Electrical impedance relates the current through a circuit to the voltage across the circuit for an AC signal in much the same way that electrical resistance describes the relationship for DC signals. Transthoracic electrical impedance is determined by placing biopotential electrodes on the thorax and measuring the electrical impedance between them. This is done by passing a very low-level current, usually less than 100 μA, through the electrodes and measuring the voltage drop across them. This voltage will be proportional to the impedance between the electrodes. Since there is an impedance associated with the polarization layer in the electrodes, it is important to minimize this impedance so that the signal will be dominated by the actual impedance in the body. This can best be done by passing a high-frequency current through the electrodes. At a frequency of 50 kHz, electrode impedance is minimal and is independent of the excitation current frequency.

The change in transthoracic electrical impedance with respiration is small, with typical changes being approximately 0.5% over the tidal volume. Thus, even at elevated frequencies where electrode impedances are minimal, they must be constant to avoid introduction of artifact. Not only this but also other sources of impedance variation in the thorax must be minimized for stable operation. Neither of these requirements can be optimally achieved in practice. Electrode impedances vary with electrode motion, and transthoracic impedance also varies with movement of the neonate. In addition, thoracic blood volume can change transthoracic electrical impedance. Indeed this can be applied to estimating cardiac output noninvasively while a subject holds his breath so that respiratory impedance variations are eliminated. Thus the typical neonatal respiration signals seen from transthoracic-impedance sensing contain three components: the respiratory component, the cardiac component, and artifact. Since only the first component is being measured, the other two can cause significant errors, especially in giving false negative apnea alarms.

The anatomy of a typical neonatal respiration monitor is shown in Fig. 19-17. These devices are primarily designed to detect apnea, and they are frequently referred to as apnea monitors. The respiration signal is sensed by one of the techniques described previously. When the electrical impedance technique is used, the same electrodes usually are employed to produce the electrocardiogram as well, and the respiration monitor also includes a cardiac monitor such as the one shown in Fig. 19-14. As with all the other electronic monitoring equipment described in this chapter, it is important to electrically isolate the sensor from the rest of the electronic system. The signal is then amplified and may be displayed directly on an oscilloscope. In monitors that carry out combined functions, all the signals can be shown on different channels of the same oscilloscope. The amplified signal also is fed to a breath detector, a circuit designed to indicate when the neonate takes a breath. This function is not easy to carry out electronically, since the neonatal respiration waveform can be quite complex. The presence of artifact makes the detection even more difficult. Once a breath is detected, a tachometer circuit is used to determine the respiration rate that is displayed on the rate indicator. These circuits are similar to the ones used in the cardiac monitor, and most respiration monitors use an averaging tachometer. An alarm circuit can be employed to indicate when the respiration rate falls outside the preset limits. The breath detector also signals an interval timer that determines the interval between breaths. In newer monitors this function is carried out as a part of the tachometer, but it is shown separately in Fig. 19-17 for clarity. The apnea alarm circuit determines when the interval between breaths reaches a preset time, for example, 20 seconds, and then activates the alarm indicator to give a visible and audible alarm.

The overall problem with neonatal apnea monitors is the frequency of false positive and false negative alarms. As was pointed out in the discussion of respiration sen-

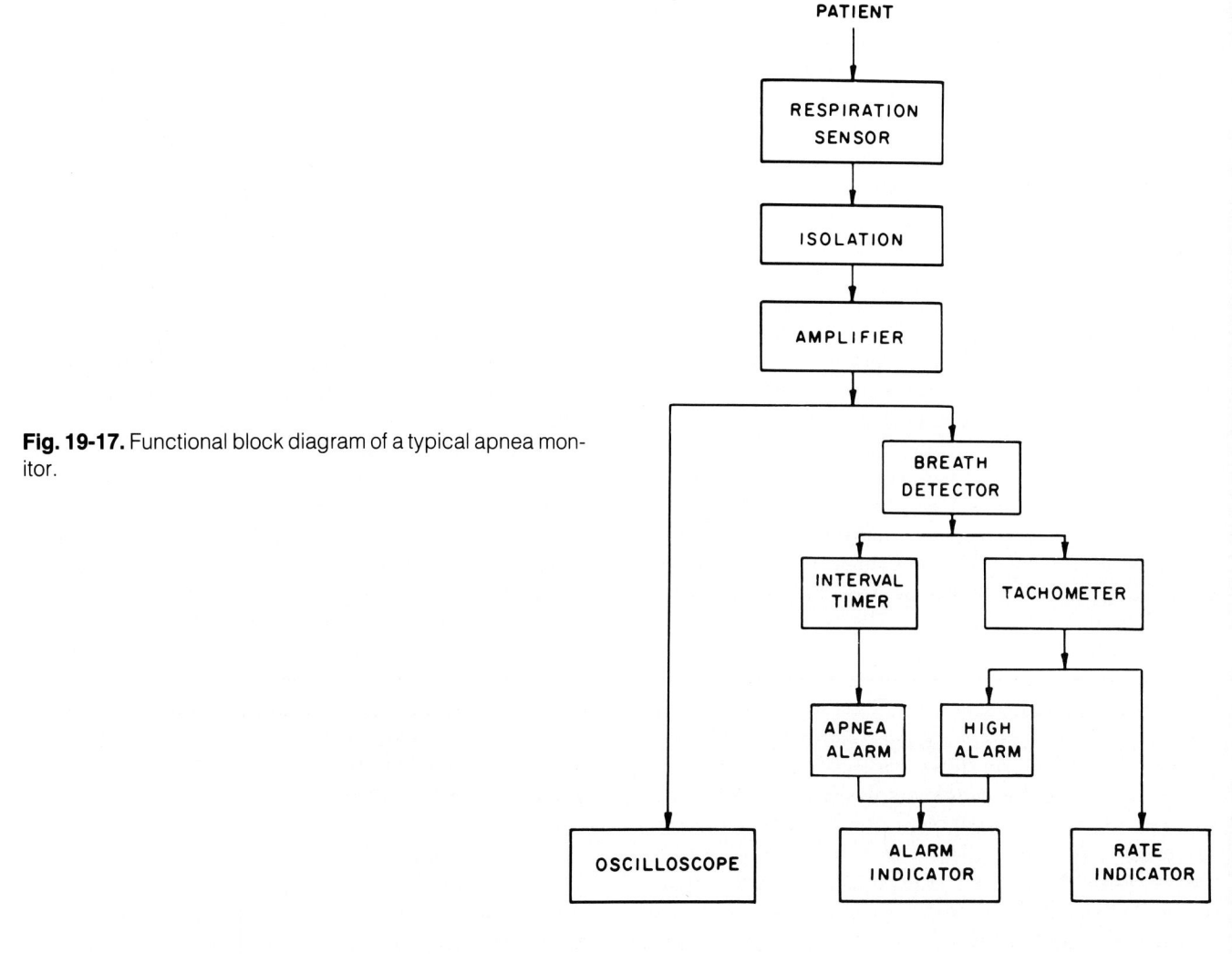

Fig. 19-17. Functional block diagram of a typical apnea monitor.

sors, motion and cardiac artifacts frequently interfere with the respiration signal. If the monitor misinterprets these artifacts as respiration, an abnormally high respiration rate will be calculated by the tachometer, and the interval timer will not measure the true interval between breaths. This, as pointed out earlier, can disable the apnea alarm when apnea is occurring, giving a false negative alarm condition.

There also can be problems with the breath detector sensing true breaths. In cases where there are large excursions in tidal volume from one breath to the next, the amplitude of the respiration signal will show similar variations. Often the smaller breaths are missed by the respiratory monitor, and this will give erroneously low values for the respiration rate and may trigger false positive apnea alarms.

A problem with all the types of indirect respiration sensors is that they are unable to detect obstructive apnea. In this case the neonate goes through respiratory efforts even though no air is exchanged, and there are chest wall movements, whole body movements, and thoracic electrical impedance changes. Only direct measurement from the airway can reliably detect this type of apnea.

In general, currently available methods for indirect respiration and apnea monitoring are not ideal. False alarms do exist in all the different type of monitors, and the clinician should be aware of conditions which produce these false alarms. Nevertheless respiration and apnea monitors have been of considerable help in neonatal intensive care, and although not currently ideal, they are certainly the best alternative.

SAFETY CONSIDERATIONS

Neonatal intensive care involves the use of many electrical, electronic, and other types of devices that have been shown to benefit the patient, yet their use also introduces a small amount of risk. Thus, to effectively apply these devices and systems in the care of the neonate, it is necessary to understand the threat they present to the patient and the clinical personnel along with their benefits. In this way necessary safety precautions can be understood and practiced when these devices are used in patient care.

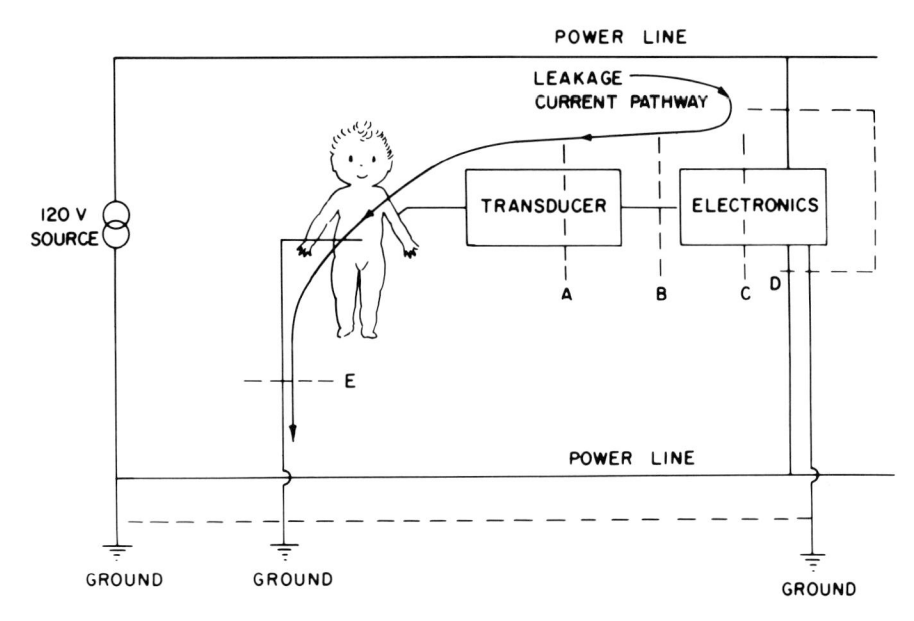

Fig. 19-18. Connection of an electronic monitor to a neonate showing a possible leakage current pathway from the power line to ground through the patient.

A major consideration in using electrical and electronic devices in the nursery is the electrical shock hazard. Unfortunately, when safety considerations in intensive care units are discussed, it is implied that the electrical problem is the only safety problem. This is certainly not the case. In neonatology there are many examples of hazards to the neonate from the use of monitoring and therapeutic devices in the nursery. For example, small air emboli introduced into the neonatal circulation through intravenous lines can severely compromise cardiac output; leaks in arterial catheter lines can result in serious bleeding; and overheating of the incubator can expose the neonate to dangerous thermal environments. These potential hazards are discussed in other sections of this text and therefore are not described in detail here, but the reader is reminded that they represent safety hazards every bit as severe as the electrical shock hazard.

The electrical shock problem is a result of the fact that the 120-V electrical power system is connected in such a way that one side of the power line is attached to the earth, or "ground." This means that if anything which is capable of conducting electrical current comes in contact with the other side of the power line and the earth or an electrical conductor connected to the earth, an electrical current can flow. An extreme example of this is a person taking a bath and reaching for an electrical appliance in the bathroom. The water in the bathtub is connected to the earth (or ground) through the metal water pipes; if in touching the electrical appliance this person inadvertently comes in direct or indirect contact with the ungrounded side of the power line because of a defective appliance, the person could experience electrical currents sufficiently high to cause cardiac arrest.

This example of a bather reaching for an electrical appliance is not so far removed from the situation of neonates and for that matter sometimes the clinical staff in the intensive care nursery. Even though these individuals are not lounging in a bathtub, often they are still connected to ground. In the case of the infant in an incubator the incubator itself is connected to the electrical power system, and its metal parts are grounded through the electrical power plug. The infant is surrounded by these metal parts, and thus it is very easy to become connected to ground either by direct contact with a metal interior part in the incubator or by having the connection made by an electrolytic solution such as spilled intravenous fluids, urine, and formula. Similarly, clinical staff members also can be grounded by touching the metal parts of devices that are grounded, such as an incubator, or by contact through the floor of the nursery itself in cases where a conductive floor and shoes are employed.

This situation is represented in Fig. 19-18. Here the neonate is connected to ground. When electronic monitoring devices are used, the neonate can be electrically connected to them through various transducers such as surface biopotential electrodes or a pressure transducer connected to an indwelling catheter. Since the electronic monitoring device is connected to the power line, it is possible for electrical leakage pathways to exist between the ungrounded side of the power line and the transducer on the patient. Thus it is possible for an electrical current to flow from the power line through the electronic circuit, the transducer, and the neonate to ground. Such a current leakage pathway usually will result in a negligibly small current. However, in circumstances where the connection of the electronic monitoring device to ground through its power source is interrupted, such as with a defective power cord, plug, or electrical outlet, the electrical current leakage pathway through the neonate is the only ground connection to the instrument, and relatively high and potentially lethal current through the patient can exist.

The possibility that an electrical current will follow the path through the patient shown in Fig. 19-18 can be greatly reduced by taking special precautions. Electrical isolation circuits incorporated into the monitors can maintain leakage currents below a critical maximum point for safe operation of the system. Such isolation can be applied to the monitoring device at any of the points indicated by dashed lines in Fig. 19-18. For example, specially designed transducers with built-in electrical isolation, such as pressure transducers used for direct monitoring of arterial blood pressure, can be used, resulting in isolation at line A in the figure. An electronic isolation circuit also can be placed between the transducer and the monitor of the electronic circuit, as indicated by the dashed line B. Similarly, isolation circuitry can be incorporated into the electronic circuit itself so that all portions of this circuitry which are connected to the power supply and hence the power line will be isolated from those portions of the circuit which are connected to the transducer and hence the patient. This isolation would interrupt the leakage current pathway at dashed line C. Isolation can be introduced between the main power line and the power connection to the medical instrument, as indicated by the dashed line D.

In this case the goal of isolation is to provide a power source to the monitoring instrument that no longer has one side connected to the ground. In this way the possibility of currents returning to ground through the patient is eliminated. Isolation transformers between the power line and the monitoring instrument are used to achieve this independence from ground. Some neonatal intensive care units have built-in isolation transformers at each patient location so that the electrical outlets are already electrically isolated from ground and from the power sources at other patient locations in the nursery.

The final method to eliminate the shock hazard is to isolate the patient from ground, as indicated by the dashed line E in Fig. 19-18. Since the neonate connection to ground is most likely to be through the incubator, the incubator itself can be disconnected from ground so that its interior metal surfaces are no longer sources of ground connections for the neonate. Of course any other piece of electrical apparatus or personnel that the neonate is likely to contact also must be isolated from ground for this system to work. This is difficult to achieve, and thus this last approach is not recommended.

THE FUTURE

Electronic instrumentation for intensive care monitoring of neonates will continue to be important in their care. Improved technology and experience in applying the technology will bring about more reliable instruments, and new sensors will allow additional physiologic variables to be monitored. Computer technology and the microcomputer will make it possible to have monitors that can critically evaluate the quality of a signal and be better able to differentiate true alarm conditions from false alarms. Computer technology also will make it possible to have automated data-recording and charting functions on the monitors as well as to combine monitored data with other clinical data from the patient. This chapter has examined electronic neonatal monitors that for the most part have enjoyed widespread clinical application. There is a wide range of other more specialized monitoring devices that have been developed for clinical research. Although most of these will never be used for routine patient care, the scientific results that they will make available will certainly affect our understanding and care of the neonate in the future.

Michael R. Neuman

BIBLIOGRAPHY
General

Hill, D.W., and Dolan, A.M.: Intensive care instrumentation, New York, 1976, Grune & Stratton, Inc.

Neuman, M.R.: The biophysical and bioengineering bases of perinatal monitoring. V. Neonatal cardiac and respiratory monitoring, Perinatol. Neonatol. 3:17, 1979.

Neuman, M.R.: The biophysical and bioengineering bases of perinatal monitoring. VI. Neonatal temperature, blood pressure and blood gas instrumentation, Perinatol. Neonatol. 3:25, 1979.

Rolfe, P.: Monitoring in newborn intensive care, Biomed. Eng. 10:399, 1975.

Rolfe, P.: Monitoring equipment for the neonate, Br. J. Hosp. Med. 1:89, 1976.

Webster, J.G., editor: Medical instrumentation—application and design, Boston, 1978, Houghton-Mifflin Co.

Cardiac monitoring

Cobbold, R.S.C.: Transducers for biomedical measurements: principles and applications, New York, 1974, John Wiley & Sons, Inc.

Delgado, J.M.R.: Electrodes for extracellular recording and stimulation. In Nastuk, W.L., editor: Physical techniques in medical research, vol. 5A, New York, 1964, Academic Press, Inc.

Ferris, C.D.: Introduction to bioelectrodes, New York, 1974, Plenum Press.

Geddes, L.A.: Electrodes and the measurement of bioelectric events, New York, 1972, John Wiley & Sons, Inc.

Miller, H.A., and Harrison, D.C., editors: Biomedical electrode technology, New York, 1974, Academic Press, Inc.

Webster, J.G.: Interference and motion artifact in biopotentials, Region 6 Conference Record, IEEE Trans. Biomed. Eng. p. 53, 1977.

Pressure measurement

Fleming, D.G., Ko, W.H., and Neuman, M.R.: Indwelling and implantable pressure transducers, Cleveland, 1977, CRC Press, Inc.

Geddes, L.A.: The direct and indirect measurement of blood pressure, Chicago, 1970, Year Book Medical Publishers, Inc.
Greatorex, C.A.: Indirect methods of blood pressure measurement. In Watson, B.W., editor: IEE medical electronics monographs 1 to 6, London, 1971, Peter Peregrinus.
Huch, A., and others: A new device for non-invasive measurement of intracranial pressure (ICP) in newborns, Med. Prog. Technol. **6**:185, 1979.
Salmon, J.H., Hajjar, W., and Bada, H.S.: The fontogram: a non-invasive intracranial pressure monitor, Pediatrics **60**:721, 1977.
Stegall, H.F., Kardon, M.B., and Kemmerer, W.T.: Indirect measurement of arterial blood pressure by Doppler sphygmomanometry, J. Appl. Physiol. **25**:793, 1968.
Vidyasagar, D., and Raju, T.N.K.: Non-invasive technique of measuring intracranial pressure in the newborn, Pediatrics (Suppl.) **59**:957, 1977.

Respiration monitoring

Baker, L.E.: Electrical impedance pneumography. In Rolfe, P., editor: Non-invasive physiological measurements, vol. 1, London, 1979, Academic Press, Inc.
Nyboer, J.: Electrical impedance plethysmography, ed. 2, Springfield, Ill., 1970, Charles C Thomas, Publisher.
Olsson, T., and others: Transthoracic impedance with special reference to newborn infants and the ratio of air-to-fluid in the lungs, Acta Paediatr. Scand. (Suppl.) **207**:1, 1970.
Rolfe, P.: A magnetometer respiration monitor for use with premature babies, Biomed. Eng. **6**:402, 1971.

PART FOUR

Care of the newborn

Newborn intensive care units (NICUs) are now considered necessities in university or large community hospitals; a need for a transitional care area has been established, and there is increasing evidence of the value of special transportation vehicles that permit care of sick infants in transit. Each hospital must realistically assess its particular needs and capabilities on the basis of regional population, staff, services, and facilities. Preliminary steps have been taken toward an ultimate goal of regionalization of care for the newborn, but until such regional centers are functional, existing services and facilities for the newborn must be continually and critically reassessed to deliver the best level of care that is possible with the available resources (see Chapter 2).

Review of the different facilities established to care for the newborn provides a basic understanding of the role of each unit as it relates to the general care of the infant as well as an appreciation of the specific medical needs of infants requiring a wide range of medical services. Following the definition of each unit and its facilities and staff, aspects of care common to all units are discussed. These suggestions are offered as *minimum standards*. Application of principles of care and definition of the physical location for the delivery of care remains the prerogative and responsibility of each hospital and its medical staff.

NORMAL NEWBORN NURSERY—TYPE I CARE
Characteristics of patients

Infants admitted to this area may include:
1. Well full-term newborns who are in the lowest mortality group by weight and gestational age. They will be 38 through 41 weeks of gestational age and 2,500 to 4,000 gm in weight (see Figs. 15-2 and 15-3).
2. Well preterm newborns who weigh 2,000 to 2,500 gm and who are at least 36 weeks' gestational age. The capacity to adequately care for these infants depends on the presence of personnel skilled in feeding.
3. Other newborns who are at a comparably low mortality and morbidity risk (once this fact has been firmly established), who do not qualify under type II care, and who are well at the time of admission.

Personnel
Registered nurses

One nurse per shift is required but does not necessarily have to be in constant attendance and may share responsibilities in an adjacent obstetric area. The nurse *must* be responsible for maintenance of all emergency equipment and know the appropriate physician to call for emergencies.

Paramedical personnel (practical nurses, aides, and others)

One individual must be attending the infants at all times (regardless of census), with a ratio of between 1:6 and 1:8 required. These individuals should be trained in routine care, pharyngeal suction, oxygen administration by mask and bag, and routine feeding. They also must understand principles of hemostasis and be able to tie an umbilical cord as an emergency measure. If rooming-in is used, at least one person trained in these procedures must be available in an adjacent area at all times.

Physicians

A specific pediatrician should be designated as the physician responsible for general, medical, and administrative policies and routines affecting these infants and should regularly review all such matters. Each infant should have a particular physician responsible for his medical care.

Facilities and services

1. Infants should be cared for in a unit near the maternity ward or in rooming-in accommodations.
2. Care may be rendered centrally in one large room with a minimum of 3 feet in all directions between bassinets and approximately 20 square feet per infant.
3. The number of bassinets should at least equal the number of postpartum beds plus 20% to 30% to allow for multiple births, prolonged maternal or infant hos-

pitalizations, and variation in the census. Because the area requires one caretaker for each 6 to 8 infants, the rooms should be designed to accommodate 6 to 8 or 12 to 16 infants.
4. Infants should be placed in close proximity to the nursing station for the first 24 hours of life to ensure more intensive observation during this period.
5. The hospital's laboratory must be able to provide on a 24-hour basis standard bacteriologic studies, urinalyses, hematocrit determinations, white blood cell counts with differentials, blood typing and cross matching, direct and indirect Coombs' tests, and microdeterminations of direct and indirect bilirubin, blood glucose, calcium, sodium, potassium, and chloride concentrations. Serology testing for phenylketonuria also should be regularly available during the day shift.
6. Roentgenologic services for the nursery should include the capability of taking portable films on a 24-hour basis.
7. Equipment should include foot-controlled sinks and soap dispensers, stethoscopes, sterile umbilical tape, examining equipment, and emergency resuscitation equipment.

Medical policy and administration

1. Hospitals in which 500 or more infants are delivered each year should provide this type of care. Hospitals with less than 500 deliveries should be encouraged to discontinue their obstetric services and concentrate these services in one regional facility.
2. Special protocols should be established for observation of infants during the first 12 to 24 hour of life.
3. Any infant who becomes ill, in whom a presumptive diagnosis of sepsis is made, or whose course requires other than routine care should be transferred to an area where type II care is available.
4. Infants who underwent unsterile or unregistered deliveries, or both, not otherwise included under type II care may be admitted to this unit and maintained in an incubator with the special observation protocols used for the first 12 to 24 hours applied throughout their hospitalization.
5. All infants should be examined by a physician within 24 hours of birth and within the 24 hours before discharge. In nurseries where babies are discharged within 3 days of birth, two examinations should be required within 72 hours.
6. Caps and masks should not be required in the nursery. Short-sleeved gowns and hand-to-elbow washing techniques should be used by all visiting personnel. Scrub gowns or freshly laundered uniforms should be worn by nurses.
7. Regular monthly bacteriologic monitoring protocols should be instituted.

8. An area for emergency resuscitation with appropriate equipment, suction equipment, and oxygen must be available in each nursery and available on a portable basis for rooming-in arrangements.

TRANSITIONAL CARE NURSERY—TYPE II CARE
Characteristics of patients

Unless also qualifying for type III care, patients admitted to this unit should include:
A. Infants of high-risk mothers
   1. Maternal toxemia, preeclampsia, and eclampsia
   2. Maternal diabetes
   3. Maternal cardiac or pulmonary disease
   4. Maternal hypertension
   5. Maternal drug addiction
   6. Prepartum mothers with fever or evidence of infection
   7. Rh-negative mothers with positive history and present evidence of sensitization
   8. Mothers under 15 or over 40 years of age
   9. Mothers whose infants were delivered by cesarean section
   10. Grand multiparas
   11. Mothers with evidence of polyhydramnios or oligohydramnios
   12. Mothers with any other major medical or surgical complication (for example, thyrotoxicosis, hepatitis, or sickle cell disease)
B. Infants with birth weights from 750 to 2,250 gm
C. Infants with birth weights over 4,000 gm
D. Infants with gestational age by last menstrual period over 42 weeks
E. Infants with birth weight below the tenth percentile or above the ninetieth percentile for gestational age

Personnel
Registered nurses

At least one registered nurse must be in attendance on each shift and should be part of the pediatric nursing service and have no nursing responsibilities other than those related to care of these infants. The overall responsibilities should include the availability and continued maintenance of all emergency equipment.

Paramedical personnel (practical nurses, aides, and others)

These additional personnel must be available to provide a final total personnel-to-patient ratio of 1:3. The nurses working in this unit must have special training in cardiopulmonary resuscitation, be proficient in cardiac and respiratory monitoring, and be able to assist with procedures, including intubation, umbilical vessel catheterization, and lumbar punctures. The nurses also must be trained to care for infants requiring assisted ventilation for 2 to 3 hours.

Pediatrician

The pediatrician in charge should have additional training in the management of high-risk infants. In coordination with the senior nursing staff, the pediatrician should establish guidelines that will determine the ultimate location of most patients admitted to this unit and review the admissions daily to monitor the appropriateness of the previous day's transfers. When questions arise about particular patients, the physician or a designee should evaluate the patient before a final disposition.

Facilities and services

1. Infants can be cared for in an area either completely separated or contiguous to the well baby nursery or the NICU. This area may be located in the delivery suite.
2. Care in this area requires 40 to 50 square feet per infant. There should be 4 feet on all sides between bassinets and/or incubators in this area. Infants requiring intermediate care can be located in a single large room or smaller rooms with sufficient space to house three infants, since this level of care requires a nurse for every three patients.
3. Since approximately 3 to 4.5 infants per 100 deliveries require the services of such a unit, a specific hospital's needs should be based on annual delivery rate and the short duration of admission. Maximum capacity should rarely exceed four beds even in the largest perinatal centers.
4. Basic equipment for this area should include all the items required for type I care, in addition to incubators, appropriate monitoring equipment, and respirators.
5. Infusion pumps should be used to control administration of fluids.
6. There should be four to six electrical outlets, two oxygen outlets, two compressed air outlets, and two suction outlets per patient care area.
7. The hospital's laboratory should provide the same support as that for type I care. In addition, it should provide acid-base, blood urea nitrogen, and PaO_2 determinations on a 24-hour basis.
8. A portable roentgen unit with trained technicians must be available to provide radiologic studies in the unit.

Medical policy and administration

1. Hospitals with more than 1,000 deliveries per year should provide this level of care.
2. Administrative policies for type I care are applicable.
3. The duration of stay depends on the functional capability of the unit. Some type II nurseries provide care only slightly more complex than a type I nursery; the duration of stay in this type of unit should be limited to less than 6 to 8 hours with subsequent transfer to type I or type III care. In other type II nurseries with capabilities approaching type III care the duration of stay may have no limitations, but guidelines should be established by the unit in conjunction with its supporting type III nursery. Premature infants with birth weights of 1,500 to 2,500 gm should be cared for in a specific area located adjacent to either the NICU or the regular nursery.
4. A transport module that provides oxygen, maintains temperature, and allows easy access to the infant should be available for transfer of infants between areas.

NEONATAL INTENSIVE CARE NURSERY—TYPE III CARE
Characteristics of patients

Infants admitted to this area should include:
1. Any infant 4 weeks or less of age who requires intensive care. Occasionally older infants who are small and have special nursing needs (for example, intravenous alimentation of a 3-month-old baby with a short bowel syndrome) may be admitted to this area and cared for in an incubator.
2. All infants with birth weights less than 1,500 gm. If such infants are otherwise normal after 24 to 48 hours, they may require less intensive observation. However, they must be cared for by a staff with skill and experience in feeding and observing low birth weight or premature infants. It may be convenient to group these infants in a subunit of the neonatal intensive care nursery.
3. Any infant less than 4 weeks of age who requires surgery (exclusive of circumcision).
4. Infants with sepsis, meningitis, pneumonia, syphylis, or other infections may remain in this area at the discretion of the director of the nursery with institution of appropriate isolation procedures.

Personnel
Registered nurses

There should be a 2:1 patient-to-nurse ratio with 1:1 ratio for the sickest infants (for example, an infant requiring mechanical ventilation). Nurses in this area should have no other assignments outside this nursery unless it is on regular rotation to a type II nursery. All nurses in this area should have a closely supervised, well-controlled orientation program with its duration suited to the needs of the particular nurse; nurses without this orientation should not work in this area.

Paramedical personnel (practical nurses and aides)

These personnel should assist in the routine aspects of care, freeing the registered nurses for more technical duties and for more intensive care of the sickest infants.

Physician

The director of this unit should be a full-time perinatologist. Twenty-four hour in-hospital coverage by a pediatric resident staff or a pediatrician is essential, and consultants must be available in all medical and surgical specialities.

Facilities and services

1. Infants must be cared for in an area that is separated from the well baby nursery, but the area may be contiguous to the transitional care nursery. In designing new units this area should be adjacent to the delivery suites if possible. Older hospitals may be unable to rearrange existing facilities to provide this access at reasonable costs.
2. A minimum of 80 square feet per infant is needed to provide this care; 100 per infant is ideal.
3. Approximately 1 to 1.5 infants per 1,000 deliveries will need intensive care.
4. This area should have all the equipment required for type II care in addition to more extensive monitoring facilities; the question of using open versus closed (incubator) care for sick infants should be resolved by the physician in charge.
5. There should be 12 to 16 electrical outlets, three to four oxygen and compressed air outlets, and three suction sources for each infant.
6. The hospital laboratory must provide all the determinations needed for type I and type II care. In addition to 24-hour service for the aforementioned, determinations of phosphorus, magnesium, and total protein levels, platelet counts, and coagulation studies should be available. Where delays in acid-base determinations and particularly Pao_2 are unavoidable because of location of the laboratories or limitation of personnel, a unit to measure pH, Po_2, and Pco_2 should be available within the nursery.
7. Roentgenographic facilities and trained personnel should be provided on a 24-hour basis for the unit.

Medical policy and administration

1. Hospitals with more than 3,000 deliveries per year should establish intensive care nurseries or have regularized means of transfer to a nearby unit.
2. Administration and medical care of patients in this area should be the responsibility of the director of the unit.
3. Provisions should be made to ensure admission for sick infants transferred from smaller services; interhospital transportation of sick infants should be done to provide regional coverage and should be closely supervised by the director of this unit.

TRANSPORT UNITS

See p. 5.

Ideally, infants at high risk should be delivered in institutions capable of providing intensive care from the moment of delivery. Nonetheless, it is estimated that 40% of neonatal problems are at present unpredictable. To provide for such emergencies, an effective transport system with specially trained nursing personnel is essential. The early transfer of unexpected high-risk infants to a special care unit significantly alters neonatal morbidity and mortality. Much can be done to protect the infant from the risks involved in such a transfer and to ensure the infant's condition during the transfer. Transport facilities capable of initiating therapy in a critically ill infant before effecting transfer to a regional special care unit may be required.

HOSPITAL UNITS
Physical facilities
Lighting

Lighting should allow easy detection of both cyanosis and jaundice and is best provided by fluorescent bulbs emitting 100 to 150 foot-candles' illuminance at the infant's bedside. This intensity also will alleviate the problem of shadows within the nursery. Spotlights may be provided in selected locations with either portable lamps containing two 150-W fluorescent bulbs or by ceiling- or wall-mounted spotlights. Such white infrared lamps provide warmth as well as light; ceiling mounting of these lamps permits procedures to be done outside the incubator without the infant losing heat to the environment. The use of blue lighting in nurseries has been limited because of frequent complaints of nausea and dizziness from personnel working in these units. (See Chapter 30 for discussion of phototherapy.)

Walls

True skin color is best seen in nurseries with walls that are beige or white; brighter tones of blue and yellow interfere with the ability to evaluate jaundice and cyanosis.

Because of problems with temperature regulation in sick infants and reports of heat loss or overwarming in selected infants, some authorities have suggested elimination of outside windows from neonatal intensive care areas. However, nurseries without windows create an additional mental strain on personnel that may negate the thermal advantages. Air insulation between two glass panes will reduce severe variations in temperature and is a compromise when windows are present. Outside awnings in parts of the country where radiant heat gain is a problem also reduce the chance of overheating.

Storage

Nursing efficiency is increased in a unit where easy accessibility to disposable supplies is guaranteed by design of the unit; modular storage walls can be effectively used to this end. Storage areas for bulky equipment, such as respirators, incubators, and phototherapy lamps, should be available near the nursery.

Temperature control and ventilation

The air temperature in nurseries should be maintained between 72° to 76° F (22° to 26° C) with the relative humidity 35% to 60%. These temperature and humidity ranges prevent excessive heat loss or gain for the infant and ensure personnel comfort.

The American Academy of Pediatrics suggests a minimum of 12 changes of room air per hour for control of infection. The fresh air input should be located either on or near the ceiling, with the exhaust outlet near the floor; the ventilation unit for the NICU should be separated from the remainder of the hospital system. A slight positive pressure differential between the unit and adjacent hallways should exist within the ventilation system. Most nurseries also incorporate an air-conditioning system within the ventilation system. Attention to filtering outside air with adherence to established standards is particularly important in urban nurseries where polluted air is an increasing ecologic problem.

Laminar flow provides direct vertical, sterile air flow more efficiently than currently used ventilation systems. Recently constructed newborn centers have successfully incorporated laminar flow systems into their units without any reported changes in the incidence of nosocomial infections.

Oxygen and compressed air

Oxygen and compressed air are generally supplied to the intensive care unit from a central source. The capability to provide mixtures of air and oxygen producing concentrations from 21% to 100% must be available. These mixtures should be available at atmospheric pressure and pressures up to 50 psi in units where positive pressure ventilators are used. Warning devices to alert personnel to falls in pressure should be part of each system. Compressed air systems require detailed planning and meticulous care once they are operational. Air should be washed, filtered, and then dehumidified before delivery into the system. All intakes must be closely checked to minimize the introduction of contaminated air. Small compressor units are unreliable and should be avoided; also compressor units should be operated pneumatically and not electrically, because of an increasing number of power failures in some urban areas.

Acoustics

Design of intensive care units should use available methods of sound dampening. Monitors, respirators, ventilation systems, and incubators all create noise, and at the present time no safe level of noise has been established. By restricting the noise level within the nursery and within the incubator to less than 75 dB, the hearing of both personnel and patients may be protected.

Electricity (p. 286)

The medical profession is often uninformed of electrical hazards (cardiac arrests, burns, and so on) related to the use of monitors, and hospitals used to have no routine safety testing procedures appropriate for patient safety. In an attempt to minimize electrical hazards, certain recommendations can be made. The use of a single ground of low-resistance wire is particularly effective when connected to all outlets in the nursery. Frequent checking of the integrity of this ground and all wiring will prevent the hazard of stray electrical currents. When more than one piece of electrical equipment is used, there must be enough outlets at each incubator to accommodate the equipment, with all units connected to a common ground. Before installation and at regular monthly intervals subsequently all electrical equipment should be tested and maintained by a qualified engineer to detect defective equipment and current leakage and to specify appropriate safety precautions. Plugs on all equipment should be hospital grade, and extension cords, adapters, and junction boxes must not be used. No piece of equipment should exceed a leakage of more than 10 μA, and a leakage of 100 μA for a combination of devices must be avoided. The amount of leakage that is safe for the newborn remains unknown.

An appropriate number of the electrical outlets in the nursery must be on the hospital's emergency circuit to maintain life support systems. In-service training programs should be maintained to educate all nursery personnel in the proper use of equipment and recognition of potential electrical hazards. All new equipment should be checked for proper insulation and approved by a qualified engineer *before* use in a clinical area, regardless of previous approvals by the manufacturer.

Wash basins

There should be a wash basin adjacent to the door in each area and one basin for each four to six incubators. All basins should have foot, knee, or remote controls for hot and cold water and soap. Scrub brushes and paper towels should be conveniently placed near each basin.

Equipment

Apnea monitors (pp. 122 and 284)

The availability of an increasing array of monitors has improved the care of the high-risk infant but has placed additional responsibilities on all personnel. The concept of a central nursing area with centralized monitoring, although quite useful in adult coronary units, has not been generally accepted in newborn units.

Most apnea monitors use the principle of impedance pneumography and present problems in proper application and maintenance of leads. The size of the electrodes, the irritation of the electrode paste or tape or both, and the lack of flat areas on the infant for application are recurrent problems for the nursery staff. The technique of applying electrodes to the arm of the sick infant provides a solution to this problem.

Cardiac monitor (pp. 119 and 277)

Cardiac monitors either record the heart rate on an established scale or display the electrocardiographic figure on an oscilloscope. Rate changes indicate both ventilation problems and cardiovascular instability. The technical problems of electrode placement and grounding are common to all cardiac monitors. The proper application of the electrode ensures conductivity at the interfaces and minimizes false alarms or alarm failures; with currently available systems, proper application of leads on the small infant is less of a problem for the nursing staff.

Blood pressure recorders (p. 126)

Continuous blood pressure monitoring by direct recording with arterial catheters through a transducer is often used in NICUs. This mode of monitoring demands an awareness of the increased hazard of blood loss, infection, and electrocution and of the need for adequate safeguards. The transcutaneous Doppler method for measuring blood pressure provides a simple, noninvasive method for monitoring blood pressure. The Doppler method detects very weak impulses that the sphygmomanometer would be unable to detect. Correlations with the direct measurement of blood pressure are firmly established, but the determinations are intermittent, which is a disadvantage in acute situations.

Incubators (p. 259)

Thermal protection, reverse isolation, and complete visual observation of high-risk infants are possible with the use of incubators. The inspired air in such units is filtered, protecting the infant from airborne infections; but the infant, if infected, can still expire contaminated air into the incubator and nursery, placing infants outside incubators in jeopardy.

Ideally incubators should permit easy access to the infant; thus the open-front incubator with a movable patient tray is superior to a unit with a back hinge and front posts in allowing immediate access to the infant. Access holes for intravenous lines, monitor wires, suction tubing, and respirator apparatus also are required.

Monitors and infusion pumps often are placed on the top of an incubator; this may damage them, impair visual observation of the infant, and cause delays in gaining access to the infant in emergencies. A shelf attached to the incubator itself or mounted on the wall above each unit should be used to avoid accidentally dislodging equipment from the hood of the incubator.

Oxygen or humidity or both may be provided by the incubator itself or by means of a head box placed within it. The hazard of waterborne organisms and the cost of nursing time to clean water traps should be carefully weighed against the benefits of and need for additional humidity. Each nursery should have a clean, warm incubator on standby at all times for unexpected admissions and emergencies. There also should be a regular check of all incubators to safeguard against electrical hazards.

Bassinets

Bassinets should allow examination and care of the infant and be easy to clean; each unit should provide a storage area beneath the bassinet for disposable items used in the routine care of infants. A complete, functional unit for each infant provides an additional safeguard against cross-infection within the nursery.

Laboratory support

Intensive care units require responsive and rapid chemistry, bacteriology, and radiology laboratory support; the closer such facilities are to the intensive care area, the more efficient and responsive they are. Continuous communication between the intensive care unit and paramedical laboratory personnel regarding the exact nature of the clinical problems ensures a more responsive laboratory and minimizes the problems asssociated with a heavy demand on the laboratory staff. Regular conferences with laboratory personnel to explain the common problems of the newborn have proved very useful in many nurseries.

Microchemical techniques should be available 24 hours a day in the intensive care facility. The availability of a blood gas analyzer within the intensive care area ensures immediate results as a basis for prompt changes in therapy. The obvious disadvantages of blood gas services provided by nonlaboratory personnel is poor quality control. Because of the legitimate need for this capability within intensive care units, clinical pathology services have assumed responsibility in some units with their own laboratory personnel.

The bacteriology laboratory should employ culture

and sensitivity techniques that allow rapid identification of pathogens and their antibiotic sensitivities. If the bacteriology laboratory is not near the unit, the provision of a microscope, appropriate stains, and a small incubator will facilitate diagnostic evaluations and improve the efficiency of the staff.

A portable roentgen unit in the intensive care area ensures immediate roentgenologic support while simultaneously avoiding the hazards of hypothermia and hypoxia, which may be involved in the transport of a sick infant to the radiology department (Chapter 39). Newer magnification techniques promise improved quality of roentgenograms and more exact definition of radiologic signs. Proper shielding of patients and personnel is vital. With modern portable collimated roentgen units, light localizers, and proper technique there should be little radiation scatter beyond the light field.

Control of environment

The establishment of stringent microbiologic environmental control has been the most significant factor in reduction of nosocomial infections in nurseries. Critical evaluation of these controls should be continued, although recent studies permit some modification of previously established standards. Before altering existing procedures and techniques, personnel must realistically compare the type of hospital (for example, university) where the study was conducted with their own institution. Many smaller hospitals have very wisely demanded the continuation of established environmental controls, acknowledging inherent differences between their own facilities and those where innovations have been initiated.

Gowning procedures in nurseries are either strict or modified. The strict version requires physicians and paramedical personnel other than the nursing staff to remove outer coats and jewelry, to scrub hand to elbow, and to gown before entering the unit; nurses change from nursing uniforms to scrub gowns. When the nursing staff leaves the unit for other parts of the hospital, they should wear long-sleeved gowns over their scrub dress and discard them on return to the nursery.

In modified gowning, personnel may enter the unit without changing their outer garments but before examination of an infant must remove their coats and vigorously scrub to the elbow. If an infant is to be removed from the incubator (his own microenvironment), the person must wear a surgical gown that is discarded after completion of the examination. Many authorities still believe that incubators should be employed if the modified gowning procedure is used, but there is disagreement on this point. However, it is mandatory that nurseries adopting modified gowning procedures supervise and strictly enforce other basic environmental controls.

Thorough hand washing eliminates the most common route of cross-infection within nurseries. It requires accessible antiseptic agents and a sufficient number and proper location of wash basins. A diluted (less than 3%) solution of hexachlorophene is frequently used for personnel, even though the iodophors are superior because of their additional effectiveness against gram-negative organisms. Proper technique for washing calls for rolling sleeves above the elbow, initially washing hand to elbow for 2 minutes and repeating the wash a second time for 15 to 30 seconds. Because of cutaneous sensitizing effects of the iodine-containing compounds, nurseries that use these compounds as the primary agent always should have a second solution readily available.

In addition to gowning and thorough hand washing, random periodic bacteriologic surveillance of intensive care units and personnel offers an additional safeguard against nursery epidemics. However, a survey that is too extensive not only overtaxes the laboratory but also provides little useful information for personnel. Spot checks, unannounced to the staff, serve as an effective method for checking efficacy of disinfectant procedures.

The cleaning of equipment requires establishment of specific, detailed guidelines that are well known to all personnel. The aim of cleaning most equipment is disinfection (killing or decreasing the number of organisms known to be the potential cause of infection), but sterilization (killing of all organisms) is mandatory for certain items, such as surgical instruments. Gas sterilization has been recommended as the ideal solution to the problems of cleaning and disinfection, but such a gas system is unavailable in most hospitals at the present time. The most commonly used disinfectants are iodophors, chlorine compounds, phenolic compounds, and glutaraldehyde. Caution must be exercised to follow directions with certain phenolic disinfectants. A recently reported increased incidence of hyperbilirubinemia in a hospital nursery was traced to excessive use of a phenolic disinfectant in greater concentrations than recommended. In addition, the nursery was inadequately ventilated; this promoted atmospheric contamination with the detergent. When ventilation defects were corrected and the disinfectant was used properly, the epidemic ceased. Before disinfection of equipment thorough cleaning is necessary to remove dust particles and grease that may partially inactivate the disinfectant. Supervisory personnel should check the disinfectant procedure itself as well as periodically culture recently disinfected equipment. Specific guidelines for cleaning various equipment used in intensive care units are available in a manual of the American Academy of Pediatrics on hospital care of newborns. Meticulous attention to details and supervision of the technique of all personnel are critical for safe, effective microbiologic control.

Temperature control (p. 259)

Appropriate temperature regulation reduces infant mortality, particulary in premature infants. Most incubators control temperature by using a fan to circulate warm air (forced convection). The air temperature in the incubator should approximate the neutral thermal state. In these units the temperature is controlled by a cutaneous thermistor, usually secured over the liver, which regulates a fan within the incubator. Careful placement of the thermistor is essential to ensure proper recording of the abdominal skin temperature and to avoid errors introduced by loose placement. Improper placement results in artifacts produced by changes in posture or introduction of moisture through bathing or urination.

There is generally some warming beyond the set point, and previous reports indicated an increased incidence of apnea during the warming phase of the incubator. For this reason some investigators have suggested a radiant heat source rather than forced convection, since the former generally provides more sustained, less oscillating heat. The predominance of the forced convection units represents the manufacturers' decisions apparently based on technical and commercial considerations.

The use of the servo controlled incubator alters the normal changes in body temperature that occur with infection. Fever interrupts the feedback loop in the servo controlled unit so that high skin temperature causes incubator cooling. For this reason incubator air temperature must be monitored carefully.

The recent introduction into many units of open radiant warmers demands meticulous attention to control infection, the increased insensible water losses, and possible cooling effects of convective air currents within the nursery. Servomechanisms must be used with these units to minimize fluctuations in body temperature.

Whether cots or incubators are used, it is possible to calculate the air temperature that provides each infant adequate warmth and simultaneously limits the caloric expenditure. Tables 19-4 and 19-5 present the recent recommendations of the American Academy of Pediatrics of useful guidelines for this often neglected aspect of newborn care.

Generally, the relative humidity in the incubator should be kept in the range of 30% to 60%. In many units the ambient humidity is sufficient to maintain the desired humidity within the incubator without use of the water reservoir. This arrangement avoids the risk of contaminating the incubator with waterborne organisms. Attention to this detail is particularly important with the very low birth weight infant. Because low humidity increases heat loss, the addition of humidity may result in easier control of air temperature within the incubator and better control of infant temperature.

Table 19-4. Incubator air temperatures—first 24 hours

Birth weight		Temperatures			
		°C		°F	
Grams	Pounds	Median	± range	Median	± range
	1	35.5	0.5	96.0	0.9
500		35.5	0.5	96.0	0.9
	2	35.0	0.5	95.0	0.9
1,000		34.9	0.5	94.9	0.9
	3	34.2	0.5	93.6	0.9
1,500		34.0	0.5	93.2	0.9
	4	33.7	0.5	92.7	0.9
2,000		33.5	0.5	92.3	0.9
	5	33.3	0.7	92.0	1.3
2,500		33.2	0.8	91.8	1.4
	6	33.1	0.9	91.6	1.6
3,000		33.0	1.0	91.4	1.8
	7	32.9	1.1	91.2	1.9
3,500		32.8	1.2	91.0	2.1
	8	32.8	1.3	91.0	2.3
4,000		32.6	1.4	90.7	2.5
	9	32.5	1.4	90.5	2.5

From Standards and recommendations for hospital care of new infants, ed. 6, Evanston, Ill., 1977, American Academy of Pediatrics, p. 90.
These tables are recommended for use as a guide when relative humidity is approximately 50%. Temperature should be higher than that in the table for lower humidity and altered in either direction, depending on various factors in the thermal environment and the individual infant's requirements.
Adapted and modified from data published by Scopes and Ahmed and Oliver.

Oxygen therapy

The administration of oxygen to newborns requires clinical judgment supported by laboratory determinations. The use of cyanosis alone as a guide to the amount of oxygen that should be administered is potentially hazardous both in terms of underestimating (hypoxic brain injury) and exceeding (retrolental fibroplasia) the oxygen demands of a sick infant. The potential complications of oxygen therapy must be weighed against the risks involved in arterial catheterization. In institutions where physicians and nurses are inexperienced with technique, where laboratory support is inadequate, and where transfer to a special care center is impossible, clinical judgment of physical signs alone must be an acceptable compromise. In such cases, by gradually lowering the ambient oxygen concentration to a point where cyanosis is clinically detectable and then increasing the concentration by 10%, the physician has a rough guideline for both preventing hypoxia and avoiding hyperoxia. Regardless of existent institutional limitations, a general knowledge of the physiologic principle governing oxygen therapy is essential for any physician caring for sick infants.

When laboratory service and technical skill with umbilical artery catheterization are available, more exact

Table 19-5. Incubator air temperatures according to age

	Birth weight							
	Under 1,500 gm (3 lb, 5 oz)				1,501 to 2,500 gm (3 lb, 5 oz, to 5 lb, 8 oz)				Over 36 weeks' gestation and over 2,500 gm (5 lb, 8 oz)	
	°C Median ± range		°F Median ± range		°C Median ± range		°F Median ± range		°C Median ± range		°F Median ± range	
Age												
1 day	34.3	0.4	93.8	0.7	33.4	0.6	92.1	1.1	33.0	1.0	91.4	1.8
2 day	33.7	0.5	92.7	0.9	32.7	0.9	90.9	1.6	32.4	1.3	90.4	2.3
3 day	33.5	0.5	92.3	0.9	32.4	0.9	90.4	1.6	31.9	1.3	89.4	2.3
4 day	33.5	0.5	92.3	0.9	32.3	0.9	90.2	1.6	31.5	1.3	88.6	2.3
5 day	33.5	0.5	92.3	0.9	32.2	0.9	90.0	1.6	31.2	1.3	88.1	2.3
6 day	33.5	0.5	92.3	0.9	32.1	0.9	89.8	1.6	30.9	1.3	87.6	2.3
7 day	33.5	0.5	92.3	0.9	32.1	0.9	89.8	1.6	30.8	1.4	87.4	2.5
8 day	33.5	0.5	92.3	0.9	32.1	0.9	89.8	1.6	30.6	1.4	87.0	2.5
9 day	33.5	0.5	92.3	0.9	32.1	0.9	89.8	1.6	30.4	1.4	86.7	2.5
10 day	33.5	0.5	92.3	0.9	32.1	0.9	89.8	1.6	30.2	1.5	86.4	2.7
11 day	33.5	0.5	92.3	0.9	32.1	0.9	89.8	1.6	29.9	1.5	85.8	2.7
12 day	33.5	0.5	92.3	0.9	32.1	0.9	89.8	1.6	29.5	1.6	85.1	2.8
13 day	33.5	0.5	92.3	0.9	32.1	0.9	89.8	1.6	29.2	1.6	84.6	2.8
14 day	33.4	0.6	92.1	1.1	32.1	0.9	89.8	1.6				
15 day	33.3	0.7	92.0	1.3	32.0	0.9	89.6	1.6				
4 weeks	32.9	0.8	91.2	1.4	31.7	1.1	89.0	1.9				
5 weeks	32.1	0.7	89.3	1.3	31.1	1.1	87.9	1.9				
6 weeks	31.8	0.6	89.2	1.1	30.6	1.1	87.1	1.9				
7 weeks	31.1	0.6	87.9	1.1	30.1	1.1	86.2	1.9				

From Standards and recommendations for hospital care of newborn infants, ed. 6, Evanston, Ill., 1977, American Academy of Pediatrics. See footnotes to Table 19-4.

determination of the oxygenation of a sick infant is possible. The transport and delivery of oxygen to the tissues is a complex process involving many factors: PaO_2, hemoglobin concentration, oxygen content, tissue perfusion, and affinity of hemoglobin for oxygen. Periodic measurement of PaO_2, hemoglobin, and pH, in addition to close clinical observation, is the most reasonable and accurate approach to minimizing the risk of both hyperoxic and hypoxic insults to a sick infant. When arterial catheterization is contraindicated, radial or brachial artery puncture can be used, but repeated sampling from these sites requires skill and experience. In infants with mild respiratory distress not requiring arterial catheterization and in infants suspected of having significant right-to-left shunts, these sites for sampling are particularly useful.

Recent advances in noninvasive techniques to monitor arterial blood oxygen tension should decrease the need for umbilical and peripheral artery catheterization. Studies have demonstrated that, with adequate skin perfusion, the correlation between arterial oxygen tension and transcutaneous oxygen tension is very close (p. 430). The obvious immediate advantage of the transcutaneous measurement is that it provides a continuous recording of oxygen tension as opposed to the intermittent values provided by the other methods. The transcutaneous method has been particularly helpful in weaning infants from ventilation and avoiding recurrent hypoxia during care. However, sick infants still require accurate monitoring of blood pressure as part of their care, thus necessitating umbilical artery catheterization. But in less acutely ill infants transcutaneous measurement of oxygen tension will prevent the risks of arterial catheterization while providing accurate recording of oxygen levels.

When it is determined that an infant requires supplemental oxygen in spite of its potential hazards, the delivery of oxygen should be carefully controlled and monitored. When small increases in ambient oxygen are required, direct delivery into the incubator often suffices. With concentrations exceeding 30% a head box within the incubator more accurately provides the correct concentration, while simultaneously limiting significant fluctuations in oxygen, especially when the incubator ports are opened. Some incubators have cut-off mechanisms to prevent administration of oxygen exceeding a preset concentration. In general, these controls cannot be relied on independently, and the ambient oxygen concentration should be checked at regular intervals by a paramagnetic oxygen analyzer or continuously monitored by means of an oxygen electrode. Orders for oxygen therapy should never be written in terms of flow (that is, liters per minute) but rather in terms of the desired ambient concentration with indicated intervals for routinely checking the concentration.

Oxygen should be humidified and warmed before delivery to a sick infant. If dry gas is administered to a patient, it will be humidified by evaporation from the respiratory mucosa. Under normal circumstances this process presents no problem; but in a sick infant, particularly with respiratory distress, difficulties arise. By drying the respiratory mucosa, the viscosity of pulmonary secretions is increased, and effective ciliary action is impaired. With these changes in major airways, airway resistance, already increased in most infants, may be further increased. Such therapy also may aggravate problems of water balance by significantly increasing insensible water losses from the respiratory tract. Oxygen that is not warmed also may present a significant cold stress to the premature infant. There is a marked increase in oxygen consumption with the delivery of cold air to the face.

Oxygen may be humidified and warmed through the use of humidifiers and, on occasion, nebulizers. Humidifiers are designed to produce a maximum amount of water vapor, whereas nebulizers produce water particles of a particular size. Infants requiring nasotracheal intubation need humidifiers in their ventilation, whereas babies who are breathing spontaneously in head boxes and who have copious secretions often are treated with nebulizers. With nebulizers exact control of humidity, condensation of water in the tubing, and difficulty of sterilization are common problems. The latter problem and the small droplet size produced by nebulizers have been suggested as possible explanations for the increased incidence of pulmonary infections in patients on respirators. Humidifiers are not difficult to sterilize and therefore are less likely to promote pulmonary infections, but they too are plagued with problems of condensation of water within gas lines and difficulty in controlling the temperature of the gas as it is delivered to the patient. Recent engineering improvements have alleviated the latter problem, but condensation remains a nuisance and demands nursing attention and time for observing and removing partial obstructions caused by condensed water.

FEEDING

The advantage of early feedings in maintaining normal metabolism and growth during the transition from fetal to extrauterine life is clear (p. 308). As soon as an infant can safely tolerate enteral nutrition, feedings should be initiated. This approach may decrease the incidence of problems such as hypoglycemia, hyperkalemia, hyperbilirubinemia, and azotemia. In the regular nursery most infants are left without feedings for the first 6 hours of life. At this time an initial feeding of sterile water is offered, and, if tolerated, the breast or formula of choice is offered subsequently. Animal studies of the pulmonary findings after aspiration have demonstrated equally severe tissue reaction to glucose water and milk formula. When there is any question about tolerance of feeding because of physical or neurologic status of the infant, feeding should be withheld and parenteral fluids substituted.

Most term infants will rapidly progress from 30 ml every 3 to 4 hours to 75 to 90 ml before discharge at 4 to 5 days of life. Vigorous premature infants may require smaller (5 to 10 ml) feedings at more frequent intervals (every 2 hours) before progressing to larger, less frequent feedings. Caution and judgment must be continuously exercised in advancing the feedings of a premature infant. Rigid feeding schedules should be avoided, and the initial small volume should be fed gradually and cautiously increased. The rate of increase that is well tolerated varies considerably from infant to infant.

Parenteral fluids

Regardless of birth weight, if the neurologic or physical status of the infant prohibits early feeding, parenteral fluid therapy, rather than starvation, is indicated (p. 308). The physician must select the intravenous route that minimizes complications and allows the infusate to be delivered with maximum efficiency. In the newborn the sites routinely used include peripheral veins on the hand or foot, scalp veins, the antecubital veins, and the umbilical vessels. If these sites have been exhausted, a venous cutdown may be performed; most frequently the saphenous vein is used. The technical expertise and previous experience of the individual physician usually determine the infusion site.

Hypodermoclysis should be abandoned as a route of parenteral therapy. If a saline-glucose solution is infused under the skin, it must enter the functional extracellular fluid to be effective. In dehydration, blood flow is reduced, and thus the rate at which the subcutaneous fluid can enter the circulation is decreased. Furthermore in some patients not only does the fluid remain in the extravascular tissue but also sodium and water leave the blood volume and enter the clysis fluid, increasing the likelihood of circulatory collapse.

Peripheral veins on the dorsal aspect of the hand or the foot, antecubital veins, and scalp veins are readily available in most newborns for routine parenteral therapy. However, veins on the flexor surfaces of the wrist and dorsum of the foot should be avoided, if possible, when peripheral alimentation solutions are used. Infiltration with these solutions, if not immediately noted, may cause cutaneous sloughing and damage to underlying tendons.

The care used in starting the infusion, the subsequent nursing care, and the contents of the infusate are factors in determining the duration of use of each infusion site. The administration of hypertonic alkaline or acid solutions through a peripheral vein diminishes the duration of the effective use of that particular site. Because the scalp generally has an abundant supply of superficial veins, these veins have become the most popular route for intravenous delivery of fluids in most nurseries. When approaching these vessels, the physician should exercise caution to avoid the fontanels, bony prominences, and small arteries. Nursery personnel should scrutinize each infusion site frequently to ensure its maximum longevity. If extravasation of acid, alkaline, hypertonic, or calcium-containing solution goes undetected, necrosis and sloughing of the involved area may occur with an increased risk of infection. In critically ill infants requiring long-term parenteral therapy a venous cutdown often is performed. In infants receiving intravenous alimentation Dudrick's method for placing a catheter in the superior vena cava has demonstrated that aseptic technique during insertion of the catheter and meticulous care thereafter will allow constant, long-term infusion of a hypertonic, acidic (pH, 5.5) solution with minimum risk of infection.

Umbilical vessels

The sick neonate receiving supportive oxygen therapy as an intrinsic part of treatment requires careful, continuous monitoring of the PaO$_2$. Even though peripheral arteries (brachial, radial, and temporal) are available, the umbilical artery allows simple insertion of a catheter for continuous monitoring of blood gases. Employing the standards of Dunn (Fig. 19-19), the physician threads the catheter to a position 1 cm above the diaphragm (or at the level of L3 below the renal arteries) and carefully secures it with suture or tape. The position then is verified radiologically. Umbilical artery catheterization demands constant observation of the umbilicus for bleeding, meticulous care of the catheter to prevent propagation of thrombus or air embolism, continuous scrutiny of the lower extremities for evidence of arterial spasm (cyanosis or blanching), and limitation of the catheterization to a period as short as the clinical course allows.

The catheter should be removed cautiously to allow proximal arterial spasm for hemostasis. The acute and chronic risks of using the umbilical artery catheter should be carefully considered and weighed against the advantages for each individual patient; this route should not be used for routine parenteral therapy.

Realizing the potential complications of the umbilical artery catheter and assuming that there is little risk in using the umbilical vein, many physicians have adopted the latter route for parenteral therapy. Accessibility, technical ease of inserting the catheter, and longevity of the umbilical vein catheter are obvious advantages to this site. However, the umbilical vein catheter may easily pass into the portal vein, and the administration of sodium bicarbonate through the catheter creates the risk of infusing a hypertonic and strongly alkaline solution directly into the liver. One necropsy series reported a significant incidence (33%) of hemorrhagic liver necrosis in patients receiving tromethamine via the umbilical vein. Umbilical vein phlebitis, pyemia, and pulmonary embolus were noted by Scott in infants whose therapy was delivered via umbilical vein catheters. Colonic perforation and peritonitis in infants following exchange transfusion via the umbilical vein also have been noted. Thus this route of intravascular therapy should be used only when no other is available.

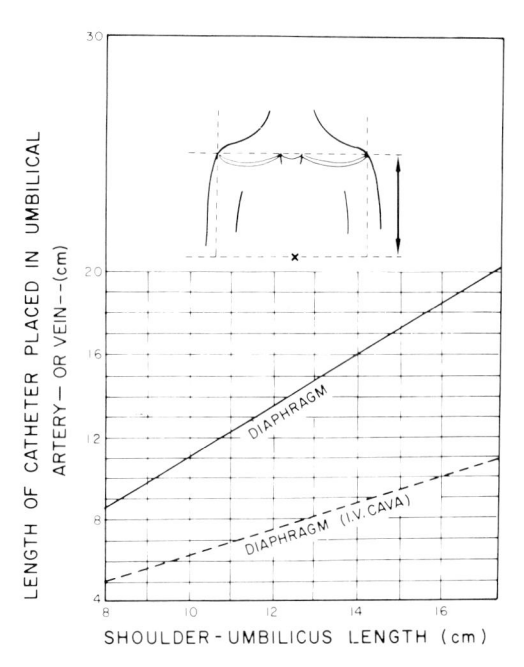

Fig. 19-19. Guide for placement of umbilical catheters.

Regardless of the route selected for therapy, certain recommendations are generally applicable. The advantages of the selected route must be weighed against its risks; there must be use of the proper technique in starting the infusion to minimize hazards, to safeguard its continuation, and to promote its longevity; proper nursing observation is required during the infusion, including maintenance of intravenous flow records and frequent inspection of the infusion site; and peristaltic pumps should be used to ensure constant flow and to minimize the chance of overhydration of a sick infant.

Gavage feeding (p. 308)

Many debilitated infants who are unable to suck and swallow adequately have evidence of active peristalsis (stools and bowel sounds). Various temporizing measures have been attempted to avoid the complications of parenteral fluid therapy and to take advantage of the infant's functioning intestinal tract. Gavage feeding is the oldest and most established of these techniques but is not entirely free of hazards. In addition to changes in heart rate and blood pressure during passage of the gavage tube, the tube itself may be an obstruction to respiration, particularly in the premature infant. The practice of passing a gavage tube before each feeding as opposed to an indwelling tube changed daily depends on the capability and experience of the nursing staff; with an experienced nurse the indwelling tube is not essential. When nasogastric feedings are used, the residual gastric aspirate should be noted before each feeding and recorded as a guide to the infant's likely tolerance of the volume of food offered.

A gastrostomy may be helpful in the postoperative period after gastrointestinal surgery. However, a controlled study has demonstrated increased mortality in premature infants routinely fed through a gastrostomy. A *Murphy drip*, an adaptation of the gastrostomy or the gavage feeding, allows slow, controlled introduction of formula into the stomach by partially occluding the feeding tube. In infants this method has been helpful primarily postoperatively. The introduction of a *nasojejunal feeding* tube allows slow infusion of formula into the jejunum and circumvents the problems of vomiting, distention, and the dumping syndrome, which may be encountered with the gastrostomy or gavage tube. The variety of complications reported to be associated with nasojejunal feedings using polyvinyl catheters has not been encountered with Silastic catheters.

Total intravenous alimentation

See Chapter 20, part two.

SKIN CARE

Most infants should be bathed with commercial soaps for their initial bath and with either the same preparation or tap water on subsequent days. Until further clarification of the hazards of hexachlorophene by federal authorities, routine use of this agent has been abandoned in infant washing. This change of policy demands close bacteriologic surveillance of nurseries to determine the existent flora and subsequent changes. Judicious use of dilute hexachlorophene (3%) on infants may be indicated for skin infections, and such use has been approved by the Food and Drug Administration.

Nursery personnel may continue to use hexachlorophene in hand washing, although other superior iodine-containing preparations currently are available. Skin irritation or allergic reaction may result from the use of these iodine preparations. A rigid requirement of washing from hand to elbow for 2 minutes in the initial wash and for 15 to 30 seconds in the second wash is needed to minimize infection and cross-contamination. Shorter but equally careful washes between handling of each infant also should be mandatory.

CHARTING

Charts should be organized in an orderly fashion so that the clinical problems, therapy, and progress of the patient are obvious to all personnel. In intensive care facilities nurses' notes, laboratory flow sheets, respirator and oxygen therapy logs, and intravenous therapy sheets should be kept at the infant's bedside. Organization of these records, allowing minimum reduplication and easy recording for the nursing staff, leads to development of concise record keeping and exact documentation of each infant's course. All too often reconstruction of a significant change in an infant's course is impossible through review of the records. Although continuous electronic recording of vital parameters is increasing, many factors require human observation and demand careful record keeping to avoid loss of valuable time when there is an urgent need to document the exact nature of the infant's course. Alternatively the value of detailed charting must be weighed against the nursing time required to complete flow sheets. The proper balance will increase the efficiency of care and will allow optimum use of time and effort by all personnel involved in delivery of care to sick infants.

PARENTS

The role of parents in any intensive care unit must be a serious concern for the team caring for each infant (Chapter 18). Maintaining strict environmental control, allaying parental anxiety, and preventing interference with patient care are no longer acceptable reasons for denying parents access to their critically ill infants. Unlimited visiting privileges for parents should be allowed in every unit, with obvious restrictions of visiting during procedures or medical emergencies; grandparents also should be allowed to see infants. More recently sibling visitation has been implemented in nurseries without increasing the risk of infection when appropriate screening for contagion is used. This change in visiting to include siblings has been particularly beneficial to families during long hospitalizations and when death of an infant is likely.

Before a policy of increased parent-child interaction is defined in a particular nursery, there should be a preliminary discussion of each person's role (the attending physician, resident, and nurses) in supporting the parents. There also should be a free exchange of ideas among the staff after implementation of such a program. Involvement of parents in the intensive care unit offers a means for personalizing what is often a stark, impersonal setting and for providing greater personal and professional motivation for the entire staff. Furthermore, without adequate access of parents to their infants, early parent-infant bonding is adversely affected with probable long-term untoward results (Chapter 18).

Under such policies the physician partially shares with paramedical personnel the previously exclusive right of talking to parents. This requires a greater degree of open communication with the nursing staff, which participates in communicating medical facts to parents. In any unit the parents' major contact is with the nurses, to whom they look for information; this relationship optimally should facilitate the care of the patient and the understanding of the parents. In such a setting the nursing staff may provide emotional support for a mother, supplementing that supplied by the physician; this support assumes significant proportions in the context of delivery of total care. The death of an infant is made more bearable to parents when the personnel consider this support a vital part of their responsibility.

Premature infants who survive a serious illness but who undergo prolonged hospitalizations should be in a nursery where parents are actively involved in routine care. Tasks that are often tedious and meaningless to paramedical personnel (such as diaper changing and washing) are cherished moments for parents who previously were separated from their infants. At the time of discharge the anxiety of parents who have been significantly involved in the care of their child, even at the worst moments, is significantly less than in those parents who have been anxious bystanders for 2 months.

John M. Driscoll, Jr.

BIBLIOGRAPHY

American Academy of Pediatrics: Hospital care of newborn infants, ed. 6, Evanston, Ill., 1977, The Academy.
Babson, S.G.: Peripheral intravenous alimentation of the small premature infant, J. Pediatr. **79**:494, 1971.
Babson, S.G.: Feeding the low birth weight infant, J. Pediatr. **79**:694, 1971.
Canadian Pediatric Society, Committee on the Fetus and Newborn: Oxygen therapy in the preterm infant, Can. Med. Assoc. J. **99**:564, 1968.
Cheek, J.A., Jr., and Staub, G.F.: Nasojejunal alimentation for premature and full-term newborn infants, J. Pediatr. **82**:955, 1973.
Chernick, V., and Raber, M.B.: Electrical hazards in the newborn nursery, J. Pediatr. **77**:143, 1970.
Desmond, M., Rudolph, A., and Phitaksphraiwan, P.: The transitional care nursery, Pediatr. Clin. North Am. **13**:651, 1966.
Duc, G.: Assessment of hypoxia in the newborn: suggestions for a practical approach, Pediatrics **48**:469, 1971.
Dunn, P.M.: Localization of the umbilical catheter by postmortem measurement, Arch. Dis. Child. **41**:69, 1966.
Gluck, L.: Design of a perinatal center, Pediatr. Clin. North Am. **17**:777, 1970.
Goldenberg, V.E., Wiegenstein, L., and Hopkins, G.B.: Hepatic injury associated with tromethamine, J.A.M.A. **205**:71, 1968.
Heird, W.C., Dell, R.B., Driscoll, J.M., Jr. Grebin, B., and Winters, R.W.: Metabolic acidosis after intravenous alimentation with amino acids, N. Engl. J. Med. **287**:943, 1972.
Heird, W.C., Driscoll, J.M., Jr., Schullinger, J.N., Grebin, B., and Winters, R.W.: Intravenous alimentation in pediatric patients, J. Pediatr. **80**:351, 1972.
Heird, W.C. Nasojejunal feedings: a commentary, J. Pediatr. **85**:111, 1974.
Hey, E.: The care of babies in incubators: recent advances in pediatrics, ed. 4, London, 1971, J. & A. Churchill.
Huch, A., and Huch, R.: Transcutaneous, noninvasive monitoring of PO_2, Hosp. Pract. **11**:43, 1976.
Kitterman, J.A., Phibbs, R.H., and Tooley, W.H.: Catheterization of umbilical vessels in newborn infants, Pediatr. Clin. North Am. **17**:895, 1970.
Klaus, M.H., Jerauld, R., Kreger, N.C., McAlpine, W., Steffa, M., and Kennell, J.H.: Maternal attachment: importance of the first postpartum days, N. Engl. J. Med. **286**:460, 1972.
Klaus, M.H., and Kennel, J.H.: Mothers separated from their newborn infants, Pediatr. Clin. North Am. **17**:1015, 1970.
Oliver, T.K., Jr.: Temperature regulation and heat production in the newborn, Pediatr. Clin. North Am. **12**:765, 1965.
Peabody, J., and others: Failure of conventional monitoring to detect hypoxia, Clin. Res. **25**:1902, 1977.
Perlstein, H., Edwards. N.K., and Sutherland, J.M.: Apnea in premature infants and incubator air temperature changes, N. Engl. J. Med. **282**:461, 1970.
Rhea, J.W., Ghazzawi, O., and Weidman, W.: Nasojejunal feeding: an improved device and intubation technique, J. Pediatr. **82**:951, 1973.
Rhea, J.W., and Kirby, J.O.: A nasojejunal tube for infant feeding, Pediatrics **46**:36, 1970.
Scott, J.M.: Iatrogenic lesions in babies following umbilical vein catherization, Arch. Dis. Child. **40**:426, 1965.
Segal, S.: Transportation of high risk infants, Vancouver, B.C., 1972, Canadian Pediatric Society.
Segal, S., and Pirie, G.E.: Equipment and personnel for neonatal special care, Pediatr. Clin. North Am. **17**:793, 1970.
Sinclair, J.C., Driscoll, J.M., Jr., Heird, W.C., and Winters, R.W.: Supportive management of the sick neonate: parenteral calories, water and electrolytes, Pediatr. Clin. North Am. **17**:863, 1970.
Spaulding, E.H.: Chemical disinfection in the hospital, J. Hosp. Res. **3**:25, 1965.
Swyer, P.R.: The regional organization of special care for the neonate, Pediatr. Clin. North Am. **17**:761, 1970.
Vengusamy, S., Pildes, R.S., Raffensperger, J.F., Levine, H.D., and Cornblath, M.: A controlled study of feeding gastrostomy in low birth weight infants, Pediatrics **43**:815, 1969.

Chapter 20

Nutrition, body fluids, and acid-base homeostasis

PART ONE
Nutritional requirements of the low birth weight infant

Until relatively recently the nutritional management of low birth weight (LBW) infants received little attention, partially because of the difficulties of providing any nutrient intake to these infants and partially because of their pressing medical problems. In fact, as few as 15 years ago, most low birth weight infants received little or no nutrient intake for the first several days of life. It then became apparent that morbidity could be reduced by provision of intravenous infusions of glucose solutions soon after birth. Subsequently, as the survival rate of premature infants improved, particularly that of small premature infants, physicians became more aware of ongoing nutritional requirements in the face of limited endogenous energy stores. The accumulating body of evidence, based primarily on animal studies, that inadequate nutrition during the period of cellular proliferation of the central nervous system (CNS) results in an irreversible deficit in the number of CNS cells, coupled with the persistently high incidence of CNS dysfunction in surviving LBW infants, further helped to increase awareness of the probable importance of adequate nutrition in this group.

Despite an increased awareness of the probable importance of nutrition, the LBW infant's requirements for most nutrients are still not known with certainty. This is largely because the optimum rate of growth for the LBW infant remains controversial. Many feel, quite logically, that the goal of nutritional management should be continuation of the intrauterine rate of growth. Others feel that the amounts of some nutrients required to achieve this goal impose an unacceptably high burden on the LBW infant's immature physiologic and biochemical mechanisms.

Since specific requirements of most nutrients are functions of the overall energy expenditure and rate of weight gain, specific nutrient requirements depend in large part on the goal chosen for growth rate. Although most agree that attempts to maintain the intrauterine growth rate are warranted, this goal is rarely achieved. Furthermore, its necessity throughout the neonatal period has never been demonstrated. Prevention of catabolism and depletion of endogenous energy stores, plus production of at least some increment in lean body mass, is a more realistic short-term goal for nutritional management of the low birth weight infant. Whether these goals are adequate for normal cellular growth of the CNS and normal development of other vital physiologic mechanisms remains to be shown.

In the foregoing discussion of specific nutrient requirements, no attempt is made to specify desirable intakes of the various nutrients. Rather, the requirements for specific nutrients are discussed with respect to the various goals that might be applicable to a particular infant. Following discussion of specific requirements is a more general discussion of the role of human milk in routine nutritional management of the LBW infant.

REQUIREMENTS FOR SPECIFIC NUTRIENTS

The intake range of various nutrients recommended for LBW infants by the American Academy of Pediatrics Committee on Nutrition is summarized in Table 20-1. Each is discussed in somewhat more detail in the sections that follow.

Table 20-1. Recommended nutrient intakes for low birth weight infants

Nutrient	Recommended intake*
Protein	1.8 gm
Fat	3.3 gm
	(300 mg essential fatty acids)
Carbohydrate	—
Sodium	20 mg
Potassium	80 mg
Calcium	50 mg
Magnesium	6 mg
Phosphorus	25 mg
Chloride	55 mg
Iron	0.15 mg
Zinc	0.5 mg
Copper	60 µg
Manganese	5 µg
Iodine	5 µg
Vitamins	
Vitamin A	250 IU
Vitamin D	40 IU
Vitamin E	0.7 IU
	(1 IU/gm linoleic acid)
Vitamin K	4 µg
Vitamin C	8 mg
Thiamin	40 µg
Riboflavin	60 µg
Niacin	250 µg
Vitamin B_6	35 µg
	(15 µg/gm protein)
Folic acid	4 µg
Pantothenic acid	300 µg
Vitamin B_{12}	0.15 µg
Biotin	1.5 µg
Inositol	4 mg
Choline	7 mg

From Committee on Nutrition, American Academy of Pediatrics: Nutritional needs of low birth weight infants, Pediatrics **60**:523, 1977. Copyright American Academy of Pediatrics 1977.
*Minimum levels of intake recommended per 100 calories. Recommended caloric intake is 110 to 150 calories/kg/day.

Calorie requirements

For decades it has been thought that the "growing" LBW infant requires a minimum of 120 Cal per kilogram per day—approximately 75 Cal/kg/day for resting expenditure and the remainder for specific dynamic action (10 Cal/kg/day), replacement of stool losses (10 Cal/kg/day), and growth (25 Cal/kg/day). The 75 Cal allotted for resting expenditure includes basal requirements (approximately 50 Cal/kg/day) plus additional requirements imposed by activity and response to cold stress. Modern nursery management has probably decreased this component of energy expenditure. Careful control of the environmental temperature, for example, reduces considerably the energy expended in responding to cold stress. In fact, studies of relatively inactive infants maintained in a strictly thermoneutral environment show maximum resting energy expenditures of 50 to 60 Cal/kg/day.

The energy expenditure for specific dynamic action (that is, the difference between resting expenditure of the fed infant and that of the fasted infant, now more frequently called the "thermic effect of food") may be a function of the composition of the diet. In general, the higher the protein content of the diet, the higher the "thermic effect" of that diet.

Some fecal loss of nutrients, primarily fat, is inevitable in both LBW and term infants. In general, these losses do not exceed about 15% of the intake.

The precise energy requirement for growth cannot be measured directly, but most recent studies suggest average values of 4 to 5 Cal per gram of tissue deposited. Since this value includes the energy cost of stored nutrients as well as the energy cost of tissue synthesis, it obviously is a function of the quality of tissue deposited. Using these estimates to calculate the energy requirement for a rate of weight gain approximating that occurring in utero between weeks 31 and 35 of gestation (that is, 1,000 gm) gives values between 75 and 95 Cal/kg/day. Provision of this energy intake does not ensure that the intrauterine growth rate will occur unless adequate amounts of all other nutrients required for growth also are provided.

Assuming a resting energy expenditure of 50 Cal/kg/day, the total energy need of the LBW infant for growth at the intrauterine rate is about 140 Cal/kg/day. An energy intake as low as 50 to 60 Cal/kg/day probably allows preservation of endogenous energy stores. Although this energy intake will help conserve endogenous protein stores, exogenous protein intake is necessary for complete preservation.

Protein requirements

Recommendations concerning protein requirements of LBW infants have generated more controversy than those for any other nutrient. This controversy began about 40 years ago with the demonstration by Gordon and associates that a protein intake higher than that available from human milk, the routine food for LBW infants at that time, resulted in greater weight gains. This study, however, did not fully differentiate between the effects on weight gain of higher protein intake and water retention secondary to the concomitantly higher electrolyte and mineral intake associated with the higher protein intake. Thus many insisted that the greater weight gain observed was merely the result of water retention. Indeed, Kagan and associates demonstrated that the calculated increase in dry weight (total weight gain minus increase in total body water) was similar in infants fed protein intakes ranging from 2 to 6 gm/kg/day.

Other clinical studies in which formulas that were

identical except for protein content were compared failed to confirm the findings of Kagan and associates. Davidson and co-workers, for example, observed better weight gain in infants fed protein intakes of 4 gm/kg/day than in those receiving 2 gm/kg/day but did not demonstrate a superiority of 6 gm over 4 gm. Babson and Bramhall did not observe greater weight gains in infants fed higher protein intakes unless these were accompanied by higher solute intakes. However, increases in both crown-rump and femur length were greater in infants fed higher protein intakes.

More recently, Raiha and associates compared both quantity and quality of protein intake in infants weighing under 2,100 gm. Subjects of this study were randomly assigned to one of five feeding regimens: (1) pooled human milk, (2) "humanized" cow's milk protein (40% casein and 60% whey), 1.5 gm/dl, (3) "humanized" cow's milk protein, 3 gm/dl; (4) cow's milk protein (82% casein and 18% whey), 1.5 gm/dl, and (5) cow's milk protein, 3 gm/dl. All infants received 117 Cal/kg/day; protein intakes were 2.25 and 4.5 gm/kg/day, respectively, from the low- and high-protein artificial formulas, and approximately 2.0 gm/kg/day from human milk. The electrolyte and mineral contents of the artificial formulas were identical and only slightly higher than those of human milk. Weight gain of the artificial formula groups was greater than that of the human milk group. However, unlike previous studies with similar protein intakes, no differences among the four formula groups were detected. Serum albumin concentrations were lower in the group fed human milk, but this group appeared to be as "well nourished" as any of the other groups. Moreover, metabolic imbalances such as elevated plasma concentrations of some amino acids, hyperammonemia, azotemia, and acidosis were absent in this group, whereas some or all were common in the formula-fed groups, particularly those fed on the high-protein regimens. The metabolic imbalances of infants fed the lower concentration of "humanized" cow's milk protein (regimen 2) differed minimally from those of infants fed human milk. The abnormal plasma aminograms were a function of both the quantity and the quality of protein intake. The concentrations of several amino acids were strikingly elevated in both high-protein groups. Blood ammonia and urea nitrogen concentrations of infants fed the higher protein intakes were elevated. However, only infants who received the unmodified cow's milk protein formulas (82% casein and 19% whey) developed metabolic acidosis, the severity of which was related to the amount of protein intake.

This latter study, as well as most of the others discussed, raises doubts concerning the adequacy of human milk for LBW infants. It also suggests that a protein intake as high as 4.5 gm/kg/day may be hazardous. In this regard it is important to consider the findings of Goldman and associates concerning the subsequent neurologic development of LBW infants fed high-protein intakes during the perinatal period. At 4 to 6 years of age the incidence of strabismus was considerably greater in those who received protein intakes of over 6 gm/kg/day than in those who received lower protein intakes. The number of children with low IQ scores was also greater in the group who received the higher protein feedings as infants.

Failure to consider protein quality may explain some of the discrepancies among studies of the protein requirements of the LBW infants. Because of the immaturity of various enzymatic processes, some amino acids that are nonessential for the adult may be essential for the premature infant. Tyrosine and cysteine are examples; premature infants lack sufficient activity of the enzymes converting, respectively, phenylalanine to tyrosine and methionine to cysteine. Histidine, and perhaps arginine also, is thought to be an essential amino acid for the premature infant. The probable need to consider protein quality can be illustrated by the following example. Human milk protein contains approximately twice the amount of cysteine per gram of protein as unmodified cow milk protein. Thus twice as much cow's milk as human milk is necessary to provide the same amount of cysteine. If the amount of cysteine delivered is assumed to be the limiting factor, growth of infants receiving 2 to 3 gm/kg/day of human milk protein (51 to 76 mg cysteine/kg/day) should be roughly equivalent to that of infants receiving 4 to 6 gm/kg/day of cow's milk protein (48 to 72 mg cysteine/kg/day).

Based on the studies just reviewed, a protein intake of 2.5 to 3.5 gm/kg/day should produce adequate growth in most premature infants, provided that the protein is of such quality as to provide sufficient amounts of all amino acids that are essential for the premature infant. Both human milk protein and humanized cow's milk protein appear to meet such requirements. Unmodified cow's milk protein, however, may not. If so, few reasons can be offered for the higher unmodified cow's milk protein intakes that may be required. In fact, provision of protein in excess of requirements merely taxes the infant's metabolic machinery for disposing of the excess.

Fat requirements

All infants, as well as adults, have an absolute requirement for certain polyunsaturated fatty acids that cannot be synthesized in vivo—namely, linoleic, linolenic, and arachidonic acids. The latter two, however, are thought to be synthesized from linoleic acid. If so, the only absolute requirement is for linoleic acid. This requirement can be met by provision of 2% to 4% of the total calories as linoleic acid. Although there is no other known requirement for lipids in the infant diet, fat has a high caloric density and accounts for 40% to 50% of the caloric content of natural milks as well as most available artificial formulas. Replacement of this fat with carbohydrate is impossible unless the osmolality of the formula is increased by 50% to 75%.

Gastrointestinal (GI) assimilation of fat by the LBW infant is poor. Although this may be caused by several factors, the LBW infant's limited bile salt pool and pancreatic lipase activity are probably the major ones. Despite these well-documented limitations, absorption of fat is a function of the quality of fat ingested. Human milk fat, for instance, is better absorbed than cow's milk fat. In part this is because its fatty acids are relatively unsaturated and because its positional distribution of palmitic acid on the triglyceride molecule is such as to enhance absorption. However, untreated human milk (in fact, any untreated milk) also contains various lipases that undoubtedly account, in part, for the better absorption of human milk fat. Nonetheless, fats with chemical properties similar to the fat of human milk are better absorbed than those with chemical properties of cow's milk fat.

Triglycerides of short- and medium-chain fatty acids pass directly into the portal blood regardless of the intraluminal bile salt and lipase activities. Thus substitution of a major portion of the fat content of infant formulas with medium-chain triglycerides results in absorption of over 90% of the total fat. This increased absorption, however, does not necessarily result in improved weight gain; thus the role of medium-chain triglycerides in routine feeding of LBW infants remains uncertain.

Carbohydrate requirements

In contrast to the LBW infant's absolute requirements for protein and certain fatty acids, no absolute requirement for carbohydrate has been demonstrated. On the other hand, metabolism of the CNS and the hematopoietic tissues is dependent to a large extent on glucose. Although glucose can be produced from either exogenous or endogenous protein (gluconeogenesis), the various glucose homeostatic mechanisms of LBW infants are not fully functional.

Approximately 40% to 45% of the total caloric content of most dietary regimens for premature infants is provided as carbohydrate. Satisfactory clinical progress has been observed with formulas containing only lactose, only sucrose, only glucose, or mixtures of these sugars. Since pancreatic amylase activity of LBW infants is limited relative to that of older children and adults, these infants would not be expected to tolerate large amounts of complex carbohydrates.

The satisfactory clinical progress of LBW infants fed formulas containing only lactose is somewhat surprising in view of these infants' relatively low intestinal lactase activity. Although this metabolic limitation may result in some carbohydrate malabsorption and greater stool water, particularly in more immature infants, some dietary lactose is probably important. This sugar is thought to support proliferation of *Lactobacillus* organisms in the intestinal tract. Growth of these organisms, in turn, may suppress growth of certain pathogenic gram-negative organisms, thus providing some protection against systemic infection with these organisms. The development of such a fermentative bacterial flora has been suggested as a responsible factor for the lower incidence of gram-negative sepsis in breast-fed infants. However, human milk contains a number of other factors (leukocytes, immunoglobulins, lysozyme, complement factors, and specific bacterial growth inhibitors) that may be of equal or even greater importance in such protection (Chapter 26).

Electrolyte requirements

The electrolyte requirements of the LBW infant are those necessary for tissue synthesis plus replacement of obligatory losses. Assuming continuation of the intrauterine growth rate, the daily requirements for tissue synthesis are the amounts that accumulate daily during gestation (Table 20-2), or approximately 1.0 mEq/kg of sodium and 0.5 mEq/kg of both potassium and chloride. These amounts, plus the usually assumed obligatory losses of approximately 0.5 mEq of both sodium and chloride and approximately 0.75 mEq of potassium per 100 calories used, represent reasonable estimates for the minimal requirements of the LBW infant. Since intestinal absorption is never 100%, dietary electrolyte intakes should exceed these minimal requirements of approximately 1.5 to 2 mEq/kg/day of sodium, 1.5 to 1.75 mEq of potassium, and 1.25 to 1.5 mEq of chloride.

In general, the requirements for potassium and chloride are met by the quantities present in both human milk and commonly used formulas. However, the sodium content of human milk may not provide adequate sodium for the LBW infant, even if all the sodium present were completely absorbed. Indeed, hyponatremia occurs frequently in LBW infants fed human milk, particularly very LBW infants who seem to have greater obligatory losses.

Mineral requirements

Although less attention has been focused on mineral requirements of LBW infants than on other nutrient requirements, considerable data are available concerning the requirements for calcium and phosphorus. The attention paid to these two minerals is attributable, primarily, to the high incidence of hypocalcemia in LBW infants (Chapter 33, part two). This condition develops more commonly in infants who receive formulas with a

Table 20-2. Intrauterine accumulation of various nutrients during the last trimester of pregnancy

Component	\multicolumn{5}{c}{Accumulation during various stages of gestation}
	26-31 weeks	31-33 weeks	33-35 weeks	35-38 weeks	38-40 weeks
Body weight (gm)*	500	500	500	500	500
Water (gm)	410	350	320	240	220
Fat (gm)	25	65	85	175	200
Nitrogen (gm)	11	12	12	6	7
Calcium (gm)	4	5	5	5	5
Phosphorus (gm)	2.2	2.6	2.8	3.0	3.0
Magnesium (mg)	130	110	120	120	80
Sodium (mEq)	35	25	40	40	40
Potassium (mEq)	19	24	26	20	20
Chloride (mEq)	30	24	10	20	10
Iron (mg)	36	60	60	40	20
Copper (mg)	2.1	2.4	2.0	2.0	2.0
Zinc (mg)	9.0	10.0	8.0	7.0	3.0

Adapted from Ziegler, E.E., and others: Growth **40**:329, 1976.
*Body weight of the 26-week fetus is 1,000 gm; that of the 40-week fetus is 3,500 gm.

high phosphorus content, specifically a low calcium/phosphorus ratio, thus explaining the emphasis placed on the calcium/phosphorus ratio of infant formulas. Experience has shown that a ratio of roughly 2:1 is satisfactory.

The requirements for calcium (and other minerals) necessary to allow continuation of the intrauterine rate of accumulation can be calculated from the data shown in Table 20-2. The calcium content of human milk is approximately 20 mEq/L; at best only 60% to 75% of the total ingested is absorbed from the GI tract. Thus it is obvious that the volume of human milk required to provide the calcium that accumulates in utero (100 to 150 mg/kg/day) is considerably greater than that commonly ingested (or, for that matter, possible to be ingested) by most LBW infants. Indeed, infants who are fed with human milk have less dense skeletons roentgenographically than do infants who receive larger amounts of calcium. The recent increase in popularity of human milk for feeding LBW infants has been accompanied by an increased incidence of skeletal mineralization problems, including multiple fractures, hypocalcemia, and hypophosphatemia. Although there is no consensus with respect to the etiology of these problems, inadequate calcium intake and possibly inadequate phosphorus intake as well are among the factors responsible.

Although magnesium deficiency has been observed in LBW infants, very little is known about absolute requirements. The recommended daily allowance is 15 to 20 mg/kg/day; however, human milk provides only approximately 10 mg/kg/day, which appears to be adequate.

Requirements for trace minerals in LBW infants have not been established. Thus most recommend provision of the same amounts thought to be required by term infants.

Human milk contains 3 to 5 mg of zinc per liter, its iodine content is 40 to 80 µg/l, and its copper content is approximately 0.4 mg/l. Thus the LBW infant fed adequate amounts of human milk (180 ml/kg/day) will not receive the recommended intakes of zinc or iodine. However, depending on absorption, zinc intake may be adequate to allow accumulation at the intrauterine rate. Infants fed human milk rarely develop zinc deficiency.

Vitamin requirements

In the absence of specific information concerning the LBW infant's requirements for many vitamins, the requirements for term infants are usually recommended (see Table 20-1). Infants receiving either human milk or artificial formulas in amounts to produce adequate growth usually receive sufficient amounts of all vitamins, although human milk may be deficient in vitamin D. Nonetheless, since the consumption of sufficient volumes of human milk or formula to satisfy vitamin requirements may not be attained for several weeks, vitamin supplements usually are recommended. Moreover, the immature infant may have special needs with regard to certain vitamins.

Deficiency of vitamin E (α-tocopherol) with enhanced erythrocyte hemolysis occurs in growing premature infants (p. 738). Vitamin E functions as an antioxidant to prevent peroxidation of polyunsaturated fatty acids in various cell membranes. The use of polyunsaturated vegetable oils in infant formulas results in an increased membrane content of these fatty acids, thus increasing the need for vitamin E. Infants fed such formulas, therefore, should receive supplements. In general, the aim should be to maintain a ratio of vitamin E to polyunsaturated fatty acids (E/PUFA ratio) of at least 1.

Folic acid functions as a coenzyme in many metabolic reactions, including the synthesis of purines and pyrimidines needed for formation of DNA. Thus it is essential for production of new cells. Studies of folate metabolism in preterm infants have shown that serum concentration falls from approximately normal adult values at birth to values below this range by a few weeks of age. The concentration persists in this range until around 3 months of age before rising again to normal adult values. This decrease in serum folate concentration can be prevented by oral supplements of 50 µg/day. Supplementation does not affect growth or hemoglobin levels, although supplemented infants have fewer hypersegmented neutrophils and higher erythrocyte folate levels. On the basis of these findings, Dallman's recommendation for supplementation of the diet of LBW infants with 50 µg/day is endorsed.

ROLE OF HUMAN MILK IN FEEDING THE LBW INFANT

Currently there seems to be a widespread movement toward establishing human milk banks to ensure its supply for feeding LBW infants. However, evidence that human milk is nutritionally superior for these infants is lacking. On the contrary, as just discussed, growth rates of LBW infants fed pooled human milk is less rapid than that of infants fed formulas of higher nutrient concentrations. This observation has been ascribed in part to the relatively low protein concentration of human milk; indeed, the maximum volumes tolerated by LBW infants provide only about 2 gm/kg/day of protein. Milk of mothers who deliver prematurely has an approximately 20% higher protein concentration and therefore may support greater growth rates, although recent reports have not confirmed this possibility. Human milk also contains insufficient amounts of other nutrients, namely calcium and phosphorus, and the concentration of fat-soluble vitamin D in human milk is also low. Even if the water-soluble vitamin D in human milk is eventually shown to be physiologically active, the fact remains that its calcium and phosphorus content is insufficient for optimum skeletal mineralization.

A distinct advantage of human milk for feeding LBW infants, at least theoretically, is its immunologic properties (p. 640). It is thought that the many cellular and humoral components of human milk may confer passive immunity or enhance immunologic maturation, thereby providing some protection against infections and necrotizing enterocolitis. There is, however, no clinical evidence that feeding human milk prevents necrotizing enterocolitis in human infants. A lower incidence of infections in LBW infants fed freshly expressed mother's milk for part of the day has been demonstrated. Others have shown some changes in stool pH and fecal flora that may be beneficial. Nevertheless, the immunologic properties of human milk are altered by storage and processing methods; cellular elements do not survive freezing (the most common mode of storage), and many of the humoral factors are heat labile and may be destroyed even at pasteurization temperatures.

Despite the possible immunologic advantages of fresh human milk, the additional steps involved in collection, storage, and dispensing of expressed human milk make inadvertent contamination likely. Thus stringent hygienic techniques and bacterial screening are mandatory. Use of donor milk raises the possibility of exposure to viruses; of major concern is the relatively common occurrence of cytomegalovirus excretion in the milk of seropositive women. Herpes and rubella viruses and hepatitis B surface antigen have also been detected in human milk, although transmission of illness via milk has not been demonstrated.

Whether human milk is provided by the infant's mother or by a donor (or donors), more research is necessary to demonstrate its superiority in the premature nursery setting. On the other hand, if an individual mother wishes to provide milk for her infant, the psychologic benefits accrued from her involvement in the infant's care, as well as for eventual success in nursing, are strong considerations for encouraging milk expression until the infant can suckle. Even in these situations, however, the infant must be carefully monitored for development of specific nutrient deficiencies involving primarily protein, calcium, phosphorus, vitamin D, and/or sodium. The same nutritional monitoring is also indicated for the premature infant receiving formula. All premature infants are at nutritional risk because of (1) poor nutritional stores, (2) increased growth rate with rapid use of nutrients, (3) immature physiologic systems, and (4) incomplete knowledge of exact nutrient requirements.

William C. Heird
Emi Okamoto
Thomas L. Anderson

BIBLIOGRAPHY

Auld, P.A.M., Bhangananda, P., and Mehta, S.: The influence of an early caloric intake with IV glucose on catabolism of premature infants, Pediatrics **37**:592, 1966.

Babson, S.G., and Bramhall, J.L.: Diet and growth in the premature infant: the effect of different dietary intakes of ash-electrolytes and protein on weight gain and linear growth, J. Pediatr. **74**:890, 1969.

Barltrop, D., and Oppe, T.E.: Dietary factors in neonatal calcium homeostasis, Lancet **2**:1333, 1970.

Bruck, K.: Temperature regulation in the newborn infant, Biol. Neonate **3**:65, 1961.

Burland, W.L., Simpson, K., and Lord, J.: Response of low birth weight infants to treatment with folic acid, Arch. Dis. Child. **46**:189, 1971.

Burr, G.O., and Burr, M.M.: A new deficiency disease produced by the rigid exclusion of fat from the diet, J. Biol. Chem. **82**:345, 1929.

Committee on Nutrition, American Academy of Pediatrics: Nutritional needs of low birth weight infants, Pediatrics **60**:523, 1977.

Dallman, P.R.: Iron, vitamin E and folate in the preterm infant, J. Pediatr. **85**:742, 1974.

Davidson, M., and others: Feeding studies in low birth weight infants: a relationship of dietary protein, fat and electrolytes to rates of weight gain, clinical courses and serum chemical concentrations, J. Pediatr. **70**:695, 1967.

Day, G.M., and others: Growth and mineral metabolism in low birth weight infants. II. Effects of calcium supplementation on growth and divalent cations, Pediatr. Res. **9**:568, 1975.

Dobbing, J., and Smart, J.L.: The quantitative growth and development of the human brain, Arch. Dis. Child. **48**:757, 1973.

Filer, L.J., Jr., Mattson, F.H., and Fomon, S.J.: Triglyceride configuration and fat absorption by the human infant, J. Nutr. **99**:293, 1969.

Fomon, S.J.: Infant nutrition, Philadelphia, 1974, W.B. Saunders Co.

Fomon, S.J., and others: Excretion of fat by normal full-term infants fed various milks and formulas, Am. J. Clin. Nutr. **23**:1299, 1970.

Friedman, G., and Goldberg, S.J.: Concurrent and subsequent serum cholesterols of breast and formula fed infants, Am. J. Clin. Nutr. **28**:42, 1975.

Goldman, H.I., and others: Clinical effects of two different levels of protein intake of low birth weight infants, J. Pediatr. **59**:951, 1961.

Goldman, H.I., and others: Late effects of early dietary protein intake on low birth weight infants, J. Pediatr. **85**:764, 1974.

Gordon, H.H., Levine, S.J., and McNamara, H.: Feeding of premature infants: a comparison of human and cow's milk, Am. J. Dis. Child. **73**:442, 1947.

Gutberlet, R.B., and Cornblath, M.: Neonatal hypoglycemia revisited, Pediatrics **58**:10, 1976.

Holt, L.E., Jr., and Snyderman, S.E.: The amino acid requirements of children. In Nyham, W.L., editor: Amino acid metabolism and genetic variation, New York, 1967, McGraw-Hill Book Co., Inc.

Hytten, F.E.: Clinical and chemical studies in human lactation. II. Variation in major constituents during a feeding, Br. Med. J. **1**:176, 1954.

Isselbacher, K.J.: Mechanisms of absorption of long and medium chain triglycerides. In Senior, J.R., et al., editors: Medium chain triglycerides, Philadelphia, 1976, University of Pennsylvania Press.

Kagan, B.M., and others: Body composition of premature infants: relation to nutrition, Am. J. Clin. Nutr. **25**:1153, 1972.

Koldovsky, O.: Development of the functions of the small intestine in mammals and man, Basel, 1969, S. Karger.

Levine, S.Z., and others: The respiratory metabolism in infancy and in childhood. VI. The specific dynamic action of food in normal infants, Am. J. Dis. Child. **33**:722, 1927.

Macy, I.C., Kelley, H.J., and Sloane, R.E.: The composition of milks: a compilation of the comparative composition and properties of human, cow, and goat milk, colostrum and transitional milk, Publication No. 254, Washington, D.C., 1953, National Academy of Science–National Research Council.

Mohen, J.A., Lev, R., and Mabry, W.: Colostral leukocyte, J. Surg. Oncol. **2**:163, 1970.

Norman, A., Strandvik, B., and Ojamae, O.: Bile acids and pancreatic enzymes during absorption in the newborn, Acta Paediatr. Scand. **61**:571, 1972.

Oski, F.A., and Barness, L.A.: Vitamin E deficiency: a previously unrecognized cause of hemolytic anemia in the premature infant, J. Pediatr. **70**:211, 1967.

Raiha, N.C.R.: Phenylalanine hydroxylase in human liver during development, Pediatr. Res. **7**:1, 1973.

Raiha, N.C.R., Rassin, D.K., and Gaull, G.E.: Milk protein quality and quantity: biochemical and growth effects in low birth weight infants, Pediatr. Res. **9**:679, 1975.

Raiha, N.C.R., and others: Milk protein quantity and quality in low birth weight infants, Pediatrics **57**:659, 1976.

Reichman, B., and others: Diet, fat accretion and growth in premature infants, N. Engl. J. Med. **305**:1495, 1981.

Roy, C.C., and St. Marie, M.: Correction of the malabsorption of the premature infant with a medium chain triglyceride formula, J. Pediatr. **86**:446, 1965.

Shaw, J.C.L.: Evidence for defective skeletal mineralization in low birth weight infants: the absorption of calcium and fat, Pediatrics **57**:16, 1975.

Shojaniu, A.M., and Gross, S.: Folic acid deficiency and prematurity, J. Pediatr. **64**:323, 1964.

Smart, J.L., and Dobbing, J.: Vulnerability of developing brain. VI. Relative effects of fetal and early postnatal undernutrition on reflex ontogeny and development of behavior in the rat, Brain. Res. **33**:303, 1971.

Snyderman, S.: The protein and amino acid requirements of the premature infant. In Jonxis, J.H.P., Vesser, H.K.A., and Telstra, J.A., editors: Metabolic processes in the fetus and newborn infant, Leiden, The Netherlands, 1971, H.E. Stenfert Kroese B.V.

Snyderman, S., Boyer, A., and Kogut, M.: The protein requirement of the premature infant. I. The effect of protein intake on the retention of nitrogen, J. Pediatr. **74**:879, 1969.

Sturman, J., Gaull, G., and Raiha, N.C.R.: Absence of cystathionase in human fetal liver: is cystine essential? Science **169**:74, 1970.

Tantibhedhyangkul, P., and Hashim, S.A.: Medium chain triglyceride feeding in premature infants: effects on fat and nitrogen absorption, Pediatrics **55**:359, 1975.

Tsang, R.C.: Neonatal magnesium disturbances, Am. J. Dis. Child. **124**:282, 1972.

Tsang, R.C., and Oh, W.: Neonatal hypocalcemia in low birth weight infants, Pediatrics **45**:773, 1970.

Watkins, J.R., and others: Bile salt metabolism in the human premature infant, Gastroenterology **69**:706, 1975.

Winberg, J., and Wessner, G.: Does breast milk protect against septicemia in the newborn? Lancet **1**:1091, 1971.

Winick, M., and Noble, A.: Cellular response in rats during malnutrition at various ages, J. Nutr. **89**:300, 1966.

Ziegler, E.E., and others: Body composition of the reference fetus, Growth **40**:329, 1976.

PART TWO

Methods of nutrient delivery for the low birth weight infant

Provision of adequate nutrients by the oral route in healthy, vigorous term infants or larger preterm infants usually presents no problems. However, successful institution of early enteral feedings in small premature infants, particularly sick or debilitated ones, remains an important problem. A poor or unsustained suck, an uncoordinated swallowing mechanism, and delayed gastric emptying are pathophysiologic factors common to many such infants. Each of these neurophysiologic deficiencies predisposes the infant to vomiting, aspiration, or both. Early intravenous fluid therapy with dextrose solution has been used in an attempt to avoid these hazards. However, such infusions fall far short of the nutritional requirements of low birth weight (LBW) infants. Until recently, experience with alternate methods of feeding was limited. During the past few years, however, methods for delivery of sufficient nutrients solely by the intravenous route (total parenteral nutrition), as well as methods for continuous infusion of feedings by the GI tract (continuous nasogastric or nasojejunal infusions), have been evaluated.

The recommended approach to delivery of nutrients to premature and sick neonates is use of a combination of all available methods. This allows an individual infant with a particular clinical problem to be the basis for selection of the primary method of nutrient delivery rather than insisting on rigid adherence to one particular method. Almost every infant should be given a trial of conventional feeding, that is, nipple or gavage feedings as tolerated plus intravenous supplementation with 5% or 10% glucose. If adequate nutrients cannot be delivered by this fashion, intravenous supplementation with glucose plus amino acids can be substituted for glucose alone. In the event that feedings are not tolerated by the GI tract, the sole use of intravenous nutrition deserves serious consideration. Up to 75 Cal/kg/day can be infused by peripheral vein without delivery of an unreasonable fluid load in most LBW infants. Use of this method is particularly relevant if it is anticipated that adequate enteral feedings can be given within a reasonable period of time. Total parenteral nutrition by means of a central vein catheter should be used only in situations associated with prolonged intolerance of GI tract feedings, that is, longer than peripheral intravenous sites can be maintained. This approach recognizes individual differences among LBW infants and should result in improved nutritional management of premature and sick neonates without imposing unnecessary risks.

Gavage feeding by a nasogastric catheter placed intermittently or left in place for a period of time and methods for maintaining intravenous infusions are discussed elsewhere (p. 298). Some of the newer methods of nutrient delivery are presented here in the context of describing the reported clinical experience with each method.

CONTINUOUS TRANSPYLORIC OR INTRAGASTRIC INFUSIONS

The first comprehensive report of the use of nasojejunal, or transpyloric, feeding in pediatric patients was that of Rhea and Kilby. Subsequently, Cheek and Staub reported extensive experience with this method of feeding in LBW infants. The method overcomes a number of problems encountered in feeding premature and sick neonates (for example, poor suck, uncoordinated swallowing, and delayed gastric emptying).

Technique

The technique of nasojejunal feeding described by Rhea and associates involves nasal insertion of a small Silastic catheter enclosed in a more rigid open-ended catheter. The infant is then placed on the right side to facilitate passage of the tube through the pylorus. A gold bead is placed at the tip of the Silastic catheter to further facilitate passage through the pylorus. Once the tube is in the correct position roentgenographically, the outer rigid tube is removed and the smaller Silastic catheter is secured in place. Formula is then infused at a continuous rate by use of a constant infusion pump.

The technique of continuous nasogastric infusion is much simpler. An appropriately sized catheter is placed through the nares into the stomach and its position confirmed. Once in correct position, the catheter is secured and formula is infused at a constant rate with a continuous infusion pump.

With both methods the volume of formula infused initially should be small but can usually be increased, depending on the infant's ability to tolerate increasing volumes. Both methods overcome the poor suck and uncoordinated swallowing so common in LBW infants. Obviously, transpyloric infusions more effectively overcome the problem of delayed gastric emptying.

Clinical experience

Cheek and Staub reported the use of transpyloric feeding in 36 infants with an average weight of 1,624 gm. Volumes of standard formulas up to 145 ml/kg were administered; weight gain averaged 17.3 gm/day. Studies comparing more than one method of nutrient delivery have rarely demonstrated advantages of continuously administered transpyloric feedings over continuously administered intragastric feedings or even over conventional gavage feedings. Roy and associates demonstrated differences in assimilation of formula delivered continuously by the transpyloric route or as two hourly bolus feedings. Neither the volumes delivered to approximately 1,300-gm infants nor their weight gains differed as a function of the method of delivery; however, stool frequency and stool fat content were greater in the group who received continuous transpyloric feedings.

Complications

A number of reports of intestinal perforation in patients receiving continuous nasojejunal feedings have appeared. Most occurred in very small infants in whom polyvinyl rather than Silastic catheters were used (polyvinyl catheters become extremely rigid once they have been in place for a short period). In addition, some of the described perforations occurred shortly after manipulation of the indwelling catheter, especially after it was moved forward. Rhea and associates have used this technique (employing Silastic catheters) in over 500 patients, and perforation has never occurred.

TOTAL PARENTERAL NUTRITION

The feasibility and nutritional effectiveness of total parenteral nutrition was first demonstrated by Dudrick and associates in 1966. By infusing a hypertonic mixture of protein hydrolysate and glucose plus minerals and vitamins through an indwelling central venous catheter, they successfully maintained positive nitrogen balance in both human and animal subjects and demonstrated that this method of nutrient delivery sustained normal growth of younger subjects. Subsequently this method of nutrition has found widespread use in many areas of medicine, including provision of nutrients to LBW infants. Nonetheless, it cannot be recommended as a routine feeding method for LBW infants. The technique may, however, prove valuable in selected infants; for this reason a discussion of the technique and the results achieved is presented.

Table 20-3 lists the general requirements for any parenteral fluid mixture that will provide sufficient nutrients to promote growth and maintain positive nitrogen balance. The major nitrogen source currently used is a mixture of crystalline amino acids. Those available provide most essential as well as nonessential amino acids, but none provides an "ideal" amino acid mixture. Any of the available crystalline amino acid mixtures at a dosage of 2.5 gm/kg/day is recommended. Although intakes of 4 gm/kg/day have been advocated, this higher intake offers no advantage in terms of either improved nitrogen balance or improved weight gain. Moreover, the lower intake is not associated with azotemia. Although the plasma concentrations of some amino acids reach high values with the lower intake, it is likely that such values are even greater with the higher intake.

Glucose is the most commonly used caloric source, but intravenous fat preparations are usually added as well, either in amounts to provide essential fatty acid requirements (0.5 gm/kg/day) or as a major source of calories (2 to 3 gm/kg/day). If glucose is used exclusively, 25 to 30 gm/kg/day are necessary to meet full caloric requirements (100 to 120 nonprotein Cal/kg/day).

Several electrolyte and vitamin additives are available for parenteral use; usually these are added to the mixture in amounts approximating established oral or intravenous maintenance requirements. The parenteral needs for minerals may be significantly different from the oral needs; thus the amounts of various minerals supplied are considerably less than the usual oral recommendations.

The composition of a suitable infusate is shown in Table 20-4. It should be prepared frequently (daily or every other day) under laminar flow. The content of each day's infusate should be determined after careful assessment of the infant's clinical and biochemical status. The

Table 20-3. Requirements for total parenteral nutrition

Requirement	Source
Amino acids	Hydrolysates of fibrin or casein; crystalline amino acid mixtures
Calories	Glucose, lipid emulsions
Electrolytes (Na, K, Cl)	Additives
Minerals (Ca, Mg, P)	Additives
Fat- and water-soluble vitamins	IV vitamin mixtures and/or individual vitamins
Essential fatty acids	Lipid emulsions
Trace minerals	Additives

Table 20-4. Composition of suitable infusate for total parenteral nutrition

Constituent	Amount
Amino acids	2.5 gm/kg/day
Glucose	20-30 gm/kg/day
Lipid emulsion	0.5-3.0 gm/kg/day
Sodium (NaCl)	3-4 mEq/kg/day
Potassium*	2-3 mEq/kg/day
Calcium (Ca gluconate)	1.5 mEq/kg/day
Magnesium (MgSO$_4$)	0.25 mEq/kg/day
Phosphorus	2.0 mmol/kg/day
Vitamins (MVI)†	1 ml/day
Total volume	125 ml/kg/day

*Two mEq/kg/day are provided as KH$_2$PO$_4$; remainder is provided as KCl.
†USV Pharmaceutical Corp., Tuckahoe, N.Y.

infusate is a chemically complex mixture with a high osmolality, necessitating slow and continuous infusion into a large central vein. In infants the infusate usually is administered through a catheter inserted into the superior vena cava via either the external or internal jugular vein (see further). Often a 0.22-μm Millipore filter is placed in the infusion line as a final filter for removal of debris and/or microorganisms. A constant infusion rate is maintained by use of an infusion pump.

In the LBW infant the initial daily infusate should deliver no more than 10 to 15 gm glucose/kg/day. The glucose content can then be increased gradually to a level of 25 to 30 gm/kg/day, depending on the dosage of fat emulsion used and in accordance with the infant's tolerance of glucose. Rarely can full caloric maintenance from a predominantly glucose infusate be achieved in less than 7 to 10 days. The LBW infant's tolerance for lipid also seems to be very variable, and dosages greater than 3 gm/kg/day cannot be recommended.

Inexperience with the technique and lack of information regarding the metabolic responses of the premature infant necessitate frequent chemical monitoring, which can be achieved only with microchemical methods. A suggested monitoring schedule is listed in Table 20-5. The clinical status of each infant should be assessed fre-

Table 20-5. Suggested chemical monitoring schedule during total parenteral nutrition

Variable	Initial period*	Later period
Plasma electrolytes, glucose	Every other day	2-3 times per week
BUN	Every other day	Weekly
Blood acid-base status	Every other day	2-3 times per week
Plasma Ca^{++}, P, and Mg^{++}	2 times per week	Weekly
Liver function studies	Weekly	Weekly
Hemogram	2 times per week	2 times per week
Total protein and A/G	Weekly	Weekly

*First 7 to 10 days or until full caloric requirement can be met without hyperglycemia.

quently with respect to feasibility and safety of beginning oral feedings. The intravenous alimentation solution can then be decreased as enteral intake increases; from a practical point of view it should not be discontinued until adequate fluid and calories can be provided solely by enteral feedings.

Catheter insertion and care

Because of the small size of the subclavian vein in infants, percutaneous subclavian puncture is difficult as well as hazardous. Thus catheters for long-term total parenteral nutrition usually are inserted through an external or internal jugular vein cutdown. After the catheter is threaded into the superior vena cava, the proximal end of the catheter is tunneled subcutaneously to exit in the parietooccipital area of the scalp. Exit of the catheter at a point distant from the phlebotomy affords added safety from infection, some freedom from the infant's wandering hands, and ease of maintenance of the catheter site. The catheter is often placed with the infant under general anesthesia in an operating room setting. However, these steps are not necessary if the child can be adequately restrained and absolute sterility can be maintained elsewhere.

Regular meticulous care of the central venous catheter is mandatory for prolonged, safe, complication-free use. At least three times per week a specially trained nurse, technician, or physician should dress the catheter exit site. The occlusive dressing must be removed and the skin area cleaned with both defatting and antiseptic (Betadine) agents. The antiseptic ointment should be reapplied, followed by a fresh occlusive dressing. With meticulous care a single catheter can be used safely for up to 90 days. However, the average life of a catheter is closer to 30 days.

Clinical experience

The efficacy of total parenteral nutrition in infants with major anomalies of the GI tract and in infants with intractable diarrheal syndromes is well established. The technique is also useful in selected LBW infants without these problems. With GI disease, total parenteral nutrition promotes weight gain and positive nitrogen balance until GI function is recovered. Although there is clinical evidence to suggest that GI histologic features may improve during total parenteral nutrition, animal studies suggest that parenterally administered nutrients do not support growth and function of the normal GI tract.

Weight gains of up to 20 gm/kg/day and nitrogen balances of as much as 250 mg/kg/day occur routinely in patients receiving total parenteral nutrition (110 to 125 calories/kg/day and 2.5 gm amino acids/kg/day). After a caloric intake of greater than 100 calories/kg/day is established, LBW infants can be expected to gain, on average, approximately 15 gm/kg/day and have positive nitrogen balances in the range of 200 gm/kg/day.

Complications

The complications related to total parenteral nutrition can be divided into three groups: septic, catheter related, and metabolic.

The infusate promotes the growth of certain bacteria and fungi; thus it must be mixed under strictly aseptic conditions to prevent contamination. A more important factor contributing to high rates of septic complications, however, is failure to maintain meticulous aseptic technique in placement and subsequent care of the catheter.

Many catheter-related complications have been reported (malposition, thrombosis, dislodgment), but most can be prevented by strict adherence to established principles of placement and maintenance of central vein catheters.

Metabolic complications, for the most part, are related to the content of the parenteral nutrient solution. The complications most frequently observed are listed in Table 20-6 along with their most common cause(s). Hyperglycemia is the most commonly encountered; however, with careful monitoring this complication can be minimized. Blood urea nitrogen concentrations exceeding 20 mg/dl (up to 50 mg/dl) occur rarely in infants receiving amino acid intakes of 2.5 gm/kg/day. Another complication that is more frequent, as well as potentially more hazardous in premature infants, is that of abnormal plasma aminograms. This phenomenon is

Table 20-6. Metabolic complications of total parenteral nutrition

Complication	Common cause
Hyperglycemia (osmotic diuresis, hyperosmolarity)	Glucose intolerance
Hypoglycemia	Sudden cessation
Hypernatremia or hyponatremia, hyperkalemia or hypokalemia, hyperchloremia or hypochloremia	Iatrogenic
Hypercalcemia or hypocalcemia, hyperphosphatemia or hypophosphatemia, hypermagnesemia or hypomagnesemia	Iatrogenic
Hyperchloremic metabolic acidosis	Certain crystalline amino acid mixtures
Azotemia	Excessive nitrogen intake
Hyperammonemia	Related to nitrogen source
Abnormal plasma aminograms	Related to nitrogen source
Hypervitaminoses or hypovitaminoses	Iatrogenic
Essential fatty acid deficiency	Omission
Zinc or copper deficiencies	Omission
↑SGOT, ↑SGPT, ↑ direct bilirubin, hepatomegaly?	Unknown

seen with use of any of the currently available amino acid mixtures.

The hepatic complications of hyperalimentation have recently received increasing attention and may comprise both a cholestatic and hepatocellular component. More subtle tests of early canalicular dysfunction such as gamma-glutamyl transpeptidase and 5'-nucleotidase may be abnormal prior to the more commonly used measures of liver injury (Table 20-6). The cause of cholestasis has not been established although amino acid excess has been most often implicated. Vileisis, in a recent prospective controlled study of two groups (low protein regimen at 2 to 3 gm/kg/day and higher protein regimen at 3 to 6 gm/kg/day), revealed no elevation of direct bilirubin (≥2 mg/dl) prior to 2 weeks of protein administration. Subsequently the higher protein group developed cholestasis earlier (27 versus 47 days) and achieved a greater peak direct bilirubin level (8.4 versus 3.2 mg/dl). Retrospective analysis of the infants who developed cholestasis revealed a greater daily dextrose intake in this group, which may also be an etiologic factor in the liver injury. The long-term significance of the transient cholestatic jaundice has not been established and requires further study.

Conclusions

Experience suggests that total parenteral nutrition, with adequate precaution, can be used in selected premature infants to produce satisfactory growth and positive nitrogen balance without undue risk. The long-term effects of this technique, however, cannot be assessed until experience with it is much greater than at present.

INTRAVENOUS NUTRIENTS BY PERIPHERAL VEIN

The ability to provide adequate nutrients solely by peripheral vein infusion presents at least two major problems: (1) the necessarily high osmolality of the infusate, if given in reasonable volumes, substantially limits the duration of individual infusion sites; (2) alternatively the increased volumes of less hypertonic solutions required to deliver adequate nutrients often exceed the infant's tolerance for fluid. Nonetheless, this method has been used with success.

Technique

The nutrient mixtures that have been used for peripheral intravenous nutrition are those administered via central vein, with the exception that glucose concentrations rarely exceed 10 gm/dl. More recently, intravenous lipid emulsions, which provide 11 calories/gm without an appreciable osmotic contribution, also have been used to increase calorie administration by peripheral vein. The nutrient mixture is usually infused into one of the peripheral veins on the dorsal aspect of either the hand or foot or into one of the superficial veins of the scalp. Caution in placement of the scalp vein needle, as well as subsequent meticulous care of the site, minimizes complications.

Clinical experience

In a controlled study conducted in infants weighing less that 2,500 gm, Anderson and associates compared peripheral intravenous administration of glucose alone and glucose plus amino acids (2.5 gm/kg/day), both regimens delivering 60 Cal/kg/day. The study, conducted in infants less than 1 week of age, included only those who received no nutrients by the enteral route. Even with this limited caloric intake, infants who received the regimen of glucose plus amino acids gained small but statistically insignificant amounts of weight (average, 2 gm/kg/day). More important, all were in positive nitrogen balance (average, 150 mg/kg/day). Infants who received only glucose, on the other hand, lost weight (approximately 12 gm/kg/day) and were in negative nitrogen balance (average, 125 mg/kg/day). This study shows that the catabolic tendency of the LBW infant during the first week of life can be reversed simply by adding amino acids to the frequently used regimen of intravenously administered glucose (10 gm/dl). The fluid volume (150 ml/kg/day) delivered by Anderson and associates was well tolerated.

Addition of small amounts of an intravenous fat emulsion to this regimen should prevent essential fatty acid deficiency and increase the total caloric intake, thereby making short-term use of such a regimen as efficacious at total parenteral nutrition by central vein catheter. The validity of this prediction is supported by a report concerning use of glucose, amino acids, and an intravenous lipid emulsion delivered by peripheral vein to neonates with surgical problems. All received amino acids (4.0 gm/kg/day), glucose (7 gm/kg/day), and an intravenuous lipid emulsion (4 gm/kg/day) in a total volume of 150 ml/kg/day providing 88 Cal/kg/day. Duration of infusion varied from 8 to 30 days, and the average daily weight gain was 19.6 gm (range 9.6 to 33.0 gm/day). The lipid emulsion particles are metabolized similarly to natural chylomicrons and result in the triglycerides being hydrolyzed by lipoprotein lipase to glycerol and free fatty acids. The latter may be oxidized to make energy or resynthesized into triglycerides. The dose of lipid tolerated by neonates varies considerably with an upper limit of approximately 3 gm/kg/day. Preterm infants who are small for gestational age appear to have less tolerance than appropriately grown infants, resulting in higher triglyceride and free fatty acid levels. Lipid emulsions should generally be infused over 24 hours and complications minimized by monitoring serum triglyceride levels. Recent data indicate that lipid infusions may result in a sustained increase in serum glucose concentration and a small transient rise in insulin values in preterm infants. The mechanism whereby lipid emulsions alter glucose homeostasis requires further study.

Complications

The metabolic complications of this method of nutrient delivery should be roughly the same as those observed with parenteral nutrition by central vein. However, fewer metabolic complications have been reported. Septic complications rarely occur, but phlebitis and local complications of fluid extravasation (such as cutaneous sloughs or superficial infections) occur frequently. However, maintenance of adequate infusion sites for any extended period is the greatest problem.

Lipid emulsions have been documented to have potential complications, the long-term significance of which remains to be determined. Free fatty acids released during lipid hydrolysis may compete with bilirubin for albumen binding sites in vitro, although there are no reports of greater bilirubin toxicity in infants administered lipid emulsions. Nonetheless, caution should be exercised in jaundiced infants (Chapter 30). Pulmonary arterial lipid deposits have been observed in the pulmonary arterial walls of infants receiving lipid infusions, and fat globules have also been noted in alveolar macrophages at autopsy.

INTRAVENOUS SUPPLEMENTATION OF TOLERATED ORAL FEEDINGS

The technique of supplementing tolerated oral feedings with intravenous infusions of various nutrients has been practiced for a number of years. In its simplest form—supplementing tolerated enteral feedings with intravenous infusions of 10% glucose—this method represents what might be considered conventional feeding of premature infants at the present time. More recently, enteral feedings have been supplemented with intravenous infusions of glucose and amino acid mixtures or mixtures of glucose, amino acids, and lipid.

Clinical experience

Although this technique has been used frequently, few controlled studies have been reported. The most impressive weight gains reported to date, approaching those expected in utero, were achieved by Cashore and associates by supplementing tolerated oral feedings with peripheral intravenous infusions of a mixture of protein hydrolysate, glucose, and an intravenous lipid emulsion. Length and head circumference also increased at approximately the in utero rates.

Complications

The complications of this technique include the usual complications of enteral feedings as well as the complications of intravenous nutrition. However, use of the combination of nutrient delivery methods is advantageous in that smaller volumes of enteral feedings can be given, thus decreasing the risk of aspiration and other complications. The most commonly encountered metabolic problem is hyperglycemia. Azotemia, reflecting an excessive nitrogen intake, was observed by Bryan and co-workers as well as by Pildes and associates. A more disturbing, but not unexpected, problem is that of abnormal plasma aminogram; this problem is likely to occur less frequently as better amino acid mixtures become available.

CONCLUSIONS

A number of methods for feeding LBW infants are available. The task of the physician caring for the LBW infant is to be aware of these various methods and their usefulness in specific clinical situations. With such an awareness it should be possible to adapt a suitable feeding regimen for all LBW infants, resulting in vastly improved nutritional management compared with present practice.

William C. Heird
Thomas L. Anderson

BIBLIOGRAPHY

Anderson, T.L., Nicholson, J.F., and Heird, W.C.: Conrolled trial of intravenous glucose vs. glucose and amino acids in premature infants, Pediatr. Res. **10**:351, 1976.

Benda, G.I., and Babson, S.G.: Peripheral intravenous alimentation of the small premature infant, J. Pediatr. **79**:494, 1971.

Black, D.D., Suttle, E.A., Whitington, P.F., and others: The effect of short-term parenteral nutrition on hepatic function in the human neonate: a prospective randomized study demonstrating alteration of hepatic canalicular function, J. Pediatr. **99**:445, 1981.

Boros, S.J., and Reynolds, J.W.: Duodenal perforation: a complication of neonatal transpyloric tube feeding, J. Pediatr. **85**:107, 1974.

Borresen, H.C., Coran, A.G., and Knutrud, O.: Metabolic results of parenteral feeding in neonatal surgery, Ann. Surg. **172**:291, 1970.

Borresen, H.C., and Knutrud, O.: Parenteral feeding of neonates undergoing major surgery, Acta Paediatr. Scand. **58**:420, 1969.

Bryan, M.H., and others: Supplemental intravenous alimentation in low-birth-weight infants, J. Pediatr. **82**:940, 1973.

Caldwell, M.D., Meng, H.C., and Jonsson, L.T.: Essential fatty acid deficiency (EFAD)—now a human disease, Fed. Proc. **33**:915, 1974.

Cashore, W.J., Sedaghtiam, R., and Usher, R.H.: Postnatal growth of low birth weight infants given early intravenous nutrition, Pediatr. Res. **7**:400, 1973.

Castro, G.A., and others: Intestinal disaccharidase and peroxidase activities in parenterally nourished rats, J. Nutr. **105**:776, 1975.

Cheek, J.A., and Staub, G.F.: Nasojejunal alimentation for premature and full-term infants, J. Pediatr. **82**:955, 1973.

Chen, J.W., and Wong, P.W.K.: Intestinal complications of nasojejunal feeding in low-birth-weight infants, J. Pediatr. **85**:109, 1974.

Coran, A.G.: The long-term total intravenous feeding of infants using peripheral veins, J. Pediatr. Surg. **8**:801, 1973.

Crump, E.P., Gore, P.M., and Horton, C.P.: The sucking behavior in premature infants, Hum. Biol. **30**:128, 1958.

Dahms, B.D., and Halpin, T.C., Jr.: Pulmonary arterial lipid deposit in newborn infants receiving intravenous lipid infusion, J. Pediatr. **97**:800, 1980.

Driscoll, J.M., Jr., and others: Total intravenous alimentation in low-birth-weight infants: a preliminary report, J. Pediatr. **81**:145, 1972.

Dudrick, S.J., Vars, H.M., and Rhoades, J.E.: Growth of puppies receiving all nutritional requirements by vein. In Fortschritte der parneteralen ernahrung, Symposion der International Society of Parenteral Nutrition, Munich, 1967, Palas.

Dudrick, S.J., Wilmore, D.W., and Vars, H.M.: Long-term venous catheterization—an adjunct to surgical care and study. In Zuidema, G.D., and Skinner, D.B.: Current topics in surgical research, vol. 1, New York, 1969, Academic Press, Inc.

Dudrick, S.J., and others: Long-term total parenteral nutrition with growth, development and positive nitrogen balance, Surgery **64**:138, 1968.

Filler, R.M., and others: Long-term total parenteral nutrition in infants, N. Engl. J. Med. **281**:589, 1969.

Fox, H.A., and Krasna, I.H.: Total intravenous nutrition by peripheral vein in neonatal surgical patients, Pediatrics **52**:14, 1973.

Greene, H.L., and others: Intractable diarrhea and malnutrition in infancy: changes in intestinal morphology and disaccharidase activities during treatment with total parenteral nutrition or oral elemental diets, J. Pediatr. **87**:695, 1975.

Gustafsson, A., and others: Nutrition in low birth weight infants. I. Intravenous injection of fat emulsion, Acta Paediatr. Scand. **61**:149, 1972.

Hallberg, D.: Studies on the elimination of exogenous lipids from the blood stream: the kinetics for the elimination of a fat emulsion studied by single injection technique in man, Acta Physiol. Scand. **64**:306, 1965.

Heird, W.C., and Driscoll, J.M., Jr.: Newer methods for feeding low birth weight infants, Clin. Perinatol. **2**:309, 1975.

Heird, W.C., MacMillan, R., and Winters, R.W.: Total parenteral nutrition in pediatrics. In Barness, L., editor: Report of First Wyeth Nutritional Symposium, Philadelphia, 1975, Wyeth Laboratories.

Heird, W.C., MacMillan, R.W., and Winters, R.W.: Total parenteral nutrition in the pediatric patient. In Fischer, J.E.: Total parenteral nutrition, Boston, 1976, Little, Brown & Co.

Heird, W.C., and Winters, R.W.: Total intravenous alimentation, Am. J. Dis. Child. **126**:287, 1973.

Heird, W.C., and Winters, R.W.: Total parenteral nutrition: the state of the art, J. Pediatr. **86**:2, 1975.

Keller, A.: Studies of motility relations of the infant stomach, Nord. Med. **38**:1141, 1948.

Levine, A.M., and others: Role of oral intake in maintenance of gut mass and disaccharide activity, Gastroenterology **67**:975, 1974.

Peden, V.H., and Karpel, J.T.: Total parenteral nutrition in premature infants, J. Pediatr. **81**:137, 1972.

Peden, V.H., Sammon, T.J., and Downey, D.A.: Intravenously induced infantile intoxication with ethanol, J. Pediatr. **83**:490, 1973.

Pildes, R.S., and others: Intravenous supplementation of L-amino acids and dextrose in low-birth-weight infants, J. Pediatr. **82**:945, 1973.

Pyati, S., Ramamurthy, R.S., and Pildes, R.S.: Continuous drip nasogastric feedings: a controlled study, Pediatr. Res. **10**:359, 1976.

Rhea, J.W., Ahmid, M.S., and Mange, E.S.: Nasojejunal (transpyloric) feeding: a commentary, J. Pediatr. **86**:451, 1975.

Rhea, J.W., Ghazzawi, O., and Weidman, W.: Nasojejunal feeding: an improved device and intubation, J. Pediatr. **82**:951, 1973.

Rhea, J.W., and Kilby, J.O.: A nasojejunal tube for infant feeding, Pediatrics **46**:36, 1970.

Roy, N., and others: Impaired assimilation of nasojejunal feedings in very low birth weight infant, Pediatr. Res. **10**:359, 1976.

Rubin, E., and Lieber, C.S.: Fatty liver, alcoholic cirrhosis produced by alcohol in primates, N. Engl. J. Med. **290**:128, 1974.

Schwachman, H., and others: Protracted diarrhea of infancy treated by intravenous alimentation, Am. J. Dis. Child. **125**:365, 1973.

VanCaillie, M., and Powell, G.K.: Nasoduodenal vs. nasogastric feeding in the very low birth weight infant, Pediatrics **56**:1065, 1975.

Vileisis, R.A., Cowett, R.M., and Oh, W.: Glycemic response to lipid infusion in the premature neonate, J. Pediatr. **100**:108, 1982.

Vileisis, R.A., Inwood, R.J., and Hunt, C.E.: Prospective controlled study of parenteral nutrition—associated cholestatic jaundice: effect of protein intake, J. Pediatr. **96**:893, 1980.

Wilmore, D.W., and Dudrick, S.J.: Growth and development of an infant receiving all nutrients exclusively by vein, J.A.M.A. **203**:140, 1968.

PART THREE

Provision of water and electrolytes

During delivery the infant is moved from the sea of the amniotic fluid to terrestrial life. The constant water loss in this new environment with its threat of dehydration necessitates the exogenous provision of water and electrolytes to replace those lost. This section is concerned with the physician's formulation of this provision.

VOLUME AND COMPOSITION OF BODY FLUIDS

At birth the percentage of body weight represented by water is approximately 75% in term infants and greater in those born prematurely (Fig. 20-1). The sharp decrease in this percentage over the first year of life is due to the accumulation of body fat, representing only 12% of body weight at birth in full-term infants but 30% by age 1 year. In addition, the relative distribution of water between the intracellular and extracellular spaces changes during this period. In an infant born at term the intracellular volume occupies 35% of body weight and the extracellular volume 40%. By age 3 months these volumes are equal, each occupying 35% of body weight. In contrast, in the older infant and child the intracellular volume represents 45% of body weight and the extracellular volume 20%.

The composition of body fluid varies with the compartment in which it is contained, the primary cation of extracellular fluid being sodium and that of intracellular fluid potassium. The vascular membrane and cell membrane separating the major body fluid subdivisions are freely permeable to water. Therefore, although the electrolyte composition varies, osmotic equilibrium is obtained between these compartments. The size of the compartments then depends primarily on the number of osmoles within, which in turn is dependent on the cellular pump for the intracellular space and on the kidney for the extracellular space. Within the extracellular space the relative distribution between the intravascular and interstitial compartments is dependent on the oncotic pressure exerted by plasma proteins, which favors expansion of vascular volume at the expense of interstitial volume, and the counteracting influence of capillary hydrostatic pressure. Osmolality of serum can be measured easily by freezing point depression (normally 285 to 295 mOsm/L), and a close approximation can be obtained by doubling the serum sodium concentration. Approximation by this method is reasonable, since sodium and an equal number of anions are nearly the sole determinants of osmolality in extracellular fluid. The osmolality of interstitial and intracellular compartments can be inferred from plasma osmolality, since osmotic equilibrium is present.

Real or apparent alterations in plasma osmolality, as estimated from the serum sodium concentration, may occur in several situations. Electrolytes are dissolved in body water (except for small amounts bound to plasma proteins). As measured in the clinical laboratory, however, the concentrations are determined not just in water but in plasma or serum, consisting of water plus the volume occupied by protein. The apparent volume in which these substances are dissolved (plasma) is greater than the actual volume of plasma water. In 1 L of plasma there are only 940 ml water; the remainder consists of 60 gm of protein. Concentrations in plasma water thus exceed those in plasma by 1,000/940, or 1.06. Although these differences in sodium concentration related to plasma protein are of little clinical significance, the differences due to elevation of plasma *lipids* may be important. A marked hyponatremia may be present when sodium is measured on a lactescent sample but disappear when lipid is extracted and the sodium concentration is measured

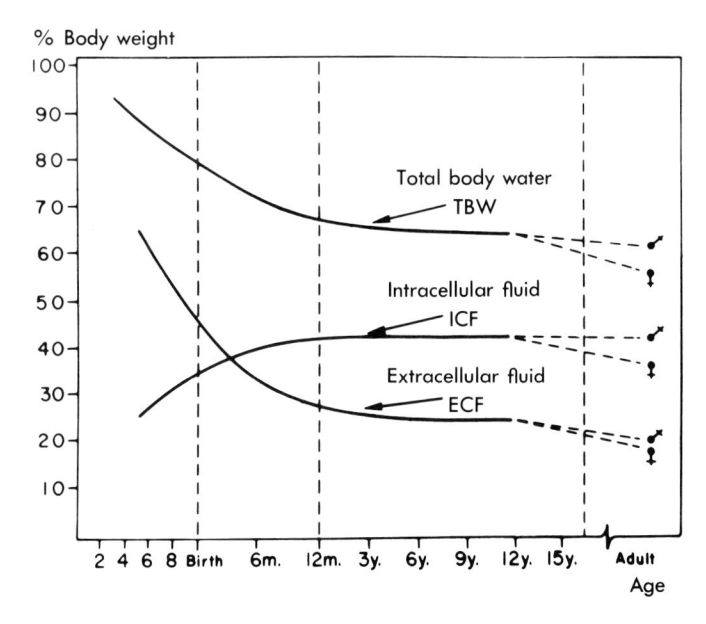

Fig. 20-1. Change with age in total body water and its major subdivisions. (Data from Friis-Hansen. From Winters, R.W., editor: The body fluids in pediatrics, Boston, 1973, Little, Brown & Co., p. 100.)

in plasma water. Such elevations of lipids are only rarely encountered in the neonatal period. Increased concentrations of glucose and urea are more often observed, however, and may lead to erroneous estimation of osmolality if calculated only from serum sodium concentration.

The molecular weight of glucose is 180. At a plasma concentration of 90 mg/dl glucose would contribute 5 mOsm/L of plasma. With marked elevation of plasma glucose levels, as in an infant of low birth weight given a parenteral infusion containing a high concentration of glucose, this substance may contribute 40 mOsm/L or more (representing plasma glucose levels of 800 mg/dl or greater). If a normal plasma osmolality were to be maintained in the presence of a plasma glucose concentration of 800 mg/dl, only 240 mOsm would be contributed by sodium and an equal number of anions, resulting in a serum sodium concentration of 120 mEq/L. The addition of glucose, which is osmotically active, to the extracellular fluid at a rate greater than maximal cellular metabolism of glucose causes water to move from the intracellular to the extracellular compartment to achieve osmotic equilibrium. The result is an expanded extracellular volume with increased osmolality and dilutional hyponatremia. This relationship has been quantified by Katz in an idealized fashion for the adult such that a decrease in serum sodium concentration of 1.6 mEq/L would be expected for each 100 mg/dl increase in serum glucose concentration over the baseline of 100 mg/dl. In the LBW infant the contraction of intracellular volume involves the potential danger of cerebral hemorrhage.

Urea readily diffuses across the cell membrane, and no osmotic gradient exists (except in acute elevations of serum urea levels). Each 28 mg of serum urea nitrogen (BUN or SUN) represent 1 mmol of urea. (Each millimole of urea contains two nitrogens with an atomic weight of 14 each). A BUN concentration of 15 mg/dl is equivalent to 5.4 mmol of urea per liter. This would contribute only 5.4 mOsm to each liter of body water. However, an infant with acute renal failure may have a BUN concentration of 100 mg/dl, which would contribute 35.7 mOsm/L. If a normal plasma osmolality of 280 mOsm/L were maintained in this setting, serum sodium concentration must be 122 mEq/L, $\frac{(280-36)}{2}$.

DETERMINATION OF ADEQUATE FLUID AND ELECTROLYTE PROVISIONS

In the older infant and child the goal of parenteral fluid therapy is the maintenance of zero balance for water and electrolytes, assuming that there are no preexisting deficits or excesses. Over the short term the positive balances necessary for growth are neglected. In the neonate the volume of body fluids that is physiologically appropriate, and thus desirable to maintain, is not entirely clear. Some weight loss over the first few postnatal days has been called "physiologic." This decrease in weight is due largely to the loss of water and sodium from the extracellular space. A reasonable goal of fluid therapy during this period would be the prevention of dehydration, although not necessarily maintenance of zero balance for water and electrolytes. Weight loss should not be greater than 10% of birth weight (or 15% of birth weight for infants weighing less than 1,500 gm). Beyond the first 3 days of life, therapy should be designed to maintain zero balance. Over the short term it is not necessary to provide sufficient calories for growth but only enough to retard catabolism. Oral or tube feedings should be instituted and progressed in volume as quickly as is feasible (p. 298).

Zero balance for fluid and electrolytes occurs when the intake of these substances is exactly equal to the output from all sources. (Intake − output = 0.) The formulation of a reasonable plan for the intake of fluid and electrolytes thus requires the accurate determination of the output of these substances. Since fluid losses are related most closely to caloric expenditure, this is the most useful and most uniformly applicable frame of reference. During the neonatal period, nongrowing infants (those receiving parenteral fluids only) expend about 75 Cal/kg/day (p. 303). Over the first 2 days of life, however, metabolic rate is approximately 25% lower. The infant receiving oral feedings may expend 120 Cal/kg/day if intake is sufficient to allow growth. Those who are small for gestational age have higher metabolic rates than those with the same weight but appropriate for gestational age.

There are four normal sources of water loss: insensible loss, urine, sweat, and fecal water. *Insensible loss* is the loss of water through the lungs during respiration and through evaporation from skin. Of the total insensible loss, about 30% is pulmonary. An average loss by this route is 40 ml/100 Cal for an infant in an environment of moderate humidity (40% to 60%). In LBW infants, particularly those with weights less than 1,250 gm, insensible loss may be up to 300% higher than that predicted for term infants. The causes of this inverse relationship between insensible water loss and gestational age are several and include increased permeability of skin to water, greater surface area per unit of body weight, and a relative increase in the vascularity of skin in infants of lower birth weight.

Wide variations in urine output are possible because of the concentrating and diluting features of the kidney. The primary determinants of urine volume and osmolality in the neonatal period are water and solute intake and the presence or absence of growth. The minimum and maximum volume of urine is determined by the amount

Table 20-7. Urinary osmolality at varying solute loads when 92 ml water/100 Cal are available for urine formation*

Renal solute load (mOsm/100 Cal)	Urinary osmolality (mOsm/L)
10	110
20	220
30	330

*92 ml water = 80 ml provided exogenously + 12 ml endogenously from water of oxidation.

of solute for excretion and the maximal renal concentrating and diluting ability. The newborn is able to dilute urine maximally to osmolalities of 30 to 50 mOsm/L and to concentrate urine maximally to 700 to 800 mOsm/L (less than the 1,200 mOsm/L seen in children and adults). Thus, if 40 mOsm must be excreted per day and the maximal concentrating ability is 700 mOsm/L, the minimum volume of urine would be 57 ml; and the maximum volume, if the diluting capacity is 50 mOsm/L, would be 800 ml. The renal solute load in infants may vary from 10 to 30 mOsm/100 Cal metabolized; the lower values are characteristic of rapidly growing infants receiving breast milk or similar commercial formulas, and the higher values are for starved infants or those fed formulas with high protein and electolyte content. A parenteral fluid regimen that is not electrolyte free should provide a solute load between these extremes. An average load for an infant on a parenteral fluid regimen containing glucose with no oral feeding would be 20 mOsm/100 Cal, approximately half from metabolism and half from added electrolyte. Using this range of values for solute excretion, one can calculate a water allowance for urine that will permit the excretion of this load within the middle range of urinary osmolalities, stressing neither the concentrating nor diluting capacities of the kidney. If 80 ml water are provided per 100 Cal, such urinary osmolalities should result (Table 20-7).

Sweat losses are generally negligible or nonexistent. LBW infants exhibit a limited or absent response to the stress of warmth; term infants, who are able to respond, are generally in a temperature-controlled environment in the modern nursery. If sweating should occur, term infants may increase evaporative loss threefold. *Fecal losses* are 0 to 10 ml/100 Cal; infants on a parenteral feeding regimen alone have the lower values.

Based on a consideration of these losses, an average parenteral fluid plan for a term infant receiving no oral feeding should provide about 40 ml of water per 100 Cal for insensible loss and 80 ml/100 calories for urine, with perhaps 5 ml/100 Cal for stool water, resulting in a total volume of 125 ml/100 Cal expended or 90 to 95 ml/kg. (Although calculation of fluid requirements based on caloric expenditure is more appropriate physiologically, it is recognized that computation of fluid administration based on body weight simplifies these calculations in a busy nursery. Therefore values will be given using both denominators.) On the first day of life this should be decreased by 25% to 30%. This volume is a first approximation and may need adjustment based on continuing clinical and laboratory evaluation and special modifying considerations discussed later.

Water allowances are calculated to avoid extremes of concentration or dilution, and electrolytes should be provided similarly to avoid maximal renal sodium reabsorption or excretion. Upper and lower levels of tolerance are not known. However, since babies historically have thrived on both human milk and cow's milk, it seems reasonable to provide an electrolyte intake somewhere between the two. Providing 2.5 mEq each of sodium and potassium per 100 Cal (2 mEq/kg) and 5 mEq chloride per 100 Cal expended (4 mEq/kg) will accomplish this. Thus the electrolytes contained in the infusion (10 mOsm/100 Cal) plus endogenous solute from energy metabolism (10 mOsm/100 Cal) result in a calculated renal solute load of 20 mOsm/100 Cal. Potassium should be omitted during the first 24 hours.

Very low birth weight infants may not be able to maintain zero sodium balance on this quantity of electrolyte because of increased renal excretion of sodium (decreased tubular reabsorption of sodium). These infants, particularly those weighing less than 1250 gm, may sometimes require up to 8 mEq sodium/kg during the first 1 or 2 weeks of life to maintain zero or slightly negative balance during the period of "physiologic" weight loss, followed by decreasing requirement thereafter.

These calculations apply to a mature infant who is fairly inactive, is in a thermoneutral environment with a relative humidity of 40% to 60%, and has adequate renal function. Metabolic rate increases with activity, illness, or decrease in ambient temperature. Additional calories are expended if the infant is fed orally or is growing. Given this number of variables, it should be clear that repeated assessment of the adequacy of any parenteral therapy plan is essential. Accurate body weight should be determined as an index of hydration, daily or more frequently. Tissue turgor is often difficult to interpret, particularly in LBW infants with little subcutaneous fat, but nonetheless it should be examined. Edema should be sought in the pretibial, presacral, and facial areas as a sign of overhydration. Oral mucous membranes in a well-hydrated infant should be moist, as assessed by an examiner's clean finger. The measurement of urine and plasma osmolality or urine specific gravity is most valuable in judging hydration. In the absence of renal disease, urinary osmolalities should be between 150 and 400 mOsm/L (specific gravity 1.006 to 1.013). Plasma osmolality is estimated from the serum sodium concentration. Variations in serum sodium more often reflect changes in water balance than in sodium balance, and in the absence of very large sodium loads hypernatremia suggests an increased need for water. Modest hyponatremia is frequent in very low birth weight infants, but values under 130 mEq/L may reflect overhydration. The rate of excretion of sodium in urine (not sodium concentration) may be useful in distinguishing true sodium depletion from dilutional hyponatremia if the intake of sodium is known. Changes in the hematocrit value and in serum concentrations of urea, and proteins are more dependent on variables other than hydration and therefore are of only ancillary value in assessing states of hydration.

MODIFIERS OF WATER AND ELECTROLYTE PROVISIONS

Since the quantitative recommendations just mentioned are predicated on a specific physiologic state, it is apparent that alterations in any of these physiologic components must change the parenteral fluid plan. An *increase in insensible water loss* over the average values just discussed is encountered primarily in two situations common in nursery units: in LBW infants and in infants undergoing phototherapy. Infants of low birth weight, particularly those less than 1,250 gm, may have relatively enormous water requirements because of increased insensible loss. Fanaroff and associates found insensible water loss in these babies to be 60 to 120 ml/kg/day (80 to 160 ml/100 Cal metabolized). In such infants water allowances for the first day of life should be increased to 120 to 140 ml/100 Cal (85 to 100 ml/kg) and rapidly increased as necessary (based on new clinical data) to 200 ml or more per 100 Cal metabolized (140 ml/kg). Although the necessity for increasing parenteral fluid allowances in LBW infants to maintain water balance has been emphasized, it should also be stressed that overestimation of the rate of fluid administration in these infants may have undesirable consequences as well. The incidence of patent ductus arteriosus and necrotizing enterocolitis appears to be higher in premature infants receiving a high rate of fluid administration than in those receiving a volume 20 ml/kg/day less. Suggested rates of fluid administration for different groups of LBW infants, based on the low-volume group in the study of Bell and others, are given in Table 20-8. Phototherapy increases both insensible water loss and stool water. The mechanism of the increased insensible loss is not known but is related most probably to elevated skin blood flow. The stool loss may be due to decreased GI transit time secondary to photodecomposition products. An additional water increment of 25 ml/100 Cal (20 ml/kg/day) is a reasonable first approximation for infants undergoing phototherapy. The use of a radiant warmer will increase insensible loss to 45 to 60 ml/kg/day. Elevation of ambient temperature by 1° or 2° within the thermoneutral zone will increase insensible water loss by about 50% (in infants weighing less than 1,250 gm by 70%). Elevation of ambient temperature outside this neutral zone will triple or quadruple the insensible loss.

Table 20-8. Fluid requirement (ml/kg/day)

Birthweight (gm)	Days 1-2	Day 3	Days 15-30
751-1,000	105	140	150
1,001-1,250	100	130	140
1,251-1,500	90	120	130
1,501-1,750	80	110	130
1,751-2,000	80	110	130

Adapted from data of Bell, E.F., and others: Lancet **2**:90, 1979.

Decreased insensible water loss occurs in infants on mechanical respirators with highly humidified air or in those exposed to a high environmental humidity. Pulmonary loss of water is often zero in infants on respirators, and water allotment should be decreased by the 10 ml/kg/day normally lost through this route. The use of a plastic heat shield can reduce insensible loss by 25% in infants weighing less than 1,250 gm.

Alterations in water allotment for urine may be necessitated by obligatory increases or decreases in urine volume. An *increase in urine volume* due to defective concentrating ability is seen in renal dysplasia, particularly that associated with posterior urethral valves (Chapter 31). Central diabetes insipidus is a potential but rare problem in neonates. Hydration is best maintained in these situations by measurement of urine volume and sodium and replacement of these losses in addition to 40 ml/100 Cal (30 ml/kg) provided for insensible loss. With marked polyuria extreme changes in hydration can occur rapidly. Careful and frequent monitoring of body weight (every 8 to 12 hours) is therefore important.

An obligatory *decrease in urine volume* occurs with renal failure; in the neonatal period this is most often secondary to hypoxia or septic shock. The maintainance of zero balance for water in this situation requires replacement of the output from insensible loss (40 ml/100 Cal (30 ml/kg), from which is subtracted the endogenous input of water from oxidation (approximately 12 ml/100 Cal), resulting in a parenteral water requirement of 25 to 30 ml/100 Cal. This is administered as 10% glucose in water. Urine volume, if any, can be replaced if one desires to maintain the present state of hydration. If there is preexisting expansion of extracellular volume, it may be preferable to allow a negative balance by not replacing urine volume until a normal state of hydration

Table 20-9. Water and electrolyte provision in the neonatal period

	ml water per 100 Cal expended	ml water per kilogram of body weight*	mEq per kilogram of body weight Sodium	mEq per kilogram of body weight Potassium
Basic maintenence requirements				
Insensible water loss	40	30		
Urinary water	80	60	2	2
Stool water	5	3		
Totals	125	93	2	2
Modifications of basic requirements				
First day fo life	−30 to 35	−22 to 25	1.5	0
Birthweight less than 2,000 gm	(See Table 20-8)		2 to 8	2
Phototherapy	+25	+20		
Obligatory increase in urine volume (concentrating defect)	+ measured volume of urine		+ measured Na$^+$ and K$^+$	
Obligatory decrease in urine volume (renal failure)	−90 to 95† + measured volume of urine	−68 to 71†	0	0
Mechanical ventilation	−14	−10		

*Based on a caloric expenditure of 75 Cal/kg.
†These figures are obtained by eliminating the 80 ml/100 Cal for urine volume plus the input from water of oxidation of 10 to 15 ml/100 Cal.

is achieved. Potassium should not be administered and sodium given only if there is sodium loss in urine and no expansion of extracellular volume.

Increased loss of stool water occurs in diarrhea. The best gauge of diarrheal losses is change in body weight. In general, these losses are isotonic and should be replaced with isotonic saline plus an additional 2 mEq of potassium per kilogram of body weight.

Ongoing losses from chest tubes and fistulas must not be overlooked. Even though losses may be small in daily volume, cumulative losses by these routes may cause serious dehydration and electrolyte imbalance. Drainage from chest tubes should be measured, and sodium and potassium content should be determined and then replaced by water and the appropriate electrolytes. Fistulous losses may be determined by weighing overlying bandages.

SPECIFIC RECOMMENDATIONS

Guidelines for the specific formulation of a parenteral fluid and electrolyte plan are given in Table 20-9. For ease of computation in practice, values are given per kilogram of body weight as well as on the more physiologic basis of calories metabolized. Changes in caloric expenditure with fever, increased activity, or cold stress will necessitate changes in fluid provisions as calculated per kilogram of body weight. The most common error in fluid and electrolyte therapy is the failure to continually reevaluate clinical and laboratory data as a basis for quantitative alterations in the original plan. Specific recommendations are estimates, and their appropriateness for a given infant must be reassessed frequently during therapy. Since these infusions do not provide sufficient calories for growth, enteral feedings should be instituted as soon as possible.

Martin A. Nash

BIBLIOGRAPHY

Bell, E.F., and others: The effects of thermal environment on heat balance and insensible water loss in low-birth-weight infants, J. Pediatr. **96**:452, 1980.

Bell, E.F., and others: High volume fluid intake predisposes premature infants to necrotising enterocolitis (letter to editor), Lancet **2**:90, 1979.

Bell, E.F., and others: Effect of fluid administration on the development of symptomatic patent ductus arteriosus and congestive heart failure in premature infants, N. Engl. J. Med. **302**:598, 1980.

Engelke, S.C., and others: Sodium balance in very low-birth-weight infants, J. Pediatr. **93**:837, 1978.

Fanaroff, A.A., and others: Insensible water loss in low birth weight infants, Pediatrics **50**:236, 1972.

Friis-Hansen, B.: Body water compartments in children: changes during growth and related changes in body composition, Pediatrics **28**:169, 1961.

Katz, M.A.: Hyperglycemia-induced hyponatremia calculation of expected serum sodium depression, N. Engl. J. Med. **289**:843, 1973.

Okken, A., and others: Insensible water loss and metabolic rate in low birth weight newborn infants, Pediatr. Res. **13**:1072, 1979.

Sulyok, E., and others: On the mechanism of renal sodium handling in newborn infants, Biol. Neonate **37**:75, 1980.

Wu, P.Y.K., and Hodgman, J.E.: Insensible water loss in preterm infants: changes with postnatal development and non-iodizing radiant energy, Pediatrics **54**:704, 1974.

PART FOUR

Disturbances of acid-base equilibrium

The newborn is subject to many common disorders that manifest acid-base disturbances ranging from respiratory distress syndrome to various renal and gastrointestinal problems. Essential to proper diagnosis and treatment of these disorders is an understanding of the principles underlying acid-base regulation, which can be viewed in general as a complex interaction between physiochemical and physiologic mechanisms.

PHYSIOCHEMICAL MECHANISMS OF ACID-BASE REGULATION

The physiochemical mechanisms regulating acid-base equilibrium are primarily the various buffer systems of body fluids. Buffers are defined as substances that can minimize changes in pH when acid or base is added to a system. In biologic systems these consist of weak acids (HB) and their conjugate bases (B^-):

$$\underset{\text{Weak acid}}{HB} \rightleftharpoons \underset{\text{Conjugate base}}{H^+ + B^-}$$

Each weak acid with its conjugate base is called a buffer pair. Strong acid added to a buffer system is converted to a weak acid by reaction with the conjugate base:

$$\underset{\text{Strong acid}}{H^+X^-} + \underset{\text{Conjugate base}}{Na^+B^-} \rightarrow \underset{\text{Neutral salt}}{Na^+X^-} + \underset{\text{Weak acid}}{HB}$$

Strong base, on the other hand, reacts with a weak acid to generate the conjugate base and water:

$$\underset{\text{Strong base}}{Na^+OH^-} + \underset{\text{Weak acid}}{HB} \rightarrow \underset{\text{Conjugate base}}{Na^+B^-} + \underset{\text{Water}}{H_2O}$$

The pH of a buffered solution is defined by the Henderson-Hasselbalch equation, simply a special case of the general dissociation equation:

$$pH = pK' + \log \frac{[\text{Conjugate base}]}{[\text{Weak acid}]}$$

This equation states that the pH is equal to a constant, pK' (characteristic for a particular buffer system), plus the logarithm of the ratio of the concentrations of the conjugate base and the undissociated acid.

Many substances in the various compartments of body fluids behave as buffers. Those in blood are better characterized than those in other fluid compartments and may be divided into two general categories of buffers: the bicarbonate system and the nonbicarbonate system (Table 20-10). The bicarbonate system exists chiefly in the plasma. Bicarbonate is the conjugate base of this system, and carbonic acid (H_2CO_3) is the weak acid. The nonbicarbonate system, present chiefly in the erythrocyte, consists largely of hemoglobin, with smaller contributions from plasma proteins as well as organic and inorganic phosphates. For convenience the nonbicarbonate buffers are designated by the symbols HBuf (the weak acid) and Buf^- (the conjugate base). If the erythrocyte membrane is disregarded and all blood buffers are assumed to exist in a homogenous medium, the following equation holds:

$$pH = pK'_{H_2CO_3} + \log \frac{[HCO_3^-]}{[H_2CO_3]} = pK'_{HBuf} + \log \frac{[Buf^-]}{[HBuf]}$$

Table 20-10. Distribution of blood buffers

Buffer system	Percent buffering in whole blood
Nonbicarbonate buffers	
Hemoglobin and oxyhemoglobin	35
Organic phosphate	3
Inorganic phosphate	2
Plasma protein	7
Total	47
Bicarbonate buffers	
Plasma bicarbonate	35
Erythrocyte bicarbonate	18
Total	53

According to the equation, the pH of blood is a function of the ratio of the two sets of buffers. This gives rise to the following implications: (1) any strong acid or base added to the blood will be buffered by both systems; (2) primary changes in one of these buffer pairs can be buffered only by the other buffer system; and (3) the physiologic mechanisms regulating pH need regulate only one buffer pair (that is, regulation of one pair automatically results in regulation of the other).

PHYSIOLOGIC MECHANISMS OF ACID-BASE REGULATION

The bicarbonate buffer system possesses several unique advantages as a physiologic regulator of pH. First, the weak acid of the system (H_2CO_3) is in equilibrium with the dissolved carbon dioxide of the plasma:

$$H_2CO_3 \rightleftharpoons H_2O + (CO_2)_d$$

At equilibrium the amount of dissolved CO_2 exceeds that of H_2CO_3 by a factor of 800:1; thus for practical purposes H_2CO_3 and $(CO_2)_d$ can be treated interchangeably. Second, the dissolved CO_2 of pulmonary capillary blood achieves equilibrium with the partial pressure of CO_2

(P_{CO_2}) in the alveolar gas phase of the lung, a relationship given by Henry's law:

$$H_2CO_3 + (CO_2)_d = S \cdot P_{CO_2}$$

In this equation, S is the solubility constant for CO_2 in plasma; its value is 0.0301 mmol $(CO_2)_d$ per liter of plasma per mm Hg of P_{CO_2}. In health, $S \cdot P_{CO_2}$ (0.0301 × 40 mm Hg) equals 1.2 mmol/L. A third biologic advantage of this buffer system is the almost unlimited supply of CO_2 available from metabolism. In addition, the plasma concentration of HCO_3^-, the conjugate base of the bicarbonate buffer system, can be regulated by the renal tubule.

As expressed by the Henderson-Hasselbalch equation, blood pH is equal to a constant plus the log of the ratio of the concentrations of bicarbonate and dissolved CO_2:

$$pH = 6.1 + \log \frac{[HCO_3^-]}{[S \cdot P_{CO_2}]}$$

Thus, if the ratio of $[HCO_3^-]/S \cdot P_{CO_2}$ is decreased, pH decreases; if it is increased, pH increases. The physiologic mechanisms for maintaining normal acid-base equilibrium, as well as for countering disorders of acid-base equilibrium, must be directed toward maintenance of this ratio.

Plasma P_{CO_2} is controlled by changes in alveolar ventilation mediated through the respiratory center of the CNS. The stimulus triggering increased alveolar ventilation is an increase in arterial P_{CO_2} or a decrease in the arterial pH or P_{O_2}. Decreased alveolar ventilation is triggered by opposite changes of these stimuli. The exact mechanism by which these stimuli bring about changes in alveolar ventilation is not known.

Plasma bicarbonate concentration is regulated through three possible renal tubular actions: (1) reabsorption of all filtered bicarbonate, (2) synthesis of new bicarbonate, or (3) reabsorption of less bicarbonate than is filtered. The normal tubule reabsorbs practically all the glomerular filtrate; thus the first of these actions scarcely affects plasma bicarbonate concentration. However, this mechanism, coupled with synthesis of new bicarbonate, can produce an increased plasma bicarbonate concentration. "New" bicarbonate is produced by the renal tubule from carbonic acid; however, hydrogen ions (H^+) must be excreted in the urine for the reabsorbed bicarbonate to be effective. Since the lower limit of urinary pH is 4.0, H^+ cannot be excreted in any appreciable amount unless buffered. This buffering is accomplished by excretion of the H^+ either as NH_4^+ or as titratable acid. For every milliequivalent of either ammonium or titratable acid excreted, 1 mEq of bicarbonate is returned to the extracellular fluid.

Neither of these two mechanisms may be fully developed in the newborn or preterm infant. Thus the newborn has a diminished physiologic renal reserve for dealing with acid-base disorders. This fact, coupled with the fact that none of the physiologic mechanisms for acid-base control ever functions at maximal efficiency (that is, to completely prevent pH changes), makes the newborn's position in the face of acid-base disturbances particularly precarious.

NET ACID BALANCE

The concept of net acid balance (NAB) as it applies to infants was primarily formulated by Kildeberg and colleagues. It is not synonymous with acid-base balance; rather, it denotes the difference between the input of net acid (NAI) and the output of net acid (NAO), that is, noncarbonic, nonmetabolized or nonmetabolizable acid:

$$NAB = NAI - NAO$$

This concept is helpful in understanding some of the more complex disorders of acid-base equilibrium as well as acid-base changes in response to a particular diet. Net acid is the only category of acid to which the balance principle can be applied, since net acid is the only acid for which the intake component can be measured independently of the output component. As with formulation of any balance, the designation of a given component as intake or output is arbitrary and depends on a sign convention. It is theoretically correct, for example, to regard the intake of any balance as a negative output. With net acid balance the problem is more complicated. By definition (Brønsted-Lowry), acid and base are in a sense reciprocal. Thus a positive intake of net acid is conceptually identical to a negative intake of net base as well as a positive output of net base. In this discussion net acid output is defined as the renal net acid excretion (NAE), and all other components (with appropriate sign) are defined as net acid input.

The first component of net acid intake concerns dietary intake. There is little preformed net acid in milk or infant formulas; rather, most milks contain appreciable quantities of potential base in the form of undetermined anion (UA), that is, the sum of the concentrations of sodium, potassium, calcium, and magnesium minus the sum of the concentrations of chloride and 1.8 times the concentration of total phosphorus. Regardless of its specific chemical species, UA must be an organic base in the Brønsted-Lowry sense; therefore it is equivalent to bicarbonate after it is metabolized. Only the UA absorbed from the GI tract is available for metabolism. Thus the UA of the diet (UA_d) must be decreased by the UA content of the feces (UA_f). The difference ($UA_d - UA_f$) gives the actual intake component, the amount absorbed (UA_{abs}). A second component of net acid intake is sulfuric acid ($H^+SO_4^=$), which is produced metabolically from nonanabolized sulfur-containing amino acids. A third component of net acid intake consists of organic acids resulting from metabolism ($H^+_{OA^-}$). The anions of these nonmetabolized or nonmetabolizable acids are excreted in the urine, leaving behind an equivalent amount of H^+, which can be eliminated only by the kidneys.

These three components of net acid or net base input are the only ones that must be taken into account in the nongrowing organism. Growth, however, introduces further complexities. First, growth involves deposition of new intracellular and extracellular body water, both containing bicarbonate. An incremental change in body water, in effect, leaves net acid stranded in the body fluids as new bicarbonate is laid down (H^+_{NBW}). This component can be estimated in short-term studies by assuming that the increment of weight gain is equivalent to the increment in total body water and that the average bicarbonate concentration of the increment of total body water is 12 mEq/L (that is, one third as extracellular fluid at 21 mEq/L plus two thirds as intracellular fluid at 8 mEq/L). Growth also entails synthesis of new cell solids. No direct information exists as to whether this process involves production or consumption of net acid. Over relatively short periods of time neither this component nor H^+_{NBW} is quantitatively significant. In addition, growth of the skeleton produces an appreciable acid burden on the kidneys. This process involves synthesis of hydroxyapatite, a process that consists essentially of deposition of a "solid base" from a neutral extracellular fluid, thereby leaving H^+ behind:

$$10\ Ca^{++} + 4.8\ HPO_4^= + 1.2\ H_2PO_4^- + 2\ H_2O \rightarrow$$
$$(Ca_3[PO_4]_2)_3 \cdot Ca(OH)_2 + 9.2\ H^+$$

This effect can be determined by measuring the calcium balance and applying the known stoichiometric relationships between calcium and phosphate (reactants) and hydroxyapatite (product). The stoichiometry of this equation demonstrates that 9.2 mmol of H^+ are produced for each 10 mmol of calcium consumed, a figure remarkably close to the results obtained with direct titration of bone mineral.

All the components just mentioned can be independently measured; thus the total input of net acid can be computed. The remaining item required to construct the balance is measurement of net acid output, which, as mentioned previously, is defined as the renal net acid excretion, that is, urinary ammonium plus titratable acid minus bicarbonate. Thus the net acid balance can be summarized in the following equation:

$$NAB = \underbrace{(H^+SO_4^= + H^+_{OA^-} + H^+_{Ca^{++}} - UA_{abs})}_{\text{Net acid intake}} - \underbrace{NAE}_{\text{Net acid output}}$$

GENERAL DISTURBANCES OF ACID-BASE EQUILIBRIUM

Acid-base disorders are classified primarily by the number and type of etiologic factors giving rise to the disorder. A "simple" acid-base disturbance is one in which only one etiologic factor is involved, whereas a "mixed" disturbance is one involving more than one primary etiologic factor. Based on the type of etiologic factors, acid-base disturbances are classified as either metabolic or respiratory disturbances. Metabolic disturbances result from either gain or loss of strong acid or base by the extracellular fluid, whereas respiratory disturbances result from a gain or loss of CO_2. Once a primary disturbance has been produced, secondary physiologic mechanisms are set in motion to ameliorate the blood pH deviation caused by that disturbance. In turn, these secondary adjustments, called compensation, effect an adjustment of the component of acid-base equilibrium not primarily affected by the primary etiologic factor. Thus for a metabolic disorder compensation is respiratory. Correction of an acid-base disturbance, as opposed to compensation, involves those physiologic mechanisms which fully correct the primary abnormality, that is, the component of acid-base equilibrium affected by the primary etiologic factor.

Metabolic acidosis

Metabolic acidosis is defined as the condition resulting from accumulation of acid other than carbonic acid by the extracellular fluid or from loss of bicarbonate from the extracellular fluid (Table 20-11). The response of the blood buffers to a gain of strong acid (HA) is as follows:

$$HA + HCO_3^- \rightarrow A^- + H_2CO_3 \rightarrow H_2O + CO_2$$
$$HA + Buf^- \rightarrow A^- + HBuf$$

These reactions are prompt, and compensatory hyperventilation begins almost immediately. Later buffering by the tissues, visualized as exchange of H^+ for cellular cations, also assumes a significant role.

Bicarbonate loss can be buffered only by the nonbicarbonate buffers; thus the buffer reactions in response to a loss of bicarbonate are different:

$$CO_2 + H_2O \rightarrow H_2CO_3 + Buf^- \rightarrow HBuf + HCO_3^-$$

After an immediate adjustment of ventilation with respect to CO_2 production, the more sustained respiratory compensation plays a role. These compensatory mechanisms against metabolic acidosis are fully operative in the newborn, provided that pulmonary function is adequate.

Metabolic alkalosis

Metabolic alkalosis results from loss of H^+ from the extracellular fluid or from gain of exogenous bicarbonate

Table 20-11. Causes of metabolic acidosis

General cause	Specific cause	Example
Gain of strong acid by extracellular fluid	Gain of exogenous acid (HCl) Incomplete oxidation of fat Incomplete oxidation of carbohydrate Gain of H_2SO_4, H_3PO_4, and (?) organic acids	NH_4Cl acidosis Diabetic or starvation ketoacidosis Organic acidosis Uremic acidosis
Loss of HCO_3^- from extracellular fluid	Renal losses GI losses	Renal tubular acidosis Diarrheal acidosis

Table 20-12. Causes of metabolic alkalosis

General cause	Specific cause	Example
Gain of HCO_3^- by extracellular fluid	Gain of exogenous HCO_3^- Oxidation of organic acids	Ingestion or infusion of HCO_3^- Ingestion or infusion of lactate, citrate, etc.
Loss of acid from extracellular fluid	Loss of HCl Renal losses of H^+ GI losses (?) Extrarenal transfer of H^+ to intracellular fluid	Vomiting of gastric juice Diuretic therapy; K^+ depletion Chloridorrhea (?) K^+ depletion

Table 20-13. Causes of respiratory acidosis

General cause	Site in respiratory system	Mechanism
Decrease in alveolar ventilation	Central nervous system	Depression of respiratory center (disease, certain drugs)
	Airways and/or lungs	Decreased ventilation or diffusion (intrinsic lung or airways disease)
	Chest wall	Loss of bellows action (structural or functional abnormalities of chest wall or muscles)

(Table 20-12). Because the source of the lost H^+ is water, the immediate consequences of this loss are equivalent to a gain of hydroxyl ions. The immediate buffer responses are as follows:

$$OH^- + H_2CO_3 \rightarrow HCO_3^- + H_2O$$

and

$$OH^- + HBuf \rightarrow Buf^- + H_2O$$

As a result of consumption of carbonic acid, P_{CO_2} decreases. Decreased ventilation persists until a normal plasma P_{CO_2} is again reached. Decreased ventilation can also be sustained, resulting in increased plasma P_{CO_2} values. However, plasma P_{CO_2} values higher than 45 to 50 mm Hg are rare.

Respiratory acidosis

Respiratory acidosis results from a decrease in alveolar ventilation relative to CO_2 production (Table 20-13). The immediate consequence is an increased alveolar P_{CO_2} and thus an increased arterial P_{CO_2} and carbonic acid. The buffer response to increased carbonic acid occurs by means of the nonbicarbonate buffers:

$$H_2CO_3 + Buf^- \rightarrow HBuf^- + HCO_3^-$$

Secondary renal compensatory responses require several days, even under the best of circumstances. These responses consist of reabsorption of all filtered bicarbonate and generation of new bicarbonate through H^+ excretion, a process that is probably limited in the newborn.

Respiratory alkalosis

Respiratory alkalosis results from increased alveolar ventilation relative to CO_2 production (Table 20-14) so that alveolar and arterial P_{CO_2} decreases. The decreased arterial carbonic acid is replaced exclusively by the nonbicarbonate buffers:

$$HCO_3^- + HBuf \rightarrow Buf^- + H_2CO_3 \rightarrow (CO_2)_d + H_2O$$

Table 20-14. Causes of respiratory alkalosis

General cause	Site in respiratory system	Mechanisms
Increase in alveolar ventilation	Central nervous system	Primary stimulation of respiratory center (central hyperventilation, certain drugs)
	Chemoreceptors	Reflex stimulation of respiratory center
	Intrathoracic stretch receptors	Reflex stimulation of respiratory center

Tissue buffering also contributes by exchange of H^+ for extracellular cations. If hyperventilation causing respiratory alkalosis is sustained, renal compensation occurs as excretion of bicarbonate, a process that probably is not limited in the newborn.

Other acid-base disturbances

Two other disorders of acid-base equilibrium should be classified as simple disturbances: dilution acidosis and contraction alkalosis. In these disturbances the primary etiologic factors are expansion and contraction of the extracellular fluid volume, respectively, without affecting the total amount of buffer in the compartment. For example, dilution of bicarbonate through infusion of saline results in dilution acidosis. Similarly, diuresis of edema fluid without bicarbonate diuresis (induced, for example, by diuretic administration) results in a decreased extracellular volume with no change in its bicarbonate content, or contraction alkalosis. Either of these may occur from time to time in the newborn. Perhaps the most common disturbances of acid-base equilibrium in the newborn period are mixed disturbances, such as combined respiratory and metabolic acidosis, as commonly seen in patients with the respiratory distress syndrome and as a result of intrapartum asphyxia.

LATE METABOLIC ACIDOSIS

The entity of late metabolic acidosis was first recognized in 1964 by Kildeberg. While examining serial determinations of blood acid-base status in preterm infants, he noted that approximately 8% showed low values of blood base excess and a tendency toward low values of plasma P_{CO_2}.

Clinical manifestations

Typically, late metabolic acidosis occurs during the second and third weeks of life in preterm infants with no other problems. These infants may or may not be symptomatic; in fact, they are usually vigorous. They develop blood base excess values in the range of −10 to −16 mEq/L. Plasma P_{CO_2} values are usually less than 40 mm Hg but do not reflect the expected respiratory response to the degree of blood base excess depression observed. Some infants recover spontaneously, but others require treatment.

Etiology

Review of the clinical courses of the infants in whom this acid-base disorder is detected reveals two common features. First, all affected infants received artificial formulas starting shortly after birth, usually formulas containing cow's milk protein (3 to 4 gm/kg/day). Second, there was a delayed onset of postnatal weight gain evident as early as the end of the first postnatal week (that is, before evidence of acidosis was detected).

Svenningsen and Lindquist studied the incidence of late metabolic acidosis as a function of both gestational age and dietary protein intake. In 334 term, appropriate for gestational age infants receiving various formulas the overall incidence of late metabolic acidosis was 4.8%. The incidence in 131 preterm, appropriate for gestational age infants, however, was 20.2%; whereas the incidence in 51 near-term but small for gestational age infants was 11.8% (not significantly different from the incidence in term, appropriate for gestational age infants). The formulas used in this study delivered 2.4, 3.3, and 5.7 gm of protein per kilogram per day. The influence of protein intake on development of late metabolic acidosis was most marked in the group of preterm, appropriate for gestational age infants. In this group, late metabolic acidosis occurred in 10.3% of those receiving the lower protein intake, in 24.5% of those receiving the intermediate protein intake, and in 37.5% of those receiving the high protein intake. Thus late metabolic acidosis is much more likely to occur in preterm infants receiving formulas of high protein content.

A more recent study suggests that the quality of the protein intake also plays a role in development of late metabolic acidosis. Raiha and associates showed that the incidence of late metabolic acidosis was much higher in infants receiving cow's milk protein than in those receiving the same amount of humanized cow's milk (60% whey proteins and 40% casein proteins instead of the usual 18:82 distribution of cow's milk). The incidence was greater in infants receiving 2.25 gm of cow's milk protein per kilogram per day than in those receiving 4.5 gm of humanized cow's milk protein per kilogram per day.

Pathogenesis

Late metabolic acidosis can best be discussed within the framework of the net acid balance concept. The condition represents a transient disproportion between the rates of endogenous acid production and renal net acid excretion, that is, a positive net acid balance. Such a disproportion can result from either an abnormally high rate of endogenous acid formation or an abnormally low rate of renal net acid excretion, or both. Although the technique of net acid balance has not been applied to patients with late metabolic acidosis, several facts are known. First, the amount of sulfuric acid produced increases as the total protein content of the formula increases. Thus this component of net acid intake would be greater in infants receiving high protein intakes. Second, the calcium content of the formula affects the calcium balance such that formulas with high calcium content result in release of more H+ to the body fluids incident to skeletal mineralization. The effect of diet on the other component of net acid intake, organic acid production, is not known. However, considering the degree of hyperaminoacidemia observed in preterm infants receiving high protein intakes, it is likely that this component also will be increased. These components of net acid intake are offset by the amount of base absorbed from the GI tract. A higher preformed base content of the diet in general results in absorption of more base from the GI tract. In this regard cow's milk protein contains a larger amount of potential base than do formulas containing less protein.

Kildeberg has determined renal net acid excretion in infants with late metabolic acidosis. Expressed on a "per kilogram" basis or on a "per gram of urea nitrogen excreted" basis, renal net acid excretion of these infants is higher than that of similar infants without late metabolic acidosis. Thus the inability of the premature kidneys to excrete a normal amount of net acid is not the sole or primary cause of late metabolic acidosis. However, the net acid excretion is obviously insufficient for the amount of endogenously produced net acid.

Treatment

This disorder is most likely to occur in patients receiving formulas containing a high protein content, especially a high casein content. In light of other recently reported metabolic disadvantages of such formulas (for example, azotemia, hyperaminoacidemia, and mild hyperammonemia), it is best to avoid such formulas as the routine nourishment for preterm infants. Cessation of formula feedings and substitution of glucose alone may be helpful in selected infants. Acidosis may require treatment with sodium bicarbonate. Once the disturbance is treated or once it has resolved spontaneously, recurrences are rare.

Prognosis

Infants with late metabolic acidosis do not display adverse signs or symptoms related to this disorder. However, the duration of hospitalization is likely to be longer for infants with poor weight gain. Infants with late metabolic acidosis do not gain as rapidly as their unaffected counterparts, but it is difficult to determine if this effect is primary or secondary. Studies by Karelitz and associates suggest that acidosis in itself inhibits growth. This effect, however, was not obvious in the patients reported by Raiha and associates; infants who developed acidosis exhibited overall weight gains similar to those who did not develop acidosis; they did not exhibit a decreased rate of weight gain during the period of acidosis.

LABORATORY FINDINGS IN ACID-BASE DISORDERS

The bicarbonate buffer system is the traditional base of reference for characterization of acid-base equilibrium, as expressed in the Henderson-Hasselbalch equation. This equation contains three unknowns (pH, HCO_3^-, and P_{CO_2}) and two constants (pK' and S). Obviously, two of these three unknowns must be measured to solve the equation. One method involves measuring the pH of blood or plasma and the total CO_2 content of plasma, that is $(CO_2)_t$, defined as $[HCO_3^-] + S \cdot P_{CO_2}$. Other methods involve electrometric measurement of plasma P_{CO_2} and blood pH or measurements of blood pH and plasma P_{CO_2} by the equilibration, or Astrup, method.

Whole-blood buffer base, defined as the sum of all conjugate bases of both the bicarbonate and the nonbicarbonate buffer systems of whole blood (that is, HCO_3^- and Buf^-), is an additional variable for characterization of blood acid-base equilibrium. The difference between the observed buffer base of any blood sample and the normal buffer base of that sample is called the *base excess*. Thus the base excess gives an accurate measure of the amount of strong acid or strong base that has been added to whole blood. For example, a base excess of 10 mEq/L indicates addition of 10 mEq of base per liter (or loss of 10 mEq of H^+ per liter). A base excess of −10 mEq/L, on the other hand, indicates addition of a similar amount of strong acid (or loss of base).

One further laboratory measurement is important in characterizing clinical acid-base disturbances: the R fraction, or anion gap, which is calculated as follows:

$$R = \text{Plasma } [Na^+] - (\text{Plasma } [Cl^-] + \text{Plasma } [HCO_3^-])$$

In the newborn the normal value for R is about 10 to 15 mEq/L. In metabolic acidosis that is a result of accumulation of strong acid other than hydrochloric acid, the value of R increases. In metabolic acidosis that is a result of accumulation of hydrochloric acid or of a loss of bicarbonate, the R fraction remains normal.

TREATMENT OF ACID-BASE DISORDERS

There are three general principles for treatment of any acid-base disorder: (1) control the process producing the primary disorder, if possible; (2) augment any deranged physiologic corrective mechanisms; and (3) attack the displacement of blood pH directly with acidifying or alkalinizing therapy. These principles are illustrated for each of the simple disturbances of acid-base equilibrium.

Metabolic acidosis

In some instances therapy of metabolic acidosis aimed at control of the primary cause of the acidosis is possible (for example, control of diarrhea in diarrheal acidosis, adequate oxygenation in lactic acidosis, insulin therapy in diabetic ketoacidosis). Nearly all patients with metabolic acidosis have concomitant deficits of sodium and water, and such deficits impair the urinary acidification mechanisms. Thus rehydration with attendant restoration of renal function is important in correcting acidosis; such therapy allows maximum excretion of hydrogen ions (as NH_4^+ and/or titratable acid), thereby returning bicarbonate to the plasma.

Despite these measures, severe degrees of metabolic acidosis may require that the low blood pH be attacked directly by administration of bicarbonate. The formula for computing the amount necessary to restore plasma bicarbonate to normal is of the following general form:

HCO_3^- needed (mEq) = HCO_3^- deficit,

or base excess (mEq/L) × HCO_3^- space (L)

Use of such a formula is limited by lack of an accurate estimate of the value for "HCO_3^- space." The various values recommended range from 20% to 60% of the body weight; the one most frequently used is 30% of the body weight. Another method of therapy is simply to administer sodium bicarbonate intravenously (2 to 4 mEq/kg) over a 4- to 6-hour period and then reassess the acid-base status. Further dosage can then be planned on the basis of this experience. This approach allows the patient, in effect, to be titrated serially according to feedback information from blood acid-base analyses (p. 185).

Late metabolic acidosis is often a self-limiting disorder requiring no specific therapy. On occasion, however, the acidosis may be of sufficient severity as to require bicarbonate therapy. In this case therapy should be designed as just discussed.

Metabolic alkalosis

Treatment of metabolic alkalosis also should be aimed at control of the primary disorder (such as vomiting or overzealous diuretic therapy). In addition, adequate amounts of sodium and/or potassium chloride should be provided to allow the corrective renal mechanism for excretion of bicarbonate to operate maximally. Occasionally, administration of acidifying salts (such as arginine hydrochloride), which yield hydrochloride when metabolized, may be necessary. The dosage of this agent can be calculated from the following equation:

Dosage of arginine hydrochloride =

(Normal plasma $[Cl^-]$ − Observed plasma $[Cl^-]$) ×

0.3 (Body weight [kg])

Alternatively, 2 to 4 mmol/kg can be administered and the acid-base status reassessed. With either approach, arginine hydrochloride should be given slowly (over a 6- to 12-hour period) with serial monitoring of blood acid-base status.

Respiratory acidosis

Therapy of respiratory acidosis should be directed primarily toward the cause of decreased alveolar ventilation. In the neonate this often means intermittent or continuous respiratory assistance. Bicarbonate or other base therapy, simply to increase the blood pH, may be undertaken as an adjunct to respiratory support in severe acidosis (plasma pH <7.20). Tris(hydroxymethyl)aminomethane (tromethamine, THAM), because it buffers CO_2, also has been advocated as an agent for increasing the blood pH in severe respiratory acidosis. At best, this effect provides only a transient decrease in plasma P_{CO_2}; amounts of tromethamine far exceeding its LD_{50} would be necessary to buffer all the CO_2 produced by metabolism over any sustained period of time. Tromethamine exerts as much or more osmotic effect per unit of buffering as sodium bicarbonate and furthermore may act as a respiratory depressant. There is no evidence for a superiority of tromethamine over sodium bicarbonate in correcting acidosis.

Respiratory alkalosis

Therapy of respiratory alkalosis also should be directed toward control of the primary cause of the disturbance (increased alveolar ventilation). Most instances of respiratory alkalosis in the newborn period are iatrogenic, secondary to central hyperventilation consequent to birth asphyxia or the result of drug administration to either mother or baby; thus the period of hyperventilation might be prolonged, depending on the infant's ability to metabolize or excrete the particular drug in question. Severe disturbances are rare, and the usual mild metabolic acidosis seen in the first hours of life helps offset the elevated pH.

William C. Heird

BIBLIOGRAPHY

Dell, R.B.: Normal acid-base regulation. In Winters, R.W.: The body fluids in pediatrics, Boston, 1973, Little, Brown & Co.

Heird, W.C.: Acid-base, fluid, and electrolyte disturbances in the newborn. In Young, D.S., and Hicks, J.M., editors: The neonate, New York, 1976, John Wiley & Sons, Inc.

Heird, W.C., Dell, R.B., and Winters, R.W.: Osmotic effects of THAM, Pediatr. Res. **6:**495, 1972.

Hunt, J.N.: The influence of dietary sulfur on the urinary output of acid in man, Clin. Sci. **15:**119, 1956.

Karelitz, S., Schell, N.B., and Goldman, H.I.: Lactic acid milk in feeding of premature infants, J. Pediatr. **54:**756, 1959.

Kildeberg, P.: Disturbances of hydrogen ion balance occurring in premature infants. II. Late metabolic acidosis, Acta Paediatr. Scand. **53:**517, 1964.

Kildeberg, P.: Clinical acid-base physiology: studies in neonates, infants and young children, Copenhagen, 1968, Munksgaard International Booksellers & Publishers Ltd.

Kildeberg, P.: Late metabolic acidosis of premature infants. In Winters, R.W., editor: The body fluids in pediatrics, Boston, 1973, Little, Brown & Co.

Kildeberg, P., Engel, K., and Winters, R.W.: Balance of net acid in growing infants: endogenous and trans-intestinal aspects, Acta Paediatr. Scand. **58:**321, 1969.

Kildeberg, P., and Winters, R.W.: Balance of net acid: concept, measurement and applications. In Barness, L.A., editor: Advances in pediatrics, vol. 25, Chicago, 1978, Year Book Medical Publishers, Inc.

Leman, J., Jr., and Lennon, E.J.: Role of diet, gastrointestinal tract and bone in acid-base homeostasis, Kidney Int. **1:**275, 1972.

Lennon, E.J., Lemann, J., Jr., and Litzow, J.R.: The effects of diet and stool composition on the net external acid balance of normal subjects, J. Clin. Invest. **46:**1601, 1966.

Lennon, E.J., Lemann, J., Jr., and Relman, A.S.: The effects of phosphoproteins on acid balance in normal subjects, J. Clin. Invest. **41:**637, 1962.

Nash, M.A., and Edelmann, C.M., Jr.: The developing kidney, Nephron **2:**71, 1973.

Raaflaub, J.: Uber die Basizitat der Knochenmineralien, Experentia **17:**443, 1961.

Raiha, N.C.R., and others: Milk protein quantity and quality in low birthweight infants, Pediatrics **57:**659, 1976.

Ranlov, P., and Siggaard-Anderson, O.: Late metabolic acidosis in premature infants: prevalence and significance, Acta Paediatr. Scand. **54:**531, 1965.

Relman, A.S., Lennon, E.J., and Lemann, J., Jr.: Endogenous production of fixed acid and the measurement of the net balance of acid in normal subjects, J. Clin. Invest. **40:**1621, 1961.

Schain, R.J., and O'Brien, K.: Longitudinal studies of acid-base status in infants with low birth weight, J. Pediatr. **70:**885, 1967.

Svenningsen, N.W., and Lindquist, B.: Incidence of metabolic acidosis in term, preterm and small-for-gestational age infants in relation to dietary protein intake, Acta Paediatr. Scand. **62:**1, 1973.

Winters, R.W., and Dell, R.B.: Regulation of acid-base equilibrium. In Yamamota, W.S., and Brobeck, J.R., editors: Physiological controls and regulation, Philadelphia, 1965, W.B. Saunders Co.

Winters, R.W., Engel, K., and Dell, R.B.: Acid-base physiology in medicine, a self-instruction program, ed. 2, Westlake, Ohio, 1969, The London Co.

Chapter 21 The sensorimotor development of the preterm infant

He who sees things from their beginnings will have the finest view of them.
Aristotle

The progressive decrease in neonatal and infant mortality during the latter half of this century has been accompanied by a surge of interest in the behavioral capabilities of the newborn infant. Until the late 1950s the human neonate was considered to be immature and disorganized and to function mainly at a brain stem level. Neurobehavioral assessment of the neonate thus was based mainly on evaluation of muscle tone and primitive reflexes. Recent studies have recognized the term newborn at birth to be a vital, responsive, and reactive being with remarkable sensory development and an amazing ability for self-organization and social interaction. The major breakthrough came with the descriptions by both Wolff and Prechtl of the behavioral states of arousal in the newborn, leading to an understanding that physiologic and neurosensory responses may vary according to the infant's state of awakeness or sleep. Of equal importance was the documentation by Fantz of the newborn's ability to fixate and visually differentiate between patterns. Additional research has documented the neonate's ability to respond selectively to sound, to mimic, to move in rhythm to the human voice, and to exhibit visual and auditory habituation. Brazelton combined many of these measures to develop a neurobehavioral method for evaluation of the newborn, which has become very useful clinically to both evaluate and demonstrate newborn behaviors.

The improved short and long-term outcomes for the very low birth weight infant (less than 1,500 gm) have led to an extension of neonatal behavioral research to this less mature population of infants.

This chapter reviews the current knowledge of preterm neurobehavioral development, including state organization, visual and auditory responsiveness, sucking, and the development of active and passive muscle tone. The development of the term infant is referred to as a basis for describing preterm behavior.

Historically there has always been a fascination for the "tiny infant." Early reports of preterm behavior are difficult to evaluate, since gestational age seldom was noted. Also very few tiny infants survived prior to the 1960s so that most behavioral descriptions were of infants born weighing more than 1,500 gm. Gesell and, later, Saint-Anne Dargassies were the first to consider gestational age in their classical naturalistic observations of preterm infants. Gesell used the appropriate term *fetal infant* for infants born in the fetal period.

The earliest descriptions of spontaneous movement and reflex responses in previable infants were by Humphrey and Hooker in 1930, who filmed fetal aborti placed in saline after birth and documented a central nervous system already functional at 7 weeks' gestation. Fetal monitoring and real-time ultrasonography more recently have provided a totally new dimension to the observations of fetal sensorimotor maturation under normal physiologic conditions in utero. Since technical advances and improvements in perinatal care have extended the period of potential viability to some weeks before the previously defined limit of 28 weeks' gestation, both fetal and preterm behaviors are reviewed. Gestational age is defined as the age from the first day of the mother's last menstrual period until birth, postnatal age is the age that has been reached after birth, and postmenstrual age is the sum of gestational and postnatal ages.

STATES OF AROUSAL

The sleep and awake states of arousal influence every physiologic and neurosensory function and must be considered in both the assessment and clinical care of the neonate.

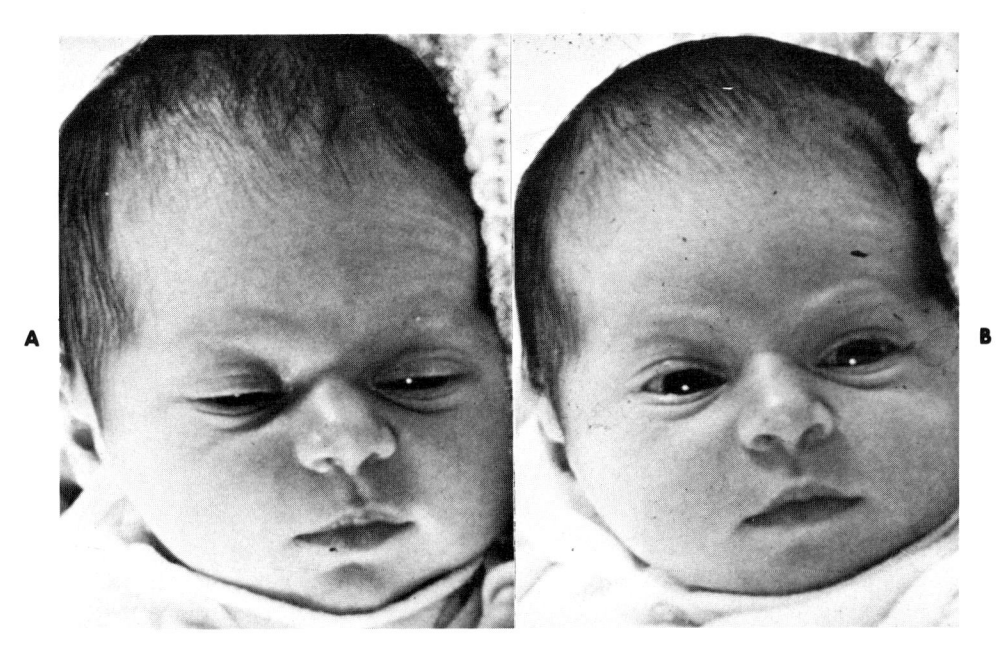

Fig. 21-1. Term infant in the drowsy **(A)** and quiet awake **(B)** states of alertness. (From The Amazing Newborn, Case Western Reserve University.)

The term infant

The observation by Aserinsky and Kleitman in 1953 of a relationship between rapid eye movement (REM) sleep and dreaming led to an explosion of research into the ontogenic development of the human awake-sleep cycles. Wolff introduced the concept of "state of arousal" and designed the first descriptive rating scale for the term infant. A state is defined as a clustering of recognizable physiologic and behavioral variables that repeat themselves.

Description and definition of states

Wolff noted that the infant has six organized patterns of behavior: two sleep states (quiet and active sleep), drowsiness, and three awake states (quiet awakeness, active awakeness, and crying).

In quiet sleep the infant is at full rest, respiration is very regular, and body movements are absent except for occasional startles or fine mouth movements. The eyelids are closed, and no eye movements are seen under the lids. In active sleep there is body activity ranging from gentle limb movements to an occasional stirring of the body, arms, and legs. Spontaneous erections occur in boys. Respiration is irregular, and facial grimaces are frequent, including smiling, frowning, mouthing, or bursts of sucking. The eyelids are closed, and occasionally rolling or rapid eye movements can be seen through the closed eye lids. The term *rapid eye movement*, or *REM, sleep* originated from these movements in active sleep.

In drowsiness, which usually occurs while waking or falling asleep, the baby may be still or moving, and smiles, frowns, or mouthing sometimes can be seen. The eyes have a dull glazed appearance and usually do not fixate, the lids are droopy, and just before closing, the eyes may roll upward. In the quiet awake state the infant is fully alert but relatively inactive. The eyes are wide open with a bright shiny appearance (Fig. 21-1). The quiet awake state is considered to be qualitatively similar to conscious attention in the adult. In this state the infant is able to fixate and focus on visual objects, to orient to sound, and to respond to social cues such as a voice, a face, cuddling, and holding. During the active awake state there is frequent motor activity of the arms, legs, trunk, and head. The eyes are open and moving, and there may be vocalization. During crying there is vigorous motor activity with the eyes open or tightly closed.

Prechtl's definitions of the various states are similar to those of Wolff; however, he thought that the behaviors constituting a state should be present for at least 3 minutes. In addition, he omitted the drowsy state, regarding it as a transition between states, and defined only five states.

Although the states seem like a continuous spectrum ranging from quiet sleep to active awakeness, they are qualitatively highly specific with a distinct type of internal organization and brain center control. These states constitute the basic rest-activity cycles of sleep and wakefulness. They are relatively stable, and with the exception of short transitional periods repeat in regular

Table 21-1. Polygraph documentation of states

	Quiet sleep	Active sleep	Awakeness
Heart rate	Regular, slower	Irregular, faster	Irregular
Respiration	Regular, slower	Irregular, faster	Irregular
Electromyogram activity	Present	Absent	Present
Eye movements (electrooculogram)	Absent	Frequent	Scanning or rapid
Electroencephalogram	Discontinuous, episodic activity	Low voltage, arrhythmic	Low voltage, slow waves

cycles during the day and night. The central nervous system control of the the various states originates at different levels of the reticular-activating system. Quiet sleep requires complex cortical integration and control and is regarded as the more mature sleep state. Active sleep is considered to be an ontogenically primitive sleep state in which dreaming occurs. Awakeness, like quiet sleep, is regulated by higher cortical centers.

The states can be described either clinically or by continuous polygraph recordings of various combinations of respiration, heart rate, eye movements, brain electrical activity, and muscle tone. These recordings provide objective quantitative information on sleep and awake states (Table 21-1). A sleep profile thus can be constructed according to the percentage of time spent in each state, the degree of organization of these states, the cycling regularity, and the number of transitions between states.

Temporal distribution of state

During the first week of life the term infant spends only 8% to 16% of the day in a state of quiet awakeness. The rest of the time is spent mainly in quiet or active sleep. A sleep cycle that includes a period of quiet and active sleep is 60 minutes long at term (range, 50 to 70 minutes), compared with 90 minutes in the adult. At term, active sleep constitutes 50% of the sleep cycle, and awakening usually follows active sleep, in contrast to adults, who waken from quiet sleep or drowsiness. Periods of awakeness usually occur at 4-hour intervals around feeding times. With increasing age there are longer periods of awakeness during the day with sleep throughout the night. The relative amount of quiet sleep also increases, so that by adulthood active sleep constitutes only 20% of total sleep, whereas the rest is quiet sleep (Fig. 21-2).

The state cycles (also thought to be present in utero) are disrupted immediately after birth so that the infant stays awake longer with periods of quiet alertness alternating with activity. This results in increased alertness during the first 24 hours at the expense of active sleep, whereas the proportion of quiet sleep remains unchanged. By the fifth day the state cycles have stabilized.

Importance of state

Practically every physiologic body function and behavior in the newborn is dependent on state. For example, heart rate, blood pressure, and oxygen consumption are lower and transcutaneous PO_2 higher in quiet sleep.

Many external or environmental changes have a modifying effect on state. The kinesthetic and vestibular effects of picking up a crying baby, soothing him, and placing him up to the shoulder can induce increased quiet awakeness and attention, as can an interesting face or change of tone of voice. State also can be affected by internal needs such as hunger or stooling and by various pathologic conditions including asphyxia, perinatal complications, and drugs given to the mother before birth.

The modifying effect of state on the various reflex responses is shown in Table 21-2. The following outline describes other important links between state, physiologic function, and the environment.

A. The influence of state on physiologic functions
1. Heart rate: regular in quiet sleep; irregular and faster in active sleep and awake states (p. 122)
2. Respiration: regular in quiet sleep; irregular and faster in active sleep and awake states; apnea and periodic breathing occur mainly in active sleep (p. 456)
3. Oxygen consumption: lowest in quiet sleep; highest in crying
4. Transcutaneous PO_2: lower in active sleep than in quiet sleep
5. Blood pressure: lowest in quiet sleep; greater variability in active sleep; higher in awake activity and crying
6. Endocrine: cortisol secretion increases with increasing arousal
7. Neurophysiologic function
   a. Visual fixation: optimal in quiet awakeness; less in drowsiness and active awakeness
   b. Habituation: state changes act as dishabituating stimuli
      (1) Heart rate response to auditory stimulation: masked by state changes
      (2) Blink reflex to light: only in quiet sleep
   c. Conditioning: masked by state changes
B. Effects of environmental factors and external stimuli on state
   1. Touch
      a. Soothing and swaddling: reduces activity during active awakeness and crying

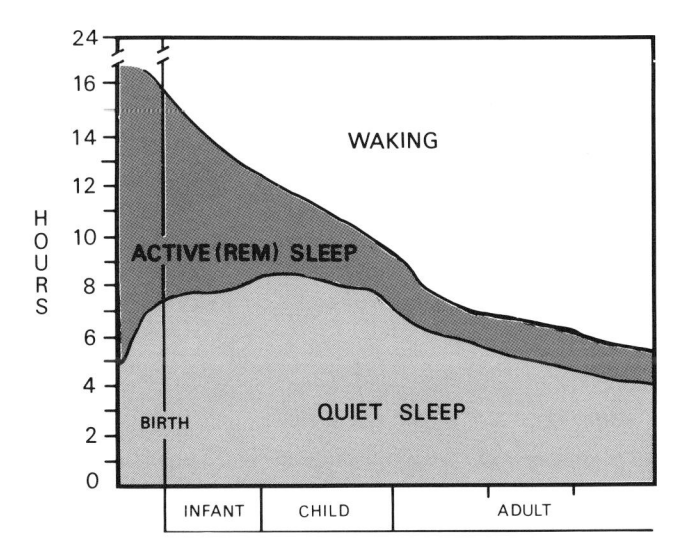

Fig. 21-2. Development of sleep and waking from infancy to adulthood. (Adapted from Roffwarg, H.P.: Science **152**:604, 1966. Copyright 1966 by the American Association for the Advancement of Science.)

Table 21-2. Effects of state on intensity of responses to sensory stimulation

	Quiet sleep	Active sleep	Quiet awake
Proprioceptive reflexes			
Knee jerk	+++	±	++
Biceps jerk	+++	±	++
Ankle clonus	+++	−	−
Moro	+++	−	++
Exteroceptive reflexes			
Tactile			
Rooting	−	−	++
Palmar grasp	−	+	++
Plantar grasp	−	+	++
Nociceptive			
Babinski	++	+++	+++
Abdominal	++	+++	+++
Inguinal	+++	+++	+++
Visual attention	−	−	+++
Auditory (hearing)	±	++	+++

Modified from Prechtl, H.F.R.:

   b. Handling (rubbing, stroking, maternal holding, etc.): induces awakeness and activity
   c. Pain and tickling: increases awakeness and activity; inactive infants most sensitive to pain
 2. Visual (pictures, objects, or faces): induces quiet awakeness in drowsy, active, or crying infants; quiet awake state prolonged by interesting visual stimuli
 3. Light
   a. Light: active sleep reduced; quiet sleep increased; reduces level of activity in fussy or crying babies
   b. Darkness: increases level of activity; shift from quiet sleep to active sleep.
 4. Auditory (sound)
   a. Variations in sound: increases activity
   b. Rhythmic sound (e.g., heartbeat): reduces activity; more sleep, less crying
   c. Continuous sound: reduces activity in crying and fussy babies; less active sleep and more quiet sleep.
 5. Vestibular (proprioceptive—putting to shoulder and rocking in upright position): induces quiet awakeness in sleeping, active awake, fussy, and crying babies
 6. Temperature
   a. Decrease: increases motor activity; decreases quiet sleep
   b. Increase: reduces activity (induces apnea?)
 7. Sucking (pacifier or finger in mouth): induces quiet awakeness in active awake and crying infants; inhibits head movements and peripheral vision
 8. Stress
   a. Circumcision: increases fussy crying; shorter latency to sleep; increases quiet sleep
   b. Laboratory conditions: decreases alertness during awake states; more drowsiness, fussiness, and crying
   c. Repeated awakening: longer awakeness; more sleep after the deprivation period
 9. Body position: increased crying and active sleep in supine position; increased quiet sleep and higher PO_2 in prone position
C. Influence of internal physiologic needs on state
 1. Hunger: increases activity, active awakeness, and crying
 2. Satiety: quietens, increases sleep
 3. Full bladder: more erections in active sleep
 4. Need to stool: waking activity
D. Effects of pathologic conditions on state
 1. Coma: complete absence of state cycles and definable sleep
 2. Asphyxia: poor sleep cycle organization; decrease in active sleep; increase in quiet sleep
 3. Drugs
   a. Meperidine (Demerol) and barbiturates: decrease in awakeness, visual alertness, and active (REM) sleep spontaneous behavior
   b. Diazepam and barbiturates: increase in a state that looks like quiet sleep; active sleep decreases
   c. Heroin: quiet sleep reduced; sleep cycles longer
 4. Jaundice: decrease in quiet awake periods; increase in sleep cycle duration and active sleep
 5. Maternal diabetes: increase in active sleep
 6. Toxemia causing intrauterine growth retardation: poor organization of sleep states; disorganized quiet sleep with irregular respirations
 7. Malformation of brain
   a. Hydrocephalus and microcephaly syndromes: increases amounts of awakeness with less sleep; poor or absent sleep organization
   b. Down's syndrome: increase in awakeness; decrease in active sleep
 8. Biochemical disturbances (hypocalcemia, hypoglycemia, hypernatremia): hyperirritability or decreased awakeness

Fetal rest-activity cycles

Sterman recorded fetal movements and documented a periodicity to fetal activity from as early as 21 weeks' gestation. Two motility cycles were found: a shorter cycle of 30 to 50 minutes' duration, which seems to be an intrinsic rhythm of the fetus, and a longer cycle of 80 to 110 minutes, which is related to the maternal sleep cycle. Dierker more recently found similar activity cycles by monitoring fetal movements, heart rate, respiration, and EEG activity. Sterman did not find a change in the periodicity of the cycles with increasing gestational age; however, Dierker noted greater stability of rest-activity cycles with increasing maturity.

The preterm infant
Description and definitions

In the very young preterm infant, sleep and wakefulness or even periods of activity and inactivity are extremely difficult to classify. Nonetheless in 1945 Gesell and Amatruda gave a marvelous description of the observable behaviors associated with developing sleep and wakefulness in maturing preterm infants. Although Gesell documented many naturalistic behaviors, he made little attempt to quantify them. More recently Parmelee and also Emde classified multiple behavioral variations of state that can be used to describe the preterm infant, although many of the states, or clusters of behaviors, are so transient that they do not meet Prechtl's requirements of 3-minutes' duration to call them true states.

The development of the sleep states

To describe the many physiologic and behavioral components of the developing sleep states, both Dreyfus-Brisac and Parmelee used polygraphic recordings of electrophysiologic measures in addition to behavioral observations. For these studies sleep was defined as whenever the infant's eyes were closed without crying or gross

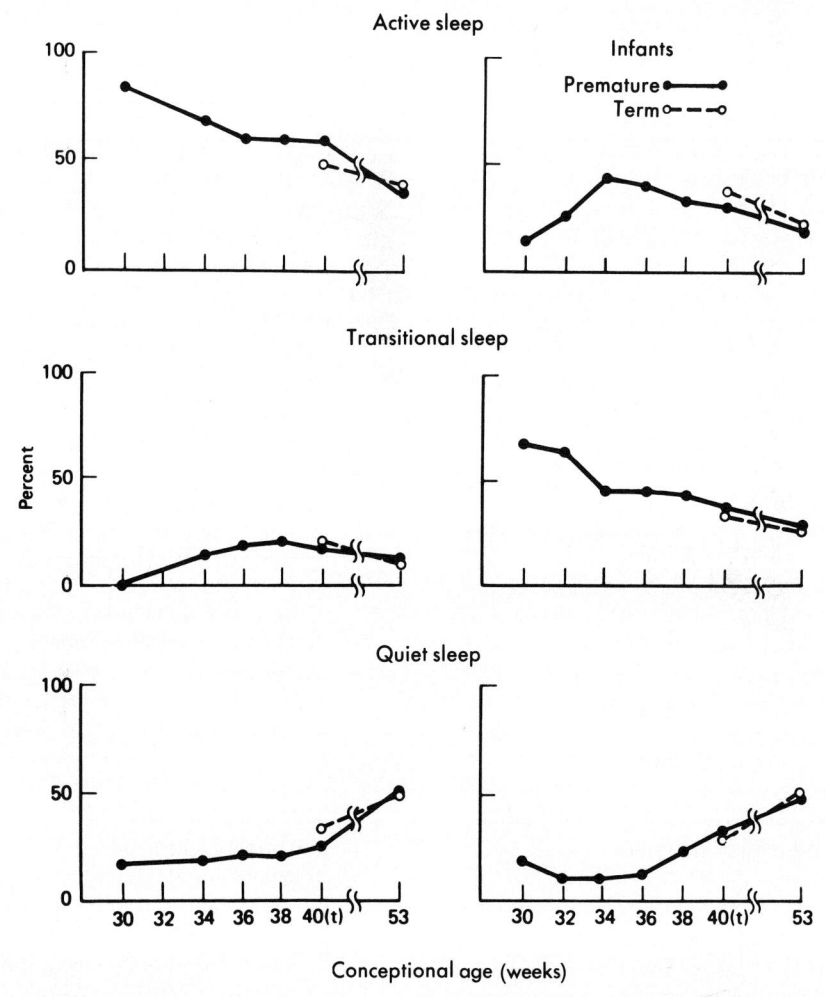

Fig. 21-3. Percentage of sleep states at each gestational age using two methods of state classification. (From Parmelee, A.H.: Dev. Med. Child Neurol. **9**:70, 1967.)

body activity. Dreyfus-Brisac described an atypical type of sleep between 24 and 27 weeks' postmenstrual age. At this time there are constant small body movements, a fairly regular heart and respiratory rate, and very few REMs, and the EEG shows a discontinuous type of activity. With increasing gestational age there is increasing inhibition of these behaviors. Brief quiet periods without body movement appear at between 28 and 30 weeks gestation. By 32 weeks 53% of sleep time is spent without motion, and this increases to 60% by term. The near absence of REMs at 24 to 27 weeks is followed by infrequent sparse eye movements at 28 to 30 weeks. These increase and appear in clusters by 32 weeks' gestation and then decrease again by term. Respiration, which is initially mainly irregular, becomes increasingly regular by term. The discontinuous EEG seen at 24 weeks gradually differentiates into patterns characteristic of active and quiet sleep from about 32 weeks.

Parmelee defined three types of sleep in preterm infants: quiet, active, and transitional sleep (Fig. 21-3). Using these definitions, Parmelee found a gradual increase in quiet sleep with a decrease in transitional and REM sleep with age. When the behaviors were classified into only quiet or active sleep, Parmelee found that most of the sleep time was spent in active sleep at 30 weeks. Thereafter there was a gradual increase in quiet sleep and a decrease in active sleep.

A primitive cycling of the sleep states appears at about

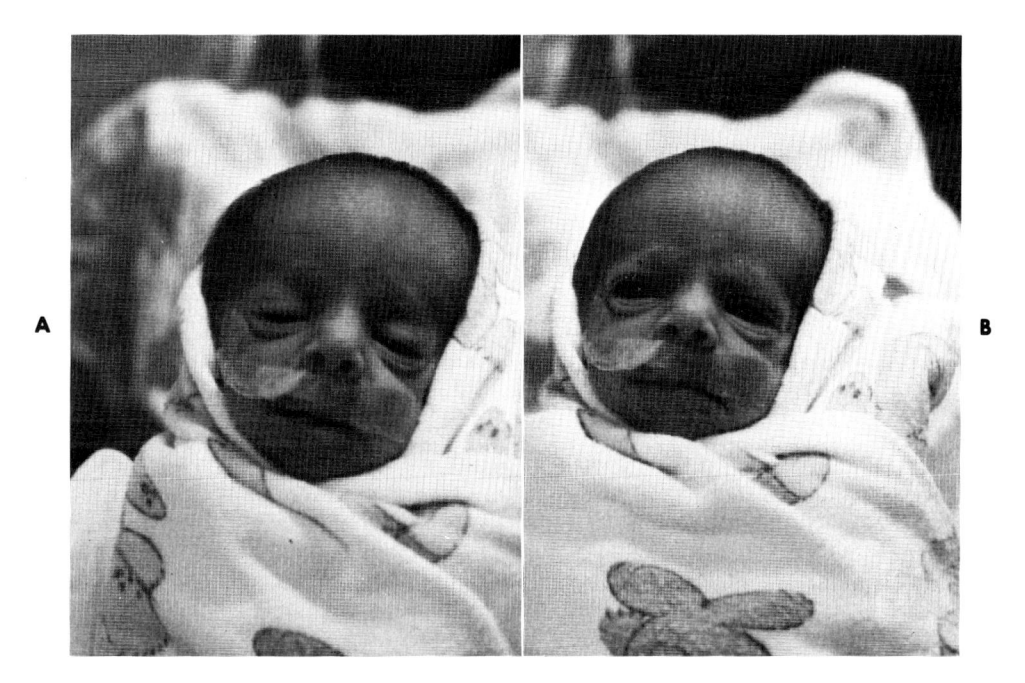

Fig. 21-4. Preterm infant (34 weeks postmenstrual age) in drowsy **(A)** and quiet awake **(B)** states of alertness. (From Hack, M.: Pediatrics **68**:87, 1981. Copyright American Academy of Pediatrics 1981.)

Fig. 21-5. Percent of time spent quiet awake or drowsy and mean total fixation time in preterm infants from 30 to 35 weeks postmenstrual age. (From Hack, M.: Pediatrics **68**:87, 1981. Copyright American Academy of Pediatrics 1981.)

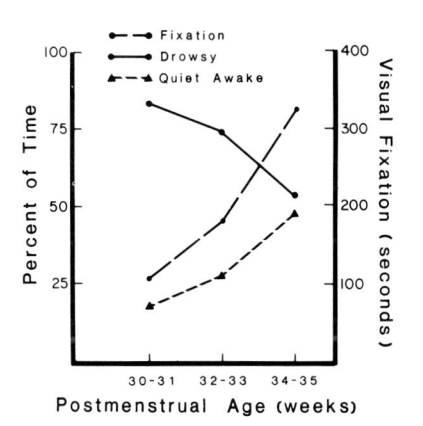

32 weeks' gestation; however, the respective periods for each state are shorter than at term. A cycle that includes active and quiet sleep is 40 minutes long at 36 weeks (range, 36 to 50) in comparison to 60 minutes at term. Most researchers report a fairly good correlation of all the behavioral parameters of active sleep by 34 to 36 weeks and of quiet sleep by 36 to 38 weeks.

There has been speculation as to the reason for the increased amount of REM activity in immature infants. Roffwarg postulated that REM sleep provides a source of endogenous stimulation needed for central nervous system growth. This is supported by the fact that cerebral circulation and brain temperature are increased in active sleep. Active sleep is also accompanied by increased protein synthesis in the brain.

The development of preterm awakeness

The development of awakeness has been far more difficult to classify than that of sleep. This is in part because of the short periods the infant spends with eyes open, and also because clinically and polygraphically it is often difficult to decide whether an immature infant with eyes open is awake or in active sleep. Awakeness, especially in the preterm infant, is best defined by behavioral observation because polygraphically many of the measures such as heart rate and respiration are similar in active sleep, as pointed out earlier. Also the EEG of the awake state can only be differentiated from that of active sleep by 36 weeks' gestation.

Saint-Anne Dargassies described "waking" with short eye-open periods from 30 weeks' postmenstrual age. By 32 weeks these periods occur spontaneously and are of longer duration. To define and describe the gradual progression of developing awakeness from 30 to 36 weeks, Hack used a rating of facial behaviors while the infant fixated on a black and white pattern. The less mature infants demonstrated mostly drowsiness, whereas quiet awakeness increased with age (Figs. 21-4 and 21-5). Uncoordinated and rolling eye movements and mouthing activity were observed in both quiet awakeness and drowsiness. These are rarely seen in awake term infants and probably indicate the lability and poor organization of awakeness in the preterm infant. It is interesting to note that the gradual increase in the ability to sustain quiet awakeness with the concomitant decrease in drowsiness parallels the relative increase in quiet sleep and decrease in active sleep during the same age period described by Parmelee (Fig. 21-3). The progressive organization of awake state control also coincided with an increase in visual attention and alertness. These developmental changes are probably dependent on the rapidly increasing complexity of dendritic interactions occurring at all levels of the maturing central nervous system at this time. They also may indicate increasing control of arousal at the reticular activating center and at higher cortical levels.

Although both the awake and sleep states reach a level of maturity close to that of the term infant by 36 to 37 weeks, there remain differences between infants born at term and preterm infants who have reached term after many weeks of extrauterine life. These include less organization and stability of the various parameters of state, less regular respiration, and also subtle EEG differences.

Modifying effects on preterm state

There is little information as to the effects of external and internal stimuli on the developing states of the preterm infant. It is known, however, that:
1. Preterm infants have more quiet sleep when they are cared for in a neutral thermal environment than in a cooler environment.
2. Infants older than 29 weeks' postmenstrual age have more awake periods when touched by their parents.
3. Preterm infants placed in the prone position have more quiet sleep, less active sleep, and higher PO_2 levels than infants in the supine position.
4. Kinesthetic and auditory stimulation provided by rocking incubators and recordings of heart beat induce quiet sleep and decrease active sleep and awakeness.
5. Stress associated with severe respiratory distress causes less quiet sleep and more active sleep in infants with respiratory distress syndrome (RDS) than in control infants without RDS. After recovery these differences disappear.
6. Painful conditions such as necrotizing enterocolitis may result in open-eye periods with a vacant type of awake staring.

Although further information still is lacking, the many additional effects on state listed earlier in the outline probably affect preterm awakeness and sleep and should be considered when providing clinical care for immature infants.

FACIAL EXPRESSION AND SOCIAL BEHAVIORS

The preterm infant lacks many of the social signals and expressions of emotion necessary for eliciting early attachment and caretaking. Despite the multitude of facial movements seen in active sleep, there is very little expression of early affect seen before 30 to 32 weeks. Preterm behaviors suggestive of social expression that could potentially elicit social responses include eye opening, grimacing, smiling, yawning, and crying. Minde rated these behaviors from 32 to 34 weeks' postmenstrual age and found no changes during this period which could be related to age or maternal caretaking.

Hack similarly documented the occurrence of behaviors such as smiling, yawning, chewing, tonguing, sucking, sneezing, or mouthing during 30-second epochs of visual fixation. No consistent patterns or coincidence of behaviors were noted.

Crying and other vocalizations

Aborti of 23 to 24 weeks' gestation may cry at birth, and infants as young as 26 weeks' gestation respond to painful stimuli by crying. Very little spontaneous crying occurs before 30 to 32 weeks' gestation. From this time the infant may demonstrate hunger by crying before feeding time. Crying is not elicited during the Moro reflex before 32 weeks' gestation, whereas after 34 weeks 80% or more of infants will cry.

Michelsson examined the pain-induced cry of preterm and term infants spectrographically and found a higher pitch in the less mature infants.

Other vocalizations occur such as grunts and squeaks. Grunting sometimes denotes fussiness and may occur instead of crying in infants from 32 to 36 weeks of age.

Smiling

Two patterns of smiling are seen during infancy: endogenous, or spontaneous, smiling, which is present at birth, and exogenous, or elicited, smiling, which occurs in response to external stimuli from about 3 to 4 weeks after term birth.

Endogenous smiling is seen only in active sleep or drowsiness. It appears as a side stretching and upturning of the corners of the mouth with the rest of the face remaining relaxed and relatively undisturbed. It is subcortical and probably mediated along with frowning, mouth movements, and other spontaneous REM-associated behaviors such as sneezes, yawns, and stretching. It usually occurs in clusters during a mid-REM period and has no relationship to feeding. It also can be elicited by auditory or tactile stimuli during the first week of life. During the first months after birth endogenous smiling diminishes in frequency and disappears by about 6 months of age.

Exogenous smiling begins gradually during the first 4 weeks after term birth and occurs mainly during quiet awakeness and sometimes during drowsiness. This type of smiling looks more like a social responsive smile. The mouth stretches further and may open, the superficial muscles of the cheeks and eyes contract, and the skin at the corners of the eyes tends to wrinkle, giving the impression that the whole face rather than the mouth alone is smiling. Exogenous smiling initially can be elicited by auditory, tactile, and nonsocial visual stimuli, but these are replaced by true social stimuli by 8 to 12 weeks of age. At this time the awake infant can respond to the caretaker's voice or moving face with an alert smile, brightening of the eyes, and a grin.

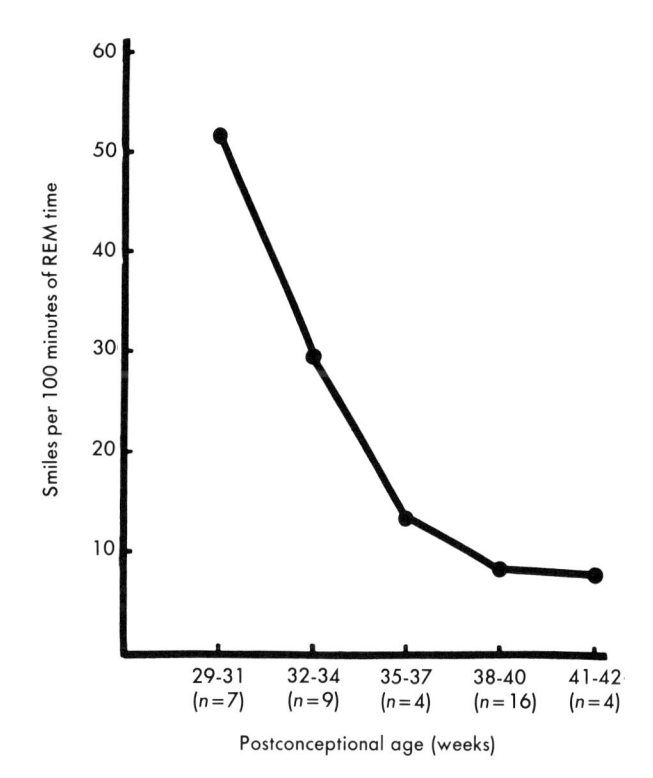

Fig. 21-6. Incidence of smiling during active (REM) sleep from 20 to 42 weeks. (From Emde, R.N., Gaesenbauer, T., and Harmon, R.: Emotional expression in infancy: a biobehavioral study. In Psychological issues, vol. 10, no. 1, monograph 37, New York, 1976, International University Press, Inc.)

The ontogeny of smiling in preterm infants has been studied by Emde who observed facial behaviors during REM periods in preterm infants ranging from 29 to 37 weeks' postmenstrual age and compared them with term infants. The preterm infants smiled more (34 smiles per 100 minutes of REM sleep versus 8.8 smiles in the term infants). The preterm smiles also tended to occur more in bursts or clusters. In preterm infants 66% of smiling occurred in clusters compared with 33% in the term infants. The increased incidence of smiling in the preterm infants tended to decrease with maturity (Fig. 21-6).

SUCKING

The sucking reflex is one of the earliest coordinated behaviors in human fetal life. It is also one of the most important means of interaction between the infant and caretaker and is essential for biologic survival. Physiologically the process of sucking involves complicated integrations of oral, respiratory, and swallowing responses, whereas psychologically sucking is gratifying in itself and tends to soothe the infant.

For the effective accomplishment of sucking several sequential coordinated behaviors need to be completed. These include rooting, opening of the mouth, grasping of the nipple, sucking, and swallowing. The sucking reflex has two components: an expression component by which the tongue applies positive pressure to the nipple by pressing it up against the hard palate and moving backward, and a suction component whereby negative intraoral pressure is produced by lowering the floor of the mouth. Sucking precedes swallowing, which inhibits respiration. These functions must all be coordinated before effective, safe oral feeding can be achieved.

The term infant

All animals have a species-specific sucking rhythm with bursts of sucking interspersed with pauses. The human sucking reflex differs from that of other mammals in that humans have both a nutritive and a nonnutritive mode of sucking, whereas animals demonstrate only nutritive sucking. Wolff has postulated that this difference between humans and other mammals represents a qualitative evolution in the central nervous system control over the sucking reflex.

In nonnutritive sucking, which can be induced by placing a nipple in the mouth without providing nutrient, there is a regularity to the burst-pause pattern. Term infants have an overall rate of two sucks per second per burst (range, 1.9 to 2.4), with a mean of eight sucks per burst (range, 4 to 13) and an interburst interval of about 6 seconds (range, 3 to 11 seconds). Rhythmic mouthing seen in infants in quiet sleep has the same temporal organization as that seen with nonnutritive sucking on a nipple. In nutritive sucking there are long bursts of sucks with a slower rate of sucking (about one suck per second). The burst-pause pattern appears mainly toward the end of the feeding period.

Nonnutritive sucking occurs in all the sleep and awake states, although less during quiet sleep and crying. Nutritive sucking is seen mainly in an awake hungry infant. Although long periods of sucking have been described in the immediate period after birth, effective sucking seems to develop gradually during the first few days of life, and many normal term infants only develop regular sucking rhythms by 4 days of age. This is probably related to perinatal factors which might affect the infant's early behavioral responses. Rooting is elicited mainly in a hungry awake infant and is less active on the first day of life.

Although sucking is a basal brain function it can be modified by higher brain centers. Its temporal organization (rhythmicity) and plasticity of response, i.e., the ability to adapt to changes in the environment, make it an ideal research tool for evaluating early conditioning and learning. The sucking response can be modified by multiple factors, although the basic burst-pause pattern usually is maintained.

Intraoral factors affecting sucking include the shape and size of the nipple, the amount of nutrient and rapidity with which it is given, as well as the taste of the fluid. (Sweeter fluids tend to increase the total amount of sucking.) Extraoral stimuli such as presenting a visual or auditory stimulus may affect the rhythmicity of sucking. Perinatally stressed and abnormal newborns also demonstrate changes in nonnutritive sucking patterns.

The fetus and preterm infant

Most of the components of sucking are noted very early in life and were originally described in detail by Hooker. Mouth opening first appears at about 7 to 8 weeks' postmenstrual age. Only at 12 to 13 weeks do the oral reflexes first appear as isolated, separate reflex responses

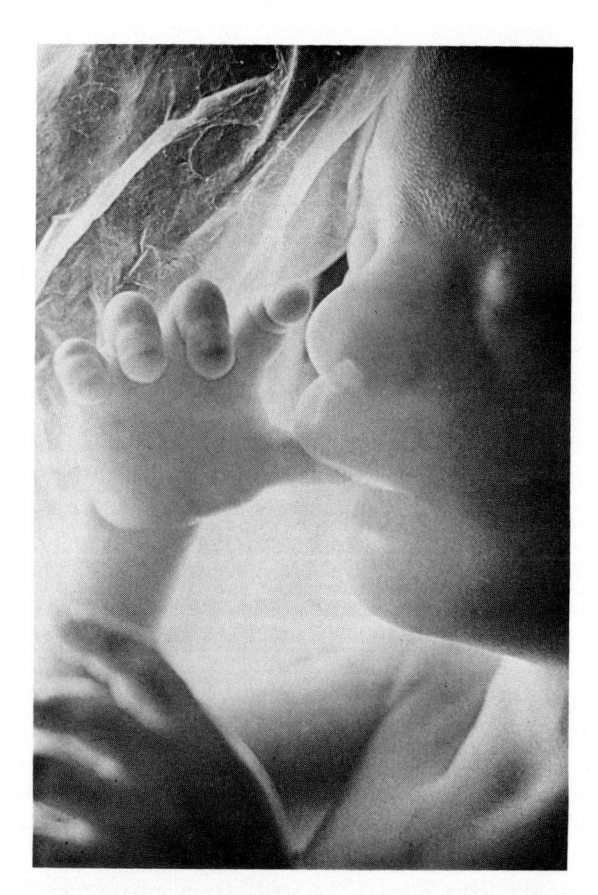

Fig. 21-7. Reflex sucking in utero. (From A CHILD IS BORN by Lennart Nilsson. English translation copyright © 1966, 1977 by Dell Publishing Co., Inc. Originally published in Swedish under the title ETT BARN BLIR TILL by Albert Bonniers Forlag. Copyright 1965 by Albert Bonniers Forlag, Stockholm. Revised edition copyright © 1976 by Lennart Nilsson, Mirjam Furuhjelm, Axel Ingerlman-Sunberg, Cales Wirson. Used by permission of DELACORTE PRESS/SEYMOUR LAWRENCE. A Merloyd Lawrence book.)

to trigeminal nerve stimulation. Other related reflexes (protrusion of the lips, mouth opening, and tongue movements) are noted at 16 weeks, and a gag reflex can be elicited at about 18 weeks. Lip puckering has been reported at 22 weeks and sucking at 24 weeks. Fetal postural changes sometimes bring the hand in contact with the mouth, and reflex finger sucking can occur (Fig. 21-7). Swallowing of amniotic fluid, noted as early as 10 to 14 weeks' gestation, plays a role in amniotic fluid turnover and is essential for normal fetal-placental development.

Although the isolated components of sucking and swallowing are all present before 28 weeks' gestation, they do not seem to be effectively coordinated for oral nipple feeding before 32 to 34 weeks, and even at this time they are immature.

Crump evaluated the sucking ability of low birth weight infants by measuring sucking rate. This was defined as the volume (milliliters) of fluid taken per second. Term infants had a sucking rate of 0.6 ml per second during the first 3 days of life, whereas low birth weight infants (mean birth weight, 2,109 gm) sucked at a rate of 0.24 ml per second. An increase in sucking rate is observed with increasing birth weight and postnatal age. Infants born after 37 weeks' gestation had a sucking rate and rhythm similar to those of term infants.

Gryboski observed nonnutritive sucking patterns and esophageal peristalsis from birth in groups of preterm infants. The infants showed irregular mouthing during the first few days after birth, the younger infants for up to 5 days and the older infants for 1 to 2 days. Thereafter an immature or a mature suck-swallow pattern was documented. The immature pattern, consisting of short sucking bursts preceded or followed by swallowing, occurred for 6 to 8 weeks in infants less than 35 weeks' gestation and only for a few days in older infants. The more mature suck-swallow pattern seen thereafter was characterized by longer bursts of sucking with multiple swallows occurring simultaneously with sucking.

In summary, although extrauterine fetal infants are able to "mouth" on a pacifier and suck repeatedly from 26 weeks' gestation, nonnutritive sucking may only assume a recognizable rhythmic pattern after 33 weeks' gestation. At this time the sucking rates per burst are slower (1.7 sucks per second per burst) and the interburst variability greater than those of term infants. A mature sucking rate and pattern are achieved by 37 weeks' gestation. Information is lacking as to whether postnatal oral experiences can accelerate this maturity.

ATTENTION AND PERCEPTION

Most of the current information on neonatal attention and perception is based on observations of responses to visual and auditory stimuli. Attention during the neonatal period is defined as a selective orientation toward some part of the stimulus environment. It is one of the prerequisites for perception and learning and is presumed to be cortically mediated. Measures of visual attention include orientation to and following of a visual stimulus and the duration of fixation on the stimulus. Other indices of attention are decreasing body movements, cessation of sucking, heart rate deceleration, and increased skin potential reactivity. Measures of perceptual ability in infancy include testing for visual preferences, measuring differential attention to familiar versus novel stimuli for early recognition memory, measuring a progressive decline in attention to a given stimulus (habituation), and measuring increased or renewed attention when a different stimulus is presented (dishabituation). These perceptual abilities in the newborn are difficult to evaluate, since changes in the state of arousal during testing may alter or mask responses and confuse results: a quiet awake infant's attention may wane if he becomes drowsy or actively awake; similarly, responses to auditory stimuli in active sleep may decrease if the infant goes into quiet sleep and increase if he wakes up.

VISUAL ATTENTION
The term infant

Before the 1950s it generally was not believed that the term neonate could see much. Observations of visual following and attention by Wolff, Stechler, Brazelton, and others together with Fantz's objective recordings of neonatal visual fixation dramatically changed this view. A normal healthy term infant in the quiet alert state will respond to a visual stimulus such as a red ball by alerting with facial awakening and eye brightening. He might also decrease body movements and change his rate of sucking while he fixates and scans the stimulus. If the ball is moved slowly, the infant will turn his eyes and head and track horizontally or vertically with conjugate eye movements. This attention increases initially but gradually decreases with either a change of state or by the infant's turning away from the stimulus. Some infants may show an obligatory type of attention during the first week or two after birth with prolonged fixation of 10 minutes or more. The newborn also blinks much less than the adult, resulting in a staring type of gaze.

The method developed by Fantz for recording visual fixation is called the corneal reflection technique. The criterion for fixation is when the corneal reflection of the stimulus overlaps the pupil and presumably also is reflected on the retina. Using this method, Fantz documented the newborn's ability to fixate on a single pattern and to show preferences between patterns, preferring patterned over plain stimuli, curved over straight contours, and patterns of a larger size over patterns with an increased number of smaller details (i.e., simple rather than complex patterns). With infrared cameras it has been shown that infants tend to scan mainly the outer contours of patterns while looking less at inner details. When looking at human faces, they tend to scan the external features such as the eyes, side of the head, or hair outline. Only by about 2 months of age do they examine more the internal features of a face or pattern. There has been some discussion in the literature as to whether the newborn has an innate ability to recognize the human face. There is, however, very little definite evidence that the infant prefers a face over other geometric patterns when they are equal in contour, density, and number and size of details.

Factors affecting visual attention

Visual fixation and following are optimum in the quiet alert state but may occur to a lesser degree during drowsiness. Lifting an infant to an upright position may facilitate the ability to attend visually, and providing a pacifier tends to inhibit diffuse body activity and improve fixation. Combined auditory and visual social cues especially draw the attention of the newborn infant. Factors that disturb the state of quiet awakeness such as asphyxia, maternal drugs, or jaundice may affect the ability to fixate and attend visually (see outline on p. 330). Prophylactic eye drops also may inhibit vision by causing periorbital edema and conjunctival irritation and are best postponed beyond the initial period of parent/infant contact.

Visual acuity

There is very little specific information on visual acuity in the neonate. An acuity ranging from 10/400 to 10/820 Snellen equivalent has been documented in term neonates using the optokinetic response, with a best result of 10/150. With the visual preference method acuity ranging from 20/300 to 20/1600 is described in term newborns. This poor acuity may explain the infants' preference for simple rather than more complex patterns. Furthermore the infant has a fixed focal length of approximately 19 cm and cannot accommodate to closer or more distant objects.

The preterm infant

Knowledge of the normal anatomic and physiologic maturation of the fetal visual system is limited. There is also very little understanding of how neural development correlates with observable visual behavior.

Anatomically all the retinal layers are present by 22 weeks' gestation. Immature rods and cones can be distinguished at 23 weeks, myelinization of the optic nerve begins at 24 weeks, and all the neurons of the visual cortex are present by 25 to 26 weeks' gestation. Between 28 and 34 weeks there is a phase of rapid dendritic differentiation and synaptogenesis, with the cortical neurons undergoing changes in cell size, axonal length, and dendritic branching and synapses. Physiologically it has been shown that visual evoked potentials can transmit impulses from the cornea to the visual cortex by 26 weeks' gestation. These are initially very immature with long latencies which decrease somewhat inconsistently with age.

Although the preterm infant has a pupillary light response and can react to light by blinking at 29 weeks' gestation, there does not seem to be any awake visual attention before 30 to 32 weeks.

Using the corneal reflection technique, Hack demonstrated fixation on a single pattern from 30 weeks' postmenstrual age and visual preference to a patterned versus a plain surface from 31 weeks. Indices of alertness and attentiveness during fixation such as widening and brightening of the eyes, visual scanning, and cessation of sucking increase progressively from 30 weeks, so that an immature drowsy look is replaced by an awake, expressive visual alertness and active scanning of the stimulus by 36 weeks' postmenstrual age.

The time spent looking at a single pattern increases with age, with more fixation occurring during quiet awakeness than during drowsiness (Fig. 21-5).

In a separate study paired stimuli were presented to infants ranging in age from 31 to 34 weeks' postmenstrual age. The infants showed strong preferences for patterns of larger size or with greater details; however, no preferences for increasing detail were found when the amount of contrast in the pattern was held constant. These preferences did not differ from those of infants born at term or who had reached term after 8 to 10 weeks' postnatal experience.

Dubowitz recently studied both visual following and pattern preferences in preterm infants and found that under 30 weeks' gestation only 1 of 10 infants studied was capable of fixating on a moving red ball; between 30 and 32 weeks 20 of 25 infants fixated or followed, and after 32 weeks 11 of 12 infants demonstrated this ability. Pattern preferences were found in very few infants less than 32 weeks' gestation and in all infants over 32 weeks.

An orienting or attentional type of sucking response to visual stimuli has been documented by Barrett in preterm infants ranging in age from 33 to 37 weeks' gestation. Evidence of visual memory in preterm infants also has been documented by Sequeland. He presented a pattern continuously until infants showed familiarity by decreasing their rate of sucking. When a different stimulus was shown, the infants increased their rate of sucking, indicating recognition or memory of differences in the two patterns shown.

Visual acuity

The only information on preterm acuity is that of Kiff and Lepard, who found a Snellen visual acuity of 20/820, and of Miranda, who found that preterm infants (mean postmenstrual age, 35 weeks) could discriminate a ¼-inch line corresponding to a Snellen fraction of approximately 20/1280.

The term versus the preterm infant

Gesell noted an advanced attentiveness in preterm infants who had reached term when compared with term infants; however, this was only temporary and passed by 4 weeks after term. Kurtzberg, however, demonstrated decreased visual following in preterm infants at term. Kopp, Sigman, and Parmelee found that preterm infants at term spent more time looking at visual stimuli than did term infants. Friedman could not confirm these results but found that preterm infants took longer to fixate on a stimulus and also longer to decrease their response, indicating a possible inability to inhibit looking in the preterm infant. These studies suggest that preterm infants gain no benefit from the early visual stimulation they receive in the nursery. In fact, it is questionable how much visual stimulation these infants actually receive, since they have very short periods of awakeness and, considering their poor visual acuity and inability to accommodate, are exposed to very few appropriate visual stimuli in the incubator.

AUDITORY ATTENTION
The term infant

The term infant is capable of responding to sound when either asleep or awake. The specific behavioral response depends on the infant's state of arousal and on the tone, frequency, and repetitiveness of the auditory stimulus. When asleep, the infant responds by eye blinking, startling, and other body movements and with changes in respiration and heart rate. This response is greater in active than in quiet sleep. The awake infant responds to sound by an alerting of facial expression, by turning of eyes and sometimes head in the direction of the sound, and by a decrease in heart rate and change in respiration. These indices of attention are noted especially when the sound is in the range of human speech (500 to 900 cycles per second). Lower and higher frequency sounds have different effects. Low-frequency sounds, especially when continuous, tend to soothe the infant and induce sleep, whereas high-frequency sounds may cause distress with cardiac acceleration and crying. Infants tend to decrease responses (habituate) to repetitive auditory stimuli and respond again (dishabituate) when the frequency of sound is changed. Cairns and Butterfield showed that the term infant has different sucking responses to human and nonhuman auditory stimuli and that infants can be conditioned to modify their sucking rate to bring on the sound of a human voice. There is also some evidence that the newborn can differentiate between maternal and other voices within a few days of birth.

Fetal responses

There have been isolated reports of fetal movement and heart rate acceleration in response to auditory stimuli from as early as 26 weeks' gestation. The human auditory apparatus is structurally complete and physiologically functional at 24 weeks' gestation, so that this is feasible. There are, however, many factors that confound the evaluation of hearing in utero. The fetus is already exposed to high levels of background noise from the maternal circulatory and digestive systems, so that any additional auditory stimuli may not be heard. In addition, there is no air in utero so that sound can be conducted only through fluid or bone. Any documented fetal responses may in part be a result of the maternal response to the auditory stimulus or the vibration associated with giving the stimulus.

Parmelee reviewed the literature on fetal auditory responsivity and concluded that there is still uncertainty as to whether the fetus can respond to external auditory stimuli presented before 34 weeks' gestation. After 34 weeks the fetus responds clearly with body movements or heart rate acceleration. It may be possible to use these auditory responses as a measure of fetal well-being in utero.

The preterm infant

The extrauterine preterm infant responds to auditory stimuli from as early as 28 weeks' gestation. Gesell reported responses to sound at 28 to 30 weeks with a decrease in response after repeated stimulation. Monod and Garma measured preterm responses to auditory click stimuli and documented motor responses 29% of the time at 30 to 31 weeks' gestation and eye blink responses only 5% of the time. With increasing age the motor responses tended to decrease in quiet sleep, whereas in active sleep the percentage of motor responses did not change. Eye blink responses to sound increased in active sleep with increasing age.

Cortical evoked auditory responses have been documented from 25 weeks' gestation. With increasing age the complexity of the wave responses increase and their latency decreases.

Auditory brain stem evoked potentials (ABR) have been studied longitudinally from 26 weeks' gestation. The ABR consists of a series of waves evoked by an auditory stimulus such as a click, and gives information on the threshold sensitivity of the peripheral auditory system (cochlea and auditory nerve) and on the velocity of conduction along the auditory fibers ascending the brain stem en route to the cortex. The latencies (conduction times) of these waves decrease with increasing gestational age and are not dependent on the state of the infant. Infants born at term have latencies similar to those of preterm infants who have reached term. The ABR has been used to assess early hearing and to document the effects of neonatal risk factors on auditory and brain stem function. The only individual risk factors that have been found to correlate with increased latencies are intraventricular hemorrhage and prolonged acidosis secondary to asphyxia, although multiple risk factors may prolong latency periods.

In summary, cortical and base of brain evoked potentials show that the auditory system is functional from 26 weeks' gestation. Inconsistent behavioral auditory responses can be obtained from 28 weeks' gestation with more consistent responses from 32 to 34 weeks' gestation. There is no evidence that the noise environment of the nursery has a measurable effect on the ontogeny of auditory perception.

MOTOR BEHAVIOR

This section reviews the development of resting posture, active and passive muscle tone, and spontaneous movement.

Fetal movements

Hooker described reflex fetal movement from 7 weeks' gestation. Initially there is a total body reflex movement in response to stroking the trigeminal perioral area. This includes flexion and later extension of the head as well as movement of the trunk and limbs away from the stimulus. Later, from 8 to 11 weeks, the reflex is toward the stimulus. With increasing age reflex movements become more localized.

With ultrasonography spontaneous movements of the fetal trunk can be seen at 8 weeks and discrete limb movements from 9 weeks' gestation. The extent and frequency of these movements increase from 10 to 20 weeks' gestation, when they can be felt as "quickening" by the mother. The movements are spontaneous but can be elicited by stimulation with a noise, coughing, or displacement of the uterus. From 24 weeks trunk movements tend to diminish, whereas those of the extremities increase. The decrease in the relative amount of amniotic fluid after 28 weeks' gestation also tends to constrain movement.

Various attempts to classify fetal movements have been made. Timor-Tritsch defined four patterns of motion by measuring pressure changes transmitted through the maternal abdomen: rolling body movements, simple short extremity movements, high-frequency movements, and breathing movements. Birnholz, using phase array ultrasonography, categorized the movement patterns shown in Fig. 21-8. Twitching is seen mainly from 7 to 10 weeks, independent limb movements from 10 to 12 weeks, and combined limb, head, and torso movements from 12 to 16 weeks. More complex hand, face, and respiratory movements are seen from 24 weeks. The earlier movements are sporadic and jerky and gradually become more regular and controlled as the fetus matures.

Fetal movement can be influenced by the rest-activity cycling of the mother as well as by smoking, hypoglycemia, other fetal distress, and maternal pathologic conditions.

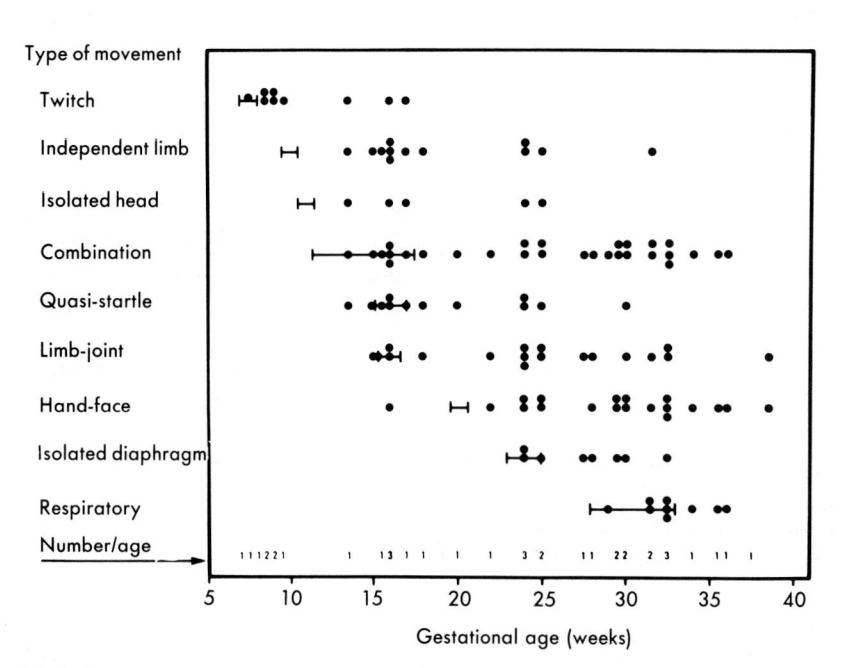

Fig. 21-8. Development of fetal movement patterns in utero. (From Birnholz, J.: Am. J. Roentgenol. **130**:537, 1978. © 1978, American Roentgen Ray Society.)

The preterm infant

After birth the forces of gravity influence both the types of movement and the postures the infant may assume.

Muscle tone

A gradual increase in active and passive muscle tone from 28 to 40 weeks' gestation originally was described by Andre Thomas and Saint-Anne Dargassies. Muscle tone develops first in the lower limbs and then progresses in a caudocephalad direction. Flexor tone develops before extensor tone. At 28 weeks muscle tone is essentially flaccid (hypotonic); an improvement in tone is noted in the lower extremities by 32 to 34 weeks and in the upper extremities by 36 to 38 weeks. Passive tone angles through which a joint can be extended at various gestational ages are shown in Fig. 21-9. Active tone is first seen as the ability to support the legs and later to support the body with righting of the trunk, and finally righting of the head occurs. By term the awake infant has good head control and supports the legs and trunk when placed in a standing position on a flat surface (Fig. 21-10) (p. 256).

Posture

Infant posture depends both on muscle tone and on the movements the infant is able to perform to achieve a certain posture. According to Saint-Anne Dargassies the 28-week-gestation infant lies with arms and legs extended and then gradually assumes a position of predominate flexion as muscle tone increases. This qualitative increase in muscle tone and flexion position with age has been used by Dubowitz and others to assess gestational age. More recent quantitative evaluations of preterm postures by both Brandt and Prechtl have not found age-related preferences for posture. Prechtl studied 14 healthy low risk infants born at 28 to 36 weeks' gestation by recording, every minute during a 2-hour period, the posture of the head, arms, and legs and clonic as well as more complex stretching movements. There do not seem to be any age-related changes in these movements before 35 weeks, although there are intraindividual differences. From 36 weeks' gestation the movements tend to become more coordinated with less tremors, clonic movements, and stretching. By term the infant can perform complex movements such as head turning in response to a light source and hand-mouth coordination.

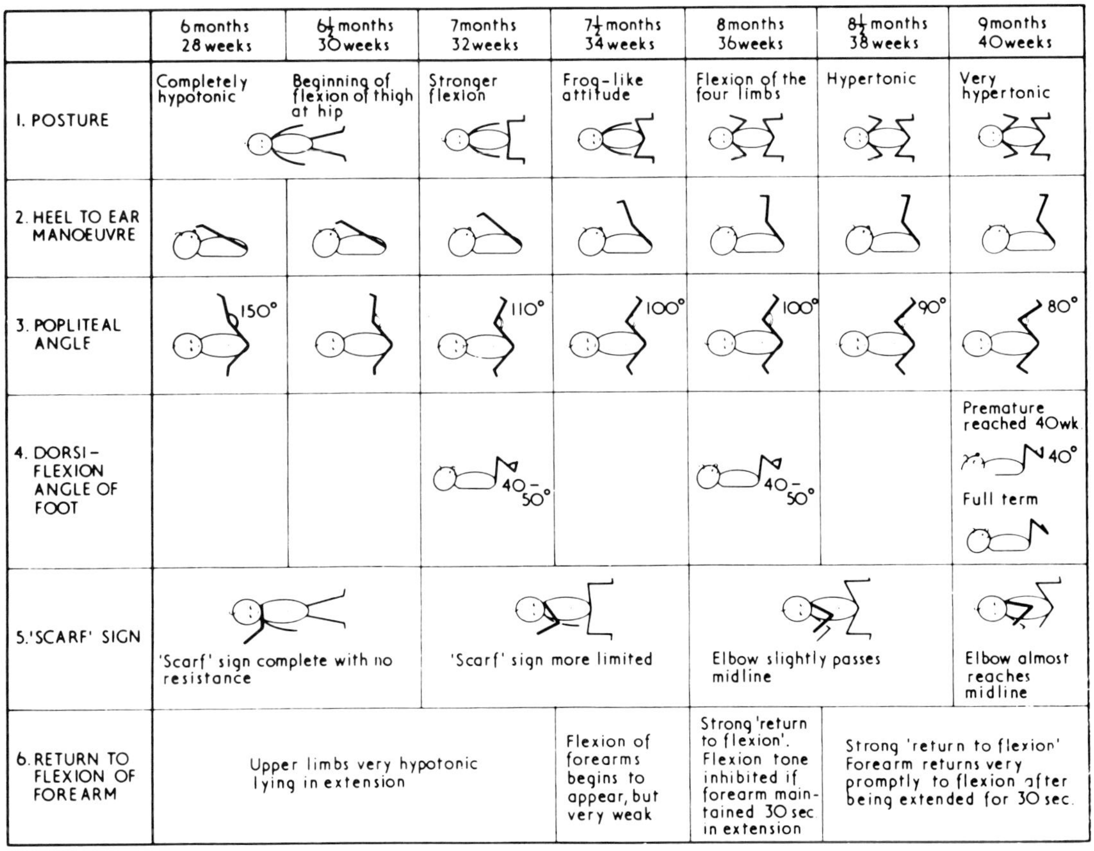

	6 months 28 weeks	6½ months 30 weeks	7 months 32 weeks	7½ months 34 weeks	8 months 36 weeks	8½ months 38 weeks	9 months 40 weeks
1. POSTURE	Completely hypotonic	Beginning of flexion of thigh at hip	Stronger flexion	Frog-like attitude	Flexion of the four limbs	Hypertonic	Very hypertonic
2. HEEL TO EAR MANOEUVRE							
3. POPLITEAL ANGLE		150°		110°	100°	100°	90°	80°
4. DORSI-FLEXION ANGLE OF FOOT				40-50°	40-50°	Premature reached 40wk 40° / Full term	
5. 'SCARF' SIGN		'Scarf' sign complete with no resistance		'Scarf' sign more limited		Elbow slightly passes midline	Elbow almost reaches midline
6. RETURN TO FLEXION OF FOREARM		Upper limbs very hypotonic lying in extension		Flexion of forearms begins to appear, but very weak	Strong 'return to flexion'. Flexion tone inhibited if forearm maintained 30 sec in extension	Strong 'return to flexion' Forearm returns very promptly to flexion after being extended for 30 sec	

Fig. 21-9. Development of posture and passive muscle tone from 28 weeks' gestation until term. (From Amiel Tison, C.: Arch. Dis. Child. **43:**89, 1968.)

	6 months 28 weeks	6½ months 30 weeks	7 months 32 weeks	7½ months 34 weeks	8 months 36 weeks	8½ months 38 weeks	9 months 40 weeks
1. LOWER EXTREMITY	—	Beginning of extension of lower leg on thigh upon stimulation of soles in lying position	Good support when standing up but very briefly (see illustration below)	Excellent righting reaction of leg →→→			
2. TRUNK	—	—	—	± transitory	Good righting of trunk with infant held in vertical suspension (see illustration below)	Good righting of trunk with infant held in walking position (see illustration below)	
3. NECK EXTENSORS Baby pulled backward from sitting position	—	—	Head begins to right itself with great difficulty	Still difficult and incomplete	Good righting but cannot hold it	Begins to maintain head which doesn't fall back for few seconds	Keeps head in line with trunk for more than a few seconds
4. NECK FLEXORS Baby pulled to sitting position from supine	Head pendulant	Head pendulant	Contraction of muscles is visible but no movement of head	Head begins to right itself but still hanging back at end of movement	At first head is hanging back, then with sudden movement head goes forward onto chest	Head begins to follow trunk, keeps in line for few seconds in upright position	Difference between Extensors and Flexors has diminished (see illustration below)
			Straightening of legs 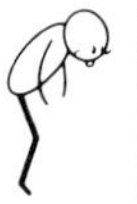		Straightening of trunk 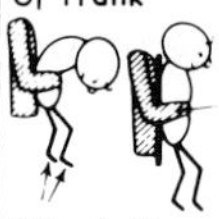 / Stimulation / arm support		Straightening of head and trunk together 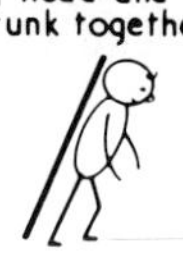

Fig. 21-10. Development of active muscle tone from 28 weeks' gestation until term. (From Amiel Tison, C.: Arch. Dis. Child. **43**:89, 1968.)

Factors affecting motor behavior

Neonatal motor behavior is largely under control of the spinal cord and medulla, although higher brain centers and especially the state of the infant are influencing factors. Factors affecting motor behavior, either directly or indirectly by changing state, include environmental temperature, electrolyte disturbances (glucose, sodium, calcium, magnesium), and various disorders such as jaundice, respiratory distress, and infection. Preterm infants tend to become hypotonic and exhibit less movement when sick. Small for gestational age infants also tend to be relatively hypotonic with less spontaneous activity for their age. Accelerated neurologic maturity with an increase in muscle tone has been documented at birth in some infants born to mothers with complicated pregnancies (toxemia, premature rupture of membranes, and antepartum bleeding). Such infants also may have accelerated pulmonary maturity.

The term versus the preterm infant

In general, there are minimal differences in preferred posture and motor behavior between preterm infants who have reached term and those born at term. Subtle differences in motor behavior, however, do distinguish these two groups. The preterm infant has not been confined to a flexed position in utero and is less hypertonic and exhibits easier passive movement of limbs and more active and varied spontaneous movements.

THE BRAZELTON NEONATAL BEHAVIORAL ASSESSMENT SCALE

The Brazelton neonatal behavioral assessment scale incorporates most of the behaviors described in this chapter. By using this method of assessment it is possible to evaluate the term newborn's behavioral capabilities and to see how the infant responds to the immediate environment. Although the full Brazelton examination seldom is used clinically by neonatologists, many of the responses are useful for evaluating an infant's interactive abilities and to demonstrate individual differences to parents. During the course of the examination 26 behavioral responses are tested and rated on a nine-point scale, and 20 neurologic responses are rated on a three-point scale.

BEHAVIORAL ITEMS

Response decrement to repeated visual stimuli
Response decrement to rattle
Response decrement to bell
Response decrement to pinprick
Orienting response to inanimate visual stimuli

Orienting response to inanimate auditory stimuli
Orienting response to animate visual stimuli: examiner's face
Orienting response to animate auditory stimuli: examiner's voice
Orienting responses to animate visual and auditory stimuli
Quality and duration of alert periods
General muscle tone, in resting and in response to being handled (passive and active)
Motor maturity
Traction responses as infant is pulled to sitting position
Cuddliness: responses to being cuddled by the examiner
Defensive movements: reactions to a cloth over face
Consolability with intervention by examiner
Peak of excitement and capacity to control self
Rapidity of buildup to crying state
Irritability during the examination
General assessment of kind and degree of activity
Tremulousness
Amount of startling
Lability of skin color (measuring autonomic lability)
Lability of states during entire examination
Self-quieting activity: attempts to console self and control state
Hand-to-mouth activity

NEUROLOGIC RESPONSES

Plantar grasp
Hand grasp
Ankle clonus
Babinski sign
Standing
Automatic walking
Placing
Incurvation
Crawling
Glabella
Tonic deviation of head and eyes
Nystagmus
Tonic neck reflex
Moro reflex
Rooting (intensity)
Sucking (intensity)
Passive movement
    Arms (R, L)
    Legs (R, L)

The best performance of every response is recorded. In addition, state changes are noted throughout the examination to assess the infant's capacity for self-organization. The examination starts with a sleeping baby and gradually works through the various responses as the infant awakens. Responses to visual, auditory, and tactile stimuli are tested as well as the ability to habituate to repeated stimuli. During the course of the examination responses to aversive stimuli such as uncovering, undressing, a pinprick, and a cloth placed over the face also are tested together with the ability for self-quieting and the ability to respond to soothing and cuddling.

The Brazelton scale has been used to evaluate the effects on neonatal behavior of maternal obstetric drugs, narcotic addiction, and various neonatal conditions such as intrauterine growth retardation, jaundice, and asphyxia.

Als recently has extended the use of the Brazelton scale to evaluate preterm behavioral organization. She has hypothesized that initially the main task for the preterm infant is to stabilize and integrate physiologic functions such as respiration, heart rate, temperature, digestion, and elimination. The motor system then gradually develops with active postural adjustments and movement. Later the awake and sleep states emerge with organization of state, and finally the alert state becomes available for social interaction. The preterm infant thus is viewed as part of a continuous organism-environment transactional system.

With this concept the assessment of preterm infant behavior provides a method for systematically documenting the infant's current status of behavioral organization along five subsystems of functioning: physiologic, motor organizational, state organizational, interactive, and self-regulation. The examiner's efforts and support necessary to bring out the infant's best performance during the course of the behavioral examination also are documented. This test is not yet readily applicable for clinical use; however, it is of great importance because it compels the caretaker to view the preterm infant as part of an environmental system rather than an isolated organism. The effects of various medical procedures always need to be viewed in this context.

CONCLUSION

The improved survival rates and greater accessibility of neonatal intensive care units to developmental psychologists have resulted in a surge of interest and research in preterm behavioral development. The various studies reported in this chapter have focused mainly on the ontogeny of isolated sensory behaviors. As yet there have been very few studies on the interrelationship between the various sensory abilities and very little attention given to viewing the preterm infant as part of an interactional system between the infant, caretaker, and nursery environment. It has been shown, however, that infants in intensive care nurseries are seldom left to rest, are subjected to multiple medical caretaking procedures, and are exposed to continuous light and auditory stimuli. It is thus surprising that despite this unnatural and disturbing type of environment the preterm infant who has reached term shows only minimal behavioral differences when compared with the term newborn. This may in part be caused by the preterm infant's relative lack of responsiveness, which protects him from the excessive stimuli of the outer world. It seems that the inherent program of biologic and structural development continues despite environmental changes and disease processes.

Maureen Hack

BIBLIOGRAPHY
General

Brazelton, B., Parker, W., and Zuckerman, B.: Importance of behavioral assessment of the neonate. In Gluck, L., editor: Current problems in pediatrics, vol. 7, no. 2, Chicago, 1976, Year Book Medical Publishers, Inc.

Condon, W.S., and Sander, L.W.: Neonatal movement is synchronized with adult speech: interactional participation and language acquisition, Science 183:99, 1974.

Dreyfus-Brisac, C.: Neurophysiological studies in human premature and full-term newborns, Biol. Psychiatry 10:485, 1975.

Friedman, S., and Sigman, M., editors: Preterm birth and psychological development, New York, 1981, Academic Press, Inc.

Gesell, A., and Amatruda, C.: The embryology of behavior—the beginnings of the human mind, New York, 1945, Harper & Row Publishers, Inc.

Gottfried, A., and Cornell, E.: Intervention with premature human infants, Child Dev. 47:32, 1976.

Humphrey, T.: Some correlations between the appearance of human fetal reflexes and the development of the nervous system, Prog. Brain Res. 4:93, 1964.

Hutt, S.G., Lenard, H.G., and Prechtl, H.F.R.: Psychophysiological studies in newborn infants, Adv. Child Dev. Behav. 4:128, 1969.

Lawson, K., Daum, C., and Turkewitz, G.: Environmental characteristics of a neonatal intensive-care unit, Child Dev. 48:1633, 1977.

Lipsitt, L.P.: The study of sensory and learning processes of the newborn, Clin. Perinatol. 4:163, 1977.

Meltzoff, A.N., and Moore, M.K.: Imitation of facial and manual gestures by human neonates, Science 198:75, 1977.

Osofsky, J.D., editor: The handbook of infant development, New York, 1979, John Wiley & Sons, Inc.

Peiper, A.: Cerebral function in infancy and childhood, New York, 1963, Consultants Bureau.

Prechtl, H.F.R.: The behavioral states of the newborn infant: a review, Brain Res. 76:185, 1974.

Saint-Anne Dargassies, S.: Neurological development in the full-term and premature neonate, Amsterdam, 1977, Exerpta Medica.

Wolff, P.H.: The causes, controls, and organization of behavior in the newborn, Psychol. Issues 5:1-97, 1966.

Wolff, P.H., and Ferber, R.: The development of behavior in human infants, premature and newborn, Ann. Rev. Neurosci. 2:291, 1979.

States of arousal
The term infant

Anders, T.F., and Chalemian, R.J.: The effects of circumcision on sleep-wake states in human neonates, Psychosom. Med. 36:174, 1974.

Anders, T.F., Emde, R.N., and Parmelee, A.H., Jr., editors: Manual of standardized terminology, techniques, and for scoring of states of sleep and wakefulness in newborn infants, Los Angeles, 1971, Brain Information Service, School of Health Sciences, University of California at Los Angeles.

Anders, T.F., and Hoffman, E.: The sleep polygram: a potentially useful tool for clinical assessment in human infants, Am. J. Ment. Defic. 77:506, 1973.

Anders, T.F., and Roffwarg, H.P.: The effects of selective interruption and deprivation of sleep in the human newborn, Dev. Psychobiol. 6:79, 1973.

Aserinsky, E., and Kleitman, N.: Regularly occurring periods of eye motility and concomitant phenomena during sleep, Science 118:273, 1953.

Biosmier, J.D.: Visual stimulation and wake-sleep behavior in human neonates, Dev. Psychobiol. 10:219, 1977.

Brackbill, Y.: Cumulative effects of continuous stimulation on arousal level in infants, Child. Dev. 42:17, 1971.

Blackbill, Y., Douthitt, T.C., and West, H.: Psychophysiologic effects in the neonate of prone versus supine placement, J. Pediatr. 82:82, 1973.

Brazelton, T.: Psychophysiologic reactions in the neonate. I. The value of observation of the neonate, Pediatrics 58:508, 1961.

Desmond, M.M., and others: The clinical behavior of the newly born, J. Pediatr. 62:307, 1963.

Emde, R.N., Swedberg, J., and Suzuki, B.: Human wakefulness and biological rhythms after birth, Arch. Gen. Psychiatry 32:780, 1975.

Emde, R.N., and others: Stress and neonatal sleep, Psychosom. Med. 33:491, 1971.

Gaensbauer, T.H., and Emde, R.N.: Wakefulness and feeding in human newborns, Arch. Gen. Psychiatry 28:894, 1973.

Korner, A.F., and Thoman, E.B.: Visual alertness in neonates as evoked by maternal care, J. Exp. Child Psychol. 10:67, 1970.

Long, J.G., Philip, A.G.S., and Lucey, J.F.: Excessive handling as a cause of hypoxemia, Pediatrics 65:203, 1980.

Martin, R.J., Okken, A., and Rubin, D.: Changes in arterial oxygen tension during active and quiet sleep in the neonate, Birth Defects 15:493, 1979.

Prechtl, H.F.R.: Patterns of reflex behavior related to sleep in the human infant. In Clemente, C.D., and others, editors: Sleep and the maturing nervous system, New York, 1972, Academic Press, Inc.

Roffwarg, H.P., Muzio, J.N., and Dement, W.C.: Ontogenetic development of the human sleep-dream cycle, Science 152:604, 1966.

Schmidt, K.: The effect of continuous stimulation on the behavioral sleep of infants, Merrill-Palmer Q. 21:77, 1975.

Theorell, K., Prechtl, H.F.R., and Vos, J.E.: A polygraphic study of normal and abnormal newborn infants, Neuropaediatrie 5:279, 1974.

Wolff, P.H.: Observations on newborn infants, Psychosom. Med. 21:110, 1959.

Fetal rest-activity cycles

Dierker, L.J., and others: Correlation between gestational age and fetal activity periods, Biol. Neonate 42:66, 1982.

Sterman, M.B., and Hoppenbrouwers, T.: The development of sleep-waking and rest-activity patterns from fetus to adult in man. In Clemente, C.D., and others, editors: Sleep and the maturing nervous system, New York, 1972, Academic Press, Inc.

Timor-Tritsch, I.E., and others: Studies of antepartum behavioral state in the human fetus at term, Am. J. Obstet. Gynecol. 132:524, 1978.

The preterm infant

Dreyfus-Brisac, C.: Sleep ontogenesis in early human prematurity from 24 to 27 weeks of conceptional age, Dev. Psychobiol. 1:162, 1968.

Dreyfus-Brisac, C.: Ontogenesis of sleep in human prematures after 32 weeks of conceptional age, Dev. Psychobiol. 8:91, 1970.

Eisengart, M., Gluck, L., and Kessen, W.: Early feeding of premature infants effect on blood sugar and gross motor activity, Biol. Neonate 17:151, 1971.

Emde, R.N., and Koenig, K.L.: Neonatal smiling and rapid eye movement states, J. Am. Acad. Child Psychiatry 8:57, 1969.

Emde, R.N., and Koenig, K.L.: Neonatal smiling, frowning, and rapid eye movement states. II. Sleep-cycle study, J. Am. Acad. Child Psychiatry 8:637, 1969.

Emde, R.N., and Metcalf, D: An electroencephalographic study of behavioral rapid eye movement states in the human newborn, J. Nerv. Ment. Dis. 150:376, 1970.

Hack, M., Muszynski, S., and Miranda, S.: State of awakeness during visual fixation in preterm infants, Pediatrics 68:87, 1981.

Holmes, G., and others: Central nervous system maturation in the stressed premature, Ann. Neurol. 6:518, 1979.

Minde, K., and others: Mother-child relationships in the premature nursery: an observational study, Pediatrics 61:373, 1978.

Parmelee, A.H., Jr.: Neurophysiological and behavioral organization of premature infants in the first months of life, Biol. Psychiatry 10:501, 1975.

Parmelee, A.H., Jr., Bruck, K., and Bruck, M.: Activity and inactivity cycles during the sleep of premature infants exposed to neutral temperatures, Biol. Neonat. 4:317, 1962.

Parmelee, A.H., Jr., and others: Sleep states in premature infants, Dev. Med. Child Neurol. 9:70, 1967.

Stern, E., Parmelee, A.H., Jr., and Harris, M.A.: Sleep state periodicity in prematures and young infants, Dev. Psychobiol. 6:357, 1973.

Facial expressions and social behaviors

Emde, R.N, Gaensbauer, T., and Harmon, R.: Emotional expression in infancy: a biobehavioral study, Psychol. Issues, vol. 10 no. 1, monograph 37, New York, 1976, International Universities Press, Inc.

Emde, R.N., and Harmon, R.J.: Endogenous and exogenous smiling systems in early infancy, J. Am. Acad. Child Psychiatry 11:177, 1972.

Emde, R.N., McCartney, R.D., and Harmon, R.J.: Neonatal smiling in REM states. IV. Premature study, Child Dev. 42:1657, 1971.

Folcy, H.: When do pre-term and light-for-dates babies smile? Dev. Med. Child Neurol. 19:757, 1977.

Hines, R., and others: Behavioral development of premature infants: an ethological approach, Dev. Med. Child Neurol. 22:623, 1980.

Michaelis, R., and others: Activity states in premature and term infants, Dev. Psychobiol. 6:209, 1973.

Michelsson, K.: Cry analyses of symptomless low birth weight neonates and of asphyxiated newborn infants, Acta Paediatr. Scand. (Suppl.) 216:1971.

Sroufe, L.A., and Waters, E.: The ontogenesis of smiling and laughter: a perspective on the organization of development in infancy, Psychol. Rev. 83:173, 1976.

Wolff, P.H.: Observations on the early development of smiling. In Foss, B.M., editor: Determinants of infant behavior, vol. 2, New York, 1963, Methuen, Inc.

Sucking

Anderson, G.C., and Vidyasagar, D.: Development of sucking in premature infants from 1 to 7 days post birth, Birth Defects, 15:145, 1979.

Crook, C.K.: The organization and control of infant sucking, Adv. Child Dev. Behav. 14:209, 1979.

Crump, E.P., Gore, P.M., and Horton, C.P.: The sucking behavior in premature infants, Hum. Biol. 30:128, 1958.

Dubignon, J.M., Campbell, D., and Partington, M.W.: The development of non-nutritive sucking in premature infants, Biol. Neonat. 14:270, 1969.

Gryboski, J.: Suck and swallow in the premature infant, Pediatrics 43:96, 1969.

Wolff, P.H.: The serial organization of sucking in the young infant, Pediatrics 42:943, 1968.

Wolff, P.H.: The interaction of state and non-nutritive sucking. In Bosma, J., editor: Third Symposium on Oral Sensation and Perception, Springfield, Ill., 1972, Charles C. Thomas, Publisher.

Visual attention
The term infant

Brazelton, T.B., Scholl, M.L., and Robey, J.S.: Visual responses in the newborn, Pediatrics 37:284, 1966.

Bruner, J.S.: Pacifier-produced visual buffering in human infants, Dev. Psychobiol. 6:45, 1973.

Cohen, L.: Infant perception: from sensation to cognition. In Salapetek, P., editor: Basic visual processes, vol. 1, New York, 1975, Academic Press, Inc.

Cohen, L., DeLoache, J., and Strauss, M.: Infant visual perception. In Osofsky, J.D., editor: The handbook of infant development, New York, 1979, John Wiley & Sons, Inc.

Fantz, R.: Pattern vision in newborn infants, Science 140:296, 1963.

Fredrickson, W., and Brown, J.: Posture as a determinant of visual behavior in newborns, Child Dev. 46:579, 1975.

Friedman, S.: Newborn visual attention to repeated exposure of redundant vs. "novel" targets, Perception and Psychophysics 12:291, 1972.

Gregg, C.L., Haffner, M.H., and Korner, F.: The relative efficacy of vestibular-proprioceptive stimulation and the upright position in enhancing visual pursuit in neonates, Child Dev. 47:309, 1976.

Haynes, H., White, B., and Held, R.: Visual accommodation in human infants, Science 48:528, 1965.

Kopp, C., Sigman, M., and Parmelee, A.H., Jr.: Neurological organization and visual fixation in infants at 40 weeks conceptional age, Dev. Psychobiol. 8:165, 1975.

Linksz, A.: Visual acuity in the newborn with notes on some objective methods to determine visual acuity, Doc. Ophthalmol. 34:259, 1973.

Salapatek, P., and Kessen, W.: Visual scanning of triangles by the human newborn, J. Exp. Child Psychol. 3:155, 1966.

Sigman, M., and others: Visual attention and neurological organization in neonates, Child Dev. 44:461, 1973.

Sigman, M., and others: Infant visual attentiveness in relation to birth condition, Dev. Psychobiol. 13:431, 1977.

Stechler, G.: Newborn attention as affected by medication during labor, Science 14:315, 1964.

Stechler, G.: Attention in the newborn: its effects on motility and skin potential reactivity, Science 151:1246, 1966.

Stechler, G., and Latz, E.: Some observations on attention and arousal in the human infant, J. Am. Acad. Child Psychiatry 5:517, 1966.

Wolff, P.H.: The development of attention in young infants, Ann. N.Y. Acad. Sci. 118:815, 1965.

The preterm infant

Barrett, T.E., and Miller, L.K.: The organization of non-nutritive sucking in the premature infant, J. Exp. Child Psychol. 16:472, 1973.

Dubowitz, L.M.S., and others: Visual function in the preterm and full-term newborn infant, Dev. Med. Child Neurol. 22:465, 1980.

Friedman, S., Jacobs, B., and Werthmann, M.: Sensory processing in pre- and full-term infants in the neonatal period. In Friedman, S., and Sigman, M., editors: Preterm birth and psychological development, New York, 1981, Academic Press, Inc.

Hack, M., Mostow, A., and Miranda, S.: Development of attention in preterm infants, Pediatrics 58:669, 1976.

Hittner, H., Hirsch, J., and Rudolph, A.: Assessment of gestational age by examination of the anterior vascular capsule of the lens, Pediatrics 91:455, 1977.

Kiff, R., and Lepard, C.: Visual response of premature infants: use of the optokinetic nystagmus to estimate visual development, Arch. Opthalmol. 75:631, 1966.

Miranda, S.: Visual abilities and pattern preferences of premature infants and full-term neonates, J. Exp. Child Psychol. 10:189, 1970.

Purpura, D.P.: Morphogenesis of visual cortex in the preterm infant. In Brazier, M.A.B., editor: Growth and development of the brain, New York, 1975, Raven Press.

Robinson, R.: Assessment of gestational age by neurological examination, Arch. Dis. Child. 41:437, 1966.

Schulte, F., and others: The ontogeny of sensory perception in preterm infants, Eur. J. Pediatr. 126:211, 1977.

Sequeland, E.: Studies of visual recognition memory in preterm infants: differences in development as a function of perinatal morbidity factors. In Friedman, S., and Sigman, M., editors: Preterm birth and psychological development, New York, 1981, Academic Press, Inc.

Auditory function
Fetal

Bradley, R., and Mistretta, C.: Fetal sensory receptors, Physiol. Rev. 55:352, 1975.

Luz, N., and others: Auditory evoked responses of the human fetus behavior during progress of labor, Acta Obstet. Gynecol. Scand. 59:395, 1980.

Read, J., and Miller, F.: Fetal heart rate acceleration in response to acoustic stimulation as a measure of fetal well-being, Am. J. Obstet. Gynecol. 129:512, 1977.

Term and preterm infant

Cairns, G., and Butterfield, E.: Assessing infant's auditory functioning. In Fridlander, B., Sterritt, G., and Kirk, G., editors: Exceptional infant, New York, 1975, Brunner/Mazel, Inc.

Despland, P., and Galambos, R.: The auditory brainstem response (ABR) is a useful diagnostic tool in the intensive care nursery, Pediatr. Res. 14:154, 1980.

Eisenberg, R.: Auditory behavior in the human neonate: methodologic problems, J. Aud. Res. 5:159, 1965.

Hammond, J.: Hearing and response in the newborn, Dev. Med. Child Neurol. 12:3, 1970.

Hutt, S., and others: Auditory responsivity in the human neonate, Nature 218:888, 1968.

Marshall, R., and others: Auditory function in newborn intensive care unit patients revealed by auditory brain-stem potentials, J. Pediatr. 96:731, 1980.

Monod, N., and Garma, L.: Auditory responsivity in the human premature, Biol. Neonate 17:292, 1971.

Parmelee, A.H., Jr.: Auditory function and neurological maturation in preterm infants. In Friedman, S., and Sigman, M., editors: Preterm birth and psychological development, New York, 1981, Academic Press, Inc.

Schulman, C.: Effects of auditory stimulation on heart rate in premature infants as a function of level of arousal, probability of CNS damage, and conceptional age, Dev. Psychobiol. 2:172, 1969.

Schulman-Galambos, C., and Galambos, R.: Brain stem auditory evoked response in premature infants, J. Speech Hear. Res. 18:456, 1975.

Starr, A., and others: Development of auditory function in newborn infants revealed by auditory brainstem potentials, Pediatrics 60:831, 1977.

Motor behavior
Fetal movement

Birnholz, J., Stephen, J., and Faria, M.: Fetal movement patterns: a possible means of defining neurologic developmental milestones in utero, Am. J. Roentgenol. 130:537, 1978.

Timor-Tritsch, I., and others: Classification of human fetal movement, Am. J. Obstet. Gynecol. 126:70, 1976.

The preterm infant

Amiel-Tison, C.: Neurological evaluation of the maturity of newborn infants, Arch. Dis. Child. 43:89, 1968.

Brandt, I.: Patterns of early neurological development. In Falkner, F., and Tanner, J., editors: Human growth, vol. 3, New York, 1979, Plenum Publishing Corp.

Dubowitz, L., Dubowitz, V., and Goldberg, C.: Clinical assessment of gestational age in the newborn infant, Pediatrics 77:1, 1970.

Gould, J., Gluck, L., and Kulovich, M.: The relationship between accelerated pulmonary maturity and accelerated neurological maturity in certain chronically stressed pregnancies, Am. J. Obstet. Gynecol. 127:181, 1977.

Howard, J., and others: A neurologic comparison of pre-term and full-term infants at term conceptional age, J. Pediatr. 88:995, 1976.

Kurtzberg, D., and others: Neurobehavioral performance of low birth-weight infants at 40 weeks conceptional age: comparison with normal full-term infants, Dev. Med. Child Neurol. 21:590, 1979.

Prechtl, H.F.R., and others: Postures, motility and respiration of low-risk pre-term infants, Dev. Med. Child Neurol. 21:3, 1979.

Saint-Anne Dargassies, S.: Neurological maturation of the preterm infant of 28 to 41 weeks' gestational age. In Falkner, F.: Human development, Philadelphia, 1966, W.B. Saunders Co.

Brazelton neonatal behavioral assessment scale

Als, H., Lester, B., and Brazelton, T.: Dynamics of the behavioral organization of the premature infant: a theoretical perspective. In Field, T., editor: Infants born at risk, New York, 1979, SP Medical & Scientific Books.

Als, H., and others: Manual for the assessment of preterm infant behavior (A.P.I.B.). In Fitzgerald, H. Lester, B., and Yogman, M., editors: Theory and research in behavioral pediatrics, New York, 1980, Plenum Publishing Corp.

Als, H., and others: Towards a research instrument for the assessment of preterm infants' behavior (A.P.I.B.). In Fitzgerald, H., Lester, B., and Yogman, M., editors: Theory and research in behavioral pediatrics, New York, 1980, Plenum Publishing Corp.

Brazelton, T.B.: Neonatal behavioral assessment scale, T.B. Brazelton Clinics in Developmental Medicine, no. 50, London, 1973, Spastics International Medical Publications.

CHAPTER 22 Central nervous system disturbances

As a result of increased knowledge in the fields of neonatal-perinatal medicine and neonatal neurology, the ability to accurately assess and treat disorders of the nervous system in infants has improved enormously over the past 20 years. Newer techniques such as computed tomography and ultrasonography have been developed or refined so that, following a thorough neonatal neurologic assessment, the physician can more accurately detect neurologic dysfunction, diagnose specific neurologic disorders, and identify neonates at increased risk for later neurologic dysfunction.

NEONATAL NEUROLOGIC ASSESSMENT

The stage of brain development in the newborn is dependent on gestational age. The birth process or extrauterine life does not appear to significantly influence the rate of growth of the developing brain. Thus determination of the level of neurologic function must be made in relation to gestational age and not only to chronologic age.

The nervous system is a heterogeneous organ with differing regional rates of growth and development. Differentiation and development of the brain are continuing at the time of birth. Myelination shows striking regional differences in rates of development and is still far from complete at 40 weeks' gestation. It is, however, much more advanced in the temporal lobes, midbrain, brain stem, spinal cord, and peripheral nerves than in the cerebral hemispheres. In the term neonate, dendritic sprouting and arborization are continuing, with the ongoing formation of interneuronal excitatory and inhibitory synaptic connections. The inhibitory synaptic connections are more numerous at this time than the excitatory ones.

The pluripotential cells originate in the germinal matrix of the developing brain, a very active cellular area located along the ventricular system, and migrate outward to populate the six layers of the cortex. The developing fetus has most of its neurons by 18 to 20 weeks' gestation. After this time reabsorption of this very vascular germinal area begins. This is usually completed by 35 to 36 weeks' gestation.

The brain capillaries are unique because of the presence of tight junctions, decreased numbers of pinocytotic vesicles, specific plasma membrane carriers, increased numbers of mitochondria, which can oxidize several different fuels, producing large amounts of ATP, and a tough basement membrane for protection of the capillaries during various types of stress. Although increasing information is being acquired about these unique characteristics, it is known that the basement membrane from isolated capillaries of developing animal brain is one fourth the thickness of that from capillaries of adult brain. The minimum capillary basement membrane may be one of the factors contributing to the occurrence of subependymal and intraventricular hemorrhage in the preterm infant.

The physiology of neuronal membranes in the newborn indicates that the neuronal pumps are less efficient and the cell membranes are more leaky than later in development. Cerebral metabolism of the newborn differs from that of the older child. The newborn is far more resistant to anoxia than the older infant and seems better able to use both ketone bodies and anaerobic glycolysis as energy sources.

Since subcortical structures of the nervous system are at a higher state of development both morphologically and neurophysiologically than cortical structures, information derived from the neonatal neurologic examination reflects primarily the functional status of subcortical structures. There is, however, increasing evidence of the neonate's cortical function as manifested by rudimentary learning ability and ability to integrate sensory stimuli (Chapter 21).

An optimum clinical neonatal neurologic assessment is outlined below.

A. History
  1. Parental history
  2. Obstetric history
     a. Past pregnancy outcome
     b. Present obstetric history
        (1) Prenatal
        (2) Intrapartum
     c. Neonatal history
B. General pediatric examination
  1. Gestational age
  2. Head size and shape
  3. Cranial sutures
  4. Fontanels
  5. Transillumination of skull
  6. Bruit
  7. Facies
  8. Minor anomalies
  9. Eye
  10. Hepatosplenomegaly
  11. Skin lesions
  12. Back
  13. Odor
  14. Contractures
C. Neurologic examination
  1. Level of consciousness
  2. Motor system
     a. Posture
     b. Tone
     c. Strength
     d. Movements
  3. Reflexes
  4. Sensory system
  5. Cranial nerve tests
     a. Fix and follow: II, III, IV, VI, Cortex
     b. Pupillary response: II, III
     c. Doll's eye: III, IV, VI, medial longitudinal fasciculus, VIII
     d. Suck: V, VII, XII
     e. Swallow: IX, X
  6. Interpretation
     a. Low risk
     b. High risk
     c. Suspect

The general mechanics of performing this assessment are explained in the following section.

History

A detailed account of the parental, obstetric, and neonatal histories is necessary for a systematic evaluation of the neonatal nervous system. The parental history should include the age and race of both parents, familial disease in both parents' families, and the mother's medical history.

A complete obstetric history should include information regarding the present pregnancy and details of all previous pregnancies and their outcome. The present obstetric history should include details of both the prenatal and intrapartum course, with complete information regarding any bleeding, infections during pregnancy, or maternal drug exposure.

Knowledge of the Apgar score at 1, 5, and 10 minutes, along with information about methods of resuscitation, is essential. Data of particular note following resuscitation are the times elapsed until return of heart rate, onset of respiration, and reappearance of normal tone.

The neonatal history should include detailed information of the nursery course. Particularly relevant clinical events include seizures, cyanotic spells, apneic episodes, diminished or absent crying, distinct and/or prolonged episodes of hypotonia, and/or decreased activity, poor suck, and prolonged requirement for gavage feedings. A list of biochemical and physiologic variables associated with suboptimum brain homeostasis is shown on p. 357. The length and severity of any of these findings during a neonate's course should be documented because they could be important in identifying an infant who may be at risk for subsequent abnormal development and/or who requires special follow-up.

General pediatric examination

The general pediatric examination is described on p. 254. There are particular findings in the general examination that are of special importance from the neurologic standpoint. The head should be examined for size, shape, status of anterior fontanel, and evidence of any trauma such as cephalhematoma or fractures. Cranial bruits should be listened for, especially in a newborn with congestive heart failure in the first 24 hours of life. Peculiar facies, associated with over 300 specific syndromes and/or other designated minor anomalies, should be identified, since the central nervous system frequently is involved with a generalized malformation. If three or more minor anomalies are identified, the chances of a major internal anomaly occurring is approximately 90% (Chapter 38). The examination of the eyes is described under the examination of cranial nerve II. Of particular importance from the neurologic standpoint is evidence of skin lesions, such as the vesicles of congenital herpes, petechiae, cutaneous lesions of other TORCH agents, hemangioma of Sturge-Weber disease, pigmented lesions of neurofibromatosis, the pale nevi of tuberous sclerosis, or the vesicles of incontinentia pigmenti (Chapter 34). Hepatosplenomegaly may occur in diseases that also involve the nervous system, such as encephalitis secondary to infection with one of the TORCH agents. Abnormalities of the back should be identified, including the finding of a small dermal sinus or tuft of hair, which may indicate either a direct channel to the subarachnoid space from the skin or a significant abnormality of the lumbosacral spinal column. Abnormalities in hair texture and swirls may be associated with underlying neurologic disorders. The particular smell of a neonate or his urine may lead to suspicion of an aminoaciduria. The location and extent of joint contractures present at birth are important to document. Fixed contractures of joints at birth, known specifically as arthrogryposis multiplex congenita, indicates a syndrome that is usually secondary to disease of the nervous system at some level but may in some patients be secondary to joint disease.

Neurologic examination

Since the functional state of the neonatal nervous system is influenced by both exogenous and endogenous factors unrelated to disease, these must be considered if an accurate neurologic assessment is to be obtained. An infant examined in the immediate postprandial state is usually sleepy with decreased responsiveness and may be hypotonic as well as hyporeflexic. That same infant examined just before a feed may be crying, irritable, hypertonic, hyperreflexic, and jittery. The optimum time to examine an infant in relation to feedings is approximately 1 to 2 hours afterward. A second major factor that can affect the functional state of the neonate's nervous system is the ambient temperature of the examining room and/or the temperature of the neonate. Hypothermia can cause depression, and hyperthermia can result in irritability, so the infant is best examined in thermal neutrality. The third factor that may alter reflexes and responsiveness is the infant's state of consciousness. The infant is best examined in the quiet alert state (p. 328). The fourth factor is the gestational age of the infant, which is best documented by maternal history and a combination of physical and neurologic criteria during the first days of life. It is important to grade the functional status of the neonate's nervous system in relation to the gestational age, not the chronologic age of the neonate. The fifth factor that can influence the findings of the neurologic examination is the degree of illness of the infant. In severely ill neonates there can be a generalized depression of the nervous system. In addition, there may be limitations on examining sick infants when they are in incubators, when they are being mechanically ventilated, and/or when they are connected to multiple monitors with several catheters in place. One must be willing to examine and reexamine a neonate to confirm the presence of significant abnormalities.

Level of consciousness

An altered state of consciousness is a major sign of neonatal neurologic impairment. The level of consciousness is determined by an evaluation of spontaneous activity and response to stimulation. Since this is affected by sleep state, it is best to test the infant in the quiet alert state for documentation of optimum function of the central nervous system (p. 328). The neonate's level of consciousness can be divided into five levels ranging from normal to abnormal. The neonate is said to be normal when in the quiet alert state he has his arms and legs flexed and exhibits symmetrical spontaneous activity that is nonstereotyped. The second level is the hyperalert state, identified in a neonate who does not sleep for extended periods of time during the first 24 hours. The eyes are wide open, possibly with a decreased blinking response as well as a decreased ability to fixate and follow. Although the activity level may be normal or decreased, it may appear increased because of the increased threshold to all types of tactile, auditory, visual, and proprioceptive stimuli. The third level is lethargy, which can be of variable degree. There is a decrease in spontaneous activity, although the threshold for responsiveness may be increased as just mentioned. Even though responses are delayed, there is a complete repertoire of responses to stimulation. The fourth level is stupor, when the infant's responses are limited to withdrawal of an extremity or decerebrate posturing in response only to strong noxious stimuli. Corneal and gag reflexes are absent, and respiratory rhythm may be abnormal. The fifth level is coma, with no response to external stimuli. In the neonate this is a relatively rare state, since the spinal withdrawal reflexes are almost never abolished. This state may be observed in infants on respirators who have had severe intraventricular hemorrhage.

Motor system

Posture. Observation of posture should be performed both before and after removing the neonates from the crib or incubator and undressing them (Fig. 22-1). Even if the neonate cannot be moved, such as when on a ventilator, much can be gained from observation of posture. When evaluating posture it is imperative to recognize the changes that occur with gestational age. With increasing age the infant's extremities normally begin to assume a much more flexed position.

Abnormalities of posture at rest include asymmetry between sides, as seen in the infant with a brachial plexus lesion; asymmetries between arms and legs, as seen with a spinal cord lesion; the frog-leg position with hips completely abducted and knees flexed, following severe asphyxia, with severe systemic disease, or with neuromuscular disease producing hypotonia or paralysis; head retraction and extensor posturing, which may occur with intracranial hemorrhage, hypoxic ischemic encephalopathy, or meningitis. The cortical thumb (a closed hand with the thumb inside the fingers) can be a normal position of the hand in the neonate (Fig. 22-2). This position

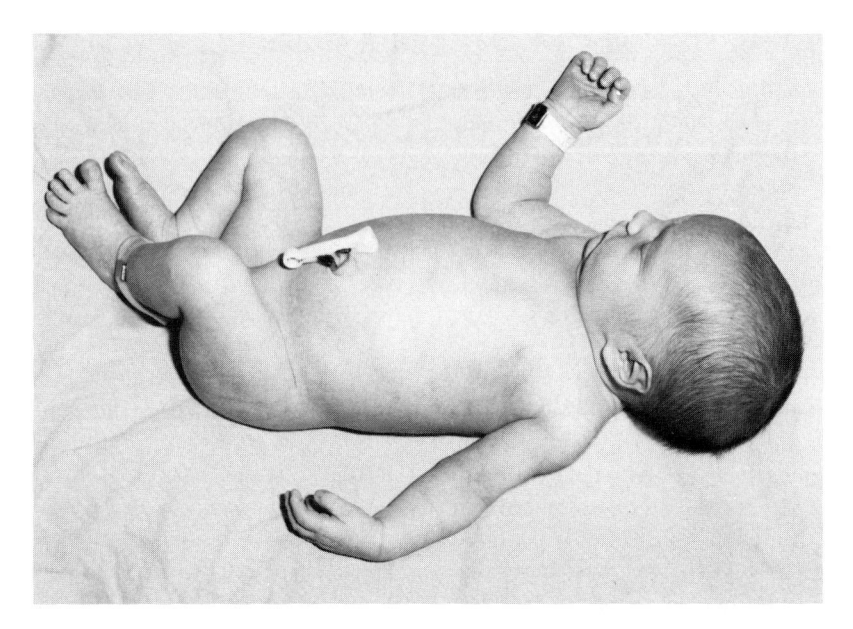

Fig. 22-1. Normal newborn at rest. Note that the posture of the arms and legs is asymmetrical. The arms are usually partially flexed; the legs are flexed at the knees and hips. Contrast this with the hypotonic infant, Fig. 22-18.

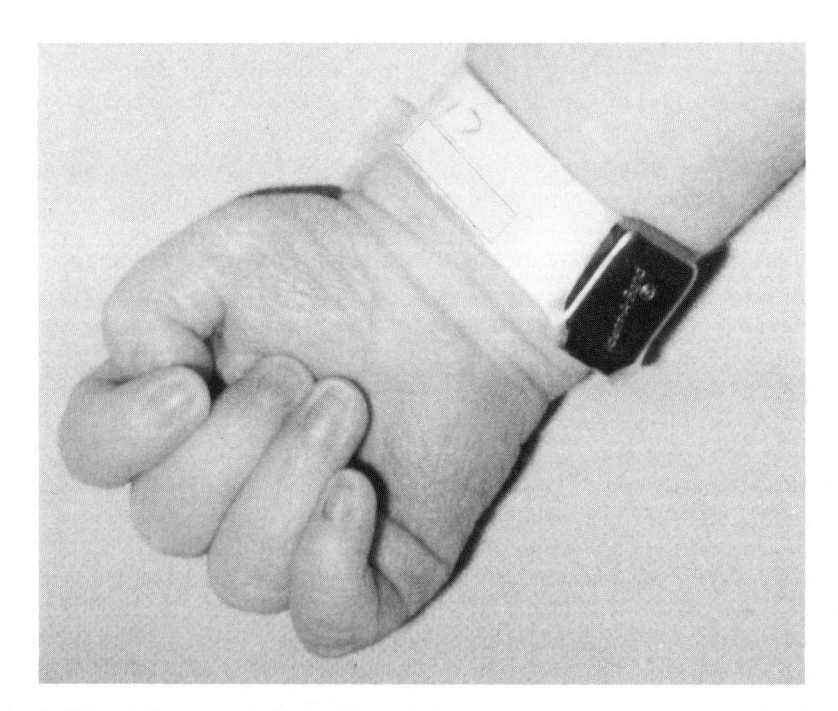

Fig. 22-2. The cortical thumb (fisting) in which the thumb is tightly enclosed within the clenched fingers. This is a common finding in the newborn but should not be persistently present. The infant should open his hand periodically (see Fig. 22-1 of the same infant). *Persistent* symmetrical or asymmetrical fisting is abnormal at any age and is often the earliest sign of cortical spinal tract damage.

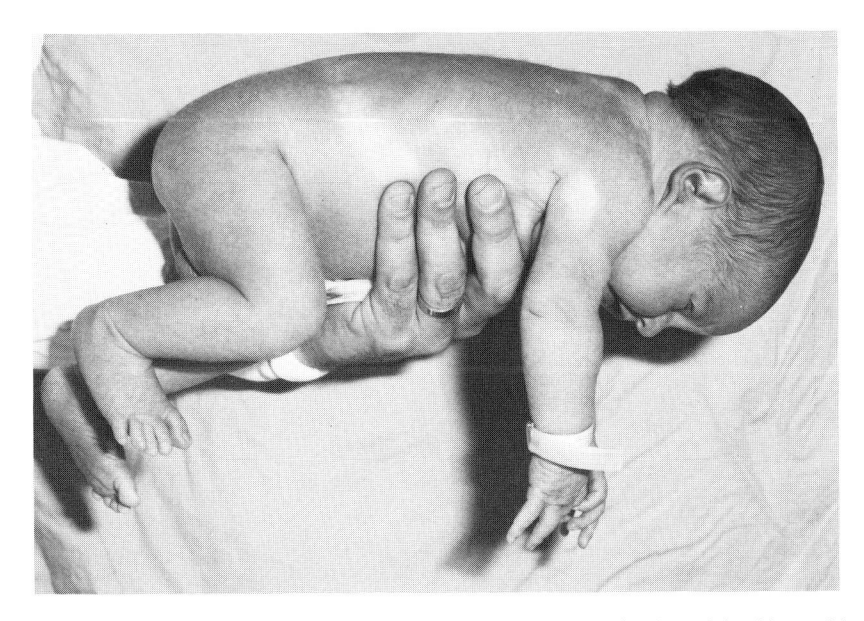

Fig. 22-3. Ventral suspension of the normal newborn. Note the flexion of the hip and knee, the slight dorsiflexion of the back, and the momentary ability to support the head. Contrast this with the hypotonic infant in Fig. 22-17.

is, however, not obligatory, and the neonate will periodically open the hand and extend the thumb. An obligatory cortical thumb is an early sign of abnormal cortical spinal tract function in the infant.

Tone. Muscle tone can be assessed by using the same maneuvers used in the gestational age assessment of the Dubowitz examination, including arm and leg recoil, popliteal angle, wrist-arm angle, foot dorsiflexion, hip flexion, shoulder adduction (scarf sign), head lag, and position in ventral suspension (p. 256). The examiner must consider the gestational age of the infant when attempting to determine whether the tone is reduced, normal, or increased. A neonate with poor head control may, for example, be considered normal if he is a preterm infant rather than a small for gestational age term infant.

An example of ventral suspension is seen in Fig. 22-3. The baby of 40 to 42 weeks should dorsiflex his back with some elevation of his head; his feet and legs remain flexed. Hypotonia, weakness, or cerebral depression may produce a baby who looks like a limp dishrag. Upright suspension with the baby supported by the examiner's hands under his arm (Fig. 22-4) provides good estimation of both tone and strength in the shoulder girdle, since an infant with decreased tone or strength can slip through the examiner's hands. Tone can also be assessed by movement of individual joints.

Strength. Strength and weakness are related to the state of alertness, to gestational age, and/or to problems in the central or peripheral nervous system as well as in the muscles. Testing muscle strength is difficult in a new-

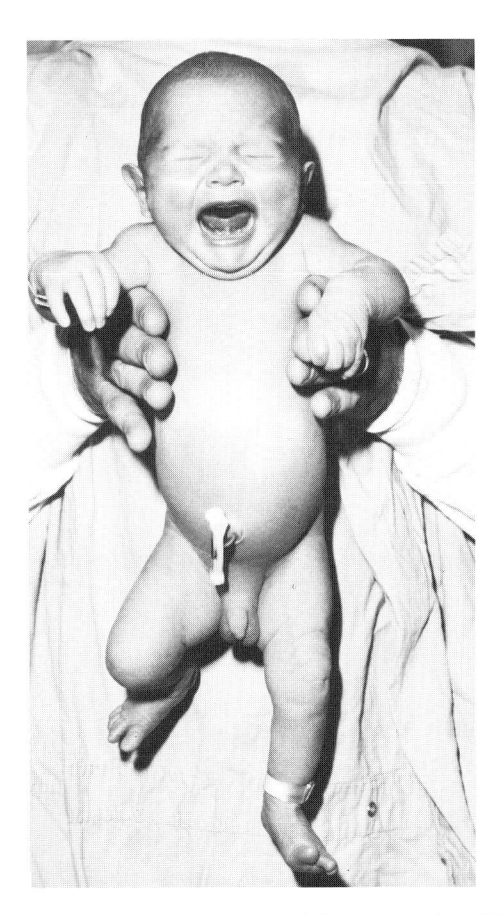

Fig. 22-4. Normal newborn in upright suspension. Most of the baby's weight is supported by the resistance of the infant's arms. There is no tendency to slide through the examiner's fingers. The examiner is not holding the child around the chest.

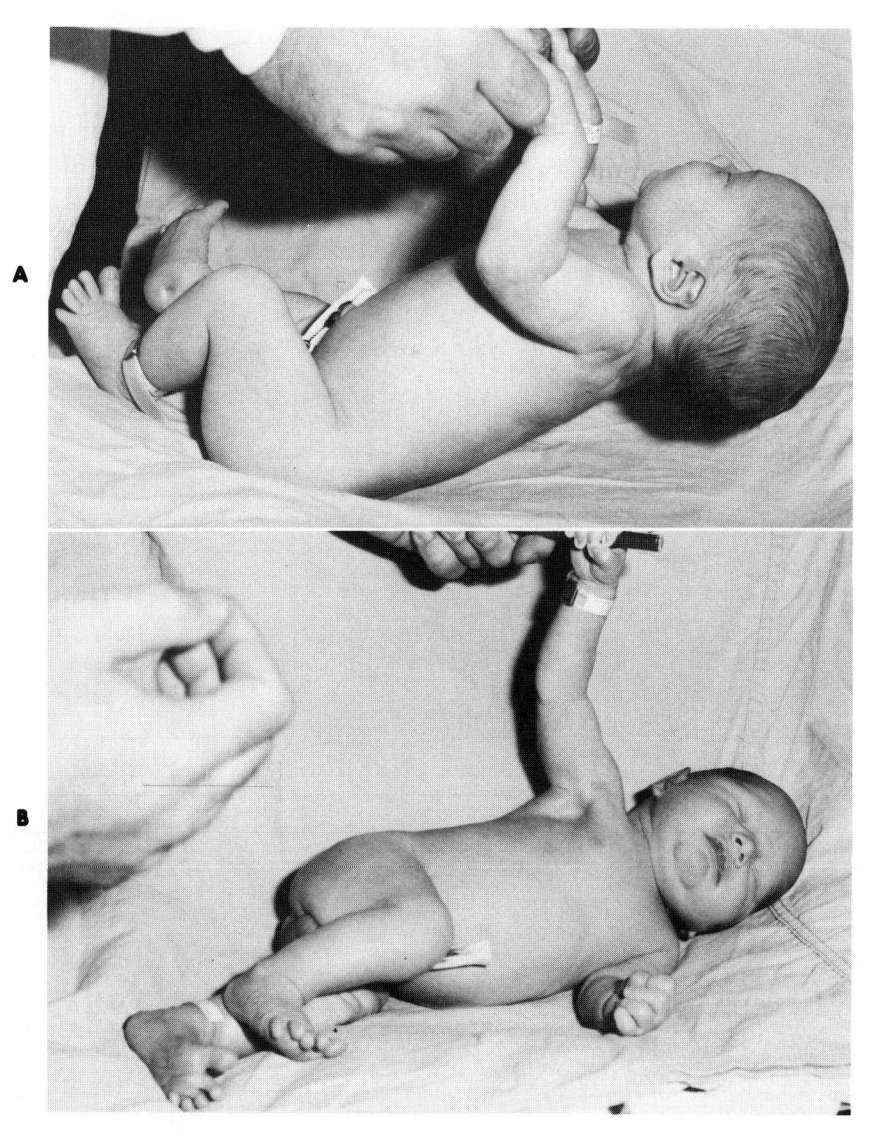

Fig. 22-5. A, Strength may be assessed by lifting the supine infant from the table. The observer's fingers are grasped by the infant; the strength of the grasp, contraction of the biceps, the shoulder girdle, and even the anterior neck muscles are seen and felt. Note this normal newborn's lack of head lag. **B,** An alternative method of testing strength in either arm is shown in this illustration. The infant is grasping a pencil. Note the tight grip and contraction of biceps as well as of the trapezius and pectorals. The infant can almost be lifted from the sheet.

born infant, and differentiating between muscle weakness and hypotonia may be impossible, since neonates who are weak are usually hypotonic or floppy. However, an adequate screening test of strength in the upper extremities and neck is through the use of the neonate's grasp. The examiner's finger is inserted into the lateral aspect of the neonate's palm, eliciting a reflex palmar grasp. With strong stimulation the strength in the hand in association with this grasp in the normal newborn should be sufficiently strong to partially support the infant's weight as he is lifted from the supine to sitting position. As the neonate is pulled up, the observer should feel contractions in the biceps and the shoulder girdle and some contraction in the sternomastoids, preventing the head from completely falling back (Fig. 22-5). Strength in the lower extremities can be assessed by observing the supporting response, the ability of the newborn to support his weight when his feet are placed on the examining table. Stepping, placing, and the crossed extensor reflexes also may be used to assess strength; asymmetries of strength should be noted.

Observations of the quality of spontaneous movements

and movements that can be elicited in response to pinprick stimulation can give considerable information about strength of specific muscle groups. This information is important in localizing the level of a lesion of the spinal cord (p. 373).

Movements. Observation of an infant prior to being touched may reveal a variety of movements. The quantity of spontaneous movement can vary from normal to excessive to decreased. The pattern of movement observed in a normal infant during spontaneous activity can be characterized as random, symmetrical, nonstereotyped movements involving all extremities.

In addition to patterned movements, the neonate may have movements that are characterized as being either tremors or jitteriness or seizures. Since neonatal seizures are usually caused by treatable conditions that if left untreated will cause brain damage, it is important to identify and differentiate an infant with this type of activity from an infant who may simply have tremor or jitteriness. Seizures can take various forms, and it should be noted that almost any bizarre alterations of the state of the neonate may represent a seizure (p. 388). The usual difficulty is in distinguishing seizure activity manifested by generalized symmetrical tonic-clonic movements from the classic tremulous movements or jitteriness. A few distinguishing clinical features can be helpful. Generalized symmetrical tonic-clonic movements are a relatively uncommon manifestation of neonatal seizures. The rhythmic movements of jitteriness or tremors that do not reflect any seizure activity are characteristically of equal amplitude and do not have a fast and slow component, as do the tonic-clonic movements of seizures. In a susceptible neonate, jitteriness or tremors are characteristically stimulus sensitive, being easily provoked by external stimuli such as a Moro reflex, noise, or simple handling, whereas seizures are not. The movements of tremors or jitteriness can usually be stopped by the examiner passively fixing the affected limb.

The specific causes of seizures are discussed in the section on seizures. Frequently, abnormalities that cause seizures may also produce jitteriness or tremors. Tremors of high frequency and low amplitude may occur with hypoglycemia or hypocalcemia or in an otherwise normal infant and disappear within the first week of life. Low-frequency, high-amplitude tremors are often seen in infants who have excessive activity and/or a low threshold Moro but who are otherwise normal. Coarse tremors occur as a sign of drug withdrawal in infants of addicted mothers (Chapter 33, part five).

Reflexes. The reflexes found to be the most useful in an initial neurologic assessment include the Moro reflex, the tonic neck reflex, the placing and stepping response, sucking, the classic deep tendon reflexes, and palmar or plantar grasp. A multitude of other neonatal reflexes have been described that, although interesting, have limited value in the clinical evaluation of the nervous system. Reflexes are primarily useful when there is a consistent asymmetry identified in association with abnormal findings gained from evaluation of tone, strength, posture, and movement. A reflex also can be useful in indicating CNS dysfunction if it is either obligatory or does not habituate. When either of these two conditions occurs, a sign of CNS dysfunction has been identified. Finally, the absence of these commonly used neonatal reflexes is indicative of abnormal neurologic function.

Sensory system

The primary sensation tested is the neonate's response to superficial pain. To optimally evaluate this sensory modality, the examiner must have the infant in a relatively quiet and preferably alert state. Testing of sensation is most important when one suspects a spinal cord, nerve root, plexus, or peripheral nerve lesion or wants to delineate the sensory level in an infant with a meningomyelocele. Fig. 22-6 is the classic adult dermatome pattern extrapolated to infants and indicates the association of specific motor responses to stimuli. The nerve conduction time in both peripheral nerves and spinal cord is greatly delayed in the newborn; with a pin, there may be a delay of as long as 2 or 3 seconds before the infant responds, if he perceives the stimulus. Perception of sensory stimuli by the infant can be manifested by crying, grimacing, alteration in respiratory pattern, change in level of consciousness, or possibly change in color. Withdrawal of the extremity is a local reflex phenomenon and does not alone necessarily imply that the sensory stimulus has reached cortical awareness. The truncal incurvation reflex (GALANT) has little value as generally applied; however, it is segmentally innervated, and local stimulation of one area of the trunk may produce local trunk incurvation, indicating that the segmental arc is intact. Therefore this reflex may be helpful in localizing a spinal cord injury.

Cranial nerves

All the cranial nerves of a neonate can be examined easily by modifying the common neurologic examination and/or by making deductions from neonatal responses involving cranial nerves.

Cranial nerve I. The olfactory nerve can be examined in the neonate but requires special procedures. This examination is not done during the screening examination, since its dysfunction is only rarely associated with neurologic disease in the neonate.

Cranial nerve II. Vision can be readily tested in the neonate (p. 337), and its presence indicates that the entire visual system is intact, including the presence of a

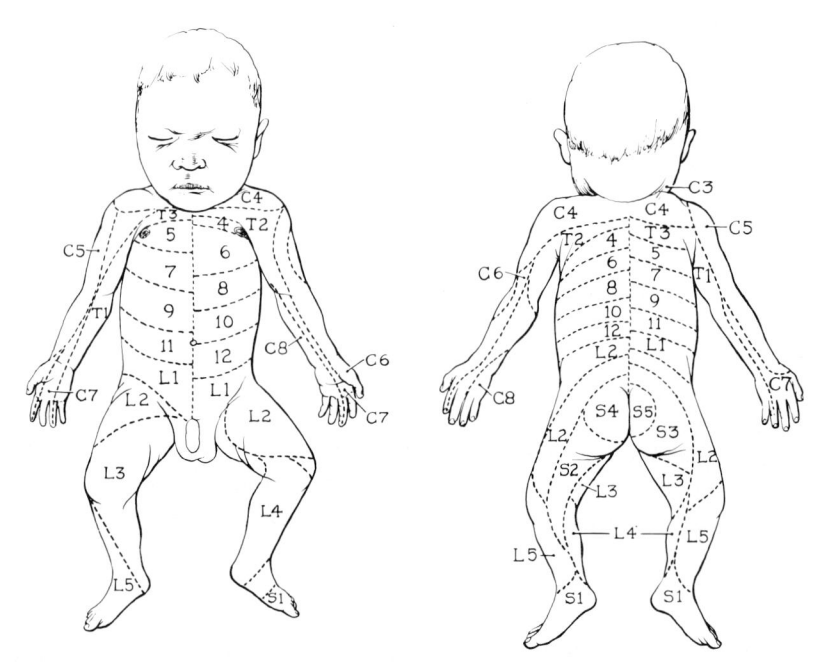

Fig. 22-6. Sensory dermatomes extrapolated from the adult to the infant. As noted on the two sides of the infant, there is considerable overlap of sensory innervation.

functional occipital cortex. Blinking in response to a light stimulus indicates only that the visual system is intact to the level of the superior colliculi and is not evidence of visual cortical function. Presence of vision is tested by observing the neonate fix and follow an object such as the human face or a red ball through an arc of approximately 60 degrees. Since the neonate is myopic, the test object should be placed within 10 to 12 inches of the infant's face. This should be included in the neurologic screening assessment of all neonates. One may elect to refine the examination of vision to determine visual acuity by producing optokinetic nystagmus (Chapter 35) by movement of a large drum with different width black and white stripes in front of the neonate's eyes. This should usually produce some following movements of the eyes and occasionally nystagmus back in the opposite direction. With gradations of distance and width of the stripes on the drum, visual acuity can be estimated. The remaining part of the evaluation of cranial nerve II involves a thorough evaluation of the external characteristics of the eye and a funduscopic examination. The external eye findings that may be associated with diseases of the nervous system include cataracts, cloudy cornea, irregular shape or asymmetrical size of the pupil, vascular hemangioma of the sclera, and microphthalmos. Funduscopic examination is difficult but is extremely rewarding, since this is the only chance for the examiner to see actual nerve cells. The ophthalmoscope should be set at −2 to −4 diopters for the best visualization of the optic fundus. Optic disc pallor may be a normal feature, so-called pseu-

dooptic atrophy of the newborn. Retinal hemorrhages, reported to occur in 8% to 50% of neonates, are not always associated with significant neurologic abnormalities; however, subhyaloid hemorrhages are usually associated with subdural hematomas in the infant. Retinal lesions of chorioretinitis secondary to toxoplasmosis, cytomegalovirus, rubella, or syphilis are only rarely seen in the neonatal period.

Cranial nerves III, IV, and VI. The third cranial nerve must be intact for normal pupil function. The pupils should be equal and respond to light even at 28 to 30 weeks of gestation. The optimum functioning of cranial nerves III, IV, and VI connected via the medial longitudinal fasciculus can be assessed by watching the conjugate eye movements while an infant is fixating and following. In addition, conjugate eye movements can be evaluated during the observation of normal doll's eye movement, assessed by holding the infant at arm's length in an upright posture and rotating him. This rotation stimulates the semicircular canals, and the impulses travel through the vestibular portion of cranial nerve VIII to the brain stem via the medial longitudinal fasciculus and innervate cranial nerves III and VI. This stimulation causes the eye to tonically deviate away from the direction of the rotation. Rotation should be performed in both directions. When it is impossible to rotate the neonate as mentioned, the semicircular canals may be stimulated by injecting cold water into the ear canal. In this maneuver the eyes deviate to the side of cold water injection. When the eyes remain in a fixed position regardless of stimulation or head movement, serious brain stem dysfunction is usually present. A loss of doll's eye movement can be seen when an excessive amount of barbiturates has been administered. A repetitive failure of the eye to move in a single direction should be noted and considered abnormal. Dysconjugate eye movements with some nystagmoid movements may not be uncommon during these maneuvers when they are performed during the first 3 weeks of life. However, when there is a repetitive failure of movement of the eyes in a single direction, persistent dysconjugate eye movements, or continuous nystagmus at rest, significant neurologic dysfunction is present.

Cranial nerves V, VII, IX, X, XI, and XII. The sensory portion of the fifth cranial nerve can be tested by eliciting the corneal reflex or using a pinprick on the face and watching for grimacing movements. In some observer's experience the corneal reflex is not a reliable test of sensation in the newborn. The motor function of cranial nerve V is judged to be intact if the infant can close the mouth through effective masseter strength. The other cranial nerves that must be intact for an effective suck to occur are cranial nerve VII for pursing of the lips and cranial nerve XII for the milking action of the tongue. The observation of effective swallowing indicates adequate function of cranial nerves IX and X. The function of cranial nerve XI can be estimated by visualization of the sternocleidomastoid muscle when the infant is held in the supine position. There should be an ability to maintain the head in an extended position for brief periods of time. Presence of any mass in the sternocleidomastoid muscle, such as a hematoma, can be observed at this time.

Cranial nerve VIII. Examination of the vestibular portion of cranial nerve VIII has been mentioned under the sections on cranial nerves III, IV, and VI. Examination of the auditory portion of this nerve can be tested in the newborn only in a gross fashion. Auditory evoked potential using electroencephalography can now be used for more accurate testing. At the bedside, evidence of the infant's hearing can be assessed by using a graded noise stimulus. This can be either in the form of an electrical noisemaker giving a graded noise or simply a small hand bell. In confirming whether the infant hears the noise, observations either of the infant being alerted from sleep or being quieted if awake can be taken as evidence that the neonate hears. Repeated examinations may be necessary, since there may be a lack of response or a variable response of the neonate to the noise stimulus.

Hearing screening. The importance of screening for hearing loss in early infancy is gaining wide recognition, particularly as the incidence of congenital hearing loss becomes more apparent. Screening procedures implemented within the hospital nursery involve detecting either a behavioral or electrophysiologic response of the infant to a sound stimulus. Mass experimental auditory screening of neonates has revealed an expected incidence of approximately 1 in 50 deaf infants in the intensive care nursery. The first of these methods to gain wide acceptance, as well as support by the Joint Committee on Infant Hearing Screening, is a five-item high-risk register. This well-researched and established register identifies infants at risk for hearing loss by means of history and physical examination. However, actual audiologic testing takes place only on a follow-up basis after hospital discharge. Application of a protocol using an arousal response criterion during the infant's light sleep state has also been recommended by the Joint Committee on Infant Hearing Screening, as a supplement to the five-item high-risk register. However, a recently developed automated screening system, known as the Crib-O-Gram, is rapidly becoming the behavioral test method of choice. It uses a motion-sensing transducer placed beneath the infant's mattress, which detects changes in neonatal motor activity coincident with the introduction of a calibrated sound stimulus. These changes are entirely integrated, analyzed, and scored by computer algorithms, thus permitting greater objectivity, ease of presentation, and usage than any other method currently available. The Brainstem Evoked Response (BSER) technique is the only one of several electrophysiologic test methods (i.e., electrocochleography, respiratory responses, cardiovascular responses) found adequate for screening purposes. Clinical application of BSER measurement has been demonstrated in premature infants, wherein consistent responses may be obtained without sedation in quiet infants. Additionally, limited muscle activity, vigilance, and sleep state have shown negligible effects on the response. Many of the abnormalities detected by screening BSER are transient. The screening method of choice should ultimately be dictated by the individual facility, available personnel, and number of infants to be served. However, any protocol is effective only when implemented as part of an overall program that also incorporates a longitudinal follow-up approach.

Interpretation of the neurologic assessment

The neurologic assessment is particularly valuable when used to detect treatable diseases, to diagnose specific neurologic disorders, and to assess gestational age. The use of the neurologic assessment for the prognostic identification of neonates at risk for later abnormal development must be interpreted with caution. Except in situations where multiple unequivocal signs indicate severe damage, considerable discretion should be used in making prognostic statements. The capacity of the developing nervous system for reorganization of connections following certain kinds of injury may account for some of our inability to accurately prognosticate from abnormal neurologic signs found in the neonatal period.

Even though definitive interpretation of neonatal signs of neurologic dysfunction should be made with caution, some positive statements can be made.

1. The full-term neonate with a negative family history, a negative prenatal, intrapartum, and neonatal history, and a normal neurologic and pediatric examination has a negligible chance of subsequent abnormal neurologic development related to perinatal causes.
2. Certain neurologic signs, even though infrequent in their occurrence, have considerable predictive power for later abnormal neurologic function and include persistent abnormalities in tone, especially hypotonia, diminished level of activity, weak cry for more than 24 hours, and an inability to suck, requiring gavage feedings. Each of these signs carries a tenfold to twentyfold increased risk of the subsequent development of cerebral palsy. A neonate with an Apgar score of 3 or less at 10 minutes and/or neonatal seizures, especially if associated with intrapartum asphyxia and/or trauma, has a greater than fiftyfold increased risk for subsequent development of cerebral palsy.
3. Combinations of abnormalities are more significant than a single abnormality.
4. A neonate with signs of neurologic dysfunction at time of discharge has a fiftyfold increased risk of having subsequent abnormal neurologic development.
5. More signs of neurologic dysfunction occur in a neonate who has acute damage to a previously normal nervous system than a neonate with long-standing absence of a part of the nervous system.
6. The total duration of the presence of an abnormal neurologic sign does not necessarily add to or detract from its significance. Clear-cut signs of neurologic dysfunction may be present only a few days and then disappear, with the child later developing signs of frank neurologic dysfunction as development progresses.
7. Asymmetrical findings are usually more significant than symmetrical findings, not so much in helping to localize the area of brain involved but simply in indicating that an underlying abnormality exists.
8. Signs of neurologic dysfunction occurring in the presence of identifiable neuropathologic lesions are more predictive of subsequent neurologic abnormality than signs with no association to a demonstrable brain lesion.

There is a need for further development of more sophisticated, noninvasive techniques for identifying pathologic changes in the neonatal brain, thus facilitating more accurate neonatal cliniconeuropathologic correlation and enhanced predictability of long-term sequelae from the findings of the neonatal neurologic examination.

At discharge an updated complete neurologic assessment should be done, including any specific laboratory or roentgenologic data relative to the nervous system. At that time the neonate should be placed in one of three categories (low risk, high risk, or suspect) regarding risk for subsequent delayed or abnormal development. This designation is for the purpose of planning for the child's optimum health supervision, specifically for detection of developmental delays. As stimulation programs are evaluated and deemed useful, the entry of a child into one of these programs is best done when the child first shows delay.

In using the findings from the neonatal neurologic examination in counseling parents regarding the risks of subsequent abnormal neurologic development, caution must be used. The physician must be honest with the parents but should not destroy all hope, since the ultimate functional state of the child cannot be predicted accurately from the neonatal discharge examination, and most children with significant neurologic dysfunction are cared for at home during the first 7 years of life. Overt neurologic dysfunction will appear during the child's development if the brain has sustained significant damage. Through optimum child health supervision this child can be helped to maximize his or her assets and minimize the deficits.

NONINVASIVE DIAGNOSTIC TOOLS
Transillumination
See p. 378.

Ultrasonography

The use of ultrasound scans has been a major advance in the definition of normal intracranial anatomy and identification of intracranial pathology. The principles of ultrasonography are discussed in Chapter 8 together with its use in the early evaluation of anatomic structures within the brain. In the postnatal period, ultrasound has been used most extensively to identify various degrees of subependymal/intraventricular hemorrhage (p. 367) and provides excellent data on the degree and distribution of ventricular dilatation (p. 375). In addition to the fact that the instrument is portable, the major advantages of ultrasonography include the apparent safety of the pulsed ultrasonic waves and the relatively low cost. A real-time sector scanner applied over the skin of the anterior fontanel can provide excellent coronal and sagittal views of the brain in experienced hands that may be at least as reliable as computed axial tomography (CAT scanning) in the identification of small as well as large subependymal, intraventricular, and intracerebral hemorrhages. CAT scans may be preferable for subarachnoid bleeds.

Computed axial tomography (CAT scanning)

CAT scanning affords an excellent means of identifying the site and extent of neonatal intraventricular hemorrhage. In addition, the size of ventricles and the presence of major parenchymal lesions may also be defined. However, despite the undeniable value of the procedure, it does require moving an infant who is often in a precarious state with regard to maintenance of ventilation, perfusion, temperature, and metabolic status. Moreover, the long-term effects of the radiation exposure from multiple studies remain unknown. Thus, when portable ultrasound is available, the need for a CAT scan is diminished considerably.

Intracranial pressure monitoring

A variety of catheters and pressure transducers have been developed for measuring neonatal intracranial pressure (ICP). These techniques are useful for monitoring an infant's ICP under special circumstances, such as hydrocephalus, brain tumors, and trauma. However, their invasive nature precludes their use in other clinical circumstances where they are needed and may be of similar clinical value.

In neonates the open anterior fontanel provides a unique site for noninvasive ICP assessment. Measurements of anterior fontanel pressure (AFP) can be obtained by applying directly on the fontanel a small, flat surface-pressure transducer; this can alternatively be accomplished by using a fluid-filled system connected to a pressure transducer or using a transducer containing a photoelectric detector and an activated bellows (p. 280).

AFP measurements have been compared to the manometric pressure of CSF obtained at the time of lumbar and ventricular punctures in humans and to ventricular pressure in experimental animals. These comparisons have demonstrated positive correlation between ventricular or CSF pressures and AFP. AFP measurement has advantages over the invasive techniques, since penetration of the dural barrier is not required, thus preventing infection and inadvertant CSF loss. The precise diagnostic role of AFP measurements in preterm infants at risk for intracranial hemorrhage or raised intracranial pressure remains to be determined.

Doppler measurement of cerebral blood flow (CBF) velocity

The study of CBF velocity by external Doppler technique may offer a new noninvasive tool to gain information related to changes in cerebral hemodynamics. This has been assessed from changes in pulsatile flow in the anterior cerebral arteries using an ultrasonic transducer placed on the anterior fontanel. The Doppler technique measures the shift in frequency of an incoming ultrasound beam created in large part by the movement of red blood cells under the instrument. The resultant changes in pulsatile flow calculated from Doppler frequency shifts have been expressed primarily as pulsatility index measurements. Preliminary data with this technique have demonstrated altered cerebral blood flow patterns during asphyxia, at the time of pneumothorax, and in association with left-to-right shunting through a patent ductus arteriosus. The relationship between intraventricular hemorrhage and altered patterns of cerebral hemodynamics in preterm infants requires further study, which may be aided by this technique.

BIRTH INJURY

Over a century ago a causal link was proposed between suboptimum perinatal events in both preterm and fullterm infants and subsequent neurologic dysfunction and brain damage. Since Little's original observations in the 1860s, numerous theories as to the etiology and pathogenesis of birth injury have been advanced.

Prior to the 1940s "birth trauma" was felt to be the overriding etiologic and pathogenetic mechanism leading to perinatal brain damage. The unreasonably important etiologic and pathogenetic role given to the mechanical forces of compression/distortion in producing fetal and neonatal brain damage during labor and delivery was probably secondary to a substantial degree of real trauma. With improving obstetric care, especially in the management of labor and delivery during the past 40 years, the mechanical forces producing birth trauma have been almost totally eliminated. In the 1940s a strong link was established between perinatal asphyxia and brain injury. This section on birth injury is divided into birth asphyxia and birth trauma in an effort to document the current state of knowledge in these two different areas.

Birth asphyxia

Although there were suggestions in classic retrospective clinical and neuropathologic studies that asphyxia was one of the etiologic factors in producing brain damage, most of our information concerning the specific effect of intrauterine asphyxia on the fetus has evolved since the development of fetal monitoring techniques. Recent human and animal studies have permitted a clearer distinction to be made between the effects of asphyxia and trauma on the fetal nervous system. It should, however, be recognized that there can be an additive effect of the usual intrapartum compression/distortion in conjunction with intrapartum asphyxia resulting in enhanced physical and physiologic compromise leading to neonatal brain insult. Following is an outline of the numerous prenatal and intrapartum conditions and the postnatal contributions to brain dysfunction and damage seen in full- and preterm infants.

A. Conditions associated with increased risk for fetal asphyxia
 1. Altered placental exchange

a. Abruption
   b. Placenta previa
   c. Postmaturity
   d. Prolapsed cord
   e. Cord around neck
   f. Intrauterine fetal growth retardation
   g. Signs of fetal distress
   h. "Placental insufficiency"
 2. Altered maternal blood flow to placenta
   a. Maternal hypotension
   b. Maternal hypertension
   c. Abnormal uterine contractions
 3. Reduced maternal arterial oxygen saturation
   a. Maternal hypoventilation
   b. Maternal hypoxia
   c. Maternal cardiopulmonary disease
B. Disorders associated with CNS dysfunction and damage
 1. Asphyxia with:
   a. Shock with redistribution of organ flow
   b. Impaired regulation of cerebral blood flow
 2. Intracranial hemorrhage
 3. Shock
 4. Hypothermia
 5. Hypoglycemia
 6. Hyperbilirubinemia
 7. Electrolyte imbalance
   a. Hyponatremia
   b. Hypernatremia
   c. Hypocalcemia
   d. Hypomagnesmia
 8. Infection
 9. Malnutrition

Three distinct sites of involvement were identified in brains of neonates who had experienced intrapartum asphyxia and were studied neuropathologically. They were the cortical and subcortical gray matter, the region of the subependymal germinal matrix, and the periventricular white matter. As babies were classified by gestational age it became apparent that there was a difference in the locus of lesions seen in preterm and full-term neonates. The pattern of damage in the full-term infant was principally located in the peripheral and dorsal areas of the cerebral cortex with the lesions involving the gyri at the depths of sulci and the neuronal nuclei of the basal ganglia. This has been identified as *hypoxic ischemic encephalopathy* (HIE) (see further). The pattern of damage in the preterm infant was principally located at the center of the hemisphere in the germinal matrix along the periventricular region with relative sparing of the cortical mantle. These lesions in the preterm infant were principally hemorrhagic and termed *subependymal germinal matrix hemorrhage/intraventricular hemorrhage* (SEH/IVH) (see further). The lesion in the white matter in the area of the periventricular region was first described by Banker and identified as *periventricular leukomalacia* (PVL) (see further). This last lesion can be seen in both preterm and full-term infants. This delineation of differences of loci of lesions and their variation by gestational age has greatly contributed to our understanding of the clinical signs of neonatal neurologic dysfunction. In addition, new theories regarding the pathogenesis of hypoxic perinatal brain damage have evolved.

Hypoxic ischemic encephalopathy (HIE)

This is a type of neonatal neurologic dysfunction seen in the full-term neonate after an episode of intrapartum asphyxia. Although the magnitude of this problem is not fully appreciated, three important observations that can help in understanding the magnitude of this problem have recently been documented. First, more full-term infants who have been asphyxiated survive than do comparable preterm infants. Second, more patients with cerebral palsy were full-term than preterm infants, even though the incidence of cerebral palsy is higher in preterm infants. The reason for this discrepancy is that even though the incidence of cerebral palsy is lower in the full-term infant, the denominator to which this low incidence applies is 92% of births in the United States.

Furthermore, the problem of HIE in the full-term neonate is accentuated by the fact that there does not appear to have been a significant reduction in the types of cerebral palsy seen in children who have been full-term neonates. A comprehensive Swedish study showed that, although there has been a decrease in the total incidence of cerebral palsy from 1954 to 1974, this has been the result of a reduction of spastic diplegia in neonates weighing less than 2,500 gm. In the United States there has been a similar reduction in the incidence of CNS sequelae in infants weighing less than 2,500 gm. No comparative data exist regarding CNS sequelae in infants who were full term.

Clinical manifestations

The full-term infant was previously thought to have a clinical course after a period of intrapartum asphyxia that primarily reflected brain insult. However, it is now known that this infant can have an unpredictable clinical course because of the variable involvement of different organ systems. The reason for the unpredictable and varied clinical course in full-term infants is not completely understood but probably relates to factors such as the ability of the fetus to redistribute blood flow in protecting vital organs, the current inability to establish accurately the length, severity, and acuteness of onset of the asphyxial episode, and as yet unidentified components of the asphyxial insult.

To appropriately manage a full-term neonate who has experienced a period of intrapartum asphyxia, identification of such a neonate must be as early as possible, preferably during the intrapartum period so as to reduce the exposure of the fetus to the noxious asphyxial environment by appropriate and timely delivery. However, since not all fetuses can be identified during the intrauterine asphyxial episode, they must be appropriately evaluated from birth in a sequential fashion.

The varied clinical course of neonatal asphyxia was documented in a retrospective study involving 6,045 consecutive deliveries. Fifty-three full-term infants from this group had Apgar scores of 5 or less at 1 and 3 minutes, which were thought to be secondary to intrapartum asphyxia. Eighteen of the 53 infants had no clinically apparent disease throughout their hospitalization. However, 35 of the 53 infants had at least one or as many as five organ systems affected (19 of the 35 infants had more than one system involved). The organ systems involved in the 35 affected infants with low Apgar scores in order of decreasing frequency were the pulmonary system, the cardiovascular system, the central nervous system, the gastrointestinal system, and the renal system. No infants demonstrated problems with the coagulation system, although this has been described in some infants from other studies. Nine of these 35 died during the neonatal period. The common cause of death was persistent fetal circulation, which occurred in four infants. No one system or group of systems appeared to be a primary target of the intrapartum asphyxial episode. Only one third of the infants had clinical signs that suggested central nervous system involvement. Of the nine infants who died, only two died from central nervous system disturbances (massive brain swelling with cortical necrosis). The nervous system, or any other organ system, could not be clinically predicted as being the affected organ from either the intrapartum course or the status of the neonate in the delivery room.

The functional state of the altered nervous system in an asphyxiated infant during the first 2 weeks of life is characteristic enough to be labeled as a separate entity, neonatal hypoxic ischemic encephalopathy. It is important to recognize that most asphyxiated neonates will have a history of an intrapartum asphyxial episode, an abnormal delivery, a low Apgar score and requirement for resuscitation, or the appearance of signs of neurologic dysfunction within the first few hours after birth. It is important, however, to recognize that not all neonates who develop HIE have low Apgar scores. The major neonatal signs of CNS dysfunction in the first few hours of life include seizures along with abnormalities in state of consciousness, tone, posture, reflexes, respiratory pattern, oculovestibular response, autonomic function, and fullness of the anterior fontanel.

Seizures have been reported in from 8% to 22% of infants with low Apgar scores and in up to 68% of infants presenting with abnormal neurologic examinations following an intrauterine asphyxial episode. Classically, the onset of seizures occurs in the 12 to 24 hours after delivery.

If signs of seizures other than tonic-clonic movements are used, the onset of seizures may be as early as 2 to 6 hours. Seizures are not invariably associated with late neurologic sequelae; however, their occurrence within the first 24 hours, the appearance of status or serial seizures, and a persistently abnormal electroencephalogram are signs of significant existing neurologic dysfunction as well as an increased likelihood of late sequelae.

Abnormalities in the level of consciousness have shown promise in delineating the severity of an asphyxial insult and in predicting which infants may have neurologic sequelae if they survive. In a recent study, full-term infants who were thought to have HIE were categorized into three clinical groups. Their distinguishing features were derived from seven categories: level of consciousness, neuromuscular control, complex reflexes, autonomic function, seizures, EEG findings, and duration of abnormality. Although the last six categories were important in delineating the stages of encephalopathy, the level of consciousness seemed to be the primary determinant. The levels of consciousness were defined as follows: stage 1—hyperalertness; stage 2—lethargy or obtundation; and stage 3—stupor. The other clearly delineated feature that had relevance regarding the severity of HIE and prediction of long-term outcome was the length of time the infant stayed in a given stage. It was concluded that infants who did not enter stage 3 and had signs of stage 2 for less than 5 days appeared to be normal later in infancy. It was also demonstrated that infants who entered stage 3 or who had signs of stage 2 for more than 7 days or whose EEG failed to revert to normal either expired or developed significant neurologic sequelae. These results have been confirmed using this same scoring system in the absence of EEG criteria. Studies such as this demonstrate the need for carefully defining signs of neurologic dysfunction, quantitating their severity, and defining the time course over which these signs are present.

When the full-term asphyxiated neonate is principally manifesting signs of neurologic dysfunction following an intrapartum asphyxial episode, three recurring rather typical outcomes can be identified based on the infant's clinical course.

The first type of clinical course in an infant with mild HIE usually occurs after a difficult but successful vaginal delivery. The neonate has an Apgar score of 3 at 5 minutes, 5 at 10 minutes, 6 at 15 minutes, and 9 at 20 minutes. During the first 2 hours of life the neonate may have increased tone in all extremities and increased reflexes with a flexion posture of all extremities. The actual activity level might be decreased, but responses to all sensory input increased such that the infant would be characterized as hyperalert. Over the next 12 to 24 hours one or two tonic-clonic seizures may occur. By 24 hours the infant is returning to normal tone with a gradual decrease in responsiveness to all sensory stimuli. By 48 hours the neonate is responding normally with a good suck and is having no further seizures. At 5 to 8 days the infant has a normal neurologic examination and subsequent development is unimpaired.

The second type of clinical course in a neonate with HIE might start similarly to that of the first neonate, but on admission to the nursery lethargy and hypotonia with decreased reflexes, frog-leg posturing, and decreased activity are noted. Seizures may develop within the first 6 hours of life and may be accompanied by periods of apnea and some increase in tenseness to the anterior fontanel. Over the second 24 hours there may be increasing seizures that can be controlled by medication. The degree of hypotonia persists even through the first week of life and, because of the infant's inability to suck, tube feedings must be started and maintained for some time. Over the next 2 weeks the neonate may not show any improvement in the return of tone, degree of activity, or posture, although seizures may decrease in frequency. This infant would be at a markedly increased risk of having significant neurologic dysfunction at subsequent developmental assessment.

The third type of clinical course involves a low-Apgar neonate who appears to be moderately well on admission to the nursery. However, if closely examined the neonate may have mild hypotonia, some lethargy, and a poor sucking response during the transitional period. The hypotonia may become more severe, and at approximately 3 or 4 hours of age episodes of lip-smacking and/or eye-blinking may be noted with the appearance of tonic-clonic seizures at 12 to 16 hours of age. At this time the anterior fontanel may be slightly tight, seizures may continue, and over the subsequent 48 hours the patient's previously tight anterior fontanel may bulge. Mild lethargy proceeds to stupor, and the neonate develops an abnormal respiratory pattern with periods of apnea and bradycardia. Pupils are noted to be fixed and dilated with a loss of oculovestibular response. Seizures during this latter period of time are very uncommon except for the cerebral posturing. Spontaneous recovery of an infant with this clinical course is extremely unlikely, and death is the usual outcome.

When the outcome of full-term neonates with a history of an asphyxial episode plus an abnormal neurologic examination during the first week of life was assessed, infants were at increased risk for early death (7%) or development of significant neurologic handicaps (28%). When abnormalities of tone were isolated as a predictor of severe handicap in full-term neonates with a clinical course compatible with asphyxia, the risk for cerebral palsy in children surviving the neonatal period was 25%. Thus an abnormal neurologic examination in a full-term infant interpreted in light of a history compatible with intrapartum asphyxia is an extremely powerful tool when predicting early death, in identifying neonates with signs of HIE, and in identifying neonates who are at increased risk for later development of neurologic sequelae.

More work is needed to refine the predictive powers of the neonatal neurologic examination. In the full-term infant with a history compatible with intrapartum asphyxia the following abnormalities are useful in predicting either an increased risk of early death or development of later neurologic dysfunction. A combination of abnormal signs is more helpful than a single sign. The most helpful signs to be used in clusters appear to include the following: an Apgar of 3 or less at 5 minutes; an Apgar score that stays below 3 for 10, 15, 20 minutes or longer; reduced levels of activity, tone, and consciousness lasting for more than a day; need for gavage feeding; multiple episodes of apnea during the first week; lethargy or stupor lasting longer than 7 days; asymmetrical neurologic signs; seizures with onset during the first day of life; and an overall impression of abnormality of brain function during the time the infant was in the nursery.

Pathologic findings

The pathologic changes in the brain of a full-term neonate who has experienced an episode of intrauterine asphyxia depend on the length of survival of the patient and the severity of the asphyxial episode. In patients dying in the first few hours after birth there may be no gross or microscopic changes, although animal studies suggest that there may be light and electron microscopic changes shortly after an asphyxial insult in both neurons and astrocytes. Those patients dying after the first 24 hours of age frequently have brain swelling and cerebral necrosis as documented in data from brain findings in 122 full-term infants dying during the neonatal period from various causes. Brain swelling was an isolated finding in as many as 39% of the cases. The observed cerebral necrosis involves the cortical gray matter (especially at depths of sulci), underlying white matter, and the gray matter of the basal ganglia. In some patients cerebral necrosis most severely involves the region of the postcentral gyrus and posterior parietal anterior occipital regions, as seen in the full-term newborn monkey following either experimentally produced perinatal asphyxia or spontaneously occurring placental abruption. Areas of petechial periventricular hemorrhage and leukomalacia can also be seen. Although germinal matrix necrosis and intraventricular hemorrhage are not usually a part of the pattern of cerebral damage seen in the full-term infant, with the advent of CT scanning these latter two findings are beginning to be found.

Those full-term infants who survive the perinatal asphyxial episode and beyond the neonatal period will have two primary neuropathologic conditions: ulegyria and status marmoratus of the basal ganglia.

Animal studies

The two animal models using the rhesus monkey that have been used to give the most comprehensive view of the pathogenesis of damage seen in the normally formed brain of a full-term infant experiencing perinatal asphyxia are termed *acute total asphyxia* and *partial prolonged asphyxia*. The data derived from experiments using these two animal models are particularly relevant to the human setting because of three unique factors. First, the experiments using these two different animal models replicate, as closely as possible, the two different types of perinatal asphyxial events that most frequently occur in the human fetus and neonate. Second, many different studies have been done using these same two models to delineate the spectrum of both short- and long-term clinical and neuropathologic findings following two different types of controlled perinatal asphyxial episodes. Third, the clinical spectrum identified using these animal models very closely replicates the findings in the human setting.

Acute total asphyxia. The first of these two animal models devised to study the effects of perinatal asphyxia on the newborn nervous system was the model of acute total asphyxia (ATA) using the full-term newborn rhesus monkey. Asphyxia in this model is similar to the asphyxia seen following complete compression of the umbilical cord in humans. There are a few examples of this type of very pure acute total asphyxia in the human setting.

The summary of changes in this form of asphyxia is outlined in Table 22-1. It is important to note that the length of the asphyxial insult cannot be more than approximately 16 minutes in most animals because of an inability to resuscitate the animal after this time. After approximately 6 to 8 minutes of asphyxia both the partial pressure of oxygen and the mean arterial blood pressure are extremely low. If the animal can be resuscitated, the neonatal course is complicated only by some mild respiratory distress. Seizures are not seen following this type of asphyxia. The brain lesions seen following ATA are confined to the neuronal nuclei in the brain stem, thalamus, basal ganglia, and spinal cord. The foci of damage in general correlate with areas of both very high metabolic rate and very high cerebral blood flow, as demonstrated in studies using both ^{14}C-labeled deoxyglucose or ^{14}C-labeled antipyrine. Although almost total cessation of

Table 22-1. Partial and total asphyxia in the full-term newborn rhesus monkey

		Partial prolonged asphyxia	Acute total asphyxia
Insult	Length	3-4 hours	13 minutes
	pH	6.9	6.9
	Po$_2$	15 mm Hg	3 mm Hg
	Pco$_2$	90 mm Hg	120 mm Hg
	Blood pressure	40 mm Hg	5 mm Hg
Clinical course	Resuscitation	Yes	Yes
	Seizures	Yes	No
	Retinal hemorrhage	Yes	No
	Survival	Variable	Variable
	Sequelae	No dysfunction detected	Spasticity Sensory loss
Pathologic aspects	Brain swelling	Yes	No
	Site of edema	Intracellular	
	Brain necrosis	Yes	Yes
	Locus of necrosis	Cerebral cortex Basal ganglia Thalamus	Brain stem Thalamus Basal ganglia Spinal cord
	Cerebral blood flow	Cortex abnormal at birth	Brain stem abnormal at birth

flow to the cerebral hemispheres following acute total asphyxia in the dog has been demonstrated, the neuropathologic finding of acute total asphyxia showed no brain swelling, cortical necrosis, or ulegyria. With the pattern of damage as described previously there is some similarity between the clinical motor deficits seen in the monkey and those seen in the patient surviving perinatal asphyxia. The monkey has essentially a spastic quadriplegia with loss of sensation in both hands and feet. Although there are some human clinical cases of patients surviving ATA associated with this pattern of brain damage, a clinical course without seizures, and a pattern of central nervous system damage excluding the cortex, this is not the most common pattern seen in asphyxiated human infants. For this reason the data from this model of ATA have obvious limitations in providing information regarding the pathogenesis of cerebral damage seen in most patients said to have experienced perinatal asphyxia as a full-term infant.

Partial prolonged asphyxia. The animal model giving insights into the pathogenesis of brain swelling and ulegyria has been the model of partial prolonged asphyxia (PPA). There have been a series of experiments using this model.

The first set of experiments was used to delineate the spectrum of both the short- and long-term clinical and

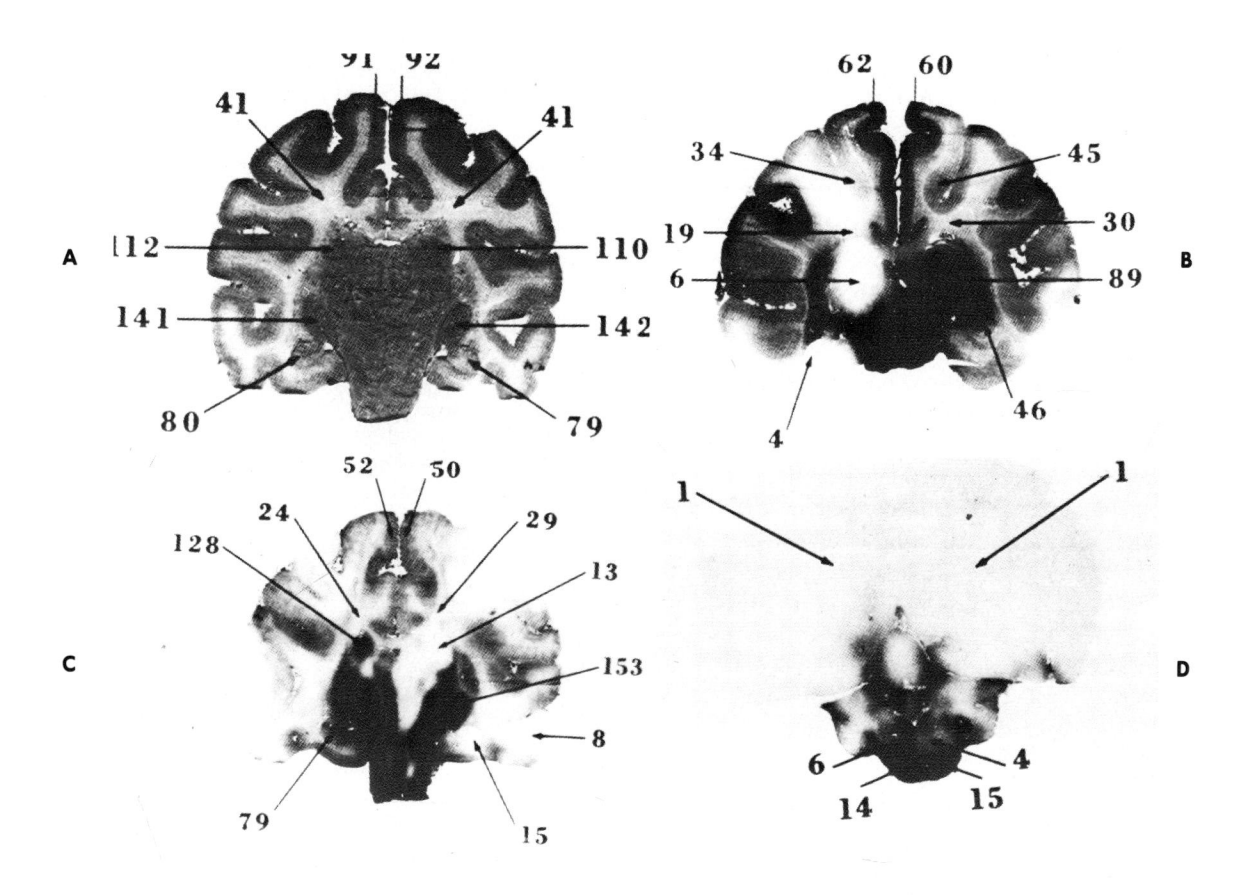

Fig. 22-7. Autoradiograms of coronal sections from full-term monkeys. **A,** Normal; **B,** mild PPA; **C,** moderate PPA; **D,** severe PPA. Numbers represent cerebral blood flow values in ml/gm/minutes.

neuropathologic findings following intrauterine PPA. After a 3- to 4-hour period of intrauterine partial asphyxia, monkeys with extremely low Apgar scores requiring resuscitation were produced. After delivery and stabilization these monkeys required oxygen for some mild respiratory distress. Approximately 50% of these monkeys developed seizures at approximately 12 to 18 hours of age. In those monkeys that were electively sacrificed because of an inability to maintain adequate vital signs at preset levels in the first 4 days of life, two groups of animals in the neonatal period were identified. The first group of animals had brain swelling at the time of birth to the extent that they could not be resuscitated; the second group, sacrificed during the 4 days of life, had autopsy evidence of brain swelling with varying degree of hemorrhagic cortical necrosis. The third group were sacrificed at 6 months of age and found to have ulegyria. These animals at time of sacrifice did not show any evidence of neurologic dysfunction. It is important to point out that the intrauterine insult, resuscitation procedure, and postdelivery care for all the monkeys in the study were essentially the same. In no way could the long-term survivors be separated from the animals that had to be sacrificed in the first 4 days of life by the severity of the intrauterine asphyxial episode. This study demonstrated a causal relationship between neonatal asphyxia and the spectrum of cerebral damage seen when fetal blood pressure was maintained in relatively normal range and fetal head trauma was eliminated. This study also suggested that cortical necrosis and possibly brain swelling were both present in the neonatal period in those surviving monkeys that ultimately developed ulegyria.

A second set of experiments using this particular animal model was done to study the changes in brain extracellular and intracellular space in the fetal monkey following an episode of PPA. Using the electron microscope method for determining the extracellular space, it was found that in normal controls this space was measured to be approximately 9.1%, while in the animals who had PPA it was 4.1%. This study indicated that there had been a translocation of brain fluid into the intracellular space. In addition, mitochondria from asphyxiated fetuses were swollen and characterized by a distended matrix. These findings suggested that the brain swelling accompanying PPA is associated with a type of edema known as cytotoxic edema, which produces intracellular swelling.

A third set of experiments using ^{14}C-labeled antipyrine was carried out to determine the pattern of cerebral blood flow in the full-term monkey fetus subjected to PPA. This was done to eliminate possible contributions of postnatal events in the production of the findings just mentioned. This determination of cerebral blood flow was performed at the end of an episode of intrauterine PPA and before any specific resuscitative efforts were done. Immediately after an injection of the ^{14}C-labeled antipyrine the animal was sacrificed. Focal and generalized reductions in cerebral blood flow occurred in the same areas of brain in which cortical and basal ganglia damage had been seen in the initial study. During this latter study the fetal mean arterial pressure was not significantly reduced, lessening the possibility that sustained systemic hypotension during the fetal insult was a significant factor in the focal, multifocal and generalized reductions of cerebral blood flow. However, the lower limits of the plateau of autoregulation of cerebral blood flow in the full-term monkey fetus is not known. In addition, fetal head compression, secondary to uterine pressure and/or vaginal delivery, was not present because intrauterine pressure showed no elevation and the animals were delivered by cesarean section. This study demonstrated that the brains had significantly altered blood flow at birth following an intrauterine asphyxial episode unaccompanied by significant fetal hypotension or head compression (Fig. 22-7).

These two animal models replicate as closely as possible the two different types of perinatal asphyxial events that most frequently occur in the human fetus and neonate—acute asphyxial episodes, as occurs with cord prolapse, and partial prolonged asphyxial episodes, as occur with an abruption. In most cases the perinatal insult in the human setting appears as a combined partial prolonged asphyxial episode with a terminal acute asphyxial episode.

Pathogenesis

On the basis of currently available human and animal data, the proposed pathogenesis for HIE and its sequelae in the full-term infant is outlined in Fig. 22-8. The extent of changes seen in the brain can vary, depending on the length and severity of the asphyxial episode. The diagram is drawn as though there was a continuum of the intrapartum asphyxial episode from top to bottom with the outcome being seen on the right side of the figure, indicating the terminal effect of the intrapartum asphyxial episode if the intrapartum status were terminated at each particular level.

The initial response of the human fetus to a period of intrapartum asphyxia, from whatever cause, is thought to be a general redistribution of organ blood flow to maintain oxygenation to vital organs while not increasing the cardiac output. Initially there is an increase in blood flow to the brain, heart, and adrenal glands with a decreased blood flow to lungs, kidneys, GI tract, and placenta (p. 2). Data to support this initial fetal response has come from work with both sheep and monkey fetuses. The exact levels at which the human fetus is prompted to redistribute blood flow is unknown. Although the levels at which this redistribution occurs are unknown, the fact that this does occur in humans seems extremely plausible, since the diseases seen following an intrauterine asphyxial episode involve organs shown to receive a reduced amount of blood in animal models.

Numerous infants born following intrapartum asphyxial episodes with low Apgar scores have had no evidence of HIE. This has been the case in asphyxiated infants who succumb because of other organ dysfunction, such as occurs in the lung with persistent fetal circulation. The lack of findings in the central nervous system could be explained by the fact that the brain received an increased percentage of cardiac output, thus maintaining tissue oxygenation and preventing the development of cytotoxic edema and tissue ischemia.

If the intrauterine asphyxial episode continues beyond the point that homeostatic mechanisms to maintain oxygenation to the brain begin to fail, data from animal studies suggest that two major alterations in brain begin to occur: alterations of brain water distribution and alterations of cerebral blood flow. Both of these are thought to act synergistically and contribute to the key finding of cerebral blood flow. Both are thought to act synergistically and contribute to the key finding of multifocal tissue ischemia, seen in Fig. 22-7. The earliest and most significant reduction of flow is seen in the brain slice in the upper right corner (B). There is a generalized reduction of flow with focal areas of almost total lack of flow. The increasing degrees of ischemia occurred with increasing degree and length of asphyxia (C and D).

An understanding of all the factors that lead to this multifocal tissue ischemia seems to be of central importance in the overall pathogenetic mechanism leading to the brain damage seen in neonatal HIE. The entire sequence of events leading to the various types of neuropathologic outcomes is not totally clear from the data currently available, although the points represented in each of the squares in the diagram have been demonstrated in animal or human material (Fig. 22-8).

The first effects of the altered distribution of brain water appear as cytotoxic edema. This redistribution of water into the cell, which can appear very quickly after the onset of hypoxia, is thought to occur secondary to failure of the ATP-dependent sodium pump within the

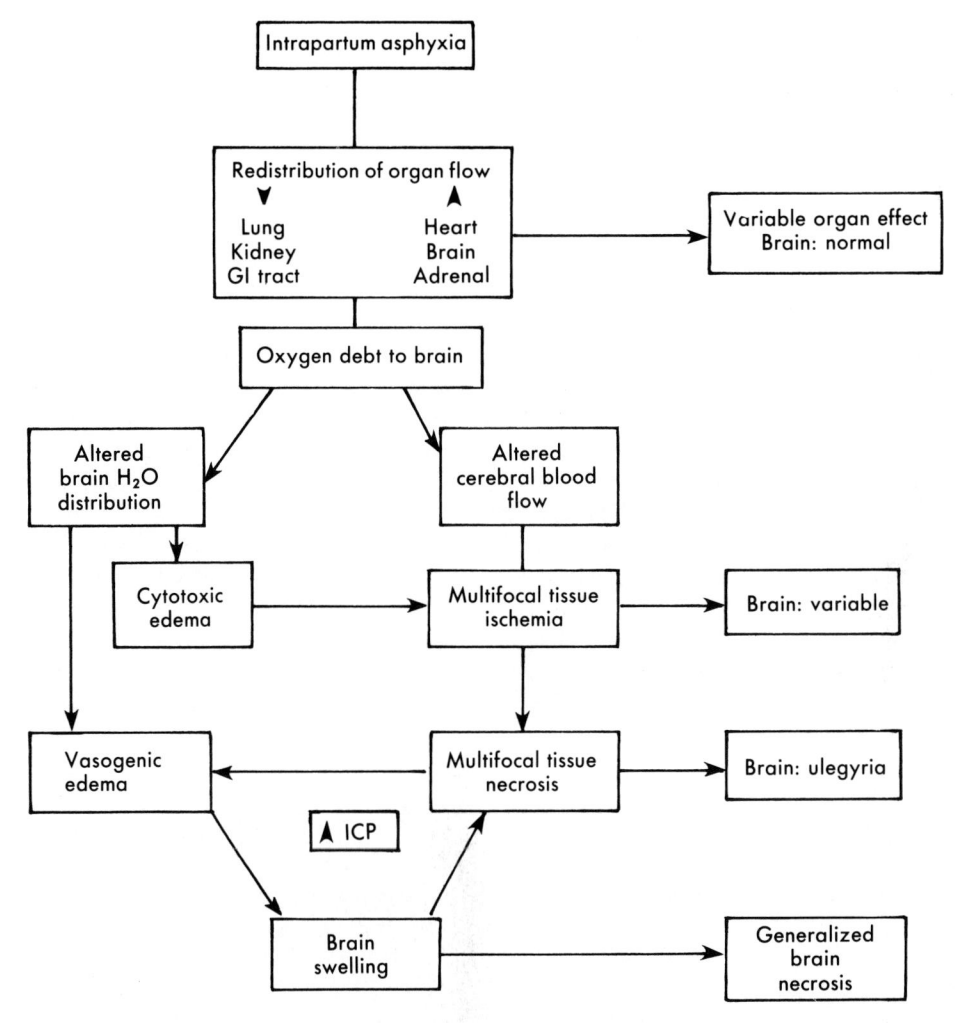

Fig. 22-8. Proposed pathogenesis for the development of hypoxic-ischemic brain damage.

brain capillary endothelial cell, as well as in adjacent astrocytes. After sodium accumulates within the cell from failure of this pump, there is a major shift of extracellular fluid into the intracellular compartment, giving rise to this specific type of edema. This early phase of cytotoxic edema may not result in any evidence of increased intracranial pressure, since there is simply a change in the site of the fluid within the cranial vault, not an increased amount of fluid initially. However, if the intrapartum asphyxia is not terminated, the cytotoxic edema can progress to the point that fluid from the intravascular space can move into the cell, giving a total increase in intracranial volume. However, a second effect of the intracellular edema of the capillary endothelial cell with swelling into the capillary lumen may be a reduction in the luminal dimensions and potentially contribute to the focal and multifocal ischemia. This point is made in Fig. 22-8 by the dotted line connecting cytotoxic edema and multifocal tissue ischemia. The phenomenon has been called the *no reflow phenomenon*. Increase in interstitial pressure is one other change that has been suggested following this type of edema. There has been some suggestion that, with increases in interstitial pressure that may follow increasing cytotoxic edema, external compression of the capillaries may also contribute to the multifocal tissue ischemia.

It is important to point out that a real controversy exists regarding whether brain edema is involved in the pathogenesis of brain injury. The second and equally important effect on the brain from increasing oxygen debt probably occurring simultaneously with the previously described alteration in brain water distribution is an alteration of cerebral blood flow probably mediated through changes in the vascular resistance of the cerebral arteriole leading to an impaired autoregulation and an altered CO_2 sensitivity. An increase in circulating catecholamines may possibly produce some cerebral vasoconstriction at the arteriolar level from an increase in

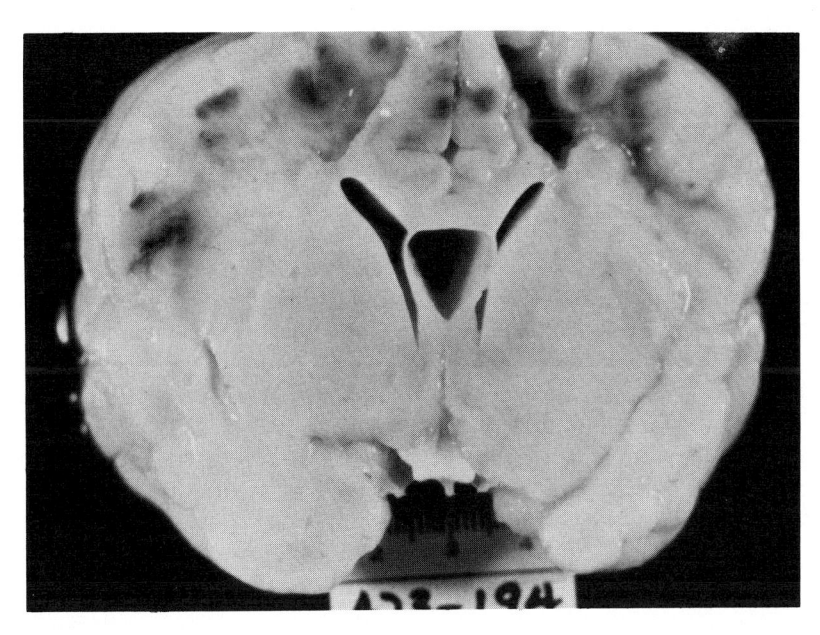

Fig. 22-9. Full-term asphyxiated infant brain with hemorrhagic cortical necrosis.

sympathetic activity. It is felt that all of these factors, in addition to the previously mentioned no reflow phenomenon and increase in interstitial pressure, could play a role in leading to the multifocal tissue ischemia.

The specific contribution of changes in local cerebral perfusion pressure (mean arterial blood pressure–intracranial pressure) to the multifocal areas of tissue ischemia is unknown. In the experimental setting the mean arterial blood pressure was not consistently low enough to have produced ischemia and especially not in the asymmetrical distribution seen. It is also unclear from the literature what length of time is required for tissue ischemia to be present before actual death of tissue occurs in the cerebral cortex. It is conceivable that, if the intrauterine asphyxial episode is relieved after the development of only mild multifocal tissue ischemia, the brain in the surviving infant could be spared any evidence of tissue necrosis.

If the intrapartum episode is severe and persists for a prolonged period, the existing tissue ischemia will lead to tissue necrosis. At about the same time that multifocal tissue necrosis is developing, it is most likely that vasogenic edema, the second type of change in brain water distribution, occurs. This type of edema develops after disruption of the tight junctions of the capillary endothelium with leakage of osmotic materials and accompanying water from the intravascular space into interstitial brain tissue. As the multifocal areas of necrotic brain begin to coalesce, significant cerebral edema and measurable increases in intracranial pressure begin to occur. From animal data it is known that, when intracranial pressure reaches one half to two thirds of the mean arterial pressure, tissue ischemia from a reduction of cerebral blood flow begins, especially in areas of cortex situated at the depths of sulci. As can be seen in Fig. 22-9, the triad of multifocal tissue necrosis, vasogenic edema, and brain swelling with increasing intracranial pressure leads to a vicious downward spiral with an ever-increasing oxygen debt to brain, leading to further tissue necrosis. In this setting the issue of adequate cerebral perfusion pressure, even within the neonate's cranial vault, does begin to play a significant role in suboptimum oxygenation of brain tissue through the role of progressive ischemia.

It is proposed that, if the intrapartum insult is not extremely severe and/or is terminated, smaller areas of multifocal tissue necrosis can occur but not to the extent that would lead to significant areas of vasogenic edema with the development of increased intracranial pressure. Through the reparative process of brain these areas of multifocal tissue necrosis are converted into areas of ulegyria. The extent and pattern of ulegyria depend on the degree and location of cerebral necrosis.

Several reasons have been proposed for the lack of cerebral edema that may be observed in all patients dying following intrapartum asphyxia. First, this may be related to the ability of the fetus to compensate with redistribution of blood flow to protect the brain, but with inadequate flow and oxygenation to the heart, lungs, kidneys, or gastrointestinal tract, which may lead to a fatal outcome. Second, the absence of edema may be related to the type and length of the asphyxial episode. There is consistently an absence of brain swelling in monkeys experiencing acute total asphyxia. However, there may be enough neuronal necrosis, principally confined to the brain stem and basal ganglia, to result in death through impaired respiratory control. Third, it is important to recognize unknown and as yet unidentified or unquantitated pathogenetic factors.

Treatment

The general guidelines for treatment of the asphyxiated neonate involve first eliminating the original hypoxia and second alleviating tissue ischemia if present. Specific management, beyond the immediate resuscitation in the delivery room, is still under considerable discussion. When a particular organ is the principal target of the asphyxial episode, such as with the lungs and persistent fetal circulation (p. 566), the kidneys and acute tubular necrosis (p. 792), or the GI tract and necrotizing enterocolitis (p. 512), the management of a specific process assumes central importance. In addition, there are other physiologic and biochemical factors that can affect brain homeostasis if left uncorrected. Most of these factors are altered in the asphyxiated full-term neonate and must be dealt with in the overall therapeutic plan. This dicussion is directed toward the management of the neonate with HIE, and other deranged organ systems will be discussed only if directly affecting brain homeostasis.

There are four unanswered questions in regard to the therapeutic management of the neonate with HIE:

1. Can the asphyxiated fetus or neonate who has a central nervous system altered enough to leave permanent damage be identified?
2. Can this asphyxiated fetus or neonate profit from any therapeutic intervention?
3. If therapeutic intervention is possible, is there a critical time after which treatment is ineffective in eliminating or significantly reducing permanent brain damage?
4. What is the appropriate intervention for this asphyxiated fetus or neonate?

The first question probably is the most important one. Current data increasingly support the position that the full-term neonate who has had a history of fetal distress, a low Apgar score requiring resuscitation, and altered tone or level of consciousness during the first 2 to 6 hours of life is manifesting early findings of HIE. Rarely have neonates presenting with an Apgar score of 7 to 10 developed neurologic findings and a clinical course consistent with HIE. It is extremely important in such cases to be sure that the neurologic dysfunction is not secondary to some other cause. It is rare for a neonate to have signs of neurologic dysfunction secondary to intrapartum asphyxia after 24 hours of age with no clinically apparent alteration in the nervous system prior to that time.

The remaining three questions most specifically concern therapy. The first two questions relate to the stage of the asphyxial process. Certainly, if the neonate is born after a prolonged intrapartum asphyxial episode and presents with advanced degrees of vasogenic edema and raised intracranial pressure, therapeutic intervention may have minimal benefit.

The therapeutic management of an infant with signs of HIE is first directed toward eliminating the hypoxic environment by immediate delivery of the fetus with institution of adequate oxygenation of the neonate. However, after birth the central role of therapy should be directed at relieving any existing brain ischemia and/or reducing the brain's metabolic requirements. The first phase of any therapeutic plan for a neonate who either has HIE or is at risk for developing HIE is the institution of a very careful monitoring system. In monitoring the course of a patient who may have brain ischemia, the monitoring system should include serial neurologic assessment by clinical examination, detection of reduced cerebral perfusion pressure through monitoring of blood pressure and intracranial pressure, structural status of the brain by either CT scan or ultrasound, and evidence of suppressed electrogenesis by electroencephalogram or evoked potentials. All these functions can be measured in the neonate with fairly standard clinical tools. An adequate monitoring system is extremely important not only in initiating therapy in a neonate who becomes abnormal but also in following the progression of any therapeutic intervention once initiated. Other systemic parameters that should be monitored continuously include arterial pH and blood gases, temperature, blood glucose levels, serum and urine electrolytes and osmolality, serum BUN, serum creatinine, and accurate fluid input and output.

Once the hypoxic environment has been eliminated, efforts should be directed at promoting adequate brain tissue oxygenation by maintaining and/or restoring cerebral perfusion in an attempt to relieve ischemia. Signs of systemic hypoperfusion should be identified by findings such as an inadequate heart rate, poor capillary refill, abnormal arterial and venous blood pressure, and urine output. The causes of hypoperfusion in the neonate may be secondary to asphyxia, hypovolemia, and/or, rarely, septic shock. Hypovolemia should be suspected in situations where the mother has vaginal bleeding (abruption or placenta previa). Peripheral vasoconstriction may result initially in normal or near normal blood pressure and hematocrit even in the presence of hypovolemia. As the acid-base status normalizes and the peripheral vascular bed opens up, blood pressure may fall. Also, the acid-base status may deteriorate as sequestered lactic acid is released into the circulation.

The neonate's blood pressure should be maintained at levels that allow adequate perfusion to all body tissues. It is more important to observe the patient's degree of peripheral perfusion and urinary output than to maintain specific levels of blood pressure as outlined in neonatal blood pressure charts (p. 127). The relationship of low cerebral blood flow to hypotension and adverse neurologic outcome has been documented. Likewise, a loss of autoregulation of cerebral blood flow has been documented, suggesting that hypertension may be equally hazardous to brain tissue as is hypotension. Volume expansion must therefore be undertaken with careful and continual monitoring of the circulatory status. Dopamine at levels of 2 to 5 µg/kg/minute may have a role in normalizing blood pressure and renal blood flow, although the efficacy and safety of this drug have not been fully explored in the newborn.

For adequate oxygen-carrying capacity to be present, a normal hematocrit level (45 to 60) should be maintained (p. 708). Patients with hematocrits greater than 65 should be considered to be polycythemic and are candidates for a partial exchange transfusion to reduce hyperviscosity and enhance tissue oxygenation.

Once adequate oxygenation is established, administration of sodium bicarbonate may be indicated with a severe, persistent metabolic acidosis documented by arterial pH and blood gases (p. 185). Rapid infusion of bicarbonate should be avoided to prevent hazardous increases in serum osmolality and the adverse effects of alkalinization on cerebral blood flow.

In the normal state it is important that the brain receive a continuous supply of both oxygen and glucose, the two primary sources of energy for neurons and glia. This is necessary because these cells do not have the capacity to store energy in any chemical form. There is a controversy concerning the appropriate levels of glucose in the brain to be maintained following an asphyxial insult. Data support both the view of increasing glucose supply to the brain, which is unable to appropriately use glucose in the postasphyxial state, as well as the opposing view, which suggests a possible deleterious effect of high glucose levels because of the potential hazard of promoting the development of local lactic acidosis, which may be associated with an increase in brain damage seen in the asphyxiated brain. At the present time I feel that a glucose infusion should be established and monitored with Dextrostix and blood glucose determinations to maintain glucose levels of 45 to 90 mg/dl, not only for cerebral but also for myocardial tissue function. Hypocalcemia may be seen in association with hypoglycemia in the asphyxiated full-term neonate, and calcium in the form of calcium gluconate may need to be given for calcium levels of <7.5 mg/dl (Chapter 33, part two).

Fluid overload can be a distinct but avoidable hazard in the treatment of an asphyxiated neonate. The status of the kidney regarding potential acute tubular necrosis and/or the presence of inappropriate secretion of antidiuretic hormone may materially affect fluid output. Fluid and elecrolyte monitoring can detect the presence of either of these conditions. While this monitoring is going on it is suggested that the asphyxiated nenoate initially be started on an electrolyte-free dextrose solution (10%) restricted to a rate of 50 ml/kg/day. Changes in fluid volume and content should be altered depending on data from continuous monitoring of serum electrolytes, serum osmolality, urine output, and body weight done as frequently as every 12 hours.

Seizures, when present, should be recognized and vigorously treated in these patients (p. 388). This is particularly important because of the known fact that cerebral oxygen use is increased almost fivefold during a seizure. In the brain with HIE the ability to autoregulate flow in response to energy requirements is altered, making it imperative to eliminate any increases in energy requirements of the brain.

At the present time the treatment of brain edema/ischemia in the asphyxiated neonate remains an area of controversy and speculation. The two phases of cerebral edema in the clinical course of HIE may require different therapeutic approaches. Therapy during the initial stage of cytotoxic edema and focal ischemia without significant increase in intracranial pressure would be directed at reducing local increases in pressure through the use of fluid restriction, osmotic agents such as mannitol, and diuretics such as furosemide. At the same time, while initial tissue ischemia is present, the use of agents that would reduce energy requirements of brain, such as the barbiturates, may have a specific role.

If the patient is seen for the first time during the second phase of HIE, when there is clinical evidence of a significant increase in intracranial pressure, a more vigorous approach to reducing intracranial pressure by fluid restriction, osmotic agents, and diuretics has been suggested. Barbiturates in large doses have been shown to reduce intracranial pressure in the adult, and their role in HIE is being studied in the neonate.

The use of steriods in cytotoxic edema initially had some appeal on theoretical grounds, but currently there is no proof of their effectiveness. In vasogenic edema characterized by breakdown of the brain capillary with disruption of the blood brain barrier, steriods have been thought to be effective, although this has not been clearly established.

SUBEPENDYMAL GERMINAL MATRIX HEMORRHAGE/INTRAVENTRICULAR HEMORRHAGE (SEH/IVH)

SEH/IVH is the most common and most serious neurologic disorder of preterm infants. Although the etiology and pathogenesis of this condition are not known, it is dicussed here because current information seems to favor asphyxia as a prerequisite in most cases. The contribution during labor and delivery of overt trauma and/or compression-distortion forces to SEH/IVH has not been established at this time.

Information regarding this type of hemorrhage has recently accumulated at a very rapid rate because of the increasing availability of computed axial tomography (CAT scanning). Prior to CAT scanning, information about SEH/IVH was derived primarily fom retrospective clinical and autopsy studies. These led to the assumptions that all hemorrhages are clinically detectable and that such hemorrhages are almost uniformly lethal. Following Larroche's description of posthemorrhagic hydrocephalus in neonates it was clear that these two assumptions were incorrect. With the advent of CAT scanning and current developments in cranial ultrasound a more accurate picture of incidence, clinical symptomatology, pathogenesis, and prognosis in SEH/IVA is evolving.

Incidence

Retrospective autopsy studies established the incidence of SEH/IVH in live-born infants as varying from 25% to 59%, primarily occuring in preterm infants. This process has been felt to be primarily an extrauterine postnatal event, since the incidence of SEH/IVH in stillborn infants has been estimated to be only about 5%. A prospective clinical study has shown that the median age at occurrence of hemorrhage is approximately 38 hours after birth. When CAT scanning was used in prospective studies to document the incidence of SEH/IVH, these hemorrhages were found in approximately 40% to 50% of infants admitted to special care units who weighed less than 1,500 gm or were less than 35 weeks' gestation. When patients were separated according to the extent of hemorrhage, it was found that 8% of the patients had subependymal hemorrhage alone, 21% had mild hemorrhage, 26% had moderate hemorrhage, and 45% had marked hemorrhage. The overall mortality for patients with hemorrhage has varied from 27% to 50%. The mortality figures from various studies are difficult to compare, but it is evident that patients with hemorrhage have a higher mortality than those who do not have hemorrhage. It is also evident that the extent of hemorrhage correlates positively with mortality, although bleeding is generally the primary cause of death only in infants with marked hemorrhage.

Clinical manifestations and diagnosis

Clinical signs of SEH/IVH in the preterm infant prior to CAT scanning have been generally described as catastrophic in onset with an abrupt deterioration of clinical status, the appearance of a bulging anterior fontanel, hypotension, apnea, severe metabolic acidosis, and in most instances rapid progression to death. A second clinical syndrome has been described as a "saltatory" or "stuttering" course in which there is sudden deterioration followed by improvement. This cycle may be repeated several times until improvement is sustained or death occurs, usually within 48 hours of the acute event.

As with data on the incidence of SEH/IVH, the definition of these clinical signs evolved from studies in which the diagnosis was made on autopsy, ventricular tap, and/or lumbar puncture findings. In two prospective studies it has been demonstrated that neither clinical signs nor lumbar puncture findings are reliable means of detecting SEH/IVH in all cases. One study specifically designed to prospectively identify the variety of clinical signs of SEH/IVH, using the CAT scan to document the bleeding prior to the patient's clinical deterioration, demonstrated the following findings: hemorrhages were correctly predicted clinically in only 54% of patients who were documented to have SEH/IVH on CAT scan. In patients with a negative scan 79% were correctly predicted not to have bled. The ability to clinically predict SEH/IVH was related to the severity of hemorrhage in that 81% of the marked hemorrhages were correctly predicted, whereas only 32% of the mild to moderate hemorrhages were correctly predicted.

In the study just mentioned four clinical signs were found to be statistically associated with proven SEH/IVH, including inappropriate fall of hematocrit level and/or failure of hematocrit level to rise with transfusion, full anterior fontanel, change in activity, and decreased tone. Abnormal eye signs and seizure activity occurred in only a few patients, but when present these signs were always associated with SEH/IVH. Thus in many of these infants the quantity of blood must be insufficient to cause clinical symptoms.

Because of the difficulties in clinical detection of SEH/IVH, CAT scanning became accepted as the most accurate and reliable method for detecting SEH/IVH in the high-risk preterm infant, for quantitating the amount of hemorrhage, and for following infants for development of posthemorrhagic hydrocephalus. However, the expense, possible radiation exposure, distance of CAT scanners from many neonatal intensive care units, and at times limited availability restricted their application as a general screening procedure. Other noninvasive techniques also have been studied for these diagnostic purposes, including determination of transcephalic impedance, cranial transillumination, blood flow determination by Doppler ultrasound, and B-mode real-time ultrasound. The latter method has the distinct advantages of bedside performance with portable equipment, minimum manipulation of the infant, and, at the energy levels and frequency currently employed with pulsed ultrasound, no hazards to the infant. Using various types of real-time ultrasound equipment, including linear array and sector scanners, various institutions have demon-

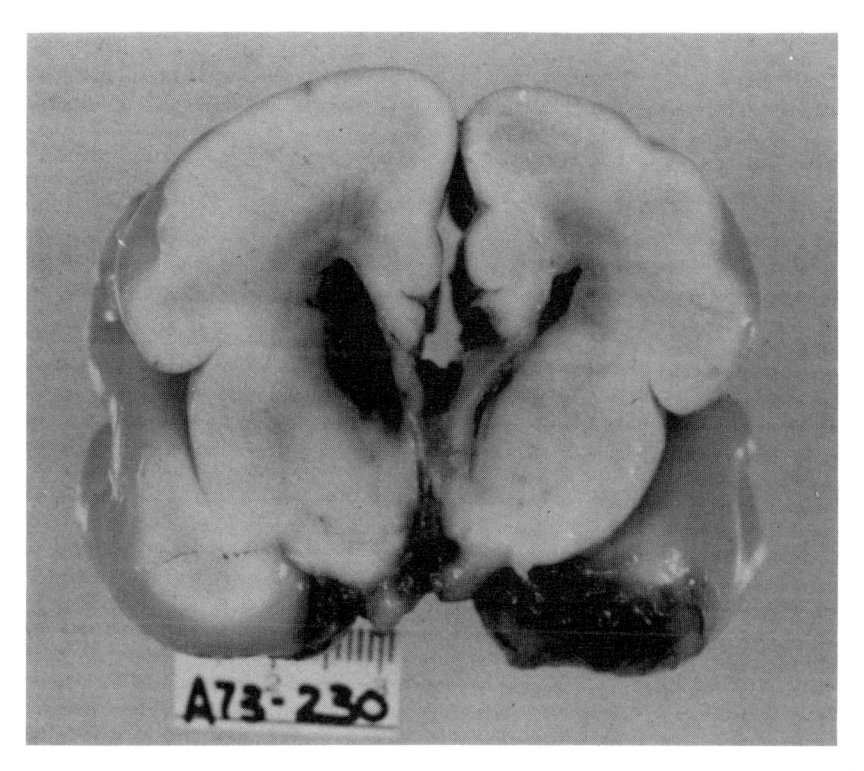

Fig. 22-10. Premature infant brain with asymmetrical subependymal germinal matrix hemorrhage and bilateral intraventricular hemorrhage.

Pathology

The pattern of cerebral damage in SEH/IVH in the premature infant involves the central areas of the hemispheres with sparing of the cortical mantle (Fig. 22-10). This pattern is in contrast to the cerebral damage seen in the full-term asphyxiated infant with hemorrhagic cortical necrosis and sparing of the central portion of brain (Fig. 22-9). This recurring central location of hemorrhage in the subependymal and periventricular region of the preterm infant's brain is related to the presence of the germinal matrix all along the anteroposterior border of the ventricular system, with the extent dependent on gestational age. The largest concentration of germinal matrix is at the level of the foramen of Monro in the region of the head of the caudate nucleus. Before 26 to 28 weeks' gestation the germinal matrix is a highly vascularized zone of the developing brain containing pluripotential cells that migrate from this region forming, among other things, the six layers of the cerebral cortex and deeper nuclear structures. Until resorption of the germinal matrix is completed around 35 weeks' gestation, this periventricular area remains highly vascularized but with poor tissue support for the remaining bed of vessels, making these susceptible to mechanical forces generated by changes in intravascular and intracranial pressure.

The high frequency of hemorrhage in this area appears to be related in part to several unique aspects of the vascular anatomy of this area at this stage of development in the preterm infant. First, there is an abundant but poorly supported capillary bed in the germinal matrix region, with veins of only a single endothelial cell's thickness at this stage of venous development and irregular capillary-vein junctions. A second determinant is the anatomic organization of the deep venous or galenic system. The central portions of the cerebral hemispheres have their venous drainage via the deep terminal, choroidal, and thalamostriate veins, all of which drain into the internal cerebral vein at a sharp angle, resulting in an abrupt change in direction of venous flow. A third anatomic feature is the extensive and rich arterial circulation to the basal ganglia area adjacent to the germinal matrix. At this stage of embryogenesis, in contrast to the much less prominent arterial supply to this same region in the more mature infant at term, cortical arterial flow predominates.

The exact site of vascular disruption in the germinal matrix has been disputed with different autopsy studies suggesting venous disruption, arterial disruption, and thrombosis. However, based on recent investigations currently using stereomicroscopic and injection techniques, the capillary bed of Hubner's artery is considered to be the primary site. Neither germinal matrix infarction nor rupture of veins or arteries was identified in this study. Confusion concerning the venous origin of SEH/IVH could have arisen because bleeding occurs contiguous to the terminal veins, often from capillaries opening at right angles to the vein.

Pathogenesis

The exact pathogenesis of SEH/IVH is not known, although many factors have been implicated. These presumed relationships were derived from retrospective studies entirely based on autopsy-identified cases of SEH/IVH. Since many infants with SEH/IVH have clinically inapparent hemorrhages, the data derived only from retrospective autopsy studies are of limited use in delineating an accurate pathogenesis of SEH/IVH or for changing care practices. Factors thought to contribute to the occurrence of IVH include obstetric trauma, hypernatremia, hyperosmolality, asphyxia, acidosis, liberal bicarbonate administration, respiratory distress syndrome (RDS), hypothermia, and hypotension. A prospective study using the CAT scan to identify the presence or absence of SEH/IVH was designed specifically to identify any positive clinical or laboratory correlations with SEH/IVH. Excessive sodium administration, early bicarbonate administration, and systemic acidosis were found to be significantly associated with hemorrhage in those patients who died. These same factors were not associated with hemorrhage in the survivors. These associations probably reflect the severity of the infant's disease along with need for aggressive treatment rather than a cause and effect relationship.

Factors in the prospective study regarding etiology and pathogenesis of SEH/IVH that were found to be associated with hemorrhage are alveolar rupture, hypercarbia, application of intermittent mandatory ventilation, high-peak inflation pressures of greater than 25 cm H_2O, prolonged inspiratory to expiratory ratios, stages 3 and 4 RDS, patent ductus arteriosus, bicarbonate administration after the first 24 hours of life, systemic hypotension, and volume expansion given in the first 24 hours of life. Of these, the presence of alveolar rupture had the most striking association with SEH/IVH. These factors significantly associated with SEH/IVH were again those which are present in the sickest preterm infants. Following further breakdown of the findings in this study and a subsequent review of the incidence of intraventricular hemorrhage in well preterm infants, the incidence of intraventricular hemorrhage is as follows: well preterm infants in the intermediate care nursery, 12% to 15%; mild to moderate RDS not requiring ventilatory support, 24%; moderate to severe RDS without alveolar rupture, 56%; moderate to severe RDS with alveolar rupture, 87%. Thus there is a baseline incidence of SEH/IVH in preterm infants in the intermediate care and intensive care nurseries that increases with the sicker infants and particularly with the very ill preterm infants with severe RDS who require mechanical ventilation and then have alveolar rupture.

As increasing evidence accumulates concerning factors that control or alter cerebral blood flow, it is apparent that autoregulation is present in the preterm infant. Autoregulation, however, may be lost or impaired with an asphyxial insult in the preterm infant. Increases in arterial blood pressure may be transmitted directly to the very small blood vessels and capillaries, especially in the germinal matrix area. The quantitative impact of the various factors affecting cerebral blood flow are not fully understood. Furthermore, it is not known whether the vessels of the germinal matrix are affected by the same factors that affect other cerebral vessels. It is clear, however, that the germinal matrix does not provide adequate tissue support for its rich vascular bed, and it is a site where factors affecting intravascular pressure and flow may exert tremendous effects on arterioles, capillaries, and venules. Fig. 22-11 shows these three segments of the vessel along with factors in each of these areas that can influence tone and/or integrity of this vascular bed and could lead to SEH/IVH. Most biologic systems are not constructed such that only one adverse event will cause damage unless that event is overwhelming. There may be a combination of factors with a cumulative effect on the vascular bed of the germinal matrix leading to hemorrhage. However, impaired autoregulation of cerebral blood flow or damage to the immature capillary bed with less than the normal amount of supporting basement membrane may have the most profound role in SEH/IVH. More research will be necessary to delineate all the factors that can impinge on the germinal matrix as well as to estimate the quantitative role that each of these hypothesized factors has on the ultimate occurrence of SEH/IVH.

Prognosis

Concerns regarding prognosis of neonates who survive SEH/IVH include progressive posthemorrhagic hydrocephalus and subsequently altered neurologic development and function. Previous data tended to indicate that progressive posthemorrhagic hydrocephalus was inevitable in infants surviving SEH/IVH. Data from prospective studies demonstrate that progressive hydrocephalus, usually of the comunicating variety caused by obliterative arachnoiditis, occurs in up to 23% of patients who survive SEH/IVH. When progressive hydrocephalus occurs, it is primarily in those infants who have had severe IVH. Progressive hydrocephalus demonstrated by CAT scan occurs some 2 to 3 weeks prior to increasing head circumference or other signs of intracranial pressure.

```
           ARTERIOLE            CAPILLARY BED           VENULE
        ▮▮▮▮▮▮▮▮▮▮▮▮▮▮▮▮━━━━━━━━━━━━━━━━━━━━━━━
        ▮▮▮▮▮▮▮▮▮▮▮▮▮▮▮▮━━━━━━━━━━━━━━━━━━━━━━━
```

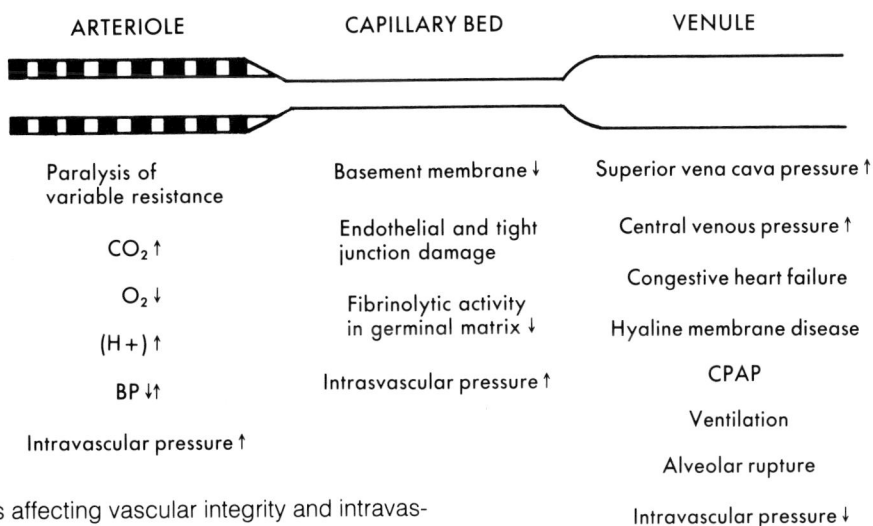

Paralysis of variable resistance	Basement membrane ↓	Superior vena cava pressure ↑
CO_2 ↑	Endothelial and tight junction damage	Central venous pressure ↑
O_2 ↓	Fibrinolytic activity in germinal matrix ↓	Congestive heart failure
(H+) ↑		Hyaline membrane disease
BP ↓↑	Intrasvascular pressure ↑	CPAP
		Ventilation
Intravascular pressure ↑		Alveolar rupture
		Intravascular pressure ↓

Fig. 22-11. Factors affecting vascular integrity and intravascular pressure.

The optimum treatment of posthemorrhagic hydrocephalus is not established. Several studies are in progress to evaluate management alternatives, including repeated lumbar puncture, pharmacologic management with both osmotic and diuretic agents, and shunt surgery. Spontaneous resolution within 2 weeks of detection of the progressive hydrocephalus following SEH/IVH does occur in a significant number of cases. It is thus important to be aware of the potential for spontaneous resolution before any therapeutic approach is undertaken.

The number of infants who have been followed long enough to determine the incidence of developmental abnormalities in survivors of SEH/IVH is not large enough to make any sweeping prognostic statements. Although there have been reports of poor outcome in survivors of SEH/IVH, there are also ongoing studies that have shown normal development in some of these children. Studies to date, however, have not been able to determine, on the basis of clinical presentation, which of these neonates will subsequently have normal or abnormal development. Until follow-up studies of infants from large prospective studies are complete, an accurate estimate of the incidence of developmental abnormalities and neurologic deficits cannot be made. In addition, the complicating problem of hydrocephalus must be accurately documented and managed to exclude the confounding secondary effects of increased intracranial pressure on developmental outcome.

PERIVENTRICULAR LEUKOMALACIA

Periventricular leukomalacia is a lesion principally occurring in the preterm infant's brain, presumably resulting from localized hypoperfusion, leading to areas of necrosis in the periventricular white matter largely in the regions adjacent to the external angles of the lateral ventricles. The lesion, as originally described, begins as areas of ischemic coagulation necrosis followed by macrophage and astrocytic proliferation and capillary endothelial hyperplasia; eventually cavitation of tissue in periventricular regions becomes apparent. Because the involved area includes white matter through which long descending motor tracts descend from the motor cortex, with the leg fibers being closest to the ventricles and therefore more likely to be damaged, the clinical sequela is most commonly spastic paresis of the legs. With lateral extension of the lesion there may also be involvement of the arms, resulting in spastic quadriplegia. Another possible sequela is visual deficits, presumably related to involvement of optic radiations. More extensive lesions involving association and commissural fibers would be expected to result in mental retardation or other specific deficits in abstract reasoning. Although this lesion occurs predominantly in the preterm infant, it has been described in term infants and is usually associated with evidence of neuronal necrosis.

The incidence of this lesion is not known, principally because there is currently no way to accurately diagnose this lesion before death. Originally it was reported in 20% of infants dying in the first month of life. Recent reports indicate that this lesion is much less common, perhaps because of increased emphasis on maintaining blood pressure and circulation in the high-risk infant. A striking decrease in the incidence of spastic diplegia has also been noted in population surveys of cerebral palsy. Both of these observations have accompanied a marked improvement in survival of low birth weight infants.

BIRTH TRAUMA

Although the frequency of overt physical traumatic injury has been significantly reduced, the same types of pathologic conditions as described in the past continue to occur. These include intracranial hemorrhage of various types (exclusive of SEH/IVH), skull fracture, cephalhematoma, spinal cord trauma, brachial plexus palsy, and facial nerve palsy. At present, brachial plexus palsy and facial nerve palsy are the only types that occur with any frequency. The life-threatening or severely handicapping disorders caused by intrapartum trauma per se have been almost completely eliminated. Each of these conditions is discussed.

Intracranial hemorrhage

All types of intracranial hemorrhage (ICH) that have been described in adults have occurred in newborn infants. However, the various types of ICH occur with different frequencies and different degrees of severity. In the newborn infant more than one type of hemorrhage can and does frequently occur in the same patient. The types of hemorrhage that are thought to be primarily associated with trauma are dealt with in this section.

Subarachnoid hemorrhage, perhaps the most frequent form of neonatal intracranial bleeding, is usually of limited degree and is rarely of clinical significance. A high percentage of newborns will have some erythrocytes (RBCs) in their cerebrospinal fluid (CSF). In one study RBCs in preterm infants ranged from 0 to 39,000/mm^3 with a median of 112/mm^3. Furthermore, small amounts of subarachnoid blood may be detected in postmortem examinations of newborns who were neither clinically symptomatic nor suspected of having suffered intracranial bleeding. Most commonly the RBCs in CSF are an incidental finding, perhaps a result of mild trauma during delivery.

The ease with which one can produce a traumatic lumbar puncture can make interpretation of bloody CSF difficult. In the evaluation of bloody CSF specimens, to distinguish subarachnoid bleeding from a traumatic lumbar puncture, it is necessary to count the number of RBCs in first and third (or fourth) tubes of CSF and also to examine centrifuged CSF supernatant for xanthochromia; the latter finding is indicative of subarachnoid blood and is not the result of a traumatic lumbar puncture.

Significant degrees of subarachnoid hemorrhage can occur with asphyxia, particularly in preterm infants; the bleeding is related to asphyxial injury of capillaries and small veins, with or without the added effect of trauma in the course of delivery. Clinically significant subarachnoid bleeding, especially in the full-term infant, can result from trauma alone. This can occur as an isolated process or in association with hemorrhage in other areas (subdural, epidural) with or without cerebral contusion. When the subarachnoid hemorrhage is associated with other types of bleeding or signs of physical injury, as documented by computed tomography or ultrasound examination, and caused by difficult delivery, the outcome is frequently poor, with either demise in the early neonatal period or profound brain damage in survivors.

The clinical presentation of the full-term infant with isolated subarachnoid hemorrhage can vary considerably. Most commonly there are no clinical signs, and the infant is totally asymptomatic and diagnosed only because of an abnormal lumbar puncture. On occasion an infant appears normal initially and then develops seizures on the second or third day of life as the only clinical manifestation. The infant may look remarkably well between seizures and subsequently have a benign course, with no apparent sequelae. In contrast, the initial clinical manifestations of neonatal subarachnoid hemorrhage may be the early onset of alternating depression and irritability with refractory seizures. It may be impossible in such an infant to establish the primary role of birth trauma or asphyxia as the cause of the subarachnoid hemorrhage and its manifestations. Such infants may develop hydrocephalus as a late complication of subarachnoid bleeding, with obstruction of CSF circulation and reabsorption as well as other later signs of neurologic impairment and delayed development.

Subdural hemorrhage has become a very rare neonatal neurologic disorder. The two principal locations of subdural hemorrhage are over the cerebral hemispheres and in the posterior fossa. When this type of bleeding has occurred, common historical events include the mother being primiparous with the total labor and delivery occurring in less than 2 or 3 hours, a difficult delivery involving high or midforceps application, and/or the infant being large for gestational age. In this type of hemorrhage the events of labor simply produce excessive molding of the calvarium with relatively sudden stretching and tearing of the superficial venous channels over the cerebral hemispheres or venous sinuses in the posterior fossa. The clinical presentation depends on the quantity and location of blood.

Subdural hemorrhage over the cerebral hemispheres occurring at the time of birth may be clinically silent, clinically apparent in the first few days after birth, or not apparent until as late as the sixth week of life. When this type of hemorrhage is manifested early, the signs are those of increasing intracranial pressure in the presence of jaundice and/or anemia. When an infant shows evidence of a convex subdural hematoma as late as the fourth to sixth week, there is usually an increasing head circumference, poor feeding and/or vomiting, failure to thrive, altered states of consciousness, and occasionally seizures. Even though an increasing head size with signs of increased intracranial pressure usually means hydrocephalus, one must always consider a subdural hematoma in the differential diagnosis, especially with the previously mentioned historical events occurring during labor and delivery. Computed tomography is a very rapid method of diagnosing this condition and quantifying the amount of blood present. Management of subdural collections of fluid usually involves watching for reabsorption of fluid. Only occasionally does management involve the use of subdural taps and/or the removal of fluid. The decision depends on the amount of fluid, the rate of evolution of the clinical syndrome, and the presence of signs of increased intracranial pressure.

Subdural hemorrhage, when occurring in the posterior fossa, is secondary to marked molding of the calvarium with tears of the falx or tentorium. This can occur in either full-term or preterm infants. Because of the limited space around the brain stem for collection of blood before function is compromised, this type of hemorrhage is usually lethal in a very short time following the onset of bleeding.

Cerebellar hemorrhage

Massive hemorrhagic destruction of the cerebellum, although infrequent, may occur in low birth weight infants in association with perinatal trauma and asphyxia. At the present time the exact etiology and pathogenesis are not fully understood. The clinical course is characterized by severe progressive apnea, a falling hematocrit level, and death.

More mildly affected infants may survive with residual damage. Infants with these sublethal retrocerebellar or intracerebellar hematomas can be suspected from changes in respiration, a high-pitched or hoarse cry, vomiting, hypotonia, and an absent Moro reflex. Rapid enlargement of the head may occur toward the end of the first week of life. Diagnosis is made by CT scan. Surgical drainage of the subdural hemorrhage may be life saving.

Epidural bleeding

This type of bleeding is extremely rare in the newborn, especially since the use of high or midforceps has been almost totally eliminated in obstetric practice. The origin of this type of bleeding is from a laceration of the middle meningeal artery following a skull fracture of the temporal bone, which usually occurs after a slippage of the forceps in a very difficult delivery. The clinical course includes signs of a rapidly appearing anemia, signs of increased intracranial pressure, and asymmetrical or focal neurologic signs. When any of these signs are present following a difficult delivery, an aggressive diagnostic approach must be taken to rule out one of the treatable forms of intracranial bleeding. Diagnosis of this condition depends on clinical suspicion, the presence of a fracture in the temporal bone, and blood confirmed by computed axial tomography. Treatment involves evacuation of blood and ligation of the site of arterial bleeding.

Cephalhematomas

See p. 218.

Fractures of the skull

See p. 220.

Spinal cord trauma

See p. 230.

Acute transection of the spinal cord may occur in difficult breech deliveries with hyperflexion or extension of the body in relation to the after-coming head. Much less frequently cord transection may occur with vertex presentation and deliveries in which there has been considerable lateral as well as direct traction. Mechanisms postulated for injury have included excessive longitudinal stretching of the cervical cord with hyperextension or excessive flexion of the neck as well as torsional forces. Transection is most common at C5 and C7 levels. Complete lesions at higher cervical cord levels may be incompatible with survival.

The infant initially appears profoundly hypotonic, with no spontaneous movements of the legs and limited movements of the arms and hands, depending on the exact level of the cervical cord injury. Respiratory movements may be entirely abdominal because of intercostal muscle paralysis. In many reports the affected infant resembles an infant with congenital Werdnig-Hoffmann disease (p. 394), but in infants with cord injury a level of sensory deficit may be determined if the examiner will carefully observe the infant's facial response, grimace, and cry on pinprick stimulation. The level of motor deficit may be determined by observation of movement of the hands and arms. Urinary and anal sphincter impairment is also evident. Spinal fluid is bloody and xanthochromic. Myelography, if performed, shows a swollen, edematous cord at the affected level. Direct observation of the cord at operation or after death reveals swelling, maceration, and hemorrhage. Use of steroids soon after injury to reduce spinal cord swelling may provide the only potential beneficial form of therapy. In the child who survives the neonatal period, attention must be directed toward care of the bladder and kidneys, as in children with meningomyeloceles. Physical therapy is useful in preventing contractures. Children with intact arm musculature may eventually be able to ambulate with a swing-through gait.

Complete spinal cord transection is a well-recognized entity, both clinically and pathologically, but is now a very rare event because of improved obstetric care. Attention is now being directed to less dramatic forms of cervical cord and brain stem injury, which are rarely recognized clinically.

Brachial plexus palsy

See p. 226.

Brachial plexus palsy is the most common nerve injury of the newborn. Damage to the upper brachial plexus (Erb's palsy) is more common than damage to the lower brachial plexus (Klumpke's palsy). This type of injury usually occurs from traction on the head and neck in a vertex delivery, not from arm traction.

In Erb's palsy the most commonly involved neural structures are the fifth and sixth cervical roots or upper trunk of the brachial plexus. Characteristic posture includes an adducted shoulder and an internally rotated arm, with the elbow extended, forearm pronated, and wrist flexed. Because of involvement of high cervical roots, from which the phrenic nerve arises, diaphragmatic paralysis on the same side may occur.

In lower plexus injury involving roots C7, C8, and T1 the weakness primarily affects the forearm and hand, particularly the flexors of wrists and fingers and intrinsic muscles of the hand. Horner's syndrome may coexist with these lower brachial plexus injuries. Rarely the entire plexus is injured, with complete paralysis of the entire arm.

The prognosis for recovery of function varies considerably, and in some infants return of motor power and recovery of tone may begin before discharge from the nursery. Onset of improvement has been noted as late as 4 to 6 weeks after birth, but with this delay a complete recovery is unlikely. Considerable argument has arisen regarding preferred positioning of the affected arm with a brachial plexus paralysis and the role of immobilization. Full range of motion exercises should be given several times daily to prevent contractures that might limit functional use of the arm if and when recovery does occur. Surgical exploration of the brachial plexus is generally not indicated.

Facial nerve palsy

See p. 222.

Congenital facial paralysis, present at birth with impaired facial movements involving the entire face, and with impaired eye closure as well as flattening of the nasolabial fold on the affected side, is generally considered to be the result of pressure. The cause of the pressure can be obstetric forceps application. An alternative explanation is pressure on the face, with facial nerve compression, in utero against the mother's sacral prominence. The alternative explanation seems necessary, since there are infants with facial nerve paralysis on delivery to whom forceps were never applied. This traumatic facial paralysis present at birth has a good prognosis, and usually complete recovery occurs spontaneously.

Another disorder of facial muscles, which is occasionally confused with peripheral facial nerve injury, is the syndrome of asymmetrical crying facies in the newborn, which may resemble congenital facial palsy at first glance. However, in this condition, which is considered to be caused by congenital absence or hypoplasia of the angular depressor muscles of the mouth on one side, there is no distortion of the nasolabial fold nor impairment of eye closure. The asymmetry of the face is evident only when the infant cries, or at a later age laughs. The corner of the mouth on the affected side is not pulled down. This may confuse the unwary examiner, who may consider the abnormal side to be that on which the corner of the mouth is pulled down when the infant cries. It is not known whether the primary pathology is absence of the depressor muscle or congenital absence of the branch of the facial nerve that innervates the muscle. This condition is occasionally familial and may also be associated with other congenital anomalies, including cardiac malformations in the so-called cardiofacial syndrome.

Weakness of facial muscles, either unilateral or bilateral, when associated with coexistent external rectus muscle palsies with restricted lateral movement of one or both eyes, is referred to as the Möbius syndrome; this condition should be distinguished from isolated facial palsy. The degree of facial paralysis may vary, with some infants having limited mobility noticeable only when the infant cries or has difficulty with feeding. Careful examination will reveal a rather flat or immobile face with limited expression, and the eyes may remain open when the infant sleeps. In the Möbius syndrome, in addition to impaired abduction of the eyes, lower cranial nerves may be involved with impaired palate and pharyngeal function. This can produce marked dysphagia, severe feeding difficulties, nasal regurgitation and possible aspiration, and speech problems at a later age. Nasogastric tube feedings or gastrostomy may be required. The pathologic basis for these multiple cranial nerve palsies is considered to be absence of their nerve nuclei in the brain stem, although pathologic studies on affected infants have varied considerably.

Congenital ptosis, caused by weakness of the levator palpebrae muscles, may occur as an isolated entity, with the site of the primary disorder being unknown. This tends to persist into later life. If, in addition to the ptosis, the infant has a smaller pupil on the same side, this is most likely congenital Horner's syndrome, which rarely can be an isolated congenital defect but is more commonly associated with a lower brachial plexus palsy and involvement of sympathetic outflow, with traction or avulsion injury affecting the upper thoracic roots.

ABNORMALITIES OF HEAD SIZE
The enlarging head

Hydrocephalus is the most common cause of an excessive rate of head growth in the neonatal period, but it must be differentiated from subdural effusions and hematomas, porencephalic cysts, megalencephaly (enlargement of the brain), and the normal rate of growth of premature and full-term infants (Fig. 22-12). Hydrocephalus is not of itself a disease but is the end result of a number of disease processes that produce an accumulation of CSF.

Pathophysiology

CSF is produced by the choroid plexus, as well as from the brain substance, at a relatively constant rate of 0.37 ml/minute (0.26 to 0.65 ml/minute). CSF produced in the lateral ventricles flows through the foramen of Monro, the third ventricle, down the aqueduct to the fourth ventricle, and exists through the foramina of Luschka and Magendie. The fluid then flows along the base, up the sylvian fissures, and over the surface of the hemispheres to be absorbed through valves along the sagittal sinus by bulk flow. The amount of spinal fluid made within the cerebral cortical substance and transported across the ependyma to the ventricles or absorbed by this route is still a matter of investigation. Studies using infusions of artificial CSF have indicated that there are variable pressures at which bulk absorption begins to occur. In most individuals the pressure required is around 60 mm of water; in others the pressure may have to reach 180 mm before bulk absorption occurs. The ability of the newborn's head to expand without reaching these higher pressures may account for some forms of hydrocephalus; the arrest of hydrocephalus may occur in some infants when the sutures close firmly enough to achieve that pressure.

In addition to the increased pressures, the undamped pulsations of the choroid plexus are felt to play an important role in the dilatation of the ventricles. With progressive ventricular dilatation, compression of the cortical mantle occurs prior to expansion of the cranium and suture separation. Thus considerable reduction in cortical mantle thickness may occur before hydrocephalus becomes evident by measureable increases in the occipitofrontal head circumference. Ventricular enlargement is not a uniform process and occurs chiefly at the expense of periventricular white matter. The gray matter, including cortex and basal ganglia, is relatively spared, with little neuronal loss until extreme thinning (less than 0.5 cm) has occurred. Following adequate treatment of moderate hydrocephalus or with spontaneous resolution the cortical mantle may be restored to its former normal thickness, and there may not be any neurologic deficit.

Etiology

Hydrocephalus was formerly classified as obstructive or communicating. however, with the exception of hydrocephalus secondary to cortical atrophy (hydrocephalus ex vacuo) and the rare hydrocephalus secondary to overproduction of CSF by a choroid plexus papilloma, all hydrocephalus is caused by an obstruction. The obstruction may lie within the ventricular system, as in aqueductal stenosis, the Dandy-Walker syndrome, or tumors; or it may lie outside the ventricular system, as with arachnoidal adhesions. Obstruction outside the ventricular system was formerly called communicating hydrocephalus because dye placed in the ventricle appeared in the lumbar subarachnoid space.

Overproduction—choroid plexus papillomas. Overproduction of CSF, although rare, is associated with papillomas of the choroid plexus and probably with no other lesion. Infants with choroid plexus papillomas have a communicating hydrocephalus. Elevated CSF protein and xanthochromia are common, and an intraventricular mass can be identified readily by computerized tomography or by air study. These can be surgically removed, with resultant cure of the hydrocephalus.

Obstruction to CSF flow
Congenital malformations

AQUEDUCTAL STENOSIS. The aqueduct is a common location for obstruction producing hydrocephalus in the neonatal period. Normally a single channel, in congenital aqueductal stenosis the aqueduct is often found to be broken into many small channels with varying degrees of occlusion but without evidence of inflammation. Previously, aqueductal stenosis was considered a developmental abnormality, but Johnson has produced identical lesions in rodents by neonatal infection with mumps, influenza, and parainfluenza viruses. No pathologic evidence of the preceding infection could be demonstrated at the time the animals developed hydrocephalus. Thus "congenital" aqueductal stenosis may in some cases be caused by unrecognized viral disease.

THE DANDY-WALKER SYNDROME. The Dandy-Walker syndrome produces a clinically recognizable form of hydrocephalus. The large cystic fourth ventricle causes a prominent occipital shelf, occipital transillumination, and elevation of tentorium and venous sinuses on roentgenographic film.

In addition to the large cystic dilatation of the fourth ventricle, there is defective development of the cerebellum with the vermis being smaller than normal and only small amounts of laterally displaced tissue thought to be remnants of cerebellar hemispheres. Despite the marked atrophy of the cerebellar vermis, infants with this syndrome are not ataxic in later life.

THE ARNOLD-CHIARI MALFORMATION. This malformation occurs in varying degrees of severity. In its most severe and

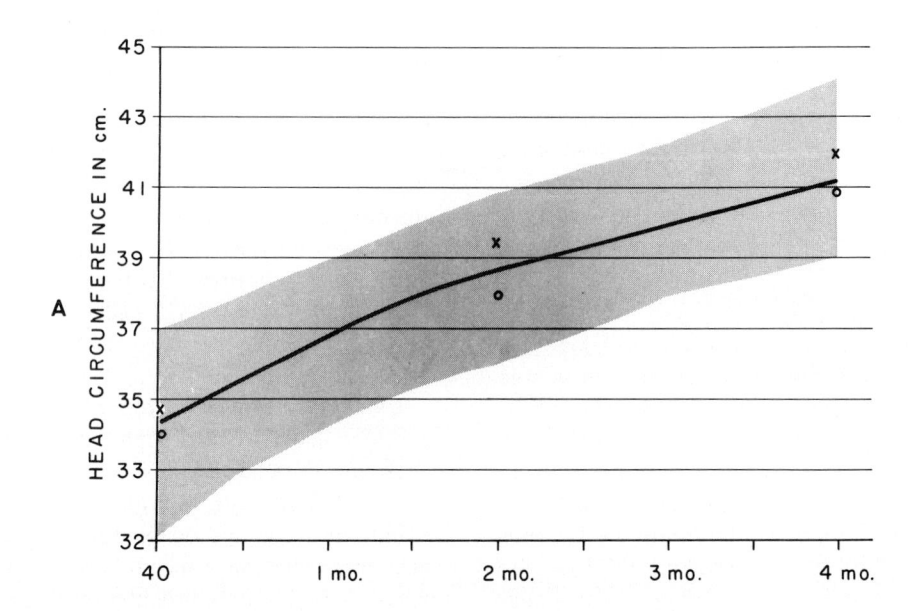

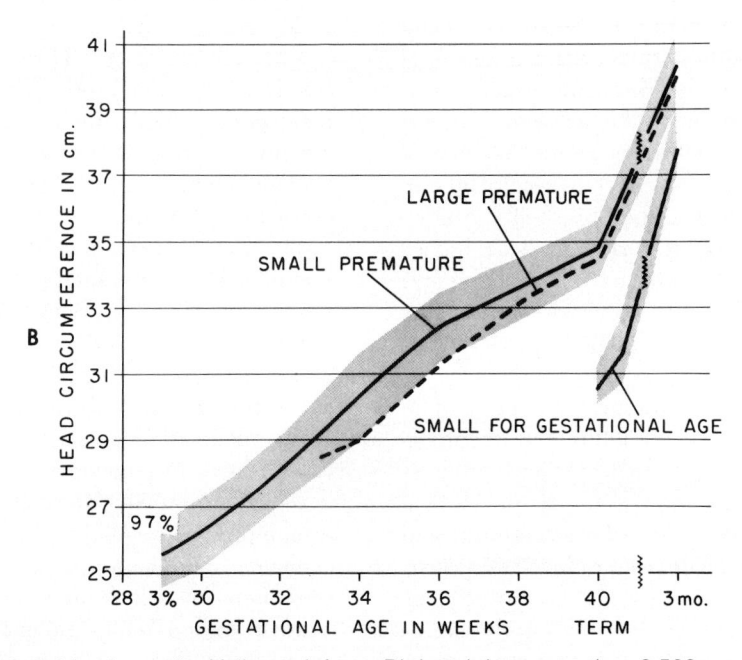

Fig. 22-12. A, Head growth of full-term infants. Birth weight greater than 2,500 gm. The solid line is a combination of males and females. (Redrawn from O'Neill, E.M.: Arch. Dis. Child. **36:**241, 1961.) *X* represents males; *O,* females. **B,** Head growth of low birth weight infants (less than 2,500 gm): the small premature of appropriate size for gestational age (27 to 29 weeks' gestation); the large premature of appropriate size for gestational age (31 to 33 weeks' gestation); and the severely underweight or small for gestational age full-term infant (gestation greater than 38 weeks, weight less than 2.0 kg). (**A** from Nellhaus, G.: Pediatrics **41:**106, 1968. **B** adapted from Babson: J. Pediatr. **77:**11, 1970.)

classic form it is characterized by downward displacement of the cerebellar tonsils through the foramen magnum, downward displacement, elongation, and folding of the medulla oblongata and fourth ventricle on the cervical cord, and downward displacement of the cervical cord. It is most commonly seen in patients with spinal dysrhaphia, such as meningomyeloceles. Aqueductal stenosis and micropolygyria are often associated with the Arnold-Chiari malformation. The etiology of this malformation is unknown; it is not caused by traction on the fixed spinal cord.

The distortion of the medulla, fourth ventricle, and CSF circulation pathways, both at the exit of the fourth ventricle and around the brain stem, may be sufficient to obstruct CSF flow and produce hydrocephalus. Therefore either this anatomic malformation or the associated malformation of aqueductal stenosis may cause hydrocephalus, which may be the only clinical manifestation of this extensive malformation of the lower brain stem, cervical cord, and cerebellum. On rare occasions lower cranial nerve palsies with vocal cord or laryngeal paralysis and respiratory obstruction may be an early manifestation of the Arnold-Chiari malformation.

VEIN OF GALEN MALFORMATIONS. Vein of Galen malformations are another rare cause of hydrocephalus. The markedly dilated vein of Galen compresses the aqueduct, producing the picture of aqueductal stenosis. This large malformation may produce heart failure in the early days or weeks of life and produces a loud bruit that may be heard over the vertex of the skull. Arteriography delineates the malformation. With neonatal cardiac failure direct attack on the malformation may be necessary despite the high mortality. If hydrocephalus is the only symptom, treatment usually consists of shunting rather than a direct attack on the malformation.

Posthemorrhagic hydrocephalus. The most common form of hydrocephalus in the newborn is posthemorrhagic hydrocephalus, occurring as a sequel to intraventricular hemorrhage. In these infants hydrocephalus is secondary to obliterative arachnoiditis in the posterior fossa, resulting from the blood, with impaired CSF flow out of the fourth ventricle or impaired flow of CSF through the subarachnoid pathways and cisterns at the level of the tentorial notch. Rarely intraventricular blood may cause aqueductal obstruction.

Inflammatory or postinflammatory processes. Fibrosis and adhesions at the exit of the fourth ventricle or along subarachnoid pathways of CSF circulation may also be the result of neonatal bacterial meningitis, with hydrocephalus occurring immediately or at a later time.

Pathology

The pathology of hydrocephalus is the progressive thinning of cortical white matter, with reduction of oligodendroglial cells and astrocytes. The neurons and axons seem quite resistant to the effects of pressure. The hydrocephalus causes greater thinning of the vertex and occipital cortex, since the basal ganglia tend to buttress the lower part of the ventricular wall. Because of the thinning at the vertex (leg area) and because fibers from the leg area undergo the greatest stretch in circumventing the dilated ventricles, patients with hydrocephalus tend to develop a paraparesis with the preservation of the arms. The compressed cerebrum shows a loss of lipids and proteins from white matter with an increase in water content. The lipid and protein loss can presumably be reconstituted with relief of the hydrocephalus. Since the neurons and axons remain intact, there may be no residual deficit.

Clinical manifestations

There are few clinical manifestations of hydrocephalus in the neonatal period other than enlargement of the head. Since the head can easily enlarge, intracranial pressure is dissipated, and the signs and symptoms of increased intracranial pressure are rarely seen. Vomiting and lethargy are uncommon, and papilledema is rarely if ever seen. Neurologic disability and seizures, if present, are usually the result of the underlying disease process rather than of the hydrocephalus.

As the head enlarges, the fontanel is tense when felt with the infant in the upright position. Suture separation occurs as the fontanel tension increases. Since the sutures of the newborn, especially the small preterm infant, may normally be widely separated, in the absence of increased intracranial pressure or ventricular dilatation it may be difficult to use the degree of suture separation, at least in the sagittal suture, as a clinical sign of pressure. However, the squamosal suture, which runs horizontally slightly above the ear in between the temporal and parietal bones, is a sensitive indicator of pressure. Separation of that suture after the first few days of life of more than a few millimeters is a useful sign of increased intracranial pressure, most commonly due to hydrocephalus.

There is prominence of the frontal bones (in contrast to the parietal bossing classically seen in subdural hematomas), and the scalp veins become prominent. The setting sun sign, the appearance of sclera above the pupil, is a moderately late sign probably caused by pressure in the region of the superior colliculi. The posterior shelf of the Dandy-Walker malformation has been described. The most significant clinical manifestation of hydrocephalus is enlargement of the head. Plotting serial head measurements on an appropriate head circumference chart is the only clinical method of diagnosing progressive hydrocephalus and is far more accurate than a single measurement.

Diagnosis

The most important element in the diagnosis of hydrocephalus is suspicion. Early detection can come only from plotting serial head circumference measurements made with a metal tape. The greatest head circumference obtained should be recorded on a standard head growth chart. Measurements should be made in centimeters; although growth from 13¼ inches to 14¼ inches does not seem great, growth from 34.9 cm to 36.2 cm is more likely to alert the physician. Head circumference measurements should be a recorded part of every baby visit in the first months of life. The diagnosis of hydrocephalus is suggested when the rate of head growth is greater than the norm (that is, when the rate is crossing percentiles). The absolute head circumference is of less significance than the rate of growth. It is just as significant if the head grows from the third percentile to the fiftieth percentile as if the growth is from the seventy-fifth to greater than the ninety-fifth percentile.

A complete history and physical examination are obviously important in the initial workup of an infant with a large head. However, unless the head circumference exceeds the ninety-seventh percentile or unless the rate of head growth is currently greater than the norm, more definitive evaluations need not be undertaken; the infant's course should be followed.

Transillumination also should be a part of the initial evaluation of a large head. Transillumination must be done in a totally dark room with a flashlight with a light-tight seal on the end. Sufficient time must be spent in the room to allow adequate adaptation to the dark. The whole head, including the occiput, should be transilluminated. Transillumination giving a ring greater than 1 cm around the seal (1.5 cm in the frontal area and in prematures) is abnormal. Abnormal transillumination is seen in chronic subdural hematomas, edema of the scalp, cortical atrophy, porencephaly, hydranencephaly, and hydrocephalus if the cortical mantle is less than 1.0 cm in thickness.

Further definitive diagnostic evaluation may include skull films, cranial ultrasonography, and computerized tomographic scanning. Intracranial pressure monitoring may be helpful in differentiating hydrocephalus from megalencephaly. Arteriograms are rarely indicated. Pneumoencephalography and ventriculography have been almost entirely replaced by CT scanning and cranial ultrasound examination. All these techniques provide high resolution of ventricular size and identification of intraventricular, intracerebral, subarachnoid, or subdural blood, as well as revealing various malformations, including localized areas of porencephaly, absence of the corpus callosum, and forebrain cleavage anomalies. CT scanning involves transport to the x-ray department and occasional sedation for scanning, and it can be repeated serially, as indicated, and provides a noninvasive method of following the progression or resolution of ventricular dilatation with or without treatment. Ultrasound examinations, which are totally without any radiation hazard and which can be performed in the special care nursery at the bedside, may provide an even more readily available, nontraumatic, and noninvasive method for obtaining the same information as does CT scanning. This has become the technique of choice.

Table 22-2. Differential diagnosis of the enlarging head in the neonatal period

Hydrocephalus	Differentiate from
Overproduction	Subdural hematomas
Choroid plexus papilloma	Hydranencephaly
Obstruction	Porencephaly
Aqueductal stenosis or occlusion	Megalencephaly
	Familial
Congenital	Canavan's disease
Viral	Alexander's disease
Vein of Galen	Normal growth of premature and full-term infant
Familial	Growth after feeding malnourished infant
Dandy-Walker syndrome	Subgaleal hematomas
Arnold-Chiari syndrome (meningomyelocele)	Achondroplasia
Obstruction at base or absorption	Normal head/dwarf body

Differential diagnosis

The differential diagnosis of an enlarging head in the neonate is between hydrocephalus and a number of other, less common causes (Table 22-2).

Subdural hematomas (p. 372) may be secondary to neonatal or postnatal trauma and are more common with bleeding disorders. The initial manifestation may be subtle, such as enlargement of the head with no other symptoms, or may include symptoms of increased intracranial pressure or failure to thrive. A boxlike head configuration with biparietal bossing may suggest that the enlargement is caused by subdural hematomas rather than hydrocephalus. Transillumination is usually abnormal in chronic subdural hematomas but may be absent during the acute phase.

The diagnosis of subdural hematoma is made by CT scanning with and without enhancement or by ultrasound examination. Subdural taps are rarely indicated, and the subdural needle should become an object of antiquarian interest in the newborn unit. If subdural blood or effusion is present, treatment by subdural taps should be reserved for those infants with focal neurologic deficits or symptoms and signs of increased intracranial pressure, such as enlarging head size, tense fontanel, or evidence of deterioration in degree of consciousness and awareness. In the absence of such findings, there is little rationale for treatment.

Hydranencephaly is a congenital absence of the brain, but with normal coverings of dura, skull, and scalp, thus differentiating it from anencephaly. It is probably caused either by bilateral carotid occlusion in utero, with resorption of the cerebral hemispheres, or by intrauterine infection. Hydranencephalic infants often appear normal at birth and demonstrate few neurologic abnormalities other than lack of fixing and following an object with the eyes. A large head is a common initial manifestation. Transillumination of marked degree serves to identify these infants on initial screening, but the entity still must be differentiated from large subdural hematomas or severe hydrocephalus.

CT scanning or cranial ultrasound examination should make the definitive diagnosis. Shunting may result in collapse of what little tissue is present, with secondary rupture of blood vessels and rapid deterioration of the infant.

Porencephaly is a cavitation of the brain that usually communicates with either the ventricle or the subarachnoid space. The caviation is commonly the result of prenatal vascular occlusion with resorption of the dead tissue. Developmental arrests at the site of fissures (schizencephaly) produce similar clinical features. Porencephaly may be associated with hydrocephalus or with subdural fluid collections. Infants may have seizures, focal neurologic deficits, or hydrocephalus. Transillumination is often localized. Treatment of the hydrocephalus is indicated; intractable focal seizures secondary to porencephaly may respond to drainage of the cyst.

Arachnoid cysts are uncommon lesions of unknown cause. Many of them appear to be the entrapment of CSF in the pia-arachnoid. They often mimic hydrocephalus but are usually asymmetrical. They may produce localized transillumination and local erosion of bone. When occurring in the posterior fossa, they may produce hydrocephalus by aqueductal compression.

Arachnoid cysts may be extremely difficult to differentiate from porencephalic cysts except by injection of air, as with pneumoencephalography or metrizamide cisternography.

With ventriculocardiac shunts the cardiac (atrial) end of the shunt may become infected and produce chronic bacteremia or septicemia. Cardiac shunts may embolize to the lungs, producing pulmonary hypertension, or may occasionally break off in the heart. All shunts may become plugged or obstructed at either end, with resultant signs of increased intracranial pressure. All shunts inserted in infancy require replacement as the infant grows, unless the hydrocephalus becomes arrested (p. 381). There are indications that shunts from the ventricle may cause aqueductal stenosis and shunt dependence.

Despite all these complications, for the infant with progressive hydrocephalus whose ventricles continue to dilate with progressive thinning of cortical mantle, there is no current alternative to shunting.

Enlargement of the head may be caused by enlargement of the brain substance, *megalencephaly*. In such patients, head growth is rarely as rapid as in hydrocephalus. Megalencephaly may be familial, with or without mental retardation, but is often associated with structural abnormalities such as overgrowth of glial cells, astrocytosis, or microgyria. Megalencephaly may be seen with storage of materials within the brain substance, as in Alexander's disease, Tay-Sachs disease in its later stages, or Canavan's disease (spongy degeneration of the white matter. However, enlargement of the brain in these diseases is not noted until after the first 6 months of age.

Differentiation from hydrocephalus may be suggested by the rate of head growth and may be confirmed by computerized tomography.

Normal growth of the head of a *premature infant* from 32 to 40 weeks is almost twice as fast as that of a full-term infant 0 to 2 months of age (Fig. 22-11). Therefore, unless the rate of head growth is plotted on an age-specific graph, the rate of head growth of small babies will appear to be excessive. This may lead to the erroneous diagnosis of hydrocephalus.

With malnutrition there is a relative sparing of the brain. However, small head size, small brain size, and retardation may result from severe malnutrition. The effect of in utero malnutrition on cerebral development is less well defined. With *feeding of malnourished infants* there may be a *rapid growth* in head circumference, with spreading of the sutures demonstrable on a skull film. This is thought to be catch-up growth secondary to increase in cell size. This catch-up growth may also be seen in the head growth of babies who are small for gestational age (SGA) (Fig. 22-11, *B*).

Achondroplasia is characterized by hypotonia, developmental delay, and an enlarged head. These infants consistently have a large head, greater than the ninety-seventh percentile. However, growth usually parallels the ninety-seventh percentile, and the infants do not exhibit a tense fontanel or dilated scalp veins characteristic of hydrocephalus. Air studies reveal only moderately dilated ventricles, and the infants rarely require shunting. Occasionally, the small foramen magnum does cause cervical cord compression and may interfere with CSF flow at the base. However, unless the rate of head growth continues to exceed the norm, the patient does not require evaluation or shunting. The marked hypotonia in these infants results in marked delay in the devel-

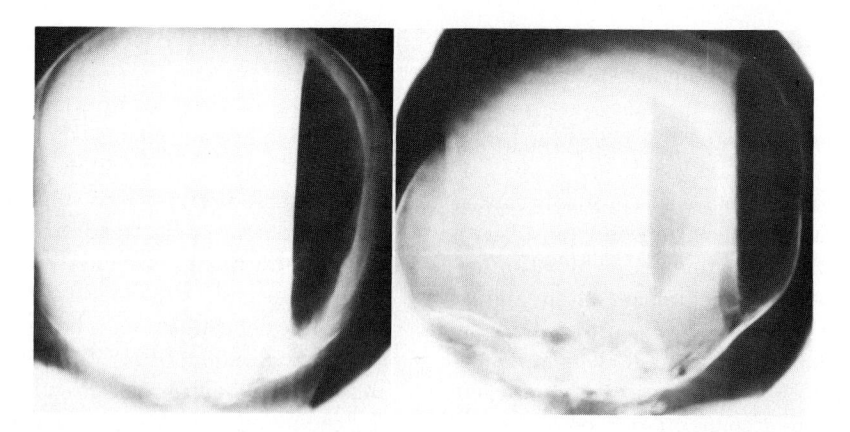

Fig. 22-13. Pneumoencephalogram of a newborn with congenital hydrocephalus. The ventricles are markedly enlarged with virtually no cortical mantle in the left parietooccipital area. The infant had aqueductal stenosis and a possible occlusion of the left posterior cerebral arteries. The infant was shunted at 2 days of age, and at 5 years had no demonstrable neurologic or psychologic deficit.

opment of motor milestones. However, these infants are rarely retarded.

Dwarfs and SGA babies may be seen in the neonatal period with what appears to be an enlarged head. It is important in these patients to measure head circumference in relation to gestational age and to follow the rate of head growth rather than rely on a single measurement.

Treatment

At the present time the definitive treatment for hydrocephalus is surgical but is less than satisfactory. It consists of shunting the fluid around the obstruction. Currently most shunts are placed from the cerebral ventricles into the peritoneum. The shunts consist of varying types of tubing, with variable types of openings at either end and several types of one-way valves.

The role of medical management of hydrocephalus is not clear at the present time, especially for posthemorrhagic hydrocephalus, which is an increasingly common problem in the infant following intraventricular hemorrhage. The exact role of serial lumbar puncture, a carbonic anhydrase inhibitor such as acetazolamide (Diamox), or osmotic agents such as sorbitol, is not clear with such infants. In view of the occurrence of spontaneous arrest and resolution of hydrocephalus in some infants, very careful observation of these infants with repeated CT scans or cranial ultrasound as well as clinical evaluations is indicated before surgical treatment is undertaken. If the hydrocephalus spontaneously arrests and ventricular dilatation subsides, further conservative care is indicated.

The success of shunting depends to a large extent on the experience and interest of the neurosurgeon. However, even in the best of hands, there are complications. The shunts may become infected at either end, although infants with thin cortical mantles may do exceedingly well (see further), infants with thicker cortical mantles do better.

Prognosis and follow-up care

Since shunting in infants with hydrocephalus carries the risks and complications just enumerated and is obviously palliative rather than curative, to estimate the prognosis one must understand the natural history of both treated and untreated hydrocephalus. Infants with uncomplicated hydrocephalus usually require shunting. In one randomized, controlled series, all but two of fifteen unoperated control patients ultimately required operation. Even those two seemed to have slowly progressive hydrocephalus. Spontaneous arrest of hydrocephalus undoubtedly does occur, but the true frequency is diffuclt to determine. Arrest of the process should be documented not by head circumference, but by ventricular size and cortical mantle thickness. Serial computerized axial tomography offers a better method of following the course of these infants and determining when true arrest occurs.

In cases of uncomplicated hydrocephalus the infants should be evaluated when the physician documents a progressive and definite increase in head circumference. At this time the ventricles are usually moderately dilated, but even marked thinning of the cortical mantle should not be a deterrent to operation. It has been shown that even when the cortical mantle is less than 10 mm in thickness, the prognosis may be good (Fig. 22-13). In one series, half the infants whose mantle was less than 10 mm in thickness at the time of operation had normal IQs.

Hydrocephalus associated with meningomyeloceles has a worse prognosis than hydrocephalus unassociated with spinal dysrhaphia. The reasons for this difference are not entirely clear. In one series, children with hydrocephalus and meningomyeloceles had only a 20% chance of reaching adulthood. The average IQ of the untreated survivors was less than 70. It is Lorber's recommendation that in hydrocephalus associated with meningomyelocele, if the cortical mantle is 26 to 35 mm in thickness, the patient should be watched, and only one third will require operation; whereas if the mantle thickness is less than 16 mm, operation urgently needs to be done.

Perhaps one of the differences between those in the meningomyelocele group and those in the uncomplicated hydrocephalus group is that the former are watched more closely. They are in the hospital from birth, and the physician is constantly following head size and performing definitive studies early. In this sense, perhaps we have been too vigorous and aggressive in the early diagnosis and treatment of complicated hydrocephalus. In uncomplicated hydrocephalus, patients are more likely to have large heads and definite ventricular dilatation.

Arrested hydrocephalus

Arrest of the hydrocephalic process after shunting has been defined as a cessation of head growth until the head reaches approximately the ninetieth percentile. Growth after that should parallel the normal curve. The fallacy in this definition is that ventricular enlargement with mild increase in pressure may occur without abnormal enlargement of the head. The cortex, therefore, may become markedly thin without evidence of increased intracranial pressure or increasing head size. children with arrested hydrocephalus often show impaired intellectual performance on reaching school age. These children may also decompensate acutely or die from infections or minor head trauma. Therefore children who have had shunts should be followed carefully with head size measurements and serial charting on appropriate graphs of head circumference; periodic computerized tomographic scanning or cranial ultrasonography also should be performed to assess the size of the ventricles and thickness of the cortical mantle. The physician also should be aware that, following the shunting procedure, collapse of the cortex may lead to subdural hematomas, which also can also produce enlargement of the head or increased pressure. In a child whose head continues to grow after shunting, subdural hematomas should be suspected.

The small head

Microcephaly, a small head, is always caused by microencephaly, a small brain, and the two terms have been used interchangeably. A small head circumference, *corrected for gestational age*, suggests the diagnosis. In the normally shaped head the occipital frontal circumference is an index of cranial volume; where the head shape is abnormal, as in certain forms of craniosynostosis, the head circumference is not a valid index of cranial volume and does not correlate with microcephaly.

Microcephaly has been defined as an occipital frontal circumference greater than 3SD below the mean, or less than the third percentile. It has generally been equated with mental retardation. The populations used in most studies of microcephaly have had mental retardation or neurologic handicap, and a correlation between the degree of microcephaly and the degree of mental handicap has been established. However, the incidence of microcephaly in the general population and the chance of an infant with a small head having a normal IQ are not known. Twenty-five percent of hypopituitary dwarfs with normal IQ were microcephalic. Normal intelligence was also measured in 40% of those infants born microcephalic after exposure to the atomic bomb as fetuses. There is also variation of head circumference with race and variation of the lower limit of normal head circumference within established norms. In one series of children seen because of neurologic or cognitive handicaps, 40% were found to be microcephalic, and 14% of the microcephalic children were found to have normal intelligence. Thus, although mental retardation is often associated with a small head, a small head does not necessarily mean retardation.

Microcephaly may be either congenital or acquired. Congenital microcephaly may follow intrauterine infections with rubella virus, cytomegalovirus, or congenital *Toxoplasma gondii* (Chapter 28). These infections may be apparent from chorioretinitis or the constellation of abnormalities seen with the rubella syndrome, or they may be inapparent and suggested by specific serologic testing for TORCH infections. Congenital microcephaly is also a part of many chromosomal abnormalities and of other syndromes.

One form of microcephaly is familial and inherited as an autosomal recessive trait. The characteristic appearance of children with this form of microcephaly consists of a normal body and face, with a markedly furrowed brow, a backward sloping of the forehead, and a very small cranial volume. This appearance usually serves to identify the familial form. Genetic counseling is indicated.

Acquired microcephaly may result from perinatal infections such as herpes simplex, from intrapartum and/or neonatal hypoxic-ischemic insults, and from metabolic causes, including aminoacidurias and hypothyroidism. In these patients the head circumference is normal at birth, but the rate of brain growth is impaired, with resultant microcephaly.

Each infant with microcephaly deserves a complete evaluation and determinations of the etiology if at all possible. This should include serologic studies for TORCH agent infections, skull x-ray films, and amino acid screening. The presence of other somatic abnormalities may lead to a chromosomal evaluation. Microcephaly must be differentiated from craniosynostosis (see further). There is no treatment for microcephaly, since it is secondary to microencephaly. In some instances, however, the microencephaly can be prevented.

ABNORMALITIES OF HEAD SHAPE

Abnormalities of head shape may occur in the newborn period and may require surgical intervention. These abnormalities include the large head with frontal bossing and distended veins seen in hydrocephalus, the large head with parietal bossing seen in chronic subdural hematomas, and the small head with furrowed brow and backward sloping forehead of familial microcephaly. The broad forehead with wide bridge of the nose and hypertelorism may suggest arhinencephaly and other disorders of midline cerebral structures. One of the most common entities causing abnormalities of head shape in the neonatal period is craniosynostosis (Chapter 38).

Craniosynostosis

Craniosynostosis is the premature closure of one or more of the cranial sutures. Since the suture closure and consequent head deformity usually occurs prenatally, diagnosis often can be made within the neonatal period. The fontanels as well as the sutures should be evaluated, since their presence or absence has great significance. The anterior fontanel normally closes between the tenth and sixteenth month of life; the posterior fontanel closes between the last 2 months before birth and the first 2 months following birth.

Etiology. The cause of primary (or congenital) craniosynostosis is unclear; it is thought to be a disorder of the membranous bones of the skull and not related to any local underlying growth failure of the brain. Postnatal or secondary craniosynostosis can result from rickets, hypophosphatasia, idiopathic hypercalcemia, or growth failure of the entire brain.

Pathophysiology. In the normal newborn the cranial bones are separate; however, during the first few hours or days of life the cranial bones override one another. This is easily detectable by palpating ridges and feeling the mobility of the bones in relation to one another. This mobility allows the circumference of the head to be molded or reduced in size as the cranial bones slide over one another during passage through the birth canal. Within several hours or days after birth the bones are no longer overriding. Soon after birth the definite sutures are established, and the edges of the flat bones are separated by fibrous tissue. Growth occurs perpendicular to the line of the suture.

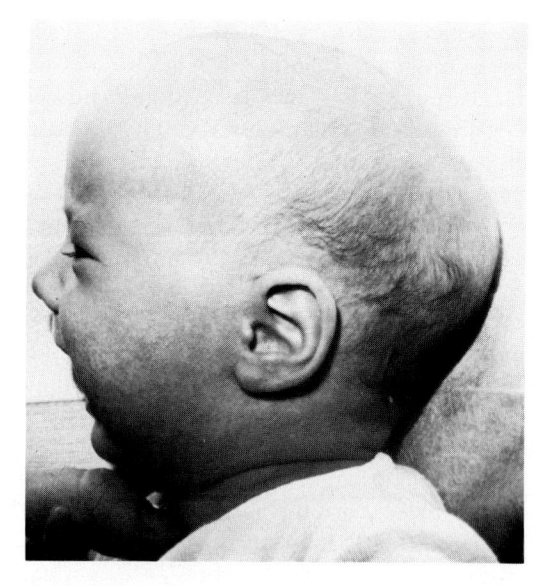

Fig. 22-14. Infant with posterior sagittal synostosis. Note the elongation of the posterior area of the skull, which was also narrow. Ridging of the posterior sagittal suture was present.

The principal sutures of the infant skull are the sagittal, coronal, lamboid, and metopic. Closure of a suture inhibits growth of the skull perpendicular to the fusion. The normal increase in brain volume requires expansion of the skull, which is forced to grow parallel to the fused suture. Deformity results from two factors: restriction of the growth of the vault at right angles to the involved suture and compensatory growth in the areas where the sutures are open. Closure of one of paired sutures results in inhibition of growth and flattening of the skull on that side. Closure of all sutures results in a marked distortion of skull shape as the brain expands through whatever fontanels are opened. Closure of sutures results in distortion of head shape if the underlying brain is normal. The small head with closed sutures whose shape is normal is the result of failure of the brain to grow. In these patients, closure of the sutures is secondary to failure of brain growth; failure of brain growth is not secondary to suture closure.

Sagittal synostosis

Sagittal synostosis is the most common form of craniosynostosis. It occurs predominantly in males and may be familial. It is seen in the neonatal period as a long, narrow head, scaphocephaly, whose circumference is often slightly greater than normal (Fig. 22-14). Sagittal synostosis is rarely associated with other somatic abnormalities and is uncommonly associated with ocular abnormalities, increased intracranial pressure, or mental retardation.

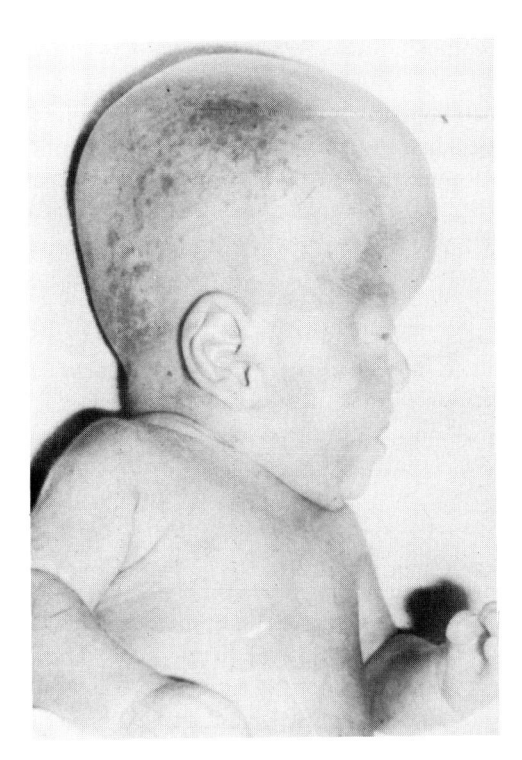

Fig. 22-15. Infant with Apert's syndrome. The shape of the head indicates closure of the lambdoid and coronal sutures. Deformities of the face are caused by closure of sutures at the base of the skull.

Operative correction (p. 384) is purely for cosmetic purposes. The time of closure of the sutures relative to the amount of cerebral growth remaining determines the degree of cosmetic deformity. Since correction is a cosmetic procedure, it is difficult to lay down firm guidelines for operation. There is also an undocumented suspicion that many scaphocephalic heads tend to assume spontaneously a more normal shape with time.

Coronal synostosis

Unilateral and bilateral coronal synostoses are approximately equal in incidence. Coronal synostosis usually is seen as a short broad head with an increase in height. The head circumference tends to be small, although the cranial volume may be normal. The orbits may be shallow and oblique, causing proptosis. Coronal synostosis occurs predominantly in females. There is a higher incidence of developmental abnormalities and associated mental retardation with this entity than with sagittal synostosis. The stenosis is commonly associated with closure of sutures at the base, giving an appearance similar to Crouzon's disease. The short anterior fossa may lead to angulation and compression of the optic nerve, with resultant optic atrophy. The cosmetic deformity produced by coronal stenosis is more severe than that with sagittal stenosis, but the operation is still cosmetic.

Unilateral coronal synostosis produces flattening of the forehead on the affected side and accentuation of the frontal bossing on the opposite side. The orbits may be at different levels, interfering with the development of binocular vision. For this reason, operation is usually indicated. Synostosis of one coronal suture may result in severe deformity with ipsilateral involvement of the face and orbit. Other complications are exophthalmos, strabismus, nystagmus, papilledema, optic atrophy, and loss of vision. Even more serious malformation and resultant complications are present in patients with bilateral coronal synotoses or in whom multiple sutures are involved.

Lambdoid stenosis

Premature closure of both lambdoid sutures produces a small, flattened occiput and often broadening and increased height of the skull. Unilateral closure produces flattening on the affected side. The flattening of the occiput in a child with unilateral closure must be differentiated from positional flattening (see further). The absence of a ridge over the lambdoidal suture and skull roentgenograms (Towne's view) should adequately differentiate these entities. Operation is cosmetic.

Metopic suture

Early closure of the metopic suture during intrauterine life may produce a keel-shaped deformity of the forehead. Operation for this deformity is purely cosmetic.

Multiple sutures

Closure of multiple sutures produces varied types of severe deformity of the head (Fig. 22-15). Since there is not sufficient room for expansion of the brain, increased intracranial pressure may occur, and operations should be carried out as early as possible. Although there is an increased incidence of mental retardation, many children with multiple suture closures have normal intelligence.

Diagnosis and treatment of craniosynostosis

Diagnosis. There are several physical findings that should alert the examining physician to suspect a diagnosis of premature craniosynostosis. These findings are an irregular or asymmetric skull, detection of one area where the overriding sutures cannot be felt, the inability of the physician to move the cranial bones in relation to one another in the early days of life, and a bony ridge along the suture line. Hypertelorism, difference in level or position of the eyes, ocular proptosis, strabismus, and optic atrophy also may be present. Signs and symptoms of increased intracranial pressure include funduscopic changes (Chapter 35), a cracked-pot percussion note of the skull too marked for age, bulging of any patent fontanel, and marked irritability.

Radiographic studies are essential to determine the status of the sutures, shape of the skull, skull base, and facial structures. The affected sutures may be totally obliterated or indicated by a thin radiolucent line. Frequently, there is thickening of bone along the suture, with bone bridging. It is important to recognize that the entire length of a given suture does not need to be involved. In the normal situation the suture closes from posterior to anterior (sagittal suture) and from lateral to medial (coronal sutures). In premature synostosis the closures occur in the same directions. Consequently, prompt diagnosis may be postponed because the portion of the suture best visualized by early radiographic examination may be normal. The *devil's eye configuration*, observed on the posteroanterior radiographic projection, results from the lateral elevation of the lesser wing of the sphenoid. This finding is a clue to unilateral (if it occurs on only one side) or to bilateral coronal synostoses. Radiographic evidence of increased intracranial pressure is manifested by excessive separation of the normal sutures or a beaten silver appearance of the skull.

The question of synostosis often arises when the anterior fontanel is thought to be too small or closed too soon. Frequently the suspicion proves to be correct. On the other hand, the anterior fontanel may be patent, even though the metopic, sagittal, or one or both coronal sutures are closed. Since the anterior fontanel is open in approximately 50% of patients with each type (sagittal and unilateral or bilateral coronal) of synostosis and with multiple suture closures, it is important not to be lulled into a false sense of security simply because the anterior fontanel remains patent.

Craniosynostosis may be an isolated defect or a component of a syndrome. When craniostenosis is suspected or proved, the pediatrician should be alerted to seek the presence of other malformations. Associated malformations include syndactyly, defects of elbow and knee joints, cardiac anomalies, and choanal atresia. Specific combinations, particularly those involving the limbs, constitute genetically distinct syndromes. The most common syndromes involving premature closure of the sutures are acrocephalosyndactyly (Apert's syndrome) and craniofacial dysostosis (Crouzon's disease). Apert's syndrome consists of acrocephaly, or pointing of the head anteriorly, irregular abnormalities of the sutures, midfacial hypoplasia, and syndactyly of the hands and, occasionally, of the feet. In this syndrome the coronal suture is primarily involved, although other sutures may be involved as well. Crouzon's disease includes shallow orbits and maxillary hypoplasia as well as premature craniosynostosis, especially of the coronal, lambdoidal, and sagittal sutures. Mental deficiency has been reported more frequently in Apert's syndrome than in Crouzon's disease.

Differential diagnosis. The differential diagnosis of the varied deformities of craniosynostosis should rarely present a problem. A small, normally shaped head with closure of the sutures always represents primary microencephaly and never requires surgery. Confusion of the distorted head shapes comes mainly from the positional flattenings. The long, narrow head of the premature infant is the result of the infant's lying on his side. The roentgenogram shows no ridging of the sagittal suture and no fusion of that suture. Unilateral occipital flattening may be the result of unilateral lambdoidal stenosis. More commonly, it is positional, resulting from an infant's lying one one side of his occiput. Torticollis and bed position relative to light and activity may play a role. Often flattening is seen when there is a lack of interest in the environment, and the infant lies on the occiput with little movement. Occipital flattening should alert the physician to the possibility of developmental delay. The absence of ridging of the sutures and x-ray studies should serve to differentiate positional flattening from lambdoidal stenosis.

Treatment. The surgery for craniosynostosis is cosmetic except where multiple sutures are involved. There is little or no indication that these patients develop increased intracranial pressure; there is no evidence that the mental retardation sometimes associated with suture closure can be prevented by operation; and there is no evidence that operation prevents the optic atrophy sometimes seen with coronal stenosis. There is general agreement that the constricting effect of total synostosis on the otherwise normal brain will cause increased intracranial pressure during the period of rapid brain growth and produce brain damage.

Cosmetic indications for surgery are difficult to evaluate, particularly since the operation should ideally be done before 6 months of age, preferably between the second and third month. The operation is thus a prophylactic cosmetic operation, and a skilled and experienced neurosurgeon can often restore normal appearance to the infant's head.

The technique of operation involves creating new sutures parallel to the fused suture. It is important that the newly created sutures cross two suture lines (that is, in coronal stenosis the new suture must cross both the sagittal and squamosal sutures). If two sutures are not crossed, then the newly created suture will not allow sufficient expansion to correct the cosmetic deformity. The new suture line must be treated with phenol or lined with an inert material to prevent refusion. In Shillito's hands the mortality at the operation was only 0.4%; there was a 14% morbidity from wound infections, cardiac arrests, leptomeningeal cysts, and anesthetic complica-

Central nervous system disturbances 385

tions. It is against these risks that the cosmetic indications must be weighed.

DEVELOPMENTAL ABNORMALITIES
Defects in closure of the neuraxis

During the third and fourth weeks of gestation, differentiation of the neural plate occurs, with invagination and dorsal closure to form the neural tube. The neural tube gives rise to the central nervous system, and neural crest cells that form during the process of closure give rise to dorsal root ganglia, sensory ganglia of cranial nerves, and autonomic ganglia. Initially the neural tube closes in the region of the medulla and then proceeds, in a zipperlike fashion, rostrally and caudally. Interruption of the process of closure results in a variety of midline defects, from the cranium down to the lowest level of spinal cord. Because mesodermal differentiation into the dura and vertebrae and cranium surrounding the differentiating neural tube occurs as an interaction of the neural tube with surrounding mesoderm, defects in closure of the neural tube involve neural elements and their coverings, including meninges and overlying bony structures. Defects in closure of the neuraxis result in the most common major structural developmental abnormalities of the newborn central and peripheral nervous systems. See Chapter 37 for prenatal diagnosis.

Classification of abnormalities of closure of the spinal cord—spina bifidas

Defects in closure of the spinal canal, termed spina bifidas, may be associated with abnormalities of the cord and meninges of varying severity. They are classified below.

Meningocele. Meningocele is a cystic dilatation of the meninges associated with spina bifida and a defect of the overlying skin. The spinal cord and nerve roots are normal. There is no neurologic deficit.

Meningomyelocele. Meningomyelocele is a lesion identical to the meningocele but with associated abnormalities of the spinal cord and nerve roots. There is neurologic deficit below the level of the lesion. The extent of the deficit depends on the location of the lesion (see further).

Myeloschisis (spina bifida aperta). This is a spina bifida with exposure of the spinal cord and roots and with no cystic covering of meninges. This defect may be small or may extend the whole length of the spinal axis. The clinical significance is identical to that of meningomyelocele.

Spina bifida occulta. This is nonfusion of one or more posterior arches of the spine, usually lumbosacral. A common abnormality found at L5 in 30% of adults, it is of consequence only when associated with underlying

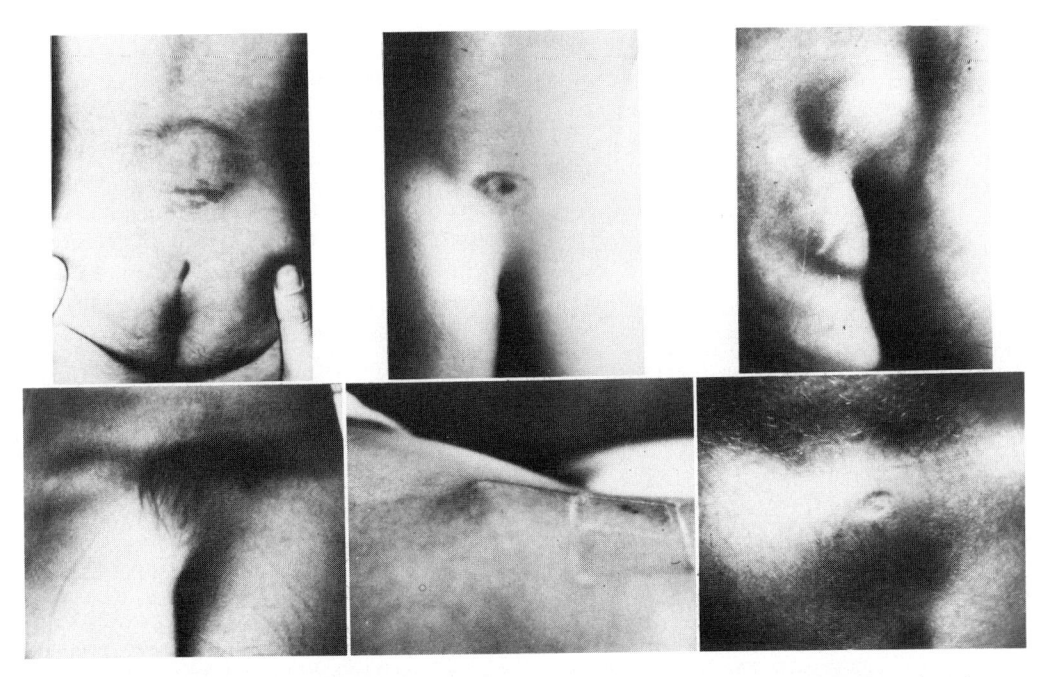

Fig. 22-16. Lesions of the back associated with spina bifida occulta and spinal cord problems. *Top: Left*, Lipoma with hairy patch above hemangioma; *center*, hemangioma; *right*, lipoma. All had tethered cords and intradural lipomas. *Bottom: Left*, Patch of fine hair; *center*, bony spur; *right*, midline scar. Defects shown at bottom left and center were associated with diastematomyelia.

abnormalities or when found at other levels. Significant associated abnormalities are usually signaled by a hemangioma, a patch of abnormal hair, a dimple, or a lipoma in the lumbosacral area (Fig. 22-16). The underlying abnormalities include diastematomyelia, spinal lipomas or dermoids, and dermal sinuses (p. 388).

Embryology

One of the more recent theories suggests that damage to ectoderm produces a bleb of fluid from the neural cleft, which results in embryonic scarring. The degree of damage to ectodermal and mesodermal tissue and the success of the healing and scarring process determine the resultant defect.

Meningomyeloceles and myeloschisis

Clinical manifestations. The degree of neurologic deficit associated with these defects is determined by the level of the lesion. Accurate diagnosis and prognosis for ambulation can be determined to a large degree at birth by careful sensory and motor testing of the infant. The sensory level, in general, gives an approximation of the motor level in these children (Table 22-3) but may be several segments lower. The prognosis can be predicted with a high degree of certainty at birth (Table 22-4), thus helping with the evolution of plans for therapy.

Table 22-3. Motor examination of lower extremities in children with meningomyeloceles

Movement	Lumbar	Sacral	Muscle
Hip			
Flexion	1, 2, 3, 4		Iliopsoas, rectus femoris
Adduction	2, 3, 4		Adductors
Adduction	4, 5	1	Gluteus medius
Extension	4, 5	1, 2	Gluteus maximus, obturator
Knee			
Extension	2, 3, 4		Quadriceps
Flexion	5	1, 2	Hamstrings
Foot			
Dorsiflexion	4, 5	1	Tibialis anterior
Plantar flexion	5	1, 2	Soleus, gastrocnemius

Treatment. A newborn with a meningomyelocele presents the pediatrician with difficult decisions about what to tell parents and whether to recommend surgical closure of the defect. Closure, although usually not technically difficult, carries significant implications. It greatly increases the chances of the infant's survival, but in doing so it initiates an obligation for total care of the child. This places a considerable emotional and financial burden on the family for the numerous operations and the rehabilitation that will be required. It also involves appreciable suffering for the infant. Furthermore, the decision to operate must be made promptly, for there is reasonable evidence to suggest that the operation should take place within the first 24 hours to prevent further deterioration of the spinal cord and roots.

Numerous factors may influence the decision. These should include the size of the lesion and the technical feasibility of closure, the location of the lesion and the prognosis for ambulation of the child, the presence or absence of associated abnormalities (such as hydrocephalus, kyphosis, or other major structural abnormalities), the presence of personnel and facilities to provide adequate care for the infant, and the infant's family structure and the attitudes of the family toward the defect and its consequences. Keeping these factors in mind, the physician must weigh the consequences of the following three possible courses of action.

1. *Immediate closure of the defect.* If the defect is closed immediately, the infant will have approximately a 90% chance of survival. The chance of developing hydrocephalus requiring repetitive shunt procedures will depend on the site of the lesion (Table 22-4). Urologic involvement will occur in about 90%. Fecal soiling can be controlled with rigorous management. Orthopedic care involving braces and transplants of muscles, tendons, and cortex will depend on the site of the lesion, as will the prognosis for ambulation. Psychologic help and social-work assistance will be required for these children. Closure of the defect obligates the physician and society to provide optimum care in each of these areas for the survivors. Despite this care, the function of the child with spinal cord involvement will only approximate nor-

Table 22-4. Deficit and prognosis of meningomyeloceles as related to site of lesion

Motor/sensory level	Maximum motor deficit	Prognosis for ambulation	Risk of hydrocephalus
L5-S1	Dorsiflexion and plantar flexion of feet, weakness of glutei	Will ambulate with or without short leg braces; outlook good	60%
L3-L4	Involvement of quadriceps and hamstrings, plus above	May be able to ambulate with long leg braces and crutches; paralytic hip dislocation	86%
L1 and L2 or above	Complete paraplegia	No functional ambulation	96%

mal, the degree of normality depending primarily on the severity of the original lesion.

2. *Passive euthanasia.* Many physicians faced with an infant with a meningomyelocele wish that the problem would go away. However, it has been said that the problem does not go away; only the physician goes away. Even if these infants receive no treatment, 15% to 30% of them will survive. Feeding, antibiotics, and care of the sac will each increase the quantity of survivors without affecting their quality. Figures on the natural history of untreated meningomyeloceles are difficult to find. One series suggests that 40% are stillborn or die within the first week of life. Forty percent of the survivors die by 2 months of age, another 30% die by 2 years of age, and 30% survive. Causes of death are not listed, but many of the late deaths are related to neurologic deterioration secondary to hydrocephalus and to renal deterioration secondary to the neurogenic bladder. Death may occur soon after birth, but for many, death occurs weeks, months, or years later. Thus lack of therapy results in fewer infants surviving while still allowing the survival of a number of infants who are less functionally able to compete than if they had received therapy.

3. *Active euthanasia.* This solution to the problem has many moral objections and is currently illegal.

Most children with a meningomyelocele should have active comprehensive therapy. The use of such therapy will not alter the degree of paralysis, but with a vigorous team approach most children will lead happy, useful lives. With normal intelligence these children can be in regular schools despite their paralysis. This course of action is better for the child, the family, and society than providing no therapy and awaiting the child's death.

Management. The quality of survival is paramount, and the preservation of existing function in the lower extremities requires early operation to close the spinal defect. Where a high lesion has produced complete paraplegia, early operation does little to improve the quality of survival; the hydrocephalus and the neurogenic bladder will require treatment at the appropriate time. Although closure of the spinal defect takes initial precedence, evaluation of the hydrocephalus and of the renal and bladder status and orthopedic consultation should all take place in the early weeks of life.

An infant born with a meningomyelocele should be transferred immediately to the care of a physician experienced in dealing with the problem. The decision of whether to operate on these infants requires someone who has worked with and followed the course of such infants. The techniques of closure and exploration of the sac may require both neurosurgeons and plastic surgeons, and an orthopedic surgeon may be needed at the initial operation to deal with spinal anomalies. Both survival itself and the quality of that survival may be determined during this neonatal period. After closure of the sac, the infant's course must be closely followed for the progression of existing hydrocephalus. Hydrocephalus may cause bulging of the wound and its breakdown, as

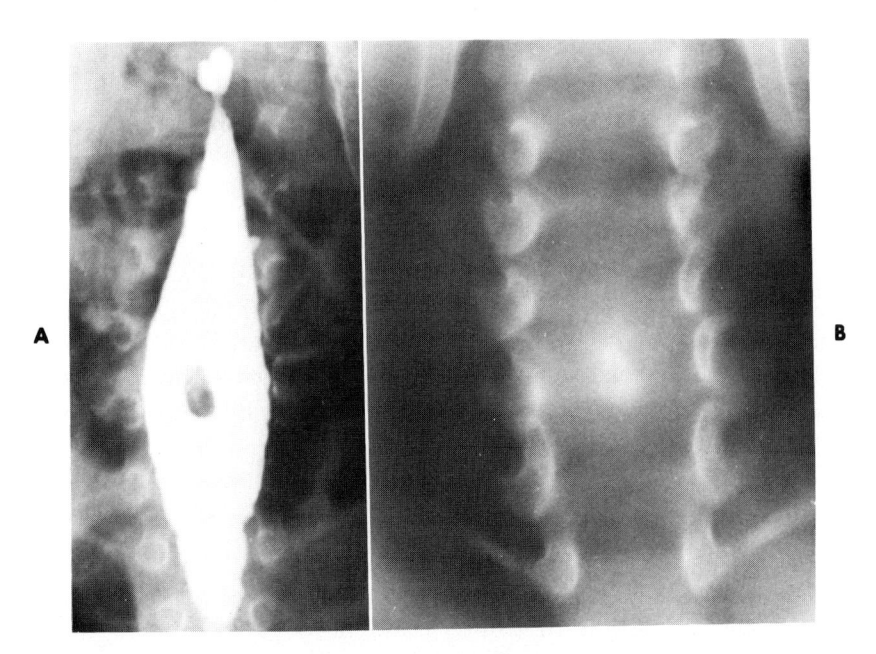

Fig. 22-17. A, Tomogram of the spine of an infant with diastematomyelia. The bony spur protruding through the spinal canal and widening of the canal at that area is shown. **B,** Myelogram of the same patient. The spinal cord split around the spur and refused. Same patient as in Fig. 22-15, bottom center. The patient was asymptomatic.

well as thinning of the cortex. Evaluation and shunting for hydrocephalus are discussed on p. 380. An intravenous pyelogram and voiding cystourethrogram also should be performed as soon as feasible in the neonatal period. Hydronephrosis may be present at birth, and urinary tract infection may be a continuing problem.

Diastematomyelia

Diastematomyelia is a division of the spinal cord or roots by a bony spicule or fibrous or cartilaginous band that pierces the cord in an anteroposterior direction. This lesion is often associated with a spina bifida occulta at one or more levels and is usually accompanied by a cutaneous lesion such as a hemangioma, a patch of long, fine hair, a lipoma, or a dimple (Fig. 22-16).

At birth there is no neurologic deficit associated with the diastematomyelia; but as the infant grows, the spinal cord is not able to ascend because of the bone. Traction on the spinal cord produces neurologic deficit. The deficit may range from persistent enuresis to a neurogenic bladder with hydronephrosis. Pain in the legs, weakness, or growth failure of a foot or leg all may be later manifestations. The cutaneous manifestations should suggest the diagnosis. Spine films show a spina bifida and usually widening of the canal. A midline bony defect confirms the diagnosis (Fig. 22-17). Infants with cutaneous lesions should be followed every 2 to 3 months. A myelogram needs to be done if any neurologic deficit appears. Treatment consists of removal of the bony spicule and release of any tethering of the spinal cord. The operation is prophylactic rather than curative; an established neurologic deficit may be permanent.

Dermal sinuses and dermoids

Dermal sinuses may occur anywhere along the midline of the back or head but are most common in the occipital area of the skull and in the lumbar region. The sinus is 1 to 2 mm in diameter and may be accompanied by hemangioma or a tuft of hair. These sinuses are to be differentiated from the common superficial dimples seen at the upper end of the gluteal crease. The dermal sinus may extend variable depths into the skin and may continue into the intraspinal space. This lesion should be ruled out on the initial newborn examination. In some cases the sinus has passed unnoticed until it shows redness and swelling associated with infection or is carefully looked for in the patient with meningitis. Roentgenograms of the spine may show a spina bifida, and there may be widening of the spinal canal if an associated dermoid or lipoma is present. If a sinus is associated with meningitis or with superficial infection or if there is neurologic deficit, the sinus must be removed. Excision should follow the sinus tract to its end. Since intraspinous hematomas may be at the end of a dermal sinus in a significant number of cases, laminectomy may be necessary to remove the tumor.

Lipomas

Lipomeningoceles are large, amorphous accumulations of fatty tissue beneath the skin that may be associated with meningeal defects and may resemble meningomyeloceles. Smaller subcutaneous lipomas may be associated with spina bifida occulta. They may occur at any level of the subcutaneous tissue and may involve the cord itself. It is the intraspinal extensions of these lipomas that become neurologically significant. Widening of the spinal canal shown on a roentgenogram or the development of a neurologic defect suggests the intraspinal process. Operation should be prophylactic, and, as in diastematomyelia, neurologic deficit may not be reversible. Therefore these infants must be followed frequently and surgery performed at the earliest sign of neurologic involvement.

Encephaloceles

Encephalocele is the name given to cranial anomalies that are similar to the spina bifidas. The term includes craniomeningoceles, encephalomeningoceles, and cranium bifidas. These lesions may occur anywhere along the midline of the head, including the nose, the nasopharynx, and the orbit, but are most common in the occipital area. It usually is not possible to determine the extent of brain involvement before surgery. The size of the lesion should not be a deterrent to surgery, since large lesions may be meningoceles, or small lesions may contain cerebral tissue. Roentgenograms of the defect, ultrasound, computerized axial tomography, and ventriculograms or pneumoencephalograms are indicated before surgery. Surgery should be undertaken as soon as feasible in the neonatal period to prevent infection and to facilitate care and feeding of the child. Operation is similar to that undertaken for closure of the back in meningomyeloceles. These children should be evaluated for other structural anomalies of the cervical spine or back and should be followed closely in the postoperative period for the development of hydrocephalus and neurologic signs or symptoms. Prognosis for encephalocele is poor.

SEIZURES

Seizures are the most frequent and distinct neurologic sign occurring in the neonatal period and result in the most requests for neurologic consultation and evaluation. They may represent primary central nervous system disease or be manifestations of systemic or metabolic insults. The incidence of seizures in the newborn varies, depending on the population, that is, full-term or preterm infants, and the time of onset, that is, first week or first month of life. Estimates of frequency of seizures in the newborn vary from as low as 0.8% of an entire nursery population to 20% in an intensive care unit of sick preterm infants. Seizures at this time represent a relative medical emergency, since they are usually the signal of a life-threatening underlying disease or disorder that can produce irreversible brain damage. Furthermore, experimental evidence suggests that seizure activity in the immediate postnatal period, a time of both active myelination and continuing cell division, may result in reduction in DNA content and brain cell number. It is therefore important to diagnose and treat neonatal seizures and their underlying causes with great dispatch.

Clinical manifestations

Seizures in the older child are classified by their clinical manifestation and at times by their site of origin, since both may have etiologic, therapeutic, and prognostic implications. Seizure phenomena in the newborn differ greatly from those observed in older infants and children in that only rarely will newborns have well-organized symmetrical generalized tonic-clonic seizures. The explanation for these differences is related to the status of the neuroanatomic and physiologic organization of the neonatal brain referred to later. Various neonatal seizure manifestations follow:

A. Abnormal movements or alterations of tone in trunk and extremities
 1. Fragmentary clonic—multifocal, migratory (non-jacksonian)
 2. Alternating hemiclonic
 3. Tonic
    a. Single extremity
    b. Extension of arms and legs (decerebrate)
    c. Extension of legs, flexion of arms (decorticate)
 4. Myoclonic—isolated or generalized
 5. Bicycling movements of legs
 6. Rowing or drum-beating movements of arms
 7. Loss of tone with generalized flaccidity
 8. Generalized tonic-clonic
B. Facial, oral, lingual movements
 1. Sucking
 2. Grimacing, twitching
 3. Chewing, swallowing, yawning
C. Ocular movements
 1. Tonic horizontal eye deviation
 2. Staring, blinking
 3. Nystagmoid jerks
D. Respiratory manifestations
 1. Apnea, usually preceded or accompanied by one of the other subtle manifestations of seizures
 2. Hyperpneic or stertorous breathing

In addition to these very specific clinical manifestations, any alteration in the state of the infant that is "on-off" in character and is repetitive or paroxysmal in occurrence may be a seizure. Such activity must be differentiated from tremors (p. 353) as well as from decerebrate or decorticate posturing indicative of progressive rostrocaudal pressure and herniation. This can be a difficult distinction, even for the experienced clinician.

Pathophysiology

A seizure requires that the synchronous firing of adjacent neurons reach a critical mass to produce clinical manifestations. Epileptic neurons recruit adjacent neurons to fire synchronously and thereby produce a seizure. Although the neonatal cortex has a relatively complete complement of neurons, there is a relative paucity of dendrites and synaptic connections, with the neuropile having not yet reached its full stage of growth and complexity. The neuronal membranes are leaky and allow sodium to enter and potassium to exit from the cell far more easily than from more mature membranes. With the level of sodium-potassium ATP well below mature levels, the cell is less able to pump out sodium efficiently and become repolarized. Thus the newborn's neurons remain relatively hyperpolarized, making it more difficult for the epileptic neuron to have rapid and repetitive firing and to permit recruitment of other neurons for synchronous discharge. These reasons primarily account for the infrequency of cortical seizures in the newborn. The temporal lobe and subcortical structures are more mature and therefore better able to sustain epileptic activity and produce a clinical seizure. This may explain the propensity of the newborn to have such temporal lobe and subcortical manifestations of seizures as grimacing, chewing, repetitive swallowing, staring, or altered respiratory rhythm.

Etiology

There are a variety of causes of neonatal seizures, and for many of the causes there is a specific treatment. Therefore determining the cause of seizures is critical. Etiologies are determined on the basis of historical data, physical findings, and clinical observations, plus a variety of laboratory tests and observation of clinical response to various therapeutic measures.

Asphyxia is the most frequent cause of seizures in the full-term infant. Seizures occur not only in those infants whose asphyxia is evident at birth, but also in infants whose asphyxia occurred prior to delivery, which may not have been documented by fetal monitoring. At times seizures caused by asphyxia may also be associated with subarachnoid bleeding, but this is not invariable. The incidence of seizures in asphyxiated infants is reported to vary between 22% and 60%. They most commonly begin early, between 6 and 18 hours of life. Seizures in severely asphyxiated infants are among the most difficult of seizures to control and in general carry the poorest prognosis of all neonatal seizures.

Intracranial hemorrhage has historically been considered the most common cause of neonatal convulsions, with the frequent implication that birth trauma was the primary event. Subarachnoid bleeding may be due to trauma but is also common with asphyxia. It is difficult to separate the asphyxial insult from the subarachnoid bleeding as the cause of seizures. Furthermore, small amounts of subarachnoid bleeding are frequently noted in infants who have a single seizure on the second or third day of life, who in all other respects appear well and who have a good prognosis. Seizures have also been reported by some to be extremely common in small preterm infants with intraventricular hemorrhage. Intraventricular hemorrhage has been cited as the cause of the vast majority of seizures in infants weighing less than 2,500 gm. In other studies, however, only 11% of infants with intraventricular hemorrhage diagnosed and documented by CT scan have had seizures; these seizures occurred almost entirely in those infants with marked degrees of hemorrhage. Abnormal movements other than seizures also may occur in the infant with intraventricular hemorrhage; decerebrate or opisthotonic posturing due to extensive rostrocaudal pressure and brain stem herniation may occur in such infants, and these movements should be distinguished from seizure activity, particularly by the other associated clinical findings. Seizures occurring in infants with subdural bleeding are not infrequent, although subdural bleeding is a rather rare event in the neonate at the present time. Seizures occurring in the infant with subdural hemorrhage are more likely to be caused by the associated traumatic cerebral contusion producing the bleeding than by the blood in the subdural space.

Infectious causes of neonatal seizures include sepsis, meningitis, TORCH agent infections, and Coxsackie B encephalitis. The mechanism by which sepsis is associated with neonatal seizures is unclear, but the association is real. Seizures occur in approximately 55% of infants with neonatal meningitis, whether caused by group B streptococci, gram-negative organisms, or *Listeria* species. Of the TORCH agents causing neonatal seizures, herpesvirus is particularly important, since it is the only TORCH agent that does not produce subclinical or silent CNS infection. Seizures in congenital herpes infection may occur with generalized disseminated herpetic infection or in association with localized infection primarily involving skin, eye, or oral mucosa, with additional involvement of brain. Infants with generalized systemic disease have evidence of multiple organ involvement in addition to seizures. The viral infection in the CNS may be associated with only a single or few herpetic vesicles on the scalp at the site of a fetal scalp monitor, on an extremity, on the buttocks in association with breech presentation, or in the eye.

Coxsackie B encephalitis may occur as an isolated infection or in neonatal epidemics resulting in seizures and at times myocarditis.

Hypoglycemia is a cause of neonatal seizures that, if untreated, may lead to acute brain damage. Transient hypoglycemia is particularly likely to occur in association with asphyxia in the stressed low birth weight infant (p. 72). In general, hypoglycemia as a direct cause of seizures is no longer a major problem in most neonatal units because of the emphasis that has been given (1) to the frequent use of Dextrostix and blood glucose determinations for detection of infants at risk prior to seizure occurrence, (2) to early provision of supplemental intravenous glucose to infants at risk, and (3) to careful monitoring of blood glucose following identification of hypoglycemia and initiation of appropriate treatment. Most important is the necessity of continuing monitoring for possible recurrence of hypoglycemia, after it has been detected and treated, because of the possiblity of hypoglycemia recurring without resultant further seizures. There are increasing numbers of infants with persisting hypoglycemia caused by identifiable disorders producing hyperinsulinism, such as nesidioblastosis or islet cell adenoma with inborn metabolic defects. Any infant who is not being weaned from intravenous glucose initiated for hypoglycemia by 7 to 10 days should be considered a candidate for one of the above-mentioned disorders.

Hypocalcemia, with serum calcium levels of less than 7.5 mg/dl and phosphorus levels greater than 8 mg/dl, may occur early in association with hypoglycemia in the stressed or asphyxiated low birth weight infant (Chapter 33, part two). Despite this association, it is rarely the cause of seizures at that time. More commonly, hypocalcemia is a cause of seizures in the older infant, after the fifth day of life, particularly in the mature formula-fed infant. Maternal hyperparathyroidism caused by parathyroid adenoma should be considered in such instances. The DiGeorge phenotype may on rare occasion be recognized in infants with hypocalcemia and seizures after the first week of life, and hypocalcemia that persists may be due to chronic idiopathic hypoparathyroidism, which can occur in infancy and which requires further laboratory tests for verification. Hypomagnesemia as a cause of neonatal convulsions is extremely uncommon and, when it does occur, is usually associated with hypocalcemia. Fewer than 10% of infants with hypomagnesemia have normal calcium levels. Hypomagnesemia as a cause of seizures should be considered in a patient whose hypocalcemic seizures did not clear after the hypocalcemia was corrected.

Hyponatremia may be a cause of neonatal seizures in infants born of toxemic mothers who were given not only salt-poor diets but also extremely hypotonic intravenous fluids during labor, such as 5% dextrose in water (p. 27). Associated symptoms in the symptomatic newborn with hyponatremia include lethargy, irritability, and tremors. The seizures may be refractory to treatment. Increasingly, hyponatremia is being identified in high-risk neonates in whom seizures are secondary to the syndrome of inappropriate secretion of antidiuretic hormone (SIADH). SIADH may occur with CNS diseases such as meningitis or asphyxial encephalopathy, with intraventricular hemorrhage, or in the presence of pulmonary atelectasis and pneumothorax.

Hypernatremia in the sick preterm infant may be seen frequently when the infant is being given care under an open radiant warmer. Evaporative fluid losses can be quite high, producing hypernatremia. In addition, hypernatremia may be a result of iatrogenic factors, such as incorrect administration of sodium-containing parenteral fluids, including sodium bicarbonate, the inadvertent substitution of mislabeled intravenous solutions, or the substitution of table salt for sugar in formula preparation.

Neonatal drug withdrawal (Chapter 33, part five) is manifested by tremulousness, irritability, and seizures. It may occur following chronic maternal administration of narcotics, including methadone and pentazocine (Talwin), analgesics such as propoxyphene (Darvon), sedatives, including ethchlorvynol (Placidyl), hydroxyzine hydrochloride (Atarax), and barbiturates. Seizures are seen less commonly than tremulousness and constant agitation and generally occur after the first 48 hours of life.

Disorders of amino acid and ketoacid metabolism that may initially manifest as seizures include maple syrup urine disease, nonketotic hyperglycinemia, and methylmalonic acidemia. Other commonly associated findings are hypotonia, feeding difficulties, and severe metabolic acidosis with ketonuria. These disorders are the only inheritable disorders that usually present in the neonatal period. Hyperbilirubinemia should now be an extremely uncommon cause of neonatal seizures because of the early diagnosis and treatment of this condition. However, seizures will occur in approximately half of infants with kernicterus. Seizures present immediately following delivery and extremely refractory to anticonvulsant therapy have been caused by intoxication of infants by maternal anesthetic agents, such as mepivacaine, that were inadvertently injected into the infant by a misplaced catheter and needle at the time of caudal anesthesia; or they were caused by high local concentrations of mepivacaine at the time of paracervical block anesthesia.

Pyridoxine dependency is a rare cause of neonatal seizures that may occur in utero or in immediate postnatal life and may be familial. The primary defect may be a deficiency in binding of the coenzyme pyridoxal phosphate to glutamic decarboxylase, the enzyme involved in the formation of gamma-aminobutyric acid (GABA). The absence of GABA, a presumed CNS inhibitor, could produce seizures. Such seizures can be immediately controlled after intravenous injection of 25 to 50 mg of pyridoxine.

Seizures caused by congenital cerebral malformations may begin in the neonatal period but rarely in the first several days. The diagnosis of the malformation may be suspected on the basis of abnormal facies, small or large head size, or multiple congenital anomalies. However, in otherwise normal appearing infants the anomalies may be evident only by special roentgenographic techniques, such as computed tomography, cranial ultrasonography, or rarely with transillumination alone.

Diagnosis

Each infant must be considered to have a potentially treatable disease, regardless of antecedent history. Important historical data should be obtained from the mother's chart and from the mother herself, and one should also be aware of the availability of illicit drugs, any drugs she may have been taking at her physician's direction, and her prior obstetric history. History of previously affected newborn infants should also be obtained. Intrapartum monitoring may provide significant data regarding the possibility of intrauterine asphyxia, although the infant at birth may not have low Apgar scores, since some infants with hypoxic ischemic encephalopathy with seizures suffer their asphyxial insult prior to birth.

The day on which seizures begin may also be a clue to etiology. For example, stressed low birth weight infants with first-day seizures are more likely to have hypoglycemia and hypocalcemia. Neonatal seizures due to intracranial infection are more frequent after the first 48 hours. Seizures due to hypoxic ischemic encephalopathy most commonly begin within 12 hours of birth and become progressively more frequent and severe during the next 24 to 48 hours. Seizures beginning after the fifth day of life are more likely related to classic hypocalcemia, congenital development defects, or TORCH infections. Such temporal relationships are not invariable but may be helpful in diagnostic evaluation.

Every infant with seizures must be screened for systemic and intracranial infection with immediate blood culture and lumbar puncture. Analysis of spinal fluid should include smear with Gram stain, glucose and protein determinations, and erythrocyte and differential leukocyte counts. Even in the presence of blood in spinal fluid, presumably the result of a traumatic tap, the fluid should be centrifuged and xanthochromia looked for, as evidence of prior subarachnoid blood. If adequate spinal

Table 22-5. Dosages of anticonvulsants for the neonate

Drug	Dosage for loading	Dosage for maintenance	Route of administration
Phenobarbital	20 mg/kg	5 mg/kg/day	IV; maintenance can be given IM or PO
Phenytoin	15-20 mg/kg	3-5 mg/kg/day	IV only; do not administer at rate faster than 50 mg/minute
Paraldehyde	4%-8% solution	Not used for maintenance	IV

fluid is obtained, erythrocyte counts should be compared in the first and third or fourth tubes.

Immediate skull roentgenograms are rarely of value. Although not every infant with seizures requires complex roentgenographic evaluation, CT scans may be helpful in revealing subependymal or intraventricular hemorrhage or subdural blood. Postasphyxial or hypoxic ischemic encephalopathy may also be manifested by striking alterations of cerebral perfusion evident on enhanced CT scans or as areas of diminished attenuation or density on nonenhanced scans obtained 5 to 7 days after the asphyxial event. CT scans also may identify intracranial calcifications caused by congenital TORCH infections, even when these are not evident on skull roentgenograms. Cranial ultrasound appears to have similar diagnostic potential in the neonate, and it is indicated, if available, for all newborns with seizures.

An electroencephalogram (EEG) may confirm the diagnosis of seizures through the correlation of the paroxysmal electrical discharge with the clinical manifestations. However, an EEG is rarely helpful in determination of the cause of seizures, except in the very rare example of pyridoxine-dependent seizures; infants with this problem with profoundly abnormal paroxysmal electrical activity on EEG will have almost immediate normalization of the EEG, as well as seizure cessation, following intravenous injection of pyridoxine. Despite the availability of EEG laboratories in almost all hospitals and recently published EEG standards in the term and preterm infant, very few EEG laboratories will have their records interpreted by knowledgeable pediatric electroencephalographers. The EEG may, however, be more helpful in determination of prognosis.

Treatment

While the physician is awaiting results of laboratory tests and reviewing historical data and physical findings, treatment should be administered. There is no reason to withhold treatment for seizures until after EEG, CT scan, or ultrasound examination has been completed. After initial determination of blood glucose level by Dextrostix, if hypoglycemia is present, 10% glucose is given intravenously, 4 to 9 ml/kg (p. 864), and this should be continued with constant pump infusion of a 10% to 15% glucose solution, depending on response to therapy and further blood glucose determinations. If hypocalcemia is documented or highly suspected, calcium gluconate is given intravenously as a 5% solution, in a dosage of 200 mg/kg or 4 ml/kg.

The dosage of anticonvulsants in the neonatal period is shown in Table 22-5. Phenobarbital is the initial drug of choice, effective not only in controlling status but also protective against recurrent seizures. The initial loading dosage of phenobarbital is 20 mg/kg to achieve effective plasma levels in the range of 20 µg/ml. Daily maintenance dosage of phenobarbital of 5 mg/kg/day will not result in excessive accumulation of phenobarbital or sedation, and this should be started within 24 hours after the initial loading dose. If phenobarbital is not effective in terminating seizures, phenytoin (Dilantin) should be administered intravenously, 15 to 20 mg/kg, at a rate of injection not to exceed 50 mg/minute. This will achieve therapeutic levels of between 10 and 20 µg/ml in the neonate. Following this the phenytoin maintenance dosage is 3 to 4 mg/kg/day. These maintenance doses must be administered intravenously, since the newborn infant does not absorb oral phenytoin with a predictable result. Intramuscular phenytoin injections not only result in unpredictable plasma concentrations because of poor absorption, but also the drug is irritating and may form crystals following intramuscular injection.

For seizures that persist despite intravenous phenobarbital and phenytoin, paraldehyde may be administered intravenously as a 4% to 8% solution. This is both safe and effective, and the limiting factor for paraldehyde is usually the volume of fluid that the infant can tolerate, rather than total quantity of undiluted paraldehyde.

Diazepam (Valium) is not recommended for neonatal seizures. It is no more effective than intravenous phenobarbital, and it cannot be used for maintaining seizure control, since plasma concentrations of diazepam are not maintained for more than 30 minutes after intravenous injection. It has the disadvantage of producing or enhancing respiratory depression and hypotension, even if given alone, and particularly if administered along with phenobarbital. Because of its sodium benzoate carrier, it may be particularly disadvantageous in the patient with or at risk for indirect hyperbilirubinemia because the sodium benzoate may take up all available albumin binding sites, increasing the infant's chance for kernicterus.

Prognosis

Prognosis of neonatal seizures is clearly related to etiology and to a lesser extent to degree of maturity of the infant. Data from the Collaborative Perinatal Cerebral Palsy Project, relating neonatal characteristics of children with later severe neurologic handicaps, compared a number of antecedent variables, including Apgar score, birth weight, and clinical and laboratory evidence of intracranial hemorrhage and seizures. Thirty percent of the severely handicapped children had seizures in the first month of life, whereas only 0.3% of the neurologically intact survivors had neonatal seizures. Thus neonatal seizures were one of the strongest predictors of later motor or intellectual deficit. Infants of less than 34 weeks gestational age with neonatal seizures have a fourfold increase in mortality as compared with full-term infants with convulsions.

Perinatal asphyxia is clearly the poorest prognostic etiology for neonatal seizures both for preterm and full-term infants. Around 80% to 85% of infants with seizures caused by perinatal asphyxia are likely to have permanent neurologic sequelae. The prognosis for infants with seizures related to intraventricular hemorrhage appears to be poor, since seizures in this group are most likely to occur in infants with marked degrees of bleeding, and these are the infants with intraventricular hemorrhage with the poorest prognosis, as compared with those with mild or moderate amount of bleeding. The infant with subarachnoid hemorrhage who has a seizure without pronounced asphyxia has a good prognosis.

Among those infants with seizures related to a primary metabolic disorder, infants with hypoglycemia and late onset hypocalcemia, if treated promptly, have a good prognosis. Preterm infants with significant and/or prolonged hypoglycemia and early onset hypocalcemia, even when treated early, may have a poor prognosis. The associated perinatal stress in the preterm infant may, however, be the more profound determinant of poor outcome. The outcome for infants with other metabolically determined seizures is related to the primary disorder, for example, maple syrup urine disease, than to the seizures. Infants with seizures related to intracranial infections generally have a poor prognosis, but outcome often depends on rapidity of diagnosis and treatment of the infection.

Prognosis can also be related to time of onset of seizures in the neonate. Early onset of seizures, in the first 24 hours, is more likely to be associated with a poorer prognosis than seizures beginning after that time. Seizure duration is also important, and those infants whose seizures persist and are recurrent for more than 24 hours are at a greater risk of later neurologic sequelae than those with a single brief or multiple seizures that cease or are controlled within 24 hours. The interictal EEG may offer significant help in predicting outcome. The presence of either a flat or periodic EEG or bilateral multifocal electrical discharges in the EEG are predictive of an unsatisfactory outcome. Those infants with a normal interictal EEG and a normal neurologic examination at time of discharge are likely to have a favorable outcome.

THE FLOPPY NEONATE

Hypotonia is one of the most comon and often nonspecific signs of illness in the newborn (Fig. 22-18). It may be related to the infant's intrauterine environment, reflecting the effects of maternal disease or drug administration on the fetus. Impaired plancental function, circulation and oxygen transport in labor resulting in fetal hypoxia, hypercarbia, and acidosis may be similarly reflected at birth or postnatally in decreased muscle tone, decreased activity, and other evidence of central depression. Sepsis, respiratory distress syndrome, and other systemic diseases may also be associated with hypotonia. The physician must therefore determine whether it is secondary to metabolic abnormalities or to cerebral disease states, including hypoxic ischemic encephalopathy (p. 358), intraventricular hemorrhage, and meningitis. Less commonly the hypotonia may be the earliest sign of neuromuscular disease. A key problem in the hypotonic neonate is determination of whether the hypotonia is associated with weakness, since even with repeated careful examination it may be difficult or impossible to make the distinction between weakness and hypotonia in the newborn.

Weakness is the result of anatomic or physiochemical events within the motor system. This motor system or pathway comprises the upper motor neuron, including the motor nerve cells in the cerebral cortex, the descending corticospinal tracts that pass through the brain, brain stem, and the spinal cord, and the motor unit, which includes the anterior horn cells of the spinal cord, the peripheral nerve, the neuromuscular junction, and the muscle. Using clinical observations of tone and movement, muscle bulk, deep tendon reflexes, and response to sensory stimuli, the physician may be able to define the site of anatomic lesions or disease in the motor pathway. Disorders of the upper motor neuron, that is, above the level of the anterior horn cell, are commonly manifested by hypotonia in the newborn rather than by spasticity, as in the older infant or child; however, even with hypotonia, deep tendon reflexes may be increased. In contrast, lesions of anterior horn cell and peripheral nerve are invariably associated with diminished or

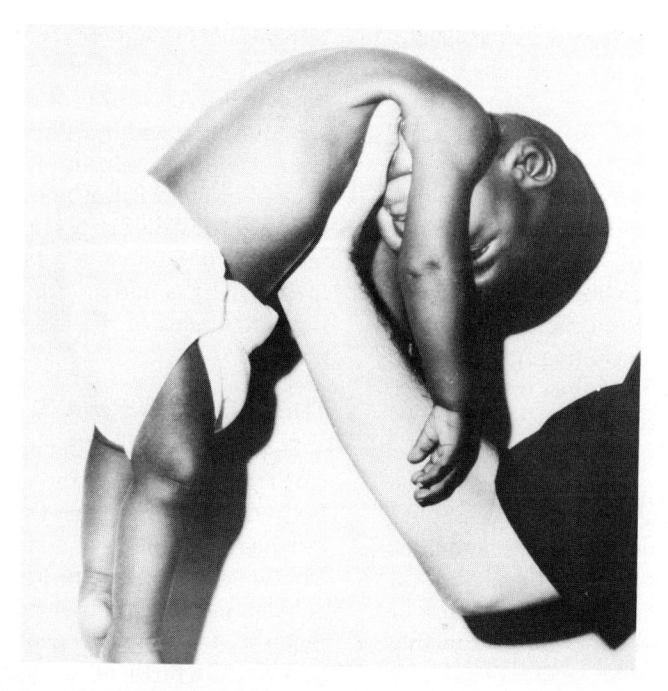

Fig. 22-18. A markedly floppy child in ventral suspension. Contrast this child with the infant shown in Fig. 22-3. This infant showed no flexion of the legs or back and no elevation of the head. The child has Werdnig-Hoffmann disease.

absent reflexes in the newborn. The deep tendon reflexes in neonates with muscle disease may rarely be present. Disorders of the neuromuscular junction are associated with normally active reflexes. Sensory responses manifested either by limb withdrawal, gross trunk movements, or, in the case of infants with profound weakness with limited trunk or extremity movement, by grimace or crying, indicate in the weak infant that sensory pathways are intact; absence of any response to sensory stimuli in the awake newborn is usually indicative of either spinal cord or peripheral nerve disease. The course of the infant's hypotonia and weakness may also be helpful in establishing a diagnosis, since weakness and hypotonia which is most pronounced at delivery and then improves is more likely the result of intrapartum events, whereas progression of the hypotonia and weakness postpartum over days or weeks may be more indicative of neuromuscular disease.

After determining that the problem is related to neuromuscular and not systemic or central nervous system disease, one attempts to localize the site of the weakness. Important signs of neuromuscular disease in the neonate, in addition to hypotonia, weakness, and altered deep tendon reflexes, are poor sucking and swallowing associated at times with aspiration or nasal regurgitation, respiratory distress related to impaired chest movement with diaphragmatic breathing, weakness of facial movements, varying degrees of ophthalmoplegia, fasiculations of the tongue, which must be distinguished from the tremulous tongue movements of the crying infant, and joint contractures.

With careful examination and serial observation of the hypotonic and inactive weak infant, with the additional help of electromyography, and with muscle biopsy with histochemical analysis, specific diagnosis of neuromuscular disorders in the newborn can be determined. Older terms such as *the hypotonic infant, floppy baby syndrome*, or *amyotonia congenita* may be discarded. Recognition of the existence of these disorders and understanding that there are many causes of neonatal hypotonia and weakness may result in the diagnosis of conditions that are perhaps treatable or that may improve with time, provided that the infant is given adequate support. Some of the conditions are severe and may be progressive and fatal. Even for these infants, diagnosis is important, not only for prognosis but also for genetic counseling.

Discussion of the differential diagnoses of the floppy or hypotonic newborn, with or without weakness due to various etiologies, follows.

Disorders with neonatal hypotonia and weakness
Spinal cord dysfunction
See Chapter 17.

Anterior horn cell disease
Degeneration of the anterior horn cell is the most common definable cause of motor unit dysfunction and is

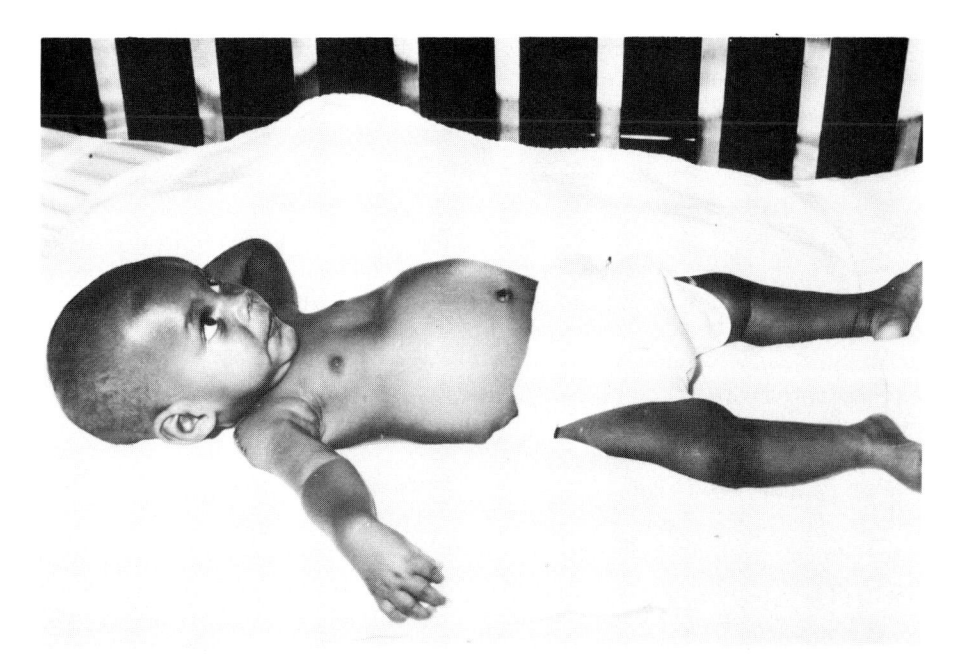

Fig. 22-19. The clinical picture of Werdnig-Hoffmann disease, or marked hypotonia of many causes. The legs are externally rotated and slightly flexed at the knees (the frog-leg position). Note the abdominal breathing and retraction of the chest. There is minimal movement of the arms, as seen by their asymmetry. Note also the alertness of the infant.

known as Werdnig-Hoffmann disease, an autosomal recessive disorder (Fig. 22-19). It is characterized by extensive widespread muscular atrophy due to progressive denervation and loss of motor neurons in spinal cord and brain stem, which usually begins in utero. There may be a maternal history of decreased fetal movements, although usually the first manifestations occur after delivery. Clinical manifestations are reported in one third of cases in the neonatal period, with more than half becoming symptomatic by 3 months of age. The disorder is usually lethal by the first year in patients with neonatal onset.

Clinical manifestations. The cardinal manifestations in the symptomatic newborn are inactivity, generalized hypotonia, weakness, and small muscle bulk, and the infant lies in the frog-leg posture. Breathing is abdominal with little or no intercostal or chest movement, and there is marked head lag. Because of weakness of bulbar musculature, impaired sucking and weak cry are noted early, as are fasciculations of the edges of the tongue. Reflexes are absent, but the infant does show response to painful stimuli.

Diagnosis. The diagnosis may be suggested by the classic history and physical findings, especially with the history of a similarly affected sibling. Confirmation requires evidence of denervation on electromyogram (EMG), and muscle biopsy shows atrophy of motor units. No methods of prenatal detection are available.

Treatment. Therapy is supportive, with attention given to feeding techniques to prevent aspiration and provide sufficient nutrition. In addition, techniques of postural drainage and suctioning are important, as is genetic counseling of the family.

Peripheral neuropathy

Peripheral neuropathies are rarely diagnosed in the neonatal period. However, a syndrome of progressive muscular weakness and wasting closely resembling Werdnig-Hoffmann disease has been described.

Clinical manifestations and diagnosis. Hypotonia, generalized weakness with decreased spontaneous movements, and arreflexia are present. Progressive feeding difficulties may occur. The finding of elevated spinal fluid protein, prolonged nerve conduction in motor nerves, and group atrophy on muscle biopsy are the bases for diagnosis.

Treatment. Neuropathies in infants tend to be chronic and may be nonprogressive. Response to steroid therapy may occur.

Neuromuscular junction disease: myasthenia gravis

Two forms of myasthenia are seen in the newborn. Transient neonatal myasthenia gravis is seen in 12% of infants whose mothers have myasthenia gravis. However, maternal myasthenia may not be clinically evident at delivery, and some of these mothers may not have required anticholinesterase medication during pregnancy. No correlation exists between the severity and duration of the mother's illness and the degree of weakness of the newborn, although the birth of one affected infant increases the likelihood of subsequent children being similarly affected. This neonatal disease is presumably caused by a circulating factor transplacentally transmitted to the infant (p. 639). A correlation with severity of disease in the newborn and antiacetylcholine receptor antibody titers in the newborn have been reported. These infants almost always show improvement and full recovery within a period of 5 to 47 days. Congenital myasthenia gravis occurs in infants of normal mothers and has a familial tendency for occurrence in other siblings but is rare. The myasthenia in these infants may be persistent, and involvement of extraocular muscles is common, with little or no generalized weakness.

Clinical manifestations. The initial features of both forms of myasthenia are similar, with feeding difficulty being the most common initial manifestation. Despite eagerness to feed, the infant's sucking quickly fatigues so that adequate intake of formula is impossible. Respiratory distress, generalized weakness, hypotonia, and a feeble cry occur and may be the first and most urgent signs of distress shortly after birth in severe cases. Weak facial movements are also common. Ocular muscle weakness is uncommon, as is ptosis in the transitory neonatal form, whereas extraocular muscles are commonly involved in the congenital form, in the absence of generalized weakness. The onset of weakness is usually noted within the first day, with rapid worsening followed by improvement, but the onset may be delayed until the third day of life; in the congenital form the diagnosis is often delayed for several weeks or months.

Diagnosis. The physician must maintain a high level of suspicion, particularly when knowledge of maternal disease, even in complete remission, is available. Infants born to known myasthenic mothers should be followed closely through the first 24 to 36 hours of age for signs just mentioned. The clinical diagnosis is made by the response to intramuscular or subcutaneous injection of neostigmine methylsulfate, 0.125 to 0.5 mg, with atropine, 0.1 mg. Within 10 minutes a measurable increase in strength, facial movements, and sucking ability should be evident. The infant's state before and after administration of neostigmine should be documented. Edrophonium (Tensilon), 0.5 to 1 mg, may also be used, but the brevity of its action makes evaluation of drug response difficult. A negative response using this drug does not rule out the disease.

Treatment. Infants responding to intramuscularly administered neostigmine should be maintained with oral administration of 1 mg neostigmine given 20 minutes before feeding. The dosage must be individually titrated. Periodic attempts to decrease the dosage, with observation of the effect on the infant, should help the physician determine duration of treatment. Supportive measures include gavage feeding and suction.

Muscle diseases

In recent years, increasing use of muscle biopsies and the application of histochemistry to muscle pathology, plus electron microscopic analysis of muscle ultrastructural changes, has resulted in the delineation of a number of congenital, inherited disorders of muscle. Some of these are nonprogressive and appeared to have a relatively good prognosis, whereas others have been found to be the cause of profound neonatal weakness and hypotonia with variable but at times fatal outcome.

Myotonic dystrophy

Myotonic dystrophy is probably the most commonly found severe congenital myopathy in the neonatal period. The mother is the affected parent in over 90% of the severely affected infants, although neonatal disease is not related to the severity of maternal disease. Polyhydramnios is a common complication of pregnancy.

Clinical manifestations. The most common clinical manifestations, present at birth, include profound hypotonia and inactivity, feeding and swallowing difficulties, and arthrogryposis involving the lower limbs, with talipes equinovarus deformities. Reflexes are either diminished or absent, and in addition to pharyngeal weakness causing feeding problems, there may be bilateral facial weakness and a characteristic tented upper lip. Smooth muscle involvement in the disease may result in abdominal distention and varying degrees of ileus. Severe chest weakness can lead to respiratory distress. With the added feature of diaphragmatic muscle weakness, diagnosis may be difficult, since electromyography rarely reveals myotonic discharge in the affected newborn, and both serum enzymes (CPK, SGOT) and muscle biopsy are normal. The most helpful clues to the diagnosis are the characteristic facial appearance in a hypotonic infant, with a mother who has the classic features of the adult form of myotonic dystrophy—myotonia, distal muscle weakness, characteristic facies, and cataracts. Treatment is limited to supportive care. At times assisted ventilation as well as parenteral hyperalimentation may be necessary.

Other muscular dystrophies

Duchenne muscular dystrophy, the most common muscle disease of childhood, is never symptomatic in the neonatal period. Not unitl 1 year is it possible to recognize the characteristic hypotonia. The other characteristics of this sex-linked recessively inherited disease are not noted until several years of age. However, in the male newborn infant at risk, that is, with affected brothers or maternal uncles, a presumptive chemical diagnosis can be made in the first week of life by determination of the CPK level, which is dramatically elevated.

Congenital muscular dystrophy is a term that has been used as a diagnosis for a poorly defined muscle disease symptomatic in infancy with weakness and flexion contractures. This does not appear to be a distinct disease with specific histologic features at present, and these cases await further clarification.

Central core disease

Central core disease, one of the first morphologically distinct congenital myopathies, was initially clinically characterized by nonprogressive weakness and hypotonia in children whose motor development was delayed and who also had kyphoscoliosis and other skeletal deformities, including hip dislocation. As the condition has been more completely delineated, it is apparent that it is a cause of congenital hypotonia present at birth or shortly thereafter. Deep tendon reflexes are usually present but may be reduced in proportion to the degree of weakness. No cranial muscles are involved. With the passage of time, delay in motor milestones is evident, as is proximal weakness. Muscle biopsy shows central areas in many but not all muscle fibers in which histochemical reactions for oxidative enzymes are absent. In many patients there is a marked predominance of type I histochemically determined muscle fibers.

Centronuclear (myotubular) myopathy

This was initially described as a disorder of children with congenital, slowly progressive weakness, whose muscle biopsies were characterized by the presence of centrally placed nuclei in muscle fibers. The condition was termed *myotubular myopathy*, with the suggestion that the abnormality in muscle fibers causing the weakness was due to arrested fiber development at the fetal myotubular stage. In addition to the originally described cases of children with slowly progressive limb weakness, ptosis, and extraocular and facial weakness, there is a form of this disease that is manifested in the immediate neonatal period by profound generalized hypotonia and weakness. The affected infants may have respiratory failure caused by a combination of intercostal and bulbar muscle weakness. These infants also have profound weakness of extraocular and facial muscles, so that eye and facial movements are absent. Tendon reflexes are absent. Diagnosis is established by the clinical presentation with histologic and histochemical description of muscle fibers with marked variation in size and many small fibers with a myotubular structure and centrally placed muscle nuclei. The neonatal weakness may be so profound as to result in a fatal outcome. However, some infants who are provided adequate care and support may survive to later infancy and childhood with a nonprogressive course, with variable degrees of persisting weakness. Only males are affected in the severe congenital disease.

Congenital muscle fiber type disproportion

Muscle fibers are characterized as either type I or type II on the basis of differing histochemical stains. There is a rather heterogeneous group of children with variable degrees of muscle weakness whose muscle biopsy reveals small type I muscle fibers and normal size type II fibers. In addition, there appears to be a homogenous group of infants with small size type I fibers, with a congenital myopathy evident at birth. Presenting characteristics are hypotonia, decreased movements, and congenital contractures of joints involving hands or feet. Congenital hip dislocations are also commonly present. Such joint contractures and deformities may be labeled as arthrogryposis. They may be the predominant clinical manifestation of this congenital myopathy, in which presumably restricted limb movements in utero have resulted in the deformed joints. Associated abnormalities in congenital muscle fiber type disproportion myopathy include short stature, high arched palate, long thin face, and kyphoscoliosis, which becomes evident as the child grows older. These infants have a nonprogressive course, and improvement can be anticipated with survival into childhood and adult life. The disorder is often familial.

Other congenital myopathies

There are other congenital muscle conditions occasionally manifested by hypotonia but no significant weakness in the first weeks or months of life. Nemaline or rod-body myopathy, one of the earliest disorders of muscle weakness with a nonprogressive course, categorized initially on the basis of histochemical and ultrastructural abnormalities, is commonly manifested by hypotonia and variable degree of weakness with delayed motor development. However, most of the children with this disease have not been symptomatic as neonates. A number of much rarer congenital myopathies, characterized strictly on the basis of morphologic changes in muscle fibers, are not well delineated as clinical entities. Multicore myopathy, fingerprint body myopathy, sarcotubular myopathy, reducing body myopathy, and at least five other different types of myopathy with unusual mitochondria have been described. Some patients may show neonatal hypotonia and weakness, but their clinical descriptions remain incomplete at present. Undoubtedly some infants with congenital hypotonia and weakness that is not progressive have these or other as yet undescribed disorders of muscle structure or metabolism. Many such infants are undoubtedly still currently described under the rubric *benign congenital hypotonia*, which appears to be a diagnostic label for children with a clinical syndrome of generalized hypotonia from birth, minimum or mild weakness, a nonprogressive course, and a normal muscle biopsy. The use of this diagnosis is at present a reflection more of our lack of knowledge than of neurologic sophistication.

Muscle biopsy, a feasible procedure in even the weakest infants, has until recently been considered primarily an investigative rather than diagnostic tool in the neonatal period. For muscle biopsy to achieve its potential as a diagnostic test in the evaluation of the hypotonic and weak infant, modern histochemical techniques and electron microscopy must be used in the pathologic examination of tissue. Used in this manner, with biopsies taken from clinically weak muscles, muscle biopsy is a low-risk procedure with great potential for the diagnosis of many neuromuscular and metabolic diseases for which the initial symptoms present in the neonate are hypotonia and weakness.

Arthrogryposis multiplex congenita

Arthrogryposis is a condition of multiple causes characterized by fixed deformity of one or more joints at birth. It is not a disease. Clubfoot, either unilateral or bilateral, may be one form of this disorder. The joint fixation is secondary to lack of movement of the joint for periods of time in utero. This could be due to fetal malposition or to intrauterine paralysis. The weakness or paralysis may be caused by anterior horn cell disease, neuropathies, or congenital myopathies such as congential fiber type disproportion and neonatal or congenital myotonic dystrophy.

ACUTE METABOLIC DISEASE

Acute metabolic disease in the neonatal period is uncommon, but its prompt recognition may determine the mental outcome of the infant or may even be life saving. The hallmark is the abrupt onset of lethargy, vomiting, and coma in a previously well infant. These findings are often accompanied by seizures. Onset may be in the first hours or days of life. This constellation of symptoms also suggests the diagnosis of sepsis, meningitis, or intracranial hemorrhage. Immediate evaluation should include blood cultures and lumbar puncture. Urinalysis for acetonuria often will lead to the diagnosis of ketoacidosis found in several of the metabolic diseases. Ketoacidosis otherwise is uncommon in the first month of life, even with starvation, vomiting, or diarrhea. Its presence should therefore suggest the possibility of a metabolic disorder. Specific diagnosis requires the prompt performance of metabolic screening procedures and chromatography of serum and urine for amino acids. For some diseases, such as hyperammonemia, chromatography will be normal, and diagnosis requires specific testing. Acute therapy in most of these diseases consists of removal of protein from the diet and the administration of glucose and intravenous fluids while awaiting the diagnosis. Exchange transfusions may occasionally be life saving. A family history of siblings or relatives with acute neonatal disease should increase suspicion of a metabolic disorder. A discussion of each of the metabolic disorders that may include seizures and other neurologic manisfestations is found in Chapter 32.

PROGNOSIS OF HIGH-RISK NEONATES

There has been a progressive reduction in the neonatal mortality as well as a decreasing incidence of central nervous system morbidity among surviving high-risk neonates. In the United States as a whole the neonatal mortality has been reduced from 12.3 deaths per 1,000 live births in 1974 to 9.9 in 1977. Although the United States ranks sixteenth in the world as regards neonatal mortality, *it has the lowest birth weight–specific neonatal mortality in the world.*

The highest neonatal mortality occurs in the lowest birth weight groups. These low birth weight groups, especially the 1,000- to 1500-gm infants, have, however, shown the greatest improvement. For most centers around the United States this particular birth weight–specific group has shown a reduction in mortality from approximately 30% to 35% in the late 1960s to approximately 10% to 15% mortality in the late 1970s. Mortality in the higher weight groups, especially term infants, has been less than 1%. Approximately 8.2% of births in this country are preterm, and this has not significantly changed in the last 10 to 20 years. Approximately 52% of deaths occur in only 1% of births, those being less than 1,000 gm. A continuing reduction in neonatal mortality over the next 20 years will require a simultaneous decline in the incidence of preterm births.

The mortality in very low birth weight infants following discharge from the hospital is also higher than that of term infants. Some of these deaths are attributable to infections or complications of chronic diseases such as bronchopulmonary dysplasia. There is also an increased incidence of the sudden infant death syndrome and child abuse.

Concomitant with the decrease in neonatal mortality there has been an improvement in long-term outcome. Neurologic and developmental handicaps in small premature babies born before 1960 ranged form 60% to 70%, whereas current morbidity ranges from 10% to 20%. This includes neurologic defects (spastic diplegia, hydrocephalus, blindness, and deafness) and/or developmental delay with an IQ below 80 (Fig. 22-20). Atraumatic deliveries, prevention of perinatal anoxia, improved methods for diagnosing, treating, and preventing Rh hemolytic disease, and improved methods of ventilation and nutrition seem to have been causally related to the reduction of severe handicap.

Infants weighing between 1,501 and 2,500 gm have a

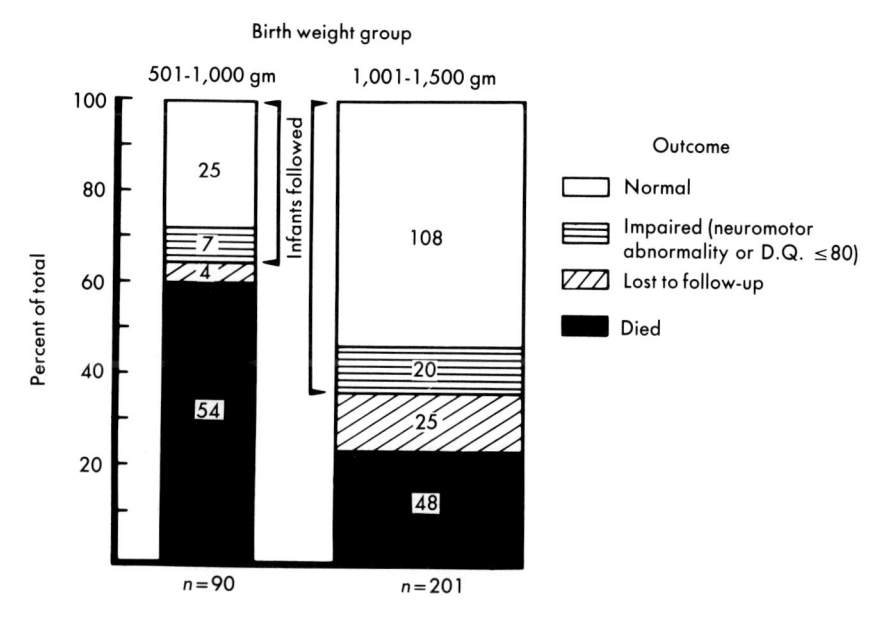

Fig. 22-20. Overall prognosis for 291 very low birth weight infants admitted to neonatal intensive care (Rainbow Babies and Childrens Hospital, University Hospitals of Cleveland) during 1975 and 1976 and followed to a mean of 2 years' conceptual age. D.Q. (developmental quotient) represents the combined results of Bayley scales (developmental quotients) in 112 infants tested at a mean age of 21 months and Stanford-Binet scales (intelligence quotients) in 48 infants tested at a mean age of 31 months. (From Hack, M., Merkatz, I.R., and Fanaroff, A.A.: N. Engl. J. Med. **301:**1162, 1979. Reprinted by permission of the New England Journal of Medicine.)

long-term prognosis similar to that of term infants. Very low birth weight infants without severe complications will also usually develop normally. Infants at highest risk for a poor outcome are those who survive clinically significant intraventricular hemorrhage, asphyxia with subsequent neurologic signs, and neonatal meningitis and infants who require assisted ventilation for severe respiratory distress syndrome or apnea of prematurity. Intrauterine growth retardation in both term and preterm infants was previously considered to result in a poorer outcome. Improved methods of care, however, have minimized the perinatal complications of intrauterine growth retardation such as asphyxia, hypoglycemia, and polycythemia, and growth-retarded infants who are born without intrauterine infections or congenital malformation now appear to do as well as appropriately grown infants of a similar gestational age.

It should be stressed that for all very low birth weight infants the effects of environment (social class and caretaker-infant interaction) have an overwhelming effect on early development, and in the absence of severe neurologic impairment they are the factors that will determine ultimate outcome. Maternal-infant separation in early infancy, as well as the understandable parental anxiety and overprotectiveness, may also foster an abnormal emotional environment for the growing infant. These may be partly ameliorated by preventing unnecessarily prolonged hospitalization and by encouraging parental visitation and participation in the nursery care of the infant (Chapter 18). Behavioral and learning difficulties appear to be more common in the children born prematurely than to those born at term, although there are few data on recent survivors.

The various types of CNS dysfunction detected in surviving children who have been high-risk neonates follow.

A. Motor deficits
   1. Spastic diplegia
   2. Spastic quadriplegia
   3. Spastic hemiplegia
   4. Choreoathetosis
B. Mental retardation
C. Disorders of abstract reasoning
D. Seizures
E. Sensory abnormalities
   1. Hearing deficits
   2. Visual abnormalities
      a. Retrolental fibroplasia
      b. Eye motility dysfunction
F. Posthemorrhagic hydrocephalus
G. Microcephaly

The changing patterns of cerebral palsy as reported from Sweden from 1954 to 1974 have shown a stepwise reduction in the incidence of cerebral palsy related to a disproportionate change in the type of cerebral palsy to decrease, with the advent of our understanding of the causes and treatment of hyperbilirubinemia. The next most significant reduction in cerebral palsy occurred with a decrease in the incidence of cerebral diplegia, seen especially in surviving low birth weight infants. It is important to note that there has not been a similar drop in Sweden in the incidence of spastic quadriplegia, which is seen primarily in children who were asphyxiated full-term neonates. Although the changes that have been documented in Sweden are also felt to have occurred in the United States, there has not been a similar population-based study of the changing incidence of various types of cerebral palsy.

It is important not to lose sight of two very important points in our continued attempt to reduce the incidence of neurologically handicapped children. As the overall incidence of CNS dysfunction from prenatal or intrapartum causes is evaluated, it is still seen that Down's syndrome and myelomeningocele, two conditions of presumed genetic and/or prenatal origin, account for more children with CNS dysfunction than do problems arising out of the intrapartum period. Major inroads are being made in prenatal detection of these two problems. The second major point to recognize is that, although there has been major success in reducing the incidence of central nervous system sequelae in children who were preterm infants, there are actually more children with cerebral palsy who were full-term than who were preterm infants. Although the incidence of cerebral palsy is approximately 3.38 in 1,000 full-term infants versus 90 in 1,000 preterm infants, it is important to recognize that the denominator from which the full-term infants come is approximately 92% of all births in this country, with preterm births making up the remaining 8%.

With continued efforts in the prenatal diagnosis of neurologic disorders, the reduction of the number of preterm births, the earlier recognition of the distressed fetus (especially in the intrapartum period), and the immediate detection of the neonate with signs of neurologic dysfunction, there can be a continued reduction in the number of children with CNS dysfunction.

Alfred W. Brann, Jr.
James F. Schwartz

BIBLIOGRAPHY
Neonatal neurologic assessment

American Speech and Hearing Association, American Academy of Ophthalmology and Otolaryngology, and American Academy of Pediatrics: Supplementary statement of Joint Committee on Infant Hearing Screening, A.S.H.A. **16:**160, 1974.

Clark, D.B.: Abnormal neurologic signs in the neonate: physical diagnosis of the newly born, In Kay, J., editor: Report of the Forty-Sixth Ross Conference on Pediatric Research, 1964.

Dubowitz, L.M.S., Dubowitz, V., and Goldberg, C.: Clinical assessment of gestational age in the newborn, J. Pediatr. **77:**1, 1970.

Hogan, G.R., and Ryan, N.J.: Neurological evaluation of the newborn, Clin. Perinatol. **4:**31, 1977.

Illingworth, R.S.: The development of the infant and young child: normal and abnormal, ed. 4, Baltimore, 1970, The William & Wilkins Co.

McFarland, W.H., Simmons, F.B., and Jones, F.R.: An automated hearing screening technique for newborns, J. Speech Hearing Disorders **45:**495, 1980.

Nelson, K.B., and Ellenberg, J.H.: Neonatal signs as predictors of cerebral palsy, Pediatrics **64:**225, 1979.

Parmalee, A.H., and others: Neurological evaluation of the premature infant, Biol. Neonate **15:**65, 1970.

Prechtl, H.: Prognostic values of neurological signs, Proc. R. Soc. Med. **58:**3, 1965.

Prechtl, H., and Bientema, D.: The neurological examination of the full term newborn infant. In Clinics in developmental medicine, no. 12, London, England, 1964, William Heinemann Ltd.

Schulman-Galambos, C., and Galambos, H.: Brainstem auditory evoked responses in premature infants, J. Speech Hearing Res. **18:**456, 1975.

Thorne, I.: Cerebral symptoms in the newborn, Acta Paediatr. Scand. (Suppl.) **9:**15, 1969.

Noninvasive diagnostic tools

Bada, H.S., and others: Noninvasive diagnosis of neonatal asphyxia and intraventricular hemorrhage by Doppler ultrasound, J. Pediatr. **95:**775, 1979.

Bejar, R., and others: Diagnosis and follow-up of intraventricular and intracerebral hemorrhages by ultrasound studies of infant's brain through the fontanelles and sutures, Pediatrics **66:**661, 1980.

Hill, A., and Volpe, J.J.: Measurement of intracranial pressure using the Ladd intracranial pressure monitor, J. Pediatr. **98:**974, 1981.

Lipman, B., Serwer, G.A., and Brazy, J.E.: Abnormal cerebral hemodynamics in preterm infants with patent ductus arteriosus, Pediatrics **69:**778, 1982.

Pape, K.E., and others: Ultrasound detection of brain damage in preterm infants, Lancet **1:**1261, 1979.

Perlman, J.M., Hill, A., and Volpe, J.J.: The effect of patent ductus arteriosus on flow velocity in the anterior cerebral arteries: ductal steal in the premature newborn infant, J. Pediatr. **99:**767, 1981.

Philip, A.G.S., Long, J.G., and Donn, S.M.: Intracranial pressure: sequential measurements in full-term and preterm infants, Am. J. Dis. Child. **135:**521, 1981.

Volpe, J.J.: Neonatal intraventricular hemorrhage, N. Engl. J. Med. **304:**886, 1981.

Birth injury

Ahmann, P.A., and others: Intraventricular hemorrhage in the high risk preterm infant: incidence and outcome. Ann. Neurol. **7:**118, 1980.

Allan, W.C., and others: Sector scan ultrasound imaging through the anterior fontanelle, Am. J. Dis. Child. **134:**1028, 1980.

Anderson, D.C., and Cranford, R.E.: Corticosteroids in ischemic stroke. In Current concepts of cerebrovascular disease-stroke, **10(1):**68, 1979.

Bada, H.S., and others: Noninvasive diagnosis of neonatal asphyxia and intraventricular hemorrhage by Doppler ultrasound, J. Pediatr. **95:**775, 1979.

Banker, B.Q.: The neuropathological effects of anoxia and hyoglycemia in the newborn, Dev. Med. Child Neurol. **9:**544, 1967.

Banker, B.Q., and Larroche, J.: Periventricular leucomalacia of infancy, Arch. Neurol. **7:**386, 1962.

Bondareff, W., Myers, R.D., and Brann, A.W.: Brain extracellular space in monkey fetuses subjected to prolonged partial asphyxia, Exp. Neurol. **28:**167, 1970.

Brann, A.W.: Effects of intrauterine asphyxia on the full-term brain: neonatal neurological assessment and outcome, Report of the Seventy-Seventh Ross Conference on Pediatric Research, 1980.

Brann, A.W., and Montalvo, J.M.: Barbiturates and asphyxia, Pediatr. Clin. North Am. 17:851, 1970.

Brann, A.W., and Myers, R.E.: Brain swelling and hemorrhagic cortical necrosis following perinatal asphyxia in monkeys (abstract), J. Neuropathol. Exp. Neurol. 28:178, 1968.

Brann, A.W., and Myers, R.E.: Chronic fetal compromise and brain damage, Neurology (Minneap.) 19:301, 1969.

Brann, A.W., and Myers, R.E.: Central nervous system findings in the newborn monkey following severe in utero partial asphyxia, Neurology 25:327, 1975.

Brann, A.W., Myers, R.E., and DiGiacomo, R.: The effect of halothane-induced maternal hypotension on the fetus. In Medical primatology 1970, Proceedings of the Second Conference of Experimental Medicine and Surgery in Primates, Basel, Switzerland, 1971, S. Karger Publishing Co.

Brock, M.: Cerebral blood flow and intracranial pressure changes associated with brain hypoxia. In Brierley, J.B., and Meldrum, B.S., editors: Brain hypoxia. In Clinics in Developmental Medicine, nos. 39-40. London, England, 1971, William Heinemann, Ltd.

Cailee, J.M., and others: Cerebral blood volume and water extraction from cerebral parenchyma by hyperosmolar contrast media, Neuroradiology, 16:579, 1978.

Clifford, S.H.: The effects of asphyxia on the newborn infant, J. Pediatr. 18:567, 1941.

Courville, C.B.: Birth and brain damage, Pasadena, Calif., 1971, M.F. Courville.

Courville, C.B., and March, C.: Neonatal asphyxia, Bull. Los Angeles Neurol. Soc. 9:121, 1944.

Cowan, W.M.: The development of the brain, Sci. Am. vol. 107, 1979.

Deonna, T., and others: Neonatal intracranial hemorrhage in premature infants, Pediatrics 56:1056, 1975.

Dykes, F.D., and others: Intraventricular hemorrhage: a prospective evaluation of etiopathogenesis, Pediatrics 66:42, 1980.

Finer, N.N., and others: Hypoxic-ischemic encephalopathy in term neonates: perinatal factors and outcome, J. Pediatr. 98:112, 1981.

Fisherman, R.A.: Brain edema, N. Engl. J. Med. 293:17, 1975.

Frederick, J., and Butler, W.R.: Causes of neonatal death. II. Intraventricular haemorrhage, Biol. Neonate 15:257, 1970.

Friedman, S.P., and Courville, C.B.: Atrophic lobar sclerosis of early childhood. (ulegyria): report of two verified cases with particular reference to their asphyxial etiology, Bull. Los Angeles Neurol. Soc. 6:32, 1941.

Ghaplin, E.R., and others: Posthemorrhagic hydrocephalus in the preterm infant, Pediatrics 65:901, 1980.

Goldstein, G.W.: Pathogenesis of brain edema and hemorrhage: role of the brain capillary, Pediatrics 64:357, 1979.

Grontoft, O.: Intracranial haemorrhage and blood-brain barrier problems in the newborn, Acta Pathol. Microbiol. Scand. (Suppl.) vol. 100, 1954.

Gruenwald, P.: Subependymal cerebral hemorrhage in premature infants and its relation to various injurious influences at birth, Am. J. Obstet. Gynecol. 61:1285, 1951.

Guggenheim, M.A., and others: Risk factors in germinal matrix hemorrhage, Ann. Neurol. 8:225, 1980.

Guyton, A.C., Granger, J.H., and Taylor, A.E.: Interstitial fluid pressure Physiol. Rev. 51:527, 1971.

Harcke, H.T., Jr., and others: Perinatal cerebral intraventricular hemorrhage, J. Pediatr. 80:37, 1972.

Holowach-Thurston, J., and others: Decrease in brain glucose in anoxia in spite of elevated plasma glucose levels, Pediatr. Res. 7:691, 1973.

James, J.E.: Methodology for the control of intracranial pressure with hypertonic mannitol, Acta Neurochir. 51:161, 1980.

Katzman, R., and others: Brain edema in stroke, Report of Joint Committee for Stroke Resources, Stroke vol. 8, 1977.

Korobkin, R.: The relationship between head circumference and the development of communicating hydrocephalus following intraventricular hemorrhage, Pediatrics 56:74, 1975.

Krishnamoorthy, K.S., and others: Neurologic sequelae in the survivors of neonatal intraventricular hemorrhage, Pediatrics 64:233, 1979.

Krishnamoorthy, K.S., and others: Neurologic sequelae in the survivors of neonatal intraventricular hemorrhage, Conference on Intraventricular Hemorrhage, sponsored by Ross Laboratories, Washington, D.C., 1980.

Kuschinsky, W., and Wahl, M.: Local chemical and neurogenic regulation of cerebral vascular resistance, Physiol. Rev. 58(3):656, 1978.

Larroche, J.C.: Post-haemorrhagic hydrocephalus in infancy: anatomical study, Biol. Neonate 20:287, 1972.

Lazzara, A., and others: Clinical predictability of intraventricular hemorrhage in preterm infants, Pediatrics 65:30, 1980.

Leech, R.W., and Alvord, E.C.: Anoxic-ischemic encephalopathy in the human neonatal period: the significance of brain-stem involvement, Arch. Neurol. 34:109, 1977.

Little, W.J.: On the influence of abnormal parturition, difficult labours, premature birth, and asphyxia neonatorum on the mental and physical condition of the child, especially in relation to deformities, Trans. Obstet. Soc. Lond. 3:293, 1862.

Lou, H.C., Lassen, N.A., and Friis-Hansen, B.: Low cerebral blood flow in hypotensive perinatal distress, Acta Neurol. Scand. 56:343, 1977.

Lou, H.C., Lassen, N.A., and Friis-Hansen, B.: Impaired autoregulation of cerebral blood flow in the distressed newborn infant, J. Pediatr. 94:118, 1979.

Lou, H.C., Skou, H., and Pederson, H.: Low cerebral blood flow: a risk factor in the neonate, J. Pediatr. 95:606, 1979.

MacDonald, H.M., and others: Neonatal asphyxia. I. Relationship of obstetric and neonatal complications to neonatal mortality in 38-405 consecutive deliveries, J. Pediatr. 96:898, 1980.

Malamud, N.: Pattern of CNS vulnerability in neonatal hypoxemia. In Schade, J.P., and McMenemey, W.H., editors: Selective vulnerability of the brain in hypoxemia, Philadelphia, 1963, F.A. Davis Co.

Marchal, C., and others: Treatment des souffrances cerebrales neonatales, Pediatrie 27:709, 1972.

Marsh, M.L., Marshall, L.F., and Shapiro, H.M.: Neurosurgical intensive care, Anesthesiology 47:149, 1977.

Meschia, G.: Supply of oxygen to the fetus, J. Reprod. Med. 23:160, 1979.

Miller, F.C., and Paul, R.H.: Intrapartum fetal heart rate monitoring, Clin. Obstet. Gynecol. 21:561, 1978.

Morris-Jones, P.H., Houston, I.B., and Evans, R.C.: Prognosis of neurologic complication of acute hypernatremia, Lancet 2:1385, 1967.

Myers, R.E.: Atrophic cortical sclerosis associated with status marmoratus in a perinatally damaged monkey, Neurology (Minneap.) 19:1177, 1969.

Myers, R.E.: Experimental models of perinatal brain damage: relevance to human pathology; intrauterine asphyxia and the developing fetal brain, Chicago, 1977, Year Book Medical Publishers.

Myers, R.E., Beard, R., and Adamson, K.: Brain swelling in the newborn rhesus monkey following prolonged partial asphyxia, Neurology (Minneap.) 19:1012, 1969.

Norman, R.M.: Late neuropathological sequelae of birth injury. In Greenfield's neuropathology, London, 1969, Edward Arnold Publishers, Ltd.

Palma, P.A., and others: Progressive hydrocephalus following intraventricular hemorrhage in infants (1800 grams), Pediatr. Res. 14:635, 1980.

Pape, K.E., and Wigglesworth, J.S.: Haemorrhage, ischaemia, and the perinatal brain. In Clinics in Developmental Medicine, nos. 67-70, Philadephia, 1979, J.B. Lippincott Co.

Papile, L., and others: Incidence and evolution of subependymal and intraventricular hemorrhage: a study of infants with birth weights less than 1,500 grams, J. Pediatr. 92:529, 1978.

Peeters, L.H., and others: Blood flow to fetal organs as a function of arterial oxygen content, Am. J. Obstet. Gynecol. 135:637, 1979.

Purves, M.J.: The physiology of the cerebral circulation, London, 1972, Cambridge University Press.

Purves, M.J., and James, I.M.: Observations on the control of the cerebral blood flow in the sheep fetus and newborn lamb, Circ. Res. 25:65, 1969.

Reivich, M., and others: Regional cerebral blood flow during prolonged arterial asphyxia, Research on the Cerebral Circulation. 217-227.

Sarnat, H.B., and Sarnat, M.S.: Neonatal encephalopathy following fetal distress: a clinical and electroencephalographic study, Arch. Neurol. 33:696, 1976.

Schub, H.S., and others: Prospective long-term follow-up of prematures with subependymal/intraventricular hemorrhage, Pediatr. Res., 1981 (in press).

Seeds, A.E.: Maternal-fetal acid-base relationships and fetal scalp-blood analysis, Clin. Obstet. Gynecol. 21:579, 1978.

Seisjo, B.K., Berntman, L., and Nilsson, B.: Regulation of microcirculation in the brain, Microvasc. Res. 19:158, 1980.

Selzer, M.E., Myers, R.E., and Holstein, S.B.: Prolonged partial asphyxia: effects on fetal brain water and electrolytes, Neurology (Minneap.) 2:732, 1972.

Sexson, W.R., and others: The multisystem involvement of the asphyxiated newborn, Pediatr. Res. 10:432, 1976.

Shulman, S.T., and others: Transection of the spinal cord, Arch. Dis. Child. 46:291, 1971.

Silverboard, G., and others: Reliability of ultrasound in diagnosis of intracerebral hemorrhage and posthemorrhagic hydrocephalus: comparison with computed tomography, Pediatrics 66:507, 1980.

Silverboard, G., and others: Comparison of lumbar puncture with computed tomography scan as indicator of intracerebral hemorrhage in the preterm infant, Pediatrics 66:432, 1980.

Terplan, K.L.: Histopathologic brain changes in 1152 cases of the perinatal and early infancy period, Biol. Neonate 11:348, 1967.

Towbin, A.: Cerebral intraventricular hemorrhage and subependymal matrix infarction in the fetus and premature newborn, Am. J. Pathol. 52:121, 1968.

Towbin, A.: Central nervous system damage in the human fetus and newborn infant: mechanical and hypoxic injury incurred in the fetal-neonatal period, Am. J. Dis. Child. 119:259, 1970.

Towbin, A.: Central nervous system damage in the premature related to the occurrence of mental retardation in physical trauma as an etiological agent. In Angle, C.R., and Bering, E.A., editors: Mental retardation, Washington, D.C., 1970, U.S. Government Printing Office.

Tsiantos, A., and others: Intracranial hemorrhage in the prematurely born infant, J. Pediatr. 85:854, 1974.

Volpe, J.J., Pasternak, J.F., and Allan, W.C.: Ventricular dilation preceding rapid head growth following neonatal intracranial hemorrhage, Am. J. Dis. Child. 131:1212, 1977.

Wilkenson, H.A., and others: Diuretic synergy in the treatment of acute experimental cerebral edema, J. Neurosurg. 34:203, 1971.

Zeigler, A.L., and others: Cerebral distress in full term newborns and its prognostic value: a follow-up study of 90 infants, Helv. Paediatr. Acta 31:299, 1976.

Abnormalities of head size

Bergman, E.W., Freeman, J.M., and Epstein, M.H.: Treatment of infantile hydrocephalus with acetazolamide and furosemide: three- to four-year follow-up, Ann. Neurol. 8:227, 1980.

Cutler, R.W.P., and others: Formation and absorption of cerebrospinal fluid in man, Brain 91:707, 1968.

DeLevie, M., and Nogrady, M.B.: Rapid brain growth upon restoration of adequate nutrition causing false radiologic evidence of increased intracranial pressure, J. Pediatr. 76:523, 1970.

Dobbing, J.: Undernutrition and the developing brain, Am. J. Dis. Child. 20:411, 1970.

Dodge, R.P., and Porter, P.: Demonstration of intracranial pathology by transillumination, Arch. Neurol. 5:594, 1961.

Gilles, F.H., and Shillito, J.: Infantile hydrocephalus: retrocerebellar subdural hematoma, J. Pediatr. 76:529, 1970.

Gold, A.P., Ransohoff, J., and Carter, S.: Vein of Galen malformation, Acta Neurol. Scand. 40:(Suppl. 11):1, 1964.

Johnson R.T., and Johnson, K.P.: Hydrocephalus as a sequela of experimental mixoviruses, Exp. Mol. Pathol. 10:68, 1969.

Lorber, J.: Medical and surgical aspects in the treatment of congenital hydrocephalus, Neuropaediatrie 2:239, 1971.

Lorber, J.: Results of treatment of myelomeningocele, Dev. Med. Child. Neurol. 13:279, 1971.

Lorber, J., and Zachary, R.B.: Primary congenital hydrocephalus, Arch. Dis. Child. 43:516, 1968.

Martin, H.P.: Microcephaly and mental retardation, Am. J. Dis. Child. 119:128, 1970.

Scarf, J.E.: Treatment of hydrocephalus: an historical and critical review of methods and results, J. Neurol. Neurosurg. Psychiatry 26:1, 1963.

Schick, R.W., and Matson, D.D.: What is arrested hydrocephalus, J. Pediatr. 58:791, 1961.

Abnormalities of head shape

Freeman, J.M., and Borkowf, S.: Craniostenosis, Pediatrics 30:57, 1962.

Shillito, J., and Matson, D.D.: Craniosynostosis, Pediatrics 41:829, 1968.

Developmental abnormalities

Freeman, J.M., editor: A practical approach to the problems of meningomyeloceles, Baltimore, 1974, University Park Press.

Haworth, J.C., and Zachary, R.B.: Congenital dermal sinuses in children: their relationship to pilonidal sinus, Lancet 2:10, 1955.

Laurence, K.M.: The survival of untreated spina bifida cystica, Dev. Med. Child Neurol. 1(suppl.):10, 1966.

Lorber, J.: The prognosis of encephalocele, Dev. Med. Child Neurol. 13(suppl.):75, 1967.

Sieben, R.L., Hamida, M.B., and Shulman, K.: Multiple cranial nerve deficits associated with the Arnold-Chiari malformations, Neurology (Minneap.) 21:673, 1971.

Seizures

Bejsovee, M., Kulenoa, Z., and Ponca, E.: Familial intrauterine convulsions in pyridoxine dependency, Arch. Dis. Child. 42:201, 1967.

Freeman, J.M.: Neonatal seizures, diagnosis and management, J. Pediatr. 77:701, 1970.

Painter, M.J., and others: Phenobarbital and diphenyldantoin levels in neonates with seizures, J. Pediatr. 92:315, 1978.

Paunier, L., and others: Primary hypomagnesemia with secondary hypocalcemia in an infant, Pediatrics 41:385, 1968.

Prichard, J.S.: The character and significance of epileptic seizures in infancy. In Kellaway, P., and Petersen, I. editors: Neurologic and encephalographic correlative studies in infancy, New York, 1964, Grune & Stratton, Inc.

Rabe, E.F.: The hypotonic infant, J. Pediatr. **64:**422, 1964.

Rose, A.L., and Lombroso, C.T.: Neonatal seizure states, Pediatrics **45:**404, 1970.

Schulte, F.J., and others: Maternal toxemia, fetal malnutrition and motor behavior in newborn, Pediatrics **48:**871, 1971.

Schulte, F.J., and Schwenzel, W.: Motor control and muscle tone in the newborn period: electromyographic studies, Biol. Neonate **8:**198, 1965.

Smith, B.T., and Masotti, R.E.: Intravenous diazepam in the treatment of prolonged seizure activity in neonates and infants, Dev. Med. Child Neurol. **13:**630, 1971.

Volpe, J.J.: Neonatal seizures, Clin. Perinatol. **4:**43, 1977.

Wasterlain, C.G.: Inhibition of cerebral protein synthesis in status epilepticus, Neurology **22:**427, 1972.

Wasterlain, C.G., and Plum, F.: Vulnerability of developing rat brain to electroconvulsive seizures, Arch. Neurol. **29:**38, 1973.

The floppy neonate

Barwick, D.D., and Walton, J.N.: Polymyositis, Am. J. Med. **35:**646, 1963.

Blattner, R.J.: Arthrogryposis multiplex congenita, J. Pediatr. **71:**367, 1967.

Dodge, P.R., and others: Myotonic dystrophy in infancy and childhood, Pediatrics **35:**3, 1967.

Dubowitz, V.: Infantile muscular atrophy, Brain **87:**707, 1976.

Dubowitz, V.: The floppy infant. In Clinics in developmental medicine, no. 31, London, England, 1969, William Heinemann, Ltd.

Landau, W.M.: Spasticity and rigidity, Recent Adv. Neurol. **6:**1, 1969.

Paine, R.S.: The future of the "floppy infant"; a follow-up study of 133 patients, Dev. Med. Child Neurol. **5:**115, 1963.

Taksuji, N., Brown, B., and Brob, D.: Neonatal myasthenia gravis, Pediatrics **45:**488, 1970.

Taskar, W., and Chutorian, A.M.: Chronic polyneuritis of childhood, J. Pediatr. **74:**699, 1969.

Zellweger, H., and others: Severe congenital muscular dystrophy, Am. J. Dis. Child. **114:**591, 1967.

Prognosis of neurologic abnormalities in the newborn

Drillien, C.M.: Etiology and prognosis of small for date babies, Pediatr. Clin. North Am. **17:**9, 1970.

Hagbert, B.: Epidemiological and preventive aspects of cerebral palsy and severe mental retardation in Sweden, Euro. J. Ped. **130:**71, 1971.

Koops, B.L., and Harmon, R.J.: Studies on long-term outcome in newborns with birth weights under 1500 grams, Adv. Behav. Ped. **1:**1, 1980.

Mulligan, J.C., and others: Neonatal asphyxia. II. Neonatal mortality and long-term sequelae, J. Pediatr. **96:**903, 1980.

National Center for Health Statistics: Advance report final mortality statistics, 1977, Monthly Vital Statistics Report, (Suppl.) **28**(1), 1977.

Vital statistics of the United States, vol. 2, Mortality, Part A, Washington, D.C., 1974, U.S. Government Printing Office.

World Health Organization: Report on social and biological effects on perinatal mortality, vol. 1, 1978, WHO.

CHAPTER 23 The respiratory system

PART ONE
The developmental biology of the lung

The lung is clearly a critical organ in early adaptation to extrauterine life. At birth, interruption of the fetal-placental circulation requires the newborn infant to immediately achieve effective gas exchange. Sufficient prenatal maturation of the respiratory system therefore is an essential aspect of intrauterine development. Differentiation of the lung requires carefully regulated coordination of anatomic, physiologic, and biochemical processes. The ultimate product of these maturational events is an organ having adequate surface area, blood supply, and metabolic capability to sustain oxygenation and ventilation during the neonatal period. Particularly important from a biochemical viewpoint is the capacity for rapid synthesis of surface-active phospholipids, which are necessary in establishing normal lung function after birth.

The elucidation of processes leading to lung maturity has depended on multidisciplinary research approaches that have been closely linked to improved clinical understanding of neonatal respiratory disorders. Information on the developmental biology of the respiratory system has provided important insights into pulmonary dysfunction after birth, as well as explanations for developmental anomalies of the lung. Indeed full appreciation of the pathophysiology of disorders such as the respiratory distress syndrome (RDS) requires one to develop a thorough understanding of the process of fetal lung maturation and the biology of pulmonary surfactant. Accordingly the purpose of this section is to review fundamental aspects of fetal lung development, including the physiology and biochemistry of surfactant. Because of the relatively high incidence and major significance of respiratory distress in neonatal-perinatal medicine, and in an effort to provide a frame of reference for the clinician, an attempt is made to relate the basic information to pertinent clinical problems of the newborn.

HISTORICAL PERSPECTIVE

Ever since pulmonary surfactant deficiency was recognized as an underlying problem in neonates with RDS, major efforts have been devoted to investigations concerning the physiology and biosynthesis of this phospholipid-rich substance which lines the respiratory epithelium. In some instances basic research approaches have paid rich dividends in enhancing care of the sick neonate. Advances that have bridged the gap from the laboratory to the bedside are the development of tests of fetal lung maturity, based on amniotic fluid analyses, and the use of corticosteroids for accelerating lung maturation in utero. Table 23-1 presents a chronologic outline of the advances in understanding surfactant and a description of the related discoveries concerning RDS.

The first 50 years were dominated by morphologic studies directed at either pulmonary hyaline membranes (PHM) or structural features of fetal lung development, particularly the glandular and canalicular phases in early gestation. In addition, during this period the effects of surface forces acting at the air-fluid interface of the lung were described by von Neergaard, providing the first experimental observation of the potential significance of pulmonary surfactant.

The next 20 years, from approximately 1950 to 1970, featured clinical studies on the pathophysiology of RDS and basic investigations on the nature and role of pulmonary surfactant. This era of research began with the recognition that PHMs represent a secondary, nonspecific phenomenon occurring because of tissue damage and

Table 23-1. Chronology of advances in understanding of pulmonary surfactant and RDS

Date	Observation
1902	Initial description of pulmonary hyaline membranes (PHM)
1923	First English description of PHM in association with neonatal pneumonia
1929	Discovery of the effects of surface forces at the air-water interface of the lung
1930-1949	Prevailing view that PHM resulted from aspirated amniotic sac contents
1936-1942	Description of structural features of fetal lung development, including three stages (glandular, canalicular, and alveolar)
1949	Proposal that an interval of air breathing was prerequisite to development of PHM
1950	Association of PHM with prematurity, fetal anoxia, maternal diabetes, and cesarean section
1950	Description of the clinical respiratory abnormalities associated with PHM
1951	PHM considered to be a secondary phenomenon resulting from tissue damage
1953-1955	Radiographic description of the reticulogranular pattern in generalized atelectasis
1954-1959	Elucidation of major pulmonary function abnormalities in RDS
1955-1957	Discovery of surfactant in pulmonary edema foam and lung extracts
1955-1958	Proposal that atelectasis is significant factor in respiratory distress with PHM
1955-1960	Clarification of the clinical pattern of RDS
1959	Demonstration of pulmonary surfactant deficiency in infants succumbing to RDS
1961	Identification of phosphatidylcholine (lecithin) as the major surfactant component
1961-1965	Lowered RDS mortality with intensive respiratory and metabolic care
1962-1967	Description of the timing of lung surfactant appearance during late gestation
1965-1967	Observation that lung phosphatidylcholine concentrations are decreased in RDS
1965-1970	Demonstration that aggressive mechanical ventilation improves survival in severe RDS but causes bronchopulmonary dysplasia
1971	Discovery of the predictability of amniotic fluid lecithin/sphingomyelin ratios, allowing prevention of *iatrogenic RDS*
1971	Improved oxygenation with continuous positive airway pressure
1971-1973	Discovery of the physiologic and biochemical effects of corticosteroids on the fetal lung
1971-1975	Demonstration of enhanced neonatal care via regionalized perinatal programs
1972	Direct demonstration by EM autoradiography of the role of type II pneumonocytes
1972	Prevention of RDS wth antenatal corticosteroid administration
1974	Clarification of pathways for de novo biosynthesis of lung phosphatidylcholine
1975	Discovery of phosphatidylglycerol as a significant component of surfactant
1975-1980	Growing interest in surfactant secretion and turnover

transudation of protein into the alveoli. Soon thereafter surfactant was "rediscovered" in pulmonary edema foam and lung extracts by Pattle and Clements, respectively. Such parallel advances culminated in the observation by Avery and Mead that lungs of immature fetuses and infants succumbing to RDS were deficient in surfactant, thus explaining the alveolar collapse and also providing a basis for more rational approaches to both research and treatment of RDS. Subsequently the timing of the appearance of surfactant in the fetal lung has been carefully defined, particularly during late gestation, when the major maturational changes take place. Improved understanding of the basis of pulmonary dysfunction in RDS and the role of surfactant also has facilitated serial improvements in techniques for mechanical ventilatory support of premature infants.

During the past decade there has been somewhat of a shift in emphasis from the anatomic and physiologic approaches to the study of fetal lung development toward biochemical studies and efforts to stimulate intrauterine lung maturation by administration of hormones and other pharmacologic agents. As a result, the metabolic regulation of surfactant production and turnover has become a major focus of research. Elucidation of the phospholipid composition of surfactant has encouraged basic scientists to concentrate their efforts on phosphatidylcholine (lecithin, or PC) and phosphatidylglycerol (PG), whereas clinicians have used measurements of these compounds in amniotic fluid for routine prenatal assessment of lung maturation. This has permitted perinatologists to better time the delivery and prevent a substantial number of premature infants from developing RDS.

THE MORPHOLOGY AND HISTOLOGY OF LUNG DEVELOPMENT
Architecture of the respiratory system

Simply stated, the respiratory system may be divided into three components: (1) the upper airways (from the nose and mouth to the trachea), which are mainly extrathoracic and of relatively large diameter, (2) the gas-distributing system of the lungs, or lower conducting airways, which begins with the main stem bronchi and extends to the terminal bronchioli, and (3) the acinar

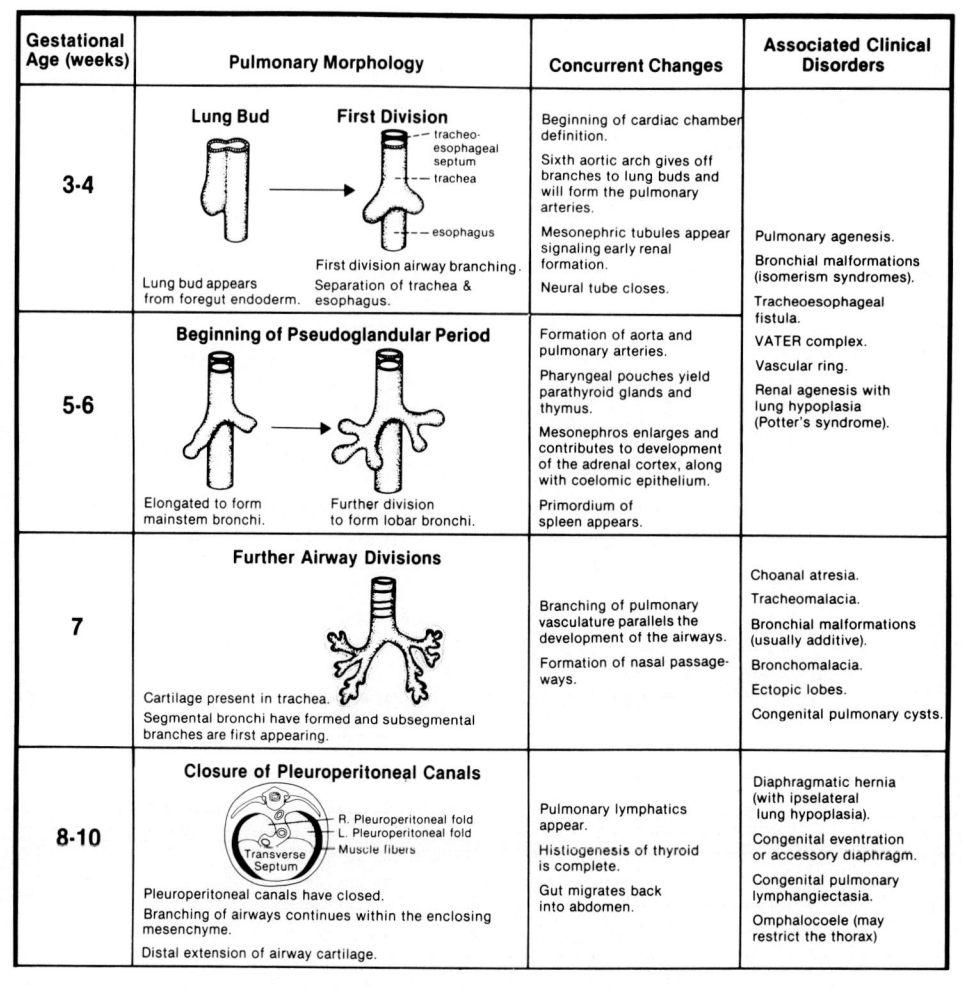

Gestational Age (weeks)	Pulmonary Morphology	Concurrent Changes	Associated Clinical Disorders
3-4	**Lung Bud / First Division** — Lung bud appears from foregut endoderm. First division airway branching. Separation of trachea & esophagus (tracheoesophageal septum, trachea, esophagus).	Beginning of cardiac chamber definition. Sixth aortic arch gives off branches to lung buds and will form the pulmonary arteries. Mesonephric tubules appear signaling early renal formation. Neural tube closes.	Pulmonary agenesis. Bronchial malformations (isomerism syndromes). Tracheoesophageal fistula. VATER complex. Vascular ring. Renal agenesis with lung hypoplasia (Potter's syndrome).
5-6	**Beginning of Pseudoglandular Period** — Elongated to form mainstem bronchi. Further division to form lobar bronchi.	Formation of aorta and pulmonary arteries. Pharyngeal pouches yield parathyroid glands and thymus. Mesonephros enlarges and contributes to development of the adrenal cortex, along with coelomic epithelium. Primordium of spleen appears.	
7	**Further Airway Divisions** — Cartilage present in trachea. Segmental bronchi have formed and subsegmental branches are first appearing.	Branching of pulmonary vasculature parallels the development of the airways. Formation of nasal passageways.	Choanal atresia. Tracheomalacia. Bronchial malformations (usually additive). Bronchomalacia. Ectopic lobes. Congenital pulmonary cysts.
8-10	**Closure of Pleuroperitoneal Canals** — (R. Pleuroperitoneal fold, L. Pleuroperitoneal fold, Muscle fibers, Transverse Septum). Pleuroperitoneal canals have closed. Branching of airways continues within the enclosing mesenchyme. Distal extension of airway cartilage.	Pulmonary lymphatics appear. Histiogenesis of thyroid is complete. Gut migrates back into abdomen.	Diaphragmatic hernia (with ipselateral lung hypoplasia). Congenital eventration or accessory diaphragm. Congenital pulmonary lymphangiectasia. Omphalocoele (may restrict the thorax)

Fig. 23-1. Major structural features of lung maturation, concurrent events in morphogenesis, and temporally associated malformations of the respiratory tract. Gestational ages listed refer to weeks of *postconceptional* development, i.e., fetal age is dated from the time of ovulation (assumed to be 2 weeks after the beginning of the the last menstrual period), as opposed to clinical gestational age, calculated from the first day of the last menstrual period. (From Perelman, R., Engle, M.J., and Farrell, P.: Lung **159:**53, 1981.)

region, which is responsible for carrying out exchange of oxygen and carbon dioxide.

The air-conducting portion of the lung is lined by ciliated epithelium. Bronchi are distinguished as airways that contain cartilage; large bronchi contain cartilage in any cross section, whereas small bronchi show less cartilage, which in fact may not be present in some cross-section histologic examinations. The most peripheral conducting airways (bronchioli) are distal to the last plate of cartilage. Clusters of three to five terminal bronchioli with their associated acini are grouped into lobules. In fully developed lungs the acinar regions feature respiratory bronchioli, alveolar ducts, and alveoli, whereas the immature lung contains saccules that originate from respiratory bronchioli. Saccules and alveoli are distinguished as narrow-walled structures with a characteristic epithelium containing both thin cells (type I) with few subcellular organelles and larger pneumonocytes (type II) with abundant mitochondria, endoplasmic reticulum, Golgi apparatus, and osmiophilic lamellar bodies known to contain surfactant.

The pulmonary vasculature is an essential component of a functional lung that allows gas exchange to take place efficiently. The mature lung has a dual arterial supply and dual venous drainage system. Branches of the pulmonary arteries supply the terminal respiratory units and most of the pleura, and bronchial arteries originating from the aorta supply the airway walls and hilar regions of the lung, including pleural surfaces and the walls of large blood vessels emerging from the mediastinum. The

Gestational Age (weeks)	Pulmonary Morphology	Concurrent Changes	Associated Clinical Disorders
16	**Beginning of Canalicular Period** Conducting Airways / Pulmonary Acinus Segmentation of bronchi is complete. Early formation of pulmonary acinus. Ciliated columnar epithelium lines the airways.	Formation of preacinar blood vessels is complete. Kidney is anatomically formed. CNS myelinization begins. Intrauterine movement is present.	Lung hypoplasia.
20	**Pulmonary Vascularization** Canalized airways lined by cuboidal epithelium. Decrease in mesenchyme. Capillaries penetrate early saccules.	Fetal "breathing" present. Pancreatic exocrine and endocrine function has been initiated. Thyroxin secretion.	Lung hypoplasia.
26	**Beginning of Terminal Sac Period** Respiratory saccules (S) appear from transitional ducts. Epithelium attenuates forming septae.	Eyelids unfused. Testes descending.	Respiratory insufficiency.
32-36	**Type II Pneumonocytes** Increased number of type II pneumonocytes with lamellar bodies. Abundant fetal pulmonary fluid present in potential airspaces.	Surfactant may be present but is often deficient. Increased adrenocorticoids. Accumulation of subcutaneous adipose tissue begins. Auricular cartilage present.	Hyaline membrane disease. Transient trachypnea. Apnea of prematurity.
Infancy to 8 Years	**Continuing Alveolar Proliferation** Alveoli (A) form and increase in both size and number (from 20×10^6 to 300×10^6 alveoli per lung).	Growth of the lungs approximates linear growth. Continued maturation of central ventilatory control mechanisms.	Cystic fibrosis. Lobar emphysema. Pectus excavatum.

Fig. 23-1, cont'd. For legend see opposite page.

systemic circulation via the bronchial arteries has relatively low flow compared with the pulmonary artery circuit and only accounts for 10% or less of the total pulmonary blood flow. Equally insignificant from a quantitative viewpoint are the bronchial veins that drain from the hila to the azygos or systemic vessels. Thus most of the venous return from the lung occurs via the pulmonary veins.

Development and growth of the airways, pulmonary vasculature, and acinar region

The cardinal features of lung maturation are presented in Fig. 23-1, together with a list of important temporally related events in fetal development. Differentiation of the respiratory system can be conveniently divided into five phases: (1) the embryonic phase, comprising the first 5 weeks after conception and leading to initiation of airways formation; (2) the glandular or pseudoglandular stage from 5 to 16 weeks of gestation, during which time the lower conducting airways are formed; (3) the canalicular phase, which begins at the seventeenth week with the "birth of the acinus" and concludes at 24 to 26 weeks of gestation; (4) the terminal sac period, during which time the first respiratory units are formed; and (5) the alveolar phase, which is initiated in the perinatal period and continues until approximately 8 years of age.

The respiratory system first appears after 3½ to 4 weeks of gestation as an outgrowth of the foregut. The lung bud then divides into two components to form the main stem bronchi. These airways subsequently branch within the enclosing mesenchyme to form the gas-conducting portion of the lung by the end of the sixteenth week after conception. Although the early stages of intrauterine lung development are defined primarily by changes in appearance of the airways, it must be emphasized that marked changes also take place in the vascular component of the lung (Fig. 23-1).

The overall pattern of formation of the respiratory system can be summarized by Reid's laws of lung development, a modified version of which follows:

1. The bronchial tree is developed by the sixteenth week of intrauterine life. Differentiation of the airways and the progressively increasing formation of cartilage occur in a centrifugal manner, i.e., from hilum to periphery.
2. The preacinar blood vessels follow the development of the airways, whereas the intraacinar arteries and veins develop parallel with the alveoli. Although the main pulmonary veins develop later than do the arteries, the adult pattern of vessels connecting heart with lungs, as well as the ductus arteriosus, are formed by the seventh week of gestation, whereas the preacinar arterial branching takes place alongside the dividing airways, and the developing veins are enveloped by mesenchyme. From 7 to 16 weeks after conception, the main feature of arterial growth is an increase in number of branches. By the sixteenth week virtually all preacinar vessels are present. Thereafter the existing vessels grow in size and length, while new vessels appear in the intraacinar region.

    The canalicular phase of lung development (after the seventeenth week) is characterized by slow invasion of the developing acinus by capillaries. This vascularization process occurs in a centripetal fashion, with the last phase being an extension to the respiratory bronchioles. During fetal life the diameter of blood vessels increases more rapidly at the proximal end than in the distal portions; this is in contrast to the similar rate of growth along an axial pathway following birth. In the fetus the arteries are more muscular than in the adult (wall thickness being higher relative to external diameter). In contrast, the walls of fetal veins have less muscle than those in the adult.
3. Alveoli develop mainly after birth, increasing in number from 20 million in the newborn to approximately 300 million at 8 years of age. There is marked expansion of the acinus after birth. For instance, by 2 months of age the length of the acinus has nearly doubled its neonatal size. A striking observation is that the alveoli develop in a centripetal direction, first on the saccules and their derivatives (the alveolar ducts), then on the respiratory bronchioles. In later childhood alveoli will develop on terminal bronchioles. The size of the alveoli continues to increase until growth of the chest wall ceases with attainment of adult thoracic size.

Cytodifferentiation of the respiratory epithelium

The lung is an extremely complex and heterogeneous organ, containing approximately 40 different cell types. Fortunately the distal respiratory epithelium responsible for gas exchange is more simplified and features mainly two distinct cells in the mature human lung. The ultrastructural features of the cytodifferentiation of the respiratory epithelium have been described for many mammals. In lower animal species, which have been studied in greatest detail, a characteristic sequence of changes has been identified. The same cellular phases of lung development also are present in the human fetus.

In early gestation the epithelial cells are simple and columnar in type and show few signs of organelle differentiation. Specific cell types are not recognizable until the canalicular stage of development. Subsequently, before surfactant is present, large quantities of glycogen accumulate within the respiratory epithelium. Finally during the last 10% to 20% of gestation in most species certain lining cells of the terminal respiratory units undergo alterations, permitting them to be distinguished as type II pneumonocytes. Although type II pneumonocytes have been identified in the human fetus between 22 and 26 weeks of gestation, these cells become more prominent at 34 to 36 weeks of gestation. The major change allowing these cells to be readily identified is the appearance of osmiophilic lamellar bodies in the cytoplasm (Figs. 23-1 and 23-8). There is a very close correlation between the presence of these lamellar inclusions and the appearance of surface-active material in lung extracts.

In addition to the lamellar bodies, other features of the type II pneumonocytes allow them to be distinguished from type I cells of the respiratory epithelium. For instance, type II pneumonocytes have abundant mitochondria, endoplasmic reticulum, polyribosomes, and Golgi apparatus, suggesting the capability for a high rate of metabolic activity. Indeed histochemical and ultrastructural autoradiographic techniques have confirmed the role of the type II pneumonocyte in the synthesis, storage, and secretion of pulmonary surfactant. These studies also have indicated that the osmiophilic lamellar bodies are the intracellular deposits of surfactant. In essence they may be viewed as secretory granules of unique morphology and composition. The synthesis of surfactant phospholipid has been traced by sequential electron microscopic analysis after administration of a radioisotopic precursor (usually, ^{3}H-choline, which labels phosphatidylcholine almost exclusively). Such studies revealed a sequence typical for exocrine cells: rapid uptake of precursor from capillaries, transfer to endoplasmic reticulum, synthesis of phospholipids, transfer via the Golgi apparatus and perhaps transfer of special proteins to the osmiophilic lamellar bodies for "packaging," and then secretion into the alveolar space.

Although more ultrastructural morphometric analysis of the developing lung is needed, it has been estimated that type II pneumonocytes normally account for no more than 15% of the lung acinar cell population.

Despite being similar in number, type I pneumonocytes cover the major part of the alveolus, by virtue of their larger size and the long cytoplasmic extensions characteristic of these cells. Because of their thin nature and proximity to capillary endothelial cells, type I pneumonocytes are ideally suited to assist in the transfer of oxygen and carbon dioxide. Therefore gas exchange occurs primarily across that portion of the respiratory epithelium comprised of type I pneumonocytes.

Clinical correlation

The intrauterine timing of pulmonary anomalies can be appreciated from the foregoing review of the sequence of changes taking place during development of the respiratory system. Fig. 23-1 lists several malformations and gives an indication of the approximate time in gestation when the abnormality originates. It is evident, for instance, that *all* malformations of the conducting airways must take place prior to 16 weeks of gestation. Thus upper airway abnormalities take place between conception and 5 weeks of gestation. Bronchial malformations, which are usually additive and lead to duplicated airways, occur between 5 and 16 weeks, whereas lung hypoplasia, characterized by inadequate development of pulmonary acini, would be evident after 16 weeks.

Knowledge about the process of fetal lung development also provides insights into the age at which the respiratory system is capable of supporting satisfactory gas exchange. Given the present limits of our clinical technology, fetal viability can be first expected at approximately 26 weeks of gestation. This is when the respiratory saccules have developed, and adequate vascularization by capillary invasion has taken place. Before 26 weeks some exchange of oxygen or carbon dioxide may take place, but generally inadequate surface area exists to support continued respiration.

THE PHYSIOLOGY OF PULMONARY SURFACTANT
Role of surfactant in respiratory mechanics

Because of the rapid development of high surface forces along the respiratory epithelium when breathing is first initiated, the availability of adequate quantities of pulmonary surfactant in terminal air spaces is of paramount importance in successful postnatal lung function. Surface forces have interested physiologists since 1929, when von Neergaard noted their effect on the pressure-volume characteristics of liquid- and air-filled lungs. From these early experiments it was theorized that the retractive tendency of air-filled lungs was not only a result of tissue elastic recoil but also of surface forces operating at the gas-liquid interface of the respiratory system. This work and subsequent investigations have defined the contribution of surface factors to the overall

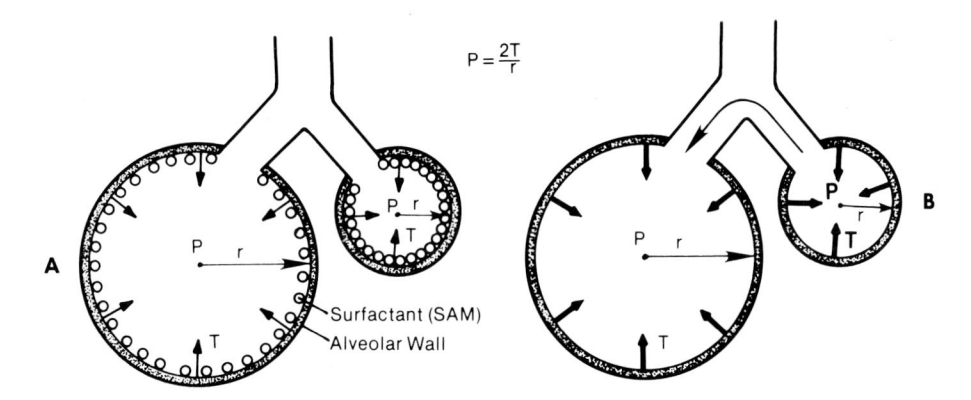

Fig. 23-2. Relationship of Laplace's law to alveolar stability in the normal and surfactant-deficient lung. Although schematically represented as spherical, terminal respiratory units tend to be polygonal in the mature lung. Laplace's law states that the pressure (P) within a sphere is directly proportional to surface tension (T) and inversely proportional to the radius of curvature (r). **A,** Normal lung. As alveolar size diminishes, surface tension is reduced in the presence of SAM, thereby decreasing the collapsing pressure to be opposed. The pressure within the small and large interconnected alveoli is equal, negating the tendency for transfer of gas. **B,** Surfactant-deficient lung. Without the surface tension lowering capacity of SAM, alveoli become unstable at low volume and tend to collapse. Some alveoli may empty into larger ones to equalize pressure between the two in accordance with Boyle's law. (Adapted from an original painting by Frank H. Netter, M.D., from THE CIBA COLLECTION OF MEDICAL ILLUSTRATIONS, copyright by CIBA Pharmaceutical Co., Division of CIBA-GEIGY Corporation.)

collapsing tendency of the lung. Of great interest is the finding that surface tension accounts for approximately two thirds of the total retractive force of the air-inflated lung. The magnitude of surface forces therefore may be viewed as a major obstacle to the neonatal lung. The early research on pressure-volume relationships also established the phenomenon of *hysteresis,* or separation of inflation and deflation curves on expansion with air but not with liquid. Contrary to expectations based on Laplace's law, experimental observations suggested that the collapsing forces of the lung normally decrease as the alveolar diameter is reduced via deflation or simulated expiration (Fig. 23-2).

Although the studies of von Neergaard led to the prediction of a surface tension–lowering substance in the alveoli, several decades passed (Table 23-1) before other investigators conclusively demonstrated surface-active material, i.e., surfactant, in pulmonary fluid (edema foam) and lung extracts. In the key experiments performed with a modified Wilhelmy surface balance it was observed that, when surface films derived from lung extracts were compressed, the surface tension decreased to very low levels and then rose rapidly on expansion. In addition, surface tension tracings during cyclic expansion and compression of the films were widely separated, thus duplicating the hysteresis loop of the intact lung.

Considered collectively, research advances have evolved a biophysical view of pulmonary surfactant as an antiatelectasis factor located in the "alveolar lining layer" that provides a low and variable surface tension and imparts hysteresis to the air-tissue interface. Surface-active material, then, is capable of performing the twofold function of (1) decreasing the pressure required to distend the lung and (2) maintaining alveolar stability over a wide range of local volumes. These functions and the importance of surfactant can be better appreciated by further discussion of relevant experimental techniques and observations.

Laboratory assessment of surfactant

In the laboratory setting pressure-volume and surface balance experiments allow physiologic assessment of surface-active material, lung stability, and distensibility, or compliance, and thus an evaluation of maturity. In its simplest form, a surface balance consists of a Teflon trough, a movable barrier, and a platinum plate (Fig. 23-3). After a surface film is layered over saline in the trough, the barrier is cycled to expand and compress the film. The surface tension is measured from the force exerted on the platinum plate, provided the angle of contact between the plate and liquid approximates zero. As shown in Fig. 23-3, pressure-volume relationships for whole lungs or isolated lung lobes are studied in a closed system by instilling air or saline from a reservoir into the

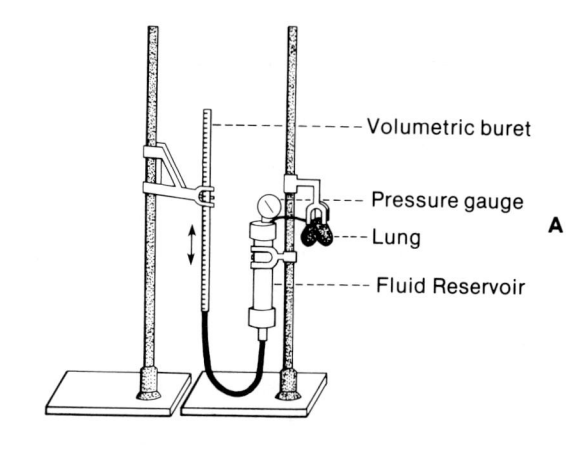

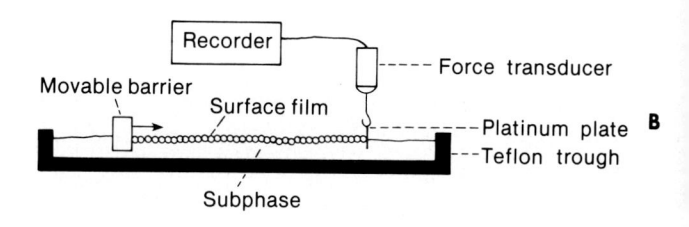

Fig. 23-3. Schematic representation of a pressure-volume apparatus **(A)** and surface balance **(B)**, the operation of which is discussed in text.

respiratory system under pressure produced by raising a fluid-filled buret. After stabilization at a maximum pressure (usually 30 or 35 cm H_2O) the buret is lowered in a stepwise fashion to empty the lung. At points of no gas flow, relating the change in pressure to change in volume (slope of the P/V curve) yields an estimate of distensibility or static compliance ($\Delta V/\Delta P = C$). As represented in Fig. 23-4, saline-filled lungs establish maximum volume at considerably lower inflation pressures than do air-filled lungs. In the absence of a gas-liquid interface the effects of surface forces are eliminated, resulting in a greater tendency to collapse on deflation and much less hysteresis. Retention of volume on deflation to zero pressure in the air-filled, mature lung is an expression of intrinsic alveolar stability. Immature lungs require considerably higher pressures to initiate air filling (opening pressure), have a lower volume at any pressure, and have little or no residual volume on deflation. Therefore maturation of the lung is associated with an increased peak volume as well as an improved capacity to retain air on deflation, i.e., deflation stability.

Appearance of surfactant and importance in the perinatal period (see p. 134)

Although some evidence suggests surfactant may appear in the human lung as early as 24 weeks of gesta-

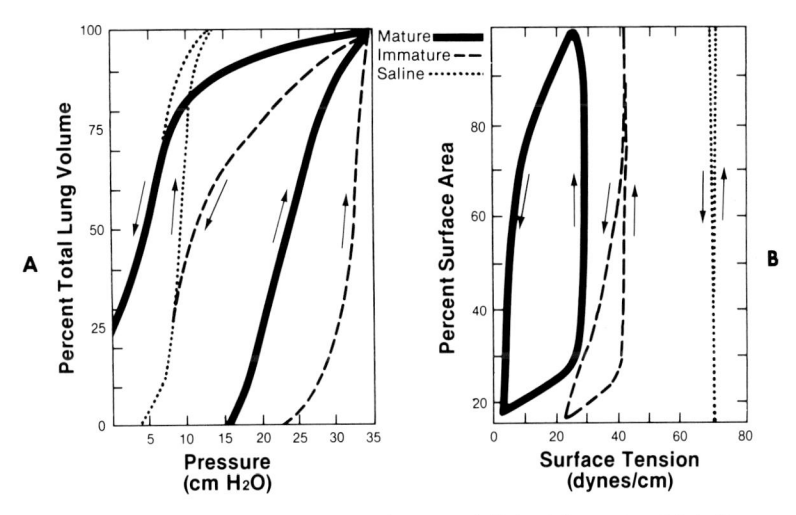

Fig. 23-4. Contrast between mature and surfactant-deficient (immature) fetal lungs as studied with the pressure-volume apparatus **(A)** and surface balance **(B)**. **A,** Representative pressure-volume curves for air-filled mature lungs (*solid line*) and for air-filled surfactant-deficient lungs (*dashed line*). Note that the mature lung shows lower opening pressure, relative stability on deflation, and maintenance of residual volume. The pressure-volume curve generated by saline filling of the mature lung (*dotted line*) is also shown and emphasizes the lack of surface forces when no air-liquid interface is present. It is further evident that less pressure is required for complete filling with saline than air and that there is less hysteresis between the inflation and deflation portions of the curve. **B,** Representative tracings resulting from cyclical compression and expansion of extracts from a mature lung (solid line) and an immature lung (dashed line). The dotted line represents a saline reference tracing. In contrast to the immature lung, mature lung extracts achieve a low surface tension value (<10 dynes/cm) at maximal compression, i.e., minimal surface area. (Adapted from Kotas, R.V., and others: J. Appl. Physiol. **43**:92, 1977.)

tion, functional surfactant is generally evident in developing mammalian lungs at 80% to 90% of gestation. When surfactant is present, it is noteworthy that deflation stability indicated by %V$_{10}$ is maximized (Fig. 23-5). These pulmonary maturational events during late gestation portend a successful transition from maternal/placental–dependent gas exchange to extrauterine ventilation.

With the onset of postnatal breathing considerable force is required to overcome the high viscosity and inertia of the fetal pulmonary fluid that fills the potential air spaces at birth. The high pressures generated in the first few breaths not only are required for expansion but are also quite important in moving lung liquid and establishing an air-liquid interface. As air enters the lung and the size of the airways diminishes in the periphery, the surface tension at the junction between lung fluid and air increases. The clearance of fluid from smaller airways may be more efficient in the presence of adequate surfactant. Since the shape of the meniscus at the air-liquid interface is dependent on the surface tension of liquid molecules at the surface, pulmonary surfactant enhances lung fluid movement by increasing the area of the air-liquid interface over which pressure can be exerted.

Therefore, if sufficient surface-active material is present, less effort is required to replace each unit of lung fluid with air.

Once the mature lung has been expanded, the surfactant film lining the alveoli and terminal bronchioles tends to increase surface tension at high lung volumes, promoting emptying, and lower it at diminished lung volumes (Fig. 23-2). Lowering surface tension as the size of terminal airspaces decreases prevents collapse at end expiration. The remaining volume of gas, termed *functional residual capacity* (FRC), acts as a reservoir that prevents wide fluctuations in blood oxygen and carbon dioxide levels during respiration. Furthermore a partially expanded airspace, i.e., the lung at FRC, requires less effort to reexpand than one that is completely collapsed.

Neonatal surfactant deficiency

The physiologic consequences of surfactant deficiency are manifested clinically in the premature neonate as RDS. The classic association of tachypnea, grunting, retractions, hypoxemia, and characteristic chest roentgenogram for the most part can be related to the changes in surface properties of the thin layer of liquid lining the

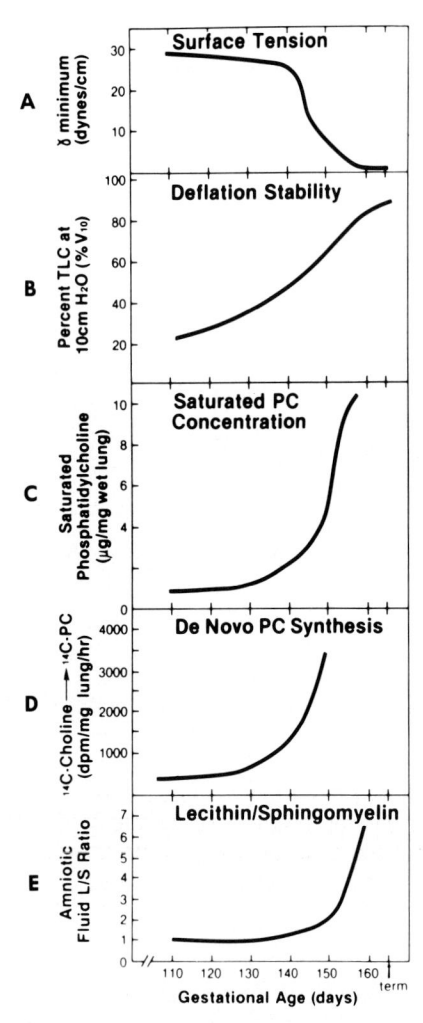

Fig. 23-5. Representative curves depicting the correlation between biochemical and physiologic events during fetal lung maturation in the rhesus monkey. **A,** Surface tension. **B,** Deflation stability. **C,** Saturated PC concentration. **D,** De novo PC synthesis. **E,** Lecithin/sphingomyelin. (Adapted from Kotas, R.V., and others: J. Appl. Physiol. **43:**92, 1977.)

air spaces. As discussed previously, in air spaces devoid of surfactant, surface forces (and therefore pressure) rise rapidly on deflation, leading to instability, further loss of volume, and consequently atelectasis. The reduced volume at end expiration not only negates the buffering capacity afforded by a normal FRC but also requires the generation of high pressures to reexpand the lung with each breath. Large pressure changes coupled with the very compliant thorax of the premature neonate result in retractions. With the stresses of increased oxygen consumption and the work of breathing, metabolic demands are markedly augmented. Because of immaturity and minimum substrate reserves, the prematurely delivered infant with RDS is ill equipped to meet these demands.

Clinical observations have revealed that grunting, a common finding in RDS, improves oxygenation. It has been suggested that the consequences of the grunt are to prolong end expiration, maintain the surfactant-deficient lung at slightly larger volumes, and afford increased time for gas exchange to take place. The clinical application of continuous positive airway pressure (CPAP) was theorized to serve the same physiologic function as the grunt.

The use of positive end expiratory pressure (PEEP) may have an effect over and above the mechanical one leading to improved gas exchange. This additional role, termed *conservation* of pulmonary surfactant, has stimulated research concerning the influence of current modes of therapy for RDS on surfactant turnover. Investigations have shown that increased ventilation can effect pulmonary surfactant and pressure-volume characteristics. Reduced compliance observed in hyperventilated lungs has been attributed to a decrease in surfactant and corroborated by reduced surface tension–lowering capacity of lung extracts. It has been suggested that ventilation enhances the movement of surfactant from alveoli into the airways, and PEEP hinders this phenomenon. According to this hypothesis the degree and rate of spread of surface-active material would depend on the volume of the alveoli at end expiration. The smaller the alveolus, the greater the flux. Other studies involving injection of various radioactive phospholipid precursors suggest that hyperventilation promotes release—then inactivation of surface-active material—and that end expiratory pressure, by preventing surface film collapse, negates these adverse effects.

Neurohumoral regulation of surfactant secretion

Evidence accumulated in recent years from multidisciplinary studies supports the concept that the autonomic nervous system or its mediators may influence pulmonary surfactant by regulating the rate of secretion or possibly by controlling in part the turnover of surface-active phospholipids. These studies have used pharmacophysiologic approaches applied primarily to mechanically hyperventilated animals. As mentioned previously, the hyperventilation model is advantageous because this system features increased release of surfactant into the air spaces. Of great interest is the observation that β-adrenergic antagonists (e.g., propranolol) can prevent this response to increased ventilation. In addition, β_2 agonists terbutaline and isoxsuprine, which are both used clinically for suppression of premature labor, have been shown to stimulate a significant increase in the amount of phospholipid recovered from lung lavages; this effect can be blocked by prior administration of propranolol. These observations suggest that adrenergic mechanisms can control surfactant concentrations in the terminal air

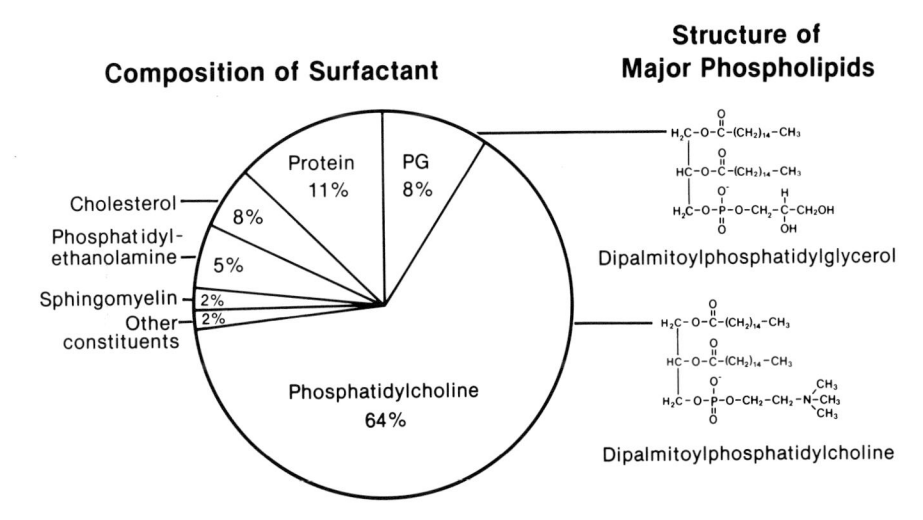

Fig. 23-6. Composition of surface-active material, obtained by lung lavage, and the structure of major phospholipids present in pulmonary surfactant. (From Perelman, R., Engle, M.J., and Farrell, P.: Lung **159**:53, 1981.)

spaces. Since other studies have demonstrated that α-adrenergic agents do not affect lung surfactant, it may be concluded that the β-adrenergic receptors are specifically involved in regulating pulmonary phospholipid metabolism.

Cholinergically mediated regulation also has been suspected for many years, ever since studies revealed evidence of decreased surfactant in lungs from vagotomized animals. Subsequent observations in such animals have demonstrated decreased numbers of lamellar bodies ("secretory granules") in type II alveolar pneumonocytes and the presence of generalized atelectasis. Administration of acetylcholine, pilocarpine, or electrical stimulation of the vagus nerve has resulted in changes implying augmented secretion of pulmonary surfactant. Prior treatment with atropine eliminated increased surfactant secretions and thus confirmed involvement of cholinergic stimulation.

Thus β-adrenergic receptors, cholinergic receptors, and (based on other more preliminary data) certain prostaglandins are potential regulators of surfactant turnover. Whether these alter surfactant metabolism during hyperventilation by increasing secretion or by slowing degradation remains unclear. The more precise delineation of the effect of the aforementioned mediators on surfactant kinetics offers an important challenge to the understanding of pulmonary phospholipid metabolism.

THE BIOCHEMISTRY OF PULMONARY SURFACTANT
Chemical composition

Because phospholipids are ideally suited as surface-active agents in interfacial films, the biophysical behavior of pulmonary surfactant provided an early clue to its composition. Studies initiated shortly after the rediscovery of surfactant indicated that the liquid obtained by lung lavage was largely composed of lipid, particularly phospholipid, with smaller amounts of protein. Accordingly, pulmonary surfactant has been defined by Farrell and Avery as "a unique lipoprotein, particularly rich in highly saturated lecithins (saturated phosphatidylcholine molecules) and containing lesser amounts of cholesterol, neutral lipid, and other phospholipids." The predominance of phosphatidylcholine is evident from the data presented in Fig. 23-6, which also illustrates the percentage of contribution from other lipids. The uniqueness of phosphatidylcholine in the respiratory system stems from its fatty acid substructure. Unlike most tissues that exhibit phosphatidylcholine molecules having a saturated fatty acid at the 1-carbon position and an unsaturated fatty acyl constituent at the 2-carbon position, lung parenchyma and bronchoalveolar fluid contain a high proportion of disaturated phosphatidylcholine. In fact, from analysis of extensively purified surfactant fraction, results have been obtained indicating that approximately 60% of the total lipid is 1,2-dipalmitoyl-phosphatidylcholine; the structure of this compound is shown in Fig. 23-6. The highly saturated nature of lung phosphatidylcholine molecules appears to be essential in the relation to the surface tension–lowering capability of the alveolar lining layer.

A second phospholipid marker of surfactant, also structurally depicted in Fig. 23-6, is phosphatidylglycerol. After a period of controversy concerning its identity this special constituent has only recently been identified unequivocally in preparations of lung tissue. In essence this compound was originally misidentified by some investigators as phosphatidyl-N, N-dimethylethanolamine, or PDME; concurrently, other investigators reported the presence of phosphatidylglycerol and the absence of significant phosphatidyl-N, N-dimethylethanolamine. The fallacious recognition of phosphatidyl-N, N-dimethylethanolamine on thin-layer chromatograms promoted an unfortunate misunderstanding of pathways for phosphatidylcholine biosynthesis. Not until recent years has this issue been resolved and the following points established: (1) phosphatidylglycerol is present in whole lung tissue, where it accounts for approximately 3% of the total phospholipid; (2) phosphatidylglycerol is enriched in bronchoalveolar fluid and accounts for approximately 8% of the total phospholipid; (3) phosphatidylglycerol, like saturated phosphatidylcholine, is actively synthesized in the lung and appears to undergo relatively rapid turnover; and (4) the fatty acid composition of phosphatidylglycerol is also similar to that of phosphatidylcholine in that it contains highly saturated constituents.

The proteins present in pulmonary surfactant are also unique. Two proteins in particular, termed *surfactant apoproteins*, seem to be essential components of the surface-active material and function as the matrix for phospholipid molecules. The specific nature of the proteins awaits indentification.

Mechanisms for production of phosphatidylcholine

Two pathways exist for the de novo synthesis of phosphatidylcholine. The first of these is the choline-incorporation mechanism or cytidine diphosphocholine pathway. As shown in Fig. 23-7, this is a three-reaction metabolic sequence, involving phosphorylation of choline, activation by conversion of choline phosphate to the cytidine diphosphate (CDP) derivative, and final transfer of the phosphorylcholine portion of the activated compound to diglyceride, yielding phosphatidylcholine. It is actually the cooperative interaction of these three reactions and the biochemical processes leading to phosphatidic acid formation and hydrolysis that finally produces phosphatidylcholine. In the second de novo mechanism, termed the *methylation pathway*, ethanolamine undergoes similar steps of phosphorylation, activation, and linkage to diglyceride to form phosphatidylethanolamine (PE), which then undergoes three successive methylations to produce phosphatidylcholine. It had been proposed at one time that phosphatidylethanolamine methylation was a major pathway in the fetal primate lung prior to term gestation. This conclusion was based on misidentification of phosphatidyl-N, N-dimethylethanolamine, several unwarranted assumptions, and erroneous interpretation of indirect evidence. Subsequently from studies using direct biochemical techniques it has been determined conclusively that the cytidine diphosphocholine pathway is the primary mechanism for biosynthesis of phosphatidylcholine in the developing mammalian lung. The evidence for this conclusion is reviewed in detail by Farrell and Hamosh.

The mechanism by which saturated phosphatidylcholine molecules are specifically formed in the mature lung has stimulated great interest in recent years. The consensus of opinion at present, based on a variety of experimental observations, is that the cytidine diphosphocholine pathway despite its predominance does not yield saturated phospholipids, but rather mixed molecules with respect to fatty acid composition. This has led to the current view that the phosphatidylcholine-lysophosphatidylcholine cycle, shown in Fig. 23-7, *F*, is the mechanism operating to control the fatty acid substructure of the final product. Thus there is evidence suggesting that either deacylation-reacylation or deacylation-transacylation reactions are important in the formation of saturated phosphatidylcholine. This question, however, has not been fully resolved. Other possibilities such as a specific transfer protein leading to enrichment of surfactant in saturated phospholipid require further study.

Appearance of increased phosphatidylcholine in the fetal lung

As shown in Fig. 23-5, fetal lung development is characterized by major biochemical changes during late gestation. Most of the studies of phospholipid concentrations and their rates of synthesis have been conducted in either lower animal species or nonhuman primates such as the rhesus monkey. This work has revealed a considerable degree of uniformity in regard to the period of gestation when biochemical changes take place. Irrespective of the total duration of a species' pregnancy, it has been found that augmented lung phosphatidylcholine production is characteristically demonstrable at 85% to 90% of gestation. For instance, in rhesus monkey fetuses increased saturated phosphatidylcholine concentration takes place at approximately 145 to 150 days of the 168-day intrauterine period; this would correspond to 34 weeks of human gestation. At this time or shortly thereafter phosphatidylcholine concentrations in amniotic fluid rise, indicating to the clinician the attainment of fetal lung maturity. As further illustrated in Fig. 23-5, there is a very close correlation between the biochemical changes and their physiologic counterparts. Therefore one can logically assume that the fetal lung is endowed with special regulatory mechanisms operating to control the timing of the biochemical maturation process. This ensures accumulation of a reservoir of phosphatidylcholine prior to delivery. Once this increased concentration of phosphatidylcholine is present, increased

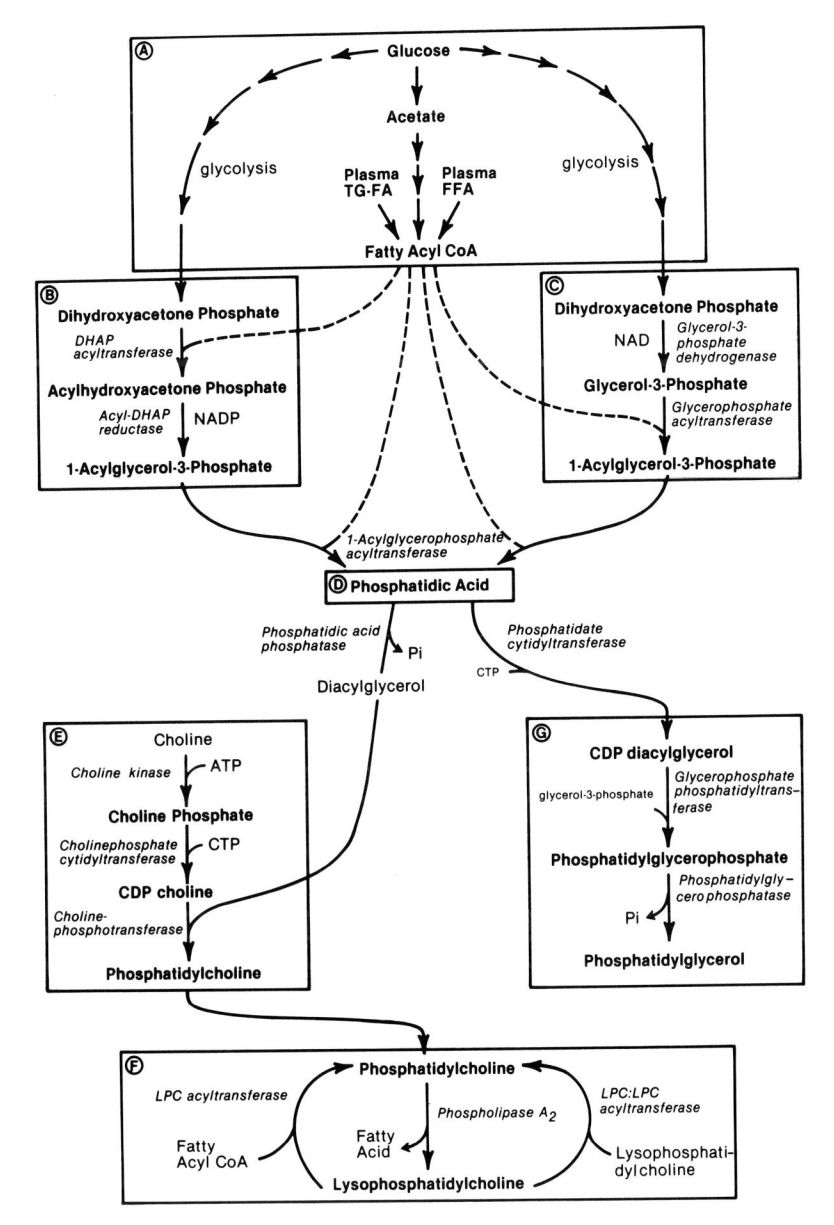

Fig. 23-7. Pathways of phosphatidylcholine and phosphatidylglycerol biosynthesis. *TG-FA,* Triglyceride fatty acids; *FFA,* free fatty acids; *DHAP,* dihydroxyacetone phosphate; *LPC,* lysophosphatidylcholine. (From Perelman, R., Engle, M.J., and Farrell, P.: Lung **159:**53, 1981.)

phosphatidylglycerol also is seen in both lung and amniotic fluid, providing further evidence of fetal lung maturity.

Regulation of phosphatidylcholine synthesis

The major emphasis of present research deals with regulatory mechanisms for phosphatidylcholine synthesis and study of pharmacologic agents that accelerate the process of fetal lung development. Fig. 23-8 presents schematically some of the factors of potential importance in controlling the turnover of surfactant phospholipid. These factors include exogenous precursors, key enzymes, and certain hormones.

Substrates

Because an abundance of precursor substrate must be supplied for phosphatidylcholine biosynthesis, the circulatory system is essential in supporting lung metabolism. Furthermore nutrients from the placenta during gestation and from the diet after birth potentially could play an important role in facilitating surfactant production. Substances of special interest in this regard are glucose,

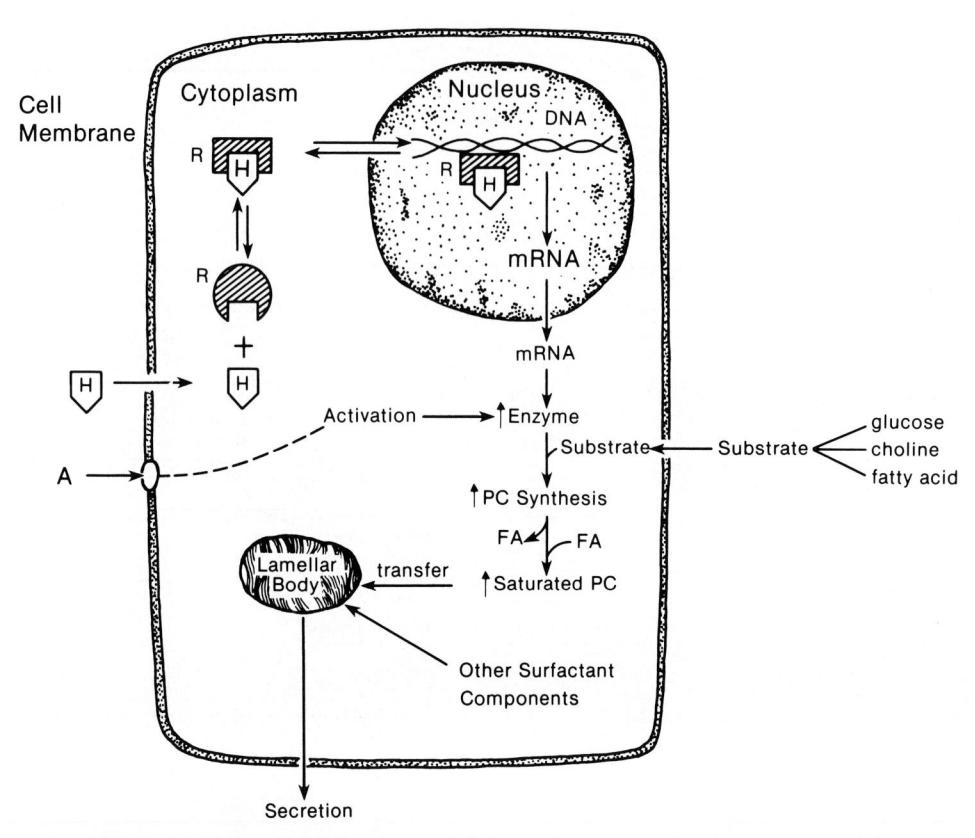

Fig. 23-8. Hypothetical scheme of the production and delivery of surfactant to the "alveolar lining layer" by a type II pneumonocyte. Various potential regulatory steps illustrate hormone-mediated control mechanisms, regulation by substrates, and the key role of enzymes in phospholipid production. *A,* Activator; *H,* hormone, particularly corticosteroid; *R,* receptor; *FA,* fatty acid; *DNA,* deoxyribonucleic acid molecule stimulated by hormone to increased "expression"; *mRNA,* messenger ribonucleic acid molecules coding for increased synthesis of specific enzymes. (Reprinted from Ballard, P.L.: Glucocorticoid receptors in the fetal lung. In Hodson, W.A., editor: Development of the lung, New York, 1977, Marcel Dekker, Inc. By courtesy of Marcel Dekker, Inc.)

fatty acid, and choline. In addition to glucose from the blood stream, there is a distinct possibility that endogenous glucose stored as glycogen in the type II pneumonocyte can contribute to the surge in phosphatidylcholine synthesis during late gestation.

Enzymes

The rate of product formation in various metabolic pathways often is governed by key enzymes. From biochemical studies of the past decade there is evidence that phosphatidylcholine biosynthesis might be regulated by some of the enzymes shown in Fig. 23-7. In particular, data have been obtained suggesting that phosphatidic acid phosphatase, choline kinase, cholinephosphate cytidyltransferase, and cholinephosphotransferase all might play a role in elevating fetal lung phosphatidylcholine levels in late gestation. The influence of enzymes on overall pathway rates may be exerted by either adjustments in enzyme concentration or by direct modulation of enzyme activity through altered kinetic properties. Increases in enzyme concentrations often are achieved by augmented protein synthesis through expression of specific genes. Thus DNA present in the nucleus of the type II pneumonocyte might initiate increased synthesis of messenger RNA, which could in turn initiate synthesis of an enzyme such as phosphatidic acid phosphatase to provide more diglyceride for phosphatidylcholine biosynthesis.

A second general mechanism—direct modulation of enzyme activity via kinetic properties—seems operative in the developing lung. For instance, the first enzyme of the cytidine diphosphocholine pathway (choline kinase) shows unique kinetic properties in lung tissue that account for the active use of this pathway rather than the methylation mechanism during fetal lung development.

Hormones

Various hormones are known to influence the rate of phosphatidylcholine biosynthesis in fetal lung cells. For instance, corticosteroids have a powerful effect on the rate of the cytidine diphosphocholine pathway. Other stimulatory agents include thyroid hormones, estrogens, and theophylline. Evidence also has been obtained suggesting that lung metabolism can be stimulated by cyclic AMP, which probably acts via enzymes as a second messenger. In addition, labor and/or oxytocin have been shown to stimulate the process of fetal lung development; it is possible that the mechanism for this effect involves endogenous corticoids secreted in increased concentrations as a response to stress. Results of recent studies further indicate that some hormones such as insulin may retard surfactant formation. This might explain the clinical observation that hyperinsulinemic fetuses (principally in gestations complicated by maternal diabetes) often show delayed lung maturation.

As shown in Fig. 23-8, hormone receptors are present in the cytoplasm and nucleus of type II pneumonocytes. The developmental pattern for lung receptors is of obvious interest in connection with corticosteroids. In this regard it appears that the presence of the receptor system is not a limiting factor in the stimulation of lung development. The cytoplasmic binding activity for steroid hormones has been detected as early as 9 weeks of gestation, and nuclear transfer of receptor-hormone complexes occurs in lungs of 16-week-old fetuses. Cytoplasmic receptors are present in the fetal lung throughout gestation and have been detected in the lungs of premature and term newborn infants. The concentration of binding sites is constant in lungs studied from 12 to 20 weeks of gestation, whereas lower levels are found between 27 and 40 weeks of gestation. The high concentration of corticosteroid receptors in type II pneumonocytes indicates that the lung is a target tissue for this class of hormones.

Biochemical role of corticosteroids

Biochemical studies dealing with the stimulatory influence of corticosteroids on the fetal lung were pursued shortly after Liggins discovered their maturational effect (based on clinical and morphologic observations on lambs) and after Kotas and Avery demonstrated the accelerated appearance of surfactant in hormone-treated rabbit fetuses. Most biochemical studies have used rats and rabbits in which cortisol analogues are directly administered to immature fetuses. Data obtained with these short gestational species support the following conclusions: (1) corticosteroids increase de novo synthesis of phosphatidylcholine, promoting accumulation of this phospholipid in the fetal lung; (2) corticosteroids specifically stimulate the cytidine diphosphocholine pathway, without altering the phosphatidylethanolamine methylation mechanism; (3) corticosteroids cause an increase in the activity of several enzymes essential to synthesis of phosphatidylcholine. Although these changes could be secondary phenomena, they probably represent primary, gene-mediated effects of hormones on type II pneumonocytes. The same effects demonstrated with rabbits and rats also have been observed with cultured human fetal lung explants incubated in the presence of cortisol. Not only have increased phospholipids been repeatedly demonstrated in lung parenchyma, but it also has been determined that fetal pulmonary fluid shows increased saturated phosphatidylcholine after steroid administration. Curiously, however, amniotic fluid phospholipids are not markedly altered after corticosteroid administration; this is probably because of a time delay after metabolic stimulation before newly synthesized phosphatidylcholine molecules can reach the amniotic cavity.

The net biochemical effect of the hormone, through an apparent induction of key enzymes, is to enhance the capacity of the fetal lung to produce the surface-active phospholipids of the respiratory system, as summarized in the following outline on the effects of corticosteroids on fetal lung development:

A. Anatomic*
 1. Increased potential air space
   a. Attenuation of alveolar cells
   b. Narrowing of septa
   c. Greater "alveolarization"
 2. Increased prominence or numbers of type II pneumonocytes
B. Physiologic
 1. Greater distensibility
 2. Greater deflation stability
 3. Earlier appearance of surfactant
C. Biochemical
 1. Increased concentration and/or degree of saturation of phosphatidylcholine in
   a. Lung parenchyma
   b. Lung lavage fluid
 2. Increased conversion of choline to phosphatidylcholine, i.e., the apparent rate of the cytidine diphosphocholine pathway is enhanced
 3. Increased activities of lipoprotein lipase, cholinephosphotransferase, lysophosphatidylcholine acyltransferase, and glycerolphosphate phosphatidyltransferase†

Because of exogenous corticosteroids, the capacity for pulmonary surfactant production is developed at an earlier time in gestation than would normally occur. The

---

*The anatomic effects of glucocorticoids on the fetal lung require further definition.
†There is a dispute in the literature regarding specific enzyme changes occurring after fetal or maternal administration of corticosteroids.

hormone therefore acts as a stimulus capable of changing the timing of fetal lung development such that the maturation process is accelerated. Although limited observations suggest that corticosteroids may be the natural inducer for biochemical maturation of the lung in late gestation, this has not been substantiated. Furthermore it has been shown that cortisol alone is not the physiologic stimulus for intrauterine lung maturation.

Further studies on the role of endogenous substances and the triggering of physiologic and biochemical processes leading to lung maturation are required.

SUMMARY

After the embryonic period of development, comprising the first 5 weeks after conception, there are three major stages of fetal lung development: the pseudoglandular, the canalicular, and the terminal sac phases.

The overall pattern of the formation of the respiratory system can be summarized by Reid's laws: (1) the conducting airways are developed by the sixteenth week of gestation; (2) alveoli develop mainly after birth, increasing in number until age 8 years and in size until growth of the thoracic cavity ceases; and (3) the preacinar blood vessels follow development of the airways, whereas the intraacinar vessels develop parallel with the alveoli.

During cytodifferentiation of the respiratory epithelium, type II pneumonocytes containing osmiophilic lamellar bodies become more prominent, implying increased levels of intracellular surfactant.

Pulmonary surface-active material (surfactant) is an antiatelectasis factor located in the "alveolar lining layer" that provides a low and variable surface tension and imparts hysteresis to the air-tissue interface. Functional surfactant decreases the pressure required to inflate the lung postnatally and maintains stability over a wide range of local volumes.

Although many substances are present in pulmonary surfactant, the predominant and functionally essential constituent is saturated phosphatidylcholine, or lecithin. Lung cells and bronchoalveolar fluid are unique in showing high concentrations of saturated phosphatidylcholine and significant amounts of phosphatidylglycerol.

The major biochemical feature of fetal lung development is an increase in the concentration of saturated phosphatidylcholine, a change that occurs by approximately 90% of term gestation. Shortly after the appearance of increased surfactant phospholipid in lung extracts and in the airways, marked changes take place in lung distensibility and deflation stability, reflecting attainment of functional maturity.

Phosphatidylcholine is synthesized de novo in the lung by the cooperative interaction of the cytidine diphosphocholine pathway and the sequence of metabolic reactions leading to formation of diglyceride through phosphatidic acid.

Regulation of phosphatidylcholine synthesis, secretion, and turnover in the developing lung involves complex mechanisms, including hormonal control of enzyme activities.

Philip M. Farrell
Robert H. Perelman

ACKNOWLEDGMENT

We wish to thank Dr. Michael Engle for helpful advice and several stimulating discussions during the planning of this section. We are also grateful to Leta Hensen for her excellent contribution to the design and preparation of illustrations used herein, and to Katie Rogge for clerical and editorial assistance.

BIBLIOGRAPHY
General

Ansell, G.B., Hawthorne, J.N., and Dawson, R.M.C., editors: Form and function of phospholipids, ed. 2, New York, 1973, Elsevier Scientific Publishing Co.

Avery, M.E., and Fletcher, B.D.: The lung and its disorders in the newborn infant, ed. 3, Philadelphia, 1974, W.B. Saunders Co.

Farrell, P.M., editor: Lung development: biological and clinical perspectives, New York, 1982, Academic Press.

Farrell, P.M., and Avery, M.E.: State of the art: hyaline membrane disease, Am. Rev. Respir. Dis. **111**:657, 1975.

Hodson, W.A., editor: Development of the lung, New York, 1977, Marcel Dekker, Inc.

Strang, L.B.: Neonatal respiration, physiological and clinical studies, London, 1977, Blackwell Scientific Publications, Ltd.

Developmental anatomy

Boyden, E.A.: Development and growth of the airways. In Hodson, W.A., editor: Development of the lung, New York, 1977, Marcel Dekker, Inc.

Burri, P.H., and Weibel, E.R.: Ultrastructure and morphometry of the developing lung. In Hodson, W.A., editor: Development of the lung, New York, 1977, Marcel Dekker, Inc.

Gilbert, E.F., and Opitz, J.M.: Genetic disorders of the respiratory system. In Jackson, L.G., and Schimke, R.N., editors: Clinical genetics: a sourcebook for physicians, New York, 1979, John Wiley & Sons, Inc.

Hislop, A., and Reid, L.M.: Formation of the pulmonary vasculature. In Hodson, W.A., editor: Development of the lung, New York, 1977, Marcel Dekker, Inc.

Landing, B.H.: Congenital malformation and genetic disorders of the respiratory tract, Am. Rev. Respir. Dis. **120**:151, 1979.

Meyrick, B., and Reid, L.M.: Ultrastructure of alveolar lining and its development. In Hodson, W.A., editor: Development of the lung, New York, 1977, Marcel Dekker, Inc.

Reid, L.: The embryology of the lung. In de Revck, A.V.S., and Porker, R., editors: CIBA Foundation Symposium on Development of the Lung, London, 1967, Churchill Livingstone.

Physiology

Avery, M.E., and Mead, J.: Surface properties in relation to atelectasis and hyaline membrane disease, Am. J. Dis. Child. **97**:517, 1959.

Brumley, G.W., and others: Correlations of mechanical stability, morphology, pulmonary surfactant, and phospholipid content in the developing lamb lung, J. Clin. Invest. **46**:863, 1967.

Clements, J.A.: Surface tension of lung extracts, Proc. Soc. Exp. Biol. Med. **95**:170, 1957.

Clements, J.A., Brown, E.S., and Johnson, R.P.: Pulmonary surface tension and the mucous lining of the lungs: some theoretical considerations, J. Appl. Physiol. **12:**262, 1958.
Faridy, E.E., Permutt, S., and Riley, R.L.: Effect of ventilation on surface forces in excised dogs' lungs, J. Appl. Physiol. **21:**1453, 1966.
Jobe, A., Kirkpatrick, E., and Gluck L.: Lecithin appearance and apparent biologic half-life in term newborn rabbit lung, Pediatr. Res. **12:**669, 1978.
Jobe, A., Mannino, F., and Gluck, L.: Labeling of phosphatidylcholine in the alveolar wash of rabbits in utero, Am. J. Obstet. Gynecol. **132:**53, 1978.
Kotas, R.V., and others: Fetal rhesus monkey lung development: lobar differences and discordances between stability and distensibility, J. Appl. Physiol. **43:**92, 1977.
Oyarzun, M.J., and Clements, J.A.: Control of lung surfactant by ventilation, adrenergic mediators and prostaglandins in the rabbit, Am. Rev. Respir. Dis. **117:**879, 1978.
von Neergaard, K.: Neue Auffassungen uber einen Grundbegriff der Atemmechanik: die Retraktionskraft der Lunge, abhangig von der Oberflachenspannung in den Alveolen, Z. Gesamte Exp. Med. **66:**373, 1965.
Wyszogrodski, I., and others: Surfactant inactivation by hyperventilation: conservation by end-expiratory pressure, J. Appl. Physiol. **38:**461, 1975.
Young, S.L., and Tierney, D.F.: Dipalmitoyl lecithin secretion and metabolism by the rat lung, Am. J. Physiol. **222:**1539, 1972.

Biochemistry

Brehier, A., and others: Corticosteroid-induction of phosphatidic acid phosphatase in fetal rabbit lung, Biochim, Biophys. Acta **46:**205, 1961.
Epstein, M.F., and Farrell, P.M.: The choline incorporation pathway: primary mechanism for de novo synthesis in fetal primate lung, Pediatr. Res. **9:**658, 1975.
Farrell, P.M., and Hamosh, M.: The biochemistry of fetal lung development, Clin. Perinatol. **5:**197, 1978.
Farrell, P.M., and Zachman, R.D.: Induction of choline phosphotransferase and lecithin synthesis in the fetal lung by corticosteroids, Science **179:** 297, 1973.
Gluck, L., and others: Diagnosis of the respiratory distress syndrome by amniocentesis, Am. J. Obstet. Gynecol. **109:**440, 1971.
Godinez, R.I., Sanders, R.L., and Longmore, W.J.: Phosphatidylglycerol in rat lung. I. Identification as a metabolically active phospholipid in isolated perfused rat lung, Biochemistry **14:**830, 1975.
Kennedy, E.P., and Weiss, S.B.: The function of cytidine coenzymes in the biosynthesis of phospholipids, J. Biol. Chem. **222:**193, 1956.
King, R.J., and Clements, J.A.: Surface active materials from the dog lung. II. Composition and physiological correlations, Am. J. Physiol. **223:**715, 1972.
Kotas, R.V., and others: Evidence for independent regulators of organ maturation in fetal rabbits, Pediatrics **47:**57, 1971.
Liggins, G.C.: Premature delivery of foetal lambs infused with glucocorticoids, J. Endocrinol. **45:**515, 1969.
Oldenborg, V., and van Golde, L.M.G.: Activity of cholinephosphotransferase, lysolecithin-lysolecithin acyltransferase and lysolecithin acyltransferase in the developing mouse lung, Biochim. Biophys. Acta **441:**433, 1976.
Schultz, F.M., and others: Fetal lung maturation. I. Phosphatidic acid phosphohydrolase in rabbit lung, Gynecol. Invest. **5:**222, 1974.
Stern, W., Kovac, C., and Weinhold, P.A.: Activity and properties of CTP: cholinephosphate cytidyltransferase in adult and fetal rat lung, Biochim. Biophys. Acta **441:**280, 1976.
Tsao, F.H., and Zachman, R.D.: Phosphatidylcholine lysophosphatidylcholine cycle pathway enzymes in rabbit lung. II. Marked differences in the effect of gestational age on activity compared to the CDP-choline pathway, Pediatr. Res. **11:**858, 1977.
Ulane, R.E., Stephenson, C.L., and Farrell, P.M.: Evidence for the existence of a single enzyme catalyzing the phosphorylation of choline and ethanolamine in primate lung, Biochim. Biophys. Acta **531:**295, 1978.
van Golde, L.M.G.: Metabolism of phospholipids in the lung, Am. Rev. Respir. Dis. **114:**977, 1976.

PART TWO

Assessment of pulmonary function

The majority of neonates requiring intensive care have respiratory problems. In recent years newer methods for evaluating pulmonary function in neonates with suspected abnormalities of the cardiopulmonary system have been developed. Whereas standard techniques for assessing pulmonary function can be applied in a healthy infant, special limitations and problems are encountered in very small or sick babies. A practical clinical approach to disordered cardiopulmonary function is presented in this section, and an attempt is made to facilitate the differentiation between heart and lung disease.

CLINICAL OBSERVATIONS

Four common presenting physical signs relay indirect information regarding pulmonary function. These are respiratory rate, retractions, grunting, and cyanosis.

Respiratory rate

Precise monitoring of respiratory rate is invaluable, since significant deviation from the normal is observed with mechanical pulmonary dysfunction, acid-base imbalances, or arterial blood gas abnormalities. A detailed discussion of respiratory control and apnea of prematurity appears on p. 456.

Fig. 23-9 shows that the work of breathing is dependent on respiratory rate and the type of pulmonary dysfunction. The total work of breathing consists of elastic and resistive components. The elastic component represents the work required to stretch the lungs during a tidal inspiration, whereas the resistive component is the work required to overcome the movement of air through the airways. As this figure suggests, infants with lung disease attempt to minimize their work of breathing by controlling the respiratory rate; nonetheless the total work of breathing is still greater than normal. The range over which respiratory rate can achieve successful gas exchange when the infants are breathing spontaneously is limited. At high rates increased dead space ventilation occurs, whereas at low rates decreased alveolar ventilation results. In patients with *respiratory distress syn-*

Fig. 23-9. Relative contributions of the elastic and resistive components of work of breathing in infants with normal pulmonary function, decreased compliance *(CL)*, and increased resistance *(RL)*.

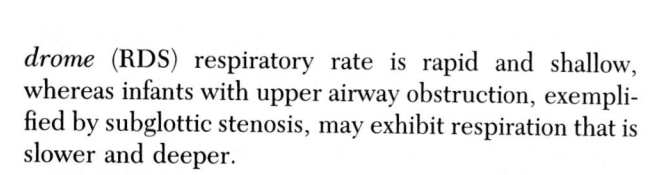

drome (RDS) respiratory rate is rapid and shallow, whereas infants with upper airway obstruction, exemplified by subglottic stenosis, may exhibit respiration that is slower and deeper.

Retractions

The diaphragm is the principal mechanical driving force for ventilation, creating a negative intrapleural pressure during inspiration (Fig. 23-10). The pressure generated is ultimately determined by a combination of (1) the force of the diaphragm; (2) the mechanical properties of the lung; and (3) the stability of the chest wall.

The neonatal chest wall is very compliant, and substernal retractions are readily observable with relatively small changes in lung mechanics. In infants with very stiff lungs and marked retractions the chest configuration resembles that seen in pectus excavatum. In neonates with respiratory distress, retractions become more apparent as the lungs become stiffer. Apart from their characteristic appearance in RDS, severe retractions also can signal complications of respiratory disease such as airway obstruction, misplacement of an endotracheal tube, pneumothorax, or atelectasis. Diminishing retractions suggest that lung compliance is improving. The significance of retractions often is overlooked when defining respiratory failure in neonates. In smaller infants (especially those weighing less than 1,500 gm) the progression of retractions should be closely monitored, since many of these infants may exhibit increased retractions even before blood gases demonstrate frank respiratory failure.

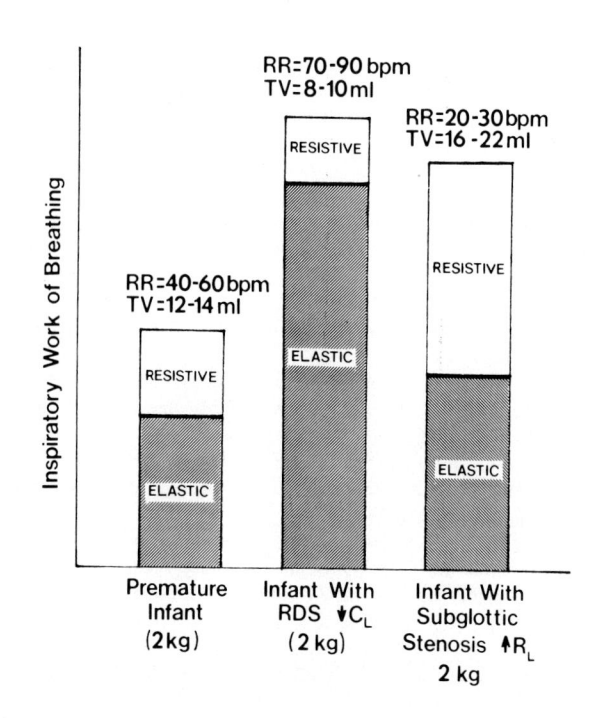

Grunting

Normally the vocal cords abduct during inspiration and adduct (without any sound) during expiration. When mechanical function is disrupted, however, the work of breathing is greatly increased, and neonates attempt to compensate by closing their vocal cords during expiration. Expiration through a partially closed glottis produces the grunting sound. Grunting may be either intermittent or continuous, depending on the severity of lung disease.

Fig. 23-11 demonstrates the change in lung volume, flow, and transpulmonary pressure that may accompany grunting. The entire expiratory phase of a grunting infant is represented by the section *A-C*. Grunting is represented by section *B-C* at the end of expiration. During the initial phase of expiration the infant closes the glottis, holds air in the lungs, and produces an elevated transpulmonary pressure in the absence of airflow. During the last third of the expiratory phase gas is expelled from the lungs, causing an audible grunt. It is not actually the grunt, then, that produces the elevated transpulmonary pressure but the ability of the infant to close the vocal cords while respiratory muscles contract. During the "Valsalva phase," when the vocal cords are closed, there is an improved ventilation/perfusion ratio because of increased airway pressure and increased lung volume, the end result being an improvement in arterial oxygenation.

Harrison, who demonstrated the significance of grunting in RDS, noted that, when grunting was abolished by endotracheal intubation, arterial oxygen tension (PaO_2) decreased. They concluded that grunting was responsi-

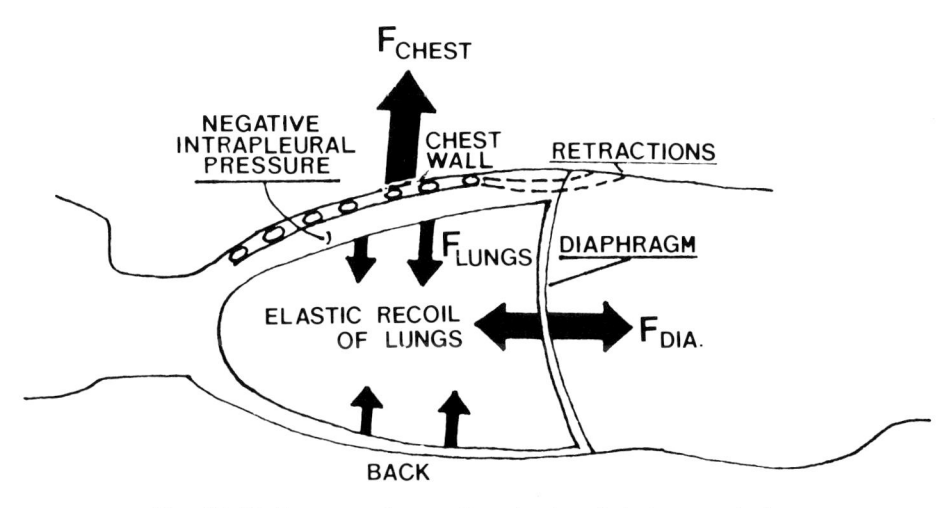

Fig. 23-10. Forces acting on the chest wall during respiration.

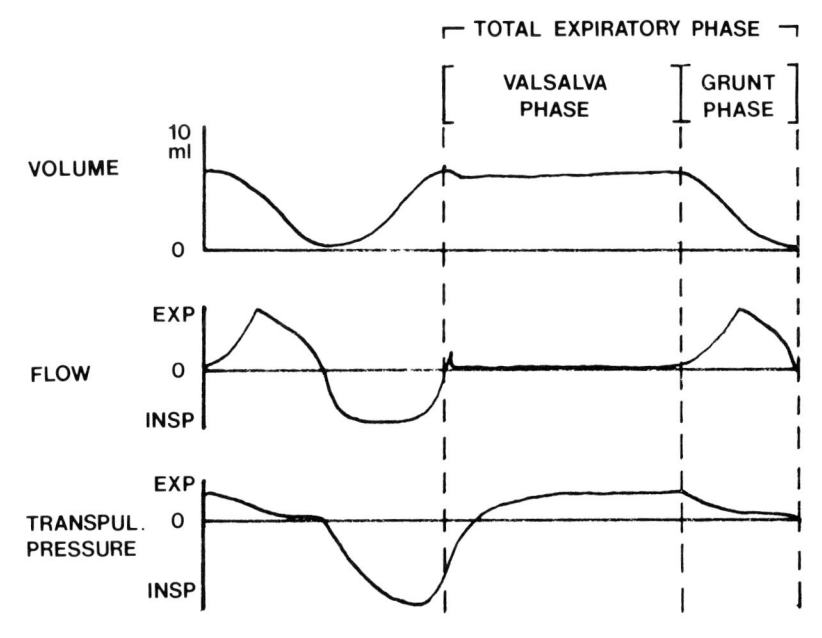

Fig. 23-11. Physiologic measurements during grunting respiration.

ble for stabilizing lung volume and improving arterial oxygenation. Other studies have suggested that the grunting mechanism can maintain a functional residual capacity (FRC) and a PaO₂ equivalent to those maintained during the application of 2 or 3 cm H₂O of continuous positive airway pressure (CPAP) (p. 434).

Cyanosis

Cyanosis, best observed by examining the lips and tongue, is an insensitive indicator of pulmonary dysfunction. Several types of pulmonary dysfunction, including airway obstruction, ventilation-perfusion inequality, intrapulmonary shunting, and, rarely, diffusion abnormalities, in addition to cardiac disease, may result in cyanosis. The clinical features of cyanosis and their significance are discussed in detail on p. 560.

BLOOD GASES

Blood gases are the most widely used clinical method for assessing pulmonary function in neonates and form the basis for diagnosis and management of infants with cardiorespiratory disease. The purpose of this section is to discuss how changes in arterial oxygen (PaO_2) and carbon dioxide ($PaCO_2$) tension reflect disordered pulmonary function in different clinical situations. Techniques of blood gas determination in infants with RDS are discussed in Part three.

Arterial oxygen tension (PaO_2)

Oxygen is carried in the blood both in chemical combination with hemoglobin and also in physical solution. The oxygen taken up from the lungs is dependent on the alveolar/capillary pressure gradient. At ambient pressures the amount of dissolved oxygen is only a small fraction of the total quantity carried in whole blood (0.3 ml of oxygen/100 ml of plasma/100 mm Hg at 37° C). Most of the oxygen in whole blood is bound to hemoglobin (1 gm of hemoglobin combines with 1.34 ml of oxygen at 37° C). The quantity of oxygen bound to hemoglobin is dependent on the partial pressure and is described by the oxygen dissociation curve (Fig. 23-12). The blood is almost completely saturated at a PaO_2 of 90 to 100 mm Hg. The flattening of the upper portion of the S-shaped dissociation curve makes it virtually impossible to monitor oxygen tension above 60 to 80 mm Hg by following arterial oxygen saturation alone. Cyanosis generally is noted only at a PaO_2 of less than 40 mm Hg in neonates. The dissociation curve of fetal (as compared with adult) blood is shifted to the left and at any PaO_2 below 100 mm Hg fetal blood binds more oxygen. The shift appears to be the result of the lower affinity of fetal hemoglobin for diphosphoglycerate. Note that pH, PCO_2, temperature, and 2,3-diphosphoglycerate (DPG) content all influence the position of the dissociation curve.

The partial pressure of oxygen in arterial blood is not only dependent on the ability of the lung to transfer oxygen as determined by alveolar ventilation but also is largely influenced by the *ventilation/perfusion relationships (V/Q ratio)* within the lung. For normal gas exchange the ventilation and perfusion should be similarly proportioned. The ratio should be very close to 1, i.e., for every milliliter of ventilated air there should be a proportionate degree of perfusion. In healthy adults this V/Q ratio is about 0.8 because of variations in the ratio in different parts of the lung. In the presence of cardiopulmonary disease the V/Q ratio may be abnormal, depending on the nature of the pulmonary pathologic condition. In cases of intrinsic pulmonary disease associated with hypoventilation the V/Q ratio will be less than 1. In cardiac anomalies with right-to-left shunt and in pulmonary disease where a large portion of the lung is ventilated but underperfused, a V/Q ratio greater than 1 will be observed.

The most common disturbance in V/Q relationships in neonates is intrapulmonary shunting, which is a consequence of atelectasis. Areas of the lung in which intrapulmonary shunting occurs are perfused but not ventilated and thus have a V/Q of 0. Areas of gas trapping that are virtually nonventilated but perfused also function essentially as a shunt. The result of intrapulmonary shunts is a decrease in PaO_2 similar to that which occurs when there is a right-to-left shunt in the heart or through

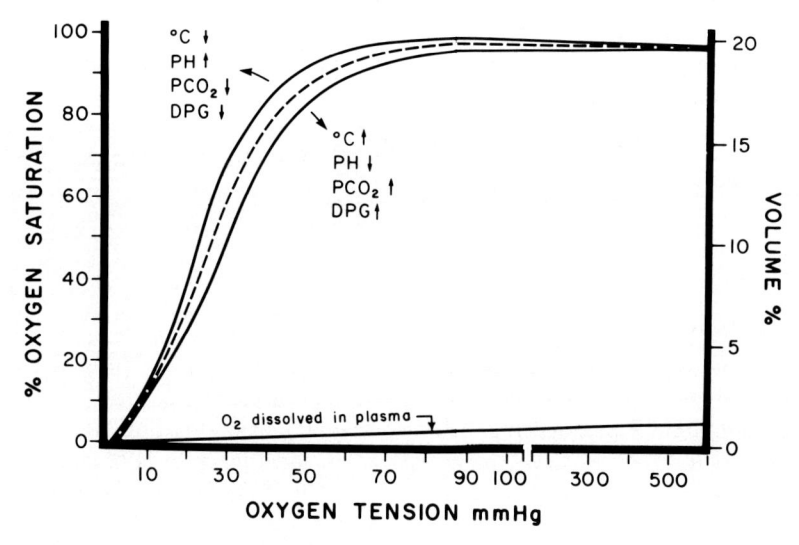

Fig. 23-12. Factors shifting the oxygen dissociation curve of hemoglobin (fetal hemoglobin is shifted to the left). (From Klaus, M., Fanaroff, A., and Martin, R.J.: Respiratory problems. In Klaus, M., and Fanaroff, A., editors: Care of the high risk neonate, Philadelphia, 1979, W.B. Saunders Co.)

a patent ductus arteriosus (PDA) with pulmonary hypertension. Similar arterial unsaturation may occur when the alveoli are well ventilated but not perfused. Right-to-left shunts may occur at three levels: interatrial through the foramen ovale, through the ductus arteriosus, or within the lung itself. In infants with RDS, V/Q abnormalities typically result from a combination of all the above mechanisms (p. 427). Preterm infants both with and without respiratory disease frequently exhibit a fall in PaO₂ during crying, which may be explained on the basis of increased right-to-left shunting resulting from the large intrathoracic pressure changes.

Arterial carbon dioxide tension (Paco₂)

PaCO₂ is a major determinant of pulmonary function in neonatal respiratory disease, directly reflecting alveolar ventilation and in most situations minute ventilation. As tissue levels of CO_2 increase above those of arterial blood, molecules diffuse into the capillaries and are transported in red blood cells and plasma. Unlike the S-shaped dissociation curve for O_2, the relationship between CO_2 content and tension is almost linear over the physiologic range. PaCO₂ is maintained in a range of 35 to 45 torr in healthy infants, although levels below this range are sometimes seen in spontaneously breathing, full-term infants with transient tachypnea or meconium aspiration syndrome. In these conditions hyperventilation is common and results in the decrease in PaCO₂. An elevated PaCO₂ level is one of the major indicators of respiratory failure.

As a determinant of pulmonary function, an increased PaCO₂ is generally secondary to one of two major abnormalities in pulmonary physiology. The first condition, atelectasis, is exhibited in RDS and associated with decreased lung compliance, increased respiratory rate, and increased work of breathing. As the infant becomes fatigued, carbon dioxide retention may occur. The second condition resulting in carbon dioxide retention is alveolar overdistention. The overaeration caused by air trapping is common in meconium aspiration syndrome and may be produced in infants with respiratory disease by the use of assisted ventilation. Alveolar overdistention causes lung stiffening, increased work of breathing, and carbon dioxide retention. In addition to measurement of PaCO₂, pH must be always determined and HCO_3^- concentration calculated to assess the status of any infant with pulmonary disease.

The initiation of ventilation with the *first breath* after normal delivery results in a rapid fall in PaCO₂ within minutes of birth. PaO₂ rises equally rapidly to levels of 60 to 90 mm Hg, although some degree of mismatching of V/Q is evident in the first 1 to 2 hours of life. This is thought to be the result of intracardiac and/or pulmonary right-to-left shunting. The effects of this sudden adaptation on the blood gases are illustrated in Fig. 23-13, which shows the rapid change in PaO₂ and PaCO₂ under normal conditions and when there is asphyxia with delayed onset of breathing. The speed with which pulmonary ventilation and perfusion are uniformly distributed is an indication of the remarkable adaptive capaci-

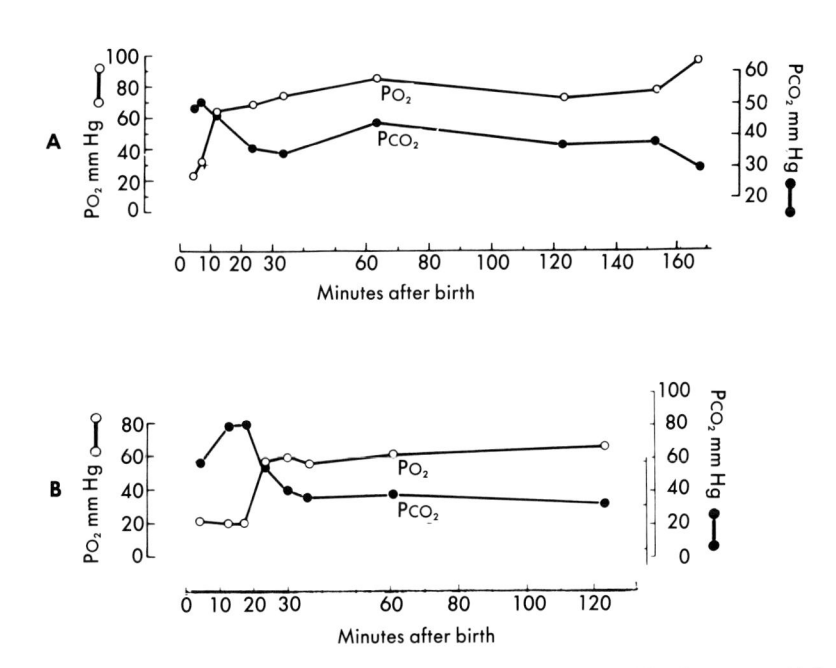

Fig. 23-13. Changes in Po₂ and Pco₂ during the first minutes after birth in a normal infant **(A)** and an asphyxiated infant **(B)** with delayed onset of respiration. (Courtesy R. Tunell, M.D.)

ties of the newborn infant for the maintenance of normal homeostasis.

Hyperoxia-hyperventilation test

The hyperoxia test was introduced approximately 10 years ago in infants with RDS to aid in prognosis for this disease. The test is performed by placing the infant in a 100% oxygen concentration for 5 to 10 minutes and then sampling arterial blood gas or monitoring transcutaneous Po_2 (p. 430). The underlying physiology for this method is that 5 to 10 minutes of oxygen exposure should diffuse oxygen even into the poorly ventilated areas and abolish any V/Q abnormalities. If hypoxia remains after 5 to 10 minutes of 100% oxygen exposure, it suggests the presence of direct right-to-left shunting. Whereas the test was used to evaluate the degree of shunting in RDS to predict outcome, its most useful current application is to differentiate between primary lung and congenital heart disease with right-to-left shunting. A modification of the hyperoxia test combining hyperoxia with hyperventilation is a possible method to distinguish between structural congenital heart disease and persistent fetal circulation (PFC), both of which have right-to-left shunting. During normal ventilation exposure to 100% oxygen in both cyanotic heart disease and PFC will result in virtually no change in PaO_2. However, by hyperventilating the infant for between 5 and 10 minutes and decreasing the Pco_2 to ranges of 18 to 25 mm Hg, infants with PFC may exhibit Po_2 levels of greater than 100 mm Hg, if only transiently. In contrast, patients with anatomically fixed right-to-left shunting and particularly those with transposition of the great vessels rarely generate a Po_2 above 40 mm Hg, even with hyperventilation.

Evaluation of ductal shunting

If right-to-left ductal shunting occurs, venous or desaturated blood from the right side of the heart enters the main pulmonary artery and crosses the ductus to the descending aorta. Since the ductus almost always enters the aorta after the origin of the right subclavian and carotid arteries (and therefore temporal arteries), blood arriving at these two sites will be well oxygenated, whereas blood samples from the left subclavian and aorta will be (relatively) less oxygenated. Preductal gases can be obtained either through the temporal arteries, right brachial artery, or right radial artery. Postductal gases are drawn through the left radial artery, femorals, or umbilical artery catheter (descending aorta). Alternatively placement of two transcutaneous Po_2 electrodes, one on the right upper chest and the other on the abdomen, accomplishes the same effect in differentiating preductal and postductal PaO_2.

A study of almost 100 patients with RDS demonstrated only a 5-torr difference between preductal and postductal gases. This indicates that in these infants the majority of right-to-left shunting was through the foramen ovale. In patients with persistent fetal circulation (persistent pulmonary hypertension) there may be right-to-left shunting through both the foramen ovale and ductus arteriosus; this can be demonstrated by either simultaneously obtained preductal and postductal arterial gases, during echocardiography, or by contrast injection at cardiac angiography.

PHYSIOLOGIC MEASUREMENTS

Tests of cardiopulmonary function performed on sick neonates ideally should involve as little additional stress to the infant as is feasible. Roentgenographic evaluation of the chest is an integral part of the diagnostic evaluation of respiratory disorders and is discussed in Chapter 39. Measurements of central venous pressure and pulmonary artery pressure are techniques that may indirectly give useful information regarding pulmonary function and are discussed in Chapter 10. Furthermore the effects of varying levels of CPAP or assisted ventilation on blood gases will provide useful insight into the specific alterations in pulmonary mechanisms in infants with respiratory disease (p. 434).

Measurement of air flow

Nasal thermistors can be sensitive enough to detect the small temperature gradients that exist between inspired and expired air. Such a qualitative determination of flow can be very useful in conjunction with standard impedance pneumography and heart rate monitoring (p. 122). In this way the careful characterization of episodes of central apnea, obstructive apnea, and bradycardia (or combinations of all three) can be readily made (p. 456).

Quantitative measurement of air flow can be obtained from an infant pneumotachometer consisting of a fine-mesh screen that provides a known resistance to the flow of air through it. Measurement of the pressure gradient across the screen will be directly proportional to air flow, and the latter then can be directly calculated and integrated into tidal volume. A variety of infant face masks, nose pieces (as for the administration of CPAP), and even endotracheal tube connectors have been fitted with screens to function as neonatal pneumotachometers.

Measurement of lung volumes

The total volume of air in the lungs can be measured and subdivided into lung volumes (Fig. 23-14). Body plethysmography and gas dilution studies are the methods usually employed for making these determinations but are cumbersome and time consuming and thus confined mainly to research. As a result, numerous attempts have been made to quantitate tidal volumes from surface

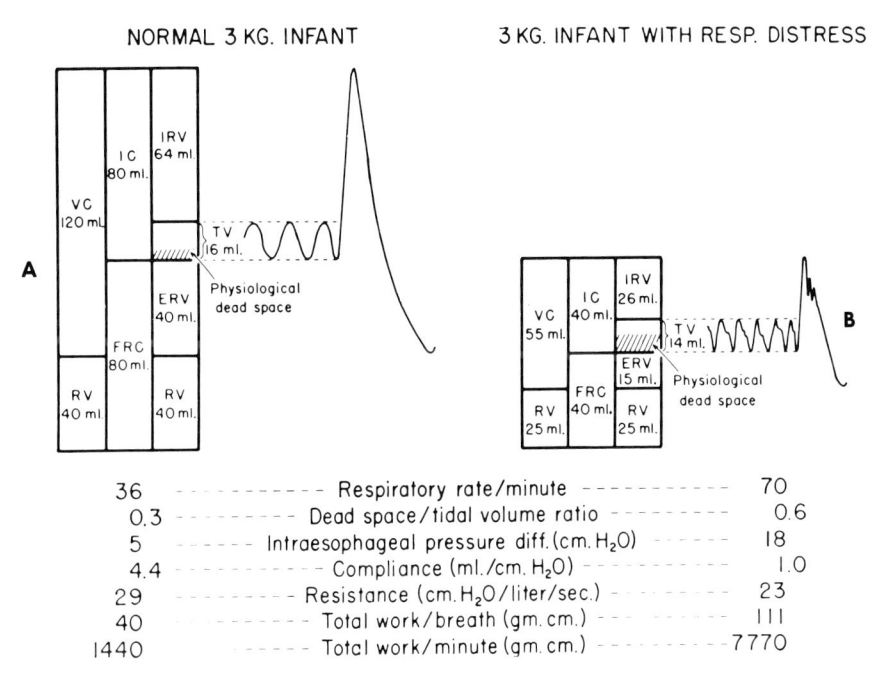

Fig. 23-14. Partitioning of lung volumes and other measures of pulmonary function in a normal infant **(A)** and one with RDS **(B)**. (From Avery, M., Fletcher, B., and Williams, R.: The lung and its disorders in the newborn infant, Philadelphia, 1981, W.B. Saunders Co.)

measurements of chest wall motion, although these techniques also require complex calibrations and have met with variable success. The size of the lung compartments is related to the height, weight, and surface area of the subjects. FRC, or volume of the gas in the lungs at end expiration, serves as a buffer of inspired gas so that large changes in alveolar gas tensions are reduced.

One of the principal functions of the first breath is to transform the fluid-filled fetal lung from an airless organ to one with an appropriate FRC. The ability of the lung to maintain a volume of gas at end expiration depends on two factors. One is the chest wall, which acts as a support for the lungs, and the other is the ability of the lung to produce surfactant to stabilize the expanded alveoli. Both these functions are less well developed in the premature infant.

The factor or factors responsible for the *first breath* are unknown. Multiple stimuli such as exposure to a cold environmental temperature and tactile changes play a role. However, the exact interrelationships of pH, Po_2, and Pco_2 that combine to induce breathing in the human neonate are still to be determined. The pressure change of the first breath must overcome the effects of viscosity of fluid in the airway, the effects of surface tension, and the effects of tissue resistance. Roentgenographic studies of the lung indicate that inflation with air occurs immediately with the first breath. FRC is rapidly established, with little change throughout the first week of life. There is some evidence for gas trapping for 2 or 3 days, which may be related to the gradual disappearance of lung fluid during this period.

Dead space is that portion of the tidal volume not involved in gas exchange, and thus it will vary with the presence or absence of areas of high V/Q. The dead space is divided into several compartments. Anatomic dead space is the constant airway volume not involved in gas exchange and is made up of the air passages from nares to terminal bronchioles. Alveolar dead space is the volume of gas in alveoli that are well ventilated but underperfused. Physiologic dead space is the sum of anatomic and alveolar dead space. In the normal newborn physiologic dead space is 6 to 8 cc; smaller values are obtained in premature infants. The relationship of dead space to tidal volume is physiologically significant and normally in the range of 0.3. It is of practical importance to minimize the dead space added by apparatus for assisted ventilation or measurement of lung function to prevent rebreathing and accumulation of carbon dioxide.

Esophageal pressure determinations

Studies have shown that measurements of esophageal pressure in infants closely reflect intrapleural pressure. Pleural pressure can be determined relatively simply by using esophageal balloons or esophageal catheters. Most balloons are made of hand-dipped latex and measure approximately 0.5 cm in diameter and 2 to 3 cm in length. The esophageal balloon is usually placed approximately 12 cm from the gum margin, and, if cardiac artifact is observed, the balloon is withdrawn until the cardiac artifact diminishes. At first esophageal tone will be increased, so the balloon should remain in place long enough for this tone to diminish before measurements are made. The balloon catheter is connected to a pressure transducer and may remain in the esophagus for extended periods without producing symptoms in the infant. In conjunction with flow and volume tracings this technique can be used to determine dynamic lung compliance (change in volume per unit change in intrapleural pressure) and pulmonary resistance (change in pressure divided by flow). Esophageal pressure also has been described as a useful technique for evaluation of optimum levels of CPAP in infants with RDS (p. 434).

Lung compliance is dependent not only on the intrinsic elasticity of pulmonary tissue but also on the level of FRC. The degree of elasticity can be estimated from specific compliance (lung compliance divided by FRC), which corrects for the absolute level of lung volume. Whereas lung compliance in the normal neonate (4 to 6 ml/cm H_2O) is comparable to that of the adult when corrected for unit body weight, compliance of the thorax is relatively much higher in infants.

In normal newborns the lung compliance is low at the initiation of the first breath; this accounts for the high pressure (frequently as high as 40 cm H_2O) required for the initiation of the first few breaths. With the establishment of respiration and with gradual clearance of lung fluid during the first 3 to 6 hours of life the FRC increases with concomitant improvement in lung compliance. Since the improvement in lung compliance is a result of improvement in FRC, the specific compliance is unchanged. Pathophysiologic factors that may increase the amount of fluid or impede the clearance of lung fluid may delay this improvement in lung compliance. Placental tranfusion with subsequent increase in the blood volume and transudation of fluid into the interstitial tissue of the lung is an example of this phenomenon. The variability of compliance values in the first 2 hours of life, in part the result of physiologic variation, also may account for the frequent observations of higher respiratory rates in some infants during this period.

If a higher respiratory rate is associated with any form of retraction, grunting, or cyanosis requiring oxygen supplementation, the infant has a pathologic condition. In distressed infants in whom lung compliance is markedly reduced, the compliant immature chest wall poses a disadvantage in that, as the infant attempts to increase negative intrathoracic pressure, the chest wall collapses (retracts). The more compliant airway of the smaller infant may predispose him to actual airway collapse during expiration and result in distal gas trapping.

Total pulmonary resistance results from air flow through the nasopharynx, trachea, and bronchi and is dependent on airway caliber, flow rate, and resistance imposed by lung tissue. In the full-term infant total pulmonary resistance is around 30 cm H_2O/L/second, approximately six times greater than that in the adult. A major site of airway resistance in the neonate is the nasopharynx. In the normal infant, airway resistance (resistance that is imposed by the breathing tubes) is approximately 18 to 20 cm H_2O/L/second and viscous resistance (the resistance caused by tissues) is 8 to 10 cm H_2O/L/second. This latter value is also larger than that in adults. Because of the higher resistances that occur in infants, respiratory apparatus that would materially increase airway resistance further must be avoided where possible.

The *work of breathing* is a measure of the energy expended in inflating the lungs and moving the chest. In general terms work is the cumulative product of pressure and the volume of air moved at each instant. In the normal infant total pulmonary work has been determined to equal an average value of 1,440 gm.cm/minute. In an infant with respiratory distress the total pulmonary work may increase as much as six times. This becomes most important when considered in terms of the oxygen cost of breathing. The neonate requires a greater caloric expenditure to breathe than does the adult, and the distressed infant requires an even greater caloric expenditure for this function. In the full-term infant the work of breathing is minimum when the infant has a respiratory rate of 30 breaths per minute.

William W. Fox
Thomas H. Shaffer

BIBLIOGRAPHY

Avery, M.E., Fletcher, B.D., and Williams, R.G.: The lung and its disorders in the newborn infant, ed. 4, Philadelphia, 1981, W.B. Saunders Co.

Berman, L.S., and others: Optimum levels of CPAP for tracheal extubation of newborns, J. Pediatr. 89:109, 1976.

Comroe, J.H.: Physiology of respiration, ed. 2, Chicago, 1974, Year Book Medical Publishers, Inc.

Chernick, V., and Avery, M.E.: The functional basis of respiratory pathology. In Kendig, E., and Chernick, V., editors: Disorders of the respiratory tract in children, ed. 2, Philadelphia, 1977, W.B. Saunders Co.

Dinwiddie, R., and Russell, G.: Relationship of intraesophageal pressure to intrapleural pressure in the newborn, J. Appl. Physiol. 33:415, 1972.

Harrison, V.C., Heese, H.deV., and Klein, M.: The significance of grunting in hyaline membrane disease, Pediatrics 41:549, 1968.

Peckham, G.J., and Fox, W.W.: Physiological factors affecting pulmonary artery pressure in infants with persistent pulmonary hypertension, J. Pediatr. 93:1005, 1979.

Scarpelli, E.M.: Concepts in respiratory pathophysiology. In Scarpelli, E.M., Auld, P., and Goldman, H., editors: Pulmonary disease of the fetus, newborn, and child, Philadelphia, 1978, Lea & Febiger.

Schlueter, M.A., and Tooley, W.H.: Right-to-left shunt through the ductus arteriosus in newborn infants, Pediatr. Res. 8:354, 1974.

Smith, C.A., and Nelson, N.M.: The physiology of the newborn infant, Springfield, Ill., 1976, Charles C Thomas, Publisher.

PART THREE

The respiratory distress syndrome and its management

Despite the enormous strides that have been made in understanding the pathophysiology of respiratory distress syndrome (RDS) and more particularly the role of surfactant in its cause, RDS, or hyaline membrane disease (HMD), as it is still commonly known, remains by far the most frequent clinical problem encountered among preterm infants. Furthermore this has persisted despite real progress made in preventing RDS either by pharmacologic inhibition of premature labor, prevention of iatrogenic prematurity (specifically that related to elective cesarean section), or accelerating pulmonary maturity. The improved outcome in RDS, which can be attributed directly to the application of many technologic advances, has raised questions as to whether it is still the major cause of death in low birth weight infants. Because the management of RDS has become more complex, there has been a dramatic increase in the complications of treatment and sequelae of the disease process. Thus autopsy studies show an increase in the incidence of air leak syndromes, bronchopulmonary dysplasia (BPD), and intracranial hemorrhage. In this section the clinical features and evaluation of infants with RDS are discussed and current therapeutic approaches outlined.

INCIDENCE

RDS continues to be one of the most important causes of mortality and morbidity in newborn babies, although lack of a precise definition necessitates cautious interpretation of statistics regarding incidence, mortality, and outcome. The diagnosis can be clearly established pathologically or by documentation of surfactant deficiency; nonetheless most series refer only to a combination of clinical, biochemical, and radiologic features. Approximately 10% to 15% of babies weighing less than 2.5 kg at birth will manifest RDS, the highest incidence being observed among the lowest birth weight groups. The greatest risk factor appears to be gestational age, whereas other risk factors include maternal diabetes, maternal bleeding, and perinatal asphyxia. The incidence varies inversely with advancing gestational age; thus only exceptional cases are encountered at 37 weeks or beyond, whereas RDS occurs in greater than 70% of newborns at 28 to 30 weeks of gestation. The disease occurs throughout the world with a slight male predominance.

PHARMACOLOGIC ACCELERATION OF PULMONARY MATURATION

If premature delivery of any infant appears probable or necessary, the ability to hasten lung maturity is now available. In recent years much attention has been focused on hormonal and other pharmacologic agents that achieve this result (p. 412). The effects of various catecholamines as well as aminophylline have been studied; however, the most promising method at this time appears to be prepartum glucocorticoid administration. Although conflicting evidence has appeared in the literature, it appears that these agents, when administered to the mother at least 24 to 48 hours before delivery, decrease both the incidence and severity of RDS. Corticosteroids appear to be only effective before 34 weeks' gestation and when administered at least 24 hours and no longer than 7 days before delivery. Furthermore, very small premature infants do not appear to benefit. Ballard's data indicate that prenatal betamethasone therapy is less effective in male than in female infants in decreasing the incidence of RDS. Similar sex differences in response to maternal dexamethasone have been reported in the Boston prospective study. This effect is not caused by sex differences in steroid levels in the fetal circulation or by effects of steroids on the fetal pituitary and requires further study to define the mechanism underlying this apparent male disadvantage. Postpartum administration of corticosteroids to the infant is of no benefit. To date, there are no proven complications of this treatment, but concern has been expressed about the possibility of increased infection in both mother and infant, as well as potential effects on the infant's later growth and development.

PATHOPHYSIOLOGY

The lungs of infants who succumb from RDS have a characteristic uniformly ruddy and airless appearance, macroscopically resembling hepatic tissue. On microscopic examination the striking feature is diffuse atelectasis such that only a few widely dilated alveoli are readily distinguishable (Fig. 23-15). An eosinophilic membrane lines the visible airspaces that usually constitute terminal bronchioles and alveolar ducts. This characteristic membrane (from which the term *hyaline membrane disease* is derived) consists of a fibrinous matrix of materials derived from the blood and contains cellular debris derived from injured epithelium. The recovery phase is characterized by regeneration of alveolar cells, including the type II cells, with a resultant increase in surfactant activity.

The development of RDS is thought to begin with impaired or delayed surfactant synthesis followed by a series of events that may progressively increase the severity of the disease for several days (Fig. 23-16). Surfactant synthesis is a dynamic process that is dependent on factors such as pH, temperature, and perfusion and may be compromised by cold stress, hypovolemia, hypoxemia, and acidosis. Other unfavorable factors such as exposure to high oxygen concentration and the effects of

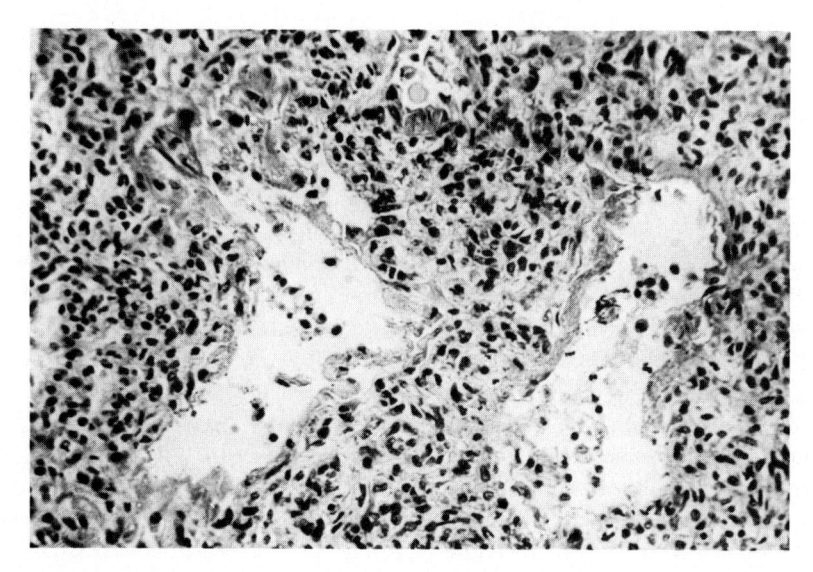

Fig. 23-15. Photomicrograph of lungs of infant with RDS. Note marked atelectasis and hyaline membrane lining the dilated alveolar ducts.

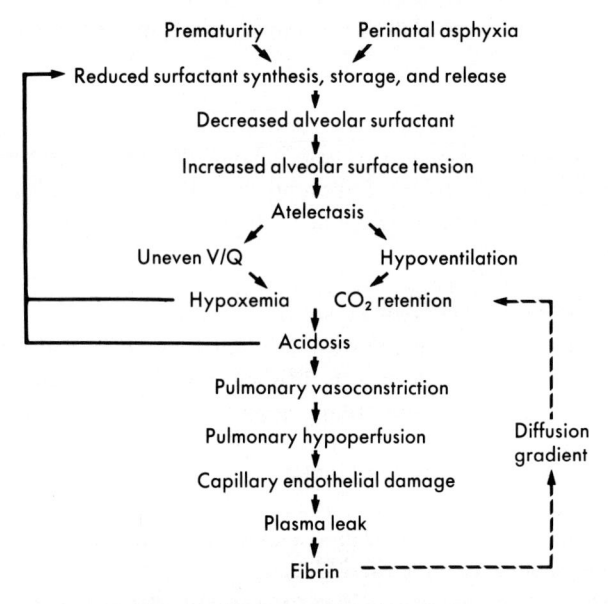

Fig. 23-16. Pathogenesis of RDS.

respirator management may further damage the alveolar epithelial lining, resulting in reduced surfactant synthesis. Deficiency of surfactant and the accompanying decrease in lung compliance lead to alveolar hypoventilation and ventilation/perfusion (V/Q) imbalance. The resultant hypoxemia and hypercarbia in turn may reduce surfactant production. Severe hypoxemia will result in lactic acidosis secondary to systemic hypoperfusion and anaerobic metabolism. Hypoxemia and acidosis also result in pulmonary hypoperfusion secondary to pulmonary vasoconstriction, and the result is further aggravation of hypoxemia secondary to right-to-left shunting at the level of the ductus arteriosus and foramen ovale and within the lung itself. The role of decreased pulmonary blood flow in reducing surfactant production after birth, however, has not been clearly established. It is important to note that the relative roles of surfactant deficiency and pulmonary hypoperfusion in the overall clinical picture of RDS will vary somewhat with each patient.

CLINICAL FEATURES

Infants with RDS characteristically are seen either immediately after delivery or within several hours of birth with the typical signs of neonatal respiratory distress, as outlined below and on p. 419. It should be emphasized that continuing close observation and careful physical examination of the infant are as essential as roentgenographic studies in evaluating the clinical status of any infant with respiratory distress. The hazards of hastily concluding that all infants with respiratory distress have RDS are discussed in Part four.

Infants with RDS typically are initially seen with a combination of tachypnea, nasal flaring, subcostal and intercostal retractions, cyanosis, and an expiratory grunt. Respiratory rate is usually regular and increased well above the normal range of 30 to 60 breaths per minute. The presence of apneic episodes at this early state is an ominous sign which may reflect thermal instability or sepsis but more often is a sign of hypoxemia and respiratory failure. Retractions are prominent and are the result of the very compliant rib cage being drawn in on inspiration as the infant generates high intrathoracic pressures to expand the poorly compliant lungs. The typical expiratory grunt is an early feature of the clinical course and may subsequently disappear. It is thought to result from partial closure of the glottis during expiration and in this way acts as a means of trapping alveolar air and maintaining the functional residual capacity (FRC) (p. 420). It should be noted that, although these signs are characteristic for neonatal respiratory distress, they may result from a wide variety of nonpulmonary causes such as hypothermia, hypoglycemia, anemia, or polycythemia (p. 460), and furthermore such nonpulmonary conditions may complicate the clinical course of RDS.

Additional clinical features include pallor, secondary to either anemia or peripheral vasoconstriction. The blood pressure must be closely monitored in infants with RDS (p. 126). Cyanosis, which may be masked by pallor, is a consequence of right-to-left shunting in RDS and is typically relieved by administering a higher concentration of oxygen. In severe respiratory distress oxygen may not relieve cyanosis (see hyperoxia test, p. 424), and ventilatory support or other measures need to be initiated. Acrocyanosis of the hands and feet is a common finding in normal infants and should not be confused with central cyanosis, which always must be investigated and treated. Peripheral edema is frequently present in RDS and of no particular prognostic significance.

Auscultation of the chest is seldom rewarding in infants, since the breath sounds are widely transmitted and cannot always be relied on to reflect pathology. In moderate to severe RDS breath sounds may be harsh or markedly decreased because of atelectasis. Unilaterally decreased breath sounds (with mediastinal shift to the opposite side) or bilaterally decreased air entry is indicative of pneumothorax, and immediate transillumination is performed (p. 448). The detection of a murmur in a cyanotic infant with respiratory distress may indicate underlying cardiac disease or reflect increased pulmonary vascular resistance. The murmur of a patent ductus arteriosus (PDA) is most frequently audible during the recovery phase of RDS when pulmonary vascular resistance has fallen below systemic levels and there is left-to-right shunting (p. 438). Distant, muffled heart sounds should alert one to the possibility of pneumopericardium or rarely a pericardial effusion. Percussion of the chest is of no diagnostic value in preterm infants.

A constant feature of RDS is the early onset of clinical signs of the disease, within the first 6 hours of delivery. Inadequate observation may lead to the impression of a symptom-free period of several hours. The uncomplicated clinical course is characterized by a progressive worsening of symptoms with a peak severity by days 2 to 3 and onset of recovery by 72 hours. When the disease process is severe enough to require assisted ventilation or complicated by the development of air leaks, significant shunting through a PDA, or early signs of BPD, recovery may be delayed for days or even weeks.

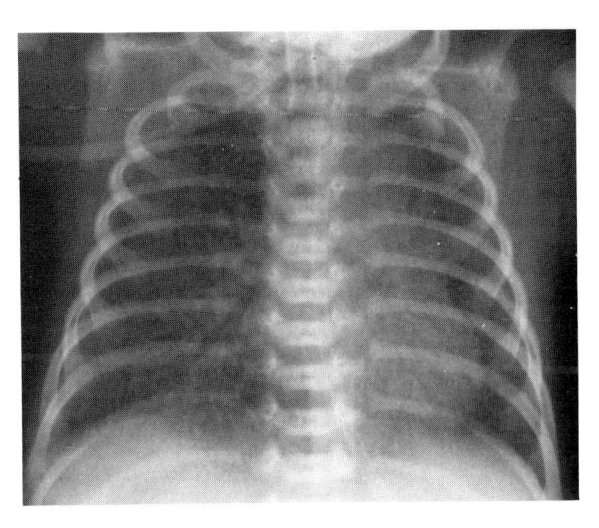

Fig. 23-17. Typical roentgenographic appearance of RDS with reticulogranular infiltrate and an air bronchogram.

RADIOLOGIC FINDINGS

See Chapter 39.

The diagnosis of RDS is based on a combination of the previously described clinical features, evidence of prematurity (including biochemical pulmonary immaturity [p. 134]), exclusion of other causes of respiratory distress (p. 460), and the characteristic radiologic appearance. The typical radiographic features consist of a diffuse reticulogranular pattern in both lung fields with superimposed air bronchograms (Fig. 23-17). The granular pattern is primarily caused by alveolar atelectasis, although there may be some component of pulmonary edema. The prominent air bronchograms represent aerated bronchioles superimposed on a background of non-aerated alveoli. An area of localized air bronchograms may be normal in the left lower lobe overlying the cardiac silhouette, but in RDS they are widely distributed particularly in the upper lobes. It is possible for the initial roentgenogram to be normal in RDS, only to develop the typical pattern after 6 hours of age. Heart size is typically normal or slightly increased. Cardiomegaly may be prominent as a consequence of birth asphyxia, in infants of diabetic mothers, or because of the development of congestive cardiac failure from a PDA. It is not uncommon for the granularity to be distributed asymmetrically throughout the lung fields in RDS with aeration most diminished on the right. It is important to note that the roentgenologic appearance of RDS, typical or atypical, cannot be reliably differentiated from that of neonatal pneumonia, most commonly caused by group B streptococci. This problem has been the major reason for the widespread use of antibiotics in the initial management of infants with RDS. The increased use of various means of ventilatory support and the enhanced survival of infants with more severe pulmonary disease have resulted in the more frequent radiographic recognition of complications such as pulmonary air leaks (p. 448) and BPD (p. 467) in the sickest infant. Recent evidence indicates that infants with RDS have a larger thymic silhouette compared with infants of comparable size without RDS. This supports the theory that patients with RDS had inadequate exposure to endogenous corticosteroids during fetal life.

Echocardiographic evaluation of infants with RDS may be of value in the diagnosis of a PDA and to quantitate elevations in pulmonary artery pressure (pp. 438 and 554).

ASSESSMENT OF BLOOD GASES

See p. 421.

The ability to accurately monitor and interpret the blood gas status of infants is essential in all cases of neonatal respiratory disease. In its most basic form this involves intermittent arterial sampling usually via an indwelling umbilical arterial catheter or less commonly a radial arterial line. Infants with acute respiratory distress requiring an increased inspired oxygen concentration or assisted ventilation should have blood gases sampled every 4 hours or more often as their clinical condition dictates to minimize morbidity from oxygen toxicity (pp. 440 and 472). The practical aspects of oxygen administration are discussed on p. 296.

Arterial sampling

The precise measurement of arterial oxygen tension (PaO_2) has been enhanced by incorporating an oxygen electrode into the tip of an umbilical arterial catheter. After appropriate in vivo calibration such an intravascular electrode allows PaO_2 to be continuously monitored while minimizing the need for arterial sampling. A closely related technique has been to fit a fiberoptic oximeter into the umbilical arterial catheter to continuously measure oxygen saturation instead of the more conventional PaO_2. The latter is customarily maintained between 60 and 90 mm Hg in infants with RDS. Even with these newer techniques intermittent arterial sampling still is required to maintain the arterial carbon dioxide tension ($PaCO_2$) at less than 55 mm Hg and the pH at least 7.25.

The technique of umbilical catheterization, its complications, and their management are discussed in detail on p. 299. It should be noted that, although umbilical arterial catheters still form the basic means of arterial sampling in infants with RDS, the list of catheter-related complications is formidable. The most frequent visible problem from an umbilical or radial line is blanching or cyanosis of part of or all the distal extremity, secondary to either vasospasm or a thrombotic or embolic incident. This complication may be reduced in the case of an umbilical catheter by high placement with the catheter tip at the level of the seventh or eighth thoracic vertebra as opposed to lower placement at the third or fourth lumbar segment just above the aortic bifurcation. Tyson and colleagues have observed thromboatheromatous complications resulting from umbilical arterial catheters in 33 of 56 neonates at autopsy. Hypertension may result if a renal artery is involved, and passage of a catheter past the origin of the superior mesenteric artery has been suggested to increase the risk of necrotizing enterocolitis. The risk of arterial thrombi appears to be reduced by the addition of small amounts of heparin to the continuous infusion and the use of Silastic catheters with decreased thrombogenicity. All these complications illustrate the importance of applying rigid criteria for the insertion and removal of indwelling arterial catheters and the need for less hazardous methods of monitoring blood gases.

Transcutaneous monitoring

Transcutaneous measurement of PO_2 ($TcPO_2$) has emerged as an important technique for indirectly determining PaO_2 in a noninvasive and continuous manner. Electrodes for $TcPO_2$ monitoring consist of modified Clark electrodes (as used in blood gas analyzers) that are attached to the skin and can be heated to a desired temperature. A good correlation between $TcPO_2$ and PaO_2 can be obtained at a skin electrode temperature of 44° C in both term and preterm infants in the presence or absence of respiratory disease and over a wide range of PaO_2 (Fig. 23-18, A). The precise reasons for the close relationship between PO_2 in the arterial blood and at the skin surface are quite complex, although it clearly depends on adequate vasodilatation of the capillary bed under the electrode with increasing temperature.

For infants with mild respiratory distress $TcPO_2$ monitoring is extremely valuable and may make it unnecessary to insert an umbilical arterial catheter, provided intermittent assessments of pH and PCO_2 are made. Generally, this is not the case in infants with moderate or severe respiratory difficulty in whom $TcPO_2$ measurement remains an important adjunct rather than a substitute for arterial blood gas sampling. In profoundly ill neonates with tissue hypoperfusion $TcPO_2$ measurements may somewhat underestimate the infant's level of PaO_2. As levels of PaO_2 exceed 100 mm Hg, $TcPO_2$ will tend to underestimate PaO_2, and the scatter between these two parameters will increase. Thus $TcPO_2$ should be maintained at less than 90 mm Hg to ensure an optimal correlation with PaO_2 and minimize the risk of hyperoxemia.

The major impact of $TcPO_2$ monitoring in these acutely ill infants has been to rapidly optimize respiratory care and drastically reduce the time required to determine optimum inspired oxygen concentrations, levels of con-

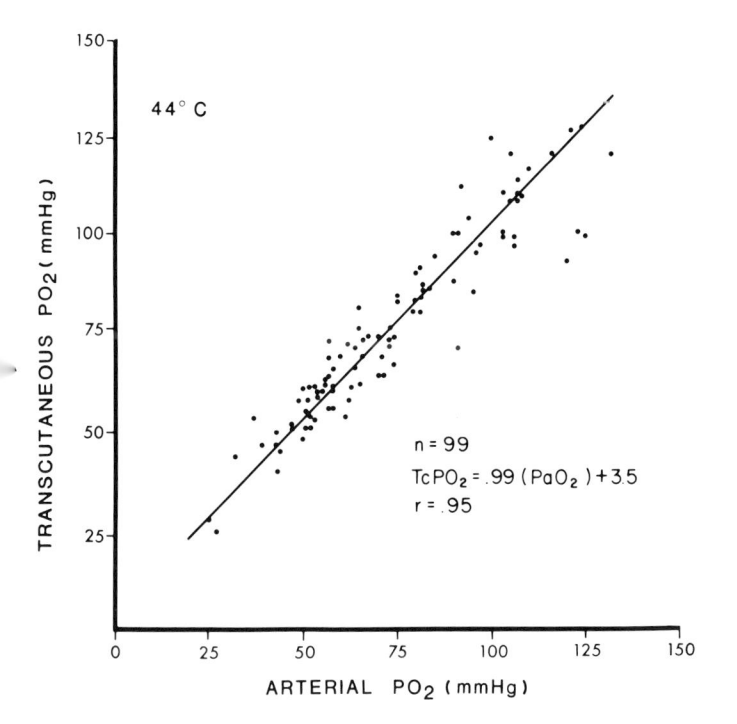

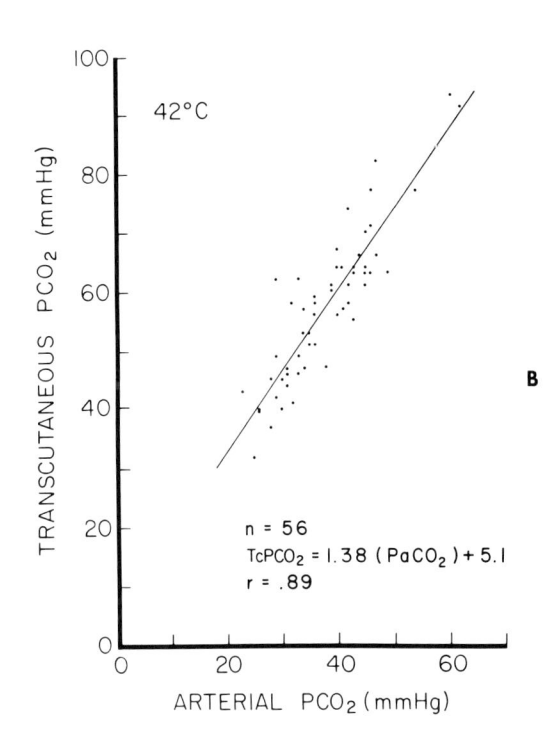

Fig. 23-18. Correlation between transcutaneous and arterial Po₂ in preterm infants with RDS **(A)**. Correlation between transcutaneous and arterial Pco₂ in preterm and term infants with cardiopulmonary disease **(B)**.

tinuous positive airway pressure (CPAP), and respirator settings. Other benefits include the ability to determine responses to all procedures. Furthermore complications such as pneumothorax, endotracheal tube dislodgment, disconnection from oxygen supply, or respirator malfunction will be rapidly recognized so that immediate corrective treatment can be initiated. A major contribution of TcPo₂ monitoring has been the repeated observation that excessive and vigorous handling of sick infants results in hypoxemia. Long and associates noted that the use of continuous oxygen monitoring resulted in a reduced amount of both hypoxia and hyperoxia and furthermore that many episodes of inappropriately low or high oxygen levels would go undetected without continuous monitoring.

TcPo₂ also has proved invaluable in the longer term care of small premature infants recovering from RDS and requiring oxygen for weeks or even months. Recently we have observed that nursing such infants in the prone rather than the supine position resulted in an increase in TcPo₂ especially in those infants who had residual cardiopulmonary disease. It should be noted that in older infants with a postnatal age in excess of 2 months TcPo₂ may underestimate Pao₂, although relative changes in oxygenation still can be readily discerned.

The temperature of the skin electrode and maximum heat output must be carefully controlled to avoid burns to the skin, and for this reason the electrode is repositioned every 4 hours. Transient areas of erythema are common and usually disappear within hours, although blister formation may occur, particularly in very sick infants with poor perfusion. Quantitation of the heat output of the skin electrode to maintain a temperature at 44° C may be a useful measure of tissue perfusion provided the electrode is properly insulated.

Transcutaneous measurement of Pco₂ offers a useful adjunct to TcPo₂ monitoring either via separate or combined electrodes. In contrast to TcPo₂ measurements, a surprisingly good correlation between TcPco₂ and Paco₂ can be obtained using an electrode heated to only 37° C. This may relate to the more ready diffusibility of carbon dioxide compared with oxygen. Nonetheless the correlation can be significantly improved when the electrode is heated to either 42° or 44° C (Fig. 23-18, *B*). The Pco₂ measured at the skin surface in this way is higher than the comparable arterial values. This appears to result from a combination of carbon dioxide production by the skin as a result of local metabolism, the anaerobic heating coefficient of blood as it is warmed beneath the electrode, and other as yet undetermined factors. Transcutaneous Pco_2 electrodes respond to changes in carbon dioxide relatively slowly with an in vivo response time of approximately 60 to 90 seconds, compared with the brisk (5 to 10 seconds) response time for $TcPo_2$. Under conditions of profound hypoperfusion and shock the elevation of $TcPco_2$ over the simultaneous value of $Paco_2$ will be further increased, presumably as a result of CO_2 accumulation in tissues. The continuous measurement of tissue pH is being evaluated in infants; however, this requires the insertion of a small needle beneath the skin. Transcutaneous measurement of O_2 saturation is being developed as an adjunct to $TcPo_2$ monitoring. Careful evaluation of these new techniques for assessing the blood gas status of neonates is imperative so they can find their appropriate place in routine neonatal respiratory care.

TREATMENT

Therapy for RDS comprises the careful application of general supportive measures supplemented by various specific means of controlling and/or assisting ventilation. Close and detailed supervision of small infants requires a dedicated, trained staff experienced and interested in problems specific to the newborn and skillful in the technical procedures involved.

Thermoregulation

Infants with respiratory difficulty require an optimum thermal environment to minimize oxygen consumption and oxygen requirements (p. 259). Infants who are hypoxic lose the ability to increase metabolic rate when cold stressed, and a fall in body temperature may be noted. Thus meticulous attention must be paid to the temperature and humidity of the infant's environment and inspired air so that the appropriate neutral thermal environment may be maintained.

Fluids and nutrition

See also Chapter 20.

The ability to supply an adequate caloric intake to the critically ill infant receiving respiratory assistance has been facilitated by the availability of intravenous amino acid–glucose and lipid solutions. The role of nutritional support for these infants cannot be overemphasized. Anderson demonstrated that premature infants receiving as little as 60 calories/kg/day with 10% of the calories provided as protein could remain in positive nitrogen balance (p. 303). In many units therefore it has become commonplace to start administration of an amino acid–glucose solution on the second or third day of life, especially for infants weighing less than 1,500 gm and receiving mechanical ventilation. Fluid balance must be closely watched, since overenthusiastic attention to calories may result in fluid overload, PDA, and congestive heart failure. Maintenance fluid requirements usually begin at 60 to 80 ml/kg/day as a 10% dextrose solution and increase gradually to 150 ml/kg/day by the fifth day of life. However, these fluid requirements will be greatly modified by many additional factors, particularly the very high insensible water loss experienced by many very low birth weight infants under radiant warmers or phototherapy and the limited concentrating ability of immature kidneys (p. 314).

Savage reported no improvement in gas exchange in a small series of infants with RDS treated with furosemide on the first day of life. Moylan, on the other hand, studied infants at or beyond 2 days of age who were in stable condition while being mechanically ventilated. He demonstrated a significant increase in PaO_2 2 to 5 hours after diuretic administration, while mean urinary output increased fourfold during the 2 hours following furosemide administration. The conclusion is that while furosemide is an excellent diuretic in the newborn, in infants with respiratory distress postnatal age, previous intake of water and electrolytes, and time of sampling after the administration of the diuretic all can influence the response. A modest diuresis frequently precedes recovery from the pulmonary disease. Edema of the pulmonary interstitium may be a significant factor affecting gas exchange in infants with RDS without specific accompanying radiographic or clinical evidence of pulmonary edema. Restriction of maintenance fluids during assisted ventilation may help minimize this problem. A clear role for diuretics has not yet been defined.

In a retrospective study Stevenson found that premature infants with RDS accompanied by a PDA had received larger volumes of fluid during the 2 days prior to the diagnosis of a PDA than did control infants without evidence of a PDA. In a prospective study using sequential analysis, Bell showed that the risk of a PDA with congestive heart failure was greater in infants receiving a high-volume regimen (169 ± 20 ml/kg/day) than those on a low-volume regimen (122 ± 14 ml/kg/day) designed to meet average estimated water requirements (p. 314). In the high-volume group 35 out of 85 (41%) developed murmurs consistent with a PDA, and 11 of these were associated with congestive heart failure. In contrast, only 9 of 85 (10%) of infants in the low-volume group had a PDA murmur, and two developed congestive heart failure. More cases of necrotizing enterocolitis also were observed in the high-volume group. This, together with other recent data, indicates that limitation of fluid intake could possibly reduce the risk of PDA, necrotizing enterocolitis, and BPD. The fluid therapy in infants with RDS is thus a critical aspect of care.

The renal inability to conserve salt together with a low sodium intake, overzealous use of diuretics, or the osmotic diuresis associated with hyperglycemia all may precipitate hyponatremia, particularly in infants weighing less than 1,500 gm. Maintenance of sodium balance usually is achieved by the administration of 2 to 4 mEq/kg/day of sodium, commencing at 24 to 48 hours, and close monitoring of serum sodium levels. Potassium balance is accomplished by adding 1 to 2 mEq/kg/day to the intravenous infusion from the second day of life.

Intravenous lipid seldom is used in the acute states of respiratory disease because the infants often have hyperbilirubinemia and because there may be a detrimental effect on arterial blood gases. Orogastric feeding is not recommended while infants are receiving nasal CPAP. Infants to whom intermittent positive pressure ventilation (IPPV) is being administered via a respirator may be fed, although studies have shown an accompanying deterioration in blood gas status, and therefore oral feedings during this time are usually withheld. In contrast, recently we have reported that, in infants who had recovered from RDS, nasogastric feeding did not change PaO$_2$.

Acid-base therapy

The need to correct acid-base disturbances should be determined by evaluation of pH, PCO$_2$, bicarbonate, and changes in buffer base (p. 320). Metabolic acidosis is most often encountered when the infant has been depressed at birth and required resuscitation. (See p. 179 for emergency treatment in the delivery room of acidosis associated with asphyxia.) A subsequent metabolic acidosis out of proportion to the degree of respiratory distress may signify sepsis or an intraventricular hemorrhage.

Respiratory acidosis may require transient or prolonged ventilation therapy (see further). Administration of sodium bicarbonate to infants with respiratory acidosis provides only transient correction at best and may further increase the PCO$_2$. It usually is not necessary to correct a respiratory acidosis if the pH is greater than 7.25 unless an infant's condition is unstable or deteriorating. Severe acidosis, respiratory or metabolic, especially when coupled with hypoxia, may result in pulmonary arterial vasoconstriction and ventilation-perfusion abnormalities or may result in arrhythmia and decreased cardiac output or both. In severe respiratory acidosis, alkali therapy should be withheld until some form of assisted ventilation has been initiated first. If this fails to improve oxygenation and raise the pH, sodium bicarbonate may be admininstered while continuing with assisted ventilation and always attempting to determine the cause of the acidosis.

Antibiotics in RDS

Neonatal pneumonia (most commonly caused by the group B streptococci) may mimic RDS both clinically and roentgenographically and thus be indistinguishable from it. Such infection usually is acquired around the time of delivery either through ascending infection or passage through a colonized genital tract. The potentially fulminant course of neonatal pneumonia and the difficulty in distinguishing it from RDS have led to the recommendation that all infants with significant respiratory distress receive antibiotics following appropriate cultures. Features suggestive of neonatal infection include maternal fever, prolonged rupture of membranes, persistent hypotension and/or metabolic acidosis, early onset of apnea, organisms in the gastric aspirate, neutropenia, and neutrophilia (Chapter 27). Nonetheless the absence of these features does not exclude the diagnosis of pneumonia. A penicillin combined with an aminoglycoside is the antibiotic regimen of choice, which may be discontinued after 72 hours if cultures are negative.

Transfusion

It is customary to maintain a venous hematocrit of 40% to 45% during the acute phase of RDS to support an adequate oxygen-carrying capacity. The use of exchange transfusion also has been proposed as a means of increasing the delivery of oxygen to tissues. Deliovria-Papadopoulos demonstrated significantly improved survival after exchange transfusion with fresh adult blood. The presumption was that provision of red cells with an increased 2,3-diphosphoglycerate content would shift the oxygen affinity curve to release more oxygen to tissues. On the other hand, there does appear to be an increase in the risk of retrolental fibroplasia following exchange transfusion. Therefore the latter has not been accepted as an established mode of therapy for RDS.

Surfactant therapy

The discovery that surfactant deficiency was key in the pathophysiology of RDS led several investigators to administer artificial aerosolized phospholipids to infants with RDS. In these studies only limited therapeutic success was encountered. In contrast, animal models in which natural surfactant compounds were used yielded more promising results. This stimulated Fujiwara to develop a mixture of both natural and synthetic surface-active lipids for use in humans. The goal was to achieve alveolar stability with less potential risk for a reaction to foreign protein than would be the case with exclusively natural surfactant. When administered to an initial group of 10 preterm infants with severe RDS who were not improving despite artificial ventilation, a single 10 ml of surfactant instilled into the endotracheal tubes resulted in a dramatic decrease in inspired oxygen and ventilator pressures. None of the infants in this uncontrolled series subsequently succumbed from RDS. Recovery, however was complicated by clinical evidence of a PDA in nine of the infants, possibly the result of a prompt fall in pulmonary vascular resistance with the resultant left-to-right shunting following surfactant therapy. This observation has been recently confirmed by Clyman in preterm lambs. The encouraging data from Japan undoubtedly will be followed by controlled clinical trials if adequate reassurance can be given that the administration of a surfactant preparation containing animal products is safe for human infants. Alternatives include the development of artificial protein-free mixtures of pure phospholipids in dry form, which have been proposed by Morley to improve the clinical course of RDS.

Continuous positive airway pressure (CPAP)

Prior to 1970 mechanical ventilation was used in the treatment of RDS when severe respiratory failure supervened despite administration of increased oxygen concentrations. Consequently the results were extremely discouraging, with only 65% survival expected for infants weighing greater than 2 kg, approximately 33% at 2 kg, and 20% if they were smaller. In 1971 Gregory introduced a new approach with the application of CPAP via head box or endotracheal tube to infants who were breathing spontaneously. The initial results were encouraging, since they not only demonstrated significant increase in PaO_2 with a resultant decrease in oxygen requirements, but the outcome data also suggested improved survival. Soon thereafter multiple reports describing different techniques of application appeared. These included a pressurized face chamber, face mask, plastic bags, and nasal prongs. Other investigators chose to indirectly produce positive transpulmonary pressure by exerting continuous negative pressure (CNP) around the chest wall either with a modified negative pressure ventilator or a chamber within the incubator to which a vacuum was applied. The purpose of all these different modes of therapy is to achieve continuous distending pressure (CDP) throughout the respiratory cycle. It should be apparent that this may be accomplished either by exerting a positive pressure on the airway (CPAP) or by exerting negative pressure around the thorax (CNP). Debate continues as to the most efficacious method by which to deliver CDP as well as the optimum time to initiate therapy; there is, however, no argument as to its benefit despite a limited number of controlled studies.

The physiologic basis for the use of continuous distending airway pressure was first suggested by Harrison, who investigated the role of grunting in RDS. He concluded that grunting (exhaling against a partially closed glottis with active contraction of the abdominal muscles) represented an attempt by the infants to overcome atelectasis (p. 420). When grunting was eliminated with endotracheal intubation, a fall in PaO_2 ensued. The grunting resumed after extubation, and PaO_2 rose promptly. Although it has been widely accepted that CPAP increases PaO_2, thereby allowing a reduction in fractional inspired O_2 concentrations (FiO_2), it is not entirely clear what physiologic factors account for these effects. It has been postulated that recruitment of previously collapsed alveoli results in better oxygenation by improving ventilation-perfusion relationships within the lungs. After application of CPAP there is an increase in FRC, which presumably decreases intrapulmonary right-to-left shunting, lending credence to this idea. However, there is a variable effect on lung compliance, which usually decreases. This suggests that, in addition to recruitment of some alveoli, there also may be overdistention of others. With application of CDP the breathing pattern becomes more regular and slower, and grunting generally ceases after CDP has been applied. Because of the rapidity with which these changes occur, it has been postulated that the changes in frequency result from modification of the Hering-Breuer reflex because of the change in the FRC (p. 456).

The optimum level of CDP may be defined as that airway pressure at which PaO_2 is maximum with minimum effect on cardiovascular function. If the pressure is increased above this level, $PaCO_2$ rises. Monitoring of esophageal pressure reveals a sharp rise when optimum CDP is achieved, suggesting recruitment of alveoli and enhanced transmission of airway pressure to the intrapleural space. The optimum level of CDP is not static in any given patient.

The initial report by Gregory described the use of either a pressurized head box or an endotracheal tube. However, an alternative to endotracheal CPAP was vigorously sought to avoid intubation and its attendant risks. The head chamber presented many difficulties: it was not easy to construct, limited access to the infant, and at times produced constriction about the neck with subsequent skin breakdown. It also required an extremely high airflow and thus produced an unacceptable noise level for the infant. Various modifications were suggested to overcome some of these problems, including a face mask that covered only the nose and mouth but required the exertion of great pressure on the head and face to maintain an adequate seal. Devices for CNP administration also were developed. However, an obvious drawback to these is that therapy must be interrupted for any procedure to be performed on the infant. In addition, with any leak in the chamber thermoregulation becomes a problem as a result of the torrential airflow.

In 1973 Kattwinkel reported a method for delivering CPAP via the now widely used nasal prongs. There are several advantages to this technique: it is relatively atraumatic, avoids the need for an endotracheal tube, allows constant access to the baby, is simple to set up and care for, and requires lower flow rates than do head or face chambers. Furthermore there are no attendant problems with thermoregulation. An alternative method to the short nasal prongs is the use of nasopharyngeal tubes placed in one or both nares. A recent study by Goldman has demonstrated a considerably higher work of breathing with nasal prongs compared with a face mask, which is thought to be a result of the resistance of the tubing. The systems for delivery of continuous distending airway pressure, therefore, continue to be modified.

Increases in the FiO_2 represent the minimum level of respiratory support that an infant with RDS may require. Such support is, however, frequently insufficient, and further assistance is required. Because CPAP almost invariably has a beneficial effect on PaO_2, hypoxemia remains the most universally accepted rationale for institution of this therapy. Specific guidelines, however, are still quite variable. In our nursery the inability of the infant to maintain a PaO_2 of greater than or equal to 60 mm Hg in an FiO_2 of 0.7 constitutes adequate indication for initiating CPAP. CPAP is applied earlier under certain circumstances, particularly in very small infants with early onset of severe RDS. The place for routine early administration of CDP to infants with RDS remains to be determined. Because CPAP has a variable effect on $PaCO_2$, one must monitor the blood gases closely, and, if respiratory failure ensues (i.e., $PaCO_2$ greater than 55 to 60 mm Hg, pH less than 7.20), endotracheal intubation with mechanical ventilation should be instituted.

In summary, CDP has proved an extremely effective tool for the management of RDS. The level and duration of high oxygen concentration required by these infants are both reduced, and the need for mechanical ventilation appears to be decreased. In addition, CPAP is extremely useful as an intermediate step in weaning infants from mechanical ventilation, and there is evidence that the duration of intubation is decreased. Several studies have additionally shown an improved outcome with decreases in both the mortality and the incidence of BPD among survivors. If the need for, and duration of, endotracheal intubation are truly decreased, this could lead to a decline in the incidence of the long-term airway problems which sometimes follow this procedure. Despite over a decade of experience, the indications for elective intervention with CDP remain controversial.

Mechanical ventilation

In 1929 Drinker introduced the negative pressure ventilator for adults, and positive pressure ventilators followed thereafter. Although sporadic reports on the use of mechanical ventilation in infants appeared as early as the 1940s, it was many years before ventilators appropriate for use with small infants were available. By the late 1960s the use of ventilators in newborns became more widespread, and in the 1970s mechanical ventilation appears to have contributed significantly to the reduction in perinatal mortality.

Despite several reports attesting to the efficacy of intermittent assisted ventilation with mask and bag, it became apparent that for many infants with RDS and respiratory failure the only chance for survival was continuous ventilatory support. Early uncontrolled trials described the use of both intermittent negative pressure ventilation (INPV) and intermittent positive pressure ventilation (IPPV). INPV was delivered initially with a ventilator-incubator combination that enclosed the infant's entire body from the neck down. The smallest babies were tossed about by the relatively large flows and changes in pressure, became bruised, developed skin breakdown beneath the seals at the neck, and also experienced significant thermal stress. Later modifications attempted to stabilize the infant's body by limiting the negative pressure chamber to extend only from the neck to the hips. Stahlman and associates reported a series of 80 patients treated with INPV. Although these patients were severely ill, exhibiting PaO_2 levels of less than 30 to 40 mm Hg, an FiO_2 of 1.0, prolonged apnea, and gasping respiration or bradycardia, the derangements of pH, $PaCO_2$, and PaO_2 were corrected in many, and 39% survived.

In simultaneously conducted controlled and uncontrolled studies employing IPPV via both pressure- and volume-cycled ventilators, the efficacy of this mode of therapy in correcting arterial blood gas status was subsequently demonstrated. Proponents of INPV were quick to point out that it eliminated the morbidity of endotracheal intubation (p. 438), still a major problem in neonatal intensive care units, and that this mode of therapy was associated with a reduced incidence of air leak syndromes and chronic lung disease. Access to the infant, however, was considerably more difficult and required interruption of mechanical ventilation, thereby limiting its usefulness, and few neonatal centers employ this mode of therapy today. Because of their greater versatility, positive pressure ventilators are used almost exclusively today, and the remainder of this discussion is confined to IPPV.

With the original positive pressure ventilators, gas flow to the patient occurred only during the inspiratory phase of the cycle. The expiratory phase was characterized by passive emptying of the lungs. Attempts at spontaneous ventilation during periods without gas flow would have entailed markedly increased work of breathing for the patient as well as inhalation of recently exhaled and therefore carbon dioxide–enriched gas. It was thus necessary to abolish spontaneous ventilation either by increasing alveolar ventilation to the point that respiratory drive was overcome or by neuromuscular blockade. The alternative concept of intermittent mandatory ventilation (IMV), during which a fresh flow of gas is delivered to the patients throughout the respiratory cycle, represented a major step forward in mechanical ventilation of neonates. This mode permits both spontaneous and artificial ventilation to occur concurrently. A further major advantage of IMV is that it has facilitated and simplified weaning from mechanical support.

The application of distending airway pressure throughout the respiratory cycle (as developed by Gregory in spontaneously breathing infants) combined with IPPV and known as positive end expiratory pressure (PEEP) followed naturally. The addition of positive pressure throughout the cycle is thought to prevent collapse of alveoli and improve oxygenation by enhancing V/Q ratios.

Despite much experience and significant success with mechanical ventilation, there is still considerable difference of opinion regarding the optimum method of ventilating infants, particularly those with persistent derangement of blood gases. Both volume- and pressure-cycled ventilators have been used, with the latter gaining more favor as attempts are made to ventilate infants with low pressures. Using a volume-cycled machine, one presets the tidal volume (generally 7 to 10 cc/kg) delivered to the patient and adjusts the flow rate to determine the time over which it is delivered, thus determining the ratio of inspiratory to expiratory time (I/E ratio). It must be recognized, however, that such ventilators will deliver these volumes irrespective of the pressure generated unless pressure limits are set. This assumes increasing importance in infants with severe RDS in whom compliance is so markedly diminished that delivery of a "normal" tidal volume requires a tremendous peak inspiratory pressure (PIP). Furthermore the high flow rates limit the adjustment of the I/E ratio. The alternative is the use of a pressure-cycled ventilator, wherein flow is delivered to the patient until the predetermined PIP is reached. At this point the pressure may be immediately allowed to return to end expiratory levels, producing a sawtooth pressure curve, or it may be maintained at peak levels for some time before the expiratory phase begins, producing a pressure curve with plateaus (Fig. 23-19). Thus the "pressure" ventilator used in this way is really time cycled and pressure limited. Within this framework the I/E ratio thus may be widely manipulated. Prolonged I/E ratios to the extent of reversal of the normal ratio (i.e., I/E > 1/1.5) usually produce an increased PaO₂ but may cause carbon dioxide retention if alveolar ventilation is impaired. Compromise of cardiac function with decreased venous return secondary to prolonged high intrathoracic pressures has not been a significant clinical problem in neonates with markedly decreased lung compliance.

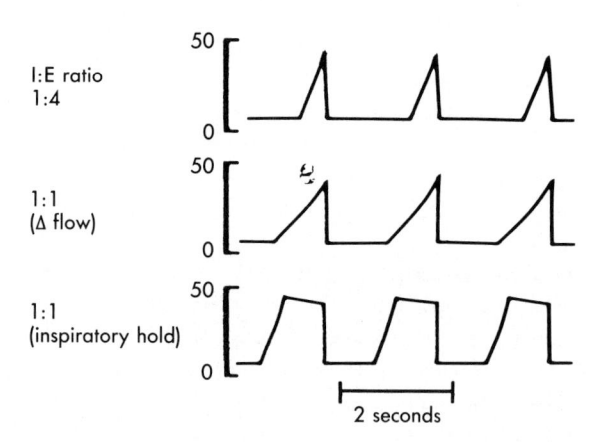

Fig. 23-19. Airway pressure waves produced by altering either I/E ratio or inspiratory flow rate. (From Boros, S.J.: J. Pediatr. **94:**114, 1979.)

Increases in PIP generally will decrease $PaCO_2$ but also may result in increased incidence of serious air leaks and chronic lung disease. It has been suggested that lower PIPs combined with higher I/E ratios may result in decreased morbidity and even mortality. Increases in the level of PEEP also tend to improve PaO_2, but one is limited in this aspect of therapy by the increased risk of air leaks as well as decreased alveolar ventilation and cardiac output. Indeed some studies suggest that mean airway pressure (MAP) is the most important determinant of oxygenation as well as complications such as air leaks and BPD.

There remains much confusion regarding the optimum rate of ventilating these infants. Although an increased rate generally results in improved alveolar ventilation and decreased $PaCO_2$, the effect on PaO_2 may be none or detrimental. Some studies suggest that the slow rates (in combination with an increased I/E ratio) are associated with decreased morbidity and mortality; however, other reports describe high survival rates using rapid ventilation at low pressures. Heicher documented a decreased incidence of pneumothoraces when it was possible to ventilate (and adequately oxygenate) infants at a rapid rate and low PIP.

Newer modes of mechanical ventilation employing very high frequencies are evolving. These comprise the use of conventional IPPV at rates of around 100 breaths/minute, high-frequency jet ventilation, and high-frequency oscillation. These last two techniques enable alveolar ventilation to occur under experimental conditions at volumes that are only a fraction of normal tidal volumes. Marchak has demonstrated that adequate gas exchange can be sustained over short periods using high-frequency oscillation at rates of up to 1,200 cycles/minute in infants with RDS. Future controlled studies are needed to demonstrate whether barotrauma can be reduced by the use of these new techniques of ventilation.

At our own institution the indications for ventilator therapy are deterioration of either blood gases or clinical condition. The infant may be unable to maintain adequate oxygenation (PaO$_2$ more than 50 mm Hg) or adequate ventilation (PaCO$_2$ less than 55 to 60 mm Hg with pH greater than 7.20) in an FiO$_2$ of 1.0 with a nasal CPAP of 10 cm H$_2$O, or he may exhibit increasing periods of apnea and/or bradycardia requiring vigorous stimulation or positive pressure bagging. We prefer to perform endotracheal intubation with tubes of 2.5 or 3 mm internal diameter to minimize damage to the upper airway (p. 438). However, as a greater number of smaller babies are being ventilated, 2.5 mm tubes are being used increasingly.

The use of neuromuscular blockade has been advocated in infants who require mechanical ventilation with high rates or pressures and become increasingly agitated when their attempts at spontaneous respiration are out of phase with the ventilator. This results in decreased effectiveness of mechanical support, and, when oxygenation has become inadequate, paralysis may improve the blood gas status of some of these infants. Neonates with or without lung disease who have persistence of the fetal circulation are particularly susceptible to the effects of agitation, and in these patients neuromuscular blockade may result in a decrease in right-to-left shunting and increased oxygenation. Generalized edema that appears to be the result of absent muscular activity and the radiologic appearance of a gasless abdomen are common complications. There remains much controversy surrounding the use of such agents, however, since there are little data available on the indications, efficacy, and complications of their use, especially in very low birth weight infants. The administration of phenobarbitone has been proposed to result in a decreased incidence of intraventricular hemorrhage in infants with RDS receiving ventilatory support, although this too requires further study.

Weaning the infant from ventilatory support is frequently as difficult a problem as the initial management. In milder cases it may easily be accomplished, but with severe disease the superimposition of iatrogenic lung disease may make the process difficult or even impossible. The approach is usually to decrease PIP as tolerated until 20 to 25 cm H$_2$O and then to direct one's attention to FiO$_2$ and IMV. It has been suggested that treatment with aminophylline to stimulate respiratory drive will facilitate the weaning process, but the evidence for this is scanty. When a low IMV of approximately 10 breaths per minute is tolerated, a short trial of endotracheal CPAP is in order. Prolonged periods of endotracheal CPAP in small infants with resolving lung disease are usually unsuccessful. This is because the infant may be incapable of sustaining the additional work of breathing associated with an increased airway resistance together with the added dead space of the endotracheal tube. Endotracheal CPAP should be maintained at 2 cm H$_2$O during the weaning process. The infant is then extubated but may benefit from nasal CPAP. Steroids are not routinely used prior to extubation, but if stridor caused by laryngeal edema develops, racemic epinephrine aerosols may be administered.

There have been some advocates of vigorous chest physiotherapy for infants with severe RDS especially while receiving assisted ventilation. Although some infants undoubtedly benefit from the therapy, many will show deterioration of blood gases. Continuous transcutaneous monitoring of Po$_2$ is recommended if physical therapy is prescribed, and, unless there is evidence of a beneficial effect, the principle of minimum handling of these fragile infants should be adhered to. During suctioning the catheter should not be inserted more than 1 cm beyond the lower end of the endotracheal tube to minimize damage to the airway (p. 438). During the accompanying bagging periods, O$_2$ concentration may be increased 10% over the infant's current requirement, and a pressure manometer must be in place to ensure that comparable pressures are maintained off the ventilator.

Extracorporeal membrane oxygenation (ECMO)

Extracorporeal membrane oxygenation (ECMO) is an innovative technique that in selected patients offers some promise as a means of supporting life. It has been suggested as an alternative or adjunct to conventional respirator therapy in the hope of decreasing acute and chronic lung damage, although at this time technical difficulties are so great that it is not considered a reasonable alternative. Perfusion and gas exchange are performed via prolonged venoarterial cardiopulmonary bypass through a membrane lung. This allows the infant's heart and lungs to recover at low ventilator settings and inspired oxygen concentrations. This experimental approach has had some encouraging results in the management of neonatal respiratory failure in a limited number of very sick infants with RDS, persistent fetal circulation, and the meconium aspiration syndrome.

COMPLICATIONS OF RDS

Complications related to RDS may occur spontaneously but are more commonly the result of well-intended therapeutic interventions. The major complications are consequent on the placement of arterial catheters (pp. 299 and 430), oxygen administration, mechanical ventilation, and the use of endotracheal tubes. The complications of assisted ventilation are the following:

1. Pulmonary air leaks: pneumothorax, pneumomediastinum, pulmonary interstitial emphysema

2. Endotracheal tube accidents: displacement, dislodgment, occlusion, atelectasis after extubation
3. Tracheal lesions: erosion, granuloma, subglottic stenosis
4. Infection: pneumonia, septicemia, meningitis
5. Chronic lung disease: BPD
6. Miscellaneous: intracranial hemorrhage, PDA, retrolental fibroplasia

The liberal use of total parenteral nutrition together with other pharmacologic interventions also has contributed to morbidity. The reader is referred to detailed discussions of these conditions in the relevant sections of this book.

Patent ductus arteriosus (PDA)

See p. 604.

Clinical features of a PDA with left-to-right shunting may be noted in infants recovering from RDS. The incidence of PDA ranges from 15% to 36% in preterm infants and is more prevalent in very low birth weight infants or those with pulmonary disease. A PDA should be suspected when there is a delay in clinical improvement from RDS and the infant still requires the respirator or is oxygen dependent. Aggressive management is indicated if a PDA is confirmed. Evaluation of the left-to-right shunting through the ductus is of fundamental importance. This may be achieved by echocardiography (measuring left atrial size, left ventricular end-diastolic dimension, or left atrial/aortic ratio) or contrast roentgenographic studies via an umbilical arterial catheter. Therapy includes fluid restriction, medical management of congestive heart failure, and either surgical or pharmacologic closure of the ductus. The PDA has been implicated in the cause of BPD because it presumably prolongs the duration of ventilatory assistance. Excess fluid intake has been associated with both BPD and PDA. Although it generally has been thought that congestive heart failure secondary to a PDA represents a complication of RDS, Jacob has suggested that infants with respiratory distress less than or equal to 1.2 kg who have a maturing surfactant pattern in their tracheal aspirate may have a silent patent ductus. The implication is that, rather than being a complicating factor in RDS, a PDA may be the cause of respiratory distress in some very low birth weight infants. Pharmacologic or surgical closure of the ductus in these infants is followed by a dramatic decrease in ventilatory and oxygen requirements. There is need for controlled data to determine the place for early PDA closure in very immature infants with RDS. Surgical ligation remains a proved and effective method of treating a PDA in the preterm infant, with a very low (less than 2%) operative mortality. Whether this should be the treatment of choice or pharmacologic closure should be initially attempted is currently under intensive investigation. Ultimate survival following ligation is estimated at about 66% and largely dependent on the severity of RDS and timing of the surgical procedure.

Infection

Early in the course of experience with mechanical ventilation infection was extremely prevalent, and mortality was high. This was most commonly associated with gram-negative organisms including *Pseudomonas* and *Klebsiella* organisms and *Escherichia coli*. More recently infection as a complication of mechanical ventilation appears to be less common. Superinfection, with *Candida organisms*, *Staphylococcus aureus*, and gram-negative organisms as the most common offenders, however, has been known to occur, particularly in infants with birth weights less than 1.5 kg who have required prolonged mechanical ventilation and multiple courses of antibiotic therapy.

In the neonate requiring mechanical ventilation careful attention must be given to aseptic technique, particularly at the time of endotracheal intubation and during suctioning. Changing all equipment related to mechanical ventilation every 24 hours is also effective. The prophylactic use of antibiotics under these conditions is of no proved value.

Endotracheal tube complications

Accidental displacement of an endotracheal tube into a main stem bronchus or into the hypopharynx or esophagus is a well-recognized and extremely hazardous complication of mechanical ventilation. The frequency with which such complications occur has been estimated to be from 2% to 40%. Accidental tube displacement usually is associated with ipsilateral hyperinflation and contralateral collapse and clinically characterized by deterioration in the patient's condition, often with cyanosis. Auscultation of the chest may suggest this complication, but roentgenographic studies may be needed to resolve the issue. Similarly, accidental extubation usually is accompanied by sudden deterioration with cyanosis, bradycardia, and respiratory collapse. It is necessary to quickly determine whether there is any mechanical failure in the ventilator and to assume manual ventilation with mask and bag. If any doubt exists, tube position should be inspected visually and the tube replaced if necessary. Note that clinical examination of the chest may be unreliable in determining tube position because of the transmission of breath sounds across the thorax in small infants. Sudden deterioration from tube displacement always must be differentiated from a pneumothorax, and immediate x-ray confirmation of tube position should be undertaken. Although it has been stated that both the quantity and tenacity of secretions increase with assisted ventilation in infants with RDS, tube occlusion because

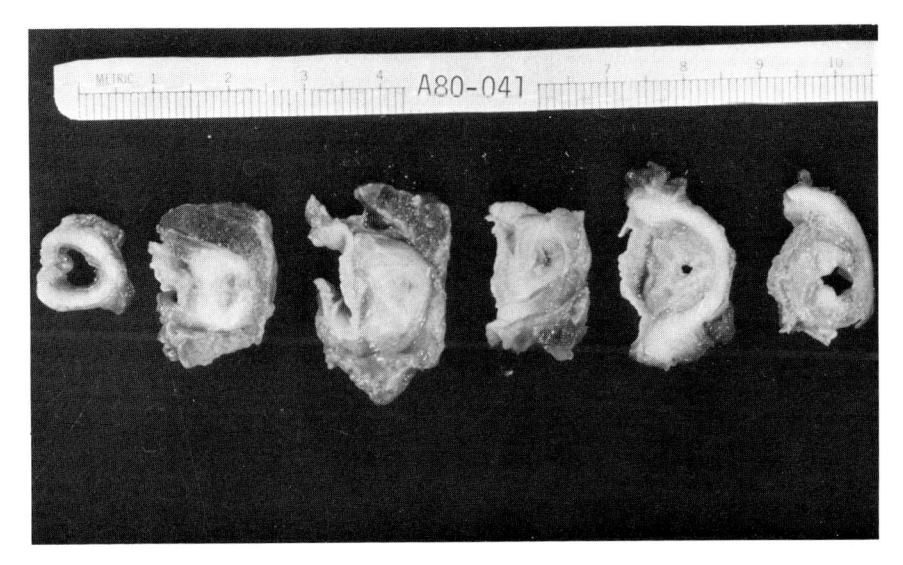

Fig. 23-20. Sequential sections taken through the larynx and upper trachea of an infant who died at 8 months following orotracheal intubation for 4 months. There is complete occlusion of the glottis by granulation tissue. (Courtesy Drs. R.E. Wood and B. Dahms.)

of secretions has become a very infrequent complication, since adequate humidification is available with current ventilators.

The frequency with which serious tracheal lesions complicate endotracheal intubation and IPPV of the newborn infant is difficult to determine. Following extubation edema of the cords may result in transient hoarseness and stridor in many infants. The use of dexamethasone prior to extubation or epinephrine-isoxsuprine inhalations has not provided universal relief, although there are strong advocates of both these measures. Both gross and histologic evidence of inflammation and epithelial erosions of the trachea has been noted at postmortem examination of infants dying after prolonged endotracheal intubation.

Furthermore fiberoptic inspection of the airways of infants who have been intubated for a significant period will reveal some pearly lesions below the cords, although most of these prove to be insignificant. More recently partial or complete occlusion of the trachea and even the main stem bronchi at the site of suction catheter injury has been noted. Recent reports have recommended the use of smaller endotracheal tubes that ensure the presence of an air leak when the tube is in place, securing the tube well so that movement of the tube within the trachea is minimum when infants are moved, careful suctioning techniques using side-hole catheters, and not allowing the catheters to go too far below the distal end of the endotracheal tube to diminish the incidence of severe tracheal lesions. Subglottic stenosis has been noted in approximately 1% of survivors of mechanical ventilation with birth weights less than 1.5 kg (Fig. 23-20).

These infants may be seen initially with airway obstruction during a superimposed respiratory infection. Tracheostomy may be necessary for this small group of infants. Whether the complications of endotracheal tubes can be reduced or eliminated by avoiding prolonged intubation and performing earlier tracheostomy in some infants remains to be proved.

Atelectasis after extubation occurs frequently in infants recovering from RDS. Clinically the infants demonstrate increased respiratory difficulty, retraction, and cyanosis; their blood gases show respiratory failure with hypoxemia and hypercarbia. Roentgenographically the right upper lobe is the most frequent site affected, and shift of the mediastinal structures is common. Previously the approach to treatment comprised physiotherapy with postural drainage and repeated endotracheal suctioning. In many of these infants, particularly those with birth weights below 1,500 gm, this regimen was often unsuccessful, and reintubation was necessary. The recent availability of the flexible fiberoptic bronchoscope has alleviated the problem, and it is possible to keep the infant well oxygenated while suctioning the bronchial tree. Mucus plugs or even bronchial casts sometimes are removed intact, and prompt clinical and roentgenographic improvement may be noted (Fig. 23-21).

Residual pulmonary disease

Residual pulmonary disease occurs in a significant number of infants surviving mechanical ventilation for severe RDS. The spectrum ranges from infants with minimum roentgenographic changes associated with slight cardiorespiratory distress to crippling cardiorespi-

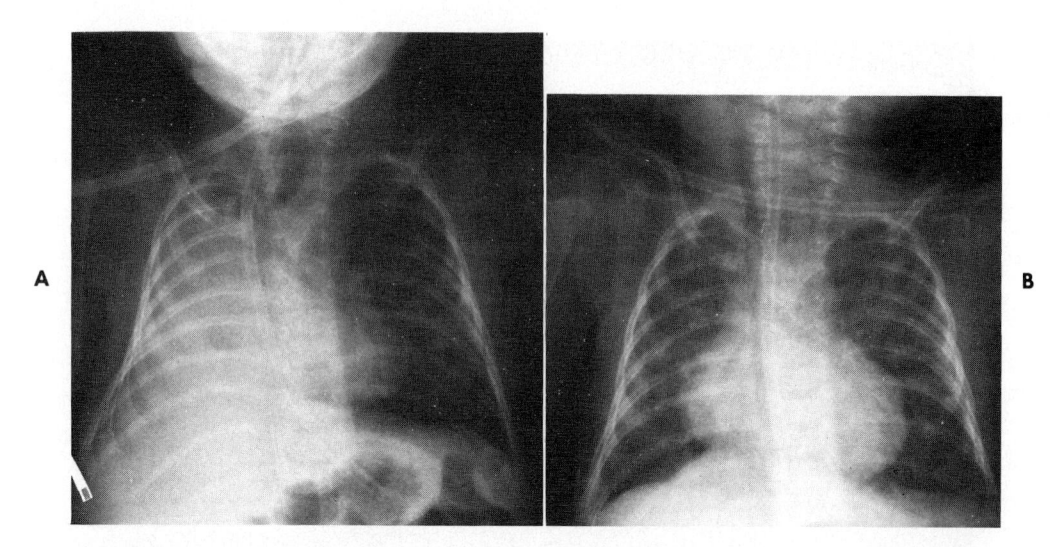

Fig. 23-21. Chest roentgenograms of a 1.1-kg infant with **(A)** massive atelectasis of the right lung following extubation and **(B)** reexpansion of the collapsed lung immediately following bronchoscopic removal of a large mucus plug from the right main stem bronchus. (Courtesy Dr. R.E. Wood.)

ratory failure seen after prolonged ventilation with high concentrations of oxygen. The infants may develop restrictive and/or obstructive lung disease, abnormal chest roentgenograms, and cor pulmonale. The pathogenesis and management of these infants are considered in Part five.

Intracranial hemorrhage

See Chapter 22.

Subependymal and/or intraventricular hemorrhage occur frequently, especially in very immature infants with severe pulmonary disease. As discussed elsewhere, numerous causes for intraventricular hemorrhage have been proposed, including neonatal asphyxia with hypotension, rapid volume expansion, changes in serum osmolarity resulting from excessive bicarbonate administration, coagulation abnormalities, hypoxemia, and hypercarbia. It is difficult to clearly establish a relationship between intracranial hemorrhage and bicarbonate administered to infants with RDS. Undoubtedly many preterm infants have received too much bicarbonate, but the proof of a relation to intracranial hemorrhage is not convincing.

Since these factors are all closely interrelated with severe RDS, it is not surprising that intraventricular hemorrhage has been further correlated with mechanical ventilation employing high peak inflation pressures, prolonged inspiratory times, and especially the development of alveolar rupture and air leaks, all of which would be expected to alter cerebral blood flow or volume by impairing venous return. Even though intracranial hemorrhage is a clearly recognized complication of RDS, it is often unclear at autopsy whether RDS or intraventricular hemorrhage is the cause of death when both are present, and this may be as much a matter of guesswork as of knowledge. The discovery that intracerebellar hemorrhage may result from tight-fitting face masks used for the administration of CPAP was first reported by Pape and associates and noted to be accompanied by extensive molding and displacement of the infants' skull. Martin subsequently reported a series of asphyxiated preterm infants with massive cerebellar hemorrhage in whom mask CPAP had not been employed. These observations further illustrate the importance of continually evaluating the role of iatrogenic factors in the cause of intracranial hemorrhage. This is especially important because recent prospective studies using ultrasound or computerized tomography (CAT scans) have demonstrated a much higher incidence of subependymal and intraventricular hemorrhage in surviving infants than was previously suspected. This trend will persist as respiratory care for infants with RDS continues to improve and less infants die from pulmonary disease per se.

Oxygen toxicity

Administration of oxygen is an essential component of the care and survival of neonates with respiratory problems. The two major manifestations of oxygen toxicity involve damage to the immature retina (Chapter 35) and lungs (p. 467). Pulmonary tissue appears particularly sensitive to the toxic effects of oxygen to which its cells are directly exposed.

There has been an ongoing argument as to the relative roles of prolonged oxygen exposure, endotracheal intubation, immaturity, and technique of assisted ventilation (positive versus negative pressure ventilators) in the genesis of chronic pulmonary disease in infants. Nonetheless there is clearly an association between oxygen therapy and the development of BPD. The goals of therapy for respiratory distress are to achieve adequate tissue oxygenation while maintaining a PaO$_2$ between 50 and 90 mm Hg, using the lowest environmental oxygen concentration, and avoiding excessive barotrauma to limit potentially damaging effects.

Follow-up evaluation

In evaluating the neurodevelopmental outcome (p. 398) of infants with RDS it is important to recognize the heterogeneity of this population. Each unit should follow their own infants and closely evaluate growth, intellectual development, vision, and hearing. Major factors influencing the outcome include the fact that the populations comprise mixtures of inborn and transported infants, infants with wide variations in birth weight and gestational age, infants with varying degrees of asphyxia, as well as differing indications and techniques of ventilation at different centers.

Stahlman, in 1973, presented a most encouraging report on the outcome of 85 infants treated for RDS. She found no difference in intelligence or handicap between ventilated and nonventilated infants of the same birth weight. No cases of cerebral palsy or hydrocephalus were identified. It should hastily be pointed out that all but three of her ventilated infants weighed greater than 1,500 gm. Today similar excellent results can be predicted for these relatively large infants at most centers, provided they have not suffered significant perinatal asphyxia.

It is the infants with birth weights below 1,500 gm who are of major concern, as documented by Fitzhardinge in her referral population. Factors associated with poor outcome include a neonatal history of seizures or intracranial hemorrhage and other severe neurologic sequelae. Twenty-nine percent of infants born between 1970 and 1973, requiring mechanical ventilation, had neurologic deficits, and 44% were handicapped on assessment at 2 years. Because of a number of changes in her nursery, including changes in techniques of ventilation and improved nutrition, survivors of mechanical ventilation between 1974 and 1975 showed only an 11% incidence of neurologic deficit, and 28% were handicapped. In 1975 and 1976 follow-up analysis of infants weighing less than 1.5 kg from our own nursery revealed an overall handicap rate of 18% (IQ less than 80, or neurologic deficit) for infants without RDS or those requiring only additional oxygen or CPAP (total of 220 infants). During this period the rate was 35% for those surviving mechanical ventilation. Thus the developmental outcome for infants with mild or moderate RDS is comparable to that of infants without RDS, whereas those requiring mechanical ventilation tend to do less well. Stahlman has followed up pulmonary function into middle and late childhood and has observed only mild abnormalities of pulmonary function that correlated with persistent respiratory symptoms in infancy.

When all infants less than 1,500 gm are considered, the overall statistics gathered in a number of studies are encouraging. However, when specific weight groups are examined, it is evident that the smallest infants (less than 1 kg) have not shared in this general improvement and that very small infants requiring extensive respiratory support continue to have a poor outcome, if they survive.

Richard J. Martin
Avroy A. Fanaroff
Mary Ellen L. Skalina

BIBLIOGRAPHY
General

Ablow, R.C., and others: A comparison of early onset group B streptococcal neonatal infection and the respiratory distress syndrome of the newborn, N. Engl. J. Med. **294:**65, 1976.

Avery, M.D., Fletcher, B.D., and Williams, R.G.: The lung and its disorders in the newborn infant, ed. 4, Philadelphia, 1974, W.B. Saunders Co.

Ballard, P.L., and others: Fetal sex and prenatal betamethasone therapy, J. Pediatr. **97:**451, 1980.

Boyle, R.J., and Oh, W.: Respiratory distress syndrome, Clin. Perinatol. **5:**283, 1978.

Bryan, M.H., and others: Pulmonary function studies during the first year of life in infants recovering from the respiratory distress syndrome, Pediatrics **52:**169, 1973.

Chu, J., and others: The pulmonary hypoperfusion syndrome, Pediatrics **35:**733, 1965.

Farrell, P.M., and Wood, R.E.: Epidemiology of hyaline membrane disease in the U.S.A., Pediatrics **58:**167, 1976.

Papageorgiou, A.N., and others: The antenatal use of betamethasone in the prevention of RDS: a controlled double-blind study, Pediatrics **63:**73, 1979.

Reynolds, E.O.R., and Taghizadeh, A.: Improved prognosis of infants mechanically ventilated for hyaline membrane disease, Arch. Dis. Child. **49:**505, 1974.

Robert, M.F., and others: The association between maternal diabetes and the respiratory distress syndrome in the newborn, N. Engl. J. Med. **294:**357, 1976.

Strang, L.B.: Hyaline membrane disease. In Neonatal respiration, ed. 1, Oxford, England, 1977, Blackwell Scientific Publications Ltd.

Tooley, W.H.: Hyaline membrane disease, Am. Rev. Respir. Dis. **115:**19, 1977.

Blood gas assessment

Conway, M., and others: Continuous monitoring of arterial oxygen tension using a catheter-tip polarographic electrode in infants, Pediatrics **57:**244, 1976.

Huch, R., and others: Transcutaneous Po$_2$ monitoring in routine management of infants and children with cardiorespiratory problems, Pediatrics **57:**681, 1976.

Long, J.G., Philip, A.G.S., and Lucey, J.F.: Excessive handling as a cause of hypoxemia, Pediatrics 65:203, 1980.

Martin, R.J., Herrell, N., and Pultusker, M.: Transcutaneous measurement of carbon dioxide tension: the effect of sleep state in term infants, Pediatrics 67:622, 1981.

Martin, R.J., and others: Effect of supine and prone positions on arterial oxygen tension in the preterm infant, Pediatrics 63:528, 1979.

Mokrohisky, S.T., and others: Low positioning of umbilical artery catheters increases associated complications in newborn infants, N. Engl. J. Med. 299:561, 1978.

Tyson, J.E., deSa, D.J., and Moore, S.: Thromboatheromatous complications of umbilical arterial catheterization in the newborn period, Arch. Dis. Child. 51:744, 1976.

Wilkinson, A.R., Phibbls, R.H., and Gregory, G.A.: Continuous measurement of oxygen saturation in sick newborn infants, J. Pediatr. 93:1016, 1978.

Fluid and nutrition

Anderson, T.L., and others: A controlled trial of glucose versus glucose and amino acids in premature infants, J. Pediatr. 94:947, 1979.

Bell, E.F., and others: Effect of fluid administration on the development of symptomatic patent ductus arteriosus and congestive heart failure in premature infants, N. Engl. J. Med. 302:598, 1980.

Fanaroff, A.A., and Klaus, M.: The gastrointestinal tract—feeding and selected disorders. In Fanaroff A.A., and Klaus, M., editors: Care of the high risk neonate, Philadelphia, 1979, W.B. Saunders Co.

Moylan, F.M.B., and others: Edema of the pulmonary interstitium in infants and children, Pediatrics 55:783, 1975.

Savage, M.O., and others: Furosemide in respiratory distress syndrome, Arch. Dis. Child. 50:709, 1975.

Stevenson, J.G.: Fluid administration in the association of patent ductus arteriosus complicating respiratory distress syndrome, J. Pediatr. 90:257, 1977.

Transfusion

Delivoria-Papadopoulos, M., and others: The role of exchange transfusion in the management of low-birth-weight infants with and without severe RDS, J. Pediatr. 89:273, 1976.

Surfactant therapy

Avery, M.E.: On replacing the surfactant, Pediatrics 65:1176, 1980.

Clyman, R.I., and others: Increased shunt through the patent ductus arteriosus after surfactant replacement therapy, J. Pediatr. 100:101, 1982.

Fujiwara, T., and others: Artificial surfactant therapy in hyaline membrane disease, Lancet 1:55, 1980.

Morley, C.J., and others: Dry artificial lung surfactant and its effect on very premature babies, Lancet 1:64, 1981.

Notter, R.H., and Shapiro, D.L.: Lung surfactant in an era of replacement therapy, Pediatrics 68:781, 1981.

CPAP

Ahlstrom, H., Jonson, B., and Svenningsen, N.W.: Continuous positive airways pressure treatment by a face chamber in idiopathic respiratory distress syndrome, Arch. Dis. Child. 51:13, 1976.

Bancalari, E., Garcia, O.L., and Jesse, M.J.: Effects of continuous negative pressure on lung mechanics in idiopathic respiratory distress syndrome, Pediatrics 51:485, 1973.

Bonta, B.W., and others: Determination of optimal continuous positive airway pressure for the treatment of RDS by measurement of esophageal pressure, J. Pediatr. 91:449, 1977.

Boros, S.J., and Reynolds, J.W.: Hyaline membrane disease treated with early end-expiratory pressure: 1 year's experience, Pediatrics 56:218, 1975.

Fanaroff, A.A., and others: Controlled trial of continuous negative external pressure in the treatment of severe respiratory distress syndrome, J. Pediatr. 82:921, 1973.

Goldman, S.L., Brady, J.P., and Dumpit, F.M.: Increased work of breathing associated with nasal prongs, Pediatrics 64:160, 1979.

Gregory, G.A., and others: Treatment of the idiopathic respiratory-distress syndrome with continuous positive airway pressure, N. Engl. J. Med. 284:1333, 1971.

Kattwinkel, J., and others: A device for administration of continuous positive airway pressure by the nasal route, Pediatrics 52:131, 1973.

Rhodes, P.G., and Hall, R.T.: Continuous positive airway pressure delivered by face mask in infants with the idiopathic respiratory distress syndrome: a controlled study, Pediatrics 52:1, 1973.

Tanswell, A.K., and others: Individualized continuous distending pressure applied within 6 hours of delivery in infants wth respiratory distress syndrome, Arch. Dis. Child. 55:33, 1980.

Yu, V.Y.H., and Rolfe, P.: Effect of continuous positive airway pressure breathing on cardiorespiratory function in infants with respiratory distress syndrome, Acta Pediatr. Scand. 66:59, 1977.

Mechanical ventilation

Bland, R.D., and others: High frequency mechanical ventilation in severe hyaline membrane disease: an alternative treatment, Crit. Care Med. 8:275, 1980.

Boros, S.J.: Variations in inspiratory:expiratory ratio and airway pressure wave form during mechanical ventilation: the significance of mean airway pressure, J. Pediatr. 94:114, 1979.

Boros, S.J., and Orgill, A.A.: Mortality and morbidity associated with pressure- and volume-limited infant ventilators, Am. J. Dis. Child. 132:865, 1978.

Daily, W.J.R., Sunshine, P., and Smith, P.C.: Mechanical ventilation of newborn infants. V. Five years' experience, Anesthesiology 34:132, 1971.

Donn, S.M., Roloff, D.W., and Goldstein, G.W.: Prevention of intraventricular hemorrhage in preterm infants by phenobarbitone, Lancet 2:216, 1981.

Drinker, P., and Shaw, L.A.: An apparatus for the prolonged administration of artificial respiration, J. Clin. Invest. 7:229, 1929.

Finer, N.N., and Tomney, P.M.: Controlled evaluation of muscle relaxation in the ventilated infant, Pediatrics 67:641, 1981.

Frantz, I.D., Stark, A.R., and Dorkin, H.L.: Ventilation of infants at frequencies up to 1800/min (abstract), Pediatr. Res. 14:642, 1980.

Heese, H.deV., and others: Intermittent positive pressure ventilation in hyaline membrane disease, J. Pediatr. 76:183, 1970.

Heicher, D.A., Kasting, D.S., and Harrod, J.R.: Prospective clinical comparison of two methods for mechanical ventilation of neonates: rapid rate and short inspiratory time versus slow rate and long inspiratory time, J. Pediatr. 98:957, 1981.

Herman, S., and Reynolds, E.O.R.: Methods for improving oxygenation in infants mechanically ventilated for severe hyaline membrane disease, Arch. Dis. Child. 48:612, 1973.

Manginello, F.P., and others: Evaluation of methods of assisted ventilation in hyaline membrane disease, Arch. Dis. Child. 53:878, 1978.

Marchak, B.E., and others: Treatment of RDS by high-frequency oscillatory ventilation: a preliminary report, J. Pediatr. 99:287, 1981.

Murdock, A.I., and others: Mechanical ventilation in respiratory distress syndrome: a controlled trial, Arch. Dis. Child. 45:524, 1970.

Pollitzer, M.J., and others: Pancuronium during mechanical ventilation speeds recovery of lungs of infants with hyaline membrane disease, Lancet 1:346, 1981.

Stahlman, M.T., and others: Negative pressure assisted ventilation in infants with hyaline membrane disease, J. Pediatr. 76:174, 1970.

Stern, L., and others: Negative pressure artificial respiration: use in treatment of respiratory failure in the newborn, Can. Med. Assoc. J. **102**:595, 1970.

ECMO

Bartlett, R.H., and Gazzaniga, A.B.: Extracorporeal circulation for cardiopulmonary failure, Curr. Probl. Surg. **15**:5, 1978.

PDA

Baylen, B.G., and others: The critically ill infant with patent ductus arteriosus and pulmonary disease—an echocardiographic assessment, J. Pediatr. **86**:423, 1975.

Friedman, W.F., and others: The patent ductus arteriosus, Clin. Perinatol. **5**:411, 1978.

Jacob, J., and others: The contribution of patent ductus arteriosus in the neonate with severe RDS, J. Pediatr. **96**:79, 1980.

Endotracheal tube complications

Wood, R.W., and Sherman, J.: Treatment of atelectasis in infants by flexible bronchoscopy, J. Pediatr. (in press).

Intracranial hemorrhage

deLemos, R.A., and Tomasovic, J.J.: Effects of positive pressure ventilation on cerebral blood flow in the newborn infant, Clin. Perinatol. **5**:395, 1978.

Dykes, F.D., and others: Intraventricular hemorrhage: a prospective evaluation of etiopathogenesis, Pediatrics **66**:42, 1980.

Finberg, L.: The relationship of intravenous infusions and intracranial hemorrhage, J. Pediatr. **91**:777, 1977.

Martin, R., Roessmann, O., and Fanaroff, A.A.: Massive intracerebellar hemorrhage in low birth weight infants, J. Pediatr. **89**:290, 1976.

Pape, K.E., and Wigglesworth, J.S.: Haemorrhage, ischaemia, and the perinatal brain, Clinics in Developmental Medicine 69/70, London, 1979, William Heinemann Ltd.

Oxygen toxicity

Boat, T.F., and others: Toxic effects of oxygen on cultured human neonatal respiratory epithelium, Pediatr. Res. **7**:607, 1973.

Ehrenkranz, R.A., Ablow, R.C., and Warshaw, J.B.: Oxygen toxicity, Clin. Perinatol. **5**:437, 1978.

Follow-up

Fitzhardinge, P.M., and others: Mechanical ventilation of infants of less than 1501 grams birth weight: health, growth and neurologic sequelae, J. Pediatr. **88**:531, 1976.

Johnson, J.D., and others: Prognosis of children surviving with the aid of mechanical ventilation in the newborn period, J. Pediatr. **84**:272, 1974.

Lindrough, M., and others: Evaluation of mechanical ventilation in newborn infants, Paediatr. Scand. **69**:151, 1980.

Rhodes, P.G., Hall, R.T., and Leonidas, A.C.: Chronic pulmonary disease in neonates with assisted ventilation, Pediatrics **55**:788, 1975.

Rothberg, A.D., and others: Outcome for survivors of mechanical ventilation weighing less than 1,250 gm at birth, J. Pediatr. **98**:106, 1981.

Stahlman, M., and others: A six-year follow-up of clinical hyaline membrane disease, Pediatr. Clin. North Am. **20**:433, 1973.

Stahlman, M., and others: Role of hyaline membrane disease in production of later childhood lung abnormalities, Pediatrics **69**:572, 1982.

PART FOUR

Other pulmonary problems

MECONIUM ASPIRATION SYNDROME

Meconium staining of the amniotic fluid or fetus is usually considered to be indicative of fetal distress. The passage of meconium in utero accompanies 8% to 20% of all deliveries and is seen predominantly in small for gestational age (SGA) and postmature infants, as well as those with cord complications or other factors compromising the in utero placental circulation. Although knowledge of the pathophysiologic stimuli in the fetus that govern the passage of meconium in response to stress is still incomplete, this phenomenon is almost never observed prior to a gestational age of 34 weeks. Many infants with meconium-stained amniotic fluid exhibit no signs of depression, although some brief period of asphyxia may well have induced the passage of meconium prior to delivery. Nonetheless the presence of meconium in the amniotic fluid necessitates careful supervision of labor and close monitoring of fetal well-being (Chapter 9). The accoucheur must be alerted to the possibility of a depressed fetus, and someone skilled in newborn resuscitation must be present in the delivery room. With appropriate management of the airway the meconium aspiration syndrome and complications thereof can be largely prevented.

Pathophysiology

The quantity of meconium will affect the appearance and viscosity of the amniotic fluid, which ranges from a green-tinged, lightly meconium-stained fluid to one with a thick, pea soup consistency. Under normal circumstances fetal respiration is associated with movement of fluid from the airways out into the amniotic fluid. With fetal distress gasping movements may be initiated in utero. Under these circumstances amniotic fluid and particulate matter contained therein may be inhaled into the large airways. The meconium inhaled by the fetus may be present in the trachea or larger bronchi and be manifested as airway obstruction at delivery. Because of the viscosity of the fetal lung fluid, it is uncommon for inhaled meconium to penetrate into the smaller air spaces prior to delivery. Nonetheless meconium and squames may be found as far as the alveoli in stillborn infants. After the commencement of air breathing, especially if accompanied by gasping respirations, there is a rapid distal migration of meconium within the lung. Roentgenographic studies by Gooding, who instilled tantalum-labeled meconium into the trachea of neonatal puppies prior to their first breath, confirmed that this can occur within 1 hour.

Pathophysiologically the pulmonary problems relate to airway obstruction and a ball valve phenomenon cre-

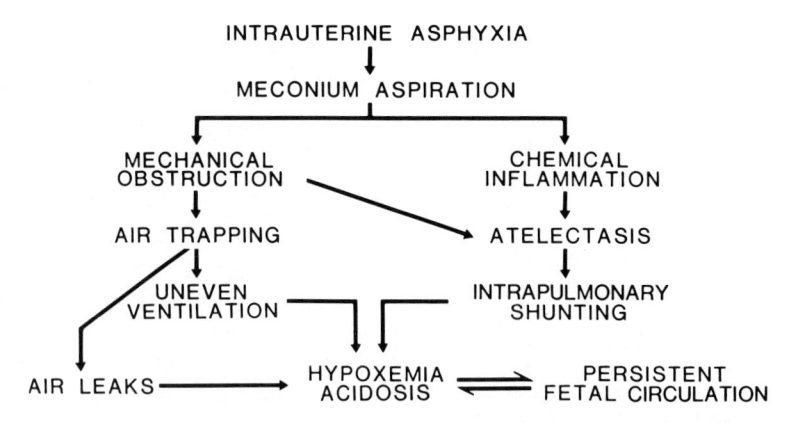

```
                INTRAUTERINE ASPHYXIA
                         ↓
                MECONIUM ASPIRATION
                    ↓         ↓
            MECHANICAL    CHEMICAL
            OBSTRUCTION   INFLAMMATION
                ↓             ↓
            AIR TRAPPING → ATELECTASIS
                ↓             ↓
            UNEVEN        INTRAPULMONARY
            VENTILATION   SHUNTING
                    ↓    ↓
     AIR LEAKS →  HYPOXEMIA  ⇌  PERSISTENT
                  ACIDOSIS      FETAL CIRCULATION
```

Fig. 23-22. Pathophysiology of meconium aspiration syndrome.

ated by the presence of meconium within the airways. Thus there are areas of atelectasis resulting from total small airway obstruction, adjacent to areas of overexpansion from gas trapping in areas with partial obstruction (Fig. 23-22). In rabbits, after insufflation of the lungs with a meconium-saline mixture, there is a consistent increase in functional residual capacity (FRC) and expiratory lung resistance. Air leaks, including pneumomediastinum and pneumothorax, frequently occur following aspiration of meconium and cellular debris. Similarly pulmonary hypertension also is noted.

Clinical features

The infant with meconium aspiration syndrome frequently exhibits the classic signs of postmaturity with evidence of weight loss together with nails, skin, and umbilical cord that are heavily stained with a yellowish pigment. The infants often are depressed at birth. In fact the initial clinical picture may be dominated by neurologic and respiratory depression secondary to the hypoxic insult precipitating the passage of meconium. Respiratory distress with cyanosis, grunting, flaring, retractions, and marked tachypnea soon ensues. Characteristically the chest acquires an overinflated appearance, and rales may be audible on auscultation. The chest roentgenogram shows coarse, irregular pulmonary densities with areas of diminished aeration or consolidation (Fig. 23-23). Pneumothorax and pneumomediastinum are noted in 21% to 50% of infants with meconium aspiration syndrome. Hyperinflation of the chest may be noted roentgenographically with flattening of the diaphragm. Massive aspiration is characterized by a "snowstorm" appearance, and cardiomegaly also may be detected. Arterial blood gases characteristically reveal hypoxemia with evidence of right-to-left shunting. Hyperventilation may result in a respiratory alkalosis, although infants with severe disease usually will have a combined respiratory and metabolic acidosis secondary to the asphyxia and

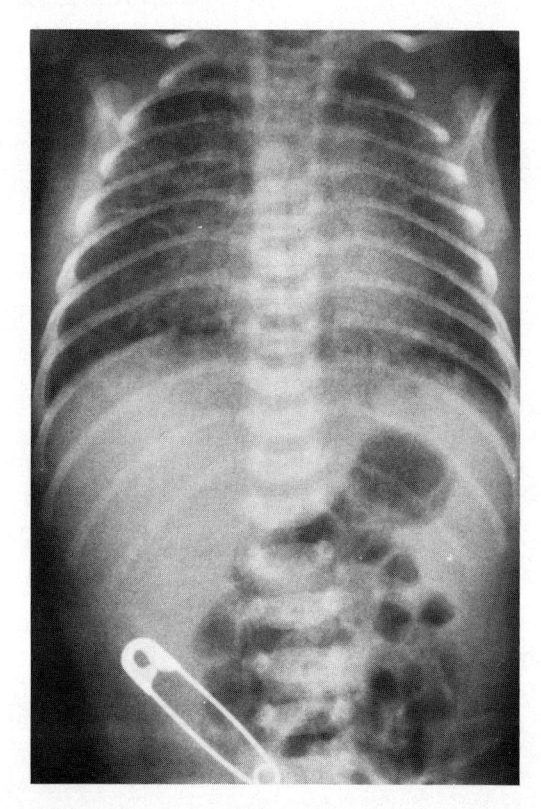

Fig. 23-23. Chest roentgenogram showing multiple linear streaks of meconium aspiration pneumonia.

respiratory failure. One should be alerted to the possible development of persistent fetal circulation (PFC) which frequently accompanies meconium aspiration syndrome (p. 566).

Management

The key to management of this disorder lies in its prevention. The presence of meconium in the amniotic fluid, however, is not an indication for panic. Although it is clear that meconium staining of the amniotic fluid may signal fetal hypoxia, if other parameters such as fetal heart rate (FHR) and pH remain in the normal range, then the outcome is usually favorable. The combination of meconium-stained amniotic fluid and ominous FHR patterns is associated with significant fetal and neonatal asphyxia with accompanying morbidity, and appropriate interventions should be instituted.

Independent studies from several centers have demonstrated clearly that a combined obstetric and pediatric approach can almost entirely eliminate this major neonatal problem. The cooperative team approach should begin with upper airway suctioning by the obstetrician after delivery of the head. The obstetrician should suction the nose and pharynx with a DeLee suction catheter. Tracheal suctioning under direct vision is ideally performed prior to the first breath and always must be completed prior to the initiation of positive pressure ventilation when resuscitating an infant. The controversy is whether all infants with meconium staining of the amniotic fluid should be suctioned. The impressive outcome data when such management is carried out argue strongly for the suctioning of all infants, a position we would advocate. Most significantly, Gregory and associates have found a 56% incidence of meconium in the trachea of meconium-stained infants, in 9% of whom meconium was visualized below the cords despite being absent in the mouth or pharynx. Retrospective data have indicated the benefits of immediate tracheal suctioning of meconium-stained infants in the delivery room with a marked reduction in morbidity and mortality from meconium aspiration syndrome. Gage documented that catheter suctioning of meconium from the airway of kittens was clearly more effective than bulb suctioning of the upper airway under experimental conditions. He furthermore observed that meconium remained in the trachea for periods exceeding 20 minutes despite spontaneous respirations. These studies underline the importance of tracheal aspiration by the most experienced person in the delivery room before positive pressure resuscitation is begun.

The subsequent management of this disorder consists of supportive respiratory therapy. Little can be done to enhance the mechanisms by which meconium is phagocytosed and removed from distal portions of the respiratory tract. Supportive management includes the use of antibiotics, because bacterial sepsis may have precipitated the passage and subsequent aspiration of meconium, and bacterial pneumonia may be indistinguishable roentgenographically from meconium aspiration syndrome. Furthermore, even though the meconium should be considered sterile, it enhances bacterial growth in vitro. Some authors have advocated the use of steroids; however, in a controlled study hydrocortisone was shown to be of no benefit in the management of this syndrome.

Ventilatory assistance is indicated when adequate levels of PaO_2 cannot be maintained in a high inspired oxygen concentration. Specific details of respiratory management are considered in Part three. Arterial oxygen tension should be maintained at the upper recommended levels, i.e., 80 to 90 mm Hg, to minimize hypoxic pulmonary vasoconstriction. Although in initial reports the use of continuous distending airway pressure (CDP) was contraindicated for meconium aspiration, some infants do indeed respond favorably. Truog studied experimental meconium aspiration syndrome in lambs and noted decreased shunting, and improved PaO_2 (without any detrimental effect on pulmonary blood flow) following early application of PEEP. Continuous positive airway pressure (CPAP) may, however, further increase the risk of air leaks, which is already high because of the many overdistended alveoli. Assisted ventilation is indicated for impending respiratory failure and may be required for a prolonged period. Infants struggling against the ventilator are usually paralyzed, although there are limited data regarding this mode of therapy. A significant mortality can be expected in those infants who require assisted ventilation. Persistence of the fetal circulation is managed with a regimen of minimum disturbance for the infant, hyperventilation (maintaining $PaCO_2$ at approximately 25 mm Hg), and pulmonary vasodilators such as tolazoline. Transcutaneous monitoring has permitted better control of these potentially unstable infants. The asphyxial complications are treated appropriately and efforts made to prevent hypoglycemia, particularly in SGA infants. The ultimate prognosis may depend not so much on the pulmonary disease as on the accompanying asphyxial insult. No specific long-term deficits in pulmonary function have been described after this disorder, although bronchopulmonary dysplasia may result from prolonged assisted ventilation (p. 467).

Other aspiration syndromes

At the time of delivery the neonate may aspirate clear amniotic fluid or fluid mixed with pus or blood. It remains unclear whether infants can aspirate a sufficient volume of clear amniotic fluid to interfere with normal ventilation. In deliveries where the amniotic fluid is purulent, the risk of bacterial pneumonia necessitates appropriate antibiotic therapy following evaluation for sepsis. Aspiration of either fetal or maternal blood requires no specific therapy and appears to resolve rapidly. Squamous debris associated with amniotic fluid aspiration may persist in the lung for some days. Unless the material is assumed to be infected, therapy should be merely supportive. Aspiration after regurgitation is most likely to be seen in preterm infants, those with disorders of swallowing, and infants with esophageal atresia with tracheoesophageal fistula. Small preterm infants are at greatest risk when fed excessive volumes per gavage. These infants may initially be seen with airway obstruction or apnea and subsequently develop respiratory distress with pulmonary infiltrates visible on roentgenograms. The severity of disease varies, and it may be indistinguishable from an inflammatory pneumonitis. Aspiration syndromes associated with disorders of the swallowing mechanisms may be suspected from the perinatal history (asphyxia), feeding history (color changes, excessive drooling, poor suck), and physical examination. The precise cause however, may not be readily apparent, and these infants require extensive neurologic evaluation. Neonates with tracheostomies or gastrostomies are at risk for aspiration. Infants with recurrent aspiration, particularly those with disorders of the swallowing mechanism, present complex management problems.

NEONATAL PNEUMONIA

See p. 659.

The lungs represent the most common site for the establishment of sepsis in the neonate. Such infection, be it bacterial or viral in origin, may be acquired prior to or at the time of birth or in the early postnatal period. Since bacterial pneumonia carries a substantial mortality in the neonate, an extremely high index of suspicion must be maintained for all infants, preterm and term alike, in whom signs of respiratory distress are observed.

Etiology

Congenital bacterial pneumonia may be acquired by the fetus via transplacental passage of organisms, although ascending infection from the genital tract prior to or during labor appears to predominate. It follows that prolonged rupture of membranes in excess of 24 hours is a major predisposing factor, although it is possible that bacteria may gain access to the fetus by ascent through intact membranes. Since bacterial contamination of the infant always occurs during vaginal delivery, neonatal pneumonia may well occur in the absence of prolonged rupture of membranes or any maternal symptoms. Gasping during delivery as a result of fetal asphyxia may predispose the infant to aspirate contaminated amniotic fluid. After admission to the neonatal nursery the risk of acquiring bacterial pneumonia will be largely influenced by the rate of nosocomial infection within the hospital environment.

Over recent years group B streptococci have emerged as the major pathogen producing neonatal pneumonia, with a mortality from 20% to 50%. The organism is characteristically acquired from the maternal genital tract during labor or delivery, and overt group B streptococcal sepsis develops in approximately 1% of infants colonized in this way. This represents an overall infection rate of approximately 1 in 300 live births. Other bacteria to be considered when pneumonia is acquired in utero or in the immediate perinatal period include *Escherichia coli*, *Klebsiella* organisms, group D streptococci, *Listeria* organisms, and pneumococci, acquired via vertical transmission from the mother. When neonatal pneumonia develops several days or even weeks after birth, in addition to these organisms, infections from *Staphylococcus* and *Pseudomonas* organisms and fungi should be considered. Although infection with *Chlamydia trachomatis* does appear to be acquired during parturition, pneumonia caused by this organism typically has a gradual onset of respiratory symptoms beyond 3 weeks of postnatal life. Viral pneumonia can be acquired by the fetus from transplacental passage of organisms, as may be the case in the congenital intrauterine infections (TORCH syndromes) (p. 692). Viruses probably also account for a substantial number of postnatally acquired pneumonias. Viral pneumonia is not frequently recognized as such in the neonate, although epidemics secondary to respiratory syncytial virus infection and adenovirus have been described with significant morbidity and mortality.

Clinical course

The nonspecific nature of the clinical signs that are characteristic of neonatal sepsis make a high index of suspicion the key to early diagnosis. In some cases of severe pneumonia the infants may be totally lacking in pulmonary symptoms and present only mild or severe neurologic depression. Other alerting features include thermal instability, apneic spells, abdominal distension, or jaundice. The presence of tachypnea, cyanosis, or other sign of respiratory distress may focus attention on the lungs in these infants. Chest roentgenogram findings range from unilateral or bilateral streaky densities, which may progress to confluent mottled opacified areas, to a diffusely granular appearance with air bronchograms. This may make it impossible to roentgenographically differentiate bacterial pneumonia from respiratory distress syndrome (RDS), particularly when caused by group B streptococci (p. 433). Problems also may be experienced in differentiating severe neonatal pneumonia on roentgenogram from the "snowstorm" appearance of meconium aspiration. The difficulty in making a definitive diagnosis of neonatal pneumonia by roentgenogram has led to the widely accepted practice of administering antibiotics to infants with respiratory distress (particularly RDS) after appropriate cultures have been obtained. White cell count with differential, platelet count, or Gram stain of tracheal aspirate is only of value if abnormal, in which case there is an increased likelihood of respiratory distress being caused by neonatal sepsis. Serologic studies should be performed if congenital intrauterine infection is suspected, and cord blood immunoglobulins should be measured, although not all infants with intrauterine pneumonia will have elevated IgM levels. Chlamydial pneumonitis may be diagnosed by culturing nasopharyngeal or tracheobronchial secretions under appropriate laboratory conditions.

Treatment almost invariably is instituted prior to identification of the pathogenic organism and determination of its antibiotic sensitivities. Broad-spectrum coverage, including a penicillin and aminoglycoside, is the initial line of treatment. For pneumonia of later onset, agents specific for staphylococcal infection should be added. Once the responsible bacteria has been isolated and antibiotic sensitivies identified, the single most effective drug should be continued for 10 days or longer depending on the infant's clinical course. Although antibiotics form the mainstay of treatment, good supportive care is essential. This must include careful fluid management, blood gas monitoring, and ventilatory assistance, as indicated. The duration of chlamydial pneumonia in the neonate appears to be shortened by a 14-day course of oral erythromycin. Early onset bacterial pneumonia, usually caused by group B streptococci, carries an overall mortality of approximately 50%, which may be even higher in preterm infants. This discouragingly high mortality may occur despite the very early administration of appropriate antibiotic therapy. Bacterial and viral pneumonias of later onset are a cause of considerable morbidity in neonatal intensive care units, but this risk of a subsequent fatal outcome is small.

PULMONARY HEMORRHAGE

Massive pulmonary hemorrhage in the newborn often is associated with RDS and in many instances may be radiologically indistinguishable from it. It is usually a preterminal event that has been reported in association with intrauterine asphyxia, neonatal cold injury, aspiration of gastric contents or maternal blood, cerebral edema, severe Rh immunization, kernicterus, congenital heart disease, oxygen administration, widespread viral infection, and bleeding disorders, in addition to RDS. Massive bleeding also may be observed as a complication of procedures to the upper airway, producing erosion or ulceration, and in most instances these will be self-evident. Esterley and Oppenheimer observed massive pulmonary hemorrhage in more than 45% of autopsied neonates with birth weights over 2,500 gm, especially in infants with evidence of intrauterine growth retardation. Frederick and Butler reported massive pulmonary hemorrhage in about 10% of neonatal autopsies, although this incidence probably has decreased because of improved neonatal care. The antecedents of pulmonary hemorrhage are mostly conditions associated with hypoxia, hypervolemia, or congestive heart failure in which an acute rise in lung capillary pressure may be expected. Cole observed that, in infants with massive pulmonary hemorrhage, the hematocrit of the fluid from the endotracheal tube was significantly lower than the venous hematocrit and usually less than 10%. Gel filtration of the proteins from the hemorrhagic fluid and plasma provided clear evidence of molecular sieving, indicating passage of molecules through a porous medium. The most likely interpretation is that massive pulmonary hemorrhage represents the buildup of the capillary filtrate in the interstitial space; when it can no longer be accommodated, it bursts through the pulmonary epithelium into the airspaces. Whereas in most instances pulmonary hemorrhage is thus a reflection of advanced pulmonary edema, in some infants it represents true hemorrhage. Under these circumstances the hematocrit of the pulmonary effluent will be close to the venous hematocrit. The likely reason for the increase in pressure is that severe asphyxia causes acute left-sided heart failure and an acute rise in filtration pressure in the pulmonary capillaries, resulting in generalized lung edema. The factors predisposing to the increased capillary pressure that occurs in neonates with hemorrhagic edema include those favoring filtration of fluid such as hypoproteinemia, overtransfusion, and those causing damage to lung tissue, such as infection, RDS, mechanical ventilation, and excessive oxygen administration. Massive bleeding into the lungs seems relatively uncommon, occurring in association with coagulation disorders, pneumonia, or direct trauma.

Clinically the onset of massive pulmonary hemorrhage is heralded by sudden deterioration of the infant with pallor or shock, cyanosis, bradycardia, and often apnea. Pink or red frothy liquid drains from the mouth and may be seen arising from the trachea between the vocal cords or suctioned through an endotracheal tube. In many infants, however, it should be noted that blood will not be observed arising from the endotracheal tube. The diagnosis has been suspected by the finding of diffuse infiltrates or opacification of the lung fields. On autopsy the lungs may appear grossly hemorrhagic and heavy and histologically may reveal intraalveolar hemorrhage.

Hemorrhagic pulmonary edema can be successfully treated by prompt institution of assisted ventilation and transfusion of fresh blood. In some instances exchange transfusion has been successful. Prevention of asphyxia at birth and episodes of asphyxia in infants with predisposing conditions is most important.

TRANSIENT TACHYPNEA

Transient tachypnea (wet lung, or type II RDS) often presents a diagnostic dilemma. The disorder is very common and has many overlapping features with respiratory distress caused by surfactant deficiency. Since the infants almost invariably recover fully, it is difficult to define pathologically transient tachypnea of the newborn. The preferred explanation for the clinical features is delayed resorption of fetal lung fluid; thus it is seen more commonly following cesarean section, ostensibly because the infant's thorax is not subjected to the same pressures as when delivery takes place per vaginum in "the big squeeze."

Milner attempted to determine whether vaginal compression did have any measurable effect on lung mechanics and lung volume in the hours immediately after birth. Lung function tests were carried out in the first 6 hours of life on 26 babies delivered vaginally and 10 delivered by cesarean section. Striking differences in the thoracic gas volume measurements were observed. The mean thoracic gas volume after vaginal delivery was 32.7 ml/kg; after cesarean section it was only 19.7 ml/kg. Chest circumferences were the same in both groups. He concluded that infants not exposed to vaginal compression have excessively high volumes of interstitial and alveolar fluid for the first few hours, so that thoracic gas volume is reduced, but overall thoracic volume remains within the normal range. In other words, liquid volume is increased, while the gaseous component is decreased.

The syndrome of transient tachypnea typically presents as respiratory distress in nonasphyxiated term infants or preterm infants who are close to term. The clinical features comprise various combinations of cyanosis, grunting, flaring, retracting, and tachypnea in the first few hours after birth. Arterial blood gases reveal varying degrees of hypoxemia, although respiratory failure is uncommon. The chest roentgenogram is the key to the diagnosis. The characteristic finding is prominent perihilar streaking and fluid in the interlobar fissures. The prominent perihilar streaking may represent engorgement of the periarterial lymphatics that appear to participate in the clearance of alveolar fluid. In most instances the roentgenographic appearance can be readily distinguished from the diffuse reticulogranular pattern with air bronchograms that is characteristic of RDS.

The "transient" nature of this disease is quite variable, and it lasts anywhere from 12 to 24 hours in its mildest form to in excess of 72 hours in severe cases. Transient tachypnea must be differentiated from other causes of neonatal respiratory distress. Initially great difficulty may be encountered in distinguishing this disorder from RDS and group B streptococcal pneumonia. Evaluation, monitoring, and basic supportive care must cover all these contingencies. Transient tachypnea of the newborn by definition is self-limiting with no risk of recurrence or residual pulmonary dysfunction.

Transient tachypnea also must be distinguished from the clinical syndrome of *cerebral hyperventilation*. This usually is seen in term infants with history of birth asphyxia. The infants are profoundly tachypneic with minimum roentgenographic changes apart from occasional asphyxia-related cardiomegaly. Respiratory alkalosis is typical and is thought to be the result of respiratory center irritation, although there may be a component of postasphyxial pulmonary edema. The prognosis is related primarily to the nature and extent of the accompanying asphyxial insult.

PNEUMOTHORAX AND OTHER AIR LEAK SYNDROMES

Pulmonary air leaks comprise a spectrum of disease that includes pneumothorax, pneumomediastinum, pneumopericardium, and pulmonary interstitial emphysema. If significant morbidity and even mortality are to be minimized with these conditions, particularly tension pneumothorax, a high index of suspicion is essential to initiate early diagnosis and aggressive management.

Incidence

Pneumothorax is far more frequent in the neonatal period than any other time of life. The incidence varies widely depending on selective features such as frequency of neonatal asphyxia, techniques of resuscitation, incidence of respiratory problems, methods of administering assisted ventilation, and even the quality of x-ray examinations and experience of personnel interpreting the films (Chapter 39). Based on numerous radiographic surveys, the overall frequency of pneumothorax approximates 1% of all live births.

The likelihood of a pneumothorax being symptomatic in an infant without underlying lung disease is small, and many of these go undetected. Several interventions and disease states markedly increase the risk of pulmonary air leaks. These include vigorous resuscitation at birth, RDS, meconium aspiration syndrome, and pulmonary hypoplasia. In infants treated with assisted ventilation the incidence of pneumothorax and other air leaks is higher in most series, with some variability according to the technique employed. An incidence of 5% to 20% has been documented in RDS both with and without the use of CPAP, increasing to greater than 40% with the use of assisted ventilation and positive end expiratory pressure (PEEP). In term infants with meconium aspiration syndrome the incidence of air leaks is reported to range from 20% to 50%, often occurring early in the course of the disease.

Pathophysiology

Macklin first described, in the overdistended cat lung, the passage of air from a ruptured alveolus, moving up the vascular sheath into the mediastinum and from there into the pleural cavity. Both uneven alveolar ventilation and air trapping would appear to figure prominently in the pathophysiology of the air leak syndromes. On the one hand, inhomogeneity of ventilation is a result of both the atelectatic alveoli in RDS and the small airway plugs of meconium aspiration syndrome. The relatively more distensible areas of the lung receiving most of the ventilation are subjected to exceedingly high transpulmonary pressures, leading to an increased risk of alveolar rupture. On the other hand, during partial airway obstruction full expiration is prevented, and with subsequent inspirations accumulation of air may rupture the alveolar space. The susceptibility to pulmonary rupture is further enhanced in the neonate by a reduction in alveolar connecting channels (pores of Kohn) that would allow air to redistribute between ventilated and nonventilated units. Finally, many cases of pneumothorax and pneumomediastinum may originate at birth as a result of the high initial pressures that may be generated with the first few breaths. If this high pressure is transmitted to units already open, they may rupture as a result of these large pressure changes. High pressures are often necessary in infants with hypoplastic lungs; thus rupture is common.

Clinical features

Extrapulmonary extravasation of air should be suspected in any infant with respiratory disease whose condition suddenly deteriorates. Tachypnea is a uniform finding and may be accompanied by grunting and increasing pallor or cyanosis. If there is a unilateral pneumothorax, the cardiac apex may be shifted away from the affected side and breath sounds decreased, although this is a less reliable sign. Some infants may develop distention of the involved hemithorax or a tensely distended abdomen from downward displacement of the diaphragm. Signs of shock may be present because of compression of the great veins and decreased cardiac output. In pneumothorax, hypoxemia results from both decreased alveolar ventilation and right-to-left shunting of pulmonary blood flow through the atelectatic areas. It should be noted that in preterm infants with RDS a pneumothorax frequently develops beyond the first days of life when the severity of disease is decreasing and lung compliance increasing. Pneumothorax also may be suspected by a precipitous fall in transcutaneous oxygen tension, diminished excursion of the arterial pressure tracing, or reduced thoracic impedance. Because of a paucity of clinical signs, pneumomediastinum without accompanying pneumothorax frequently escapes clinical detection but is readily identified roentgenographically. Pneumopericardium is a rare complication that may accompany a pneumomediastinum, possibly because of air tracking along pleural reflections around the great vessels. Although it is frequently stated that pneumomediastinum in the neonate precedes pneumopericardium, there is no good evidence to substantiate this. Pneumopericardium may be asymptomatic or present as a cardiac tamponade with reduced stroke volume and venous return. Thus there is a fall in systolic blood pressure, and the heart sounds are absent or muffled. A friction rub is rarely audible. Pneumoperitoneum secondary to passage of air from the chest through the diaphragmatic apertures is an extremely rare occurrence that needs to be differentiated from free intraabdominal air secondary to a perforated viscus.

Large bilateral pneumothoraces often are observed in infants with the hypoplastic lungs accompanying renal agenesis (Potter's syndrome), other forms of renal dysplasia, or congenital diaphragmatic hernia. The presence of otherwise unexplained extrapulmonary air in the early neonatal period should raise the question of underlying renal malformations, and a thorough physical examination together with the appropriate investigations should be promptly undertaken (p. 787).

Recent data have revealed an association between the occurrence of a pneumothorax and intraventricular hemorrhage in preterm infants. Hill has reported a marked increase in anterior cerebral artery blood flow (using a noninvasive Doppler technique) followed by hemorrhage in infants after the development of a pneumothorax. Thus it is proposed that a pneumothorax may increase the risk of intraventricular hemorrhage by impairing venous return to the heart and increasing cerebral arterial blood flow secondary to hypercarbia and raised systemic diastolic pressure.

Diagnosis

Transillumination of the chest is an extremely useful technique for immediate diagnosis of pneumothorax and is invariably positive if the pneumothorax is large. Its principle benefit is to detect sudden life-threatening air leaks, which require immediate therapy prior to obtaining a definitive roentgenographic diagnosis. The technique involves the use of a fiberoptic light probe at the end of a flexible tube that is placed on the infant's chest wall while the nursery is darkened. In the presence of a large pneumothorax the entire hemithorax on the affected side lights up, while the opposite side shows diminished transillumination because of lung compression on that side. Decompression should be accomplished without awaiting roentgenographic confirmation. When there are lesser or questionable areas of abnormal transillumination and the infant's condition is stable, roentgenographic confirmation is indicated prior to therapeutic intervention. This will allow precise localization of the pneumothorax and differentiation from a pneumomediastinum or pneumopericardium.

Good roentgenographic techniques (Chapter 39) are basic to the accurate localization of accumulations of extrapulmonary air in the neonate. A large tension pneu-

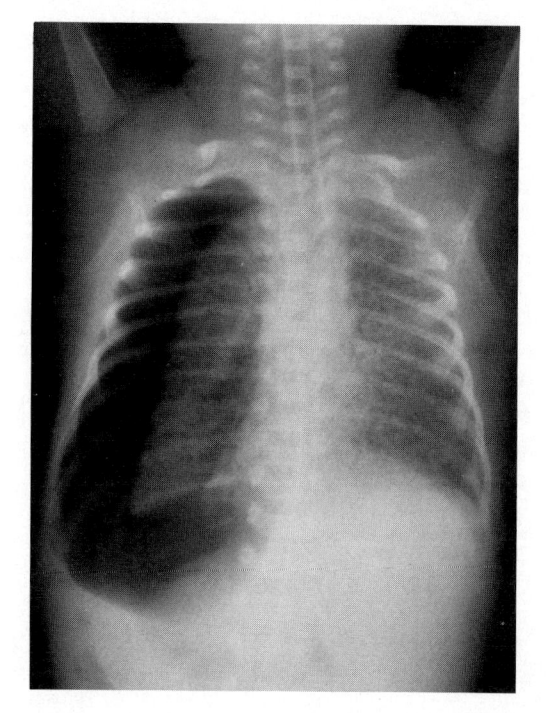

Fig. 23-24. Tension pneumothorax on the right and pulmonary interstitial emphysema in both lungs. An endotracheal tube is in place.

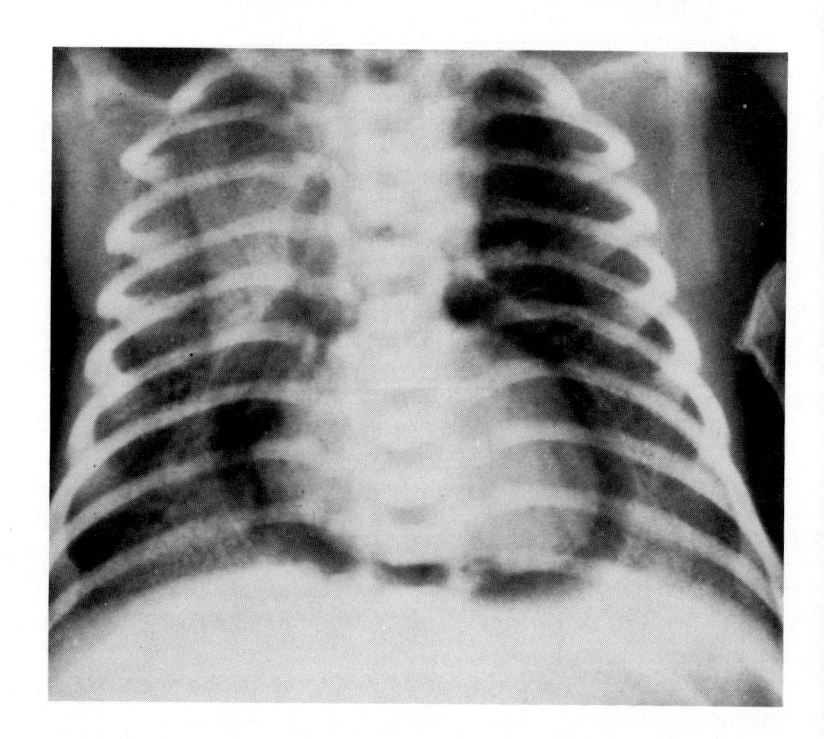

Fig. 23-25. Pneumopericardium in a newborn.

mothorax is readily diagnosed by the presence of air in the pleural cavity separating the parietal and visceral pleura, collapse of the ipsilateral lobes, displacement of the mediastinum to the contralateral side, and downward movement of the diaphragm (Fig. 23-24). Because of the decreased compliance of the lung in infants with severe RDS, total collapse is not seen even with a tension pneumothorax, and there may be only minimal shift of the mediastinal structures. A useful roentgenologic sign of pneumothorax is a prominent curvilinear marking above the heart that reflects displacement of the bulging mediastinal pleura across the midline to the contralateral side. The classic roentgenographic appearance can be readily overlooked in an anteroposterior film taken with the patient in the supine position if a large amount of the intrapleural air is situated just anterior to the sternum. In such instances a horizontal-beam lateral film with the infant supine will identify the retrosternal accumulation of air. If an isolated pneumomediastinum is present on anteroposterior film, there will be a hyperlucent rim of air lateral to the cardiac borders and thymus, elevating the latter away from the pericardium in a characteristic crescent or "spinnaker sail" configuration. This must be roentgenographically differentiated from a pneumopericardium in which air completely surrounds the heart, including its inferior border (Fig. 23-25).

Management

In an infant who does not have any underlying pulmonary disease, no specific management is necessary for an asymptomatic pneumothorax. The presence of an isolated pneumomediastinum requires close observation of vital signs and frequent clinical assessment, since this may progress to a pneumothorax at any time. In infants with lung disease the presence of a pneumothorax accentuates the respiratory difficulty and requires prompt if not urgent intervention. This consists of the placement of a large-bore, multiple-holed chest tube into the pleural space, preferably anterior to the lung. Anterior placement in the pleural space is best achieved by insertion of the tube into the chest at the first to third intercostal space on or just lateral to the midclavicular line. This should be connected to an underwater seal at a suction pressure of from 10 to 20 cm H_2O, since reaccumulation of air may occur if suction is not applied. The chest tube should be introduced under sterile conditions and secured with a pursestring suture. A high incidence (35%) of lung perforation has been described at autopsy in infants who required pleural drainage for pneumothorax. Such iatrogenic lung perforation may well prolong the period of recovery from pulmonary disease or even contribute to the mortalitiy in these infants (Fig. 23-26). Great care therefore must be exercised during chest tube insertion, with curved mosquito clamps used rather than a trocar to guide the catheter into the pleural space. Dramatic improvement in color and circulation follows the relief of a tension pneumothorax, which can be confirmed by repeat transillumination. The ease with which the lung can be reexpanded depends to a large extent on the compliance of the underlying pulmonary tissue. Expansion is particularly slow in infants with hypoplastic lungs associated with a congenital diaphragmatic hernia. Fluid intake may need to be reduced during the acute phase of a pneumothorax, since an increase in vasopressin release has been documented at this time, as assessed by urinary excretion of the hormone. Suction should be maintained until fluctuation of air in the tube and active bubbling have ceased. At this time the tube should be clamped and removed within 24 hours if there has been no reaccumulation of air in the pleural cavity.

Infants who are symptomatic from a large pneumomediastinum may benefit from decompression via an anteriorly placed chest tube, although this is rarely necessary. Conservative therapy is followed in isolated cases of pneumopericardium, although, if there is an accompanying gas tamponade, pericardiocentesis may be life saving. Recent data from experimentally induced pneumopericardium in puppies suggest that a reduction in cardiac size is indicative of drastic hemodynamic compromise, requiring immediate pericardiocentesis.

Pulmonary interstitial emphysema

Pulmonary interstitial emphysema is primarily a roentgenographic and pathologic diagnosis made when air ruptures from alveoli into the perivascular tissues of the lung. Pathologic examination reveals irregular air-filled cysts varying in diameter from 0.1 to 1 cm, localized to interlobular septa, and extending radially from the hilum. Initial reports on pulmonary interstitial emphysema reflected a greater frequency in term infants, who acquired their disease secondary to aspiration or pneumonia. More recently pulmonary interstitial emphysema has been seen predominantly in preterm infants who require the prolonged use of positive pressure ventilation.

The administration of CPAP or PEEP may encourage the continuous escape of air into the interstitium from alveoli maintained in a partially expanded state. This process could produce a vicious cycle by causing compression atelectasis of the adjacent lung, necessitating a further increase in ventilatory pressure and permitting still more escape of air into the interstitial tissues. From this location air may further progress into the mediastinum and pleural space, although it is uncommon for air to move into the neck during the neonatal period.

Two forms of pulmonary interstitial emphysema are characteristically described: a diffuse variety and a localized variety, although their causes do not appear to differ. Diffuse pulmonary interstitial emphysema usually has been associated with prolonged artificial ventilation and a high incidence of bronchopulmonary dysplasia (BPD) (Part five). From a review of our own patient population we observed a high mortality (90%) when pulmonary interstitial emphysema was noted in the first 24 hours of life. The high mortality in this early onset group is undoubtedly a reflection of the severity of their lung disease, which necessitated early intervention with ventilatory support. When infants first developed pulmonary interstitial emphysema after 24 hours, the results were much more favorable. Sixty percent of these infants had bilateral diffuse disease. In those with unilateral disease the left and right sides were involved with equal frequency. Infants with a later onset of pulmonary interstitial emphysema had a 73% survival rate, and only 16%

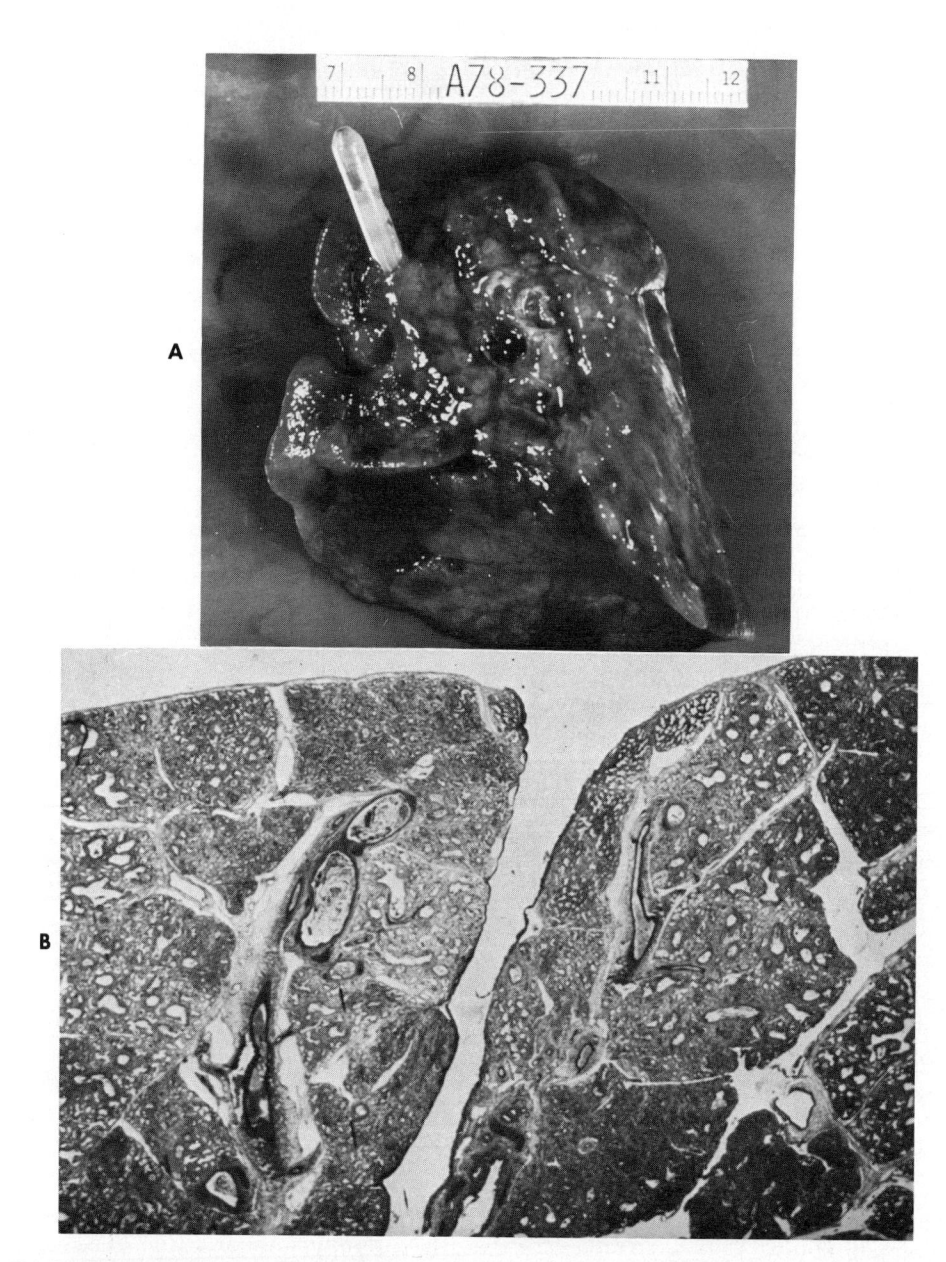

Fig. 23-26. Perforation of the lung associated with insertion of chest tube by means of trocar and cannula. **A,** Gross appearance. **B,** Histologic features demonstrating tract into the lung.

of the survivors developed distinct clinical and roentgenographic evidence of BPD, whereas the remainder had complete resolution of their disease. No specific management is indicated for diffuse pulmonary interstitial emphysema apart from every attempt being made to maintain mechanical ventilatory pressures at a safe minimum.

The localized form is characterized on roentgenogram by discrete involvement of one or more lobes and is usually accompanied by mediastinal shift to the opposite side. The severity of symptoms will depend on the size of the uninvolved area and the ability of the uninvolved lung to adequately meet the infant's ventilatory needs. Both forms of pulmonary interstitial emphysema frequently show spontaneous regression over time. Localized pulmonary interstitial emphysema has been successfully treated by selective intubation of the main stem bronchus on the uninvolved side, and this may hasten resolution in as little as 24 hours. This procedure always should be attempted prior to any surgical intervention. Lobectomy will be indicated in a small number of cases of localized pulmonary interstitial emphysema when spontaneous regression is not occurring and medical management has failed. Although clear guidelines for surgical intervention are difficult to establish, it should be reserved for infants in whom the risks of recurring complications outweigh those of surgery.

Pseudocysts represent a form of localized pulmonary interstitial emphysema within the pulmonary parenchyma situated beneath the visceral pleura or along fissure lines. They appear roentgenographically either as single or multiple circular areas of lucency with a well-demarcated wall comprising compressed alveoli. Harris reported pseudocysts in 6% of infants with RDS treated with continuous distending airway pressure. All recovered without surgical intervention, mostly within 2 weeks, although the period of roentgenographic resolution ranged from 3 days to 3 months after appearance of the cysts.

DEVELOPMENTAL ANOMALIES
Pulmonary hypoplasia
Pathophysiology

Bilateral pulmonary hypoplasia represents a broad spectrum of anatomic malformations ranging from total bronchial and parenchymal agenesis to mild pulmonary parenchymal hypoplasia. Complete pulmonary agenesis is almost always unilateral (usually involving the left lung) and is frequently accompanied by other congenital anomalies. The lung on the opposite side is typically hypertrophied and often herniates across the midline to occupy part of the affected hemithorax.

Pulmonary hypoplasia, on the other hand, may be either unilateral or bilateral. It may be seen as an isolated entity (so-called primary pulmonary hypoplasia) or be secondary to lesions restricting lung growth. A classification of neonatal pulmonary hypoplasia is as follows:
A. Primary
   1. Pulmonary agenesis (unilateral) with or without other malformations
   2. Idiopathic pulmonary hypoplasia (bilateral)
B. Secondary
   1. Congenital diaphragmatic hernia (unilateral)
   2. Oligohydramnios
      a. Chronic amniotic fluid leak (bilateral)
      b. Renal agenesis and dysplasia (bilateral)
   3. Skeletal and neuromuscular disease (bilateral)

The result of pulmonary hypoplasia is a decreased number of alveoli, peripheral bronchioles, and arterioles, the latter often leading to medial muscular hypertrophy. A histologic diagnosis involves the demonstration of a low ratio of lung to body weight and/or a decreased radial alveolar count. The diagnosis of primary pulmonary hypoplasia implies a lack of any specific pathophysiologic process that could cause fetal lung compression. Nonetheless it has been proposed that decreased fetal respiratory movement, as might result from hypoxia, neuromuscular disease, or chest wall abnormalities in utero, could result in some degree of functional lung compression and hypoplasia. Another possible explanation of primary pulmonary hypoplasia is that, for as yet unknown reasons, morphologic development of the lungs simply progresses at a slower than normal rate in some infants.

The severity of secondary pulmonary hypoplasia depends on the degree to which thoracic size is reduced. A modest degree of lung restriction results in a histologically normal but undersized lung, whereas severe restriction additionally causes a significant reduction in the extent of bronchiolar branching. The association between unilateral pulmonary hypoplasia and congenital diaphragmatic hernia has been well documented and appears to result from the presence of bowel within the thorax, mechanically restricting lung growth (p. 488). In this situation the affected lung may exhibit severe immaturity as well as being small, although the reason for this interruption of pulmonary maturation is unclear. The characteristic increase in pulmonary vascular resistance is the result of a decrease in size of the total pulmonary vascular bed, an increase in pulmonary arterial smooth muscle, and a decrease in the number of vessels per unit of lung. After hernia repair the number of airway branchings and alveoli remains reduced, whereas the pulmonary blood vessels show a persistently increased muscularity for several months. Pulmonary hypoperfusion on the affected side has been demonstrated to persist for years in these infants.

Bilateral pulmonary hypoplasia commonly occurs in association with oligohydramnios caused by either renal disease in the fetus or chronic leakage of amniotic fluid. The presence of pulmonary hypoplasia in infants with bilateral renal agenesis was first recognized by Potter in 1946. It has since become apparent that a similar picture of lethal pulmonary hypoplasia is seen in conjunction with bilaterally dysplastic kidneys with or without cyst formation. Characteristic features include premature birth in the breech position, a typical facial appearance, limb malformations, and severe respiratory insufficiency often complicated by air leaks and invariably resulting in a fatal outcome (p. 793). In cases of renal agenesis the reduction in lung volume and number of alveoli is greater than in renal dysplasia, where these changes are more variable in their severity. Infants subjected to oligohydramnios secondary to a chronic leakage of amniotic fluid over many weeks may similarly exhibit a variable degree of pulmonary hypoplasia. Oligohydramnios may act by compressing the fetal thorax or altering the dynamics of lung fluid so that expansion of the lungs cannot be maintained. Recent pathologic findings by Hislop imply that an interference in normal lung growth has occurred prior to 16 weeks' gestation in these infants. Since the contribution of fetal urine to amniotic fluid becomes important relatively late in pregnancy, oligohydramnios is unlikely to be the sole cause of the hypoplastic lung. Thus renal agenesis appears to have some direct but as yet unidentified effect on early pulmonary maturation. During fetal development the kidney appears to be an important source of proline, and this has been proposed to contribute to the formation of collagen and mesenchymal tissue in the developing pulmonary parenchyma. Further insight is needed into the interaction between early renal and pulmonary maturation in the fetus.

Clinical course

In infants with unilateral pulmonary agenesis the diagnosis may be suspected by unilaterally decreased breath sounds and displacement of the mediastinum to the affected side. Some breath sounds, however, may be audible over the affected side if a portion of normal lung has herniated across the midline. The roentgenographic appearance of a radiopaque hemithorax will help confirm the diagnosis, and accompanying vertebral defects are not uncommon. Treatment is largely of symptoms and prognosis will depend on the presence or absence of other anomalies.

The diagnosis of bilateral primary pulmonary hypoplasia may be readily overlooked. Swischuk recently reported on eight infants with hypoplastic lungs that did not appear to be accompanied by other organ system disease. These infants were seen with characteristic features of respiratory distress immediately after birth, associated with hypoxemia, hypercarbia, and acidosis. They exhibited clinical evidence of persistent fetal circulation, and all demonstrated small but clear lung fields on chest roentgenogram, accompanied by a pneumothorax in seven out of eight infants. Two infants survived, indicating that a favorable outcome is possible if pulmonary hypoplasia is not pronounced. This entity should be considered in infants with persistent fetal circulation who have the previously stated roentgenographic criteria of bilateral pulmonary hypoplasia.

The clinical course and outcome of infants with pulmonary hypoplasia secondary to congenital diaphragmatic hernia are dependent largely on the degree of herniation and ability to accomplish adequate surgical repair in addition to the extent of the pulmonary hypoplasia and accompanying increase in pulmonary vascular resistance. In classic Potter's syndrome bilateral renal agenesis will always result in the infant's demise. A favorable outcome is possible when renal dysplasia is less severe or pulmonary hypoplasia is associated with oligohydramnios of shorter duration.

Congenital lobar emphysema

Congenital lobar emphysema is characterized by overdistention of one or more lobes of an infant's lung caused by trapping of air within the affected area. The relative frequency of involvement of the various pulmonary lobes

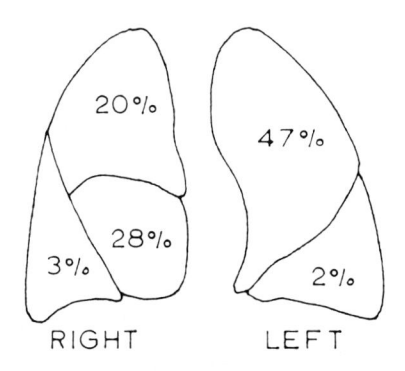

Fig. 23-27. Distribution of congenital emphysema by percentage of lobar involvement. (From DeLuca, F.G.: Clin. Perinatol. **5**:377, 1978.)

is illustrated in Fig. 23-27. A variety of conditions, as outlined subsequently, may contribute to this inability of the affected lung to deflate normally, although frequently a specific cause cannot be established. Partial intraluminal bronchial obstruction may result from a deficiency of bronchial cartilage restricted to one lobe or even from inflammatory exudate or aspirated mucus. Similarly bronchial compression may be caused by adjacent vascular structures such as blood vessels or mediastinal and intrapulmonary masses. Finally, partial airway collapse has been proposed to result from the high compliance of the airways of the neonate. It can be seen that congenital lobar emphysema generally cannot be attributed to a single cause but should be considered as a symptom complex rather than a specific disease entity.

The severity of symptoms depends on the size of the overinflated lobe and the resultant compression of surrounding lung tissue and degree of mediastinal shift. These infants may exhibit symptoms soon after birth, but more commonly symptoms begin at 1 or 2 months of age. Respiratory distress frequently is accompanied by wheezing. Physical findings include hyperresonance to percussion, decreased breath sounds over the affected lobe, and shift of the apical heart beat to the contralateral side. Chest roentgenogram clearly demonstrates a hyperinflated lobe that may have herniated across the midline and caused mediastinal shift and compression of the adjacent lung. Roentgenologic differentiation from lung cysts or even a pneumothorax may be difficult but will be aided by the presence of linear bronchovascular and alveolar markings within the emphysematous lobe. Angiography may be indicated in increased incidence of coexistent congenital heart disease and to visualize adjacent pulmonary vascular structures.

Treatment should begin with bronchoscopy in an attempt to identify and remove any cause of airway obstruction. Excision of the affected lobe is generally indicated if the infant remains symptomatic following bronchoscopy and may be life saving if respiratory failure is severe. If symptoms are minimal or the infant is asymptomatic, conservative management probably should be attempted. After removal of an emphysematous lobe, ventilation rapidly improves with expansion of the previously collapsed lobes. The long-term prognosis is thought to be excellent, although adequate follow-up studies of the effects of lobectomy performed in the neonatal period are not yet available.

Lung cysts

Congenital lung cysts are a rare cause of respiratory distress in neonates that should be readily differentiated from acquired cystic lesions. The latter are typically the result of severe RDS that has required prolonged assisted ventilation or has been complicated by the development of an air leak syndrome (p. 448). Acquired cysts or pneumatoceles rarely result from staphylococcal or other bacterial pneumonia in the neonate and may be large and persist for several months.

There is still considerable controversy concerning the cause of congenital lung cysts. Their presence in stillborn infants, albeit rare, indicates that they truly may be congenital. Nonetheless they are almost never associated with cystic disease in other organs or with any other specific malformation. Congenital lung cysts commonly are located at the periphery of the lung and may represent a disorder of bronchial development occurring in later fetal life. The infants may be seen initially with respiratory distress caused by overdistention of a cyst, recurrent infection, or wheezing secondary to partial airway obstruction. The diagnosis is made roentgenologically by recognizing round or oval translucent areas within the pulmonary parenchyma. It should be noted that cysts arising from bronchi may change in size depending on the degree of bronchial obstruction, and on the first day of life they may not even be apparent on roentgenogram because of the presence of fetal lung fluid within the cyst. Multiple cysts must be distinguished roentgenographically from a diaphragmatic hernia (p. 488) where air-filled loops of bowel within the thorax may present a similar appearance.

Conservative therapy is appropriate if the infant is asymptomatic. Operative resection of congenital lung cysts, however, will be indicated as a result of complications from pressure effects on adjacent areas of normal lung. Urgent surgical intervention may be needed if pulmonary function is acutely compromised. Surgical resection usually is indicated for the rare case of cystic adenomatoid malformation, which is a form of congenital cystic lung disease generally confined to a single lobe. These infants show a roentgenographic density (which probably represents a hematoma) surrounded by scattered radiolucent areas and progressive compression of the surrounding lung.

Chylothorax

Chylothorax is an extremely unusual entity in the neonate that usually is associated with nonspecific respiratory symptoms in the first days of life. The cause is unknown although presumably related to either traumatic injury of the thoracic duct at delivery or some congenital malformation of the duct wall. Other lymphatic vessels in the body tend not to be affected in most cases. Since chylothorax is typically unilateral, there may be decreased breath sounds over the side of the effusion and mediastinal shift to the contralateral side. The characteristic roentgenographic appearance is of a large pleural effusion depressing the adjacent diaphragm and displacing the mediastinum. The definitive diagnosis is made by thoracentesis, which will reveal clear fluid rich in lymphocytes during the first day, changing to markedly opalescent fluid with a high protein and fat content following the introduction of milk feeding. The majority of infants recover completely after single or multiple thoracenteses. If continuous drainage of chyle via a chest tube is required, this may result in severe malnutrition, and under these circumstances administration of total parenteral nutrition is indicated. During the administration of intravenous hyperalimentation a marked decrease in the fat content of the pleural fluid has been observed. Although it has been recommended to feed a formula rich in medium-chain triglycerides, this does not appear to significantly reduce the triglyceride and fatty acid content of the fluid accumulating in the pleural space.

Mediastinal masses

Mediastinal masses are rare in the newborn, and, when present, they are usually cystic structures that represent some congenital remnant or malformation. They must be clearly differentiated roentgenographically from a normal thymus, which frequently occupies a prominent place in the anterior mediastinum of neonates. Lesions causing narrowing or significant displacement of the mediastinal trachea will be associated with wheezing, and in addition to the mass noted on roentgenogram, the lung fields may appear hyperinflated.

Miscellaneous intrapulmonary malformations

It has been customary to subdivide congenital lobar malformations within the pulmonary parenchyma into accessory and sequestered lobes. Accessory lobes may reflect an early defect in lung development in which pulmonary tissue has separated from the rest of the lung, although connections with an airway or portion of the gut may persist. These lobes characteristically produce no symptoms but present uncertainty as to their identity when they appear on chest film. Sequestered lobes, on the other hand, are intralobar structures that probably originate from an anomaly in the blood supply to that area of the lung. They do not have any connection to bronchi or the gastrointestinal tract but do have their own independent blood supply arising from the aorta. Respiratory symptoms attributable to a sequestered lobe are unlikely to occur in infancy. They may be confused roentgenographically with an area of atelectasis or pneumonia.

Congenital pulmonary lymphangiectasia is a rare entity in which there is congenital dilatation of the lymphatic channels in the lung. The lungs are bulky at autopsy with visible lobulation caused by diffuse dilatation of subpleural lymphatics and thickening of interlobular septa. The cause of this disorder appears to be an early cessation of growth of the lymphatic trunks in the septa, leading to the diffuse pattern of cystic lymphatic spaces seen microscopically. These infants typically are seen at term with respiratory distress that progresses to a fatal outcome. There may be coexistent lymphedema in other areas of the body, and congenital cardiac malformations frequently are found at autopsy. Chest roentgenograms reveal a variable pattern of hyperinflation and diffuse granularity with prominent interstitial markings. It follows that diagnosis of this rare condition is not easy, since the roentgenologic and clinical picture simulates those of the common causes of respiratory distress in the neonate.

Pulmonary arteriovenous fistula is an extremely rare cause of repiratory distress in the newborn that may be associated with hemangiomas in other areas such as the skin. This is a potentially curable disorder with single or multiple communications between pulmonary arteries and veins that require surgical intervention.

RESPIRATORY CONTROL AND APNEA OF PREMATURITY

Preterm infants normally exhibit varying patterns of breathing that range from regular respiration to frequent pauses or apneic episodes. The pathophysiology of apnea of prematurity remains one of the most poorly understood problems in the care of low birth weight infants, and a disproportionate amount of time in neonatal intensive care units is spent evaluating, monitoring, and treating apneic episodes. The extent of the problem is illustrated by the fact that more than 50% of all surviving infants from our neonatal intensive care unit with birth weights of less than 1.5 kg require either respiratory support or pharmacologic intervention for recurrent prolonged apneic episodes. Nonetheless a greater awareness of the influence on the immature respiratory center of various components of respiratory control such as chemoreceptors and pulmonary stretch receptors is slowly emerging (Fig. 23-28). A more complete understanding will permit a rational approach to the management of problems related to respiratory control in the neonate.

Maturation of chemical and reflex control of breathing

Spontaneous and sustained breathing movements alternating with episodes of apnea have been well documented in the human fetus. Recent studies have further established that in mature fetal lambs breathing efforts increase in response to elevated levels of arterial P_{CO_2} (Pa_{CO_2}). Both full-term and preterm infants increase minute ventilation in response to small increases in inspired carbon dioxide concentration. Earlier studies suggested that neonates exhibit increases in ventilation to carbon dioxide (when corrected per kilogram body weight) that are quantitatively comparable to those of adults. The weight of recent evidence, however, indicates that carbon dioxide responsiveness, which reflects predominantly central chemoreceptor activity and is a traditional measure of respiratory drive, is progressively less well developed in the more immature infant. Infants of less than 33 weeks' gestational age exhibit reduced ventilatory responses to inspired carbon dioxide. It is unclear whether this reduced ventilatory response to

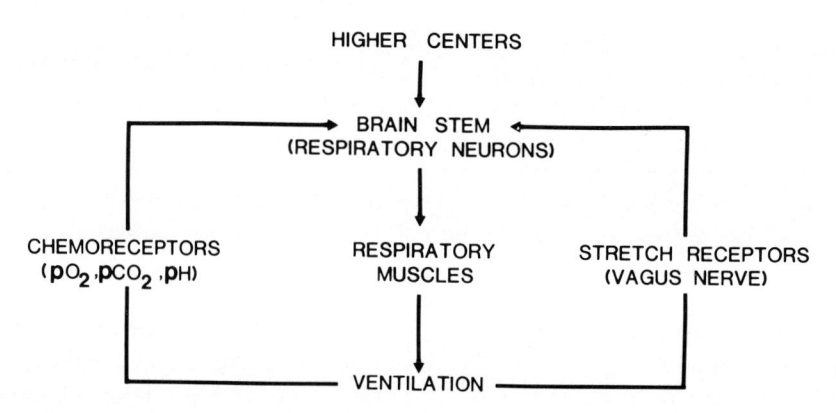

Fig. 23-28. Simplified diagrammatic representation of the various afferent inputs to the neonatal respiratory center.

carbon dioxide in small preterm infants is primarily the result of decreased central chemosensitivity or mechanical factors preventing an appropriate increase in ventilation. It has been proposed that the carbon dioxide response curve has a decreased slope (indicating less respiratory drive) in preterm infants who exhibit apnea, but a cause and effect relation between decreased carbon dioxide responsiveness and apnea of prematurity has not been clearly established. In older infants beyond the immediate neonatal period Shannon observed impaired carbon dioxide responsiveness in those at risk for sudden infant death, although other investigators have not confirmed these findings.

Rigatto observed that preterm infants respond to a fall in inspired oxygen concentration with a transient increase in ventilation over approximately 1 minute, followed by a sustained depression of ventilation (Fig. 23-29). In term infants a similar response has been observed during the first week of life. This biphasic response to hypoxemia in the neonate is in marked contrast to the ventilatory response in adults, where a low oxygen concentration results in a sustained increase in ventilation. The characteristic response to low oxygen in infants has been proposed to indicate initial peripheral chemoreceptor stimulation followed by overriding depression of the respiratory center as a result of hypoxemia. Consistent with these findings is the observation that a progressive decrease in inspired oxygen concentration causes a significant flattening of carbon dioxide responsiveness in preterm infants (Fig. 23-30). The magnitude of the fall in PAO_2 necessary to depress ventilation remains to be determined. Nonetheless this unstable response to low inspired oxygen may play an important role in the cause of neonatal apnea.

The effects of pulmonary stretch receptors in altering the timing of respiration at varying lung volumes are much more readily elicited in the newborn than in the adult. During the first days of life sudden lung inflation results in an initial gasp (Head's reflex) followed by prolonged apnea (the so-called Hering-Breuer inflation reflex). Similarly a small but sustained increase in lung volume (as with the administration of CPAP) causes a significant prolongation of expiratory time and a concomitant decrease in respiratory rate. The ease with which this apparent reflex activity can be elicited in the term neonate suggests that it may play an important role in stabilizing respiratory control at this age. The Hering-Breuer deflation reflex, consisting of an increase in respiratory rate in response to a diminished lung volume, is probably of significance in preterm infants, who invariably develop areas of atelectasis. The increase in breathing rate is primarily caused by a shortening of expiratory time and may assist in maintaining an adequate FRC in these infants. Pulmonary irritant reflexes also have been elicited in the neonate. Direct stimulation of the tracheal wall with a fine catheter threaded through the endotracheal tube of intubated infants results in augmented respiratory efforts. Such a response is rarely present prior to 35 weeks' gestational age. This is suggestive of a functional immaturity of pulmonary irritant receptors at an earlier gestational age, which may be a factor in the increased risk of aspiration in small preterm infants.

Patterns of respiration

Respiration in immature infants is characterized by a wide spectrum of breathing patterns ranging from regular respiration to frequent and even prolonged pauses. Periodic breathing, defined as recurrent sequences of

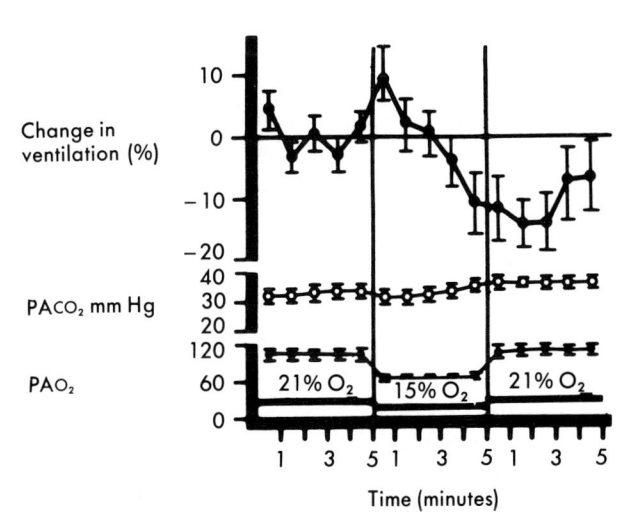

Fig. 23-29. Changes in ventilation and alveolar gas concentrations in response to 15% oxygen exposure. (From Rigatto, H., and Brady, J. P.: Pediatrics **50:**219, 1972. Copyright American Academy of Pediatrics 1972.)

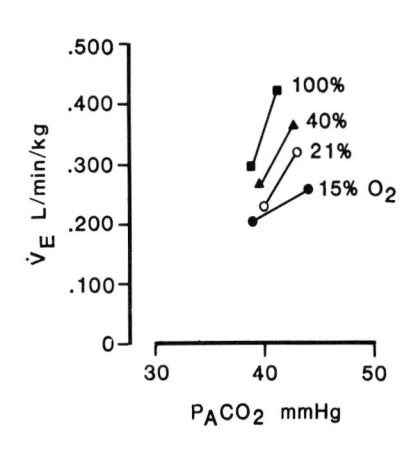

Fig. 23-30. Steady-state carbon dioxide response curves at different inspired oxygen concentrations. The more hypoxic the infant, the flatter the response to carbon dioxide. (From Rigatto, H., de la Torre Verduzco, R., and Cates, D. B.: J. Appl. Physiol. **39:**896, 1975.)

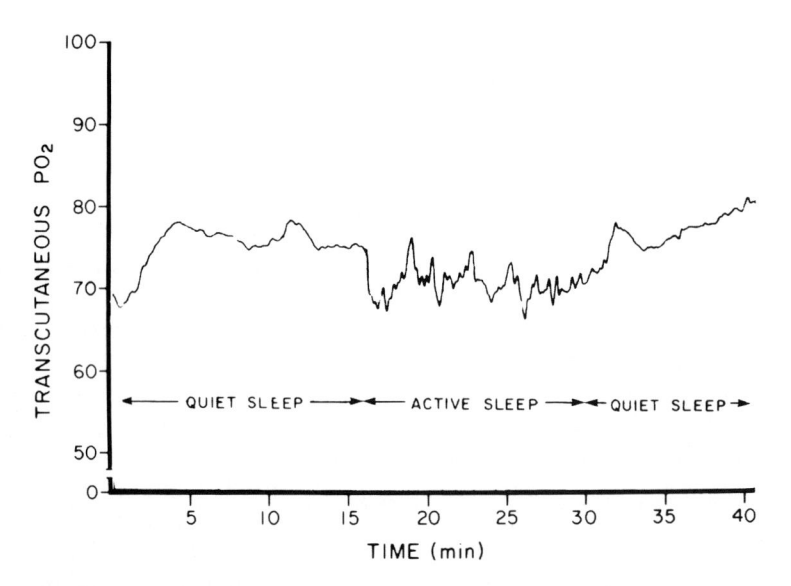

Fig. 23-31. Continuous recording of TcPo$_2$ in an infant during quiet and active sleep.

pauses in respiration lasting 5 to 10 seconds and followed by 10 to 15 seconds of rapid respiration, is so common as to be considered normal in preterm infants. It can be abolished by increasing environmental oxygen, but in view of the fact that periodic breathing is considered harmless, this is *not recommended*. It is still unclear whether there is a close etiologic relation between periodic breathing in premature infants and the periodic respiratory pattern of Cheyne-Stokes breathing that may exist in adults suffering from various pathologic conditions.

Apneic episodes generally are defined as periods during which there is cessation of respiration for at least 10 to 15 seconds, frequently complicated by cyanosis, pallor, hypotonia, or bradycardia. Small preterm infants exhibit these functional changes more readily than do more mature infants, even when the apnea is of shorter duration. Since a fall in heart rate frequently occurs very early in the apneic episode, bradycardia may result primarily from vagal influences on central cardiorespiratory control. The problem of recurrent apneic episodes increases both in incidence and severity with decreasing gestational age.

In preterm infants apnea is predominantly central, which is defined as simultaneous cessation of both respiratory movements and airflow at the mouth or nose. Pure obstructive apnea, on the other hand, defined as absence of airflow while respiratory movements continue, is uncommon in the premature infant unless there is extreme flexion of the neck. Recently Thach has documented that a high proportion of apneic spells are mixed episodes consisting largely of central apnea accompanied by one or more obstructed inspiratory efforts. In infants beyond the neonatal period pure obstructive apnea, however, has been frequently documented and may predispose the infant to the sudden infant death syndrome.

Respiratory control and sleep state

There has been considerable recent interest in the relation between sleep state and respiratory control in the neonate. Although discrepancies exist in defining criteria for the determination of sleep state, apnea occurs predominantly during active (or REM) and indeterminate (or transitional) sleep in both preterm and term infants. It is uncommon for prolonged apnea to be observed during quiet sleep, when respiration is characteristically regular with little breath-by-breath change in tidal volume or respiratory frequency, although periodic breathing may be seen in quiet sleep.

Several mechanisms have been proposed to explain the high incidence of apnea during active sleep. Chest wall movements are predominantly out of phase (or paradoxical) during active sleep, in contrast to quiet sleep when these are almost never observed in term infants (although they may be seen in preterm infants during quiet sleep as well). In other words, abdominal expansion during inspiration is almost always accompanied by inward movement of the rib cage during active sleep, whereas during quiet sleep rib cage and abdomen expand together. These paradoxical chest wall movements during active sleep appear to be the result of decreased intercostal muscle activity and are more common in preterm than term infants. We determined the effect of sleep state on Pao$_2$ in an attempt to correlate any changes in Pao$_2$ with altered chest wall movements. In all 10 infants studied, Pao$_2$ was consistently lower (6 to 10 mm Hg) and more variable during active sleep than

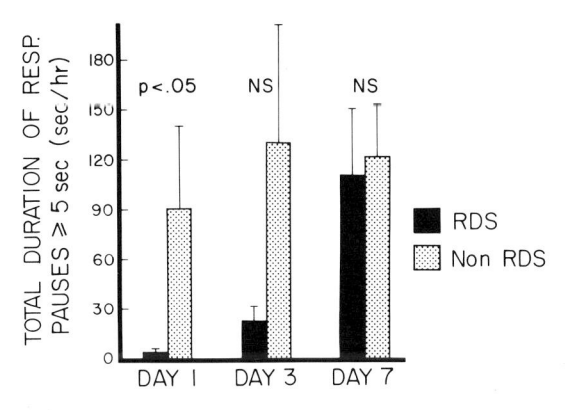

Fig. 23-32. Comparison of the total duration of respiratory pauses (≥5 seconds) in two comparable groups of preterm infants with and without RDS over the first week of life. (From Carlo, W.A., and others: Am. Rev. Resp. Dis. **126:**103, 1982.)

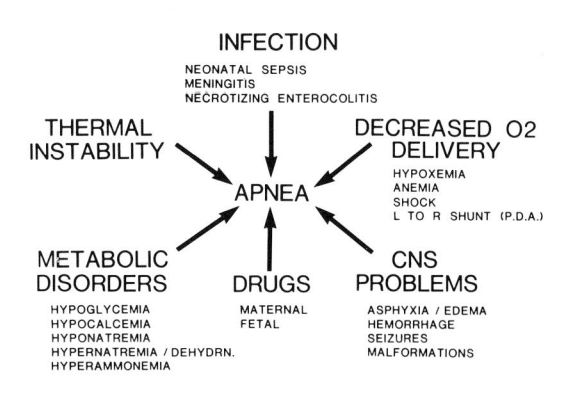

Fig. 23-33. Specific causes of apnea.

during quiet sleep (Fig. 23-31). A fall in FRC also has been observed in infants during active sleep, and this, together with the decrease in PaO_2 during active sleep, would be expected to increase the infant's vulnerability to apneic episodes. Furthermore it has been proposed that electromyographic changes suggestive of diaphragmatic fatigue accompany these paradoxical chest wall movements in normal preterm and term infants without evidence of pulmonary disease. Ventilatory responses to increased carbon dioxide and decreased oxygen concentrations have been compared during active and quiet sleep, and preliminary data would indicate that steady state carbon dioxide responses are unaffected by sleep state, whereas the depression of ventilation observed in response to hypoxia is accentuated during active sleep. Nonetheless the relative influences of chest wall movements, neurochemical control, and central respiratory rhythmicity on respiratory control during sleep remain to be unraveled.

Causes of apnea

Recurrent apnea occurs predominantly in preterm infants who weigh less than 1.5 kg and manifest no other overt abnormality. Designated *idiopathic apnea of prematurity* in these infants, this disorder probably involves incomplete organization and interconnections among the respiratory neurons within the brain stem. Nonetheless the cause of neonatal apnea is multifactorial, and a variety of specific causes may be operative. Apneic episodes and shorter respiratory pauses are infrequently observed in infants with RDS over the first days of life and if present at this time should suggest a specific problem that needs to be evaluated (Fig. 23-32). Some of the pathophysiologic disorders associated with apnea of prematurity are tabulated in Fig. 23-33. These all must be considered and appropriate diagnostic tests performed before a label of "idiopathic apnea" is affixed. When apnea is seen shortly after birth, the history may indicate a traumatic delivery or excessive maternal drug administration. Under these circumstances an EEG, CAT scan, or measurement of drug levels may be appropriate. It is not uncommon for a septic infant to develop apnea as the sole or major presenting symptom. A history of prolonged rupture of membranes, foul-smelling amniotic fluid, or maternal fever might suggest such an infectious origin. The thermal environment should be carefully evaluated, since Perlstein has clearly documented that apneic episodes are frequently preceded by rises or falls in the environmental temperature. During the physical examination special note must be taken of clinical evidence for decreased oxygen delivery such as pallor, shock, or left-to-right shunting through a patent ductus arteriosus. Apnea associated with metabolic disturbances, such as hypoglycemia, may be eliminated by simple measures to correct the metabolic abnormality. In some instances, e.g., hypocalcemia, the metabolic disturbance may be an incidental finding, in which case correction thereof may not diminish the apneic episodes. The clinical status of the infant, time of onset, and degree of severity of the apneic episodes determine the extent of metabolic evaluation and septic workup. Sound clinical judgment and experience together with continuous surveillance of the infant are necessary.

Management of idiopathic apnea

The principle that should be followed in managing infants with recurrent idiopathic apnea is to commence with that therapy which carries the least potential for short- or long-term side effects. In general, the following steps in management should be followed when apneic episodes do not resolve with gentle tactile stimulation but require vigorous stimulation or intermittent mask and bag ventilation to reinitiate respiration.

A variety of different modes of sensory stimulation have been shown to decrease apnea in preterm infants, notably intermittent tactile stimulation and the use of a water bed. The latter can be simulated by connecting a ventilator to an inflatable air mattress. The mechanism whereby apnea is reduced by these means is unclear, although it is tempting to speculate that the neonatal respiratory center responds to a variety of nonspecific sensory inputs such as vestibular or proprioceptive stimulation. Oscillating water beds do not appear to significantly alter the amount of time spent in quiet sleep, active sleep, or wakefulness.

A low CPAP of 3 to 5 cm H_2O, most simply administered via the nasal route, decreases the incidence of apnea in the majority of preterm infants. The main disadvantage of this technique is that it becomes cumbersome over a prolonged period and makes gavage feeding difficult because of the increased risk of aspiration. The precise means by which apnea is decreased on CPAP is unclear. Proposed mechanisms include the stabilization of PaO_2 by increasing FRC, an effect on the stretch receptor influence on respiratory timing, or possible splinting of the upper airway. It should be noted that with or without the use of CPAP any increase in inspired oxygen concentration beyond 21% must be accompanied by close monitoring of PaO_2 via either intermittent sampling or the transcutaneous route.

The increased use of xanthine drugs (e.g. theophylline and caffeine) has had a major impact on the management of neonatal apnea. Despite the widespread use of these drugs, information on their mechanism of action remains scanty. The recommended dose of theophylline (the most widely used drug) is a 5.5 mg/kg loading dose followed by 1.1 mg/kg every 8 hours to achieve an adequate therapeutic plasma level of approximately 10 μg/ml. This is substantially lower than the originally described dose because of the slow elimination of xanthines by preterm infants compared with older individuals. More recently it has been proposed that caffeine may be superior to theophylline because of slower excretion, less toxicity, and the fact that theophylline is metabolized to caffeine in substantial amounts in the neonate. At high dosage levels carbon dioxide responsiveness is increased in the neonate, but at the currently recommended dose, carbon dioxide responses appear to be unaffected by theophylline despite a beneficial therapeutic effect. Whether the increased level of 3',5'-cyclic AMP (which results from the xanthine-induced inhibition of phosphodiesterase) plays a role in increasing respiratory drive in these infants is also unclear. Care must be taken to avoid short-term toxicity, notably tachycardia or a diuresis. Long-term sequelae of theophylline or caffeine administration have not appeared, although the duration of these studies leaves these data far from complete. Concerns about cerebral vasoconstriction induced by the methylxanthines have not been clinically substantiated.

EXTRAPULMONARY CAUSES OF RESPIRATORY DISTRESS

In a newborn infant manifesting respiratory embarrassment there is a tendency to conclude that underlying pulmonary parenchymal disease is present. However, the differential diagnosis of respiratory disease in the newborn is extensive. Disorders of the major airways, chest wall, central nervous system, cardiovascular system, and musculoskeletal system, together with hematologic or metabolic problems, easily may be confused with lung disorders. To avoid serious diagnostic and therapeutic errors, a broad and flexible approach encompassing extrapulmonary causes of respiratory distress in the etiologic considerations is essential. The time-tested approach includes review of historical information related to pregnancy, delivery, and neonatal transition, meticulous observation and careful physical examination of the infant, and analysis of simple laboratory data, including blood gases, hematocrit, and blood sugar, together with appropriate roentgenographic studies. An approach to the classification of extrapulmonary causes of respiratory distress is as follows:

A. Neuromuscular disorders
   1. Brain: asphyxia, drugs, hemorrhage, infection
   2. Spinal cord: trauma, Werdnig-Hoffmann disease
   3. Nerves: injury (phrenic nerve)
   4. Myasthenia gravis
   5. Muscular dystrophies
B. Mechanical-restrictive problems
   1. Airway obstruction
   2. Rib cage abnormalities
      a. Thoracic dystrophies
      b. Generalized bone disease
   3. Diaphragmatic disorders
      a. Phrenic nerve injury; congenital eventration of diaphragm
      b. Congenital diaphragmatic hernia
      c. Pleural effusion or chylothorax
      d. Abdominal distension
C. Hematologic disorders
   1. Anemia
   2. Polycythemia
D. Disturbances of acid-base equilibrium: metabolic acidosis
E. Cardiovascular disorders
   1. Congenital heart disease
   2. Congestive heart failure and/or pulmonary edema
   3. Persistent fetal circulation

Central nervous system

In the newborn, respiratory distress based on intracranial pathology is most commonly secondary to cerebral edema or intracranial hemorrhage, usually as a consequence of anoxia or birth trauma. These infants present a wide range of respiratory symptoms, including apnea, cyanosis, irregular respiration, and tachypnea, which may be accompanied by grunting, flaring, and retractions. The respiratory symptoms usually resolve, and ultimate prognosis depends on the severity of the hypoxic insult. Medications administered to the mother may have a significant depressant effect on the infant's respiratory center (p. 459), and infants of drug-addicted mothers demonstrating withdrawal symptoms also may initially exhibit primarily respiratory symptoms (Chapter 33, part five).

Spinal cord injury

See pp. 230 and 373.

Injury to the spinal cord occurs predominantly with breech deliveries or with shoulder dystocia. Vigorous traction on the infant's trunk while the head is firmly engaged in the mother's pelvis may result in fractures of the vertebrae with transection of the cord. Initially it may be impossible to distinguish neurologically between hemorrhage and edema of the cord and transection. There is complete paralysis below the level of the injury, which often is the level of the seventh cervical vertebra.

Infants are depressed at birth, often being seen initially with delayed or absent respiratory excursions, shock, respiratory failure, and absence of spontaneous movement. Some withdrawal responses mediated by a spinal reflex distal to the site of injury may be elicited after painful stimuli, and this may confuse the clinical picture. The infants otherwise are flaccid and immobile with absent tendon reflexes. Associated neurologic features are dependent on the level of the lesion. High lesions are associated with phrenic nerve injury and result in diaphragmatic paralysis, producing cyanosis, feeble cry, and irregular respiration. The abdomen does not bulge with inspiration, and roentgenologically the diaphragm will be noted to be markedly elevated. Therapy is largely supportive.

Neuromuscular disease

See Chapter 22.

In the newborn, respiratory failure caused by muscle weakness may be secondary to abnormalities of the nervous system or muscles or deformity of the chest wall itself. To recognize these entities, which in and of themselves are all rare, it is necessary to have a high index of suspicion.

The transition to extrauterine life for infants with neuromuscular disorders often is characterized by depression with low Apgar scores and even failure to establish spontaneous respiration. The subsequent lethargy, hypotonia, diminished spontaneous activity, difficulty with feeding, and weakness then may be attributed to the accompanying perinatal asphyxia. However, telltale signs, including short stature, limb deformities, arthrogryposis, muscle wasting, fasciculation of the tongue, absent tendon reflexes, ptosis, or facial diplegia, may focus attention on a primary neuromuscular disorder. Specific steps then can be taken to establish the primary diagnosis.

Werdnig-Hoffmann disease (infantile spinal muscular atrophy) is a hereditary disease associated with degeneration of anterior horn cells of the cord, resulting in symmetric muscular atrophy (p. 394). In its severe forms the bulbar motor nuclei also are involved, and the onset may be early, often in utero, with the mother observing a cessation or pronounced reduction of previously active movements. The infants show generalized hypotonia and paralysis of the limbs and trunk, although the face is spared. Bulbar weakness results in difficulty in sucking and swallowing with noisy respiration caused by an accumulation of mucus in the pharynx, and death from aspiration penumonia is thus common. Fasciculation of the tongue is diagnostic but may be difficult to ascertain in the newborn.

Respiratory involvement, when seen in infants during the first month, is severe. Diaphragmatic pull results in retraction and abdominal distention, and intercostal muscle function is ineffective. Cunningham and Stocks studied pulmonary function in nine infants with Werdnig-Hoffmann disease. Because of diminished fetal movement and hypotonia at birth, five infants were considered to have had intrauterine onset of the disease. These infants demonstrated significantly reduced thoracic gas volumes, whereas infants with postnatal onset had normal lung volume. The reduction in lung volume correlated only with time of onset of disease, not with duration or degree of muscle weakness. Their findings suggest that fetal breathing is a prerequisite for normal fetal lung development, which is supported by data from Wigglesworth (p. 453). There is no specific therapy, and respiratory failure is frequently precipitated by infection.

Myasthenia gravis is rare in the newborn infant and appears in two forms (p. 395). Neonatal myasthenia gravis is a transient illness that occurs only in children born to mothers with myasthenia gravis. There has been no correlation between the severity of neonatal myasthenia and the severity or duration of the mother's illness. The second form is congenital myasthenia gravis, which is a rare persistent illness occurring in children of normal mothers. Neonatal myasthenia gravis begins shortly after birth and disappears within 6 to 8 weeks. It has been repeatedly suggested that this form may be caused by placental transmission of a neuromuscular blocking substance.

The incidence of symptomatic neonatal myasthenia gravis in babies born to myasthenic mothers is approximately 12%. The dominant clinical manifestations include feeding difficulty, generalized weakness, respiratory difficulty, feeble cry, and facial weakness, including ptosis. Respiratory difficulty occurs in two thirds of the patients and appears to be a result of weakness of their respiratory muscles and inability to handle pharyngeal secretions. Respiratory failure plays a dominant role in those infants who die, and at autopsy examination atelectasis, pulmonary congestion, and evidence of bronchial obstruction or pneumonia may be observed. The diagnosis is based on the observation of weakness in the newborn offspring of a mother with myasthenia gravis and alleviation of the weakness following administration of an anticholinesterase compound. The diagnostic test is best carried out with neostigmine, since edrophonium (Tensilon) has too short a period of action. A positive test is characterized by increase in tone and strength, often detectable as improved suck, stronger respiratory activity, and relief of ptosis.

The neonatal form of *dystrophia myotonica* (p. 396) is now recognized as a clinical entity that is quite different from the adult form of the disease. The clinical picture consists of extreme hypotonia and generalized muscle atrophy combined with polyhydramnios, insufficient respiratory activity after birth, joint deformities, and facial diplegia, resulting in a tent-shaped mouth. It should be noted that all infants who are diagnosed in the neonatal period have respiratory problems and that there is a high mortality (50%). The main presenting features in the newborn period are generalized hypotonia together with poor suck and difficulty with swallowing. In addition, the infants exhibit respiratory insufficiency, joint deformities, facial diplegia, and edema most noticeable on the limbs and head with sparing of the trunk. Mental retardation is a common feature of the neonatal form of dystrophia myotonica. Because the baby fails to breathe adequately immediately after birth and usually the mother is not known to have dystrophia myotonica, the diagnosis usually is made when the baby has already been mechanically ventilated. It is a difficult moral and ethical problem to decide whether and to what extent treatment should be continued. Infants who survive the first few weeks of life show gradual improvement in respiration followed by improved swallowing and muscle tone. Subsequent development is slower than normal, and the long-term prognosis is poor. There is little hope of an independent life because of the combination of severe mental retardation and muscle weakness.

Airway obstruction

In the neonate upper airway obstruction occurs infrequently; however, the presentation is often dramatic, and significant respiratory distress may occur. The characteristic clinical presentation depends on the degree and site of obstruction. The following is an anatomic approach to the causes of airway obstruction in the newborn:

A. Nose
  1. Choanal atresia
  2. Drugs: reserpine
  3. Infection: syphilis
  4. Iatrogenic: tubes or tape
B. Mouth and jaw
  1. Pierre Robin syndrome
  2. Hypoplastic mandible
  3. Tongue: enlargement and/or paralysis
  4. Cysts: thyroglossal; gingival
C. Larynx
  1. Floppy epiglottis
  2. Laryngeal web
  3. Cord paralysis
  4. Reflex: laryngospasm
D. Trachea and bronchi
  1. Tracheomalacia
  2. Tracheal stenosis
  3. Tracheal cyst
  4. Bronchostenosis
  5. Bronchomalacia
  6. Lobar emphysema
E. Extrinsic
  1. Goiter
  2. Vascular ring
  3. Aberrant vessels
  4. Hemangiomata
  5. Cystic hygroma
  6. Teratoma
  7. Tracheoesophageal fistula
  8. Mediastinal masses

Developmental anomalies affecting the larynx and trachea have initial symptoms of noisy respiration and often a high-pitched inspiratory stridor, whereas wheezing is more likely with lesions of the mediastinal trachea. Since the newborn infant is an obligate nose breather, infants with nasal obstruction will manifest severe respiratory difficulty, including cyanosis and retractions. The diagnosis is easily established by inability to advance a catheter through the nose into the pharynx. Examination of the size and motion of the tongue also may give a clue as to the cause of upper airway obstruction. Infants with the Pierre Robin syndrome, Möbius syndrome involving cranial nerve palsies, and macroglossia all may be seen to have respiratory difficulty. Stridor, hoarseness, and the character of the cry may alert the examiner to the location of the airway obstruction.

External pressure on the airway, as with goiters, cystic hygromas, hemangiomas, and other masses, all may result in airway obstruction. When upper airway obstruction is suspected clinically, roentgenograms of the chest should include the facial region and neck; specific coned views of the neck and facial soft tissue may be required to establish the diagnosis. One always should carefully inspect the airways on the chest film, looking particularly for displacement or narrowing. Fluoroscopic examination of the airway may be necessary to establish the cause of upper airway obstruction. The recent development of a fiberoptic bronchoscope suitable for preterm and term infants permits direct visualization of the upper respiratory tract without compromising oxygenation of the infant. This technique is ideal for evaluation of stridor in the newborn as well as identifying vocal cord deformities.

A normal cry generally rules out lesions affecting the vocal cords. If the newborn is aphonic or hoarse, this suggests a congenital laryngeal abnormality or involvement of the recurrent laryngeal nerve. Unilateral vocal cord paralysis is commonly caused by birth trauma, whereas bilateral paralysis is commonly secondary to brain damage; prolonged endotracheal intubation also may damage the vocal cords (p. 438). Lesions causing narrowing or significant displacement of the mediastinal trachea usually are characterized by hyperaeration of the lung fields. A vascular ring will be noted to produce an anterior indentation of the trachea. The lesion then can be precisely defined anatomically with angiocardiography.

Congenital choanal atresia

Choanal atresia is a rare malformation; the reported incidence is 0.02% to 0.04% of live births with two thirds of the cases being unilateral. The anomaly is twice as frequent in girls as in boys and involves the right side twice as often as the left. Most cases of choanal atresia occur sporadically. Associated congenital anomalies occur as frequently as 50% of the time and include defects of the heart, eyes, and gastrointestinal tract or syndromes such as Apert's or Treacher Collins.

In view of the fact that newborn infants up to the third to sixth week of life are obligate nasal breathers, bilateral choanal atresia is first seen as an acute picture with respiratory distress and cyanosis. The diagnosis usually is established by probing both sides of the nose with a firm catheter. These infants are at great risk of suffocation until they have learned mouth breathing. They require close observation and monitoring during the first weeks of life, and an oral airway should be established. Early surgical treatment now is recommended with transendonasal perforation of the atretic membrane. In approximately 90% of cases of choanal atresia there is an osseous wall, and only 10% are membranous.

Unilateral choanal atresia, in contrast to the severe life-threatening symptoms of the bilateral variety, may escape detection for many years. Infants may initially have mucous or foul-smelling secretions from the affected side. Many are seen with respiratory distress associated with upper respiratory tract infections. Hall reported a series of 17 patients in whom choanal atresia was associated with multiple anomalies, including mental retardation, hypogonadism (males), small ears, cardiac defects, micrognathia (hypoplastic mandible), postnatal microcephaly, and ocular coloboma. The prognosis for these infants was poor.

Pierre Robin syndrome

The Pierre Robin syndrome comprises micrognathia, cleft of the soft palate, and upper airway obstruction caused by the tongue falling back into the hypopharynx. The infants are seen initially with varying degrees of respiratory difficulty from none to retractions, cyanotic spells, poor feeding, and failure to thrive. Subsequently cyanosis and cor pulmonale may supervene. An airway can be maintained by nursing the infants when they are prone with the head down; this allows the tongue to fall forward and thus prevent obstruction of the airway. Many infants, however, cannot be successfully maintained this way and continue to have frequent bouts of cyanosis and aspiration.

Some investigators have established an airway by positioning an endotracheal tube through a nostril into the hypopharynx. Suturing the tongue forward also has been recommended but is often unsuccessful, with the suture tearing out. Tracheostomy may be necessary, particularly if there is difficulty in maintaining the airway, and gastrostomy also may be indicated. With time the mandible develops, and the muscles of the jaw become strong enough to keep the tongue forward.

Rib cage abnormalities

Thoracic cage and skeletal abnormalities are a rare group of conditions that may cause respiratory distress by restriction of thoracic volume. They include a number of entities incompatible with life. In this group of diseases are those with hypoplasia of the ribs and thorax, including asphyxiating thoracic dystrophy (Jeune's syndrome), thanatophoric dwarfism, achondrogenesis, homozygous achondroplasia, osteogenesis imperfecta (severe form), Ellis–van Creveld syndrome (chondroectodermal dysplasia), hypophosphatasia, spondylothoracic dysplasia, and rib-gap syndrome.

Respiratory distress caused by structural abnormalities of the chest wall should be readily apparent; however, with marked narrowing of the thorax attention may focus on what appears to be a distended abdomen, and the respiratory problem may be erroneously attributed to an intraabdominal pathologic condition. The presence

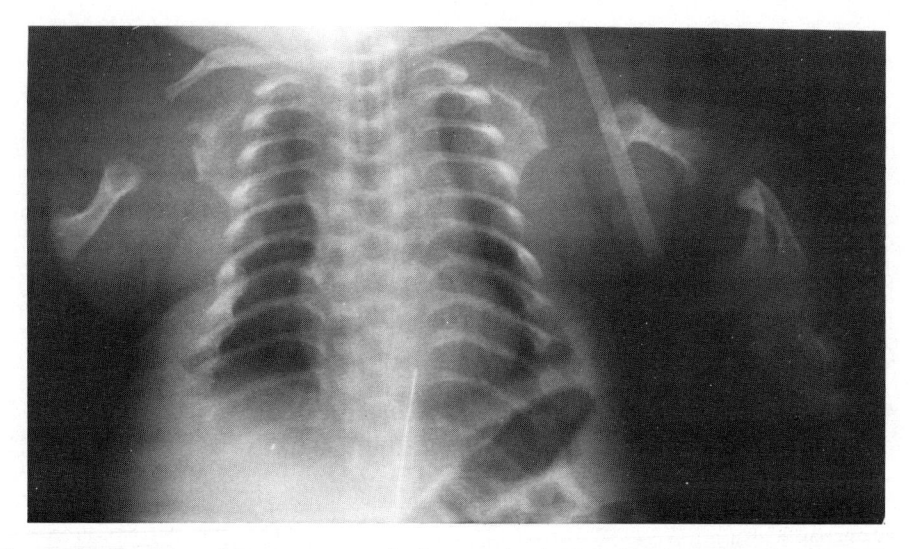

Fig. 23-34. Radiographic appearance in thanatophoric dwarfism showing the narrow thorax, low diaphragm, and foreshortened humeri.

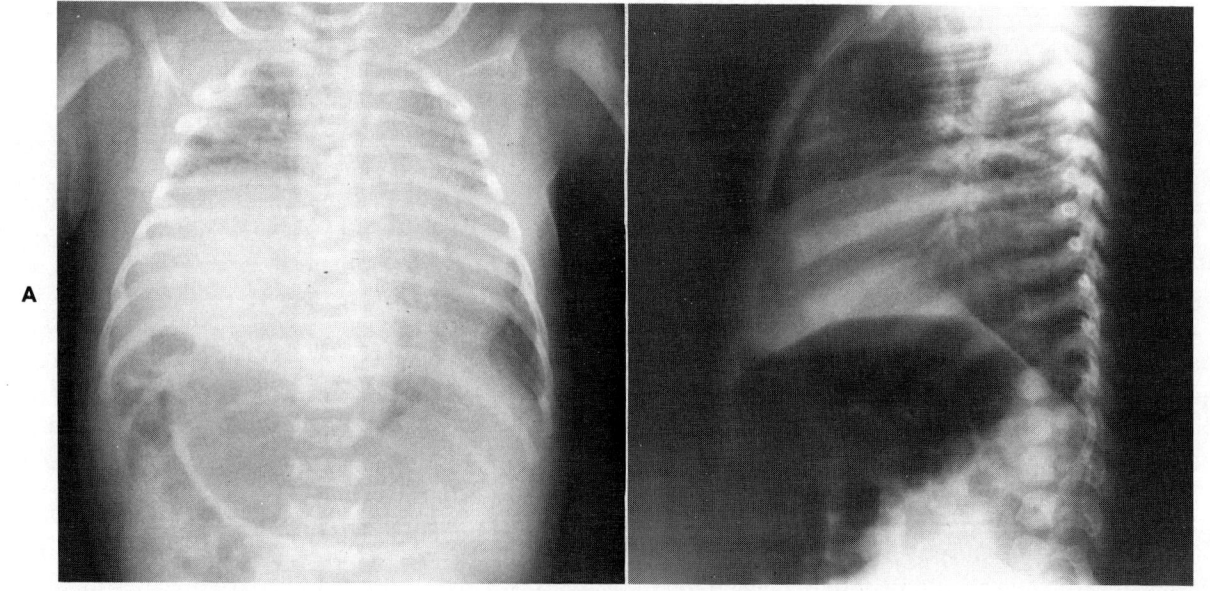

of other associated anomalies, e.g., short-limbed dwarfism, together with close observation of respiratory excursions, examination of the bony thorax, and measurement of the circumference of the chest, will establish the diagnosis even before a review is made of the thoracic and skeletal roentgenograms.

With structural abnormalities of the chest wall, asphyxia and respiratory distress are present from birth. The infants are blue and tachypneic and demonstrate severe retractions and characteristically a virtually immobile chest. Diaphragmatic excursions are prominent; thus respiration appears entirely abdominal. Pulmonary hypoplasia accompanies the thoracic dystrophy, and roentgenographically the lungs may appear airless.

Infants with asphyxiating thoracic dystrophy, thanatophoric dwarfism, achondrogenesis, homozygous achondroplasia, or Ellis–van Creveld syndrome have chests with a squared-off appearance, and the posterior rib arcs all appear the same length. The clavicles appear very high, and the diaphragms are low (Fig. 23-34). The transverse diameter of the thorax may appear diminished in comparison with the vertical diameter. On a lateral view the ribs are very short and may appear clubbed anteriorly. The anteroposterior diameter of the thorax is decreased.

The lungs may be poorly aerated, infiltrates are frequently present, and the heart may appear enlarged. Differentiating between the various syndromes of thoracic cage and skeletal abnormalities usually is accomplished by means of skeletal survey. Multiple fractures and bone demineralization are characteristic of osteogenesis imperfecta and hypophosphatasia.

Asphyxiating thoracic dystrophy

The hallmarks of asphyxiating thoracic dystrophy are extreme constriction and narrowing of the thorax, short ribs, and short-limbed dwarfism with abnormalities of the bones of the pelvis and extremities. Associated anomalies include polydactyly and deformed teeth. Renal abnormalities may be present, and renal failure may occur later. The syndrome is inherited as an autosomal recessive trait. As mentioned previously, the chest appears narrow with prominence of the sternum. The thorax is relatively immobile, and the ribs are horizontally directed and short and have bulbous ends. In addition to the thoracic abnormalities, the infants have trident iliac bones with a double-notch appearance of the acetabula.

Thanatophoric dwarfism

Thanatophoric dwarfism was differentiated from achondroplasia in 1967. The disorder has been uniformly fatal in the perinatal period and probably is the most common form of lethal neonatal dwarfism. Appearance at birth is characteristic and includes striking micromelia in association with a normal trunk, a large head, and a narrow thorax. The radiographic findings include severely flattened vertebral bodies with markedly widened intervertebral disk spaces, small iliac rings, and flaring of the metaphyses of the long bones. There is a high incidence of polyhydramnios, and the infants often present in the breech position. The condition is inherited as an autosomal recessive trait, occurring more frequently in the black population.

Diaphragmatic disorders
Phrenic nerve paralysis

See p. 228.

Phrenic nerve injury with paralysis of the diaphragm is an unusual cause of respiratory distress. It is most commonly present on the right side and follows birth trauma; thus an associated brachial plexus injury or Horner's syndrome may coexist in approximately 75% of the patients. The injuries are observed in large for gestational age infants, particularly those larger than 4 kg, following shoulder dystocia or difficult breech extractions. Fractures of the humerus or clavicle frequently are observed and attest to a violent delivery. The nerve roots of C3 to C5 are stretched, with lateral hyperextension and traction on the neck. Recovery is dependent on the degree of injury; avulsion is obviously permanent, and diaphragmatic eventration secondary to muscle atrophy will ensue.

Lesser injury or edema of the nerve roots results in a spectrum of respiratory symptoms, which may include cyanosis, weak cry, tachypnea, or apnea, and decreased movement is noted on the affected side. On x-ray examination the involved hemidiaphragm is elevated, and atelectasis frequently is observed on that side. The heart and mediastinum are shifted away from the affected side (Fig. 23-35). Fluoroscopically the paralyzed hemidiaphragm is seen to elevate with inspiration and descend on expiration (paradoxical movement), contrasting with the normal diaphragmatic descent on inspiration. Congenital eventration of the diaphragm also results in an elevated hemidiaphragm with paradoxical movement. The major complication to be anticipated is pneumonia superimposed on the atelectasis, which accounts not only for the major morbidity but for the mortality as well. Treatment of phrenic nerve palsy initially is supportive, and in the absence of avulsion spontaneous resolution is to be expected. Surgical plication of the diaphragm may be indicated for selected infants with avulsion. Congenital diaphragmatic hernia is discussed on p. 488.

Avroy A. Fanaroff
Richard J. Martin

BIBLIOGRAPHY
Meconium
Fox, W.W., and others: The therapeutic application of end-expiratory pressure in the meconium aspiration syndrome, Pediatrics 56:214, 1975.

Gage, J.E., and others: Suctioning of upper airway meconium in newborn infants, J.A.M.A. 246:2590, 1981.

Gooding, C.A., and others: An experimental model for the study of meconium aspiration of the newborn, Radiology 100:137, 1971.

Gregory, G., and others: Meconium aspiration in infants—a prospective study, J. Pediatr. 85:848, 1974.

Matthews, T.G., and Warshaw, J.B.: Relevance of the gestational age distribution of meconium passage in utero, Pediatrics 64:30, 1979.

Ting, P., and Brady, J.: Tracheal suction in meconium aspiration, Am. J. Obstet. Gynecol. 122:767, 1975.

Tran, N., and others: Sequential effects of acute meconium obstruction on pulmonary function, Pediatr. Res. 14:34, 1980.

Truog, W.E., and others: Effects of PEEP and tolazoline infusion on respiratory and inert gas exchange in experimental meconium aspiration, J. Pediatr. 100:284, 1982.

Vidyasagar, D., and others: Assisted ventilation in infants with meconium aspiration syndrome, Pediatrics 56:208, 1975.

Yeh, T.F., and others: Hydrocortisone therapy in meconium aspiration syndrome: a controlled study, J. Pediatr. 90:140, 1977.

Pulmonary hemorrhage
Cole, V., and others: Pathogenesis of hemorrhagic pulmonary edema and massive pulmonary hemorrhage in the newborn; Pediatrics 51:175, 1973.

Esterley, J., and Oppenheimer, E.: Massive pulmonary hemorrhage in the newborn. I. Pathologic considerations, J. Pediatr. 69:3, 1966.

Frederick, J., and Butler, N.: Certain causes of neonatal death. IV. Massive pulmonary hemorrhage, Biol. Neonate 18:243, 1971.

Transient tachypnea
Avery, M.E., Gatewood, O.B., and Brumley, G.: Transient tachypnea of the newborn: possible delayed resorption of fluid at birth, Am. J. Dis. Child. 111:380, 1966.

Kuhn, M.P., Fletcher, B.C., and deLemos, R.A.: Roentgen findings in transient tachypnea of the newborn, Radiology 92:751, 1969.

Milner, A.D., Saunders, R.A., and Hopkin, I.E.: Effects of delivery by cesarean section on lung mechanics and lung volume in the human neonate, Arch. Dis. Child. 53:545, 1978.

Air leaks
Allen, R.W., Jung, A.L., and Lester, P.D.: Effectiveness of chest tube evacuation of pneumothorax in neonates, J. Pediatr. 99:629, 1981.

Brooks, J.G., and others: Selective bronchial intubation for the treatment of severe localized pulmonary interstitial emphysema in newborn infants, J. Pediatr. 91:648, 1977.

Gregoire, R., and others: Natural history of pulmonary interstitial emphysema in the preterm infant, Pediatr. Res. 13:495, 1979.

Harris, H.: Pulmonary pseudocysts in the newborn infant, Pediatrics 59:199, 1977.

Higgins, C.B., and others: The hemodynamic significance of massive pneumopericardium in preterm infants with respiratory distress syndrome. Radiology 133:363, 1979.

Hill, A., Perlman, J.M., and Volpe, J.J.: Relationship of pneumothorax to occurrence of intraventricular hemorrhage in the premature newborn, Pediatrics 69:144, 1982.

Kuhns, L., and others: Diagnosis of pneumothorax or pneumomediastinum in the neonate by transillumination, Pediatrics 56:355, 1975.

Macklin, C.C.: Transport of air along sheaths of pulmonic blood vessels from alveoli to mediastinum, Arch. Intern. Med. 64:913, 1939.

Madansky, D.L., and others: Pneumothorax and other forms of pulmonary air leaks in newborns, Am. Rev. Respir. Dis. 120:729, 1979.

Moessinger, A.C., Driscoll, J.M., and Wigger, H.T.: High incidence of lung perforation by chest tube in neonatal pneumothorax, J. Pediatr. 92:635, 1978.

Stern, P., LaRochelle, F.T., and Little, G.A.: Vasopressin and pneumothorax in the neonate, Pediatrics 68:499, 1981.

Developmental anomalies
Askenazi, S.S., and Perlman, M.: Pulmonary hypoplasia: lung weight and radial alveolar count as criteria of diagnosis, Arch. Dis. Child. 54:614, 1979.

Avery, M.E., Fletcher, B.D., and Williams, R.G.: The lung and its disorders in the newborn infant, ed. 4, Philadelphia, 1981, W.B. Saunders Co.

Deluca, F.G., and Wesselhoeft, C.W.: Surgically treatable causes of neonatal respiratory distress, Clin. Perinatol. 5:377, 1978.

Hislop, A., Hey, E., and Reid, L.: The lungs in congenital bilateral renal agenesis and dysplasia, Arch. Dis. Child. 54:32, 1979.

Levin, D.L.: Morphologic analysis of the pulmonary vascular bed in congenital left-sided diaphragmatic hernia, J. Pediatr. 92:805, 1978.

Potter, E.L.: Bilateral renal agenesis, J. Pediatr. 29:68, 1946.

Swischuk, L.E., and others: Primary pulmonary hypoplasia in the neonate, J. Pediatr. 95:573, 1979.

Wohl, M.E.B., and others: The lung following repair of congenital diaphragmatic hernia, J. Pediatr. 90:405, 1977.

Respiratory control and apnea of prematurity
Aranda, J., and others: Pharmacokinetic aspects of theophylline in premature newborns, N. Engl. J. Med. 295:413, 1976.

Bryan, A.C.: Diaphragmatic fatigue in newborns, Am. Rev. Respir. Dis. 119:143, 1979.

Fleming, P.J., Bryan, A.C., and Bryan, M.H.: Functional immaturity of pulmonary irritant receptors and apnea in newborn preterm infants, Pediatrics 61:515, 1978.

Frantz, I.D., and others: Maturational effects on respiratory responses to carbon dioxide in premature infants, J. Appl. Physiol. 41:41, 1976.

Kattwinkel, J.: Neonatal apnea: pathogenesis and therapy, J. Pediatr. 90:342, 1977.

Martin, R.J., Okken, A., and Rubin, D.: Arterial oxygen tension during active and quiet sleep in the normal neonate, J. Pediatr. 94:271, 1979.

Martin, R.J., and others: Effect of lung volume on expiratory time in the newborn infant, J. Appl. Physiol. 45:18, 1978.

Perlstein, P., Edwards, N., and Sutherland, J.: Apnea in premature infants and incubator air temperature changes, N. Engl. J. Med. 282:461, 1970.

Rigatto, H., and Brady, J.P.: Periodic breathing and apnea in preterm infants. II. Hypoxia as a primary event, Pediatrics 50:219, 1972.

Rigatto, H., de la Torre Verduzco, R., and Cates, D.B.: Effects of O_2 on the ventilatory response to CO_2 in preterm infants, J. Appl. Physiol. 30:896, 1975.

Schulte, F.J., Busse, C., and Eichhorn, W.: Rapid eye movement sleep, motorneuron inhibition, and apneic spells in preterm infants, Pediatr. Res. 11:703, 1977.

Shannon, D.C., Kelly, D.H., and O'Connell, K.: Abnormal regulation of ventilation in infants at risk for sudden infant death syndrome, N. Engl. J. Med. 297:747, 1977.

Thach, B.T., and Stark, A.R.: Spontaneous neck flexion and airway obstruction during apneic spells in preterm infants, J. Pediatr. 94:275, 1979.

Extrapulmonary causes of respiratory distress

Berdon, W.E., and Baker, D.H.: Vascular anomalies and the infant lung: rings, slings and other things, Semin. Roentgenol. 7:39, 1972.

Carpenter, R.J., and Neil, H.B.: Correction of congenital choanal atresia in children and adults, Laryngoscope 87:1304, 1977.

Cremin, B.J.: Infantile thoracic dystrophy, Br. J. Radiol. 43:199, 1970.

Cunningham, M., and Stocks, J.: Werdnig-Hoffmann disease: the effects of intra-uterine onset on lung growth, Arch. Dis. Child. 53:921, 1978.

Denson, S.E., Taussig, L.M., and Pond, G.D.: Intraluminal tracheal cyst producing airway obstruction in the newborn infant, J. Pediatr. 88:521, 1976.

Gibson, G.J., and others: Pulmonary mechanics in patients with respiratory muscle weakness, Am. Rev. Respir. Dis. 115:389, 1977.

Hall, B.D.: Choanal atresia and associated multiple anomalies, J. Pediatr. 95:395, 1979.

Harper, P.S.: Congenital myotonic dystrophy in Britain. I. Clinical aspects, Arch. Dis. Child. 50:505, 1975.

Jesarty, R.M., Huzar, R.J., and Basu, S.: Pierre Robin syndrome: cause of respiratory obstruction, cor pulmonale and pulmonary edema, Am. J. Dis. Child. 117:710, 1969.

Kohler, E., and Babbitt, D.P.: Dystrophic thoraces and infantile asphyxia, Radiology 94:55, 1970.

Langer, L.O., Jr., and others: Thanatophoric dwarfism, Radiology 92:285, 1969.

Mamba, T., Brown, S.B., and Grob, D.: Neonatal myasthenia gravis: report of two cases and review of the literature, Pediatrics 45:488, 1970.

Mellins, R.B., and others: Respiratory distress as the initial manifestation of Werdnig-Hoffmann disease, Pediatrics 53:33, 1976.

Pagtakhan, R.D., and Chernick, V.: Intensive care of respiratory disorders. In Kendig, E.L., Jr., and Chernick, V., editors: Disorders of the respiratory tract in children, ed. 3, Philadelphia, 1977, W.B. Saunders Co.

Pearse, R.G., and Howeler, C.J.: Neonatal form of dystrophia myotonica, Arch. Dis. Child. 54:331, 1979.

Simpson, K.: Neonatal respiratory failure due to myotonic dystrophy, Arch. Dis. Child. 50:569, 1975.

Wesenberg, R.L.: The newborn chest, Baltimore, 1973, Harper & Row, Publishers, Inc.

Wigglesworth, J.S., Winston, R.M.L., and Bartlett, K.: The influence of the central nervous system on fetal lung development: an experimental study, Arch. Dis. Child. 52:965, 1977.

Yang, S.S., and others: Lethal short limbed chondrodysplasia in early infancy. In Rosenberg, H.S., and Boland, R.P., editors: Perspectives in pediatric pathology, Chicago, 1976, Year Book Medical Publishers, Inc.

PART FIVE

Chronic pulmonary diseases of the neonate

Prolonged respiratory difficulty in infants is a relatively new and challenging problem in neonatal intensive care. The increased incidence of chronic respiratory disease can be directly related to the more aggressive respiratory management and increased survival of small preterm infants. Fortunately most infants with acute pulmonary disease in the first days of life make a rapid and complete recovery and subsequently have normal lungs. Nonetheless a substantial number of survivors are left with persistent pulmonary sequelae, the precise cause of which remains to be elucidated.

Bronchopulmonary dysplasia (BPD) is the major form of chronic pulmonary disease in neonates. In 1967 Northway introduced the term *BPD* to describe chronic pulmonary insufficiency following severe respiratory distress syndrome (RDS) in infants who had been treated with artificial ventilation and prolonged high oxygen concentrations. Subsequent reports have described a similar disorder after prolonged assisted ventilation for meconium aspiration syndrome, persistent fetal circulation, and various forms of congenital cardiopulmonary disease. Although this section focuses primarily on BPD, prolonged pulmonary disease is not limited to infants who have received assisted ventilation. Chronic aspiration syndromes caused by functional or structural abnormalities of the gastrointestinal tract are a cause of persistent respiratory distress (p. 491). Infants with pulmonary hypoplasia secondary to a diaphragmatic hernia frequently exhibit chronic pulmonary problems postoperatively. Pulmonary infections caused by viruses or *Candida* or *Chlamydia* organisms may result in a prolonged course of respiratory symptoms, whereas cystic fibrosis may be seen rarely in early infancy. The following is the radiographic differential diagnosis of BPD[*]:

1. Wilson-Mikity syndrome
2. Meconium aspiration syndrome
3. Pulmonary interstitial emphysema
4. Pulmonary edema
5. Viral pneumonia (especially cytomegalovirus)
6. Total anomalous pulmonary venous return (type III)
7. Pulmonary lymphangiectasia
8. Recurrent pneumonitis or aspiration (immune deficiency, gastroesophageal reflux, H-type tracheoesophageal fistula, etc.)
9. Cystic fibrosis
10. Idiopathic pulmonary fibrosis (Hamman-Rich syndrome)

Krauss first described a clinical syndrome of delayed and/or prolonged respiratory distress in infants weighing less than 1.25 kg. This has come to be known as chronic pulmonary insufficiency of prematurity. These infants demonstrate a fall in functional residual capacity (FRC) of unknown cause late in the first week of life (Fig. 23-36). The slowly progressive atelectasis is accompanied by hypoxemia, hypercarbia, apneic episodes, and a requirement for supplemental oxygen. Roentgenograms performed during this period may be normal or show only

---

[*]From Edwards, D.K.: J. Pediatr. 95:823, 1979.

468 Behrman's neonatal-perinatal medicine: diseases of the fetus and infant

Fig. 23-36. Functional residual capacity (FRC) determined by helium dilution versus age in days in infants with chronic pulmonary insufficiency of prematurity (CPIP), nondistressed premature infants less than 1,250 gm at birth, and nondistressed infants weighing 1,500 to 2,000 gm at birth. (From Kraus, A.N., Klain, D.B., and Auld, P.A.M.: Pediatrics **55**:55, 1975. Copyright American Academy of Pediatrics 1975.)

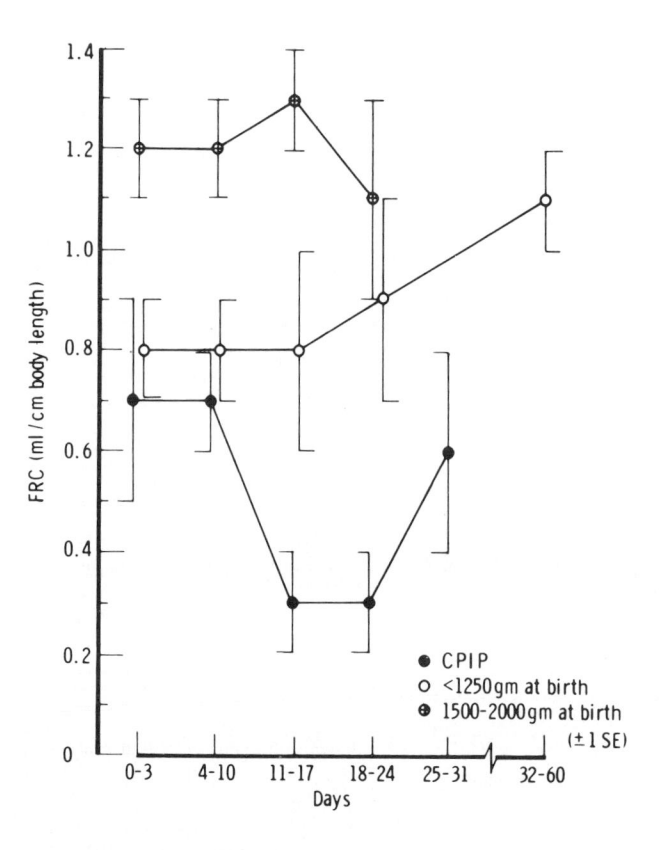

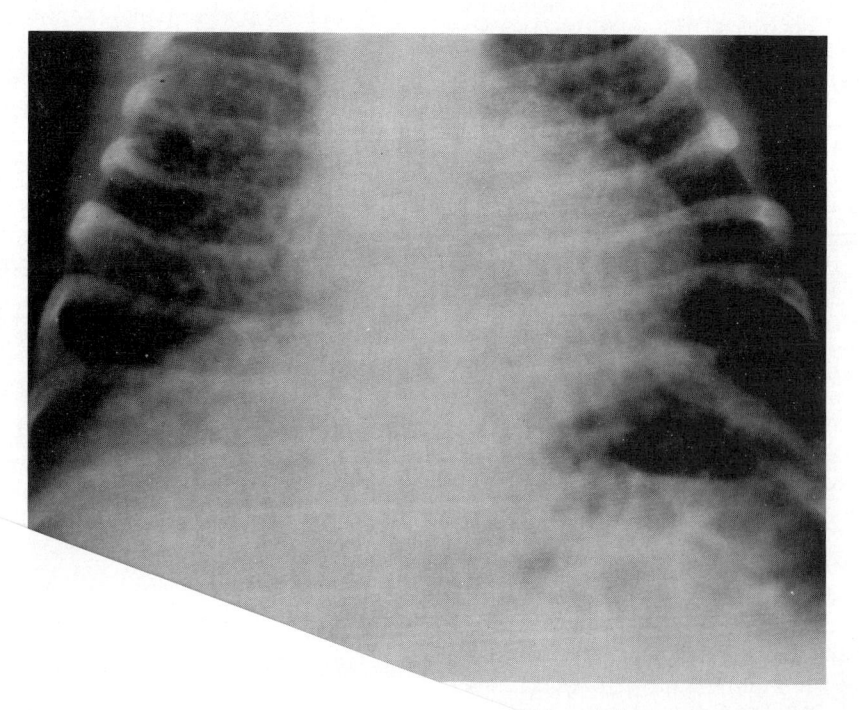

minimum haziness. Gradual resolution can be expected during the third to fourth week of life.

Of all the differential diagnostic possibilities, Wilson-Mikity syndrome has probably engendered the greatest confusion with BPD (Fig. 23-37). The roentgenographic similarities have caused some investigators to associate the two conditions, although compelling differences exist in terms of their clinical course. Patients with Wilson-Mikity syndrome generally have an initially benign course, frequently with normal early chest roentgenograms, and an insidious onset of respiratory difficulty and roentgenographic abnormalities. In contrast, patients who develop BPD initially have severe respiratory disease (usually RDS) and a need for high inspired oxygen concentrations and assisted ventilation. Thus, even though the roentgenographic appearance of the two can be indistinguishable, the characteristic clinical histories usually will permit easy distinction of these conditions. For unknown reasons there has been a dramatic decline in the incidence of the Wilson-Mikity syndrome in recent years, and in its typical form this entity is rarely seen.

CLINICAL AND ROENTGENOGRAPHIC FEATURES

BPD has been estimated to occur in approximately 5% of all infants admitted for neonatal intensive care and requiring intermittent positive pressure ventilation (IPPV). Epidemiologic studies, however, do vary widely in defining precise diagnostic criteria and appropriate neonatal population denominators for comparative studies. Hodson reported an overall incidence of 18% in infants weighing less than 1,500 gm, whereas Tooley observed chronic lung disease in 35% of survivors of RDS who were less than 1,500 gm. Most of these infants, however, had only minimal abnormalities when compared with the roentgenographic findings originally described by Northway.

BPD is a disease of varying severity that encompasses a relatively broad spectrum of pulmonary complications. At one end are the mildest cases that typically consist of premature infants recovering from RDS who may demonstrate a plateau in both ventilator settings or inspired oxygen requirements during weaning. This plateau phase may be relatively short (24 to 48 hours) and associated with roentgenographic findings of mild pulmonary infiltrates. Some clinicians would still classify these babies as having severe RDS, whereas others would call it early or mild BPD. At the other end of the spectrum BPD is characterized by severe cystic emphysema. BPD is not specifically confined to preterm neonates but may develop in large term or postterm infants with meconium aspiration syndrome or persistent fetal circulation. These babies usually require higher ventilator settings or more prolonged inspired oxygen exposure to develop the disease than do premature infants. In addition, after surgery some infants such as those recovering from repair of a diaphragmatic hernia, tetralogy of Fallot, and omphalocele may be ventilated for extended periods and develop BPD.

Nearly all reported cases of BPD have occurred in infants who required some form of IPPV. The development of BPD often is suspected when substantial ventilator and oxygen dependence extends beyond 7 days. Nonetheless definitive roentgenographic features do not typically develop until later in the course, usually around the third week of life. The roentgenographic progression of BPD through the sequence of four stages originally described by Northway is no longer commonly seen. The roentgenographic appearance of stage I is essentially indistinguishable from that of uncomplicated RDS. Dense parenchymal opacification, as seen in stage II BPD, may commonly simulate another process, such as congestive heart failure from a patent ductus arteriosus (PDA), fluid overload, or pulmonary hemorrhage. The bubbly pattern of stage III BPD is not necessarily seen, and when it does appear, it may not follow a period of parenchymal opacity. Finally, the roentgenographic development of chronic lung disease (stage IV) may be more insidious than originally described. The characteristic picture of chronic lung disease ultimately appears at around 20 to 30 days of age. The major features of stage IV disease include hyperinflation and nonhomogeneity of pulmonary tissues, together with multiple fine lacy densities extending to the periphery (Fig. 23-38).

Complete or partial roentgenographic healing is the usual course of infants who survive the acute phases of their disease. BPD typically runs a protracted course punctuated by a variety of complications that lead to acute exacerbations of respiratory symptoms. Cor pulmonale frequently is observed, presumably secondary to pulmonary hypertension resulting from extensive parenchymal disease and chronic hypoxia. Episodes of congestive heart failure will be seen with increasing respiratory distress and hepatomegaly and may be associated with roentgenographic enlargement of the cardiac silhouette. Absolute cardiomegaly, however, is observed infrequently because of pulmonary hyperexpansion, and changes in the pulmonary vasculature may be obscured by the parenchymal disease. Pneumonia commonly complicates the course of BPD during the first months of life. These pulmonary infections are usually nonspecific in appearance and location and frequently related to the aspiration of feedings. Recurrent atelectasis is a frequent problem in patients with BPD. Subsegmental or segmental collapse may occur anywhere in the lungs, although the left lower lobe is frequently involved. Atelectasis may be distinguished from consolidation by com-

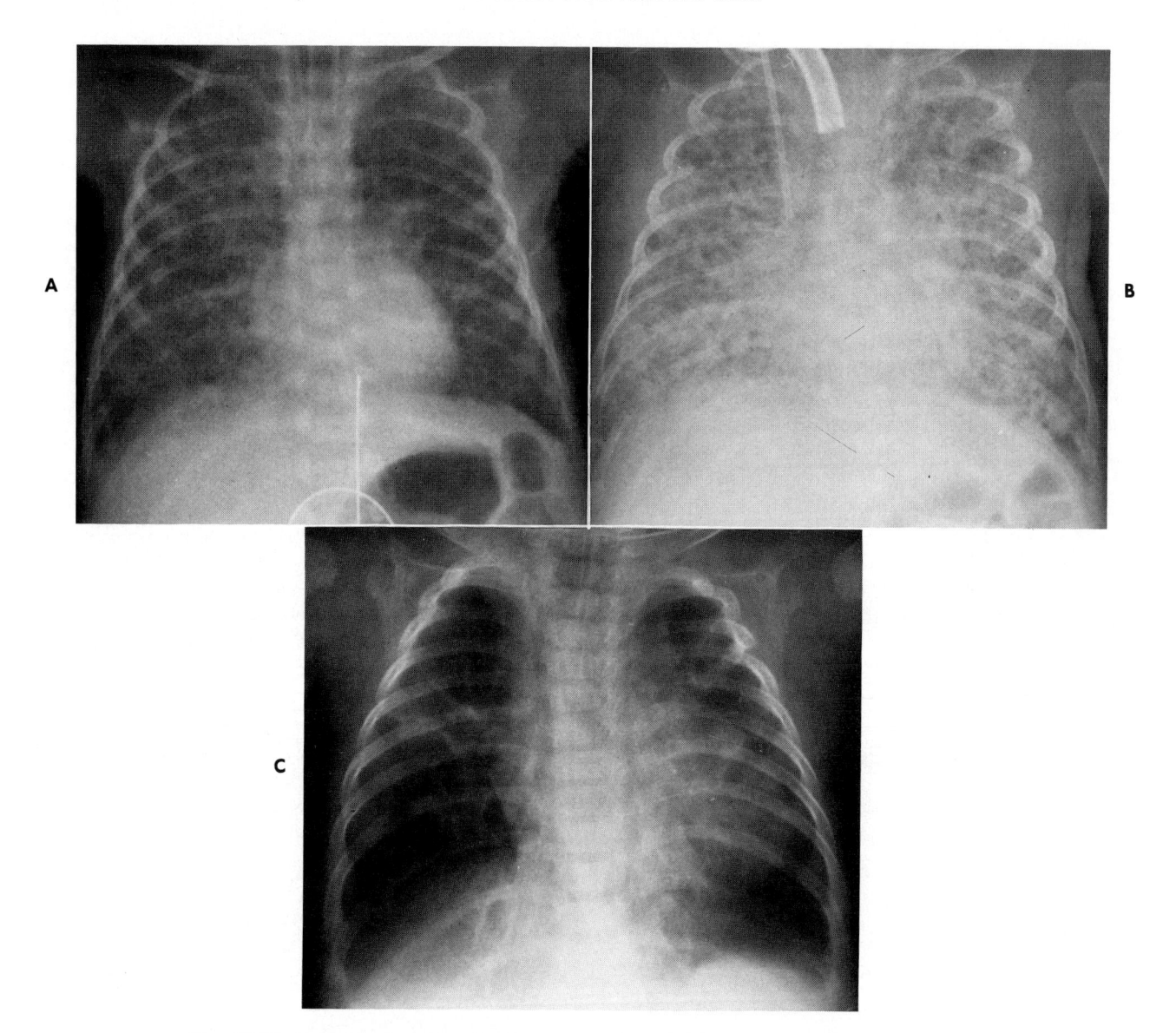

Fig. 23-38. Typical roentgenographic progression of BPD from early BPD **(A)**, through stage III **(B)**, and later stage IV disease **(C)**.

pensatory emphysema of the remaining lung and a change in the position of fissures. Absence of an air bronchogram in the affected portion of the lung suggests an obstructive cause of the atelectasis. Active intervention, including fiberoptic bronchoscopy, may be indicated (p. 438).

PATHOPHYSIOLOGY

Several pathogenetic mechanisms are thought to be responsible for the structural changes that characterize BPD. The term *bronchopulmonary dysplasia* appears to imply a disorder of growth accompanied by abnormal histologic features. A detailed account of the various maturational changes in the developing premature lung is given elsewhere (p. 404). In addition to the degree of pulmonary immaturity, Reid has proposed that an understanding of the process of healing after RDS is key to understanding the development of BPD. After resolution of RDS intraalveolar exudate is cleared to leave a normal lung; the exudate is absorbed into the alveolar wall, resulting in interstitial fibrosis, or organized in situ so that there is an obliteration of the alveolar space. The lung also may become airless and solid because of simple alveolar collapse. In either case the lung is not contributing to gas exchange. Nonaerated regions may reaerate or, if they continue airless, will form scars of condensed lung tissue and fibrose. The bronchiolar mucosa is markedly abnormal with dysplasia and peribronchiolar inflammation. There is bronchiolar muscular hypertrophy and fibrosis of structural portions of the pulmonary lobule.

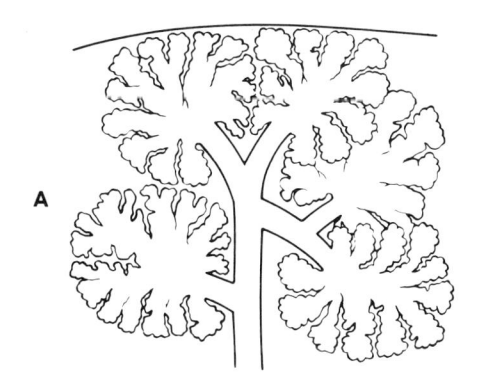

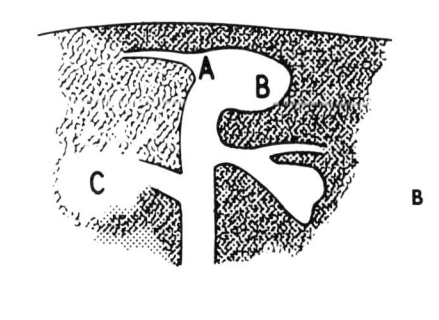

Fig. 23-39. Mechanism whereby inflammatory scarring can lead to alternating regions of scarring and emphysema. *A,* Obliterated bronchiolus; *B,* cyst (bronchiolar); *C,* cyst (alveolar). **A,** Normal lobule. **B,** After fibrosis. (From Reid, L.: J. Pediatr. **95:**836, 1979.)

Arterioles are variably hypertrophic, and there is significant involvement of lymphatic and perilymphatic areas. There seems to be a stage when shadows on roentgenographic examination represent transudate/exudate or collapse, but this stage is transient and thus reversible. When the fleeting shadows give way to a static picture, the pattern of scarring may be established (Fig. 23-39).

The typical macroscopic appearance in BPD is a coarse pattern of scarring mixed with regions of emphysema. The emphysema arises in at least three ways: (1) scarring means that the emphysema of the intervening lung arises in part from overinflation, or can be considered compensatory; (2) there is a failure of multiplication of the alveoli within at least some units, which indicates that there is also a hypoplastic form of emphysema; (3) inflammation and destruction of the alveolar wall or of its capillary bed lead to a destructive form of emphysema; this is particularly relevant to the damage done by high levels of oxygen. Reid notes that the emphysema in BPD arises from these three processes. Parts of the vascular bed are condensed in the scars, and these arteries develop smaller than normal arterial diameters and thicker muscular walls. Since the latter encroaches on the lumen, the vascular bed is further reduced in volume. In the intervening aerated regions the arteries grow but receive an abnormally large part of the cardiac output. Their growth is also abnormal and will be compensating to some extent for the changed hemodynamic state.

Watts has examined pulmonary function in a group of 10 preterm infants with severe BPD (stages III and IV of Northway). The most striking finding was a severe maldistribution of ventilation in these infants, as determined by nitrogen washouts. The BPD group had a pulmonary clearance delay of 223% versus 60% for a comparable group of preterm infants who also had been ventilated but subsequently developed no signs of BPD. Minute volumes were normal in the infants with BPD, with increased respiratory frequency, decreased tidal volume, and hypercarbia with a mean $PaCO_2$ of 55 mm Hg. Other studies have additionally documented hypoxemia, diminished specific compliance, increased FRC, and decreased effective capillary blood flow in patients with BPD. Airway obstruction appears to play a role in the chronic disease process, although this has not been clearly quantitated.

ETIOLOGY

Several clinical factors have been implicated in the etiology of BPD. Most discussions of etiology have focused on the relative effects of oxygen toxicity and mechanical ventilators on the disease process, whereas the importance of pulmonary immaturity has not received enough attention. The smallest infants have poorly developed surfactant systems, decreased pulmonary stability, and ill-defined structures of both interstitium and alveoli, placing them at highest risk. The lungs of these infants are still developing and require less extrinsic airway pressure or toxic gas exposure to produce significant pulmonary changes. One developmental factor that probably has major significance in the disease is that a neonate of 7 months' gestational age has inadequately developed elastic and connective tissue elements. Stress to these structural elements may be important in the production of emphysema. A clinical comparison can be made to long-time smokers with chronic lung disease and emphysema, in whom elastic tissue is the first pulmonary tissue element to be disrupted.

The role of infection in the origin of BPD is not clear. Pneumatoceles and cystic lung disease occur in neonatal lungs secondary to infections by *Escherichia coli* or *Pseudomonas, Klebsiella,* or *Staphylococcus* organisms. If these infections are chronic, they might result in bronchitis or small airway disease. Recurrent infections appear, on the other hand, to be a common complication of long-term BPD. Birth asphyxia may be an important factor in predisposing infants to development of BPD.

Asphyxia causes two problems that result in higher oxygen and ventilator requirements. Disruption of surfactant synthesis results in more severe atelectasis and acidosis, whereas hypoxemia predisposes the infant to increased pulmonary vascular resistance and right-to-left shunting. Interstitial emphysema is a diffuse form of alveolar air leak in which small bubbles of air move along the interstitial spaces of the lung. This condition has been reported to predispose infants to BPD, but the cause and effect relation between these two conditions is not fully established (p. 448).

Oxygen toxicity

Clinical and experimental evidence has suggested that pulmonary oxygen toxicity is a major factor in the cause of BPD. Although many body tissues can be injured by sufficiently high oxygen concentrations, the lung is exposed directly to the highest partial pressure of inspired oxygen. The precise concentration of oxygen that is toxic to the lung probably depends on a large number of variables, including maturation, nutritional and endocrine status, and duration of exposure to oxygen and other oxidants. Although a safe level of inspired oxygen has not been established, concentrations in excess of 50% carry a substantial risk of lung damage when administered over a period of many days. The pathogenesis of oxygen toxicity, according to studies in both animals and human beings, is nonspecific and consists of atelectasis, edema, alveolar hemorrhage, inflammation, fibrin deposition, and thickening and hyalinization of alveolar membranes. There is early damage to capillary endothelium in animals, and plasma leaks into interstitial and alveolar spaces. Pulmonary surfactant may be altered, adding to the formation of atelectasis. Type I alveolar lining cells also are injured early, and bronchiolar and tracheal ciliated cells can be damaged by 80% to 100% oxygen. The contribution of the alveolar macrophage to pathologic effects in the lung is not clear. Total resolution after oxygen toxicity is possible if the initial exposure is not overwhelming. It is presumed that cellular pathologic processes similar to those in animals also occur in humans.

The contribution of the alveolar macrophage to pathologic effects in the lung is not clear. Continued exposure to high O_2 is accompanied by an influx of polymorphonuclear leukocytes containing proteolytic enzymes. In addition, Bruce has observed that the antiproteinase defense system is significantly impaired in infants exposed to greater than 60% inspired O_2 for 6 or more days. Therefore proteolytic damage of structural elements in alveolar walls may be an important pathogenetic factor.

Although the cellular basis for oxygen toxicity has not been completely elucidated, the principal mechanisms involve the univalent reduction of molecular oxygen and formation of free radical intermediates. The latter can

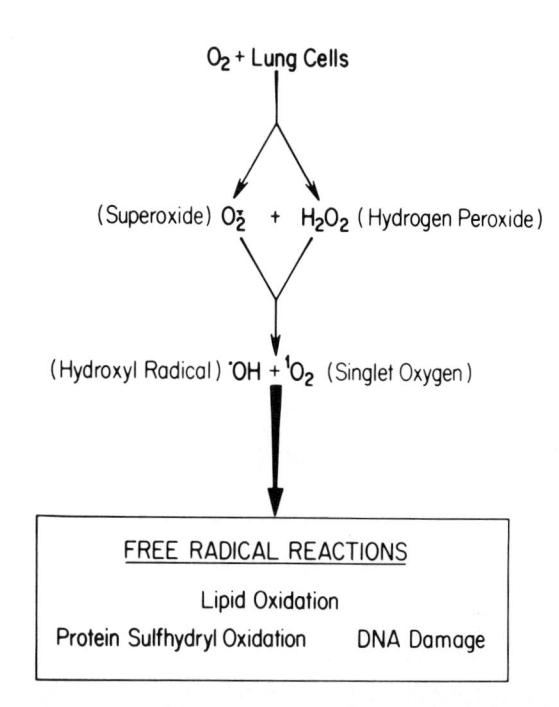

Fig. 23-40. Chemical mechanisms of oxygen toxicity. (From Deneke, S.M., and Fanburg, B.L.: N. Engl. J. Med. **303**:76, 1980. Reprinted by permission of the New England Journal of Medicine.)

react with intracellular constituents and membrane lipids, thus initiating chain reactions that may result in tissue destruction. An oxygen-radical mechanism of toxicity is consistent with the known chemical reactivity of oxygen, hydrogen peroxide, and superoxide radical. Chemical interactions between oxygen and various radicals can result in singlet excited oxygen formation. Singlet excited oxygen is a highly reactive, electronically excited state of molecular oxygen that is toxic to many biologic systems. At present hydrogen peroxide, superoxide radical, hydroxyl radical, and singlet excited oxygen all are considered possible agents of hyperoxic tissue damage. The term *oxygen radical* sometimes is used very loosely to mean any of these species, since all have been implicated in lipid peroxide formation and subsequent free-radical chain reactions (Fig. 23-40).

To resist the detrimental effects of oxygen toxicity, the body has evolved various antioxidant enzymes such as superoxide dismutase, which eliminates the superoxide radical, whereas other compounds such as vitamin E and selenium also may offer endogenous antioxidant protection. Studies designed to enhance antioxidant protection in the neonate, as by the administration of high doses of vitamin E, however, have failed to demonstrate any sustained beneficial effect.

The natural susceptibility of animals to oxygen varies widely among species. The response also seems to be age dependent, since immature animals survive continuous oxygen exposure longer than do adults of the same spe-

Oxygen concentration, %	Number of experiments	Cessation of all ciliary movement, hr	Cessation of particle transport, hr
20	6	Did not cease	Did not cease
80	6	72-96	48-96

Fig. 23-41. Effect of 80% oxygen on ciliary function of cultured human tracheal epithelium. (From Boat, T.F., and others: Pediatr. Res. **7**:607, 1973.)

cies. Loss of mucociliary function may be an additional pathogenetic component of BPD, since exposure to 80% oxygen has resulted in a cessation of ciliary movement after 48 to 96 hours in cultured human neonatal respiratory epithelium (Fig. 23-41). Further understanding of the role of maturation in the response of the lung to high oxygen concentrations should offer greater insight into both the harmful and protective influences on pulmonary oxygen toxicity.

Assisted ventilation

In their initial observations Northway and associates concluded that administration of high concentrations of oxygen was the major agent responsible for the production of BPD. Nonetheless they indicated that the use of intermittent positive pressure respirators and endotracheal intubation also may contribute to the pathologic state. Clinical experience with newborn infants, however, has not borne out the role of oxygen alone in the pathogenesis of this syndrome. This is supported by the observation that BPD is virtually unheard of in infants treated with negative pressure ventilation without the use of endotracheal tubes, despite high concentrations of oxygen being administered. Furthermore BPD is infrequently observed as a complication of nasal CPAP despite prolonged oxygen requirements.

It has become generally accepted that barotrauma resulting from high pressures used in assisted ventilation is the major culprit in the development of BPD. The role of the endotracheal tube itself may be difficult to separate from those of either the oxygen or the respirator under these circumstances. Endotracheal tubes would appear to hinder the drainage of tracheal secretions. They further increase both the dead space and the resistance to airflow and may cause a diminution in arterial Po_2 by preventing closure of the glottis when the tube is in place.

Peak inspiratory pressure (PIP) is one of the major factors now implicated in the cause of BPD. With the current "pressure" type of mechanical ventilators the inspiratory pressure is adjusted to deliver an adequate tidal volume to the infant for maintenance of normal $Paco_2$. Most clinicians attempt to use a PIP of less than 30 cm H_2O and, after the acute disease reaches peak severity, attempt to lower PIP to prevent BPD. The role of PIP in causing BPD is not entirely clear because, if ventilator rates are rapid (more than 60 breaths per minute), or if the inspiratory phase is short, the PIP may not have time to be transmitted to the alveoli, and alveolar damage may not result.

Mean airway pressure (MAP) also may be an important factor in the cause of BPD. Four factors are major determinants of MAP. These include (1) PIP, (2) the length of time this inspiratory pressure is applied (determined by either inspiratory time or inspiratory:expiratory ratio), (3) waveform, which determines how long during inspiration the airways are exposed to the PIP, and (4) end expiratory pressure. At the present time there are few clinical data to quantitate the role of MAP causing BPD. It is possible that, if oxygen is indeed largely responsible for the changes described as BPD, there must be the additional presence of IPPV via an endotracheal tube for this response to occur. Finally, the duration of both assisted ventilation and oxygen therapy may be a key etiologic factor. This is difficult to substantiate, since it is impossible to separate the time factor from the initial severity of the underlying disease. The more severe the disease, the longer the time required for assisted ventilation.

Fluid therapy

The precise relationship between fluid therapy, PDA, and BPD has not yet been completely established. Bell has demonstrated that the incidence of both PDA and congestive heart failure in low birth weight infants is increased when high volumes of maintenance fluids are used. Recent evidence by Brown indicates that the presence of a PDA complicating the course of RDS increases the risk of BPD. Spitzer has proposed that the time taken for maximum urinary output to occur during recovery from RDS is related to the time in an increased O_2 environment and may predict the development of BPD.

MANAGEMENT

Prevention of prematurity and the major causes of neonatal respiratory distress would probably eliminate BPD as a clinical problem. Since this has not yet been accomplished, all our attention should be directed toward the difficult task of reducing the concentration of supplemental oxygen and minimizing ventilator pressures within the constraints of appropriate management for acute respiratory distress. In spite of our best efforts at prevention, BPD remains a clinically significant problem. Successful treatment of severe BPD may require a long-term multidisciplinary commitment, since some infants require care for as long as 2 years.

Respiratory support

A rational approach to the respiratory care of infants with BPD requires an understanding of the abnormalities of pulmonary function inherent in the disease. In infants with BPD the low dynamic lung compliance and high airway resistance result in an increased work of breathing. Hypercarbia will result, since the neonate cannot sustain an appropriately high level of minute ventilation. Intermittent mandatory ventilation (IMV) is a form of assisted ventilation that allows the infant to breathe spontaneously between a set number of mechanical breaths per minute. This technique is of particular value in infants with BPD who may require prolonged ventilatory support. An IMV rate is selected that allows $PaCO_2$ to be maintained in a high normal range. A PEEP of 2 to 4 cm H_2O is used to stabilize lung volume. An increased inspired oxygen concentration is required to maintain a PaO_2 in the 50 to 70 mm Hg range. Adequacy of gas exchange should be monitored by arterial blood gases at intervals dictated by the child's clinical condition. During times of stability transcutaneous PO_2 measurements are satisfactory, whereas $PaCO_2$ can be approximated from venous samples, which will average 5 mm Hg above arterial values.

Long-term mechanical ventilation requires the presence of a secure airway. If the use of such support is for 1 to 2 months or less, a well-secured endotracheal tube is sufficient, provided that attention is given to fit. An appropriately sized endotracheal tube will leak when 30 cm H_2O positive pressure is applied to the airway. If no leak occurs, the endotracheal tube is too large and should be replaced with a smaller tube. If mechanical ventilation is required for more than 1 to 2 months, tracheostomy is a more appropriate form of airway control. Prolonged use of oversized endotracheal tubes may result in a high incidence of subglottic stenosis (p. 438).

Inspired gases must be humidified to prevent damage to the respiratory tract mucosa that may be caused by exposure to dry gas. Chest physiotherapy is performed at variable intervals (depending on secretions) in an attempt to prevent atelectasis and the pooling of secretions. This generally includes chest percussion and vibration, followed by airway suctioning and finally maximum hyperinflation of the lungs. Meanwhile every effort should be made to keep the inspired oxygen concentration and PIP as low as possible to prevent further pulmonary oxygen toxicity.

Weaning from IMV may be a long, slow process taking many months in extreme cases. Intercurrent illnesses such as upper or lower respiratory tract infections, bronchospasm, or congestive heart failure may interrupt the weaning process and should be treated aggressively. After IMV has been discontinued, the infant may benefit from endotracheal CPAP for 1 to 2 weeks. Weaning from oxygen should progress concurrently and with even greater caution. Reduction in inspired oxygen of as little as 2% may result in a profound change in the infant's clinical condition and requires constant reassessment. Halliday has documented echocardiographic evidence suggesting a mild increase in pulmonary vascular resistance with similar small decreases in inspired O_2.

Nutritional management

Adequate nutrition is a key aspect of care for the infant with BPD, who may have a 25% increase in resting O_2 consumption over controls. Malnutrition will delay somatic growth and the development of new alveoli, making weaning from mechanical ventilation almost impossible. The malnourished patient is also more prone to infection. For these reasons an aggressive approach should be taken toward supplying a parenteral or oral caloric intake that is adequate for growth. High-calorie formulas and supplements may be used to maximize the intake of calories while restricting fluid intake to prevent congestive heart failure. If for any reason enteral nutrition is precluded for more than 3 or 4 days, peripheral hyperalimentation with glucose, amino acids, and subsequently fat should be substituted until the gastrointestinal tract again becomes available. Adequacy of nutrition should be closely monitored, and growth charts for height, weight, and head circumference need to be kept. Other means of assessment include arm anthropometry to determine muscle mass and fat deposits and measuring serum levels of albumin. Rib fractures noted on routine chest roentgenograms together with generalized bone demineralization are not infrequently observed in BPD and are usually a manifestation of rickets. Their cause may relate to dietary or parenteral deficiency of calcium or vitamin D. Another contributing factor might be the calciuria resulting from chronic furosemide therapy, and extra calcium and vitamin D intake are indicated (Chapter 33, part two).

Fluid management

Many infants with severe BPD have roentgenographic, electrocardiographic, and echocardiographic evidence of cor pulmonale, which appears to resolve as lung function improves. These infants may have fewer problems with fluid overload and congestive heart failure if they are digitalized until evidence of cor pulmonale disappears. In addition, infants with BPD are particularly susceptible to pulmonary edema, perhaps because of abnormal lymphatic drainage or the deleterious effects of right-sided heart failure on left ventricular function. The importance of left ventricular hypertrophy in these infants has additionally been confirmed by both echocardiographic and pathologic studies without accompanying elevation of pulmonary vascular resistance. Fluids are restricted as much as possible, considering the need for a high caloric intake, and chronic diuretic therapy is instituted with a thiazide or a loop diuretic such as furosemide. Parameters that need frequent monitoring include intake and output, electrolytes, urine specific gravity, body weight, rales, peripheral edema, and liver enlargement.

Control of infection

Even though many types of infection can have serious consequences for the child with BPD, pneumonia generally results in the most profound setback. As a result, the child needs to be closely watched for early evidence of infection. Tracheal secretions are obtained biweekly for culture and Gram stain, or more often if a change in the quality and quantity of secretions indicates possible infection. A complete blood count, blood culture, and chest roentgenogram are obtained if pneumonia is suspected. Although it is difficult to distinguish between colonization of the airway and true infection, this distinction is important because overtreatment with antibiotics may result in the emergence of more virulent organisms. Selection of antibiotics is based on the sensitivity of the implicated organism, and treatment is continued for a minimum of 1 week or until the infection has been controlled. Clinical measures to prevent pulmonary superinfection are important. These include changing tracheostomy tubes twice weekly and careful hand washing prior to handling the infant.

Bronchodilator therapy

Infants with both subacute and chronic forms of BPD may exhibit clinical elements of bronchospasm. Mechanical ventilation and oxygen therapy during the early stages of disease result in hypertrophy of peribronchiolar smooth muscle and increase in airway resistance in addition to the decrease in lung compliance. Rooklin reported that theophylline therapy produced a trend toward decreased pulmonary resistance and increased dynamic compliance at 2 and 24 hours after treatment in infants with BPD who were less than 30 days of age. Older infants in this study demonstrated no improvement in pulmonary function following bronchodilator therapy, possibly because higher doses were required or because there was a greater degree of fibrosis. Nevertheless we recommend a trial of bronchodilators in all patients with BPD who exhibit clinical signs of bronchospasm.

Infant stimulation

The infant with severe BPD may be ventilator dependent for many months and thus deprived of normal parental stimulation. Developmental delays are the invariable result, which are compounded if any gross neurologic handicap exists. A well-organized program of infant stimulation may help the infant achieve maximum potential. Such a program will instruct the caretakers in helping the infant with various social, language, cognitive, and motor skills. As the child grows, speech therapy is useful in teaching communication skills, especially important for children with a tracheostomy. Beanbag chairs, strollers, and other adaptive tools are employed to mobilize the child and teach gross motor skills. Progress is monitored by periodic developmental evaluations, and emphasis is placed on areas where delay is evident.

Parental support

The parents of an infant with severe BPD lose considerable control of their child to the hospital staff, particularly in areas related to medical care. Parental participation in other aspects of child care is critical for the child's development and for establishment of normal relationships. Therefore parents are encouraged to visit as frequently as possible and to participate in the day-to-day care of their child. They are educated about relevant medical equipment and procedures. In time many are able to assume complete responsibility for procedures such as chest physiotherapy and tracheal suctioning in addition to holding and playing with their child. During the prolonged hospitalization every effort must be made to assign a consistent physician and nursing team to oversee the child's care and be available for continuing parental support.

OUTCOME

During the first year of life the mortality of infants with severe BPD is high (30% to 40%), usually as a result of respiratory failure, sepsis, and/or intractable cor pulmonale. Eighty percent of these deaths occur during the initial hospitalization. Nonetheless, with adequate nutrition, somatic growth, and control of infection and heart failure, pulmonary function may gradually improve, along with resolution of cor pulmonale and radiographic healing.

Lower respiratory tract infections are common during the first year of life in patients with BPD, although their exact incidence is difficult to ascertain from the literature. Frequently no specific organisms are isolated, and the disease resolves with broad-spectrum antiobiotic therapy. Among survivors of BPD, hospitalization for episodes of wheezing suggestive of bronchiolitis or asthma is common during the first 2 years of life. Acute roentgenographic evidence of hyperinflation may be difficult to appreciate in infants with BPD, who generally already are hyperinflated. Such episodes of bronchiolitis may be accompanied by focal, transient areas of atelectasis.

Northway has reported the follow-up analysis of a group of infants surviving with stage IV BPD. Thirty-seven percent were clinically normal by 3 years of age, 29% had minor handicaps in somatic growth or cardiopulmonary function or an IQ in the 80 to 90 range, and 34% had significant handicaps, including cerebral palsy, mental retardation, deafness, or blindness. This incidence of handicaps, however, was not significantly different from that in a group of infants with a history of severe RDS requiring IPPV who did not develop BPD. Markestad also observed in 20 survivors of BPD that at 2 years the prognosis for future development compared favorably with that of ventilated infants without BPD. Pulmonary function studies of infants with a history of BPD indicate that pulmonary function may be impaired beyond 2 years in many cases, even though the infants may be asymptomatic. Smyth observed a high incidence of obstructive airway disease at 8 years in a small group of BPD survivors. Data on longer term follow-up studies of pulmonary function in larger numbers of these infants are currently unavailable, although these clearly will be very important to ascertain in the future.

William W. Fox
Jeffrey P. Morray
Richard J. Martin

BIBLIOGRAPHY
General

Bryan, M.H., and others: Pulmonary function studies during the first year of life in infants recovering from respiratory distress syndrome, Pediatrics **52**:169, 1973.

Edwards, D.K., Dyer, W.M., and Northway, W.H., Jr.: Twelve years experience with bronchopulmonary dysplasia, Pediatrics **59**:839, 1977.

Halliday, H.L., Dumpit, F.M., and Brady, J.P.: Effects of inspired oxygen on echocardiographic assessment of pulmonary vascular resistance and myocardial contractility in bronchopulmonary dysplasia, Pediatrics **65**:536, 1980.

Hodson, W.A., and others: Bronchopulmonary dysplasia: the need for epidemiologic studies, J. Pediatr. **95**:848, 1978.

Krauss, A.N., Klain, D.B., and Auld, P.A.M.: Chronic pulmonary insufficiency of prematurity (CPIP), Pediatrics **55**:55, 1975.

Markestad, T., and Fitzhardinge, P.M.: Growth and development in children recovering from bronchopulmonary dysplasia, J. Pediatr. **98**:597, 1981.

Melnick, G., and others: Normal pulmonary vascular resistance and left ventricular hypertrophy in young infants with bronchopulmonary dysplasia: an echocardiographic and pathologic study, Pediatrics **66**:589, 1980.

Northway, W.H., Jr.: Observations on bronchopulmonary dysplasia, J. Pediatr. **95**:815, 1980.

Northway, W.H., Jr., Rosan, R.C., and Porter, D.Y.: Pulmonary disease following respiratory therapy of hyaline membrane disease: bronchopulmonary dysplasia, N. Engl. J. Med. **276**:357, 1967.

Reid, L.: Bronchopulmonary dysplasia—pathology, J. Pediatr. **94**:836, 1979.

Rooklin, A.R., and others: Theophylline therapy in bronchopulmonary dysplasia, J. Pediatr. **94**:882, 1979.

Smyth, J.A., and others: Pulmonary function and bronchial hyperreactivity in long-term survivors of bronchopulmonary dysplasia, Pediatrics **68**:336, 1981.

Spitzer, A.R., Fox, W.W., and Delivoria-Papadopoulos, M.: Maximum diuresis—a factor in predicting recovery from respiratory distress syndrome and the development of bronchopulmonary dysplasia, J. Pediatr. **98**:476, 1981.

Tooley, W.H.: Epidemiology of bronchopulmonary dysplasia, J. Pediatr. **95**:851, 1979.

Watts, J.L., Ariagno, R.L., and Brady, J.P.: Chronic pulmonary disease in neonates after artificial ventilation: distribution of ventilation and pulmonary interstitial emphysema, Pediatrics **60**:273, 1977.

Weinstein, M.R., and Oh, W.: Oxygen consumption in infants with bronchopulmonary dysplasia, J. Pediatr. **99**:958, 1981.

Wilson, M.G., and Mikity, V.G.: A new form of respiratory disease in premature infants, Am. J. Dis. Child. **99**:489, 1960.

Workshop on Bronchopulmonary Dysplasia, J. Pediatr. (Suppl.) **85**:815, 1979.

Etiology

Bell, E.F., and others: Effect of fluid administration on the development of symptomatic patent ductus arteriosus and congestive heart failure in premature infants, N. Engl. J. Med. **302**:598, 1980.

Boat, T.F., and others: Toxic effects of oxygen on cultured human neonatal respiratory epithelium, Pediatr. Res. **7**:607, 1973.

Brown, E.R., and others: Bronchopulmonary dysplasia: possible relationship to pulmonary edema, J. Pediatr. **92**:982, 1978.

Bruce, M., and others: Proteinase inhibitors and inhibitor inactivation in neonatal airways secretions, Chest, **81**:44S, 1982.

Deneke, S.M., and Fanburg, B.L.: Normobaric oxygen toxicity of the lung, N. Engl. J. Med. **303**:76, 1980.

Merritt, T.A., and others: Newborn tracheal aspirate cytology: classification during respiratory distress syndrome and bronchopulmonary dysplasia, J. Pediatr. **98**:949, 1981.

Stern, L., and others: Negative pressure artificial respiration: use in treatment of respiratory failure of the newborn, Can. Med. Assoc. J. **102**:595, 1970.

Taghizadeh, A., and Reynolds, E.O.R.: Pathogenesis of bronchopulmonary dysplasia following hyaline membrane disease, Am. J. Pathol. **82**:241, 1976.

CHAPTER 24 The gastrointestinal system

PART ONE

Development

To understand some of the physiology and pathophysiology of the gastrointestinal (GI) tract, one must appreciate the changes that occur in the digestive system during development. Following fertilization the developing organism undergoes a series of sequential and coordinated changes in morphology and metabolism that result in the formation of organized arrangements of specialized cells. The GI tract develops from the entoderm and a mesoblastic mesenchymal layer, which together are called the splanchnopleure; the epithelial lining and glandular epithelia are derived from the entoderm, and the muscular, vascular, and serosal elements are derived from the mesodermal layer. The development and differentiation of the digestive tract depend on the intimate association of the epithelial and mesenchymal components. From studies of animals it appears that the epithelium and mesenchyme must be derived from the same organ tissue for normal epithelial development to occur in most areas of the GI tract. In other organ systems, heterologous mesenchymal tissue will allow the epithelial growth and proliferation to develop normally. In a third situation, epithelial growth initially requires homologous mesenchyme, but once differentiation has started, any mesenchymal component will allow it to continue. Actual cellular contact between these two components must occur for normal development to progress.

Table 24-1 summarizes the major events that occur during the development of the GI tract. By 3½ weeks' gestation the foregut and hindgut as well as the liver buds are discernible. By 4 weeks the intestine remains as a simple tube, pancreatic buds are beginning to appear, and liver cords, ducts, and the gallbladder begin to form. Over the next 1 to 2 weeks the intestine elongates more rapidly than does the embryo itself and forms a loop that protrudes along the yolk stalk into the umbilical cord. Between 6 and 8 weeks, while the greatest portion of the intestine is still in the umbilical cord, the small intestine rotates around the axis of the superior mesenteric vessels in a counterclockwise fashion. The duodenum and the splenic flexure of the colon do not enter into the cord but are held in position by mesenteric bands. Over the next 2 weeks the small intestine continues to grow and coil inside the cord; and at 10 weeks of gestation the intestine reenters the abdominal cavity, with the jejunum leading the way and filling the left portion of the abdominal cavity. The ileum follows and fills the right half of the abdominal cavity; then the colon reenters. The cecum becomes fixed close to the iliac crest, and the ascending and transverse colon come to lie in their respective positions. The mechanisms by which the intestine herniates into the cord and then reenters the abdominal cavity are unknown. The reentry may be due in part to the increased capacity of the abdominal cavity to accept the intestine because of the absorption of the mesonephros and the decreased rate of growth of the liver. Abnormalities of exit or return of the intestine lead to various types of nonrotation or malrotation. From the fifth to the fortieth week of gestation the intestine grows approximately 1,000-fold; at term the length of the small intestine is approximately three to four times the crown-heel length.

Initially the mucosal surface of the small intestine is

This work was supported in part by grants from the U.S.P.H.S., HD 02147 and HD 00049, from the National Institutes of Health, and by grant RR-81 from the General Clinical Research Centers Program of the Division of Research Sources, National Institutes of Health.

Table 24-1. Development of the human gastrointestinal tract

Age (weeks)	Crown-rump length (mm)	Stage of development
2.5	1.5	Gut not distinct from yolk sac
3.5	2.5	Foregut and hindgut present Yolk sac broadly attached at midgut Liver bud present Mesenteries forming
4	5.0	Intestine present as a single tube Esophagus and stomach distinct Liver cords, ducts, and gallbladder forming Omental bursa forming Pancreatic buds appear as outpouching of gut
5-6	8.0-12.0	Intestine elongates into a loop and rotates Stomach rotates Parotid and submandibular buds appear
7	17.0	Circular muscle layer present Duodenum temporarily occluded Intestinal loops herniate into cord Villi begin to develop
8	23	Villi lined by single layer of cells Small intestine coiling within cord Taste buds appear Microvilli short, thick, and irregularly spaced Lysosomal enzymes detected
9-10	30-40	Auerbach's plexus appears Intestine reenters abdominal cavity Crypts of Lieberkühn develop Active transport of glucose appears Dipeptidases present Microvilli of enterocytes more regular and glycocalyx present Mitochondria numerous below microvilli

Adapted from Arey, L.B.: Developmental anatomy: a textbook and laboratory manual of embryology, ed. 7, Philadelphia, 1965, W.B. Saunders Co.

covered by four layers of stratified epithelia; however, by the seventh week of intrauterine life, villi begin to form in the duodenum and proximal jejunum. The duodenum becomes occluded with rapidly growing cells but becomes recanalized once again by the ninth to tenth week of intrauterine life. Although similar, rapid proliferation occurs distal to the duodenum, the lumen of the rest of the small intestine does not become totally occluded. Characteristically, during intestinal ontogenesis, differentiation and maturation progress from the proximal to the distal portions of the digestive system. Villi are present in the jejunum by 9 weeks and in the entire small intestine by 14 weeks' gestation, at which time they are lined by a single layer of cells with centrally placed nuclei. Primitive crypts of Lieberkühn begin to appear by 10 to 12 weeks, and by 19 weeks of gestation, well-developed villi and crypts are found even in the ileum. The enterocytes develop microvilli by 8 to 10 weeks of intrauterine life. These are initially short and irregularly spaced, demonstrate different stages of maturity, and have a partially developed glycocalyx. By the tenth week of intrauterine life the microvilli are regular, and many mitochondria are present beneath the microvilli. The structures resembling lysosomes are not yet present, although enzymes that are usually contained within lysosomes are readily detected. The microvilli have core microfilaments present, and these tend to be well developed by 12 weeks of intrauterine life. The crypt cells have less well defined microvilli and tend to lag behind the development of the cells of the villi, but mature as they progress up the villus. Many of these cells have ribosomes but decreased amounts of smooth and rough endoplasmic reticulum.

CELLULAR PROLIFERATION

Most of the data on cellular proliferation are obtained from animals, and very few data are available in humans. In the adult the turnover time for a cell of the crypt to reach the tip of the villus is approximately 48 to 72 hours. In the suckling animal, however, this rate of migration is

Table 24-1. Development of the human gastrointestinal tract—cont'd

Age (weeks)	Crown-rump length (mm)	Stage of development
12	56	Parietal cells present in stomach Muscular layers of intestine present Alkaline phosphatase and disaccharidases detectable Active transport of amino acid present Mature taste buds present Enterochromaffin cells appear Pancreatic islet cells appear Bile secretions begin Colonic haustra appear Coelomic extension into umbilical cord obliterated
13-14	78-90	Meissner's plexus appears Circular folds appear Peristalsis detected Lysosomes detected ultrastructurally
16	112	Pancreatic lipase and tryptic activity detected Meconium present Lymphopoiesis present Peptic activity present
20	160	Peyer's patches present Muscularis mucosa present Mesenteric attachments complete Zymogen granules present and well developed in pancreas
24	200	Paneth's cells appear Maltase and sucrase and alkaline phosphatase very active Ganglion cells detected in rectum Amylase activity present
28	240	Lactase activity increasing Esophageal glands present
32	270	Circular folds present Hydrochloric acid found in stomach
34	290-300	Sucking and swallowing become coordinated Esophageal peristalsis rapid, nonsegmental contraction occurs
36-38	320-350	Maturity of GI tract achieved

markedly decreased; the rate of migration in the young rat may be two or three times longer than that of the adult. The infant villi are decreased in length as compared with those in the adult animal; the crypts are shallow, and the mitotic index is also decreased. At the time of weaning, cellular migration and proliferation increase rapidly and even exceed the values of adults. There are very few data for human neonates, but the rate of cellular migration and proliferation may be decreased as well. Studies of the small intestine of stillborn infants or of infants expiring soon after birth reveal broad villi that are shorter than those found in the adult and crypts that are not as deep as those found in the older child or adult. These factors may explain the clinical impression that there is a delay in healing after a severe insult to the intestine of the infant as compared with that of the adult. The activities of enzymes involved in pyrimidine biosynthesis, thymidine kinase, dihydroorotase, aspartate transcarbamylase, and uridine kinase correlate well with the rate of cellular proliferation and migration in animals.

ENZYMATIC DEVELOPMENT

In the human intestine the activity of alkaline phosphatase, adenosine triphosphatase (ATPase), and aminopeptidase is present in the 7- to 8-week fetus. These enzymes are active in the ileum from about the fourteenth week onward, and by 23 weeks of gestation all of these enzymes are very active. The disaccharidases are detectable in very low activity in the 12- to 14-week fetus. The activities increase rapidly so that by 24 weeks of gestation these enzymes have reached significant levels of activity. The activity of lactase, although detectable in early fetal life, seems to lag behind the development of the other disaccharidases. Often the increase in lactase activity is not detected until 28 to 30 weeks of gestation. Although preterm babies may have low activity of lactase, lactose intolerance is an uncommon clinical problem.

In suckling animals the activity of sucrase, isomaltase, maltase, and alkaline phosphatase may be affected by steroids and thyroxine. The effects of these and other stimuli have not been evaluated in the human fetus or infant. In human adults the activity of the α-glucosidases is affected by the type of carbohydrate ingested, demonstrating that these enzymes may be altered by diet. However, it appears that lactase is an enzyme that cannot be altered by dietary manipulation. In animals, the activity of lactase seems to be greatest around the time of birth and decreases during weaning to reach very low levels in adulthood. In humans a similar developmental pattern probably occurs so that in various populations the activity of lactase is very low by the time the child reaches 4 to 5 years of age. Studies in Nigeria revealed that infants in that area tend to lose lactase activity by the time they are 12 to 13 months old, whereas studies in American blacks and American Indians demonstrate that the activity decreases at the age of 5 years. Many adults, especially those of Scandinavian and English descent, tend to retain the activity of lactase throughout their adult lives.

A variety of dipeptidases are present and active beginning at 11 or 12 weeks of gestation. The activities of these enzymes seem to increase slowly. The dipeptidases and total proteolytic enzymes of the fetal intestine are active by the second trimester of gestation.

Cells in the crypts tend to mature as they migrate onto the villus. The activities of the peptidases, disaccharidases, and alkaline phosphatase increase markedly as the cell migrates onto the villus. However, the various lysosomal enzymes tend to remain unchanged. The factors that affect or alter enzymatic activity as the cell migrates up the villus are not understood at this time.

PANCREATIC ENZYMES

Zymogen granules are well developed in fetal acinar cells by 20 weeks' gestation. Lipase, which is detectable in the 16- to 18-week fetus, increases in activity by 28 weeks. After birth there is an increase in the activity of this enzyme, which continues during the first 9 months of life. However, there is an adequate quantity of lipase present to hydrolyze fat in the term infant.

Amylase activity is detectable by 22 weeks of gestation. It increases during gestation but remains low in activity even after birth. Fetal pancreatic amylase has been detected in amniotic fluid as early as 16 weeks of intrauterine life. Although the baseline level of pancreatic amylase is low in the neonate, the activity can be increased markedly following the infusion of secretin-pancreozymin. Tryptic activity is also detectable early, at approximately 16 weeks of gestation, and increases markedly after 28 weeks. If enterokinase is added, marked activity of trypsin can be achieved even at 24 weeks of gestation. The activity of enterokinase is first detected at 26 weeks; at term it is 20% of that of older children.

FUNCTIONAL DEVELOPMENT OF THE INTESTINE
Protein absorption

There is controversy about whether the human fetus and newborn can absorb whole protein (antibodies) intact. If any protein is absorbed intact, it occurs by pinocytotic activity; and studies in subhuman primates suggest that the ileum is the major site capable of absorbing proteins intact.

It is known that breast-fed infants have a much lower incidence of intestinal and respiratory tract infections than do formula-fed infants. This is probably not a result of intestinal absorption of intact immunoglobulins but rather the many host resistance factors that are present in human colostrum and milk that prevent the overgrowth and attachment of various bacteria and viruses to the enterocytes. The fetal intestine is able to transport amino acids readily, and this ability does not seem to change during development. In the fetus, as in the adult, dipeptides and tripeptides are absorbed and subsequently hydrolyzed more rapidly than are amino acids. The activities of the pancreatic proteolytic enzymes and of the intestinal peptidases are adequate for the digestion and absorption of protein in most prematurely born infants. However, in the immature infant of 28 weeks or less the activities of the proteolytic enzymes are such that incomplete protein hydrolysis may occur, and protein malabsorption may result.

Fat absorption

Lipid can be absorbed from the intestine of a 12-week-old human fetus and is accomplished by pinocytosis. Data from studies in premature infants indicate that the intraluminal phase of lipid absorption is not completely developed, and these infants absorb most fats poorly. The preterm infant secretes lingual as well as pancreatic lipase, but even at term the infant possesses only 10% to 20% of the lipase activity found in older children. However, the limiting factor in lipolysis in premature infants appears to be the decreased pool and rate of biosynthesis of bile acids. There is a possibility that the rate of absorption of bile acids in the terminal ileum may also be decreased. The biosynthesis of bile acids increases rapidly over the first several months of extrauterine life. Interestingly, if a mother has received either phenobarbital or steroids just prior to parturition, the bile acid pool and rate of synthesis of these compounds increase markedly.

The concentration of bile acids in duodenal secretions

correlates well with the infant's capability to absorb lipid when fed various formulas. However, the preterm infant absorbs vegetable fats very well and the fats found in human milk almost completely, even in the absence of adequate concentrations of bile acids. The presence of naturally occurring lipases in human milk facilitates the absorption of fats in these preterm infants, and processing of the milk by pasteurization or sterilization inactivates these lipases.

An intracellular intestinal protein that binds unsaturated fatty acids more readily than saturated fatty acids has been characterized. The role of the protein in fat absorption during development must be investigated to understand fully the deficiencies of fat absorption in the preterm infant.

Carbohydrate absorption

Except for lactase, the activities of the other disaccharidases are adequate for digestion of their respective sugars by 24 to 28 weeks of gestation. In studies using breath hydrogen analysis as a measure of carbohydrate malabsorption, most preterm and even some term infants have been found to have lactose malabsorption for several weeks after delivery. Such malabsorption is usually of little clinical significance even in the most immature infant because the amount of milk that they can ingest is limited. In addition, lactose behaves as a natural laxative in infants who often have poor intestinal motility and is important in the diet of preterm infants because it facilitates the absorption of calcium.

Except in the case of lactose, the rate-limiting step in carbohydrate absorption is the ability of the infant's intestine to transport glucose rapidly. The fetal intestine can transport glucose aerobically and anaerobically by 10 to 12 weeks of gestation. By the second trimester the intestine can transport glucose only under aerobic conditions, but the transport capabilities increases over the first year of the infant's life. Even at 12 months of age, the K_m for glucose absorption is approximately 5.8 mmol, whereas in the adult it is 20 mmol or more.

Despite the decreased activities of intestinal lactase and pancreatic amylase and the decreased capability of the intestine of the preterm infant to transport glucose readily, carbohydrate malabsorption is not a major clinical problem even in the immature infant. Obviously, if feedings contain large quantities of starch or lactose or if the intestine is damaged from hypoxia or ischemia, carbohydrate malabsorption may become a major clinical problem.

Development of motility

The factors involved in the motility of the GI tract also develop in a craniocaudal manner. Auerbach's plexus is detectable by 9 weeks of gestational age, and Meissner's plexus by 13 weeks. The muscular layers of the intestine and colonic haustra appear by 12 weeks of gestation. The muscularis mucosae is present at 20 weeks, and the normal distribution of ganglion cells is found in the 24-week fetus, at which time the cells have reached the rectum. The ganglion cells progress from an apolar neuroblast to a bipolar stage and eventually to a multipolar stage. There is a gradual and steadily progressive maturation of ganglia from early embryonic life throughout childhood. Early immaturity of the cells is physiologic, and maturation takes place gradually over the first several years of life.

Swallowing occurs in the human fetus such that by 16 to 17 weeks of intrauterine life the fetus swallows 2 to 7 ml of amniotic fluid every 24 hours. By 20 to 21 weeks this is increased to 16 ml per day, and at term the infant swallows approximately 450 ml of amniotic fluid per day. Although there is marked variation, the coordination of sucking and swallowing is not well developed before 34 weeks of gestation (Chapter 21).

Esophageal motility also is poorly developed in the preterm infant, and there is poor coordination in response to deglutition, rapid peristaltic waves, and simultaneous nonperistaltic contractions along the entire length of the esophagus. The lower esophageal sphincter pressures are also decreased. Gastric emptying time is delayed and may be related to the amount of hydrochloric acid the infant can secrete. After delivery, gastric emptying time is greatly influenced by the infant's position. As the fetus matures, there is an increased rate of GI motility. Contrast material reaches the cecum of the 32-week premature infant in 9 hours, and of the term infant in 4 to 7 hours. The immature muscular layers of the GI tract, the incoordination of peristaltic waves, the increased numbers of antiperistaltic waves, and possibly decreased hormonal secretions all may lead to the prolonged transit time encountered in the preterm infant. We have noted that preterm infants rarely pass meconium in utero even when subjected to severe asphyxia, whereas term and postterm infants pass meconium readily, even if the asphyxial episode is brief. Preterm infants, especially those with respiratory distress, have an absent or impaired rectosphincteric reflex and behave similarly to patients with Hirschsprung's disease. Many of these infants act as if they have a functional obstruction.

Development of immunologic function

Lymphopoeisis is present in the 15-week-old fetus (Chapter 26), and Peyer's patches are well developed by 20 weeks of intrauterine life. The patches increase in size and number and reach a plateau by the time the child is 10 years of age.

In utero there is a lack of stimulation and an absence of local immune response in both premature and term infants. Soon after birth, term infants develop local immunity with a secretory immunoglobulin-A response.

Little response occurs for about 14 days, but by 28 days after delivery almost 100% of term infants will demonstrate secretory antibodies. Prematurely born infants develop a less effective immune response to oral stimulation. In addition, many other local host defense mechanisms of the GI tract may not function well in the preterm infant, and thus penetration of sensitizing antigens, bacteria, and viruses may result.

Summary

The GI tract is capable of adapting readily to extrauterine life by 36 to 38 weeks of gestation. The activity of the various enzymes, the ability to transport nutriments, and the ability to respond to antigenic stimuli are present in the term infant. In the preterm infant, however, the GI tract may not have reached full functional capacity. This may make the preterm infant vulnerable to the development of necrotizing enterocolitis, enteric infections, and GI malfunction, and to delayed growth or development. Following is an outline of factors that interfere with normal gastrointestinal function in preterm infants:

A. Poor coordination of sucking and swallowing
B. Incompetent gastroesophageal sphincter
C. Delayed gastric emptying time
   1. Decreased gastric acidity (?)
   2. Decreased pepsinogen production
D. Decreased absorption of fat
   1. Decreased bile acid production
   2. Decreased micellar formation
E. Incomplete digestion of protein
F. Decreased activity of lactase (transitory)
G. Decreased or poorly coordinated GI motility
H. Decreased secretions of immunoglobulins and decreased immunologic response
I. Decreased rate of cellular proliferation and migration

Philip Sunshine
Frank R. Sinatra
Charles H. Mitchell
Thomas V. Santulli

BIBLIOGRAPHY
General

Anderson, C.M., and Burke, V.: Paediatric gastroenterology, Oxford, 1975, Blackwell Scientific Publications, Ltd.

Bloom, S.R., editor: Gut hormones, London, 1978, Churchill-Livingstone.

Gryboski, J.: Gastrointestinal problems in the infant, Philadelphia, 1975, W.B. Saunders Co.

Koldushy, O.: Digestion and absorption. In Stave, U., editor: Perinatal physiology, ed. 2, New York, 1978, Plenum Medical Book Co.

Roy, C.C., Silverman, A., and Cozzetto, F.J.: Pediatric gastroenterology, ed. 2, St. Louis, 1975, The C.V. Mosby Co.

Development

Aaronson, I., and Nixon, H.H: A clinical evaluation of anorectal pressure studies in the diagnosis of Hirschsprung's disease, Gut 13:138, 1972.

Arey, L.B.: Developmental anatomy: a textbook and laboratory manual of embryology, ed. 7, Philadelphia, 1965, W.B. Saunders Co.

Auricchio, S., Rubino, A., and Mürset, G.: Intestinal glycosidase activities in the human embryo, fetus and newborn, Pediatrics 35:944, 1965.

Bernfield, M.R.: Developmental mechanisms of congenital malformations: biological and clinical aspects of malformations, Mead Johnson Symp. Perinat. Dev. Med. 7:14, 1976.

De Belle, R.C., and others: Intestinal absorption of bile salts: immature development in the neonate, J. Pediatr. 94:472, 1979.

Deren, J.J.: Development of intestinal structure and function. In Code, C.F., editor: Handbook of physiology, vol. 3, Baltimore, Md., 1968, Waverly Press, Inc.

Ferguson, A., Maxwell, J.D., and Carr, K.E.: Progressive changes in the small intestinal villous pattern with increasing length of gestation, J. Pathol. 99:87, 1969.

Grand, R.J., Watkins, J.B., and Torti, F.M.: Development of the human gastrointestinal tract: a review, Gastroenterology 70:790, 1976.

Ito, Y., Donahoe, P.K., and Hendren, W.H.: Maturation of the rectoanal response in premature and perinatal infants, J. Pediatr. Surg. 12:477, 1977.

Johnson, J.D., Kretchmer, N., and Simoons, F.J.: Lactose malabsorption: its biology and history, Adv. Pediatr. 21:197, 1974.

Katz, L., and Hamilton, J.R.: Fat absorption in infants of birth weight less than 1300 gm, J. Pediatr. 85:608, 1974.

Kelley, R.O.: An ultrastructural and cytochemical study of developing small intestine in man, J. Embryol. Exp. Morphol. 29:411, 1973.

Koldovský, O.: Development of the functions of the small intestine in mammals and man, Basel, Switzerland, 1969, S. Karger.

Koldovský, O., Sunshine, P., and Kretchmer, N.: Cellular migration of intestinal epithelia in suckling and weaned rats, Nature (London) 212:1389, 1966.

Lev, R., and Orlic, D.: Uptake of protein in swallowed amniotic fluid by monkey fetal intestine in utero, Gastroenterology 65:60, 1973.

Lindberg, T.: Intestinal dipeptidases: characterization, development and distribution of intestinal dipeptidases of the human foetus, Clin. Sci. 30:505, 1966.

MacLean, W.C., Jr., and Fink, B.B.: Lactose malabsorption by premature infants: magnitude and clinical significance, J. Pediatr. 97:458, 1980.

McLain, C.R., Jr.: Amniography studies of the gastrointestinal motility of the human fetus, Am. J. Obstet. Gynecol. 86:1079, 1963.

Ockner, R.K., and Manning, J.A.: Fatty acid-binding protein in small intestine: identification, isolation and evidence for its role in cellular fatty acid transport, J. Clin. Invest. 54:326, 1974.

Petit, J.C., Ealinha, A., and Salomon, J.C.: Immunoglobulins in the intestinal content of the human fetus with special reference to IgA, Eur. J. Immunol. 3:373, 1973.

Sunshine, P., and others: Adaptation of the gastrointestinal tract to extrauterine life, Ann. N.Y. Acad. Sci. 176:16, 1971.

Walker, W.A.: Host defense mechanisms in the gastrointestinal tract, Pediatrics 57:901, 1976.

Watkins, J.B., and others: Bile-salt metabolism in the newborn: measurement of pool size and synthesis by stable isotope technique, N. Engl. J. Med. 288:431, 1973.

Younoszai, M.K.: Jejunal absorption of hexose in infants and adults, J. Pediatr. 85:446, 1974.

PART TWO
Gastrointestinal emergencies

INTESTINAL OBSTRUCTION
See also p. 501.

Prenatal factors

Certain characteristics of prenatal and family history frequently will help identify neonates who are at increased risk to develop GI obstruction. The most important of these factors is polyhydramnios. Neonates with upper GI obstruction are unable to ingest and absorb an appropriate amount of amniotic fluid, and this results in maternal polyhydramnios. Although maternal factors, such as toxemia and diabetes mellitus, and fetal disorders, such as multiple gestation and anencephaly, also can be associated with polyhydramnios, all neonates with excessive amounts of amniotic fluid should be observed carefully for evidence of esophageal atresia or obstruction of the proximal intestine. Esophageal patency should be confirmed by the passage of a nasogastric tube. A family history of cystic fibrosis also may help identify neonates at increased risk for intestinal obstruction. In addition to meconium ileus, neonates with cystic fibrosis have an increased incidence of intestinal atresia. Familial occurrence of multiple intestinal atresias as well as Hirschprung's disease also has been described.

Clinical manifestations

Lesions of the GI tract producing intestinal obstruction can be divided into high and low lesions, depending on the level of obstruction. A high GI obstruction is considered to exist when the lesion is proximal to the midportion of the jejunum. These disorders are characterized by the early onset of vomiting. The vomitus is colorless in lesions proximal to the ampulla of Vater, such as pyloric atresia and some cases of duodenal obstruction, but is bile stained and alkaline with more distal lesions. The presence of bilious vomiting in a neonate is always abnormal; although it may be caused by nonsurgical disorders, such as sepsis, it must always be regarded as a surgical lesion until proved otherwise. A very early sign of obstruction that may even precede the onset of vomiting is the finding of a gastric aspirate that is either bile stained or present in excess of the normal 15 ml. Abdominal distension may not be marked in proximal obstruction and is often confined to the epigastric region. Massive distension can be seen, however, in high intestinal obstruction following perforation.

Low lesions causing GI obstruction often will have delayed onset of vomiting, which is usually preceded by progressive abdominal distension. The distension may be massive even in the absence of perforation and is greatest in the more distal lesions. The vomiting is almost always bilious and may have a fecal odor. In addition to abdominal distension and vomiting, newborns with distal intestinal obstruction often have little or delayed passage of meconium. Delayed passage of meconium occasionally may be seen in nonsurgical disorders, such as sepsis, prematurity, maternal narcotic administration, hypothyroidism, and hypermagnesemia.

Physical examination of a neonate with intestinal obstruction may provide important clues to the cause of obstruction. Infants with Down's syndrome have an increased incidence of both duodenal atresia and Hirschprung's disease. The presence of an abdominal mass in addition to signs of obstruction may indicate meconium ileus, malrotation with midgut volvulus, or intestinal duplication. The classic auscultatory findings associated with intestinal obstruction in older children and adults are not found in neonates, and bowel sounds may be either absent, normal, or hyperactive. Abdominal wall tenderness, induration, and erythema usually indicate that peritonitis has developed as a complication of perforation. Careful examination of the perineum and genitalia also may reveal the cause of obstruction in cases of anorectal anomalies or incarcerated inguinal hernias.

Laboratory manifestations

Roentgenographic studies of the abdomen provide the most important diagnostic information in the evaluation of a neonate with suspected intestinal obstruction. The initial abdominal roentgenograms should include supine, upright, and lateral decubitus views (Chapter 39). In proximal lesions, these studies are usually sufficient to define the level of obstruction. Air normally reaches the colon by 8 hours of age; however, in cases of intestinal obstruction air is absent distal to the area involved. In duodenal obstruction dilatation of both the stomach and the first or second portion of the duodenum produces the "double bubble" sign (Fig. 24-1). Although this finding is usually associated with duodenal atresia, it also may be seen with any lesion causing duodenal obstruction, such as malrotation, annular pancreas, or a preduodenal portal vein. High jejunal obstruction will have a few additional loops of dilated bowel with air-fluid levels. Contrast studies of the upper GI tract are not indicated in cases where the roentgenograms reveal clear evidence of high intestinal obstruction and are necessary only in patients with incomplete upper intestinal obstruction.

Numerous loops of dilated bowel with air-fluid levels suggest distal small intestinal or colonic obstruction and indicate the need for a barium examination of the rectum and colon. Contrast studies of the colon will determine the position of the cecum in cases of suspected malrotation and will help define the level of obstruction by showing either a normal or unused colon. An unused colon ("microcolon") is seen with obstructions of the distal

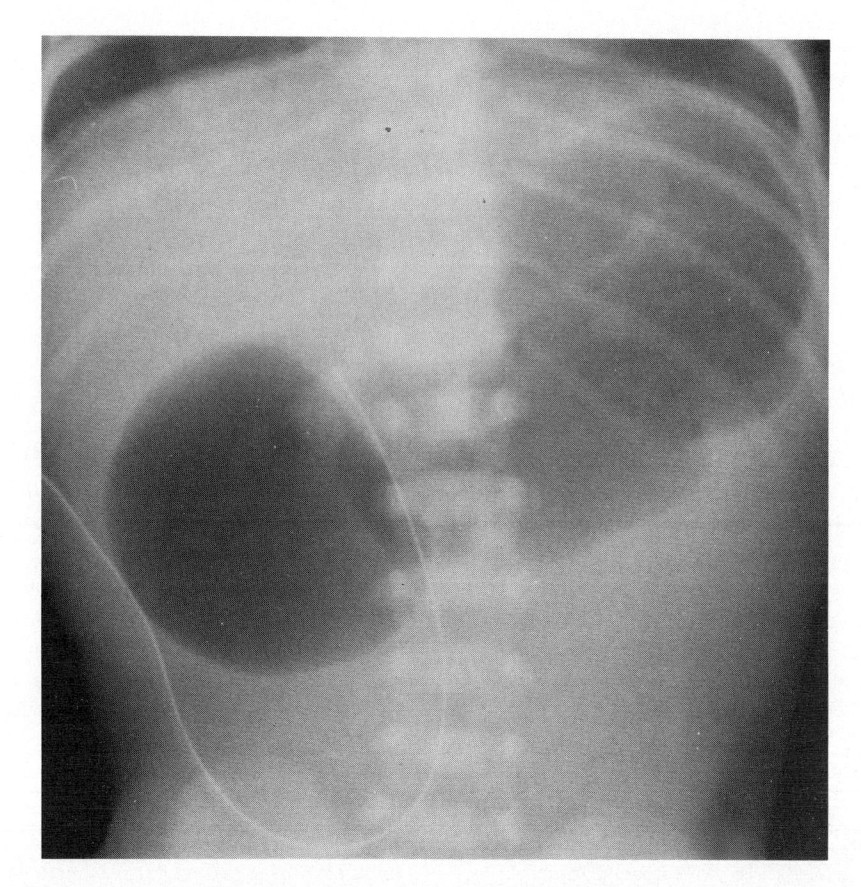

Fig. 24-1. Newborn with duodenal atresia: large air-filled stomach and duodenum, the "double bubble" sign, and absence of intestinal gas throughout the remainder of the abdomen.

small bowel, such as ileal and distal jejunal atresias or meconium ileus. In addition, the characteristic features of meconium plug syndrome or Hirschsprung's disease may be seen at the time of the lower bowel contrast study. Calcifications in abdominal roentgenograms of a neonate with intestinal obstruction indicate that meconium was present in the peritoneal cavity at some time in the past and are most often seen in association with ileal atresia.

The infant with suspected intestinal obstruction should be evaluated in a carefully organized manner to definitely establish the presence of a surgical lesion before operation. If the roentgenographic studies indicate a high intestinal obstruction, intraperitoneal calcifications, malrotation, or the presence of a microcolon, the decision to operate is not difficult. Problems arise, however, in the infant with evidence of low intestinal obstruction in whom the barium enema is interpreted as being normal, demonstrating a meconium plug syndrome or Hirschsprung's disease. In each of these instances a mucosal biopsy of the rectum may be indicated. The presence of ganglion cells in the submucosa will eliminate the diagnosis of Hirschsprung's disease and perhaps save the infant from an unnecessary colostomy.

Treatment

Once a neonate is suspected of having intestinal obstruction, all feedings are immediately discontinued and the bowel is decompressed by means of a nasogastric tube. This not only decreases further distension of the stomach but also prevents aspiration of GI contents. The infant's fluid and electrolyte status must be carefully monitored, with both maintenance and replacement requirements given by intravenous infusion. It is also essential to replace the fluid and electrolytes lost during gastric suctioning to prevent severe hypokalemic, hypochloremic alkalosis. Once the patient is medically stable, surgery should be performed. The unique group of disorders encountered in this age group demands the skill of an experienced pediatric surgeon. Morbidity and mortality are markedly increased by delays in diagnosis and treatment because of increased rates of perforation, peritonitis, and GI ischemia.

A useful classification of the causes of obstruction is shown in the following outline.

A. Mechanical (occlusive)
   1. Congenital
      a. Intrinsic
         (1) Atresia and stenosis
         (2) Meconium ileus
         (3) Hypertrophic pyloric stenosis
         (4) Meconium plug syndrome
      b. Extrinsic
         (1) Malrotation (with or without midgut volvulus)
         (2) Segmental volvulus (without malrotation)
         (3) Peritoneal bands
         (4) Incarcerated hernia—inguinal, diaphragmatic, internal
         (5) Annular pancreas
         (6) Duplication
         (7) Meconium peritonitis
   2. Acquired
      a. Intrinsic
         (1) Intussusception
         (2) Milk curd obstruction
      b. Extrinsic
         (1) Adhesions—bacterial peritonitis, after bowel perforation, postoperative
B. Nonmechanical (nonocclusive)
   1. Congenital
      a. Neurogenic
         (1) Congenital aganglionosis
      b. Functional
         (1) Prematurity
         (2) Unknown
   2. Acquired
      a. Neurogenic—paralytic ileus from cerebral injury
      b. Functional
         (1) Infection
         (2) Peritonitis—bowel perforation
         (3) Respiratory distress syndrome
         (4) Maternal drugs
         (5) Metabolic—electrolyte, hormonal

GASTROINTESTINAL PERFORATION AND PERITONITIS

Perforation of the GI tract with the subsequent development of peritonitis is a lethal complication of neonatal GI disease leading to an overall mortality exceeding 80%. Although perforation may occur anywhere in the GI tract and is seen in several clinical situations, the mode of presentation and subsequent course are similar regardless of location or etiology.

Pathogenesis and clinical manifestations

GI perforation may occur prenatally or at any time following birth. Most cases of intrauterine perforation are caused by distal intestinal obstruction due to atresia, meconium ileus, or volvulus. Meconium escapes into the peritoneal cavity and induces a severe chemical peritonitis followed by calcification of the meconium. Soon after birth the infant develops signs and symptoms of intestinal obstruction. Meconium is sterile during intrauterine life but rapidly becomes colonized with bacteria following birth. Continued intraperitoneal leakage of meconium in the neonatal period through an unsealed perforation will result in a bacterial as well as chemical peritonitis. In the neonate, peritonitis rapidly becomes generalized because of the infant's limited ability to effectively "wall off" the inflammatory processes.

Postnatal perforation of the GI tract is also most commonly the result of an underlying intestinal obstruction. In addition to the usual signs of intestinal obstruction, the diagnosis often is suggested by massive, rapidly developing abdominal distension. The abdomen becomes uniformly tympanitic to percussion, and the normal area of liver dullness is lost. Distension is often so severe that respirations become compromised and dyspnea and cyanosis develop. The diagnosis is made by abdominal roentgenograms that demonstrate the presence of free intraperitoneal air (Fig. 24-2).

Although intestinal obstruction is the most common cause, it accounts for less than 50% of the reported cases of GI perforation in the neonatal period. Iatrogenic causes, such as rectal perforation following the use of thermometers, enemas, and sigmoidoscopes as well as colonic perforations following exchange transfusion, have been reported. Perforations also are seen as a complication of necrotizing enterocolitis and following GI surgery when anastomotic or stomal leaks occur.

In almost 25% of patients with neonatal GI perforation, no identifiable underlying cause is found. These so-called spontaneous GI perforations present a remarkably similar clinical picture. Typically the infant has been asphyxiated at birth, often in association with severe maternal complications. The infant may then develop signs of intestinal perforation at any time during the first 2 weeks of life. The most widely accepted theory of pathogenesis is that there is selective ischemia of the GI tract following an episode of asphyxia. During periods of hypoxemia, blood supply is normally shunted away from less vital areas, such as the GI tract, and preferentially maintained in the brain and myocardium. Spasm of intramural arterioles results in ischemic necrosis and subsequent perforation. The majority of "spontaneous" perforations of the GI tract occur in the stomach and are usually found along the anterior margin of the greater curvature. For many years the perforation was thought to be secondary to a muscular defect in the wall of the stomach, but recent evidence suggests an ischemic process. Gastric perforation is a particularly lethal form of intesti-

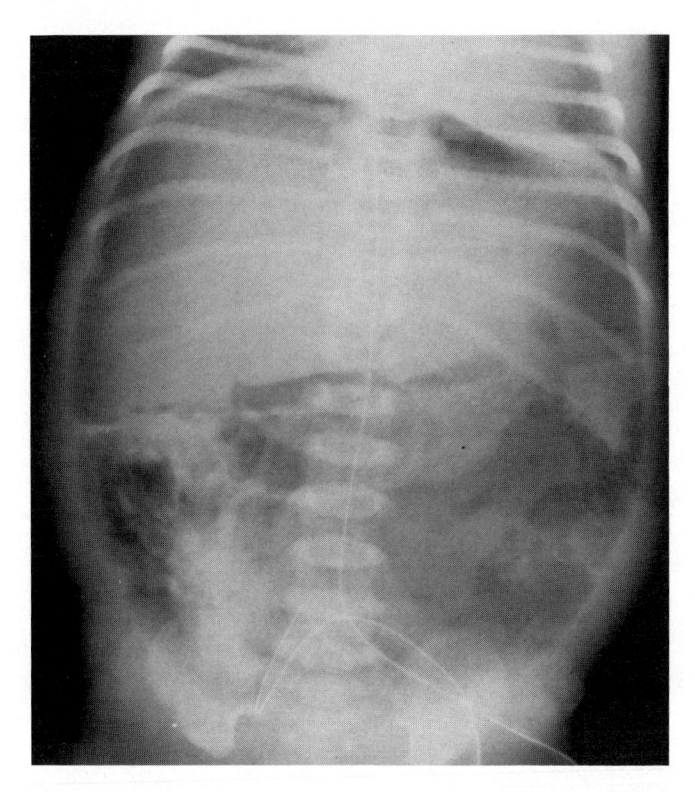

Fig. 24-2. Newborn with perforation of stomach. Roentgenogram of abdomen taken in supine position demonstrating pneumoperitoneum, with air outlining the liver.

nal perforation because of the added insult of hydrochloric acid spillage into the peritoneal cavity. The infants develop severe abdominal distension, respiratory distress, and often profound shock.

Treatment

Regardless of etiology, therapy is similar. Abdominal decompression by nasogastric suction and correction of fluid and electrolyte abnormalities must be initiated immediately. Often blood, plasma, or albumin must be infused to correct hypovolemia and shock. Appropriate cultures are obtained and parenteral therapy with antibiotics started. In patients where massive abdominal distension results in respiratory compromise, emergency intraabdominal decompression by means of a paracentesis tube attached to an underwater seal may be necessary. Surgical exploration and repair should be performed as soon as possible. Survival rates are decreased when surgery is delayed for more than 12 hours following the onset of symptoms. This is especially true in infants with gastric perforation. At surgery a careful search should be made for multiple sites of perforation and areas of stenosis or atresia. The use of a gastrostomy is of great help in the postoperative management of these infants.

GASTROINTESTINAL HEMORRHAGE

Although GI bleeding in the neonate may be massive and the cause often undetermined, the overall prognosis is good in an otherwise healthy infant. The diagnostic possibilities differ from those encountered in older children; therefore the approach to therapy is somewhat modified.

Pathogenesis and clinical manifestations

Over 50% of neonates who present with GI bleeding have no identifiable cause (Fig. 24-3). The typical infant is often an apparently normal newborn who develops GI bleeding between the first and fourth days of life. The amount of bleeding is severe enough to require transfusion in over half the infants in this group. Roentgenographic and hematologic evaluation fails to reveal a cause for the bleeding, and spontaneous remission without recurrence is the rule. The mortality in this group is extremely low as long as adequate blood replacement and monitoring are provided during the acute period. Although stress ulcerations of the stomach or duodenum are thought to be responsible for much of the bleeding, the actual etiology remains speculative.

Vomiting of bright red blood during the first day of life is frequently due to swallowed maternal blood. The rapid transit time seen in newborns, however, also may result in hematochezia. Confirmation of the origin of such bleeding may be made by performing the Apt test, in which fetal hemoglobin appears pink and adult hemoglobin brown after exposure to 1.0 ml of a 0.25M solution of sodium hydroxide. The test cannot be performed on tar-

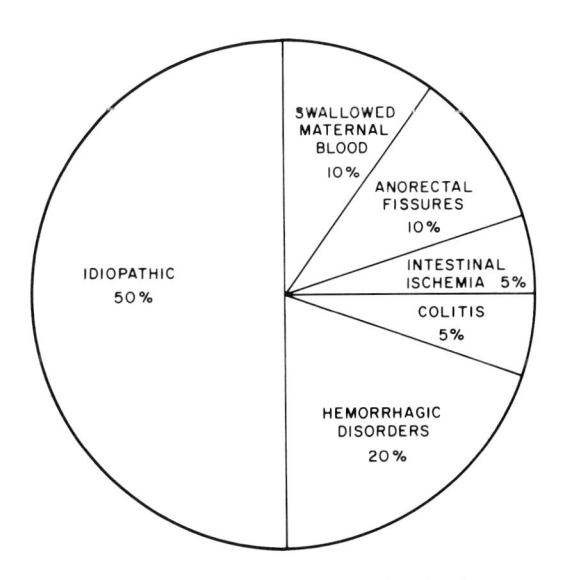

Fig. 24-3. Common causes of GI bleeding in the neonate.

ry stools in which the conversion of oxyhemoglobin to hematin has already taken place.

Coagulopathies secondary to hemorrhagic disease of the newborn may present as GI bleeding and require parenteral therapy with vitamin K. Other bleeding disorders such as disseminated intravascular coagulation and congenital coagulation defects also may cause hematemesis or hematochezia in the neonate. The presence of superficial bleeding into the skin or prolonged bleeding at venipuncture sites often will alert the physician to these disorders.

Anorectal fissures are common causes of bright red rectal bleeding or blood-streaked stools. The amount of blood lost is small, and transfusions are not required. The lesion is easily demonstrated on careful proctoscopic examination.

Gross or occult blood is often present in the stools of neonates with various disorders associated with GI ischemia. The majority of these conditions accompany other signs and symptoms, which aid in their recognition. Malrotation with midgut volvulus, intussusception, and intestinal duplications may cause rectal bleeding, but the predominant findings are usually those of intestinal obstruction or an abdominal mass. Likewise, necrotizing enterocolitis often is associated with rectal bleeding but is usually accompanied by abdominal distension, diarrhea, lethargy, and pneumatosis intestinalis.

Various forms of colitis may cause bloody diarrhea in the neonate. Common entities included in this group are infectious colitis especially that caused by enterotoxigenic *E. coli*, and the colitis associated with cow's milk or soy protein allergy. Rare instances of chronic ulcerative colitis with onset in the neonatal period also have been reported. Appropriate cultures and proctoscopic examination will distinguish this group from other patients with rectal bleeding. On rare occasions a breast-fed infant may have gastrointestinal bleeding secondary to factors in the mother's diet, the most common of which is cow's milk. Removal of the offending substance from the mother's diet is all that is needed to alleviate the symptoms.

Common causes of GI hemorrhage in older infants and children, such as Meckel's diverticulum, polyps, and esophageal varices, are extremely rare in the newborn period.

Treatment

Initial therapy in a neonate with GI bleeding consists of restoring the circulating blood volume and providing adequate tissue perfusion. These are usually accomplished by the administration of fresh whole blood or fresh frozen plasma or both. Careful monitoring of fluid, electrolyte, and hematologic status as well as quantitation of ongoing blood loss will prevent many of the complications of both shock and postinfusion hypervolemia. With severe bleeding this monitoring may require the insertion of a central venous catheter to more accurately estimate fluid requirements. If the hematologic evaluation reveals defective coagulation, appropriate replacement is started immediately. These studies are especially important in neonates with evidence of bleeding elsewhere. A nasogastric tube is inserted and periodically irrigated to observe for the presence of upper GI bleeding. Stool should be examined for the presence of white blood cells and tested for maternal and occult blood.

Improvements in fiberoptic endoscopy with the development of smaller caliber instruments now makes it possible to perform esophagoscopy and gastroscopy even in preterm neonates. Endoscopy may be performed safely in the newborn intensive care unit without anesthesia. As expertise increases with this technique, the number of infants with "idiopathic" upper GI hemorrhage, as well as the number of infants undergoing laparotomy for superficial ulceration or gastritis, will decrease.

The incidence of surgically correctable lesions in the absence of signs of obstruction, necrotizing enterocolitis, or an abdominal mass is very low in this age group. Careful physical examination and abdominal roentgenograms are usually sufficient to rule out the majority of these disorders. Even when massive, most instances of GI hemorrhage in a neonate without other GI symptoms will stop spontaneously following adequate supportive care. In patients with uncontrolled, continuing hemorrhage, however, laparotomy is often necessary. Such intervention should not be undertaken until an adequate trial of conservative therapy has failed. Significant morbidity and mortality have been reported in infants undergoing laparotomy for unexplained GI bleeding.

DIAPHRAGMATIC HERNIA

Division of the body cavity into its abdominal and thoracic components is normally completed between the eighth and tenth weeks of fetal life with the closure of the posterolateral portion of the diaphragm. Failure to close this pleuroperitoneal canal, or foramen of Bochdalek, results in the most common form of congenital diaphragmatic hernia. These hernias involve the left leaf of the diaphragm in over 75% of cases and generally occur without a true hernial sac. Herniated GI contents consist of stomach and both large and small bowel; liver, spleen, kidney, and pancreas also may be found. Since herniation may occur before the tenth fetal week when normal rotation of the gut takes place, incomplete rotation with band formation is seen in up to 60% of the cases. Other associated anomalies include cardiac defects, such as patent ductus arteriosus and coarctation of the aorta, and Meckel's diverticulum. In addition, the herniated viscera interfere with normal growth and differentiation of the lung buds, resulting in pulmonary hypoplasia on the involved side. The severity of pulmonary hypoplasia is dependent on the amount of herniated viscera; it tends to be increased with left-sided defects, since in general the degree of herniation is greater on the left. The presence of the liver may limit the degree of herniation in right-sided defects.

Clinical manifestations

The onset and severity of symptoms usually depend on the amount of herniated abdominal contents. The neonate may be extremely ill at birth, may develop symptoms after the first days of life, or may remain asymptomatic until later in infancy or childhood. Those infants with symptoms immediately after birth often require resuscitation, have severe respiratory distress, and are often in respiratory failure with hypoxemia, hypercarbia, and severe acidosis. Instead of improving with assisted ventilation, the infant's condition will worsen as air begins to fill the herniated loops of bowel, causing the mediastinum to shift further to the unaffected side of the thorax, compressing the contralateral lung. The maximal cardiac impulse is shifted to the side opposite the hernia. Breath sounds are absent over the involved side and, as the disease progresses, may become decreased over the uninvolved side as well. The abdomen is scaphoid, and the normal abdominal respirations are replaced by rocking thoracic respiratory efforts. The diagnosis is confirmed by roentgenograms of the chest, which reveal gas-filled bowel within the pleural space (Fig. 24-4). Barium contrast studies are seldom necessary in the neonatal period.

The infants who do not immediately develop symptoms appear normal at birth and may not have any respi-

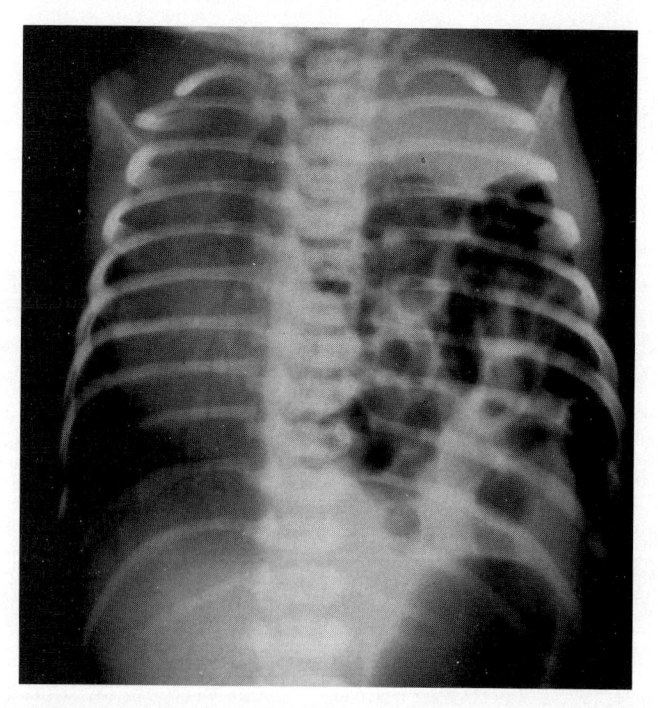

Fig. 24-4. Neonate with left-sided posterolateral diaphragmatic hernia (Bochdalek type) showing air-filled loops of bowel in the left hemithorax and shifting of the mediastinal structures to the right.

ratory distress for several days. This usually occurs when the hernia is on the right and the liver prevents the other abdominal viscera from herniating into the thorax. Often the infants are thought to have pneumonia, segmental collapse of the lung, a pleural effusion, or multiple lung cysts. Roentgenograms of the chest are usually adequate for diagnosis, but on occasion, fluoroscopic examination is necessary to document absence of the normal diaphragmatic excursion. When this condition is diagnosed later in childhood, it is often discovered by incidental or routine roentgenographic examination.

Treatment

Once the diagnosis is suspected, nasogastric decompression should be initiated immediately in an attempt to limit the amount of distension of the herniated bowel. Following roentgenographic confirmation, every effort should be made to reduce the herniated viscera as soon as possible. In those infants who demonstrate respiratory distress soon after birth, assisted ventilation is almost always required, and care must be taken to use the minimum amount of pressure necessary to establish effective perfusion and ventilation and yet avoid causing a pneumothorax in the contralateral lung. Although appropriate measures to improve ventilation and to correct acidosis and hypoxia should be instituted in preparation for surgery, any unnecessary delay in surgical intervention will serve to increase morbidity and mortality. It is difficult to establish effective ventilation or to correct the severe respiratory and metabolic acidosis until surgical reduction has been accomplished. However, it is imperative that the surgery be performed in a center where the patient can receive optimum postoperative management, and thus surgery might have to be delayed until the infant is transported to such a center. Surgery is generally accomplished through an abdominal incision that also allows correction of any associated anomalies, such as intestinal malrotation. One should not attempt to expand the ipsilateral hypoplastic lung beyond its state of development, since it will only lead to alveolar rupture and subsequent air leaks. A ventral silon pouch or secondary closure of the fascia and peritoneum may be necessary in patients when primary closure would result in increased intraabdominal pressure or in compromised blood supply to the liver or GI tract.

Postoperatively, continuous intercostal catheter suction is maintained until the pleural cavity is fully obliterated. Continuous intestinal decompression usually by gastrostomy helps prevent the complications of vomiting, aspiration, and insults to the respiratory tract. Despite prompt and effective therapy, most of the infants who develop distress immediately after birth will continue to have respiratory failure with poor ventilation and perfusion of their "normal lung." Pulmonary hypertension and shunting of blood from right to left through the foramen ovale, the patent ductus arteriosus, or both, are encountered frequently. The vasculature of this supposedly normal lung has been found to be abnormal, and the resultant pulmonary hypertension has been difficult to manage. A pulmonary vasodilator, such as tolazoline, has been used as an adjunct in the postoperative management of these infants. Initial reports noting the success of such treatments have been followed with reports that tolazoline has not been as effective as anticipated. The use of prostaglandins (PGE_1) as an adjunct in attempting to decrease pulmonary vascular resistance has been advocated as well. However, PGE may maintain the patency of the ductus arteriosus and lead to congestive heart failure, especially if fluid management is not precise. Thus ligation of the ductus arteriosus may also be necessary. Previously, attempts to manage patients with diaphragmatic hernias by prophylactically ligating the patent ductus arteriosus at the time of the initial surgery were not successful, since the patients often developed intractable right-sided heart failure. With the use of PGE, this approach to therapy will have to be reevaluated. In addition, ventilator therapy with very rapid rates (100 to 150 per minute) and very low pressures with short inspiratory times has been effective in the management of these infants (p. 566). Recently the use of extracorporeal membrane oxygenation has been associated with an increased rate of survival in these infants (p. 437).

Prognosis

Mortality in the neonatal period continues to be very high, especially if the infant develops symptoms soon after birth. Patients with the combination of severe hypoxia, right-to-left shunting, and pulmonary hypertension have had a consistently poor outcome. However, with the use of pulmonary vasodilators and appropriate ventilatory management the survival rate should improve significantly.

Other sites of herniation

Although rarely obvious in the newborn period, intestinal herniation through the esophageal hiatus or Morgagni's foramen occurs. Small defects in closure of the pleuroperitoneal folds may result in hernias as well. Small defective areas of the diaphragm closed by only pleura and peritoneum may serve as a hernial sac, producing localized eventrations.

Eventration of the diaphragm

This defect is caused by incomplete development of the diaphragm wherein the pleural and peritoneal layers are present, but the muscular layer between them is absent or dysplastic. The diaphragm does not function and is easily stretched, and abdominal viscera can ascend into the hemithorax. The eventration can occur on either side, but partial defects are more common on the right and complete eventration is more common on the left side. Often other congenital malformations are present as well. The phrenic nerve is usually intact, but stimulation of the nerve does not cause contraction of the diaphragm because of the absence of the muscle layer.

Approximately half of the patients have symptoms of respiratory distress and cyanosis in the neonatal period. Symptoms that occur later include recurrent respiratory tract infections, wheezing, and dyspnea. Symptoms relating to the GI tract occur more commonly when the eventration is on the left side.

Roentgenograms of the chest will usually demonstrate the smooth elevation of the hemidiaphragm, but fluoroscopic examination may be necessary to document the paradoxical movement of the diaphragm.

In asymptomatic patients with small defects, no treatment is needed. In patients with large defects or in those who are symptomatic, plication of the diaphragm is indicated. Occasionally a prosthesis may have to be used to correct a large defect.

Philip Sunshine
Frank R. Sinatra
Charles H. Mitchell
Thomas V. Santulli

BIBLIOGRAPHY

Allen, M.S., and Thomson, S.A.: Congenital diaphragmatic hernia in children under one year of age: a 24-year review, J. Pediatr. Surg. **1**:157, 1966.

Boles, E.T., Schillia, M., and Weinberger, M.: Improved management of neonates with congenital diaphragmatic hernias, Arch. Surg. **103**:344, 1971.

Collins, D.L., and others: A new approach to congenital posterolateral diaphragmatic hernia, J. Pediatr. Surg. **12**:149, 1977.

Dibbins, A.W.: Neonatal diaphragmatic hernia: a physiologic challenge, Am. J. Surg. **131**:408, 1976.

Emanuel, B., Zlotnick, P., and Raffensperger, J.G.: Perforation of gastrointestinal tract in infancy and childhood, Surg. Gynecol. Obstet. **146**:926, 1978.

Fonkalsreed, E.W., Ellis, D.G., and Clatworthy, H.W., Jr.: Neonatal peritonitis, J. Pediatr. Surg. **1**:127, 1966.

Franken, E.A.: Gastrointestinal bleeding in infants and children: radiologic evaluation, J.A.M.A. **229**:1339, 1974.

Grob, M.: Intestinal obstruction in the newborn infant, Arch. Dis. Child. **35**:40, 1960.

Grosfeld, J.L., and Ballantine, T.V.M.: Esophageal atresia and tracheoesophageal fistula: effect of delayed thoracotomy on survival, Surgery **84**:394, 1978.

Holder, T.M. and Ashcraft, K.W.: Congenital diaphragmatic hernia. In Ravitch, M.M., and others, editors: Pediatric surgery, ed. 3, Chicago, 1979, Year Book Medical Publishers, Inc.

Lloyd, J.R.: The etiology of gastrointestinal perforations in the newborn, J. Pediatr. Surg. **4**:77, 1979.

Mulligan, D.W.A., and Levison, H.J.: Lung function in children following repair of tracheoesophageal fistula, J. Pediatr. **95**:23, 1979.

Naeye, R.L., and others: Unsuspected pulmonary vascular abnormalities associated with diaphragmatic hernia, Pediatrics **58**:902, 1976.

Schwalb, E., Coryllos, E., and Wrener, M.: Ischemic intestinal perforation in newborns: management of multiple ileal perforations following intrapartum shock, Clin. Pediatr. **10**:30, 1971.

Sherman, N.J., and Clatworthy, H.W., Jr.: Gastrointestinal bleeding in neonates: a study of 94 cases, Surgery **62**:614, 1967.

Shields, R.: The absorption and secretion of fluid and electrolytes by the obstructed bowel, Br. Med. J. **52**:774, 1965.

Simpson, J.S.: Ventral silon pouch: method of repairing congenital diaphragmatic hernias in newborns without increasing intra-abdominal pressure, Surgery **66**:798, 1969.

Spencer, R.: Gastrointestinal hemorrhage in infancy and childhood: 476 cases, Surgery **55**:718, 1964.

Stanley-Brown, E.G., and Stevenson, S.S.: Massive gastrointestinal hemorrhage in the newborn infant, Pediatrics **35**:482, 1965.

Stauffer, U.G., and Rickham, P.P.: Acquired eventration of the diaphragm in the newborn, J. Pediatr. Surg. **7**:635, 1972.

Wayne, E.R., and others: Eventration of the diaphragm, J. Pediatr. Surg. **9**:643, 1974.

PART THREE

Gastrointestinal disorders

DISORDERS OF SUCKING AND SWALLOWING

Although the sucking response has been elicited by the sixteenth week of intrauterine life and the fetus has been documented to swallow at about the same time during development, the ability of the fetus to coordinate and integrate sucking, swallowing, and breathing is not well developed until 33 to 34 weeks of gestation (p. 335). Significant individual variation exists in the onset of this coordinated mechanism, which usually persists until the infant is about 6 months of age. When first fed, the mature infant will have short bursts of 3 to 5 sucks followed by single swallows. After the first day or two, the sucking pattern evolves to consist of 10 to 30 sucks followed by swallowing; in this mature response the lips and jaws exert pressure on the nipple and, combined with negative intraoral pressure, bring milk into the mouth. The dorsum of the tongue is elevated against the soft palate to form a seal preventing milk from entering the pharynx and also forcing milk that is in the posterior pharynx into the esophagus. At this point, the mouth is separated from the pharynx, and the infant can breathe during this phase of swallowing. The tongue then brings the milk to the back part of the pharynx; the muscles of the soft palate contract and bring the palate upward and backward to close the connection with the nose; the epiglottis closes the entry to the larynx; and together these mechanisms inhibit breathing. The tongue then comes forward, the epiglottis rises, and the infant can breathe once again. Once the milk passes the posterior pharynx into the esophagus, the pharyngoesophageal sphincter relaxes and then closes to initiate peristalsis in the esophagus. The normal esophageal peristaltic wave is large and monophasic, but in premature infants the wave may be

Table 24-2. Conditions associated with or causing disorders of sucking and swallowing

Absent or diminished suck	Mechanical factors interfering with sucking	Disorders of the swallowing mechanism (not including esophageal abnormalities)
Maternal anesthesia or analgesia	Macroglossia	Choanal atresia
Anoxia or hypoxia	Cleft lip	Cleft palate
Prematurity	Fusion of gums	Micrognathia
Trisomy 21	Tumors of mouth or gums	Postintubation dysphagia
Trisomy 13	Temporomandibular ankylosis or hypoplasia	Palatal paralysis
Hypothyroidism		Pharyngeal tumors
Neuromuscular abnormalities		Pharyngeal diverticula
Kernicterus		Familial dysautonomia
Werdnig-Hoffmann disease		
Neonatal myasthenia gravis		
Congenital muscular dystrophy		
Infections of the CNS		
Toxoplasmosis		
Cytomegalovirus infection		
Bacterial meningitis		

Adapted from Gryboski, J.: Gastrointestinal problems in the infant, Philadelphia, 1975, W.B. Saunders Co.

biphasic and there also may be nonperistaltic segmental contractions of the esophagus.

Although the infant has a well-developed and intricate mechanism for sucking and swallowing, when semisolid foods are first given, the infant will often force the foods back out of the mouth and not swallow them. Abnormalities of the sucking and swallowing reflexes occur in premature infants, may be secondary to maternal analgesia and anesthesia, may be found in infants who were anoxic or hypoxic at birth, or may be the first manifestation of central nervous system (CNS) disorders. Also, infants who have prolonged orotracheal or nasotracheal intubation will have transitory incoordination of sucking and swallowing. The conditions that are associated with or cause disorders of sucking and swallowing are listed in Table 24-2.

DISORDERS OF THE ESOPHAGUS

The esophagus develops from the foregut by 4 weeks of gestation, and by 7 weeks of intrauterine life has attained its normal position as the stomach has descended into the abdomen. By 13 weeks of intrauterine life, the longitudinal muscle layers and the muscularis mucosa are well formed, and the ganglion cells are differentiated, although they are not evenly distributed until 18 or 19 weeks of gestation. The epithelial lining is initially columnar and then becomes ciliated; by the fifth to sixth month of intrauterine life, stratified squamous epithelium is present. The esophagus is the only part of the digestive system that has neither digestive nor absorptive function; its role is to act as a conduit for food from the mouth to the stomach and to act as a barrier against gastric reflux. Also, the esophagus never acquires a true mesentery or serosa. Disorders of the esophagus in the neonate usually present with vomiting, dysphagia, choking, cyanosis, respiratory distress, or combinations of these signs.

Esophageal duplications and cysts

Esophageal duplications usually present as expanding posterior mediastinal masses and cause cyanosis and respiratory difficulties. As they enlarge, the infant has intermittent vomiting and discomfort with feedings or may develop recurrent episodes of pneumonia. The cysts usually have a muscular wall and are lined with ciliated or squamous epithelium. At times they are lined with gastric epithelium, which can cause esophagitis, bleeding, or erosion into a bronchus or lung. Abnormalities of the cervical or upper thoracic vertebrae, intrathoracic anomalies such as agenesis of a lung or tracheoesophageal fistulas, and intraabdominal cysts have been associated with these duplications. The diagnosis is almost always made roentgenographically with the aid of a barium swallow and with views of the patient in the lateral and oblique positions. The differential diagnosis should include bronchogenic cysts, tumors of neurogenic origin, teratomas, and abscesses. Treatment is surgical removal of the abnormality with care taken to search for communication with intraabdominal cysts.

Gastroesophageal reflux and esophageal dysmotility

Gastroesophageal reflux is a very common problem in newborns, especially in preterm babies. Normally, the distal esophagus possesses a physiologic sphincter called the esophageal vestibule, the proximal end of which lies in the thorax, the midportion in the esophageal hiatus of the diaphragm, and the distal end in the abdomen. It is

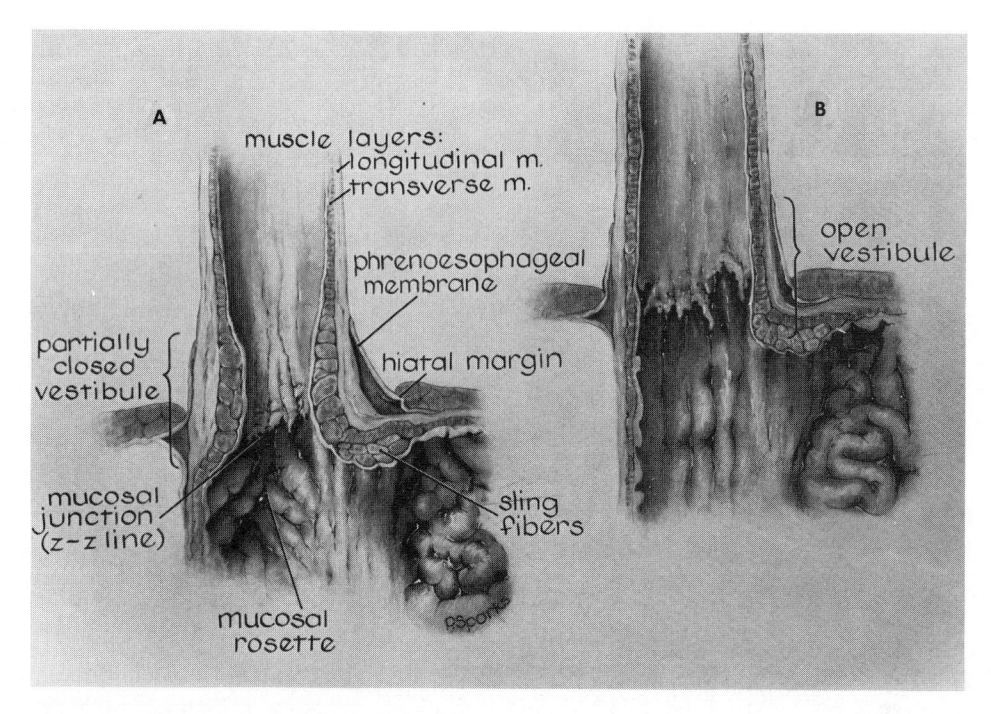

Fig. 24-5. Anatomy of the esophagogastric junction in infants and children. **A,** Vestibule partially closed. **B,** Vestibule open. (From Friedland, G.W., and others: Am. J. Roentgenol. Radium Ther. Nucl. Med. **120:**305, 1974.)

0.5 cm long in the infant, which is much shorter than the vestibule of older children and adults. The mucosa in this area is lined by columnar epithelium, which is resistant to acid-pepsin digestion, has no acid- or pepsin-secreting cells, and is firmly attached to the underlying muscle. The cuff of muscle enclosing the mucosa is joined to the diaphragm by the phrenoesophageal membrane. This cuff and the "mucosal choke" permit opening and closing of the vestibule and prevent retrograde flow of gastric contents into the esophagus (Fig. 24-5). This segment of terminal esophagus has a higher pressure than that of the stomach below and of the esophagus above. The lower esophageal sphincter (LES) pressure falls after deglutition, and the opening of the vestibule is related to deglutition and not necessarily to the stripping peristaltic wave of the esophagus. The vestibule opens from above downward and closes in the same manner, and both occur very rapidly in the infant. The interval between swallowing and the opening of the vestibule is very short (0.12-0.20 second) and increases with age so that it is 0.3 second at 2 years and 2.25 seconds at 11 years.

The LES pressure in term infants is usually less than 2.5 mm Hg. It remains low during the first 2 weeks and increases markedly between 2 and 4 weeks of age to reach adult pressure measurements by 1 to 2 months of age (5.6 ± 3 mm Hg). Because of lowered LES pressure, the prolonged relaxation of the sphincter, and the poor coordination of esophageal motility in the neonate, over 40% of normal infants will have some regurgitation of their feedings, which can be documented roentgenographically. The frequency of regurgitation is greater in preterm infants, and it may be several weeks to several months before the gastroesophageal sphincter is able to prevent regurgitation. Often those infants who have had prolonged orotracheal intubation for assisted ventilation have the greatest difficulty with reflux.

Persistent regurgitation, which leads to discomfort, poor weight gain, and/or aspiration, must be recognized and specific therapy must be initiated. There is a great deal of debate as to whether a patient with persistent regurgitation has gastroesophageal reflux (GER) or actually has a hiatal hernia. GER can occur in the absence of a roentgenographically demonstrable hiatal hernia and can also occur when the LES is normal. Thus documentation of GER becomes the important factor and not the absolute documentation of a concomitant hiatal hernia, which may or may not be roentgenographically or endoscopically evident. Since we believe that most, if not all, patients with significant GER have a hiatal hernia, we will discuss the problem from this biased point of view.

Hiatal hernia
Pathophysiology

In patients with a hiatal hernia, the vestibule is located in the thorax, and the ability of the "mucosal choke" to work effectively is markedly diminished (Fig. 24-6). Nor-

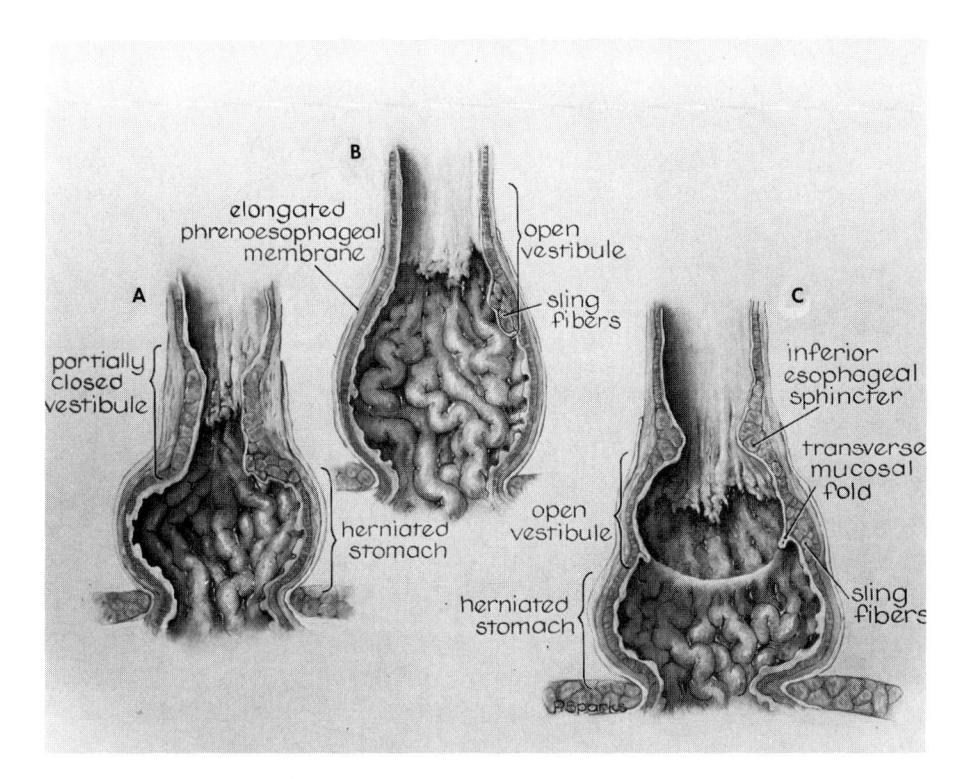

Fig. 24-6. Anatomy of a sliding hiatal hernia. **A,** Infant, vestibule closed. **B,** Infant, vestibule open. **C,** Adult, vestibule open, inferior esophageal sphincter contracted. The latter produces a rounded ring at the proximal end of the vestibule on an esophagram. The transverse mucosal fold forms a thin, ledgelike ring deformity at the distal end of the vestibule on an esophagram. These landmarks are rarely seen in infants and young children. (From Friedland, G.W., and others: Am. J. Roentgenol. Radium Ther. Nucl. Med. **120:**305, 1974.)

mally, when there is an increase in intraabdominal pressure from an exogastric source, as occurs in crying, the pressure is transmitted equally to the vestibule and to the stomach so that retrograde flow from the stomach to the esophagus is inhibited. When the vestibule is in the thorax, it lies in an area of lowered pressure and is subjected to greater opening forces so that free reflux can occur. Those patients with small hernias often will have the greatest difficulties with gastroesophageal reflux. In those patients with a large hiatus, there may be enough pressure on the phrenoesophageal membrane so that reflux is diminished.

Incidence and etiology

The incidence of hiatal hernia in infants is difficult to assess. For years, the incidence in the United States was reported to be much less than that reported in England and Canada. However, this difference was probably due to the fact that patients in the United States were not as carefully evaluated by cineradiography. As these techniques have been adopted in the United States, more infants with hiatal hernias are being recognized.

The etiology of the hernias is incompletely understood, but most authorities believe that it is a congenital anomaly. The shortened esophagus may be of developmental origin or may be secondary to esophagitis, scarring, or stricture formation.

Clinical manifestations

The symptoms of hiatal hernia are vomiting and, often, failure to thrive. Over 85% of the patients have onset of vomiting during the first week of life, and an additional 10% have the onset between the first and sixth week of age. Although many normal infants have some vomiting during infancy, the infants with hiatal hernia have persistent vomiting that may continue throughout the first 12 to 18 months of life. In infants and children the sliding type of hiatal hernia is the most common. Infants with hiatal hernias may have marked irritability, arching of their backs, and discomfort during feedings; in addition, some have torsion "spasms" of their head and neck. In the older infant or child, such torsion and bizarre posturing have been termed *Sandifer's syndrome*, which may be a reflex mechanism to alleviate the pain or spasm cre-

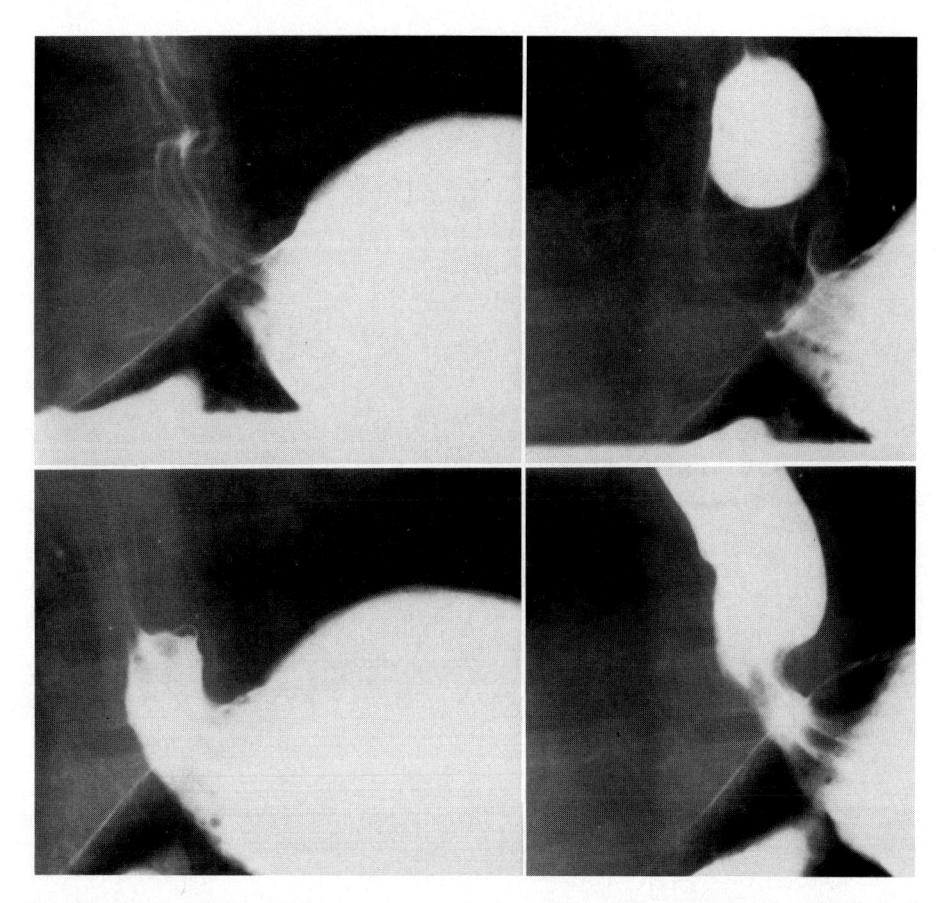

Fig. 24-7. Roentgenograms of patient with hiatal hernia. Herniated stomach is seen with thick rugal folds above the diaphragm. Lower right figure demonstrates the vestibule closing between the barium-filled esophagus above and herniated stomach below.

ated by the gastroesophageal reflux. Some patients also may develop secondary or reflex pylorospasm and have projectile vomiting that resembles pyloric stenosis (Roviralta's syndrome). A few patients have had exploratory surgery for pyloric stenosis, but either no pyloric tumor was found or pylorotomy did not decrease the vomiting. Such infants should be carefully evaluated for evidence of a hiatal hernia. Older infants and children may also demonstrate protein-losing enteropathy, clubbing of fingers, unremitting asthma, or the "rumination syndrome."

Laboratory manifestations

Because the opening and closing of the vestibule are very rapid in infants, routine fluoroscopy is a poor technique by which to document hiatal hernia. A cineesophagram on videotape or a 70-mm camera should be used to evaluate the gastroesophageal junction. Also, the infant should be examined in the flat, upright, and Trendeleburg positions. The diagnosis is made when the vestibule is found in the thorax and when it closes with the barium-filled esophagus above and the herniated tubular-like pouch of the stomach below. The diaphragm also may compress the stomach at the hiatus as the stomach slides from the abdomen to the thorax, and the stomach may be visualized (numerous thickened folds having a rugal appearance are seen in the thorax). If the infant is given barium by bottle and nipple, the infant usually will cry when the nipple is removed and thus increase the abdominothoracic pressure difference. The hernia often is seen at this time and gastroesophageal reflux visualized (Fig. 24-7). An esophageal stricture also will be recognized.

As an adjunct to the cineesophagrams, gastroesophageal scintiscan using technetium (^{99m}Tc) sulfur colloid has been used to document GER. Even the most experienced radiologists using both the scintiscan and cineesophagrams will detect less than two thirds of patients with GER. The use of the acid reflux test (Tuttle and Grossman test) has proved to be the most valuable and precise technique to document GER in infants and children, especially if continuous monitoring of the distal esophageal pH is carried out over a 4- to 24-hour period. A very small caliber tube, to which a pH electrode is attached, can be passed into the distal esophagus and can remain in position for long periods with minimal, if any, discomfort to the patient.

The diagnosis of esophagitis has been documented by radiographic techniques, but endoscopic examination and biopsy are probably superior to cineesophagrams in confirming the diagnosis.

Complications include stricture formation secondary to esophagitis, anemia secondary to chronic blood loss, and pulmonary infection secondary to vomiting and aspiration.

Treatment

The medical management includes maintaining the infant in an upright position during and following feedings; some infants must be maintained in at least a 60-degree upright position during most of the 24 hours. An infant seat can be used to keep the infant upright, or the parent can carry the infant about in a Snugli (Fig. 24-8). Feedings thickened with cereals may help a great deal. The use of antacids is controversial but has been of help in certain infants. We prefer to use the antacids containing alginic acid, especially during the time that the infant has upper or lower respiratory tract infections, because at these times the infant swallows a great deal and reflux occurs more frequently.

Surgery is reserved for patients who continue to vomit a great deal and fail to gain weight appropriately after a 2- to 3-month course of medical management. Severe anemia, continued blood loss, and the development of strictures are other indications for surgery. Gastropexy has been used with success in some infants, but the Nissen fundoplication should be used in those infants with severe disease or complications. Future roentgenographic evaluation may be facilitated if a clip is placed at the gastroesophageal junction.

Prognosis

Medical treatment in over 75% of the patients will completely correct their difficulties; another 10% to 15% of the patients will require prolonged medical management, and 10% to 15% will require surgery. Although 85% to 90% of the patients respond to medical management, follow-up studies of these infants reveal that one third to one half still have roentgenographic evidence of the hernia at a time that they are asymptomatic. Roentgenography following surgery reveals that the hernia is corrected in most cases. However, the LES pressure is unchanged from preoperative values.

Chalasia

Most patients with chalasia probably have a sliding hiatal hernia. Carré found that patients with hiatal hernia or partial thoracic stomach outnumber infants with chal-

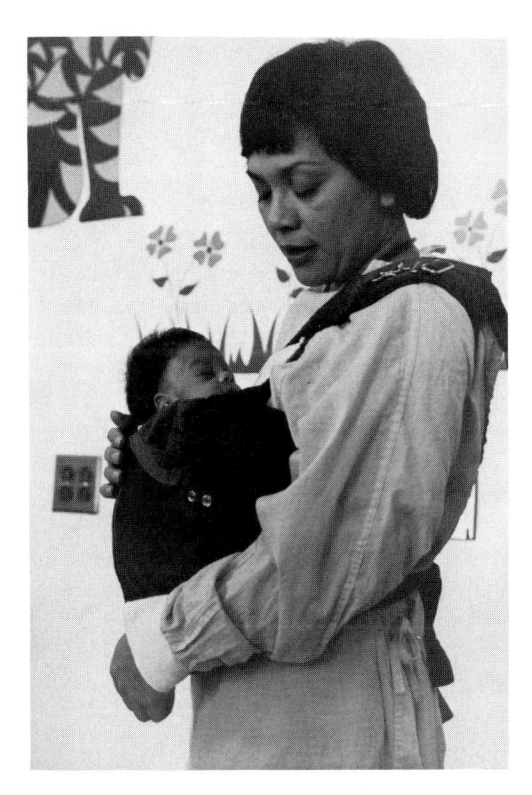

Fig. 24-8. Infant with hiatal hernia being maintained in an upright position with the use of a Snugli.

asia 14 to 1. The diagnosis of chalasia is made when gastroesophageal reflux is demonstrated, but the hernia is not visualized roentgenographically. A number of infants with free gastroesophageal reflux have CNS abnormalities such as mental retardation, spastic diplegia, or quadriplegia. Infants with urinary tract infection or chronic renal disease also often show this form of "secondary chalasia." Treatment is the same as outlined for hiatal hernia.

Achalasia is characterized by failure of the lower esophageal sphincter to relax with deglutition. It is extremely rare in infants and is thought to be secondary to either congenital absence or degeneration of the ganglion cells in Auerbach's plexus. Symptoms usually result from megaesophagus and do not become evident until later childhood or early adult life.

Familial dysautonomia (Riley-Day syndrome) may be the cause of uncoordinated sucking and swallowing, with pooling of secretions in the pharynx. Esophageal dysmotility is present, especially when the infant or child is in the supine position. Other portions of the intestinal tract may demonstrate dysmotility as well. The patients also may have hypotonia, excessive salivation, labile blood pressure, postural hypotension, absent or decreased lacrimation, decreased sensation to pain and taste, and blotching of the skin. The diagnosis often can be made in the neonatal period because of absence of the circumvallate papillae of the tongue. Also, the patients do not demonstrate a normal skin flare and wheal when histamine is injected intradermally.

Neonatal esophageal rupture (Boerhaave's syndrome)

Esophageal rupture is an extremely rare catastrophe in the neonate. The usual history is that of a normal full-term infant who has vomiting and becomes dyspneic and cyanotic. There may be a history of intubation. Feedings tend to increase the respiratory distress. A roentgenogram of the chest shows a tension pneumothorax or hydropneumothorax and filamentous ringlike areas on the side of the pneumothorax. Thoracentesis reveals serosanguineous fluid; often milk will be present if the infant has been fed. Pneumomediastinum is not commonly found. The treatment is immediate surgical repair, and at operation, longitudinal tears with ragged or friable edges are encountered. Usually the rupture will occur into the right pleural cavity, an area not supported by the aorta. Despite vigorous therapy, the mortality is still close to 40%, and esophageal stricture may develop in surviving infants.

Vascular rings

See Chapter 25.

Although vascular rings and anomalies of the aortic arch produce symptoms related to the respiratory tract, they may, on occasion, produce dysphagia. This is especially true of infants with an anomalous subclavian artery. Barium swallow will demonstrate the indentations on the esophagus, especially if observed in the lateral views. Surgical correction of the lesion is usually undertaken when respiratory problems are encountered.

Esophageal atresia and tracheoesophageal fistula
Incidence and etiology

The incidence of these defects is approximately 1 in 3,000 live births, and there is no sex predilection. The etiology is unknown, but it is speculated that the defects may be caused by vascular abnormalities, with reduced blood supply to areas of the foregut, which then become atretic. The development of the anomaly appears to take place between the fourth and sixth week of intrauterine life. The various types and the frequency of the abnormalities are demonstrated in Fig. 24-9. About one third of the infants with tracheoesophageal fistula weigh less than 2,500 gm, and two thirds of these are thought to be small for gestational age. More than 50% of the infants who have associated cardiovascular abnormalities weigh less than 2,500 gm at birth. Polyhydramnios occurs in many mothers of affected infants; the incidence varies from 14% to 90%.

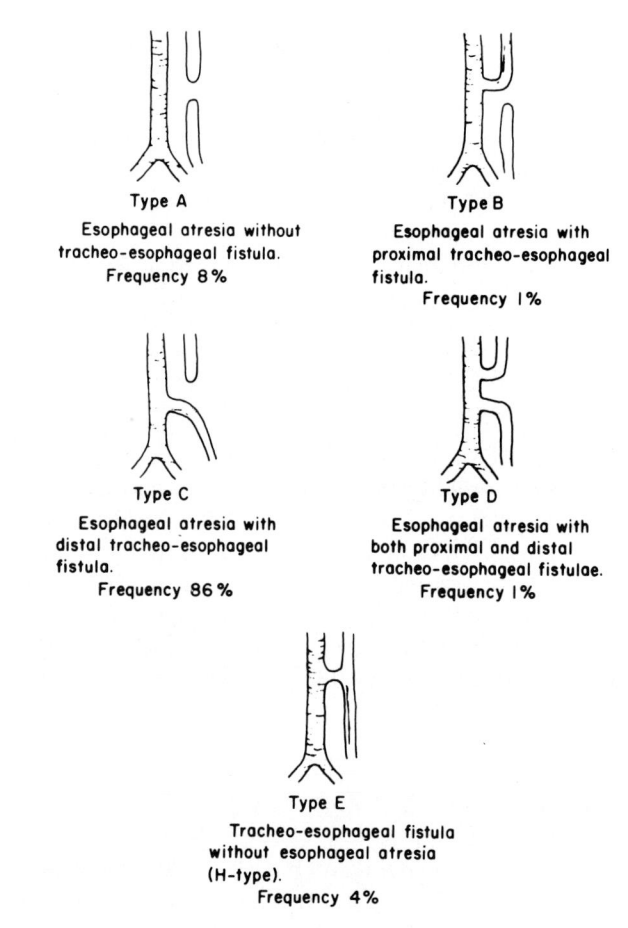

Fig. 24-9. Tracheoesophageal anomalies: type and incidence.

Type A — Esophageal atresia without tracheo-esophageal fistula. Frequency 8%
Type B — Esophageal atresia with proximal tracheo-esophageal fistula. Frequency 1%
Type C — Esophageal atresia with distal tracheo-esophageal fistula. Frequency 86%
Type D — Esophageal atresia with both proximal and distal tracheo-esophageal fistulae. Frequency 1%
Type E — Tracheo-esophageal fistula without esophageal atresia (H-type). Frequency 4%

Clinical manifestations

The appearance of polyhydramnios should suggest the possibility of an upper GI obstruction in the neonate, especially in low birth weight infants. Although the infant may appear well at birth, increased secretions and mucus are soon present in the upper airway. The infant may have coughing or choking or become cyanotic, especially after a feeding. True regurgitation is not found because forceful vomiting is not possible when the esophagus and stomach are not connected. After feedings with water or formula these materials will run out of the mouth. Some abdominal distension occurs as air passes from the trachea into the stomach, especially during crying episodes. In those infants with esophageal atresia but without fistula formation, the abdomen is scaphoid. Examination of the chest reveals rhonchi, rales, or even decreased breath sounds if segments of the lung are collapsed. Pulmonary damage occurs as gastric secretions reflux up the lower esophageal segment into the respiratory tree.

The diagnosis can be made readily by passing a radiopaque catheter via the nose into the pouch. In most

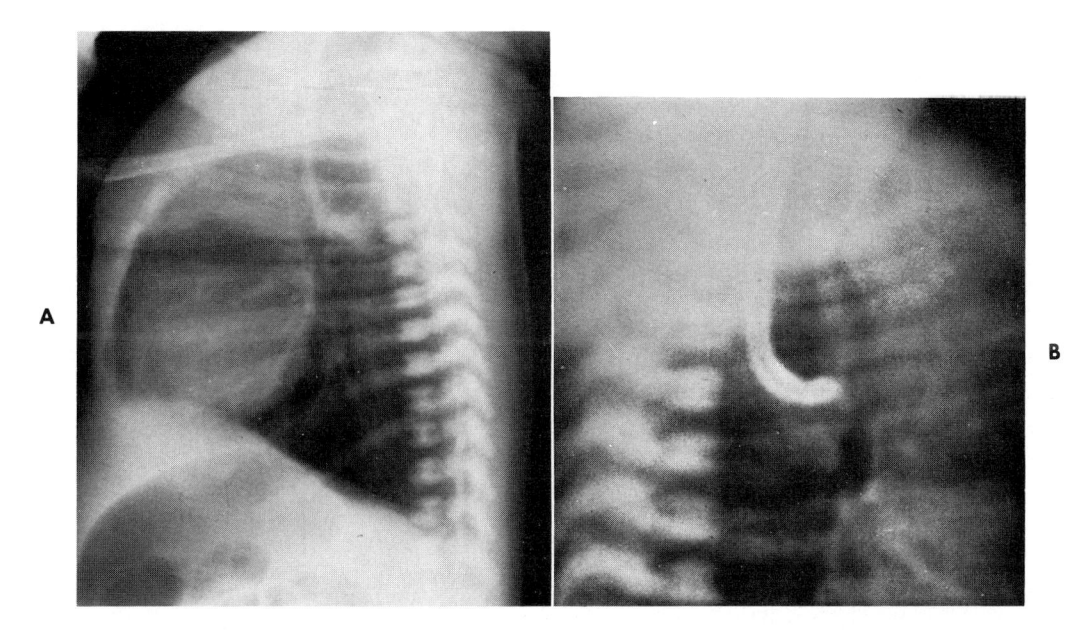

Fig. 24-10. Esophageal atresia and distal tracheoesophageal fistula. **A,** Roentgenogram of chest taken in the lateral position reveals blind air-filled esophageal pouch. **B,** Radiopaque catheter is seen curled in the blind esophageal pouch.

cases, resistance will be met, and aspiration reveals contents that are alkaline and not acidic. Occasionally, the catheter will curl on itself, and no resistance is felt. We have experienced situations where, following a cesarean section, the nasogastric tube curled in the esophageal pouch, and 15 to 30 ml of amniotic fluid was removed. In most situations, roentgenograms of the chest reveal the catheter curled in the esophagus (Fig. 24-10), and there is almost never a need to instill radiopaque material such as barium or a water-based contrast material into the esophagus to make the diagnosis. Occasionally, the latter material may have to be used to demonstrate a proximal-type fistula, but it should be instilled via a tube in place under fluoroscopy and with the infant in the prone position. After the study, the material should be removed.

Associated anomalies are listed in Table 24-3. These data are based on a study of the Surgical Section of the American Academy of Pediatrics. Several other series have demonstrated different incidences of associated anomalies, but the most common are GI (20%-40%), congenital heart disease (19%-35%), and genitourinary (10%-50%).

Treatment

Surgical repair is the treatment of choice, and with experienced pediatric surgeons the survival rate has increased markedly. Careful attention paid to details of preoperative and postoperative management is imperative. The infant must be kept in thermoneutrality, given appropriate antimicrobial agents, kept in a semi-Fowler

Table 24-3. Abnormalities associated with esophageal atresia and tracheoesophageal fistula

Abnormality	Incidence
Low birth weight	33%
GI anomalies	22%
Imperforate anus (9.3%)	
Intestinal atresia	
Malrotation	
Meckel's diverticulum	
Congenital heart disease	19%
Atrial septal defect	
Patent ductus arteriosus	
Ventricular septal defect	
Anomalies of pulmonary or aortic valves	
Coarctation of aorta	
Genitourinary anomalies	10%
Musculoskeletal anomalies	8.5%
Anomalies of the face	5%
CNS anomalies	3.3%

Adapted from Holder, T.M., and others: Esophageal atresia and tracheoesophageal fistula, Pediatrics **34:**642, 1964.

position to lessen gastroesophageal reflux, and have the upper pouch suctioned to prevent aspiration. Adequate oxygenation, ventilatory support, and infusion of appropriate fluids and electrolytes are mandatory. Postoperative support, especially with parenteral nutrition, also has lessened morbidity and mortality.

Initial surgical management consists of a gastrostomy with the infant under general or local anesthesia after the pulmonary status and overall condition are stable. A delayed extrapleural thoracotomy is performed with ligation of the fistula and, if possible, reanastomosis of the esophagus. In infants with esophageal atresia without fistulas, the distance between the upper and lower segment may be too great for approximation. Several techniques have been used to manage these patients. The first is to exteriorize the upper pouch, perform a gastrostomy, and later attempt to bring the ends together. If this is not possible, interpositioning of a segment of colon may be necessary. Another technique used is to leave the upper pouch intact and attempt to stretch it with the use of mercury bougies to elongate the upper esophageal segment.

Complications and prognosis

With early recognition and institution of prompt and effective therapy, the prognosis has greatly improved. Factors that have an adverse effect include prematurity and its complications, severe pulmonary disease, and other severe congenital malformations. Over 85% of infants weighing more than 2,500 gm will survive. Almost all will survive in this weight group if no other major abnormalities or pneumonitis is present. Survival in preterm infants has increased from 15% to over 70% in some series. Late complications of the disease include leaking at the site of anastomosis, stricture formation, recurrence of fistulas, dysmotility of the lower esophageal segment, hiatal hernia, and unilateral diaphragmatic paralysis.

Recent evaluations of pulmonary function in long-term survivors suggest a high incidence of abnormal pulmonary function thought to result from recurrent aspiration secondary to gastroesophageal reflux.

Tracheoesophageal fistula without atresia

The H-type fistula (type E) is rare; it usually occurs as a single fistula but may have more than one tract. The diagnosis is often difficult to make but should be suspected in an infant who has repeated episodes of coughing, choking, bouts of pneumonia, or persistence of a collapsed pulmonary segment. The diagnosis is made roentgenographically; a tube is placed in the stomach, filled with an oily contrast material, and gradually withdrawn while the infant is prone. Lateral views will demonstrate the fistula, which usually runs cephalad from esophagus to trachea.

Diagnosis can also be made at bronchoscopy, during which time methylene blue is introduced into the esophagus. The subsequent appearance of the dye in the trachea will identify the site of the fistula. Often the fistula can be repaired surgically through the neck.

DISORDERS OF THE STOMACH

The stomach develops from the foregut and is distinct by the fourth week of intrauterine life. By the seventh week it has descended into the abdomen and has elongated and rotated in such a manner as to attain its mature anatomic position. The muscular and glandular elements develop between 8 and 13 weeks of gestation. Peptic activity has been found as early as 16 weeks but increases rapidly from 28 to 40 weeks of intrauterine life. Pepsin secretion continues to increase after birth and reaches adult values when the infant is about 2 years of age. Hydrochloric acid is rarely found in the fetal stomach before 32 weeks gestation, but production of the acid increases during the latter part of gestation. Although decreased during the first 4 to 6 hours of age, the term infant's basal secretion of hydrochloric acid is the same as that of a child when the rate of secretion is calculated on the basis of body weight. The relationship between the production of hydrochloric acid in the neonate and the finding of hypergastrinemia, which normally persists for at least the first 8 hours of life, is unclear. Similarly, the relationship of hydrochloric acid production and gastric emptying time is also unclear, but it is evident that preterm infants have a marked delay in gastric emptying. If these infants are kept right-side down after feedings, the stomach empties more rapidly.

Abnormalities of the stomach in the newborn period include gastric hypoplasia, diverticula, duplications, tumors, volvulus, and hypertrophic pyloric stenosis. Vomiting, abdominal pain, and on occasion bleeding are the symptoms most commonly encountered in these abnormalities.

Volvulus of the stomach

Abnormalities of fixation during development may lead to volvulus of the stomach with pathologic rotation of the organ around one of two axes. The more common is the organoaxial volvulus about the cardiopyloric line, whereas the less common is about the long axis of the gastrohepatic omentum, the mesenteroaxial volvulus, or the upside-down stomach. The disorder may be associated with other anomalies, such as eventration of the diaphragm or diaphragmatic herniae. Many of the patients show symptoms during infancy and have severe abdominal pain, which is often, but not always, relieved by vomiting. Distension in the epigastrium, abdominal pain, vomiting, and difficulty in passing a nasogastric tube should alert the physician to the diagnosis. Contrast studies with barium should confirm the diagnosis, but, if the studies are performed when the patient is asymptomatic, abnormalities may not be seen. Abnormal positioning of the stomach, mucosal edema, and an eventration of the diaphragm may be present even if the volvulus is not detected. Medical therapy of frequent small feedings, smooth muscle relaxants, or sedation is usually not effective. Surgical reduction of the volvulus and anterior gastropexy are usually curative.

Congenital hypertrophic pyloric stenosis
Incidence and etiology

The incidence is variously reported as 2 to 5 per 1,000 live births. There is a familial tendency, and an infant with an affected parent has about a 7% chance of being affected. If the mother has been affected, the risk is fourfold greater than if the father has had pyloric stenosis. It is more common in males and does not necessarily affect the firstborn. Neither the type nor the amount of feeding seems to affect the incidence.

The etiology of the disorder is unknown, but several interesting theories have been proposed. A diminution in number or alteration of the structure of ganglion cells of the pylorus has been suggested as a cause of the disorder. However, careful electron microscopic examinations of the parasympathetic ganglia of the pylorus of affected infants have demonstrated no such abnormalities. Hypergastrinemia and/or hypersecretion of hydrochloric acid have also been suggested as a cause of pyloric stenosis, but data to substantiate this hypothesis are controversial at best. Whatever the etiology, the pyloric circular smooth muscle fibers, which are continuous with those of the stomach, become hypertrophied and may increase two or three times their normal width. This results in a firm, thickened, elongated mass, the so-called olive.

Clinical manifestations

Symptoms characteristically begin between the second and sixth week of life, although cases have been found during the first week. Vomiting, which begins intermittently, progresses in frequency to occur after every feeding. The vomitus is without bile and is expelled with great force. The infants continue to be eager feeders but become anxious and irritable. Less and less food passes the pylorus; as a consequence, the passage of stool may become less frequent, and weight loss occurs. On examination, the pyloric mass, or olive, may be palpated just right of the midline in the right upper quadrant. It is best felt when both the infant and examiner are relaxed and when the stomach is empty, as after vomiting. When the stomach is full, the pylorus tends to be displaced posteriorly. In such situations the infant should be examined in a sitting position, and the examiner can often bring the pylorus forward to palpate the tumor. During or shortly after feeding, peristaltic waves may be seen progressing from the left upper quadrant toward the obstructing mass.

In the premature infant, symptoms usually occur later, and the onset is more insidious. Preterm infants usually begin to have symptoms when they have attained the age and weight of a term infant. Because of the thinner, more poorly developed abdominal musculature, the pyloric mass is easily palpated, and peristaltic waves are more easily seen. Peristaltic waves are not diagnostic, since they may be seen in normal premature infants.

It is often difficult to diagnose those infants with pyloric stenosis who are being breast-fed exclusively. The vomiting may be intermittent, and the disease may not be manifested until the infant is 3 or even 4 months of age.

The vomiting of acid secretions leads to metabolic alkalosis, followed by dehydration and relative starvation. Correction of acid-base and electrolyte imbalances is essential before the infant is taken to surgery. Surgery causes an increased aldosterone effect, which tends to perpetuate the alkalosis, and inadvertent hyperventilation during anesthesia also can aggravate the alkalosis and may produce tetany. An unexplained observation has been the occurrence of indirect hyperbilirubinemia and decreased hepatic glucuronyl transferase activity in some patients with congenital hypertrophic pyloric stenosis. Decreased activity of glucuronyl transferase has also been found in some patients with hypergastrinemia.

The differential diagnosis of pyloric stenosis must include congenital adrenal hyperplasia, prepyloric web or diaphragm, and gastroesophageal reflux associated with pylorospasm. Patients with severe pylorospasm may have roentgenographic signs similar to those of patients with pyloric stenosis, but the spasm can be relieved with intravenous glucagon. The glucagon has little, if any, effect on pyloric stenosis.

Laboratory manifestations

Roentgenologic evaluation may be necessary to confirm the diagnosis. The study is best done after the gastric contents have been aspirated with a nasogastric tube. With the tube in place, barium is instilled under fluoroscopic control. The elongated pyloric canal contains compressed invaginated folds of mucosa, giving a "string" (Fig. 24-11) or "double-track" sign. These are among the most helpful findings, and the latter differentiates pyloric stenosis from pylorospasm. The canal itself swings upward and to the left, giving a vertical orientation. The pyloric mass may protrude into the duodenal bulb, causing the barium to outline the contours of the mass, the "umbrella sign." The "beak sign" is caused by a stream of barium entering the narrow proximal canal. The "nipple sign," or "pyloric tit," best seen on fluoroscopy, occurs when a peristaltic wave approaches the pyloric mass on

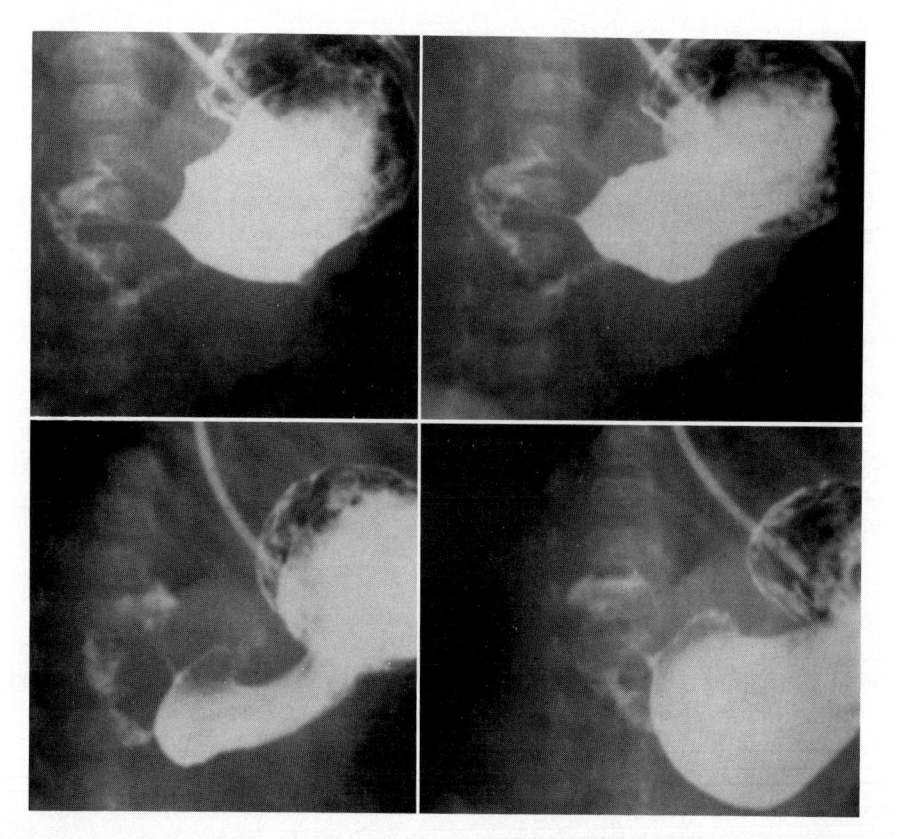

Fig. 24-11. Multiple views of an upper GI barium study of a patient with hypertrophic pyloric stenosis. Note the "string sign" of the narrowed pyloric canal, the "beak sign" as the barium enters the pyloric canal, the "umbrella sign" as the barium fills the duodenal bulb outlining the pyloric mass, and the "tit sign" caused by indentation of the pyloric mass on the prepyloric area.

the lesser curvature and a sharp angulation occurs. Delayed gastric emptying is a constant finding..

Treatment

Therapy consists of pyloromyotomy following correction of dehydration and associated electrolyte disturbances. Feedings of clear liquids may be given 4 to 6 hours after surgery if the infant is alert and sucking well. Full-strength formula may be given by the second day. If the duodenum is inadvertently entered at the time of surgery, gastric decompression and intravenous fluid therapy may have to be continued for several days before oral alimentation is initiated.

Prepyloric gastric antral webs

The exact mechanism by which these diaphragms, webs, membranes, or pyloric atresias develop is not well delineated. Numerous theories have been proposed, including intrauterine vascular accidents, inflammation, incomplete recanalization, and local endodermal proliferation with subsequent redundancy. If the web or diaphragm is complete, signs of gastric outlet obstruction are evident soon after birth. If the web is incomplete, there may be variability in age of onset and symptoms. Over 70% of the patients have symptoms within the first 6 months of life, and almost all have vomiting, which may be bilious. Older children may have abdominal pain, eructation, or poor weight gain. The diagnosis is usually made roentgenographically with barium contrast, and delayed gastric emptying is noted. The web or diaphragm may not be seen unless specifically searched for and is evident as a thin radiolucent line, often called a *gray-wire sign*. In older infants and children, endoscopy has led to the diagnosis readily.

The treatment of the condition is surgical, at which time the gastric outlet is enlarged. Coexistent congenital anomalies, including cardiac lesions, may be present and were encountered in 50% of the patients reported by Bell and co-workers.

Peptic ulcer disease

Acute peptic ulcer disease in neonates occurs in both the stomach and duodenum and is usually secondary to severe perinatal asphyxia or hypoxia. The ulcers also occur in those infants who have received assisted ventilation for prolonged periods of time and who have had intermittent episodes of hypoxia or hypercarbia and in infants with neonatal sepsis or meningitis. The ulcers are usually multiple and superficial; they may cause severe bleeding and at times perforation. Microscopically the ulcers are superficial, and little if any thickening of the bowel is found. There is often absence of an acute inflammatory reaction. Roentgenographic examination of the stomach with contrast media frequently fails to demonstrate the superficial ulcerations. Treatment is outlined under the section on GI emergencies.

Lactobezoars

Although lactobezoars had been previously encountered infrequently in the neonate, recent reports have indicated that they may not be an uncommon complication of feeding high-calorie formulas to small preterm infants. Most of the patients described had birth weights of 1,500 gm or less and had received a formula containing 24 calories/oz, wherein 40% to 50% of the fat content is medium-chain triglycerides and 50% of the carbohydrate is corn syrup solids. The feedings were usually initiated during the first week or two of life, and the infants became symptomatic 3 to 12 days later. The presenting symptoms usually included abdominal distension, increased gastric residuals, vomiting, diarrhea, and heme-positive stools. Several infants have been asymptomatic, and the diagnosis was made by palpating an abdominal mass or by routine roentgenogram taken of the abdomen.

The diagnosis is usually made by palpating a mass in the left upper quadrant of the abdomen and confirmed by an abdominal roentgenogram, which demonstrates a well-formed intraluminal cast surrounded by air. Often the injection of 2 to 3 ml/kg of air into the stomach will outline the lactobezoar quite well. Contrast studies with barium or Gastrografin are not needed.

The etiology of the lactobezoars is unknown but could be related to many factors, such as the delayed gastric emptying time of a sick premature infant, decreased gastric acidity, the higher caloric density of the milk, the calcium content of the formula, or the quality and quantity of the fat and protein.

Treatment for the lactobezoar is to place the infant on parenteral feedings only for a period of 24 to 48 hours, or until the lactobezoar is no longer evident on abdominal roentgenograms. Nasogastric decompression and lavage have not been necessary in the management of the infants. At least two infants have had gastric perforations associated with the lactobezoars, so it is not an innocuous disorder. Delaying the introduction of the 24 calories/oz formulas until the infant is at least 2 to 3 weeks of age has been advocated as a method to prevent lactobezoar formation. Unfortunately, the disorder has also been encountered in premature infants receiving 20 calories/oz formulas as well.

Bezoars have also been identified in patients who have received antacids as therapy for acute gastritis or for upper gastrointestinal tract hemorrhage. Treatment is the same as just outlined.

DISORDERS OF THE SMALL INTESTINE
Congenital duodenal obstruction

Duodenal obstruction in the neonate may be caused by both intrinsic and extrinsic lesions that may result in complete or partial obstruction. Complete obstruction is most often secondary to congenital duodenal atresia, whereas partial obstruction may be due to a wide variety of both intrinsic and extrinsic lesions, including duodenal stenosis or diaphragm, annular pancreas, malrotation, and preduodenal portal vein.

Etiology

Duodenal atresia accounts for over half of all cases of congenital intrinsic duodenal obstruction. This malformation appears to result from failure of recanalization of the GI tract during the second month of fetal life and is often found in association with several anomalies, including Down's syndrome (30%), intestinal malrotation (20%), congenital heart disease (17%), tracheoesophageal anomalies (7%), and renal anomalies (5%). Annular pancreas, secondary to persistence of the left bud of the ventral pancreas, is described in over one fifth of all patients with congenital intrinsic duodenal obstruction. Although controversy exists, it is our impression that, when patients with annular pancreas have symptoms in the neonatal period, the entity is generally associated with an intrinsic stenosis or atresia of the duodenum. Patients with annular pancreas alone are often asymptomatic. Over 50% of infants with duodenal obstruction are of low birth weight, and 40% develop hyperbilirubinemia.

Clinical manifestations

The earliest clue to the possible existence of duodenal obstruction is maternal polyhydramnios, occurring in almost 50% of all cases. Since 80% of the lesions are located in the postampullary region of the duodenum, most affected infants will have the onset of bilious vomiting during the first 24 hours of life. Abdominal distension tends to be localized to the upper abdomen. Respiratory distress secondary to abdominal distension is rare, and meconium is normally passed in over 50% of cases.

Partial obstruction may lead to delayed onset of symptoms, which are intermittent and difficult to diagnose. Roentgenographs of the abdomen may resemble the "double-bubble" appearance of duodenal atresia (Fig.

24-1), but there is scattered air throughout the rest of the GI tract. A barium enema may be helpful in identifying those patients with malrotation and partial duodenal obstruction secondary to fibrous band formation. Occasionally, contrast studies of the upper GI tract will be necessary to document the presence of an incomplete duodenal obstruction. Rare malformations such as a preduodenal vein are often impossible to diagnose before surgery.

Treatment

This consists of nasogastric suction, fluid and electrolyte replacement, and surgical creation of a duodenoduodenostomy or duodenojejunostomy. Attempts should not be made to resect annular pancreatic tissue.

Prognosis

Over 60% of infants with this group of malformations will survive with proper therapy; the majority of deaths result from complications of the associated anomalies. Many of these associated malformations are potentially correctable if recognized and treated early.

Malrotation

Failure of normal rotation and fixation of the GI tract results in a group of varied and potentially lethal clinical disorders. The complications of malrotation are largely due to intestinal obstruction and vascular compromise.

Pathology

Arrest of the cecum in the upper abdomen results in fibrous band formation between the cecum and the posterior peritoneum, which causes partial duodenal obstruction (Ladd's bands) (Fig. 24-12). In addition, posterior fixation of the small intestinal mesentery occurs around the superior mesenteric artery on an abnormally narrow and horizontal base, allowing the development of midgut volvulus. Malrotation may occur as an isolated anomaly or in association with other malformations of the GI tract, such as omphalocele, gastroschisis, diaphragmatic hernia, or duodenal atresia.

Clinical manifestations

Almost 80% of infants with intestinal malrotation have symptoms during the first month of life. Although band formation may produce symptoms on the first day of life with a clinical syndrome resembling duodenal atresia, most neonates appear normal for the first few days. Signs of intestinal obstruction begin shortly thereafter. The sudden onset of bilious vomiting in a previously well neonate is evidence of malrotation with volvulus formation until proved otherwise. Barium enema will confirm the presence of the abnormally placed cecum (Fig. 24-13).

Volvulus formation results in severe midintestinal ischemia and bilious vomiting, rectal bleeding, and shock. Barium enema reveals obstruction to retrograde flow at the level of the midtransverse colon. Midgut volvulus is an acute surgical emergency requiring immediate operative intervention.

As in other causes of partial duodenal obstruction, malrotation without volvulus formation may present a difficult diagnostic problem. Infants may have a protracted course with intermittent episodes of vomiting and abdominal pain. Barium swallow will help identify this group of patients by demonstrating a dilated duodenum and the presence of jejunal loops in the right side of the peritoneal cavity.

Treatment

Surgical correction of malrotation includes lysis of peritoneal bands, fixation of the cecum and terminal ileum in the left side of the abdomen, and counterclockwise reduction of the midgut volvulus. If large segments of ischemic bowel are identified, resection is not performed at the initial laparotomy. The bowel is reexamined in 24 to 48 hours, and obviously infarcted bowel is then resected. This technique results in maximal preservation of functional bowel and in improved long-term survival. If extensive intestinal resection is mandatory at the second operation, short bowel syndrome is a frequent complication. Prolonged periods of total parenteral nutrition are often required postoperatively.

Congenital jejunoileal obstruction
Etiology

Clinical and experimental data suggest that congenital atresias of the jejunum and ileum result from intrauterine vascular accidents occurring late in fetal life. Intussusception, strangulating obstruction, or volvulus during the intrauterine period produces avascular necrosis and eventual resorption of the involved segment of bowel. Since early fetal development is not affected, associated extraintestinal anomalies are seldom seen. This is in striking contrast to congenital duodenal obstruction, in which there is an embryologic failure during early fetal life resulting in both intraintestinal and extraintestinal anomalies. Associated malformations seen in patients with jejunoileal obstruction are mainly confined to the GI tract; malrotation and meconium ileus are the most common.

Clinical manifestations

Bilious vomiting and abdominal distension are present in over 80% of patients. Jaundice and failure to pass meconium are other very common clinical features. Distension is most marked in distal ileal lesions, in which case vomiting may be delayed in onset and is often fecal

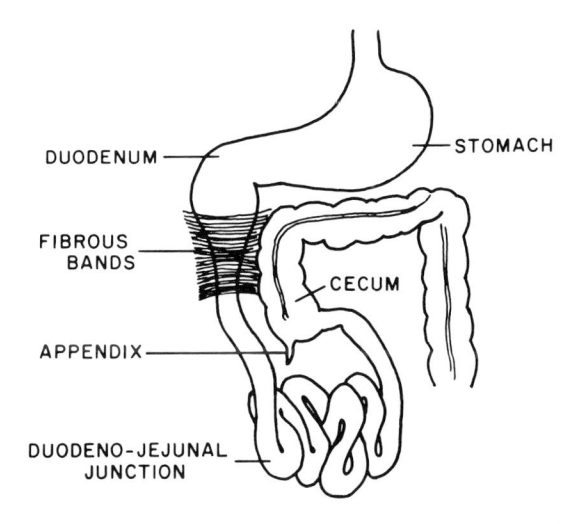

Fig. 24-12. Diagram of duodenal obstruction caused by fibrous bands (Ladd's bands) in a patient with malrotation. (Adapted from Snyder, W.H., Jr., and Chaffin, L.: Malrotation of the intestine. In Mustard, W.T., and others, editors: Pediatric surgery, ed. 2, Chicago, 1969, Year Book Medical Publishers, Inc.)

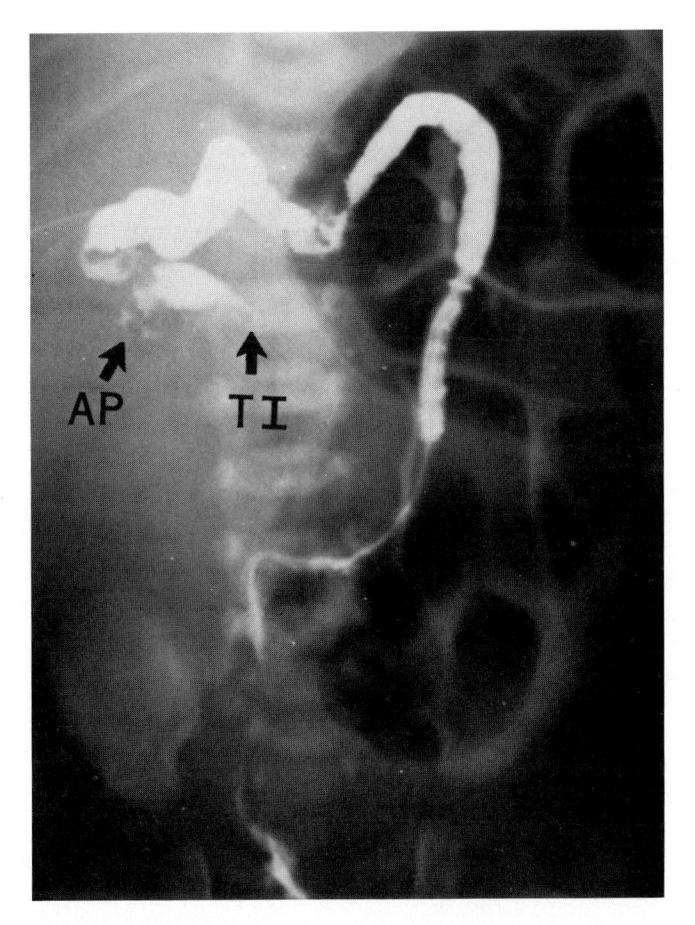

Fig. 24-13. Infant with distal ileal atresia and malrotation. Note the dilated air-filled loops of small intestine, the presence of a "microcolon," and the abnormal position of the appendix *(AP)* and terminal ileum *(TI)*.

in character. Diagnosis is usually confirmed by roentgenograms of the abdomen, which reveal dilated loops of bowel and air-fluid levels proximal to the level of obstruction. Relatively few loops are noted in cases of high jejunal atresia, whereas numerous air-fluid levels are seen in distal ileal obstruction. Intraperitoneal calcifications may be observed in up to 10% of cases and indicate the presence of meconium peritonitis secondary to antenatal intestinal perforation. Barium enema is performed to document the presence of an unused microcolon (Fig. 24-13) and to determine the location of the cecum. Malrotation has been described in up to 25% of cases.

Treatment

Surgical management consists of resecting a short segment of the dilated proximal bowel and performing an end-to-end anastomosis. End-to-side anastomosis also has been effectively used. A Mikulicz enterostomy may be necessary in critically ill infants as a temporary measure. Poor postoperative peristalsis may be due to inadequate blood supply of the terminal portion of the dilated proximal segment. Sepsis, respiratory failure, and anastomotic complications are largely responsible for the 35% overall mortality.

Gastrointestinal duplications

Enteric duplications may occur in any part of the GI tract; the clinical presentation is primarily dependent on the area involved. The distal small intestine is the most common site, involved in approximately 40% of cases. Other abdominal sites account for an additional 40% and the remaining lesions are either esophageal or thoracoabdominal in origin.

Pathology

The cysts vary in size, shape, and mode of attachment, but all are found in direct contact with the GI tract and are lined with mucosa similar to that of the adjacent normal bowel. Occasional cysts also will have ectopic gastric mucosa that is capable of hemorrhage and perforation. Most are spherical and noncommunicating, but cysts with both proximal and distal communications are seen. Small intestinal duplications are found on the mesenteric side and share a common wall and blood supply. The origin of these lesions is unkown, but vascular accidents and failure of separation between primitive notochord and entoderm have been proposed as possible explanations. The latter theory also has been used to explain the common association of vertebral anomalies.

Clinical manifestations

Although patients with enteric cysts may remain asymptomatic, over 75% present in the first week of life and most of the remainder by the end of the first month, with symptoms of intestinal obstruction in association with an abdominal mass. Vomiting is the most common mode of presentation. Obstruction occurs secondary to extrinsic compression, volvulus formation, or intussusception. Acute pancreatitis and obstructive jaundice are rare complications seen in association with duodenal duplications. Abdominal roentgenograms and appropriate contrast studies often suggest the correct diagnosis. However, a roentgenologic diagnosis is made in less than 50% of small intestinal duplications.

Treatment

Resection and primary anastomosis of the involved area of bowel are preferred treatments. In patients in whom the involvement is extensive or anatomically not resectable, an internal drainage procedure with removal of ectopic gastric mucosa is used. Overall survival is around 80%; most deaths are related to associated anomalies or complications of perforation.

DISORDERS OF THE COLON
Colonic atresia and stenosis

The colon is the least likely site for intestinal atresia and accounts for less than 10% of all bowel atresias. The pathogenesis is thought to be secondary to vascular compromise with ischemia, necrosis, and fibrosis. Atresias occur equally in areas supplied by the superior and inferior mesenteric arteries. The atretic segment is often membranous or consists of a fibrous diaphragm, with the serosal side of the bowel appearing normal.

Clinically there is abdominal distension, obstipation, and vomiting that eventually becomes bilious and occasionally fecal in nature. Abdominal roentgenograms demonstrate dilated loops of bowel, and a barium enema delineates the area of atresia or stenosis and the presence of an unused microcolon (Fig. 24-14). Treatment consists of a colostomy followed at a later time with resection of the atretic segment and end-to-end anastomosis.

Congenital aganglionic megacolon (Hirschsprung's disease)
Incidence

Hirschsprung's disease accounts for 20% to 25% of patients with intestinal obstruction in the neonatal period. The incidence is 1 in 3,000 to 1 in 5,000 live births and occurs up to five times more frequently in males and three times more frequently in Caucasians than in blacks. A familial incidence of about 8% has been noted and is greater in those with long aganglionic segments. About 3% of patients have Down's syndrome. The infant is usually full term and of normal weight, whereas a majority of patients with intestinal atresias are of low birth weight.

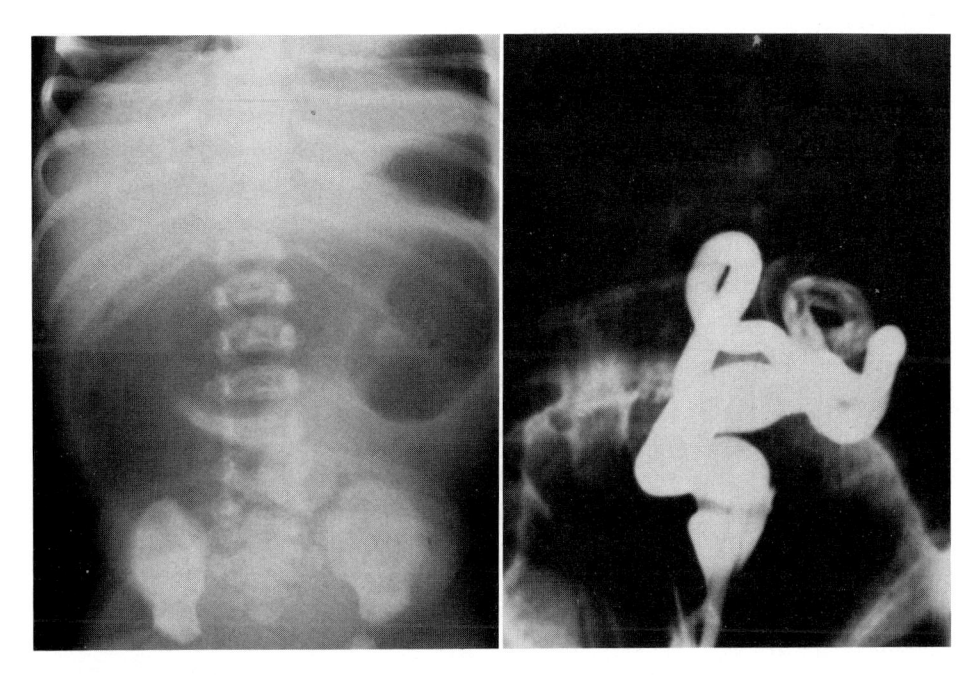

Fig. 24-14. Roentgenograms of the abdomen of a neonate with colonic atresia demonstrating air-filled loops of dilated colon and small intestine. Barium enema demonstrates small caliber of distal bowel and the inability of barium to pass proximal to the atretic segment.

Pathology

There are no ganglion cells in Meissner's plexus (submucosal) or Auerbach's plexus (myenteric). This is probably secondary to the failure of normal aboral migration of ganglion cells from the neural crest. Consequently, the preganglionic parasympathetic axons have no ganglia for a terminus and become hyperplastic. The aganglionic tissue often contains a great deal of acetylcholinesterase. Aganglionic intestine is aperistaltic and remains in a state of contraction. The proximal segment, which has normal innervation and peristalsis, develops work hypertrophy and eventually becomes dilated (megacolon). Between the two segments, a funnel-shaped transitional zone develops (Fig. 24-15). Eighty percent of patients have aganglionosis limited to the rectosigmoid region, and 3% have aganglionosis of the entire colon. Rarely, the disease also may involve the small intestine. Because of the embryology of innervation, skip lesions are rarely, if ever, seen.

Clinical manifestations

Infants with Hirschsprung's disease appear normal at birth. Only 6% pass meconium in the first 24 hours; more than half do not pass meconium for more than 48 hours. Conversely, of all infants who have delayed passage of meconium, 10% to 15% will have Hirschsprung's disease. Abdominal distension and constipation are the most frequent initial symptoms and may begin during the first few days of life. Bilious vomiting may shortly ensue and is the most consistent symptom of total colonic aganglionosis. The clinical picture may be indistinguishable from meconium ileus, ileal atresia, or large bowel obstruction. The obstruction may lead to perforation; in any infant with colonic, ileal, or appendiceal perforation, the diagnosis of Hirschsprung's disease should be excluded.

Some newborns will have relief of symptoms with digital rectal dilatation and pass a large volume of stool and flatus. These infants may return in 4 to 6 weeks with failure to grow, diarrhea or constipation, hypoproteinemia, and in some patients edema. There may be distension and vomiting, the latter leading to dehydration. A careful rectal examination will reveal a tight anal sphincter and absence of stool in the rectal ampulla.

Enterocolitis may occur at any age and is the major cause of death. The etiology is unclear but may be related to progressive dilatation, venous stasis, mucosal edema, and ischemia. The infant may or may not be toxic appearing with diarrhea and fever. Decompression with gentle enemas of isotonic electrolyte solutions followed by a colostomy or ileostomy, proximal to the aganglionic area, may be life saving.

Diagnostic evaluation

Diagnosis may be made by roentgenologic studies, biopsy, and anorectal manometry. Upright roentgenograms of the abdomen may show gaseous distension of the colon and multiple fluid levels. Classically, the barium enema demonstrates a narrowed aganglionic seg-

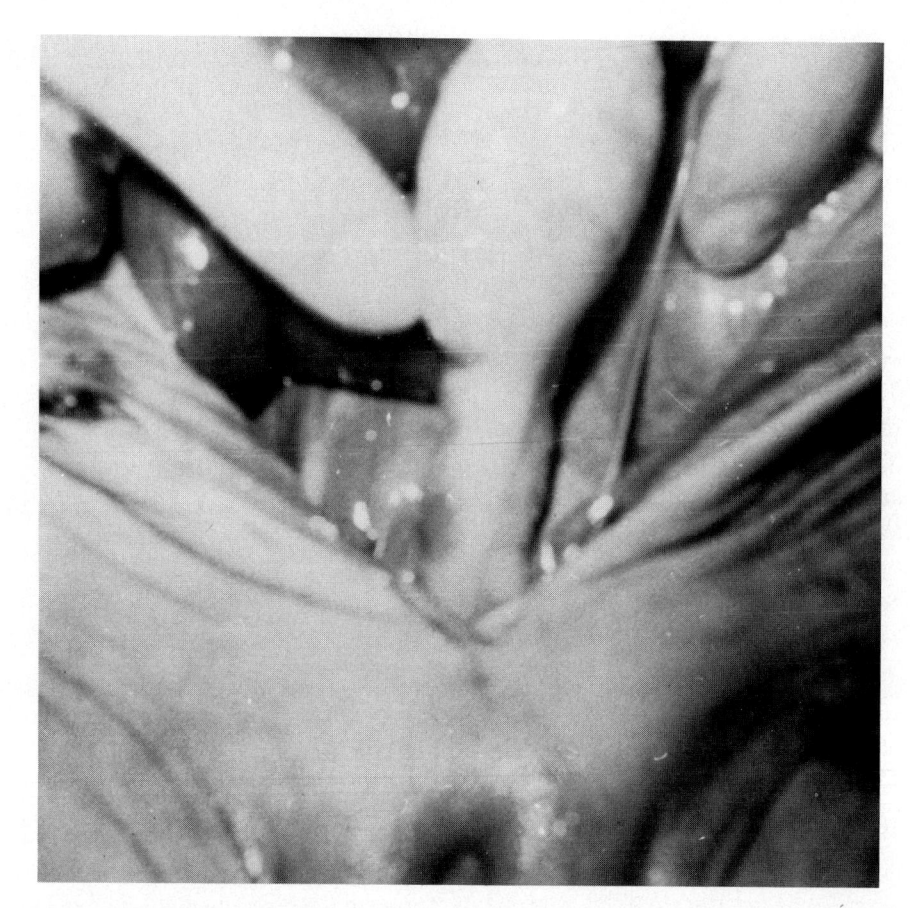

Fig. 24-15. Postmortem findings in an infant with Down's syndrome who developed severe abdominal distension and alternating diarrhea and constipation. Hirschsprung's disease was found at postmortem examination, and the figure illustrates the classic contracted short segment with hypertrophy and dilatation of the proximal segment.

ment that opens into a funnel-shaped transition zone and then into a dilated innervated segment (Fig. 24-16). In the newborn period the caliber of the rectum may appear normal, and the innervated segment may not have undergone dilatation. To avoid missing a short aganglionic segment, the catheter tip should be inserted no more than 2 cm beyond the anal verge. The barium must be allowed to run in slowly, with no more than 5 to 10 ml of contrast material used at a time and with careful fluoroscopic observation of the initial filling. A short, narrowed rectal segment is best seen on lateral view. In total colonic aganglionosis the colon caliber may be normal, but it is characteristically foreshortened, and there are rounded splenic and hepatic flexures. Irregular sawtooth contractions may be seen as well. Barium remaining in the colon after 24 hours is also highly suggestive of Hirschsprung's disease. Unfortunately, a normal barium study has been reported in as many as 23% of neonates with Hirschsprung's disease.

Rectal tissue may be easily obtained with a suction biopsy. It is important to take the biopsy specimen at least 2 cm above the mucocutaneous junction because a hypoganglionic area normally exists below that level. Suction pressures of 5 to 10 mm Hg are adequate and safe. The presence of ganglion cells excludes the diagnosis of Hirschsprung's disease, and the absence of ganglia is highly suggestive of the diagnosis. The presence of large numbers of nerve fibers, as well as the histochemical demonstration of acetylcholinesterase activity in suction biopsy specimens, adds further accuracy to the diagnosis of the disorder. At the time of surgery, biopsies are taken to determine the length of the aganglionic segment.

Anorectal manometry using three miniaturized balloons may facilitate diagnosis. An internal balloon causes acute distension of the rectum and initiates the reflex, and balloons positioned within the internal and external sphincters measure the responses. A normal reflex results in relaxation of the internal and contraction of the external sphincter. In addition, the normal internal sphincter has intermittent contractions; the aganglionic patient has continuous rhythmic contractions. Often pre-

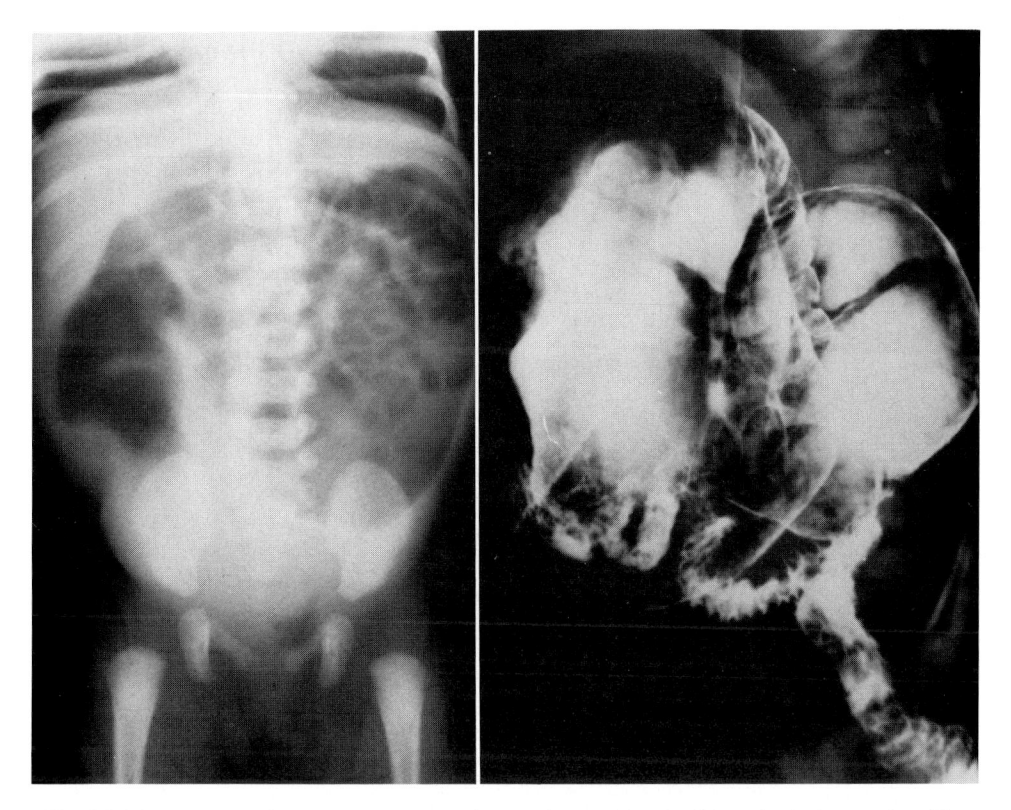

Fig. 24-16. Abdominal roentgenograms of a newborn with distal intestinal obstruction. The diagnosis of Hirschsprung's disease is suggested by the relative absence of air in the rectum. A lateral view taken during a barium enema reveals a narrowed aganglionic rectum leading into a markedly dilated sigmoid colon.

mature infants, especially those with respiratory distress, have an abnormal manometric pattern, with little if any response of the internal sphincter.

Treatment

The treatment of choice in the neonate is a colostomy performed proximal to the aganglionic segment, with multiple biopsies taken to identify the level of involvement. An ileostomy must be performed in patients with total colonic aganglionosis. A definitive repair done by either a Swenson, Duhamel, or Soave procedure may be performed by an experienced pediatric surgeon in the latter part of the first year.

Meconium plug syndrome

A meconium plug is typically a light-colored, gelatinous, firm mass composed of mucus and other intestinal secretions and located in the lower colon and rectum. It lacks the usual flow characteristics of normal meconium. About 25% of meconium plugs occur in premature infants. Abnormal motility, either from immaturity or other pathophysiologic mechanisms, is probably responsible for the syndrome. Meconium ileus, ileal atresia, and Hirschsprung's disease may present a picture similar to meconium plug. The infant does not pass stool for more than 24 hours and develops signs of low intestinal obstruction with distention and bilious vomiting. Bowel sounds are hyperactive. The anal canal may seem small and tight on rectal examination. The digital examination may result in the passage of the plug and flatus. As with any low bowel obstruction, there is the risk of perforation, especially in the cecum.

Roentgenograms of the abdomen are compatible with low intestinal obstruction. Barium enema performed slowly under low pressure may reveal a normal-sized colon with meconium appearing as multiple elongated filling defects (Fig. 24-17). If the barium does not cause evacuation of the mass, a water-soluble contrast material, such as meglucamine diatrizoate (Gastrografin), may be used to facilitate passage of the plug. Only in rare patients is surgery necessary. All patients should undergo a rectal biopsy to exclude Hirschsprung's disease, since 10% to 15% of these patients will also have aganglionosis.

The neonatal small left colon syndrome is probably a variant of the meconium plug syndrome. Forty percent to 50% of these infants are delivered of insulin-dependent diabetic mothers. The meconium plug invariably

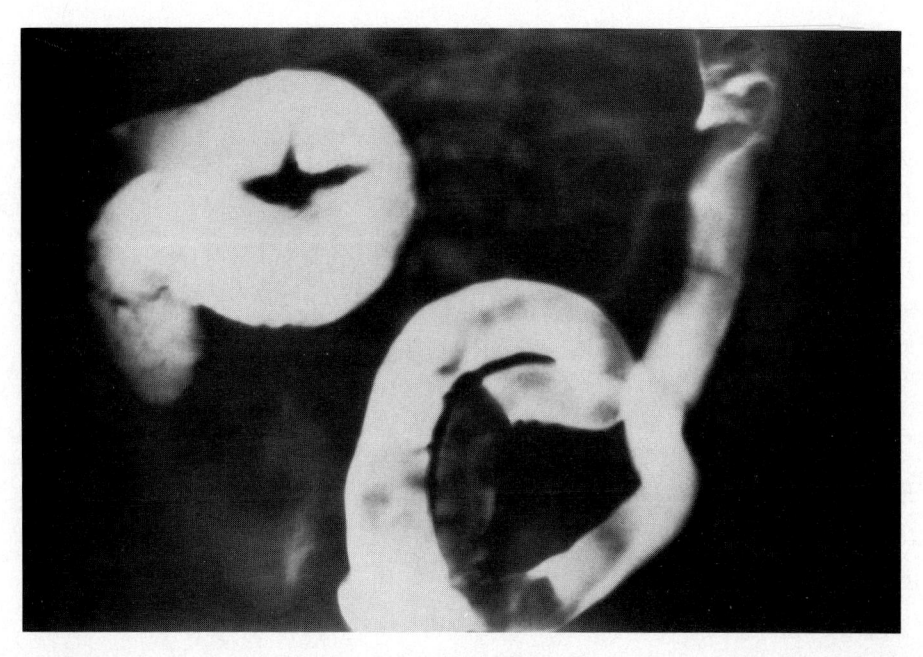

Fig. 24-17. Barium enema of an infant with the meconium plug syndrome. Colon is of normal caliber, and numerous filling defects are visualized.

extends to the splenic flexure, and initially the distal colon appears to be of small caliber on contrast enema. As with other meconium plugs, the enema may be therapeutic both in relieving the meconium plug and dilating the colon.

Inspissated milk syndrome

Once thought to be a rare cause of intestinal obstruction in preterm infants, this syndrome is being encountered with greater frequency as more infants are fed hypercaloric and hyperosmolar formulas. The infant begins to have obstipation or constipation between 5 and 14 days of age and develops abdominal distension and vomiting. Often a mass is felt in the right lower quadrant of the abdomen, and small ropelike pellets are felt throughout the colon. Roentgenographic examination of the abdomen usually reveals dilated loops of bowel, few if any fluid levels, and intraluminal masses often surrounded by a halo of air. Perforation rarely occurs. The diagnosis is often confused with meconium ileus, meconium plug syndrome, Hirschsprung's disease, or necrotizing enterocolitis. The halo of air differentiates this problem from the meconium ileus syndrome because in the latter the meconium clings to the bowel wall and prevents gas from passing around it. A contrast study with barium or meglucamine diatrizoate reveals a normal or slightly narrowed colon with numerous small filling defects. Often the meglucamine diatrizoate enema will facilitate the passage of the milk curds and "cure" the infant. On occasion, surgery is necessary to remove the inspissated material.

Intussusception

Intussusception is rare in the neonatal period. The ileocecal type of intussusception is most common; and if an enteroenteric type is found, a specific associated lesion, such as Meckel's diverticulum, should be sought. Vomiting, usually bile stained, and blood in the stool are the most frequent symptoms. It is uncommon to find a palpable mass, and bowel sounds may be normal. Abdominal roentgenograms followed by contrast studies of the colon will often clarify the diagnosis, but in many neonates the diagnosis is made only at surgery.

Anorectal anomalies
Incidence and etiology

The incidence of anorectal malformations is about 1 in 5,000 live births. The incidence in males is one and a half times that of females. There is usually no familial history, but patients have been reported suggesting subgroups with both recessive and dominant inheritance. Among the latter is a syndrome of imperforate anus, triphalangeal thumbs, bony anomalies, and sensorineural deafness. Associated anomalies are found in one third to one half of patients with anorectal anomalies; esophageal atresia and skeletal, cardiovascular, and genitourinary anomalies occur most frequently.

Anorectal anomalies result when there are variations in the normal progression of development; the urorectal septum, the anal tubercles, and/or the anal membrane fail to differentiate appropriately. Of clinical importance is the location of the anorectal anomaly in relation to the puborectalis sling. This anatomic location is the basis for the suggested international classification of the anomalies.

ANORECTAL ANOMALIES: A SUGGESTED INTERNATIONAL CLASSIFICATION*

A. Low (translevator)
  1. At normal anal site
    a. Anal stenosis
    b. Covered anus—complete
  2. At perineal site
    a. Anocutaneous fistula (covered anus—incomplete)
    b. Anterior perianal anus
  3. At vulvar site (female)
    a. Anovulvar fistula
    b. Anovestibular fistula
    c. Vestibular anus
B. Intermediate
  1. Anal agenesis
    a. Without fistula
    b. With fistula
      (1) Rectobulbar (male)
      (2) Rectovestibular (female)
      (3) Rectovaginal—low (female)
  2. Anorectal stenosis
C. High (supralevator)
  1. Anorectal agenesis
    a. Without fistula
    b. With fistula
      (1) Rectourethral (male)
      (2) Rectovesical
      (3) Rectovaginal—high (female)
      (4) Rectocloacal (female)
  2. Rectal atresia
D. Miscellaneous
  1. Imperforate anal membrane
  2. Cloacal exstrophy
  3. Others

Clinical manifestations

The most important diagnostic study is the careful examination of the perineum. Any perineal fistula, no matter how small, is indicative of a low lesion. Every skin dimple or fold, especially along the midline raphe, should be gently explored with a small lacrimal duct probe. As the raphe extends posteriorly over the site of the anus, a bulge (or "bucket handle") may be seen. Anal dimples and puckering secondary to skin stimulation of the anal area should be noted (Figs. 24-18 and 24-19).

Laboratory manifestations

Roentgenologic studies help determine the level of atresia and the presence of a fistula. In the past the pubococcygeal line, drawn from the lower part of the pubis to the inferior margin of the lower sacral segment, has been used to delinate high from low lesions. This line, however, is usually above the puborectalis sling. A more satisfactory level can be found by determining the M (muscle) point on the ischium. The M point is at the junction of the upper two thirds with the lower third of the pear-shaped ischium (Fig. 24-20). Air in the rectum can help determine the distal extent of the proximal rectum, but pitfalls do exist. First, it may take 24 hours or longer for air to traverse the intestine to the rectum. Second, air may escape via a fistula; this may lead to air in the bladder and be indicative of a rectovesicular fistula. Third, meconium may prevent air from reaching the limit of the proximal bowel. To obtain the best possible roentgenograms, the infant should be held in a steep Trendelenburg position for 20 minutes, then in a completely inverted position for 10 minutes. This will allow air to percolate through any meconium present. The hips must be well flexed and the x-ray tube centered in a true lateral position over the buttocks. A fixed marker should be used to locate the anus. Associated sacral anomalies should be noted because they may presage neurologic deficiency.

In high or intermediate anomalies, fistulas are common. In males they are usually rectourethral or rectovesicular; in females they join the vaginal vault or the lower vagina. Contrast studies with the use of a water-soluble medium may help identify the fistula. Cystourethrography may be done in males; in females, a no. 5 Fr. Foley catheter may be inserted into a cloacal opening or urogenital sinus, if present, and contrast medium injected.

Treatment

Initial management of the high or intermediate types is colostomy. Subsequently, a contrast medium may be injected into the distal loop (loopogram) to determine accurately the extent of anomaly and any associated fistula. Later repair is by abdominal approach, preserving sphincter function. Low types may be repaired perineally.

Prognosis

The overall mortality is about 10%; surgical procedures to correct the malformations account for 1% of the deaths, prematurity and associated anomalies for the remainder. Almost all the patients with low anomalies should be continent. The functional results in the high anomaly depend on the type of anomaly, the surgical procedures used to correct it, and any associated neurologic deficits. Long-term follow-up is essential in assessing the results in high anomalies. Overall, in our experience with high anomalies, 60% of the patients have normal anal function, 20% satisfactory, and 20% unsatisfac-

---

*From Santulli, T.V., Kiesewetter, W.B., and Bill, A.H.: J. Pediatr. Surg. **5:**281, 1970. Based on a classification proposed by the Paediatric Surgical Congress, Melbourne, Australia, 1970.

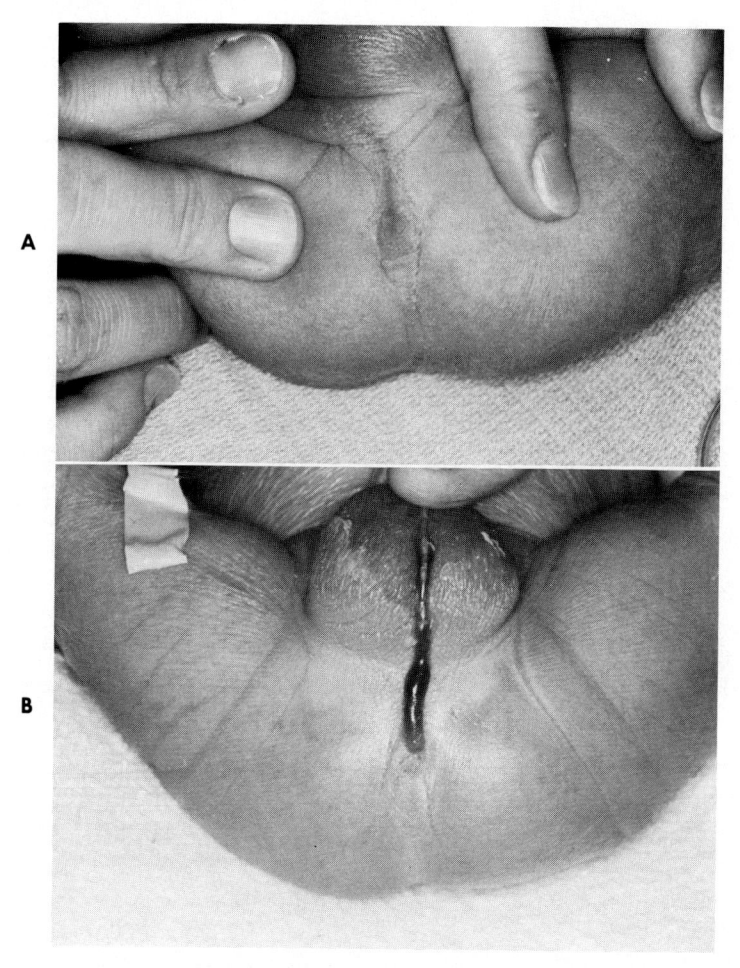

Fig. 24-18. Imperforate anus, male. **A,** There is no visible fistula. The anal dimple is fairly well defined. This boy had a high form of the anomaly with a rectourethral fistula. **B,** Low form of imperforate anus with anocutaneous fistula. The anus is covered by the thickened skin. The fistula is represented by the tract of meconium, which has "dissected" its way up the perineal raphe just beneath the epithelium.

tory (total or near total incontinence, frequent fecal impactions, or permanent colostomy).

Anal fissure

Anal fissure is the most common cause of rectal bleeding in infancy frequently presenting as a small amount of bright red blood on the exterior of a hard, large stool. Diarrheal stools may be irritating and cause fissuring and bright red blood streaking. In either case, the passage of stool may be painful, and stool holding may result. In the newborn and young infant the fissures occur primarily in the lateral and anterior anal areas. They initially are slit-like with smooth edges extending to the mucocutaneous junction. If they become chronic, the edges may thicken and have a puckered appearance. Treatment consists of softening the stools and cleaning the anus carefully after defecation. Mineral oil or diocytyl sodium sulfosuccinate, 5 mg/kg/day, may be used. The uncommon chronic fissure may be cauterized with silver nitrate and dilated with a lubricated finger cot.

Anorectal abscess and fistula

Anorectal abscess is caused by infection of the glands and ducts that drain into the crypts of Morgagni. The infection spreads to the perianal skin, forming a rounded, red, indurated mass that eventually may become fluctuant. Painful defecation is usual but not universal. An intermittent discharge may occur. In about half the patients a fistula is established between the perianal skin and anal canal or rectum. The lesion is ten times as common in males as in females. A fistula or fluctuant abscess should be incised, drained, and treated with warm soaks. A firm abscess may be treated initially with soaks alone. In all patients the stools should be softened.

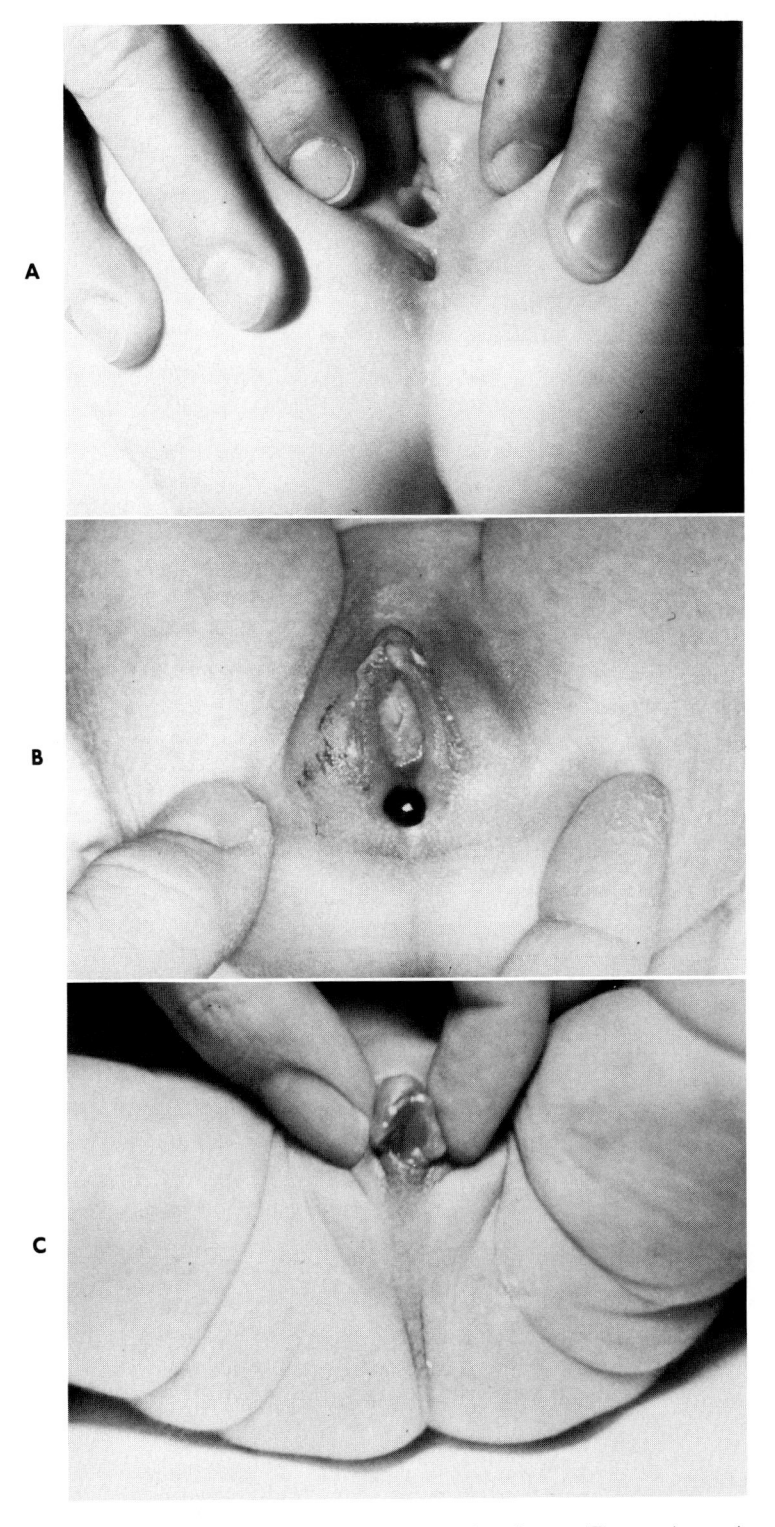

Fig. 24-19. Imperforate anus, female. **A,** Ectopic perineal anus. The anal opening is in the perineum between the fourchette and the anal dimple. It resembles a normal anus except for its anterior position. **B,** Low imperforate anus with anovulvar fistula. There is meconium at the fistula, which is at the fourchette, the junction of the labia majora. This is the most common form of the anomaly in the female. **C,** High anomaly. A single small orifice, typical of a urogenital sinus with imperforate anus. The fistula (rectocloacal) was high in the posterior wall of a urogenital sinus, the common passageway for urethra and vagina. This is the most serious anomaly in the female. (**A** from Santulli, T.V., and others: Surg. Clin. North Am. **45:**1264, 1965.)

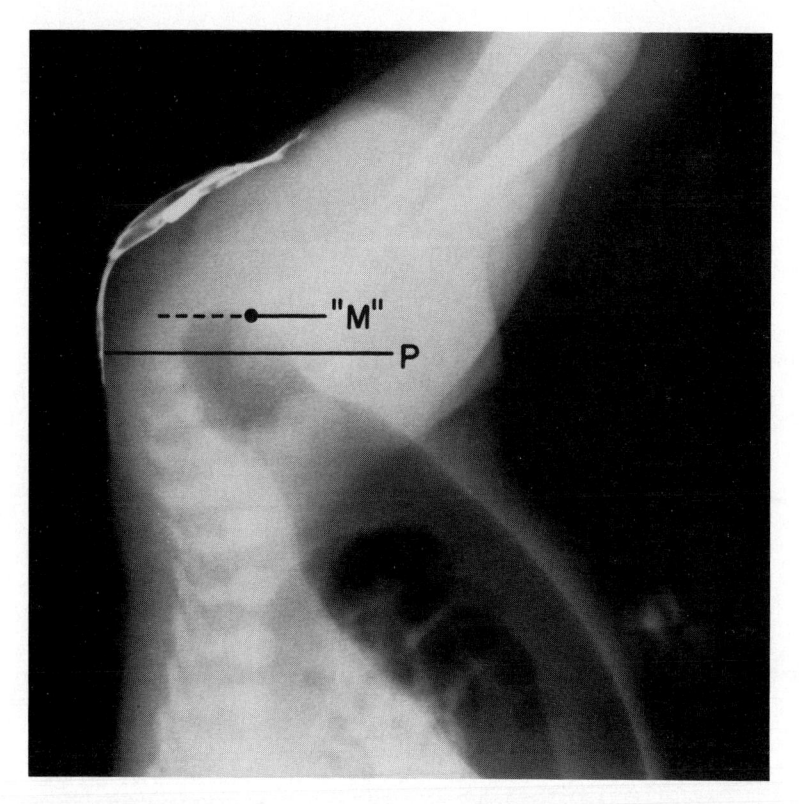

Fig. 24-20. Inverted lateral view of a roentgenogram of the lower abdomen of an infant with rectal atresia (imperforate anus). Barium placed at the anal area is used to estimate the length of the atretic segment. *P*, Pubococcygeal line; "*M*", muscle point.

Constipation and obstipation

Constipation and obstipation are common in the newborn. The failure to pass meconium is often the first symptom of Hirschsprung's disease, meconium plug, low atresias or stenosis, and anorectal anomalies. After the immediate neonatal period the stools may become less frequent and hard because of dietary changes. This is especially seen after the addition of solid food, such as cereal or yellow vegetables. A change from breast milk to formula or to whole milk may be accompanied by a change to firm or hard stools. One of the most common causes of constipation is stool holding secondary to an anal fissure. Constipation may be an early symptom of endocrine or metabolic disorders. Congenital hypothyroidism, the lipidoses, diabetes insipidus, renal tubular acidosis, and hypercalcemia have been associated with constipation.

Constipation may be treated by increasing the sugar content and therefore the intestinal osmotic load of the formula. If the bowel is dilated and hypotonic, an initial oil retention enema may be required, followed the next day with a pediatric enema (3 ml/kg). Mineral oil is effective and easily given orally in a dosage of 3 to 5 ml/kg initially, and increased until the stools are soft.

NECROTIZING ENTEROCOLITIS (NEC)

Although NEC has been described and recognized for over 100 years, it was not until the mid 1960s that physicians in the United States became more cognizant of its varied clinical manifestations. The incidence of NEC is approximately 1% of all admissions to neonatal units, although in some centers it may approach 7.5% of admissions and may account for 2% to 5% of all deaths.

Etiology and pathogenesis

Ischemia of the intestinal tract and invasion of the mucosa with enteric pathogens are the two most important causative factors. Others follow:
1. Prematurity, especially if the infant weighs less than 1,500 gm and is appropriate for gestational age
2. Perinatal asphyxia or hypoxia
3. Multiple gestation
4. Respiratory distress
5. Umbilical artery or venous catheters
6. Exchange transfusions
7. Polycythemia
8. Patent ductus arteriosus
9. Hyperosmolar feedings
10. Increased colonization of nursery with either *Klebsiella*, *E. coli*, or *Clostridium* organisms (Chapter 27)

11. Premature rupture of membranes

The very small and asphyxiated preterm infant is at greatest risk of developing the disease. However, full-term infants as well as SGA babies can develop NEC.

Bowel ischemia probably occurs secondary to the vascular insufficiency that may occur as a result of perinatal hypoxia or asphyxia when blood is shunted away from the intestine and other "nonvital organs" to perfuse the heart and brain. Studies in fetal sheep have demonstrated that, during asphyxic periods, over 80% of the blood that usually perfuses the GI tract is shunted to other organs. Because of poor GI motility and stasis, an increased incidence of sepsis, and poor immunologic response of the preterm infant, bacteria may readily invade the mucosa. A vicious chain of events ensues, with overgrowth of bacteria, mucosal damage, and secondary invasion of other layers of the bowel, with resultant perforation and peritonitis. It is our impression that the disease occurs much more commonly in nurseries where there is an increased rate of colonization with certain strains of *Klebsiella*, *E. coli*, or *Clostridium*. Other factors implicated as predisposing infants to develop NEC are plasticizers, which are leeched out of the plastic containers used to infuse blood and blood products, and hyperosmolar feedings, especially those with elemental diets. The hyperosmolality in the intestinal lumen causes the mucosa to become relatively ischemic when intestinal secretions are increased to render the formula isotonic.

Pathology

Although all portions of the GI tract except the duodenum may be involved in NEC, the right colon, cecum, and especially the terminal ileum are primarily involved. The affected bowel is usually dilated, hemorrhagic, and often has a brown or blue-gray hue. Air is often seen in the bowel wall (Fig. 24-21). An exudative film covers the peritoneal surfaces. Microscopically, the most common findings include mucosal edema and hemorrhage and complete necrosis of the mucosa with extension through the submucosa and the muscle layers (Fig. 24-22). Villi and crypts are absent, and although some bacteria are seen, the inflammatory response is often delayed for several days. Thrombi of the mesenteric capillaries, arteries, and veins may occur. Pneumatosis is a common finding, with air dissecting into the serosal layers of the intestine. Single or multiple perforations and evidence of peritonitis also may be present.

Clinical manifestations

Less than two thirds of the patients have either gross or microscopic blood in the stools, and less than half have diarrhea. The most common presenting symptoms include apnea, temperature instability, and abdominal distension (Table 24-4). The usual time of onset is between 4 and 10 days, but infants may show signs as early as 4 hours and as late as 30 days, and the disease may occur in patients who have never been fed.

Laboratory manifestations

Roentgenographic abnormalities include loss of the normal diamond or polygonal bowel segments. There is usually sausage-shaped dilatation of the intestine, which progresses to marked distension and pneumatosis intestinalis (Fig. 24-23), air in the portal circulation, or free air in the abdomen following perforation. In the initial stages of disease, pneumatosis intestinalis may be absent; it may never appear if judicious and intensive medical therapy is initiated. Anemia, leukopenia, leukocytosis, and electrolyte imbalances also may complicate the picture. Those patients with the most severe disease often have evidence of coagulopathy with thrombocytopenia and prolongation of partial thromboplastin time. Organisms often have been cultured from blood and occasionally urine, but bacteremia or septicemia may not be a prominent finding early in the course of the illness.

Treatment

Early recognition and aggressive therapy of the disease are critical for survival. The patient should be given nothing by mouth; intravenous fluids should be initiated and the intestine decompressed by nasogastric drainage once the diagnosis is suspected. Repeated and frequent cultures of blood, stool, and urine and correction of fluid and electrolyte balance are indicated. Antibiotics, including ampicillin and aminoglycosides, are usually given intravenously for presumptive sepsis. Treatment with oral kanamycin or gentamicin has also been advocated, but the data regarding the efficacy of oral antibiotics remain controversial.

Coagulation factors should be monitored and abnormalities corrected. Roentgenograms of the abdomen should be taken every 4 to 8 hours to immediately identify those infants in whom perforation has taken place. Left lateral decubitus films are particularly helpful in detecting perforations.

Surgery is indicated for those infants in whom perforation has occurred and in whom edema and erythema of the anterior abdominal wall suggest perforation and peritonitis. Surgery is also indicated for those patients who are deteriorating rapidly or who show no improvement after medical management for 4 to 12 hours. Surgery usually includes resection of the necrotic bowel and exteriorization of the proximal and distal ends. An attempt to perform a primary anastomosis often leads to disastrous complications.

The time at which oral feedings should be instituted following medical or surgical management and the desirability of using human milk are controversial. We do not initiate oral feedings for at least 7 days after the diagnosis has been made and the medical management instituted.

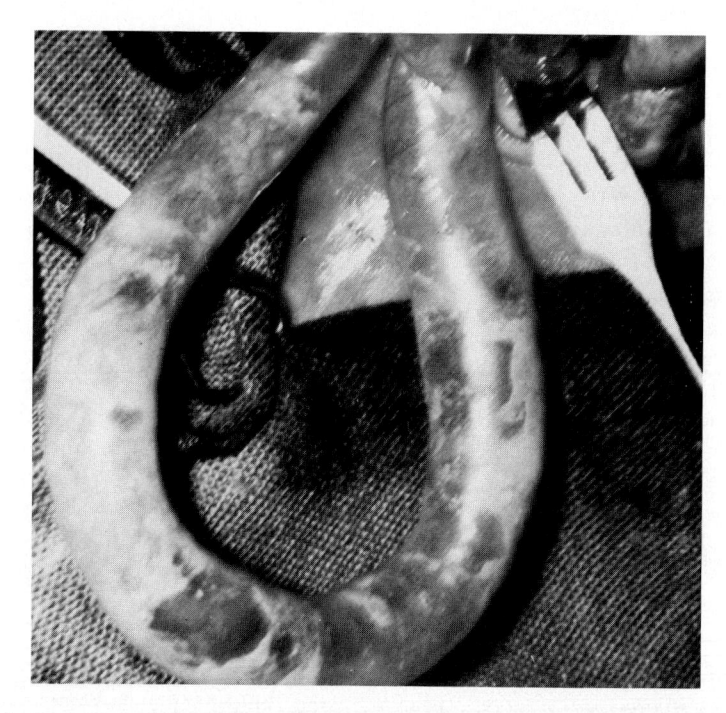

Fig. 24-21. Segment of ileum in a patient with necrotizing enterocolitis, demonstrating dilatation and pneumatosis intestinalis.

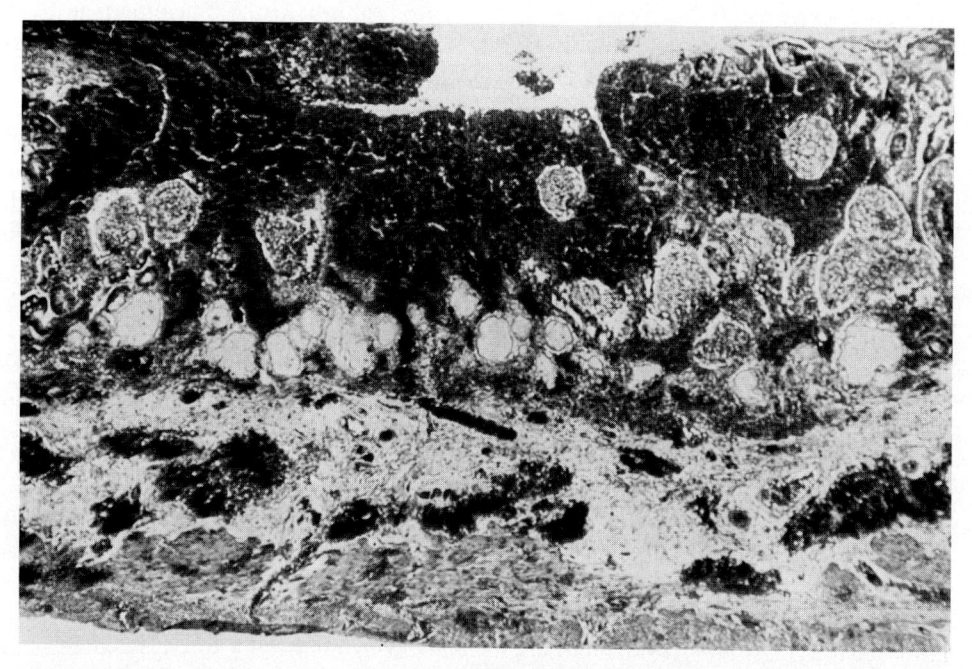

Fig. 24-22. Photomicrograph of the ileum of a patient with necrotizing enterocolitis. The necrotic mucosa and submucosa are replaced with a hemorrhage. (×40.)

Table 24-4. Clinical manifestations of patients with necrotizing enterocolitis

	Percent of patients	
Signs	Review of literature (Hodson)	Experience at Stanford University Medical Center (40 patients)
Lethargy	84	86
Abdominal distension	90	100
Apnea	66	86
Vomiting	70	67
Diarrhea	—	43
Temperature instability	81	—
Hematochezia	39	33
Microscopic blood in stools	24	30
Air in bowel wall	79	86
Air in portal circulation	24	30
Free air in the peritoneal cavity	20	36

Adapted from Hodson, W.A.: Diagnosis and clinical criteria for recognition. In Moore, T.D., editor: Necrotizing enterocolitis in the newborn infant (report of the Sixty-eighth Ross Conference in Pediatric Research), Columbus, 1975, Ross Laboratories, pp. 19-23.

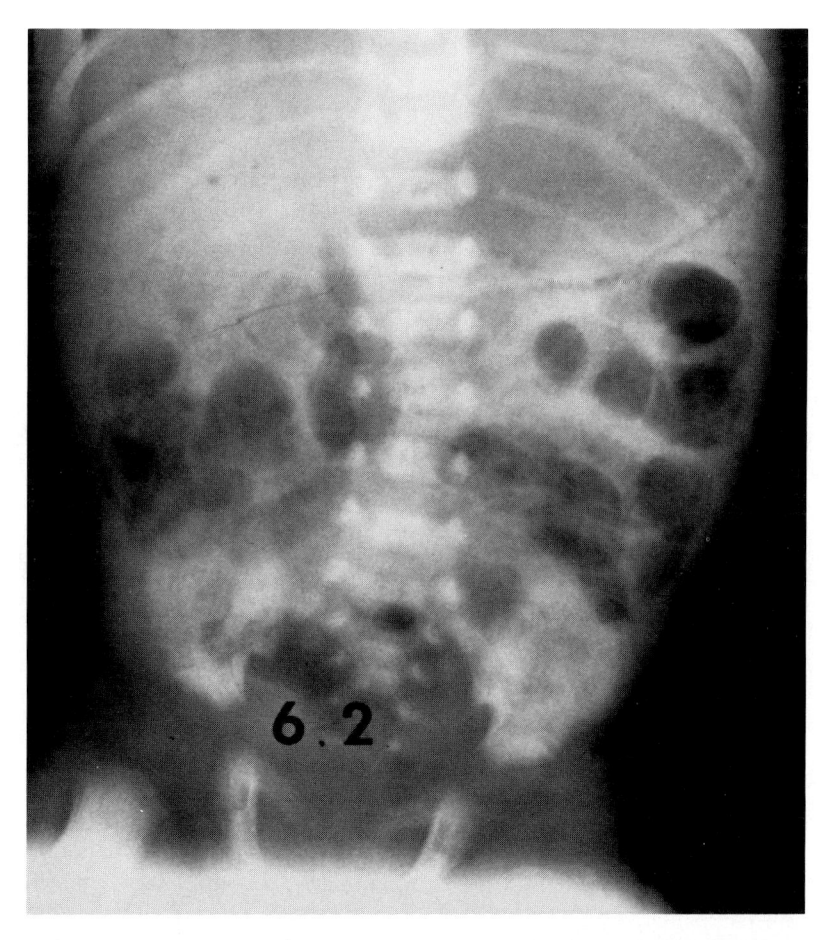

Fig. 24-23. Abdominal roentgenogram of a 4-day-old infant with neonatal necrotizing enterocolitis. Intramural air is noted in the stomach and the intestine. Air is also noted in the liver. This patient was treated medically, and the following day the air in the portal venous system and the pneumatosis intestinalis had disappeared.

After one or two feedings of plain water, we provide a dilute human milk formula and gradually increase the concentration and amount over 2 to 3 weeks. We initiate a synthetic formula only when we are unable to continue feedings with human milk.

Prevention

There have been numerous reports of techniques to prevent NEC or at least to decrease the incidence of the disorder. Prophylactic use of oral aminoglycosides was initially hailed as a means of prevention, but subsequent studies have not supported this. In addition, the use of oral gentamicin in animals that had been asphyxiated resulted in decreased activities of lactase and may interfere with the normal digestive and absorptive processes. Delay in the initiation of enteral feedings in the small premature infant or in the infant who has suffered perinatal asphyxia or shock has also been recommended as a preventive measure. Such infants are given nothing by mouth for 7 to 21 days and fed parenterally. Enteral feedings are then initiated slowly, but at the first sign of abdominal distension, increasing gastric residuals, or regurgitation, enteral feedings are stopped and not reinitiated for several days to weeks. These techniques have been successful in decreasing the incidence of NEC, but prolonged intravenous infusions of hypertonic solutions of glucose and amino acids may predispose the infant to other complications.

The use of human milk, especially fresh unprocessed milk, for the high-risk infant has been advocated by many to decrease the incidence of NEC. Unfortunately, the incidence of NEC has not been altered by the feeding of either processed or unprocessed milk, although the severity of the disease may be lessened.

Prognosis

Most centers now recognize and treat the disease early and report an overall mortality of about 20% to 40%, decreased from a rate of 85% in the early 1960s. Although the finding of air in the liver was believed to be an ominous sign that indicated a lethal outcome, now many infants with air in the portal circulation survive without surgical therapy. Late strictures and adhesions occur but with a surprisingly low incidence.

DISORDERS OF THE PANCREAS

The pancreas develops as one dorsal and two ventral outpouchings of the primitive midgut beginning in the fourth week of fetal life. A few secretory granules are detected by the twelfth week, but it is not until the sixteenth week of intrauterine life that the activities of pancreatic lipase and trypsin are detected. By the twentieth week of fetal life the zymogen granules are well developed, and the activities of the digestive enzymes begin to increase slowly. Although the neonate has markedly decreased activities of these enzymes as compared with the older infant, the enzymes are present in adequate amounts to allow the digestive-absorptive process to proceed adequately. The endocrine pancreas is histologically and functionally mature at birth.

In the infant, as in the older child and adult, the pancreas lies retroperitoneally hidden behind the stomach with its head nestled in the curve of the duodenum, its body arched over the upper lumbar vertebrae, and its tail extending toward the hilum of the spleen. Although the newborn's pancreas may elicit concern because of functional insufficiency, congenital anomaly, or injury, with the exception of cystic fibrosis, pancreatic problems are rare in this age period.

The mature pancreas primarily secretes water, bicarbonate, digestive enzymes, and small amounts of immunoglobulin A and secretory piece. The enzymes include α-amylase, lipase, and various proteases. α-Amylase splits the α-1,4-glycoside linkages of starch and other polysaccharides, yielding maltose (glucose-glucose), maltotriose (glucose-glucose-glucose), and mixed dextrins with α-1,6 branches. Lipase is secreted with colipase and phospholipase. It hydrolyzes triglycerides to 2-monoglycerides and free fatty acids. Both α-amylase and lipase are secreted in active form. The proteases (trypsin, chymotrypsin, carboxypeptidases A and B, and elastase) are secreted in an inactive precursor form and are activated in the small intestine. Enterokinase, a peptidase in the small intestinal mucosa activates trypsin from trypsinogen; trypsin in turn activates the other proteases. General enzyme secretion is stimulated by the small intestinal hormone cholecystokinin-pancreozymin (CCK-PZ). Specific small intestinal secretagogues may cause selective zymogen secretion. Chymodenin is such a hormone and causes selective secretion of chymotrypsinogen. Secretin, another mucosal hormone, stimulates water and bicarbonate secretion.

In the neonate, lipase and proteases are adequate for the digestion of milk, which contains little polysaccharide. Amylase activity remains decreased until after 3 to 6 months. The initial enzyme concentrations decrease in the first 24 hours after feeding but rise at the end of the first week. Over the next 2 years the enzymes increase gradually to mature levels of activity. Pancreatic insufficiency in the newborn manifests itself with diarrhea and steatorrhea, beginning shortly after birth. There is maldigestion of carbohydrate and protein, but the increased fat may make the stool characteristically pale, greasy, bulky, and offensively malodorous. Early in infancy, watery diarrhea may predominate.

Direct measurement of pancreatic function may be made with the pancreozymin-secretin stimulation test. This is technically more difficult in the small infant than

Table 24-5. Pancreatic function after secretin-pancreozymin tests

	Birth	24 hours after feedings	1 week	1 month	Normal children	Cystic fibrosis	Pancreatic insufficiency
Volume (ml/kg/50 min)						0.3-2.7	1.8-3.9
Premature	4.4 (4-15)	5.9 (1.5-9.8)	8.2 (1.6-16.8)	8.96 (3.4-18.7)	3.9 (1.8-81)		
Term	5.39 (1.6-9.7)	3.29 (9.6-80)	4.3 (9.6-10.4)				
HCO$_3^-$ (mEq/L/50 min)				0.19	0.001-0.04 (0.08-0.37)	0.008-0.19	
Trypsin (µg/kg/50 min)						0-450	0.9-320
Premature	60 (0-482)	43.1 (1.6-148)	233.3 (5-660)	196.1 (0.9-660)	765 (215-2,100)		
Term	66.1 (1.2-350)	26.3 (5-67.8)	96.6 (5-230)				
Lipase (IU/kg/50 min)						0-270	0-68
Premature	77.4 (3-343)	65.9 (2.4-209)	328.8 (7.2-1,249)	283.6 (11-730)	1,464 (350-5,000)		
Term	143.9 (2.2-785)	31.7 (4.9-67.4)	39.9 (6.2-125)				
Chymotrypsin (µg/kg/50 min)					860 (252-1,900)	0-126	0-105
Amylase (IU/kg/50 min)						0-117	0-31
Premature	0.88 (0-3.6)	0.62 (0.2-1.4)	2.07 (0.2-8.2)	1.67 (0-4.6)	665 (160-2,150)		
Term	3.20 (0.1-9.8)	0.38 (0.2-0.5)	1.29 (0.1-3.0)				
Carboxypeptidase A (IU/kg/50 min)					724 (141-2,480)	0-204	0-149

From Gryboski, J.: Gastrointestinal problems in the infant, Philadelphia, 1975, W.B. Saunders Co., p. 452.

the more easily done 72-hour fat collection for steatorrhea or the sweat test for cystic fibrosis. When results of the latter two tests are equivocal, the direct measurement may be essential for correct diagnosis. After a 4-hour fast, the pancreozymin-secretin test may be done with the use of two separate sump tubes, one into the duodenum, the other into the stomach to prevent dilution by gastric contamination, which may falsely decrease the results. A special two- or three-lumen tube may be used. A resting sample is collected for 10 to 20 minutes; then CCK-PZ, 1.5 units/kg, is given slowly intravenously or intramuscularly. Two 10-minute collections are made; then secretin, 1.5 units/kg, is similarly given, and three more 10-minute collections are made. Skin tests should be done before giving the secretagogues systemically, and pulse and blood pressure should be monitored during the test. The samples are measured for volume, pH, and bicarbonate. The sample is then immediately deep frozen for enzyme determination. Results are expressed in individual values per kilogram per 50 minutes (Table 24-5). Functional insufficiency of the pancreas may be selective or generalized.

Enterokinase deficiency

Enterokinase is secreted by the duodenal mucosa. When it is deficient, trypsinogen, and consequently the proteases, are not activated. Unless the duodenal aspirate is incubated with normal duodenal mucosa or porcine enterokinase, pancreatic function studies will resemble generalized protease deficiency. Amylase and lipase are normal unless the protein deficiency has been severe enough to prevent amylase and lipase synthesis. Treatment is supplementation with pancreatic enzymes.

Trypsinogen deficiency

The diagnosis of trypsinogen deficiency is confirmed when the pancreatic function test indicates little, if any, activity of proteases. The addition of trypsin to the sample will activate the other proteases. The infants usually have anemia, hypoproteinemia, edema, and failure to thrive. Treatment consists of pancreatic enzyme replacement and the feeding of a protein hydrolysate formula. Whether this is a distinct entity or is identical to enterokinase deficiency has not yet been ascertained.

Lipase deficiency

The few children with lipase deficiency have not had marked growth retardation, and their protein anabolism is essentially unimpaired. They do have marked steatorrhea with oily, leaky stools. Treatment is with high doses of pancreatic enzyme replacement. A low-fat diet with medium-chain triglycerides also may be helpful. This abnormality may represent the initial stages of a generalized pancreatic exocrine insufficiency.

Pancreatic insufficiency and bone marrow dysfunction

Together these are referred to as Schwachman's syndrome; the patients have diarrhea, neutropenia, bone marrow hypoplasia, and marked growth retardation. Metaphyseal dysostosis is found in 10% to 15% of the patients. The pancreatic insufficiency is primarily an enzyme deficiency with normal water and bicarbonate secretion. The neutropenia, which may be cyclic, also may be associated with anemia and thrombocytopenia. The exocrine pancreatic tissue is replaced by fatty tissue with preservation of the ductular system and islets of Langerhans. Symptoms commonly begin in infancy but are rare in the newborn period. Although the patients may have a good appetite, they have diarrhea and failure to thrive. The sweat test is normal. Treatment is with oral pancreatic replacement, which can be decreased as the patients mature. Unfortunately, even with adequate replacement and an adequate diet, these patients grow poorly, and most remain below the third percentile for height and weight.

Cystic fibrosis

The manifestations of cystic fibrosis are protean, but pulmonary and GI disorders count for most of the clinical problems.

Incidence

Cystic fibrosis is inherited as an autosomal recessive trait. The overall incidence is about 1 in 2,500 live births in white populations, but with great geographic variability. It is rare in black populations, American blacks accounting for less than 2% of cases. The heterozygote incidence is approximately 1 in 25 and represents the most common lethal genetic disease in Caucasian children.

Etiology and pathogenesis

The primary defect is unknown, but of clinical importance is the presence of thick, viscid mucus, which becomes inspissated within the lumens of ductular structures. Pancreatic insufficiency is present in 80% of affected newborns. The pancreatic interlobular fibrous bands become larger, and small cysts may be seen. There may be marked fatty replacement of the parenchyma as atrophy progresses. The islets of Langerhans are not affected early in the patient's life. The neonate may have early signs of liver pathology, with prominent portal tracts and numerous bile ducts. Focal biliary cirrhosis has been found within the first few days of life. Prolonged neonatal obstructive jaundice also has been reported. The intestine maintains a normal villus pattern but with increased goblet cells. The various glandular structures, including those of the appendix, may be dilated and inspissated with mucoid material.

Clinical manifestations

Meconium ileus is the most common manifestation of cystic fibrosis in the newborn. Ten percent to 20% of affected children will become obstructed from thick, tenacious intraluminal material that cannot pass the terminal ileum (Fig. 24-24). The meconium contains increased amounts of albumin, but the quantity does not correlate with the likelihood of obstruction, since the highest levels are found in those patients without obstruction. The viscosity is due to an increase in mucoproteins and the formation of an insoluble calcium glycoprotein. Associated intestinal atresia may be found in 20% to 30% of those affected and may be due to in utero obstruction, with resulting volvulus and intramural cicatrization. Symptoms usually begin within the first 24 to 48 hours, with failure to pass meconium, abdominal distension, and vomiting that eventually becomes bilious. The abdomen may have a doughy consistency, and indentation of small mobile masses may be possible. On rectal examination the ampulla contains scanty or no meconium, but sphincter tone is normal.

The patient who does not have meconium ileus may return at 4 to 6 weeks of age with diarrhea, edema, hypoproteinemia, and failure to thrive. Often a nonspecific skin rash similar to that seen in patients with protein malnutrition is found. These symptoms are seen most often in infants on breast milk or soy formulas possibly because of the lower protein content. Vitamin K malabsorption with secondary hypoprothrombinemia may lead to a hemorrhagic diathesis and be the initial clinical manifestation of cystic fibrosis. Hypocalcemia may result from the saponification of calcium with unabsorbed fats; however, vitamin D deficiency is not a problem. Vitamin E, another fat-soluble vitamin, may become deficient and lead to deposition of ceroid pigment in the intestinal serosa, the "brown bowel syndrome."

As the infant matures, signs of malabsorption occur. Thereafter, pulmonary complications are of prime concern, although they may occur rarely in the neonatal period. Later complications include biliary cirrhosis, peptic ulcer disease, lactose maldigestion, rectal prolapse, nasal polyps, increased intracranial pressure, and

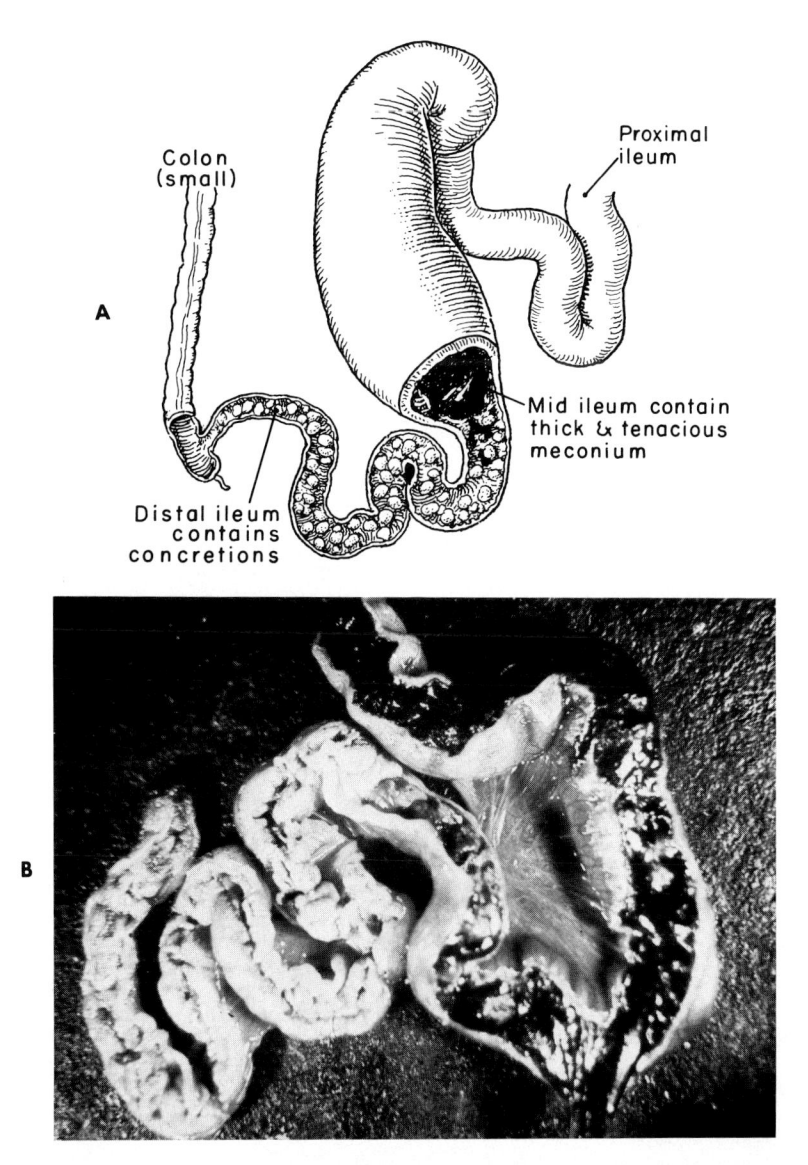

Fig. 24-24. A, Simple meconium ileus. Obstruction of distal ileum is due to concretions of inspissated meconium. **B,** Specimen showing whitish concretions in distal ileum and tenacious tarry meconium proximally. (From Santulli, T.V.: Meconium ileus. In Mustard, W.T., and others, editors: Pediatric surgery, vol. 2, ed. 2, p. 852. Copyright © 1969 by Year Book Medical Publishers, Inc., Chicago. Used by permission.)

the pulmonary complications of infection, fibrosis, and cor pulmonale.

Laboratory manifestations

Roentgenograms of the abdomen reveal dilated loops of bowel of varying size, few air-fluid levels relative to the amount of dilatation, and a bubbly, granular appearance due to meconium mixed with air (Fig. 24-25). Barium enema may show the presence of a microcolon. In 25% of cases there may be evidence of volvulus, atresia, or perforation. Calcification, especially scrotal, indicates antenatal perforation and meconium peritonitis (Chapter 39) (Fig. 24-26). Abnormal metaphyseal bands have been reported in roentgenograms of bones and are commonly seen in the iliac crest and femur. A sweat test should be performed to confirm the diagnosis. Unfortunately, getting the necessary minimum of 40 mg of sweat may be difficult at this age. In addition, the presence of hypoproteinemia and edema may result in a falsely reduced concentration of sodium and chloride in sweat. Testing of the first meconium passed with test strips such as BM-test or Albustix may indicate increased albumin. About 10% to 15% of patients will have a normal test, but these may be infants with normal pancreatic function. Premature

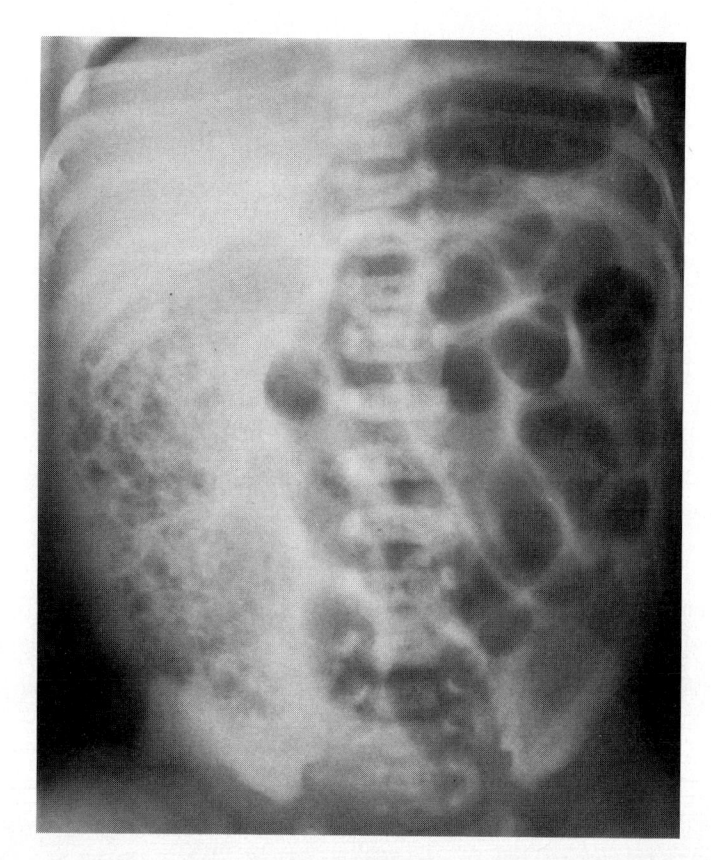

Fig. 24-25. Abdominal roentgenogram of an infant with meconium ileus. Note the bubbly ground-glass appearance of air mixed with inspissated meconium in the right side of the abdomen.

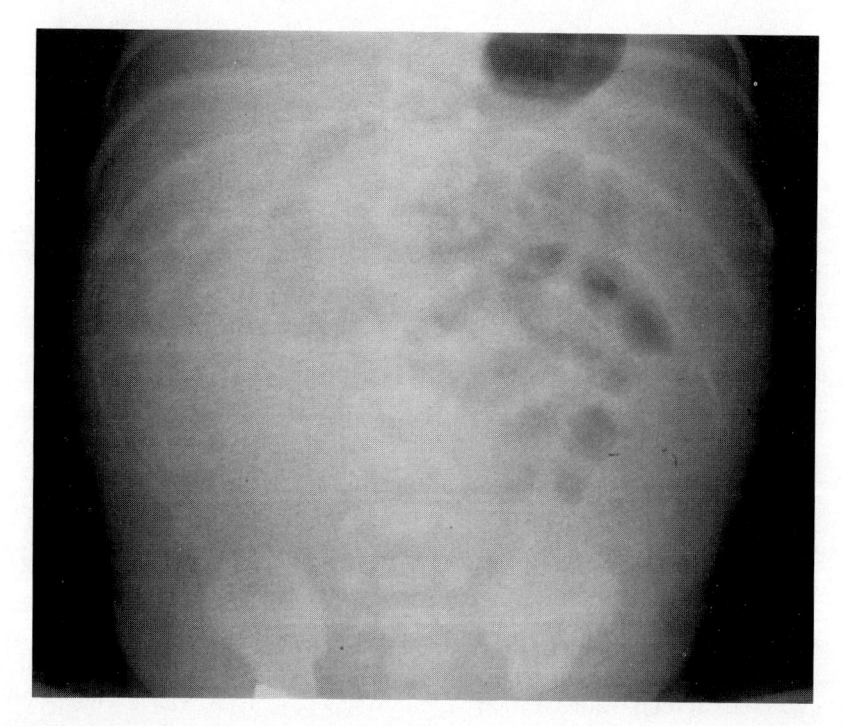

Fig. 24-26. Infant with cystic fibrosis, ileal atresia, and meconium peritonitis. Note the presence of tubular loops of bowel, the paucity of distal intestinal gas, and extensive intraperitoneal calcification.

infants with their relative pancreatic insufficiency may also show increased albumin in their meconium.

Treatment

In the rare patient who may have a mild form of obstruction, nonoperative treatment consisting of acetylcysteine enemas and the feeding of pancreatic enzymes (pancreatin, viokase, pancrepilase [Cotazyme]) by nasogastric tube may be successful. When the obstruction is complete, it may be relieved by the use of meglucamine diatrizoate (Gastrografin) enemas in selected patients. This procedure should be used only in patients with uncomplicated meconium ileus; the infant should be well prepared with adequate fluid and electrolyte replacement. The success of this procedure is attributed to the hypertonicity of the meglucamine diatrizoate solution, which is used as an enema under fluoroscopic control so that the medium is seen to pass through the ileocecal valve into the terminal ileum to disimpact the tenacious meconium.

Operative correction may be accomplished in several ways, including ileotomy with irrigation of the inspissated meconium, resection with end-to-end anastomosis, or some form of enterostomy. We prefer limited resection with side-to-end anastomosis and proximal enterostomy. If a volvulus is present, reduction is accomplished and the viability of the bowel carefully evaluated. Operations for pseudocysts, calcified meconium peritonitis, and intestinal atresia secondary to meconium ileus are usually extremely difficult, and in these instances primary anastomosis is usually avoided; a temporary gastrostomy is also done.

Prognosis

This is one of the most difficult forms of neonatal obstruction to treat. The future of the individual patient who recovers from obstruction is unpredictable. It depends primarily on the lung involvement, and this does not seem to have any relation to the degree of obstruction or the severity of the pathologic findings at operation.

MALABSORPTION AND DIARRHEA

Digestion and absorption proceed as a cascade of coordinated events beginning with ingestion, mastication, and swallowing, and terminating with the transport of nutrients from the intestinal cell into the organism. The initial aspect of digestion occurs when the food is mixed with saliva and the carbohydrates come into contact with salivary amylase. The stomach secretes hydrochloric acid, pepsin, and mucus to initiate the breakdown of lipids, protein, and to some extent carbohydrates. In addition to acting as a reservoir, the stomach delivers an isotonic mixture to the small intestine. The acidic content of

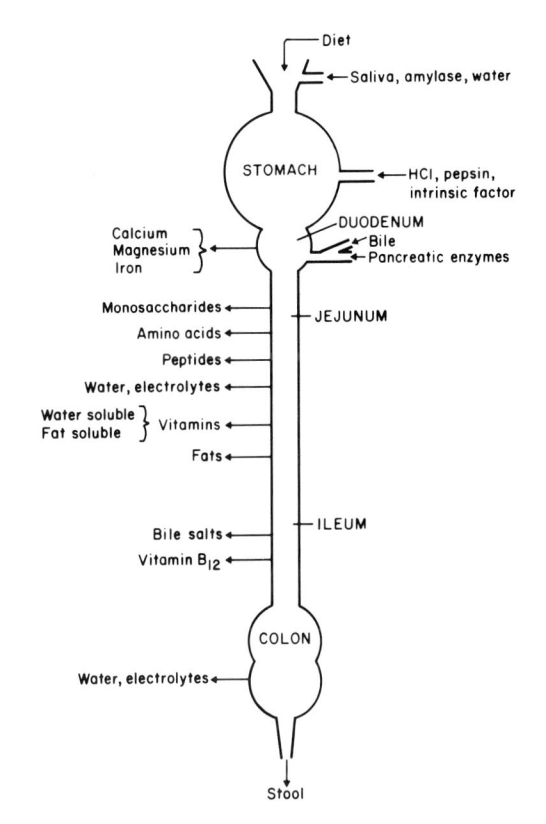

Fig. 24-27. Sites of secretion and absorption in the GI tract. (Adapted from Hamilton, J.R.: Mod. Med. **38**:131, 1970, and Booth, C.C.: Fed. Proc. **26**:1583, 1967.)

the mixture stimulates the duodenum to secrete CCK-PZ, secretin, and enterokinase. These hormones in turn stimulate the release of pancreatic enzymes, or their precursors, and bile into the intestinal lumen.

Protein is broken down primarily by trypsin, chymotrypsin, carboxypeptidases A and B, and aminopeptidases to peptides and amino acids. Dipeptidases and tripeptidases, in the brush border of the enterocytes, further hydrolyze the compounds, and the resultant amino acids are transported across the intestinal cell to the bloodstream.

Fats are digested in the presence of bile acids and lipase to form glycerol, monoglycerides, and fatty acids, which then enter the mucosal cell in a micellar phase. The transport of micelles does not seem to be energy dependent. Once inside the mucosal cell, the monoglycerides and fatty acids are reesterified to triglycerides, which in turn are enveloped by lipoproteins, phospholipids, and cholesterol to form chylomicrons. The chylomicrons then are transported across the intestinal cell to the lymphatics. Short- and medium-chain triglycerides are absorbed intact and transported across the cell to the portal venous system.

Carbohydrates are attacked initially by salivary amylase and then by pancreatic amylase. Disaccharides are further hydrolyzed by the disaccharidases in the brush border of the enterocyte to their constituent monosaccharides, which are then transported across the enterocyte by an active process. There is more rapid hydrolysis and transport if the sugar enters the brush border as a disaccharide rather than in the form of a monosaccharide. Fig. 24-27 illustrates the various areas in which absorption takes place in the GI tract. Hormones elaborated by the GI tract coordinate secretion, motility, and activation of digestive enzymes for normal digestive-absorptive function to proceed (Table 24-6).

Any abnormality that interferes with this concert of coordinated events can lead to suboptimal digestion or

Table 24-6. Hormones of the GI tract: site of origin, factors that stimulate secretion, and actions

Hormone	Origin	Stimuli	Actions
Gastrin*	Gastric antral mucosa, duodenal mucosa(?), cells of pancreatic islets	Products of intragastric protein digestion; vagal stimulation, gastric distension, hypercalcemia	Exists in 3 pairs of peptides: big gastrin (G-34), little gastrin (G-17), and mini-gastrin (G-14); stimulates secretion of hydrochloric acid, pepsinogen, insulin, glucagon, and calcitonin; stimulates growth of GI mucosa and pancreatic parenchyma
Secretin	Mucosa of duodenum and upper jejunum	Acid entering duodenum	Stimulates secretion of water and bicarbonate by pancreas; stimulates biliary secretion, gastric secretion of pepsin, and secretion of Brunner's glands
Cholecystokinin-pancreozymin (CCK-PZ)*	Mucosa of duodenum and upper jejunum	Amino acids, especially tryptophan, phenylalanine, valine, and methionine; fatty acids, C>10 carbon chains, calcium ions	Stimulates secretion of exocrine pancreatic enzymes and bicarbonate, contraction of gallbladder, hepatic bile flow, secretion of glucagon; augments secretin, increases gastric and intestinal motility; inhibits absorption of fluid, sodium, potassium, and chloride from jejunum and ileum
Gastric inhibitory peptide	Mucosa of small intestine	Carbohydrates, fats, and amino acids	Stimulates secretion of insulin, glucagon, and intestinal secretions; inhibits gastric secretion and motility
Vasoactive intestinal peptide*	Throughout GI tract and in pancreas	Unknown	Stimulates secretion of small intestine, pancreatic secretion of water and bicarbonate; augments action of secretin and CCK-PZ; inhibits secretion of gastric acid, pepsin, and histamine; inhibits gastric motility
Human pancreatic polypeptide	Pancreas	Foods, especially protein meals	Physiologic role in humans remains to be elucidated
Motilin	Duodenal mucosa	Ingestion of fat, acidification of duodenum	Stimulates contraction of LES and motor activity in stomach without affecting acid secretion
Chymodenin	Mucosa of small intestine	Unknown	Stimulates secretion of chymotrypsinogen from pancreas
Gut glucagon-like immunoreactants	Pancreatic glucagon, pancreas; gut glucagon, distal small intestine, and colon	Oral and intraintestinal hypertonic glucose and triglycerides	Two types: pancreatic glucagon and gut glucagon; stimulates insulin secretion, increases superior mesenteric artery blood flow and GI motility; is glycogenolytic, lipolytic, and gluconeogenic
Somatostatin*	D cells of pancreas	Acidification of duodenum	Inhibits secretion of insulin, gastrin, glucagon, secretin, GIP, CCK-PZ, VIP, and motilin
Urogastrone*	Brunner's glands of duodenum	Ingestion of fat	Inhibits secretion of gastric acid and intrinsic factor
Bombesin-like peptides*	Stomach and upper small intestine	Standard meal	Regulates gastrin release, involved in control of gallbladder contraction and pancreatic enzyme secretion; depresses intestinal motility; stimulates release of HPP

*Found both in GI tract and brain.

malabsorption. In infants this problem is especially critical because not only is the infant deprived of necessary nutriments, but the infant also tends to lose large amounts of fluid as well and can become profoundly dehydrated. Since damaged mucosal cells are not replaced as rapidly as they are in the adult, attempts to refeed the infant may actually perpetuate the malabsorptive state and lead to many secondary aspects of malabsorption, including intractable diarrhea. Older infants and children with malabsorption may have normal, bulky, or watery stools, but the neonate will have almost exclusively watery diarrhea and, on occasion, vomiting. The causes of maldigestion in the neonate also are somewhat different from the causes in older infants and children[*]:

A. Abnormalities of intestinal mucosa
  1. Infectious diarrhea
     a. Toxigenic *E. coli*
     b. *Salmonella*
     c. *Shigella*
     d. Staphylococci
     e. Enteroviruses
     f. Cytomegaloviruses
  2. Physical, chemical, or toxic agents
     a. Antibiotics
        (1) Ampicillin
        (2) Tetracycline
        (3) Neomycin
     b. Increased concentrations of nitrates or sulfates in water
     c. Diarrhea encountered during heroin or methadone withdrawal
  3. Enzymatic or biochemical abnormalities
     a. Monosaccharide malabsorption
        (1) Congenital
        (2) Acquired
     b. Disaccharide malabsorption
        (1) Congenital
        (2) Acquired
     c. Congenital chloridorrhea
     d. Primary hypomagnesemia
     e. Acrodermatitis enteropathica
     f. Abetalipoproteinemia
     g. Wolman's disease
     h. Amino acid malabsorption
        (1) Phenylketonuria
        (2) Maple syrup urine disease
        (3) Hartnup disease
        (4) Oasthouse urine disease
        (5) "Blue diaper" syndrome
     i. Specific vitamin malabsorption
        (1) Vitamin B_{12} malabsorption
        (2) Folic acid malabsorption
     j. Primary bile acid malabsorption

  4. Acquired defects of the bowel
     a. Massive resection of the small bowel
     b. Necrotizing enterocolitis
B. Abnormalities of pancreatic secretions or stimulators
  1. Cystic fibrosis
  2. Pancreatic achylia
  3. Enterokinase deficiency
C. Abnormalities of liver function
  1. Neonatal hepatitis
  2. Biliary atresia
  3. Congenital cholestatic syndromes
D. Congenital anomalies of the intestine
  1. Hirschsprung's disease
  2. Malrotation
  3. Congenital stenosis
  4. Duplications
E. Immunologic disorders
  1. Wiskott-Aldrich syndrome
  2. Immunodeficiency with thymic dysplasia
F. Hormonal abnormalities
  1. Adrenogenital syndrome
  2. Neural crest tumors
  3. Thyrotoxicosis
G. Allergic gastroenteropathy
  1. Cow's milk protein sensitivity
  2. Soy-protein sensitivity
H. Miscellaneous
  1. Renal abnormalities and/or infection
  2. Intestinal lymphangiectasia

Loose stools in normal infants

Loose stools are commonly encountered, especially in the preterm infant. These may be due to a transitory intolerance to various milks or in rare situations to "overnutrition"; excessive calories induce the diarrhea. The loose stools usually disappear quickly, often with little therapy other than decreasing the quantity of formula ingested.

Infectious diarrhea

Infectious diarrhea is probably the most common cause of severe diarrhea and malabsorption in the neonatal period (p. 662). Enterotoxic *E. coli* is the most common organism incriminated in outbreaks of diarrhea in newborn nurseries. Diarrhea caused by *Salmonella* organisms is seen much less frequently, and that caused by *Shigella* organisms or staphylococci is only rarely encountered. Other organisms, such as *Pseudomonas* or *Klebsiella*, also may cause enterocolitis in a susceptible host. Although enteropathogenic *E. coli* is not identified by specific serotyping, these organisms may elaborate an endotoxin and cause severe diarrhea. In many situations, a specific bacterial organism may not be isolated, and a viral etiology, especially an enterovirus, is suspected. Most organisms cause diarrhea by direct invasion of the intestinal mucosa, especially in the ileum and colon, with resultant inflammation, ulceration, and outpouring of

---

[*]Adapted from Sunshine, P.: Current problems in pediatrics, vol. II, no. 8, Chicago, 1972, Year Book Medical Publications, Inc.

fluid, blood, and mucus. In some situations an enterotoxin is elaborated that stimulates adenyl cyclase to increase intestinal secretions markedly. This results in the loss of diarrheal fluid with markedly increased sodium and potassium content. In some situations a severe and intractable diarrhea that is resistant to the usual form of antimicrobial therapy may ensue. The diagnosis and treatment of these disorders are outlined in Chapter 27. Although parasites such as *Giardia* and *Entamoeba histolytica* may cause diarrhea in older infants, they are almost never responsible for diarrhea in the neonate.

Physical and chemical agents

Antimicrobial agents, especially ampicillin and tetracycline given orally, not infrequently lead to a diarrheal state in the newborn. Often the diarrhea will cease when the antibiotic is discontinued, but in some situations the infant may have to be treated with a carbohydrate-free forumula for a period of time. Diarrhea and malabsorption also have been reported in infants whose formula is made with well water containing increased concentration of nitrates or sulfates.

Carbohydrate malabsorption

Next to infectious diarrheas, primary or secondary carbohydrate intolerance is the most common form of malabsorption seen in the neonate. Acquired forms of carbohydrate malabsorption are much more common than congenital forms and are usually secondary to other disease states that may damage the intestinal mucosa. Because the sugar fails to undergo hydrolysis, it remains in the intestinal lumen. Small quantities of disaccharide, however, are passively absorbed and excreted unchanged in the urine. The bulk of the sugar then passes through the intestinal tract, where it may act as an osmotic hydrogogue. In the colon, bacteria act on the sugar to produce both organic acids, such as lactic acid, and hydrogen gas. This increases the osmotic diarrhea in the colon and also exerts an irritative effect and stimulates the passage of more fluid. Many infants have abdominal distension and profuse vomiting as well. Carbohydrate tolerance tests, using 2 gm/kg of the sugar and measuring glucose in blood at 0, 20, 40, 60, and 90 minutes, are an effective way to diagnose these disorders. A normal infant should have a rise of 20 mg/dl or more above the fasting level, whereas the affected patient has little if any rise in blood glucose level and also develops abdominal pain and diarrhea. The offending sugar and increased concentrations of organic acids are found in the stool. A low stool pH is often encountered, but this also may be found in infants who ingest milk with a high lactose concentration, such as breast milk. Some infants do not have a normal increase in blood glucose following a carbohydrate-loading study because of delayed gastric emptying time. This is especially true for lactose tolerance tests. Direct measurement of intestinal disaccharidase activity in mucosa obtained by peroral jejunal biopsy may be necessary to confirm the diagnosis. Recently the measurement of hydrogen in expired air has been used to detect carbohydrate malabsorption. This noninvasive technique is very reliable in older infants and children but may not be as accurate in infants. The relationship of hydrogen gas excretion and colonic colonization rates remains to be elucidated.

Lactose malabsorption

Congenital lactose malabsorption is rare, but secondary intolerance is a relatively common form of sugar malabsorption. In most situations where mucosal damage has occurred, lactase is one of the first enzymes to decrease in activity and one of the last enzymes to return to normal activity during the healing process. Treatment consists of removing lactose from the diet for periods up to 2 or 3 months.

Sucrose-isomaltose malabsorption

Sucrose-isomaltose malabsorption is due to a congenital absence or a marked decrease in activity of both sucrase and isomaltase. It is unusual for a neonate to be diagnosed as having this disorder because sucrose and starch are not introduced into the diet until later in infancy. This congenital abnormality is much more common than congenital lactose malabsorption, and over 100 cases have been described. It is one of the rare genetic disorders in which two enzymes are involved, and it may be that the activities of the two are located at independent sites on the same protein molecule. Secondary sucrose intolerance has been found following severe enteritis and other defects involving the small intestine. Treatment consists of placing the patient on a diet that eliminates sucrose as well as dextrins and starches. As the infant matures, small amounts of sucrose are tolerated.

Glucose-galactose malabsorption

Congenital glucose-galactose malabsorption also is rare; approximately 25 patients have been reported with this familial, autosomal recessive disorder. The basic defect is the inability of the microvilli to bind either glucose or galactose. Sodium absorption, sodium activation of sucrase, sodium-potassium–dependent ATPase activity, and the transport of *l*-amino acids are all normal. The renal tubular cell also is affected, and glucosuria is present. These patients are able to absorb fructose normally. Treatment consists of providing specially prepared formulas with fructose as the only source of carbohydrate. This is one of the most difficult of all the sugar intolerances to treat, often because the diagnosis is not appreciated and many attempts are made to feed the infant with glucose water. Although the mucosa is normal early in the course of the disease, significant changes do occur if the diarrhea continues unabated. As the infants mature, they often tolerate small amounts of glucose and sucrose but still may have episodes of abdominal cramps, diarrhea, and flatulence if large amounts are ingested.

Transient malabsorption of monosaccharides also has been encountered in infants and usually follows severe gastroenteritis or massive resection of the small intestine. These infants cannot tolerate even a 1% or 2% glucose solution and at times cannot tolerate fructose as well. If appropriate intravenous therapy is given and the basic pathophysiologic process corrected, the infants regain their ability to tolerate monosaccharides, although a prolonged period of time may be necessary for this to occur.

Congenital chloridorrhea

Congenital alkalotic diarrhea is thought to be secondary to an inability of the infant to absorb chloride, especially in the ileum and colon. The infant usually has severe diarrhea in the first weeks of life, with massive losses of water and electrolytes, especially potassium and chloride. This loss, despite replacement, may lead to hypovolemia, secondary hyperaldosteronism, high urinary excretion of potassium, and a resultant hypochloremic, hypokalemic alkalosis. The infants are usually preterm and have hydramnios. Often there is delayed passage of meconium, suggesting that the infants may have had diarrhea in utero. Abdominal distension and hyperbilirubinemia complicate the disease. The diagnosis is made by finding increased concentrations of chloride in stool, absent to very low concentrations of chloride in urine, and a hypochloremic, hypokalemic alkalosis. As the infant matures, growth retardation, secondary hyperaldosteronism, urinary tract infection, and degenerative renal changes ensue. Prompt treatment can reverse many of the complications of the disease and consists of providing supplemental potassium chloride to maintain normal serum electrolyte concentrations and blood pH. The infants require between 2 and 14 mEq/kg/day of potassium and chloride. A secondary chloride-losing diarrhea also has been reported following bowel surgery.

Absence of β-lipoprotein in blood

Abetalipoproteinemia is a rare disease inherited as an autosomal recessive trait. In contrast to most of the other malabsorptive states in the neonate, these patients have bulky, fatty diarrhea, which usually begins during the first weeks of life. This progresses to abdominal distension, poor weight gain, and hypotonia. The basic defect is due to decreased ability to synthesize the β-lipoprotein molecule from normal precursors. The synthesis of chylomicrons, therefore, is markedly reduced. The patients also have neurologic degeneration, retinitis pigmentosa, and acanthocytosis. A low-fat diet with supplementary medium-chain triglycerides decreases steatorrhea and improves weight gain. Whether this form of therapy has any effect on the neurologic damage to the infant remains speculative. In some infants with severe diarrhea and malabsorption due to other causes, hypolipoproteinemia, hypocholesterolemia, and acanthocytosis may be secondarily encountered.

Pancreatic and liver function abnormalities

Pancreatic disorders causing malabsorption, such as cystic fibrosis, pancreatic achylia, enterokinase deficiency, and lipase deficiency, are discussed on p. 516. Abnormalities of liver function that cause malabsorption include neonatal hepatitis, biliary atresia, and congenital cholestatic syndrome (Chapter 30).

Immunologic disorders

GI symptomatology in the neonatal or early infancy period is associated with immunodeficiency with thrombocytopenia and eczema (*Wiskott-Aldrich syndrome*) and immunodeficiency with *thymic dysplasia*. Both these disorders are inherited as X-linked recessive traits. Patients with the Wiskott-Aldrich syndrome usually present with bleeding episodes associated with thrombocytopenia and then develop severe eczema, recurrent bacterial and viral infections, and bloody diarrhea. Patients with thymic dysplasia have watery diarrhea of early onset, and often an etiologic agent is not cultured from the stool. The diarrhea is refractory to therapy and progresses to include signs of secondary malabsorption as well. These entities are discussed in Chapter 26.

Hormonal abnormalities

Patients with salt-losing *congenital adrenal hyperplasia* (CAH) have vomiting, often projectile in nature, at the end of the first or beginning of the second week of life (Chapter 33, part four). This may simulate pyloric stenosis except that the infant also often has diarrhea. Patients with salt-losing CAH may have virilization and hyperkalemia instead of the hypokalemia seen in patients with pyloric stenosis.

Neural crest tumors, especially ganglioneuroma or ganglioneuroblastoma, may cause severe watery diarrhea that is refractory to the usual therapy. Initially, it was thought that the increased secretions of catecholamines produced intestinal vasoconstriction resulting in watery diarrhea. Recently, it has been demonstrated that some tumors secrete vasoactive intestinal peptide, a hormone that may be responsible for the loose stools.

Neonatal thyrotoxicosis (Chapter 33, part three), which is almost always a transient disease caused by transplacental passage of either long-acting thyroid stimulator (LATS) or an antibody to the microsomal fraction of the gland, can be associated with watery diarrhea. Although the infant may actually have symptoms of hyperthyroidism, such as tachycardia, in utero, some infants will not develop thyrotoxicosis until 5 to 10 days old.

Allergic gastroenteropathy

The most common allergic gastroenteropathy in the neonatal period is *cow's milk–protein allergy*. *Soy protein allergy* is also increasingly recognized. The infants may have a wide variety of signs and symptoms, including eczema, rhinitis, diarrhea, vomiting, colic, fever, leukocytosis, and thrombocytopenia. Milk-protein allergy occurs in between 3 to 10 per 1,000 live births; symptoms may begin as early as the first or second day or as late as 4 to 5 months of age. Often there is a strong family history of allergy, but the mode of inheritance is unknown at present. Infants with mild symptoms usually respond rapidly when the formula is changed to a non-cow's milk or hydrolyzed protein, but some infants continue to have severe diarrhea with blood loss, anemia, hypoproteinemia, and edema, which may resemble an infantile form of ulcerative colitis. The diagnosis is often difficult to document because skin testing or assay for antibodies against milk proteins in serum has been confusing or uninterpretable. Coproantibodies to milk protein have been detected in freshly spun stools from infants with milk-protein allergy; however, these antibodies also are present in the stools of normal infants or infants with gastroenteritis. Many, but not all, infants have peripheral eosinophilia. At present, the diagnosis is made when a patient has remission of symptoms following elimination of cow's milk protein from the diet, and exacerbation of symptoms with leukocytosis when the offending protein is reintroduced. If this diagnostic study is attempted in very young or very sick infants, severe diarrhea or GI hemorrhage may ensue. We prefer not to reintroduce cow's milk protein for at least 3 or 4 months and at that time to introduce only 1 or 2 tablespoons at a time, preferably in a hospital setting with intravenous fluids at the bedside. A majority of infants will be able to tolerate milk by the time they are 2 years of age or older. Unfortunately, many will go on to develop other food allergies, hay fever, asthma, or allergic dermatitis. Transient intolerance to milk or other proteins also is encountered following episodes of severe gastroenteritis in older infants.

Parenteral diarrhea

Mild to severe diarrhea may accompany systemic infections, especially if the genitourinary tract is involved. The mechanism for the production of the diarrhea is unknown.

Intestinal lymphangiectasia

Intestinal lymphangiectasia is characterized by dilatation and abnormalities of the lymphatics of the intestine, marked GI protein loss, and unilateral or bilateral lymphedema. Abnormalities of the inguinal, pelvic, and retroperitoneal lymph nodes also are found. On occasion, the only abnormality found in the neonatal period is lymphedema of a single extremity. In early to late infancy, diarrhea, abdominal distension, ascites, and generalized edema may be found. Signs and symptoms may not develop until the child is 5 years of age or older. The diagnosis is usually made with the use of intravenous infusion of ^{51}Cr-labeled albumin to demonstrate increased protein loss in stools. The measurement of α-1-antitrypsin in stool to quantitate enteric protein loss may supplant the ^{51}Cr technique in the near future. Small bowel biopsy or lymphangiography also may be necessary to confirm the diagnosis. Therapy consists of placing the patient on a low-fat diet containing medium-chain triglycerides.

Other specific causes of intestinal malabsorption are listed in Table 24-7.

Massive resection of the small bowel

One of the most difficult problems is the management of the neonate who has had massive resection of the small intestine. Although some adults have survived with as little as 10% of their small intestine intact, the removal of even a small section of intestine in the neonatal period may result in severe diarrhea and failure to thrive. The judicious use of fluids and electrolytes has led to marked improvement in morbidity and mortality in the immediate postsurgical period, and the introduction of total parenteral nutrition has been of immense help in rehabilitating these infants to their maximum "functional" GI capabilities.

The important factors influencing the ability of the intestine to adapt appropriately and the subsequent ability of the infant to survive massive resections of the small intestine are included in the following list.
1. The maturity of the infant
2. The length of intestine remaining
3. Is the remaining intestine proximal or distal small bowel?
4. Presence of the ileocecal valve
5. Presence of an intact colon
6. Intactness of pancreatic and liver function
7. General condition of infant prior to and following resection
8. Presence and severity of other congenital malformations

Although the jejunum is the primary site at which the

Table 24-7. Specific defects of intestinal absorption

Defect	Comment
Phenylketonuria	Inability to absorb tryptophan in the presence of increased serum concentrations of phenylalanine
Maple syrup urine disease	Inability to absorb tryptophan in the presence of increased serum concentrations of branched-chain amino acids
Oasthouse urine disease	Inability to absorb methionine
Cystinuria	Defect in absorption of cytine, ornithine, lysine, arginine, cysteine, and homocystine
Hartnup disease	Defect in absorption of monoamino and monocarboxylic amino acids
Folic acid malabsorption	Megaloblastic anemia, mental retardation, and seizures; inability to absorb folic acid from intestine or to transport folic acid from blood to CSF
Familial vitamin B_{12} malabsorption	Normal gastric HCl and intrinsic factor; associated with hyperpigmentation and proteinuria
Fructose intolerance	Defect in fructose-1-phosphate aldolase, hepatomegaly, vomiting, and abdominal distension following ingestion of fructose or sucrose
Acrodermatitis enteropathica	Suspected defect in absorption of zinc; diarrhea and mucocutaneous lesions; suspected autosomal recessive transmission
Wolman's disease	Deficiency of an intracellular lipase that leads to accumulation of lipid intracellularly

Adapted from Sunshine, P.: Current problems in pediatrics, vol. II, no. 8, Chicago, 1972, Year Book Medical Publishers, Inc.

digestive-absorptive process takes place, infants with resection of the jejunum tend to fare much better than those in whom the ileum is removed. The ileum is the primary site for bile acid absorption and, if lost, will interfere with the absorption of lipid. Unabsorbed bile acids can also irritate the colon and exaggerate fluid and electrolyte loss. The ileum tends to become more hyperplastic following the resection of the jejunum than does the jejunum following ileal resection. In addition, the ileum contains more lymphoid tissue than does the jejunum, and the presence of this tissue may be an important factor in adaptation following resection.

If the ileocecal valve remains intact, it tends to delay intestinal transit time, allows the digestive-absorptive process to proceed more efficiently, and also acts as a barrier to prevent overgrowth of colonic bacteria in the distal small intestine. Similarly, if the large intestine is left intact, greater absorption of water and electrolytes will take place.

The minimum length of small intestine required for survival is not known, but patients with as little as 15 cm of small intestine remaining have survived; in these patients, however, the ileocecal valve was intact. If the valve is lost, then patients with less than 40 cm of small intestine remaining adapt poorly, if at all.

Factors that tend to regulate intestinal adaptation include the exposure of the residual bowel to nutriments, stimulation of the mucosa by biliary and pancreatic secretions, and the effects of enteric and other hormones. Nutriments in the intestinal lumen stimulate mucosal growth, whereas nonnutritive or bulk agents do not. Patients who are nourished by total parenteral nutrition do not have as extensive cellular hyperplasia as patients fed some nutriments enterally, even if the caloric intake and weight gain are adequately maintained. Nutriments in the intestinal lumen may also stimulate biliary and pancreatic secretions, which tend to enhance intestinal cellular hyperplasia. The effect of hormones such as gastrin, secretin, cholecystokinin-pancreozymin, and glucagon may also be very important in stimulating intestinal hyperplasia.

Although these adaptive factors have been documented as occurring in the adult human as well as in the adult laboratory animal, they have not been documented in the developing intestine. We know little of the rates of cellular proliferation and migration in the human infant, but the intestine does have shallow crypts and short villi. It appears that the infant's intestine may not adapt as readily as that of the older child or adult, and it may take weeks or even months for the infant to be able to digest and absorb adequate calories, even when less than 50% of the intestine is resected.

Gastric hypersecretion is another complication of the short bowel syndrome and may be secondary to either increased secretion or decreased catabolism of gastrin. This hyperacidity leads to edema and ulceration of the upper small intestine and also inactivates pancreatic lipase and micellar formation, resulting in decreased absorption of fat and other nutriments. The hypersecretion can be treated with antacids or cimetidine and usually resolves after several weeks to months. If blind loops or stasis develops, secondary bacterial overgrowth occurs, which results in both bile salt inactivation and decreased vitamin B_{12} absorption.

Treatment of the short-gut syndrome in infancy is difficult and often frustrating. Total parenteral nutrition must be initiated soon after surgery and continued through the prolonged phase of refeeding. Enteral feedings are introduced slowly with very gradual increases in concentration and volume to prevent distension, vomiting, and diarrhea. We have found that the feeding of dilute human milk is of great benefit in the management of patients with the short bowel syndrome. The milk, especially freshly expressed human milk, contains many host resistance factors and possibly an intestinal growth-promoting factor. Thereafter, other hypoosmolar foods can be added to the infant's diet. Successful feeding with elemental diets has also been reported, but these may increase the solute load presented to the intestine and perpetuate the diarrhea.

With extensive ileal resection, bile salts may be poorly absorbed. The salts, which are irritants to colonic mucosa, cause the large intestine to excrete large amounts of both fluid and electrolytes. We have found that 1 to 2 gm of cholestyramine three times a day greatly decreases the irritative effect of the bile salts and reduces the diarrheal losses. Medications such as diphenoxylate, paregoric, and codeine have been used with varying degrees of success.

A recently recognized complication following massive resection of the small intestine is the development of severe metabolic acidosis. It has been shown that, with bacterial overgrowth, the unabsorbed carbohydrate can be converted to lactic acid by bacteria in the colon or distal small intestine. The lactic acid is D-lactic acid and is not metabolized and excreted as readily as is L-lactic acid. Therapy consists of nonabsorbable antibiotics and correction of any blind loop or stagnant section of bowel.

Intractable diarrhea

Intractable or protracted diarrhea of infancy is a life-threatening disorder. Initial reports noted a mortality of over 70%, and in most patients the primary etiologic factor was never identified. The infants were thought to have a severe form of a nonspecific enterocolitis, which in many was resistant to therapy that included the use of corticosteroids and ileostomies. In addition to this idiopathic "syndrome," several specific diarrheal disorders of infancy may cause protracted diarrhea in the neonate. Many of these disorders can be treated specifically and effectively, and their early recognition will markedly reduce morbidity and mortality. Following is a list of conditions that may initiate the intractable diarrhea syndrome of infancy:

1. Complications secondary to severe infectious diarrhea
2. Severe cow's milk– or soy milk–protein sensitivity
3. Cystic fibrosis
4. Glucose-galactose malabsorption
5. Congenital chloridorrhea
6. Immunodeficiency with thymic dysplasia
7. Increased secretion of gastrin, vasoactive intestinal peptide, or human pancreatic polypeptide
8. Abetalipoproteinemia
9. Pseudomembranous colitis
10. Primary bile salt malabsorption
11. Familial enteropathy with hypoplastic villus atrophy
12. Renal tubular acidosis
13. Hirschsprung's disease with enterocolitis
14. Massive resection of the small intestine
15. Intestinal lymphangiectasia

Clinical manifestations

A prolonged diarrheal state in the neonate rapidly leads to severe malnutrition with emaciation, dehydration, acidosis, anemia, hypoproteinemia, and marked electrolyte disturbances. The infants remain unresponsive to repeated episodes of intravenous fluid therapy; attempts to refeed these infants often result in severe exacerbation or perpetuation of the diarrhea. The inability to provide adequate protein and calories during this period not only delays GI repair and regeneration but also predisposed the infant to infection and the subsequent development of generalized sepsis. An extremely difficult situation is created in which both feeding and the severe malnutrition that follows the prolonged periods of fasting serve to perpetuate the diarrheal state.

Laboratory manifestations

A vigorous diagnostic approach in the early stages of this syndrome, before rehydration and the establishment of improved nutrition and positive nitrogen balance, is poorly tolerated and may hasten the infant's death. Our initial approach to diagnosis (listed below) is an attempt to exclude specific causes for the diarrhea without the extensive use of invasive techniques. Frequent and repeated cultures of blood, stool, and urine are obtained for bacterial, viral, and parasitic agents. Careful monitoring of serum electrolytes is mandatory to ensure that the patient is kept in normal fluid and electrolyte balance. Examination of stool and urine for chloride is performed to identify those patients with congenital chloridorrhea. Evaluation of red blood cell morphology is helpful in identifying patients with abetalipoproteinemia in whom large numbers of acanthocytes are seen on peripheral smear. Urine pH determination as well as blood pH and serum bicarbonate concentration will identify the rare patients with renal tubular acidosis who present with intractable diarrhea.

INITIAL LABORATORY STUDIES TO EVALUATE PATIENTS WITH INTRACTABLE DIARRHEA

1. Complete blood count, including smear for red blood cell morphology and platelet count
2. Urinalysis
3. Repeated and frequent bacterial and viral cultures of blood, urine, and stool
4. Serum electrolytes and chemistries
5. Sweat chloride determination
6. Analysis of chloride in urine and stool

7. Serum immunoglobulins
8. Twenty-four-hour urine collection for amino acids and catecholamine metabolites

In the vast majority of patients with intractable diarrhea, total parenteral nutrition must be initiated to improve the infant's clinical condition and to repair nutritional deficiencies. After the patient responds to parenteral nutrition, a more extensive and definitive evaluation may be attempted (see list below). Proctosigmoidoscopy and rectal biopsy are of considerable help in identifying cases of allergic (milk-induced) colitis.

FOLLOW-UP STUDIES TO EVALUATE PATIENTS WITH INTRACTABLE DIARRHEA

1. Proctosigmoidoscopy and rectal biopsy
2. Small bowel biopsy for morphology and disaccharidase activities
3. Upper GI series and small bowel follow-through
4. Barium enema
5. Analysis of pancreatic secretions
6. Assay of serum gastrin and vasoactive intestinal peptide
7. Serum lipoprotein electrophoresis
8. Glucose and disaccharide tolerance tests
9. Analysis of bile acids in stool

A small group of infants appear to have a secretory diarrheal state in which the diarrhea continues in spite of prolonged periods of total parenteral nutrition and complete rest of the GI tract. Such patients should be evaluated not only for the presence of endotoxins but also for the excessive production of gastrin, vasoactive intestinal peptide, or other GI hormones capable of inducing a secretory diarrheal state. These patients have profuse watery diarrhea that may exceed 100 ml/kg/day at a time that they are receiving *nothing by mouth*.

Pathology

Patients with severe milk-induced colitis and those with cow's milk–protein sensitivity probably represent a spectrum of the same pathophysiologic process. Because the mucosa has been repeatedly damaged, edema, ulceration, and friability often are seen at proctoscopy. Microscopic examination of the tissue reveals edema, hemorrhage, and often infiltration of the mucosa with eosinophils and plasma cells; these findings often will differentiate severe allergic colitis from cases of infantile onset of idiopathic ulcerative colitis. The mucosa of the small intestine reveals hypertrophy of the crypts with diffuse necrosis and edema of the villi, often with changes similar to those seen in older infants with severe celiac disease. Eosinophilic infiltration of the mucosa may be encountered, and in some patients a fibrinous exudate overlying the necrotic mucosa is seen. Specific abnormalities of the small intestinal mucosa may be seen in patients with intestinal lymphangiectasia, abetalipoproteinemia, familial villus atrophy, and certain immunodeficiency disorders.

Treatment

The management of idiopathic intractable diarrhea is difficult, time consuming, and often very frustrating. The early use of total parenteral nutrition has markedly improved the prognosis. If a specific intestinal disease is found, either surgery or specific dietary therapy is initiated. In patients in whom a specific diagnosis cannot be made, we attempt to gradually introduce dilute human milk or a predigested non-lactose-containing formula over a period of 3 to 4 months, after which the gradual introduction of other hypoallergenic foods is attempted. Although this approach has improved the outcome of patients with protracted diarrhea, morbidity and mortality are still significant.

ABDOMINAL WALL DEFECTS

Although recent studies seriously question the traditional separation of gastroschisis and omphalocele on a developmental basis, it remains a useful clinical distinction, and the two entities will therefore be discussed separately. Clinical differential diagnostic points are summarized in Table 24-8.

Gastroschisis

Gastroschisis consists of herniation of intraabdominal contents through a paraumbilical defect in the abdominal wall. These defects are thought to result from a primary failure of abdominal wall closure or from intrauterine rupture of the amniotic membrane at the base of the umbilical cord during the period of normal umbilical herniation of the midgut.

Clinical manifestations and pathology

There is no covering sac, and the umbilical cord remains in its normal medial position with an intact umbilical ring. The defects are generally right sided and vary between 3 and 15 cm in size. The eviscerated organs consist primarily of small and large intestine and seldom include solid viscera, such as the liver and spleen. All patients have some degree of incomplete intestinal rotation as well as shortening and poor posterior fixation of the small intestine. The herniated abdominal contents are often covered with a thick gelatinous material, resulting in adherent loops of edematous bowel. This is seen most commonly with early intrauterine evisceration and prolonged exposure of the viscera to the amniotic fluid and is associated with a hypoplastic peritoneal cavity. Those with mild serosal reaction and normal peritoneal cavities are thought to represent perinatal evisceration. Gangrene may occur in the herniated loops of bowel, especially with small defects. Over half of the patients

Table 24-8. Gastroschisis and omphalocele: comparative clinical features

	Gastroschisis	Omphalocele
Incidence	1/50,000 births	1/5,000 births
Location of defect	Right paraumbilical	Central abdominal
Covering sac	Absent	Present
Umbilicial ring	Present	Absent
Umbilical cord insertion	Normal	Apex of sac
Herniation of the liver	Rare	Common
Associated extraintestinal anomalies	Rare	Common

with gastroschisis are born prematurely; approximately 10% have associated intestinal atresias.

Treatment

Initial measures should be concerned with preventing infection and maintaining body temperature and fluid balance. These steps are particularly important if the newborn is to be transported for specialized care. After careful inspection for torsion and severe angulation, the exposed viscera should be covered with warm saline dressings. A nasogastric catheter is inserted to minimize gastric distension and to help prevent aspiration of GI contents. Intravenous fluids are used to maintain normal fluid and electrolyte status, and antibiotics are begun following appropriate cultures. Following manual stretching of the abdominal wall, many smaller defects with adequate peritoneal cavities may be repaired by primary closure. Larger defects may require a staged repair through the use of a prosthetic pouch.

During the recovery period after surgery, a prolonged period of GI dysfunction and absent peristalsis is common and may last between 10 and 60 days. Total parenteral nutrition is necessary during this time to prevent the complications of severe malnutrition (p. 310). When feedings are instituted, a non-lactose-containing predigested formula is most easily tolerated. A gastrostomy is helpful during this time in limiting gastric distension, preventing pulmonary aspiration, and monitoring early attempts at feeding. Careful attention must be paid to the problems of both early and late sepsis as well as to the complications of associated prematurity. In addition, patients with gastroschisis or ruptured omphalocele may be at increased risk for the development of hypoalbuminemia and hypogammaglobulinemia.

Prognosis

Although recent mortality has been as high as 60%, a steady improvement in survival has been noted, especially since parenteral nutrition has become available. Follow-up studies show return of normal GI function in survivors after 6 months of age.

Omphalocele

Omphaloceles develop between the eighth and tenth weeks of fetal life and result from failure of the intestines to return to the abdominal cavity from their extraabdominal position in the umbilical coelom.

Clinical manifestations and pathology

They may vary from a small bulge at the base of the umbilicus to a huge sac containing most of the GI tract as well as liver and spleen. There is no intact umbilical ring, and the umbilical cord inserts at the apex of the covering sac. In patients in whom the sac has ruptured prenatally, the bowel may appear edematous and adherent and may be very difficult to distinguish from gastroschisis (Fig. 24-28). As in gastroschisis, omphaloceles are associated with a high incidence of malrotation and poor posterior fixation of the mesentery. In addition, omphaloceles are commonly seen in association with cardiac, genitourinary, and other extraintestinal anomalies. The syndrome of macroglossia and giantism in association with omphalocele (Beckwith's syndrome) must be recognized early to prevent the complications of the associated severe hypoglycemia (Chapter 33, part one).

Treatment

Early treatment to prevent infection, dehydration, and hypothermia is similar to that outlined for gastroschisis. Small defects may be closed primarily, but controversy surrounds the treatment of large intact omphaloceles. Whereas several pediatric surgical centers have favored the use of topical agents, such as Mercurochrome, to promote peripheral epithelialization, others have advocated early surgical exploration and staged reduction through the use of a ventral synthetic pouch. The latter group considers the high incidence of associated GI atresias sufficient cause for abdominal exploration. The staged repair allows control of intraabdominal pressure and prevents the complications of respiratory embarrassment and compromised intestinal venous return. Parenteral alimentation is used to maintain nutrition during the postoperative period.

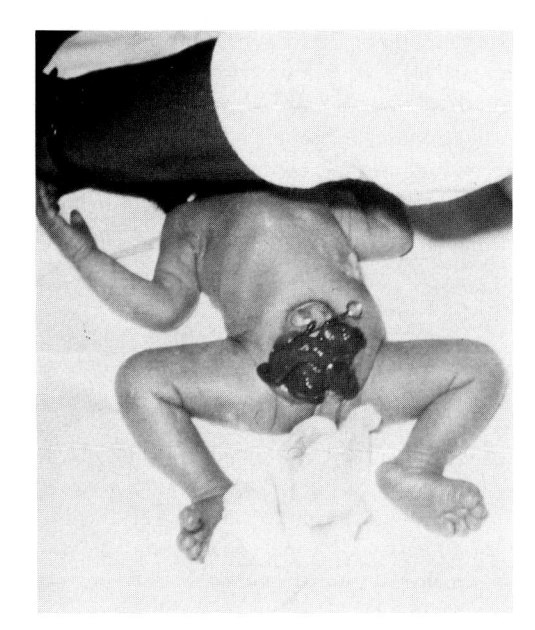

Fig. 24-28. Preterm infant with a ruptured omphalocele.

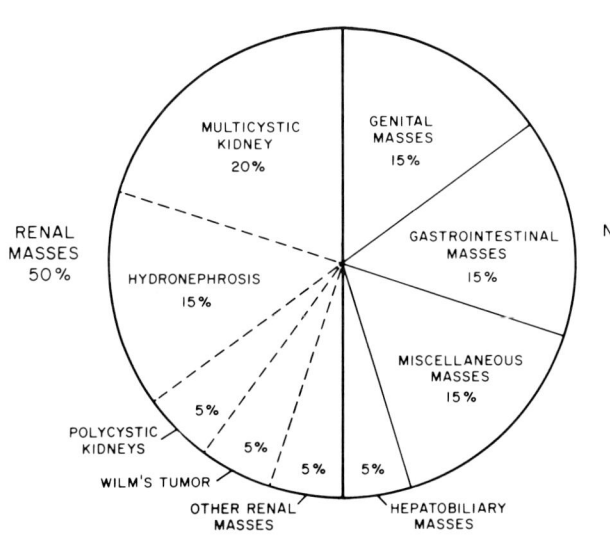

Fig. 24-29. Common causes of abdominal masses in the neonate.

Prognosis

Survival has recently increased to as high as 70% in some studies. Mortality is primarily dependent on the size of the defect and the severity of associated anomalies.

ABDOMINAL MASSES

A neonate presenting with a palpable abdominal mass is an infrequent but not rare event in an active newborn nursery. The differential diagnostic approach differs, and the prognosis, because of the relatively low incidence of malignancy, is generally better than at any other time in life. Half of all masses in this age group are renal in origin, and less than one fifth primarily involve the GI tract (Fig. 24-29).

Differential diagnosis
Renal masses

Unilateral multicystic kidney is the most common cause of an abdominal mass in the neonatal period, accounting for over 20% of all cases (p. 795). In contrast to infantile polycystic disease, they are composed almost entirely of large cysts, are unilateral, are not associated with cystic changes of other organs, and are not familial. The multicystic kidney is often associated with a hypoplastic or atretic ureter. The mass is usually asymptomatic, without urinary tract abnormalities, and may be corrected by surgical removal, although many centers now oppose surgery. *Hydronephrosis* is second only to multicystic kidney as a cause of abdominal masses in the neonate and is usually secondary to obstruction at the ureteropelvic junction or ureterovesical junction or is due to the presence of posterior urethral valves (Chapter 31). Although the infant is often asymptomatic during the first few days of life, secondary infection and subsequent sepsis are common. Less common causes of renal masses include *infantile polycystic disease*, *Wilms' tumor*, and *renal vein thrombosis*.

Genital masses

Female neonates must be carefully examined to exclude the presence of *hydrocolpos* or *hydrometra*. These masses are secondary to uterine, vaginal, or hymenal obstruction and are often associated with complex genitourinary tract anomalies. The lesions present as firm, fixed lower midline masses and often may be recognized following careful examination of the perineum. *Ovarian cysts* also may be responsible for large abdominal masses in female neonates and can reach sufficient size to extend into the upper abdomen.

GI masses

Lesions of the GI tract are rare causes of asymptomatic abdominal masses. *Intestinal duplications* are the most frequent and often are associated with symptoms of GI obstruction or hemorrhage. They are predominantly of small intestinal origin, are mobile, are often cystic in nature, and may not be palpable in the immediate neonatal period. *Mesenteric cysts* generally are seen in later childhood but have been described in the neonatal period. They are often of sufficient size to cause signs of intestinal obstruction, either by extrinsic compression or by volvulus formation. *Meconium ileus* and *intestinal malrotation with volvulus* also may present with a palpable abdominal mass in the neonatal period, but in both instances the signs and symptoms of intestinal obstruction are prominent.

Hepatobiliary masses

Disorders of the liver and gallbladder account for only 5% of all neonatal abdominal masses; *solitary hepatic cysts*, *choledochal cysts*, and *hepatic neoplasms*, such as hemangiomas and hepatoblastomas, are most frequent.

Miscellaneous masses

Neuroblastoma is the most common tumor of the neonate and may be found within the abdomen, arising from the adrenal gland or in the retroperitoneal area below the kidney (in approximately 35% of patients). Over half the tumors detected in neonates have metastasized by the time the diagnosis has been made; the liver is the most common site of spread. Nevertheless, the overall prognosis is good in this age group, and a high rate of spontaneous disappearance has been observed. *Teratomas* in the neonate are usually sacrococcygeal in origin and often are palpable only on rectal examination but may present as abdominal masses. The diagnosis is frequently made by an abdominal radiograph in which calcified bone or teeth are seen within the mass. Other rare causes of abdominal masses in the neonate include *splenic cysts*, *subcapsular splenic hematoma*, and *adrenal hemorrhage*.

Approach to diagnosis and management

The great majority of neonatal abdominal masses require early surgical exploration for both diagnosis and treatment. Nevertheless, a carefully organized preoperative evaluation can be completed in a very short time and is often of great help to the surgeon. In addition to helping locate and characterize the mass, physical examination may provide enough information to make an accurate preoperative diagnosis, as in cases of infantile polycystic disease and hydrometrocolpos. Since over half of all neonatal abdominal masses either directly or secondarily involve the kidneys, an intravenous pyelogram is the most helpful diagnostic procedure. When this procedure is performed through a foot vein, one can also obtain a simultaneous inferior vena cavagram, which may further help in arriving at the correct diagnosis. If hydronephrosis is demonstrated or suspected, a voiding cystourethrogram may be necessary. Ultrasonography may prove to be of great value, and the use of computerized axial tomography also may be extended to facilitate the diagnosis and approach to abdominal masses in the neonate. Unless evidence of intestinal obstruction is present, contrast studies of the GI tract are of limited value in this age group and generally are not necessary. Symptoms of intestinal obstruction strongly point to the alimentary tract as the etiology of the mass, since even huge extraintestinal masses rarely cause obstruction in the newborn. In addition to studies designed to define the lesion from an anatomic standpoint, urinalysis, urine culture, and blood urea nitrogen and serum creatinine determinations should be obtained before surgery. Urine also should be collected and stored for determination of catecholamine metabolites in the event that the mass proves to be a tumor of neural crest origin.

ASCITES

Although ascites in the older infant and child is most often a complication of liver disease and occasionally is secondary to severe congestive heart failure, such is not the case in the neonate. Lower urinary tract obstruction is the most common cause of ascites in the neonate and is usually due to posterior urethral valves, ureteroceles, or urethral atresia. The ascites may develop from extravasation of urine from the dilated renal pelvis into the subcapsular space and then into the peritoneal cavity. Rarely, rupture of a perinephric cyst also will produce ascites. A voiding cystourethrogram will demonstrate the lesion and often the extravasation of dye into the peritoneum. If the dye contains an aminoglycoside, such extravasation may lead to rapid absorption of the antibiotic from the peritoneum and cause respiratory arrest in the infant. Initially, it was thought that infants with ascites on a renal basis had a very poor prognosis; but often the ascites develops before irreversible renal damage has occurred. Early recognition of the disorder and institution of appropriate therapy lead to an improved outcome. In fact, some of these infants are being diagnosed correctly in utero by ultrasound and are being treated by fetal surgical techniques to prevent irreversible renal damage (pp. 86 and 797).

Other causes of ascites are included in the following outline, but it should be noted that fetal or neonatal hepatitis is an extremely rare cause of neonatal ascites. In most situations the ascites and abdominal distension are noted at birth and may be severe enough to have caused the mother to have uterine dystocia. If the condition is severe enough, fetal paracentesis must be performed before delivery can be accomplished. When ascites is found in a neonate, diagnostic paracentesis is indicated and will often clarify the type of abnormality that may be present.

A. Obstructive uropathy
B. Meconium peritonitis
C. Chylous ascites
D. Bile ascites
E. Intraperitoneal cysts
F. Hydrometrocolpos
G. Acute peritonitis with or without fetal or neonatal hepatitis
   1. Bacterial infection, including syphilis
   2. Viral infection (cytomegalovirus)
   3. Toxoplasmosis
H. Associated with generalized edema or anasarca
   1. Hemolytic disease of the newborn
   2. α-Thalassemia (homozygous)
   3. Twin-twin or fetal-maternal hemorrhage
   4. Severe cardiopulmonary malformations
      a. Pulmonary lymphangiectasia
      b. Cystic adenomatoid malformation of the lung
   5. Congenital nephrosis
   6. Chorioangioma of the placenta
   7. Infantile Gaucher's disease
   8. Syndrome of hyperplacentosis
      a. Hydramnios
      b. Edematous placenta
      c. Hydrops fetalis
      d. Toxemia of pregnancy

Meconium peritonitis usually occurs as a result of ileal atresia or volvulus and secondarily as a result of meconium ileus due to cystic fibrosis. The perforation probably occurs during the last trimester of intrauterine life, and the sterile meconium initiates a chemical reaction that can lead to intraabdominal calcifications and at times scrotal calcifications (see Fig. 24-26). Often marked induration and edema of the abdominal wall are encountered. Therapy consists of GI decompression, fluids and electrolytes, antibiotics, and general supportive measures to prepare the infant for surgery. The prognosis depends on the maturity of the infant, the amount of bowel removed, and whether bacterial invasion has occurred in utero.

Chylous ascites has been reported in fewer than 65 infants and is twice as common in males as in females. Lymphatic obstruction is felt to be secondary to congenital malformations, tumors, chronic inflammatory process, and only rarely secondary to trauma or intrathoracic surgical complications. The onset is usually insidious, with abdominal distension and ascites, which may then lead to generalized edema. There also may be chylothorax and, rarely, unilateral or bilateral lymphedema of the extremities. Inguinal hernias are commonly found. The concentration of protein and fat in ascitic fluid is markedly increased (15 gm/dl or more), and after the infant has been fed, the fluid becomes milky. A majority of patients respond to conservative management with feedings of formula containing medium-chain triglycerides. Repeated infusions of plasma proteins and frequent paracentesis also may be necessary. About 20% of patients require surgery, and half these patients will continue to accumulate ascitic fluid.

Bile ascites is another rare condition in the neonate. The onset is insidious and often follows a period in which the infant is fussy, colicky, and irritable. Fluctuating jaundice, intermittent acholic stools, dark urine, and inguinal hernias are frequently encountered. Bile-stained ascitic fluid with an increased protein content (2 to 4 gm/dl) is found. Early in the illness the fluid may not be bile stained, and the diagnosis is made by finding ^{131}I-labeled rose bengal in the fluid after this compound has been given intravenously. Since the disease is a result of perforation of the biliary tree with a stone or is a result of a congenital stenosis or choledochal cyst, surgical exploration and repair of the perforation are indicated.

Infectious peritonitis occurs as a result of perforation of the GI tract and is the manner in which most neonates present with *acute appendicitis*. Hematogenous or lymphatic bacterial spread from the respiratory or genitourinary tract accounts for the majority of patients with primary peritonitis where no intraperitoneal source of infection is found. Primary peritonitis is most commonly found in males and has an excellent prognosis in most cases. Secondary peritonitis is more complex, and adhesions, necrotic bowel, and fibrinous exudate complicate surgical therapy.

Philip Sunshine
Frank R. Sinatra
Charles H. Mitchell
Thomas V. Santulli

BIBLIOGRAPHY
Disorders of sucking and swallowing and disorders of the esophagus

Arasu, T.S., and others: Gastroesophageal reflux in infants and children—comparative accuracy of diagnostic methods, J. Pediatr. 96:798, 1980.

Ashcroft, K.W., and others: Early recognition and aggressive treatment of gastroesophageal reflux following repair of esophageal atresia, J. Pediatr. Surg. 12:317, 1977.

Berdon, W.E., and Baker, D.H.: Vascular anomalies and the infant lung: rings, slings, and other things, Semin. Roentgenol. 7:39, 1972.

Boix-Ochoa, J., Lafuente, J.M., and Gil-Vernet, J.M.: Twenty-four hour esophageal pH monitoring in gastroesophageal reflux, J. Pediatr. Surg. 15:74, 1980.

Carré, I.J.: Disorders of the oro-pharynx and oesophagus. In Anderson, C.M., and Burke, V., editors: Paediatric gastroenterology, Oxford, 1975, Blackwell Scientific Publications, Ltd.

Carré, I.J., Astley, R., and Langmead-Smith, R.: A 20-year follow-up of children with a partial thoracic stomach (hiatal hernia), Aust. Paediatr. J. 12:92, 1976.

Chrispin, A.R., and Friedland, G.W.: Functional disturbance of hiatal hernia in infants and children, Thorax 22:422, 1967.

Friedland, G.W., and others: The apparent discrepancy in incidence of hiatal herniae in infants and children in Britain and the United States, Am. J. Roentgenol. 120:305, 1974.

Friedland, G.W., Sunshine, P., and Zboralske, F.F.: Hiatal hernia in infants and young children: a 2 to 3 year follow-up study, J. Pediatr. 87:71, 1975.

Friedland, G.W., Yamate, M., and Marinkovitch, V.A.: Hiatal hernia and chronic unremitting asthma, Pediatr. Radiol. 1:156, 1973.

German, J.C., Mahour, G.H., and Woolley, M.W.: Esophageal atresia and associated anomalies, J. Pediatr. Surg. 11:299, 1976.

Greenwood, R.D., and Rosenthal, A.: Cardiovascular malformations associated with tracheoesophageal fistula and esophageal atresia, pediatrics 57:87, 1976.

Harell, G.S., and others: Neonatal Boerhaave's syndrome, Radiology 95:665, 1970.

Herbst, J., Friedland, G.W., and Zboralske, F.F.: Hiatal hernia and "rumination" in infants and children, J. Pediatr. 78:261, 1971.

Herbst, J.J., Johnson, D.G., and Oliveros, M.A.: Gastroesophageal reflux with protein-losing enteropathy and finger dubbing, Am. J. Dis. Child. 130:1256, 1976.

Holder, T.M., and others: Esophageal atresia and tracheoesophageal fistula: a survey of its members by the surgical section of the American Academy of Pediatrics, Pediatrics 34:542, 1964.

Johnson, D.G., and others: Evaluation of gastroesophageal reflux surgery in children, Pediatrics 59:62, 1977.

Koop, C.E., Schnaufer, L., and Broennie, A.M.: Esophageal atresia and tracheo-esophageal fistula; supportive measures that affect survival, Pediatrics 54:558, 1974.

Disorders of the stomach

Bell, M.J., and others: Antral diaphragm—a cause of gastric outlet obstruction in infants and children, J. Pediatr. 90:196, 1977.

Benson, C.D.: Infantile hypertrophic pyloric stenosis. In Ravitch, M.M., and others, editors: Pediatric surgery, ed. 3, Chicago, 1979, Year Book Medical Publishers, Inc.

Bleicher, M.A., and others: Extraordinary hyperbilirubinemia in a neonate with idiopathic pyloric stenosis, J. Pediatr. Surg. 14:527, 1979.

Campbell, J.B., Rappaport, L.W., and Skerker, L.B.: Acute mesentero-axial volvulus of the stomach, Radiology 103:153, 1972.

Cole, B., and Dickinson, S.J.: Acute volvulus of the stomach in infants and children, Surgery 70:707, 1971.

Erenberg, A., Shaw, R.D., and Yousefzadeh, D.: Lactobezoar in the low-birth-weight infant, Pediatrics 63:642, 1979.

Euler, A.R., and others: Basal and pentagastrin-stimulated acid secretion in newborn human infants, Pediatr. Res. 13:36, 1979.

Grosfeld, J.L., and others: Acute peptic ulcer in infancy and childhood, Am. Surg. 44:13, 1978.

Jona, J.Z.: Electron microscopic observations in infantile hypertrophic pyloric stenosis (IHPS), J. Pediatr. Surg. 13:17, 1978.

Rogers, I.M., and others: Plasma gastrin in congenital hypertrophic pyloric stenosis: a hypothesis disproved? Arch. Dis. Child. 50:467, 1975.

Disorders of the small intestine

Bower, R.J., Sieber, W.K., and Kiesewetter, W.B.: Alimentary tract duplications in children, Ann. Surg. 188:669, 1978.

deLorimier, A.A., Fonkalsrud, E.W., and Hays, D.M.: Congenital atresia and stenosis of the jejunum and ileum, Surgery 65:819, 1969.

Favara, B.E., Franciosi, R.A., and Akers, D.R.: Enteric duplications: thirty-seven cases; a vascular theory of pathogenesis, Am. J. Dis. Child. 122:501, 1971.

Fonkalsrud, E.W., deLorimier, A.A., and Hays, D.M.: Congenital atresia and stenosis of the duodenum: a review compiled from the members of the Surgical Section of the American Academy of Pediatrics, Pediatrics 43:79, 1969

Grosfeld, J., O'Neill, J., and Clatworthy, H.W., Jr.: Enteric duplications in infancy and childhood: an 18 year review, Ann. Surg. 172:83, 1970.

Hayes, D.M., Greaney, E.M., and Hill, J.J.: Annular pancreas as a cause of acute neonatal duodenal obstruction, Ann. Surg. 153:103, 1961.

Jackson, J.M.: Annular pancreas and duodenal obstruction in the neonate, Arch. Surg. 87:379, 1963.

Louw, J.H.: Jejunoileal atresia and stenosis, J. Pediatr. Surg. 1:8, 1966.

Nixon, H.H., and Tawes, R.: Etiology and treatment of small intestinal atresia: analysis of a series of 127 jejunoileal atresias and comparison with 62 duodenal atresias, Surgery 69:41, 1971.

Rees, J.R., and Redo, S.F.: Anomalies of intestinal rotation and fixation, Am.J. Surg. 116:834, 1968.

Snyder, W.H., Jr., and Chaffin, L.: Malrotation of the intestine. In Mustard, W.T., and others, editors: Pediatric surgery, ed. 2, Chicago, 1969, Year Book Medical Publishers, Inc.

Spencer, R.: The various patterns of intestinal atresia, Surgery 64:661, 1968.

Stewart, D.R., Colodny, A.L., and Daggett, W.C.: Malrotation of the bowel in infants and children: 15-year review, Surgery 79:716, 1976.

Tibboel, D., van Nie, C.J., and Molinaar, J.C.: The effects of temporary general hypoxia and local ischemia on the development of the intestine: an experimental study, J. Pediatr. Surg. 15:57, 1980.

White, J.J., and others: Changing concepts in the management of intestinal atresia, Surg. Clin. North Am. 50:863, 1970.

Young, D.G., and Wilkinson, A.W.: Abnormalities associated with neonatal duodenal obstruction, Surgery 63:832, 1968.

Disorders of the colon

Asch, M.J., and others: Total colon aganglionosis, Arch. Surg. **105**:74, 1972.

Berdon, W.E., Koontz, P., and Baker, D.H.: The diagnosis of colonic and terminal ileal aganglionosis, Am. J. Roentgenol. Radium Ther. Nucl. Med. **91**:680, 1964.

Bill, A.H., Jr., and Chapman, N.D.: The entero-colitis of neonatal Hirschsprung's disease, Am. J. Surg. **103**:70, 1962.

Clatworthy, H.W., Jr., Howard, W.H.R., and Lloyd, J.: The meconium plug syndrome, Surgery **39**:131, 1956.

Cremin, B.J.: The radiological assessment of anorectal anomalies, Clin. Radiol. **22**:239, 1971.

Davis, W.S., and others: Neonatal small left colon syndrome, Am. J. Roentgenol. Radium Ther. Nucl. Med. **120**:322, 1974.

deVries, P.A., and Friedland, G.W.: The staged sequential development of the anus and rectum in human embryos and fetuses, J. Pediatr. Surg. **9**:755, 1974.

Ellis, D.G., and Clatworthy, H.W., Jr.: The meconium plug syndrome revisited, J. Pediatr. Surg. **1**:54, 1966.

Frieldand, G.W., Rush, W.A., Jr., and Hill, A.J.: Smythe's "inspissated milk" syndrome, Radiology **103**:159, 1972.

Lake, D.B., and others: Hirschsprung's disease: appraisal of histochemically demonstrated acetylcholinesterase activity in suction rectal biopsy specimens as aid to diagnosis, Arch. Pathol. Lab. Med. **102**:244, 1978.

McGovern, B.: Occult perineal fistula in male infants with imperforate anus, Am. J. Dis. Child. **123**:26, 1972.

Passarge, E.: The genetics of Hirschsprung's disease, N. Engl. J. Med. **276**:138, 1967.

Phillippart, A.I., Reed, J.O., and Georgeson, K.E.: Neonatal small left colon syndrome: intramural not intraluminal obstruction, J. Pediatr. Surg. **10**:733, 1975.

Poole, C.A., and Rowe, M.I.: Distal neonatal intestinal obstruction: choice of contrast material, J. Pediatr. Surg. **11**:1011, 1976.

Puchner, P.J., Santulli, T.V., and Lattimer, J.K.: Urologic problems associated with imperforate anus, Urology **6**:205, 1975.

Santulli, T.V., Kiesewetter, W.B., and Bill, A.H., Jr.: Anorectal anomalies: a suggested international classification, J. Pediatr. Surg. **5**:281, 1970.

Santulli, T.V., and others: Imperforate anus: a survey from the members of the Surgical Section of the American Academy of Pediatrics, J. Pediatr. Surg. **6**:484, 1971.

Schuster, M.M.: Diagnostic value of anal sphincter pressure measurements, Hosp. Pract. **8**:115, 1973.

Sokal, M.M., and others: Neonatal hypermagnesemia and the meconium-plug syndrome, N. Engl. J. Med. **286**:823, 1972.

Swenson, O., Sherman, J.O., and Fisher, J.H.: Diagnosis of congenital megacolon: an analysis of 501 patients, J. Pediatr. Surg. **8**:587, 1973.

Swenson, O., and others: The treatment and postoperative complications of congenital megacolon: a 25 year follow-up, Ann. Surg. **182**:266, 1975.

Talwalker, V.C.: Intussusception in the newborn, Arch. Dis. Child. **37**:203, 1962.

Townes, P.L., and Brocks, E.R.: Hereditary syndrome of imperforate anus with hand, foot, and ear anomalies, J. Pediatr. **81**:321, 1972.

Woodhurst, W.B., and Kliman, M.R.: Neonatal small left colon syndrome: report of two cases, Am. Surg. **42**:479, 1976.

CHAPTER 25   # The cardiovascular system

Congenital cardiovascular disease is a major health problem in the neonatal period. The newborn with a severe cardiac malformation usually will have difficulties in this period or at least in the first 6 months of life. If he survives this critical period without problems, it is likely that he will remain asymptomatic for many years, as in patients with mild pulmonic or aortic stenosis, or decades, as in patients with an atrial septal defect (ASD).

The practice of pediatric cardiology thus tends to be partitioned, on the one hand, into care of the older child with easily identifiable, electively correctable heart disease—such as ASD and ventricular septal defects (VSD), patent ductus arteriosus (PDA), aortic and pulmonic stenosis, postductal coarctation of the aorta, and most cases of tetralogy of Fallot—and, alternatively, into care of the newborn with life-threatening malformations such as transposition of the great arteries, hypoplastic left-heart syndrome, preductal coarctation of the aorta, and a host of complex malformations. In general, the outlook for the older child with one of the seven most common malformations just noted is now excellent, whereas the prognosis for the sick neonate with cardiac disease may vary from excellent (as in infants with transposition of the great arteries with low pulmonary arterial pressure or severe isolated pulmonic stenosis) to bad (as in infants with a hypoplastic left ventricle with diminutive aorta). This chapter discusses those severe lesions which present problems in the first month of life. However, the majority of infants born with heart disease manifest no problem in the neonatal period, and recent advances in diagnosis and corrective surgery allow survival with normal life expectancy in the majority of children with congenital heart disease.

INCIDENCE OF STRUCTURAL CONGENITAL HEART DISEASE

Precise figures of the incidence of structural congenital heart disease probably will never be attainable. Some cardiac defects (such as VSD and PDA) close spontaneously, whereas others (such as ASD) may not become manifest until late in childhood. In other disorders (such as endocardial fibroelastosis and muscular hypertrophic subaortic stenosis) a congenital origin is in doubt. A recent study of 56,109 infants monitored for an average of 3 years after birth disclosed an incidence of 8.14 infants with congenital heart disease per 1,000 births. Approximately a third of all infants born alive with a congenital heart defect die within the first month of life. However, many of these infants have multiple cardiac defects together with congenital defects of other organ systems.

ETIOLOGY OF CONGENITAL HEART DISEASE

Although several causes of congenital heart disease have been firmly identified, in the majority of patients no antecedent factor can be determined. Some cardiac malformations (such as PDA) are more common in girls, whereas others (such as aortic stenosis) are more common in boys; the overall sex ratio is approximately 1:1. Prematurity, calculated by both gestational age and weight, is approximately 2½ times more frequent in infants born with heart disease. However, it has been suggested that infants with transposition of the great arteries tend to be heavier than average, but this finding has been questioned.

Factors known to be associated with congenital heart disease include maternal ingestion of thalidomide and possibly other chemicals, such as dextroamphetamine, phenytoin (Dilantin), phenobarbital, lithium carbonate, ethyl alcohol, and progestogens, maternal infection with rubella virus and possibly with other viruses, season of the year, high altitude (PDA only), major chromosomal disorders such as Down's syndrome and Turner's syndrome, disorders of connective tissue such as Marfan's syndrome and Ehlers-Danlos syndrome, and maternal diabetes. The influence of ionizing radiation is unknown.

Recently McCue and associates have described an association between complete congenital atrioventricular (AV) heart block in the fetus and neonate and maternal connective tissue disease, especially systemic lupus erythematosus. It appears likely that antinuclear antibodies of the IgG class cross the placenta and affect the fetal cardiac conduction tissues.

Common major chromosomal disorders

The incidence of structural congenital heart disease is high in infants with major chromosomal disorders. For trisomy 13 syndrome the incidence is approximately 90%; for trisomy 18 it is greater than 95%. Heart disease is also common in Down's syndrome (50%) and in Turner's syndrome (approximately 30%). In Down's syndrome the heart defect is frequently severe (for example, common AV canal). Since the mental and life-span prognosis is unpredictable in neonates with these syndromes, we have evolved a policy of investigation and treatment identical to that used for the chromosomally normal infant. Such infants withstand cardiac catheterization and cardiac surgery well. Occasionally a Turnerlike syndrome (Noonan's syndrome) is encountered. In this instance the child has the phenotypic features of Turner's syndrome but no demonstrable chromosomal abnormality; heart disease, especially pulmonic stenosis, is common.

Heart disease caused by maternal rubella

The frequency of fetal infection from mothers having rubella during the first trimester is about 50% (p. 695). The heart may be affected in a variety of ways; PDA, peripheral pulmonary artery stenosis, systemic arterial stenosis, and myocarditis are common. Recognition that cardiovascular disease is a part of a general disorder is paramount to the multidisciplinary approach necessary for the adequate management of associated mental retardation, deafness, cataract, and glaucoma, although, in general, the presence of other system malformations does not alter the treatment of the cardiovascular problem.

Infantile hypercalcemia and vascular disease

A broad maxilla, full prominent upper lip, and small anteverted nose characterize the infant with idiopathic infantile hypercalcemia. The hypercalcemia, when detected, is generally present only in infancy, and the association with vascular disease is based on the observation that a number of children with supravalvular aortic stenosis (stenosis of the ascending aorta) or peripheral pulmonary artery stenosis or both have a very similar facial appearance. The disease can occur in siblings, but it remains to be established whether treatment of idiopathic hypercalcemia in infancy will prevent the occurrence of arterial stenoses or the associated mental retardation.

Hereditary disorders of connective tissue

The cardiac defects associated with Marfan's syndrome (aortic regurgitation and aortic aneurysm) do not usually lead to problems in infancy. Similarly neonatal problems are unusual with Ehlers-Danlos syndrome. Spontaneous rupture of a renal artery has been described in a 6-day-old infant with osteogenesis imperfecta.

Glycogen storage disease

Pompe's disease is the only type of glycogen storage disease causing cardiac symptoms in the newborn period. The disease is suggested by a positive family history, large tongue, hepatosplenomegaly, and muscular hypo-

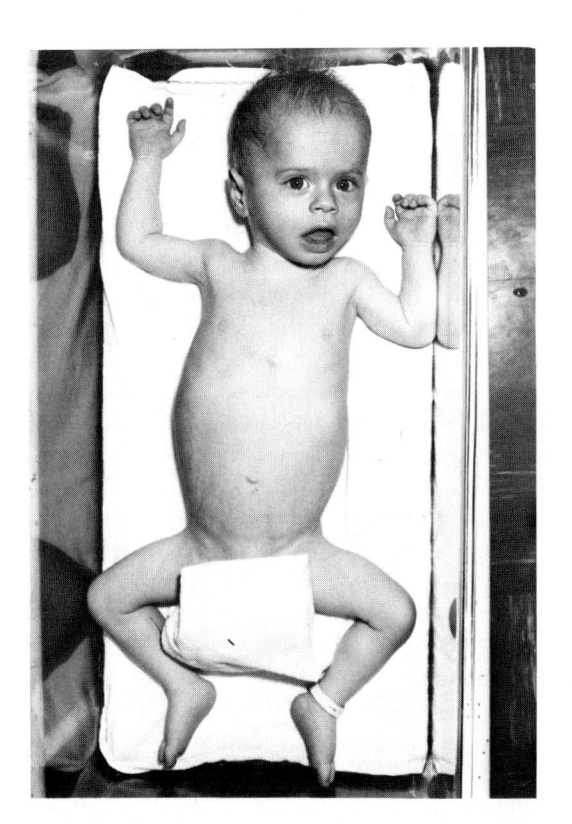

Fig. 25-1. Three-month-old infant with glycogen storage disease (Pompe's disease). Note hypotonic posture and large tongue. There was considerable hepatomegaly.

Table 25-1. Less common syndromes sometimes associated with cardiovascular abnormality

Syndrome	Congenital heart defect
VATER	VSD, tetralogy of Fallot
Cerebrohepatorenal	PDA with or without septal defect
Holt-Oram	ASD and other types of congenital heart disease
Hurler's	Cardiomyopathy
Friedreich's ataxia	Cardiomyopathy
XXXXX	PDA
Carpenter's	PDA, VSD, transposition
Cornelia de Lange's	Variable
Cri du chat	Variable
Ellis–van Creveld	Septal defects
Radial aplasia and thrombocytopenia	Variable
XXXXY	PDA
Laurence-Moon-Biedl-Bordet	Tetralogy of Fallot

Table 25-2. Reasons for study of 100 neonates proved by cardiac catheterization and angiocardiography to have cardiovascular disease*

Condition	Number
Cyanosis	66
Heart failure	7
Cyanosis and heart failure	23
Cardiogenic shock	2
Arrhythmia (complete heart block)	1
CNS abnormality (arteriovenous fistula)	1

*The overwhelming indication was cyanosis with or without heart failure. Analysis of the reasons for cardiac catheterization of infants in the 2- to 4-month age range reveals a much higher incidence of heart failure (mostly from left-to-right shunts) and of failure to thrive.

tonia. The left ventricle is grossly enlarged. Definitive diagnosis can be made by biochemical and enzymatic examinations of the skeletal muscle (Fig. 25-1).

Other syndromes associated with cardiovascular disease

In addition to the syndromes already referred to, a number of cardiac anomalies are associated with recognizable patterns of human malformation (Table 25-1).

Genetics and congenital heart disease

The question frequently asked of the pediatrician is what the risk is of a malformed heart when a first-degree relative (mother, father, sibling, or child of index case) has congenital heart disease. The question is even more pertinent now that many patients who previously would have died before reproductive age undergo successful surgery. Nora studied the children of 308 adults with ASD or VSD, most of whom had had surgical correction. Parents with ASD had 2.6% of their children affected with ASD, which is 37 times greater than the estimated population frequency. For VSD 3.7% of the children of parents with this heart defect were similarly affected. The data approximate closely with predictions of the multifactorial inheritance hypothesis. This states that the incidence in first-degree relatives of an individual with a malformation transmitted by multifactorial inheritance approaches the square root of the population frequency of that lesion (for example, if the population frequency is 0.001 [1 per 1,000], the increase is to $\sqrt{0.001}$, [0.032, or 32 per 1,000]). For ASD the number of offspring affected is very close to the multifactorial prediction; for VSD the 3.7% of children with cardiac malformations approximates the 4.2% prediction. In the future more marriages will occur between adults who both have corrected or uncorrected congenital heart disease. The risk presumably will be further increased, as has been shown to occur in the case of cleft lip and palate.

Despite the multiple factors known to be associated with congenital heart disease, in approximately 75% of infants afflicted no cause is evident: the family history is negative, pregnancy has been uncomplicated, and no other disease exists in the baby. In the majority therefore the disease is unexpected and is not repeated in siblings. Environmental factors such as ionizing radiation or undiagnosed fleeting infections during embryogenesis also influence the incidence of congenital heart disease. The question frequently asked by the mother who has just given birth to a heart-diseased infant is, naturally, what the risk is for future infants. At the present state of our knowledge a general answer should be that the risk is approximately 1:25, unless there are additional first- or second-degree relatives with congenital heart disease, in which case an assessment cannot be given. There are occasional families in which congenital heart disease occurs at a rate greatly exceeding the multifactorial inheritance hypothesis prediction.

SIGNS OF SERIOUS CARDIOVASCULAR DISEASE IN THE NEONATE

The presence of cyanosis or the signs of heart failure are the most frequent reasons for suspecting serious heart disease in the newborn. Less commonly heart disease appears as a shocklike picture, with pallor, flaccidity, and hypoactive arterial pulses; occasionally the presenting abnormality is an arrhythmia, especially supraventricular tachycardia (SVT) or complete heart block.

Uncommon signs of serious neonatal heart disease include isolated tachypnea, isolated liver enlargement, a loud cardiac murmur in a temporarily asymptomatic infant, "failure to thrive," prenatal stethoscopic detection of a loud heart murmur or arrhythmia, hyperdynamic cardiac impulse, abnormal cardiac pulses, systemic hypertension, unsuspected electrocardiogram (ECG) or x-ray film abnormality, and central nervous system symptoms secondary to a cerebral arteriovenous fistula or cerebral hypoxia. Bacterial endocarditis is almost nonexistent in the newborn. An analysis of the symptoms of 100 consecutive heart-diseased neonates undergoing cardiac catheterization in our institution is given in Table 25-2.

PHYSICAL EXAMINATION OF THE INFANT SUSPECTED OF HAVING CARDIOVASCULAR DISEASE
History

The family history should be reviewed for evidence of congenital heart disease, connective tissue disorder, glycogen storage disease, hypercalcemia, or unusual heritable disease. Questions relating to the present pregnancy should include inquiries about rubella, Coxsackie virus infection, unusual radiation exposure, or threatened abortion.

General appearance

The pedigree, history, and general appearance of the infant may reveal evidence of a major chromosomal defect, hypercalcemia, rubella, connective tissue disorder, glycogen storage disease, or rare syndrome. Early recognition that heart disease is but one manifestation of a complex disorder is essential to proper management.

Behavior of the infant

A general appraisal of the infant's spontaneous activity and response to stimuli often provides insight into the seriousness of the disease. A baby with reduced oxygen delivery to the tissues—whether from cyanotic heart disease or from heart failure—may show little spontaneous movement, presumably in an attempt to conserve available oxygen for basal metabolic requirements. In the extreme case a newborn with severe heart failure from prenatal asphyxia, myocarditis, or the hypoplastic left-heart syndrome may be flaccid and apathetic and show almost no response to external stimuli.

Breathing patterns

Tachypnea, altered depth of respiration, intercostal retractions, flaring of the alae nasi, grunting, stridor, and apneic spells all may be observed in infants with cardiovascular disease. It cannot be assumed that the presence of these respiratory symptoms automatically implies that there is primary lung disease. Severe heart failure may mimic pulmonary disease in this regard (p. 460).

Arterial pulses and measurement of blood pressure (Table 25-3)

See also p. 126.

The radial, posterior tibial, and dorsalis pedis pulses are readily palpable in the normal newborn. Feeling one strong foot pulse that is synchronous with the radial is sufficient to rule out significant adult-type postductal coarctation. In contrast, it *is* necessary to feel both radial pulses, since supravalvular aortic stenosis, aortic isthmus stenosis, and juxtaductal coarctation all may lead to an increased pressure in the right arm when compared with pressure in the left. A reasonable approach therefore is for the physician to feel both radial (or brachial) pulses simultaneously and then to palpate a radial and foot pulse simultaneously, feeling for evidence of pulse delay in the leg (characteristic of mild or moderate coarctation). The more common form of coarctation found in sick neonates is the juxtaductal or preductal form, in which the lower half of the body is perfused with blood originating from the right ventricle. In this situation the femoral and foot pulses are often normal, and one should be able to observe cyanosis of the feet compared with the appearance of the hands. In practice this sign often is missed until after the angiocardiogram has disclosed the true anatomy. If hyperactive pulses are suspected, one may move peripherally and feel the palmar pulses or even the digital pulses (not normally palpable).

If the pulses are adjudged equal in arm and leg, it is necessary to measure only brachial blood pressure. Arm blood pressure usually can be measured with a 1- to 2-inch cuff and with a stethoscope over the brachial artery; however, the Doppler technique is a significant advance in the accurate measurement of systolic blood pressure in sick neonates, premature babies, and infants in neonatal intensive care units. A major advantage of this technique is that one can easily detect systolic blood pressures with accuracy in the 20- to 40-mm Hg range. The flush technique for measurement of blood pressure remains useful for the detection or confirmation of postductal coarctation. The normal blood pressure (descending aorta) was found by Moss to average 72/47 mm Hg for the resting full-term infant and 64/39 mm Hg for the premature. Crying caused an elevation of approximately 20 mm Hg in both systolic and diastolic measurements. Therefore a baby in whom coarctation is being considered should be quiet while upper and lower limb pressures are measured.

Venous pressure

See also p. 128.

Assessment of venous pressure is of very limited diagnostic aid. Burnell compared a group of infants not in heart failure with a group in clinical right-sided heart failure (hepatomegaly) undergoing cardiac catheteriza-

Table 25-3. Peripheral arterial pulse abnormalities (excluding arrhythmias)

Condition	Characteristics
Full-term infants resting	72/47 mm Hg (aortic); brachial, femoral, radial, and dorsalis pedis pulses easily felt when baby is warm and still
Premature infants resting	64/39 mm Hg (aortic); brachial and femoral pulses easily felt; radial and dorsalis pedis pulses felt with difficulty when baby is warm and still
PDA Aortopulmonary window Peripheral arteriovenous fistula Truncus arteriosus Hyperthyroidism Aortic regurgitation	Widened pulse pressure; typical value 90/30 mm Hg; radial and foot pulses bounding; palmar and digital pulses often palpable
Severe aortic stenosis Hypoplastic left-heart syndrome Cardiogenic shock (especially myocarditis) Hemorrhagic or endotoxin shock Advanced heart failure	Narrowed pulse pressure; typical value 55/45 mm Hg; foot and wrist pulses impalpable; brachial and femoral pulses barely palpable; Doppler technique may be only accurate noninvasive method for obtaining blood pressure
Postductal coarctation (adult type)	Arm pulses normal or increased; typical value 90/50 mm Hg; leg pulses absent, diminished, or delayed; flush or Doppler technique usually necessary for lower limb (foot); typical value 60/50 mm Hg; adequacy of collaterals, as well as severity of coarctation, determines gradient
Preductal coarctation Juxtaductal coarctation	Arm and leg pulses may be normal if ductus is open; right ventricular blood perfuses descending aorta; differential cyanosis present but hard to recognize; when ductus is closed, pressure is as with postductal coarctation; absolute values depend on length of coarcted segment, degree of heart failure, and presence of associated lesions (frequent)
Supravalvular aortic stenosis Aortic isthmus stenosis	Right arm pressure may be higher than left arm pressure; typically 80/50 (right) versus 65/50 (left) mm Hg
Juxtaductal coarctation with aberrant right subclavian artery	Left arm pressure may be higher than right arm pressure
Pericardial tamponade Constrictive pericarditis	Pulsus paradoxus; arterial pressure falls by more than 10 mm Hg during inspiration (Doppler technique needed); very rare in infancy; tamponade more likely to be suggested by rapidly increasing venous pressure and liver size
Left ventricular failure	Pulsus alternans; strong pulses alternating with weaker ones; reflects rapidly failing left ventricle; occasionally observed in infants with myocarditis and terminal congenital heart disease

tion. The group in heart failure had a central venous pressure of approximately 6 mm Hg, whereas the group not in heart failure had a mean pressure of 3 mm Hg. The newborn liver appears to act as a readily distensible sponge, giving rise to gross hepatomegaly rather than allowing much rise in central venous pressure. Occasionally one may observe distended neck veins in the upright infant and rarely a prominent A wave, suggesting obstruction to right atrial emptying (for example, tricuspid atresia or Ebstein's anomaly of the tricuspid valve).

Liver size

Normally the liver may be palpable 2 or sometimes 3 cm below the right costal margin, measured in the nipple-umbilicus line. The size of the liver is a highly reliable index of the severity of right-sided heart failure; in this condition it is frequently 5 or 6 cm below the costal margin. Liver enlargement occurs in a number of other neonatal conditions, including sepsis, congenital rubella, toxoplasmosis, cytomegalic inclusion disease, metastases of neuroblastoma, and hemolytic anemias. However, the observation of an enlarged liver should lead to a strong consideration of heart failure even in the absence of cyanosis or heart murmur. A centrally placed or left-sided liver, if associated with levocardia, frequently is associated with complex congenital heart disease.

Spleen

Splenic enlargement is not a sign of heart failure; however, congenital absence of the spleen, when associated with an abnormally placed liver and evidence of heart disease, frequently portends a complex inoperable abnormality. Congenital absence or hypoplasia of the spleen is suggested by excessive numbers of Heinz bodies within the red cells. Heinz bodies, however, are seen in a variety of situations in the newborn, and their presence especially in the premature infant should be interpreted with caution (p. 734)

Peripheral edema

Occasionally the backs of the hands and dorsum of the feet may show pitting edema as a consequence of heart failure. Rarely there is more widespread edema, with sacral pitting and puffy eyelids. In general, however, the lack of a major rise in central venous pressure in infants with congestive heart failure appears also to preclude the development of marked edema, presumably because the high systemic capillary pressures occurring in adult congestive heart failure are not found in infancy. Severe widespread peripheral edema is, accordingly, a more ominous sign in infants than in adults. Etiologic possibilities in "nonimmune" hydrops fetalis (pp. 532 and 732) include prenatal paroxysmal supraventricular tachycardia (SVT), α-thalassemia, disseminated intravascular coagulation with sepsis, cystic adenomatoid malformation of the lung, and congenital nephrosis. Ultrasonography of the fetus may reveal ascites or pleural effusion. The lymphedema characteristic of Turner's syndrome, especially if associated with organic heart disease, may give the erroneous impression of heart failure.

Ascites and pleural and pericardial effusion

If ascites is observed in the newborn, heart failure is an unlikely cause because of the rarity of high systemic capillary pressures. Before ascribing ascites to heart failure, one should give careful consideration to primary liver disease, primary kidney disease, chylous ascites, and peritonitis. Similarly pleural effusion should prompt consideration of chylothorax or lung disease rather than heart failure. Pericardial effusion or pericarditis in the newborn period is rare and is usually caused by bacterial sepsis.

Precordial impulse and thrills

Considerable information can be gained by laying a warm hand over the left side of the infant's chest. The cardiac impulse of a normal full-term baby is barely palpable, so that if the impulse is readily felt, ventricular volume overloading as from a left-to-right shunt or valvular regurgitation is likely. Right ventricular enlargement and overactivity is indicated by a hyperdynamic quality at the cardiac apex. A hypodynamic or impalpable heart suggests tetralogy of Fallot if the infant is not in heart failure. If heart failure exists, the observation of a hypodynamic impulse may simply reflect low cardiac output.

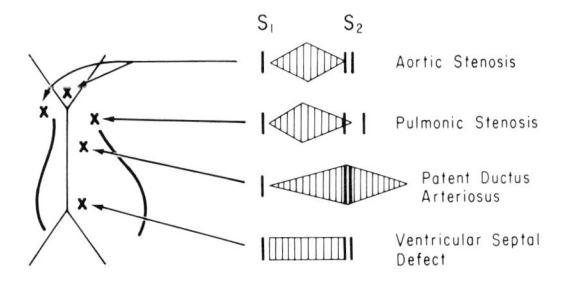

Fig. 25-2. Site, location, significance, and timing of the four most common systolic thrills felt in the newborn.

A number of thrills are diagnostically very useful in the newborn. Fig. 25-2 indicates the site, location, significance, and timing of the four most common systolic thrills. A pulmonic stenosis thrill occurs with tetralogy of Fallot and a VSD thrill with tricuspid atresia. Isolated diastolic thrills are uncommon in the newborn period but occasionally may be felt with congenital valvular regurgitation, especially of the pulmonary valve. A continuous or near-continuous thrill suggests a PDA; the thrill and its accompanying murmur may be maximum in the second, third, or fourth left intercostal space. When the pulmonary artery pressure is sufficiently low to cause a continuous runoff of blood from the aorta through a PDA, the continuous murmur or thrill is nearly always accompanied by bounding arterial pulses.

Heart rate and regularity in normal infants

See also p. 119.

The heart rate in quiet full-term infants averages 130 beats per minute, but the range may vary from 70 to 180 beats per minute during the first week of life. A mild sinus arrhythmia occurs in most newborns and is more pronounced in premature infants. The use of long-term ECG recordings in full-term newborns has revealed the existence of clinically unsuspected and presumably benign arrhythmias. A study of 56 full-term infants revealed isolated sinus arrest in one baby, a few premature supraventricular beats in three, and premature ventricular beats in two, one of whom had a premature ventricular beat every fourth beat but a normal ECG by age 14 days. A similar study of 20 premature infants revealed sinus bradycardia in eight and very marked sinus bradycardia (rate below 50 beats per minute) with nodal escapes in an additional five. All infants with birth weights below 1,500 gm had one or more periods of marked sinus bradycardia with or without nodal escape; none of the 50 full-term infants studied by the same group had sinus bradycardia (below 70 beats per minute) or had a nodal rhythm.

The finding therefore of an occasional premature beat

or of a short period of sinus bradycardia or sinus tachycardia is not in itself ominous. However, in the presence of severe heart disease such arrhythmias may portend serious trouble. The introduction of long-term ECG tape recording and the use of continuous ECG monitors equipped with a memory loop, whereby the minute preceding and including an arrhythmia can be printed out, have greatly facilitated the unraveling of intermittent arrhythmias in newborns. In instances where an arrhythmia is infrequent and the parents live at a distance from a medical center, use of transtelephonic ECG transmission (Cardiotel program) has been useful.

Heart sounds

The diaphragm side of the stethoscope is usually preferable for auscultation of both heart sounds and murmurs, since it is not necessary for the whole diaphragm (in contrast to the bell) to make contact with the chest wall. There is no advantage to use of the pediatric size stethoscope, but it is of help always to use the same type of stethoscope, preferably one of longer length, to manipulate through incubator portholes.

Infant heart sounds have a ticktock quality because of the more equal duration of systole and diastole (with faster heart rates), the presence of slight pulmonary hypertension (for the first few days), and the proximity of semilunar valves to the chest wall. Compared with that in older children, the infant's apical first sound is particularly well heard, and the small size of the chest allows simultaneous assessment of first and second sounds with the stethoscope at the lower left sternal border. In the normal infant splitting of the first sound should lead one to suspect that one is hearing either a fourth sound (atrial sound) plus a first sound or a first sound plus an ejection click (as in aortic or pulmonic stenosis). A third possibility is that the extra sound is a mitral midsystolic click, suggesting congenital mitral valve prolapse or prolapse associated with Marfan's syndrome. Narrow splitting of the second sound is apparent in most babies; widening and narrowing of the second sound with respiration is usually apparent when the respiration rate is normal. An unusually obvious persistent wide splitting of the second sound may indicate an ASD or total anomalous pulmonary venous return.

Ejection clicks, although uncommon, are useful physical signs, since when loud and obvious they are characteristic of aortic and pulmonic valvular stenosis. Soft ejection clicks sometimes are heard in normal babies. The ejection click is heard at the onset of an ejection murmur and resembles in timing, although not in character, a widely split first heart sound. The two may be distinguished, if necessary, by the recording of a simultaneous ECG and phonocardiogram; the ejection click is characteristically at least 0.09 seconds after the Q wave of the ECG, whereas the first heart sound (mitral and tricuspid valve closure) finishes earlier.

Cardiac murmurs

Certain murmurs are of major diagnostic help in the newborn period; however, the frequent presence of "innocent" murmurs and of transient ductus arteriosus murmurs renders their interpretation more difficult and more subject to error than in the older child. The situation is complicated by the fact that there are no absolute criteria for loudness, and the fast heart rate of babies sometimes makes it difficult to differentiate ejection from pansystolic murmurs. Characteristic heart murmurs of common heart defects appearing as problems in the neonatal period are discussed later in this chapter when specific lesions are considered. Serious heart disease may exist without any murmur, and conversely a grade 5 or 6 murmur may indicate a benign closing VSD. An organic systolic murmur present at the initial physical examination is more likely to be caused by an obstructive lesion such as aortic stenosis, pulmonic stenosis, or coarctation, whereas a murmur that is first heard at 2 or 3 months of age suggests a septal defect or ductus arteriosus, since the left-to-right shunt "opens up" as pulmonary vascular resistance falls in the first days and weeks of life.

Chest roentgenogram

Every newborn suspected of having a serious heart disease requires a well-centered anteroposterior chest roentgenogram and preferably a lateral film in addition. The lateral film may disclose left atrial enlargement or an unsuspected pathologic condition in the lung that is not evident on the anteroposterior film. The chest roentgenogram serves two broad purposes: (1) to evaluate the type and severity of heart disease and (2) to detect some of the many simulators of heart disease, including a wide variety of primary lung diseases and mechanical interference with lung function (Chapter 39). In the evaluation of heart disease the following features should be considered.

1. *Expansion of the lungs.* Atelectasis or hypoventilation may give the spurious impression of cardiomegaly; correspondingly, overaerated lungs (as in lobar emphysema) may disguise cardiac enlargement.
2. *Heart size.* Unfortunately no firm criteria exist with which to assess cardiomegaly, and except in extreme situations (such as a cardiothoracic ratio greater than 0.75) pronouncements are mostly intuitive. A normal-sized heart is compatible with serious heart disease (such as transposition of the great arteries in the first day of life or anomalously draining pulmonary veins, with obstruction of the common pulmonary vein collecting trunk). A very large heart may be present without heart disease, as is the case in hypoglycemia

or high hematocrit syndrome, or the heart may appear spuriously large because of the thymus gland.
3. *Shape of the heart.* The shape is often of considerable help, as in the "egg-on-side" heart of transposition, the boot-shaped heart of tetralogy of Fallot, the globular heart of Ebstein's anomaly, or the "snowman" heart of total anomalous pulmonary venous return into the left superior vena cava. Usually, however, the heart is simply large; useful signs such as prominence of the ascending aorta (aortic stenosis), prominence of the main and left pulmonary artery (pulmonic stenosis), square-shaped heart of tricuspid atresia, and the high origin of the pulmonary arteries (truncus arteriosus) often have not had time to develop or are obscured by the thymus gland.
4. *Pulmonary vascularity.* Three basic abnormalities can be recognized: oligemic lungs, hyperemic lungs, and lungs in which there is obstruction to pulmonary venous return. The pulmonary venous distension of this last category may lead to a "ground-glass," "snowstorm," or reticulated pattern (Fig. 25-3). It is quite different from the pulmonary hyperemic appearance where prominent large vessels appear to emanate from a single source, the hilum, and reflect a different spectrum of pathologic conditions (mitral valve disease, total anomalous pulmonary venous return with obstruction, or cor triatriatum).
5. *Specific appearances.* In the scimitar syndrome, one lung, usually the right, is supplied by systemic arteries, and a single large pulmonary vein (the "scimitar" on the roentgenogram), joins the inferior vena cava just below the diaphragm (Fig. 25-4). Usually the affected lung is hypoplastic, and the heart is shifted to the right (dextroposition).

The electrocardiogram

The neonatal ECG and especially the ECG taken during the first 24 hours of life show great variability within the range of normal. The changes probably are secondary to the rapidly changing circulation (closing foramen ovale and ductus arteriosus, removal of the placenta for the systemic circulation, and the falling pulmonary artery pressure). Other influences are the infant's gestational age, pH, and levels of sodium, potassium, and calcium. Despite the wide variability of the normal newborn ECG, it is still an extremely useful diagnostic tool; and since it is such a simple noninvasive procedure, it is mandatory in the assessment of any neonate suspected of having cardiovascular disease.

The QRS complex

The newborn's ECG exhibits prominent and prolonged anterior forces resulting in a tall and broad R

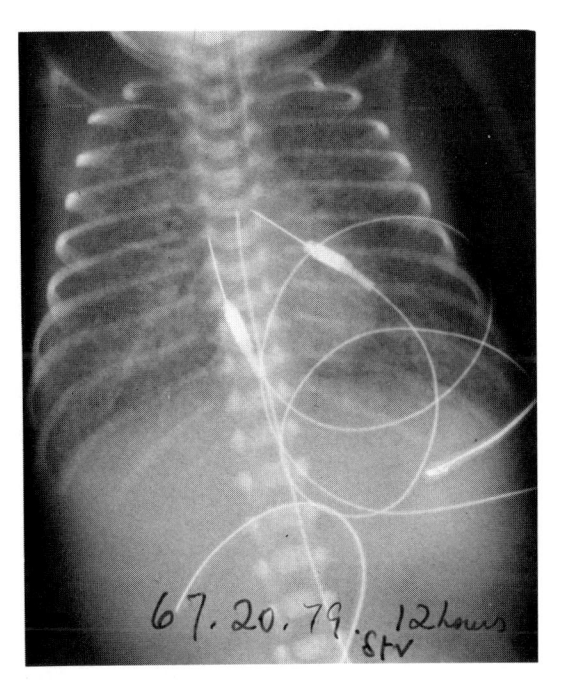

Fig. 25-3. Anteroposterior chest film of neonate with total anomalous pulmonary venous return to portal vein. Note small heart and "reticulated" lung fields, both caused by obstruction to pulmonary venous return.

wave in the right chest leads and often a deep S wave in the left chest leads. The leftward vector in the newborn is small; consequently the R wave in the left precordium has low amplitude initially, but this increases rapidly in the first few months. The posterior vector, although variable, is frequently small in the newborn period and appears late. Thus the S wave in leads V_1 and V_2 is small.

The initial, or septal, vector may be to the left in the newborn period (less so in the premature infant). Rarely this may result in a qR complex in lead V_{4R} or even in V_1 and absent or small Q waves in the left chest leads. With aging, the initial vector extends further to the right, and the Q wave increases in the left precordium. The terminal rightward force is prominent in the newborn and gradually decreases over months to years. This explains the deep S wave in the left chest leads, which decreases with age. The newborn's ECG almost invariably demonstrates clockwise rotation in the frontal plane and usually (but less often) also in the horizontal plane.

The QRS patterns in the chest leads are classified into the following:
1. Adult R/S progression: S wave has higher amplitude than R wave in right chest leads and smaller than R wave in left chest leads.
2. Partial reversal of R/S progression: R wave amplitude is higher than that of S wave in both right and left chest leads.

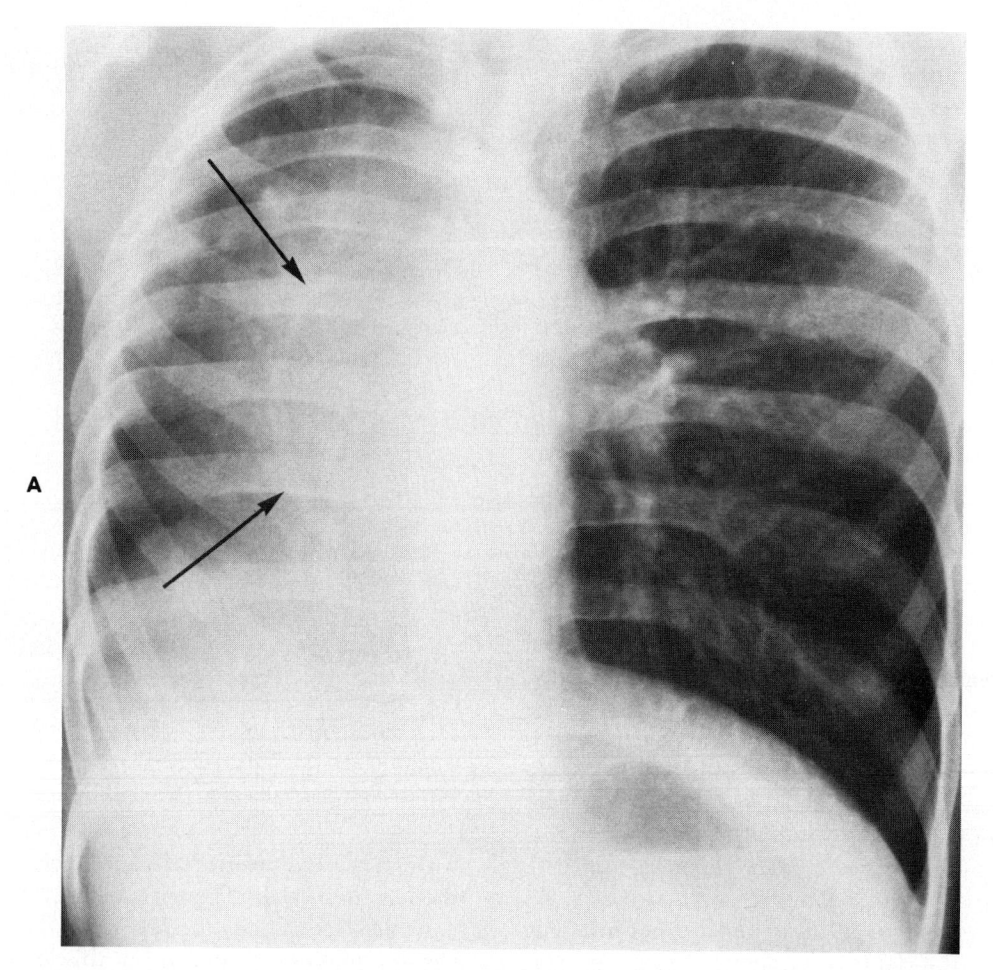

Fig. 25-4. "Scimitar" sign. **A,** With hypoplastic right lung. **B,** In an older child with normal right lung. In both cases the "scimitar" *(arrows)* represents the conjoined right pulmonary veins curving downward to enter the inferior vena cava below the diaphragm.

3. Complete reversal of R/S progression: R wave is larger than S wave in the right and smaller than S wave in the left chest leads (Fig. 25-5).

The newborn has either complete (50%) or partial reversal (50%) of R/S progression in the precordial leads, but no adult progression (with rare exceptions) of the R/S ratio is seen. By 1 month of age complete reversal disappears, and adult R/S progression is common. A pure R wave in lead V1 is rare, and a qR is only exceptionally seen in newborns.

T vector

Major changes occur in the T vector following birth. Within the first 5 minutes following birth this vector is oriented to the left anteriorly and minimally inferiorly; by 1 to 6 hours it has shifted much more inferiorly and to the right. Over the next several days the vector rotates markedly to the left and eventually becomes oriented to the left and posteriorly. In the series of Hastreiter and Abella during the first 24 hours the T vector was still oriented to the left anteriorly and inferiorly; at 2 to 7 days it was oriented to the left posteriorly and inferiorly. These changes explain the upright T in lead V_1 and the negative or flat T in lead V_6 that are characteristic of the very early neonatal period.

Electrocardiographic time intervals

Fast paper speeds (100 or 200 mm/second) increase the accuracy of the measurement of the short time intervals found in the newborn. However, the standard 25 mm/second is usually adequate. At birth the average heart rate is 140 beats per minute, but the rate drops to approximately 120 in the quiet infant during the first several hours. Premature infants have slightly higher heart rates. Although variations in heart rate from 70 to 200 beats per minute are compatible with a normal cardiovascular system, extremes should prompt ECG confirmation that the rhythm is sinus tachycardia or bradycardia. In general, one should be concerned if the *resting* rate is below 90 or above 170 beats per minute. The PR

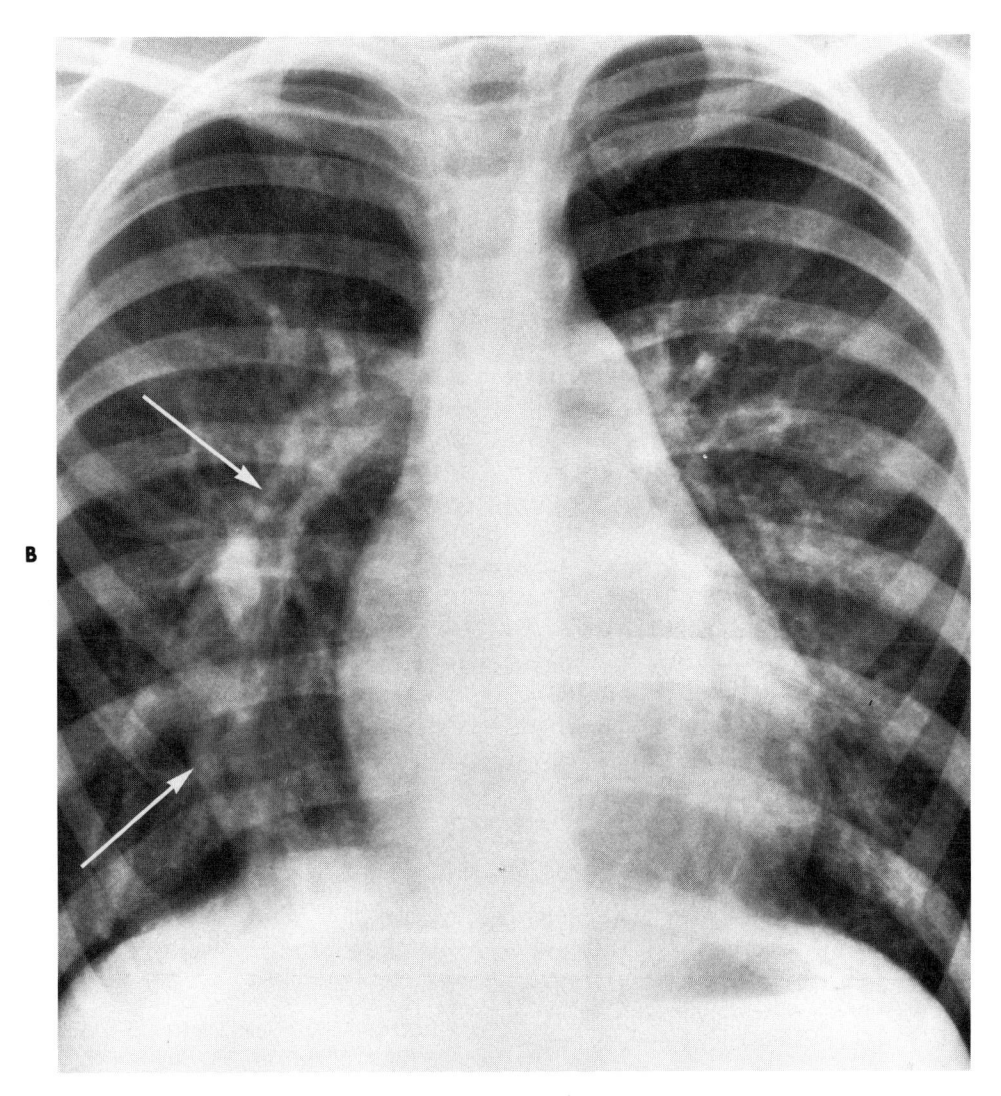

Fig. 25-4, cont'd. For legend see opposite page.

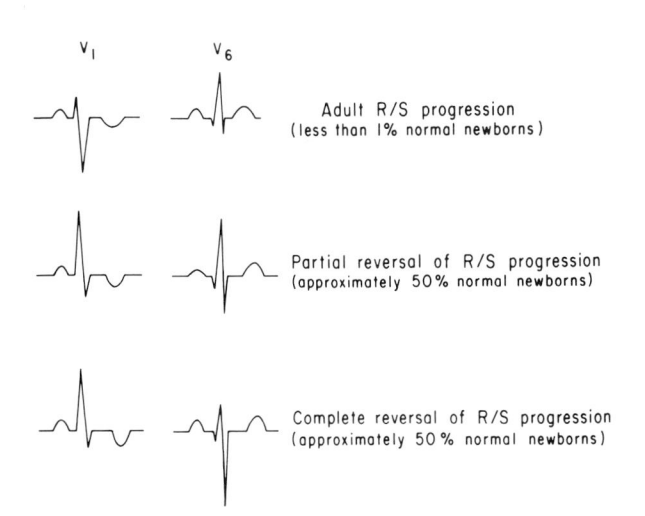

Fig. 25-5. QRS patterns in V₁ and V₆ of normal newborns. Note that adult R/S progression is sufficiently unusual to prompt consideration of left ventricular hypertrophy (or underdevelopment of the right ventricle).

- Adult R/S progression (less than 1% normal newborns)
- Partial reversal of R/S progression (approximately 50% normal newborns)
- Complete reversal of R/S progression (approximately 50% normal newborns)

interval should be recorded as the longest observable in a standard or unipolar limb lead (usually the longest is lead II). The normal range is between 0.07 and 0.12 second, influenced slightly by heart rate and the time of cord clamping. The QRS duration averages 0.065 second at birth, falls to about 0.055 second at the end of the first week, and gradually increases to 0.068 second at 12 months. The QT interval is greatly influenced by heart rate and therefore is expressed as QT observed or QT_c (QT corrected to a heart rate of 60). At birth the average observed QT interval is relatively long (0.30 second), decreasing to 0.24 second at 3 weeks and to 0.27 at 1 year. The QT_c is much more constant, averaging 0.40 second.

Electrical axes of the newborn heart

A consideration of the frontal plane QRS axis (assessed from the standard and unipolar limb leads) can be of considerable diagnostic help. The normal newborn has a

QRS axis of approximately +35 to +180 degrees. The normal P-wave axis should lie between 0 and +90 degrees (that is, upright in leads I and aV$_F$). The T-wave axis in the frontal plane is much more labile after birth than is the P or QRS axis. The T axis averages +7 degrees at 1 to 5 minutes after birth, then shifts to +115 degrees at 2 to 4 hours after birth; this is followed by a gradual return to approximately the previous level (+10 degrees) during the following 2 to 7 days. From the first week to the beginning of the third month of life the frontal T-wave axis gradually increases to reach a maximum of +60 degrees. The T wave therefore always should be upright in lead I except for a brief period in the first 24 hours of life, when it may be biphasic or on rare occasion inverted. The T waves are frequently of low amplitude during the first week of life. In the horizontal plane (that is, the precordial leads V$_{4R}$ through V$_6$) the mean QRS axis has an average value of +130 degrees during the first day of life and decreases gradually to about +110 degrees at the end of the first week; it remains stationary throughout the first month. Thus in all but an occasional infant the QRS axis is a predominantly positive deflection in the right precordial leads. The T wave is usually negative in V$_1$ immediately after birth but becomes positive in this lead at 2 to 6 hours, after which it usually becomes negative successively in V$_1$, V$_2$, V$_3$, and V$_4$. On occasion the T wave may be partially negative (biphasic) in V$_5$ and V$_6$. This characteristic has been correlated with a left-to-right shunt through the ductus arteriosus in the first 10 hours of life. After the first month of life the T wave always should be upright in V$_6$. A clearly negative T wave in V$_5$ or V$_6$ should suggest an abnormality such as myocarditis, left ventricular hypertrophy, conduction abnormality, or electrolyte disturbance. Whatever the cause of a negative T wave in V$_6$, follow-up ECGs are indicated.

The ECG of the premature and postmature infant

A number of comprehensive studies have failed to resolve the question of whether the premature infant's ECG has characteristic features different from those of a mature newborn. In part this is because the premature newborn's ECG shows even more variability than that of the full-term infant. Generally, however, there is less right ventricular dominance (also lower right ventricle–to–left ventricle weight ratio) in the ECG of the premature and more right ventricular dominance in the postmature infant.

The ECG in diagnosis during the newborn period

The newborn's ECG is most useful in the unraveling of an arrhythmia, the detection of gross atrial and ventricular hypertrophy, and the occasional almost pathognomonic finding such as myocardial infarction, indicating an anomalous left coronary artery (Fig. 25-56), or left axis deviation and left ventricular hypertrophy typical of tricuspid valve atresia (Fig. 25-46). The ECG plays a supportive role in the detection and assessment of severity of electrolyte disorders and myocardial disorders (Figs. 25-6, and 25-52 and 25-53). The major area of uncertainty is in the diagnosis of right ventricular hypertrophy. This is related to the rapidly changing hemodynamics and individual right/left ventricle weight ratios. Later in infancy and in childhood (when the left ventricle far outweighs the right) the opposite is found: the ECG is a sensitive indicator of right ventricular hypertrophy, but the voltage criteria for left ventricular hypertrophy are unreliable.

Diagnosis of atrial hypertrophy. The diagnosis of atrial hypertrophy is relatively straightforward. A P wave that is peaked and more than 3 mm (0.3 mV) in any standard or unipolar lead indicates probable right atrial hypertrophy (P pulmonale); if the P wave is 4 mm, right atrial hypertrophy is certain. Left atrial hypertrophy is characterized by broadening and notching of the P wave, so that the duration (in a limb lead) is 0.10 second or greater, and the Macruz index (the ratio of P-wave duration to the remainder of the PR interval) is increased (greater than 1.6:1).

Diagnosis of ventricular hypertrophy. The following outline shows the criteria for the diagnosis of ventricular hypertrophy. No single measurement is diagnostic; all values are possible in normal newborns, but many are statistically unlikely.

CRITERIA FOR RIGHT AND LEFT VENTRICULAR HYPERTROPHY IN THE NEWBORN

A. Right ventricular hypertrophy
 1. An R in lead aV$_R$ of greater than 7 mm
 2. A qR pattern in V$_1$
 3. An RV$_1$ greater than 28 mm
 4. SV$_6$ greater than 13 mm
 5. A pure R wave (no q or S) in V$_1$ of 10 mm or greater
 6. Positive T in V$_1$ after day 5
B. Left ventricular hypertrophy
 1. R in aV$_L$ greater than 9 mm
 2. R in V$_6$ greater than 17 mm in first week
 3. R in V$_6$ greater than 25 mm in first month
 4. Inverted TV$_6$ or T$_1$ with voltage changes
 5. Adult R/S progression; that is, SV$_1$ greater than RV$_1$ and RV$_6$ SV$_6$ (before day 3)

Electrolytes and the ECG in the neonatal period

Although abnormal serum calcium and serum potassium levels sometimes are associated with characteristic ECG abnormalities, undue reliance should not be placed on the ECG to *detect* electrolyte disturbances, since intracellular as well as extracellular electrolyte levels are responsible for the disordered waveform. Magnesium

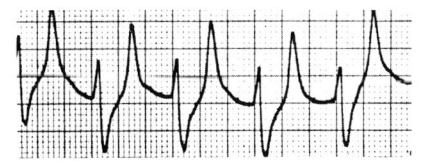

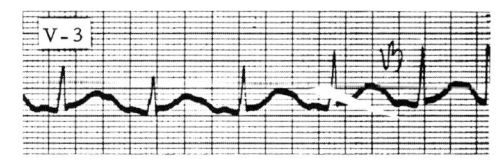

Fig. 25-6. ECG changes of advanced hyperkalemia (lead II). Note tall "tented" T waves, ST depression, and barely visible P waves on downslope of T wave. In the example of hypokalemia (lead V₃) there is a prominent U wave—the second component of what appears to be a double-peaked T wave. In other examples there would be P wave prolongation or prominence, ST depression, or low-voltage T waves. The changes of hypokalemia are much less distinctive than those of hyperkalemia.

and sodium ion levels and pH disturbances are not generally considered primary determinants of the ECG waveform but are thought to act predominantly by their effects on the intracellular and extracellular levels of potassium.

Hyperkalemia produces a succession of changes in the ECG, with tall, narrow, "tented" T waves progressing to ST segment depression, QRS widening, and a lengthened PR interval (Fig. 25-6). Finally, with severe hyperkalemia the QRS blends with the T wave to produce the "sine-wave" effect. This type of ECG often is observed in the dying neonate, especially following external cardiac massage. *Hypokalemia* leads to ST depression, low-voltage T waves, and development of a prominent U wave (Fig. 25-6). The PR interval may be prolonged with prominent P waves. The changes are much less apparent than those of hyperkalemia.

Serum calcium changes. It is now realized that the levels of intracellular and extracellular calcium ions are basic determinants of the speed of myocardial depolarization and repolarization. Hypocalcemia lengthens the QT interval, whereas hypercalcemia shortens it.

Significance of common electrocardiographic abnormalities in the neonate

Sinus arrhythmia may be obvious in the full-term neonate and very marked in the premature infant. Marked sinus arrhythmia requires ECG confirmation.

Tachycardia (rate over 170 beats per minute) may reflect fever, hyperthyroidism, or excessive activity or may on occasion be physiologic. Sinus tachycardia rates up to 200 beats per minute in the full-term infant and 210 beats per minute in the premature infant have been described. These rates (over 170 beats per minute) necessitate an ECG to distinguish between sinus tachycardia, paroxysmal SVT, atrial flutter with 2:1 AV conduction, and paroxysmal ventricular tachycardia. The major problem that arises is the distinction between paroxysmal SVT and sinus tachycardia (p. 576).

Bradycardia is when the rate is under 90 beats per minute. Rates down to 90 beats per minute in the full-term infant and 70 beats per minute in the premature infant have been found in the absence of disease. Even lower rates occur during defecation and breath holding with crying. The ECG will distinguish pathologic sinus bradycardia (from apneic spells, pathologic conditions of the central nervous system, gross hypoxia, and so on) from specific bradycardia (such as complete heart blocks, second-degree AV block, and atrial flutter or SVT with a high degree of AV block). Bradycardia and tachycardia may be seen in infants with sinus node dysfunction (sick sinus syndrome) (see Fig. 25-32).

Prolongation of the PR interval indicates first-degree AV block. If the PR interval is constant, no treatment is required; but one should be alerted to the possibility that first-degree AV block may progress to second-degree AV block, especially if digitalis is being administered. Hyperkalemia, hypokalemia, and acidosis also should be considered. In most instances no abnormality exists, and the condition is a benign variant. *Shortening of the PR interval* indicates an ectopic atrial pacemaker (close to the AV node) or the Wolff-Parkinson-White syndrome (short PR, broad QRS).

Variation of the PR interval with equal atrial (P) and ventricular (QRS) rates may indicate premature atrial beats or, if the PR interval has three or more different durations with P waves or varying forms, the benign "wandering pacemaker." *Absence of the P wave* usually indicates an AV nodal pacemaker.

Variation of the PR interval with the atrial rate faster than the ventricular rate (a P-wave rate in excess of the QRS rate), when there is no relationship between the two, indicates complete heart block (third-degree AV block), incomplete AV dissociation with ventricular captures, or second-degree heart block.

Variation of the PR interval with the atrial rate slower than the ventricular rate is a rare situation (sometimes called AV dissociation by interference) which implies that a lower pacemaker (usually AV nodal) beats somewhat faster than the sinoatrial (SA) pacemaker. Thus the ventricular rate is rarely as slow as in complete heart block. The most common causes are digitalis intoxication and myocarditis.

A *wide QRS* indicates right or left bundle branch block, complete AV block, or the Wolff-Parkinson-White syndrome. Random wide QRS complexes indicate ventricular ectopic beats or supraventricular beats with aberrant ventricular conduction. Hyperkalemia, hyponatremia, acidosis, and drugs such as quinidine and phenytoin may broaden the QRS.

A *shortened QT_c interval* is characteristic of hypercalcemia and of digitalis effect. Hyponatremia also may cause slight QT_c shortening. A *lengthened QT_c interval* is characteristic of hypocalcemia, hypokalemia, drug intoxication (especially from quinidine and phenothiazine derivatives), and patients with cerebrovascular disease. QT_c prolongation also is seen in children with congenital deafness, a heritable form of QT_c prolongation associated with syncopal spells and sudden death.

Right axis deviation (+90 to +180 degrees) is a normal finding in the first month of life. An axis between +35 and +90 degrees may be normal in the newborn period, and axes between 0 and +35 degrees occasionally are seen in a newborn. *Left axis deviation (0 to −90 degrees* is very rare in a normal infant and is highly suggestive of endocardial cushion defects (ostium primum ASD, common AV canal) and tricuspid atresia. A northwest axis (−90 to −180 degrees), if close to −90 degrees, usually represents extreme left axis deviation; if closer to −180 degrees, it is usually extreme right axis deviation. Clockwise inscription of the vector loop in the frontal plane implies the latter, counterclockwise inscription the former.

Right atrial hypertrophy is common with tricuspid atresia and Ebstein's anomaly. It is less common with transposition, tetralogy of Fallot, pulmonary hypertension, and any situation where the right ventricle is operating at systemic pressure. Right atrial hypertrophy also is seen where pulmonary hypertension is secondary to lung disease or when heart failure is present, as in SVT. *Left atrial hypertrophy* is common with mitral insufficiency and may occur with left ventricular failure (especially secondary to isolated aortic stenosis). *Right ventricular hypertrophy* is demonstrated in the ECG in a wide variety of conditions in which the right ventricle operates at systemic pressure. It also is seen in many neonates with pulmonary disease. Extreme right ventricular hypertrophy suggests isolated pulmonic stenosis. *Left ventricular hypertrophy* strongly supports a diagnosis of tricuspid atresia (especially if there is associated left axis deviation) or isolated severe aortic stenosis. Secondary T-wave changes (inverted TV_6 or T_1 or both) may be present with either diagnosis.

The Wolff-Parkinson-White syndrome may be a chance finding and in most cases indicates no underlying heart disease. There is, however, a strong association with SVT and with a pathologic condition of the central nervous system. A wide variety of organic heart diseases may be associated, but especially common are Ebstein's anomaly and corrected levotransposition (*l*-transposition).

A *myocardial infarction pattern* (abnormal Q waves) is almost diagnostic of anomalous origin of the left coronary artery from the pulmonary artery. Endocardial fibroelastosis on rare occasions may produce the ECG pattern of infarction, secondary to widespread myocardial fibrosis.

Echocardiography in the neonate

Ultrasound is defined as sound waves that are above the frequency audible by humans (20,000 cycles/second, or 20,000 Hz). For standard cardiac diagnostic purposes frequencies of 2 million to 5 million cycles/second (2 to 5 MHz) are used. Electrical energy is fed into the transducer for very brief periods, or pulses, which are repeated 1 to 2,000 times per second. Ninety-nine percent of the time the transducer acts as the receiver for the sound waves, which are reflected from the objects on which they have impinged. The short pulse duration, with a long interval between each, allows for a low energy level. This makes pulsed reflected ultrasound well within all known limits of safety for biologic tissues.

The M-mode image usually is recorded on a moving paper chart recorder so that many cardiac cycles can be recorded for future study. This method of recording for M-mode echo has now almost completely replaced the Polaroid camera method.

The standard single-element (also called M-mode) echocardiogram is obtained by angling the transducer so that the heart is transected at three levels (Fig. 25-7). Area I in the figure transects the heart at the level of the aortic valve and left atrium. Here the aortic root and left atrial size may be measured. The aortic valve cusps can be seen in the center of the aorta and form a boxlike configuration when open (Fig. 25-8). The aorta moves anteriorly with systole.

Area II transects the heart at the level of the mitral valve (Figs. 25-7 and 25-9). At the onset of ventricular diastole (point *D* in Fig. 25-9) the mitral valve opens, and the anterior and posterior leaflets move in opposite directions. The E point represents the maximum anterior excursion of the anterior leaflet during early diastole. Following the rapid filling phase the leaflets tend to close (point F_O in Fig. 25-9) as ventricular filling slows. With atrial systole the leaflets again open (A wave in Fig. 25-9) as blood flows from the atrium to the left ventricle. An A wave (atrial systole) should be identifiable in both the anterior and posterior leaflets. Normally the anterior

The cardiovascular system 549

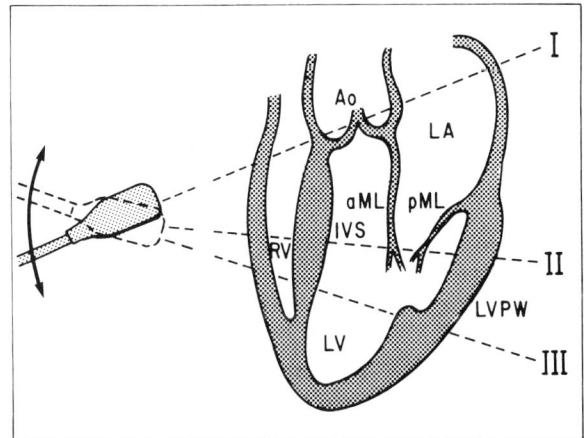

Fig. 25-7. Diagramatic cross section of heart. Echo transducer transects heart at levels I, II, and III for the three standard M-mode echo views. For M-mode sweep (as in Fig. 25-11), transducer is rotated, as shown, through three levels during recording. *A*, Aorta; *RV*, right ventricle; *aML*, anterior mitral valve leaflet; *pML*, posterior mitral valve leaflet; *LV*, left ventricle; *LVPW*, left ventricular posterior wall; *LA*, left atrium; *IVS*, interventricular septum. (Modified from Roelandt, J.: Practical echocardiography, Portland, 1977, Research Studies Press. Copyright 1977. Reprinted by permission of John Wiley & Sons, Ltd.)

leaflet motion is the mirror image of that of the posterior leaflet. In mitral valve stenosis the two leaflets have a parallel motion, and the A wave is not identifiable in the posterior leaflet.

The third area is at the left ventricular cavity (Figs. 25-7, area *III*, and 25-10) and transects the anterior heart wall, right ventricular cavity, interventricular septum, left ventricular cavity, some part of the chordae tendineae or papillary muscle apparatus, left ventricular posterior wall, and pericardium. The anterior heart wall echoes are usually diffuse and difficult to define. This makes the right ventricular cavity measurement frequently unreliable. Fig. 25-10 identifies the measurements usually made in this view. The left ventricular cavity internal dimension is measured in systole and diastole. The percentage change in cavity dimension is called the fractional shortening and is obtained by subtracting the left ventricular systolic dimension (*LVS*) from the diastolic dimension (*LVD*) and dividing by the diastolic dimension. Normally this should be at least 25%.

The thickness of the interventricular septum and left ventricular posterior wall (*LVPW*) is measured in systole (*S*) and diastole (*D*) (Fig. 25-10). Normally the interventricular septum moves posteriorly with systole, and the left ventricular posterior wall moves anteriorly. Abnormal septal motion, either flat or paradoxical, occurs in some pathologic states such as right ventricular volume

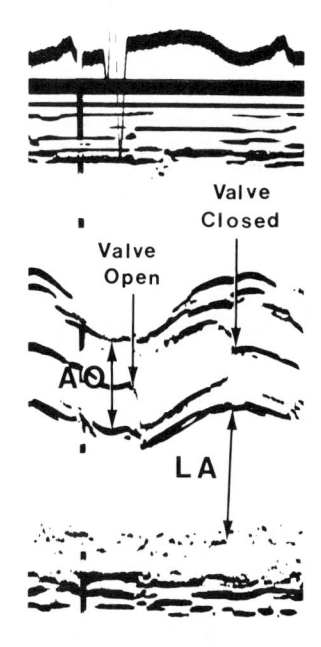

Fig. 25-8. Aorta *(AO)*, left atrium *(LA)* study; corresponds to level I in Fig. 25-7. Aorta is measured at onset of QRS, as shown with double arrow. Left atrium is measured at completion of ventricular systole (when left atrium has been filling), as shown with double arrow.

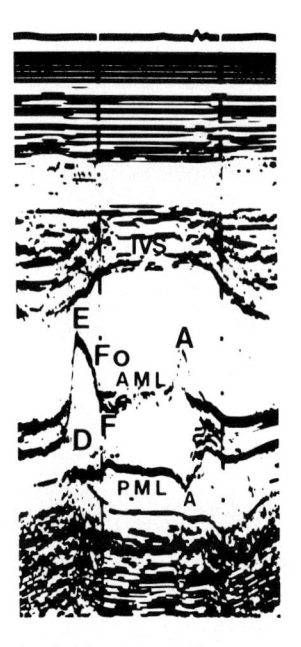

Fig. 25-9. Normal mitral valve study; corresponds to level II in Fig. 25-7. *AML*, anterior mitral leaflet; *PML*, posterior mitral leaflet; *IVS*, interventricular septum; *Fo*, rapid early closure of mitral valve.

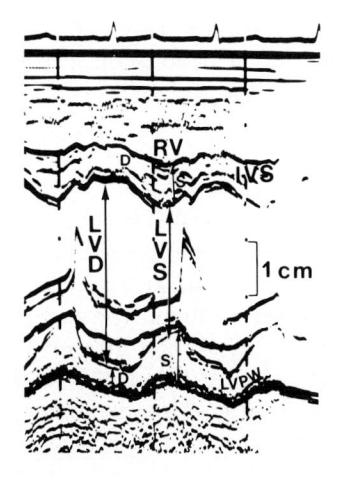

Fig. 25-10. Left ventricular study; corresponds to level III in Fig. 25-7. *LVD*, left ventricular internal dimension in diastole, measured as shown by double arrow; *LVS*, left ventricular internal dimension in systole, measured as shown by double arrow; *LVPW*, left ventricular posterior wall, measured in diastole, *D*, and systole, *S*; *IVS*, interventricular septum, measured in diastole, *D*, and systole, *S*; *RV*, right ventricle.

overload, myocardial dysfunction, and pulmonary hypertension. When the ventricular muscle function is normal, it thickens with systole.

There is normally minimal space between the epicardium and pericardium so that these structures are seen as a single echo. When a pericardial effusion occurs, there will be a space between these structures, usually more visible posteriorly than anteriorly (Fig. 25-19).

In addition these three areas being recorded individually, a sweep is made, rotating the transducer through all three levels (Fig. 25-7) and recording this on paper (Fig. 25-12). The transducer will pass through area I, identifying aorta (*AO*) and the left atrium (*LA*). As the transducer moves into the mitral valve (area *II*) and left ventricle (area *III*), the anterior aortic wall is seen to be continuous with the interventricular septum and the posterior aortic wall with the mitral valve (Fig. 25-11). The normal anterior aorta–interventricular septum relationship is lost in conditions such as tetralogy of Fallot where the aorta overrides the interventricular septum and the interventricular septum (*IVS*) comes in at the level of the aortic valve cusps (Fig. 25-21). The normal posterior aortic continuity with the mitral valve is lost in conditions such as when there is a double-outlet right ventricle and transposition of the great arteries.

The following are the usual measurements made in the three standard views:

Fig. 25-11. M-mode scan (sweeping from level *I* to *II* to *III* in Fig. 25-7), showing continuity of anterior aortic wall with interventricular septum *(IVS)* and continuity of posterior aortic wall with mitral valve. *LA*, left atrium; *RVOT*, right ventricular outflow tract; *AO*, aorta; *LVPW*, left ventricular posterior wall.

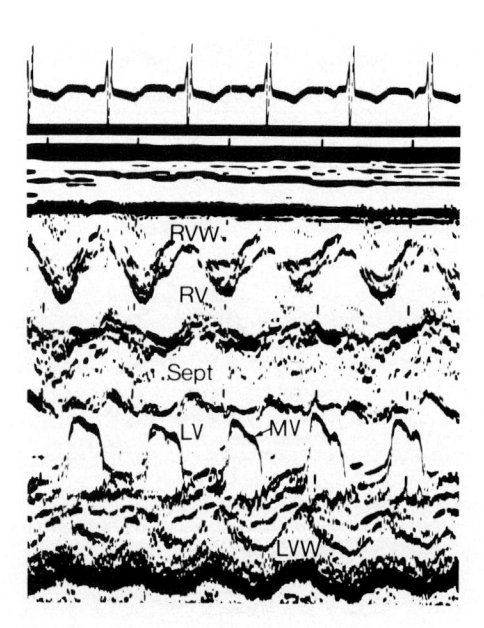

Fig. 25-12. M-mode echocardiogram from 3-day-old infant of diabetic mother. There is generalized thickening of cardiac walls; however, septum *(SEPT)* is thickened to much greater degree than left ventricular wall *(LVW)*. *LV*, left ventricle; *MV*, mitral valve; *RV*, right ventricle; *RVW*, right ventricular wall. (Courtesy Drs. R. Snider and N. Silverman.)

A. Aorta–left atrium (Fig. 25-8)
   1. The aortic root dimension (*AO*) is measured at end-diastole (onset of QRS).
   2. The left atrial cavity (*LA*) is represented as the echo-free space behind the posterior wall of the aorta. The echo identifying the left atrial posterior wall at times may be difficult to define. The left atrium is measured at end-systole (at aortic valve closure).
B. Mitral valve (Fig. 25-9)
   1. Amplitude of opening or excursion is measured from point D to E; normally this is greater than 20 mm.
   2. E-F_O slope; or early diastolic closing rate, is normally 70 mm/second or greater.
   3. Mitral valve motion: normally the two leaflets have opposite directions of motion. With mitral stenosis this may become parallel. The A wave should be identifiable in the posterior leaflet; its absence may indicate mitral stenosis.
C. Ventricles (Fig. 25-10)
   1. Right ventricular internal dimension (*RV*) is measured at end-diastole onset of QRS complex) from anterior heart wall to the right side of the interventricular septum. Because of the difficulty in accurately defining the anterior heart wall, this measurement may be unreliable.
   2. Left ventricular end-diastolic dimension (*LVD*) is the distance between the left side of the interventricular septum and the endocardial surface of the left ventricular posterior wall at end-diastole (onset of QRS).
   3. Left ventricular end-systolic dimension (*LVS*) is the distance between the left side of the interventricular septum and the endocardium of the left ventricular posterior wall at end-systole.
   4. Fractional shortening is normally at least 0.25%, or LVD − LVS/LVD.
   5. Interventricular septum thickness is measured at end-diastole (D-IVS) and end-systole (S-IVS). Normally systolic thickness is at least 30% greater.
   6. Left ventricular posterior wall thickness is measured at end-systole (S-LVPW) and end-diastole (D-LVPW). Normally systolic thickness is at least 30% greater than end-diastolic.

Table 25-4 lists standard values in normal full-term newborns. Table 25-5 lists standard values in preterm infants without evidence of heart or lung disease.

SPECIFIC APPLICATIONS OF SINGLE-ELEMENT ECHOCARDIOGRAPHY IN NEWBORNS
Infants of diabetic mothers

The infant of a diabetic mother has been known to be at increased risk for cardiac defects and other heart disease (p. 25). The recent literature documents in these infants the occurrence of a cardiomyopathy which may

Table 25-4. Echocardiographic values in normal newborns based on seven published studies (633 patients, age 1½ hours to 1 month and weighing 1.9 to 4.9 kg)

	Number of studies	Range (mm)
Aortic root diameter	540	7-13.6
Left atrial dimension	540	4-13.5
Interventricular septal thickness (diastole)	440	1.8-4.5
Left ventricular posterior wall (systole)	200	2.5-6
Left ventricular posterior wall (diastole)	440	1.6-4.6
Left ventricular dimension (systole)	211	8-18.6
Left ventricular dimension (diastole)	351	12-24.1
Right ventricular dimension (systole)	200	5.5-11.4
Right ventricular dimension (diastole)	540	6.1-17.7

Modified from Moss, A.J., Gussoni, C.C., and Isabel-Jones, J.: Echocardiography in congenital heart disease, West. J. Med. **124**:102, 1976.

Table 25-5. Left atrial dimension (LAD) and left ventricular internal diastolic dimension (LVID) in normal premature infants

Weight (gm)	LAD Mean (cm)	LAD Normal range (±2 SD)	LVID Mean (cm)	LVID Normal range (±2 SD)
600-900	0.60	0.5-0.7	1.07	0.9-1.2
901-1,200	0.65	0.5-0.8	1.08	0.9-1.3
1,201-1,500	0.69	0.5-0.9	1.18	1.0-1.3
1,501-1,800	0.79	0.6-1.0	1.37	1.2-1.5
1,801-2,200	0.88	0.7-1.1	1.39	1.1-1.6

From Meyer, R.A.: Pediatric echocardiography, Philadelphia, 1977, Lea & Febiger.

be associated with respiratory symptoms and congestive heart failure. The cardiomyopathy occurs in infants of class A, C, and D diabetics. Recent echocardiographic studies by Gutgesell and co-workers, Way and co-workers, and Mace and co-workers document abnormal thickness of the right ventricular wall and interventricular septum in infants of diabetic mothers when compared with normal babies of comparable gestational age. This was not explainable by the increased size of the infants, since the same measurements in large for gestational age normal infants were significantly smaller. In the study by Way and co-workers of 11 infants of diabetic mothers with congestive heart failure and/or respiratory symptoms, all had disproportionate thickening of the interventricular septum, although not all had evidence of left ventricular outflow obstruction. This is comparable to the autosomal dominant disease of idiopathic hypertrophic subaortic stenosis in which the interventricular septum is asymmetrically hypertrophied with respect to the left ventricular posterior wall. (Normally the interventricular septum/left ventricular posterior wall does not exceed 1.3.) In the hypertrophic cardiomyopathy of infants of diabetic mothers the interventricular septum/left ventricular posterior wall may range from 1.3 to greater than 2 and has been called disproportionate septal hypertrophy (Fig. 25-12). Obstruction, demonstrated by cardiac catheterization or by echo, may or may not be present.

Symptoms may be worsened by treatment with digitalis, and improvement may occur with propranolol administration. For this reason an echocardiogram probably is indicated in all infants of diabetic mothers. The natural history appears to be benign and the abnormality usually resolves in 3 to 12 months.

Left-to-right shunts

Persistent patency of the ductus arteriosus is common in premature infants. Usually clinical problems do not arise as a result of this lesion, and generally the PDA closes at or near term. The large left-to-right shunt that may occur as a result of the low pulmonary vascular resistance in the preterm infant can cause congestive heart failure. RDS thus may be complicated by patency of the ductus arteriosus in the premature infant. Echocardiography has made it possible in most cases to assess noninvasively the magnitude of the left-to-right shunt through the PDA.

The absolute left atrial size determined by echo does not always correlate well with the size of the left-to-right shunt found at cardiac catheterization because of transducer angle and differences in infant size. It has been helpful to relate the left atrial size to that of the aorta, which is positioned in front of the left atrium. Normally

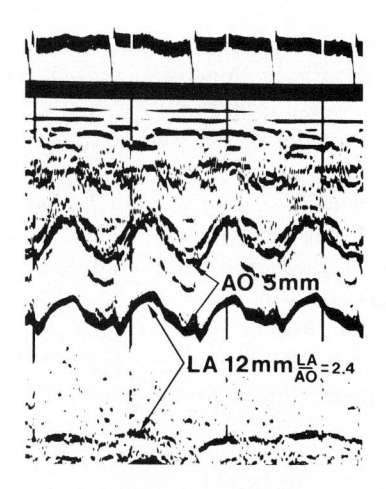

Fig. 25-13. Premature infants weighing 1,200 gm, with RDS and PDA. There is left atrial enlargement (12 mm versus normal of 9 mm). The left atrium/aorta ratio (LA/AO) is 2.4 (normal not greater than 1.3).

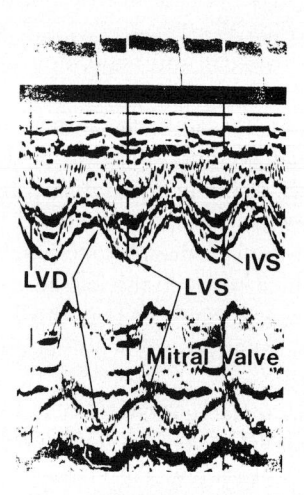

Fig. 25-14. Same infant shown in Fig. 25-13. Left ventricle in diastole (LVD) is 19 mm, normal up to 14. Fractional shortening is normal (37%) (LVD−LVS/LVD, or 19−12/19). Left ventricular enlargement and normal fractional shortening are compatible with large left-to-right shunt.

these structures have equal dimensions when the aorta is measured at the end of ventricular diastole and the left atrium is measured during ventricular systole (Fig. 25-13). In normal premature infants the ratio of the left atrial dimension to the aortic dimension has been shown to be 1 or less. In the series, reported by Silverman and co-workers, of premature infants with a clinically significant PDA, requiring surgery, the mean left atrium/aorta ratio was 1.38 ± 0.19. After surgery the ratio returned to normal levels (0.87 ± 0.12).

Figs. 25-13 and 25-14 show an echocardiogram from an

infant with RDS with an echocardiogram that showed a left atrium/aorta ratio of 2.4 and increased left ventricular diastolic dimension with normal fractional shortening. After surgery these measurements became normal.

The findings of left atrial and left ventricular enlargement by echo are characteristic of a large left-to-right shunt, such as VSD and PDA. These findings are not specific for either, and the echo must be used in conjunction with clinical evaluation of the patient.

The physical findings and general condition

In the premature infant with the physical findings of PDA, echo findings of left atrial and/or left ventricular enlargement provide a noninvasive assessment of the size of the left-to-right shunt, previously obtainable only by the invasive measures of cardiac catheterization and single-film aortography.

Echocardiographic measurement of systolic time intervals

Systolic time intervals are measurements of the components of electromechanical systole (Fig. 25-15). These consist of the preejection period (PEP) and the ventricular ejection time (VET). Measurement of the systolic time intervals of the left ventricle has been accomplished noninvasively using the indirect carotid arterial pulse, the ECG, and the phonocardiogram. Abnormal systolic time intervals, measured this way, have been found in left ventricular dysfunction and aortic stenosis.

Echocardiographically it is possible to record both the opening and closing of both the pulmonary and aortic valves. This, combined with the ECG, makes it possible to measure both right- and left-sided heart systolic time intervals. A good correlation exists between the left-sided heart systolic time intervals measured by echo and carotid pulse. Hirschfeld and co-workers have shown a good correlation between echo and pulmonary artery pressure analysis for the right-sided heart systolic time intervals.

The echocardiographic systolic time intervals that are measured include the following (Fig. 25-16):
1. Preejection period (PEP): measured from the onset of the QRS complex to semilunar valve opening
2. Ventricular ejection time (VET): measured from semilunar valve opening to semilunar valve closing
3. PEP/VET: ratio of the preejection period to the ejection time

These intervals are measured for both ventricles. High-quality recordings, where both the opening and the closing of the semilunar valve may be clearly identified, are necessary for the systolic time intervals to be measured by this method. The opening and closing of the aortic valve usually are recorded without difficulty.

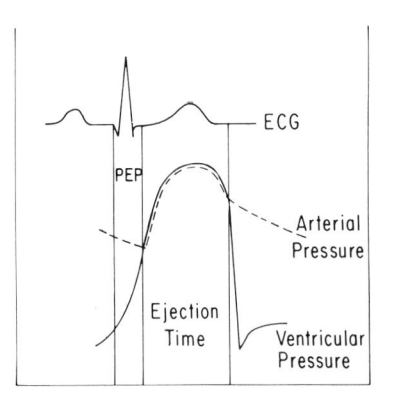

Fig. 25-15. Systolic time intervals. During PEP the ventricle develops sufficient pressure to equal that in great artery (point where ventricular pressure crosses arterial pressure). At this point semilunar valve opens, and ejection phase begins. During ejection time, semilunar valve is open, and flow occurs from ventricle to great artery. When ventricular pressure drops below that in great artery (point where pressures again cross), semilunar valve closes, and ejection phase ends. (See Fig. 25-16.)

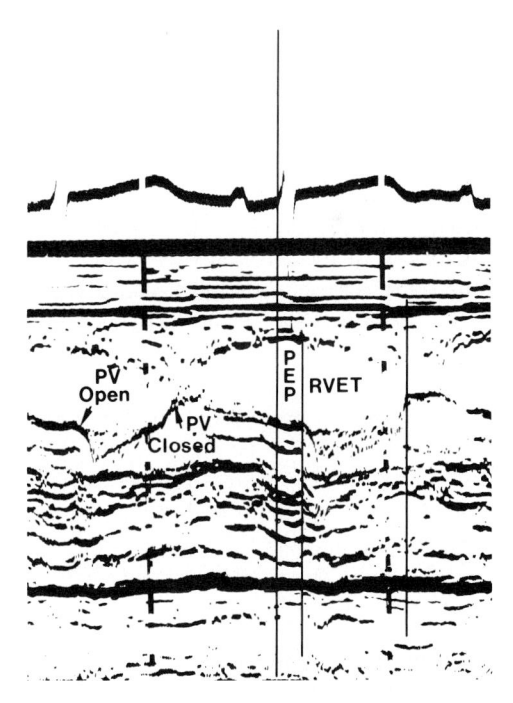

Fig. 25-16. Right-sided heart systolic time intervals. PEP is measured from onset of QRS complex to pulmonary valve opening. Ejection time (RVET) is measured from valve opening to valve closing. This figure is from normal preterm infant. RVPEP=50 msec, RVET=220 msec, and RVPEP/RVET=0.23. (See Fig. 25-15.)

Table 25-6. Systolic time intervals

Systolic time intervals	All Infants	Age <5 days	Age ≥5 days	p Value
Preterm infants				
Left ventricle				
Heart rate (beats per minute)	131 ± 14	137 ± 13	143 ± 16	<0.025
PEP (msec)	63 ± 12	66 ± 11	55 ± 9	<0.005
VET (msec)	183 ± 16	187 ± 15	175 ± 15	<0.005
PEP/VET	0.34 ± 0.07	0.36 ± 0.07	0.32 ± 0.06	<0.005
Right ventricle				
PEP (msec)	57 ± 9	60 ± 8	51 ± 7	<0.005
VET (msec)	197 ± 21	201 ± 21	186 ± 18	<0.005
PEP/VET	0.29 ± 0.05	0.30 ± 0.05	0.28 ± 0.04	<0.025
Full-term infants				
Left ventricle				
Heart rate (beats per minute)	132 ± 18	131 ± 19	141 ± 13	<0.01
PEP (msec)	69 ± 10	70 ± 10	65 ± 7	<0.005
VET (msec)	194 ± 17	196 ± 17	185 ± 14	<0.005
PEP/VET	0.36 ± 0.05	0.36 ± 0.05	0.36 ± 0.04	NS
Right ventricle				
PEP (msec)	67 ± 11	69 ± 10	57 ± 8	<0.005
VET (msec)	203 ± 18	203 ± 19	206 ± 19	NS
PEP/VET	0.33 ± 0.06	0.34 ± 0.06	0.28 ± 0.05	≤0.005

From Halliday, H., and others: Pediatrics **62**:317, 1978. Copyright American Academy of Pediatrics 1978.

High-quality echocardiograms, recording both the opening and closing of the pulmonary valve, are less consistently recorded. Halliday and co-workers have been able to record both the opening and closing of the posterior pulmonary valve leaflet in 70% to 80% of infants and 50% to 60% of children (Table 25-6).

In normal children the PEP of the right ventricle is shorter than that of the left ventricle, and the ejection time of the right ventricle is longer than that of the left ventricle. In the absence of disorders of contractility the pressure in the great artery determines the systolic time intervals. A rise in the diastolic pressure in the great artery usually results in prolongation of the PEP and thus in an alteration of the ratio between the PEP and VET (PEP/VET). These relationships have resulted in the application of systolic time interval measurements to the evaluation of pulmonary artery hypertension, persistence of the fetal circulation (PFC), and dextrotransposition (d-transposition) of the great arteries.

Echocardiographic systolic time intervals in pulmonary hypertension

Increase in the pulmonary vascular resistance has been shown to be associated with alterations in the right-sided heart systolic time intervals. Accurate prediction of the level of pulmonary artery pressure using the systolic time intervals has not been possible. However, there has been some correlation between the ratio of the pulmonary to systemic vascular resistance and the ratio of the right-sided heart to left-sided heart systolic time intervals. In some studies a ratio of 0.3 or greater for right ventricle PEP/VET ratio has been associated with a pulmonary artery diastolic pressure of 30 mm Hg or higher.

Echocardiographic systolic time intervals in persistence of the fetal circulation

In the fetus right-to-left shunting occurs at atrial and ductal levels. When these right-to-left shunts persist after birth, in the absence of significant structural heart disease, the syndrome is called persistence of the fetal circulation (PFC). At times it may be difficult by the usual clinical means to differentiate this from heart disease, and on occasion an infant without structural heart disease may be subjected to cardiac catheterization. Riggs and co-workers studied 17 infants with normal hearts but with severe elevation of the pulmonary vascular resistance. The PEP was prolonged in these infants, and the right ventricle PEP/VET ratio was increased. As the infants improved, the right ventricle and the PEP/VET ratio both increased until they became normal. When it is possible to obtain satisfactory echo recordings of the pulmonary valve, serial determinations of the right-sided heart systolic time intervals may help distinguish between PFC and structural heart disease and may be used to indicate improvement in an infant with PFC.

Echocardiographic systolic time intervals in d-transposition of the great arteries

In d-transposition of the great arteries the pulmonary valve is in a posterior position and arises from the left ventricle, and the aortic valve is anterior and arises from the right ventricle. Since the right ventricle now must overcome the systemic vascular resistance for semilunar valve opening with ejection into the systemic circulation, and the left ventricle now works against the lower pulmonary vascular resistance, some alteration in the systolic time intervals might be expected. Studies by Hirschfeld and co-workers and Gutgesell and co-workers have shown that in d-transposition of the great arteries, using the anterior semilunar valve recording for the right-sided heart systolic time intervals and the posterior semilunar valve recording for the left ventricular systolic time intervals, the right ventricular PEP increases, and the right VET shortens (similar to that of the normal left ventricle), and the left ventricular PEP shortens, and left VET lengthens.

Echocardiographic evaluation of left ventricular function

Ventricular function may be reduced in structural heart disease with congestive heart failure, endocardial fibroelastosis, anomalous origin of the left coronary artery, and cardiomyopathy. In the newborn a cardiomyopathy may occur as part of an infectious process, either intrauterine or postnatally acquired; it may be secondary to generalized hypoxia during the perinatal period and occurs in the infant of a diabetic mother. Echocardiographic demonstration of reduced left ventricular function provides a noninvasive method of diagnosing a cardiomyopathy and may eliminate the need for subjecting an already compromised infant to cardiac catheterization. The echocardiographic finding of reduced left ventricular function before cardiac catheterization contributes important information for directing the study, when the infant's course and clinical findings warrant an invasive procedure.

The following echocardiographic abnormalities indicate reduced left ventricular function (Fig. 25-17):

1. *Fractional shortening* (below 25%). Fractional shortening is the percentage change of the left ventricular cavity dimension with systole.
2. *Left ventricular enlargement.* The left ventricular diastolic cavity dimension usually will be increased.
3. *Left atrium.* Left atrial enlargement usually will be present.
4. *Mitral valve motion.* The E-F$_O$ slope may be reduced; because of the raised end-diastolic pressure in the left ventricle, there is a reduced rate at which the mitral valve drifts to the closed position following the passive filling phase and prior to atrial systole.

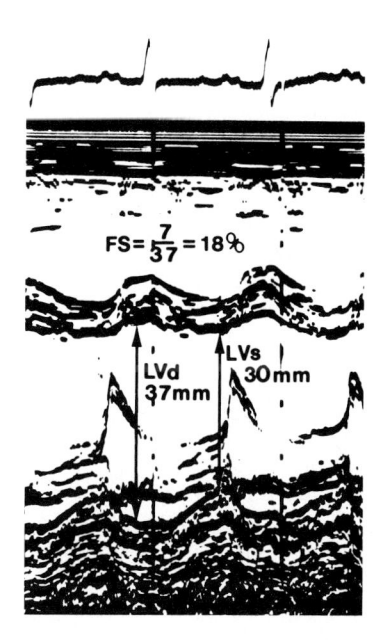

Fig. 25-17. Cardiomyopathy in 1-month-old infant. There is left ventricular enlargement (left ventricle internal dimension, diastole [LVD], 37 mm; normal to 25 mm). Fractional shortening *(FS)* is reduced to 18% (normal 25% or greater). *LVS,* left ventricle internal dimension, systole.

This is a nonspecific finding and also is present in mitral stenosis.

5. *Septal motion.* Normally the motion of the interventricular septum is toward the left ventricular posterior wall in systole. Frequently with reduced left ventricular function septal motion is flattened.
6. *Left ventricular wall muscle thickening.* Normally with systole the muscle of the interventricular septum and left ventricular posterior wall thickens. In a study of 50 normal newborns by St. John Sutton and co-workers the average percentage change in wall thickness was 95% ± 40% for the interventricular septum and about 130% for the left ventricular posterior wall. With left ventricular dysfunction there is reduced muscle thickening with systole.

Contrast echocardiography

The microbubbles that occur with a small injection of saline into a peripheral vein reflect ultrasound and thus will be recorded by the ultrasound transducer. This technique is used to identify vessels and chambers by the sequential appearance of the saline "contrast" and also to identify intracardiac shunts (Fig. 25-18).

Pericardial effusion

Echocardiography has become the most sensitive and reliable method for detecting pericardial effusion. The pericardium produces the brightest echo of the cardiac structures. Normally it is adherent to the epicardium,

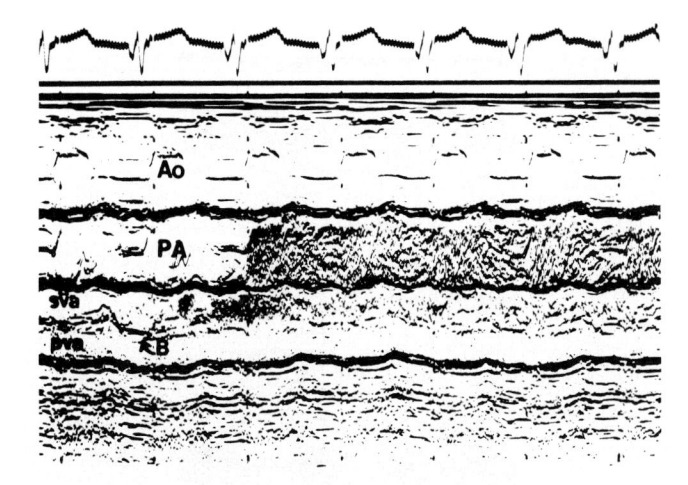

Fig. 25-18. Infant with d-transposition who has undergone interatrial baffle procedure. Five ml saline has been injected into peripheral vein. Saline contrast can be seen appearing in systemic venous atrium *(sva),* then in pulmonary artery *(PA).* None appears in pulmonary venous atrium *(pva)* or aorta *(AO),* indicating there is no leak in baffle *(B).* (Courtesy Dr. G. Michael Nichols, Portland, Ore.)

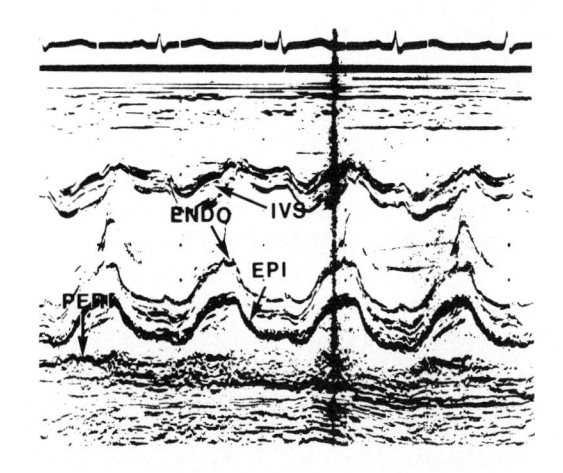

Fig. 25-19. Pericardial effusion in infant. Space between pericardium *(PERI)* and epicardium *(EPI)* contains effusion. *ENDO,* Endocardium; *IVS,* interventricular septum.

and no space appears between the two structures. When there is fluid in the pericardial sac, an echo-free space appears between the pericardium and epicardium (Fig. 25-19). Pericardial effusion may occur in the newborn with heart failure and septic pericarditis. Pneumopericardium may occur when there is pneumothorax and also will be seen as an echo-free space between the pericardium and epicardium.

Hypoplastic left-heart syndrome

The echocardiogram may be helpful in distinguishing underdevelopment of the left side of the heart from critical aortic stenosis and other causes of circulatory collapse in the newborn. The echocardiographic findings may not always be sufficient, however, to establish the diagnosis of hypoplastic left-heart syndrome; other studies, for example, an aortogram through the umbilical artery, may be indicated. Classically in hypoplastic left-heart syndrome the left ventricular wall is symmetrically thickened, the left ventricular cavity is extremely small or not identifiable, and the mitral valve is either not identified or has an excursion of less than 5 mm (Fig. 25-20). Sometimes a diminutive aortic root is visualized.

Cyanotic congenital heart disease
Truncus arteriosus

The truncus arteriosus is a large truncal root that overrides the ventricular septum (Fig. 25-21). Left atrial enlargement usually will be present. Mitral continuity with the aorta (truncus) is generally present.

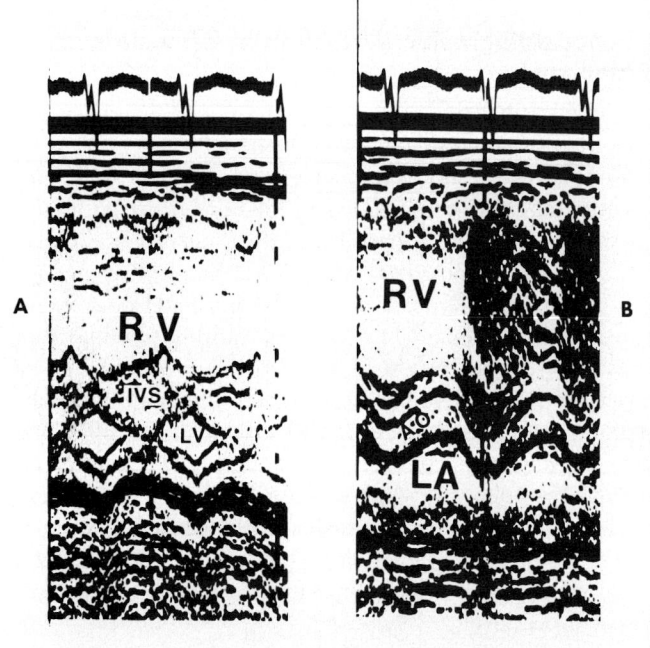

Fig. 25-20. Hypoplastic left-heart syndrome. **A,** Left ventricular cavity *(LV)* is small (4 mm). Interventricular septum *(IVS)* is thick. Right ventricle *(RV)* is large. **B,** Peripheral vein saline injection results in appearance of contrast in right ventricle. Aorta *(AO)* is very small (2 mm). *LA,* Left atrium.

Total anomalous pulmonary venous return

Right ventricular enlargement may be present. In addition, the echo may be helpful in determining left atrial and left ventricular size, since these structures may be smaller than normal in this condition. Occasionally it may be possible to identify the confluence of the pulmonary veins behind the heart (Fig. 25-22).

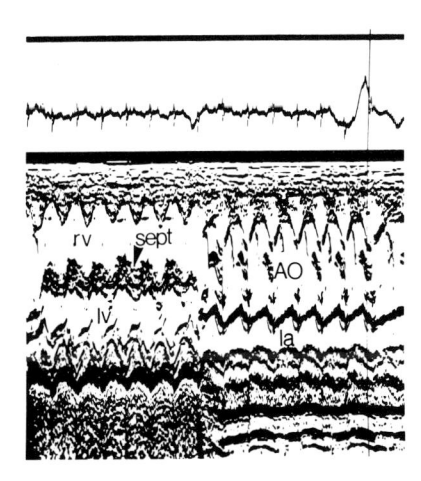

Fig. 25-21. M-mode echocardiogram sweep of left ventricle *(lv)* in newborn infant with tetralogy of Fallot. Aorta *(AO)* is seen overriding ventricular septum. VSD is evident. Left atrial cavity is small. *la,* Left atrium; *rv,* right ventricle; *sept,* interventricular septum. (Courtesy Dr. Rebecca Snider, San Francisco.)

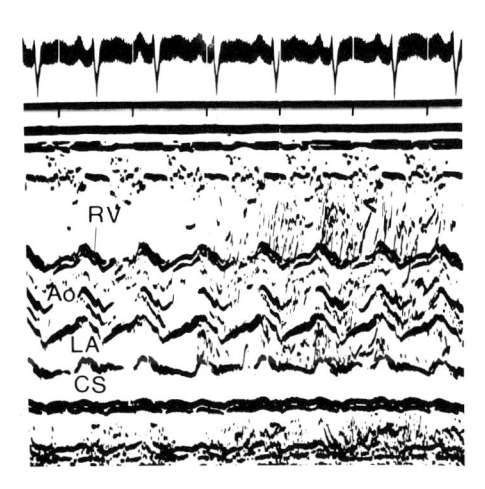

Fig. 25-22. Contrast M-mode echocardiogram from 1-day-old infant with total anomalous pulmonary venous connection to coronary sinus *(CS)*. Contrast is seen appearing in right ventricle *(RV)* and left atrium *(LA)* nearly simultaneously because of obligatory right-to-left atrial shunting. Contrast appears in subsequent beat in aorta *(Ao)* because of forward flow from left atrium. Coronary sinus is only structure that remains free from contrast echos because it is receiving the total pulmonary venous return. Structure filling deep to coronary sinus probably represents descending aorta. (Courtesy Dr. Rebecca Snider, San Francisco.)

Transposition of the great arteries

The routine M-mode echo may not be very helpful in this condition. If it is possible to record the systolic time intervals for both ventricles, then the echo may be supportive of this diagnosis. The two-dimensional echo is proving extremely helpful (Fig. 25-23).

Tricuspid atresia

Findings in tricuspid atresia are absent tricuspid valve echo and a small right ventricle. These two findings are in contrast to the usual newborn echocardiogram in which the tricuspid valve and right ventricle are easily identified.

Tetralogy of Fallot

Overriding aorta and absence of the pulmonic valve echo are characteristic of tetralogy of Fallot. Distinction between truncus arteriosus and tetralogy of Fallot may not be possible by echo (Fig. 25-21).

Other lesions where echocardiography may be extremely useful

Intracardiac tumors

Echocardiography has proved to be diagnostic of left atrial myxoma. Right atrial myxoma also has been demonstrated by M-mode echo. Allen and co-workers report the demonstration by echocardiography of a right ventricular tumor in a newborn.

Pulmonary arteriovenous fistula

Hernandez and co-workers describe diagnosis of a pulmonary arteriovenous fistula using contrast echocardiography. Normally injection of saline, with its reflective microbubbles, into the pulmonary artery would clear in the lungs and not appear in the left atrium. With a pulmonary arteriovenous fistula, pulmonary artery injection of saline would result in the appearance of reflective microbubbles in the left atrium.

Infective endocarditis

Infective endocarditis occurs infrequently in children under 2 years of age. Weinberg and Laird report the echocardiographic demonstration of valvular vegetation caused by group B streptococcal endocarditis in a 4-week-old infant, and Bender and co-workers report the diagnosis of bacterial endocarditis with mitral valve vegetations in a neonate.

Two-dimensional echocardiography

Clinical application of two-dimensional cardiac imaging is a development of the late 1970s. Real-time, two-dimensional imaging of the heart is accomplished by steering the ultrasonic beam through an arc of between 30 and 90 degrees, depending on the instrument used. The sector scan of the heart is made either by a mechanical scanner, which consists of a single crystal transducer that is made to rotate rapidly through an arc by an electric motor, or by an electronic instrument that uses phased element excitation.

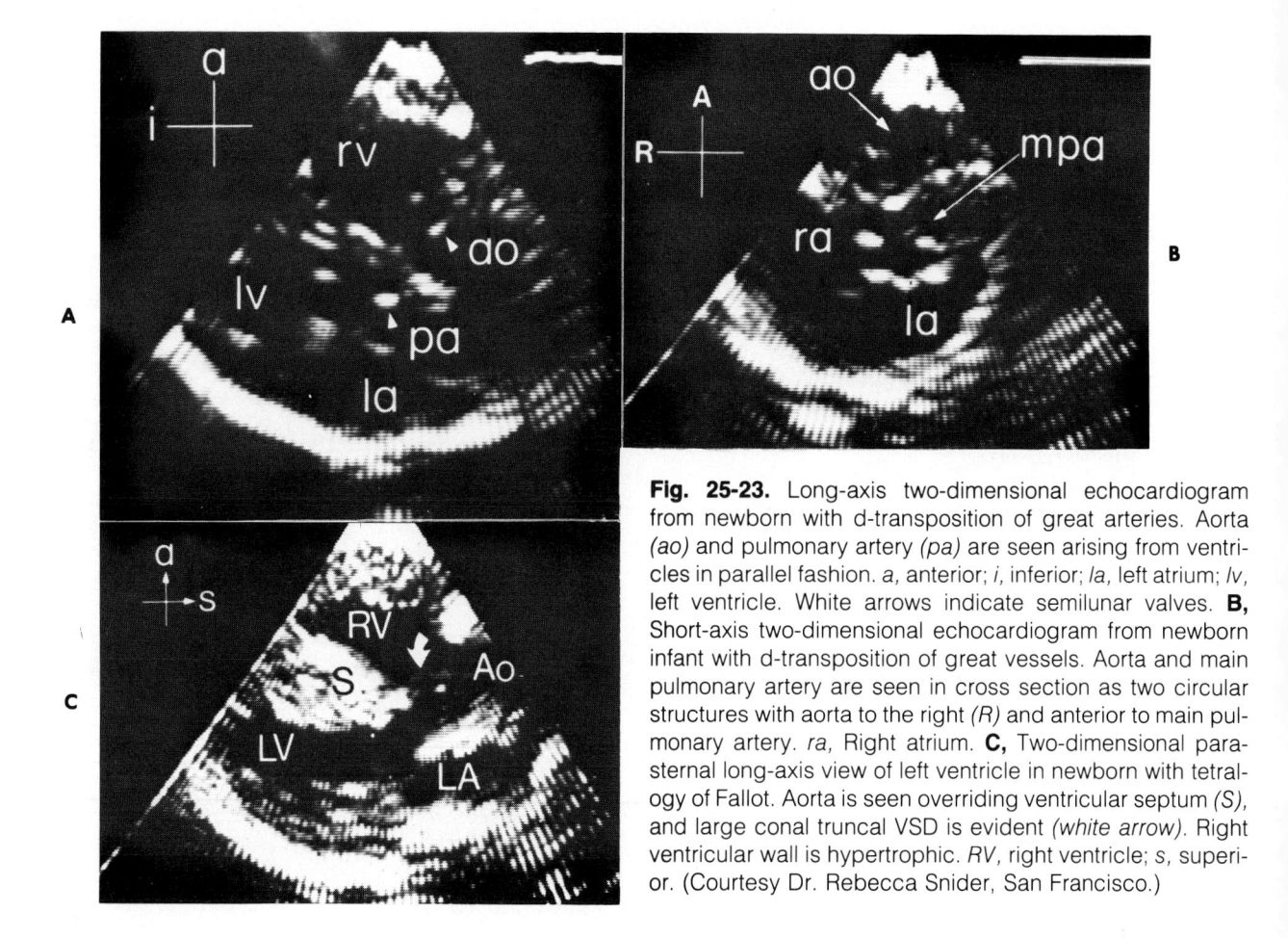

Fig. 25-23. Long-axis two-dimensional echocardiogram from newborn with d-transposition of great arteries. Aorta *(ao)* and pulmonary artery *(pa)* are seen arising from ventricles in parallel fashion. *a,* anterior; *i,* inferior; *la,* left atrium; *lv,* left ventricle. White arrows indicate semilunar valves. **B,** Short-axis two-dimensional echocardiogram from newborn infant with d-transposition of great vessels. Aorta and main pulmonary artery are seen in cross section as two circular structures with aorta to the right *(R)* and anterior to main pulmonary artery. *ra,* Right atrium. **C,** Two-dimensional parasternal long-axis view of left ventricle in newborn with tetralogy of Fallot. Aorta is seen overriding ventricular septum *(S),* and large conal truncal VSD is evident *(white arrow).* Right ventricular wall is hypertrophic. *RV,* right ventricle; *s,* superior. (Courtesy Dr. Rebecca Snider, San Francisco.)

The two-dimensional echo instrument has the advantage that a sector of the heart is seen in two dimensions, in real-time, in a visual image that resembles an angiogram. Frequently all four chambers of the heart may be seen, along with the great arteries and veins. The relationships of the great arteries to the cardiac chambers and septa are frequently more apparent than by M-mode echo. This makes it possible to diagnose or suspect conditions such as d-transposition of the great arteries, double-outlet right ventricle, tetralogy of Fallot, and truncus arteriosus. Good visualization of the cardiac septa often makes it possible to identify ASD and VSD. Visualization of the appearance and motion of the valves is generally excellent, which further aids in identifying ASD, VSD, and conditions in which there are abnormalities in AV valve appearance and function, including endocardial cushion defects, Ebstein's malformation of the tricuspid valve, tricuspid and mitral valve atresia, and conditions in which one or two AV valves enter a single ventricle.

As with single-element echo, saline contrast peripheral vein injection may be used to identify right-to-left shunts and abnormalities of systemic venous return.

In the newborn two-dimensional echocardiography may be helpful in diagnosing d-transposition of the great arteries (Fig. 25-23, *A* and *B*), double-outlet right ventricle, tricuspid atresia, tetralogy of Fallot (Fig. 25-23, *C*), anomalous pulmonary venous return, hypoplastic left-heart syndrome, endocardial cushion defect, and Ebstein's anomaly of the tricuspid valve.

During the next decade, with rapidly advancing technology in the area of real-time two-dimensional echo, there probably will be a reduced need for invasive studies in many clinical situations.

Arterial blood gases and pH

Estimation of arterial P_{CO_2}, P_{O_2}, and pH aids in the quantitative assessment of the seriousness of the condition of infants suspected of having heart disease. If the infant's heel is warm and blood is free flowing, a heel prick provides a worthwhile estimate of arterial P_{CO_2} and pH. Measurement of P_{O_2} from capillary blood is less

Table 25-7. Blood gases in the three common mechanisms for arterial unsaturation*

Mechanism	Pao₂ room air (mm Hg)	Paco₂ room air (mm Hg)	Pao₂ 100% O₂ (mm Hg)
Alveolar hypoventilation	Decreased (< 60)	Increased (> 50)	Normal (> 200)
Right-to-left shunt	Decreased (< 60)	Normal† (35 to 45)	Decreased (< 100)
Ventilation/perfusion unevenness	Decreased (< 60)	Normal† (35 to 45)	Normal (> 200)

*Pao₂ (room air) provides an estimate of the severity of the problem. A diminished Paco₂ (room air) implies alveolar hypoventilation, and failure of the Pao₂ to increase significantly with 100% O₂ implies right-to-left shunting as the problem.
†Rises slowly with prolonged right-to-left shunting or ventilation/perfusion unevenness.

accurate, since the oxygen tension of blood rapidly increases on exposure to room air. However, if the sample can be collected from the center of drops of blood, one may obtain a rough indication of oxygen tension. In the evaluation of the effect of 100% O₂ breathing on Po₂ it is necessary to sample arterial blood (see hyperoxia test, p. 424). In the newborn period this usually can be obtained from the umbilical artery, but in older infants the right brachial artery is preferable. Arterial blood collected from anywhere distal to the ductus arteriosus may be "contaminated" by right-to-left ductal shunting and consequently does not accurately reflect pulmonary function. To obtain truly "arterial" blood, it is necessary to sample a pulmonary vein, since in many cyanotic babies the right-to-left shunt is at the atrial level.

Certain deductions may be made from a consideration of the arterial Pco₂ and Po₂ while the infant is breathing room air and from the Po₂ while the infant is breathing 100% O₂ (Table 25-7). Diffusion problems may be ignored, since they do not exist in infants with heart disease. Measurement of transcutaneous Po₂ (TcPo₂) has proved a valuable noninvasive alternative to arterial blood sampling in neonates with suspected cyanotic heart disease (p. 430). It is commonly stated that, if an infant becomes pink with oxygen administration the hypoxemia is pulmonary in origin, whereas if he remains blue, it is cardiac (that is, the problem is a right-to-left shunt). Unfortunately this is an oversimplification. First, there are large intrapulmonary and foramen ovale right-to-left shunts in many neonates with lung disease, who therefore fail to achieve high arterial Po₂ with 100% O₂ (especially in RDS). Second, an infant with an isolated PDA may be cyanotic from heart failure, alveolar transudate, and obstructed small air passages. He will become pink in 100% O₂ because the mechanism of his hypoxemia is alveolar hypoventilation; yet heart disease (PDA) is his problem. Finally, if an infant with transposition is very cyanotic in room air but becomes less cyanotic in 100% O₂, the explanation is not that the cause of his cyanosis is pulmonary but that 100% inspired O₂ has lowered his pulmonary vascular resistance, allowing better mixing through an existing foramen ovale or patent ductus or both. He may clinically appear to become pink, but his arterial Po₂ will never approach 150 mm Hg. Blood gases and the response to 100% O₂ breathing therefore only suggest the disordered pathophysiologic mechanism and the seriousness of the problem rather than identify the problem as pulmonary or cardiac.

Measurement of the arterial or capillary pH is also of value as an estimate of the severity of the problem. Correction of severe acidosis may be partially achieved by the use of sodium bicarbonate. It should be remembered, however, that the use of sodium bicarbonate adds to the total body stores of sodium and of carbon dioxide. Temporary and partial correction of acidosis, however, is often, indicated as a prelude to cardiac catheterization and surgery; sodium bicarbonate, 2 to 6 mEq/kg, should be administered over a 2- to 5-minute period into as large a venous pool as possible. Frequently we have used this method of pH adjustment at the beginning of a cardiac catheterization; the usual indication is a sinus bradycardia in a dying infant, and pH is usually 7.1 or lower.

Other laboratory tests
Hypoglycemia

The initial evaluation should include a screening test for hypoglycemia (Dextrostix); when the Dextrostix is low, true blood glucose should be determined. Hypoglycemia may simulate structural congenital heart disease very closely, with cardiomegaly and cyanosis. Hypoglycemia frequently also complicates serious neonatal heart disease, especially the hypoplastic left-heart syndrome. It also is associated with PFC (p. 566). The hypoglycemia should be treated with intravenous glucose while investigation and treatment of the underlying heart disease are proceeding.

Serum electrolytes

Serum sodium, potassium, and chloride levels should be measured both because electrolyte abnormalities can occur in the infant with serious neonatal cardiovascular disease and because adrenal insufficiency may closely mimic heart disease. Sommerville and colleagues reported on three neonates and one 6-week-old baby (all male) with congenital adrenal *hypoplasia* in whom cyanosis and cardiac arrhythmias simulated heart disease.

Methemoglobinemia

Congenital or acquired methemoglobinemia may closely simulate cyanotic congenital heart disease. The infant appears a peculiar lavender or slate blue, and blood from a heel prick appears chocolate colored. Blood from an infant with methemoglobinemia fails to become pink when placed on a glass slide and exposed to room air. The diagnosis can be confirmed by spectroscopy (a characteristic absorption peak at 634 mµ) and by the rapid response to intravenous methylene blue (1 to 2 mg/kg). For long-term medication ascorbic acid (300 to 500 mg/day) administered orally may be preferable but is sometimes less completely effective.

Vectorcardiography

The study of vectorcardiography (VCG) has contributed enormously to our understanding of the scalar ECG (normal 12- or 13-lead ECG). The scalar ECG depicts in two dimensions what is actually a three-dimensional event—the P loop, followed by the QRS and T loops. The small amount of additional information gained from the VCG does not warrant its routine use in the diagnosis of the neonate suspected of having serious heart disease.

Phonocardiography

In the newborn period good phonocardiograms are hard to record because of the rapid respiratory rate of the newborn and because the frequency content of diastolic sounds is similar to that of background electronic noise. In the neonate with faster heart rate and lack of easily observable reference pulses (carotid or jugular pulse), a phonocardiogram with simultaneous recording of the ECG, carotid pulse, or respiration may be necessary to resolve a problem. We have found the phonocardiogram most useful in the unraveling of multiple additional sounds in the cardiac cycle and on occasion in the demonstration that a second sound has a constant fixed split or that a murmur is "pansystolic" or "ejection" in timing.

CYANOSIS OF THE NEWBORN*

A blue or dusky hue in the newborn frequently is brought to the physician's attention by an experienced nurse. Since the causes may vary from trivial to life threatening, rapid evaluation is essential; those newborns who have persistent central cyanosis usually deteriorate rapidly.

Recognition of cyanosis

Clinical cyanosis is chiefly dependent on the *absolute* concentration of reduced hemoglobin in the blood rather than on the ration of reduced hemoglobin to oxygenated hemoglobin. Central cyanosis implies significant arterial unsaturation, whereas "peripheral" cyanosis alone implies normal arterial saturation. In the latter, cyanosis is visible only in the skin of the extremities where a wide arteriovenous oxygen difference leads to a "capillary" reduced hemoglobin content of greater than 4 to 6 gm/dl of blood. It is sometimes stated that it is necessary to have 5 gm of reduced hemoglobin in *arterial* blood before central cyanosis is detectable visibly; clinical experience indicates that this provides a very coarse basis for detection of arterial unsaturation. Were this the case, an infant with a total hemoglobin content of 15 gm/dl of blood would be visibly cyanotic only at an arterial saturation of 67% or less, whereas central cyanosis is detectable by inspection of the tongue and mucous membranes at arterial saturations of 75% to 88% in the presence of about 3 gm of reduced hemoglobin in arterial blood (Fig. 25-24).

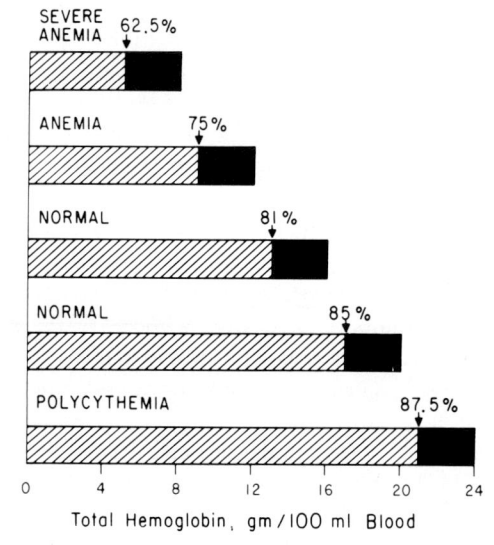

Fig. 25-24. The percentage arterial saturation of blood (diagonally lined portion of each column) when cyanosis will be detected at different total hemoglobin concentrations in the presence of 3 gm/dl of reduced hemoglobin. Central cyanosis is detectable at higher arterial saturations when the total hemoglobin concentration is high. With severe anemia, as for example 8 gm/dl of hemoglobin, central cyanosis may not be apparent until arterial saturation falls to nearly 62%.

---

*Adapted from Lees, M.H.: Cyanosis of the newborn infant, J. Pediatr. 77:484, 1970.

Central versus peripheral cyanosis

Infants suspected of being cyanotic are best inspected when they are quiet or sleeping in a thermoneutral environment under a white light, preferably daylight. Central cyanosis is defined as cyanosis of the tongue, mucous membranes, and peripheral skin in the presence of 3 gm or more of reduced hemoglobin in arterial blood. It may be physiologic or pathologic. Peripheral cyanosis is defined as blue discoloration or duskiness confined to the skin of the extremities; it too may be physiologic or pathologic, but the arterial blood will be normally saturated (that is, greater than 94%). There are intermediate conditions in which arterial saturation may be in the range of 90% (for example, 2 gm of reduced hemoglobin out of a total of 20 gm of hemoglobin), and the tongue may appear pink and the extremities cyanotic. Such a baby clinically has peripheral cyanosis as a result of a central disturbance. The clinical distinction of central from peripheral therefore is not always absolute, and elucidation frequently requires the measurement of arterial oxygen saturation or oxygen tension (PaO_2).

Clinical confirmation that cyanosis of extremities is peripheral in origin often may be obtained by immersing the baby's foot in a pan of 100° F water of 5 minutes; vasodilatation will occur, and the foot will become pink. Reflex vasodilation also may occur in the other foot. Significant arterial unsaturation (central cyanosis) should be considered to be present if the PaO_2 is below 60 mm Hg at 24 hours of age or if the arterial oxygen saturation is below 94%. This does not imply that a PaO_2 of 60 mm Hg or less necessarily represents a pathologic state, but it does mean that the infant either has alveolar hypoventilation or has an alveolar-arterial oxygen difference of about 40 mm Hg.

Peripheral cyanosis

Peripheral cyanosis is common in the neonate and may persist for hours to weeks. It usually is ascribed to "vasomotor instability" and may come and go in an unpredictable fashion. In some instances peripheral cyanosis is clearly caused by cold environment, a high total hemoglobin content, or local venous obstruction (for example, cord around the neck). In other instances the cause is obscure. The most bizarre expression is that of the "harlequin" infant, in whom one quadrant or one side of the body may be cyanotic while the rest is pink; the hands and feet feel warm despite their appearance. Peripheral cyanosis with cold extremities in a relatively warm environment suggests the possibility of peripheral vasoconstriction caused by shock or heart failure. "Differential" cyanosis, that is, pink upper half and blue lower half of the body or vice versa, always is indicative of serious heart disease.

Physiologic central cyanosis

An arterial saturation of less than 94% usually is regarded as abnormal in the awake healthy adult or older child breathing atmospheric air at sea level. However, the critical level of saturation for a newborn depends on the postnatal age, the proportion of adult to fetal hemoglobin, and whether he is crying when the blood sample is taken. Normal newborns have a PaO_2 of around 50 mm Hg by 5 to 10 minutes of postnatal life. The great majority of infants therefore would not be expected to manifest physiologic central cyanosis later than 20 minutes after birth, and many would have a pink tongue and mucous membranes before 10 minutes. An occasional normal (by other criteria) full-term infant may require a longer time to achieve a PaO_2 of 60 mm Hg.

The ratio of fetal to adult hemoglobin varies from infant to infant, and the proportions of each hemoglobin affect the oxygen saturation resulting at any given PaO_2 (p. 422). Thus, if a baby with a pH of 7.4 and a temperature of 37° C has mostly adult hemoglobin, central cyanosis (arterial saturation 75% to 85%) will be observed at a PaO_2 of 42 to 53 mm Hg, whereas if the baby has mostly fetal hemoglobin, central cyanosis will be observed at a PaO_2 of 32 to 42 mm Hg. *Thus the newborn with a high proportion of fetal hemoglobin may have a serious reduction in oxygen tension before central cyanosis is*

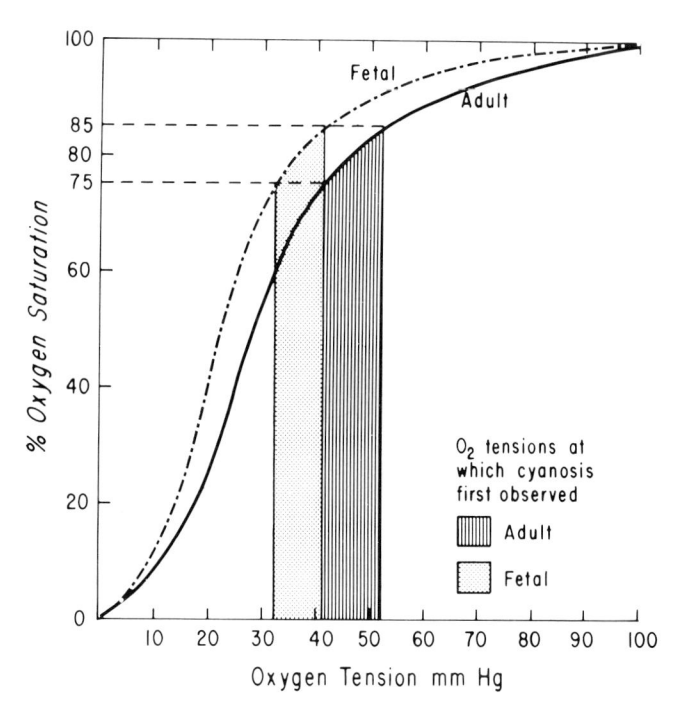

Fig. 25-25. Fetal and adult hemoglobin—O_2 dissociation curves. Note that infant with high proportion of fetal hemoglobin will have a very low PaO_2 (33 to 42 torr) before cyanosis is observed.

Table 25-8. Elucidation for cause of cyanosis from clinical signs and simple laboratory tests*

Category and pathophysiology	Common underlying disorder	Activity and respiratory pattern	100% O₂ breathing
1. Congenital heart disease Right-to-left shunt; decreased pulmonary blood flow	Tetralogy of Fallot; pulmonary atresia; tricuspid atresia; extreme pulmonary stenosis; Ebstein's anomaly	Respirations 20-50/min; increased tidal volume; total ventilation and alveolar ventilation both increased	No response because pulmonary capillary blood is almost completely saturated
2. Congenital heart disease Right-to-left shunt; increased pulmonary blood flow	Transposition; left-sided heart hypoplasia; preductal coarctation; TAPVR;* truncus arteriosus; very large VSD; AV canal	Respirations 30-60/min; tidal volume normal; total ventilation and alveolar ventilation normal or moderately increased	No response because pulmonary capillary blood is almost completely saturated
3. Congenital heart disease Severe heart failure; shunt or no shunt; alveolar hypoventilation	All in category 2; isolated PDA: isolated VSD; severe aortic stenosis; postductal coarctation; paroxysmal atrial tachycardia	Flaccid with severe heart failure; cyanosis moderate; respirations 40-120/min with rales and rhonchi; decreased tidal volume; total ventilation usually normal with greatly reduced alveolar ventilation, i.e., increased dead space/tidal volume	Usually good response because increasing alveolar oxygen tension to 650 mm Hg overcomes pulmonary capillary unsaturation secondary to alveolar hypoventilation
4. Primary lung disease Alveolar hypoventilation; intrapulmonary right-to-left shunt; V̇/Q̇ unevenness; diffusion barrier (RDS)	Atelectasis; atypical RDS; aspiration syndrome; pulmonary hemorrhage; pneumonia; Wilson-Mikity syndrome; lymphangiectasia; pulmonary agenesis; adenomatoid malformation; bronchopulmonary dysplasia	Respirations 30-120/min; typically there is distress, with flaring of alae nasi, grunting, and intercostal and sternal retraction; with severe pathosis, tidal volume and alveolar ventilation are greatly decreased; decreased compliance increases work of breathing	Response unpredictable; lack of response indicates intrapulmonary or intracardiac right-to-left shunting as a major factor
5. Mechanical interference with lung function Alveolar hypoventilation	Mucous plugs; lobar emphysema; diaphragmatic hernia; pneumothorax; chylothorax; abnormal thoracic cage; vascular ring; tracheoesophageal fistula; bronchogenic cyst; choanal atresia; Pierre Robin syndrome; mediastinal masses	May closely mimic primary lung disease if lung tissue is compressed; when the airway is partially obstructed, stridor and intercostal retractions are prominent; unreliability of signs underscores need for x-ray film in every infant with cyanosis	Usually good response because alveolar hypoventilation is often the major mechanism of cyanosis
6. Pulmonary hypertension PFC syndrome; gross V̇/Q̇ unevenness; intrapulonary right-to-left shunt; ductal right-to-left shunt	Cause often undetermined; consider meconium aspiration pneumonia and multiple pulmonary thromboses or emboli; alveolar proteinosis; oxygen toxicity; PFC	Hyperventilation with increased tidal volume and rate is usual; much of the ventilation is wasted, since it is to underperfused or unperfused alveoli	Variable response depending on the degree of V̇/Q̇ unevenness (good response) and intrapulmonary right-to-left shunt (no response); PFC syndrome may respond to oxygen, to intravenous tolazoline, or to induced alkalosis
7. Central nervous system disease Alveolar hypoventilation	Intracerebral hemorrhage; subdural hemorrhage; gross intracranial malformation; meningitis or encephalitis; primary seizure disorder	Apneic spells alternating with periods of normal breathing, or there may be continuous hypoventilation with small tidal volume or bradypnea or both; infant is often apathetic and unresponsive; seizures common	Good response, provided tidal volume is appreciably greater than anatomic dead space and frequency of breathing is not too slow

*Categories 1, 2, 3, and 6 usually require catheterization and angiography for definitive anatomic diagnosis.
†*TAPVR*, Total anaomalous pulmonary venous return; *RVH*, right ventricular hypertrophy; *RVSTI*, right ventricle systolic time interval.
‡Heart may be normal in size in certain varieties of TAPVR.

Heel-prick blood exposed to air	Dextrostix, hematocrit	Arterial pH, arterial Pco$_2$	Chest x-ray film	ECG and echocardiogram
Dark; becomes pink in air	No abnormality	pH normal unless hypoxemia is extreme; Paco$_2$ normal or low	Decreased pulmonary vascular markings; heart may be large or normal	Both usually abnormal
Dark; becomes pink in air	Hypoglycemia may be present especially with hypoplastic left-heart syndrome	pH normal unless hypoxemia is extreme; Paco$_2$ normal	Increased pulmonary vascular markings; heart may be of normal size at first but after a few days is almost always enlarged‡	Both usually abnormal
Dark; becomes pink in air	Hypoglycemia is frequent, especially with hypoplastic left-heart syndrome	Acidosis and elevated Paco$_2$ reflect increasing airway obstruction and alveolar hypoventilation	Enlarged heart; increased vascular markings; often pneumonia	Both usually abnormal
Dark; becomes pink in air	May be hypoglycemia if glycogen reserves are becoming depleted	Acidosis and elevated Paco$_2$ characterize most of the conditions and indicate severity	Each condition has a rather characteristic x-ray appearance, but exceptions occur	ECG normal or RVH*; echo usually normal but may show abnormal RVSTI*
Dark; becomes pink in air	Normal	Elevated Paco$_2$ that may or may not be compensated; in severe instances acidosis is present	Characteristic x-ray film in most instances; contrast visualization studies may be needed	ECG normal or RVH; echo usually normal but may show abnormal RVSTI
Dark; becomes pink in air	Normal	Elevated Paco$_2$ usually because of a large arterial-alveolar CO$_2$ difference caused by the presence of overventilated but underperfused areas; pH depressed	Generally have "snowstorm" or "ground-glass" appearance; heart usually normal in size; x-ray film may be normal with PFC syndrome	ECG normal or RVH; echo usually shows abnormal RVSTI
Dark; becomes pink in air	Normal	Elevated Paco$_2$; combined respiratory and metabolic acidosis is usual	Normal or may show pneumonia	Both usually normal

Continued.

Table 25-8. Elucidation for cause of cyanosis from clinical signs and simple laboratory tests—cont'd

Category and pathophysiology	Common underlying disorder	Activity and respiratory pattern	100% O_2 breathing
8. Methemoglobinemia Reduced oxygen-carrying capacity of blood because of abnormal hemoglobin	Specific enzyme deficiency; abnormal hemoglobin	Infants, although lavender blue, show little distress until over 50% of hemoglobin is methemoglobin; in severe cases tachypnea and hyperventilation closely mimic heart disease	No response
9. Hypoglycemia Probably right-to-left shunting through foramen ovale; hypoventilation	Infant of diabetic mother; small for date baby; idiopathic heart failure, especially from hypoplastic left-heart syndrome	May be apathetic and limp; jitteriness or seizures common; infant may have moderate tachypnea or repetitive apneic spells	Good response to hypoventilation component of cyanosis; variable response to right-to-left shunt
10. High hemoglobin content Increased absolute amount of reduced hemoglobin; arterial blood normally saturated, but increased viscosity and stagnant capillary flow may produce apparent central cyanosis	Maternofetal transfusion; twin-to-twin transfusion; high hematocrit value plus unusually large "placental transfusion"	Usually normal behavior and respirations, but myoclonic jerking, moderate tachypnea, or apneic spells have been reported	Good response because of almost total saturation of hemoglobin when alveolar Po_2 is raised to 650 mm Hg
11. Shock and sepsis Alveolar hypoventilation; $\dot{V}/\dot{Q}$ unevenness	Blood loss; septic shock; septicemia; myocarditis; adrenal insufficiency	Apathetic, hypotonic, and underresponsive to stimuli; respirations rapid and shallow or frequent apneic spells (hypoventilation); low pulmonary artery pressure and blood flow ($\dot{V}/\dot{Q}$ unevenness)	Good response unless hypoventilation or $\dot{V}/\dot{Q}$ disturbance or both are extreme

clinically apparent. Therefore measurement of oxygen tension is considerably more discriminatory than measurement of oxygen saturation (Fig. 25-25).

The effect of crying on the arterial saturation of the newborn must be considered. Infants age 1½ hours to 3 days have variable responses: 66% have a decrease in oxygen saturation, 27% an increase, and 6.8% no change. Older infants between 4 to 9 days of age respond differently: 21% have a decrease in saturation, 59% an increase, and 22.4% no change. Right-to-left shunting through the ductus arteriosus or foramen ovale is the most likely explanation.

Pathologic mechanisms of central cyanosis

When a resting or sleeping newborn has central cyanosis that persists longer than 20 minutes after birth, an explanation is required. Categories of disease that should be considered are (1) congenital heart disease with right-to-left shunting and diminished pulmonary blood flow, (2) congenital heart disease with right-to-left shunting and increased pulmonary blood flow, (3) congenital heart disease with alveolar hypoventilation secondary to heart failure, (4) primary lung disease, (5) mechanical interference with lung function, (6) PFC syndrome (primary or secondary), (7) central nervous system disease, (8) methemoglobinemia, (9) hypoglycemia, (10) a high hemoglobin level, (11) shock and sepsis, and (12) miscellaneous conditions. There are five mechanisms whereby arterial unsaturation may occur in a patient who is breathing atmospheric air and is not at high altitude: (1) alveolar hypoventilation, (2) diffusion impairment, (3) right-to-left shunting, (4) ventilation/perfusion unevenness, and (5) inadequate transport of oxygen by hemoglobin.

A diagnostic approach to central cyanosis

Once it is decided that an infant has central cyanosis (by examination of the tongue, $TcPo_2$, ear oximeter, or direct measurement of arterial Po_2 or O_2 saturation), it is necessary to determine the cause, since the responsible disease process is rarely self-limited. The examination of the cyanotic neonate should proceed along the lines discussed earlier in this chapter, with particular emphasis on the respiratory pattern, spontaneous movement, response to 100% O_2 breathing, arterial pH, Po_2, and Pco_2, chest roentgenogram, and ECG. Use of heel-prick blood to screen for hypoglycemia (Dextrostix) and methemoglobinemia (failure of blood to become pink in air) takes but a moment and rules out two immediately cor-

Heel-prick blood exposed to air	Dextrostix, hematocrit	Arterial pH, arterial Pco$_2$	Chest x-ray film	ECG and echocardiogram
Chocolate-colored blood; does not become pink in air or oxygen	Normal	Normal pH; Paco$_2$ may be slightly decreased if infant hyperventilates	Normal	Both usually normal
Dark; becomes pink in air	dextrostix indicates extreme hypoglycemia; confirm by another method	Paco$_2$ frequently elevated secondary to hypoventilation; pH variable	Mild to massive cardiomegaly	ECG normal; echo shows ventricular enlargement
Dark; becomes pink in air	High hematocrit value (65%-86%)	Normal	Normal or mild cardiomegaly	ECG normal or mild RVH; echo normal
Dark; becomes pink in air	Normal hematocrit value; hypoglycemia is frequent; hyperglycemia also may occur	Elevated Paco$_2$ and acidosis common	Cardiomegaly frequent	ECG may show ST-T wave abnormalities; echo may show chamber enlargement

rectable causes of central cyanosis. Measurement of serum electrolytes may reveal hyperkalemia, raising the possibility of adrenal insufficiency or unsuspected sodium or chloride abnormality. If heart disease appears likely, M-mode and two-dimensional echocardiography is very helpful.

Certain clinical patterns may suggest one of the twelve groups of conditions detailed below. However, the clinical signs are capricious, and infants sometimes do not manifest typical findings. The following associations of clinical signs may be helpful (see also Table 25-8); however, cardiac catheterization and angiocardiography are almost always required for the precise anatomic diagnosis of congenital heart disease. An aggressive diagnostic approach is justified, since in the majority of instances treatment is available.

Miscellaneous conditions producing generalized cyanosis or differential cyanosis

Cyanosis occasionally may be caused by alveolar hypoventilation secondary to respiratory depression from drugs given to the mother during labor or to the newborn. Transient tachypnea of the newborn occasionally may cause mild cyanosis in addition to extreme tachypnea (p. 447). Neuromuscular disorders, such as Werdnig-Hoffmann disease or incoordination of swallowing with aspiration, may be present with cyanosis. Anomalous systemic venous return to the left atrium produces cyanosis; classically there are no other symptoms. A pulmonary arteriovenous fistula may be responsible for marked arterial unsaturation; such fistulas are frequently multiple and are usually visible on the chest roentgenogram. A bruit is often but not always present.

Preductal coarctation of the aorta with the right ventricle supplying the descending aorta with venous blood via a PDA is the most common cause of cyanosis restricted to the lower half of the body. The less frequent opposite pattern, that is, cyanosis restricted to the upper half of the body, usually occurs in association with d-transposition, a PDA, and pulmonary hypertension.

Clinical spectrum of generalized cyanosis

The spectrum of diseases producing cyanosis, obvious and severe enough to lead to a provisional diagnosis of cyanotic congenital heart disease, is presented in Table 25-9. Clearly experience will differ greatly in different hospitals. The 56 infants analyzed here represent consecutive newborns weighing 2,500 gm or more for whom a

Table 25-9. Final diagnoses of 56 newborns of more than 2,500 gm suspected of having structural cyanotic congenital heart disease with right-to-left shunt

Diagnosis	Number
Heart disease	
Transposition of great arteries	13
Hypoplastic left-heart syndrome	7
Left-to-right shunt with left-sided heart failure (PDA or VSD)	6
Tetralogy of Fallot	4
Isolated pulmonary stenosis	3
Double-outlet right ventricle	3
Tricuspid atresia	3
Preductal coarctation	2
Truncus arteriosus	1
Total	42
No structural heart disease	
PFC	3
Wilson-Mikity syndrome	3
Atypical RDS	2
Hypoglycemia	3
High hematocrit	1
Myocarditis and cardiogenic shock	1
Septicemia	1
Total	14

cardiology consultation was obtained because a physician considered cyanotic congenital heart disease to be present. Obvious cases of RDS, pneumonia, diaphragmatic hernia, and identifiable noncardiac lesions therefore are excluded for the most part. Nevertheless only 36 (64%) of the infants proved to have cyanotic congenital heart disease with right-to-left shunt (that is, the referral diagnosis). Six had left-to-right shunts (PDA or VSD), with heart failure and alveolar hypoventilation causing cyanosis, and 14 had no structural abnormality of the heart. The relative incidence of the various categories listed in Table 25-9 will vary greatly according to whether small infants are included and whether the consultant is a neurologist, cardiologist, neonatologist, or specialist in pulmonary disease.

LUNG DISEASE VERSUS HEART DISEASE

The problem of differentiating lung and heart disease is frequent in the neonatal period; certain clinical and laboratory findings are helpful (Table 25-10). However, the signs are capricious, and sometimes cardiac catheterization and angiography are necessary to resolve the issue. Particularly difficult is the distinction between PFC syndrome and preductal coarctation of the aorta. There is right-to-left ductal shunting and pulmonary hypertension with both diagnoses, and distinction frequently requires aortography, since urgent surgery is usually required if a juxtaductal coarctation is present.

Persistence of the fetal circulation (PFC syndrome)

This term is applied to the combination of pulmonary hypertension, right-to-left shunting (largely at the foramen ovale but also the ductus arteriosus), and a structurally normal heart. The PFC syndrome may be idiopathic (primary) or secondary to hyperviscosity of blood, aspiration pneumonia (especially meconium aspiration) (p. 443), neonatal sepsis, hypoglycemia, or neonatal pulmonary disease (particularly RDS). The primary form tends to occur in full-term or postmature infants. The cause is unknown, but it is theorized that the condition results when the normal mechanisms that cause a decline in pulmonary vascular resistance and ductus closure are inadequate. It has been proposed that one cause of PFC syndrome is prenatal transplacental exposure to prostaglandin synthetase inhibitors such as aspirin or indomethacin.

Neonates with PFC syndrome are tachypneic and cyanotic. Right-to-left ductal shunting (when present) may result in a higher PaO_2 in the right arm than in the descending aorta or legs. This may produce differential cyanosis and be documented by simultaneous placement of two transcutaneous PO_2 electrodes over the right upper chest and abdomen. The pulmonary closure sound is loud, and there is no diagnostically useful murmur. The ECG characteristically shows mild right ventricular hypertrophy, and the chest x-ray film may be normal or show moderate cardiac enlargement. The infants may have increased total and alveolar ventilation and increased tidal volumes. There is a large arterial-alveolar CO_2 difference, caused by the presence of many overventilated, underperfused alveoli. The cyanosis frequently responds to 100% O_2 breathing initially, with a large increase in pulmonary vein oxygen saturation and a decrease in pulmonary artery pressure. Echocardiographic assessment of systolic time intervals is an extremely useful diagnostic tool in PFC (p. 553).

An infant with a presumptive diagnosis of PFC may tolerate diagnostic catheterization poorly, and this is generally contraindicated. It must be stressed that these infants are exquisitely sensitive to manipulation with a detrimental effect on oxygenation, and thus any invasive therapeutic procedures should be undertaken with great caution. The presence of an end-hole umbilical catheter may enable an aortogram to be performed, and this will opacify the entire thoracic aorta and rule out coarctation.

The infant with PFC syndrome and worsening blood gases despite assisted ventilation may benefit from scalp vein or pulmonary artery tolazoline infusion at a rate of 2 mg/kg/hour, with observations of the effect on transcutaneous or upper and lower limb blood gases. Tolazoline is a systemic vasodilator as well as a pulmonary vasodilator;

Table 25-10. Clinical and laboratory findings common with primary heart disease or with primary lung disease

Clinical and laboratory findings	Favors heart disease	Favors lung disease
Prematurity, postmaturity, or small for gestational age		X
Fetal distress, especially meconium staining; birth asphyxia; low Apgar scores		X
Flaccid, apathetic infant with little spontaneous movement; apneic spells	X	X
Tachypnea without other signs of respiratory distress; deep sighing respirations	X	
Respiratory distress, i.e., tachypnea with intercostal retractions, grunting, or flaring of alae nasi		X
Marked generalized cyanosis; $PaO_2 < 25$ mm Hg but with normal or reduced $PaCO_2$	X	
Generalized cyanosis with $PaO_2 < 35$ mm Hg and $PaCO_2 > 45$ mm Hg		X
Acidemia, pH < 7.2	X	X
Differential cyanosis or brachial artery PaO_2 > umbilical artery PaO_2	X	X
Cardiomegaly, hepatomegaly, obvious cardiac murmur	X	
Low PaO_2 on room air; $PaO_2 < 150$ mm Hg on 100% O_2	X	
Low PaO_2 on room air; $PaO_2 > 150$ mm Hg on 100% O_2		X
Improvement in pH and umbilical artery PaO_2 following IV tolazoline infusion		X
Hypoglycemia or high hematocrit (>65)	X	X
Chest x-ray film shows clearly ↑ or ↓ pulmonary vascular markings	X	
Chest x-ray film shows "snowstorm," reticulogranular pattern		X
Chest x-ray film shows blotchy appearance of lung fields consistent with aspiration	X	X
Moderate right ventricular hypertrophy on ECG	X	X
Gross ECG abnormality	X	
Abnormal echocardiogram, e.g., chamber enlargement, abnormal great artery position, or small left venticle	X	

it may be necessary to combat systemic hypotension with albumin or blood or pharmacologically (e.g., dopamine). Respirator-induced respiratory alkalosis often proves useful in causing pulmonary vasodilatation. Recently multiple pulmonary arterial thromboses have been noted in infants dying of PFC syndrome. These infants do not respond to vasodilator therapy.

In the management of the critically sick infant, therapeutic decisions may be aided by observing the effect of interventions on the directly recorded pulmonary artery pressure (p. 130) or by observing changes in the right ventricular systolic time intervals (echocardiogram). The search continues for a therapeutic agent that will cause selective pulmonary arteriolar vasodilatation; at this time prostaglandin D_2 appears the most promising compound.

HEART FAILURE IN THE NEONATAL PERIOD

During the first days of life heart failure may simulate disease of other organs or systems, and conversely other disease entities may have some of the clinical signs of heart failure. Although heart failure is usually the result of structural congenital heart disease or of myocardial disease, it may on occasion be secondary to arrhythmia, respiratory disease, central nervous system disease, anemia, high hematocrit, systemic or pulmonary hypertension intrapartum asphyxia, or septicemia. Thus, when heart failure is diagnosed, it is necessary to determine whether primary structural heart disease is responsible or whether the heart failure is secondary to some other disease.

Recognition of heart failure

Heart failure may be defined as a state in which the heart does not maintain a circulation adequate for the needs of the body despite a satisfactory venous filling pressure. In the newborn, heart failure gives rise to a distinctive clinical syndrome. Common symptoms and signs are feeding difficulties, tachypnea, tachycardia, rales and rhonchi, liver enlargement, and cardiomegaly. Less common manifestations include measurable increase in systemic venous pressure, peripheral edema, ascites, pulsus alternans, gallop rhythm, and inappropriate sweating. Pleural and pericardial effusions resulting from heart failure are exceedingly rare. The distinction between left-sided heart failure (characterized by tachypnea, tachycardia, pulmonary rales, and cardiomegaly) and right-sided heart failure (characterized by liver enlargement, tachycardia, and cardiomegaly) is less obvious in the newborn than it is in the older child or adult. This difference is caused in part by the fact that many of the lesions producing failure give rise first to left ventricular failure, the results of which are elevated left atrial pressure and secondary pulmonary arterial hypertension, which in turn causes right ventricular failure. On occasion one observes "pure" right-sided failure, for example, the newborn with severe isolated pulmonic stenosis, or "pure" left-sided failure, as in the early stages of heart failure associated with aortic stenosis. The signs and symptoms of heart failure in the newborn are considered here in the approximate order of their frequency of occurrence and reliability.

Physical signs of heart failure

Tachypnea. The earliest sign of left-sided heart failure is an increase in respiratory rate to above 50 breaths per minute. It is important that respirations be counted while the baby is sleeping, since the slightest movement or agitation will temporarily elevate the respiratory rate. There is no increase in the depth of respiration (tidal volume), and the baby is not distressed; that is, there is no grunting, flaring of the alae nasi, or intercostal retraction. When a respiratory infection coexists, or when cardiac failure has resulted in the accumulation of pulmonary transudate, the signs of respiratory distress often appear.

Tachycardia. An increase in the resting heart rate to 140 to 180 beats per minute is characteristic of heart failure. The rate tends to be constant, and the RR interval on the ECG varies little. A rate of over 180 beats per minute suggests the possibility of SVT.

Liver enlargement. Liver enlargement is best assessed if one measures the distance between the liver edge and the right costal margin in a line joining the right nipple and umbilicus. When measured in this way, the normal liver may extend as much as 2 cm below the costal margin, but in heart failure it is frequently 3 to 5 cm or more below the costal margin.

Cardiomegaly. The silhouette of the heart as seen on the chest roentgenogram must be carefully interpreted. In the normal newborn the cardiac diameter may seem to be as much as 75% of the thoracic diameter. A large thymus gland interferes with an evaluation of heart size. In addition, cardiomegaly is not present in all neonates with heart failure; for example, the heart is frequently small when the failure is caused by total anomalous pulmonary venous drainage with obstruction to pulmonary venous return (Fig. 25-3; p. 602).

Pulmonary rales and rhonchi. In the early stages of the formation of a pulmonary transudate fine crepitant rales are present at the lung bases. As left-sided heart failure progresses and the transudate reaches the bronchioles, the clinical signs often change to those of obstructive airway disease with rhonchi and sometimes with audible wheezing. If the baby is first seen at this stage, the clinical pattern may simulate that of bronchiolitis.

Feeding difficulties. At birth the infant with severe heart disease usually appears well nourished, since the fetal circulation often minimizes the effect of structural heart disease as long as the infant is in utero. After birth, however, the increasing tachypnea and exhaustion of heart failure make it difficult for the infant to suck, and calorie and fluid intakes are below the daily requirements. Mothers frequently say that the infant tires or goes to sleep after the first 1 to 2 ounces, and experienced nurses quickly recognize the poor feeding performance and exhaustion of the newborn with heart disease.

Peripheral edema. Systemic edema may appear as puffiness on the backs of the hands, on the dorsum of the feet, or around the eyes. Sometimes pitting edema also may occur over the tibia or sacrum, but it is unusual for edema to become widespread.

Elevated systemic venous pressure. Because of the short squat conformation of the infant's neck, elevation of venous pressure is not easily detected by inspection of the jugular veins. When venous pressure is extremely high, the scalp veins occasionally may appear distended with the infant in the sitting position. Measurements of venous pressure made during cardiac catheterization indicate that it is rarely more than 7 or 8 mm Hg even in the presence of gross liver enlargement from congestive heart failure.

Inappropriate sweating. Inappropriate sweating at normal room temperature occasionally is observed in the newborn. It probably is caused by the excessive production of catecholamines associated with heart failure.

Gallop rhythm. A diastolic gallop rhythm (accentuated third or fourth heart sound) is suggestive of primary myocardial disease, especially myocarditis, but it also is observed late in the course of left ventricular failure from a variety of other causes.

Pulsus alternans. Alternate strong and weak peripheral pulses are usually evidence of severe left ventricular failure and are particularly common in primary myocardial disease.

Ascites. Ascites caused by heart failure in the newborn is uncommon, and when it does occur, the amount of fluid in the peritoneal cavity is usually small.

Electrocardiogram. The ECG may be helpful in supplying supportive evidence of heart failure, but no single electrocardiographic sign is pathognomonic. Tall peaked P waves (greater than 0.3 mV in the standard limb leads) are common in right-sided heart failure but also are found in situations such as tricuspid atresia, where the right atrium is hypertrophied but heart failure is not present. Wide notched P waves (in the standard limb leads) often are associated with left-sided heart failure but also are seen with mitral regurgitation (as in the endocardial cushion defect complex) when heart failure, as judged by other criteria, is not present.

Echocardiogram. Under appropriate circumstances left atrial enlargement, left ventricular enlargement and reduced contractility, and right ventricular enlargement may supply valuable evidence to support a diagnosis of heart failure.

Advanced, near-terminal heart failure

Heart failure may progress very rapidly in the first hours and days of life. The delay of long-distance transportation, suboptimal environmental temperature, aspiration pneumonia, and other complications may lead to the hospital admission of a near-moribund infant in heart failure. Frequently there is no heart murmur, and the clinical picture is more one of advanced cardiogenic shock, with pallor, apathy, minimal spontaneous movement, greatly diminished peripheral pulses, bradycardia, and diminished heart sounds. The respiratory rate may be very rapid with widespread rales, or the infant may have become exhausted with slow respirations or apneic periods. The liver is usually very large, and the spleen also may be enlarged. Sometimes there is peripheral edema. The clinical picture may closely simulate that of septicemia, meningitis, or pneumonia. However, the presence of a very large liver and gross cardiomegaly usually indicates that heart failure is the major problem.

Heart failure without structural congenital heart disease

The following are situations in which heart failure occurs without structural congenital heart disease.

Myocarditis. See p. 609.
Endocardial fibroelastosis. See p. 610.
Glycogen storage disease. See p. 611.
Congenital heart block. See p. 580.
Paroxysmal supraventricular tachycardia. See p. 576.
Intrapartum asphyxia. See p. 574.
Other arrhythmias. Atrial fibrillation (p. 578), atrial flutter (p. 578), and second-degree AV block (p. 580) also may be associated with neonatal heart failure.
Respiratory disease with PDA. (See p. 434.) Heart failure may occur early or late in the course of RDS. One sequence is for hypoxia and acidosis, secondary to the respiratory disease, to produce pulmonary vasoconstriction. The greatly increased pulmonary vascular resistance may cause right-sided heart failure or right-to-left shunting, or both through the foramen ovale or ductus arteriosus. Another sequence is for heart failure to develop in association with left-to-right ductal shunting, often when the infant is 10 to 45 days old and has recovered from RDS. Duct ligation may be indicated when left-to-right ductal shunting with consequent intractable left-sided heart failure is a major component of the infant's problem. However, it must be stressed that, when bronchopulmonary dysplasia is a major factor, duct division usually is not indicated, since it will not significantly alter the underlying pathophysiology. Spontaneous closure can be anticipated in virtually all undergrown infants. Both the single-film aortogram and the echocardiogram have been useful in assessing the degree of shunting without resorting to conventional cardiac catheterization. Pharmacologic closure of the ductus arteriosus by the use of indomethacin (a prostaglandin synthetase inhibitor) has been reported by Heymann and associates and by Friedmann and associates. The use of indomethacin is discussed on p. 605.

Central nervous system disease. Heart failure may be a consequence of pulmonary hypertension secondary to alveolar hypoventilation or apneic periods or both that are caused by cerebral hemorrhage or other major central nervous system disease. An intracranial arteriovenous fistula may cause heart failure with or without clinical evidence of central nervous system disease (p. 367).

Anemia. Severe anemia (hemoglobin level less than 3.5 gm/dl) occasionally causes heart failure because of the sustained attempt to maintain an increased cardiac output. The most common example is hydrops fetalis caused by Rh incompatibility.

High hematocrit value. Infants with very high hematocrit values may manifest some of the signs of heart failure, with cardiomegaly, slight liver enlargement, and tachypnea; venesection with volume replacement should be performed (p. 741).

Systemic hypertension. See p. 617.

Pulmonary hypertension. Pulmonary hypertension may result from many disease entities. The clinical picture and hemodynamic findings may be secondary to multiple small pulmonary emboli originating from peripheral venous thromboses, to thrombi building up on a Spitz-Holter valve (used in the treatment of hydrocephalus), or to emboli that are septic in origin. Pulmonary hypertension also may be secondary to the acidosis and hypoxia associated with obstructive airway disease (for example, choanal atresia and tracheomalacia), to multiple peripheral pulmonary artery stenosis (common in the rubella syndrome), or to obstructive disease of the left side of the heart (for example, cor triatriatum or mitral stenosis). Occasionally the cause of pulmonary hypertension cannot be determined even at autopsy, or, depending on the pathologist's interpretations, death may be attributed to oxygen toxicity, pulmonary alveolar proteinosis, Hamman-Rich syndrome, pulmonary lymphangiectasia, or other assumed causes. In severe cases of pulmonary hypertension not only is the baby in heart failure, but he is also usually deeply cyanotic as the result of right-to-left shunting through the ductus arteriosus or foramen ovale.

Septicemia. (See p. 650.) Septicemia may be responsible for heart failure in the neonatal period by infection of the myocardium or by the effects of bacterial toxins on the myocardium. The liver and spleen are usually grossly enlarged; the baby is pale and apathetic and may have apneic spells. If the baby is first seen in the near-moribund state, the distinction between heart failure caused by structural heart disease and heart failure caused by septicemia may be especially difficult. Blood culture, white blood cell count, and chest roentgenography may resolve the issue, but often it is necessary to institute aggressive medical treatment for both septicemia and heart failure. When the baby's condition continues to deteriorate and death seems inevitable, a rapid hemodynamic and angiocardiographic study is warranted if there is a clinical suggestion of existing structural congenital heart disease that might be treated by surgical correction.

Management
General considerations: indications for cardiac catheterization

When clinical evidence indicates that structural heart disease is the cause of heart failure in a newborn, medical treatment should be initiated immediately, and preparations should be made for diagnostic cardiac catheterization and angiocardiography. Rarely is medical treatment alone sufficient to produce permanent improvement or is it possible to be so certain of the diagnosis from clinical signs that surgical treatment can be confidently planned without special studies. The timing of diagnostic studies is therefore critically important. The objective is to perform such studies when the infant is in the best possible condition. Fortunately optimal timing is usually age related. If heart failure occurs during the first 2 or 3 days of life, the course is usually relentlessly downhill, and, if the responsible lesion is to be surgically corrected, diagnostic studies should be performed within a few hours.

The infant with structural congenital heart disease who develops heart failure for the first time at 3 or 4 weeks of age has already demonstrated his viability. Commonly at this time heart failure appears to be precipitated by an episode of pneumonia, dehydration, or some other untoward event. Correct management of the older neonate includes a rapid assessment of whether the baby's condition is improving, deteriorating, or stable. The accurate charting of physical signs is most helpful in this respect. Continuing deterioration during the first 12 to 24 hours of medical management is usually an indication for immediate cardiac catheterization; a classic example is the 3- or 4-week-old infant with a large PDA, pneumonia, and heart failure. In this situation thoracotomy and ductus ligation represent lesser risks than continued intensive medical treatment.

An occasional infant in severe heart failure has such classic clinical signs (for example, transposition of the great arteries, coarctation of the aorta, large PDA) and is so sick that immediate surgery without diagnostic studies is indicated. Usually, however, foreknowledge of the precise anatomy is essential for informed effective surgery.

When heart failure is clearly identified as being the result of some nonstructural cause, such as SVT or myocarditis, appropriate medical treatment is indicatd rather than hemodynamic studies.

Routine measures

Chart. A chart for recording the baby's major physical signs and drug dosages at 4-hour intervals is of great assistance in evaluating the response to medical treatment. Respiratory rate (basal or sleeping), heart rate, liver size (centimeters), weight, rales (+ to +++), dose of digoxin (Lanoxin) (oral or parenteral), doses of other drugs, and other pertinent physical signs such as gallop rhythm, puffy hands or feet, and intercostal retractions should be recorded. The development of apneic periods or apathy and lethargy in a baby with heart failure usually indicates that he is becoming exhausted, probably from the additional work of respiration and lack of sufficient oxygen transfer across the lungs to maintain necessary oxidative metabolism. It is also possible that the glycogen reserve in the diaphragm becomes exhausted, as has been described in RDS.

Digitalis. Infants with heart failure should receive digitalis, unless the heart rate is below 100 beats per minute or the underlying lesion contraindicates it. The preferred preparation is digoxin. This drug is available in a pediatric elixir and in a parenteral solution. The 24-hour digitalizing dose depends on the age and maturity of the infant (Table 25-11). The newborn and especially the premature infant are more liable to digitalis toxicity than is the older infant. Any suspicion of digitalis intoxication (arrhythmia, tachycardia, or bradycardia) is an indication for an ECG, for a digoxin blood level determination, and possibly for temporarily withholding the drug and then reducing the dose of it.

Incubator. An incubator aids in the management of a neonate in heart failure in several ways. The baby can be clothed only in a diaper so that his chest movements can be observed from across the room. He can be easily positioned to lie on a 10- to 30-degree head-up incline. The oxygen-enriched atmosphere necessary to minimize cyanosis can be provided, and at the same time heat loss and oxygen consumption can be minimized by controlling the environmental temperature in a neutral thermal range. The incubator also allows maintenance of optimal humidity, protects the infant from nursery infections, and facilitates the use of intravenous infusions and of cardiac and respiratory monitoring equipment.

Table 25-11. Twenty-four-hour digitalizing dose (oral digoxin)*

Age	Digitalizing dose (oral digoxin) first 24 hours (mg/kg)
Premature infants 0-2 weeks	0.03
Premature infants 2-4 weeks	0.04
Term newborns 0-1 week	0.05
Term newborns 1-4 weeks	0.06

*The parenteral dose should be two thirds of the oral dose. The 24-hour maintenance dose is approximately one fourth of the digitalizing dose. For urgent digitalization give half the digitalizing dose initially, followed by two doses of one fourth each after 8 hours and 16 hours, respectively. The schedule will be safe in at least 95% of infants, but frequent clinical and electrocardiographic examinations are mandatory to detect signs of toxicity such as second-degree AV block, sinus bradycardia of less than 100 beats per minute, and multiple ectopic beats. Digitalis toxicity is potentiated by hypokalemia. Because of individual variations in the amount of digitalis that is required to be effective, increases in the projected digitalizing dose will be needed in many instances.

Monitoring. Infants who have bradycardia or arrhythmia or who have had apnea or a cardiac arrest require continuous electrocardiographic monitoring.

Feeding. Infants who tire easily often benefit by being fed smaller volumes every 3 or even every 2 hours. Moderately sick infants find even short periods of feeding difficult because of dyspnea, and they may aspirate milk. Gavage feeding is often useful to lessen this danger. A low-salt milk may be used for a few days, but there is a danger of salt depletion from continued use of such formulas. A good compromise between high- and low-salt formulas is a milk moderately low in mineral content, such as Similac PM 60/40 (Ross Labs). Increasing the concentration to 24 calories per ounce (30 ml) may be desirable to increase caloric intake. Frequently even gavage feeding provokes vomiting and aspiration. Under these circumstances it is important for the baby to receive his fluid requirements intravenously even though his caloric intake will fall short of normal daily requirements; the goal is to approach daily basal requirements. Severely ill infants should be given intravenous infusion initially.

Posture. Young infants in heart failure should lie on a 10- to 30-degree incline inside the incubator. This allows venous blood to pool in the legs and probably decreases the work of breathing by lessening the compression of the diaphragm by the abdominal contents. If the slope is steeper, it may be necessary to put tape from the axillae to the mattress to avoid sliding.

Oxygen. The infant with heart failure may benefit considerably from breathing an oxygen-enriched atmosphere, generally 30% to 35%. Even if pulmonary venous and arterial blood is fully saturated, additional dissolved oxygen can be carried in physical solution in plasma, thus decreasing the circulatory needs by a small factor. In the premature infant this additional advantage must be weighed against the risk of retrolental fibroplasia. Arterial blood PO_2 should be monitored and maintained between 60 and 70 mm Hg.

Treatment of anemia. The oxygen-carrying capacity of blood will be increased by correcting anemia. The optimal hematocrit value for the acyanotic baby with heart failure is probably between 40% and 50%. A transfusion usually is indicated if the hematocrit reading is below 30% when the infant's state of hydration is normal. Exchange transfusions should be given very slowly as packed cells in increments of 10 ml/kg, while continuously and carefully observing the response (respirations, heart rate, and liver size). Heart failure can be aggravated by hypervolemia from transfusion.

Diuretics (Table 25-12). Furosemide is used in infants and children with congestive heart failure. The suggested dose is 0.5 to 3 mg/kg. Where a rapid response is mandatory, intravenous furosemide is the diuretic of choice. Serum potassium should be monitored and, if necessary, potassium chloride supplied orally.

Long-term diuretic administration is rarely indicated in the management of the newborn; however, hydrochlorothiazide (Hydrodiuril) may be useful occasionally. Infants under 6 months of age require 0.5 to 0.75 mg/kg/day in two doses. Hypokalemia may be a complication. Patients on long-term thiazide therapy also should have determination of hematocrit, white blood cell, and platelet counts repeated at monthly intervals. The principal indication for the use of hydrochlorothiazide is the infant with chronic congestive heart failure for whom nothing surgical can be done or for whom surgery at best would be temporarily palliative. Spironolactone (Aldactone) is an aldosterone antagonist. It causes decreased sodium and water retention, whereas potassium is retained. It sometimes is useful in long-term management at a dosage of 1 to 3 mg/kg/day.

Fluid and electrolytes. Despite heart failure, the newborn has continued need for fluid to replace insensible and urinary water losses and for electrolytes to maintain normal body fluid tonicity. Serum sodium, potassium, and chloride levels should be measured as soon as possible; the amount and type of fluid administered intravenously will depend on serum electrolyte concentrations and the estimated degree of fluid retention. In general, fluid restriction should not be as aggressive as in the older child or adult with heart failure. The problem of prolonged intravenous fluid therapy does not often arise, because the newborn with heart failure who is sick enough to require intravenous fluids generally requires rapid hemodynamic assessment and often surgery. Approximately 80 to 100 ml/kg/24 hours of fluid will be

Table 25-12. Drugs useful in the treatment of heart failure in the neonatal period (for digitalis see Table 25-11)

Drug	Administration	Dosage	Frequency	Indications, response, complications
Spironolactone (Aldactone)	Oral (in divided doses)	1-3 mg/kg/day	Suitable for long-term therapy	For diuresis; 4- to 16-hour response; risk of hyperkalemia and of hyponatremia; contraindicated in renal dysfunction, anuria, or hyperkalemia
Furosemide	IV over 2 minutes	0.5-3 mg/kg	Can be repeated after electrolyte check	For diuresis; 1- to 1½-hour response; risk of deafness if renal failure present
Hydrochlorothiazide (Hydrodiuril)	Oral (in 2 divided doses)	0.5-0.75 mg/kg/day	Suitable for long-term therapy	For diuresis; slow response; risk of hypokalemia
Sodium bicarbonate	IV over 12-hour period	Desired bicarbonate concentration (usually 23 mEq/L) minus existing bicarbonate concentration × 0.6 × body weight (kg) = mEq bicarbonate dosage	Usually given once before planned therapy	For partial correction of metabolic acidosis; risk of hypernatremia, water retention, and alkalosis
Sodium bicarbonate	Large vein (umbilical) or intracardiac; over ½-1 minute	2-5 mEq/kg	Administer one time	Last resort as a resuscitative procedure in cardiac arrest or extreme bradycardia
Tromethamine buffer	IV into large vein, over 5-10 minutes	2-5 ml/kg as a 0.3M solution in 5-10% glucose at pH 8.4	Administer one time usually before planned surgery if hypernatremia contraindicates sodium bicarbonate	For partial correction of metabolic acidosis; an alternative to sodium bicarbonate when hypernatremia is present; risks of hypoglycemia, respiratory depression, and severe local irritation at site of administration
Morphine sulfate	Subcutaneously	0.1-0.2 mg/kg/dose	Rarely administered more than once	Useful where signs of left-sided heart failure predominate and the baby is very restless and agitated; risk of respiratory depression
Epinephrine	IV or intracardiac	1 ml of 1:10,000 solution	One time	Last resort for cardiac arrest or extreme bradycardia
Isoproterenol	IV infusion by pump	0.1-0.4 µg/kg/minute	Continuous administration during cardiogenic shock	Cardiogenic shock or severe failure especially when associated with bradycardia; requires slow weaning
Dopamine (Intropin)	IV infusion by pump	2-5 µg/kg/minute	Continuous administration during cardiogenic shock	For cardiogenic shock or severe heart failure; may provoke ectopic beats, bradycardia, or tachycardia
Calcium chloride or calcium gluconate	Intracardiac	1-2 ml of 10% solution	One time	Last resort for cardiac arrest or extreme bradycardia

required. The requirement for sodium will vary from 1 to 4 mEq/kg/24 hours and that for potassium from 0 to 3 mEq/kg/24 hours, depending on the serum electrolyte levels. The neonate in heart failure cannot tolerate sudden increases in circulating blood volume. If these daily requirements are distributed evenly throughout the 24 hours and a careful check is made on the presence of pulmonary rales, the liver size, systemic edema, and weight, their administration will not worsen the baby's heart failure by producing hypervolemia and hyponatremia and will prevent him from developing hypernatremia from too severe water restriction. If the baby is first seen when heart failure is in an advanced state with evidence of peripheral edema and widespread pulmonary rales, then intravenous administration of fluid should be reduced to 40 to 80 ml/kg/24 hours pending the baby's improvement from medical measures or following surgery.

With mild heart failure there is commonly no disturbance of pH or $PaCO_2$, but there may be some lowering of PaO_2 owing to intrapulmonary right-to-left shunting or to uneven perfusion of the lung. When a baby is in severe heart failure, a combined metabolic and respiratory disorder may be encountered.

Antibiotics. Some neonates with heart failure have increased pulmonary perfusion, which makes them more susceptible to respiratory tract infections. It is often difficult to be certain whether pulmonary infection is present. Antibiotics may be commenced while awaiting culture results.

Rotating tourniquets. Medical venesection by tourniquets placed around the upper arms and thighs can be a life-saving measure. The major indication is pulmonary edema. A tourniquet is applied tightly to three of the extremities to obstruct venous but not arterial circulation, and one of these tourniquets is moved every 10 minutes so that the circulation of each limb is unobstructed for 10 out of every 40 minutes.

Infusion of β-adrenergic drugs. Infants with severe heart failure from left-to-right shunts may improve temporarily following infusion of catecholamines. These agents act by direct inotropic effect. Isoproterenol (Isuprel) is a suitable β-adrenergic stimulator and may be particularly useful when bradycardia is present in advanced cardiogenic shock. The initial dose is approximately 0.1 μg/kg/minute, increasing to 0.4 μg/kg/minute until a heart rate of approximately 140 to 160 beats per minute is achieved. Isoproterenol should be continued throughout anesthesia until the underlying cause of heart failure has been corrected. It is then discontinued slowly during monitoring of the blood pressure and recording of the ECG. Dopamine is also useful in the treatment of cardiogenic shock and refractory heart failure. The drug is diluted in 5% dextrose and infused at a rate of 2 to 5 μg/kg/minute. Dopamine increases cardiac output, blood pressure, and urine flow in patients unresponsive to other catecholamines.

Resuscitative measures. These measures are a last resort when extreme bradycardia or cardiac arrest occurs in an infant who has an operable heart lesion. Usually they will take place on the operating table while the surgeon is preparing for the operation. They are external cardiac massage, pulmonary ventilation via an endotracheal tube, intracardiac injection of epinephrine (1 ml of 1:10,000 solution), and intracardiac injection of calcium chloride or calcium gluconate (1 to 2 ml of 10% solution).

Morphine sulfate. Morphine sulfate is indicated in instances where a baby is in heart failure, that is, extremely restless and agitated. Such occasions are more likely to occur in a 3- to 4-week-old infant in whom signs of left-sided heart failure predominate. The dose is 0.1 to 0.2 mg/kg given subcutaneously. A risk of respiratory depression must be considered.

CARDIOGENIC SHOCK

The term *cardiogenic shock* implies acute primary failure of the heart as a pump, although the distinction between cardiogenic shock and severe heart failure is somewhat arbitrary; yet the two do appear as different clinical pictures. In the neonate the clinical picture of cardiogenic shock is encountered infrequently, but it is most common with intrapartum asphyxia, myocarditis, and overwhelming septicemia.

Pathogenesis

The evidence that primary failure of the heart as a pump is the cause of shock is (1) the elevation of systemic venous pressure to 10 to 15 cm H_2O, as compared with the low venous pressure associated with endotoxin and hemorrhagic shock, (2) the presence of a triple or quadruple rhythm, (3) enlarged liver or pulmonary rales, (4) gross cardiomegaly evident on the chest roentgenogram, (5) low-voltage QRS complexes, indicating rapid dilation of the heart, (6) primary T-wave abnormalities on the ECG, and (7) severe acidosis.

Clinical manifestations

Arterial pulses are almost impalpable; the infant is bradycardic and tachypneic, and blood flow through the blanched skin is extremely slow. Often the whole skin has a mottled blue-white appearance. The liver may be enlarged, and there may be rales in the lungs, but these signs of heart failure may be absent if the heart has failed very rapidly and peripheral circulatory failure with deficient tissue blood flow is extreme. The picture then is dominated by evidence of greatly reduced tissue perfusion rather than the signs of traditional heart failure. The resemblance to endotoxic shock and to hemorrhagic shock is close.

Differential diagnosis

The need for urgent treatment of the bradycardic, mottled, dying baby precludes a complete diagnostic evaluation. Cardiogenic shock often is caused by viral myocarditis, but the differential diagnosis also should include the following possibilities: (1) bacterial sepsis with myocarditis and pericarditis, (2) end-stage left ventricular failure from congenital heart disease, (3) anomalous left coronary artery arising from the pulmonary artery, causing myocardial infarction, (4) adrenal insufficiency, especially that caused by congenital adrenal hyperplasia, (5) extreme hypoglycemia with or without heart disease, (6) bacterial or viral myocarditis, (7) primary thoracic conditions such as bilateral pneumothorax or congenital lobar emphysema, (8) hemorrhagic shock with concealed bleeding, as in ruptured spleen, and (9) complete heart block with very slow rate.

Intrapartum asphyxia and cardiogenic shock

A recent report by Cabal and associates has emphasized that cardiogenic shock may occur secondary to severe perinatal asphyxia. There are three major clinical presentations. Some infants show evidence of marked fetal acidemia with abnormal fetal heart rate patterns during labor, depressed fetal scalp pH, and elevated neonatal serum lactic acid values. At birth these infants may have reduced arterial pulses, tachypnea, pulmonary rales, hepatomegaly, and gallop rhythm. There is usually raised central venous pressure, lowered arterial blood pressure, and the radiologic observations of cardiomegaly and pulmonary vascular congestion.

In other infants cardiomegaly and massive tricuspid insufficiency caused by papillary muscle infarction dominate the picture; there is frequently a raised creatine kinase MB fraction.

Still other infants with myocardial dysfunction have had a relatively mild prenatal and immediate postnatal course but have developed cyanosis, tachypnea, and heart failure during the first 24 hours of life. In these infants it has been postulated that the disorder is one of impaired coronary perfusion to portions of the right and left ventricular myocardium through increased work demands created by unusually severe pulmonary vasoconstriction from hypoxia. This postulate was strengthened by electrocardiographic evidence of ischemia and by poor myocardial uptake of thallium 201. In all groups an association with hypoglycemia has been noted.

Treatment

The following plan is suggested for the emergency room management of the moribund infant with the clinical diagnosis of cardiogenic shock.

Record the ECG to rule out complete heart block and to monitor heart rate. Insert a central venous catheter (umbilical vein or femoral vein to right atrium). Measure the central venous pressure (expressed in centimeters of water). Withdraw blood for immediate Dextrostix test, and send sample for blood glucose and serum electrolyte determination. Blood culture (bacterial and viral), hematocrit reading, complete blood count, blood urea nitrogen level, pH, P_{CO_2}, blood type, and crossmatch also should be obtained. If the venous pressure is low (less than 4 cm H_2O), give blood or blood substitute. In endotoxic or hemorrhagic shock very large volumes (up to 40 ml/kg) may be needed to raise the central venous pressure and increase cardiac output. If the venous pressure is high (over 12 cm H_2O in a neonate), cardiogenic shock is probably present, in which case digitalize the baby and start an isoproterenol infusion. (Dose is highly variable.) Mix 1 mg in 100 ml of 5% dextrose to give 10 μg/ml. This solution then can be infused by pump at 0.1 ml/minute or 1 μg/minute (0.4 to 1.0 μg/kg/minute). A satisfactory response is indicated by a falling venous pressure and a rise in heart rate to 100 to 140 beats per minute. Dopamine also may be effective in patients refractory to isoproterenol (p. 628). The place of dobutamine (a $β_1$ agonist) has not yet been determined in neonates. If the blood glucose level is low, infuse 10% dextrose in addition to maintenance fluid. A high serum potassium or low sodium level is highly suggestive of adrenal insufficiency. These findings may require treatment with rehydration, salt replacement, and the administration of adrenocorticoids (Chapter 33, part four). Take a chest and abdominal film as soon as possible to exclude diagnoses such as pneumothorax and peritonitis with free air in the peritoneal cavity. A lumbar puncture may be indicated, depending on whether there is a strong possibility of meningitis. Correction of acidosis may require assisted ventilation rather than alkali therapy. Myocarditis, if present, is usually of viral origin. However, once the cultures have been taken, if myocarditis is presumptively diagnosed, antibiotic treatment for sepsis is indicated because of the possibility of a bacterial cause. The death rate from viral myocarditis appearing as a shocklike state in the neonate is approximately 75%. If one is faced with an obviously dying infant, corticosteroids such as hydrocortisone sodium succinate (Solu-Cortef), 50 mg/kg, may be tried; and if the heart rate is slow (below 80 beats per minute), transvenous pacing should be considered. If anomalous origin of the left coronary artery is a possible diagnosis, consider an emergency aortogram.

Ligation of the anomalous vessel at its site of origin into the pulmonary artery can be a life-saving maneuver. Alternatively, reconstructive coronary artery surgery can be performed.

ARRHYTHMIAS IN THE NEONATAL PERIOD

Considerable evidence indicates that after birth there is continued development of the cardiac conduction system and an increase in the sympathetic innervation of the heart. These factors may account for the observed heart rate variability and for the frequency of benign arrhythmias in the newborn. Premature supraventricular and ventricular beats, brief periods of sinus arrest, ectopic atrial rhythms, and wandering atrial pacemaker all have been observed during electrocardiographic monitoring of asymptomatic newborn infants.

Before embarking on the treatment of a tachycardia, bradycardia, or irregular heart beat, one must decide if the arrhythmia is benign and likely to resolve spontaneously or if it is potentially dangerous. Sometimes an arrhythmia indicates underlying extracardiac disease such as central nervous system disease, sepsis, hypoglycemia, drug toxicity (especially digitalis), severe tissue hypoxia, adrenal insufficiency, or electrolyte and acid-base abnormalities. One also must decide if the treatment is likely to be more dangerous than the arrhythmia. In deciding to treat or not to treat, major consideration should be given to whether the ventricular rate and rhythm are compatible with a normal cardiac output.

Mechanisms of arrhythmias

Most arrhythmias are thought to arise either from a disorder of automaticity or impulse formation or from alterations in impulse conduction within the heart. Both mechanisms may be combined.

The SA node, AV node, and His-Purkinje system are pacemaker tissues because they are capable of spontaneous depolarization during electrical diastole (phase 4 of the action potential). The SA node is normally the pacemaker for the heart because it has the fastest rate of spontaneous depolarization. Dysrhythmias caused by altered automaticity may occur when the inherent rate of phase-4 depolarization of the SA node falls below that of other latent pacemaker tissue in the heart. Thus "escape" rhythms will occur when sinus bradycardia is present and the junctional tissue of the AV node depolarizes faster than that of the SA node.

Arrhythmias also result when the automaticity of "ectopic" pacemaker tissue and of pacemakers below the SA node is enhanced, which is promoted by hypoxia, acidosis, digitalis toxicity, sympathetic nerve stimulation, increased wall tension, and altered electrolyte concentrations, particularly sodium, potassium, and calcium.

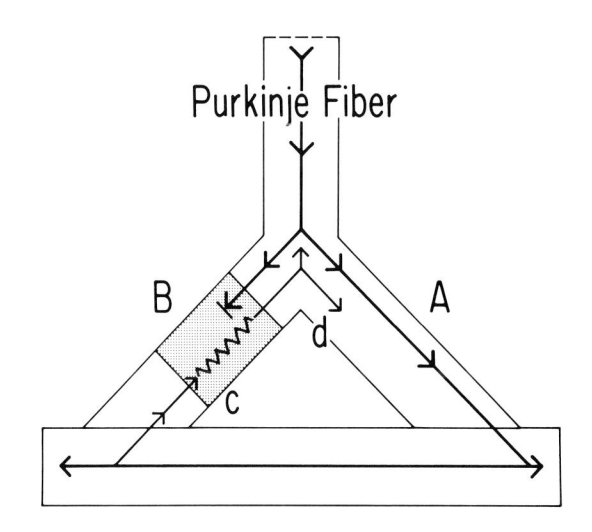

Fig. 25-26. Mechanism of unidirectional block and reentry. Impulse is propagated through Purkinje system and encounters Y-shaped fiber with its two branches terminating on ventricular muscle. Zone of unidirectional block is present in branch B. Impulse traverses branch A and is propagated through ventricular muscle. The impulse reaches distal end of block in B and is propagated slowly, retrogradely through it *(C)*. Branch A now has become sufficiently repolarized to be depolarized by reentering impulse *(D)*. One such reentrant circulation of impulses may produce premature beat. Repetition of this sequence in circuit produces reentrant tachycardia.

When local membrane characteristics are altered, as by stretch deformation (increased wall tension), thermal injury, scarring and fibrosis, or a previous premature beat, then disturbances of conduction can occur. Such activity is promoted by (1) cardiac enlargement, (2) nonhomogeneity of recovery from refractoriness in the cell population, (3) shortened refractory periods, and (4) slowed conduction. When a propagating impulse reaches the area of altered conduction (Fig. 25-26, *B*), propagation will be through an alternate pathway (area *A*). The impulse having traversed an alternate route now may reach the distal end of the previously blocked pathway, and the original pathway *(B)* is now sufficiently recovered to permit the impulse to be propagated retrogradely through it, setting up a reentrant activation front.

Drug therapy

Drug therapy for arrhythmias is based on the ability of certain drugs to alter or affect electrophysiologic properties of the cardiac tissue.

Many antiarrhythmic drugs act directly to alter the electrophysiologic properties of single fibers, usually resulting in decreased automaticity because the rate of rise of diastolic depolarization is slowed. In addition, because of altered membrane characteristics, the conduction velocity and refractory period will be affected, resulting at times in interruption of reentry pathways. Examples of such drugs are quinidine, procainamide (Pronestyl), lidocaine (Xylocaine), and phenytoin.

Other drugs act on arrhythmias by affecting directly or indirectly autonomic nervous system activity. Thus vagal tone may be directly increased by cholinergic agents such as edrophonium (Tensilon) chloride or neostigmine (Prostigmin) bromide or reflexly increased following the rise in blood pressure induced by sympathomimetic α-agonists such as phenylephrine (Neo-synephrine) hydrochloride. Propranolol hydrochloride (Inderal) is a β-adrenergic blocker. Digoxin exerts part of its chronotropic action via the sympathetic and parasympathetic nervous system, although its inotropic action is independent of the autonomic nervous system.

Benign arrhythmias
Sinus bradycardia, sinus tachycardia, and sinus arrhythmia

Healthy full-term and premature neonates have heart rates that range from 90 to 195 beats per minute. Rates above and below this range which are sustained for 15 seconds or more should have electrocardiographic documentation of the rhythm.

Transient periods of sinus bradycardia may occur during straining, micturition, or crying (Valsalva). Up to 35% of normal premature infants have been noted during monitoring to have brief periods of sinus bradycardia. The bradycardia that occurs with cord clamping or compression of the anterior fontanel may be caused by parasympathetic stimulation. Some maternal medications, such as reserpine or propranolol, may result in bradycardia in the newborn (p. 120).

Sinus tachycardia occurs with periods of increased activity and crying and also with fever and hyperthyroidism (p. 120).

Sinus arrhythmia is a phasic variation in the heart rate that may or may not be associated with respiration.

Pathologic arrhythmias
Supraventricular tachycardia

Supraventricular tachycardia (SVT) is the most common tachyarrhythmia in the newborn. It may be caused by dual AV nodal pathways with antegrade conduction down one pathway and the completion of a circle by retrograde conduction up the other (Fig. 25-26). It may be caused by rapid conduction through an accessory bundle (Wolff-Parkinson-White syndrome) or by the existence of an ectopic atrial focus with an automaticity faster than that in the SA node. There is an increased incidence of the Wolff-Parkinson-White syndrome with SVT in Ebstein's anomaly of the tricuspid valve and also with l-transposition of the great arteries. Gillette has investigated the mechanism of this disorder by electrophysiologic studies during cardiac catheterization of 35 children. These studies demonstrated at least seven different mechanisms, most involving some form of reentry. Between 8% and 26% of infants and children with SVT are estimated to have congenital heart disease.

Intrauterine SVT, although uncommon, is associated with severe congestive heart failure at birth and may be lethal. Newburger and Keane described 37 infants with intrauterine SVT. Five of the 37 had preexcitation syndrome (Wolff-Parkinson-White), and 11% had myocarditis or structural heart disease. Twenty-three of the 37 infants had severe congestive heart failure within the first hours of life, with symptoms that included cyanosis, tachypnea, edema, and ascites. Thirteen of 37 converted to normal sinus rhythm at delivery or shortly after birth. Sixteen of the 37 had recurrences within the first month, and there were three deaths, all occurring in infants with underlying heart disease. Those without underlying heart disease generally had a benign course after the newborn period. The identification of fetal SVT calls for an aggressive approach. Fetal edema can be assessed by ultrasound, and fetal lung maturity can be defined by the amniotic fluid lecithin/sphingomyelin ratio (L/S). If the L/S ratio is favorable and the gestation over 34 weeks (which it usually is), immediate delivery is indicated. If the gestational period and L/S ratio are unfavorable, betamethasone may be administered to induce surfactant production. Conversion with maternally administered propranolol or digoxin has been reported to be successful.

Newborns with SVT are either those in whom the arrhythmia is discovered during the first few days after birth when they are relatively asymptomatic or those who are brought to the hospital in heart failure having had the arrhythmia for several days.

The history usually reveals that the infant has become anxious, restless, tachypneic, or "not well" 1 to 2 days before there is serious concern. Neonates then usually become "wheezy," and at this stage it is easy for both parent and physician to diagnose a lower respiratory tract infection. As the SVT persists, the infant becomes pale, apathetic, and obviously very sick, with signs of congestive heart failure (pulmonary rales, hepatomegaly) and poor skin perfusion. Even at this stage it is possible for one to overlook, because of noisy respiration, the fact that the heart is beating at 280 beats per minute.

In the absence of AV block the ventricular rate may be very rapid. With AV block the ventricular rate will be variable.

The time taken for an infant to develop heart failure depends mainly on the ventricular rate (180 to 300 beats per minute) and the presence or absence of structural heart disease. An infant with serious cyanotic heart dis-

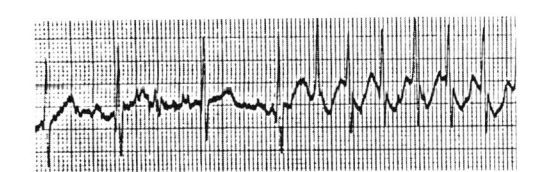

Fig. 25-27. Onset of PAT. Tracing obtained by telemetry. The rate increases from 75 to 200 beats per minute. Note the unchanging RR interval in the last six complexes and that the P waves are masked by the preceding T waves. (Courtesy Dr. Herbert Semler.)

ease who develops SVT during the course of cardiac catheterization may seriously worsen in a few minutes, whereas an infant with a normal heart may tolerate a rate of 220 beats per minute indefinitely.

Recognition of SVT is based on (1) a persistent ventricular rate of over 180 beats per minute, (2) a fixed or almost fixed RR interval on the ECG (Fig. 25-27), (3) abnormal P-wave shape, P-wave axis, or PR interval or total absence of P waves, and (4) little change in heart rate with activity, crying, or breath holding. The surface ECG may provide clues to the underlying mechanism. Thus, if no P waves are seen, a reentry mechanism is likely. If P waves are seen and there is one-to-one AV conduction, a reentry mechanism is also likely. SVT caused by an ectopic atrial pacemaker often is characterized by unconducted atrial beats, and SVT from an accessory pathway usually will show the typical Wolff-Parkinson-White abnormality on the after-tachycardia ECG. There is rarely any difficulty in diagnosis when the rate is over 210 beats per minute, but frequently the question arises as to whether a tachycardia is sinus or paroxysmal supraventricular when the rate in 180 to 210 beats per minute. Slight variations in the RR interval favor the diagnosis of sinus tachycardia. The QRS complex may at times be wide because of aberrant conduction, and the tracing may resemble that of ventricular tachycardia.

Treatment

Countershock. If the infant's condition is critical, DC countershock provides the most immediate method of terminating the attack. In more elective situations drug therapy can be used. Whichever method is chosen, acidosis, electrolyte abnormalities, hypothermia, and hypoxemia should be corrected as far as possible. Vagal stimulation maneuvers are generally unsuccessful and may waste valuable time.

DC countershock (5 to 25 W-seconds) usually will be successful for cardioversion. It is advisable to start at the lower dose and increase by 5 W-seconds. This may be repeated two or three times. After cardioversion, digitalization is begun orally or parenterally depending on the infant's condition.

Drug therapy

Digoxin. If countershock is unsuccessful, or if the infant is not critically ill, conversion may be accomplished by parenteral digitalization, giving half the digitalizing dose by slow intravenous push. The next two doses, each a fourth the digitalizing dose, may be given 4 to 8 hours after the preceding dose, depending on the response. Administration of digoxin should be continued for maintenance. When renal function is impaired, the digoxin dose should be reduced considerably, since the compound is eliminated almost entirely unchanged by the kidney. Serum digoxin levels and ECG monitoring are the best guides.

Propranolol hydrochloride. Propranolol is a β-adrenergic blocking agent that may be administered orally or intravenously. Intravenous administration should be reserved for emergency control of an arrhythmia at a dose 0.1 to 0.01 of the oral dosage. The drug is almost completely metabolized in the liver, with less than 2% excreted by the kidneys unchanged; however, reduced doses are still recommended in individuals with impaired renal function. β-Blocking agents should be used with caution in patients with heart failure, since maintenance of adequate cardiac output is dependent on circulating catecholamines in these patients. Atropine sulfate and isoproterenol should be immediately available to treat propranolol-induced bradycardia or hypothermia.

Quinidine and procainamide. Quinidine and procainamide are currently the third and fourth drug choices for treating SVT, after digoxin and propranolol. Both drugs have classic membrane effects but in addition have some vagolytic action that may result in an increased rate of sinus node discharge and enhancement of AV nodal conduction. Quinidine generally is administered orally in divided doses at 6-hour intervals. Depression of cardiac function may be a significant side effect, particularly if the drug is given parenterally. Procainamide may be administered parenterally or orally; however, orally this drug must be given every 3 to 4 hours.

Verapamil. Verapamil is a new drug that acts by blocking the slow inward current of calcium, in contrast to most antiarrhythmic drugs, which block the rapid influx of sodium into cells. Verapamil has been reported to be highly effective in slowing the ventricular response of adults with atrial flutter and fibrillation and also in converting SVT to sinus rhythm. The drug must be used with caution in patients with sick sinus syndrome and is contraindicated in patients receiving β-blocking agents.

Soler-Soler and co-workers report the use of verapamil in converting SVT in 14 infants age 5 days to 18 months. The drug was administered intravenously over 30 seconds, at a dosage of 1 mg in infants weighing less than 5 kg, 1.5 mg in infants weighing 5 to 10 kg, and 2 mg in infants weighing more than 10 kg. Stable sinus rhythm was obtained within 60 seconds in 28 of 29 attacks. These authors concluded that verapamil is at least as effective as digitalis in the conversion of SVT. Its advantages include rapid action and lack of undesirable side effects.

Overdrive pacing. Overdrive pacing, which is pacing the heart at a rate faster than that of the tachyarrhythmia, requires introduction of a pacing wire, usually transvenously, and a pacemaker that is capable of pacing at rates up to 600 beats per minute. This technique has been used successfully in adults for conversion of tachyarrhythmias. Garson and co-workers report the successful use of this technique for cardioversion in four of the five patients in whom it was tried.

Resistant cases. If therapy proves difficult and recurrences are common, it is sometimes necessary to determine the exact mechanism of the SVT by intracardiac electrography. Different mechanisms are more likely to be suppressed by different drugs.

Surgical treatment. The majority of cases of SVT in infants and children are successfully managed medically. Gillette and co-workers report nine pediatric patients ranging in age from 6 months to 14 years who underwent surgical division of an accessory connection, or Kent's bundle, for medically unresponsive SVT. There was one death. The survivors have experienced no complications.

Maintenance treatment. A newborn who has had one attack of SVT has an approximately 20% recurrence risk, and continued maintenance of digoxin for 6 months after the last attack is indicated. Recurrences are more likely in those with underlying Wolff-Parkinson-White syndrome, and in these patients continued maintenance of digoxin, sometimes supplemented by quinidine or propranolol, may be indicated.

Prognosis. Nadas and associates have divided infants into prognostically useful clinical groups. The first group consists primarily of boys under 4 months of age without structural heart disease; the second group is composed of older infants of both sexes with or without heart disease. Recurrences after the age of 1 year are unlikely with the first group, but recurrences are frequent with the second group, particularly if the Wolff-Parkinson-White syndrome is present.

Atrial flutter and fibrillation

Atrial flutter is infrequent in the neonate and is likely to be associated with organic heart disease, especially mitral valve disease, endocardial fibroelastosis, Ebstein's malformation of the tricuspid valve, pulmonary atresia, VSD, coarctation, and complex heart defects. Atrial flutter has been diagnosed in utero.

Atrial flutter is diagnosed when (1) the atrial rate is 220

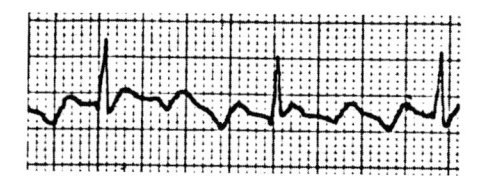

Fig. 25-28. Atrial flutter with 3:1 ventricular response. Ventricular rate is 80, atrial rate 240. The flutter waves have a "sawtooth" appearance.

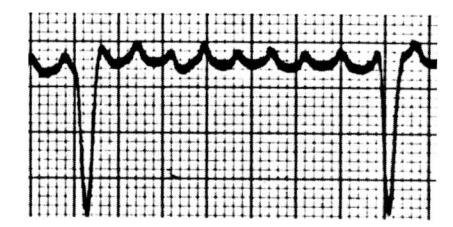

Fig. 25-29. Atrial fibrillation (12-year-old child). Ventricular rate 50 per minute, atrial rate ("f" waves) 400 per minute. On a long tracing it would be seen that the ventricular response is totally irregular.

to 400 beats per minute; (2) the atrial mechanism is regular; and (3) there is a characteristic sawtooth pattern of the flutter wave in leads II and III (Fig. 25-28). There is usually some degree of AV block. The ventricular rate will depend on the degree of AV block. If the AV block is fixed, the ventricular rate will be regular; if it is variable, the ventricular rate will be irregular.

Atrial fibrillation is rare in the newborn (Fig. 25-29). It is likely to be associated with serious organic heart disease, especially those conditions associated with left atrial enlargement. The arrhythmia may appear clinically as a tachycardia, but it is more likely to be recognized as a chaotic rhythm. The ECG shows characteristic fibrillation f waves and an irregular QRS response.

The clinical picture is similar to that of SVT, and the congestive heart failure may be life threatening, as in SVT.

Treatment is the same as in SVT. DC countershock is usually the most rapid method for cardioversion and should be followed by digoxin maintenance. Occasionally other drugs, such as propranolol hydrochloride, procainamide, or quinidine, may be necessary for cardioversion and/or maintenance. Verapamil has had success in infants with SVT and might be successful in treating atrial flutter or fibrillation.

Preexcitation syndrome (Wolff-Parkinson-White syndrome)

This syndrome (short PR interval and initial slurring and widening of the QRS) is caused by early excitation of

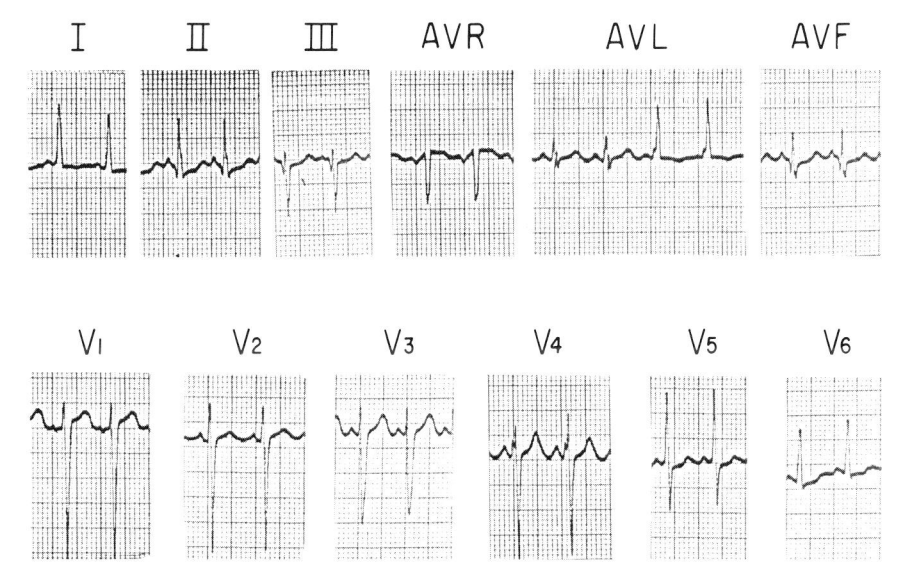

Fig. 25-30. Wolff-Parkinson-White syndrome in the neonate. PR interval is shortened (evident in most leads). QRS is slightly prolonged to 0.08 second leads II, III, and aV$_F$), and there is a slurred upstroke in the R wave (lead I). The first two complexes in aV$_L$ show normal ventricular excitation, while the next two show Wolff-Parkinson-White (ventricular preexcitation) syndrome.

the ventricles by an anomalous conducting bundle that conducts faster than the AV node, which it bypasses (hence the short PR interval). Recognition of the syndrome is important because of (1) the high incidence of SVT, and (2) the frequent misinterpretation of the ECG as left bundle branch block, left ventricular hypertrophy, myocardial infarction, or ventricular tachycardia. Wolff-Parkinson-White syndrome may be transient and may alternate with normal conduction (intermittent Wolff-Parkinson-White) (Fig. 25-30). The syndrome may be associated with congenital heart disease, particularly Ebstein's malformation, corrected transposition of the great arteries, dextrocardia, and complex malformations. The treatment for this condition is that of the symptomatic arrhythmias which may occur.

Ventricular tachycardia

Ventricular tachycardia in neonates most commonly occurs in the presence of organic heart disease but is rare, except as a complication of cardiac surgery, anesthesia, or cardiac catheterization.

With the type of tracing shown in Fig. 25-31 there are four possibilities: (1) ventricular tachycardia, (2) SVT with bundle branch block (unlikely in the neonatal period), (3) aberrant ventricular conduction complicating SVT, and (4) Wolff-Parkinson-White syndrome with SVT. Hyperkalemia also may account for markedly widened QRS complexes. If doubt exists, it is best to proceed directly to DC countershock (unless digitalis toxicity is thought to be present) of 5 to 25 W-seconds in a

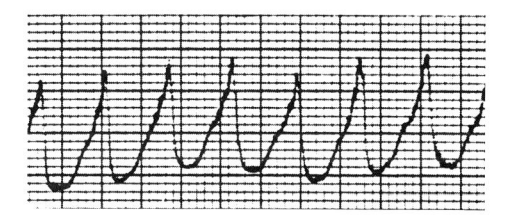

Fig. 25-31. Ventricular tachycardia. Rate is 200 per minute, and there is grossly abnormal ventricular conduction with wide bizarre QRS complexes. (For differential diagnosis, see text.)

newborn. Lidocaine may be tried at a dosage of 1 to 2 mg/kg as a single rapid infusion at 20 to 30 μg/minute with continuous cardiac monitoring to warn of premature ventricular contractions or a recurrence of the ventricular tachycardia. Oral phenytoin, propranolol, bretylium tosylate, and Tocainide (a lidocaine analogue) all have been used, but the major experience is in adults.

Stevens and co-workers report four cases of ventricular tachycardia in the neonatal period. One case was detected in utero. All patients survived, two with asymptomatic episodes of ventricular ectopia on long-term follow-up analysis. In their review of the literature, of a total of 45 cases of ventricular arrhythmia in the perinatal period, nine were detected in utero, three persisted beyond the perinatal period, and two resulted in death with associated disorders.

Ectopic beats

Ectopic beats are common in healthy newborn infants, with a reported incidence of between 21% and 31% for healthy premature infants and of up to 23% for full-term newborns. Supraventricular ectopic beats are more common than ventricular ones and may arise in the atrium or AV junctional tissue. They usually are identified by a P wave of abnormal configuration, appearing earlier than the expected PP interval. The QRS that follows may be widened because of aberrancy and because the His-Purkinje system may not be fully repolarized from the preceding normal beat.

Multiple ectopic beats usually pose no threat to life unless they occur within the framework of organic heart disease. Thus the infant with tight valvular pulmonic stenosis may develop heart failure when multiple ectopic beats develop; the relative inefficiency of the ectopic beats leads to a lowered cardiac output. By contrast, normal infants may have alarming runs of ectopic beats and by asymptomatic.

Ventricular ectopic beats should be regarded more seriously than atrial ectopic beats, especially if they are multifocal, or if there are short runs of ectopic beats, since these may portend the development of ventricular tachycardia or fibrillation. Treatment of ectopic beats in the asymptomatic infant is usually not indicated because the antiarrhythmic drugs have a negative inotropic action and because ventricular tachycardia is a rare complication.

When heart disease is present and it appears likely that ectopic beats are compromising cardiac output, an attempt should be made to suppress them with drugs. The drugs most likely to be successful are phenytoin, propranolol, and quinidine.

Sinoatrial node disorders

SA node disorders are rare in newborns and children and, when they occur, are usually the result of surgery. When there is failure of impulse formation within the sinus node or of transmission of the sinus node impulse to the rest of the atrium, the heart rhythm will be dependent on the escape rhythm arising in the AV junctional tissue. Symptoms from sinus node disease therefore only result when there is also disease in the conducting tissue beyond the sinus node. Sick sinus syndrome has been divided into type I, characterized by periods of bradycardia and sinus arrest, and type II, with paroxysmal tachycardia.

Yabek and co-workers performed electrophysiologic studies on 18 children with sinus node dysfunction and were able to identify at least three different mechanisms. Lev and co-workers studied the conduction system in two children who had prolonged sinus node dysfunction and found degeneration and fibrosis of the approaches to the SA and AV nodes and atrial preferential pathways in one child and fatty infiltration of these areas in the other.

Management consists of appropriate treatment for the tachyarrhythmias. However, sometimes pacemaker implantation is necessary because the bradycardia becomes life threatening. We have seen one newborn with intermittent symptomatic bradyarrhythmias with sinus arrest and paroxysmal tachyarrhythmias (Fig. 25-32). She was treated with prophylactic pacemaker implantation. A previous child in the family had been the victim of sudden infant death syndrome (SIDS).

Atrioventricular block

AV block in newborns is unusual, but when it occurs, it is usually asymptomatic. It may be secondary to digitalis administration or viral infections. Some types of congenital heart disease have an increased incidence of AV block. These include corrected transposition of the great arteries, ASD, Ebstein's anomaly of the tricuspid valve, and complex cyanotic cardiac defects.

When the PR interval is prolonged, first-degree AV block is said to be present. In normal newborns the PR interval may range from 0.08 to 0.12 seconds. The most common cause of first-degree heart block in the newborn is digitalis effect.

Second-degree AV block is present when not all atrial beats are conducted to the ventricle. The most common form was first described by Wenkebach and is also called Mobitz type I. In Mobitz type I the PR interval progressively lengthens until an atrial beat fails to be conducted to the ventricles and there is a dropped beat. Mobitz type II block also occurs in the newborn (Fig. 25-33). In this form of second-degree AV block, ventricular beats are dropped without preceding PR-interval prolongation. The PR interval for conducted beats usually is constant.

Third-degree heart block (complete heart block) in the newborn is most often congenital (Fig. 25-34). In an international cooperative study on congenital complete heart block it was estimated that 1 in 20,000 live-born infants has congenital complete heart block.

There is an association with various forms of congenital heart disease, the most common of which is corrected transposition of the great arteries. Familial clusterings have been reported, and in the cooperative study there were 599 patients, among whom were 14 families with two siblings affected. Approximately a third (181 of 599) of the patients in the study had complicating heart disease.

For those without complicating heart disease the risk of death was greatest in early infancy. Approximately three fourths passed their fifth birthday, and a third were older than 10 years. Ninety-two percent of the 418 sub-

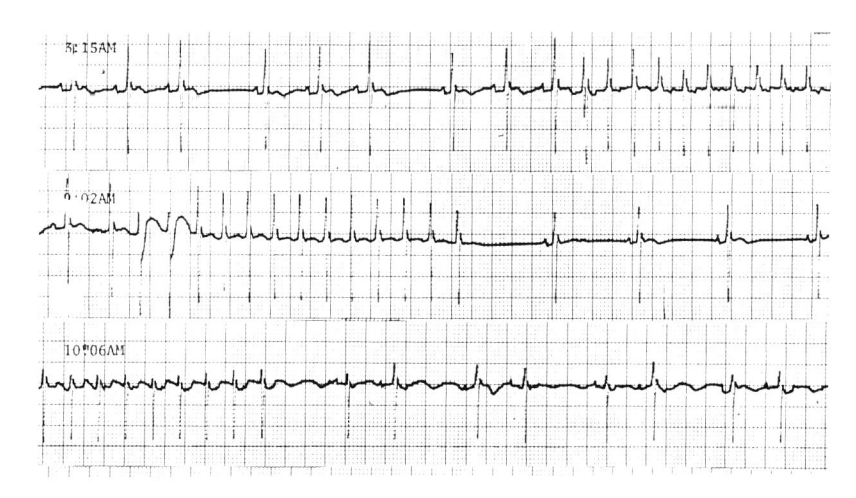

Fig. 25-32. Sinus node dysfunction (sick sinus syndrome) in 2-day-old infant. Note periods of sinus bradycardia and periods of SVT. This child was treated with pacemaker for periods of sinus bradycardia that were frequent and symptomatic. Another child in the family was a victim of SIDS.

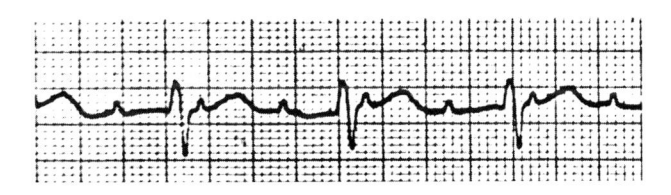

Fig. 25-33. Second-degree AV block (Mobitz type II). Every second P wave gives rise to a QRS complex after a long PR interval.

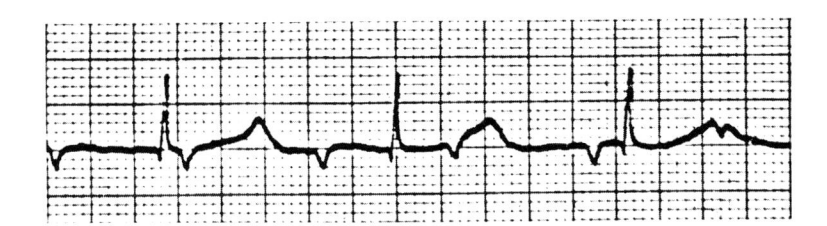

Fig. 25-34. Complete (third-degree) AV block. Note that the P wave rate exceeds the QRS rate and that there is no constant PR interval.

jects without complicating heart disease were alive at last examination.

For those patients with associated congenital heart disease the prognosis was not as good, with the risk of dying highest in early infancy. Of 181 patients, 71% were alive at the last examination. Thirty of the 36 deaths were in the first week of life.

In addition to associated heart disease, the risk factor most prevalent for early death was slow ventricular rate and rapid atrial rate. The prognosis was better for infants whose ventricular rate was greater than 55 and whose atrial rate was less than 140 beats per minute.

Recently the occurrence of congenital complete heart block in infants of women with connective tissue disorders has been recognized. McCue and co-workers report 22 children with congenital complete heart block, of whom 14 were born to 11 mothers with clinical or laboratory evidence of connective tissue disorder, primarily lupus erythematosus. This association has been further documented by other groups.

Drug treatment to increase the heart rate, such as with atropine and isoproterenol, has had only limited success. Pacemaker therapy, particularly before congestive heart failure occurs, has been the most successful intervention.

The judgment regarding timing of pacemaker implantation remains difficult, particularly since in the absence of associated heart disease the individual who survives infancy with congenital complete heart block probably will do well for many years. Benrey and associates reviewed the indications for and results of pacemaker implantation in children at Baylor. The indications included symptoms of cerebrovascular insufficiency and congestive heart failure and, in a newborn, a ventricular rate below 50 and an atrial rate over 150 beats per minute.

Levy and associates monitored 20 children with congenital complete heart block and found many with bradyarrhythmias, particularly during sleep. These authors recommend that all children with complete heart block have electromagnetic tape recordings at fairly frequent intervals.

CARDIAC ARREST AND EXTREME BRADYCARDIA

Apparent cardiac arrest—that is, lack of audible heartbeat, cardiac impulse, or peripheral pulse—usually is caused by ventricular asystole or extreme bradycardia rather than by ventricular fibrillation (Fig. 25-35). Either of these two events may be the result of primary respiratory failure. Ventricular asystole and ventricular fibrillation can be distinguished by an ECG. However, it is essential that treatment be started immediately without losing valuable minutes locating an ECG machine and attaching leads. In many neonates there is no doubt as to whether cardiac arrest has occurred. The majority of sick neonates are already having their heart rates monitored, and the alarm is set to sound at a rate of 80 beats per minute. By the time someone reaches the baby, the rate may have fallen to 60 and be continuing to decrease. Treatment should be initiated without waiting for the infant to deteriorate further. It first needs to be determined whether bradycardia or cardiac arrest is primary or is secondary to respiratory failure. In many immature and sick infants bradycardia is secondary to respiratory arrest, and prompt respiratory resuscitation takes first priority and often restores the heart rate to normal. When respirations cease, heart rate and cardiac output fall. In other instances the neonate has become too hypoxemic and acidotic for respiratory resuscitation alone to restore the heartbeat. In this situation cardiac resuscitation is required. Pupillary dilatation begins within 45 seconds after circulation stops and is complete by about 1 minute 45 seconds.

Cardiac resuscitation of the neonate

Bradycardia with a heart rate falling to 40 beats per minute or below is the most frequent indication for cardiac resuscitation in the neonate. Ventricular asystole

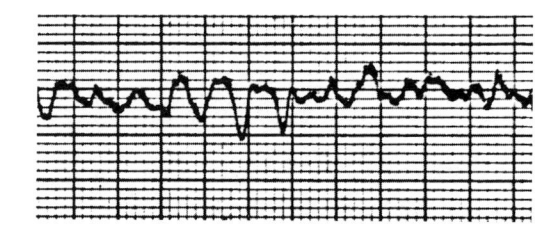

Fig. 25-35. Ventricular fibrillation. Chaotic electrical ventricular activity associated with complete ineffectiveness of ventricular contraction.

without prior bradycardia is unusual, and ventricular fibrillation is rarely observed except in the terminal stages of advanced heart disease.

The following guidelines assume that pulmonary ventilation is being assisted either by face mask or endotracheal tube and that the heart rate is either inaudible or below 50 beats per minute. Check for audible heart sounds. The hearing of regular heart sounds, however slow, rules out ventricular fibrillation. Flick the precordium over the midsternum, and listen again (equivalent to the chest "thump" in adults). If the heart rate is still inadequate, immediately start external massage. If two people are present, try to alternate cardiac massage and ventilation (40 seconds of cardiac massage to 20 seconds of ventilation). Examine ECG to distinguish ventricular asystole (straight line or occasional bizarre QRS complexes), ventricular fibrillation (irregular chaotic line) (Fig. 25-35), and complete heart block (Fig. 25-34). Precordial compression causes an obvious artifact. If ventricular fibrillation is present, defibrillate with external DC countershock until conversion (usually 10 to 25 W-seconds). If an acceptable rhythm with evidence of adequate cardiac output does not occur, resume cardiac massage. After 4 or 5 minutes of cardiac arrest and reduced cardiac output during external massage, the blood will be acidotic; sodium bicarbonate should be given intravenously (2 to 6 mEq/kg). If there has been no response after 5 to 10 minutes of ventilation, external cardiac massage, and alkali therapy, consider the use of pharmacologic agents and cardiac pacing. The pharmacologic agents that may be tried include:

1. Epinephrine: 0.2 ml/kg of a 1:10,000 solution, intravenous or intracardiac.
2. Isoproterenol: 0.1 to 0.4 μg/kg/minute by intravenous infusion or single doses of 1 μg/kg by intravenous or intracardiac route every 5 minutes.
3. Calcium chloride: 0.5 to 1 ml of 10% solution administered intravenously or by intracardiac route every 5 minutes.
4. Atropine may be indicated if second or third-degree AV block is present; intravenous dose of 0.01 mg/kg.
5. Lidocaine may be indicated in the rare instance where

ineffective contraction is caused by ventricular arrhythmias that are resistant to DC countershock alone; in infants 0.5 to 2.0 mg/kg may be given immediately before countershock and repeated every 10 to 15 minutes.

If effective cardiac contraction cannot be restored with one of these agents, it is advisable to pause and determine whether brain damage is irreversible and resuscitation should be stopped or whether an attempt at cardiac pacing is warranted.

Cardiac pacing

Indications for cardiac pacing include bradycardia, cardia arrest, digitalis intoxication, and complete heart block. The temporary bradycardia associated with the salt-losing crisis of congenital adrenal hyperplasia or any other condition from which it is possible for the infant to recover may warrant pacing. By contrast, a neonate with bradycardia from the terminal stages of RDS or the hypoplastic left-heart syndrome would not be a candidate for a pacemaker.

External pacing is rarely effective. Internal transvenous pacemaker catheters may be placed via the external jugular vein, with the tip lodged in the trabeculations of the right ventricle or, if the AV node is functional, in the right atrium. An alternative short-term route is the femoral vein (usually it is not possible to enter the right ventricle from the umbilical vein). The pacing rate should be 100 to 140 beats per minute. Usually a current of 0.5 to 1.0 MA is necessary to obtain a response. Because electrical response is no guarantee of mechanical response, heart sounds and pulses should be checked before it is concluded that the heart is actually propelling blood. The Doppler ultrasound flowmeter is particularly useful for this purpose. If temporary transvenous pacing is successful and the source of the bradycardia is not removed (as in complete AV block), it will be necessary to implant long-term epicardial or myocardial pacemaker wires.

COMMON CARDIOVASCULAR DISORDERS PRODUCING SERIOUS DISEASE IN THE NEONATE

A classification of the structural disorders more commonly encountered in neonatal practice is offered in the outline below.

A. Transposition of the great arteries
   1. D-transposition
   2. L-transposition
B. Left-sided heart obstruction
   1. Hypoplastic left-heart syndrome
   2. Congenital aortic stenosis
   3. Preductal and juxtaductal coarctation of the aorta
   4. Postductal coarctation
C. Right-sided heart obstruction
   1. Pulmonary atresia or extreme pulmonic stenosis with intact ventricular septum
   2. Pulmonary atresia with open ventricular septum, and severe tetralogy of Fallot
   3. Peripheral pulmonary artery stenosis
   4. Tricuspid atresia with and without transposition
   5. Ebstein's anomaly of the tricuspid valve
D. Lesions that produce common mixing of venous and arterial blood
   1. Truncus arteriosus
   2. Single ventricle
   3. Double-outlet right ventricle without pulmonic stenosis
   4. Total anomalous pulmonary venous return
E. Left-to-right shunts
   1. PDA
   2. VSD
   3. Combined PDA and VSD
   4. Common AV canal
   5. Systemic arteriovenous fistula
F. Myocardial disorders
   1. Myocarditis
   2. Endocardial fibroelastosis
   3. Anomalous left coronary artery
   4. Glycogen storage disease
G. Miscellaneous
   1. Absent pulmonary valve
   2. Tricuspid insufficiency
   3. Cor triatriatum
   4. Dextrocardia

Transposition of the great arteries
Incidence

Transposition accounts for 15% to 30% of neonates undergoing cardiac catheterization and for at least 16% of deaths caused by congenital heart disease at all ages in childhood. The incidence of transposition is between 0.022% and 0.047% of live births (1:2,130 to 1:4,500). Transposition is a common defect, and early recognition is of major importance; hundreds of neonates born with complete transposition of the great arteries have had the defect corrected and are leading normal lives. Males outnumber females 2 to 1, and there is some evidence that they have a higher-than-average birth weight.

Pathology

The aorta arises anteriorly and from the venous ventricle, whereas the pulmonary artery arises posteriorly and from the arterial ventricle. With dextrotransposition (d-transposition) the aortic valve is to the right of the pulmonary valve, whereas with levotransposition (l-transposition) the aortic valve is to the left of the pulmonary valve (Fig. 25-36). There is a well-developed muscular subaortic infundibulum, in contrast to the muscular subpulmonary infundibulum characteristic of the normal heart.

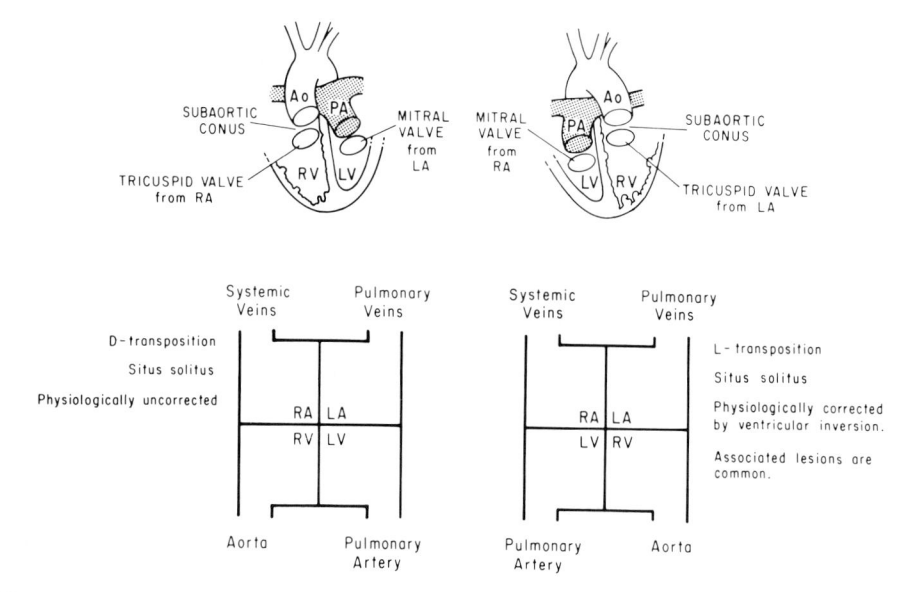

Fig. 25-36. The two most common types of transposition of the great arteries leading to problems in the neonatal period. In both types the aortic valve is high and anterior and arises from the coarsely trabeculated right (venous) ventricle. d-Transposition (left panel) is the common transposition causing problems in the newborn period.

D-transpositions outnumber l-transpositions as a cause for major concern in the newborn period by at least 10 to 1. As a generalization, one can say that d-transposition is a relatively "pure" lesion usually associated only with patent foramen ovale, PDA, and VSD. L-transposition, by contrast, often is associated with dextrocardia, situs inversus, and asplenia when it appears in the newborn period. When it appears in older infants and children, it is usually physiologically "corrected," most commonly by ventricular inversion; unfortunately there are almost always additional lesions present, such as mitral regurgitation, VSD, and subpulmonic stenosis.

Transposition of the great arteries is sometimes associated with a very large VSD or common ventricle, in which case the fact that the great vessels are transposed becomes of secondary importance. The association of tricuspid atresia and transposition is not unusual and leads to common mixing at the left atrial level. The adequacy of systemic (aortic) flow then depends on the size of an associated VSD or PDA.

The major emphasis in this section, then, is on the common d-transposition with situs solitus (normal location of the heart and viscera). Brief mention is made of the most common form of l-transposition—the physiologically corrected (by ventricular inversion) transposition in which the frequently associated VSD and mitral regurgitation may give rise to heart failure in the neonate.

D-transposition of the great arteries

D-transposition with intact ventricular septum and small or absent ductus arteriosus. Neonates with transposition and intact ventricular septum are extremely cyanotic and usually die in the first few days of life as the ductus arteriosus closes. Conversely, if the ductus arteriosus remains open, there is better mixing of venous and arterial circulations but usually at the expense of pulmonary artery hypertension. If there is only a foramen ovale or ASD, it is necessary for bidirectional shunting to occur at the atrial level; whereas if the duct also is open, a common sequence is for right-to-left shunting to occur at the atrial level and for there to be left-to-right (aorta to pulmonary artery) shunting at the ductal level. The latter situation might seem hemodynamically acceptable; but unfortunately the ductus is frequently very large, and pulmonary artery pressure is at systemic levels.

Clinical manifestations. Cyanosis is present from birth, although the temporary patency of the ductus arteriosus may allow some shunting, and the recognition of cyanosis may be delayed. The breathing rate is characteristically increased to 45 to 80 breaths per minute; there are usually no signs of respiratory distress unless the infant has associated respiratory tract infection. The peripheral pulses are normal. The cardiac impulse is often normal for the first hours or days but thereafter becomes hyperdynamic. The heart sounds are normal, and frequently there is no cardiac murmur. If a heart murmur is audible, it is likely to be nondescript and grade 3 or less in intensity, probably representing the murmur of a closing ductus. As time passes, the neonate becomes progressively more cyanotic; and when arteriovenous mixing is inadequate over a prolonged period, respiratory and metabolic acidosis ensues. Finally the infant dies from a combination of hypoxemia and acidosis during the first or second

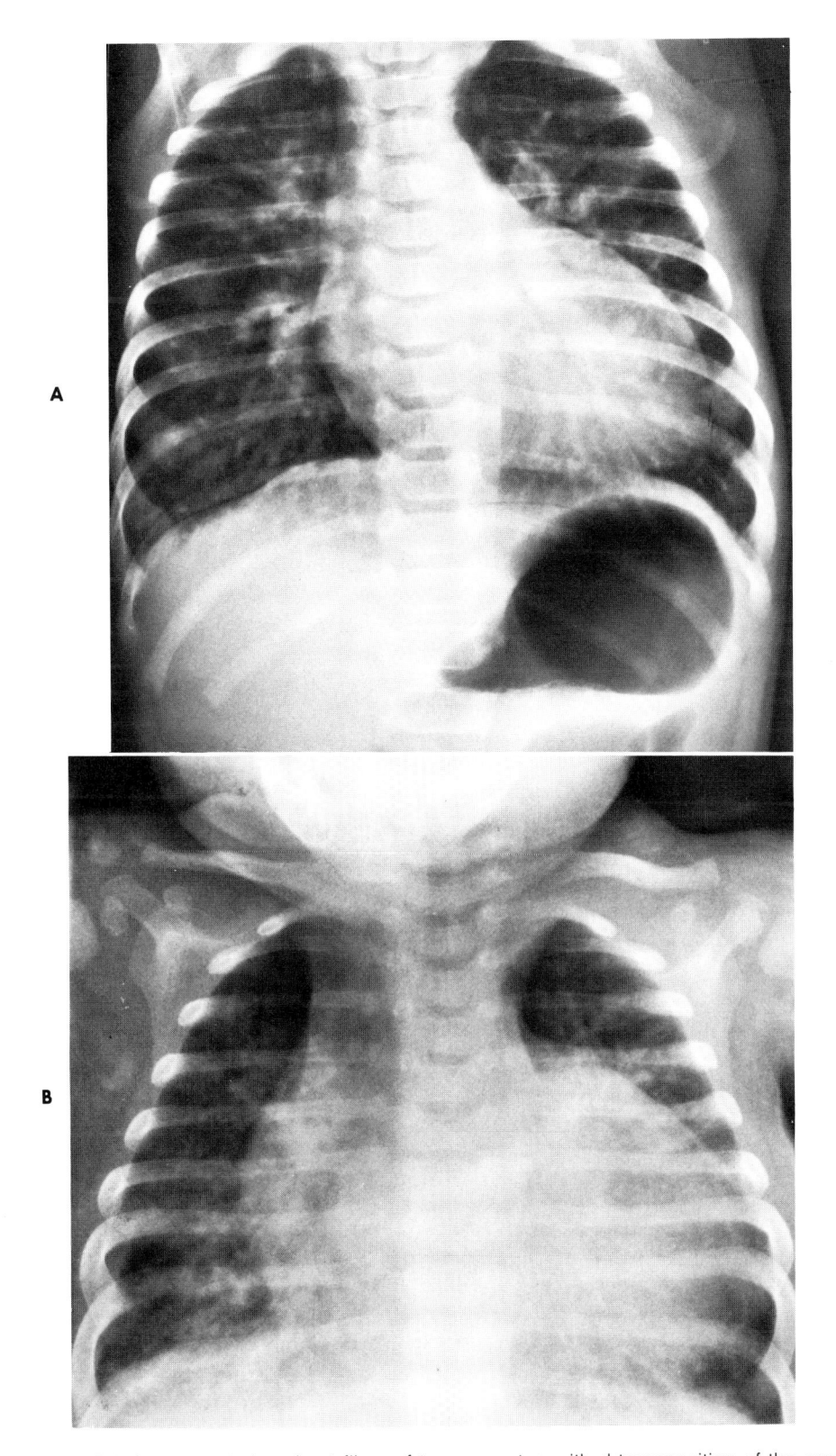

Fig. 25-37. Anteroposterior chest films of two neonates with d-transposition of the great arteries. **A,** Note narrow mediastinum, "egg-on-side" appearance, cardiomegaly, and pulmonary plethora. **B,** Note massive cardiomegaly caused by heart failure.

week of life if there is only a patent foramen ovale for exchange of arterial and venous blood.

Diagnosis. Initially the chest roentgenogram may appear normal. However, as time passes, it becomes apparent that the heart is abnormally large and somewhat eggshaped and that the pulmonary vascular markings are increased (Fig. 25-37). The classic roentgenogram of transposition shows, in addition, a narrow mediastinum when viewed anteroposteriorly and a widened mediastinum when viewed laterally. There is usually nothing diagnostically helpful in the ECG tracing. Almost always a mild degree of right ventricular hypertrophy is present, similar to that seen in a wide variety of cardiac and pulmonary diseases in which the right ventricle is working at systemic pressure.

The arterial oxygen saturation while the infant is breathing room air is usually in the 30% to 70% range, corresponding to a PaO$_2$ of approximately 15 to 30 mm Hg. The PaCO$_2$ may remain normal or even decreased for surprising periods because of some alveolar hyperventilation. The PaCO$_2$ usually rises on the second or third day of life to 50 or 60 mm Hg, higher in the very severely hypoxemic baby. Similarly the arterial pH may remain normal for a time (because of an increase in plasma bicarbonate level), but it inevitably declines in the severely sick infant because of a combination of the accumulation of the products of anaerobic metabolism and the failure of the lungs to eliminate adequate CO$_2$. Although the total lung blood flow is increased in infants with transposition, the effective pulmonary blood flow (that fraction derived from the systemic venous return) is decreased.

In most infants 100% O$_2$ breathing will increase arterial PO$_2$ by only a few millimeters of mercury (because of the slightly increased O$_2$ content of pulmonary capillary blood). An occasional infant with transposition, however, shows a much more dramatic response to 100% O$_2$, with arterial PO$_2$ increasing from 30 to 70 mm Hg and the infant changing from cyanotic to acyanotic. This change is the result of the effect of oxygen on pulmonary arterioles, causing a fall in pulmonary vascular resistance and allowing an existing ductal or ventricular shunt to become exclusively left to right, while an existing atrial shunt becomes exclusively right to left. The net effect is greater crossover between venous and arterial circuits. In this situation measurements of arterial O$_2$ saturation will give the spurious impression of absence of right-to-left shunt; however, measurement of arterial O$_2$ tension will reveal the true situation—for example, a PaO$_2$ of only 70 mm Hg versus an expected PaO$_2$ of at least 150 mm Hg with a normal circulation.

HEMODYNAMICS AND ANGIOCARDIOGRAPHY. The major problem is lack of communication between pulmonary and systemic circulations after birth. Transposition is of little consequence while the baby is in utero. Infants with transposition are typically large, well-nourished infants and frequently give no cause for concern during the first minutes and hours of life. The deterioration of the infant thereafter corresponds to gradual constriction of the ductus arteriosus. The low PO$_2$ perfusing this structure appears to lose its vasodilating effect within hours to a day or two after birth. When the ductus arteriosus closes, the infant is totally reliant on a foramen ovale or ASD for

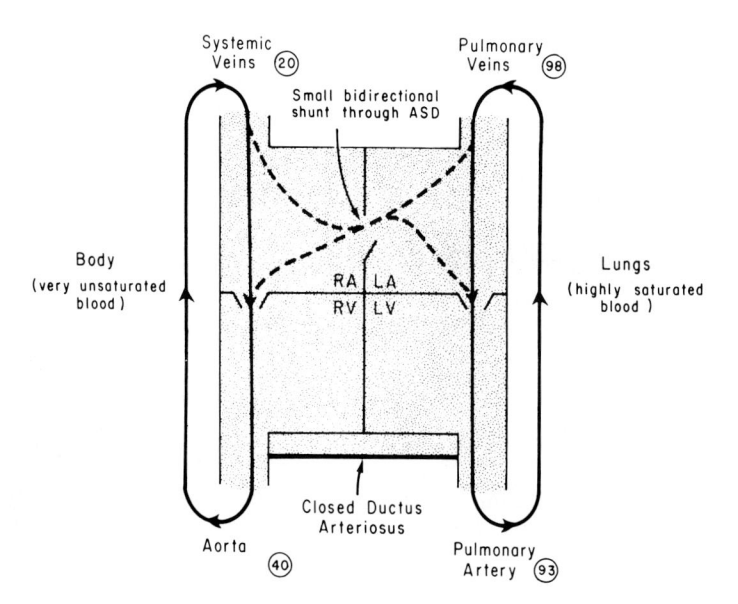

Fig. 25-38. The course of the circulation in d-transposition with intact ventricular septum. Typical oxygen saturations are circled. Small bidirectional shunts of equal magnitude across the atrial septum allow insufficient oxygen to reach the tissues for the maintenance of adequate oxidative metabolism.

the exchange of venous and arterial blood; unless the ASD is large, death will rapidly ensue from hypoxemia, hypercapnia, and acidosis (Fig. 25-38).

The major abnormal hemodynamic findings are a right ventricular pressure that is at systemic level and a left ventricular pressure (left ventricle supplies the pulmonary artery) that may be high or low, depending on the pulmonary blood flow and pulmonary vascular resistance (assuming there is no pulmonic stenosis). Aortic oxygen saturation is lower than pulmonary artery saturation; arterial oxygen saturations of about 30% to 40% are not uncommon. The catheter passes easily from the inferior vena cava to the right atrium, right ventricle, and out into the anteriorly placed aorta. In the majority of cases it also can be passed easily across the foramen ovale into the left atrium and left ventricle.

Right ventricular angiography in the lateral projection reveals the high, anterior location of the aortic valve and the presence or absence of a VSD. Left ventricular angiography discloses the posteriorly located pulmonary artery.

ECHOCARDIOGRAPHY Introduction of two-dimensional echocardiography has been of considerable assistance in the management of infants with d-transposition of the great arteries. The great arteries may be identified; subpulmonic stenosis identified, and septal defects visualized by the passage of saline contrast from right to left after peripheral vein injection.

Treatment. The advent of balloon septostomy has allowed definitive treatment frequently to commence during the course of cardiac catheterization. The pressure gradient between the left and right atrium is measured; the larger the gradient, the smaller the foramen ovale or ASD. Patients with a demonstrable gradient will benefit from enlargement of the communication, and even those without a gradient may obtain some beneficial effect from balloon septostomy. The exact indications for balloon septostomy are still controversial. Our policy has been to proceed with septostomy whether or not a gradient is demonstrable. Opening of the atrial septum by balloon is achieved by placing the tip of a balloon catheter in the left atrium, inflating it with 2 to 3 ml dilute contrast agent, and rapidly pulling it back across the atrial septum to rupture the thin "membrane" covering the foramen ovale and in some cases to tear the adjacent interatrial septum. Several results may follow balloon septostomy.

1. Balloon septostomy may be dramatically successful in some babies. Arterial O_2 saturation increases from a moribund 40% to a respectable 80%, and the improvement is maintained. The infant survives and can be operated on by the interatrial baffle (Mustard) procedure at the age of 6 to 24 months.
2. The balloon septostomy may be partially successful. The baby's arterial saturation remains satisfactory for days or weeks, but then increasing cyanosis recurs. A second balloon septostomy after the age of 6 weeks is not usually beneficial. The choice is surgical removal of part of the atrial septum versus repair by means of the Mustard procedure (switching of the venous return to match the transposed arteries). The choice depends on the weight of the infant (although total repair is now possible at 3 kg) and the experiences and preferences of the surgeon. Our general approach is atrial septectomy (followed a year later by the Mustard procedure) for those infants under 5 kg or who are under 1 month old or both and the primary Mustard procedure for those over 5 kg. In cases of doubt a recatheterization to measure pulmonary artery pressure is justified, since correction in a small infant with pulmonary artery pressure of more than 50% systemic pressure carries a higher mortality; for this group atrial septectomy to allow increased oxygen delivery to the tissues and accelerated growth represents a lesser risk.
3. The balloon septostomy may be totally unsuccessful; early atrial septectomy or baffle procedure is desirable.

The Mustard procedure is not totally corrective in as much as the right ventricle is required to perform systemic work for the rest of the child's life. Early attempts at an arterial switch operation (Jetane's procedure) were fraught with high mortality often caused by the unpreparedness of the left ventricle to work against the systemic vascular resistance. There is now a resurgence of interest in the arterial switch operation because of the concept of "preparing" the left ventricle by prior (2 to 3 months) pulmonary artery banding.

In instances where falling arterial pH and deteriorating blood gases suggest a closing ductus arteriosus, the infant with d-transposition of the great arteries may improve temporarily by the infusion of prostaglandin E_1 (PGE_1) into the aortic end of the ductus (umbilical artery line) or, if the situation is critical, into a scalp vein. PGE_1 dilatation of the ductus is especially useful to stabilize the infant's condition prior to balloon septostomy.

D-transposition with open ventricular septum. The presence of a moderate or large VSD might appear to be advantageous to the baby with transposed great arteries because of the better mixing of venous and arterial streams. Any small advantage, however, is more than offset by the greater frequency of pulmonary hypertension and heart failure. In addition, surgical correction is more difficult.

Clinical manifestations. The symptoms tend to be those of right- and left-sided heart failure rather than severe cyanosis. Neonates with transposition and large VSD frequently appear only mildly cyanotic. The cardiac impulse is hyperdynamic; the signs of heart failure are present; and a loud lower left sternal border pansystolic murmur suggests a VSD.

Diagnosis. This condition may simulate a large VSD, common ventricle, or even truncus arteriosus. On the roentgenogram the heart is seen to be large and the pulmonary vasculature increased. The ECG shows right ventricular hypertrophy and is frequently helpful.

HEMODYNAMICS. The large interventricular communication usually results in both pulmonary hypertension and greatly increased lung blood flow. The latter leads to a raised left atrial pressure, whereas the former is associated with the rapid onset of pulmonary vascular obliterative disease. Right and left ventricular pressures are equal. Pulmonary arterial saturation is higher than aortic saturation.

CARDIAC CATHETERIZATION AND ANGIOCARDIOGRAPHY. The catheter course may proceed from the inferior vena cava to the right atrium, to the right ventricle, and to the aorta, or it frequently crosses the VSD to enter the posteriorly placed pulmonary artery. The lateral angiocardiogram reveals the VSD.

Treatment. The neonate with transposition, a large VSD, pulmonary hypertension, and increased pulmonary vascular resistance may make good progress during the neonatal period at the expense of progressive pulmonary vascular obliterative disease. Neonates with transposition appear to do fairly well yet almost invariably develop rapidly advancing pulmonary vascular resistance. One approach is pulmonary artery banding (to reduce distal pulmonary artery hypertension) with or without atrial septectomy, followed by baffle procedure at the earliest possible time. An alternative approach is that of early total correction (by Jetane procedure) before pulmonary vascular obliterative disease has advanced too far.

D-transposition with other anomalies. PDA is common with transposition, and life expectancy is reduced in infants with these conditions when compared with those having similar transposition but without PDA. Pulmonic stenosis is also common but usually is recognized only in the older infant or child. The site of obstruction is commonly below the pulmonary valve, and it is a progressive lesion. Relief of subpulmonic stenosis is surgically difficult. Recent experience indicates that the Mustard correction of venous inflow, leaving the subpulmonic stenosis intact, may be the optimal treatment for infants. If subpulmonic stenosis is severe, an anterior (Waterston) shunt may be indicated.

L-transposition of the great arteries

The presence of a VSD or mitral regurgitation complicating l-transposition (the common form of "corrected" transposition) may lead to heart failure in the newborn period. As in "uncorrected" transposition, pulmonary vascular disease appears to advance at a faster rate than is the case with normally placed great arteries. On occasion a newborn is encountered with corrected transposition, a VSD, and pulmonary hypertension leading to heart failure. These infants may require pulmonary artery banding to limit pulmonary artery blood flow in an attempt to prevent the progress of pulmonary vascular disease. An alternative approach to the infant with l-transposition of the great arteries with VSD and evidence of early onset of pulmonary vascular obliterative disease is that of early surgical closure of the VSD; however, the defects tend to be large, and mortality from corrective surgery in infancy is high.

Left-sided heart obstruction

Left-sided heart obstructive disease is a frequent cause of death in the neonatal period. The designation left-sided heart obstruction is misleading, since various lesions frequently coexist. The following fairly distinctive entities are the most commonly encountered: (1) hypoplastic left-heart syndrome, (2) isolated valvular aortic stenosis, (3) preductal and juxtaductal coarctation of the aorta, and (4) postductal coarctation.

Hypoplastic left-heart syndrome

The term hypoplastic left-heart syndrome covers a group of left-sided heart defects commonly associated with each other. The major components are mitral valve atresia, underdevelopment of the left ventricle (small cavity), aortic valve atresia, and hypoplasia of the ascending aorta. A clinical diagnosis of the syndrome is often possible, but exact delineation of the anatomy requires angiocardiography. Angiocardiography is important to distinguish those patients who have a reasonably normal ascending aorta and arch from those with hypoplasia of these structures. The presence of a good aorta makes palliative surgery possible, whereas with hypoplasia of the aorta (which is usually extreme) surgical correction is controversial at the present time. The hypoplastic left-heart syndrome has some overlap with the preductal coarctation syndrome; however, we shall consider the latter diagnosis to apply only to those cases with a normal-sized left ventricular cavity and normal ascending aorta.

Clinical manifestations. The age at diagnosis ranges from 1 to 21 days. The signs and symptoms are most often those of left-sided heart failure and varying degrees of cyanosis. The typical infant is apathetic and has reduced skin blood flow. Central cyanosis is present, and the arterial pulses are of reduced volume. Doppler measurement of blood pressure commonly is about 60/30 mm Hg in all limbs. The infant breathes rapidly, and frequently there are rales. The precordial impulse is slight-

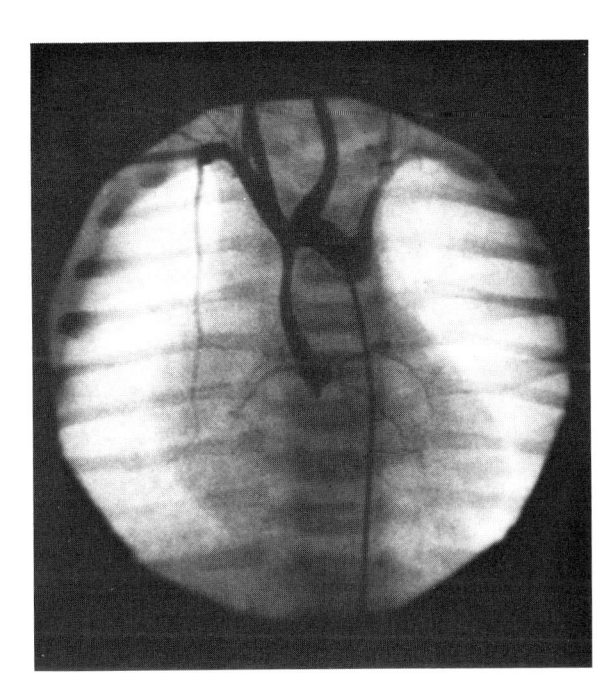

Fig. 25-39. Aortogram in hypoplastic left-heart syndrome. Note diminuitive aortic valve and ascending aorta. There is aortic valve atresia and inadequate coronary flow that is received retrogradely from PDA.

ly overactive unless the neonate is in the final cardiogenic shock phase of his disease. Auscultation most frequently reveals normal timing of the heart sounds but a pulmonary closure sound of increased intensity. Gallop rhythms are common.

Diagnosis. The chest roentgenogram shows that the heart is large, but the contour is not usually diagnostically helpful. If mitral atresia is dominant, the characteristic vascular pattern of pulmonary venous engorgement may be present. The ECG frequently shows a right ventricular hypertrophy pattern (accentuated by the small-sized left ventricle). There may be signs of left, right, or biatrial hypertrophy.

Echocardiography has become a valuable diagnostic tool for noninvasive visualization of the hypoplastic left ventricle. The characteristic pattern is that of a large right ventricle, small left ventricle, and failure to visualize mitral and/or aortic valves (Fig. 25-39). Many centers now regard the typical echocardiogram as obviating the need for cardiac catheterization. Our own approach is to supplement the echocardiogram with an aortogram using the umbilical artery catheter for injection. The stringlike hypoplastic ascending aorta is easily recognized (Fig. 25-39). If the diagnosis is in doubt following these studies, a diagnostic cardiac catheterization may be necessary.

The pH is usually normal unless hypoxemia is extreme. The $PaCO_2$ is normal until left-sided heart failure has produced alveolar transudate and alveolar hypoventilation. Initially there is little response to oxygen breathing because pulmonary capillary blood is almost completely saturated; however, when left-sided heart failure ensues, the hypoxemia caused by alveolar hypoventilation is abolished, whereas that caused by right-to-left shunting remains. Hypoglycemia is frequent, and its recognition and correction improve the chances for survival.

Hemodynamics. The hemodynamics are variable. With mitral atresia it is necessary for blood to flow from left to right across the atrial septum; it then regains the systemic circulation either by way of a VSD or PDA. If aortic atresia is present, a ductal right-to-left shunt is necessary to ensure brachiocephalic artery perfusion and, most important, coronary artery perfusion. In aortic atresia, perfusion of the upper half of the body requires the pulmonary artery pressure to be at systemic levels. The poor prognosis is probably most immediately related to inadequate coronary perfusion.

Treatment. Infants with hypoplastic left-heart syndrome are frequently hypoglycemic as well as acidotic and may benefit from infusion of glucose and sodium bicarbonate in addition to the usual management of heart failure. If mitral atresia or mitral stenosis is a dominant lesion, balloon atrial septostomy during cardiac catheterization may increase left-to-right shunting at the atrial level and allow the left atrial pressure to fall.

The major defect is usually hypoplasia of the left ventricle, and for this there is no direct therapy. Complex palliative surgical procedures have been reported; however, there has been no breakthrough in the treatment of this severe disorder.

Congenital aortic stenosis

It is unusual for this lesion to produce symptoms in the neonate. However, the clinical picture is distinguishable from that of the hypoplastic left-heart syndrome and must be differentiated because of its operability. Isolated congenital aortic stenosis producing serious illness in the neonatal period is practically always valvular, and usually no other cardiac or systemic abnormality is present.

Clinical manifestations. Failure of the left side of the heart leads to tachypnea, inappropriate sweating, and pulmonary rales. Right-sided heart failure with liver enlargement follows, but characteristically pulmonary symptoms continue to predominate. The infant may have surprisingly normal arterial pulses, but Doppler measurements reveal a pulse pressure of only 25 to 30 mm Hg. A systolic murmur is usually obvious and loudest to the right of the sternum or in the suprasternal notch; an accompanying thrill may or may not be present. A gallop rhythm (presystolic) is common. The second sound is usually single, and an aortic ejection click is frequently heard.

Diagnosis. In contrast to the older child, the infant with critical aortic stenosis almost always has conspicuous left ventricular and left atrial enlargement, as shown on a chest roentgenogram. The lung fields appear passively congested. Severe left ventricular hypertrophy with secondary T-wave changes is apparent in most patients. This characteristic helps distinguish the condition from the hypoplastic left-heart syndrome and also provides an index of severity (secondary T-wave changes indicate critical obstruction).

The combination of an ejection systolic murmur maximal at the upper right sternal border, cardiac enlargement, and an ECG showing severe left ventricular hypertrophy is very suggestive of critical congenital aortic stenosis. Myocarditis usually gives rise to low ECG potentials, where as with endocardial fibroelastosis murmurs are not so obvious. Occasionally endocardial fibroelastosis with secondary obstruction to left ventricular outflow may closely simulate congenital aortic stenosis. The presence of pathologic Q waves on the ECG favors a diagnosis of anomalous origin of the left coronary artery from the pulmonary artery rather than aortic stenosis.

The echocardiogram is frequently helpful by showing multiple aortic valve echos or evidence of subvalvular obstruction and by allowing assessment of left atrial size and of left ventricular size and contractility.

The neonate with heart failure from aortic stenosis usually has alveolar hypoventilation from alveolar transudate. The $PaCO_2$ is raised and the PaO_2 lowered. The PaO_2 while the infant is breathing 100% O_2 should increase to above 150 mm Hg unless right-to-left intrapulmonary shunting is occurring through areas of pneumonia or atelectatic lung.

Hemodynamics. Critical aortic stenosis becomes worse with the passage of time. It is difficult to measure left ventricular pressure, since the foramen ovale is often functionally sealed by the raised left atrial pressure, and entry through the aortic valve, even when technically possible, is hazardous. Accordingly, if the left ventricle cannot be entered, an aortogram should be performed. This angiogram will reveal the caliber of the ascending aorta and an indirect assessment of aortic valve area from the diameter of the stream of unopacified blood coming from the left ventricle. In cases of real doubt direct transthoracic needle puncture of the left ventricle may be necessary.

Treatment. Surgery for aortic stenosis in infancy is difficult when compared with that for severe pulmonic stenosis. Residual obstruction and some aortic insufficiency are frequent. If the infant can be brought through the first critical years, further surgery involving the use of valved conduits to bypass the obstruction may be possible.

Preductal coarctation of the aorta

The syndrome of preductal coarctation encompasses a wide spectrum of anatomy. The narrow aortic segment may be discrete and located immediately adjacent to or just above the entry of the ductus (juxtaductal or discrete preductal), or, as is often the case, the obstructed segment may be long and involve the aortic arch. If the *ascending* aorta is hypoplastic, the condition is usually classified as hypoplastic left-heart syndrome. Infants with preductal coarctation almost always have an open ductus so that blood flow to the lower half of the body is from the right ventricle by way of the ductus arteriosus. This would not of itself be dangerous were it not for the fact that right-to-left ductal shunting necessitates extreme pulmonary hypertension and consequent damage to the pulmonary vascular bed. The lungs of the baby with preductal coarctation are faced with a double problem; not only are they subjected to a high vascular pressure, but also the flow through them is reduced (the right-to-left ductal shunt acting as a "runoff" from the pulmonary artery).

Clinical manifestations. The syndrome is quite common (approximately 4%) in infants having cardiac catheterizations. There is a high incidence of associated defects; PDA is almost always present, and VSD, transposition of the great arteries, and complex lesions are common. Neonates with preductal coarctation usually develop tachypnea and cyanosis in the first to third weeks of life. It may be possible to recognize differential cyanosis (for example, blue legs and pink arms). The femoral pulses are frequently palpable and may be entirely normal. This characteristic reflects the normal perfusion of the lower limbs via the patent ductus at normal systemic artery pressure. In some neonates the femoral pulses come and go, presumably secondary to variations in the pulmonary artery pressure. Usually there is either normal pulmonary artery pressure and deficient blood flow to the lower half of the body or high pulmonary artery pressure and normal blood flow to the lower half of the body. The latter is more common and preserves adequate kidney perfusion. Eventually the infant with severe preductal coarctation (and usually associated cardiac anomalies) develops right-sided heart failure. One may hear the characteristic murmur of a coarctation, and sometimes, if hypoplasia of the arch involves the left but not the right subclavian artery, the right arm blood pressure may be higher. Often the signs of an associated VSD predominate.

Diagnosis. The clinical diagnosis is suggested by a neonate who has a loud pulmonary closure sound, a murmur suggestive of a VSD, and signs of left-sided, or left- plus right-sided, heart failure. If the baby shows diminished or varying femoral pulses, the diagnosis is strengthened; and if differential cyanosis is observed, it is virtually certain. The heart is usually slightly enlarged, and the pulmonary arteries appear enlarged (secondary to pulmonary hypertension) on the roentgenogram. The ECG almost always indicates right ventricular hypertrophy. The echocardiogram is useful in the assessment of associated lesions; however, the area of the coarctation cannot be visualized because of the adjacent lung. Preductal coarctation may closely simulate PFC syndrome, and invasive studies may be required to distinguish the two conditions.

Typically the $PaCO_2$ (blood sampled from the right arm) is 50 to 60 mm Hg, and the PaO_2 is 30 to 40 mm Hg. When blood is sampled from the femoral or umbilical artery, the PaO_2 is further lowered by right-to-left ductal shunting to 15 to 30 mm Hg, whereas the $PaCO_2$ is increased only by 2 or 3 mm Hg above that of the right arm sample (because of the small arteriovenous PCO_2 difference). This wide difference is PaO_2 between the right arm and leg and the narrow difference in $PaCO_2$ can be used as a test for right-to-left ductal shunting.

Hemodynamics. Cardiac catheterization of the neonate with uncomplicated preductal coarctation reveals severe right ventricular and pulmonary hypertension. The catheter passes from the pulmonary artery to the descending aorta by way of the usually present PDA. Contrast visualization of the right ventricle discloses filling of the pulmonary artery system and of the descending aorta (via the ductus). Increasing degrees of aortic arch atresia are associated with contrast agent also filling the brachiocephalic arteries, and in the extreme case of aortic valve hypoplasia the coronary arteries will fill from the right ventricular injection. However, at this stage the condition is best regarded as hypoplastic left-heart syndrome rather than preductal coarctation syndrome.

The left ventricle usually can be entered by the foramen ovale and mitral valve, and opacification of this structure will define the aortic valve, coronary arteries, and aorta up to the point where the contrast agent meets the stream of right ventricle—derived blood. Most characteristically the brachiocephalic arteries fill from the left ventricle, and the descending aorta fills from the right; but the pattern in each patient is dependent on the aortic arch anatomy and the vascular resistance in the various organs of the body (Fig. 25-40).

Treatment. The extreme manifestation of preductal coarctation is complete interruption of the aortic arch. In this condition flow to the descending aorta is governed by patency of the ductus arteriosus. If the ductus begins to close, renal failure, acidemia, and other complications rapidly ensue. The infusion of PGE_1 into the pulmonary artery end of the ductus or intravenously has brought about major improvement in renal and metabolic status, allowing surgical intervention to be much more successful.

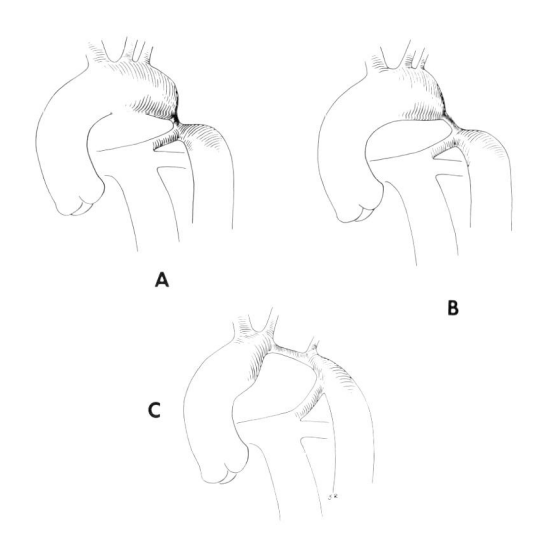

Fig. 25-40. Preductal coarctation of the aorta. Three of the more common variants are (A) juxtaductal localized coarctation, (B) preductal long-segment coarctation with hypoplasia of the left subclavian artery, and (C) aortic isthmus hypoplasia with hypoplasia of the left brachiocephalic arteries. Many other anatomic variations occur, but the physiology is usually that of a "systemic" right ventricle, whereby the descending aorta receives "venous" blood and the pulmonary artery pressure is usually at systemic levels.

Medical treatment of the neonate with preductal coarctation usually results in only temporary improvement. Surgical repair depends on the extent of aortic arch hypoplasia and the presence of associated anomalies. In most cases it is possible to bring down the left subclavian artery and anastomose it directly to the descending aorta (the ductus tissue is usually too friable for this purpose); in other cases an end-to-end anastomosis or Dacron graft replacement is possible. The ductus is divided. Unfortunately pulmonary hypertension may remain (especially if there is an associated VSD); however, in others it is completely reversible. Those infants who survive surgery are usually the ones with short-segment juxtaductal coarctation.

Postductal coarctation of the aorta (with closed ductus arteriosus)

Isolated postductal aortic coarctation sometimes causes problems in the neonatal period. Problems are most commonly encountered when other lesions, especially VSD and PDA, coexist. Infants with simple coarctation of the aorta often can be brought out of heart failure by medical means; operation can be deferred until the infants are of an appropriate age. An infant with absent femoral pulses and heart failure and who is deteriorating requires urgent hemodynamic and angiographic assessment; experience indicates that such infants nearly always have complicating lesions, such as aortic arch hypoplasia or VSD.

Clinical manifestations. The neonate with isolated coarctation of the aorta usually has moderately severe, predominantly left-sided heart failure. Occasionally hypertension may be the initial sign. Physical examination reveals the usual signs of heart failure. A diagnosis of coarctation is suggested by a late systolic ejection murmur heard well posteriorly and is made virtually certain by the absence of palpable femoral pulses. In lesser degrees of coarctation or where a good collateral circulation exists, the femoral pulses may be palpable, but there is a time lag between the brachial and the femoral pulse (normally synchronous). The diagnosis can be strengthened by a comparison of arm and leg systolic pressures with the Doppler technique, and in rare instances the coarctation can be visualized by the imprint of prestenotic and poststenotic dilatation on the barium-filled esophagus. Usually there is little doubt about the diagnosis; the only doubt is whether other lesions coexist.

Diagnosis. The heart is enlarged, and the lung fields frequently show the appearance of pulmonary venous engorgement. Right ventricular hypertrophy is usual. It is unusual to find left ventricular hypertrophy from isolated aortic coarctation before the infant is 6 months of age. The echocardiogram is useful in the assessment of coexisting lesions but cannot be used to directly visualize the coarctation because of lung superimposition. Left-sided heart failure causes an alveolar transudate and impairment of respiratory gas exchange because of alveolar hypoventilation. The breathing of 100% O_2 increases PaO_2 to above 150 mm Hg, but $PaCO_2$ is unchanged.

Hemodynamics. Frequently there is systemic hypertension above the coarctation. In the presence of heart failure right-sided heart pressures are slightly elevated. The coarctation may be delineated in several ways: by left ventricular opacification, by right ventricular opacification and subsequent levocardiogram phase, or, if necessary, by aortography. If the infant is less than 10 days old, the umbilical artery may be used; in older neonates the femoral artery can be located by the Doppler technique and entered percutaneously. A third alternative is the right brachial artery. The objective of hemodynamic study is usually not only the delineation of the coarctation but also the search for a PDA, VSD, bicuspid aortic valve, hypoplastic aortic arch, and so on.

Treatment. The infant with uncomplicated coarctation often responds excellently to medical management. Occasionally a neonate will have a systolic arm blood pressure of 150 mm Hg or higher, and the question arises as to whether antihypertensive treatment is indicated. Current practice is to regard systemic hypertension as an indication for operative relief. If antihypertensive medications are used, they must be used with great caution and with careful observation of the effect on urine production, serum creatinine, and blood urea nitrogen. Drugs that may be used are discussed on p. 619. Use of the right subclavian artery to swing down and patch the obstructed area has greatly diminished the need for second operations later in childhood. An alternative approach is "patch" angioplasty if the right subclavian artery is small or too distant from the coarctation site.

Right-sided heart obstruction

Classification of obstructive disease of the right side of the heart is somewhat arbitrary. The following are the more common entities that produce life-threatening illness in the neonatal period: pulmonary atresia with intact ventricular septum, pulmonary atresia with open ventricular septum (pseudotruncus arteriosus, extreme tetralogy of Fallot), tetralogy of Fallot, isolated valvular pulmonic stenosis, multiple peripheral pulmonary arterial stenosis, tricuspid atresia, and Ebstein's anomaly of the tricuspid valve.

Pulmonary atresia or extreme pulmonic stenosis with intact ventricular septum

Pulmonary atresia with intact ventricular septum is relatively common and is probably underestimated, since afflicted infants may die rapidly after birth. The only sources of blood to the lungs are the ductus arteriosus and the bronchial arteries. In most instances the ductus closes on the first, second, or third day of life even though it is being perfused by blood of low oxygen tension. In a few instances the ductus remains patent (perhaps predestined to be a PDA); consequently older children occasionally are encountered with complete pulmonary atresia and associated ductus arteriosus. The incidence in a series of sick neonates is 9% to 13%. Since the conditions of severe pulmonic stenosis and pulmonary atresia are closely related clinically, hemodynamically, and therapeutically, they are considered here as a single entity. A baby who angiographically appears to have pulmonary atresia sometimes is found at surgery to have a pinhole pulmonary valve orifice.

Clinical manifestations. Neonates with pulmonary atresia show early evidence of distress, presumably corresponding to closure of the ductus arteriosus. Cyanosis is marked. The respirations are characteristically deep, and alveolar ventilation is greatly increased in an unsuccessful attempt to attain physiologic respiratory gas tensions in arterial blood. The infants usually have a good Apgar score, but their color and breathing are noticed to be abnormal a few hours after birth. The cardiac impulse and peripheral pulses are normal, and frequently there is a loud, blowing, systolic murmur at the lower

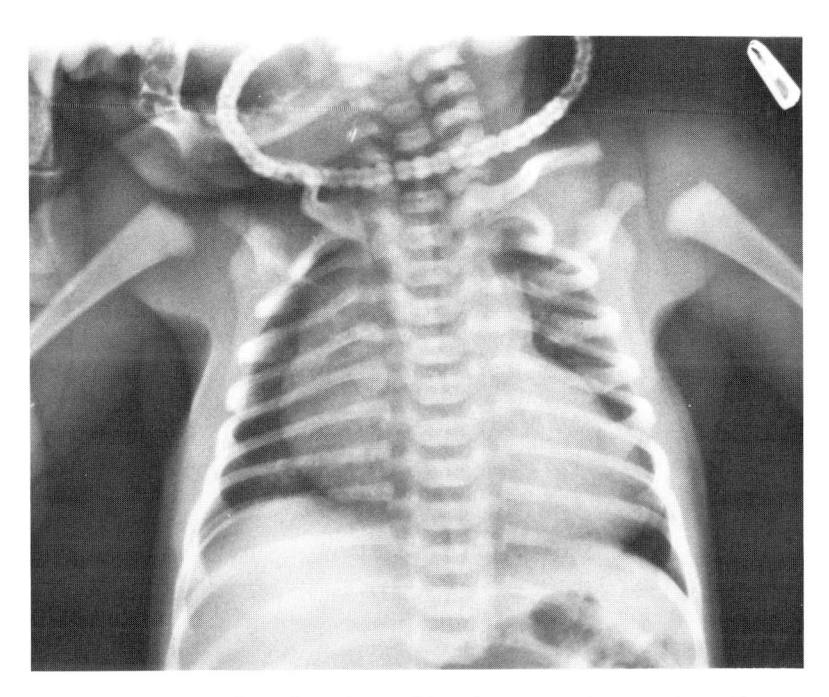

Fig. 25-41. Posteroanterior film of newborn with pulmonary valve atresia and intact ventricular septum. Note large heart and marked decrease in pulmonary vascular markings.

left sternal border, probably representing massive tricuspid regurgitation. A separate continuous murmur of a PDA is frequently heard. The second heart sound is single.

Diagnosis. The most striking finding on the chest roentgenogram is decreased pulmonary vascularity. The heart may be large and often appears egg shaped because of right atrial enlargement; there may be radiologic absence of the main pulmonary artery (Fig. 25-41). Cardiac enlargement is mainly a function of time; the heart may be normal in size during the first hours and days, whereas it is usually greatly enlarged in the occasional infant who survives beyond the neonatal period. There is a spectrum of right ventricular size so that the ECG may show marked right ventricular hypertrophy in those with a large right ventricular cavity, or it may show left ventricular hypertrophy if the right ventricle is hypoplastic, as is frequently the case. Electrocardiographic evidence of right atrial hypertrophy is usually present. Echocardiography is useful in assessing cardiac chamber size and location of the great arteries.

Increased alveolar ventilation results in a pulmonary vein P_{CO_2} of about 25 mm Hg and a pulmonary vein P_{O_2} of about 90 mm Hg. The gross right-to-left atrial shunt results in an arterial P_{CO_2} of about 31 mm Hg and a greatly reduced arterial oxygen saturation. There is no response to oxygen breathing. The arterial pH is often surprisingly normal until the infant is too exhausted to continue the high rates of ventilation necessary to maintain a normal Pa_{CO_2}.

Hemodynamics. The hemodynamics of pulmonary atresia and extreme pulmonic stenosis are similar. The right atrial pressure is moderately raised, and the right ventricular pressure is usually in the 70 to 100 mm Hg systolic range (only slightly above normal for age). Lack of marked elevation of the right ventricular pressure appears to be caused by the gross tricuspid insufficiency that is often present in infants with pulmonary atresia. Right ventricular angiography is pathognomonic; there is often gross tricuspid regurgitation and either complete absence of pulmonary artery filling or very minor opacification of this structure. The size of the right ventricle can best be assessed angiographically. Many appear hypoplastic, but both the ECG and angiogram can be deceptive in the assessment of the adequacy of the right ventricle as a pumping chamber.

Treatment. The treatment has been revolutionized by the use of PGE_1. At the time most infants are referred for diagnosis (6 to 72 hours), the ductus is in the process of closing. Following angiocardiography a catheter is placed through the umbilical artery with its tip at the aortic origin of the ductus. PGE_1 is infused at 0.05 to 0.1 µg/kg/minute. After 10 or 15 minutes the ductus dilates, allowing an increase in pulmonary blood flow and an increase in Pa_{O_2} from about 20 mm Hg to 35 to 40 mm Hg; arterial pH increases, and after a period of several hours the infant is in sufficiently good metabolic condition to allow a surgical shunt to be performed with minimal risk. PGE_1 is almost as effective if given by intravenous infusion.

The outcome of surgery depends to a major extent on the adequacy of the right ventricle. However, in our opinion no neonate should be turned down for surgery because of a hypoplastic right ventricle. In those rare infants with an adequate right ventricle and isolated critical valvular pulmonic stenosis, a pulmonary valvotomy (transventricular or transpulmonary-arterial) is dramatically successful. Those infants with right ventricular hypoplasia often will require a right pulmonary artery–to-aorta shunt (Waterston procedure) instead of, or in addition to, relief of right ventricular outflow obstruction. Although mortality is still significant at the present time, the use of PGE_1 and greater alertness and speed at every stage of referral, combined with surgical advances, are steadily improving the prognosis.

Pulmonary atresia with open ventricular septum and severe tetralogy of Fallot

Pulmonary atresia with open ventricular septum may be thought of as the extreme form of tetralogy of Fallot; there is complete obstruction to right ventricular outflow. It has been referred to at times as pseudotruncus arteriosus, or type IV truncus arteriosus, since the source of lung blood flow is the aorta (bronchial arteries). The distinction between severely symptomatic tetralogy of Fallot (that is, continuity between right ventricular outflow tract and pulmonary arteries) and complete pulmonary atresia with open ventricular septum usually is not possible to make clinically. It is readily made by right ventricular angiography.

Clinical manifestations. Infants are cyanotic from birth but usually do not cause concern until a few hours after birth, because temporary patency of the ductus arteriosus allows adequate pulmonary artery blood flow. On the first or second day of life the ductus closes, and the neonate becomes strikingly symptomatic with deep, sighing respirations, increasing central cyanosis, and lethargy. The cardiac impulse is hypodynamic, or one may feel a right parasternal tapping impulse. The second heart sound is single and maximal at the second right interspace (aortic valve closure), and there is frequently an aortic ejection click. There may be no murmur, or there may be a short ejection murmur of tight infundibular stenosis at the third left interspace.

Diagnosis. The heart is small or normal in size (in contrast to most other cyanotic lesions) and the pulmonary vasculature strikingly diminished. Even on the first day of life the heart may have the characteristic *coeur en sabot* shape of tetralogy (Fig. 25-42, *A*). Moderate right atrial and right ventricular hypertrophy is usual but is not diagnostically helpful. The echocardiogram frequently is helpful by showing aortic override. Alveolar hyperventilation produces a high pulmonary venous PO_2 and low pulmonary venous PCO_2; when pulmonary venous blood is admixed with systemic venous blood (at atrial and ventricular levels), hypoxemia and hypercapnia result in acidosis. In the first hours after birth surprisingly normal arterial blood gases can be found; but as the infant tires, ventilation falls, and acidosis results. There is no response to the breathing of 100% O_2, since hypoxemia is secondary to right-to-left shunting.

Hemodynamics. Diminished pulmonary blood flow leads to diminished left atrial pressure, with consequent right-to-left atrial shunting across the foramen ovale. Blood enters the right ventricle and, in the case of total outflow tract obstruction, leaves to enter the aorta (in systole) and the left ventricle (in diastole). The only source of lung blood flow is via bronchial arteries and in some instances a ductus arteriosus. Clearly the baby's survival is unlikely unless bronchial artery flow is excessive or the ductus remains open. Right ventricular systolic pressure is at systemic level, and the catheter usually enters the aorta readily (across the VSD). Diagnosis is confirmed by angiocardiography (Fig. 25-42, *B*).

Treatment. A neonate with pulmonary atresia and open ventricular septum considered sick enough to require diagnostic heart catheterization is practically always going to require palliative surgery. In the critical time between diagnosis and surgery the use of PGE_1 to dilate the ductus usually proves lifesaving (p. 623). Total correction in the neonatal age group has proved difficult, since reconstruction of the outflow tract and atretic pulmonary valve and artery requires the use of a homograft or synthetic conduit. In many centers the Waterston procedure (anastomosis of ascending aorta to right pulmonary artery) or the Goretex shunt (U-shaped prosthesis between aorta and pulmonary artery) has supplanted the Blalock and Potts shunt as the first choice for increasing

Fig. 25-42. Severe tetralogy of Fallot. **A,** Note normal-sized heart with marked decrease in pulmonary vascular markings. There is a slight "coeur en sabot" configuration to the heart. **B,** Right ventricular angiogram in pulmonary atresia with open ventricular septum. Note hypoplastic right ventricle *(RV)*, blind-ending right ventricular infundibulum *(RVI)*, and greatly enlarged aorta *(Ao)* receiving right ventricular contents.

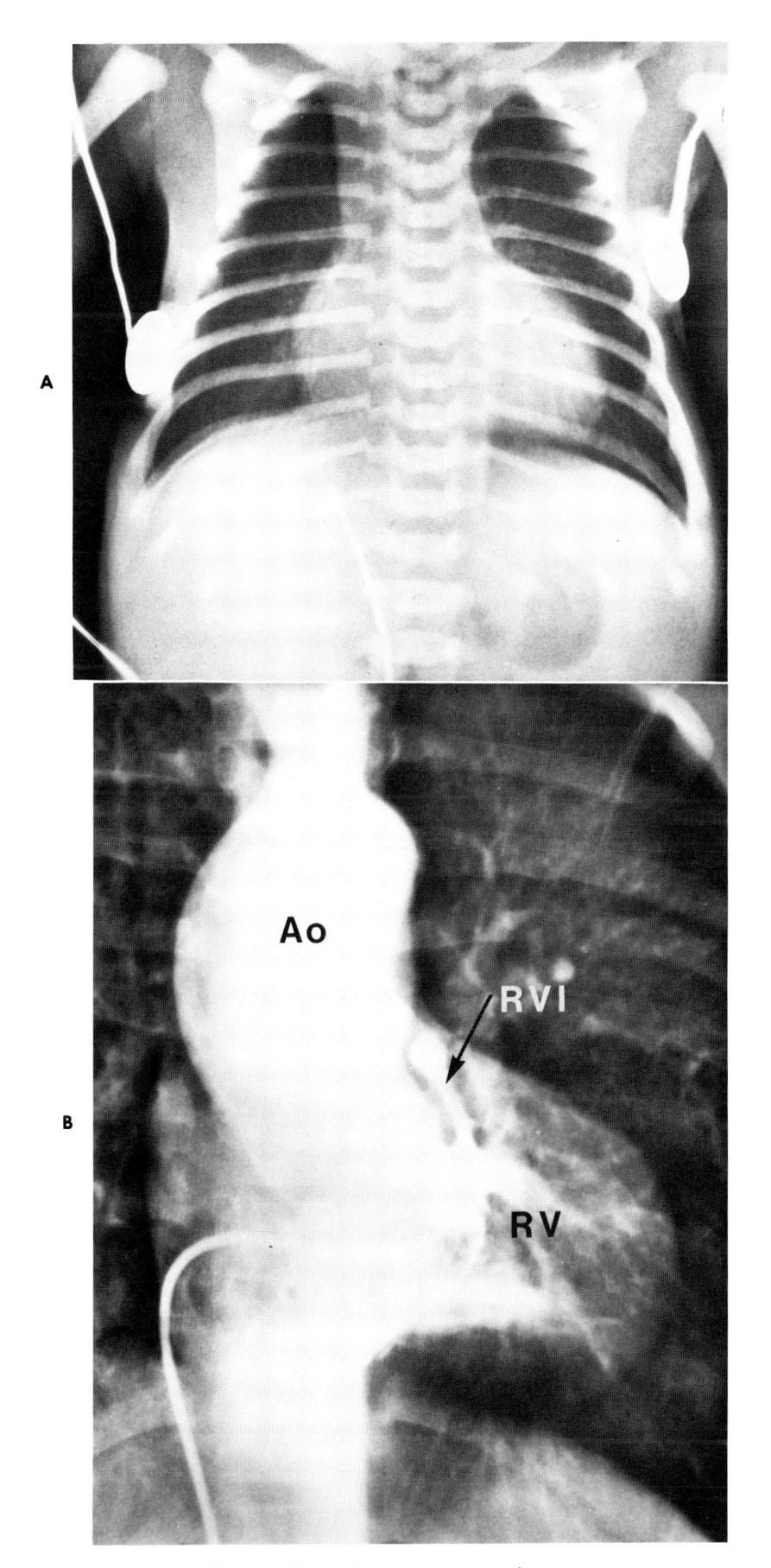

Fig. 25-42. For legend see opposite page.

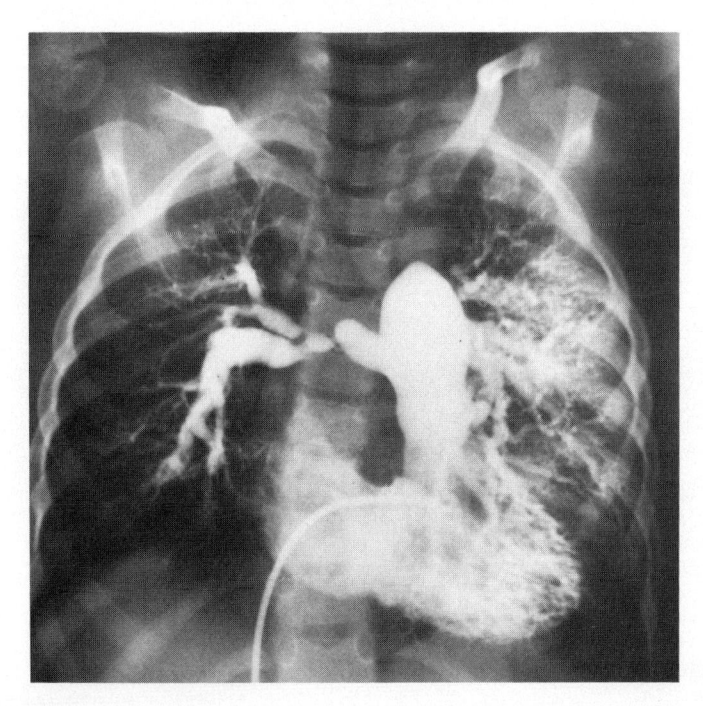

Fig. 25-43. Angiographic appearances in multiple peripheral pulmonary artery stenoses. In this particular case, Ehlers-Danlos syndrome was present, and there were associated abnormalities of systemic arteries. The left lung had been operated on, but many areas of stenosis remain in the right lung.

the pulmonary blood flow in the newborn. In selected cases, where an adequate-sized main pulmonary artery exists, a Brock procedure (transventricular "reaming out" of infundibular obstruction) may be preferable. At the time of surgery the presence and size of the main pulmonary artery are noted, since this structure will be hard to visualize later in the child's life and a knowledge of its size is mandatory before plans are made for total correction in early childhood. It is important to note that infants with numerous systemic-pulmonary collateral arteries (SPCAs) will often appear only slightly cyanotic yet require central surgical shunt procedures to cause growth of the central pulmonary arteries and allow ultimate total correction. The results of palliative surgery for pulmonary atresia with open ventricular septum are complicated by the fact that there is frequently coexistent right ventricular hypoplasia and hypoplasia of the pulmonary arterial system. Rudolph and associates have reported the use of formalin infiltration of the walls of the ductus arteriosus in neonates as a palliative technique for maintaining pulmonary blood flow when suitable vessels for a shunt procedure cannot be found.

Multiple peripheral pulmonary arterial stenoses

The most frequent cause of important pulmonary arterial stenoses giving rise to symptoms in the neonate is intrauterine rubella infection (p. 701). A familial incidence of peripheral pulmonary arterial stenosis also has been recognized, and there is evidence that idiopathic hypercalcemia of infancy is frequently associated with combined pulmonary arterial and supravalvular aortic stenosis. On occasion peripheral pulmonary artery stenosis is associated with various forms of congenital heart disease, especially tetralogy of Fallot. Cases of cutis laxa (generalized elastolysis), Ehlers-Danlos syndrome, arteriohepatic dysplasia, and Takayasu's disease all have been reported in association with peripheral pulmonary arterial stenosis.

Clinical manifestations. The symptoms are those of predominant right-sided heart failure unless there is a PDA (as is frequently the case), in which case right-to-left ductal shunting leads to cyanosis. In severe cases the lungs are underperfused so that there is an increase in pulmonary ventilation similar to that seen in severe tetralogy or pulmonic stenosis. Classically, continuous murmurs are heard in several areas of the chest; however, in many instances only nondescript systolic murmurs are heard. The pulmonary closure sound may be very loud, since, although there are peripheral areas of obstruction, central pulmonary arterial pressure is greatly increased.

Diagnosis. The areas of stenosis are associated with poststenotic dilatation (Fig. 25-43). These may be visible occasionally on the plain film and may give a spurious impression of adequate or even increased vascular markings. The heart is usually small, unless it has dilated from right-sided heart failure. Right ventricular hypertrophy, often of severe degree, is typical. As the child grows and the obstruction becomes relatively more severe, right ventricular hypertrophy increases and is a useful measurement of progress or deterioration. Signs of right atrial hypertrophy are common. Alveolar hyperventilation without right-to-left shunting produces lowered $PaCO_2$ and increased or normal O_2 saturation. Ductal right-to-left shunts are frequent, in which case cyanosis, unresponsive to 100% O_2 breathing, is present.

Determination of IgM fraction and rubella antibody titer is indicated. If a generalized disorder, such as cutis laxa or Ehlers-Danlos syndrome, is suspected, a skin biopsy may be worthwhile. Serum calcium and phosphorus levels should be determined because of their association with hypercalcemia.

Hemodynamics. Very high (200 mm Hg) right ventricular and central pulmonary arterial pressures may be found. Right atrial pressure rises as a consequence of raised right ventricular end-diastolic pressure, and right-to-left shunting through the foramen ovale is common. Definitive diagnosis can be made by observing pressure gradients within the pulmonary arterial system, but pulmonary angiography is essential if surgery is contemplated. Selective angiography defines the exact location and length of stenotic areas and determines the feasibility of corrective surgery.

Treatment. Total correction is rarely possible, since almost invariably the stenotic areas are very numerous. Occasionally a single stenosis in the main pulmonary artery or a small number of stenoses in primary, secondary, and tertiary divisions can be patch grafted. Such a patient is illustrated in Fig. 25-43. Although the surgery is time consuming, one advantage is that cardiopulmonary bypass usually is not necessary, since one lung may be operated on while the other serves for gas exchange.

Tricuspid atresia

Atresia of the tricuspid valve may occur with normally placed great arteries; tricuspid atresia without transposition is invariably associated with right ventricular hypoplasia and frequently with pulmonary valve hypoplasia. The presence of a VSD or PDA is necessary for blood to gain access to the pulmonary artery. Because the coexistence of transposed great arteries produces a very different clinical picture from that in patients with normally positioned great arteries, tricuspid atresia and tricuspid atresia with transposed great arteries are considered separately in the following sections.

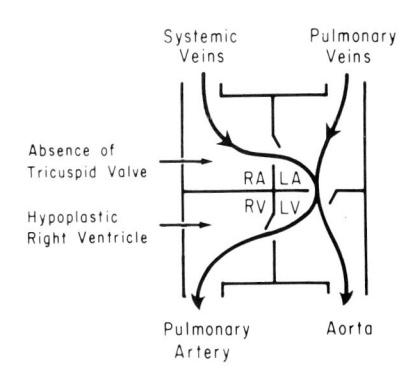

Fig. 25-44. The circulation in tricuspid atresia with patent foramen ovale and VSD.

Tricuspid atresia with ventricular septal defect and normally positioned great arteries

Clinical manifestations. Cyanosis is present from birth. Infants with a small VSD have greatly diminished pulmonary blood flow, whereas those with a large VSD may have increased pulmonary blood flow. Diminished lung blood flow is more frequent; and it tends to diminish further with time, since there is evidence that the VSD becomes progressively smaller with growth. A further limitation to pulmonary blood flow is the size of the foramen ovale or ASD (Fig. 25-44). Pulmonary underperfusion leads to hyperventilation; and the respirations, although not unduly rapid, are increased in tidal volume. The cardiac impulse is quiet; frequently a thrill caused by a VSD is present at the lower left sternal border. The arterial pulses are normal. The second sound is frequently single, and a loud grade 4 pansystolic VSD murmur is heard maximally at the fourth left interspace. The clinical findings suggest a VSD, except that the infant is cyanotic.

Diagnosis. A few infants have a characteristic square-shaped heart, but the radiologic appearances are very variable and are influenced by the size of the ASD and VSD. In the majority of cases pulmonary vasculature is obviously diminished (Fig. 25-45). The ECG is of major diagnostic significance. In over 80% of the cases both left axis deviation and left ventricular hypertrophy are present. T-wave inversion in leads V_5 and V_6 is frequent. A typical ECG is shown in Fig. 25-46. The echocardiogram, especially the sector scan, is useful in defining chamber size.

Pulmonary underperfusion and overventilation produce a low PCO_2 and high PO_2 in pulmonary vein blood. However, since there is almost complete mixing at the left ventricular level, the final arterial blood gas tensions depend largely on the ratio of pulmonary venous to systemic venous return. The pH and $PaCO_2$ are usually normal, although the PaO_2 is greatly reduced because of the very wide arteriovenous PO_2 difference.

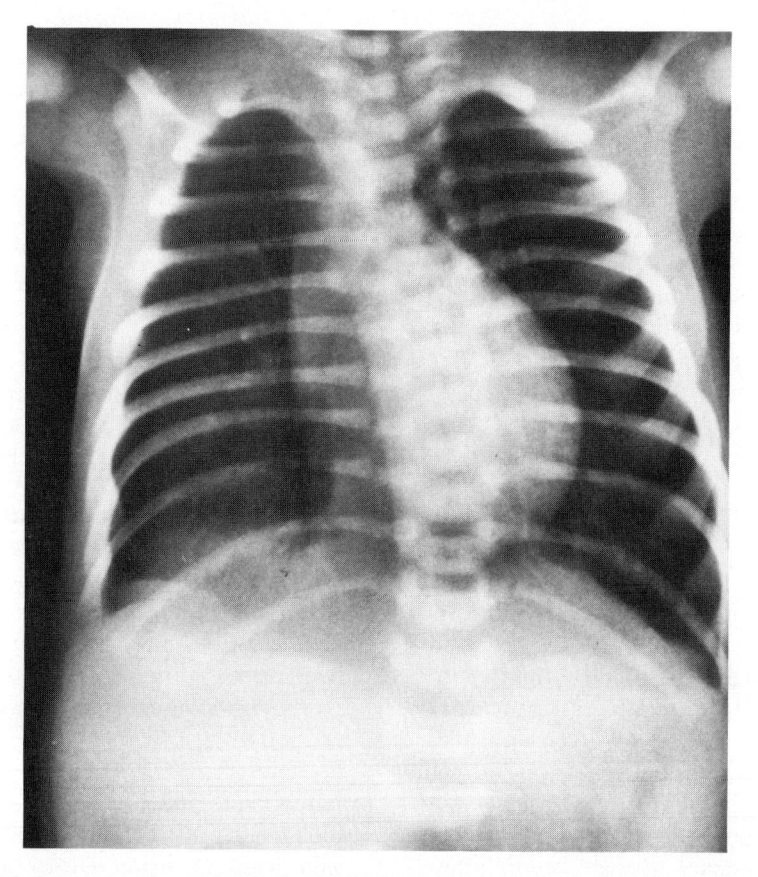

Fig. 25-45. Posteroanterior chest film of a neonate with tricuspid atresia. Note small heart, straight right cardiac border, and decreased pulmonary vascular markings. The plain chest film in tricuspid atresia shows considerable variation in the cardiac contour between patients.

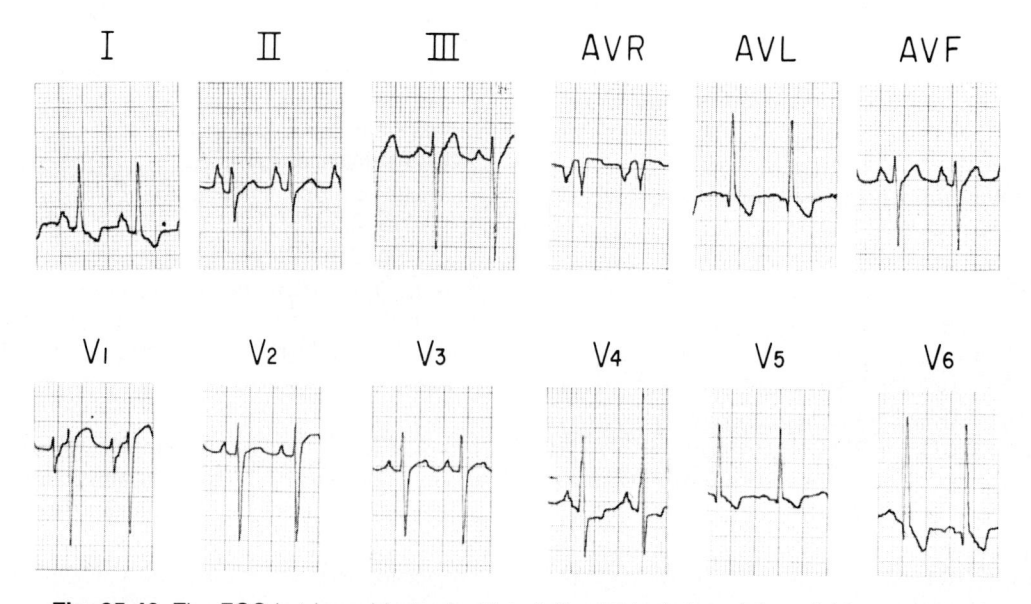

Fig. 25-46. The ECG in tricuspid atresia. Note left axis deviation, right atrial hypertrophy, and left ventricular hypertrophy with "strain" (negative T waves in leads I, V_5, and V_6).

The breathing of 100% O_2 has almost no effect on arterial P_{O_2}.

HEMODYNAMICS. The diagnosis is usually obvious before cardiac catheterization, and the hemodynamics are very characteristic. It is impossible to direct the catheter tip into the right ventricle (ordinarily accomplished without delay). Instead the catheter passes immediately from the right atrium into the left atrium and can be manipulated into the pulmonary veins and left ventricle. Right atrial angiography reveals the sequence of right atrium, left atrium, left ventricle, and then simultaneous filling of the aorta and pulmonary artery. There may be an unopacified wedge (especially apparent in the frontal projection) corresponding to the hypoplastic right ventricle. On occasion the pulmonary artery can be entered (across a VSD); the pressure is low unless the defect is substantial. The aorta usually can be entered with a flow-guided catheter and is easily visualized by contrast opacification of the left ventricle.

Treatment. There is no definitive correction for tricuspid atresia at the present time. The limiting factor is the hypoplastic right ventricle. There are, however, various palliative maneuvers. If a gradient is found between the right and left atria, a balloon septostomy may aid systemic venous return and lower right atrial pressure. Palliative surgery is designed to increase pulmonary blood flow by means of an ascending aorta–to–right pulmonary artery shunt (Waterston shunt). The Fontan procedure, whereby a conduit is placed between the right atrium and pulmonary artery, is gradually becoming technically feasible in neonates.

Tricuspid atresia with transposed great arteries. The neonate with this condition usually has also a large ventricular defect. The problem is not so much hypoxemia as pulmonary overcirculation and pulmonary hypertension. The defect may become apparent on the first day of life or after the neonatal period.

Clinical manifestations. Neonates with transposition and tricuspid atresia are cyanotic but usually not as blue as those without transposition. Respirations are rapid but of small or normal volume, typical for the infant with overperfused lungs. The cardiac impulse is hyperdynamic, and the arterial pulses are normal. If pulmonary overcirculation is marked, the signs of left-sided heart failure appear, followed by those of right-sided failure. In severe cases there are pulmonary rales, and the infant dies from hypoxemia, hypercapnia, and acidosis.

Diagnosis. The heart is frequently very large and similar to that of uncomplicated transposition. The pulmonary vascular markings are increased. Some infants show the classic left axis deviation and left ventricular hypertrophy of uncomplicated tricuspid atresia. Others display normal axis or right axis deviation. The echocardiogram is useful in defining chamber and great vessel localization. $PaCO_2$ is usually normal. PaO_2 is decreased and unresponsive to the breathing of 100% O_2. Initially the arterial pH is normal, but when heart failure supervenes and $PaCO_2$ rises, acidosis develops.

HEMODYNAMICS. The catheter course follows the right atrium, left atrium, left ventricle route. Left ventricular angiography, when filmed in the lateral projection, reveals the transposed great arteries. The aorta frequently can be entered by passage of the catheter from the left ventricle across a large VSD. Most patients have severe pulmonary hypertension and greatly increased pulmonary blood flow.

Treatment. Tricuspid atresia with transposed great arteries is one of the more difficult entities to treat. Theoretically pulmonary artery banding should limit pulmonary blood flow and protect the lungs from developing vascular obliterative changes. In practice, however, the small hemodynamic advantage gained from pulmonary artery banding does not offset the hazard of thoracotomy in a small, sick infant, and the immediate mortality is very high. Long-term management should be directed toward ensuring that the pulmonary vascular resistance stays low enough for the pulmonary arteries to accept a Fontan (right atrium to pulmonary artery) conduit.

Ebstein's anomaly of the tricuspid valve

The tricuspid valve is malformed and is attached partly to the anulus fibrosus and partly to the right ventricular endocardium. The posterior leaflets, which are often grossly malformed and sometimes vestigial or absent, are usually displaced downward. The resulting tricuspid valve is usually both stenotic and incompetent and is displaced deeply into the right ventricular cavity, dividing it into two chambers. The area of the right ventricle proximal to the valve is abnormally thin and sometimes aneurysmal.

Incidence. Ebstein's anomaly is uncommon (about 1 in 50,000 to 1 in 100,000), but its clinical recognition is important, since, if it is discovered in the neonatal period, one should be cautious in considering cardiac catheterization because of the risk involved in precipitating an arrhythmia. Spontaneous improvement in the first months of life is not unusual. Congenital Ebstein's anomaly often is undetected in the neonatal period, and such infants have no symptoms unless there is a bout of SVT.

Clinical manifestations. The initial symptom in the neonatal period is usually cyanosis. This is caused by right-to-left shunting across a patent foramen ovale or ASD secondary to raised right atrial pressure. Frequently there is a triple or quadruple rhythm caused by third or fourth heart sounds. A systolic murmur of moderate intensity is heard at the middle or lower left sternal border, and a presystolic murmur is often present. The pres-

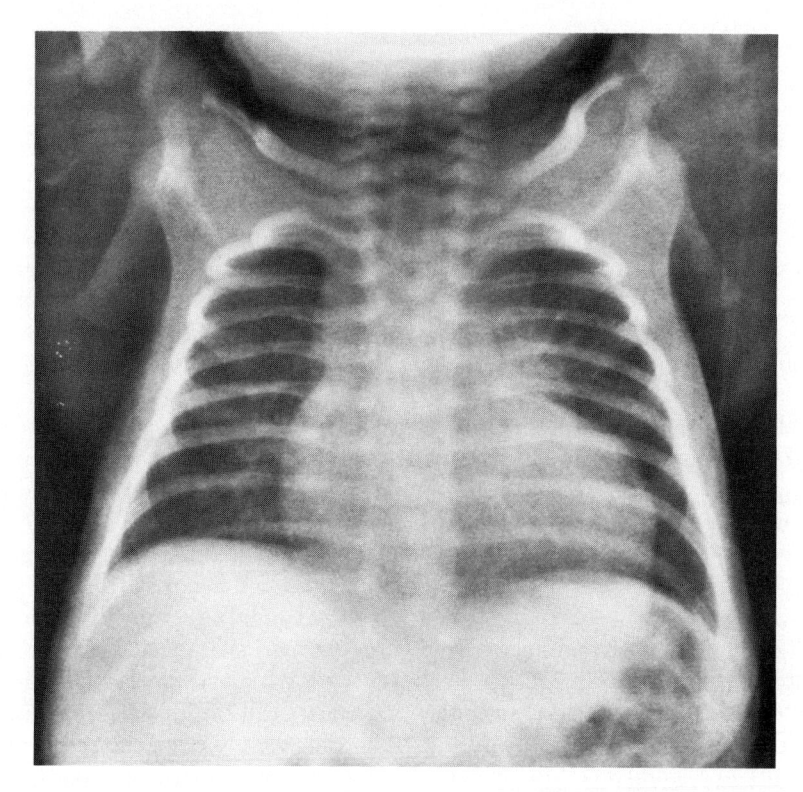

Fig. 25-47. Posteroanterior chest film from a neonate with Ebstein's anomaly of the tricuspid valve. There is cardiomegaly and decreased pulmonary vascular markings.

ence of multiple heart sounds and murmurs when combined with the rapid heart rate of the neonate leads to a confusing auscultatory picture. Phonocardiographic analysis may be of great diagnostic help. Although the right atrial pressure may be raised slightly, congestive heart failure is uncommon, since right-to-left shunting limits the elevation of right atrial pressure. Where the foramen ovale is small, however, congestive heart failure may ensue.

Diagnosis. The classic findings are those of gross cardiomegaly with pulmonary undercirculation, as shown by a chest roentgenogram. The right atrium accounts for most of the cardiac enlargement. In symptomatic neonates the right atrium usually is enlarged; however, the roentgenogram may closely simulate that of pulmonic stenosis or pulmonary atresia with intact ventricular septum (Fig. 25-47). Arrhythmias are frequent; ectopic beats, SVT, atrial flutter, and atrial fibrillation are all common; nodal rhythm and AV dissociation are less common. The Wolff-Parkinson-White syndrome occurs in approximately 9% of cases. Many infants have electrocardiographic evidence of right atrial hypertrophy, and some have prolongation of the PR interval. Right bundle branch block is common in older children and, although uncommon in the neonate, is very suggestive of Ebstein's anomaly. The symptomatic newborn with Ebstein's anomaly invariably has right-to-left atrial shunting, and the blood gases reflect the situation. The $PaCO_2$ and pH are normal, but the PaO_2 is low and is not significantly increased by the infant's breathing 100% O_2. The echocardiogram results may be pathognomonic, with large excursion and delayed closure of the tricuspid valve.

Hemodynamics. It is sometimes possible to make a firm diagnosis of Ebstein's anomaly in the neonate, based on physical signs with characteristic roentgenographic and ECG findings. Unless the neonate is critically sick, hemodynamic study is best deferred, since spontaneous improvement is common, and catheterization may precipitate an arrhythmia. If the infant's condition is deteriorating, cardiac catheterization is indicated because there are very characteristic findings and surgical treatment is possible. By cardiac catheterization the diagnosis is suggested by a high right atrial pressure, evidence of right-to-left atrial shunting, and difficulty or inability to cross the tricuspid valve. If the tricuspid valve can be crossed, there is a characteristic short ejection phase on the right ventricular pressure tracing; the intracardiac ECG may demonstrate that, although the catheter tip is in the right atrium, a right ventricular intracavitary ECG is being recorded (because of the prolapse of the atrium into the ventricle). Angiocardiography is very helpful in disclosing the anatomy of tricuspid valve.

Treatment. Treatment is rarely required in the neonatal period and can be deferred until the child is large enough to undergo replacement of the anomaly with a prosthetic valve or to undergo tricuspid valvuloplasty. If treatment in the neonatal period is essential for survival, consideration should be given to the use of tolazoline (Priscoline) to lower pulmonary vascular resistance.

Lesions that produce common mixing of venous and arterial blood

The four most important lesions that produce common mixing of venous and arterial blood are truncus arteriosus, very large VSD or common ventricle, double-outlet right ventricle without pulmonic stenosis, and total anomalous pulmonary venous return. A single atrium produces common mixing but rarely gives rise to serious illness in the neonate. Patients with these lesions tend to have certain features in common: mild cyanosis, a hyperactive cardiac impulse, cardiomegaly with increased pulmonary blood flow, and pulmonary hypertension. The cyanosis may go undetected, since the volume of well-oxygenated pulmonary vein blood exceeds that of the systemic vein blood. The resulting admixed arterial saturation is closer to pulmonary vein levels than it is to systemic vein levels. Frequently the saturation is 88% to 90%, and cyanosis will be obvious only when the hematocrit value is high.

Persistent truncus arteriosus

Two percent to 4% of severely sick neonates with heart disease have this lesion. The recognition of truncus arteriosus, although a relatively uncommon lesion, has become important since the advent of palliative and corrective surgery.

Pathology. The designation *truncus arteriosus* implies that only one artery arises from the heart and that this artery (the truncus arteriosus) gives rise to coronary arteries, pulmonary arteries, and the aorta. The truncus arteriosus almost always overrides a large VSD. The fact that the pulmonary arteries are of normal size necessitates the existence of severe pulmonary hypertension or greatly increased pulmonary blood flow; usually both are present. Various anatomic subtypes exist, depending on the exact point of origin of the pulmonary arteries from the truncus arteriosus. The so-called pseudotruncus, or type IV truncus, in the Collet-Edwards classification is now classified as tetralogy of Fallot with pulmonary atresia, the blood supply to the lung being bronchial-arterial rather than pulmonary-arterial.

Clinical manifestations. The major problem facing neonates born with a persistent truncus arteriosus is gross pulmonary overperfusion and pulmonary hypertension (usually at systemic artery pressure). In rare instances the pulmonary arteries are somewhat hypoplastic, allowing near-normal pulmonary blood flow and pulmonary artery pressure. Neonates with truncus arteriosus appear only *mildly cyanotic;* respirations are rapid but not deep. When left-sided heart failure supervenes, the signs of respiratory distress appear. The cardiac impulse is hyperactive, and the peripheral arterial pulses are bounding. The second heart sound is single and loud; there is commonly a loud, pansystolic murmur of a VSD at the lower left sternal border and on occasion a loud, continuous murmur at the upper left sternal border or an early diastolic murmur of truncal insufficiency. The general picture resembles that of a neonate with a large PDA (a neonate with a large PDA is frequently cyanotic from alveolar hypoventilation secondary to left-sided heart failure).

Diagnosis. The heart size is frequently massive, and the pulmonary vascular markings are very prominent. The sign of "high" origin of the pulmonary artery is not useful in the newborn period. Right ventricular hypertrophy is almost always present, and sometimes there is biventricular hypertrophy. The echocardiogram characteristically shows override of the aorta. Arterial pH and Pco_2 are normal unless the neonate is in heart failure. Pao_2 is low and unresponsive to the infant's breathing of 100% O_2. If heart failure supervenes, that part of the Pao_2 depression caused by hypoventilation is improved by 100% O_2 breathing.

Hemodynamics. There is right ventricular hypertension, and the catheter passes from the right ventricle into the truncus arteriosus. That the pulmonary arteries can usually be entered from the common trunk suggests the diagnosis, which is confirmed by contrast visualization of the truncus arteriosus. The lateral view is useful in defining the exact site of origin of the pulmonary artery (Fig. 25-48).

Treatment. Many neonates respond well to medical measures. However, the response is at the expense of increasing pulmonary vascular resistance. Our policy has been to treat the neonate medically and then, in consultation with the thoracic team, to make a decision as to whether the baby will grow rapidly enough to allow a total correction in the first year or two of life. If, as is often the case, the baby gains weight extremely slowly, banding of the pulmonary artery is necessary to lower pulmonary blood flow, reduce distal pulmonary artery pressure, and allow the infant to grow faster. Definitive surgical repair consists essentially of closing the VSD, disconnecting the pulmonary artery from its truncal ori-

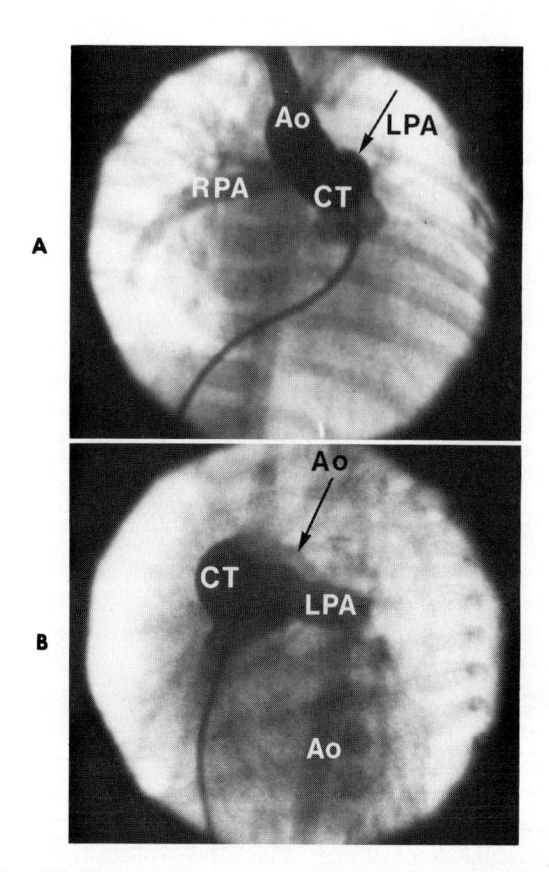

Fig. 25-48. Truncus arteriosus. Single frames taken from cineangiogram. **A,** Anteroposterior projection. Note right *(RPA)* and left *(LPA)* pulmonary arteries arising from the common trunk *(CT)*. Some truncal valve regurgitation is evident. **B,** Lateral projection showing the left pulmonary artery arising from the posterior aspect of the trunk. The trunk continues as the aorta *(Ao)*.

gin, and joining the pulmonary artery to the edges of the right ventriculotomy by means of a woven Dacron graft or aortic homograft. A prosthetic heart valve is sutured inside the tubular graft, where it functions as a pulmonary valve (Rastelli procedure).

Single ventricle

A single ventricle is very commonly associated with other anomalies: pulmonic stenosis, common atrium, ASD, and endocardial cushion defects. Thirty-five percent to 40% of neonates with this anomaly die in the first week of life.

Clinical manifestations. Mild to moderate cyanosis is present depending on the ratio of pulmonary to systemic blood flow. There is usually no murmur, or there is a nondescript left parasternal systolic murmur. Most infants without pulmonic stenosis have greatly increased pulmonary blood flow so that respirations tend to be rapid. If heart failure ensues, other signs of respiratory distress appear.

Diagnosis. The heart is large, and pulmonary vascularity is increased. Usually the ECG signs of biventricular hypertrophy are present. In the majority of cases normal Q waves are seen. The echocardiogram confirms absence of the septum.

Hemodynamics. Common mixing occurs at the ventricular level so that arterial saturation is in the 88% to 92% range. If no other lesions are present, there is increased pulmonary blood flow and pulmonary hypertension. The large number of associated lesions makes selective angiography mandatory for detailed diagnosis.

Treatment. Surgical treatment is possible by converting the single ventricle to a systemic ventricle and providing pulmonary blood flow with a Fontan conduit. In the neonatal period banding of the pulmonary artery may be required to allow survival to the age for definitive repair.

Double-outlet right ventricle without pulmonic stenosis

Double-outlet right ventricle occurs in 2% to 3% of neonates with congenital heart disease. The lesion almost always is associated with anomalies of the aortic arch and with VSD. Extracardiac defects are common, and there is an association with trisomy 18 syndrome.

Clinical manifestations. Mild cyanosis is present. The obligatory increase in pulmonary artery pressure and pulmonary blood flow rapidly produces tachypnea followed by right-sided heart failure. The outcome often is determined by the degree of hypoplasia of the aortic arch and by the location of the VSD. The murmur of a VSD is usually present.

Diagnosis. Gross cardiomegaly and increased pulmonary vascular markings are characteristic. There is usually combined ventricular hypertrophy. The diagnosis rests on angiographic evidence of the great artery origins. The aortic and pulmonary valves both arise from the right ventricle (anterior ventricle) and at the same level (normally the pulmonary valve is higher). Frequently there is hypoplasia of the aortic arch.

Treatment. Infants may benefit from pulmonary artery banding to allow survival to the age of 2 to 3 years, at which time definitive repair can be undertaken. The VSD patch is positioned in such a way as to incorporate the aortic origin into the left ventricle. Double-outlet right ventricle *with* pulmonic stenosis is rarely observed in the neonatal period; the obstruction is often subvalvular in location.

Total anomalous pulmonary venous return

Total anomalous pulmonary venous return implies the return of all pulmonary venous blood directly or indirectly to the right atrium and requires the presence of an ASD in order that blood may reach the left atrium, left ventricle, and systemic circulation. The lesion is important, since it is frequently surgically correctable. The incidence is 2% to 4%.

Clinical manifestations. The lesion appears at all ages in childhood. The most important determinant of the time of presentation appears to be the degree of obstruction to pulmonary venous return. Infants with total anomalous pulmonary venous return, who become seriously sick in the newborn period, almost always have a degree of obstruction to the return of pulmonary venous blood. There is increased pulmonary vein pressure, increased pulmonary capillary pressure, and increased pulmonary artery pressure. When the pulmonary veins drain directly into the right atrium and there is a large ASD, the hemodynamics are very similar to those of an ASD. The mild arterial unsaturation that is present may go unnoticed for many years. They usually have drainage of the anomalous veins below the diaphragm and into the liver or into the superior vena caval system, with inadequate caliber of the left innominate vein.

Clinically there is marked tachypnea, and pulmonary rales are heard if pulmonary venous pressure is elevated. Less commonly the signs of right-sided heart failure develop secondary to raised right atrial pressure. The infants are mildly or moderately cyanotic. A gallop rhythm is frequently present, and there is marked right ventricular overactivity. Commonly there is no murmur. If present, the murmur often resembles that of an ASD with a midsystolic ejection component at the upper left sternal border and a flow murmur of relative tricuspid stenosis at the lower left sternal border. Frequently the second heart sound is widely split and fixed with regard to respiration.

Pathology. There are four main types, according to the mode of entry of the pulmonary veins into the right side of the heart: (1) drainage of pulmonary veins into the right atrium, directly or via the coronary sinus, (2) drainage into the right superior vena cava or azygos vein, (3) drainage into a persistent left superior vena cava, which then empties into the left innominate vein, and (4) drainage of a common pulmonary venous collecting trunk below the diaphragm into the portal vein or ductus venosus. There are a large number of variations of these four basic types.

Diagnosis. The radiographic contours considered characteristic of the condition (figure-of-eight and so on) are not often seen in the newborn, presumably because insufficient time has elapsed for superior vena caval distension to occur. In the newborn the observation of a small heart with the pattern of pulmonary *venous* congestion is very suggestive of total anomalous pulmonary venous return with obstruction (see Fig. 25-3). In those without obstruction but with overwhelming pulmonary blood flow there is cardiomegaly and an increase in pulmonary *arterial* markings. The ECG shows moderate right ventricular hypertrophy. There is usually complete reversal of R/S progression in the precordial leads. Signs of right atrial hypertrophy are frequent. The arterial pH and Pco_2 are usually normal unless heart failure is present. The Pao_2 is inevitably lowered, although cyanosis may not be clinically apparent (arterial saturation 88% to 92%). The Pao_2 will not exceed 200 mm Hg during oxygen breathing, since hypoxemia is caused by right-to-left shunting. The echocardiogram shows right ventricle or diastolic volume overload and often an echo-free space posterior to the left atrium, representing the common pulmonary vein confluence.

Hemodynamics. The hemodynamics are extremely variable and are dependent on the presence of obstruction to pulmonary vein return, the adequacy of the ASD, and the presence of additional defects. Typically right atrial pressure is slightly elevated; and if the anomalous pulmonary collecting trunk can be entered with the catheter (which it frequently can), a rise in pressure can be demonstrated as the catheter advances retrogradely toward the pulmonary capillary bed. The point of entry of pulmonary venous blood into the right side of the heart frequently can be identified by a sudden rise in oxygen saturation. Pulmonary arterial saturation is generally about 2% higher than systemic arterial saturation (because of streaming effects within the right atrium); the degree of pulmonary hypertension is variable, depending on the pulmonary blood flow and pulmonary vein pressure.

Angiography is essential for detailed diagnosis. Ideally the anomalous pulmonary vein trunk can be carefully opacified; a second choice is opacification of the main pulmonary artery or right ventricle, with filming of the levocardiogram phase (Fig. 25-49). It is important to determine the exact relationship between the collecting trunk and the left atrium if surgery is contemplated. If the infant has not received excessive contrast agent, opacification of the left atrium and left ventricle is desirable, since these structures frequently are undersized and may determine the surgical outcome.

Treatment. The presence of a significant gradient across the atrial septum is an indication for a balloon septostomy, and this alone sometimes will decompress the right atrium sufficiently to allow the infant to thrive until weight gain decreases the risks associated with open-heart surgery. Vigorous treatment of heart failure is indicated; but, if the infant is deteriorating, thoracic surgical consultation should be sought and plans made for immediate correction. In the majority of instances the anomalous pulmonary venous collecting trunk runs immediately behind the left atrium so that surgery consists of performing an anastomosis between these two structures.

Prognosis. The mortality is high because the infants are small and frequently very sick, and open-heart surgery may have to be performed under emergency

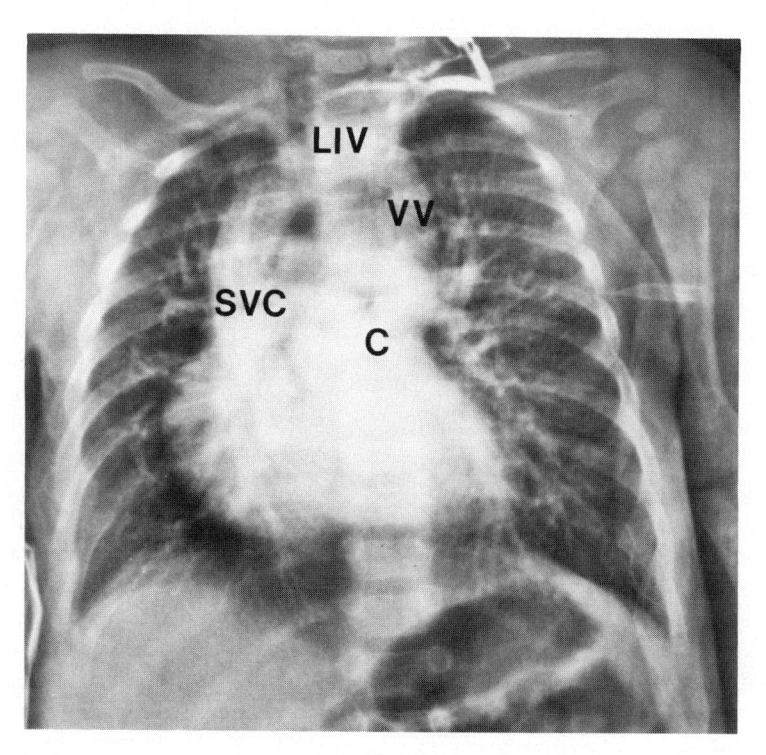

Fig. 25-49. Total anomalous pulmonary venous return. Contrast agent has been injected into a peripheral vein. The levocardiogram phase shows the confluence of pulmonary veins *(C)* ascending via a vertical vein *(VV)* into the left innominate vein *(LIV)* to enter the superior vena cava *(SVC)*.

conditions. The mortality in infants is approximately 30% compared with about 5% to 10% in children 2 to 10 years old. The mortality is similar regardless of the anatomy. A major determinant appears to be the adequacy of the left ventricle to handle the additional volume load and avoid pulmonary edema following surgical repair.

Left-to-right shunts

Four types of left-to-right shunts are considered in the following sections: PDA, VSD, combined PDA and VSD, endocardial cushion defect (common AV canal), and systemic arteriovenous fistulas. ASDs are present in the newborn period but rarely cause symptoms. Total anomalous pulmonary venous return is considered as a "common mixing" lesion rather than a left-to-right shunt. Infants with left-to-right shunts have certain clinical characteristics in common. The neonates are acyanotic, the cardiac impulse is hyperactive, and the chest roentgenogram shows cardiac enlargement with an increase in pulmonary vascular markings.

Patent ductus arteriosus

See also Chapter 23, part three.

Indirect evidence indicates that the normal human ductus arteriosus undergoes fairly rapid initial constriction during the first few hours after delivery of the baby, followed by a more gradual final functional closure over 1 to 8 days. In premature infants closure of the ductus may be delayed up until the time of full gestational age and beyond. Thus surgical closure of a PDA is not indicated in the asymptomatic premature infant, since spontaneous closure can be anticipated in most instances. PDA ligation sometimes is indicated in the premature infant who has recovered from RDS but in whom a large left-to-right shunt is causing heart failure unresponsive to medical management, including a trial of indomethacin.

Clinical manifestations. In the neonate it is common to hear a soft inconstant systolic murmur at the upper left sternal border in the first 10 hours of life. The closure of the ductus arteriosus is strongly influenced by the P_{O_2} of the blood perfusing it. However, there are paradoxes; thus the ductus arteriosus remains widely patent in infants with severe RDS but unfortunately does not always remain open in infants with pulmonary atresia and hypoxemia, even though arterial and ductal P_{O_2} may be at fetal levels.

A widely patent ductus arteriosus is an important and fairly frequent cause of serious illness in the neonate. Such neonates may be in serious heart failure and frequently have associated pneumonia. Neonates with symptomatic ductus arteriosus are tachypneic and later exhibit pulmonary rales and the signs of right-sided heart failure. In advanced left-sided heart failure they are cyanotic from alveolar hypoventilation. The peripheral pulses are bounding, and the cardiac impulse is hyperdynamic. There is usually no thrill, but a harsh multifrequency systolic murmur is evident at the left sternal border. The murmur resembles that of a VSD but is slightly higher in location and more "grating" in character. The "swishing" continuous murmur heard in some neonates with PDA requires a low pulmonary artery pressure; such infants are rarely in serious trouble in the neonatal period.

Diagnosis. The heart is enlarged, and the pulmonary vascular markings are increased. The classic roentgenographic contour is that of left ventricular and left atrial enlargement; however, in most cases the cardiomegaly is nonspecific. The ECG is almost always abnormal in seriously sick neonates. Both right ventricular hypertrophy and biventricular hypertrophy are seen. Significant left-to-right shunting is reflected in left atrial enlargement, which is usually apparent by echocardiography (left atrial/aorta dimension ratio of greater than 1.3). Flow reversal in the descending aorta, representing diastolic runoff down the PDA, can be detected and quantitated by the directional Doppler. The infant in heart failure from a PDA is frequently hypoxemic from alveolar hypoventilation and mistakenly may be thought to have a right-to-left shunt. The pH is usually normal (compensated respiratory acidosis), the $PaCO_2$ elevated, and the PaO_2 depressed. Since the depressed PaO_2 is caused by hypoventilation, the breathing of 100% O_2 should result in a level of 150 mm Hg or greater.

Hemodynamics. The diagnosis is easily and rapidly confirmed by right-sided heart catheterization. There is usually right ventricular and pulmonary arterial hypertension, and the catheter readily traverses the patent ductus to enter the descending aorta. There is a step-up in O_2 saturation at the pulmonary artery level and left-to-right shunting. Often the catheter enters the left atrium across a foramen ovale; the left atrial pressure and left ventricular end-diastolic pressures are raised. When necessary (chiefly to rule out other lesions, such as VSD or aortic arch hypoplasia), left ventricular angiography filmed in the left anterior oblique projection visualizes the ductus and excludes the aforementioned complicating lesions. If doubt exists as to the status of the left ventricle and proximal aorta, occasionally it may be necessary to perform retrograde arterial catheterization using the transfemoral approach or the umbilical artery (if the infant is less than about 7 days of age).

Treatment. Medical treatment of heart failure and pneumonia should be pursued vigorously, since the majority of full-term infants with isolated PDA survive the neonatal period, and surgery can be performed electively when the infant reaches age 1 or 2. In a minority, symptoms progress, and ligation of the ductus is indicated. The cause of the heart failure and pneumonia is totally removed by surgery. A neonate may appear to be in irreversible pulmonary edema, yet with careful medical management before surgery and with the operation performed by an experienced surgeon, the infant's recovery is rapid.

Reports of pharmacologic constriction or closure of the symptomatic PDA by inhibition of prostaglandin synthesis with indomethacin have indicated that this approach is a useful alternative to surgical ligation in alleviating left-to-right shunting in critically ill, very preterm (<30 weeks' gestation) infants. Oral dosages have been 0.2 mg/kg given by nasogastric tube, repeated if necessary for up to three doses at 8-hour intervals. Intravenous lyophilized indomethacin sodium at a dosage of 0.2 mg/kg has also been used by Merritt and co-workers. In general, infants who have shown the highest incidence of successful indomethacin ductus closure have been less than 30 weeks of gestational age and less than 10 days chronologic age, although older or later responders are not unusual.

Contraindications to the use of indomethacin are the following: (1) total serum bilirubin >10 mg/dl, (2) blood urea nitrogen >25 mg/dl, (3) serum creatinine >1.2 mg/dl, (4) platelet count <50,000/mm^3, and (5) signs of necrotizing enterocolitis or any evidence of internal or external bleeding.

Ventricular septal defect

Isolated VSD is not a common cause of serious illness in the neonate. This is because of the relatively high pulmonary vascular resistance at birth and the probability that the normal postnatal fall in pulmonary vascular resistance in those infants with large VSDs may be delayed or slow. The infant destined to develop heart failure from a large isolated VSD typically develops heart failure at 6 weeks to 4 months of age. Nevertheless about 3% of sick neonate will have serious heart failure from an isolated VSD.

Incidence. VSD is an extremely common lesion in asymptomic newborns and frequently is assoociated with other congenital heart lesions. A VSD probably is present in at least 1 of every 1,000 newborns. The natural history of isolated VSD has been greatly clarified over recent years, and it is now clear that spontaneous closure can be anticipated in approximately one third, a few closures occurring as late as the fifth decade of life. This realization has greatly influenced management and has resulted in the application of stricter criteria before advising surgical closure in asymptomatic children.

Clinical manifestations. The neonate who becomes severely symptomatic from an isolated VSD usually has a

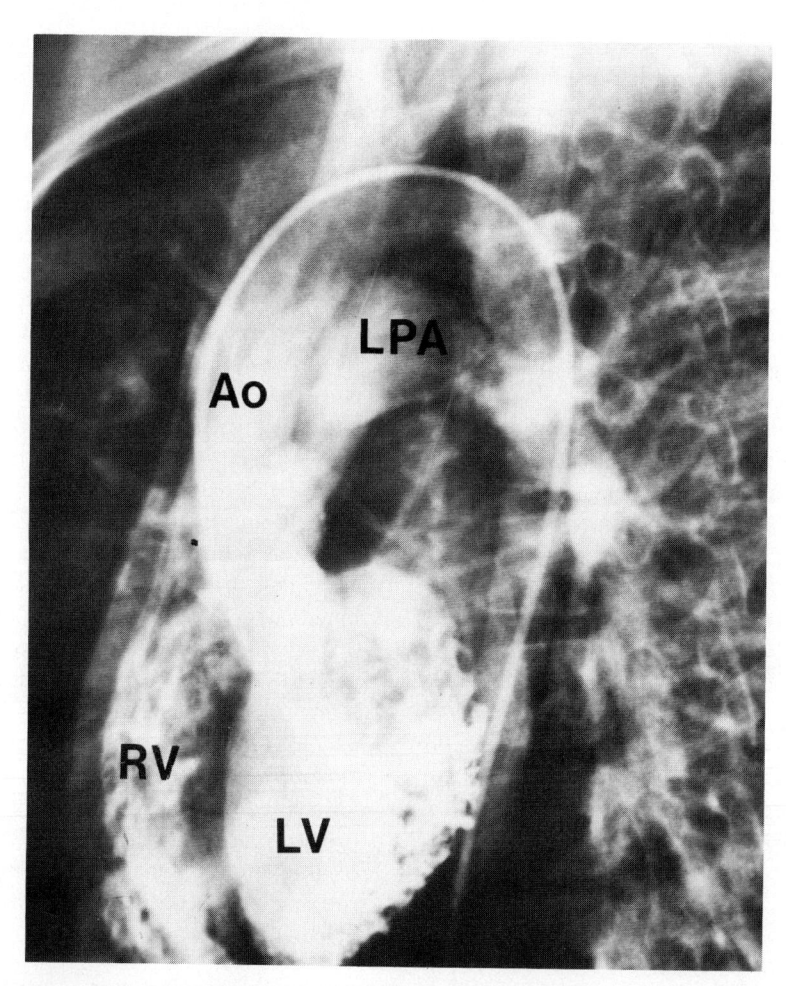

Fig. 25-50. Angiographic appearances of VSD. The catheter is in the left ventricle *(LV)*. Contrast passes through a high VSD into the right ventricle *(RV)* and fills the aorta *(Ao)* and pulmonary artery *(LPA)*.

very large defect and typically develops heart failure in the third or fourth week of life. There is usually common mixing of venous and arterial blood at the ventricular level, resulting in a mildly cyanotic infant. The physical signs of mild cyanosis, an overactive precordium, and a loud pulmonary closure sound sometimes are accompanied by a typical VSD murmur at the lower left sternal border. However, in other neonates the systemic and pulmonary vascular resistances are almost balanced, and there is little or no murmur. Thus the condition may mimic transposition with VSD, truncus arteriosus, and other "common mixing" situations.

Diagnosis. The heart is large, but the contour usually is not diagnostically helpful. The barium swallow may reveal left atrial enlargement. The pulmonary vasculature is increased. Broad notched P waves indicative of left atrial enlargement are frequent. There may be right or combined ventricular hypertrophy. The neonate with a large VSD who has severe symptoms usually is cyanotic from a combination of alveolar hypoventilation (alveolar transudate) and right-to-left shunting (at the ventricular level). Typically there is a mild compensated respiratory acidosis: the PaO_2 is depressed, and only that fraction of the depression caused by alveolar hyperventilation is responsive to the breathing of 100% O_2. The echocardiogram is useful in defining chamber size. Large VSDs are often visible on the two-dimensional study, and right-to-left shunting may be seen following peripheral vein saline contrast injection.

Hemodynamics. The neonate with heart failure from a large VSD has rather different hemodynamics from his older-infant counterpart. The VSD is large, somtimes approaching "single ventricle." In addition, there may be multiple defects, and frequently the muscular part of the septum is involved. At cardiac catheterization the venous approach reveals right ventricular and pulmonary arterial hypertension. The increase in O_2 saturation in the right ventricle may be quite small because of near-equalization of pulmonary and systemic vascular resistances and ventricular pressures. When the left atrium can be entered, the pressure is usually increased, the degree being proportional to the pulmonary blood flow.

Definitive diagnosis rests on angiocardiography; it is important to know not only the size and location of the VSD but also the existence of other cardiac anomalies. Left ventricular opacification in the lateral or left anterior oblique projection is most useful (Fig. 25-50); but if the left ventricle cannot be entered via the foramen ovale (as is frequently the case), right ventricular angiography can outline the ventricular septum. If there is a right-to-left shunt, the left ventricle and aorta also are visualized. Occasionally transarterial catheterization may be necessary to visualize the left ventricle.

Treatment. Medical treatment of heart failure is indicated; but if there is not obvious and sustained improvement within 2 or 3 days, serious consideration should be given to early surgical banding of the pulmonary artery. The aim of pulmonary artery banding is not only to relieve the neonate of his heart failure but also to protect the lungs from the long-term effects of increased blood flow and pressure. There is some evidence that neonates who develop heart failure with isolated VSD are likely to have an accelerated onset of pulmonary vasuclar obliterative disease. This is especially true of those with left atrial and pulmonary vein hypertension (who are likely to have pulmonary rales). Since this group of neonates is likely to have large or multiple VSDs, banding and later total repair appear to offer less risk compared with attempts at early one-stage total correction or prolonged medical management with the risks of progressive pulmonary vascular obliterative disease. When the VSD is well visualized angiographically, and particularly when the defect is single, the use of hypothermia with limited bypass for one-stage early correction is preferred.

Combined patent ductus arteriosus and ventricular septal defect

The lesions of PDA and VSD frequently are combined and cause symptomatic disease in the neonate. Either lesion may predominate, although frequently the calculated left-to-right shunts through each are approximately equal.

The physical signs are those of a left ventricular hyperdynamic cardiac impulse, bounding pulses (if the PDA component is substantial), and a systolic thrill and murmur at the third or fourth left interspace. The signs vary somewhat according to which lesion is dominant; it is unusual, however, to hear the typical continuous murmur of a PDA. The chest roentgenogram discloses a large heart with increased pulmonary vascularity. The ECG reveals left or combined ventricular hypertrophy except if significant pulmonary hypertension is present, in which case isolated right ventricular hypertrophy may be seen. At cardiac catheterization the ventricular defect is detected by the step-up in oxygen saturation at the right ventricular level, and commonly the catheter crosses the ventricular septum to enter the aorta. When necessary, left ventricular angiography secures the diagnosis. The presence of a PDA usually is demonstrated by catheter passage through it into the descending aorta, and the quantitation of left-to-right shunting is assessed by further increase in oxygen saturation at the pulmonary arterial level. If doubt exists, aortography or left ventriculography is indicated to settle the issue.

It is important to try to determine (by oximetry and angiography) which of the lesions is causing the greater left-to-right shunt. The calculations can be misleading because, if a large VSD is present, pulmonary artery pressure may be raised and the ductal shunting reduced (because of a lesser pressure gradient than would exist without the VSD). When both lesions are equally present, division of the ductus usually does not improve the situation. In the case of the neonate in heart failure it seems that the best surgical treatment is division of the ductus, accompanied by banding of the main pulmonary artery, followed by closure of the VSD and unbanding of the pulmonary artery at the appropriate age (usually 1 to 4 years.) If the VSD is single and easily accessible, early primary closure is often now preferred.

Common atrioventricular canal

Common AV canal is virtually the only type of endocardial cushion defect that causes serious problems in the newborn period. There is a large AV septal defect of an elliptic configuration, and the aortic leaflet of the mitral valve and the septal leaflet of the tricuspid valve are both cleft. The result is that all four cardiac chambers are in communication with one another, and additionally there is regurgitation of varying degrees through the cleft mitral and tricuspid valves. The association with Down's syndrome is well known; however, neonates without chromosomal anomaly also may have endocardial cushion defects.

Clinical manifestations. The severity of the hemodynamic abnormality usually results in symptoms appearing in the first or second week of life. The major variable is the degree of valvular regurgitation present, especially mitral regurgitation. A few children remain asymptomatic for many years; such children often turn out to have a major atrial component to their lesion, with a small VSD and minimal valvular regurgitation. Neonates with a common AV canal tend to rapidly develop tachypnea and liver enlargement. They may be mildly cyanotic from right-to-left shunting. The precordial impulse is hyperdynamic; the pulmonary closure sound is loud. Murmurs are variable. The most frequent finding is a loud pansystolic murmur at the lower left sternal border and a more blowing apical decrescendo pansystolic murmur; the former arises from the VSD, the latter from mitral insufficiency. Frequently there is a middiastolic apical murmur caused by increased mitral valve diastolic flow.

Diagnosis. The heart is enlarged, and the pulmonary vasculature is increased, but the contour is nonspecific. Left axis deviation is present in the majority of patients and is a most helpful diagnostic finding. Biatrial enlargement and right or combined ventricular hypertrophy are also frequent and depend mainly on whether valvular regurgitation or shunting is dominant. The echocardiogram may show right ventricular enlargement and mitral valve abnormalities. "Septal dropout," indicating contiguity of the mitral and tricuspid valves, is especially characteristic. The two-dimensional sector scan echo has proved especially helpful in providing detailed anatomic definition of the various types of AV canal. Most infants are in mild heart failure so that a compensated respiratory acidosis with elevated $PaCO_2$ and normal pH is present. The PaO_2 is depressed from right-to-left shunting and is not responsive to 100% O_2 breathing.

Hemodynamics. Studies of severely symptomatic neonates usually demonstrate raised atrial and right ventricular pressures. The catheter characteristically can be advanced from the right atrium to the left atrium to the left ventricle and then on withdrawal enters the right ventricle, demonstrating continuity between all four chambers. There is pulmonary artery hypertension and evidence of left-to-right shunting, usually at both the atrial and the ventricular levels. It is important to determine whether the major step-up is at the atrial level or at the ventricular level. Mitral and tricuspid valve regurgitation can best be assessed by left and right ventricular angiography.

Treatment. Medical treatment allows the infant to gain sufficient weight for total correction to be attempted. The results of total correction of the common AV canal have been disappointing because of the gross distortion of normal anatomy, the frequent presence of pulmonary vascular disease, and the risk of postoperative heart block. In many centers the trend is toward total correction at the age of 2 to 4 months, an age at which pulmonary vascular disease should not have progressed far. A small number of infants may benefit from pulmonary artery banding in infancy; these are infants in whom the major shunt is at the ventricular level and AV valve regurgitation is minimal.

Prognosis. The child with common AV canal who fares best following corrective surgery appears to be the one in whom the major shunt is at the atrial level (ostium primum ASD) and in whom the ventricular component is small. Such children are likely to have a near-normal pulmonary artery pressure. The existence of gross mitral or tricuspid valve regurgitation greatly worsens the prognosis both for palliative surgery (pulmonary artery banding) and for total correction.

Systemic arteriovenous fistula

Systemic arteriovenous fistulas are relatively uncommon as a cause of severe illness in the neonate; but their recognition is important because some are treatable, and, if they go untreated, they may cause death early in the neonatal period. The most common sites associated with severe heart failure appear to be the brain and the liver. Serious consideration should be given to the possibility of a systemic arteriovenous fistula whenever heart failure of obscure cause occurs in a neonate.

Intracranial arteriovenous fistula. Cerebral malformations involving the great vein of Galen are the most frequent intracranial arteriovenous fistulas. The clinical presentation includes tachypnea, pallor, dyspnea, and cyanosis. Signs of respiratory distress and congestive heart failure may be prominent. A cranial bruit usually but not invariably is heard. Skull measurements and transillumination may be normal. The cardiac impulse is often hyperdynamic and maximal at the lower left sternal border. There may be a systolic regurgitant murmur. The liver edge usually is enlarged below the right costal margin when congestive heart failure occurs.

The chest roentgenogram may show massive cardiac enlargement as well as active and passive pulmonary vascular engorgement. The ECG may suggest right ventricular hypertrophy. CT scan and ultrasonography of the head usually reveal the lesion. Hemodynamic studies may reveal systemic pressures in the pulmonary artery and right ventricle and oxygen saturation as high as 94% in the superior vena cava. Cineangiography with injection of contrast material into the left ventricle shows an intact ventricular septum and normal aortic root. Following opacification of the aortic arch and brachiocephalic vessels there can be extremely rapid recirculation of the ontrast agent so that the jugular veins, superior vena cava, and right atrium become rapidly and densely opacified. The mean left atrial and left ventricular end-diastolic pressures may be elevated, confirming the impression of left ventricular failure. Cerebral angiography confirms the diagnosis (Fig. 25-51).

These infants may respond satisfactorily to medical management. However, most infants with intracranial arteriovenous fistulas deteriorate rapidly. Some have medically irreversible heart failure, whereas in others central nervous system symptoms predominate. Occasionally surgical clipping of feeding arteries has been successful.

Giant hemangioma of the liver. Giant hemangioma of the liver may cause heart failure in the newborn period.

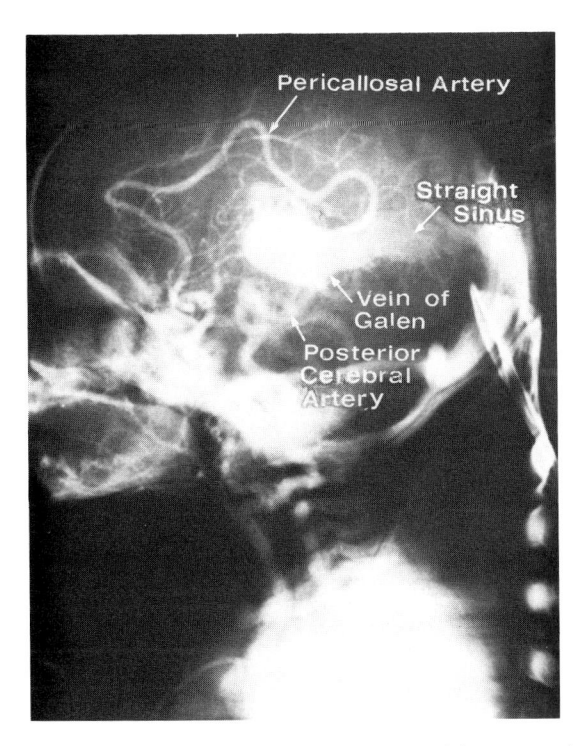

Fig. 25-51. Arteriovenous fistulas; intracranial communication. Right innominate artery injection demonstrates aneurysmal vein of Galen, which is fed directly by the right posterior cerebral artery and an enlarged, tortuous pericallosal artery. A markedly dilated straight sinus is seen draining from the vein of Galen into the transverse sinus.

There is a hyperactive cardiac impulse, gross hepatomegaly, and cardiac failure of obscure origin. Cardiac catheterization reveals highly saturated blood in the inferior vena cava. The blood supply (portal vein or hepatic artery) can be determined by selective angiography, and the lesion can be successfully removed, with resolution of heart failure.

Other systemic arteriovenous fistulas. Many variants occur and give rise to "high output" heart failure. They often can be surgically corrected. Occasionally a cutaneous hemangioma is large enough to cause death from congestive heart failure in the neonatal period.

Myocardial disorders

The more common conditions giving rise to neonatal heart failure through primary myocardial dysfunction are myocarditis, endocardial fibroelastosis, glycogen storage disease (type II, or Pompe's disease), and anomalous origin of the left coronary artery from the pulmonary artery. The latter condition is actually a form of structural cardiovascular disease, but the clinical presentation is frequently that of a myocardiopathy. A large number of rare conditions may produce myocardial dysfunction both as primary disorders (such as tumors of the heart) and as disorders secondary to systemic disease (such as muscular dystrophy). Anomalous left coronary artery, endocardial fibroelastosis, and glycogen storage disease usually appear in infants in the second to sixth month of life. The neonatal series underrepresents the true incidence.

Myocarditis

Neonatal myocarditis may be viral, bacterial, or protozoal (*Toxoplasma gondii*). Viral myocarditis is the most common, although frequently it is not possible to grow any organism from body tissues. The most common responsible viruses are the Coxsackie virus B group, the rubella virus, and cytomegalovirus (p. 700). The newborn may have active rubella myocarditis with or without other stigmata of intrauterine rubella infection. Coxsackie virus myocarditis can occur in epidemics during the neonatal period. Septic (bacterial) myocarditis has been rarely encountered since the widespread use of antibiotics. In the past bacterial myocarditis has been especially associated with pneumonia and diphtheria. *Toxoplasma* organisms may cause myocarditis by direct invasion of the heart by the parasite.

Clinical manifestations of viral myocarditis. The neonate may appear in a critical state of peripheral circulatory collapse, although in some the onset is more insidious. Frequently there is a history of a viral infection in the mother during the last 2 weeks of pregnancy. Characteristically the infant is normal at birth but rapidly develops the signs and symptoms of heart failure at 3 to 20 days of age. Auscultation usually reveals a gallop rhythm but no murmur. Sometimes the heart sounds are pathologically quiet.

Diagnosis. In the majority the heart is enlarged, and the lungs show the pattern of pulmonary venous congestion. Characteristically the QRS voltages on the standard leads are reduced (Fig. 25-52), and the T waves are frequently inverted or flattened in the left precordial leads. Although the diagnosis may seem obvious, it is important to rule out septic myocarditis (by blood culture). Any suggestion of anomalous coronary artery (infarct pattern on the ECG or appearance of a mitral regurgitation murmur) may warrant sector scan echo visualization of the coronary arteries or aortography. *Toxoplasmosis* or cytomegalovirus is suggested by abnormal head size, microphthalmia, and chorioretinitis.

Treatment. The mortality from viral myocarditis is very high. Heart failure should be treated and the infant given antibiotics to cover the possibility of septic myocarditis, at least until negative blood cultures are certain. Digitalis should not be given if the infant's heart rate falls below 100 beats per minute. Great attention should be paid to achieving a neutral thermal environment to minimize metabolic needs. The critically sick infant should receive his total nutritional support intravenously. Occasionally

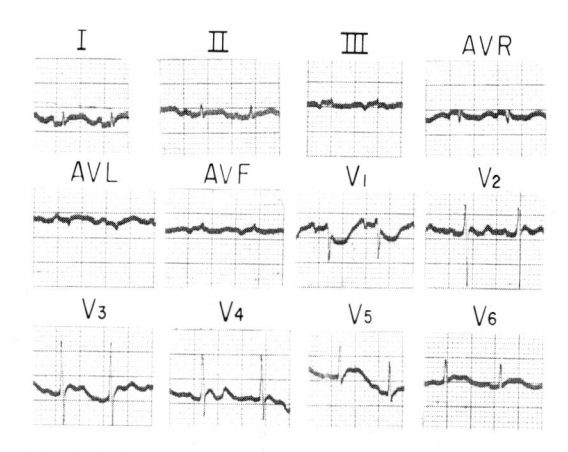

Fig. 25-52. ECG of a baby with proved Coxsackie virus myocarditis. At 1 month of age there is low QRS amplitude and ST depression (V$_1$). By 2 years of age the cardiogram had returned to normal.

one is confronted with a moribund bradycardic infant as a result of myocarditis. In this situation the use of isoproterenol (0.1 to 0.4 μg/kg/minute or sufficient to raise the heart rate to 120 beats per minute) administered intravenously seems justified. Dopamine, 1 to 10 μg/kg/minute in 5% dextrose, has been used, with encouraging results.

Endocardial fibroelastosis

Endocardial fibroelastosis occurs both as a primary condition, where the cause is unknown, and as a secondary phenomenon, particularly in association with left-sided heart obstruction. A smooth, glistening, yellowish membrane lines the left ventricle, with varying degrees of encroachment into the mitral and aortic orifices. The left atrium and very rarely the right atrium occasionally are involved. Usually the left ventricle is greatly dilated, but a contracted type of ventricle does occur, especially in the newborn. Theories of causation include genetic determination by an autosomal recessive gene, a form of end-stage myocarditis caused by Coxsackie virus or mumps virus, and a theory that the condition may be caused by a primary metabolic defect of cardiac muscle such as carnitine deficiency. Primary endocardial fibroelastosis has been seen much less frequently in recent years, for unknown reasons.

Clinical manifestations. Most infants with endocardial fibroelastosis are referred to diagnostic centers at 2 to 4 months of age with an admission diagnosis of "failure to thrive," heart failure, or cardiomegaly of unknown origin. The history usually reveals that the infant was abnormal during the neonatal period, but the absence of cardiac murmur commonly delays recognition of heart disease. The symptoms and signs of the primary form of endocardial fibroelastosis are characteristic. Infants are undernourished and show evidence of predominantly left-sided heart failure with tachycardia, tachypnea, and inappropriate sweating. The peripheral pulses are normal, and the heart is not hyperdynamic (although it may be large). The heart sounds are normal; some have no murmur, whereas others have the murmurs of mitral or aortic valve disease.

Diagnosis. There is often gross cardiac dilatation (except the contracted form), and evidence of pulmonary venous congestion is usually present. Marked left ventricular hypertrophy is almost always present. This is manifested not only by the voltage changes but also by secondary T-wave changes (Fig. 25-53). On occasion pathologic Q waves are present. The echocardiogram will show a dilated left ventricle and poor left ventricular function; serial studies will help evaluate the response to therapy.

Differential diagnosis. Endocardial fibroelastosis is usually distinguishable from acute viral myocarditis by the shorter history and by the ECG. Neonates with glycogen storage disease (type II) are hypotonic, have large tongues, and frequently have a positive family history. Skeletal muscle biopsy shows a greatly raised glycogen content in type II glycogen storage disease. The most important differential diagnosis is that of an anomalous left coronary artery arising from the pulmonary artery. This produces a clinical picture and a chest roentgenogram almost identical to those of endocardial fibroelastosis. The diagnosis of anomalous left coronary is strongly suggested by an infarct pattern on the ECG and by the murmur of mitral regurgitation (caused by papillary muscle infarction). Since the anomalous left coronary artery can be surgically treated and mimics endocardial fibroelastosis very closely, it has become our policy to perform an aortogram on every infant with a clinical diagnosis of endocardial fibroelastosis.

Hemodynamics. The left ventricle is large and fails to empty adequately. Left ventricular end-diastolic pressure is raised, and, if there is mitral valve involvement, there is frequently a diastolic gradient across the mitral valve, with greatly raised left atrial pressure. Right-sided heart pressures are elevated secondary to left-sided heart pressure elevation. If the patient is undergoing diagnostic studies, it is important to confirm the presence of two normally placed coronary arteries either by left ventricular or aortic root angiography. The cardiac output is frequently low and is reflected by a widened arteriovenous oxygen content difference.

Prognosis. Manning and associates reported 31 of 56 infants surviving over 2 years, although many survivors had large hearts and abnormal ECGs. The rapid reversion of the abnormal T waves was a favorable prognostic sign. Since the diagnosis of endocardial fibroelastosis (primary form) is essentially a pathologic one and it is

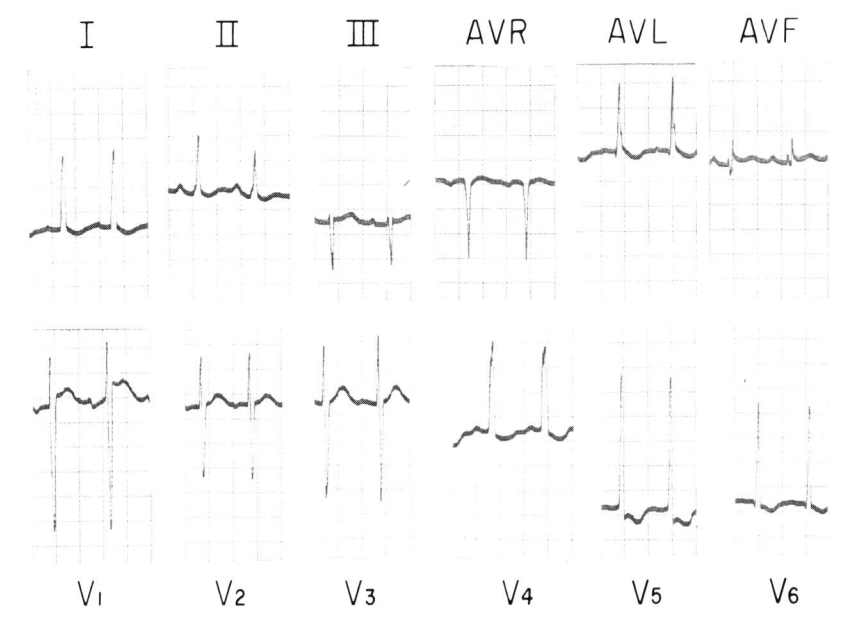

Fig. 25-53. ECG of an infant with endocardial fibroelastosis. All leads are recorded at half standard. There is marked left ventricular hypertrophy with secondary T wave changes (leads I, V₅, and V₆).

likely that it is a disease of multifactorial causes, it is extremely difficult to provide parents with a reliable prognosis.

Treatment. There is no specific therapy except where carnitine or other metabolic deficiency can be shown. Heart failure should be treated and the metabolic needs of the critically sick infant minimized by intravenous feeding and the careful maintenance of thermoneutrality. Digitalis is paticularly important, and some infants demonstrate an unusual degree of dependency on digitalis.

Glycogen storage disease

See also p. 839.

The only type of glycogenosis in which the heat is involved to a major extent is type II (Pompe's disease). In this condition there is a defect in the enzyme α-1,4-glucosidase, resulting in the accumulation of glycogen in heart, liver, and skeletal muscle. The disease is usually lethal within the first year.

Clinical manifestations. Infants affected with Pompe's disease display a very characteristic clinical picture with failure to thrive, muscular hypotonia, hepatomegaly, and large tongue (see Fig. 25-1). Usually there is no cardiac murmur or a nondescript systolic murmur that may reflect outflow tract obstruction. Affected infants lie quietly, usually supine and in the hypotonic frog-leg position. The respirations are rapid.

Diagnosis. The heart is large, and the lung fields may show passive pulmonary venous engorgement. A characteristic but not pathognomonic ECG has been described (Fig. 25-54). The PR interval is short, the QRS voltages are greatly increased, and deep Q waves over the left precordium are frequently seen. In some cases there is T-wave inversion in leads V₅ and V₆. The diagnosis may be confirmed by the finding of greater than 1.5% glycogen by wet weight in skeletal muscle biopsy; levels of 8% to 10% are not unusual.

Treatment. No definitive treatment is available; the major contribution the pediatrician can make is in counseling and alerting the parents to the possibility of diagnosis early in the gestation of future offspring by means of examination of the amniotic fluid for α-1,4-glucosidase activity.

Anomalous origin of the left coronary artery from the pulmonary artery

Early recognition of the anomalous left coronary artery is important; if the condition is untreated, the mortality in infancy is high, and both palliative surgery and corrective surgery are available. The incidence is 0.4 to 0.5% of patients with congenital heart disease. The condition often is not recognized in the neonatal period, but symptoms tend to become obvious at age 2 to 4 months. Occasionally the lesion escapes recognition until later childhood or even adult life.

Clinical manifestations. The major symptoms are failure to thrive and the manifestations of left ventricular failure. Occasionally parents will observe episodes that could be interpreted as angina pectoris or coronary

Fig. 25-54. ECG of an infant with type II glycogen storage disease. The PR interval is short. There is left axis deviation, right ventricular hypertrophy, and left ventricular hypertrophy with "strain" (inverted T waves in leads V₅, V₆, and I).

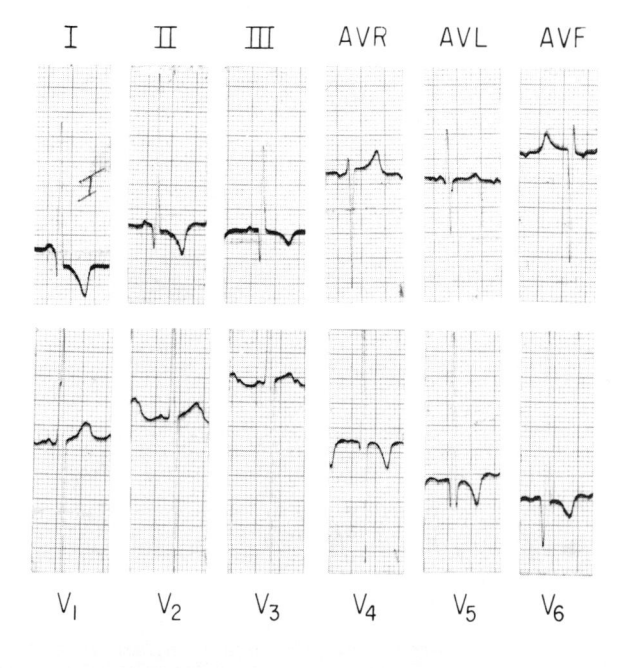

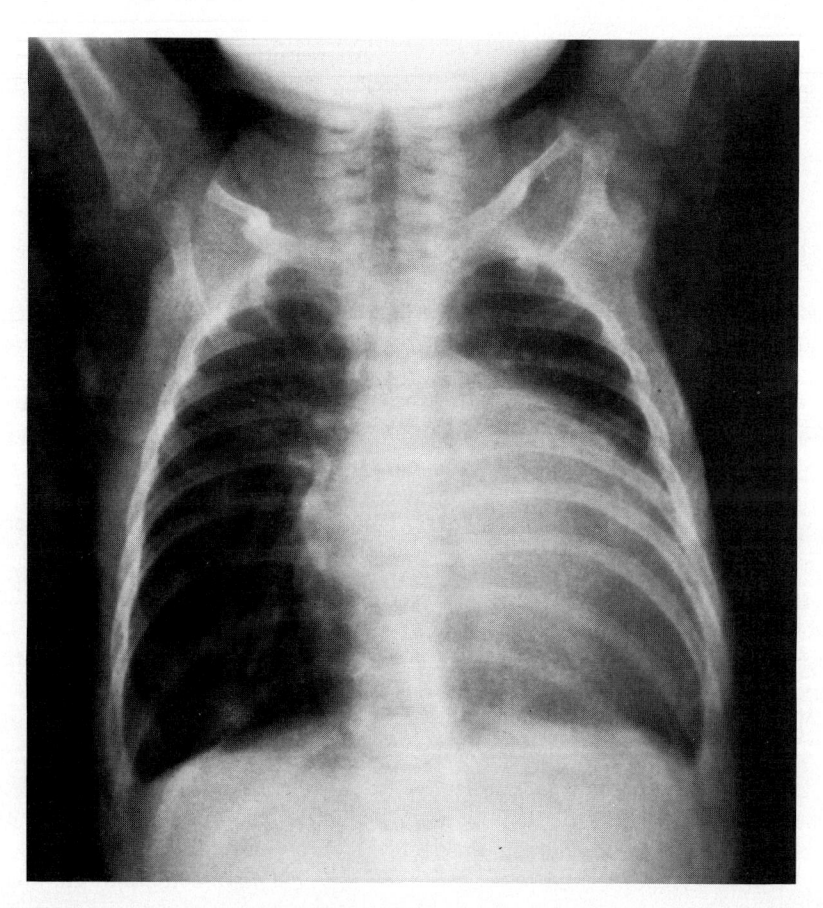

Fig. 25-55. Chest film of an infant with anomalous origin of the left coronary artery from the pulmonary artery. Note extreme cardiomegaly. Fluoroscopically the heart changed very little in volume between systole and diastole.

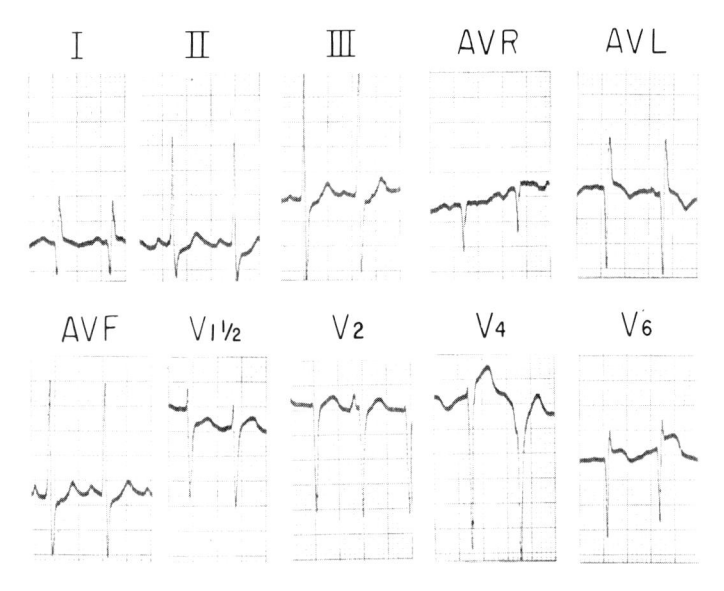

Fig. 25-56. Anomalous origin of the left coronary artery from the pulmonary artery, producing myocardial infarction. Note pathologic Q waves in leads I, aV$_L$, and V$_6$. At surgery (ligation of anomalous coronary) the apex and posterior wall of the left ventricle showed widespread infarction.

occlusion, but in the majority of infants the symptoms differ little from those of endocardial fibroelastosis. There may be no murmur, or the apical systolic murmur of mitral insufficiency may be present. Mitral insufficiency is probably secondary to infarction of the papillary muscles of the mitral valve.

Diagnosis. The heart is characteristically large and empties poorly with each systolic contration (Fig. 25-55). The most characteristic ECG is that of myocardial infarction (Fig. 25-56). However, in some the appearance is that of ischemia; in a small number only the voltage changes of left ventricular hypertrophy are present.

Hemodynamics. The hemodynamics are greatly influenced by the size and number of anastomoses between the right and left coronary arterial systems and by the pulmonary arterial pressure. Thus infants with many anastomoses and low pulmonary artery pressure have a left-to-right shunt from the aorta to the pulmonary artery by means of the anomalous left coronary artery. This "runoff" into the pulmonary artery compromises coronary capillary–filling pressure and myocardial blood flow to all areas of the heart. Temporary elevation of the pulmonary artery pressure may account for the rarity of diagnosis during the neonatal period. It is important therefore to measure pulmonary artery pressure, assess the degree of the left-to-right shunt, and visualize the coronary arterial system. The typical infant shows rapid opacification of the normal right coronary artery, followed by opacification of the anomalous left coronary artery and pulmonary artery.

Treatment. Management is controversial at the present time. Most cardiologists favor medical treatment of the infant with high pulmonary artery pressure, little or no left-to-right shunt, and a stable clinical course. Prolonged survival of these infants is possible, and the anomalous left coronary artery can be anastomosed to the ascending aorta by means of a saphenous vein graft when the child is larger. The sick infant with low pulmonary artery pressure and left-to-right shunting presents a dilemma. Simple ligation of the anomalous coronary artery improves myocardial perfusion but carries some risk. It has been claimed that prolonged medical management can extend the life of these infants to an age at which saphenous vein grafting is feasible. The opposite view favors early ligation in those with left-to-right shunting. It is hoped that infants can survive with or without ligation of the anomalous vessel until saphenous vein autografts or Dacron tube grafts can be placed and prove to be adequate long-term conduits. Recently direct attachment of the anomalous coronary artery to the aorta, in both types, during infancy has been reported to be successful.

Miscellaneous congenital heart conditions

A large number of rare heart lesions may produce symptomatic disease in the neonate. Four of these conditions are mentioned briefly in the following sections: absence of the pulmonary valve, isolated tricuspid insufficiency, cor triatriatum, and dextrocardia.

Isolated congenital absence of the pulmonary valve

Absence of the pulmonary valve is rare as an isolated anomaly and occasionally is associated with tetralogy of

Fallot. Diagnosis of the isolated lesion is suggested by a diastolic murmur, heard maximally at the second left interspace, that is slightly delayed in onset after the pulmonic closure sound. There is an associated systolic murmur because of increased systolic pulmonary valve flow. Pulmonary insufficiency characteristically produces very marked dilatation of the main pulmonary arteries. The diagnosis is confirmed by the absence of a diastolic gradient across the pulmonary valve and by pulmonary artery angiography. The disease either has a rather benign course, or the patient dies soon after birth. The poor outcome in some newborns may be because of associated physiologic pulmonary hypertension, causing a significant backward driving force from pulmonary artery to right ventricle and an impairment of adequate right ventricular emptying.

Isolated congenital tricuspid insufficiency

This is rare and appears to be caused by congenital short chordae tendineae or by papillary muscle infarction secondary to coronary and myocardial hypoxemia. The closure of apparently adequate valve cusps is prevented. Occasionally tricuspid insufficiency has been reported in association with the PFC syndrome or secondary to papillary infarction from profound fetal asphyxia and hypoxemia. The diagnosis is suggested by cyanosis (from right-to-left atrial shunting), a loud pansystolic murmur at the lower left sternal border, evidence of grossly raised venous pressure, hepatomegaly, and a large heart with an especially large right atrium. Catheterized neonates have had greatly raised right atrial pressures, and right ventricular angiography has disclosed massive tricuspid regurgitation. When the condition is secondary to fetal asphyxia, there is often spontaneous improvement or complete resolution, but when the condition appears life threatening, the lowering of pulmonary vascular resistance (by increasing inspired oxygen tension or administering vasoactive drugs such as tolazoline into the pulmonary artery) might allow improved right ventricular emptying.

Cor triatriatum

The division of the left atrium into an inner chamber receiving the pulmonary veins and an outer chamber leading to the mitral valve constitutes cor triatriatum. The communication between the two left atrial chambers is inadequate for the free efflux of pulmonary vein blood, so that pulmonary venous pressure rises, and the infant dies with the signs of left ventricular failure; failure of the accessory left atrial chamber would be a more accurate description of the hemodynamics.

The condition is rare but important because it is surgically correctable. The first sign is tachypnea, followed by pulmonary rales. Pulmonary hypertension ensues, with a loud pulmonic closure sound. The ECG shows right ventricular hypertrophy. The chest roentgenogram discloses a somewhat enlarged heart with the vascular pattern typical of pulmonary venous engorgement, a lacy pattern throughout the lung fields, often with the Kerley B lines of engorged lymphatics. The echocardiogram may be pathognomonic with visualization of the accessory chamber. There is usually no murmur so that the condition mimics PFC and a variety of primary respiratory conditions, including pulmonary lymphangiectasia and atypical RDS. The condition also mimics other causes of left-sided heart obstruction, especially total anomalous pulmonary venous return with obstruction to pulmonary venous return, pulmonary vein stenosis, and mitral atresia.

Diagnosis is confirmed by cardiac catheterization. There is a discrepancy between pulmonary artery wedge pressure (reflecting the inner chamber) and left atrial pressure. Occasionally the catheter can be passed across the diaphragm connecting the two left atrial chambers, and the gradient can be demonstrated. The anomalous left atrial septum also can be demonstrated angiographically following pulmonary artery contrast agent injection. Surgical relief is possible early in life by excision of the anomalous septum.

Dextrocardia and levocardia with situs inversus

Dextroposition of the heart is to be distinguished from true dextrocardia. With dextroposition other noncardiac conditions are responsible for rightward displacement of the heart. In these situations careful appraisal of the lungs and gastrointestinal tract reveals the true nature of the problem. If there is true dextrocardia or true levocardia with situs inversus (that is, no pathologic condition present to cause mediastinal shift), then it is likely that the child will have associated structural congenital heart disease.

Neonates who have either dextrocardia or levocardia with situs inversus account for less than 3% of congenital heart malformations discovered in the newborn period. Dextrocardia with abdominal situs inversus is not infrequently associated with cyanotic cardiac lesions. Neonates with dextrocardia and normally placed viscera or partial situs inversus have a very high incidence of complex cyanotic congenital heart disease, particularly if there is splenic agenesis or polysplenia. Similarly those with splenic agenesis and levocardia frequently have complex heart disease, whether or not there is abdominal situs inversus.

In management of the neonate with apparent dextrocardia one should consider the following:
1. The possibility of dextroposition being caused by movement of the mediastinum secondary to lung agenesis, lobar emphysema, diaphragmatic hernia,

and so on should be ruled out. Pulmonary arteriography may be required.
2. An increase in the number of Howell-Jolly and Heinz bodies and an elevated reticulocyte count suggest splenic agenesis. Splenic agenesis may be confirmed by aortography or by an abnormal spleen scan.
3. An abnormal P axis (such as negative P wave in lead I) may indicate atrial inversion. It also may be caused by an ectopic atrial pacemaker (sometimes in the left atrium).
4. Cardiac catheterization and angiocardiography are usually necessary for precise chamber localization. The venous atrium and sometimes other chambers are easily reached. There is a high incidence of systemic venous anomalies that may complicate cardiac catheterization.
5. Other congenital defects, especially gastrointestinal and genitourinary tract anomalies, should be looked for.

Treatment. Infants with dextrocardia and levocardia with situs inversus tend to have complex heart disease. This is particularly true if the spleen is absent or rudimentary. If surgical treatment is required, it usually can be only palliative and most often consists of decreasing or increasing pulmonary blood flow by pulmonary artery banding or aortopulmonary shunt.

OTHER CARDIOVASCULAR CONDITIONS
Vascular rings

The incidence of symptomatic vascular rings is not known. Out of 6,647 children recorded in the Toronto Heart Registry, 0.95% had vascular rings or allied aortic arch anomalies. The overwhelming majority of the estimated 900,000 persons in the United States with an anomalous origin of the right subclavian artery arising from a left descending aorta are asymptomatic and have no positive physical signs. The more important lesions to be considered in the symptomatic newborn are double aortic arch, right aortic arch with left ligamentum arteriosum, anomalous innominate artery, anomalous origin of the right subclavian artery, and anomalous origin of the left pulmonary artery. Most clinically significant vascular rings (for example, double aortic arch and right aortic arch with left ligamentum arteriosum) encircle both the trachea and the esophagus. Some (for example, anomalous origin of the right subclavian artery) give rise to only partial encirclement. The anomalous left pulmonary artery runs between the trachea and esophagus, partially compressing both structures.

Clinical manifestations

Neonates with significant constriction usually have respiratory difficulty, often in the first few days of life. Stridor, wheezing, and intercostal retractions all indicate airway obstruction and give rise to hypoventilation, with arterial hypoxemia and hypercapnia when the obstruction is critical. Symptoms related to esophageal compression are usually present and cause aspiration pneumonia. However, it is not usually obvious that the baby has a swallowing difficulty until he takes solid foods. Vascular rings may mimic many other causes of respiratory distress.

Diagnosis

Contrast esophagograms should be performed by an experienced radiologist because of the risk of aspiration. Radiologists frequently choose a thin barium mixture, and many prefer to record the swallow on videotape for later repeated viewing. Each lesion has rather characteristic features. The double aortic arch produces a constant compression deformity at the level of the aortic arch, with marked posterior indentation and lesser left and right indentations (Fig. 25-57). The features of the right aortic arch with left ligamentum arteriosum are similar, but the indentation on the left side is nonpulsating and sharper (ligamentum arteriosum). The anomalous right subclavian artery produces an oblique or spiral indentation on the posterior esophageal wall, pointing upward and to the right. The anomalous innominate artery arises to the left of the midline and passes in front of the trachea to compress the trachea; the barium swallow is normal. The anomalous left pulmonary artery arises from the main pulmonary trunk just to the right of the midline. It then proceeds anterior to the esophagus and behind the trachea to compress both structures. An anterior indentation on the esophagus is therefore highly suggestive of an anomalous left pulmonary artery (Fig. 25-58). If the trachea shows signs of posterior compression or narrowing, the diagnosis is virtually certain. Frequently the esophagogram is pathognomonic, and no further studies are necessary. In cases of doubt aortography resolves the issue, although several projections may be necessary. A pulmonary arteriogram usually discloses the anomalous left pulmonary artery. However, a 40-degree angle anteroposterior projection may be necessary to spatially separate the main and branch pulmonary arteries.

Treatment

Neonates with symptomatic double aortic arch, those with right aortic arch with left ligamentum arteriosum, and those with anomalous left pulmonary artery almost always require surgical correction. Occasionally a neonate with a large retroesophageal right subclavian artery has respiratory symptoms (usually caused by repeated aspiration pneumonia) sufficiently severe to warrant surgical division of the aberrant vessel. The treatment of the anomalous innominate artery is controversial; it has been suggested that occasionally it may be associated with

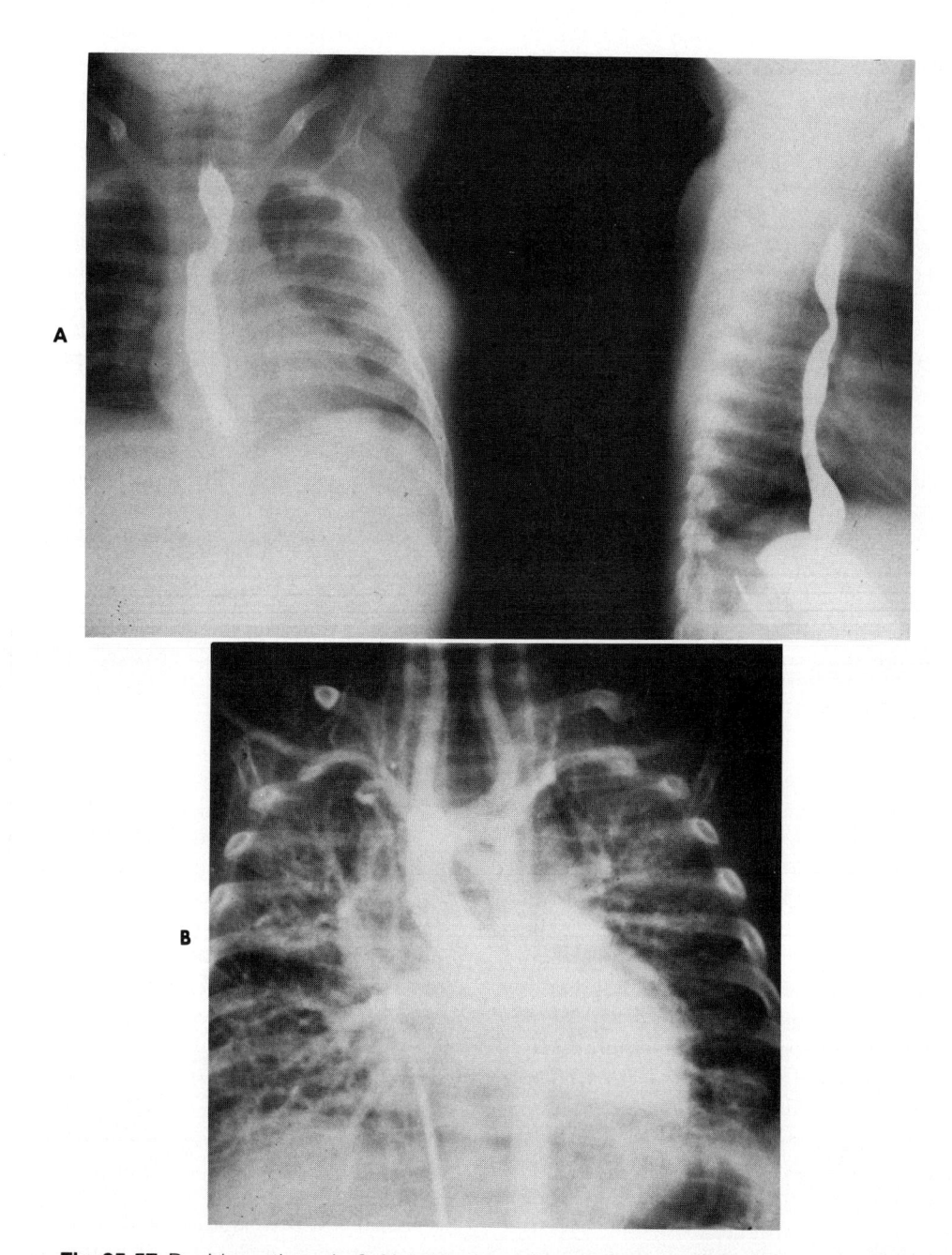

Fig. 25-57. Double aortic arch. **A,** Note imprint of posterior aortic arch on posterior and right aspect of esophagus. **B,** Angiogram discloses double arch. Anterior arch gives rise to left subclavian artery, whereas the other three brachiocephalic arteries arise from the posterior arch. (Courtesy Dr. John R. Campbell.)

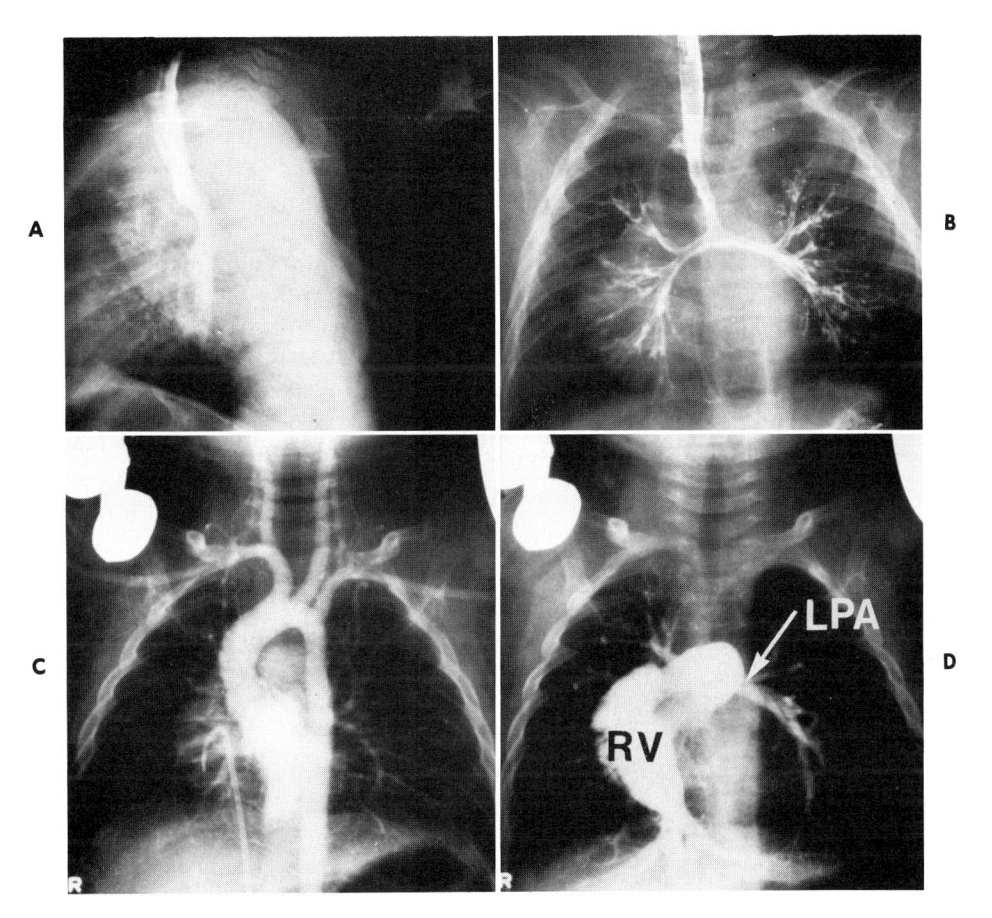

Fig. 25-58. Anomalous left pulmonary artery. The left pulmonary artery proceeds rightward as it leaves the heart. To regain the left lung, it loops leftward between the esophagus and trachea. **A,** Anterior indentation on esophagogram. **B,** Diffuse tracheal narrowing secondary to posterior compression. **C,** Normal levocardiogram. **D,** Right atrial injection. The heart is dextroposed; the right ventricle *(RV)* is in end-systole and has filled an abnormal pulmonary artery (the right ventricle and right atrium are overlapped in this projection). The left pulmonary artery *(LPA)* appears to arise from behind the main pulmonary artery rather than as the usual direct continuation. A more caudally angled and anteroposterior projection is necessary to spatially separate the main and branch pulmonary arteries.

reflex bouts of apnea. Gross has achieved surgical correction of this anomaly by pulling the vessel forward and attaching it to the sternum. It is, however, a common anomaly and, like the aberrant right subclavian artery, produces no symptoms in the vast majority of patients.

Systemic hypertension

Although rarely an emergency, systemic hypertension in a neonate always requires an explanation and usually requires treatment. Even though antihypertensive treatment may be needed urgently to combat heart failure or minimize the risk of cerebrovascular accident, the cause must be established even if the hypertension can be successfully controlled with drugs. (See also pp. 127 and 1098.)

Etiology

Hypertension in the neonate is now being more frequently recorded, and it seems clear that the increased incidence is a result of increased use of umbilical artery catheterization. Thus catheters with the tip located between T4 and T12 are above the level of origin of the renal arteries, and unilateral or bilateral renal artery thrombi are more common than previously realized. Nephrogenic hypertension also may be caused by congenital renal artery stenosis, renal vein thrombosis, polycystic kidneys, and a wide variety of congenital and acquired renal diseases. Coarctation of the aorta remains an important treatable cause. Less likely possibilities include pheochromocytoma, Cushing's syndrome, congenital adrenal hyperplasia, primary hyperaldosteronism, and neuroblastoma (secretion of catecholamines or partial obstruction to the renal artery).

Diagnosis

The accurate estimation of systemic blood pressure has been much improved by the Doppler reflected ultrasound technique. In many neonates the indwelling umbilical artery or radial artery line can supply direct measurements. For both Doppler and direct auscultation methods the cuff width should be approximately 50% of the extremity circumference; for most full-term newborns this will mean a bladder 2.5 to 4 cm wide and 5 to 10 cm in length. It is very easy to gain a spurious impression of hypertension from using too small a cuff. The leg pressure should be within 20 mm Hg of arm pressure; if it is significantly higher, it suggests that too small a cuff is being used on the leg. Brachial and femoral pulses should be felt simultaneously to be sure they are synchronous.

Examination of the urinary sediment may reveal evidence of underlying acute or chronic renal disease, either of which may be associated with hypertension. Blood urea nitrogen, creatinine, sodium, potassium, and bicarbonate levels should be obtained. A coagulation profile should be obtained if there is reason to suspect a hypercoagulable state. A 24-hour urine sample can be collected for vanillylmandelic acid (VMA), metanephrines, urinary steroid excretion, and, if appropriate, pregnanetriol. A clinical diagnosis of renal disease should be followed by intravenous urography and if necessary, by renal angiography. If an umbilical artery catheter is present, it may be both suspected as causative (possible renal artery thrombosis) and used for aortography. Many nephrologists consider persistent hypertension of unknown cause to necessitate the estimation of plasma renin activity (to rule out primary hyperaldosteronism) and renal biopsy (to rule out the possibility of occult underlying renal disease). Renal scans are sometimes useful for comparing the function of the two kidneys and are useful for comparative follow-up studies.

Table 25-13. Systolic blood pressure in newborns

Age	Number	State	Blood pressure (mm Hg) (SEM)
4-6 days	469	Sleeping	70.7 ± 0.3
5-7 weeks	144	Sleeping	89.7 ± 0.9
5-7 weeks	252	Awake	96.8 ± 0.6

Modified from deSwiet, M., Fayers, P., and Shinebourne, E.A.: Br. Med. J. **2**:9, 1976.

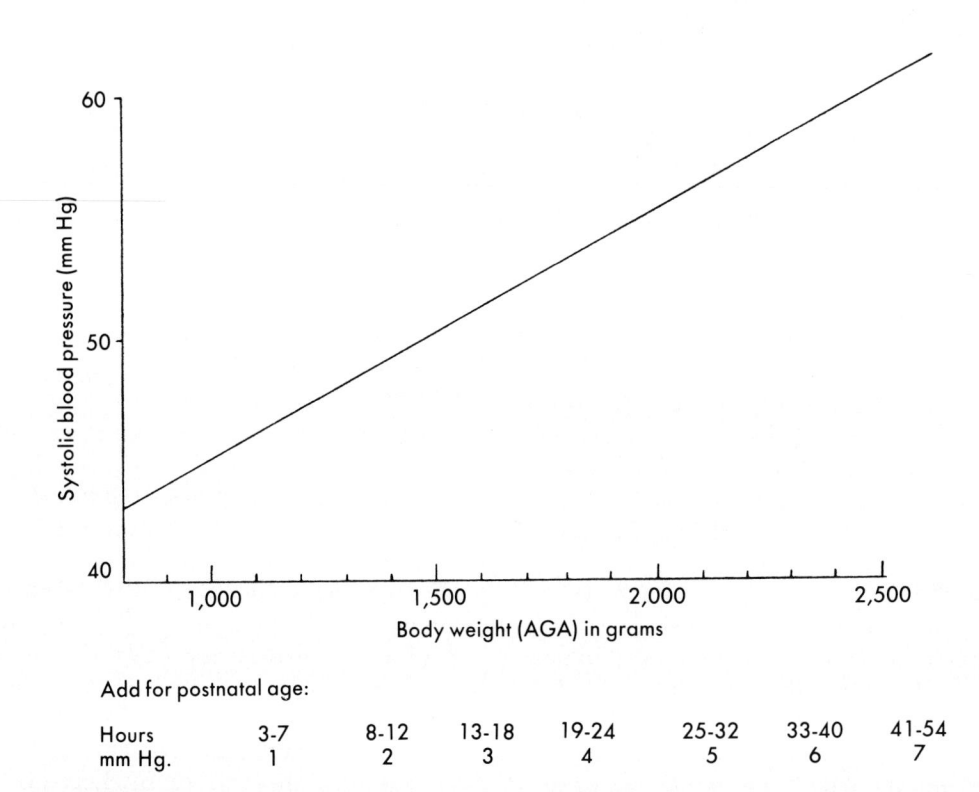

Fig. 25-59. Systolic blood pressure in AGA underweight newborns. (Courtesy Dr. Stephen Alexander; data from Bucci, G., and others: Acta Paediatr. Scand. [Suppl.] **299**:5, 1972.)

Normal blood pressure

Systolic blood pressure in the arm was measured in infants at the ages of 4 to 6 days and 5 to 7 weeks by deSwiet and co-workers using the Doppler ultrasound technique (Table 25-13).

In 391 infants in whom measurements were made on both occasions, blood pressure at 4 to 6 days was significantly related to blood pressure at 5 to 7 weeks. Fig. 25-59 was constructed by Dr. Stephen Alexander from the data of Bucci and associates relating to preterm infants. Note that a factor is added for postnatal age, that is, a 2,000-gm infant 30 hours of age would be expected to have a systolic blood pressure of 60 mm Hg. (See also p. 126 and Fig. 10-8.)

Management

An initial decision needs to be made as to whether the hypertension is imminently life threatening. If immediate control is necessary, a sodium nitroprusside drip at a dose of 2.5 to 5 µg/kg/minute is recommended. Mild hypertension frequently responds to diuretics (chlorothiazide or furosemide) whereas with severe hypertension therapy usually should begin with hydralazine.

In resistant situations multiple-drug therapy involving various combinations of furosemide, hydralazine, and methyldopa has been successful.

The question of nephrectomy for unilateral renal involvement is controversial. Plumer and co-workers reported that their hypertensive neonates generally responded poorly to medical management and suggested nephrectomy for unilateral renal involvement if blood pressure was not controlled within 24 hours. Adelman and associates successfully managed all of 17 hypertensive neonates with diuretics and anti-hypertensive agents, often with rather high drug dosages (Table 25-14).

Cyanotic spells and central nervous system problems

Neonates with cyanotic heart disease, especially those with tetralogy of Fallot or pulmonary atresia with open ventricular septum, may develop cyanotic spells that, if severe, can lead to death. Usually these spells follow crying or bowel movement or occur soon after awakening. They are quite different from the apneic spells of immaturity. Typically the child becomes progressively more cyanotic and develops deep, sighing respirations. If the condition is unrelieved, acidosis and hypoxemia lead to circulatory and respiratory depression with pallor, flaccidity, bradycardia, and on occasion convulsions, cardiac arrest, and death. The underlying heart disease is often surgically treatable, and the occurrence of even minor spells always should lead to hospital admission.

Treatment

If the spell is mild, the baby should be comforted to stop the crying. Oxygen should be given by face mask if this can be done without further upsetting the infant. If the spell is more severe, with bradycardia or impairment of consciousness, morphine sulfate (0.1 to 0.2 mg/kg body weight) should be administered subcutaneously. If the infant is profoundly depressed and has a very slow heart rate, sodium bicarbonate (2 to 8 mEq/kg over a 2-minute period) should be administered intravenously and external cardiac massage initiated to try to improve the coronary circulation. Ventilation with oxygen (face mask or endotracheal tube) is indicated if respiration is depressed. Most neonates will recover from this latter

Table 25-14. Drugs useful in the management of neonatal hypertension

Drug	Dose range per 24 hours	Dose mean per 24 hours (mg/kg)	Comments
Chlorothiazide	20-50 mg/kg PO	45	Diuretic; suitable for mild hypertension
Furosemide	1-4 mg/kg IV, PO	1.5	Diuretic; suitable for mild and moderate hypertension
Hydralazine	1-9 mg/kg IV, PO	5.7	Vasodilator; moderate and severe hypertension
Methyldopa	5-50 mg/kg IV, PO	35	Central acting; used in combination with other drugs
Diazoxide	5 mg/kg/dose IV	5	Vasodilator; rapid action; for severe hypertension
Propranolol	0.5-2.0 mg/kg PO	1.65	β-adrenergic blocker; seldom indicated in neonates
Sodium nitroprusside	2.5-5 µg/kg/minute IV		Vasodilator; rapid action; for severe hypertension

Modified from Adelman, R.D., and others: Pediatrics **62**:71, 1978.

situation. However, spells of the severe type are always multiple and progressive, unless appropriate surgery to improve pulmonary blood flow is performed. An exception is the infant who is anemic relative to his degree of unsaturation. Thus an infant with an arterial saturation of 70% is anemic if he has a hematocrit value of 40%. Sometimes the spells can be completely abolished by treating the anemia, but most often surgery is required. Phenylephrine has been used to increase bronchial collateral blood flow and propranolol to decrease β-adrenergic activity. It should be emphasized that the occurrence of spells always indicates the need for action, and usually this action is in the form of total repair or an aortopulmonary anastomosis.

Other central nervous system emergencies associated with cyanotic heart disease

Brain abscess is very uncommon in infants under 2 years of age but should be considered, especially if the baby has the potential for paradoxical embolism, for example, passage of septic material right to left across the VSD in tetralogy of Fallot. Cerebral thrombosis is also rare but occasionally may occur with a very high hematocrit value. Immediate treatment consists of venesection, 10 to 15 ml/kg, with replacement of blood by plasmanate or 5% dextrose. Anticoagulation with heparin (0.5 mg/kg given intravenously) may be considered. Anoxic brain damage is far more common in the neonate than is brain abscess or cerebral thrombosis.

Digitalis toxicity

Cardiac glycosides are excreted in an exponential fashion. Digoxin is the most commonly prescribed agent, but ouabain and digitoxin also are used in pediatrics. Toxicity caused by digitoxin is particularly dangerous because of its long biologic half-life (9 days) as compared with that of digoxin (38 hours) and ouabain (22 hours). Ouabain has very little advantage over digoxin. It starts to act slightly faster (3 to 10 minutes as opposed to 5 to 30 minutes for digoxin). However, digoxin is recommended for neonates in need of a cardiac glycoside.

Digitalis toxicity in infants and children is mainly manifested by arrhythmias, but vomiting, lethargy, or anorexia sometimes will call attention to digitalis overdose, and with massive digitalis poisoning there may be convulsions, apnea, or sudden death. A digitalis-induced arrhythmia usually is characterized by bradycardia associated with SA node or AV node inhibition. A variety of arrhythmias occur: (1) marked sinus arrhythmia with a rate variation greater than 50 beats per minute, (2) sinus arrest with escape beats, (3) AV nodal rhythm, (4) second-degree AV block, (5) complete AV block or AV dissociation, (6) atrial or ventricular premature beats, bigeminal rhythm, (7) PAT with or without AV block, and (8) ventricular tachycardia or ventricular fibrillation.

Probably the most common arrhythmias warning of digitalis intoxication are SA block, second-degree AV block, or multiple ectopic beats.

Digitalis toxicity is especially likely if there is renal disease or hypothyroidism. Certain pathologic states (myocardial disease, hypokalemia, hypomagnesemia, hypercalcemia, anoxia, and alkalosis) sometimes potentiate the action of digitalis and can result in toxicity with "normal" circulating levels of digoxin.

Digitalis toxicity should be differentiated from digitalis effect. *Digitalis effect* consists of slight slowing of the heart rate, prolongation of the PR interval, shortening of the QT interval, a shift of the ST segment, or a change in the direction of the U wave. These signs merely indicate that digitalis is fixed in the myocardium and do *not* indicate that dosage should be reduced.

Treatment

Treatment of digitalis toxicity involves the following steps.
1. Gastric lavage or emesis is indicated if oral ingestion is recent.
2. Digitalis administration should be stopped and an attempt made to increase the rate of digitalis excretion by fluids given orally or intravenously.
3. The child should be placed in an intensive care unit; the ECG should be monitored and serum electrolyte levels determined frequently.
4. Correction of any acid-base or electrolyte disturbance should be attempted. If the serum potassium level is low (as after thiazide diuretic administration), potassium chloride (1 gm/10 kg/day) may be given orally. If the situation is urgent, potassium chloride (0.5 mEq/kg) may be given intravenously in not less than 1 hour, as a solution of 40 mEq (3 gm) potassium chloride in 500 ml 5% dextrose. Potassium should be given intravenously only with a physician present and with constant ECG monitoring and frequent serum potassium determinations. McNamara and associates have suggested that potassium should not be administered routinely to patients with digitalis intoxication, because toxic doses of digitalis inhibit the transfer of extracellular potassium into the cell, and the resulting high concentration of serum potassium produces myocardial depression.
5. There is a possible source of danger in the misplacement of a decimal point when giving intramuscular doses. If the mistake is realized within a few minutes, it may be possible to drain the site of injection or excise the tissue.
6. Specific arrhythmias require specific treatment. The ease of transvenous pacing even in the newborn has revolutionized the treatment of digitalis poisoning. Slow rates associated with digitalis-induced bradycardia or heart block are common and respond very

effectively to temporary insertion of a transvenous endocardial catheter pacemaker and to control of the heart rate by electrical stimulation. Propranolol (0.05 to 0.2 mg/kg) may suppress ventricular arrhythmias.

7. Exchange transfusion, hemodialysis, and peritoneal dialysis have not been fully evaluated, but on theoretical grounds they are of limited value, since so much of the digitalis is rapidly fixed in tissues.

8. The use of disodium EDTA to lower the serum calcium level is based on the synergistic action between calcium and digitalis, but it probably should be used only if other measures fail. A suitable intravenous dose is 15 mg/kg/hour in 5% dextrose in water (maximum dose 60 mg/kg/day).

9. "Overdrive" pacing to break an arrhythmia, followed by transvenous ventricular pacing at a rate of 140 to 160 beats per minute, should be considered even when the problem is a tachyarrhythmia rather than a bradyarrhythmia.

Pericardial effusion and cardiac tamponade

The term *cardiac tamponade* or *acute cardiac compression* denotes an interference with the diastolic filling of the heart and with cardiac contraction because of an increase in intrapericardial pressure. Both pericardial effusion and cardiac tamponade are rare in the newborn period but are most likely to occur as a complication of septic pericarditis. Pericardial tamponade also may be caused by gas in the pericardial space. This is likely to occur with high-pressure respirator settings. Stroke output is diminished because the elevated pericardial pressure compresses the right atrium and interferes with the venous inflow from the great veins. A normal cardiac output is temporarily maintained by a compensatory tachycardia, and the blood pressure at first is sustained by peripheral vasoconstriction. At a critical level of intrapericardial pressure (10 to 15 cm H_2O) there is a sudden reduction in stroke volume and cardiac output, and there is a fall in blood pressure.

Diagnosis

Physical signs include (1) rising venous pressure to 20 cm H_2O or above (considerably higher than the pressure found in heart failure), leading to liver enlargement and neck vein engorgement, (2) falling arterial pressure with narrowed pulse pressure, (3) usually tachycardia and peripheral vasoconstriction, (4) pulsus paradoxus, a distinct diminution in pulse amplitude by 10 to 20 mm Hg during inspiration, (5) quiet heart, and (6) a reduced urine output.

The important step is to suspect the diagnosis. Fluoroscopy may reveal a double contour or reduced or absent cardiac pulsations. Echocardiography has become

Table 25-15. Syndrome complexes and diagnostic possibilities

Syndrome complex	Possible diagnoses	Syndrome complex	Possible diagnoses
1. Marked cyanosis during first days of life Increased pulmonary blood flow	Transposition of great arteries Hypoplastic left-heart syndrome Preductal coarctation of aorta	4. Early heart failure with or without cyanosis secondary to hypoventilation	Arteriovenous fistula (especially cerebral) Severe aortic stenosis, aortic arch hypoplasia, or long-segment aortic coarctation Large PDA Absent pulmonary valve SVT
2. Cyanosis during first days of life Reduced pulmonary blood flow	Pulmonary atresia with open ventricular septum Pulmonary atresia or extreme pulmonic stenosis with intact ventricular septum Tricuspid atresia Ebstein's anomaly of tricuspid valve Transposition with pulmonic stenosis	5. Heart failure at 1 to 4 weeks Insidious onset Murmur present	Large VSD PDA Common AV canal Postductal coarctation Double-outlet right ventricle Truncus arteriosus
3. Mild cyanosis Increased pulmonary blood flow	Truncus arteriosus Large VSD or common ventricle Total anomalous pulmonary venous return Double-outlet right ventricle and variants Transposition of great arteries with large VSD Common AV canal	6. Heart failure Large heart Acyanotic No murmur	Primary myocardial disorder Myocarditis Endocardial fibroelastosis Anomalous left coronary artery Glycogen storage disease
		7. Heart failure with small or normal-sized heart Roentgenogram of pulmonary venous engorgement	Total anomalous pulmonary venous return with obstruction (for example, drains below diaphragm into liver) Cor triatriatum

the major noninvasive method for detecting and quantitating pericardial effusions. Angiocardiography is rarely necessary.

Treatment

Pericardiocentesis may be indicated to confirm the diagnosis, determine the causative agent, or relieve the symptoms. The central venous pressure should continue to be monitored as an index of successful treatment. The line may be used for rapid blood replacement, as well as for drug therapy. Pericardiocentesis should be performed under strict sterile conditions with a 3-inch short-bevel 18- or 20-gauge needle to which is attached the V electrocardiographic lead. If the ventricle is touched by the exploring electrode, there is great amplification of existing recorded QRS complexes, or ventricular ectopic beats are provoked. If needle pericardiocentesis is unsuccessful, it is usually because the fluid is too thick for aspiration. In that case surgical therapy involving pleuropericardial drainage of chronic pericardial effusions or pericardiectomy is indicated.

Bacterial endocarditis

Bacterial endocarditis is rare in the neonatal period. When it does occur, it is likely to be part of an acute generalized overwhelming septicemia; the classic signs of subacute endocarditis do not occur.

Syndrome complexes

Despite careful attention to the history, physical examination, ECG, echocardiogram, and roentgenogram, it is often not possible to make a precise anatomic diagnosis. This is not a reflection of diagnostic inadequacy but a result of the changing fetal-to-newborn circulation, the presence of heart failure or pulmonary hypertension, and the nonspecificity of some signs. The usual result is that although one may make an intelligent guess at the structural abnormality, one is left with three or four conditions with which the signs are compatible. Certain syndrome complexes emerge, based on the presence or absence of major physical signs. Cardiac catheterization combined with selective angiocardiography is essential for accurate diagnosis except in very rare instances where signs are pathognomonic and the correct treatment is obvious. The syndrome complexes shown in Table 25-15 are intended only to indicate the more likely possibilities.

INDICATIONS FOR CARDIAC CATHETERIZATION AND ANGIOCARDIOGRAPHY

Categorical indications for hemodynamic and angiographic study of the neonate cannot be laid down, but the following are offered as guidelines.

Central cyanosis believed to be of cardiovascular origin and persisting for more than a few hours after birth may be an indication. In some patients there may be cause for procrastination, especially if the infant is cold, acidotic, or anemic or has other remediable complications. However, most newborns with obvious cardiovascular central cyanosis become steadily worse and should have a firm diagnosis established at the earliest opportunity.

Heart failure is a less common indication than cyanosis. In general, the earlier the onset, the worse the prognosis and the more urgent the need for diagnostic investigation. In the older neonate who already has demonstrated viability, a more elective approach with a trial of intensive medical treatment may be justified. At 6 weeks to 4 months of age heart failure is more common, and the approach usually can be more elective.

Various *arrhythmias* may be another indication for hemodynamic angiographic study. Cardiac catheterization may be required for the placement of a temporary transvenous pacemaker in the treatment of complete heart block or digitalis toxicity. The recording of an intracardiac electrogram may be necessary occasionally for the diagnosis of a specific arrhythmia.

Uncertainty of diagnosis may be resolved by cardiac catheterization and angiocardiography. Certain pulmonary diseases may closely mimic heart disease, and on occasion diagnostic study is the only way of resolving the issue.

Elucidation of the anatomy of a severe vascular ring causing life-threatening airway obstruction is another indication for hemodynamic and angiographic study.

Other uncommon indications include a suggestion of pericardial tamponade, pulmonary arteriography, and instillation of short-acting pharmacologic compounds directly into the pulmonary artery.

Risks and hazards of cardiac catheterization

The risk of death during or immediately following hemodynamic study is approximately 5%. Many neonates are in critical condition before and during study and in most instances would not survive if investigation and treatment were not undertaken. The major complications occurring during catheterization and leading to death are hypotension and bradycardia, perforation of the heart, arrhythmias, and the hemodynamic effects of contrast agents. Other hazards include the provocation of hypoxic spells, excessive blood loss, obstruction of a semilunar valve orifice or coronary artery by the catheter, acidosis and hypothermia, damage to arteries used in retrograde catheterization, thrombophlebitis, bacteremia, and renal damage probably related to the osmotic effects of contrast agents.

Risks may be minimized by the avoidance of sedative medication in the very sick infant, prompt replacement of excessive blood loss, careful maintenance of body temperature (by use of a water-circulating heating pad under the baby, plus radiant heat if necessary), correction of acidosis by sodium bicarbonate, tromethamine, or assisted ventilation, use of cardioactive drugs (such as isoproterenol) when indicated, strict aseptic technique, the careful balance of the risks of extensive study against the value of the potential information to be gained (for example, pulmonary artery catheterization is not necessary in a neonate with angiographically obvious tetralogy of Fallot), and limiting the use of contrast agent to the minimum amount necessary to establish the diagnosis.

There is literally no neonate with structural heart disease who is too sick to warrant hemodynamic study. The only exception is in patients where improvement with medical management can be reasonably anticipated (as in coexistent sepsis). Rarely a neonate has the typical findings of structural heart disease (such as severe tetralogy of Fallot with gross radiologic pulmonary ischemia) and is obviously in need of urgent surgery. Under these circumstances after appropriate consultation one may conclude that operation (such as an aortopulmonary shunt) without prior diagnostic study represents the least risk for the baby.

In most instances it is possible to reach all chambers of the heart from the percutaneously entered femoral vein (because of patency of the foramen ovale). If a retrograde arterial catheterization is necessary, the umbilical artery often can be used in neonates up to 10 days of age. Use of the brachial or femoral artery fortunately is rarely necessary in the neonatal period but is sometimes justified when access to the aorta and left ventricle is mandatory.

Care of the neonate after cardiac catheterization

When the neonate returns to the nursery or intensive care unit after cardiac catheterization, he should be treated as an intensive care patient and monitored closely for respirations, heart rate and arrhythmias, blood loss, urine output, blood pressure (Doppler technique), circulatory condition of the limb used, "arterialized" capillary pH and PCO_2, and general responsiveness. Deterioration and death can occur in neonates several hours after they have returned from the diagnostic laboratory in seemingly good condition.

TALKING WITH PARENTS
Explanation of the baby's specific condition

Many parents do not understand the spoken anatomic description, and statements such as "hole in the heart" often are misinterpreted. A box diagram of the four heart chambers and two great arteries is readily understood by all and can be kept by the parents when they are called on to explain the situation to other relatives. An excellent booklet entitled *If Your Child Has a Congenital Heart Defect* is available from local heart associations and from the American Heart Association at 44 East 23rd St., New York, N.Y. 10010.

The natural history of the lesion should be indicated so that a strong case can be made for or against surgery. The risks of cardiac catheterization of the sick neonate vary from less than 1% for the infant with a straight forward PDA to over 10% for an infant with anoxic bradycardia caused by heart disease. Surgery is even more hazardous, not only because of intraoperative problems but also because of recovery room death on the first days after surgery. Such postoperative deaths usually are caused by low-output states and respiratory complications (atelectasis, airway obstruction, and intrapulmonary right-to-left shunting).

Genetic counseling

The overall incidence of structural heart disease can be stated as being approximately 1%. For parents who already have one affected child, the risk increases to 3% or 4%. These odds are more easily understood if one states that 24 out of 25 times the next child will have a normal heart. If two first-degree relatives are affected, or if multiple second-degree relatives are affected, one would be unwise to quote odds, since an unusual heritable tendency already has been demonstrated.

CARE OF THE NEONATE AFTER CARDIOVASCULAR SURGERY

Recent advances in medical management (such as balloon septostomy for d-transposition of the great arteries and PGE_1 for maintaining patency of the ductus arteriosus) combined with recent advances in surgical techniques (such as subclavian flap operation for severe coarctation) have resulted in the majority of neonates with serious heart disease undergoing successful palliative or reparative heart surgery.

In many of the infants severe hypoxemia and myocardial catecholamine depletion have led to myocardial dysfunction; lack of fluid intake has led to electrolyte imbalance; and hypoglycemia and hypocalcemia may have further added to the precarious state of the infant. The surgical procedure may proceed satisfactorily from a technical point of view, but careful postoperative management is critically important.

The decision as to whether the infant should be cared for in a neonatal or cardiac intensive care unit will depend on local expertise, particularly the experience of nurses and staff. For an in-depth review of the subject the reader is referred to the monograph by Sade and associates.

Postoperative monitoring
Cardiac function

The standard surface ECG is displayed on an oscilloscope with simultaneous display of heart rate. The occurrence of bradycardia, tachycardia, or irregularity triggers an alarm and also activates a printout from a "memory loop" (a magnetic tape of the ECG of the preceding minute continuously updated). After open-heart surgery temporary atrial and ventricular pacing wires are left in place so that immediate control of a rate or rhythm problem is possible. Temporary pacing wires also facilitate the diagnosis of complex arrhythmias, as well as allow electronic control of the heart rate.

After closed heart surgery it is usually sufficient to leave pacing wires in only if a conduction disturbance or rhythm problem is anticipated, since the atrial and ventricular epicardium often is not visualized (for example, coarctation repair and PDA ligation).

Blood pressure in the postoperative period usually is monitored by means of an indwelling radial artery line, an umbilical artery catheter, or, in the more stable infant, by transcutaneous Doppler technique. We regard the lower limits of normal for systolic pressure as 45 mm Hg for the 1,500-gm infant, 60 for the 2,500-gm infant, and 65 for the 3-kg infant (Fig. 25-59).

Right atrial pressure (central venous pressure). It is necessary at times to raise right and left atrial pressures to high levels to ensure adequate ventricular filling and cardiac output. Thus, in the neonate who has undergone total repair of tetralogy of Fallot, a right atrial pressure of 12 to 15 mm Hg is sometimes necessary, and after aortic commissurotomy a left atrial pressure of 15 to 16 mm Hg may be required. When maintenance of adequate filling pressures is critical, it is common practice to leave indwelling lines through the right and left atrial appendages, through widely placed mattress sutures. These lines are pulled out through the chest wound on the second to fifth postoperative day. Central venous pressure also may be monitored from a line inserted into the umbilical vein and advanced through the ductus venosus to the inferior vena cava.

Pulmonary artery pressure. At times it may be desirable to monitor pulmonary artery pressure and have access to a source from which mixed venous blood can be withdrawn. A pulmonary artery line can be inserted through the free wall of the right ventricle at the time of open-heart surgery.

Cardiac output. Most postoperative deaths are caused by low output. The ability to accurately monitor systemic blood flow is advantageous, yet a simple technique is hard to achieve. Current methods include arteriovenous oxygen difference with assumed oxygen consumption, thermodilution measurements with a thermistor-tipped catheter, temporary electromagnetic flow probe placed around the main pulmonary artery or aorta at surgery, echocardiographic determination of changes in ventricular volume, and measurement of blood flow velocity in the ascending aorta by pulsed Doppler.

Pulmonary function

Almost every neonate who has undergone palliative or corrective cardiac surgery requires temporary ventilator support. Even if the infant was previously free breathing, the effect of anesthesia and of surgery is to depress chemoreceptor function, impair the production of pulmonary surfactant protein, allow the overproduction of bronchial secretions, disturb the ventilation/perfusion ratios, and decrease lung compliance secondary to increased lung water. The use of appropriate respirator settings is guided principally by pH and arterial blood gases.

Blood gases should be maintained close to the physiologic range by adjustments of the respirator settings, the intention being to produce favorable gases with minimal positive pressure because of the risk of pneumothorax and extrapulmonary air.

Temperature requirements

Maintenance of a neutral environmental temperature (at which oxygen consumption is minimum) greatly aids the infant postoperatively by allowing every milliliter of oxygen transferred to be used in maintaining vital body functions rather than being wasted in keeping the infant warm or in satisfying a febrile infant's hypermetabolic state. Usually this environment is achieved by skin servocontrol in an incubator or overhead radiant heat warmer; typically an abdominal skin temperature of 97° F is optimal.

Fluid and electrolyte requirements

In general, greater fluid restriction is necessary after cardiopulmonary bypass (60 ml/kg) than after nonpump procedures (100 ml/kg). This is because of the tendency to retain sodium and water from the pump prime. Hyponatremia is common and is usually caused by disproportionate retention of water and usually will respond to fluid restriction or diuretics. If serum sodium declines below 125 mEq/L, there is a risk of seizures. Hypernatremia may be seen in neonates who have received large amounts of sodium bicarbonate. Treatment is by sodium restriction and liberalization of fluids.

Hypokalemia is frequent after cardiac surgery and potentiates the action of digitalis. It can be treated by administration of potassium at 1 mEq/hour for a 3-kg neonate until serum levels reach 4 to 4.5 mEq/L. Hyperkalemia occurs as a result of renal failure. Careful watch also needs to be kept for the development of hypoglycemia and of hypocalcemia.

Table 25-16. Recommended doses of cardioactive drugs in postoperative period

Drug	Intravenous dose (μg/kg/minute)	Effect
Isoproterenol	0.1-0.5	Predominantly β-adrenergic agonist
Dopamine	2.0-20	May act at special dopamine receptors
Sodium nitroprusside	0.5-8	Arteriorlar vasodilator

Chest x-ray examinations

A portable chest film should be obtained as soon as possible after the surgical procedure to check position of the endotracheal tube and to recognize intrathoracic complications such as bleeding, pneumonia, pneumothorax, and pericardial effusion.

Use of cardioactive drugs in the postoperative period

Most infants who have undergone cardiovascular surgery require temporary sympathomimetic drug support. Despite increased biosynthesis of catecholamines by the adrenal glands, the myocardium of the patient in serious heart failure is depleted of catecholamines. An increase in cardiac output sometimes can be obtained by the use of sodium nitroprusside to reduce systemic vascular resistance. The combination of isoproterenol or dopamine to augment ventricular contractility and sodium nitroprusside to diminish afterload is especially effective. The following recommended doses are given in Table 25-16, although there is wide variation in response.

The postoperative use of PGE_1 deserves special mention. This drug acts to maintain patency of the ductus arteriosus and sustains pulmonary blood flow in lesions such as pulmonary atresia. Postoperatively it is often useful to continue infusion of the drug into the aortic end of the ductus or intravenously until it is definitely clear that the surgical aorto-pulmonary shunt is widely and usefully patent. Typically the infant may be weaned from PGE_1, 1 to 2 days after surgical shunting.

TREATMENT OF SPECIFIC POSTOPERATIVE COMPLICATIONS
Blood loss and blood replacement

The guides to blood replacement are the blood pressure, left and right atrial pressures, cardiac output, hematocrit, loss from chest tubes, and skin circulation. Blood volume should be maintained at equal to or 5% over normal values and hematocrit at at least 35% in acyanotic patients and 45% in those who have residual cyanotic heart disease. It is important to use the right blood product: whole fresh blood for bleeding, platelet transfusions for low platelet counts, and packed cells when the hematocrit is to be raised.

Renal failure

Renal failure after neonatal heart surgery is usually the result of a low-output state. The diagnosis is first suggested by a urine output falling to less than 1 ml/kg/hour and is further suspected by a rising urine sodium (greater than 60 mEq/L) and low urine/plasma osmolarity ratio (less than 1.2). A test dose of furosemide, 1 to 5 mg/kg, confirms the diagnosis if urine output does not rise significantly. Occasionally polyuric renal failure is seen with low specific gravity (less than 1.010) and rising serum creatinine and blood urea nitrogen. Treatment of renal failure in the neonate is disussed on p. 792.

Cardiac tamponade

Tamponade is suspected when there is hypotension, especially when accompanied by a rising central venous pressure. The suspicion is heightened by the x-ray finding of a widening mediastinum, pulsus paradoxus, or gallop rhythm. Since tamponade is usually caused by an intrapericardial bleed, immediate treatment is imperative with pericardiocentesis or thoracotomy in the cardiac recovery room, if necessary, but usually in the operating room.

Increased chest drainage

The maximum allowable upper limit for drainage in the immediate postoperative period is 5% of blood volume per hour. Blood should be replaced hourly with the appropriate blood product. Greater volumes of blood loss usually require reexploration unless a coagulation defect, such as thrombocytopenia, can be identified.

Continued deterioration with no obvious cause

Most deaths in the postoperative period are caused by low cardiac output. In the problem patient with a seemingly adequately operated lesion and without severe hypoxemia or arrhythmia, the following should be considered: pericardial tamponade, concealed bleeding, hypoglycemia, hypocalcemia, heart failure from hypervolemia, and overwhelming infection.

Failure to establish a positive diagnosis for low-output failure is an indication for hemodynamic and angiocardiographic study. Sometimes this can be accomplished in the recovery room, using the indwelling lines and contrast echocardiography to detect shunts and obstructions. When there is reason to believe than an undiagnosed major hemodynamic lesion is present, the patient should be transferred to the cardiac catheterization laboratory for formal study; a prosthetic patch may have torn loose, a valve inadvertently been rendered incompetent, or other unsuspected complications developed.

DRUGS USEFUL IN THE TREATMENT OF CARDIOVASCULAR DISEASE IN NEONATES

Antiarrhythmic drugs

A. *Atropine*
  1. Dosage: minimum 0.15 mg regardless of weight; 0.01 mg/kg/dose SC may be given IV; may repeat every 4 to 6 hours
  2. Preparation: check bottle, since there are many concentrations available; usual concentration is 0.5 mg/ml.
B. *Digoxin* (Lanoxin)
  1. Therapeutic range: 0.8 to 2.0 ng/ml
  2. PO digitalizing dosage
     a. Premature (birth to 3 months): 0.03 mg/kg (0.02 mg/kg parenteral)
     b. Term newborn (to 2 years): 0.05 mg/kg to 0.08 mg/kg
     c. Over 2 years: 0.04 mg/kg to 0.06 mg/kg
  3. Parenteral digitalization: two thirds of oral dosage
  4. Maintenance: a fourth to a third of digitalizing dosage, in two divided doses (q12h)
  5. Digitalization
     a. Half the calculated digitalizing dosage initially, a fourth in 8 hours and a fourth in another 8 hours; start maintenance 12 hours after last digitalizing dose
     b. Digitalis toxicity may not be manifested by vomiting; arrhythmias on ECG best way to assess possible toxicity
  6. Renal excretion unchanged: 60%
  7. Preparations
     a. Elixir: 0.05 mg/ml
     b. Ampules: 0.25 and 0.10 mg/ml
     c. Tablets, scored: 0.125, 0.25, 0.375, and 0.50 mg
C. *Lidocaine*
  1. IV initial dosage: 0.5 to 1.0 mg/kg q 20 to 60 minutes prn
  2. IV maintenance dosage: 10 to 50 µg/kg/minute
  3. Half-life: 15 to 30 minutes
  4. Preparations: 1% or 2% solution
D. *Phenytoin* (Dilantin)
  1. Oral dosage: 2 to 5 mg/kg/day
  2. IV initial dosage: 1 to 5 mg/kg slow push
  3. Slow gastrointestinal absorption
  4. Half-life: 24 hours
  5. Metabolism: liver
E. *Procainamide* (Pronestyl) hydrochloride
  1. IV dosage: 3 to 8 mg/kg over 5 minutes, to 500 mg
  2. IV maintenance dosage: 20 to 80 µg/kg/minute
  3. Oral dosage: 15 to 50 mg/kg/24 hours, divided into 4 to 6 doses
  4. Oral absorption: 75% to 95%
  5. Metabolism: liver
  6. Renal excretion unchanged: 50% to 60%
F. *Propranolol* (Inderal)
  1. IV initial dosage: 0.05 to 0.15 mg/kg, slowly over 10 minutes
  2. Oral dosage: 0.2 to 4 mg/kg/day
  3. Half-life: 2 to 3 hours
  4. Metabolism: liver
G. *Quinidine*
  1. Oral dosage: 15 to 60 mg/kg/day in 4 or 5 doses
  2. Gastrointestinal absorption: greater than 95%
  3. Metabolism: liver
  4. Renal excretion unchanged: 20% to 50%
H. *Verapamil*
  1. IV dosage, over 30 seconds
     a. Infants less than 5 kg: 1 mg
     b. Infants 5 to 10 kg: 1.5 mg
     c. Infants over 10 kg: 2 mg
  2. Reflex conversion of SVTs requires agents that increase blood pressure, resulting in reflex bradycardia, which may be very prominent; atropine should be available if severe bradycardia results
I. *Methoxamine hydrochloride* (Vasoxyl)
  1. Causes increase in peripheral vascular resistance with elevation of systolic and diastolic blood pressure that persists for 60 to 90 minutes
  2. Cardiac output unchanged or decreased
  3. Renal blood flow decreased
  4. Reflex bradycardia prominent
  5. Blood pressure should not be raised over 160 mm Hg systolic (125 mm Hg in the neonate)
  6. Preparation: ampules, 10 or 20 mg/ml
  7. Dosage: 0.25 mg/kg IM or 0.1 mg/kg IV
J. *Phenylephrine* (Neo-Synephrine) *hydrochloride*
  1. Vasoconstrictor and pressor chemically related to epinephrine
  2. For conversion of SVT, rapid IV infusion is recommended
  3. Dosage: 1 ml of the drug contains 10 mg; for use in infants the drug should be appropriately diluted
     a. Infants: 0.005 to 0.02 mg/kg IV, slowly
     b. Adults: 0.15 to 0.8 mg IV push
K. *Edrophonium chloride* (Tensilon)
  1. Short-acting anticholinergic agent that results in reflex bradycardia, which responds to atropine
  2. Advantages
     a. Rapid acting (within 30 to 60 seconds)
     b. Brief duration of action (lasts average of 10 minutes)
  3. Dosage for difficult diagnosis of myasthenia gravis or conversion of SVT: IV, may be repeated
     a. Children up to 75 pounds: 0.1 ml (1 mg)
     b. Children more than 75 pounds: 0.2 ml (2 mg)
     c. Infants: 0.1 to 0.2 mg/kg (single dose)
  4. Cardioversion—range of doses
     a. First correct acidosis
     b. SVT
        (1) Premature, newborn, infant: 5 to 25 W-seconds
        (2) Child: 15 to 25 W-seconds
        (3) Start at lower dose
     c. Ventricular tachycardia or fibrillation: higher energy levels may be required

Antihypertensive drugs

A. *Methyldopa* (Aldomet)
  1. Oral dosage: 10 mg/kg/24 hours, divided into 2 or 3 doses

a. Increase or decrease to effect
   b. Increase at 2-day or more intervals to not more than 65 mg/kg/24 hours
  2. IV dosage (crises): 20 to 40 mg/kg/24 hours, divided into four doses IV, then same dosage continued orally when controlled
  3. Preparation
   a. Tablet: 250 mg
   b. Solution (injection): 50 mg/ml
 B. *Diazoxide* (Hyperstat)—Dosage: 2.5 to 5 mg/kg/dose
  1. Initiate therapy at the low dose and give as bolus in peripheral IV (not intracardiac) over a 30-second period
  2. May repeat in half hour; then q 2 to 5 hours
 C. *Hydralazine* (Apresoline)
  1. Oral dosage: 0.75 mg/kg/day, divided into four doses
  2. Parenteral dosage alone: 1.7 to 3.5 mg/kg/day q6h
 D. *Magnesium sulfate*
  1. IM dosage: 0.1 gm/kg of 20% to 50% solution, repeated q4h if necessary
  2. IV dosage: 2 mg/kg of 3% solution; no more than 75 to 100 mg/hour
 E. *Sodium nitroprusside*
  1. Fast onset, potent hypotensive agent, quickly reversible
  2. Mechanism: peripheral vasodilatation by direct effect on peripheral vessels, independent of autonomic control
  3. Administration: IV drip only in D5W
  4. Dosage: 0.5 to 8 µg/kg/minute IV drip
  5. Preparation: 50 mg vial of desiccated nitroprusside: dissolve in 2 to 3 ml D5W, then dilute in 250, 500, or 1,000 ml D5W for infusion
   a. 50 mg in 250 ml = 1 mg/5 ml = 200 µg/ml
   b. 50 mg in 500 ml = 1 mg/10 ml = 100 µg/ml
   c. 50 mg in 1,000 ml = 1 mg/20 ml = 50 µg/ml
  6. Monitor blood pressure and heart rate closely; if severe hypotension develops, stop IV drip, and blood pressure will increase in 1 to 10 minutes
 F. *Atropine sulfate:* see Antiarrhythmic drugs
 G. *Calcium chloride* (27% calcium)
  1. Intracardiac dosage: 10 mg/kg diluted with 1.1 saline; use cautiously if patient is digitalized
  2. IV dosage: 10 mg/kg
  3. Preparation: ampules, 100 mg/ml (10% solution)
 H. *Calcium gluconate* (9% calcium)—Dosage: 200 mg/kg/dose IV

Diuretics

 A. *Chlorothiazide* (Diuril)
  1. Dosage: 20 mg/kg/24 hours, divided into two doses, oral
  2. Preparations
   a. Tablets: 250 to 500 mg
   b. Syrup: 250 mg/5 ml
 B. *Furosemide* (Lasix)
  1. IV dosage: 0.5 to 1.5 mg/kg
  2. Oral dosage: 1 to 4 mg/kg/day
  3. Preparations:
   a. Tablets, scored: 40 mg
   b. Ampules: 20 mg/2 ml
 C. *Hydrochlorothiazide* (Hydrodiuril)
  1. Dosage: tenth of chlorothiazide dosage
  2. Preparation: Tablets, scored, 25 and 50 mg
 D. *Mannitol*
  1. For treatment of oliguria and anuria
  2. Test dosage: 0.2 gm/kg; 6 gm/m^2; single IV dose given within 3 to 5 minutes
  3. Dosage for edema, ascites: 2 gm/kg; 60 gm/m^2 of 15% to 20% solution given over 2 to 6 hours IV
  4. Preparation: injection of 50, 100, 150, 200, and 250 mg/ml (5%, 10%, 15%, 20%, and 25%)
  5. CAUTION: circulatory overload, electrolyte imbalance, tremors and convulsions (hyponatremia), headache, nausea, chills, dizziness, tachycardia, intraocular hemorrhage, death in organic central nervous system disease, and pulmonary hypertension; don't mix with infused blood
 E. *Spironolactone* (Aldactone)—1.5 to 3.0 mg/kg/day in two to three doses

Miscellaneous

 A. *Morphine sulfate*—IM or IV dosage: 0.1 to 0.2 mg/kg
 B. *Nalorphine* (Nalline)—dosage: 0.01 mg/kg
 C. *Pancuronium bromide* (Pavulon)
  1. Neuromuscular blocking agent
  2. Dosage: 0.04 to 0.05 mg/kg
 D. *Prostaglandin* E$_1$
  1. For maintaining ductal patency
  2. Dosage: 0.1 µg/kg/minute; 500 µg (0.5 mg) (1 vial) in 50 ml; 10 µg/ml
 E. *Sodium bicarbonate*—IV dosage: 3 to 5 mEq/kg/dose
 F. *Succinylcholine*
  1. Dosage for intubation: 1 mg/pound IM
  2. Takes two minutes for patient to become paralyzed
 G. *Tolazoline* (Priscoline)
  1. Action: vasodilator
  2. Indications: pulmonary vasoconstriction
  3. Dosage:
   a. At cardiac catheterization, to evaluate pulmonary hypertension: 1 mg/kg bolus to pulmonary artery
   b. For PFC: 1 to 2 mg/kg push initially, 1 to 4 mg/kg/hour, drip
 H. *Diazepam* (Valium)
  1. Oral dosage: 0.12 to 0.8 mg/kg/24 hours, divided into 3 or 4 doses
  2. IM or IV dosage: 0.2 to 0.5 mg/kg single dose; given slowly

Sympathomimetics

 A. *Dobutamine* (Dobutrex)
  1. Synthetic catecholamine
  2. β-receptor stimulator that is more selective for the heart
  3. Has mild chronotropic effects
  4. Helpful in treatment of cardiac decompensation
  5. Administration: IV only
  6. Rate of infusion: 2.5 to 10 µg/kg/minute

B. *Dopamine* (Intropin)
   1. Pharmacologic properties: increased cardiac output, increased blood pressure, increased renal blood flow, useful for shock
   2. Preparation: ampules, 5 ml (40 mg/ml) (total: 200 mg)
   3. Dosage: 5 to 15 μg/kg/minute IV drip
   4. Dilution
      a. 2.5 cc/1,000 ml = 100 μg/ml
      b. 5.0 cc/500 ml = 400 μg/ml
   5. Monitor heart rate, blood pressure, central venous pressure, and urine output
C. *Epinephrine*
   1. Alpha ++, beta ++
   2. Intracardiac dosage: 0.3 to 2.0 cc diluted 1:10,000 (0.1 ml/kg)
D. *Isoproterenol* (Isuprel) (beta only)
   1. Range of recommended dosages includes 0.1 to 0.4 μg/kg/minute IV drip
   2. Should be given by infusion pump
   3. Dosage: 1 ml (200 μg) in 200 ml = 1 μg/ml
   4. Monitor heart rate, blood pressure, central venous pressure, and urine output

Martin H. Lees
Cecille O. Sunderland

BIBLIOGRAPHY
General

Ainger, L.E., Lawyer, N.G., and Fitch, C.W.: Neonatal rubella myocarditis, Br. Heart J. **28**:691, 1966.

Beuren, A.J., and others: The syndrome of supravalvular aortic stenosis, peripheral pulmonary stenosis, mental retardation, and similar facial appearance, Am. J. Cardiol. **13**:471, 1964.

Capitanio, M.A., and Kirkpatrick, J.A.: Roentgen examination in the evaluation of the newborn infant with respiratory distress, J. Pediatr. **75**:896, 1969.

Graham, T.P., Atwood, G.F., and Boucek, R.J.: Use of prostaglandin E_1 for emergency palliation of symptomatic coarctation of the aorta, Cathet. Cardiovasc. Diagn. **4**:97, 1978.

Hohn, A.R., Lowe, C.U., Sokal, J.E., and Lambert, E.C.: Cardiac problems in the glycogenoses with specific reference to Pompe's disease, Pediatrics **35**:313, 1965.

Lambert, E.C., Canent, R.V., and Hohn, A.R.: Congenital cardiac anomalies in the newborn; a review of conditions causing death or severe distress in the first months of life, Pediatrics **37**:343, 1966.

Lees, M.H., Burnell, R.H., Morgan, C.L., and Ross, B.B.: Ventilation/perfusion relationships in children with heart disease and diminished pulmonary blood flow, Pediatrics **40**:259, 1967.

Lown, B., and Kosowsky, B.D.: Artificial cardiac pacemakers, N. Engl. J. Med. **283**:907, 1970.

McNamara, D.G., Brewer, E.J., Jr., and Ferry, G.D.: Accidental poisoning of children with digitalis, N. Engl. J. Med. **271**:1106, 1964.

Manning, J.A., Sellers, F.J., Bynum, R.S., and Keith, J.D.: The medical management of clinical endocardial fibroelastosis, Circulation **29**:60, 1964.

Mehrizi, A., and Drash, A.: Birth weight of infants with cyanotic and acyanotic congenital malformations of the heart, J. Pediatr. **59**:715, 1961.

Messer, J.V.: Management of emergencies. XIV. Cardiac arrest, N. Engl. J. Med. **275**:35, 1966.

Mitchell, S.C., Korones, S.B., and Berendes, H.W.: Congenital heart disease in 56,109 births; incidence and natural history, Circulation **43**:323, 1971.

Neill, C.A.: Development of the pulmonary veins; with reference to the embryology of anomalies of pulmonary venous return, Pediatrics **18**:880, 1956.

Nora, J.J.: Multifactorial inheritance hypothesis for the etiology of congenital heart diseases; the genetic-environmental interaction, Circulation **38**:604, 1968.

Nora, J.J., and others: Medical and surgical management of anomalous origin of left coronary artery from pulmonary artery, Pediatrics **42**:405, 1968.

Olley, P.M., Coceani, F., and Bodach, E.: E-type prostaglandins; a new emergency therapy for certain cyanotic congenital heart malformations, Circulation **53**:728, 1976.

Ongley, P.A.: Heart sounds in total anomalous pulmonary venous return and in Ebstein's anomaly, Circulation **16**:431, 1957.

Rowe, R.D., and Uchida, I.A.: Cardiac malformation in mongolism; a prospective study of 184 mongoloid children, Am. J. Med. **31**:726, 1961.

Rudolph, A.M.: Complications occurring in infants and children. In Braunwald, E., and Swan, H.J.C., editors: Cooperative study in cardiac catheterization, Monograph no. 20, 1968, American Heart Association; Circulation, vols. 37 and 38, (Suppl. 3), 1968.

Tripp, M.E., and others: Systemic carnitine deficiency presenting as familial endocardial fibroelastosis: a treatable cardiomyopathy, N. Engl. J. Med. **305**:385, 1981.

Valdes-Dapena, M., and Miller, W.H.: Pericarditis in the newborn, Pediatrics **16**:673, 1955.

Electrocardiogram

Hastreiter, A.R., and Abella, J.B.: The electrocardiogram in the newborn period. I. The normal infant, J. Pediatr. **78**:146, 1971.

Hastreiter, A.R., and Abella, J.B.: The electrocardiogram in the newborn period. II. The infant with disease, J. Pediatr. **78**:346, 1971.

Michaelsson, M.: Electrocardiographic studies in the healthy newborn, Acta Paediatr. Scand. **48**:108, 1959.

Echocardiography

Allen, H.D., and others: Echocardiographic demonstration of a right ventricular tumor in a neonate, J. Pediatr. **84**:854, 1974.

Bass, J.L., Ben-Schachar, G., and Edwards, J.E.: Comparison of M-mode echocardiography and pathologic findings in the hypoplastic left heart syndrome, Am. J. Cardiol. **45**:79, 1980.

Baylen, B.G., and others: The critically ill premature infant with patent ductus arteriosus and pulmonary disease—an echocardiographic assessment, J. Pediatr. **86**:423, 1975.

Bender, R.L., and others: Echocardiographic diagnosis of bacterial endocarditis of the mitral valve in a neonate, Am. J. Dis. Child. **131**:746, 1977.

Bierman, F.Z., and Williams, R.G.: Subxiphoid two-dimensional imaging of the interatrial septum in infants and neonates with congenital heart disease, Circulation **60**:80, 1979.

Bierman, F.Z., and Williams, R.G.: Prospective diagnosis of d-transposition of the great arteries in neonates by subxiphoid two-dimensional echocardiography, Circulation **60**:1496, 1979.

Cohn, H.E., and others: Cardiovascular responses to hypoxemia and acidemia in fetal lambs, Am. J. Obstet. Gynecol. **120**:817, 1974.

Cotton, R.B., and others: Medical management of small preterm infants with symptomatic patent ductus arteriosus, J. Pediatr. **92**:467, 1978.

Donnelly, W.H., Bucciarelli, R.L., and Nelson, R.M.: Ischemic papillary muscle necrosis in stressed newborn infants, J. Pediatr. **96**:295, 1980.

Edmunds, L.H., and others: Surgical closure of the ductus arteriosus in premature infants, Circulation **48**:856, 1973.

Fiegenbaum, H.: Echocardiography, ed. 2, Philadelphia, 1976, Lea & Febiger.

Gersony, W.M., Morishima, H.O., and Daniel, S.S.: The hemodynamic effects of intrauterine hypoxia: an experimental model in newborn lambs, J. Pediatr. **89**:631, 1976.

Gittenberger-de Groot, A.C., and others: The ductus arteriosus in the preterm infant; histologic and clinical observations, J. Pediatr. **96:**88, 1980.

Gutgesell, H.P., Speer, M.E., and Rosenberg, H.S.: Characterization of the cardiomyopathy in infants of diabetic mothers, Circulation **61:**441, 1980.

Gutgesell, H.P., and others: Transient hypertrophic subaortic stenosis in infants of diabetic mothers, J. Pediatr. **89:**120, 1976.

Gutgesell, H.P., and others: Left and right ventricular systolic time intervals in the newborn, Br. Heart J. **42:**27, 1979.

Halliday, H., and others: Respiratory distress syndrome; echocardiographic assessment of cardiovascular function and pulmonary vascular resistance, Pediatrics **60:**444, 1977.

Halliday, H., and others: Echocardiographic ventricular systolic time intervals in normal term and preterm neonates, Pediatrics **62:**317, 1978.

Hernandez, A., and others: Diagnosis of pulmonary arteriovenous fistula by contrast echocardiography, J. Pediatr. **93:**258, 1978.

Hirschfeld, S., and others: Measurement of right and left ventricular systolic time intervals by echocardiography, Circulation **51:**304, 1975.

Hirschfeld, S., and others: The echocardiographic assessment of pulmonary artery pressure and pulmonary vascular resistance, Circulation **52:**642, 1975.

Hirschklau, M.J., and others: Echocardiographic diagnosis; pitfalls in the premature infant with a large patent ductus arteriosus, J. Pediatr. **92:**474, 1978.

Jacob, J., and others: The contribution of PDA in the neonate with severe RDS, J. Pediatr. **96:**79, 1980.

Kitterman, J.A., Edmunds, L.H., and Gregory, G.A.: Patent ductus arteriosus in premature infants; incidence, relation to pulmonary disease and management, New Engl. J. Med. **287:**473, 1972.

Lees, M.H.: Perinatal asphyxia and the myocardium, J. Pediatr. **96:**675, 1980.

Lendrum, B., and others: Echocardiographic (echo) studies in infants of diabetic mothers, Pediatr. Res. **12:**385, 1975.

Lester, L.A., and others: An evaluation of the left atrial/aortic root ratio in children with ventricular septal defect, Circulation **60:**364, 1979.

Liebman, J., Borkat, G., and Hirschfeld, S.: The heart. In Klaus, M.H., and Fanaroff, A.A., editors: Care of the high risk neonate, ed. 2, Philadelphia, 1979, W.B. Saunders Co.

Mace, S., and others: Echocardiographic abnormalities in infants of diabetic mothers, J. Pediatr. **95:**1013, 1979.

Meyer, R.A.: Pediatric echocardiography, Philadelphia, 1977, Lea & Febiger.

Meyer, R.A., and Kaplan, S.: Noninvasive technique in pediatric cardiovascular disease, Prog. Cardiovasc. Dis. **15:**341, 1973.

Moss, A.J., Gussoni, C.C., and Isabel-Jones, J.: Echocardiography in congenital heart disease, West. J. Med. **124:**102, 1976.

Nanda, N.C., and others: Echocardiographic evaluation of pulmonary hypertension, Circulation **50:**575, 1974.

Nelson, R.M., and others: Serum creatine phosphokinase MB fraction in newborns with transient tricuspid insufficiency, N. Engl. J. Med. **298:**146, 1978.

Pieroni, D.R., and others: Echocardiographic diagnosis of septic pericarditis in infancy, J. Pediatr. **82:**689, 1973.

Riemenschneider, T.A., and others: Disturbances of the transitional circulation: spectrum of pulmonary hypertension and myocardial dysfunction, J. Pediatr. **89:**622, 1976.

Riggs, T., and others: Neonatal circulatory changes: an echocardiographic study, Pediatrics **59:**338, 1977.

Riggs, T., and others: Persistence of fetal circulation syndrome: an echocardiographic study, J. Pediatr. **91:**626, 1977.

Roelandt, J.: Practical echocardiology, Portland, 1977, Research Studies Press.

Sahn, D.J., and others: Cross-sectional echocardiographic diagnosis of total anomalous pulmonary venous drainage, Circulation **60:**1317, 1979.

St. John Sutton, M.G., and others: Cardiac function in the normal newborn; additional information by computer analysis of the M-mode echocardiogram, Circulation **57:**1198, 1978.

Setzer, E., and others: Papillary muscle necrosis in a neonatal autopsy population; incidence and associated clinical manifestations, J. Pediatr. **96:**289, 1980.

Shabetai, R., and Davidson, S.: Asymmetrical hypertrophic cardiomyopathy simulating mitral stenosis, Circulation **45:**37, 1972.

Silverman, N.H., and Hoffman, J.I.: Echo assessment of pulmonary vascular resistance, Circulation **54:**525, 1976.

Silverman, N.H., and Snider, A.R.: Prediction of pulmonary hypertension from right ventricular systolic time intervals in ventricular septal defects, Circulation **60:**11, 1979.

Silverman, N.H., and others: Echocardiographic assessment of ductus arteriosus shunt in premature infants, Circulation **50:**821, 1974.

Snider, A.R., Ports, T.A., and Silverman, N.H.: Venous anomalies of the coronary sinus: detection by M-mode, two-dimensional and contrast echocardiography, Circulation **60:**721, 1979.

Spooner, E.W., and others: Estimation of pulmonary/systemic resistance ratios from echocardiographic systolic time intervals in young patients with congenital or acquired heart disease, Am. J. Cardiol. **42:**810, 1978.

Tajik, A.J., and others: Two dimensional real-time ultrasonic imaging of the heart and great vessels, Mayo Clin. Proc. **53:**271, 1978.

Thibeault, D.W., and others: Patent ductus arteriosus complicating the respiratory distress syndrome in preterm infants, J. Pediatr. **86:**120, 1975.

Way, G.L., and others: Echocardiographic assessment of ventricular dimensions and myocardial function in infants of diabetic mothers, Pediatr. Res. **9:**273, 1975.

Way, G.L., and others: The natural history of hypertrophic cardiomyopathy in infants of diabetic mothers, J. Pediatr. **95:**1020, 1979.

Weinberg, A.G., and Laird, W.P.: Group B streptococcal endocarditis detected by echocardiography, J. Pediatr. **92:**335, 1978.

Weissler, A.M., Harris, W.S., and Schoenfeld, C.D.: Bedside technics for the evaluation of ventricular function in man, Am. J. Cardiol. **23:**577, 1969.

Weissler, A.M., Lewis, R.P., and Leighton, R.F.: The systolic time intervals as a measure of left ventricular performance in man, Prog. Cardiol. **1:**155, 1972.

Weyman, A.E., and others: Echocardiographic patterns of pulmonic valve motion with pulmonary hypertension, Circulation **50:**905, 1974.

Cyanosis

Gatti, R.A., and others: Neonatal polycythemia with transient cyanosis and cardiorespiratory abnormalities, J. Pediatr. **69:**1063, 1966.

Goetzman, B.W., and others: Neonatal hypoxia and pulmonary vasospasm; response to tolazoline, J. Pediatr. **89:**617, 1976.

Gootman, N.L., Scarpelli, E.M., and Rudolph, A.M.: Metabolic acidosis in children with severe cyanotic congenital heart disease, Pediatrics **31:**251, 1963.

Lees, M.H., and Jolly, J.: Severe congenital methaemoglobinaemia in an infant, Lancet **2:**1147, 1957.

Oliver, T.K., Jr., Demis, J.A., and Bates, G.D.: Serial blood-gas tensions and acid-base balance during the first hour of life in human infants, Acta Paediatr. Scand. **50:**346, 1961.

Roberton, N.R.C., Hallidie-Smith, K.A., and Davis, J.A.: Severe respiratory distress syndrome mimicking cyanotic heart disease in term babies, Lancet **2:**1108, 1967.

Sommerville, R.J., and others: Adrenal insufficiency mimicking heart disease in infancy, Pediatrics **42:**691, 1968.

Wood, J.L.: Plethora in the newborn infant associated with cyanosis and convulsions, J. Pediatr. **54:**143, 1959.

Persistence of the fetal circulation

Arcilla, R.A., Thinelius, D.G., and Ranniger, K.: Congestive heart failure from suspected ductal closure in utero, J. Pediatr. **75**:74, 1969.

Corby, D.G.: Aspirin in pregnancy; maternal and fetal effects, Pediatrics **62**:930, 1978.

Csaba, I.P., Sulyok, E., and Ertle, T.: Relationship of maternal treatment with indomethacin to persistent fetal circulation syndrome, J. Pediatr. **92**:484, 1978.

Gersony, W.B.: Persistent fetal circulation; a commentary, J. Pediatr. **82**:1103, 1973.

Haworth, S.G., and Reid, L.: Persistent fetal circulation; newly recognized structural features, J. Pediatr. **88**:614, 1976.

Korones, S.B., and Eyal, F.G.: Successful treatment of "persistent fetal circulation" with tolazoline (abstract), Pediatr. Res. **9**:367, 1975.

Levin, D.R., Perkin, R.M., and Weinberg, A.G.: Pulmonary microthrombi in newborn infants with unresponsive persistent pulmonary hypertension (abstr.), Pediatr. Res. **16**:102A, 1982.

Manchester, D., Margolis, H.S., and Sheldon, R.E.: Possible association between maternal indomethacin and primary pulmonary hypertension of the newborn, Am. J. Obstet. Gynecol. **126**:467, 1976.

Soifer, S.J., and others: Developmental changes in the effect of PGD$_2$ on the pulmonary circulation in the newborn lamb (abstr.), Pediatr. Res. **16**:308A, 1982.

Heart failure

Benzing, G., and others: Simultaneous hypoglycemia and acute congestive heart failure, Circulation **40**:209, 1969.

Berdon, W.E., and Baker, D.H.: Giant hepatic hemangioma with cardiac failure in the newborn infant; value of high-dosage intravenous urography and umbilical angiography, Radiology **92**:1523, 1969.

Burnell, R.J.: Venous pressure in congestive heart failure in infancy, Arch. Dis. Child. **45**:360, 1970.

Goldberg, L.I.: Dopamine; clinical uses of an endogenous catecholamine, N. Engl. J. Med. **291**:707, 1974.

Rudolph, A.M., Mesel, E., and Levy, J.M.: Epinephrine in the treatment of cardiac failure due to shunts, Circulation **28**:3, 1963.

Cardiogenic shock and perinatal asphyxia

Bucciarelli, R., and others: Serum creatine phosphokinase MB fraction in newborns with transient tricuspid insufficiency, N. Engl. J. Med. **298**:146, 1978.

Cabal, L.A., and others: Cardiogenic shock associated with perinatal asphyxia in preterm infants, J. Pediatr. **96**:705, 1980.

Driscoll, D.J., and others: Hemodynamic effects of dobutamine in children, Am. J. Cardiol. **43**:581, 1979.

Finley, J.P., and others: Transient myocardial ischemia of the newborn infant demonstrated by thallium myocardial imaging, J. Pediatr. **94**:263, 1979.

Lees, M.H.: Perinatal asphyxia and the myocardium, J. Pediatr. **96**:674, 1980.

Rowe, R.D., and Hoffmann, T.: Transient myocardial ischemia of the newborn infant; a form of severe cardiorespiratory distress in full-term infants, J. Pediatr. **81**:243, 1972.

Arrhythmias

Benrey, J., and others: Permanent pacemaker implantation in infants, children and adolescents; long-term follow-up, Circulation **53**:245, 1976.

Berube, S., and others: Congenital heart block and maternal systemic lupus erythematosus, Am. J. Obstet. Gynecol. **130**:595, 1978.

Chameides, L., and others: Association of maternal systemic lupus erythematosus with congenital complete heart block, N. Engl. J. Med. **297**:1204, 1977.

Etches, P.C., and Lemons, J.A.: Non-immune hydrops fetalis; report of 22 cases including 3 siblings, Pediatrics **64**:326, 1979.

Ferrer, P.L.: Arrhythmias in the neonate. In Roberts, N., and Gelband, H., editors: Cardiac arrhythmias in the neonate, infant and child, New York, 1977, Appleton-Century-Crofts.

Garson, A., Jr., Gillette, P.C., and McNamara, D.G.: Supraventricular tachycardia in children: clinical features, response to treatment and long term follow-up in 217 patients, Am. J. Cardiol. **45**:430, 1980.

Gelband, H., Myerburg, R.J., and Bassett, A.L.: Management of cardiac arrhythmias. In Roberts, N., and Gelband, H., editors: Cardiac arrhythmias in the neonate, infant and child, New York, 1977, Appleton-Century-Crofts.

Gettes, L.S.: The electrophysiologic effects of antiarrhythmic drugs, Am. J. Cardiol. **28**:526, 1971.

Gettes, L.S.: On the classification of antiarrhythmic drugs, Mod. Concepts Cardiovasc. Dis. **48**:13, 1979.

Gillette, P.C.: The mechanisms of supraventricular tachycardia in children, Circulation **54**:133, 1976.

Gillette, P.C., and others: Surgical treatment of supraventricular tachycardia in infants and children, Circulation **60**:111, 1979.

Hayes, A.H.: The pharmacology of cardio-active drugs. In Engle, M.A., and Brest, A.N., editors: Cardiovascular clinics, vol. 4, Philadelphia, 1972, F.A. Davis Co.

Krikler, D.M.: A fresh look at cardiac arrhythmias; cardiac electrophysiology, Lancet **1**:851, 1974.

Krikler, D.M.: A fresh look at cardiac arrhythmias; pathogenesis and presentation, Lancet **1**:913, 1974.

Krikler, D.M.: A fresh look at cardiac arrhythmias; electrocardiographic diagnosis, Lancet **1**:974, 1974.

Krikler, D.M.: A fresh look at cardiac arrhythmias; therapy, Lancet **1**:1034, 1974.

Lev, M., and others: The anatomic substrate for the sick sinus syndrome in adolescence, Circulation **60**:113, 1979.

Levy, A.M., Camm, A.J., and Keane, J.F.: Multiple arrhythmias detected during nocturnal monitoring in patients with congenital complete heart block, Circulation **55**:247, 1977.

McCue, C.M., and others: Congenital heart block in newborns of mothers with connective tissue disease, Circulation **56**:82, 1977.

Michaelsson, M., and Engle, M.A.: Congenital complete heart block: an international study of the natural history. In Engle, M.A., and Brest, A.N., editors; Cardiovascular clinics, vol. 4, no. 3, Philadelphia, 1972, F.A. Davis Co..

Nadas, A.S., and others: Paroxysmal tachycardia in infants and children, Pediatrics **9**:167, 1952.

Newburger, J., and Keane, J.F.: Intrauterine supraventricular tachycardia, J. Pediatr. **95**:780, 1979.

Pearl, W.: Cardiac malformations presenting as congenital atrial flutter, South. Med. J. **70**:622, 1977.

Podrid, P.J., and Lown, B.: Long term therapy with tocainide, Am. J. Cardiol. **45**:452, 1980.

Rosen, M.R., and Hordoff, A.J.: Mechanism of arrhythmias. In Roberts, N., and Gelband, H., editors: Cardiac arrhythmias in the neonate, infant and child, New York, 1977, Appleton-Century-Crofts.

Soler-Soler, J., and others: Effect of verapamil in infants with paroxysmal supraventricular tachycardia, Circulation **59**:876, 1978.

Stevens, D.C., and others: Fetal and neonatal ventricular arrhythmia, Pediatrics **63**:771, 1979.

Williams, D.O., Tatelbaum, R., and Most, A.S.: Effective treatment of supraventricular arrhythmias with acebutolol, Am. J. Cardiol. **44**:521, 1979.

Yabek, S.M., Swensson, R.E., and Jarmakani, J.M.: Electrocardiographic recognition of sinus node dysfunction in children and young adults, Circulation **56**:235, 1977.

Transposition of great arteries

Liebman, J., Cullum, L., and Belloc, N.B.: Natural history of transposition of the great arteries; anatomy and birth and death characteristics, Circulation 50:237, 1969.

Rashkind, W.J., and Miller, W.W.: Creation of an atrial septal defect without thoracotomy; a palliative approach to complete transposition of the great arteries, J.A.M.A. 196:991, 1966.

Hypoplastic left-heart syndrome

Deely, W.J., and others: Hypoplastic left heart syndrome; anatomic, physiologic and therapeutic considerations, Am. J. Dis. Child. 121:168, 1971.

Aortic stenosis

Feldman, B.H., and Scott, L.P., III: Aortic stenosis in infancy, Pediatrics 33:931, 1964.

Coarctation

Freundlich, E., Engle, M.A., and Goldberg, H.P.: Coarctation of aorta in infancy; analysis of a 10-year experience with medical management, Pediatrics 27:427, 1961.

Tricuspid atresia

Edwards, J.E., and Burchell, H.B.: Congenital tricuspid atresia; a classification, Med. Clin. North Am. 33:1177, 1949.

Truncus arteriosus

Collett, R.W., and Edwards, J.E.: Persistent truncus arteriosus; classification according to anatomic types, Surg. Clin. North Am. 29:1245, 1949.

PDA

Danilowicz, D., Rudolph, A.M., and Hoffman, J.I.E.: Delayed closure of the ductus arteriosus in premature infants, Pediatrics 37:74, 1966.

Friedman, W.F., and others: Pharmacologic closure of patent ductus arteriosus in the premature infant, N. Engl. J. Med. 295:526, 1976.

Halliday, H.L., Hirata, T., and Brady, J.P.: Indomethacin therapy for large patent ductus arteriosus in the very low birth weight infant; results and complications, Pediatrics 64:154, 1979.

Heymann, M.A., Rudolph, A.M., and Silverman, N.H.: Closure of the ductus arteriosus by prostaglandin inhibition, N. Engl. J. Med. 295:530, 1976.

Kitterman, J.A., and others: Patent ductus arteriosus in premature infants, N. Engl. J. Med. 287:473, 1972.

McCarthy, J., and others: Failure of indomethacin to close the ductus arteriosus (abstract), Pediatr. Res. 11:395, 1977.

Merritt, T.A., and others: Early closure of the patent ductus arteriosus in very low-birth-weight infants: a controlled trial, J. Pediatr. 99:281, 1981.

Neal, W.A., and others: Patent ductus arteriosus conplicating respiratory distress syndrome, J. Pediatr. 86:127, 1975.

Rudolph, A.M., and Heymann, M.A.: Medical treatment of the ductus arteriosus, Hosp. Pract. 12:57, 1977.

Rudolph, A.M., and others: Formalin infiltration of the ductus arteriosus; a method for palliation of infants with selective congenital cardiac lesions, N. Engl. J. Med. 292:1263, 1975.

Serwer, J.A., Armstrong, B.E., and Anderson, P.A.W.: Continuous wave Doppler ultrasonograph IC quantitation of patent ductus arteriosus flow, J. Pediatr. 100:297, 1982.

Thibeault, D.W., and others: Patent ductus arteriosus complicating the respiratory distress syndrome in preterm infants, J. Pediatr. 86:120, 1975.

VSD

Campbell, M.: Natural history of ventricular septal defect, Br. Heart J. 33:246, 1971.

Hoffman, J.I.E., and Rudolph, A.M.: The natural history of ventricular septal defects in infancy, Am. J. Cardiol. 16:634, 1965.

Common ventricle

Van Praagh, R., and others: Diagnosis of the anatomic types of single or common ventricle, Am. J. Cardiol. 15:345, 1965.

Arteriovenous fistula

Hall, R.J., Nelson, W.P., and Blake, H.A.: Massive pulmonary arteriovenous fistula in the newborn; a correctable form of "cyanotic heart disease," an additional cause of cyanosis with left axis deviation, Circulation 31:762, 1965.

Myocarditis

Hosier, D.M., and Newton, W.A., Jr.: Serious Coxsackie infection in infants and children, Am. J. Dis. Child. 96:251, 1958.

Macauley, D.: Acute endocarditis in infancy and early childhood, Am. J. Dis. Child. 88:715, 1954.

Rosenberg, H.S., and McNamara, D.G.: Acute myocarditis in infancy and childhood, Prog. Cardiovasc. Dis. 7:179, 1964.

Cor triatriatum

Jegier, W., Gibbons, J.E., and Wigglesworth, E.W.: Cor triatriatum—clinical, hemodynamic and pathological studies; surgical correction in early life, Pediatrics 31:255, 1963.

Vascular ring

Fearon, B., and Shortreed, R.: Tracheobronchial compression by congenital cardiovascular anomalies in children, Ann. Otol. Rhinol. Laryngol. 72:949, 1963.

Stewart, J.R., Kincaid, O.W., and Edwards, J.E.: An atlas of vascular rings and related malformations of the aortic arch system, Springfield, Ill. 1964, Charles C Thomas, Publisher.

Hypertension

Adelman, R.D.: Neonatal hypertension, Pediatr. Clin. North. Am. 25:99, 1978.

Adelman, R.D., and others: Nonsurgical management of renovascular hypertension in the neonate, Pediatrics 62:71, 1978.

Blaufox, M.D.: Systemic arterial hypertension in pediatric practice, Pediatr. Clin. North Am. 18:577, 1971.

Bucci, G., and others: The systemic systolic blood pressure of newborns with low weight, Acta Paediatr. Scand. (Suppl.) 229:5, 1972.

de Swiet, M., Fayers, P., and Shinebourne, E.A.: Blood pressure survey in a population of newborn infants, Br. Med. J. 2:9, 1976.

Finnerty, F.A., Jr., Davidow, M., and Kakaviatos, N.: Hypertensive vascular disease, Am. J. Cardiol. 19:377, 1967.

Lum, L.G., and Jones, M.D., Jr.: The effect of cuff width on systolic blood pressure measurements in neonates, J. Pediatr. 91:963, 1977.

Plumer, L.B., Kaplan, G.W., and Mendoza, S.A.: Hypertension in infants—a complication of umbilical arterial catheterization, J. Pediatr. 89:802, 1976.

Postoperative care

Sade, R.M., Cosgrove, D.M., and Castenada, A.R.: Infant and child care in cardiac surgery, Chicago, 1977, Year Book Medical Publishers, Inc.

CHAPTER 26 **Immunology**

For the human newborn, extrauterine existence is contingent on a delicate balance between hostile microorganisms in the environment and the infant's host defense mechanisms. During the 9 months of gestation the fetus develops in a highly protective environment, whereas during the birth process and thereafter the infant is exposed to a wide variety of microorganisms. Although the antimicrobial defense mechanisms have begun to develop early in gestation, at the time of delivery many of these mechanisms do not function as efficiently as in older children or adults. The relatively high incidence of infectious disease in the perinatal period bears testimony to the fact that the host-parasite balance is precarious in many neonates. Thus there is an increased incidence of neonatal infectious diseases often caused by microorganisms generally considered to be of low pathogenicity.

Host defense mechanisms may be divided into nonspecific and specific categories. Nonspecific mechanisms function effectively without requiring prior exposure to a microorganism or its antigens. These include physical barrier (e.g., intact skin and mucous membranes) and chemical barriers (e.g., gastric acid, digestive enzymes, bacteriostatic fatty acids of the skin) as well as phagocytic cells and the complement system. In contrast, specific host defense mechanisms such as cell-mediated and antibody-mediated immune responses function most effectively if there has been prior exposure to the infecting agent or its antigens (i.e., immunization).

NONSPECIFIC HOST DEFENSE MECHANISMS
Phagocytic mechanisms

The most primitive of the host defense mechanisms involves the ingestion and killing of bacteria and other microorganisms by phagocytic cells. Although polymorphonuclear leukocytes (PMNs) are the most important phagocytic cells, monocytes and the nonmobile phagocytic cells of the reticuloendothelial (RE) system contribute substantially to the function of this system. Protection provided by the nonmobile phagocytes of the RE system is strikingly demonstrated by intravascular microbial invasion in patients with congenital asplenia.

Effective elimination of invading microorganisms by mobile phagocytic cells such as PMNs requires (1) movement of the PMN to the site of infection, (2) adherence of the microorganism to the phagocyte's membrane, (3) ingestion, and (4) killing. Specific defects in some of the phases of phagocytic function have been identified in the normal neonate as well as in disorders such as chronic granulomatous disease and hyper-IgE immunodeficiency (Job's syndrome).

In the neonate, movement of PMNs toward a site of infection (chemotaxis) is defective. The neonatal PMN has a decreased chemotactic response to chemoattractant factors generated from normal adult serum. Moreover, neonatal serum does not generate chemoattractant factors as readily as adult serum. Membrane deformability is closely related to phagocyte movement. The membranes of neonatal PMNs are less deformable (i.e., more rigid) than adult PMN membranes, and this also appears to contribute to the movement disorder of the neonatal PMN. In contrast, neonatal monocytes have no chemotactic defect, and membrane deformability is normal.

Adherence of bacteria to the phagocyte's cell membrane is a prerequisite for ingestion and killing of the invading microorganism. This is an inefficient process in the absence of specific antibody and complement, since many bacteria have polysaccharide capsules that impede their adherence to PMN membranes and impair ingestion. In adult serum diluted to less than 10% ingestion of bacteria by neonatal PMNs is significantly less efficient than by adult PMNs. However, at high serum concentrations ingestion of bacteria by neonatal and adult PMNs is comparable.

Ingestion results in the formation of a phagocytic vacuole within the PMN. Occurring simultaneously with this event is an oxygen-requiring metabolic burst. Normally the enzyme nicotinamide adenosine dinucleotide phosphate oxidase (NADPH oxidase) catalyzes the production of superoxide anion ($.O_2^-$) from NADPH and O_2. Additionally highly reactive products are generated by related enzymatic reactions. These include singlet oxygen, hydrogen peroxide, and hydrogen radicals. Hydrogen peroxide is thought to play a major bactericidal role by interacting with halide (iodide or chloride) ions in the presence of myeloperoxidase (MPO), resulting in the halidation of the ingested microorganism. The reaction of hydrogen peroxide with halide in the presence of MPO causes the release of light (i.e., chemiluminescence), which is closely correlated with the microbial killing activity of PMNs. Fusion of lysosomes and other intracytoplasmic granules with the phagocytic vacuole occurs, adding lysozyme, lactoferrin, cationic proteins, and other bactericidal and bacteriostatic materials to the contents of the phagocytic vacuoles.

In chronic granulomatous disease there is defective microbial killing, which appears to be due to a defect in the triggering of NADPH oxidase activity. PMNs from neonates show a decreased chemiluminescence response on ingestion of bacteria or other particles, suggesting a diminished bactericidal capacity. Neonatal PMNs kill bacteria as well as adult PMNs do when the bacterium to phagocyte ratio is 1:1; however, when the bacterium to phagocyte ratio is increased to 100:1, neonatal neutrophils demonstrate a markedly depressed bactericidal capacity. Thus, when stressed, the neonatal phagocytic cells perform less well than adult cells under the same conditions.

The complement system

The complement system consists of 17 plasma proteins that participate in both specific and nonspecific host defense mechanisms. The complement system has two pathways by which its major effector functions can be initiated: the classic pathway and the alternative pathway or properdin system (Fig. 26-1). Activation of either pathway results in the sequential cleavage of complement proteins with the generation of enzymatically active products required for subsequent steps in the complement cascade, as well as biologically active fragments and complexes (Table 26-1). Fragments of C3 and C5 (C3a and C5a) increase vascular permeability and are potent chemoattractants for PMNs, whereas another fragment of C3 (C3b) promotes phagocytosis by adhering to the surfaces of bacteria or other cells. PMNs have specific receptors for C3b that avidly bind to C3b on the bacterial cell wall. Most of the biologically significant effector functions of the complement system begin at the C3 cleavage step, the point at which the classic and alternative pathways converge. Activation of the complement system via the classic pathway requires the interaction of C1 with antibody-antigen complexes. Only complexes containing IgM or IgG antibody can activate the complement cascade via the classic pathway. However, the classic pathway also may be activated by complexes of C-reactive protein (CRP) and polysaccharides. The alterna-

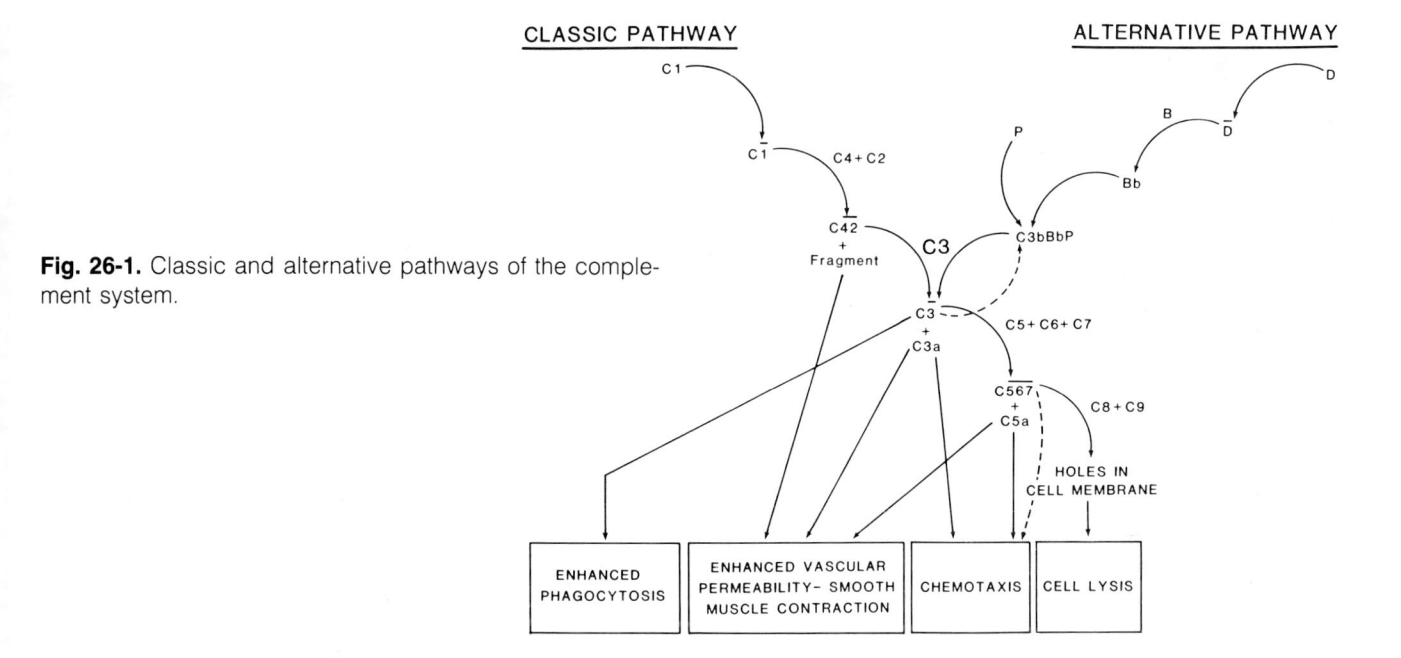

Fig. 26-1. Classic and alternative pathways of the complement system.

Table 26-1. Biologically active complement fragments

Fragment	Biologic activity
C3a	Leukocyte chemotaxis, increased vascular permeability, anaphylatoxin
C3b	Opsonization, immune adherence
C5a	Leukocyte chemotaxis, increased vascular permeability
C5b	Opsonization
C567	Leukocyte chemotaxis
C8, C9	Lysis

tive pathway may be activated in the absence of specific antibody by bacterial or mammalian cell surfaces. Activation requires the interaction of properdin factors B and D with small amounts of C3b. The adherence of C3b to a cell surface, as well as to properdin itself, serves to stabilize this reactive complex, which then cleaves more C3. The alternative pathway is a means of activating the complement system without specific antibody but also serves to increase C3 cleavage when the complement system has been activated via the classic pathway with antibody-antigen complexes.

The components of the classic complement system, as well as their functional activity, measured by total hemolytic complement (CH_{50}) assay, in full-term neonates is comparable to those of normal adults. In earlier studies in which neonates were compared to their mothers, significant deficiencies in complement components were reported. These studies did not take into account that the concentration of complement components in maternal serum is significantly elevated when compared with that of other normal adults. However, preterm neonates have significantly decreased concentrations of C1q, C4, C3, and CH_{50} activity compared with term neonates. Moreover, there was a statistically significant correlation between increasing birth weight or gestational age and serum concentrations of these components. Studies by Johnson and co-workers have shown that the functional activity of the classic pathway (CH_{50}) and the C3 concentration were below the normal adult range in 51% and 63%, respectively, of term newborns. Thus, within the population of term newborns, there are infants with normal and abnormal concentrations and function of the classic pathway components.

Concentrations of factor B of the alternative pathway in newborn serum vary from 35% to 60% of normal adult values and are abnormal in 15% to 30% of infants. There is no correlation between factor B concentration and gestational age. In contrast, properdin concentrations are significantly lower in preterm infants compared with term neonates. Stossel reported defective alternative pathway function in 15% of term neonates using an endotoxin particle opsonization assay. Other studies of alternative pathway function have shown defective function in 75% of term newborns and a significant correlation between increased function and gestational age. Johnston studied function of both the alternative and classic pathways in 27 term newborns. Eighty-one percent of these infants had defective alternative pathway function, 51% had abnormal classic pathway activity, 37% had defects in both pathways, and in only 11% were both pathways functionally normal.

Whether deficiencies in the complement system predispose the neonates to infection has not as yet been established. It is likely that defects in the complement system and the alternative pathway, in particular, will ultimately be found to play a role in susceptibility to infection, especially in preterm infants. Newborns have a limited armamentarium of circulating antibody transmitted across the placenta; they receive IgG, no IgM, and very little antibody to the entire range of gram-negative bacteria. Thus the classic pathway has relatively little value at and shortly after birth. It follows that, in the absence of specific antibody, nonspecific activation of the biologically active fragments and complexes of the complement system via the alternative pathway becomes an extremely important defense mechanism for neonates during their first encounter with many bacteria. In a majority of neonates the functional deficiency of the alternative pathway, in conjunction with impaired function of neutrophils, is likely to be clinically relevant.

SPECIFIC HOST DEFENSE MECHANISMS

The two major specific host defense mechanisms are the antibody-mediated and cell-mediated immune systems. Antibody-mediated immunity is related to B lymphocytes, plasma cells and their products, immunoglobulins, and antibodies. Cell-mediated immunity is largely the function of T lymphocytes of various types and their soluble products, the lymphokines.

Antibody-mediated immunity

Specific antibody may be produced in response to direct exposure to infection or immunization by an almost infinite spectrum of antigens (e.g., proteins, carbohydrates, bacteria, viruses, fungi, drugs). Antibodies are synthesized and secreted by plasma cells residing in the lymph nodes, spleen, mucosal linings of the gastrointestinal and respiratory tracts, and the bone marrow. The plasma cells arise from B-lymphocytes after antigenic stimulation.

Antibodies comprise a unique family of proteins termed *immunoglobulins* (Ig). There are five major classes of human immunoglobulins: IgG, IgA, IgM, IgD, and IgE. The basic structure of the immunoglobulin molecule, as illustrated by IgG, is shown in Fig. 26-2. The IgG molecule is composed of four polypeptide chains,

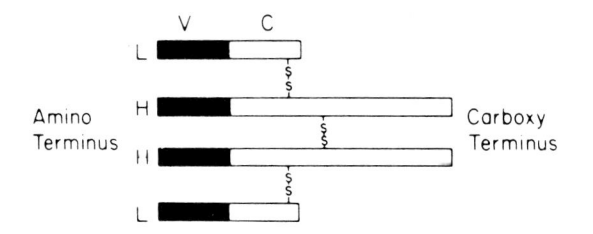

Fig. 26-2. Structure of the immunoglobulin G (IgG) molecule.

Table 26-2. Chemical and biologic properties of human immunoglobulin classes

	IgG	IgA	IgM	IgD	IgE
Heavy chains	γ	α	μ	δ	ε
Molecular weight (daltons)	150,000	160,000	900,000	180,000	190,000
		400,000*			
Biologic half-life (days)	21	5	5	2	2
Adult serum concentration(mg/dl)	1,000	250	100	2.3	0.01
Placental transfer	+	0	0	0	0
Binds complement (classic pathway)	+	0	+	0	0
Reaginic activity	0	0	0	0	+
Mucosal immunity	+	+++	+	0	++

*Secretory IgA.

two heavy chains and two light chains, held together by covalent disulfide bonds as well as by noncovalent forces. In a given IgG molecule the two heavy chains and two light chains have identical amino acid sequences. The different immunoglobulin classes are distinguished by antigenic and amino acid sequence differences in their heavy chains (Table 26-2). Some of the immunoglobulin classes are composed of subclasses, for example, IgG has four subclasses—IgG_1, IgG_2, IgG_3, and IgG_4—which result from antigenic differences in the heavy chains. In addition to these differences between the immunoglobulin classes and subclasses, there are antigenic and amino acid sequence differences among molecules from the same class and subclass. This molecular heterogeneity is due to amino acid sequence variation in the amino terminal portions of the heavy chains and light chains in the so-called variable regions. The variable regions make up portions of the antibody conbining sites of immunoglobulin molecules, and it is the structural variability in this region that permits different antibody molecules to react specifically with different antigens. In contrast, the amino acid sequences of the carboxy terminal portions of the heavy and light chains do not vary between molecules of the same immunoglobulin class or subclass and are termed the *constant regions*. Whereas the variable regions of immunoglobulin molecules confer the antigen-binding specificity, the constant regions are responsible for the biologic functions of the immunoglobulin molecules. Since the structure of the constant regions of the various immunoglobulin classes differs, their biologic properties and functions vary as well. For example, only IgM and IgG activate the complement system via the classic pathway, and only IgG can be actively transported across the placenta.

The chemical characteristics and biologic properties of the immunoglobulin classes are summarized in Table 26-2. IgG is the major immunoglobulin in the serum and interstitial fluid and has a relatively long half-life (20 to 30 days). It is responsible for immunity to bacteria (particularly gram-positive bacteria), bacterial toxins, and viral agents. IgG antibodies can neutralize viruses and toxins, as well as facilitate the phagocytosis and destruction of bacteria and other particles to which they are bound. This property is termed *opsonization*. Bacteria to which IgG is bound adhere to the surface membranes of neutrophils and monocytes (macrophages) by means of membrane receptors for a portion of the IgG heavy chain. IgG can activate the complement pathway, increase the inflammatory response, and increase neutrophil chemotaxis and complement-mediated opsonization.

IgA is the second most abundant immunoglobulin in serum, but it is the predominant immunoglobulin in the gastrointestinal and respiratory tracts as well as in human colostrum and breast milk. In secretions, IgA occurs as a dimer joined by a J-chain and bears an additional polypeptide chain termed the *secretory component*. This moiety endows the molecule with resistance against degradation by proteolytic enzymes. Secretory IgA is thus uniquely suited for functioning in the secretions of the respiratory and gastrointestinal tracts. IgA provides local mucosal immunity against viruses and limits bacterial overgrowth on mucosal surfaces. It may also limit

Table 26-3. Normal values for immunoglobulins at various ages

Age	IgG (mg/dl)	IgA (mg/dl)	IgM (mg/dl)
Newborn	600-1,670	0-5	5-15
1-3 months	218-610	20-53	11-51
4-6 months	228-636	27-72	25-60
7-9 months	292-816	27-73	12-124
10-18 months	383-1,070	27-169	28-113
2 years	423-1,184	35-222	32-131
3 years	477-1,334	40-251	28-113
4-5 years	540-1,500	48-336	20-106
6-8 years	571-1,700	52-535	28-112
14 years	570-1,570	86-544	33-135
Adult	635-1,775	106-668	37-154

From Buckley, R.H., and others: Pediatrics **41**:600, 1968. Copyright American Academy of Pediatrics 1968.

absorption of antigenic dietary proteins. IgA does not activate the classic complement pathway but can activate an alternative pathway.

IgM antibodies exist in serum primarily as pentamers joined together by a J-chain. IgM provides protection against blood-borne infection. It occurs in only small quantities in interstitial fluids and secretions. IgM antibodies are potent bacterial agglutinins and activate the classic complement sequence. Most serum antibodies to gram-negative bacteria are of the IgM type. Intrauterine and neonatal infections elicit the formation of predominately IgM antibodies. Since IgM does not cross the placenta, the presence of specific IgM antibody in cord blood to spirochetes, rubella, cytomegalovirus, or other microorganisms can be taken as reliable evidence for intrauterine infection with these agents. The absence of IgM does not, however, exclude the possibility of congenital intrauterine infection.

IgE antibodies are present in very small quantities in serum and secretions. These antibodies play a major role in allergic reactions of the immediate hypersensitivity type. IgE antibodies bind to the cell membranes of basophils (mast cells) via a receptor for the carboxy terminal portion of the heavy chain. Binding of antigen (allergen) to the IgE fixed to the basophil results in the liberation of histamine, slow-reacting substance of anaphylaxis (SRS-A), and other pharmacologic mediators of immediate allergic reactions. IgD is present in low concentration in serum but is present on the surfaces of B lymphocytes. The role of surface membrane IgD is discussed later.

Levels of immunoglobulins in the serum of newborns change dramatically during the first 2 years of life. Interpretation of normal serum immunoglobulin values requires comparison with age-matched controls. Table 26-3 shows normal immunoglobulin levels for infants and children.

Cell-mediated immunity

Cell-mediated immunity refers to a group of immunologic responses in which T lymphocytes play a central role; serum immunoglobulins and antibodies cannot produce these reactions or transfer them to another individual. The cutaneous delayed hypersensitivity reaction is a classic example of a cell-mediated immune reaction. An individual who has been exposed to tubercle bacilli or immunized with BCG has T lymphocytes that are sensitized to tuberculin. When such an individual is injected intradermally with turberculin (PPD), sensitized T lymphocytes are activated to divide as well as to secrete a variety of soluble factors known as lymphokines. Some of these lymphokines have chemoattractant properties and cause monocytes (macrophages) and neutrophils to accumulate at the site where sensitized T cells are interacting with antigen. Macrophage inhibitory factor (MIF) causes macrophages to remain at that site and *incites* these cells to extreme phagocytic and metabolic activity; these cells are termed *activated*, or "angry," *macrophages*. Antigen-stimulated T cells also secrete lymphokines, which cause nonsensitized T cells to divide (mitogen factors), and in this way these cells are nonspecifically recruited into the reaction. The accumulation of macrophages, lymphocytes, and neutrophils and the attendant inflammatory reaction at the site of tuberculin injection are what we perceive clinically as a positive delayed hypersensitivity reaction. Granuloma formation is essentially a delayed hypersensitivity reaction initiated by a particle (e.g., tubercle bacillus or fungus) rather than a soluble protein. The extensive tissue damage in the middle of a granuloma is due to indiscriminate destruction of normal tissue by "angry" macrophages. The basic scheme of cell-mediated immune reactions is that T cells are activated by antigens to which they have been sensitized (i.e., exposed), and these cells liberate lymphokines that modify the behavior of other cells such as macrophages, neutrophils, and other lymphocytes. A list of important lymphokines and their properties is found in Table 26-4.

Other cell-mediated reactions include the killing of tumor cells or virus-infected cells by direct contact of a cytolytic T cell with the target cells, the liberation of a lymphocytotoxin by the T cell, which kills the target cells, or by recruitment of non-T killer cells via a lymphokine. Moreover, T cells liberate interferon, which inhibits intracellular viral replication.

T lymphocytes also regulate antibody formation to many antigens. A subpopulation of T lymphocytes induces B lymphocytes to differentiate into plasma cells after exposure to antigen. These cells are termed *inducer* or *helper* T cells. B-cells differentiation can be inhibited by other subpopulations of T cells, termed *suppressor* T cells. Some suppressor T cells also have cytotoxic properties.

Table 26-4. Lymphokines

Target cell or tissue	Factor	Effect
Macrophages	Migration-inhibiting factor (MIF)	Inhibits macrophage migration in vitro; may lead to accumulation of macrophages
	Activating factor (MAF)	Increases phagocytosis, glycolysis, oxygen consumption
Neutrophils	Leukocyte-inhibiting factor (LIF)	Inhibits migration of neutrophils
	Chemotactic factor	Attracts neutrophils
Lymphocytes	Mitogenic factor (MF) or blastogenic factor (BF)	Provokes proliferation of normal lymphocytes
	Transfer factor (TF)	Transfer of specific reactivity to uncommitted lymphocytes
	Helper and suppressor factors	Modulate T and B cell responses
Mammalian cells of the same species	Interferon	Inhibits viral replication; may act as immunosuppressive or enhancing agents
Mammalian cells: tumor cells, some bacteria and yeasts	Lymphotoxin (LT)	Inhibition of cell proliferation or frank cell cytotoxicity
Skin	Skin reactive factor (SRF)	Augments capillary permeability in vivo; contributes to infiltration with mononuclear cells

Development of T and B lymphocyte populations

Both the T and B lymphocyte populations are derived from pluripotent hematopoietic stem cells arising from the intraembryonic mesenchyme. These cells migrate to the blood islands of the yolk sac, thence to the fetal liver, and later in embryonic life to the bone marrow, where they reside throughout extrauterine life.

Cells destined to become T lymphocytes, the prothymocytes, migrate from the fetal liver or bone marrow to the thymus, entering at the cortex. As these thymocytes migrate toward the thymic medulla, they undergo numerous cycles of cell division as well as differentiation into functionally different classes of T lymphocytes (e.g., helper-inducer cells, suppressor cells, cytotoxic cells). The thymic microenvironment plays a key role in this differentiation process, and thymic hormones continue to influence T cells even after they have left the thymic microenvironment.

The thymus comprises both epithelial and lymphoid elements. The epithelial components of the thymus are derived from the third and fourth pharyngeal pouches and migrate into the anterior superior mediastinum. The parathyroid glands arise from the same region. The thymic lymphoid cells come from the stem cells just mentioned and first appear in the embryonic thymus at approximately 8 weeks of gestation. T lymphocytes can be detected in the thymus after 11 weeks of gestation and begin to appear in the peripheral blood, spleen, and lymph nodes by 16 to 18 weeks of gestation. By 30 to 32 weeks of gestation the fetus has a near normal (adult) number of circulating T lymphocytes. Thus at birth normal newborns and many infants born prematurely will have normal numbers of T lymphocytes detectable in their peripheral blood.

B lymphocytes are the precursors of immunoglobulin secreting (antibody-secreting) plasma cells. B lymphocytes are derived from the same stem cells that give rise to T cells, but B cell differentiation occurs in a different inductive microenvironment. In birds, B cell differentiation occurs in the bursa of Fabricius, an anatomically distinct lymphoepithelial organ in the wall of the hindgut. In humans and other mammals there is no bursa of Fabricius, and the development of B cells occurs first in the fetal liver and subsequently in the bone marrow. B cell differentiation is represented schematically in Fig. 26-3. The first identifiable cells of the B cell line arise from stem cells in the fetal liver at 8 weeks of gestation. These cells, termed *pre-B cells*, contain small amounts of low molecular weight (8S) IgM in their cytoplasm. At this stage of differentiation the development of clones of cells with different antibody specificities has already begun, i.e., different pre-B cells are producing IgM with different variable regions. At approximately 10 weeks of gestation the first "true" B cells can be identified in the liver. These cells synthesize surface membrane IgM (sIgM) only. These B cells, which have been called immature B cells, are exquisitely sensitive to inactivation following contact with antigens. The ease with which these cells may be inactivated is thought to be closely related to the well-established phenomenon of immunologic tolerance in neonatal animals. The immature sIgM + B cells proliferate, and some of their progeny begin to produce other immunoglobulin classes and display them on their membranes. B cell clones emerge

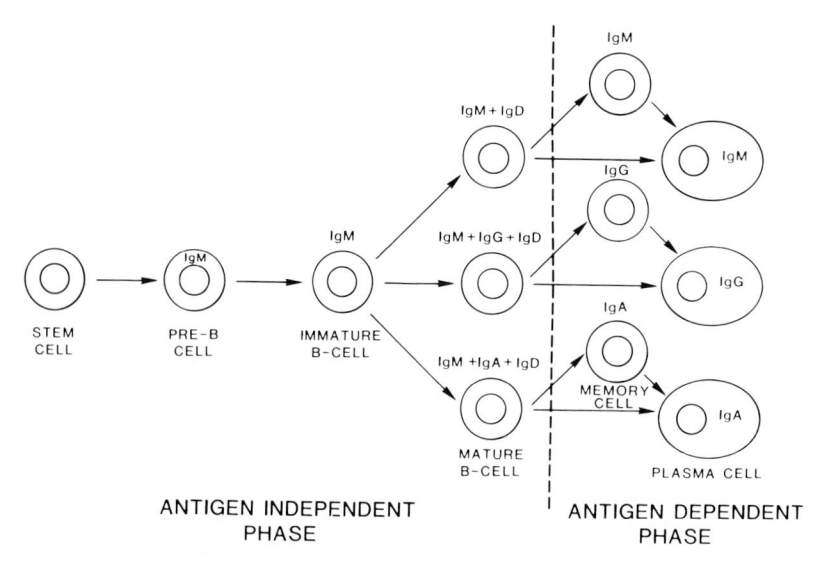

Fig. 26-3. Sequence of B lymphocyte differentiation.

bearing IgM + IgG + IgD, IgM + IgA + IgD, and IgM + IgD. By the fifteenth week of gestation the normal fetus has levels of circulating B lymphocytes that are as high or higher than those of normal adults. Unlike the immature B cells, B cells bearing surface IgD cannot be readily inactivated by antigen but can be triggered to differentiate into immunoglobulin-secreting plasma cells when exposed to antigen in the presence of helper or inducer T cells. The development of the different B cell clones and antibody diversity occurs in the absence of antigen and is termed the *antigen-independent phase of B cell differentiation*. Differentiation of B cells to plasma cells depends on the presence of antigen and is regulated by inducer and suppressor T lymphocytes; this is the *antigen-dependent phase of B cell differentiation*.

Specific immunity in the neonate

The appearance of specific antibodies or a population of sensitized T cells directed against a specific antigen requires exposure (i.e., immunization or infection) and immunocompetence. For example, in utero the fetus is normally exposed to very few foreign antigens and makes little or no antibody. At birth the only antibodies present are the IgG antibodies transferred from the mother via the placenta, unless there has been a congenital infection when IgM antibodies against the infecting agent are usually detectable. Thus an active immune response requires exposure to antigen.

Second, an infant or fetus must be developmentally capable of responding to an antigen at the time the antigen is presented. The ability to mount antibody or cell-mediated immune responses to specific antigens is acquired sequentially during the course of embryonic development. Early in gestation, fetuses can respond to certain antigens, whereas other antigens will elicit anti-

Table 26-5. Appearance of immunologic responses in the fetal lamb

Antigen	Days after conception
Bacteriophage	<40
Ferritin	56
Allogenic skin grafts	75
Simian virus 40	90
Ovalbumin	120
Lymphocytic choriomeningitis virus	140
Birth	150
Diphtheria toxoid	>190

Modified from Silverstein, A.M.: Ontogeny of the immune response: a perspective. In Cooper, M.D., and Dayton, D.H., editors: Development of host defenses, New York, 1977, Raven Press.

body production or cell-mediated immune reactions only after birth. This sequential development of antigen-specific immunocompetence was first described by Silverstein in the fetal lamb (Table 26-5) and has been observed in other mammalian species. The well-known inability to induce antibodies to the polysaccharides from *Pneumococcus* and *Haemophilus* organisms in children under 18 months of age is a clinically important example of the sequential acquisition of antigen-specific immunocompetence in humans.

Antibody responses of the fetus and premature and full-term newborn differ from those of older children and adults. They do not respond to some antigens (e.g., pneumococcal polysaccharide), and the antibody responses to other antigens (rubella, cytomegalovirus, toxoplasma) are predominately of the IgM type. The T lymphocyte population of newborns contains a relatively large number of suppressor cells for B cell differentiation. In addition, the B cells of newborns differentiate predominately into IgM-secreting plasma cells, whereas adult B cells will produce IgG- and IgA-secreting plasma cells as well. The adult pattern of B cell differentiation develops during the first year of life.

There are also deficiencies in cell-mediated immunity in premature and full-term neonates. T cells have reached normal levels by 30 to 32 weeks of gestation and are capable of proliferating at adult levels in response to phytohemagglutinin (PHA), concanavalin A (Con A), and allogeneic cells (mixed lymphocyte reaction). However, T lymphocytes from premature and full-term neonates show markedly reduced ability to secret migration-inhibiting factor (MIF) or immune interferon and to kill tumor or virus-infected cells when compared with those of normal adults. Cutaneous delayed hypersensitivity reactions are decreased even when there is evidence of adequate exposure. Infants with oral or cutaneous candidiasis may show only weakly reactive *Candida* skin tests, whereas their in vitro lymphocyte proliferation responses to *Candida* may be comparable to those seen in adults. This discrepancy is due to the decreased inflammatory reactions seen in infants. In general, the recognition, or afferent, phase of cellular immune responses in the neonate is comparable to that seen in the adult whereas the efferent, or effector, limb of these responses is diminished.

IMMUNOLOGIC ASPECTS OF THE MOTHER-CHILD RELATIONSHIP

Passive immunity is the acquisition of specific antibody or sensitized lymphocytes from another individual and represents a means by which specific immunity may be acquired without prior exposure to antigen or the mounting of a specific immune response. Such immunity is transient but nonetheless may provide sufficient antimicrobial protection during a vulnerable period of life. The development of an antibody response to an antigen seen for the first time requires 7 to 14 days. Thus active antibody-mediated immunity is of little value during the crucial first few days of an infection with a new microorganism. The presence of circulating specific antibody to that organism (i.e., passive immunity) permits the mobilization of multiple host defense mechanisms (i.e., complement system, neutrophils) to eliminate the invading microorganism as well as limit its colonization. In humans the major avenues for the acquisition of passive immunity are the transfer of IgG across the placenta and the transfer of secretory IgA via colostrum and breast milk.

Placental transport of IgG antibodies

Although B lymphocytes are present in the fetus by the end of the first trimester, there is very little active fetal immunoglobulin production, since this process depends on exposure to antigens. Serum immunoglobulin levels in the fetus are extremely low until 20 to 22 weeks of gestation, at which time an accelerated active transport of IgG across the placenta begins. Only maternal IgG is transported; IgA, IgM, IgD, and IgE are not. The specificity of this transport process is due to the presence of specific receptors on the heavy chain of the IgG molecule. The transport of IgG is an active placental process, and the neonate's serum IgG concentration at birth is 5% to 10% higher than that of the mother. Prematurely delivered infants have lower IgG levels than those delivered at term. Moreover, small for gestational age (SGA) infants have lower IgG levels than their appropriately grown (AGA) peers at any gestational age. Fetal weight loss in utero is often due to placental dysfunction, which reduces the nutrient supply and limits transfer of IgG as well. This phenomenon is further manifested by the progressive decrease in IgG transport after 44 weeks of gestation, a period when the placenta is known to become increasingly dysfunctional.

Elevated levels of IgM or IgA in cord blood usually indicate that the infant has been exposed to antigen in utero and has synthesized antibody itself. Congenital infections with syphilis and rubella characteristically produce elevation of the cord blood IgM concentration, and specific fetal antibody of the IgM type directed against the infecting agent can be detected. Elevated levels of both IgM and IgA may also be found if a maternal-to-fetal transplacental bleed has occurred.

The transfer of IgG antibodies from mother to child across the placenta provides the newborn with a portion of the mother's immunologic experience. Antibodies to viral agents, diphtheria, and tetanus antitoxins, which are usually of the IgG class, are efficiently transported across the placenta and attain protective levels in the fetus. In contrast, antibodies to agents that evoke primarily IgA or IgM antibody responses are transported poorly or not at all, leaving the neonate unprotected against those organisms (Table 26-6). Moreover, an infant cannot be protected against agents to which the mother has not made significant amounts of antibody.

Placental transfer of IgG antibody may have deleterious as well as beneficial effects. Hemolytic disease of the newborn is produced by placental transfer of IgG antierythrocyte antibodies usually directed against Rh or ABO blood group antigens. Transient neutropenia, thrombocytopenia, myasthenia, or hyperthyroidism are also produced in approximately 20% of infants born to mothers with systemic lupus erythematosus, idiopathic thrombocytopenic purpura, myasthenia gravis, or hyperthyroidism by IgG transported across the placenta. These disorders, as well as the protective effects of maternal IgG, are transient, since IgG has a half-life of 20 to 30 days.

Table 26-6. Relationship of antibody type with transplacental transfer

Good passive transfer (IgG)	Poor passive transfer (IgA)	No passive transfer (IgM)
Diphtheria antitoxin	*Haemophilus influenzae*	Enteric somatic (O) antibodies (*Salmonella, Shigella, E. Coli*)
Tetanus antitoxin	*Bordetella pertussis*	
Antierythrogenic toxin	*Shigella flexneri*	
Antistaphylococcal antibody	Streptococcus MG	Skin-sensitizing antibody
Salmonella flagella (H) antibody		Heterophile antibody
Antistreptolysin		Wassermann antibody
All antiviral antibodies present in maternal circulation (rubeola, rubella, mumps, poliovirus)		
VDRL antibodies		

Immunologic properties of human breast milk

Specific and nonspecific protective factors transferred to the neonate via the breast milk are listed in Table 26-7. Even though all immunoglobulin classes can be detected in colostrum, secretory IgA comprises the vast majority of the immunoglobulins in human breast milk. Secretory IgA consists of two "serum" IgA subunits, a J-chain and a secretory component, rendering it resistant to digestion by trypsin and pepsin as well as hydrolysis by gastric acid. There is no evidence that immunoglobulins present in breast milk enter the systemic circulation of the human neonate in significant quantities.

The levels of IgA, IgM, and IgG have been studied serially in milk. The IgG concentration is relatively constant during the first 180 days of lactation, whereas the IgM and IgA are highest in colostrum, decrease during the first 5 days of lactation, and then remain relatively constant during the next 175 days. Breast milk contains antibodies to a broad spectrum of enteric bacteria and viruses (e.g., polio, ECHO, Coxsackie), and the antibody titers to these agents decrease in parallel to the fall in concentration of IgA in the milk.

The majority of immunoglobulins present in human breast milk are thought to be produced by plasma cells located within the breast itself, and very little milk immunoglobulin is derived from maternal serum immunoglobulins. Moreover, milk antibodies are directed predominately against enteric bacterial and viral antigens; the concentration of such antibodies is much higher in colostrum than in maternal serum. Thus the antibody composition of breast milk in part compensates for the deficiency of antibodies directed against enteric antigens in placentally transferred IgG. This unique spectrum of antibody specificity is achieved by the "homing" of B lymphocytes sensitized in the mother's gastrointestinal tract to her mammary glands. B cells stimulated by enteric bacterial or viral antigens in Peyer's patches of the small intestine migrate to the mucosal linings of the lactating mammary gland where they differentiate into plasma cells and secrete their antibodies. Antigens introduced into the gastrointestinal tract will stimulate the development of antibodies in the breast milk while antibodies to these antigens do not develop in the serum. Thus a mother will transfer to her baby via breast milk antibodies specific for microbial agents present in her own gastrointestinal tract. As the neonate is being freshly colonized, these antibodies limit bacterial growth in the gastrointestinal tract and protect against overgrowth.

The cellular components of human breast milk consist of macrophages, T and B lymphocytes, neutrophils, and epithelial cells. The cellular content of colostrum or early

Table 26-7. Human milk protective elements

Component	Comment
Cellular factors	
Macrophage	Phagocytosis
	Produces lysozyme, lactoferrin, and complement
	May regulate B lymphocyte immunoglobulin production
Lymphocyte	
B cells	Humoral immunity; IgA synthesis
T cells	Cellular immunity
	Partially regulate humoral immunity
Growth-promoting factors	
DNA synthesis and cell division in vitro	Functional in both animal and human fibroblasts
DNA synthesis and growth by mucosal cells	Described in laboratory animals
Bifidus factor	Nitrogen-containing polysaccharides that specifically enhance the growth of *Lactobacillus bifidus*
Lactoperoxidase	Functions in conjunction with hydrogen peroxide and cyanide to form an in vitro antibacterial system

Immunology 641

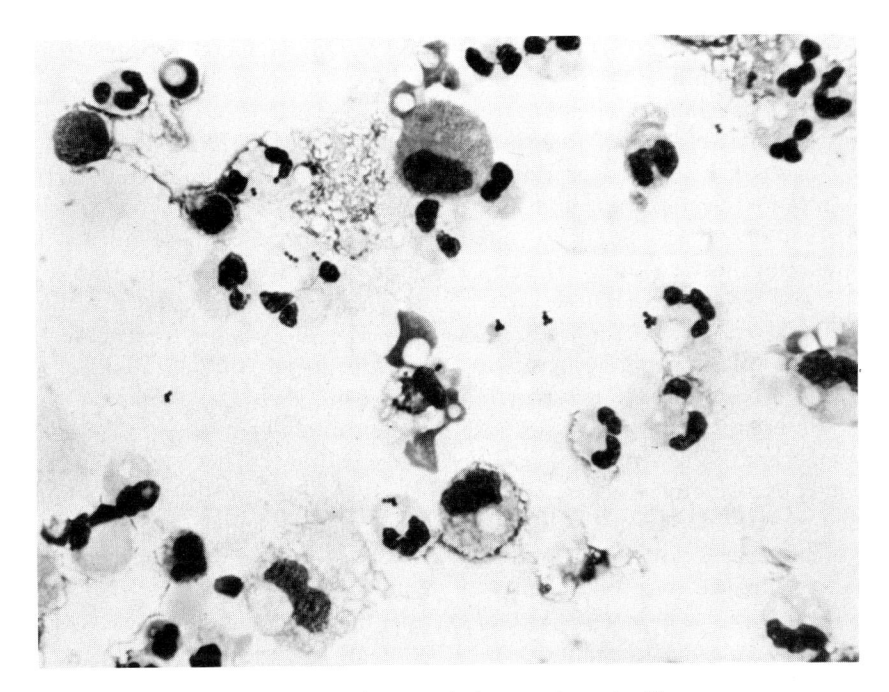

Fig. 26-4. Leukocytes in human breast milk.

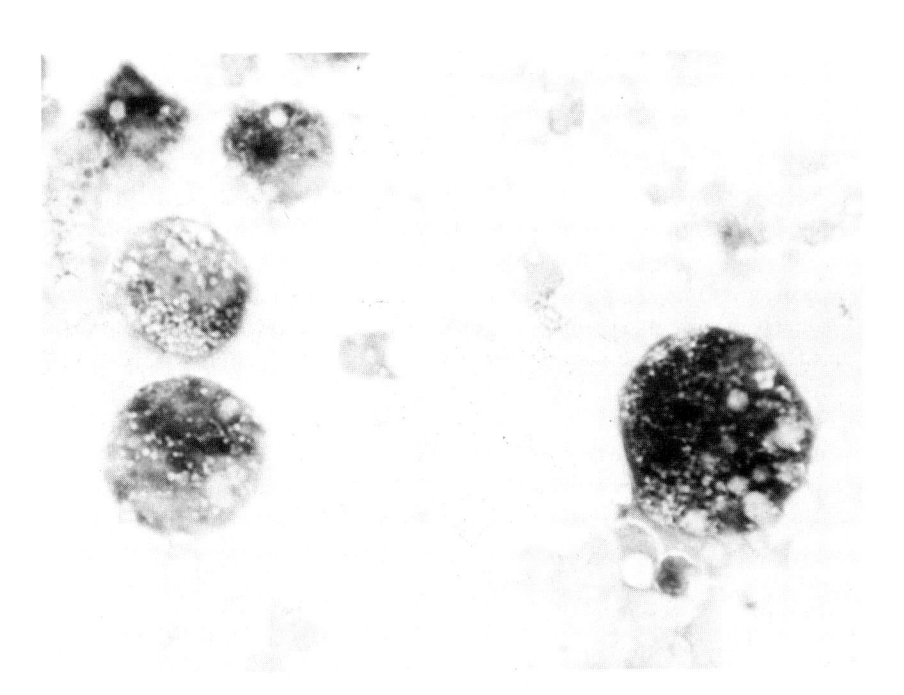

Fig. 26-5. Breast milk macrophages.

milk is higher than that of later milk and varies greatly between women. Neutrophils are present in significant numbers early in lactation, and their presence may be related to breast engorgement during the initial days of lactation. Although the function of the breast milk neutrophil is unclear, its presence does not necessarily imply infection. Epithelial cells occasionally present in milk may originate from the skin of the nipple.

The breast milk macrophage is a mononuclear phagocytic cell that comprises approximately 80% of the leukocytes in milk (Fig. 26-4). This is an active phagocytic cell that contains large amounts of intracytoplasmic lipid and IgA, bears cell surface receptors for IgG and C3b, and synthesizes several important host resistance factors including lysozyme, C3 and C4 complement components, and lactoferrin (Fig. 26-5). Milk macrophages are capable of phagocytizing and killing both gram-positive and gram-negative bacteria and appear to interact with the lymphocytes present in breast milk.

The host defense factors that the breast milk macrophage synthesizes provide important nonspecific antimicrobial protection for the neonate. Lysozyme is capable of lysing the cell walls of many bacteria. This enzyme is synthesized by the milk macrophage, and its concentration in human milk is 300 times that found in cow's milk. It is stable in an acid environment comparable to that of the gastric contents. Lactoferrin is an iron-binding protein that is present in many external secretions. It is synthesized by the milk macrophage, and its concentration in breast milk is higher than in any other body fluid. Lactoferrin's antimicrobial activity derives from its ability to chelate iron, thus depriving bacteria of a cofactor important for their growth. The growth of both *Staphylococcus* organisms and *E. coli* is limited by lactoferrin. The C3 and C4 complement components are also actively synthesized by breast macrophages. The function of these proteins in milk is unclear, since there is relatively little IgG and IgM or the early complement components, C1 and C2, which are necessary for activation of C3 to its biologically active forms. IgA may activate C3 via the alternative pathway; however, it is not known whether this occurs in milk. IgA is present in highest concentrations within the breast macrophage itself. However, this macrophage-associated IgA is not synthesized by the macrophage. Viable macrophages have been shown to release this IgA slowly, and this has led to the hypothesis that the breast macrophage may represent a vehicle for immunoglobulin transport down the neonate's gastrointestinal tract.

Viable T and B lymphocytes are present in human breast milk. T lymphocytes represent as much as 50% of the milk lymphocytes early in lactation and fall to less than 20% as lactation progresses. Breast T cells can be stimulated by Con A and PHA to undergo blast transformation and DNA synthesis. The spectrum of responses of the breast T cells differs from that of the peripheral blood T cells from the same donor. For example, milk T cells are often unresponsive to *Candida albicans* antigen, whereas the peripheral blood T cells from the same donor are highly reactive. In contrast, milk T cells respond well to the K_1 capsular antigen of *E. coli*, whereas peripheral blood lymphocytes responses to K_1 are minimal or absent. This phenomenon may be related to the previously described homing of lymphocytes sensitized in the gastrointestinal tract to mammary glands. The transfer of cell-mediated immunity from tuberculin-sensitive mothers to their breast-fed infants has recently been reported. If these reports are substantiated, this form of passive transfer of cellular immunity could be of major clinical significance. It is unlikely that intact T lymphocytes are passing from the mother's milk across the mucous membranes of the infant's gastrointestinal tract. It is more likely that a soluble T cell factor, e.g., transfer factor, might be involved. The B lymphocytes present in milk have IgG, IgA, IgM, and IgD on their surfaces. However, these cells synthesize IgA almost exclusively. The role of B cells in milk is as yet unclear.

Breast milk constituents may interact with the neonate's immune system in ways other than those already mentioned. A significant increase in the secretory IgA content of nasal and salivary secretions has been observed in breast-fed versus formula-fed newborns during the first few days of life. It is postulated that this may reflect the influence of a soluble factor in milk acting to stimulate the mucosal immune system of the breast-fed infant. Factors enhancing IgA synthesis by B cells and epithelial cell growth have also been reported to be produced by milk macrophages.

Many nurseries have tried to take advantage of the antibody content and other antimicrobial properties of human milk by using a variety of breast milk banking systems. All too often these programs either freeze the milk, which destroys the viable cells, or pasteurize the milk, which destroys both the cellular and immunoglobulin content. Other banking systems refrigerate whole "fresh" breast milk for variable periods of time with no milk "treatment." This will preserve intact the antibody content, but cellular viability falls significantly by 24 hours, and the numbers of both macrophages and neutrophils significantly decrease secondary to either cytolysis or adherence to the walls of the storage container. Thus, although human milk banking may make a significant contribution to infant nutrition, its immunologic contribution following storage is uncertain at best.

EVALUATION OF HOST DEFENSE MECHANISM FUNCTION IN THE INFANT

Some disorders of immunologic function may become clinically apparent in the neonatal period or first year of life. Because of differences in the developmental status of the newborn's host defense mechanisms and the lack of exposure to antigens, the evaluation of the function of host defense mechanisms in the infant is somewhat different from that performed for older children and adults. Infants who have experienced two or more significant bacterial or fungal infections should be suspected of having a defect in their host defense mechanisms. Patients with unusual infections (e.g., from *Pneumocystis carinii*) or infections that respond incompletely to therapy and recur are also suspect. Growth failure, chronic diarrhea, chronic dermatitis, hepatosplenomegaly, and recurrent abscesses commonly occur in immunologically deficient infants. Infants having a sibling (and in the case of X-linked disorders a maternal uncle) with a known immunologic defect should receive an appropriate laboratory evaluation even if there has not as yet been any episode of infection.

In evaluating a patient for a possible host defense mechanism defect, all host defense systems, i.e., phagocytic, complement, antibody, and cell-mediated immunity, should be considered. The evaluation should be divided into initial screening tests and definitive tests that allow one to establish a specific diagnosis. Whereas screening tests should be obtainable by physicians at all hospitals, definitive tests may be available only at major medical centers. The laboratory tests appropriate for evaluation of host defense mechanisms of the infant are listed in the following material. Those tests considered to be initial screening tests are indicated by an asterisk (*).

A. Phagocytosis
  *1. White blood cell count and differential
  *2. Nitroblue tetrazolium (NBT) dye reduction test (qualitative)
  3. Ingestion of endotoxin-coated Oil Red O particles; quantitative NBT reduction; NBT reduction:ingestion ratio
  4. Quantitative bacterial killing
  5. Chemotaxis analysis using a Boyden chamber
B. Complement
  *1. Total hemolytic complement assay (CH_{50})
  *2. Measurement of C3 by radial diffusion
  3. Measurement of individual components of the classic and alternative complement pathways by radial diffusion
  4. Functional measurement of the alternative pathway
  5. Functional assay for C5 (yeast phagocytosis)
C. Antibody-mediated immunity
  *1. Quantitation of serum IgG, IgA, and IgM by radial diffusion; serum immunoelectrophoresis
  *2. Measurement of specific antibodies after immunization (e.g., DPT-Schick test)
  *3. Isoagglutinin titer (anti-A and anti-B)
  4. IgE radioimmunoassay
  5. Quantitation of B cells in blood by immunofluorescent techniques with specific anti-immunoglobulin antibodies
  6. B cell differentiation to plasma cells in vitro using pokeweed mitogen stimulation
D. Cell-mediated immunity
  *1. Total lymphocyte count
  *2. Delayed hypersensitivity skin tests to common antigens
  *3. Lymphocyte responses to mitogens (PHA, Con A)
  4. Lymphocyte responses to antigens (*Candida*) and allogeneic cells (mixed lymphocyte reaction)
  5. Quantitation of circulating T lymphocytes by sheep erythrocyte (E) rosette technique
  6. In vitro assays of T cell function: migration-inhibiting factor (MIF), cytotoxicity

Phagocytic function

Neutropenia is the most common abnormality related to phagocytic function and may be readily detected by white blood cell count and differential. Neutropenia may be due to bacterial or viral infection, antigranulocyte antibodies, as in SLE, or be part of a primary congenital disorder. Persistent neutropenia should prompt bone marrow examination. Disorders revealing morphologic abnormalities, such as Chediak-Higashi syndrome, in which there are giant cytoplasmic granules, may be readily detected by examining the blood smear.

Chronic granulomatous disease (CGD) may present during the first few months of life. This disorder can be detected by the NBT dye reduction tests. Neutrophils from patients with CGD do not undergo the normal increase in oxidative metabolism that occurs during phagocytosis of particles. NBT reduction occurs concomitantly with particle ingestion in normal individuals but does not occur in patients with CGD. If the NBT test shows reduced or absent dye reduction, suggesting a neutrophil metabolic defect like CGD, a more accurate determination quantitating the amount of NBT reduction for the number of particles ingested (NBT reduction:ingestion ratio) should be performed. This quantitative test is helpful in detecting variants of CGD.

A variety of defects in neutrophil chemotaxis have been described, particularly in patients with recurrent abscesses. Chemotaxis can be evaluated by measuring the movement of neutrophils using a chamber divided by a micropore filter (Boyden chamber). Normally neutrophils will move through a micropore filter toward a chemoattractant produced by incubating endotoxin with fresh serum. Through this method intrinsic defects in neutrophil chemotaxis, as well as defects in the ability of patients serum to produce appropriate chemoattractant factors, may be identified. The hyper-IgE syndrome

(Job's syndrome) is an example of a neutrophil chemotactic defect that can become clinically apparent during the first year of life.

Complement system

Both transient and persistent deficiencies of serum complement components have been reported. The total hemolytic complement test (CH_{50}) measures the ability of patient's serum to serve as a complement source to permit lysis of sheep red blood cells (SRBC) by rabbit antibody to SRBC. This method will detect defects in the classic complement pathway and particularly in the earlier components of that pathway (C1, C4, C2, C3, C5). The CH_{50} test is the best single screening test for complement deficiencies; however, this does not detect deficiencies in the alternative pathway. Individual components of the classic and alternative pathways can be measured by radial diffusion techniques in many laboratories. Functional analyses of the alternative pathway and of the C5 component, important in Leiner's syndrome, are available in relatively few laboratories.

Antibody-mediated immunity

Analysis of antibody-mediated immunity begins with quantitation of serum immunoglobulins (IgG, IgA, and IgM) by radial diffusion. Results must be compared with matched normal values, as shown in Table 26-3. Immunoelectrophoresis is helpful in determining whether the immunoglobulins present are normal; homogenous proteins similar to those seen in multiple myeloma are sometimes seen in patients with congenital infections and certain immunodeficiency diseases. In general, analysis of immunoglobulins has limited value in the first 3 to 4 months of life, since most of the infant's serum immunoglobulin is maternal IgG. However, elevation of IgM in the cord blood may indicate intrauterine infection; elevation of both IgM and IgA suggests maternofetal bleeding. At all ages serum IgG values should be greater than 200 mg/dl, and the presence of IgG values below this level requires more extensive investigation. In patients who have received routine immunizations, antibody titers to diphtheria and tetanus toxoids and polio may be studied. The Schick test is clinically useful in determining the presence of diphtheria antitoxin. Diluted diphtheria toxin is injected intradermally, and, if the patient lacks antitoxin, a brawny red spot appears within 2 days and persists for more than 5 days; if no reaction is seen, antitoxin is present. To assess antibody responses before and after immunization, serum samples should be tested. Immunization with DPT and Salk killed polio vaccine is useful for this purpose. In children suspected of being immunodeficient, live virus vaccines should be avoided. Cases of paralytic polio from vaccine strains have been reported in immunodeficient children, as have fatal vaccinia and disseminated infections from BCG immunization.

In infants with immunoglobulin deficiency, studies of circulating B lymphocytes should be performed. B lymphocytes are identified using immunofluorescent techniques for the presence of immunoglobulins (mostly IgM and IgD) on their cell membranes. Even in newborns, 5% to 15% of circulating lymphocytes are B cells. B cells are characteristically *lacking* in male infants with X-linked agammaglobulinemia and in most patients with severe combined immunodeficiency disease. Some patients who cannot make immunoglobulins have circulating B cells, but those cells cannot differentiate into plasma cells and secrete immunoglobulins or antibodies. This is characteristic of patients with common variable immunodeficiency (formerly called acquired agammaglobulinemia). Such patients may be evaluated using in vitro B cell differentiation studies. However, normal children show little B cell differentiation in vitro until approximately 6 months of age. Moreover, common variable immunodeficiency is very rare during the first year of life.

Cell-mediated immunity

T lymphocytes comprise 60% to 80% of the peripheral blood lymphocyte population; thus lymphopenia ($<1,200/mm^3$) is characteristic of disorders in which the number of T cells is reduced. In contrast, in B cell deficiency disorders lymphopenia is usually not detectable, since B cells normally comprise only 5% to 15% of the peripheral blood lymphocyte population. Delayed hypersensitivity skin reactions cannot be elicited in patients with cell-mediated immunodeficiencies. Positive delayed hypersensitivity skin tests require both an intact T cell system and exposure to specific antigens. Since neonates have been exposed to very few antigens capable of inducing specific cell-mediated immunity, even delayed hypersensitivity tests to common antigens are normally negative during the first 6 months of life. For this reason screening of infants for delayed hypersensitivity to detect defects in cell-mediated immunity has only limited value. However, normal infants who have had oral candidiasis for more than 1 week or have had a repeated episode will usually have a positive skin test to *Candida* antigen (1:10 dilution). A child with persistent or recurrent candidiasis and a negative delayed hypersensitivity skin test should have additional evaluation of cell-mediated immune functions.

Because of the limited value of delayed hypersensitivity skin testing for detection of cell-mediated immune deficiencies, in vitro lymphocyte responses play an important role in the evaluation of cellular immunity in this age group. Mature T lymphocytes will proliferate and synthesize DNA when incubated with plant lectins such as PHA or Con A. These responses are quantitated by measurement of DNA synthesis in PHA- or Con A–stimulated cultures using tritiated thymidine incorporation into cellular DNA. These studies may be performed on as little as 0.25 ml of whole blood obtained from a finger or heel puncture, making such studies feasible for even very small infants. Thymidine incorporation is absent or reduced in patients who are deficient in T cells (e.g., DiGeorge syndrome and severe combined immunodeficiency disease). Ability to respond to specific antigens such as *Candida* and the ability to recognize foreign (allogeneic) cells are also T cell functions and can be measured using similar methods. In patients with lymphopenia or reduced in vitro lymphocyte responses to PHA or Con A, the number of circulating T cells should be determined. T lymphocytes form rosettes with sheep red blood cells and can be easily identified under a light microscope. Other tests of T lymphocyte function, such as lymphokine production (MIF test) or cellular cytotoxicity, require specially trained personnel and may be available only in major medical centers.

HOST DEFENSE MECHANISM DISORDERS IN EARLY INFANCY
Neutropenia

Neutropenia is present when less than 1,200 neutrophils/mm^3 are present in the peripheral blood. Some of the causes of neutropenia in the neonate are listed in Table 26-8. The patient's prognosis is related to the underlying cause for the neutropenia; however, most neutropenias in the neonatal period are transient and have a good prognosis, unless there is overwhelming neonatal sepsis.

Chronic granulomatous disease

Chronic granulomatous disease (CGD) is a disorder of white blood cell bactericidal activity. Neutrophils from patients with CGD do not increase their oxidative metabolic activity on ingestion and phagocytosis of bacteria or other particles. Hydrogen peroxide, superoxide, and other reactive radicals necessary for neutrophil bactericidal activity are not produced. In patients with CGD, bacteria may remain viable within the neutrophils for many hours, whereas bacteria ingested by normal neutrophils are quickly killed.

CGD is a hereditary disease with an X-linked recessive pattern of inheritance. However, an autosomal recessive pattern of inheritance and affected females have been reported. The autosomal recessive form of the disease is often less severe than the X-linked form. Children with X-linked CGD generally have recurrent infections during the first few months of life. Infections are predominantly due to catalase-positive bacteria *(Staphylococcus, E. coli, Serratia marcescens)* and fungi *(Candi-*

Table 26-8. Causes of neutropenia in the newborn

	Example
Infection (sepsis)	
Maternal autoimmune disease	Systemic lupus erythematosus
Isoimmunization	Antibody to neutrophil antigen
Genetic agranulocytosis	
Neutropenia and malabsorption	Schwachman syndrome
Drug induced (often associated with thrombocytopenia)	Thiazides Phenytoin sodium (Dilantin) Amidopyrine Propylthiouracil Phenothiazines Trimethadione Sulfa drugs
Cyclic neutropenia	
Inborn errors of metabolism	Ketotic hyperglycinemia Methylmalonic acidemia Isovaleric acidemia Propionic acidemia Chronic tyrosinosis Maple syrup urine disease

da, Aspergillus). These children frequently have adenopathy, draining lymph nodes, or pneumonias that respond slowly to therapy. Hepatosplenomegaly is a common finding and may be associated with liver abscesses. Persistent dermatitis, diarrhea, perianal abscesses, osteomyelitis, and ulcerative stomatitis occur frequently in this disorder.

The neutrophils of patients with CGD are unable to reduce NBT dye on phagocytosing particles. Killing of catalase-positive bacteria is also abnormal. Neutrophil counts are normal or elevated, cell-mediated immunity and antibody-mediated immunity are normal, and serum immunoglobulins become elevated as the children become older. The mothers of CGD patients have intermediate defects in NBT reduction and bacterial killing so that carriers of X-linked CGD may be detected. There is no specific therapy to correct the neutrophil defect in CGD. Individual infections require appropriate antibiotic therapy and frequent prolonged courses of therapy. The prophylactic use of antibiotics in CGD patients is controversial.

X-linked infantile agammaglobulinemia

Children unable to synthesize immunoglobulin or antibodies usually do not suffer from infection before 5 or 6 months of age. During the first 6 months of life maternal IgG antibodies are sufficient to protect the infant from infection provided that the phagocytic, complement, and cell-mediated immune systems are intact. After the first 6 months of life these children suffer repeated infection, particularly with gram-positive encapsulated bacteria (*Pneumococcus*, *Streptococcus*, *Staphylococcus*) and some gram-negative encapsulated bacteria (*Haemophilus* and *Meningococcus*); *Pneumocystis carinii* pneumonitis may also occur. Patients with X-linked agammaglobulinemia usually have repeated episodes of pneumonia and otitis media. Sepsis, meningitis, cellulitis, and septic arthritis also are common in this disorder. A fatal meningoencephalitis caused by ECHO virus has been reported in older children with X-linked agammaglobulinemia.

The serum of patients with X-linked agammaglobulinemia lacks all immunoglobulin classes; IgG is less than 100 mg/dl, and IgA, IgM, IgD, and IgE are usually undetectable. They are unable to synthesize antibodies, and B cells are absent from their peripheral blood. Pre-B cells are present in their bone marrow, suggesting that this disorder is the result of a defect in differentiation of pre-B cells to B cells. Normal numbers of T cells are present, and delayed hypersensitivity and other cell-mediated immune functions are intact. Treatment consists of immunoglobulin replacement by injections of immune serum globulin (0.7 mg/kg IM every 3 weeks) or plasma infusions (10 ml/kg IV every 3 weeks) using a group of three to five well-screened matched and monitored plasma donors ("buddy system").

Transient hypogammaglobulinemia of infancy

Transient hypogammaglobulinemia of infancy is a frequently mentioned but rarely documented entity in which the postnatal decline in serum immunoglobulins is accentuated and there is a delay in the onset of immunoglobulin synthesis. A recent study and review of the world literature identified only 16 infants with infection associated with transient depression of immunoglobulins below the normal range for age. None of these patients suffered from recurrent infections after 6 months of age. All patients showed an increase in serum immunoglobulin levels, and most patients achieved values in the normal range by 2 years of age. All patients were found to have isoagglutinins (anti-A or anti-B) and produced antibody in response to their DPT immunizations. Circulating B cells were present in normal numbers, as were T cells, and cellular immunity was also intact. Thus this entity may be easily distinguished from X-linked infantile agammaglobulinemia by the ability of these patients to make antibody and by the presence of B cells. Their serum immunoglobulin levels are also much higher than those normally seen in X-linked agammaglobulinemia. Transient hypogammaglobulinemia of infancy resolves spontaneously, and infection is not usually seen after 6 months of age, even if serum immunoglobulins are still depressed. Immunoglobulin replacement by immune serum globulin injections or plasma transfusions is not recommended.

Asymptomatic transient hypogammaglobulinemia of infancy occasionally occurs in the siblings of patients with severe combined immunodeficiency disease. There is no explanation for this phenomenon at the present time. These children do not suffer from repeated or severe infections and do not require immunoglobulin replacement therapy.

Common variable immunodeficiency (formerly acquired agammaglobulinemia) is very rarely seen under the age of 2 years. Serum immunoglobulins are depressed but usually not as low as in X-linked agammaglobulinemia. These patients are unable to synthesize antibodies in response to immunization and continue to suffer infections after 6 months of age. These features distinguish it from transient hypogammaglobulinemia. B cells may or may not be absent in this disorder.

Wiskott-Aldrich syndrome

The Wiskott-Aldrich syndrome is an X-linked recessive disorder consisting of the clinical triad of eczema, thrombocytopenia, and increased susceptibility to infection. The pathogenetic basis of this disorder is unknown. Patients with Wiskott-Aldrich syndrome present in early infancy with gastrointestinal bleeding due to thrombocytopenia. These patients characteristically have reduced or absent isoagglutinins and do not produce antibodies after immunization with polysaccharides. Infections by bacteria with polysaccharide capsules (e.g., *Pneumococcus* and *Haemophilus*) are a persistent problem. Serum IgM levels are often depressed while serum IgA levels become elevated. These immunoglobulin abnormalities are difficult to detect in early infancy. Antibody-mediated and cell-mediated immunity are relatively normal early in life, but patients with Wiskott-Aldrich syndrome characteristically lose immunologic function as they grow older. Histocompatible bone marrow transplantation has resulted in immunologic reconstitution and is the treatment of choice for this otherwise fatal disease.

Thymic hypoplasia with hypocalcemia (DiGeorge syndrome)

DiGeorge described the association of thymic hypoplasia with hypoparathyroidism. Patients with this syndrome, DiGeorge syndrome, have congenital hypocalcemic tetany, cardiac anomalies, abnormal facies, and increased susceptibility to infection due to defects in T cell function. Both the thymus and the parathyroid glands are derived from epithelial evaginations from the third and fourth pharyngeal pouches. The aortic arch has its origin in the same area. It is likely that a developmental abnormality involving the third and fourth pharyngeal pouch region during the sixth and eighth week of gestation results in this syndrome. This disorder is usually not familial and is variable in the severity of its clinical expression.

Patients with DiGeorge syndrome most frequently

present with severe hypocalcemic tetany within a few days of birth. This is due to congenital hypoparathyroidism. In addition, over 90% of infants with this syndrome have cardiac anomalies, usually involving the aortic arch. These include interrupted aortic arch, truncus arteriosus, tetralogy of Fallot, and right-sided aortic arch. Facial anomalies include micrognathia, a "fish mouth" appearance, notched pinnae accompanied by the appearance of backward-rotated ears, and hypertelorism. If patients survive the newborn period, recurrent infections with bacteria, viruses, and fungi, particularly *Candida*, become apparent, and chronic diarrhea and failure to thrive are common. Nephrolithiasis has also been reported in these patients.

Immunologic defects in DiGeorge syndrome are related to defective T cell development and function. At autopsy the thymus is either absent or markedly reduced in size (less than 5% normal for age); however, if any thymus tissue is present, it is histologically normal. Patients with DiGeorge syndrome usually have reduced numbers of lymphocytes capable of forming rosettes with sheep red blood cells (T cells), and in vitro lymphocyte responses to PHA, Con A, allogeneic cells, and antigens (e.g., *Candida*) are reduced. Delayed hypersensitivity reactions to antigens to which the patients have been exposed are also absent. The severity of the defects in cell-mediated immunity is variable and is inversely proportional to the amount of residual thymus tissue present. Serum immunoglobulins are present in normal amounts, and serum IgE may be elevated. Antibody responses in DiGeorge syndrome patients are usually poor, since many antigens require T cell help for optimum antibody synthesis.

Fetal thymus transplantation is the treatment of choice for patients with DiGeorge syndrome. This procedure results in extremely rapid restoration of T cell function, suggesting that thymic hormonal factors may play an important role in this process. However, treatment with thymosin, a thymic hormone, has not been successful in reconstituting cell-mediated immunity in DiGeorge syndrome patients with more severe T cell defects. Some patients with this disorder may have sufficient residual thymic tissue to increase their cell-mediated immunity as they become older. These patients usually have less severe cellular immune defects at diagnosis and may not require fetal thymus transplants.

Patients with this syndrome are at risk for development of graft-versus-host reaction (see further) if they are transfused with viable nonhistocompatible lymphocytes. If blood transfusion is necessary, blood should be irradiated with 3,000 rad prior to administration.

Severe combined immunodeficiency disease

The term *severe combined immunodeficiency disease* (SCID) refers to a group of disorders characterized by the absence of both antibody-mediated and cell-mediated immunity. Some forms of SCID have an autosomal recessive pattern of inheritance, whereas other forms show X-linked recessive inheritance. Deficiency of the enzyme adenosine deaminase (ADA) is responsible for SCID in approximately 30% of patients with autosomal recessive SCID.

The absence of both antibody-mediated and cell-mediated immunity results in profound susceptibility to a broad spectrum of bacterial, viral, and fungal infections. Onset of infections is usually within the first 3 months of life, and, if immunologic reconstitution is not possible, these infants will usually succumb to infection within the first year of life. Because the infants lack cell-mediated immunity, maternal antibodies are insufficient to completely protect SCID infants from infection. Cytomegalovirus pneumonia is common, progressive, and often fatal. Progressive fatal poliomyelitis may result from routine immunization with live polio vaccine as can disseminated fatal vaccinia infections from contact with smallpox vaccine or other vaccinated individuals. Measles and chickenpox infections are usually fatal. Administration of BCG often produces a disseminated and fatal infection with this "attenuated" mycobacterium.

Infections with gram-negative bacteria, especially *E. coli* and *Pseudomonas* species, predominate in early infancy, although there is some protection from *Pneumococcus* and *Streptococcus* species due to maternal IgG. *Pneumocystis carinii* pneumonitis occurs very frequently in SCID patients, and SCID must be suspected in any infant with pneumocystis infection. Most SCID patients will develop oral candidiasis, which usually progresses to involve the gastrointestinal tract and perineal area. These candidal infections usually do not respond well to conventional therapy. *Aspergillus* infections also occur in these infants. Failure to thrive, chronic diarrhea, and a variety of skin rashes often accompany or precede the onset of infections.

The clinical and immunologic picture of SCID may result from (1) absence of lymphoid stem cells, (2) enzyme deficiencies impairing stem cell or T cell development (e.g., ADA deficiency), or (3) thymic abnormalities (e.g., thymic dysplasia) interfering with T cell development; impairment of B cell function is secondary to the primary T cell defect. As just mentioned, SCID is a group of disorders, and it is likely that these pathogenetic mechanisms occur in different forms of the disease.

The diagnosis of SCID may be made at birth or even prenatally in patients with ADA deficiency by measurement of ADA activity in amniotic fluid cell cultures. SCID patients have markedly reduced lymphocyte counts ($<1,200/mm^3$) and usually less than 10% are T cells as measured by sheep red blood cell rosetting. Lymphocytes from SCID patients will not respond to PHA, Con A, allogeneic cells, or antigens. Delayed hypersensitivity to *Candida* is absent, even in the face of prolonged *Candida* infection. Defects in antibody-mediated immunity are often difficult to diagnose during the first 3 months of life because of the relatively low level of immunoglobulin synthesis that normally occurs at this age. Most SCID patients will make no immunoglobulins or antibodies of their own and will lack circulating B cells. Sometimes abnormal monoclonal immunoglobulins can be found in these infants. Some patients with SCID may have serum immunoglobulin as well as B cells. This immunologic picture has been termed the *Nezelof syndrome* and is a variant of SCID. Some patients with Nezelof syndrome lose their immunoglobulins and B cells and become indistinguishable from classic SCID patients. This type of progressive immunologic involution occurs commonly in ADA-deficient patients.

The treatment of choice for severe combined immunodeficiency is bone marrow transplantation from a related histocompatible donor matched with the patient by HLA typing and mixed leukocyte reaction testing. Unmatched bone marrow transplants are not successful and produce fatal graft-versus-host (GVH) reactions. GVH reactions occur when histoincompatible immunocompetent lymphocytes (the graft) are infused into an immunoincompetent host such as an SCID patient. Donor cells attack the patient's skin, gastrointestinal tract, liver, lungs, kidneys, bone marrow, and even central nervous system. Symptoms appear in approximately 7 to 14 days after transplantation and may include fever, maculopapular rash, hepatosplenomegaly, diarrhea, and tachypnea. The skin rash may progress to exfoliation, and diarrhea often becomes bloody. Neutropenia, thrombocytopenia, anemia, and increased infections are also common. In their severe form GVH reactions are usually fatal. GVH reactions may also be initiated by transfusing an SCID patient (or DiGeorge syndrome patient) with blood products. This may be avoided by irradiating the blood products with 3,000 rad.

When a histocompatible bone marrow donor is not available, other forms of therapy may be attempted. Some patients with the ADA-deficient form of SCID have shown clinical and immunologic improvement after enzyme replacement therapy using glycerolized (frozen) irradiated normal red blood cells as an enzyme source. Enzyme replacement is performed as a partial exchange transfusion at monthly intervals; care must be taken to avoid iron overload in these patients. Administration of thymosin in addition to enzyme replacement therapy has been beneficial for some ADA-deficient patients. Fetal liver is a source of stem cells; fetal liver transplantation without histocompatibility matching has been attempted for SCID patients. This procedure has been successful in some patients but has produced fatal GVH reactions in others. Transplantation of cultured thymic epithelium has been attempted in some SCID patients, particularly if a primary thymic defect is suspected. Some successes and some failures have been reported. Further studies of this form of therapy are needed.

Immunodeficiency associated with malnutrition

Children with protein calorie malnutrition have an increased susceptibility to severe fungal, viral, and gram-negative bacterial infections. The morbidity and mortality from tuberculosis and measles in malnourished children is significantly greater than in well-nourished controls. This spectrum of infection is similar to that seen in patients with cell-mediated immunodeficiencies. Indeed, diminished delayed hypersensitivity, decreased numbers of T lymphocytes, and decreased responses to PHA and Con A have been observed. Serum immunoglobulins are usually normal, but antibody responses to specific antigen are often diminished in malnourished children. Infants with intrauterine growth retardation have decreased numbers of circulating T cells and depressed lymphocyte responses to PHA. These deficiencies in cell-mediated immunity may be related to the increased susceptibility to infection observed in these infants. Malnutrition in early postnatal life secondary to a complicated perinatal course is likely to result in cell-mediated immunodeficiency and increased morbidity from infection in this high-risk patient population.

Developmental immunodeficiency of the neonate

In summary, the cell host defense mechanisms in the neonate function less efficiently than those of the older child or adult. For example, neutrophil chemotaxis and intracellular bactericidal activity are diminished compared with those of adults. The function of the alternative pathway of the complement system is decreased in the majority of both premature and full-term neonates. The neonate cannot make antibody to as many antigens as adults can, and immunoglobulin synthesis appears to be blunted by the presence of suppressor T cells and immature neonatal B cells. Neonatal T cells are also deficient in their effector functions, such as secretion of migration-inhibiting factor and immune interferon. The conclusion that the human neonate is immunodeficient and that multiple host defense mechanisms are operating suboptimally is inescapable. If the infant is sufficiently stressed or the natural barriers are breached, one or more of these mechanisms will fail and infection may result. To prevent this, provision of a protected environment is necessary for the newborn, particularly in the presence of perinatal complications.

Stephen H. Polmar
Ricardo U. Sorenson
William B. Pittard III

Bibliography
General

Fudenberg, H.H., and others: Basic and clinical immunology, Los Altos, Calif., 1980, Lange Medical Publications.

Miller, M.E., and Stiehm, E.R.: Host defense mechanisms in the fetus and neonate, Pediatrics **64**:705, 1979.

Stiehm, E.R., and Fulginiti, V.A.: Immunologic disorders of infants and children, ed. 2, Philadelphia, 1980, W.B. Saunders Co.

Wara, D.W., and Ammann, A.J.: Immunologic disorders of childhood. In Rudolph, A.M., Barnett, H.L., and Einhorn, A.H., editors: Pediatrics, New York, 1977, Appleton-Century-Crofts.

Development of specific and nonspecific host defense mechanisms

Cooper, M.D., Lawton, A.R., and Kincade, P.W.: A two-stage model for development of antibody-producing cells, Clin. Exp. Immunol. **11**:143, 1972.

Hayward, A.R., and Lydyard, P.M.: B-Cell function in the newborn, Pediatrics, **64**:758, 1979.

Hayward, A.R., and Lydyard, P.M.: Suppression of B-lymphocyte differentiation by newborn T-lymphocytes with an Fc Receptor for IgM, Clin. Exp. Immunol. **34**:374, 1979.

Johnston, R.B., Jr., and others: Complement in the newborn infant, Pediatrics **64**:781, 1979.

Owen, J.J.T., Cooper, M.D., and Raff, M.C.: *In vitro* generation of B-lymphocytes in mouse foetal liver: a mammalian "bursa equivalent," Nature **249**:361, 1974.

Pyke, K.W., and Gelfand, E.W.: Detection of T-precursor cells in human bone marrow and foetal liver, Differentiation **5**:189, 1976.

Raff, M.D., and others: Differences in susceptibility of mature and immature mouse B-lymphocytes to anti-immunoglobulin in induced immunoglobulin suppression in vitro: possible implications for B-cell tolerance to self, J. Exp. Med. **142**:1052, 1975.

Reinherz, E.L., and others: Discrete stages of intrathymic differentiation: analysis of normal thymocytes and leukemia lymphoblasts of T-cell lineage, Proc. Natl. Acad. Sci. **77**:1588, 1980.

Silverstein, A.M.: Ontogeny of the immune response: a perspective. In Cooper, M.D., and Dayton, D.H., editors: Development of host defenses, New York, 1977, Raven Press.

Stiehm, E.R., Winter, H.S., and Bryson, Y.J.: Cellular (T-cell) immunity in the human newborn, Pediatrics **64**:814, 1979.

Stossel, T.P., Alper, C.A., and Rosen, F.S.: Opsonic activity in the newborn: role of properdin, Pediatrics **52**:134, 1973.

Immunologic aspects of the mother-child relationship

Ahlstedt, S., and others: Antibody production by human colostral cells, I. Immunoglobulin class, specificity, and quantity, Scand. Immunol. **4**:535, 1975.

Alford, C.A., Jr.: Immunoglobulin determinations in the diagnosis of fetal infections, Pediatr. Clin. North Am. **18**:99, 1974.

Goldblum, R.M., and others: Antibody forming cells in human colostrum after oral immunization, Nature **257**:797, 1975.

Heird, W.D., and Hansen, I.H.: Effects of colostrum on growth of intestinal mucosa, Pediatr. Res. **11**:406, 1972.

Klagsbrun, M.: Human milk stimulates DNA synthesis and cellular proliferation in cultured fibroblasts, Proc. Natl. Acad. Sci. **75**:5057, 1978.

Parmely, M.J., Beer, A., and Billingham, K.: *In vitro* studies on the T-lymphocyte population of human milk, J. Exp. Med. **144**:358, 1976.

Pittard, W.B.: Breast milk immunology: a frontier in infant nutrition, Am. J. Dis. Child. **133**:83, 1979.

Pittard, W.B., Polmar, S.H., and Fanaroff, A.A.: The breast milk macrophage: a potential vehicle for immunoglobulin transport, J. Reticuloendothel. Soc. **22**:597, 1977.

Udall, J.N., and others: The effect of early nutrition on intestinal maturation, Pediatr. Res. **13**:409, 1979.

Host defense mechanism disorders in early infancy

Chandra, R.K.: Fetal malnutrition and post-natal immunocompetence, Am. J. Dis. Child. **129**:450, 1975.

Cleveland, W.W., and others: Foetal thymic transplant in a case of DiGeorge syndrome, Lancet **2**:1211, 1968.

Cooper, M.D., and others: Primary antibody deficiencies, Springer Semin. Immunopathol. **1**:265, 1978.

DiGeorge, A.M.: Congenital absence of the thymus and its immunologic consequences: concurrence with congenital hypoparathyroidism. In Bergsma, D., and Good, R.A., editors: Immunologic deficiency disease in man, New York, 1968, The National Foundation.

Ferguson, A.C.: Prolonged impairment of cellular immunity in children with intrauterine growth retardation, J. Pediatr. **9**:52, 1978.

Hitzig, W.H., Dooren, L.J., and Vossen, J.M.: Severe combined immunodeficiency diseases, Springer Semin. Immunopathol. **1**:283, 1978.

Polmar, S.H.: Metabolic aspects of immunodeficiency. In Meischer, P.A., and Jaffee, E.R., editors: Seminars in hematology, vol. 17, New York, 1980, Grune and Stratton, Inc.

Polmar, S.H., and others: Enzyme replacement therapy for adenosine deaminase deficiency and severe combined immunodeficiency, N. Engl. J. Med. **295**:1337, 1976.

Tiller, T.L., Jr., and Buckley, R.H.: Transient hypogammaglobulinemia of infancy: review of the literature; clinical and immunologic features of 11 new cases and long-term follow-up, J. Pediatr. **92**:347, 1978.

CHAPTER 27 Postnatally acquired infections

Infectious diseases continue to be one of the most significant causes of fetal wastage and of neonatal morbidity and mortality. This chapter discusses bacterial, viral, fungal, and parasitic infections during the first month of life. Infections acquired in utero or at the time of delivery due to cytomegalovirus (CMV), *Toxoplasma gondii*, rubella virus, herpes simplex virus, or the hepatitis viruses are discussed in Chapter 28.

NEONATAL SEPTICEMIA
Incidence and mortality

Neonatal septicemia refers to a generalized bacterial infection that has been documented by positive blood culture during the first month of life. Septicemia may be a prelude to infection of specific organ systems (such as meningitis or osteomyelitis) or occasionally may follow unrecognized or inadequately treated localized infection. It has been estimated that neonatal septicemia affects between 1 in 500 and 1 in 1,600 newborns. The incidence of septicemia will be influenced markedly by the quality of intrauterine life, host factors, and environmental factors. In the preantibiotic era mortality from neonatal septicemia exceeded 90%, but with the availability of antibiotics it has fallen to between 13% an 50%. The incidence of neonatal septicemia and the mortality have not decreased during the past decade and may even have increased because of the development of life support techniques that have permitted the survival of the extremely premature or otherwise high-risk neonate.

Etiology

A significant proportion of neonatal infections are opportunistic in that the host is infected by organisms that can be cultured readily from the cervix or vaginal canal of normal pregnant women, from the external environment, or from the skin or gastrointestinal (GI) tract of normal individuals. In this setting, a tabulation of microbial agents that may be responsible for neonatal sepsis is inappropriate, since any microorganism can produce disease in an appropriate host. Saprophytic microorganisms recovered from the blood of a neonate should not be assumed to be contaminants. In the following sections, emphasis will be placed on the recognition of specific situations that should permit the clinician to anticipate the possibility of neonatal infection in general and to predict the possibility of disease due to specific infectious agents, thereby permitting the rapid initiation of appropriate diagnostic, therapeutic, and supportive procedures.

Sources of infection

Transplacental acquisition of bacteria during the course of maternal bacteremia is difficult to establish but has been documented in patients infected with *Listeria monocytogenes* and *Treponema pallidum*. Transplacental acquisition of fungal infection also has been proved in neonates with cryptococcal disease and has been suggested by finding elements resembling *Candida* organisms in calcified brain lesions of neonates with hydrocephalus. Late in pregnancy, transplacental transmission of Coxsackie viruses and polioviruses has been demonstrated.

Neonatal infection may follow aspiration of infected amniotic fluid, an occurrence that is favored by prolonged rupture of the fetal membranes or contamination of amniotic fluid during the course of a difficult delivery. In some patients, amniotic infection may be found in the presence of intact membranes. Occasionally, septicemia may occur after direct invasion of the chorionic vessels on the placental surface. With ruptured fetal membranes, infection with gram-negative enteric microorganisms, *Staphylococcus aureus*, group B β-hemolytic streptococci (*S. agalactiae*), *Streptococcus faecalis*, and infection by anaerobic microorganisms should be anticipated. Systemic infection occurs in 1% to 4% of infants born to mothers whose amniotic fluid is infected.

Infection also may be acquired during delivery. In these patients, organisms that are inhabitants of the vaginal canal, including *S. agalactiae, L. monocytogenes, Mima polymorpha, Haemophilus influenzae,* and *Neisseria meningitidis,* should be considered as possible causative agents.

Following birth, bacterial or viral infection may be acquired in the delivery room or newborn nursery via the respiratory and GI tract or by invasion of bacteria through the umbilical stump. Occasionally, bacterial invasion may be secondary to an infected circumcision or may result from a cutaneous wound. Infection also may follow the route of an umbilical or peripheral intravenous catheter. The neonate who is exposed to resuscitation or inhalation therapy equipment or who lives in an environment of nebulizers and waterfilled Isolettes has an increased risk of infection due to *Flavobacterium meningosepticum, Serratia marcescens, Proteus* species, and *Pseudomonas aeruginosa.* The newborn whose skin is bypassed by the use of indwelling umbilical catheters may develop septicemia with *Staphylococcus epidermidis, S. aureus, Pseudomonas, Bacteroides, Serratia, Citrobacter, Candida,* and *Torulopsis.* Bacteremia may be induced in 10% of children during exchange transfusions but only rarely leads to septic complications.

Direct contamination of the newborn by the hands of nursery personnel or by other adults generally occurs when hand-washing techniques are inadequate. Epidemic neonatal infection due to *S. aureus* almost always is transmitted in this manner. Discontinuation of routine hexachlorophene bathing of neonates has been followed by recurrences of epidemic neonatal staphylococcal disease in many nurseries. The role of hand contamination of personnel in the epidemiology of gram-negative neonatal infections due to *Escherichia coli, Klebsiella pneumoniae, Enterobacter* species, *Serratia marcescens, Proteus mirabilis,* and *Pseudomonas* species also has been emphasized. *Salmonella* and *Shigella* infections also have been initiated in neonates by acquisition of these organisms from a maternal carrier followed by infant-to-infant spread due to inadequate hand-washing by medical personnel. In addition, direct contamination of the newborn has been associated with neonatal infection due to *Bacillus subtilis, Pasteurella multocida, Citrobacter* species, and *Campylobacter fetus.*

Infection may be introduced into an intensive care nursery by the admission of newborns whose infection was acquired in the community. Although this represents a potential threat in referral centers, these infants infrequently serve as a source of infection to others if appropriate precautions are observed.

Maternal factors influencing the development of sepsis

The socioeconomic status, race, and vaginal flora of the mother may influence the likelihood of septicemia in the newborn. In New York City the incidence of neonatal infection in poor families is approximately twice that in the most prosperous families, and the rate in blacks exceeds that in white or Puerto Rican populations. Some studies suggest that these differences reflect differing standards of prenatal care; others have shown that different economic and racial groups receiving care in the same prenatal clinic had different rates of antenatal and neonatal infection.

Symptomatic bacteriuria during pregnancy is associated with premature births, and treatment of bacteriuria during pregnancy has been followed by a significant decrease in the number of low birth weight babies. Asymptomatic bacteriuria during pregnancy may be associated with prematurity, but this association has not been confirmed by all investigators. Since both prematurity and low birth weight are associated with an increased risk of neonatal infection, symptomatic bacteriuria during pregnancy may be a factor that indirectly influences the development of sepsis in the neonate. Smoking during pregnancy also has been associated with low birth weight and thus also may indirectly influence the development of neonatal sepsis.

Mycoplasma hominis, T-mycoplasmas (T-strains), and *M. fermentans* have been isolated from the genitourinary system, and colonization by genital mycoplasmas has been associated with low birth weight. The association of low birth weight with T-mycoplasma colonization of the maternal birth canal is highly significant but not necessarily related to premature delivery. Colonization of the birth canal with T-strains or with *M. hominis* has not been related to a history of previous premature births, stillbirths, abortions, or to the development of toxemia or bleeding in the third trimester of pregnancy. However, it is more prevalent among black women than white women and more common among poor patients in both groups. Mycoplasmas have been isolated more frequently from infertile than fertile couples. They also have been recovered from the fetal membranes of spontaneous abortuses and from the viscera of aborted fetuses and stillborn infants. Colonization of neonates with mycoplasmas may be associated with neonatal *Mycoplasma* infection. *Mycoplasma hominis* has been associated with cervical lymphadenitis as well as with meningitis and brain abscess in the newborn infant. Maternal colonization by mycoplasmas may influence the development of neonatal sepsis, however, to the extent that low birth weight plays a role in increasing the risk of septicemia. Genital mycoplasmas have been isolated from the blood of patients with fever following abortion and delivery, but bloodstream infection of the fetus or newborn appears to be infrequent.

Factors operative at or near the time of delivery

Infants born to mothers with septicemia or viremia or with infections of the urinary tract, vagina, or cervix have an increased incidence of infection. An increase in neonatal infections also has been observed in infants born to febrile mothers even when the specific focus of maternal infection cannot be identified. An increased risk of neonatal infection accompanies rupture of the fetal membranes for more than 24 hours before delivery. Excessive bleeding from placenta previa or abruptio placentae, excessive manipulation, and a prolonged second stage of labor and fetal distress during delivery also are factors that have been associated with an increased incidence of neonatal infection. Cephalhematomas (p. 218) have been followed by the development of osteomyelitis of the underlying skull or by sepsis and meningitis. Fetal monitoring in utero has been associated with the formation of scalp abscesses in up to 7% of deliveries in which monitoring has been utilized.

Host factors

Male infants are infected more frequently and have a greater risk of neonatal death than female infants, even allowing for the greater number of male births. A possible exception may be in the risk of infection with group B β-hemolytic streptococci. An increasing number of differences between newborns and older children in their capacity to resist infection have been delineated (p. 636). Defects in the response of neonatal leukocytes to chemotactic factors, impaired phagocytosis, and impaired bactericidal capacity have been reported. Deficiencies of several serum complement components including C1q, C3, and C5, deficient opsonic activity of neonatal sera, and low levels of serum properdin also have been observed. IgA and IgM immunoglobulins are not acquired transplacentally; thus most neonates have very low levels of IgA and IgM globulins at birth. Despite transplacental acquisition of IgG globulin, specific antibodies to certain antigens, such as pertussis or varicella, may be lacking because they are absent from maternal blood. The frequency of neonatal infection in general and the incidence of disease due to organisms indigenous to the host or environment suggest that these infections reflect the deficits in host immunity that have been observed. This fact is highlighted by recent observations that early onset group B streptococcal disease primarily afflicts newborns who are deficient in group B Ia plasma factor and who also lack phagocytic ability and type-specific agglutinins to group B Ia streptococcal organisms.

Other factors

Bottle feeding may increase the risk of neonatal infection in comparison with infants who are breast-fed, although no in vivo protective effect has been demonstrated. Human colostrum contains agglutinins against gram-negative bacteria; they may be passed along the intestinal tract and provide some local protective effect in the GI tract. Human milk also contains large quantities of iron-binding proteins that are known to exert a powerful bacteriostatic effect on *E. coli*. It also contains macrophages and lymphoctyes that may play a role in local immunologic defense (see Chapter 26).

Clinical manifestations

Septicemia may occur at any time during the first month of life; onset within the first 2 days of life is associated more frequently with prenatal or perinatal predisposing factors, whereas onset after 48 to 72 hours of age more frequently reflects disease acquired at or subsequent to delivery.

The evolution of signs and symptoms differs from patient to patient; the course may be fulminant, leading to death in several hours, or it may be more protracted. The earliest clinical signs of neonatal septicemia are characterized by lack of specificity and include lethargy, irritability, poor feeding, or only the suggestion by the nursing staff or the mother that the newborn is not doing as well as previously. Since these signs also may accompany noninfectious neonatal problems, such as anemia, cardiac decompensation, central nervous system (CNS) disorders, or metabolic problems including hypoglycemia, the physician must supplement these clinical findings with additional clinical and laboratory information that may support the possibility of neonatal septicemia. If a diagnosis of septicemia cannot be excluded or an alternative explanation for the findings is not established, appropriate cultures must be obtained and therapy initiated.

Additional clinical manifestations of neonatal septicemia may reflect primary or secondary involvement of any organ system. Fever may be present but is often absent; hypothermia is as common as hyperthermia, particularly in premature infants who frequently experience irregular fluctuations of body temperature. Tachypnea, cyanosis, apnea, tachycardia or bradycardia, and hypotension may be noted. Although these findings may suggest that the patient is in the terminal stages of septicemia, one should not necessarily infer that septicemia has been of long duration, since the infection may become fulminant in a short period of time. The presence of focal neurologic signs, tremors, seizures, or a full fontanel may be noted even in septic neonates without neonatal meningitis. Vomiting, abdominal distension, diarrhea, hepatomegaly, splenomegaly, jaundice, pallor, petechial or purpuric lesions, or bleeding may occur. The onset of jaundice in the first 24 hours of life in the absence of a primary hemolytic disorder always should suggest the possibility of septicemia. Studies of icteric infants with septicemia have revealed that a preponderance of cases are associated with gram-negative bacilli, particularly *E. coli*. The hypothesis for this includes both hemolysis of red blood cells sensitized by bacterial polysaccharides and liver cell destruction or impairment of the bilirubin excretory functions of the liver. Rapidly developing diffuse erythema of the skin in the absence of a discrete eruption, accompanied by sudden development of anemia and leukocytosis in an infant born to a mother with premature rupture of the membranes, should suggest the possibility of *Clostridium perfringens* septicemia. The skin discoloration in these patients has been attributed to deposition of hemoglobin released from erythrocytes by lecithinase, a potent hemolysin elaborated by this organism.

Infections that may precede or accompany septicemia include omphalitis, conjunctivitis, soft tissue or skin abscesses, impetigo, otitis media, meningitis, or osteomyelitis. When cellulitis is found, infection with streptococci should be considered. The presence of impetigo or abscesses should suggest staphylococcal disease. If necrotic skin lesions with a purple hue are noted, infection with *P. aeruginosa* or *Aeromonas hydrophila* may exist.

Differential diagnosis

The nonspecificity and wide range of signs and symptoms that may be observed in neonates with septicemia frequently suggest a number of alternative diagnoses. These may include hemolytic anemia, hypovolemic shock, intracranial hemorrhage, respiratory distress syndrome, pneumonia, primary disease of the GI tract, thrombocytopenic purpura, leukemia, hypocalcemia, hypoglycemia, or other metabolic disorders.

Laboratory evaluation

A specific diagnosis can be confirmed only by the presence of a positive blood culture. When septicemia is suspected, two or more blood cultures should be obtained. If the patient is critically ill, one culture is adequate.

Since focal infections may precede or follow septicemia, cultures of other body fluids or orifices may help to establish an etiologic diagnosis. When septicemia is suspected, both urine and cerebrospinal fluid (CSF) should be examined and cultures obtained. Specific morphologic and chemical CSF findings that may suggest the presence of bacterial meningitis are discussed subsequently (neonatal meningitis). If skin lesions or soft tissue abscesses are present, these should be aspirated for smear and culture. When infection is localized in a joint, fluid should be aspirated, examined, and cultured. Stool cultures may be helpful in establishing a diagnosis of septicemia due to *Shigella*, *Salmonella*, *Campylobacter*, and infrequently *S. aureus*. Cultures of gastric aspirate or of cord blood from infants who are clinically well but who were born 24 hours or more after rupture of the membranes are not likely to be of diagnostic value and may be misleading. However, I recommend that two or more blood cultures be obtained from different peripheral venous sites in these infants as a means of screening for the possibility of significant bacteremia.

Neonatal sepsis has been associated with chorioamnionitis (p. 208). The incidence of umbilical cord neutrophilic infiltrates, however, far exceeds the number of proven cases of fetal or neonatal infection. Their presence, therefore, does not serve to separate definitively the infected from the uninfected neonate but may help to identify a high-risk group of infants. Routine prophylactic antibiotic treatment of all infants with umbilical cord vasculitis is not warranted. The presence of three or more polymorphonuclear leukocytes per high-power field demonstrable on a smear of the trapped amniotic fluid or other debris in the external auditory canal also correlates significantly with the ultimate demonstration of septicemia. The presence of organisms on Gram stain or recovered by culture of the same material is less specific, but in some patients the organisms that are obtained are identical to those recovered from the blood of the same patient. A smear of the buffy coat should be examined for bacteria by Gram stain.

The white blood cell count should be obtained in newborns with possible septicemia. Leukopenia (<3,500 white blood cells/mm^3) or leukocytosis (>25,000 white blood cells/mm^3) supports a diagnosis of infection. A differential white blood cell count may be of even greater assistance, particularly in septic full-term neonates whose total white blood cell counts are within the normal range. A comparison between the absolute number of band neutrophils found in normal and infected neonates reveals that in infants with bacterial infection (including those with normal neutrophil counts) the band counts are increased significantly beyond the normal range (Table 27-1). A depression in platelet count (<150,000 platelets/mm^3) may be noted during septicemia; however, a normal platelet count does not exclude the diagnosis. Similarly, a peripheral smear that suggests a hemolytic process may be found in neonates with septicemia but is also seen in many neonates who are not infected. An erythrocyte sedimentation rate greater than 5 mm/hour within the first 24 hours of life may suggest septicemia.

Serologic studies, described subsequently, may help to establish a diagnosis of syphilis or infection with various viral, fungal, or parasitic agents. An elevated serum IgM concentration (>17 to 20 mg/dl) during the first week of life suggests that infection has occurred in utero

Table 27-1. Absolute number of bands/mm^3 of blood of 169 normal full-term infants

Time of sampling	Mean	Standard deviation	Skewness	Median	Range for 95% Low	Range for 95% High
Birth	358	419	1.371	155	0	1,410
Day 1	531	664	1.771	306	0	2,220
Day 5	282	345	1.948	189	0	1,240

From Akenzua, G.I., and others: Pediatrics **54:**38, 1974.

or perhaps at birth. However, infants dying of bacterial infection during the first several days of life may do so with normal serum IgM levels. Conversely, elevated serum IgM concentrations may occur in newborns who have never been infected, because of contamination caused by maternal bleeding into the fetal circulation. If elevated serum IgM has been caused by admixture of fetal with maternal blood, a rapid fall in serum IgM concentration will ensue during the first week of life.

Countercurrent immunoelectrophoresis (CIE) may be effective in establishing the etiologic diagnosis of septicemia or meningitis due to *Haemophilus influenzae* (type b), *Streptococcus pneumoniae*, and *Neisseria meningitidis* within 30 minutes of the time that blood or CSF samples have been received in the laboratory. It also has been possible to establish a diagnosis of septicemia or meningitis due to group B streptococci or K1 strains of *E. coli* utilizing countercurrent immunoelectrophoresis, but appropriate antisera for these diagnostic studies are available at present only in selected research laboratories.

Hypoglycemia and hyponatremia may accompany septicemia in the newborn. Hypoglycemia has been noted during septicemia with gram-negative bacilli with much greater frequency than during infection with gram-positive organisms. Infection in normal children and adults is accompanied by an increased peripheral resistance to insulin, by increased elaboration of corticosteroids, growth hormone, glucagon, and epinephrine, and by increased glycogenolysis and gluconeogenesis. All these factors tend to promote hyperglycemia rather than hypoglycemia during active infection. Increased peripheral utilization of glucose, perhaps due to enhanced insulin sensitivity and lack of glycogen stores, has been suggested as a possible contributing factor for hypoglycemia during neonatal sepsis. Decreased corticosteroid activity has not been documented even when adrenal hemorrhage is found post mortem. Hyponatremia during septicemia probably reflects inappropriate retention of fluid in excess of solute, resulting in dilutional hyponatremia. It also may reflect changes in total body sodium concentration as a result of diarrhea, vomiting, excessive sweating, or insufficient intake. Symptoms of hyponatremia include irritability, lethargy, and seizures, signs that are indistinguishable from those noted in patients with septicemia. Measurement of serum electrolytes should be made in infants with possible or proven septicemia, since the results obtained may support the diagnostic impression, have differential diagnostic value, and are essential in designing specific regimens of supportive care for each infant.

Complications

The complications of septicemia in the neonate are similar to those which accompany this disease in older children and adults. These include congestive heart failure, shock, and disseminated intravascular coagulation. The incidence of mild disseminated intravascular coagulation in neonates with septicemia may be as high as 66%. Focal infection in one or more organ systems also may occur.

Treatment

The neonate with suspected sepsis must be treated immediately after appropriate diagnostic studies have been initiated and before the etiologic agent is identified or its susceptibility to antimicrobial agents established. The course of neonatal septicemia may be so rapid that the threat to life is greater than the possibility that undesirable side effects may accompany the use of antibiotics in some patients who subsequently prove to be uninfected. The choice of antibiotics must be based on (1) consideration of the type of microorganisms that may be encountered, (2) the sensitivity of those organisms to the antibiotic employed, (3) the likelihood of achieving bactericidal concentrations of antibiotics at the site of infection, and (4) consideration of possible adverse effects of therapy with specific antibiotic agents. Since the sensitivity of various microorganisms to antimicrobial agents may change with time and differs from institution to institution, it is imperative that physicians be aware of the sensitivity pattern of bacteria isolated in their own hospital and community. In addition, immaturity of renal and hepatic function precludes the use of certain drugs entirely and requires that dosage schedules for preferred drugs be adjusted depending on the gestational age, birth weight, and postnatal age of the infant. The dosage recommendations in Table 27-2 are based on consider-

Table 27-2. Antibiotics that may be employed for treatment of neonatal sepsis or meningitis

Agent	First week of life or premature Dosage	Route	Schedule	Full-term infant over 1 week of age Dosage	Route	Schedule	Comment
Penicillin	50,000-100,000 units/kg/day	IM, IV	q8h or q12h	50,000-300,000 units/kg/day	IM, IV	q6h or q8h	Use highest dosage in meningitis
Ampicillin	50-100 mg/kg/day	IM, IV	q12h	150-200 mg/kg/day	IM, IV	q8h	Use highest dosage in meningitis Use 100 mg/kg/day in premature infants between 1 and 4 weeks of age with sepsis
Methicillin	100 mg/kg/day	IM, IV	q8h	200 mg/kg/day	IM, IV	q6h	Give q12h on first day of life
Nafcillin	100 mg/kg/day	IM, IV	q12h	200 mg/kg/day	IM, IV	q6h	
Oxacillin	100 mg/kg/day	IM, IV	q12h	200 mg/kg/day	IM, IV	q6h	
Cephalothin	50 mg/kg/day	IM, IV	q8h	50-100 mg/kg/day	IM, IV	q6h	
Carbenicillin	225 mg/kg/day	IM, IV	q8h	300 mg/kg/day	IM, IV	q6h	Give loading dose of 100 mg/kg to all patients Full-term infants may be given 300 mg/kg/day even during first week of life
Kanamycin	15 mg/kg/day	IM, IV	q12h	25 mg/kg/day	IM, IV	q8h or q12h	When used IV, infuse over 30 minutes Recent pharmacologic studies suggest that these dosage recommendations may require revision upward, but clinical studies to support lack of toxicity at increased dosages not available
Gentamicin	5 mg/kg/day	IM, IV	q12h	7.5 mg/kg/day	IM, IV	q8h	When used IV, infuse over 30 minutes Intraventricular therapy also may be required in patients with meningitis
Tobramycin	4 mg/kg/day	IM, IV	q12h	5 mg/kg/day	IM, IV	q6h or q8h	If used IV, infuse over 30 minutes
Polymyxin B	3 mg/kg/day	IM, IV	q12h	4 mg/kg/day	IM, IV	q8h	If used IV, infuse over 30 minutes Intrathecal administration also required if used in treatment of meningitis
Neomycin	50-100 mg/kg/day	PO	q6h	50-100 mg/kg/day	PO	q6h	Use only if lack of systemic absorption can be ensured
Colistimethate	5 mg/kg/day	IM	q12h	8 mg/kg/day	IM	q8h	
Chloramphenicol	25 mg/kg/day	IV	q8h	50 mg/kg/day	IV	q6h	If used, serum concentrations should be monitored
Nystatin	200,000-400,000 units	PO	q6h	200,000-400,000 units	PO	q6h	Do not use for systemic infections
Amikacin	15 mg/kg/day	IM, IV	q12h	22.5 mg/kg/day	IM, IV	q8h	When using IV, infuse over 30 minutes
Clindamycin	20 mg/kg/day	IV	q8h	30 mg/kg/day	IV	q6h	Do not use in patients with meningitis
Moxalactam	100 mg/kg/day	IV	q12h	150 mg/kg/day	IV	q8h	Do not use as the only drug for unknown sepsis or meningitis

ation of pharmacokinetic information presently available concerning the use of antimicrobial agents in the newborn period. Although general recommendations can be given, specific dosages required by infants may change from day to day. Ideally, serum concentrations of antibiotics should be monitored to ensure therapeutic efficacy while minimizing toxicity.

When septicemia is suspected in the first 72 hours of life and the etiologic agent is unknown, the combination of ampicillin and an aminoglycoside should be used. Ampicillin provides effective coverage for all gram-positive organisms except penicillinase-producing staphylococci and is also of value in treating infection with most strains of *H. influenzae*, some strains of *E. coli, Salmonella, Shigella, Proteus mirabilis*, and many strains of *L. monocytogenes*. A synergistic inhibitory effect has been demonstrated in vitro when ampicillin and kanamycin or gentamicin have been tested for activity against various strains of *E. coli, Listeria*, and enterococci. Kanamycin and gentamicin are the aminoglycoside drugs used most frequently; choice of one or the other should be dictated by the sensitivity of the enteric organisms found in each community. Gentamicin, however, offers effective coverage for most strains of *Pseudomonas*, whereas kanamycin does not. Tobramycin sulfate recently has been approved for use in neonatal sepsis, and it also offers broad coverage of gram-negative organisms, including *Pseudomonas*; experience with this antibiotic has been limited. Amikacin is another useful alternative.

When septicemia is suspected after 3 days of age, specific consideration must be given to providing coverage of organisms that may have been acquired from the environment. Consideration should be given to the addition of a penicillinase-resistant penicillin to the regimen until an organism has been identified or, perhaps, the substitution of methicillin for ampicillin. Methicillin is preferred on my service for coverage of penicillin-resistant staphylococci because it is bound to protein to a much lesser extent than is nafcillin or oxacillin; thus the risk of displacing bilirubin from albumin-binding sites is reduced.

Following identification of the causative agent, a single antibiotic can be employed in most cases. Although specific therapy should be based on the results of antibiotic sensitivity testing, an appropriate choice usually can be made before such results are available. In Table 27-2 are listed the more commonly used antibiotics and suggested specific indications for their use. The toxicity of these drugs and additional comments, including important pharmacologic considerations, are included.

Antibiotic treatment of neonatal septicemia generally is continued for 7 to 10 days; a longer period of treatment may be required, depending on the clinical response of the patient. Meticulous observation and other supportive measures are indicated. Electronic monitoring is important but cannot be substituted for frequent assessment by skilled nurses and physicians. Oral feeding should be discontinued to decrease the likelihood of aspiration and to permit more precise monitoring of fluid intake. Gastric suction may be required intermittently to prevent or treat gastric dilatation. Appropriate quantities of fluids, electrolytes, and glucose should be provided intravenously (p. 316). Antibiotics may be provided by the intravenous route but when added to intravenous solutions should be administered within 1 hour. Two or more antibiotics should not be administered concomitantly, and antibiotics should not be placed in solutions containing other drugs or vitamins (the latter may inactivate the antibiotic before infusion). The infant's environment should be adjusted to maintain a rectal temperature of 37° to 38° C and a skin temperature of 36° to 37° C. Sponge baths with tepid water and, rarely, antipyretics may be required if temperature exceeds 39.5° C. Oxygen should be provided to relieve hypoxemia if it is present. Hyponatremia should be treated by fluid restriction if there is evidence of inappropriate secretion of antidiuretic hormone. If sodium losses are excessive, sufficient sodium should be given to relieve symptoms of hyponatremia and to raise the serum sodium concentration to 130 mEq/L. Sodium bicarbonate (2 to 3 mEq/kg) or glucose (as required) should be given to counteract profound acidosis and hypoglycemia.

Septic shock should be treated by volume expansion. Optimally, whole blood (10 to 20 ml/kg stat.) should be provided. Hydrocortisone sodium succinate (10 to 20 mg/kg) has been utilized as an immediate dose in critically ill infants with persistent hypotension and may be continued at 5 mg/kg every 6 hours in some patients. There is little evidence that steroid administration is beneficial, but individual patients may improve after administration of steroids. Disseminated intravascular coagulation may occur; treatment with heparin (1 mg/kg stat. and q4h) is recommended (p. 720). Although heparin is indicated, specific treatment of the septic disease process or shock is more important. Initially, administration of fresh heparinized whole blood may be indicated. There has been limited experience recently with the use of white cell transfusions for septic newborns with neutropenia. This technique appears promising, particularly when neutropenia reflects severe bone marrow depletion of neutrophils.

INFECTION OF ORGAN SYSTEMS
Neonatal bacterial meningitis
Incidence

Bacterial meningitis is responsible for between 1% and 4% of neonatal deaths and develops in approximately 1 of every 2,500 live births. Meningitis is probably more common during the first month of life than in any succeeding month.

Etiology

The same organisms that are responsible for neonatal septicemia cause neonatal meningitis. Preliminary results of the most recent collaborative study suggest that *E. coli* remains the organism recovered most frequently, followed by group B β-hemolytic streptococci. In some institutions, meningitis due to group B streptococci is more common than that due to *E. coli*. *L. monocytogenes* and *F. meningosepticum* have a predilection for the meninges of newborns, and *F. meningosepticum* tends to produce epidemic disease. Mixed bacterial meningitis and mixed viral and bacterial meningitis also have been reported in the neonatal period.

Pathology

A subarachnoid inflammatory exudate generally is present and is more common at the base of the brain than over the convexity. During the acute stages of the disease the brain may be swollen and hyperemic, and the ventricles may be small. Herniation of cerebral or cerebellar tissue is uncommon. Hydrocephalus occurs frequently, and the degree of ventricular enlargement tends to increase with the duration of disease. Ventriculitis has been mentioned with increasing frequency in necropsy reports of patients dying of neonatal meningitis; it may be noted in some patients with acellular and sterile CSF. In the first week of disease, polymorphonuclear leukocytes are the predominant cells within both the subarachnoid space and the ventricular system. During the second and third weeks macrophages, histiocytes, and lymphocytes are the predominant cells found in the exudates. Vasculitis is common, and both thrombosis and infarction may occur. A glial reaction is noted in areas directly subjacent to the inflammatory exudate, and a diffuse encephalopathy characterized by karyorrhexis and loss of nerve cells may be noted. Hemorrhagic cerebral necrosis occurs commonly in newborns who die of enterobacterial meningitis; this type of reaction is particularly characteristic following *Proteus* infection.

Pathogenesis

The complications of pregnancy and delivery that predispose the newborn to septicemia also increase the risk of meningitis, since in most patients the meninges are seeded hematogenously. Neonatal skin infections, pneumonia, otitis media, and urinary tract infections are also frequently accompanied by bacteremia with the subsequent development of meningitis. Meningitis may be associated with one third of the cases of septicemia and is more common in premature than in full-term infants. This risk of meningitis also is increased in infants with meningomyelocele.

Factors referable to the microorganism itself may be associated with an increased risk of meningitis. Whereas early-onset group B streptococcal septicemia usually is related to infection by organisms of subgroups I or II, meningitis (early or late onset) often is associated with infection by organisms of subgroup III. Similarly, meningitis due to *L. monocytogenes* is usually due to type IV organisms. Recent studies have shown that most neonatal meningitis due to *E. coli* is the result of infection by strains containing K1 capsular polysaccharide, an antigen that is immunochemically identical or very similar to meningococcal group B capsular polysaccharide. Thus certain microorganisms appear to possess certain antigens that confer on the organisms specific invasive potential.

Clinical manifestations

Any of the clinical manifestations of neonatal septicemia may herald the presence of neonatal meningitis. Thus in most patients an appropriate diagnostic evaluation for the newborn with possible septicemia includes lumbar puncture. Poor feeding, vomiting, respiratory distress, irritability, and temperature instability are common, and convulsions, paralysis of various cranial nerves, abnormal Moro reflex, abnormal cry, or focal neurologic signs may be seen. A bulging fontanel and stiff neck are late signs; when they appear before initial diagnosis and therapy, the outlook is dismal. Subdural effusions, coma, and hydrocephalus may occur.

Laboratory manifestations

Specific diagnosis is dependent on a careful evaluation of the CSF and ultimately depends on demonstration of organisms on a Gram-stained smear of the CSF and their growth on culture. The number and type of cells and the protein concentration in normal newborns differ from accepted norms in older children. A study of CSF obtained from 117 high-risk newborns who had no evidence of bacterial or viral infection of the CNS revealed an average CSF cell count of 8.4 cells/mm^3 with a range of 0 to 32 cells/mm^3. Approximately 60% of the CSF white blood cells were polymorphonuclear leukocytes. Protein concentration within CSF of normal full-term infants varies from 20 to 170 mg/dl with a mean value of 90 mg/dl. CSF protein concentrations in premature infants vary between 65 and 150 mg/dl during the first 2 weeks of life. The values in premature infants are related inversely to birth weight.

The CSF cell count in newborns with bacterial meningitis may reach 10,000 or more cells/mm^3, but meningitis may be found in the presence of cell counts that are normal. Protein concentration may be elevated or normal. In the presence of meningitis, CSF glucose concentration may be less than half of the blood glucose concentration obtained at the time of lumbar puncture. Occasionally, CSF glucose concentrations of 10 mg/100 ml or less may occur; however, they also occur in newborns who have hypoglycemia or intracranial hemorrhage but not meningitis. A Gram-stained smear of the CSF should be examined by an experienced observer. The CSF should always be cultured even if it appears to be crystal clear or a bloody tap has been obtained. CSF, serum, and urine also can be evaluated by countercurrent immunoelectrophoresis, which may permit an etiologic diagnosis within 30 minutes. Blood cultures should be obtained and are positive in 50% to 60% of cases.

Treatment

Until a definitive diagnosis has been made, antibiotic treatment should be initiated with ampicillin and either kanamycin or gentamicin, utilizing dosage schedules shown in Table 27-2. Once a specific pathogen has been identified and its susceptibilities are known, the best drug or combination of drugs should be employed (Table 27-3). Penicillin G would be preferred for group B streptococcal disease; ampicillin for infection with enterococci, *Listeria*, or *P. mirabilis;* methicillin for staphylococcal infection; and carbenicillin plus gentamicin for *Pseudomonas* infection. Treatment of coliforms with both ampicillin and an aminoglycoside may be preferred, since the combination may be synergistic against some strains of *E. coli*. In patients with unknown or ampicillin-resistant gram-negative bacterial meningitis, the use of chloramphenicol also should be considered.

Regimens for the treatment of gram-negative neonatal meningitis have not been particularly effective in promptly sterilizing the CSF. Ventriculitis with sequestration of microorganisms within the ventricular system in infants with gram-negative meningitis is a relatively common occurrence. Aminoglycosides administered intrathecally do not diffuse over the surface of the brain or into the ventricles in a uniform manner.

A collaborative two-phase study of neonatal meningitis has shown no decrease in mortality when therapy with intrathecal or intraventricular aminoglycosides was coupled with their parenteral administration, compared with parenteral therapy alone. For this reason, neither intrathecal nor intraventricular aminoglycosides can be recommended. Some centers have employed chloramphenicol for the treatment of gram-negative neonatal meningitis using initial dosages as listed in Table 27-2. I support this approach, provided that the patient is being treated in an institution in which measurement of serum chloramphenicol concentration can be performed rapidly using colorimetric, enzymatic, or radioimmunoassay. If a colorimetric assay is used, it is important to absorb the serum with charcoal prior to determination of chloramphenicol concentration to prevent bilirubin from interfering with assay results.

Recent advances in antimicrobial therapy have resulted in the availability of moxalactam, a drug that is effective for the treatment of gram-negative organisms other than *Pseudomonas*. It is not recommended for the treatment of infection due to gram-positive organisms. Transport of this drug across the blood-brain barrier is excellent. At present, ampicillin plus moxalactam is being compared with ampicillin plus amikacin in a collaborative study of gram-negative neonatal meningitis. Early results in this study, plus numerous individual reports, suggest that moxalactam will play an important role in the treatment of gram-negative meningitis in the future. The dosage of moxalactam that may be employed is shown in Table 27-2. Newer third-generation cephalosporins also are being tested to determine their efficacy in the treatment of neonatal sepsis and meningitis. Data are inadequate at present to determine the specific efficacy of these compounds in the treatment of neonatal infection.

Meningitis due to gram-positive organisms should be treated for 14 days, but treatment may be indicated for a more extended period of time if the clinical situation dictates. When disease is caused by gram-negative organisms, therapy is continued for 2 weeks after the CSF has been proved sterile or for a minimum of 3 weeks, whichever is longer. Examination and culture of CSF should be repeated 1 or 2 days after discontinuation of antibiotic therapy.

Supportive care of the newborn with meningitis is similar to that described for the septic neonate. In particular, the possibility of inappropriate secretion of antidiuretic hormone with development of dilutional hyponatremia is best treated by fluid restriction. Seizures may be controlled with phenobarbital (5 to 8 mg/kg) administered intramuscularly or intravenously or with phenytoin (5 to 8 mg/kg as a loading dose). Phenobarbital and phenytoin can be administered in the same total dosage as above but over a 24-hour period for maintenance control of seizures. Diazepam (0.1 to 1.0 mg) can be administered slowly intravenously until seizures are controlled; this drug may displace bilirubin from albumin-binding sites.

Prognosis

Mortality for newborns with meningitis remains between 35% and 60%, a rate that, in part, is dependent on the gestational age of the infant, the type of microorganisms producing the disease, the duration of disease before initiation of antibiotic therapy, and the sensitivity of the microorganisms to various antimicrobial drugs. The quantity of *E. coli* capsular polysaccharide material to which the host is exposed is also correlated with outcome. The greater the concentration of K1 antigen and the longer it can be detected in the CSF, the worse the prognosis. Many survivors of neonatal meningitis experience significant permanent sequelae resulting in significant neurologic damage.

Pneumonia

Incidence

Pneumonia is the most common form of neonatal infection and one of the most important causes of perinatal death. In the 1920s and 1930s pneumonia was found at autopsy in 20% to 30% of stillborn and newborn infants; more recently, intrauterine pneumonia has been reported in 5% to 35% of autopsies.

Etiology

Pneumonia may follow infection with the same organisms responsible for neonatal sepsis. When the disease is acquired in utero or at the time of delivery, infection with *E. coli, Klebsiella, Listeria, H. influenzae, Treponema pallidum, Enterobacter, Staphylococcus, Streptococcus pneumoniae, S. agalactiae,* or *Proteus* may be suspected. When disease is acquired shortly after birth, the same organisms may be responsible, but infection with *S. aureus, Pseudomonas, Serratia,* and *Candida* should be considered. Viral pneumonia may be noted at or shortly after birth, and epidemic disease has been reported to follow introduction of respiratory syncytial, ECHO, and adenovirus into the newborn unit. *Pneumocystis carinii* pneumonia has been reported in debilitated premature and full-term infants; it also has been observed in a small number of healthy full-term babies. Epidemic pneumonitis due to *Pneumocystis* appears to be more prevalent in Europe than in the United States. *P. carinii* pneumonia has been observed as an incidental finding at necropsy of infants who had been healthy but died unexpectedly.

Pathogenesis and pathology

Pneumonia may be acquired (1) transplacentally in utero, (2) by inhalation of contaminated amniotic fluid before or at the time of delivery, (3) by aspiration of infected materials during or after delivery, (4) by inhalation of aerosols that contain infectious microorganisms in the newborn nursery, or (5) hematogenously from another focus of infection or during the course of septicemia. Intrauterine pneumonia frequently follows prolonged rupture of the membranes (p. 206). All fetuses swallow amniotic fluid; thus the oropharynx or GI tract may serve as portals of entry for microorganisms. Gasping may be induced as a result of asphyxia, prompting aspiration of infected amniotic fluid. Intrauterine pneumonia acquired transplacentally has been associated with maternal pneumococcal septicemia and with viremia. When intrauterine pneumonia occurs, the process is diffuse, and the alveoli are filled with polymorphonuclear leukocytes and microorganisms. Amniotic debris may be found; this suggests that disease has followed aspiration rather than hematogenous dissemination of microorganisms.

Aspiration during or following delivery may lead to bronchopneumonia, which may be associated with hemorrhage and with evidence of pleural inflammation. Abscesses, empyema, and pyopneumothorax may be found when infection is due to *S. aureus*, although these findings are not restricted to infection with this organism. Pneumatocele formation, found so commonly in association with infection due to *S. aureus*, also has been noted in the newborn with pneumonia due to *E. coli, Klebsiella, Enterobacter,* or anaerobic organisms. *Pseudomonas* pneumonia may follow septicemia or use of contaminated resuscitation or inhalation therapy equipment. The inflammatory response in these individuals may be perivascular and characterized by necrosis of vessel walls and of alveoli.

Clinical manifestations

Intrauterine pneumonia should be suspected when respiratory distress develops in any infant, but suspicions should be heightened if antecedent problems referable to pregnancy and delivery have been noted. The infant who has acquired pneumonia in utero or during delivery may be ill at birth, and the initial cry may be delayed. Spontaneous respirations may not occur or may be established with difficulty. If respirations are established, tachypnea, moderate retractions, and an expiratory grunt may be observed. Fever may or may not be noted. In most cases there is no cough. Cyanosis may be constant or intermittent, and respirations may be irregular and punctuated by periods of apnea. Dullness to percussion, decreased breath sounds, and rales may be present, but at times these findings are absent throughout the entire course of the disease. Congestive heart failure manifested by cardiac enlargement, hepatomegaly, and tachycardia may complicate the pneumonic process. Neurologic abnormalities also may appear; they include hypotonia, flaccidity, hypertonia, tremors, and convulsions. When neurologic findings are present, the prognosis generally is poor. At necropsy of some newborns with pneumonia who have had neurologic findings, no gross intracranial lesions are found.

Postnatally acquired pneumonia may develop at any time. Symptoms are similar to those occurring in children with pneumonia immediately after birth; the onset may be abrupt or gradual. Chlamydial pneumonia patients classically exhibit a staccato cough; they are afebrile, and frequently they gain weight slowly.

Diagnosis

Roentgenograms are required to support the diagnosis of pneumonia and to distinguish it from other causes of respiratory distress (p. 1066). In some patients no abnormality will be found if roentgenographic studies have been performed early following the onset of symptoms,

Table 27-3. Indications, pharmacology, and toxicity of antibiotics

Antibiotic	Indications	Pharmacology	Toxicity	Comments
Amikacin	May be used for gram-negative organisms; I prefer to limit its use to kanamycin- and gentamicin-resistant species	Renal excretion; crosses blood-CSF barrier poorly; not absorbed from GI tract in normal host	Possible ototoxicity, nephrotoxicity, and neuromuscular blockade	Toxic reaction in neonate rare if appropriate dosage used and renal function and/or blood levels of antibiotic monitored
Ampicillin	Initial treatment of neonatal sepsis and meningitis; gram-positive organisms except penicillin-resistant staphylococci; may be used for sensitive strains of H. influenzae, Salmonella, Shigella; use for gram-negative infection only on basis of sensitivity test results or for synergistic effect with an aminoglycoside	Renal excretion primarily	Rash, elevated transaminase, eosinophilia; may produce seizures or neuromuscular irritability when administered in high dosages; nephritis may occur rarely	
Carbenicillin	Treatment of Providencia; may be used with an aminoglycoside for Pseudomonas infections or susceptible strains of Proteus	Renal excretion	Rash, elevated transaminases, nausea, vomiting, diarrhea	
Cephalosporins	Not the drug of choice for any known infection; alternative drug for treatment of penicillinase-producing staphylococci	Renal excretion; clearance of cephaloridine affected more markedly than cephalothin by renal insufficiency; crosses blood-CSF barrier poorly if at all	Rashes, urticaria, neutropenia (rare); Coombs' test may become positive during therapy; renal tubular damage may occur (more common with cephaloridine)	Phlebitis common during IV administration; use with caution if sensitivity to penicillin has been documented; produce brownish black color of urine when tested with Clinitest tablets
Clindamycin	May be used in selected neonates with B. fragilis septicemia or peritonitis		Pseudomembranous enterocolitis in adolescents and adults—rare in children; little experience in neonates	
Chloramphenicol	Salmonella sepsis with ampicillin-resistant strain; H. influenzae sepsis or meningitis with ampicillin-resistant strains; may be required in certain cases of anaerobic sepsis (e.g., with B. fragilis) or in certain cases of sepsis due to Serratia	Blocks protein synthesis acting on ribosomal site; metabolized by liver and conjugated with glucuronide for excretion	Gray baby syndrome characterized by anorexia, vomiting, abdominal distension, followed by hypothermia, shallow irregular respirations, development of ashen gray cyanosis, and death; syndrome related to immature hepatic function and characterized by high blood levels of unconjugated chloramphenicol	Dose-related reversible anemia generally develops when administered for more than 7-10 days
Erythromycin	Penicillin-resistant staphylococcus, Chlamydia, pertussis	Crosses blood-brain barrier poorly; excreted in urine, stool, and biliary system	No significant toxicity	
Gentamicin	May be used in initial treatment of neonatal sepsis or meningitis; use for Pseudomonas, hospital-acquired K. pneumoniae, Enterobacter, Serratia, and kanamycin-resistant coliform or-	Inhibits glucuronyl transferase in higher dose therapeutic dosages; crosses placental barrier; crosses blood-CSF barrier poorly	Possible ototoxicity, nephrotoxicity, and neuromuscular blockade	Toxic reaction in neonate rare if appropriate dosage used and renal function and/or blood levels of antibiotic monitored

	meningitis; treatment of gram-negative organisms except *Pseudomonas* and kanamycin-resistant coliforms	blood-CSF barrier poorly; not absorbed from GI tract in normal host	icity, and neuromuscular blockade	if appropriate dosage used and renal function and/or blood levels of antibiotic monitored
Methicillin Oxacillin Nafcillin	Penicillin-resistant *Staphylococcus aureus* infections	Renal excretion; methicillin protein bound only 20%; oxacillin 88% and nafcillin 92% protein bound	Nephrotoxicity; eosinophilia may precede renal damage	Monitor BUN, creatinine, and observe for hematuria and proteinuria; low protein binding suggests potential advantage for methicillin in neonates with hyperbilirubinemia with regard to minimizing risk of kernicterus
Moxalactam	Septicemia, meningitis, ventriculitis caused by *E. coli*, *Klebsiella*, *Serratia*, *H. influenzae*	Crosses blood-brain barrier; 60% to 90% excreted by kidneys	Eosinophilia, neutropenia (reversible), disturbances in vitamin K–dependent clotting function	Studies to determine definitive role for this drug in neonatal sepsis and meningitis presently being pursued
Neomycin	Bacterial diarrhea, enteropathogenic *E. coli*	Not absorbed from normal GI tract	Ototoxic, nephrotoxic, neuromuscular blockade	Do not use parenterally
Penicillin G	*Streptococcus pyogenes*, gram-positive anaerobes, including gram-positive bacilli; *S. pneumoniae*, nonpenicillinase *S. aureus*, *S. agalactiae*, *Neisseria gonorrhoeae*, *N. meningitidis*, *Bacteroides* except *B. fragilis*, *Pasteurella multocida*, *Fusobacterium*, *Treponema pallidum* (syphilis), *Actinomyces israeli*, and leptospires	Renal excretion	Rare nephrotoxicity, rare neuromuscular toxicity	May be used in initial treatment of neonatal septicemia or meningitis in conjunction with an aminoglycoside; however, this combination may not provide effective coverage for infection with *H. influenzae*, *Salmonella*, or enterococci
Polymyxin B and colistin (polymyxin E)	Effective against *Pseudomonas* and kanamycin-resistant *E. coli*	Renal excretion; dose not cross blood-CSF barrier; not absorbed from GI tract in normal host	Painful injection, ataxia, drowsiness, peripheral neuropathy; neuromuscular blockade may occur; nephritis and azotemia	Polymyxin B may be given intrathecally
Streptomycin	*Mycobacterium*, *Francisella tularensis*, and *Pasteurella pestis*	Renal excretion	Cardiovascular collapse, vestibular and auditory damage	Employed infrequently in neonates; if used, provide as 30 mg/kg/day IM q12h
Tobramycin	Broad coverage of gram-negative organisms including *Pseudomonas*	Renal excretion	Possible nephrotoxicity and ototoxicity	Approved for use in neonatal septicemia recently; experience to date has been limited
Nitrofurantoin	Contraindicated in newborn; may cause hemolytic anemias in patients with glucose-6-phosphate dehydrogenase deficiency			
Sulfonamides	Contraindicated in newborn, predisposes to kernicterus by displacing bilirubin from albumin-binding sites; maternal ingestion of sulfamethoxypyridazene (Kynex) may be followed by hemolysis and jaundice in newborns with glucose-6-phosphate dehydrogenase deficiency			
Tetracyclines	Contraindicated in newborn; administration to pregnant women or newborns may produce permanent brown-yellow or gray-black dental discoloration of deciduous or permanent teeth; may cause enamel hypoplasia; may inhibit bone growth in normal premature infants; may cause increased intracranial pressure (pseudotumor cerebri)			

but by 24 to 72 hours a diagnosis should be possible. In other patients an area of radiopacification is present but may be attributed to atelectasis. Roentgenograms may reveal bilateral homogeneous consolidation when pneumonia is acquired in utero or diffuse bronchopneumonia when disease has been acquired postnatally. Pneumatoceles may be observed, and occasionally hemothorax or pleural effusions are present. The radiograph of segmental or lobar atelectasis is unlike that of congenital or postnatal pneumonia. Where lobar atelectasis occurs, consolidation of an entire lobe or segment may be noted, but rarely is an entire lung involved. The involved hemithorax is smaller than the opposite side, the diaphragm may be elevated, and the heart is shifted toward the area of presumed atelectasis. In contrast, it may be extremely difficult to distinguish the roentgenogram of pneumonia from that of massive meconium aspiration. In meconium aspiration, opacities may be distributed in the same manner as in bronchopneumonia, but the roentgenographic changes tend to be maximal early and disappear rapidly during the ensuing period of several days. In contrast, the patchy opacifications noted in bronchopneumonia tend to be minimal early and become more impressive during the subsequent period of several days.

Pneumonia caused by the group B streptococci may be indistinguishable roentgenographically from respiratory distress syndrome. Pneumonia due to *Chlamydia trachomatis* may produce roentgenographic findings of hyperinflation of the lung associated with diffuse bilateral pulmonary infiltrates.

Tracheal aspirate cultures may not be particularly helpful in establishing an etiologic diagnosis, since they often reveal the same kind of flora as found in the vaginal canal. The presence of polymorphonuclear leukocytes on a tracheal aspirate smear suggests an infectious process, and recovery of *S. aureus* or *Pseudomonas* organisms from the tracheal aspirate may affect the choice of antibiotic therapy. Blood cultures should be obtained in infants with pneumonia; when positive, they establish an etiologic diagnosis. The white blood cell count and differential appear to be of little value generally, but in individual patients they may reveal a striking leukocytosis (25,000 white blood cells/mm^3) or leukopenia (<3,500 white blood cells/mm^3).

Treatment

When a diagnosis is established, treatment should be prompt. If the diagnosis is supported by historical and clinical findings but initial roentgenograms fail to confirm the clinical impression, treatment should not be delayed and should be continued until a chest roentgenogram at 72 hours fails to confirm the diagnosis. Treatment with antibiotics should be directed toward coverage of the same organisms as those which produce neonatal septicemia; thus ampicillin and kanamycin in dosages similar to those used for septicemia are indicated (Table 27-2). When infections with *S. aureus* or *P. aeruginosa* are suspected, treatment must be altered. Staphylococcal infection is best treated with methicillin, whereas *Pseudomonas* infections can be treated with gentamicin, which will cover other gram-negative organisms as well. Pneumonia due to *Chlamydia* or *Pertussis* responds best to treatment with erythromycin. Erythromycin can be given in a dosage of 40 mg/kg/24 hours in four divided oral doses. Treatment should be continued for 7 to 10 days or longer as dictated by the clinical course of the patient. Adequate fluids and oxygen as required to treat hypoxemia should be administered. If, during the course of the disease, sudden deterioration with tachypnea and cyanosis is noted, pneumothorax should be suspected and promptly relieved.

Prognosis

Intrauterine pneumonia is not necessarily fatal; however, the more critically ill infants are prone to die in utero or within the first 2 days of life despite meticulous care and administration of appropriate antibiotics. The prognosis is worse for premature than for full-term infants. In the absence of other problems, the prognosis for full-term infants who acquire pneumonia postnatally is good.

Gastroenteritis
Incidence

Gastrointestinal tract infections can occur sporadically or as a result of an epidemic outbreak of disease. The incidence varies even within the same nursery from year to year.

Etiology

The agents that have been associated with both epidemic and sporadic diarrheal disease include enteropathogenic strains of *E. coli* (EPEC), *Salmonella, Shigella, Yersinia, Campylobacter,* and on rare occasions *Pseudomonas, Klebsiella, Enterobacter,* and *C. albicans*. An epidemic of enterocolitis recently was attributed to infection by group A β-hemolytic streptococci. In many cases the etiologic agent is not identified, and viruses are assumed to be responsible despite negative viral and serologic studies. Rotavirus recently has been identified in several newborn infants by means of immune fluorescent microscopy.

E. coli may be subdivided into a number of serogroups depending on their antigenic composition. The somatic O antigen is associated with the cell body, whereas the H antigen is associated with the flagellae. Serogroup A strains, particularly serotypes O55:B5 and O111:B4, have been associated with epidemic disease more frequently than serotypes of group B. EPEC organisms have been recovered from infants with severe diarrheal disease but also may be found in the stools of certain infants who are asymptomatic or who have mild disease. More recently, diarrhea has been reported in association with colonization by *E. coli* that are not considered enteropathogenic. The frequency with which these enterotoxigenic strains produce neonatal gastroenteritis is unknown. Strains of *E. coli* considered to be enterotoxigenic may elaborate a heat-labile or heat-stable toxin that activates adenyl cyclase and produces a secretory diarrhea. Some strains of *E. coli* produce diarrhea by invasion of the gut wall; these strains may be toxin producers as well. Recently, strains of *E. coli* that adhere to but that neither invade nor produce toxin have been associated with diarrhea.

Pathology

When diarrhea is associated with EPEC, there may be no lesion in the GI tract; in some patients small ulcerations of the bowel with a scant inflammatory reaction have been noted. *Salmonella* gastroenteritis may be accompanied by superficial mucosal ulceration and occasionally be deeper ulcers, which may be associated with gross bleeding and perforation. Mesenteric lymphadenitis also may be found. *Shigella* gastroenteritis tends to be a superficial mucosal disease with shallow ulcers occasionally associated with fibrinous superficial exudates that coalesce to form pseudomembranes. *Salmonella* gastroenteritis is associated with bacteremia and the development of distant foci of infection more frequently than is infection by *Shigella* or EPEC. *Campylobacter* diarrhea also is accompanied frequently by bacteremia; the course may be rapidly fatal. Meningitis is a frequent complication of this type of infection in the premature infant.

Pathogenesis

The GI tract is colonized initially by organisms that enter the oropharynx at delivery. Maternal carriers of *Salmonella, Shigella, Campylobacter,* and EPEC serve as the initial source of these pathogens in the nursery. Subsequently, infection may spread from patient to patient as a result of inadequate hand-washing by personnel. Asymptomatic personnel who are carriers of these organisms have proved to be the source of several major epidemics. Fomite transmission has been observed, and in rare instances infection has followed ingestion of contaminated milk, water, or materials used for roentgenographic evaluation of the GI tract.

Clinical manifestations

GI tract colonization by microorganisms associated with gastroenteritis may be followed by no symptoms or by severe diarrhea with fever, vomiting, and abdominal distension. Bloody diarrhea containing mucus should suggest *Shigella, Yersinia,* or *Campylobacter* gastroenteritis, but melena and hematochezia have been observed in neonates with gastroenteritis due to *Salmonella* or EPEC. A blue discoloration of the stools or diaper may be found in some patients where *Pseudomonas* species predominate in the stool. Dehydration, acidosis, electrolyte disturbances, and hypotension may occur during the course of disease.

Diagnosis

Stool cultures should be obtained from all infants with gastroenteritis. Recovery of EPEC, *Shigella, Yersinia, Campylobacter,* or *Salmonella* organisms from the stool of an infant with diarrhea is presumptive evidence that disease is due to one of these pathogens. EPEC organisms are indentified on the basis of serologic studies in which specific antisera are employed to agglutinate *E. coli* in the laboratory. Ten to 20 colonies of *E. coli* should be typed before a negative report for EPEC leaves the laboratory. Fluorescent antibody studies also have been employed in screening stool samples for EPEC. Serotyping *E. coli* can be helpful in tracing the course of epidemic disease due to this organism but may be of no value in discerning the etiology of diarrhea in an individual patient. Techniques to ascertain elaboration of *E. coli* toxins are available; they are expensive, time consuming, and generally not used in community hospitals. A stool smear for polymorphonuclear leukocytes also may be of value. Diarrhea due to EPEC, *Yersinia, Campylobacter, Salmonella,* or *Shigella* may be associated with fecal leukocytes; fecal leukocytes generally are not found in patients with nonspecific or viral gastroenteritis. Blood cultures may be helpful in establishing a diagnosis of salmonellosis or *Yersinia* or *Campylobacter* infection and may be positive in rare cases of EPEC and shigellosis.

Treatment

Diarrhea due to EPEC should be treated by oral administration of neomycin in a dosage of 50 to 100 mg/kg/day divided into four doses for 5 days. Polymyxin B or colistimethate sulfate may be given orally if the organisms are resistant to neomycin. *Salmonella* infections that are mild and are not associated with positive blood culture require no antibiotic treatment. If septicemia occurs, ampicillin (as for sepsis) may be provided. Chloramphenicol can be used if *Salmonella* strains prove to be resistant to ampicillin. *Shigella* infections should be treated with ampicillin orally or with a nonabsorbable oral antibiotic. Kanamycin, colistin, or neomycin may be employed as determined by the sensitivity of the *Shigella* isolate. In many centers *Shigella* species have become resistant to ampicillin; chloramphenicol or kanamycin may be required if systemic therapy is necessary. Amoxicillin should not be substituted for ampicillin even if the *Shigella* isolate proves to be sensitive to ampicillin. *Campylobacter* and *Yersinia* infections can be treated with kanamycin; chloramphenicol can be provided if meningitis follows localized disease. Fluids should be administered intravenously as necessary for treatment of dehydration or maintenance of adequate hydration.

Prevention and prognosis

Infants born to mothers with diarrhea should be isolated until the results of maternal and infant stool cultures are available. Personnel with diarrhea should be excluded from the nursery. Overcrowding must be avoided and proper hand-washing techniques employed. If formulas are prepared in the hospital, use of appropriate procedures to ensure sterility is essential. If epidemic disease due to EPEC occurs, the nursery should be closed to new admissions and all infants treated with neomycin. The nursery may be reopened 48 hours after neomycin has been initiated and no new cases have appeared. Mortality has varied from 0% to 37% during the course of epidemics due to EPEC.

Necrotizing enterocolitis (NEC)

Although not primarily a diarrheal disease, enterocolitis associated with necrosis and ulceration of the GI tract has been noted in some children with diarrhea due to *E. coli, Klebsiella, Enterobacter, Shigella, Clostridia,* and *Salmonella* organisms. Pathologic similarity of pneumatosis intestinalis to gas gangrene of the bowel has suggested the possibility that toxin production plays a significant role in the pathogenesis of necrotizing enterocolitis. Epithelial surfaces of the mucosa are sloughed, and submucosal hemorrhaging may be present. Vomiting, abdominal distension, GI bleeding, peritonitis, and shock may be found. Intramural air or free air within the peritoneal cavity may be noted on abdominal roentgenograms. Blood cultures frequently are positive in affected infants; however, it is likely that septicemia is a secondary event. An infectious etiology for NEC has been postulated because the disease occurs in clusters. Several studies have documented a predilection for colonization of the GI tract with *Klebsiella* and *Enterobacter* species. These results prompted the use of oral aminoglycosides in attempts to treat or prevent NEC. The prophylactic administration of aminoglycosides has been proposed for all infants at high risk for NEC by a number of investigators. Others, however, have been concerned about the possibility that widespread use of these antibiotics would lead to the emergence of organisms resistant to these drugs. Recent reports have suggested that toxin *C. difficile* may play a role in some of these cases. A more detailed discussion of necrotizing enterocolitis is found in Chapter 24.

Otitis media

Incidence

Retrospective postmortem studies have demonstrated a high (about 70%) incidence of otitis media in premature infants; this suggests that otitis media may play a major role in neonatal mortality, particularly in premature infants. Prospective clinical studies indicate that otitis media develops in a minimum of 0.6% of all live births during the first month of life and that the rate may reach 2% to 3% in premature infants.

Etiology

The organisms producing otitis media in the newborn infant are similar to organisms that cause otitis media in older children. Recent studies of infants under 6 weeks of age have shown that *S. pneumoniae* was the causative organism in 19% to 30% of cases. *Haemophilus influenzae* was recovered in 14% to 25% of cases and β-hemolytic streptococci (groups A and B) were recovered in 5% of cases. Gram-negative organisms (*E. coli, Enterobacter, Klebsiella,* and *Pseudomonas*) were found in 7% to 18% of neonates with otitis media. In all studies, between 40% and 50% of cultures obtained by needle tympanocentesis have been sterile or deemed to be nonpathogenic. However, included among the "nonpathogenic" have been organisms such as *S. aureus, S. epidermidis,* and *Neisseria catarrhalis;* these organisms have been shown to be pathogenic in a selected group of older children. It is likely, therefore, that they may be responsible for purulent otitis media in some newborn infants. Moreover, strict anaerobic culture techniques were not employed in most studies; thus a number of "sterile isolates" may have contained anaerobic microorganisms. Viral infection also has been associated with neonatal middle ear disease.

Pathogenesis and pathology

Otitis media is more common in premature than in full-term infants. This increased risk of infection may be related to the small size of the eustachian tube, with resultant obstruction and secondary infection. Aspiration of infected amniotic fluid is probably the leading cause of otitis media in newborns. The disease increases in frequency in bottle-fed babies, a finding that may be related to the supine position of such infants during feeding or to the possibility that local immunity may be conferred from the IgA in breast milk.

Clinical manifestations

Rhinorrhea is the most common manifestation of otitis media in the newborn period. Irritability, lethargy, vomiting, poor feeding, cough, diarrhea, or fever also may be present. Erythema, dullness, and bulging of the pars flaccida of the tympanic membranes may be noted, and pneumatic otoscopy may reveal a decreased mobility of the tympanic membrane.

Diagnosis

The nonspecificity of clinical signs and symptoms coupled with difficulties in visualizing the tympanic membrane early in life probably accounts, in part, for the discrepancy between incidence figures derived from prospective clinical studies and figures from retrospective postmortem studies. Specific diagnosis should be made by culture and smear of purulent middle ear fluid obtained after perforation or by myringotomy or needle tympanocentesis. Cultures of the nasopharynx may yield the same organism in some cases but cannot be relied on in any individual patient to provide the type of information that may be used to select a specific antibiotic. Blood cultures may be helpful in patients with concomitant septicemia. Lumbar puncture should be performed to exclude meningitis. Meningitis that was not suspected before examination of CSF has been noted in a number of newborns with otitis media, but the specific frequency with which these two problems occur concurrently is unknown.

Treatment

A combination of ampicillin and kanamycin or gentamicin will provide effective treatment for most newborns with otitis media. When culture results are known, antibiotic therapy can be altered appropriately. Treatment should be continued for 14 to 21 days, utilizing the dosages employed for septicemia (Table 27-2).

Prognosis

Recurrent or persistent disease is not uncommon. Careful follow-up evaluation for infection and hearing loss is important. The insertion of plastic tubes may be indicated to ensure adequate drainage of the middle ear.

Omphalitis
Incidence

Omphalitis occurs in many neonates who develop purulent or serosanguineous drainage about the umbilical stump. Umbilical phlebitis and even arteritis may develop spontaneously or follow catheterization of umbilical vessels. Tetanus may follow contamination of the umbilical stump but is rarely encountered in societies that practice routine immunization for tetanus and asepsis at the time of delivery.

Etiology

Any organisms that are found on the skin or that may be introduced into the umbilical vessel by catheterization can produce omphalitis.

Pathogenesis

Direct bacterial invasion of the umbilical cord and surrounding skin is common. Bacteria may invade the umbilical artery and spread along its lumen, necrosing the loose connective tissue of the arterial wall. If both the umbilical and iliac ends are occluded, a septic loculated focus of infection may be found. When the umbilical end remains patent, purulent material may drain through the umbilicus. If the connective tissue of the artery is extensively involved, peritonitis may develop, or the infection may extend along its course and present as a scrotal or deep thigh abscess. If the iliac end of the artery is patent but the umbilical end is sealed, septicemia may ensue.

Clinical manifestations

Purulent drainage may be noted from the umbilical stump at its base of attachment to the abdominal wall or from the navel after the cord has separated. The discharge may be foul smelling. Periumbilical erythema and induration may be noted.

Diagnosis

When the umbilical stump discharges purulent material, it should be smeared and cultured. When a loculated periarterial abscess is present, material obtained at the time of drainage also should be cultured. Whenever septic umbilical arteritis is suspected, blood cultures should be obtained.

Treatment

In most patients omphalitis without purulent discharge responds to local application of antibiotic ointments containing neomycin, polymyxin, and bacitracin. Oral or parenteral administration of antibiotics may be indicated if a purulent discharge is noted or periumbilical inflammation is present. In such cases, methicillin and gentamicin are logical choices until a specific organism has been identified.

Ophthalmitis

See p. 983.

Incidence

Conjunctivitis most commonly is due to chemical irritation that follows the prophylactic institution of silver nitrate into the conjunctival sac. Chemical conjunctivitis may be found in almost 100% of infants so treated. Chemical conjunctivitis due to erythromycin or penicillin occurs much less frequently but does occur in some newborns. The incidence of other forms of conjunctivitis is difficult to assess. However, the incidence of gonococcal ophthalmitis has increased in recent years despite presumably effective and mandatory regimens of prophylactic eye care.

Etiology

Neisseria gonorrhoeae and *Chlamydia trachomatis* are the most important causes of conjunctivitis in the newborn period. Other bacteria, including *S. aureus*, group B hemolytic streptococci, *Pseudomonas*, *Streptococcus pneumoniae*, and Koch-Weeks bacillus, also are common causes of this disease.

Pathogenesis

Conjunctivitis due to *N. gonorrhoeae*, *C. trachomatis*, or *S. agalactiae* generally is initiated by infection with microorganisms acquired during passage through the birth canal. Infection with *S. aureus*, *Pseudomonas*, or other organisms more commonly reflects infection acquired during the neonatal period.

Clinical manifestations

Chemical conjunctivitis usually is noted soon after birth and becomes less prominent after 2 days of age. Bacterial conjunctivitis is most prominent during the first week of life but may occur at any time during the neonatal period. Inclusion conjunctivitis has been noted as early as 24 hours but generally develops during the second week of life. The signs of bacterial conjunctivitis in the newborn are similar to those observed in older individuals. A purulent ocular discharge, erythema and edema of the lids, and injection or suffusion of the conjunctiva or sclera may be found. If the infection is untreated, corneal involvement may occur and will be characterized by punctate corneal epithelial erosions. In the case of disease with *N. gonorrhoeae*, large punctate superficial lesions may be seen, which coalesce and progress to corneal perforation. When staphylococcal conjunctivitis is complicated by corneal involvement, the lower portion of the cornea is infected more frequently than the upper half, and marginal corneal infiltrates with peripheral vascularization may be seen. When a chlamydial agent is involved, inflammatory changes may be barely detectable, or there may be intense inflammation, swelling, and a yellow discharge in association with pseudomembrane formation. The cornea is affected rarely. Necrosis of the cornea has been observed followed by fibrosis and scarring of the lid margin. Chlamydial infections generally are bilateral, whereas unilateral disease is common when staphylococcal disease is present. When chlamydial conjunctivitis is not treated, inflammation persists for 1 or 2 weeks. A subacute phase follows with slight injection of the conjunctiva and an accumulation of purulent material along the lid margins. Occasionally, chronic disease develops.

Diagnosis

The clinical appearance of the patient, coupled with Gram stain and culture of the purulent discharge, establishes a diagnosis. Gram-negative diplococci within leukocytes suggest a diagnosis of gonococcal disease. When gonococcal disease is suspected, purulent material should be plated at the bedside on Thayer-Martin media or placed in special transport media and immediately sent to the bacteriology laboratory. Other organisms are less fastidious, and a swab of purulent material, cultured promptly, is sufficient to establish a diagnosis.

Chlamydial infections can be documented by performing Giemsa stains on material obtained by gently but firmly scraping the lower portion of the palpebral conjunctiva with a blunt spatula or wire loop. Cotton and Calgonite swabs have not proved adequate.

Care must be taken not to injure the conjunctiva during culture. The smears obtained in this manner may reveal a predominance of neutrophils with smaller numbers of lymphocytes and monocytes. Leber cells (macrophages containing cellular debris) and inclusion-bearing epithelial cells are characteristic. The inclusions are composed of elementary bodies that appear adjacent to the nucleus. Larger inclusions may appear in the form of a cap indented by the nucleus. In many patients inclusion-bearing cells are difficult to find. For this reason it has been suggested that purulent conjunctivitis that develops after day 5, from which no pathogenic bacteria are recovered, and that fails to respond to topical application of neomycin/polymyxin ophthalmic ointment, be treated as chlamydial conjunctivitis whether or not inclusions have been demonstrated.

Treatment

Gonococcal ophthalmitis should be treated parenterally with aqueous penicillin G in a dosage of 50,000 units/kg daily in two divided doses for 7 days. The conjunctival sac should be irrigated with sterile isotonic saline. Antibiotics containing various combinations of bacitracin, neomycin, and polymyxin, administered topically as an ophthalmic ointment or solution several times a day for a period of 7 to 10 days, have been recommended for other forms of bacterial conjunctivitis. Inclusion conjunctivitis should be treated with 10% sulfacetamide ophthalmic suspension or ointment or 1% tetracycline ointment applied six to eight times per day. Erythromycin ophthalmic ointment also may be used. Reduction in erythema and discharge usually follows within 24 hours. The proper duration of treatment is not known, but 14 days is sufficient in most cases. Recurrences and reinfection have been noted, and if this occurs, treatment must be repeated. Since chlamydial pneumonia may accompany or follow chlamydial conjunctivitis, use of erythromycin (40 mg/kg/day in four divided oral doses) should be considered in addition to the topical therapy.

Prevention and prognosis

In most patients prompt recognition and treatment eradicate conjunctival disease. If bacterial conjunctivitis is not treated, corneal involvement with eventual opacification, keratectasia or staphyloma formation, and perforation may ensue. A 1% solution of silver nitrate properly instilled into the conjunctival sac at birth generally will prevent gonococcal ophthalmitis. Topical application of erythromycin or tetracycline ointments also provides effective prophylaxis.

Osteomyelitis and septic arthritis

Incidence

Osteomyelitis is a relatively rare but potentially lethal neonatal infection. A referral center may be called on to evaluate and treat two or three newborns per year. Septic arthritis is frequently concomitant, probably reflecting spread of infection via blood vessels that penetrate the epiphyseal plate.

Etiology

S. aureus is the leading cause of osteomyelitis and septic arthritis in the newborn; however, the group B streptococcus has been the predominant organism in some institutions. Other infrequent but important causative agents include *E. coli*, *H. influenzae*, *P. mirabilis*, group A β-hemolytic streptococci, *Pseudomonas*, *N. gonorrhoeae*, *Serratia*, and *Salmonella*.

Pathology

Osteomyelitis usually affects the metaphyseal regions of long bones. However, involvement of the small bones of the hands and feet, the vertebrae, and the ribs has been noted. Multiple foci of osteomyelitis may be seen more frequently in the newborn period than in older individuals; between 10% and 40% of newborns have more than a single locus of infection. The cortical bone is thin, permitting infection to extend readily into soft tissues. Involucrum formation is common, but sequestration is rare if the process is recognized and treated promptly. Infection may extend through the metaphyseal plexus of veins into the joint. The position of the metaphyses of the hip and elbow with relation to the joint capsule permits direct spread into the joint. Destruction of cartilage, dislocations, and pathologic fractures may occur and permanently affect bone growth.

Pathogenesis

Osteomyelitis almost invariably follows hematogenous dissemination of microorganisms. Infection of the skin, omphalitis, umbilical catheterization, and occasionally improperly performed femoral venipunctures are predisposing factors in some cases. Complications of pregnancy have been reported in up to 41% and complications of delivery in 48% of newborns with osteomyelitis. In the majority of cases, some antecedent illness can be identified. Occasionally, osteomyelitis may follow direct extension of a soft tissue infection to bone; this has been noted in neonates with osteomyelitis of the maxilla.

Clinical manifestations

Destructive changes in bone due to osteomyelitis may be quite advanced by the time a definitive diagnosis is made, because of the failure to recognize the subtlety of the initial signs and symptoms. In many patients the disease is not accompanied by systemic signs or symptoms. Fever is absent or is a very late and intermittent finding. Most frequently, swelling, tenderness, and decreased motion of an extremity are the findings that prompt initial appraisal by a physician. In one patient with osteomyelitis of the clavicle, an incomplete Moro reflex was the only finding on physical examination. Localized tenderness, local erythema, and regional lymphadenopathy also may be noted. Heat and fluctuance are rare early in the disease. In some patients, an acute onset of illness with fever, icterus, hemorrhagic manifestations, and hypotension occurs.

Diagnosis

When the history and physical examination suggest the possibility of osteomyelitis, roentgenograms should be obtained. Roentgenographic changes develop 7 to 10 days after the onset of infection; those obtained early may reveal only soft tissue swelling. Later, periosteal thickening, cortical destruction, irregularities of the epiphysis, and periosteal new bone formation may be found. Additional findings may include localized areas of rarefaction, periosteal elevation, a widened joint space, and subluxation or dislocation of the bone from the joint. Since multiple sites of osteomyelitis are not infrequently found, roentgenographic skeletal surveys are warranted in newborns after a single site of osteomyelitis has been confirmed, although other sites are not suggested by the clinical findings. This type of survey should be delayed for 7 to 10 days after initiation of treatment to maximize the likelihood of defining all possible sites of infection. Fig. 27-1 depicts the roentgenographic findings in a newborn with multiple sites of disease due to *S. aureus*.

Aspiration of soft tissues and of bone is indicated; Gram-stained smears and cultures of this material should be obtained. Blood cultures are essential and in my experience yield the causative agent in 60% of cases. Joint fluid obtained from patients with joint involvement should be smeared and cultured as well. Syphilis, tuberculosis, scurvy, and deep cellulitis are disorders that must be considered in the differential diagnosis.

Treatment

Until the specific etiology has been clarified by culture, treatment should be initiated with methicillin and gentamicin parenterally. When the specific organism and its sensitivity have been identified, treatment should

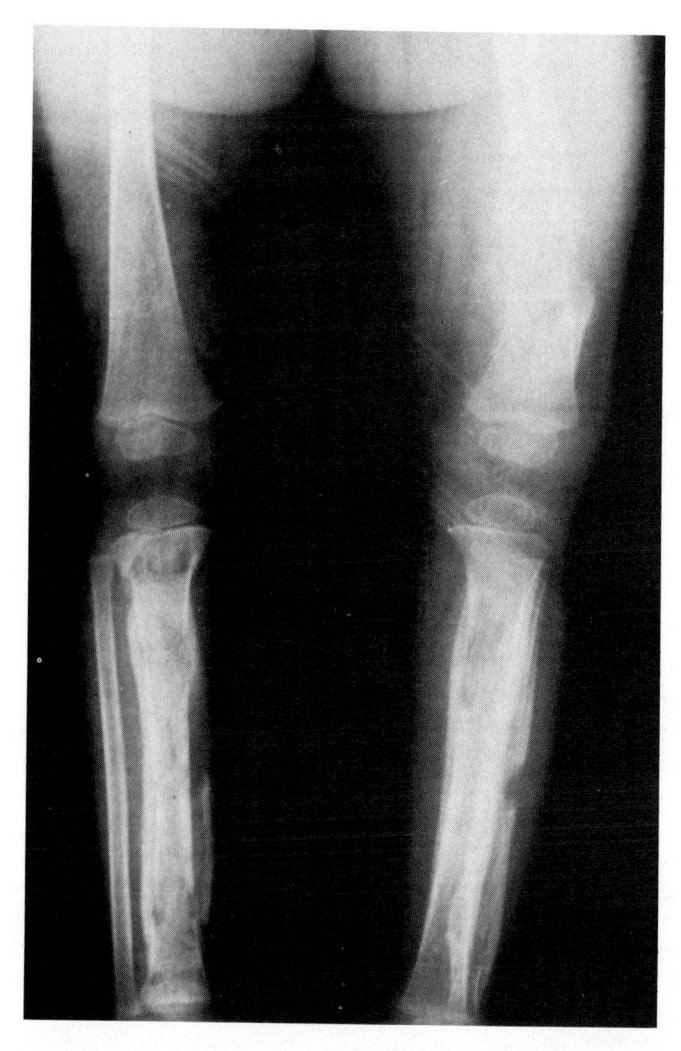

Fig. 27-1. Multiple sites of osteomyelitis in an infant due to *S. aureus* infection are demonstrated. Clinical evidence of infection became apparent at 2 weeks of age. Osteolytic lesions can be seen in the right femur, right tibia and fibula, and left tibia. Periosteal new bone formation is visible in many areas.

be continued utilizing an appropriate antibiotic (Table 27-3). The dosages employed should be those used for treatment of septicemia or meningitis (Table 27-2). Parenteral therapy should be continued for 3 to 6 weeks followed by oral therapy until healing is ensured. Intraarticular administration of antibiotics is not indicated; there is no evidence that such administration is necessary or hastens recovery. Surgical decompression may be required if pus is aspirated from the site of involvement. Generally, drilling of bone or windowing to drain medullary collections of pus is not necessary. When the hip joint is involved, prompt surgical decompression and drainage are required.

Prognosis

The degree of residual damage depends on the extent of disease before effective treatment. Permanent disability is more common when joint involvement has occurred. Growth disturbances may result from destruction of the epiphyseal plate. The number of foci of osteomyelitis in a patient who is treated effectively does not appear to correlate specifically with the extent or likelihood of permanent disability. Chronic osteomyelitis is relatively infrequent. Overall, residual effects may be anticipated in 25% of neonates with infection of the bones or joints.

Urinary tract infections

Infection of the urinary tract is discussed in detail in Chapter 31. Most infections of the urinary tract in the newborn occur in association with neonatal septicemia or serve as a focus of infection for the development of septicemia and meningitis. The organisms causing this disease are virtually identical to those which cause neonatal septicemia. Infection with *E. coli* is most common, and epidemics of septicemia and urinary tract infections have been traced to this organism. Infection with other gram-negative organisms, as well as with *S. aureus* and *S. epidermidis*, is not infrequent. Infection is more common in males than females and in association with obstructive abnormalities of the genitourinary system. Symptoms referable to the genitourinary system are rare, and in most patients the symptomatology is nonspecific, similar to that found in neonates with septicemia. In some patients, only poor feeding, weight loss, or diarrhea may be noted. Initial treatment should include ampicillin and an aminoglycoside, parenterally.

Infections of the skin and mucous membranes
Incidence

Infection of the skin and mucous membranes is common and may result from infection with bacteria, viruses, or fungi.

Etiology

Colonization of the skin begins at birth, and the organisms that are acquired reflect those in the environment. During the period of time that hexachlorophene bathing of newborns was a common practice, colonization with gram-negative flora was prevalent. Cessation of hexachlorophene bathing has been accompanied by increases in both the rate of colonization and infection due to *S. aureus*. Cutaneous or mucocutaneous lesions also may result from infection due to group A β-hemolytic streptococci, *P. aeruginosa*, *T. pallidum*, herpesvirus hominis, vaccinia virus, variola virus, rubeola virus, and *C. albicans*.

Pathology

Abscesses, pustules, or bullous lesions are caused by *S. aureus* and occasionally by streptococci. Histologic examination of the skin of patients with bullous impetigo may show intraepidermal bullae filled with polymorphonuclear leukocytes. Ritter's disease, a disorder associated with toxin-elaborating staphylococci, is characterized by a severe bullous eruption and by shedding of the epidermis. Histologic examination of the skin reveals an intraepidermal blister, cellular death and acantholysis, and a striking absence of inflammation. *Pseudomonas* or *Aeromonas hydrophila* infections cause ecthyma gangrenosum, which is characterized by the development of yellow-green pustules that progress rapidly to form hemorrhagic and necrotic ulcers.

Pathogenesis

Infection generally develops as the result of infection through a small break in the skin and is caused by organisms with which the patient has been colonized. Scalp abscesses may follow intrauterine monitoring of the delivery with scalp electrodes. Nursery personnel or other infants can serve as a source of infection of the neonate with *T. pallidum* or by various viruses. *C. albicans* infection generally follows colonization of the buccal mucosa or GI tract by *Candida* or contamination of the diaper area by *Candida* within stools.

Clinical manifestations

Skin and soft tissue infections should be discovered promptly, since clinical findings generally are apparent to even the casual observer. Bullous lesions that appear after the second day of life generally suggest staphylococcal disease, in contrast to noninfectious blistering diseases that may be manifest at birth (p. 947). The blisters range in size from small vesicles to larger bullae filled with straw-colored material. When these lesions rupture, an erythematous denuded area is found. In Ritter's disease the epidermis may be shed in sheets, and intact bullae are frequently sterile. A diagnosis of *Pseudomonas* or *Aeromonas* infection should be suspected in patients with ecthyma gangrenosum. Congenital syphilis may be suggested by the presence of maculopapular lesions, and in some cases bullae have been noted at birth, particularly on the palms and soles. The blisters develop on an erythematous base and may contain cloudy or hemorrhagic fluid that contains spirochetes. When the blisters rupture, a macerated area remains on which crusts form. *Candida* infection may be localized to the oral cavity or the diaper area. Paronychia may be seen in infants who suck their thumbs. The early cutaneous lesions are vesicular with a surrounding area of erythema. Pustules may develop, and a confluent erythematous moist erosion is soon noted. Oral moniliasis or thrush is characterized by the appearance of white cheesy material that clings to the oral, buccal, and even pharyngeal mucosa. Variola, vaccinia, herpes simplex, and herpes zoster viruses produce vesicular lesions that initially may be similar in appearance to each other, both clinically and histologically.

Diagnosis

A specific diagnosis should be based on smear and culture of the lesion. In patients with Ritter's disease, however, microorganisms may not be present within the intact bullous lesions. Blood cultures should be obtained and may be positive in neonates with cutaneous staphylococcal or streptococcal disease. *Candida* can be demonstrated by use of a potassium hydroxide preparation that shows pseudomycelia and may be cultured on Sabouraud's medium. Dark-field examination of bullous lesions may reveal *T. pallidum* in patients with congenital syphilis; when this diagnosis is suspected, appropriate serologic studies (p. 674) should be performed. Fluid obtained by aspiration of vesicles may permit identification of disease caused by various viral agents.

Treatment

Bacterial infections of the skin should be treated by systemic administration of antibiotics. Methicillin is appropriate for susceptible strains of staphylococci, penicillin G for streptococci or *T. pallidum,* and gentamicin for ecthyma gangrenosum. Intravenous fluid therapy may be required to maintain hydration in patients with Ritter's disease; specific attention also should be paid to maintenance of adequate hemoglobin and serum albumin concentrations and to maintenance of body temperature. Incision and drainage will be required if abscesses are found. Oral *Candida* infections (thrush) respond well to administration of nystatin (Table 27-2), and *Candida* dermatitis can be treated with saline soaks or with 1:5,000 benzalkonium chloride washes and with nystatin cream.

Mastitis

Neonatal mastitis or breast abscess is attributed generally to infection with gram-positive organisms, usually staphylococci. Other organisms, however, may be responsible for mastitis, and cases due to *E. coli, Pseudomonas, Proteus, Salmonella,* and group B streptococci have been described. The incidence is low; in one large center only 22 cases of neonatal mastitis were seen in a 9-year period.

Mastitis rarely develops during the first week of life but is seen more frequently during the second and third weeks after birth. Infection probably results from invasion of the duct system of the breast by skin flora. The breast may be erythematous, enlarged, and tender but is more likely to be firm than fluctuant. The disorder must be distinguished from enlargement that is physiologic and hormonally induced; the latter more likely will produce swelling bilaterally. Aspiration of the infected area for smear and culture and blood cultures are indicated. Methicillin should be used to treat staphylococcal disease and kanamycin or gentamicin for infection due to gram-negative microorganisms.

Parotitis

Suppurative parotitis is a rare disease in the newborn period; approximately 100 cases have been reported since 1878. Infection is caused by the ascent of microorganisms through Stensen's duct or may occur hematogenously. Typically, pregnancy and delivery are normal. Seven to 14 days after birth, parotid gland swelling and fever may be noted. Facial paralysis may be present. The swollen parotid gland is accompanied by an area of erythema in the overlying skin; the gland may be tender, warm, firm, or fluctuant. Purulent material may drain spontaneously from Stensen's duct or may be expressed. Septicemia may accompany localized infection, and dehydration occurs preceding the onset of disease in some patients. Staphylococci are implicated most frequently, but *Pseudomonas* and *E. coli* may be offending agents.

Diagnosis should be made by smear and culture of purulent material obtained from Stensen's duct. Blood cultures should be obtained. Incision and drainage should be performed if the lesions are fluctuant. Systemic antibiotic treatment should be provided, and initial therapy should include coverage for *S. aureus* and *Pseudomonas*. The disease must be differentiated from infections of the maxilla and from lymphangiomas, hemangiomas, lipomas, and adenomas.

Adrenal abscess

Adrenal abscesses have been reported on several occasions, usually following localization of microorganisms during an episode of septicemia. *E. coli, Bacteroides,* and group B streptococci have been isolated. This rare lesion must be distinguished from adrenal hemorrhage, suprarenal hematoma, neuroblastoma, and nephroblastoma. Abdominal ultrasonography may be helpful in suggesting the diagnosis.

Meningoencephalitis

Infection of the brain and meninges due to viruses and fungi or protozoal parasites also may be noted during the neonatal period. Transplacental infection with cytomegalovirus, rubella virus, and *Toxoplasma gondii* and perinatal infection with herpes simplex viruses are discussed in Chapter 28. Poliovirus, Coxsackie virus, ECHO virus, varicella-zoster virus, and Epstein-Barr virus (EBV) may be acquired before, at, or following the time of delivery. Disorders caused by these agents, as well as tuberculosis and syphilis, are discussed in greater detail later.

Aseptic CNS infections vary in severity; some infants may have devastating disease and die of their infections, whereas in others no symptoms are apparent. In symptomatic infants, signs and symptoms identical to those found in newborns with septicemia or bacterial meningitis occur. Examination of CSF may reveal a pleocytosis that (after the first several days) will be predominantly lymphocytic. The CSF protein concentration may be elevated, but the glucose concentration generally is not depressed when compared with the blood glucose concentration. Etiologic diagnosis depends on isolation of virus from the throat, urine, stool, or CSF and demonstration of a significant rise in antibody titer to the virus that has been isolated. There is no antiviral compound for effective specific treatment of viral meningitis.

INFECTION BY SPECIFIC MICROORGANISMS
Anaerobic infection
Incidence

Chow and associates noted an incidence of anaerobic bacteremia of 1.8 cases per 1,000 live births; anaerobic microorganisms accounted for 26% of all cases of neonatal bacteremia. The relative frequency with which anaerobes were recovered from these newborns reflects, in part, their recovery from cord blood cultures; clinically significant anaerobic bacteremia in the neonatal period may be less frequent.

Pathogenesis

Prolonged rupture of the membranes, maternal amnionitis, prematurity, fetal distress, foul odor at birth, and respiratory distress are commonly associated with anaerobic infection. That these conditions might predispose to anaerobic septicemia is consistent with observations that *Bacteroides* and anaerobic streptococci are prevalent inhabitants of the genital tract at or near term and that a variety of anaerobic microorganisms are recovered toward the end of the first week of life from the oropharynx of the normal neonate. Anaerobic septicemia and meningitis also may follow or accompany anaerobic peritonitis in newborns with GI tract obstruction of necrotizing enterocolitis. Anaerobic microorganisms frequently may be recovered from gastric aspirates of newborns of mothers who have had ruptured membranes for more than 24 hours, but their recovery is associated infrequently with clinical disease. Bacteroidaceae, *Clostridium*, *Peptococcus*, *Peptostreptococcus*, and *Veillonella* are isolated most frequently from peritoneal fluid. Isolation of more than one anaerobe or of aerobes and anaerobes from the same specimen is common.

Clinical manifestations

The signs and symptoms of anaerobic septicemia or peritonitis are indistinguishable from those described for other forms of neonatal septicemia or in patients with peritonitis. Necrotizing enterocolitis is a common finding in neonates with anaerobic peritonitis.

Diagnosis

Anaerobic infection may be overlooked unless cultures employing special media and appropriate fermentative and gas-liquid chromatographic procedures are used. The cost of such techniques is high and warranted only in selected tertiary care centers. Where such techniques are available, blood cultures should be inoculated at the bedside into evacuated tubes containing media appropriate for isolation of anaerobic microorganisms.

Treatment

The choice of antibiotic treatment for anaerobic infection ideally should be based on accurate sensitivity data. Sensitivity determinations are difficult to perform with anaerobic organisms and are frequently unreliable indicators of therapeutic response in vivo. In general, penicillin is effective against virtually all gram-positive anaerobic microorganisms and against most gram-negative organisms. A prominent exception is *B. fragilis*, which is resistant to penicillin in most cases. Since this organism is commonly isolated from peritoneal fluid in newborns with intestinal perforation or necrotizing enterocolitis, consideration must be given to adding chloramphenicol or clindamycin to the therapeutic regimen. Clindamycin should not be used in patients with meningitis. The dosages employed should be those given for septicemia. (Table 27-2).

Prognosis

Mortality secondary to neonatal anaerobic septicemia varies from 4% to 37%.

Listeria monocytogenes

Incidence

Although infection with *L. monocytogenes* may produce disease in normal healthy individuals, infection is more prevalent in the neonatal period or in adults with underlying disease.

Etiology

Listeriosis is caused by *L. monocytogenes*, a nonspore-forming, short gram-positive rod. It can be confused with diphtheroids on the basis of colonial morphology, and for this reason it is likely that the frequency with which it is isolated is underestimated. These bacteria may appear to be gram-negative because they decolorize readily during the Gram-staining procedure.

Pathogenesis

Listeriosis may develop at birth or may begin late in the neonatal period. Disease with early onset is acquired transplacentally from a mother with subclinical or clinical infection. Infection acquired early in pregnancy may lead to abortion and, if acquired later, to stillbirth or premature delivery. *L. monocytogenes* may be recovered from the vaginal canal or cervix of pregnant women; thus infection may be acquired at the time of delivery by aspiration or ingestion. *Listeria* organisms are isolated with great frequency from mothers of infants who develop *Listeria* infection during the first 5 days of life (early onset disease). Early onset disease is likely to be associated with maternal fever or other signs of maternal infection and with premature delivery. The development of late onset neonatal disease generally is not associated with maternal illness or maternal carriage of the organism. The distribution of *Listeria* serotypes from neonates with early and late onset disease also differs. Early onset disease is predominantly associated with recovery of serotypes Ia and Ib and occasionally with IVb from the blood of infected infants. Late onset disease is associated primarily with recovery of serotype IVb from the blood and CSF; it is predominantly a meningitic rather than septicemic infection.

Clinical manifestation

The initial symptoms of listeriosis in both early and late onset disease are quite variable. Anorexia, lethargy and vomiting, jaundice, respiratory distress, cyanosis, petechial rashes, and evidence of myocarditis all have been noted. A high proportion of newborn infants with early onset listeriosis are meconium stained at birth, even if they are preterm. Signs referable to the CNS are more commonly associated with late onset disease. In some instances initial symptoms are absent, and in a few patients cultures of the meconium have grown *Listeria* without the development of overt infection. Hepatosplenomegaly and granulomas of the skin or posterior pharynx have been noted in some affected infants.

Diagnosis

Blood, CSF, and urine cultures should be obtained in all patients. Cultures of the vagina or cervix may support the diagnosis if *Listeria* organisms are recovered from the mothers of infants with early onset disease. A higher index of suspicion of infection due to *L. monocytogenes* should exist if the maternal history includes prior stillbirth or repeated spontaneous abortions. CSF findings in cases of *Listeria* meningitis are identical to those observed in patients with other bacterial meningitides, with a predominance of polymorphonuclear leukocytes, an elevated protein concentration, and a depressed CSF glucose concentration. The organism may be seen on smear. Organisms also may be recovered from amniotic fluid or meconium.

Treatment

Ampicillin is effective in most cases; however, therapy should be guided by sensitivity studies.

Prognosis

Mortality may be close to 100% in early onset infection but varies between 20% and 50% if disease develops between the fifth and thirtieth days of age.

Group B β-hemolytic streptococci (*Streptococcus agalactiae*)

Incidence

An increasing number of reports of neonatal sepsis and meningitis due to *S. agalactiae* have appeared. Franciosi and associates reported an incidence of 2 cases per 1,000 live births.

Etiology

Group B streptococcal infection is caused by organisms that are gram-positive cocci that grow on solid media and in broth aerobically. Identification as a group B organism can be suggested by CAMP test and confirmed by specific precipitin or immunofluorescent methods.

Pathogenesis

S. agalactiae may be responsible for disease at or shortly after birth (early onset) or may be associated with infection that develops after 7 days of age. Hood and associates reported that of 151 mothers who had group B streptococci in their genital tracts, 56 (37%) experienced abortion, perinatal infant death, premature births, or serious illness in their infants. Other investigations have not confirmed these findings. Although colonization by group B streptococci was noted in 254 per 1,000 women during the third trimester and in 262 per 1,000 newborns, Baker and associates found that the attack rate for neonatal infection was only 2.9 per 1,000 newborns.

Early onset group B streptococcal disease is acquired during passage through the birth canal of colonized women. The subtypes of group B streptococcal organisms isolated from infants with early onset disease are similar to those of the maternal vagina; group BI is the principal offender. In contrast, group BIII was the only subtype isolated by Franciosi and associates from infants with delayed onset disease; this subtype usually is not found in the mother but has been isolated from nursery personnel. Thus early onset disease is acquired intrapartum, whereas delayed onset infection generally is acquired from environmental sources.

The group B streptococcal serotype and its interaction with the host also determine the clinical expression of disease. Klesius and associates reported the presence of nonspecific opsonins for serotypes BIb, BIc, BII, and BIII in 95% of human sera, but only 10% of the population tested had specific BIa opsonizing antibody. These findings suggest a basis for the pathogenic potential of serotype BIa in the early neonatal period; this serotype is a frequent cause of early onset fatal septicemic disease. Type III isolates are the predominant cause of both early and late onset meningitis; this suggests that type III strains possess properties that permit meningeal invasion. The capsule of type III, group B streptococci contains a high content of sialic acid. This moiety apparently is capable of preventing activation of the alternate pathway for complement metabolism. In the absence of type-specific circulating antibody, failure of activation of the alternate pathway for complement metabolism results in inefficient opsonization of the type III, group B streptococcus. Poor opsonization leads to persistence of bacteremia and predisposes to a higher frequency of meningitis.

Clinical manifestations

Two distinct clinical syndromes are seen: an early septicemic form of disease or an illness whose onset is delayed and that is primarily meningitic in type. Early onset disease frequently is associated with obstetric complications. This form of the disease commonly includes acute respiratory distress and is characterized by other signs and symptoms of septicemia. Death occurs within hours to days in most patients and usually is related to pulmonary involvement. In most instances group B streptococci can be seen within and cultured from the lung. Late onset disease generally develops after 7 days of age, and meningitis is frequently noted. In these cases, clinical findings are those of bacterial meningitis. In some patients, usually with late onset disease, otitis media, septic arthritis, osteomyelitis, ethmoiditis, facial cellulitis, necrotizing fasciitis, and conjunctivitis have occurred. Asymptomatic bacteremia with group B streptococci also has been documented.

Diagnosis

Blood and CSF should be cultured and examined. Where appropriate antisera are available, a rapid diagnosis may be made by examination of blood, CSF, or urine by countercurrent immunoelectrophoresis.

Treatment

Penicillin G or ampicillin should be given as described for septicemia or meningitis. Prophylactic treatment of maternal carriers is not indicated. Use of intravenous ampicillin during delivery of women with positive vaginal, cervical, or rectal cultures for group B streptococci at term has been associated with a significant decrease in colonization of their newborn infants with this organism. The efficacy of this approach in preventing neonatal disease, however, has not been documented to date. At least one well-controlled large study suggests that administration of aqueous penicillin G at birth was associated with a decreased incidence of group B streptococcal disease as well as a decrease in disease due to all penicillin-susceptible organisms. Since a concomitant increase in infection with gram-negative organisms may accompany this approach, it cannot be recommended for general implementation at this time.

Prognosis

Mortality from early onset disease varies from 70% to 100%. Mortality from delayed onset meningeal disease varies from 18% to 45%; survivors may experience hydrocephalus or other neurologic sequelae.

Neisseria gonorrhoeae (gonococcal disease)
Incidence

Gonorrhea is the most commonly reported communicable disease in the world; 100 million new cases are identified each year. In the United States it has been estimated that 2 million unreported cases and 1 million reported cases occur yearly. The incidence of gonococcal infection in pregnant women has ranged from 2.5% to 7.3% in recent studies. In this setting it is not surprising that infection of the neonate by *N. gonorrhoeae* occurs frequently.

Etiology

N. gonorrhoeae is an aerobic gram-negative diplococcus that is fastidious but that grows well on selected media.

Pathogenesis

Gonococcal infection may be acquired in utero as a result of orogastric contamination of an infant with *N. gonorrhoeae* following premature rupture of the membranes in an infected mother. The gonococcus also may invade mucosal surfaces, including the conjunctiva, rectal mucosa, and pharynx. Thus when maternal gonococcal infection is present, the neonate may acquire infection during delivery. Gonococcal infections also may be acquired postnatally from an infected adult or carrier.

Clinical manifestations

The most common neonatal form of disease is ophthalmitis (p. 665). Neonatal gonococcal arthritis and septicemia or meningitis also occur. Disseminated infection is more likely to occur when maternal gonococcal disease is symptomatic and associated with premature rupture of the membranes. Gonococcal vaginitis and scalp abscess have been reported in the newborn infant.

Diagnosis

Evaluation and treatment of neonates with possible gonococcal ophthalmitis have been discussed. Diagnosis of other forms of localized or disseminated gonococcal disease is dependent on identification of the organism on smear or cultures of blood, pharynx, or localized lesions. Blood should be cultured at the bedside. Cotton swabs free from fatty acids should be used for collection of other specimens. When cultures are obtained, they should be plated on Thayer-Martin media and incubated in a 2% to 10% carbon dioxide atmosphere.

Treatment

Arthritis and septicemia should be treated by administration of aqueous penicillin G in a dosage of 75,000 to 100,000 units/kg/day in three divided doses for 7 days. Meningitis should be treated with aqueous penicillin G (100,000 units/kg/day in three divided intravenous doses for at least 10 days). Gonococci with increased resistance or complete resistance to penicillin have been recovered; in these cases, treatment must be guided by the specific sensitivity of the organism involved.

Management of a neonate born to a mother with gonococcal infection

All pregnant women should have endocervical cultures examined for gonococci near term as a routine part of prenatal care. Specific measures to prevent gonococcal ophthalmitis are indicated (p. 667). Orogastric and rectal cultures should be obtained from all patients of infected mothers, and blood should also be cultured if septicemia is suspected. Any positive gonococcal culture should be considered as presumptive evidence of disseminated gonococcal infection, and penicillin treatment as described for gonococcal septicemia should be initiated. Asymptomatic culture-negative infants should be treated with single doses of aqueous penicillin (50,000 units for full-term infants and 25,000 units for preterm infants). Mothers of these infants should observe them carefully following discharge from the nursery for signs and symptoms of arthritis or generalized infection.

Syphilis
Incidence

In recent years, congenital and neonatal syphilis has resurfaced as a significant problem. The incidence in the United States is currently higher than in other Western countries.

Etiology

Syphilis is caused by *T. pallidum*, a thin spirochetal organism that varies from 5 to 20 μm in length. It is killed by heat (40°-42° C), by drying, by soap, and by water. It has not been cultured in vitro.

Pathogenesis and pathology

Syphilis in the newborn is a transplacental infection. Spirochetes rarely are found in fetal tissue before 18 weeks of intrauterine life, probably because the well-developed Langhans layer of the chorion presents a barrier to infection. After the sixteenth week of pregnancy, this layer atrophies, and fetal infection may follow. It has been suggested more recently that infections of the fetus may take place much earlier but that pathologic changes in the tissues do not occur until after the fifth month as the fetus becomes increasingly immunocompetent and inflammatory cells are found.

Spirochetemia may cause fetal wastage or death; stillbirths occur in about one fourth of pregnancies in untreated mothers. Normal children are born to only 30% of women who have had an untreated late syphilitic infection and to practically no untreated women who are infected during the first 7 months of pregnancy. The extent of disease in the newborn will depend on the time during gestation that a diagnosis of syphilis was made, the extent of disease in the mother, and the effectiveness of maternal treatment. Treatment of the mother before the eighteenth week of gestation almost always prevents signs of infection in the fetus, whereas treatment after the eighteenth week may cure fetal spirochetemia but will not always prevent the development of late stigmata of congenital syphilis. Since significant infection occurs after the first trimester of pregnancy, organ development is not affected, but all organ systems may be involved. Inflammatory and destructive changes may involve the liver, spleen, lung, bone, bone marrow, kidneys, and adrenal glands. Involvement of the CNS, teeth, and cornea may occur early but may not become apparent until late in infancy. Examination of the placenta in cases of congenital syphilis will reveal focal villitis and endovascular and perivascular proliferation in villous vessels (p. 211). Spirochetes may be visible.

Clinical manisfestations

Infants who are severely affected may be born hydropic, a finding reported in up to 40% of cases in some recent series. Severe consolidated pneumonia may be present at birth. Profound anemia and hepatosplenomegaly, which may be related to extramedullary hematopoiesis, are relatively constant findings in these patients. In other patients there are no clinical findings for 1 to 3 weeks. Poor feeding initially and fever may be noted, and snuffles (syphilitic rhinitis) may appear. The nose becomes obstructed and discharges a clear, serosanguineous material. Purulent drainage may reflect secondary infection with streptococci or staphylococci. Cutaneous lesions have been reported at birth but usually are noted after 7 days of age. They are copper-colored maculopapular lesions that characteristically are distributed on the palms and soles and about the perioral, perinasal, and diaper areas. The rash may become vesicular and confluent in areas and may progress to involve the trunk and extremities. Perianal condylomata may form, and mucocutaneous lesions may develop. The lips may be roughened and cracked, and these lesions may evolve into radiating scars known as rhagades. Moist mucous membrane patches, exfoliation of nails, loss of hair, iritis, and choroiditis may occur. Syphilitic hepatitis with jaundice, generalized lymphadenopathy, pancreatitis, orchitis, colitis, and renal involvement characterized by the development of nephrotic syndrome may be noted. CNS involvement probably occurs early but is asymptomatic in most cases. Pleocytosis and increased CSF protein concentration may be found. Pseudoparalysis of the limbs may be observed but is relatively uncommon in comparison with the frequency with which involvement of bone can be noted roentgenographically.

Roentgenograms of the bones may show osteochondritis at the metaphyses and periostitis in over 90% of infants by 3 months of age. A radiolucent area may appear at the medial aspect of the proximal tibial metaphysis; this is called Wimberger's sign (Fig. 27-2). Sub-

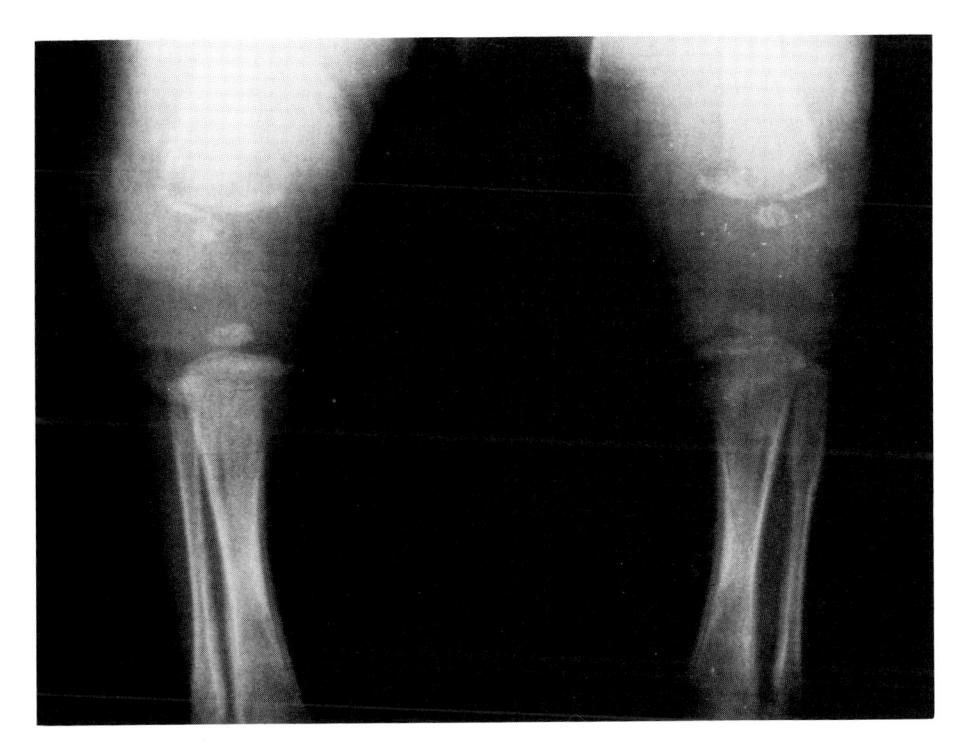

Fig. 27-2. Osteochondritis and periostitis of the bones in both lower extremities in a patient with congenital syphilis. Radiolucent area at the medial aspect of the proximal tibial metaphyses (Wimberger's sign) is present. Zone of translucency is visible proximal to the epiphyseal ends of both tibias (Wegner's sign).

epiphyseal fractures or epiphyseal dislocations may occur. Roentgenograms may reveal a dense band at the epiphyseal ends, below which is a band of translucency. The line may be smooth or serrated; a serrated appearance is known as Wegner's sign and represents points of calcified cartilage aimed at the nutrient cartilage canal. Bone lesions may be present despite prenatal treatment but generally disappear with or without postnatal therapy by 10 months of age.

Diagnosis

It is possible to make a diagnosis of congenital syphilis by dark-field examination and/or direct fluorescent antibody staining of organisms obtained by scraping the skin or mucous membrane lesions or the umbilical cord. More commonly, diagnosis is suggested by the clinical and roentgenographic findings and confirmed by serologic testing. Invasion by *T. pallidum* results in the development of antibodies known as reagins that are not specific for the *Treponema* organism as well as antibodies to the *Treponema* organism itself. Nontreponemal antigens produce two types of antibodies: univalent antibodies that may be detected by complement fixation tests (Kolmer and Wassermann) and bivalent antibodies detectable by flocculation tests (Kahn, RPR, and VDRL). If transplacentally acquired antibody is responsible for a positive test in an uninfected infant, a reduction in infant titer of at least 50% occurs during the first month of life, and the titer returns to normal by 3 months.

Specific treponemal antigen tests include the *T. pallidum* immobilization (TPI) test, the fluorescent treponema antibody absorption test (FTA-ABS), and the FTA-ABS IgM test. Antibodies that react in the TPI and FTA-ABS tests cross the placenta; these tests are specific for infection with *T. pallidum* in the mother, but a single positive test does not document neonatal infection. The FTA-ABS IgM test initially appeared to be a promising diagnostic tool that suggested specific neonatal infection by *T. pallidum*. More recently, evidence has shown that the fetal IgM is directed against maternal IgG rather than against *T. pallidum*. For this reason, false positive results are not uncommon. A positive FTA-ABS or TPI test at or near the time of birth must be repeated at 1 and 2 months of age to determine whether the antibody titer is falling (reflecting maternal but not neonatal infection) or is increasing (suggesting active congenital syphilis). When clinical or serologic tests suggest congenital syphilis, CSF should be examined and a CSF FTA-ABS test performed. Treatment is indicated if any specific antibody test is positive and the physician is uncertain about cooperation with regard to follow-up serologic examinations.

Treatment

Asymptomatic congenital syphilis without CNS involvement (normal CSF) can be treated with an injection of benzathine penicillin G in a single dose of 50,000 units/kg intramuscularly. Symptomatic congenital syphilis or neurosyphilis should be treated with aqueous crystalline penicillin G, 50,000 units/kg/day in two doses intramuscularly or intravenously for 10 days, or aqueous procaine penicillin G, 50,000 units/kg/day intramuscularly for 10 days.

Febrile reactions (Herxheimer's reactions) have been reported following initiation of treatment. Effective treatment is followed by disappearance of clinical signs, but roentgenographic findings may persist for 3 to 6 months. Blood and CSF serologic tests will become negative in several months.

Complications

When prenatal syphilis is not prevented or is unrecognized, late congenital syphilis may develop. Furthermore, the treatment of congenital syphilis after birth will not always prevent the late complications of the disease; only 60% of infants will have a positive serologic test for syphilis. Complications include interstitial keratitis, which may appear at any time but which generally appears during the second decade of life, deafness, neurosyphilis, Hutchinson's teeth (notched central incisors), mulberry molars, bone and joint involvement (saber shins, Clutton's joints), depressed nasal bridge, fissures about the nose and mouth, and gummas of the skin and other organs.

Prevention

A serologic test for syphilis should be performed early (first trimester) and late (third trimester) to ensure maximum possible protection of the fetus. If an FTA-ABS test performed on maternal serum is positive, maternal treatment should be instituted. Following therapy, the pregnant patient with syphilis should be followed with monthly titers to ensure that they fall as anticipated.

Chlamydia trachomatis
Incidence

Inclusion conjunctivitis and chlamydial pneumonia have been reported with increasing frequency. The number of pregnant women who are vaginally colonized with *Chlamydia* varies from 2% to 13%. In one study, conjunctivitis was reported in 35% and pneumonia in 20% of infants born to colonized mothers.

Etiology

C. trachomatis is an unusual organism with an intracellular and an extracellular phase; only the latter is infectious. The intracellular phase is necessary for survival of the organism, since chlamydiae cannot synthesize ATP. The organism can be grown in cell culture using McCoy cells, although this technique is available only in selected centers. Presumptive diagnosis can be made by finding inclusion bodies within epithelial cells obtained from conjunctival scrapings and processed using a Giemsa stain.

Pathogenesis

Chlamydial infections are acquired by passage through an infected birth canal. Inclusion conjunctivitis has been noted on the first day of life, suggesting that ascent of the organism may cause infection in utero. Chlamydiae also may be recovered from pharyngeal and rectal cultures.

Clinical manifestations

The most common neonatal form of disease is inclusion conjunctivitis. An afebrile pneumonia syndrome occurring between 2 and 12 weeks of age has been reported with increasing frequency. Chlamydiae also have been incriminated as a cause of otitis media in the newborn infant.

Diagnosis

Chlamydial conjunctivitis is suggested if purulent bilateral conjunctivitis is present from which no organisms are recovered using routine cultures. Identification of inclusion bodies on a Giemsa-stained smear of conjunctival scrapings strongly suggests this diagnosis. If the child has pneumonia, hyperinflation noted on a chest roentgenogram, a staccato cough, eosinophilia, and elevated serum immunoglobulins support the diagnosis of chlamydial infection.

Treatment

Pneumonia should be treated with erythromycin orally in a dosage of 40 mg/kg/day. The necessity for systemic treatment in conjunctivitis is controversial.

Tetanus
Incidence

Neonatal tetanus is usually seen where hygiene is poor. Twenty to 30 cases occur in the United States yearly.

Etiology

Clostridium tetani is a slender, gram-positive, anaerobic spore-forming bacillus that is not invasive. It produces disease by elaboration of a soluble exotoxin. Two toxins are produced: tetanospasmin and tetanolysin. Tetanospasmin produces muscular spasms and convulsions; tetanolysin causes hemolysis of red blood cells in vitro but does not have this effect in humans.

Pathology

No specific pathologic lesions are attributed to this infectious agent, although changes in the brain and spinal cord have been described in patients dying of tetanus. Death generally is due to asphyxia, either as a result of laryngeal spasm, prolonged seizures, direct effect on the medullary center and the brain stem, or as a result of a secondary pulmonary infection.

Pathogenesis

The umbilical stump that is contaminated by soil or by feces or skin lesions may serve as a portal of entry for the organism. When toxin elaboration occurs, it probably reaches the CNS by progressing up the trunks of motor nerves. Muscular contractions are produced by its effect on the neuromuscular end-plates and on the anterior horn cells of the CNS. When toxin becomes fixed to nervous tissue, it cannot be neutralized by antitoxin. Antitoxin crosses the placenta; thus infants born to mothers whose tetanus immunizations are current will have adequate antitoxin levels.

Clinical manifestations

The incubation period ranges from 2 to 10 days. Initial symptoms include difficulty in feeding and excessive crying, and within a brief time trismus is observed, followed shortly by generalized muscle spasms, rigidity, and seizures. Deep tendon reflexes may be absent during spasms or may be increased. Opisthotonos may be extreme but may also be absent. Fever and cardiorespiratory difficulties, including tachycardia, tachypnea, cyanosis, or apnea, may be observed.

Differential diagnosis

When all of the characteristic clinical findings are present, a diagnosis is apparent. Trismus generally is not observed in neonates with meningitis, intracranial hemorrhage, or kernicterus. Hypocalcemia and hypomagnesemia may be associated with seizures, tremors, and laryngospasm, but generalized rigidity and trismus are absent. Phenothiazine derivatives can produce spasms of the muscles of the neck and back, trismus, and dysphagia, but phenothiazine toxicity should be excluded by history or by metabolic studies of blood and urine. The rapid tonic seizures of tetanus are not found in individuals suffering from phenothiazine intoxication.

Treatment

The maintenance of a clear airway and provision of adequate ventilation are most important. Meticulous care must be exercised to decrease the likelihood of secondary bacterial pulmonary infections; this includes frequent suctioning under sterile conditions. Diazepam as required (0.1 to 2.0 mg) is the most effective agent in controlling seizures and rigidity in patients with tetanus. Barbiturates may be indicated as an adjunct to therapy and may help to sedate the patient. Penicillin G should be given intravenously to eradicate *Clostridium* that may continue to elaborate toxin. The bladder may need to be catheterized if it does not empty spontaneously. Although there is little evidence that tetanus antitoxin is efficacious if administered after clinical symptoms are apparent, it is recommended. Human tetanus–immune globulin (1,500 units) should be given intramuscularly. Active immunization against tetanus is still required, since recovery from tetanus does not confer permanent immunity.

Prevention

A well-immunized mother offers the best protection against tetanus neonatorum. Aseptic obstetric and neonatal care minimizes the likelihood of introduction of *Clostridium* organisms.

Tuberculosis

Incidence

Clinical tuberculosis is rare during the first month of life; however, management of the infant born to a mother who has tuberculosis is not an uncommon problem. Tuberculosis that becomes apparent during the first month of life may be congenital in etiology or acquired at or after the time of delivery by aspiration or inhalation.

Etiology

Mycobacterium tuberculosis var. *hominis* is the usual cause of congenital or neonatal disease. Infection with bovine strains of *M. tuberculosis* or with atypical *Mycobacterium* species is rare but has been reported.

Pathology

When disease is acquired via the umbilical vein, a primary complex forms in the porta hepatis of the liver, and miliary tubercles may be found in the spleen, bone marrow, lung, kidney, adrenal glands, and brain and on serosal surfaces. Gross or microscopic placental lesions may be detected. If the primary complex is located in the lungs, it is assumed that infection followed aspiration of amniotic fluid or vaginal secretions contaminated with tubercle bacilli or by inhalation.

Pathogenesis

Most cases of congenital tuberculosis are acquired hematogenously. Although the mother generally has miliary tuberculosis, congenital tuberculosis has been diagnosed in infants born to mothers with endometrial or cervical disease who have no pulmonary involvement and who also have negative tuberculin tests. Uninfected infants have been born to mothers who have miliary disease. Placental tuberculosis may be present without neonatal disease. Proof of congenital tuberculosis requires demonstration of active disease in the mother and child with no postpartum contact between the two and demonstration of a primary complex in the liver. Rupture of a caseating placental or endometrial granuloma may contaminate amniotic fluid, and the neonate may acquire disease by aspiration. Tuberculosis also can be contracted after delivery from other individuals with active pulmonary infection. In these cases, symptoms in the infants generally are delayed beyond 1 month of age.

Clinical manifestations

Symptoms of tuberculosis in the neonatal period may be nonspecific and include poor feeding, vomiting, weight loss, and fever. Respiratory symptoms may be absent, or cough and severe respiratory distress may develop. Hepatosplenomegaly, generalized lymphadenopathy, and pneumonia may be found. Obstructive jaundice, meningitis, and osteomyelitis are more common in neonates who acquire disease at or after birth than in patients with congenital tuberculosis. Otitis media may be seen, particularly in infants who aspirate infected amniotic fluid. Tuberculous otitis media frequently results in perforation of the tympanic membrane and commonly is associated with deafness and facial nerve paralysis.

Diagnosis

Examination of the placenta should be performed in every mother with possible tuberculosis. If tuberculous granulomas are noted, tuberculosis in the child should be suspected; however, they have been noted in some cases in which no disease developed in the newborn. Demonstration of acid-fast organisms on tracheal or gastric aspirate smears also aids in making a presumptive diagnosis. Gastric washings, urine specimens, and material obtained by aspiration of bone marrow or lymph nodes should be cultured for *Mycobacterium*. Chest roentgenographs may suggest pulmonary tuberculosis. A positive tuberculin test using PPD intermediate strength, Tween 80 stabilized material in an infant who has not received BCG vaccine is diagnostic. Generally, the tuberculin test is not positive for 4 to 6 weeks, even in neonates who are infected in utero. The tuberculin test may remain negative in the face of active disease. Lumbar puncture should be performed and CSF examined and cultured to exclude CNS involvement.

Treatment

Active neonatal tuberculosis should be treated initially with isoniazid (INH) in a dosage of 30 mg/kg/day in two divided doses orally and streptomycin at 20 to 30 mg/kg/day in two divided doses intramuscularly. Streptomycin therapy should be continued for 3 or 4 months. Therapy with isoniazid is continued for 18 to 24 months, and para-aminosalicylic acid (PAS) may be substituted for streptomycin when it is discontinued. Ethambutol and rifampin have not been evaluated in the neonatal period. When necessary because of infection with mycobacteria that are resistant to isoniazid, rifampin may be given in a dosage of 20 mg/kg/day. Ethambutol can be administered in a dosage of 25 mg/kg/day for 2 months followed by reduction in dosage to 15 mg/kg/day. Retrobulbar neuritis with loss of visual acuity is a prominent side effect of ethambutol; hence its use in the neonate whose visual acuity cannot be tested is not recommended unless no alternatives are available. Kanamycin in appropriate dosage may be substituted for streptomycin. Corticosteroids have been used in critically ill infants, particularly in those with CNS infection who have an actual or impending blockage to the flow of CSF or in patients with respiratory distress as a result of endobronchial disease.

Management of the newborn whose mother has tuberculosis

Infants born to mothers known to have active tuberculosis should be separated immediately from their mothers. Appropriate diagnostic studies should be performed to determine the possibility of active turberculosis in the infant. Treatment with isoniazid also should be initiated in therapeutic dosage. If neonatal tuberculosis is confirmed, streptomycin should be added and treatment carried out as indicated above. If neonatal tuberculosis is excluded, the isoniazid dosage should be decreased to 10 mg/kg/day and treatment continued with this single drug for a period of 1 year. Alternatively, isoniazid therapy may be provided for only 3 months. At the end of this period, if a chest roentgenogram and tuberculin test are still negative, isoniazid may be discontinued, and BCG vaccine may be administered. If this mode of therapy is chosen and if active disease in the mother is still present, the infant must be isolated from the mother until the tuberculin test becomes positive (about 6 weeks) or until she is no longer considered to have active disease.

When maternal pulmonary tuberculosis has been treated for at least 1 week, and if compliance with regard to maternal therapy is ensured, infant and maternal contact can be permitted provided that isoniazid prophylaxis of the infant also is ensured. In cases of maternal pulmonary tuberculosis that become apparent during pregnancy but for which treatment has been provided and in which the sputum no longer contains *Mycobacterium* organisms, isoniazid at 10 mg/kg/day should be prescribed for the infant for a period of 1 year; a period of separation from the mother is not necessary.

When maternal tuberculosis is active and/or where other cases of tuberculosis are known to be present in the household but compliance with regard to treatment of the adults cannot be ensured, the following are recommended:
1. The baby should be separated from the mother and other household contacts with active disease.
2. Active tuberculosis of the neonate must be excluded by chest roentgenogram and tuberculin testing before BCG administration, unless administration of BCG is carried out before 2 weeks of age.
3. Immunization with BCG should be provided.
4. When the tuberculin test becomes positive as a result of BCG immunization, the infant may be returned to the family setting if, in the interim, efforts have been made to ensure treatment of adults with active disease.

It is also important to observe infants who have received BCG, since BCG failures have been reported, and the infant might have acquired tuberculosis before immunization.

Most commonly, the physician is faced with the delivery of an infant born to a mother with a history of treated tuberculosis who has not received therapy for a number of years before pregnancy and delivery. The possibility of relapse is greatest just after delivery, and the relapse rate is greatest in individuals whose disease has been arrested for less than 5 years. The risk to such an infant is dependent on the likelihood of reactivation of maternal disease; thus frequent examinations of the mother are imperative. Postpartum chest roentgenograms obtained at 1, 3, and 6 months after delivery are indicated. The infant should be tuberculin-tested at 6 weeks of age and at intervals of 3 months during the first year of life. If there is any question with regard to reactivation, treatment of the mother and infant with isoniazid is indicated.

Coxsackie viruses

Incidence

The incidence of infection with Coxsackie virus in the newborn period is unknown. Both Coxsackie A and B viruses have been recovered from newborns; however, infection with Coxsackie B viruses has been documented more frequently.

Etiology

Coxsackie viruses are enteroviruses that are members of the picornavirus family. These are RNA viruses 15 to 30 μm in size that withstand freezing and are inactivated by heating for 30 minutes at 60° C. There are 23 Coxsackie A and 6 Coxsackie B viruses (B1-B6). The latter group has been associated with encephalomyocarditis in the newborn period.

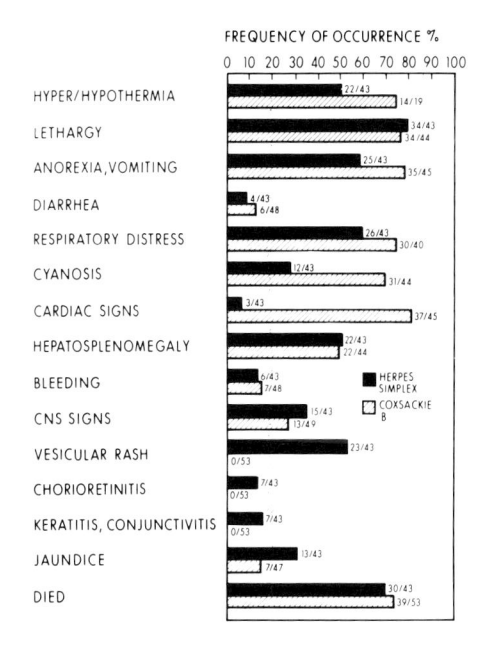

Fig. 27-3. Manifestations of disseminated herpes simplex and Coxsackie B viral infections in the neonatal period. (From Overall, J.C., Jr., and Glasgow, L.A.: J. Pediatr. **77:**315, 1970.)

Pathogenesis

These agents may be acquired during passage through the birth canal and from personnel or other infants in the newborn nursery. Transplacental transmission of Coxsackie B viruses has been reported.

Clinical manifestations

Coxsackie B viruses have been recovered from newborns who were asymptomatic, had mild illnesses, or died of severe, fulminant disease. When symptoms are apparent, poor feeding, vomiting, diarrhea, and fever or hypothermia may be seen. Asymptomatic cardiac enlargement or signs of congestive heart failure, tachycardia, hypotension, and cardiac arrhythmias can occur (Fig. 27-3). Meningeal involvement is frequent, but the patient may be asymptomatic. The signs and symptoms may simulate those of neonatal sepsis. Lethargy or seizures may be observed. The CSF reveals a lymphocytosis, but polymorphonuclear leukocytes may be seen early. Elevated CSF protein concentrations may be found. Pneumonia may contribute to the picture of cardiorespiratory distress. Hepatomegaly with jaundice, abnormal liver function tests, and a prolonged prothrombin time may be associated with bleeding into the skin and various organs of the body. Pancreatitis with elevated serum amylase concentration also may be noted. Fatalities are not infrequent, but complete recovery can ensue. Recent postmortem studies suggest that neonatal or intrauterine Coxsackie B viral infection may be associated with an increased incidence of stillbirth, congenital anomalies, and with sudden unexpected death in infancy. In addition, some cases of idiopathic myocarditis in childhood may be related to neonatal Coxsackie B viral infection of the myocardium. Coxsackie A viruses have been recovered from neonates with diarrhea, meningitis, herpangina, jaundice, and hepatosplenomegaly.

Diagnosis

The concurrence of myocarditis and meningoencephalitis in any neonate with negative bacterial cultures suggests infection with Coxsackie B virus. The diagnosis may be supported by a history of birth to a mother who is febrile at delivery and who has pleurodynia or myalgia. Diagnosis is confirmed by recovery of the virus from the pharynx and stool and demonstration of a rise in neutralizing antibody titer to the virus, which has been recovered from the blood or from various organs in fatal cases.

Treatment

No specific antiviral therapy is available. Seizures and congestive heart failure should be treated with appropriate agents.

ECHO viral infection
Incidence

The frequency of neonatal infection due to ECHO viruses is unknown.

Etiology

Any of the ECHO viruses may be associated with clinical disease. One or more cases of infection by ECHO viruses in the neonatal period have been reported with ECHO types 1, 6, 7, 9, 11, 11', 14, 15, 18, 19, 22, and 31. Transplacental transmission of ECHO virus occurs, but disease most commonly follows exposure at or following delivery. Epidemic ECHO viral infection in the nursery has been reported.

Clinical manifestations

ECHO viruses have been recovered from asymptomatic infants as well as from neonates who have succumbed to fulminant disease characterized by hepatic necrosis, aseptic meningitis, adrenal and renal hemorrhage, and disseminated intravascular coagulation. The initial clinical symptoms may be indistinguishable from those of bacterial septicemia and have included poor feeding, irritability, hypotonia, hypothermia, respiratory distress with cyanosis, apneic episodes, vomiting diarrhea, jaundice, thrombocytopenia, widespread hemorrhages, maculopapular rashes, and myocarditis.

Diagnosis

A lumbar puncture should be performed in an attempt to exclude bacterial meningitis as well as to identify possible aseptic CNS disease. Viral cultures should be obtained from the throat, stool, and CSF. Acute and convalescent serum specimens should be obtained for complement-fixing and neutralizing antibody titers in the event that a virus is isolated. The virus may be cultured from various organs post mortem.

Prognosis

In addition to death or survival without apparent sequelae, it is possible that neonates who survive ECHO viral disease in the neonatal period and who have had CNS involvement may suffer permanent residual effects. A recent study of children who have recovered from CNS enteroviral (including ECHO virus) infection acquired during the first year of life revealed significantly smaller head circumferences and depressed language and speech skills in comparison with controls.

Poliomyelitis
Incidence and etiology

Poliomyelitis rarely occurs in the neonatal period. Polioviruses are picornaviruses; three subtypes, designated I, II, and III, all can produce human disease.

Pathology and pathogenesis

The newborn may acquire infection in utero during periods of maternal viremia as well as at or shortly after birth as a result of contact with fecal material that contains poliovirus. Infection may result in fetal death, and virus has been recovered from fetal blood and tissues and from the placenta. The incubation period is 7 to 10 days. Disease that becomes manifest after the first week of life probably has been acquired postnatally. Antibodies to polioviruses can be acquired transplacentally, providing protection during the first few months of life. When paralytic disease occurs, destruction of the gray matter of the spinal cord, brain stem, and basal ganglia is prominent. Neuronal necrosis, focal and diffuse leukocytic infiltration, and perivascular cuffing may be noted.

Before the advent of poliovirus immunization, more than 80% of neonates had poliovirus antibodies at birth. It is important to stress that only by maintenance of a well-immunized adult population can we hope to continue this level of protection in the newborn period. Infection in susceptible pregnant women may occur; in most cases they will be asymptomatic or associated with nonspecific signs and symptoms, but the viremia that occurs may produce fetal infection.

Clinical manifestations

Poor feeding, irritability, vomiting, and diarrhea may be noted. Focal neurologic signs or seizure activity may suggest the presence of encephalitis. A flaccid paralysis may develop, and although involvement may be spotty and asymmetric in some cases, an ascending paralysis that mimics the manifestations of Guillain-Barré syndrome may be noted. Paralysis of respiratory muscles may occur. When disease occurs in the first month of life, death is common; however, recovery with a residual neurologic deficit has been reported. Asymptomatic neonatal infection has been documented.

Diagnosis

Viral cultures of the throat and stool should be obtained. Serologic tests on both maternal and neonatal blood may support or confirm the diagnosis.

Treatment

No specific therapy is available. Disease should be prevented by immunization of the population as recommended during infancy and childhood. Potentially susceptible women should not be immunized during pregnancy except in rare epidemic situations.

Myxovirus infections

Mumps and rubeola viruses may cross the placenta. Maternal rubeola has been asociated with an increased incidence of stillbirth and abortions as well as with an increase in prematurity, which may be due to early onset of labor. A possible relationship between mumps and either fetal death or congenital malformations remains controversial. In one study, an increase in fetal deaths has been related to mumps infection during the first trimester of pregnancy. Aqueductal stenosis and hydrocephalus were noted to follow mumps infection of suckling hamsters in every case, but similar malformations have not been definitively related to infections with mumps in humans, either in utero or postnatally. Other studies have documented an association between a positive skin test to mumps antigen and the presence of endocardial fibroelastosis, suggesting that the latter may be a result of previous exposure to mumps virus. When studies designed to evaluate this relationship employed 15 mm of erythema (the recommended standard for mumps skin test) as indicative of a positive skin test result, no relationship between delayed hypersensitivity to mumps skin test antigen and endocardial fibroelastosis could be established.

An increased incidence of congenital malformations of the CNS was reported in children of mothers who were between the third and ninth weeks of development during an epidemic of Asian influenza viral infection in Finland. Other factors, however, including increased use of drugs by women afflicted with influenza, may have accounted for the observed association; thus conclusive evidence of direct viral effect on the fetus is lacking.

Etiology

Rubeola, mumps, and influenza are caused by myxoviruses. Rubeola and mumps viruses appear to be relatively stable, but antigenic changes in influenza virus occur readily, accounting for the existence of multiple epidemic strains.

Pathogenesis

Transplacental passage of rubeola virus is well established, and measles rashes have been recognized in the fetus and newborn. Maternal and fetal disease are not always at the same stage concomitantly. Mumps virus has been recovered from the placenta after maternal viremia, but transplacental passage is poorly documented. Parotitis in a newborn has followed maternal parotitis, but evidence that mumps virus was the causative agent in such patients is lacking. Transplacental passage of influenza virus has been documented once and resulted in the death of the mother and her 30-week-old fetus during the third trimester of pregnancy. Measles, mumps, and influenza viruses may be acquired after birth in susceptible neonates. Of these, influenza viral infection of the neonate is most uncommon; the first documented cases in the neonatal period were reported in 1973. In the preimmunization era, protection of the newborn against measles generally was afforded by acquisition of antibody from the mother who had had measles during childhood. It has been assumed that immunization after 1 year of age will protect against active disease and presumably provide similar protection of the newborn, but confirmation of this supposition is lacking at present.

Clinical manifestations

Rubeola in the neonatal period may be similar to that in older individuals or may be mild, perhaps as a result of modification but not prevention by maternally acquired antibody. Prodromal symptoms of rhinorrhea, cough, conjunctivitis, and fever are followed by the appearance of Koplik's spots and a morbilliform rash. Congenital measles occurs within the first 10 to 12 days after birth, and infants generally survive.

Mumps in the neonatal period is generally mild, and parotitis has been the principal clinical manifestation.

Influenza A, which has been reported in newborns who were in intensive care nurseries, was associated with nasal congestion and drainage and marked respiratory distress and cyanosis. Illness lasted about 4 days, and all infants recovered. Disease affected only infants at high risk because of underlying disease and apparently was acquired from personnel who were infected.

Diagnosis

Diagnosis of mumps, rubeola, or influenza rests on recovery of these viruses from the blood or nasopharyngeal secretions. Acute and convalescent sera should be obtained for neutralizing, hemagglutination inhibition, and complement-fixing antibody titers. In mumps viral infection, differential S and V complement-fixing antibody titers are most helpful. Development of specific IgM antibody responses to measles and mumps infection can be demonstrated.

Treatment

No specific treatment is available for rubeola or mumps. Antiviral therapy for influenza has not been studied in the neonatal period. Secondary bacterial infections, particularly otitis media and pneumonia, should be treated appropriately. Women exposed to rubeola during pregnancy should be given 0.25 ml/kg of gammaglobulin if they have not had measles or measles immunization previously. If the neonate is exposed to measles after birth, gammaglobulin should be administered in a dosage of 0.25 ml/kg.

Varicella-zoster and Epstein-Barr virus (EBV)

Incidence

Varicella-zoster viral infection has been reported in the neonatal period.

A congenital syndrome that has been attributed to varicella during pregnancy also has been described by several investigators. The frequency of this syndrome in infants born to mothers who have had varicella during pregnancy is unknown.

Etiology

The DNA viruses producing chickenpox and herpes zoster are identical and belong to the same family as herpes simplex virus and cytomegaloviruses. EBV is also a herpeslike virus and is the agent responsible for infectious mononucleosis.

Pathology and pathogenesis

Varicella-zoster viral infection is associated with skin lesions characterized by epithelial cell hyperplasia with intranuclear inclusion bodies. Lesions progress to vesiculation and encrustation. Lesions similar in type also may be noted in the GI tract, and focal necrosis has been seen in the liver, spleen, pancreas, lungs, bone marrow, thymus, and adrenal and renal cortices.

Varicella-zoster virus may cross the placenta at any time during pregnancy, and intrauterine infections have been documented in infants of women who have had varicella during the second or third trimester of pregnancy. Varicella also may be acquired at or after birth by direct contact with infected lesions or by inhalation of fomites. Varicella viral infection induces long-lasting immunity; however, the disease may reoccur as herpes zoster even in individuals with serum antibodies to the virus. Presumably, virus resides in the nerve cells of such individuals, and reactivation represents migration of virus along the nerve to the periphery. Transplacental passage of antibody occurs but appears to be more variable and imparts an immunity that is more transient than that to rubeola. Transplacental acquisition of EBV antibody occurs and probably accounts for the absence of well-documented clinical disease due to EBV in the newborn period.

Clinical manifestations

Infants born to mothers who have had varicella during the first trimester of pregnancy have exhibited the following characteristics: intrauterine growth retardation, limb reduction defects, microcephaly, psychomotor retardation, skin defects including cicatrization, and ocular defects. Affected infants do not invariably demonstrate each clinical feature of this syndrome.

Infants born to mothers who have had varicella during pregnancy may develop congenital varicella without teratogenic defects. These neonates may develop a rash at birth or at any time during the newborn period.

When disease is noted before the tenth day of life, congenital infection is assumed. These infants have a poorer prognosis with a higher incidence of disseminated disease. In mild cases, only a few vesicles may be present, and no systemic symptoms are apparent. In some cases the vesicular lesions seem to follow nerve roots and may suggest the diagnosis of herpes zoster. In other newborns, fever, jaundice, poor feeding, respiratory distress, pneumonia, vomiting, melena, and hematuria may be noted. Mortality as high as 30% has been noted.

Diagnosis

Varicella in the newborn generally is noted in association with maternal varicella, and the diagnosis is suggested on the basis of epidemiologic considerations. The skin lesions may be similar to those of herpes simplex, but the latter disease tends to run a more severe and fulminant course. In addition, varicella lesions are smaller and less likely to become confluent than those of herpes simplex. Isolation of the virus from the lesions or from the nasopharynx and serologic studies will provide a definitive diagnosis.

Treatment

There is little evidence that pooled gammaglobulin given at birth in doses of 0.4 to 0.6 ml/kg to infants of women with varicella prevents neonatal varicella, but it may modify the disease. Herpes zoster–immune globulin modifies the disease and is preferable to the pooled gammaglobulin. In severe cases, cytosine arabinoside or idoxuridine therapy may be tried, but controlled studies with regard to their efficacy are not available; these drugs may have serious untoward effects.

Variola and vaccinia

Variola (smallpox), according to the World Health Organization, has been eradicated. Infection during pregnancy is associated with a high rate of abortion, stillbirth, and congenital infections. Vaccinia is a disease related to vaccination against smallpox. Although recommendations for discontinuation of routine vaccination have been accepted, vaccinia still may occur, since the immunization is recommended for certain groups of individuals, including those in the health care professions. Vaccination during pregnancy also may produce abortion, stillbirth, and congenital infection.

Etiology

Variola is a DNA virus in the herpes group. Vaccinia is a virus derived from variola and cowpox strains. The vaccine is prepared from the vesicles of vaccinated calves.

Pathology and pathogenesis

Histologic examination of the cutaneous lesions reveals focal necrosis and mononuclear cell infiltration. In variola, Guarnieri's bodies (intracytoplasmic inclusions) and intranuclear inclusion bodies may be seen. All organs of the body may be infected following hematogenous dissemination. In vaccinia, intracytoplasmic inclusion bodies are seen, but intranuclear inclusions are absent.

Transplacental infection with variola is common and may occur in the absence of clinical disease in the mother, a finding that may be related to maternal acquisition of cellular immunity to variola from a proven vaccination or infection but an absence of humoral immunity. Smallpox also may be acquired after delivery and has an incubation period of about 12 days. In some cases, maternal infection with vaccinia has followed acquisition of virus from other vaccinated contacts.

Clinical manifestations

Smallpox in the newborn is characterized by the appearance of vesicles that vary in size and that tend to have a central depression. The infant is critically ill and pneumonia is common. Mortality exceeds 90%.

Diagnosis

In addition to pertinent epidemiologic and clinical findings, diagnosis is made by recovery of virus from the vesicular fluid. Scraping of the vesicles may reveal multinucleated cells with intracytoplasmic inclusions in patients with variola. Neutralizing IgM antibody can be demonstrated following congenital infection.

Treatment

Methisazone and vaccinia-immune glubulin may alter the course of variola and vaccinia in children and adults. Experience with these agents in the neonatal period is limited. Vaccination with vaccinia virus during pregnancy should be avoided.

Adenovirus

Adenovirus infection is rare; most infants are born with antibodies to adenovirus that have been acquired transplacentally. Neonatal adenoviral infection has been associated with an abrupt onset of signs and symptoms suggestive of generalized septicemia, including respiratory distress, fever, hepatosplenomegaly, and jaundice as early as the second day of life; these signs suggest maternally transmitted infection or, possibly, contact with virus at birth. The virus has been recovered from the pharynx, from material obtained by lung aspiration, and from stool and urine in the newborn, as well as from the lung, kidneys, and liver post mortem.

Candida

Incidence

Mucocutaneous, cutaneous, and disseminated candidiasis all have been reported in the newborn. Oral candidiasis (thrush) is common.

Etiology

Candida organisms are yeastlike fungi that produce pseudomycelia and spores. *C. albicans, C. tropicalis, C. pseudotropicalis,* and *C. stellatoidea* are but a few of the species that have been proved pathogenic for man.

Pathology and pathogenesis

Systemic candidiasis may cause disease in any organ system. *Candida* abscesses have been described in the liver, spleen, lung, brain, kidney, and heart. Superficial infection of the skin and GI tract is even more common and is characterized by invasion of epithelium by hyphae, with penetration of the basement membrane. In some patients, pseudomembranes form. If the infection penetrates the walls of veins, thrombosis and hematogenous infection will develop. Thrush frequently is complicated by esophagitis and GI tract colonization; the latter may develop in the absence of thrush. In general, *C.*

albicans has a predilection for stratified epithelium, whereas columnar epithelium resists infection. The umbilical cord and fetal membranes may be involved in patients with congenital candidiasis.

C. albicans may be acquired from the vaginal flora of the mother at delivery, and person-to-person transmission may occur. The increasing use of intravenous and intraarterial catheters has been accompanied by an increased incidence of systemic candidiasis. Superficial and systemic candidiasis has followed congenital infection, which has been reported both in the presence and absence of intact membranes.

Clinical manifestations

Oral thrush begins as a small papular lesion that may be associated with or evolve into vesicles. These coalesce to form cheesy white patches that may cover the buccal mucosa, gingiva, and tongue. These membranes may be quite adherent to underlying tissue. No systemic symptoms are apparent. *Candida* esophagitis may be associated with poor feeding, regurgitation, vomiting, and hematemesis. Diarrhea may suggest the presence of candidiasis, but it is necessary to demonstrate mycelial forms in the stool before attributing this symptom to the presence of *Candida* infection. Systemic candidiasis may present with symptoms that are indistinguishable from those of generalized septicemia and may include pneumonitis, endophthalmitis, meningitis, shock, and disseminated intravascular coagulation. Cutaneous lesions usually are restricted to the diaper area but may be noted in any moist warm area, including the neck, axilla, and the antecubital and popliteal fossae. Generalized cutaneous lesions have been noted at birth in congenital cutaneous candidiasis, which is characterized by maculopapular lesions that become vesicular and rupture, leaving denuded skin with well-defined, raised, scaling borders.

Diagnosis

Thrush and cutaneous candidiasis usually are diagnosed on the basis of their clinical appearance, but the diagnosis can be confirmed by examination and cultures of scrapings. Cultures of blood, urine, and CSF should be obtained when systemic candidiasis is suspected. A pure culture of *Candida* obtained by bronchoscopy suggests the diagnosis of *Candida* pneumonia.

Treatment

Oral moniliasis responds to nystatin (Mycostatin) suspension (1 to 2 ml) provided four times each day for 5 to 10 days. Cutaneous candidiasis will respond to nystatin ointment three times a day for 7 to 10 days; in some cases, secondary bacterial infection requires treatment with another topical or systemic antibiotic. Nystatin with a corticosteroid (Mycolog cream or ointment) may be used in severe cases of *Candida* dermatitis.

Systemic candidiasis should be treated with amphotericin B intravenously. Treatment should be initiated at 0.1 mg/kg in a single daily dose infused over a 4- to 6-hour period. In some patients, responses to relatively low-dosage therapy (0.1 to 0.3 mg/kg/day) is dramatic, whereas in others a dosage of 1 mg/kg/day will be required. Dosages should be adjusted on the basis of the sensitivity of the organism and the blood level of amphotericin B that is achieved. Treatment is continued for 4 weeks. It is important to carefully monitor patients receiving amphotericin B for cardiac arrhythmias and to provide potassium supplementation as needed to replace the increased urinary potassium losses that will occur. Serum electrolyte, blood urea nitrogen, and creatinine levels should be monitored and treatment temporarily discontinued if the blood urea nitrogen reaches abnormally high levels. Intrathecal amphotericin B may be required in *Candida* meningitis if it does not respond to intravenous therapy.

Coccidioidomycosis
Incidence

Coccidioidomycosis occurs only rarely in the newborn period.

Etiology

Coccidioides immitis is the fungal agent that produces this disease and may be found in tissues as a spherule that has a doubly refractile capsule that contains endospores. On culture media the sporangia develop septate hyphae that are disseminated readily by the aerosol route.

Pathology and pathogenesis

Coccidioidomycosis may be a disseminated granulomatous disease. Multiple small abscesses may develop following hematogenous spread to the lungs, liver, spleen, meninges, and brain. Infection can be acquired by inhalation of spores or by their entry through lacerations or abrasions of the skin. Transplacental passage of the fungus has been reported. Placental lesions have been described in pregnant women who have disseminated coccidioidomycosis, and infection following aspiration of contaminated amniotic fluid also has been documented. Coccidioidomycosis is endemic in the southwestern portion of the United States as well as in Mexico, Argentina, Venezuela, and Paraguay. Disease, however, may occur in any geographic location, since individuals who have been exposed to the disease in an endemic area may develop reactivation of their infection at any time after the initial exposure.

Clinical manifestations

The incubation period ranges from 1 to 3 weeks. Specific signs and symptoms depend on the initial route of infection. When infection is acquired by the aerosol route, pneumonia is common. If the disease becomes disseminated, lesions will appear in the skin, bone, lymph nodes, liver, spleen, and meninges. Fever, respiratory distress, and jaundice frequently accompany neonatal coccidioidomycosis.

Diagnosis

When this disorder is suspected, tracheal and gastric aspirates, urine, CSF, blood, and bone marrow should be examined and cultured for *C. immitis*. Materials should be plated on blood agar and on Sabouraud's medium and Mycocel slants and should be cultured both at room temperature and at 37° C. Skin and serologic tests are available but may not be helpful in the initial neonatal period. Complement-fixing antibody may cross the placenta; thus a rise in the infant's titer must be demonstrated to document neonatal infection. A complement-fixing antibody titer of 1:8 or greater generally indicates disseminated disease. Thus if the maternal titer reaches this level, systemic coccidioidomycosis should be considered in the mother and anticipated as a possibility in the infant.

Treatment

Disseminated coccidioidomycosis is a fatal disease that must be treated with amphotericin B intravenously for 4 weeks or longer. Intrathecal administration is necessary if meningitis is present and fails to respond to intravenous medication. Generally, a dosage of 1 mg/kg/day administered as a single daily dose over a period of 4 to 6 hours intravenously is efficacious.

Cryptococcosis
Incidence

Cryptococcal infection is rare in the newborn period. The CNS is involved primarily, but any organ system may be affected. Neonatal infection has been shown to result from transplacental passage of *Cryptococcus*.

Etiology

C. neoformans is a ubiquitous saprophytic fungus that may produce disease. Both in tissues and in culture it appears as a nonsporulating, yeastlike, nonmycelial fungus with a broad capsule. It can be found on the skin as well as in the pharynx, GI tract, and vaginal tract of healthy individuals.

Pathology and pathogenesis

In the presence of underlying or debilitating illness, hematogenous dissemination may occur, and any organ system may be infected. Pathologic findings vary from minor inflammatory responses to abscess formation. Granulomas have been noted, and hepatitis and cirrhosis of the liver are common findings. Meningitis frequently leads to obstructive hydrocephalus. Granulomas of the brain have been reported; they may calcify. Calcifications may be visible on roentgenograms obtained at birth in neonates who have developed intrauterine cryptococcal disease. The fetus can be infected transplacentally, or the organisms may be acquired at or following delivery.

Clinical manifestations

Congenital cryptococcosis frequently is associated with premature birth. Newborns fail to thrive, feed poorly, and may show signs of CNS infection. Lethargy, irritability, and vomiting may be noted initially; this may be followed by seizures, opisthotonic posturing, or hydrocephalus. Chorioretinitis, cataracts, and endophthalmitis all have been reported. Interstitial pneumonia may be present and produce symptoms referable to the respiratory system. Hepatosplenomegaly, jaundice, ulcerative skin lesions, thrombocytopenia, and petechial or purpuric hemorrhages also have been noted. Thus the initial presentation may be identical to that of infants with infection due to cytomegalovirus or rubella virus. In addition, calcific densities may appear along the margins of dilated ventricles, suggesting cytomegalic inclusion disease or, less commonly, toxoplasmosis.

Laboratory manifestations

The CSF may contain between 100 and 1,000 cells/mm^3, but lymphocytes will predominate after the first week of infection. The protein concentration is elevated and the CSF glucose level is depressed compared with the blood glucose level. Organisms may be demonstrable on India ink preparation; however, caution must be exercised in suggesting a diagnosis of cryptococcosis solely on this basis, despite the competence of the observer.

Cultures of CSF, blood, and other body tissue should be obtained. A latex agglutination test for the detection of cryptococcal antigen in CSF has proved to be a rapid and, when properly controlled, effective test for establishing a diagnosis of cryptococcosis. The organism can be grown on blood agar and on Sabouraud's medium. Blood, sputum, abscess cavities, and bone marrow also serve as materials that frequently yield a positive culture.

Treatment

Amphotericin B should be administered as for *Candida*; however, if the patient is critically ill, treatment may be initiated with a dosage of 0.25 mg/kg/day.

Histoplasmosis

Incidence

Histoplasmosis is a disorder that is rare in the neonatal period. When it occurs, disseminated disease is common and is generally fatal unless treated.

Etiology

Histoplasma capsulatum is the fungus that produces histoplasmosis; it grows in tissues in a yeast phase and is encapsulated.

Pathogenesis

Fungus enters the body through the skin, mucous membranes, and respiratory or GI tract. Focal infections tend to seed the bloodstream, leading to formation of abscesses and granulomas in many organs. Transplacental infection has been suspected in infants born to mothers who have disseminated histoplasmosis during pregnancy. There is little evidence of human-to-human or animal-to-human transmission. Histoplasmosis is endemic in the Mississippi River Basin but has been reported in individuals throughout the United States.

Clinical manifestations

Signs and symptoms of respiratory distress may be noted early. Irritability, poor feeding, failure to thrive, and fever are common. Hepatosplenomegaly and generalized lymphadenopathy may be present. Osteomyelitis and meningitis have been reported.

Laboratory manifestations

CSF will reveal 1 to 1,000 white blood cells/mm^3 that are predominantly lymphocytes after the first several days of illness. The protein concentration will be increased and the glucose concentration depressed. Patients are frequently anemic and may be leukopenic and thrombocytopenic as well.

Diagnosis

Smears and cultures of sputum, blood, bone marrow, and CSF or biopsies of the affected organ may reveal the fungal organisms. Giemsa or Wright's stain is satisfactory, but the use of special silver stains or fluorescent microscopy may facilitate the diagnosis. Complement fixation tests may be employed but can be confused by the presence of maternal antibodies. Both yeast and mycelial phase antibodies should be measured; an elevated yeast phase antigen generally is associated with acute infection.

Treatment

Disseminated histoplasmosis should be treated with amphotericin B as indicated for the treatment of candidiasis. Intrathecal administration will be required in patients with meningitis who fail to respond to intravenous treatment.

Malaria

Incidence

Malaria remains an important cause of abortion, stillbirth, and neonatal death in many parts of the world. Sporadic cases occur each year in inhabitants of North America. Congenital malaria is well documented.

Etiology

Malaria is caused by a protozoal parasite of the genus *Plasmodium*. Neonatal infection has been recorded with all species, including *P. vivax, P. malariae, P. ovale,* and *P. falciparum*.

Pathology and pathogenesis

Malarial parasites invade erythrocytes, which subsequently adhere to and occlude blood vessels. Red blood cells that are disintegrating accumulate and may blockade the reticuloendothelial system. Anemia is the result of hemolysis. Parasites may be found in other organs of the body, including the intestinal tract, liver, spleen, lung, and brain. The placenta is involved in most women who suffer from malaria during pregnancy. Transplacental transmission of parasites is documented and may take place during the course of symptomatic maternal malaria or may occur many years after women have left an endemic area. In the latter situation, parasitemia may be subclinical; thus congenital malaria may occur without a history of a malarial attack during pregnancy. Mosquito-borne disease may occur in newborns just as in older children or in adults. When malaria occurs in pregnant women, intrauterine infection does not always ensue. In the face of parasitemia the infant may acquire malarial parasites during labor and delivery due to contamination of the infant's blood with that of the mother. Blood donated by individuals with malaria may serve as a source of malarial parasites. Neonatal malaria is rare, since IgG antibody to the malarial parasite crosses the placenta, providing some protection for the newborn. This antibody specifically aids in the phagocytosis of merozoites and infected erythrocytes, but it does not alter the hepatic phase of malaria.

Clinical manifestations

If congenital malaria has occurred, disease may become manifest in the early days of life. Malaria acquired postnatally may appear at any time between 8 and 30 days after delivery. The incubation period is dependent on the specific species involved, the size of the inoculum, and the immune status of the host. Congenital malaria may appear relatively late. Specific signs and symptoms can vary from irritability, weight loss, and low-grade fever to devastating disease. Fever, diarrhea, vomiting, tachypnea, cyanosis, and meningeal findings may be present. Anemia and jaundice, which may occur acutely, suggest hemolysis. Hepatosplenomegaly is common, and renal function may be impaired.

Diagnosis

The diagnosis is dependent on demonstration of parasites in the bloodstream. Thick smears should be prepared and examined on several different occasions to maximize the possibility of parasite detection.

Treatment

Chloroquine is indicated for the treatment of acute malaria in a dose of 5 mg/kg diluted in a multiple electrolyte solution containing glucose. This dose may be repeated once in 12 to 24 hours. Chloroquine also can be provided orally in an immediate initial dose of 10 mg/kg followed by a dose of 5 mg/kg at 6, 24, and 48 hours. For strains of *P. falciparum* that are resistant to chloroquine, quinine can be provided orally in a dosage of 20 to 30 mg/kg/day in three divided doses for 7 to 10 days or may be given intravenously in a dose of 10 mg/kg diluted in a multiple electrolyte solution containing glucose and repeated once after 24 hours. Because of the extreme toxicity of this drug, the oral route is preferred.

Pneumocystis carinii
Incidence

Pneumonia may be caused by *P. carinii* in newborns whose host resistance is impaired. Rarely, it is associated with pneumonia in healthy normal neonates.

Etiology

P. carinii is a protozoan that has only recently been cultivated in vitro. Morphologic appearance of the cysts in pathologic specimens is so characteristic that diagnosis can be made morphologically.

Pathology and pathogenesis

Pathologic changes are limited to the lungs. Infection begins in pulmonary alveolar spaces, and the exudate that develops contains lymphocytes, plasma cells, polymorphonuclear leukocytes, and histiocytes. An eosinophilic lacelike appearance may be found on stains with periodic acid–Schiff reagent. Cysts can be demonstrated readily by use of methenamine silver stains. Specific modes of transmission are unclear, but nursery epidemics of *Pneumocystis* infection have occurred and suggest an airborne route. In a few patients, intrauterine infection has been described, suggesting the possibility of transplacental transmission. The specific association of *P. carinii* infection with the debilitated host suggests that disease results from some impairment in host-parasite relationships. Nutritional deprivation may be accompanied by *Pneumocystis* infection that clears with nutritional repletion.

Clinical manifestations

The incubation period is approximately 3 weeks. The onset is insidious, and over a short period of time tachypnea, cough, and cyanosis are noted. Rales are unusual, and fever is relatively infrequent. Roentgenograms demonstrate bilateral diffuse infiltrates that tend to extend from the hilus of the lung to the periphery. Frequently, the degree of pulmonary involvement detected clinically and by pulmonary function studies is in excess of that which can be accounted for by the roentgenographic appearance of the lungs.

Diagnosis

Roentgenographic studies may suggest this disease but are not diagnostic. Diagnosis depends on demonstration of *Pneumocytosis* cysts. Although *P. carinii* organisms have been demonstrated in material obtained from tracheal aspirate, gastric aspirates, or by needle biopsy of the lung, the likelihood of establishing a definitive diagnosis is greatest if open lung biopsy is performed. This also minimizes the risk of pneumothorax in comparison with needle biopsy.

Treatment

Pentamidine isethionate is effective when given as a single daily dose of 4 mg/kg intramuscularly for 10 to 14 days. It can be obtained from the Centers for Disease Control in Atlanta, Georgia when a diagnosis of *Pneumocystis* infection is highly suspected or confirmed. *Pneumocystis* infection is best treated in children over 2 months of age and in adults with trimethoprim-sulfamethoxazole (Bactrim, Septra). There is no reason to believe that this drug combination would be any less effective in the newborn infant. It is well known, however, that sulfa drugs displace bilirubin from albumin-binding sites, predisposing infants to kernicterus at relatively low levels of serum bilirubin. Moreover, the potential for toxicity of trimethoprim in the newborn infant is unknown. For these reasons, although this drug combination is the preferred treatment for *Pneumocystis* infections beyond the newborn period, it cannot be recommended for neonates until additional pharmacologic studies have been performed.

PREVENTION OF INFECTION IN THE NEONATAL UNIT
Barrier nursing technique

Several controlled trials have demonstrated that the use of masks and gowns by nursery personnel affected neither staphylococcal carriage rates nor infectious illness in infants but tended to keep personnel away from their patients. Virtually all controlled clinical trials have demonstrated that effective hand-washing is responsible for the absence of nosocomial infection in nursery units. Conversely, ineffective hand-washing techniques frequently have been associated with epidemic disease. Hexachlorophene (3% as a liquid soap or cream) has proved to be extremely effective in preventing infection by gram-positive bacteria, and various iodinated preparations, including chlorhexidine (0.5%), are effective against gram-negative organisms. These agents have a cumulative effect when used repeatedly for hand-washing. *P. aeruginosa* has been recovered from both types of germicidal solution; thus attention must be paid to sterilization of the containers from which these materials are dispensed. Even a quick dip and rinse followed by the mechanical process of drying the hands with a paper towel is extremely effective in reducing the transmission of organisms from the hands of personnel to patients.

Routine hexachlorophene bathing of infants

Intensive or extensive exposure to hexachlorophene produces vacuolation in myelinated regions of the animal brain stem and cerebellum. Toxic encephalopathy was reported among infants in France attributable to the accidental incorporation of excessive amounts of hexachlorophene in baby talcum powder. Possible neuropathologic effects have been attributed to the use of three or more daily baths in 3% hexachlorophene, primarily in infants who weighed 1,400 gm or less at birth and who lived in the nursery environment for more than 3 days. Infants receiving fewer than three baths with 3% hexachlorophene or infants bathed in a 100-fold dilution of 3% hexachlorophene were at a much lower risk of disease. None of the infants in the studies reported who weighed more than 1,400 gm and who were bathed fewer than three times in 3% hexachlorophene or who were bathed in a 100-fold dilution of 3% hexachlorophene demonstrated neuropathologic lesions. Clinical correlates of these pathologic findings have not been established in most cases. It is possible that the neuropathology may even be self-limiting or reversible following withdrawal of hexachlorophene.

These findings, however, prompted the recommendation that routine hexachlorophene bathing of neonates be discontinued. Subsequently, some hospital nurseries have experienced an increased incidence of staphylococcal infection. In view of these events, the following recommendations can be made. In the absence of infection, prophylactic bathing with hexachlorophene should not be performed. Rather, emphasis must be placed on reliable surveillance of neonatal disease, prompt isolation and treatment of infected infants, and adequate hand-washing. Hexachlorophene should still be used as an antibacterial agent by personnel working in the neonatal unit. Crowding should be avoided, and cohort nursing techniques should be employed wherever possible. When these practices are inadequate for infection control, antibacterial bathing regimens employing hexachlorophene should be initiated temporarily. If hexachlorophene bathing is utilized, infants should be rinsed carefully to ensure that no residual hexachlorophene remains on the surface of the skin. Hibiclens, which is absorbed, has been used for this purpose by some centers.

Antibiotic prophylaxis

There is no evidence that infection is prevented by giving antibiotics to high-risk infants who are not infected. There is also no evidence that antibiotic prophylaxis is required for patients with respiratory distress syndrome or for neonates during and subsequent to exchange transfusion. Prophylaxis, however, is indicated for the prevention of gonococcal ophthalmitis.

Artificial bacterial colonization

The deliberate introduction of a nonvirulent strain of a microorganism to prevent colonization with virulent strains has been recommended and in some nurseries has proved effective in aborting epidemic bacterial infection in the newborn. Deliberate introduction of nonvirulent strains of coagulase-positive staphylococci in the nose and colonization of the umbilicus shortly after birth have been utilized. Infections have been reported that were related to the nonvirulent staphylococci introduced in this manner, suggesting that application of this technique may be hazardous and should be limited to selected and carefully controlled situations.

Care of the umbilicus

The umbilicus is a direct portal of entry to the bloodstream and also serves as a site from which other areas of the skin may become contaminated or colonized. In instances where the cord will not be used for arterial or venous catheterization, the application of triple dye to reduce bacterial colonization is recommended.

Resuscitation and ventilation equipment

Gram-negative microorganisms, particularly *Pseudomonas*, *Aeromonas*, and *Serratia*, have produced both sporadic and epidemic infection in the neonatal unit. Culturing of medications, nebulizers, and inhalation therapy equipment should be performed routinely, and equipment should be changed frequently to prevent such infections. Use of umbilical, arterial, and venous catheters as well as intravenous catheters for parenteral alimentation also has been accompanied by an increased risk of opportunistic infection. Meticulous care is

required in the preparation of solutions for use in total parenteral alimentation and in the insertion and care of catheters. Administration of fluids should be discontinued if signs of inflammation, thrombosis, or purulence are observed. When bacteremia related to intravenous therapy is noted, discontinuation of therapy is imperative; continued infusion of the suspect infusate under coverage of antimicrobials has not altered the course of infection. All apparatus used for intravenous administration should be replaced daily and when infusion devices are changed to decrease the hazard of extrinsic contamination.

Ralph D. Feigin
Deborah L. Callanan

BIBLIOGRAPHY
Neonatal septicemia

Baker, C.J., and others: Suppurative meningitis due to streptococci of Lancefield group B: a study of 33 infants, J. Pediatr. **82**:724, 1973.
Blanc, W.A.: Pathways of fetal and early neonatal infection, J. Pediatr. **59**:473, 1961.
Bobo, R.A., and others: Nursery outbreak of *Pseudomonas aeruginosa*: epidemiological conclusions from five different typing methods, Appl. Microbiol. **25**:414, 1973.
Eichenwald, H.: Antibiotics and the newborn, Hosp. Pract. **2**:51, 1967.
Fetter, B.F., Klintworth, G.H., and Hendry, W.S.: Mycoses of the central nervous system, Baltimore, 1967, The Williams & Wilkins Co.
Geil, C.C., Castle, W.K., and Mortomer, E.A., Jr.: Group A streptococcal infections in newborn nurseries, Pediatrics **46**:849, 1970.
Gotoff, S.P., and Behrman, R.E.: Neonatal septicemia, J. Pediatr. **76**:142, 1970.
Hable, K.A., and others: *Klebsiella* type 33 septicemia in an infant intensive care unit, J. Pediatr. **80**:920, 1972.
Kaplan, J.M., and others: Pharmacologic studies in neonates given large doses of ampicillin, J. Pediatr. **84**:571, 1974.
Knittle, M.A., Etizman, D.V., and Baer, H.: Role of hand contamination of personnel in the epidemiology of gram-negative nosocomial infections, J. Pediatr. **86**:433, 1975.
Laurenti, F., and others: Polymorphonuclear leukocyte transfusion for the treatment of sepsis in the newborn infant, J. Pediatr. **98**:118, 1981.
Lee, Y., and others: The genital mycoplasmas: their role in disorders of reproduction and in pediatric infections, Pediatr. Clin. North Am. **21**:457, 1974.
McCracken, G.H., Jr., Chrane, D.F., and Thomas, M.L.: Pharmacologic evaluation of gentamicin in newborn infants, J. Infect. Dis. **124**:8214, 1971.
McCracken, G.H., Jr., and Eichenwald, H.F.: Antimicrobial therapy: therapeutic recommendations and a review of newer drugs. II. The clinical pharmacology of penicillin in newborn infants, J. Pediatr. **82**:692, 1973.
McCracken, G.H., and Mize, S.G.: A controlled study of intrathecal antibiotic therapy in gram-negative enteric meningitis of infancy, J. Pediatr. **89**:66, 1976.
Okada, D.M., Chow, A.W., and Bruce, V.T.: Neonatal scalp abscess and fetal monitoring: factors associated with infection, Am. J. Obstet. Gynecol. **129**:185, 1977.
Overbach, A.M., Daniel, S.J., and Cassady, G.: The value of umbilical cord histology in the management of potential perinatal infection, J. Pediatr. **76**:22, 1970.
Pryles, C.V., and others: A controlled study of the influence on the newborn of prolonged premature rupture of the amniotic membranes and/or infection in the mother, Pediatrics **31**:608, 1963.
Yeung, C.Y., Lee, V.W.Y., and Yeung, M.B.: Glucose disappearance rate in neonatal infection, J. Pediatr. **82**:486, 1973.

Specific infectious diseases

Bazay, G.R., and others: *Pneumocystis carinii* pneumonia in three full-term siblings, J. Pediatr. **5**:767, 1970.
Bland, R.D.: Otitis media in the first six weeks of life: diagnosis, bacteriology, and management, Pediatrics **49**:187, 1972.
Edwards, M.S., and others: An etiologic shift in infantile osteomyelitis: the emergence of the group B streptococcus, J. Pediatr. **93**:578, 1978.
Esterly, N.B., and Solomon, L.M.: Neonatal dermatology. II. The blistering and scaling dermatoses, J. Pediatr. **77**:1075, 1970.
Forshall, I.: Septic umbilical arteritis, Arch. Dis. Child. **32**:25, 1957.
Goscienski, P.J.: Inclusion conjunctivitis in the newborn infant, J. Pediatr. **77**:19, 1970.
Haltalin, K.C.: Neonatal shigellosis: report of 16 cases and review of the literature, Am. J. Dis. Child. **114**:603, 1967.
Kaslow, R.A., and others: Enteropathogenic *Eschericia coli* infection in a newborn nursery, Am. J. Dis. Child. **128**:797, 1974.
Kohl, S.: *Yersinia enterocolitica*: a significant "new" pathogen, Hosp. Pract. **13**:81, 1978.
Leake, D., and Leake, R.: Neonatal suppurative parotitis, Pediatrics **46**:203, 1970.
McCracken, G.H., Jr., and Sarff, L.D.: Current status and therapy of neonatal *E. coli* meningitis, Hosp. Pract. **10**:57, 1974.
Naeye, R.L., Dellinger, W.S., and Blanc, W.A.: Fetal and maternal features of antenatal bacterial infections, J. Pediatr. **9**:733, 1971.
Nelson, J.D.: Antibiotic concentrations in septic joint effusions, N. Engl. J. Med. **284**:349, 1971.
Overall, J.C., Jr.: Neonatal bacterial meningitis, J. Pediatr. **76**:499, 1970.
Pederson, P.V., and others: Necrotising enterocolitis of the newborn—is it gas gangrene of the bowel? Lancet **2**:715, 1976.
Pittard, W.B., Thullen, J.D., and Fanaroff, A.A.: Neonatal septic arthritis, J. Pediatr. **88**:621, 1976.
Prophylaxis of gonococcal ophthalmitis, The Medical Letter **12**:37, 1970.
Robbins, J.B., and others: *Escherichia coli* K1 capsular polysaccharide associated with neonatal meningitis, N. Engl. J. Med. **290**:1215, 1974.
Sarff, L.D., Platt, L.H., and McCracken, G.H., Jr.: Cerebrospinal fluid evaluation in neonates: comparison of high risk infants with and without meningitis, J. Pediatr. **88**:473, 1976.
Shurin, P.A., and others: Bacterial etiology of otitis media during the first six weeks of life, J. Pediatr. **92**:893, 1978.
Tetzlaff, T.R., Ashworth, C., and Nelson, J.D.: Otitis media in children less than 12 weeks of age, Pediatrics **59**:827, 1977.
Torphy, D.E., and Bond, W.W.: *Campylobacter fetus* infections in children, Pediatrics **64**:898, 1979.
Ulshen, M.H., and Rollo, J.L.: Pathogenesis of *E. coli* gastroenteritis in man—another mechanism, N. Engl. J. Med. **302**:99, 1980.
Weissberg, E.D., Smith, A.L., and Smith, D.H.: Clinical features of neonatal osteomyelitis, Pediatrics **53**:505, 1974.

Specific bacterial infections

Albritton, W.L., Wiggins, G.L., and Feeley, J.C.: Neonatal listeriosis: distribution of serotypes, J. Pediatr. **88**:481, 1976.
Alexander, R.R.: Chlamydia: the organism and neonatal infection, Hosp. Pract. **14**:63, 1979.
Baker, C.J.: Group B streptococcal infections in neonates, Pediatr. **64**:P1R5, 1979.

Baker, C.J., and others: Suppurative meningitis due to streptococci of Lancefield group B: a study of 33 infants, J. Pediatr. **82:**724, 1973.

Chow, A.W., and others: The significance of anaerobes in neonatal bacteremia: analysis of 23 cases and review of the literature, Pediatrics **54:**736, 1974.

Franciosi, R.A., Knostman, J.D., and Zimmerman, R.M.: Group B streptococcal neonatal and infant infections, J. Pediatr. **82:**707, 1973.

Handsfield, H.H., Hodson, W.A., and Holmes, K.K.: Neonatal gonococcal infection, J.A.M.A. **225:**697, 1973.

Holder, W.R., and Knox, J.M.: Syphilis in pregnancy, Med. Clin. North Am. **56:**1151, 1972.

Hood, M., Janney, A., and Dameron, G.: Beta-hemolytic streptococcus Group B associated with problems of the perinatal period, Am. J. Obstet. Gynecol. **82:**809, 1961.

Horn, K.A., and others: Group B streptococcal neonatal infection, J.A.M.A. **230:**1165, 1974.

Horn, K.A., and others: Neurological sequelae of group B streptococcal neonatal infection, Pediatrics **53:**501, 1974.

Howard, J.B., and McCracken, G.H., Jr.: The spectrum of group B streptococcal infections in infancy, Am. J. Dis. Child. **128:**815, 1974.

Kendig, E.L., Jr.: The place of BCG vaccine in the management of infants born to tuberculous mothers, N. Engl. J. Med. **281:**520, 1969.

Klesius, P.H., and others: Cellular and humoral immune response to group B streptococci, J. Pediatr. **83:**926, 1973.

Koutsoulieris, E., and Koslaris, E.: Congenital tuberculosis, Arch. Dis. Child. **45:**584, 1970.

Litt, I.F., Edberg, S.C., and Finberg, L.: Gonorrhea in children and adolescents: a current review, J. Pediatr. **85:**595, 1974.

McCracken, G.H., Jr., Dowell, D.L., and Marshall, F.N.: Double blind trial of equine antitoxin and human immune globulin in tetanus neonatorum, Lancet **1:**1146, 1971.

McCracken, G.H., Jr., and Kaplan, J.M.: Penicillin treatment for congenital syphilis, J.A.M.A. **228:**855, 1974.

Pinheiro, D.: Tetanus of the newborn infant, Pediatrics **34:**32, 1964.

Ray, C.G., and Wedgwood, R.J.: Neonatal listeriosis, Pediatrics **34:**378, 1964.

Rosen, E.V., and Richardson, J.N.: A reappraisal of the value of the IgM fluorescent treponemal antibody absorption test in the diagnosis of congenital syphilis, J. Pediatr. **87:**38, 1975.

Russell, P., and Altshuler, G.: Placental abnormalities of congenital syphilis, Am. J. Dis. Child. **128:**160, 1974.

Siegel, J.D., and others: Single-dose penicillin prophylaxis against neonatal group B streptococcal infections, N. Engl. J. Med. **303:**769, 1980.

Yow, M.D., and others: Ampicillin prevents intrapartum transmission of group B streptococcus, J.A.M.A. **241:**1245, 1979.

Specific viral infections

Angella, J.J., and Connor, J.D.: Neonatal infection caused by adenovirus type 7, J. Pediatr. **72:**474, 1968.

Bauer, C.R., and others: Hong Kong influenza in a neonatal unit, J.A.M.A. **223:**1233, 1973.

Berkovich, S., and Smithwick, E.M.: Transplacental infection due to ECHO virus, type 22, J. Pediatr. **72:**94, 1968.

Burch, G.E., and others: Interstitial and Coxsackie B myocarditis in infants and children, J.A.M.A. **20:**55, 1968.

DeNicola, L.K., and Hanshaw, J.B.: Congenital and neonatal varicella, J. Pediatr. **94:**175, 1979.

Gear, J.H.S.: Coxsackie infections of the newborn, Prog. Med. Virol. **15:**42, 1973.

Gersony, W.M., Katz, S.L., and Nadas, A.S.: Endocardial fibroelastosis and the mumps virus, Pediatrics **37:**430, 1966.

Hakosalo, J., and Saxen, L.: Influenza epidemic and congenital defects, Lancet **2:**1346, 1971.

Johnson, R.T., and Johnson, K.P.: Hydrocephalus following viral infection: the pathology of aqueductal stenosis developing after experimental mumps virus infection, J. Neuropathol. Exp. Neurol. **27:**591, 1968.

Joncas, J., and others: Epstein-Barr virus infection in the neonatal period and in childhood, Can. Med. Assoc. J. **110:**33, 1974.

Newman, C.G.H.: Perinatal varicella, Lancet **2:**1159, 1965.

Overall, J.C., Jr., and Glasgow, L.A.: Virus infections of the fetus and newborn infant, J. Pediatr. **77:**315, 1970.

Sells, C.J., Carpenter, R.L., and Ray, C.G.: Sequelae of central nervous system enterovirus infections, N. Engl. J. Med. **293:**1, 1975.

Sharma, R., Sharma, R., and Jagler, D.K.: Congenital smallpox, Scand. J. Infect. Dis. **3:**245, 1971.

Siegel, M.: Congenital malformation following chickenpox, measles, mumps, and hepatitis: results of a cohort study, J.A.M.A. **226:**1521, 1972.

Yahn, D.H., Pyeatte, J.C., and Joseph, J.M.: Transplacental transfer of influenza virus, J.A.M.A. **216:**1025, 1971.

Specific fungal infections

Dvorak, A.M., and Gavaller, B.: Congenital systemic candidiasis: report of a case, N. Engl. J. Med. **274:**540, 1966.

Emanuel, B., and others: *Cryptococcus* meningitis in a child successfully treated with amphotericin B, with a review of the pediatric literature, J. Pediatr. **59:**577, 1961.

Holland, P., and Holland, N.H.: Histoplasmosis in early infancy, Am. J. Dis. Child. **112:**412, 1966.

Hyatt, H.W.: Coccidioidomycosis in a 3-week-old infant, Am. J. Dis. Child. **105:**93, 1963.

Kozinn, P.J., and Taschdjian, C.L.: Enteric candidiasis: diagnosis and clinical considerations, Pediatrics **30:**71, 1962.

Kozinn, P.J., and others: Neonatal candidiasis, Pediatr. Clin. North Am. **5:**803, 1958.

Schirar, A., and others: Congenital mycosis (*Candida albicans*), Biol. Neonate **24:**273, 1974.

Smale, L.E., and Waechter, K.G.: Dissemination of coccidioidomycosis in pregnancy, Am. J. Obstet. Gynecol. **107:**356, 1970.

Specific parasitic infections

Covell, G.: Congenital malaria, Trop. Dis. Bull. **47:**1147, 1950.

Harvey, B., Remington, J.S., and Sulzer, A.J.: IgM malaria antibodies in a case of congenital malaria in the United States, Lancet **1:**333, 1969.

Robbins, J.B.: Immunological and clinicopathological aspects of *Pneumocystis carinii* pneumonitis. In Bergsma, D., and Good, R.A., editors: Immunologic deficiency diseases in man, New York, 1968, The National Foundation, p. 219.

Williams, A.I.O., and McFarlane, H.: Distribution of malarial antibody in maternal and cord sera, Arch. Dis. Child. **44:**511, 1969.

Prevention of infection

Drutz, D.J., and others: Bacterial interference in the therapy of recurrent staphylococcal infections: multiple abscesses due to the implantation of the 502A strain of *Staphylococcus*, N. Engl. J. Med. **275:**1161, 1966.

Ehrenkranz, N.J.: Bacterial colonization of newborn infants and subsequent acquisition of hospital bacteria, J. Pediatr. **76:**839, 1970.

Geil, C.C., Castle, W.K., and Mortimer, E.A.: Group A streptococcal infections in newborn nurseries, Pediatrics **46:**849, 1970.

Gezon, H.M., and others: Hexachlorophene bathing in early infancy: effect on staphyloccal disease and infection, N. Engl. J. Med. **270:**379, 1964.

Gluck, L., and Wood, H.F.: Effect of an antiseptic skin-care regimen in reducing staphylococcal colonization in newborn infants, N. Engl. J. Med. 265:1177, 1961.

Hurst, V., and Grossman, M.: The hospital nursery as a source of staphylococcal disease among families of newborn infants, N. Engl. J. Med. 262:951, 1960.

Light, I.J., and others: Ecologic relation between *Staphylococcus aureus* and *Pseudomonas* in a nursery population: another example of bacterial interference, N. Engl. J. Med. 278:1243, 1968.

Lockhart, J.D.: How toxic is hexachlorophene? Pediatrics 50:229, 1972.

Mortimer, E.A., Wolinsky, E., and Hines, D.: The effect of rooming-in on the acquisition of hospital staphylococci by newborn infants, Pediatrics 37:605, 1966.

Shuman, R.M., Leech, R.W., and Alvord, E.C.: Neuropathology in newborn infants bathed with hexachlorophene, Morbid Mortal. 22:93, March 17, 1973.

Williams, C.P.S., and Oliver, T.K.: Nursery routines and staphylococcal colinization of the newborn, Pediatrics 44:640, 1969.

CHAPTER 28 # Viral and protozoal perinatal infections

Although the fetus and newborn are highly susceptible to a number of viral and protozoal infections, relatively few of the hundreds of viruses and several protozoa that parasitize humans are transmitted to the fetus or are a significant cause of morbidity or mortality in the neonatal period. However, it is increasingly apparent that certain viruses and protozoa do have a predilection for the fetus and may cause abortion, stillbirth, intrauterine infection, congenital malformations, acute disease during the neonatal period, or chronic infection with subtle manifestations that may be recognized only after a prolonged period. It is important to recognize the manifestations of viral and protozoal infections in the neonatal period not only to diagnose the acute infection but also because of the potential implication for the subsequent growth and development of the infant. Furthermore, chemotherapeutic agents for some viruses and therapy for toxoplasmosis are being developed or are undergoing clinical trials. In addition, compounds may become available in the not too distant future that offer hope for amelioration of other viral infections of the newborn. It is evident that appropriate treatment will require specific etiologic and diagnostic studies of the infection.

PATHOGENESIS OF INFECTIONS DURING PREGNANCY

During gestation the fetus depends on the sterile environment of the uterus and the integrity of the placenta to provide protection from infection. Maternal infections are the primary source of exposure for the human fetus and in many circumstances for the newborn. The viral or parasitic agents that have been associated with fetal and infant morbidity or mortality are summarized in Table 28-1. Although some of these agents may produce a recognized clinical illness in the mother, others cause only a subclinical, asymptomatic maternal infection. Fig. 28-1 illustrates the interaction of the virus, mother, and fetus or newborn and the possible outcome of this interaction. Most maternal viral infections are confined to the surface of the respiratory or gastrointestinal tract. These limited infections are not associated with viremia, infection of the placenta, or involvement of the fetus. The fact that the majority of the viral illnesses acquired by pregnant women fall into the category of a mild, localized infection probably explains the low frequency of identifiable intrauterine viral disease. On the other hand, both a clinically recognized infection such as rubella or a subclinical one such as cytomegalovirus (CMV) may spread systemically, infect and replicate in or cross the placenta, and then spread to involve the fetus. A similar situation exists with toxoplasmosis, where the majority of maternal infections are also subclinical, but the organism can be found in the placental tissues of involved fetuses.

Transplacental passage of the parasite is strongly suggested in most infections where disease is found in the infant at the time of or shortly after delivery. The development of methods for identifying IgM antibody produced by the fetus against a specific agent and present in the newborn at delivery has provided a means of documenting intrauterine spread of the maternal viral infection. Furthermore, evidence suggests that direct infection and replication of the parasite in the placenta are the likely sequence of events in the pathogenesis of rubella, vaccinia, varicella, *Toxoplasma* organism, and CMV infections. At present there is no identifiable characteristic of a virus that can be associated with its capacity to cross the placenta. Although Monif has pointed out the similarities in the group of viruses that may initiate infection in the fetus and the central nervous system (CNS), this analogy is limited; CMV, for example, rarely crosses

Table 28-1. Viral and parasitic agents associated with fetal and infant morbidity or mortality

Pathogen	Fetus	Neonatal disease	Congenital defects	Late sequelae
Cytomegalovirus	—	Low birth weight, anemia, thrombocytopenia, hepatosplenomegaly, jaundice, encephalitis	Microcephaly, microphthalmia, retinopathy	Deafness, psychomotor retardation, cerebral calcifications
Rubella virus	Abortion	Low birth weight, hepatosplenomegaly, petechiae, osteitis	Heart defects, microcephaly, cataracts, microphthalmia	Deafness, mental retardation, thyroid disorders, diabetes, degenerative brain tissue, autism
Hepatitis B virus	—	Asymptomatic HB Ag–positive infection, low birth weight, rarely acute hepatitis	—	Chronic hepatitis, persistent HB Ag positive, fulminant hepatitis
Toxoplasma gondii	Abortion	Low birth weight, hepatosplenomegaly, jaundice, anemia	Hydrocephalus, microcephaly	Chorioretinitis, mental retardation
Varicella-zoster virus	—	Low birth weight, chorioretinitis, congenital chickenpox or disseminated neonatal varicella, possibly zoster	Limb hypoplasia, cortical atrophy, cicatricial skin lesions	Fatal outcome because of secondary infection
Picornaviruses				
Coxsackie virus	Abortion	Aseptic meningitis, disseminated disease	Possible association with congenital heart disease, myocarditis	
ECHO virus	—	Multiple organ involvement (CNS, liver, heart), gastroenteritis		
Poliovirus	Abortion	Congenital poliomyelitis		
Herpes simplex virus	Abortion	Disseminated disease, multiple organ involvement (lung, liver, CNS), vesicular skin lesions, retinopathy	Microcephaly, retinopathy, intracranial calcifications	Neurologic deficits
Western equine encephalitis virus	—	Congenital encephalitis	—	
Measles virus	Abortion	Congenital measles	—	
Vaccinia virus	Abortion	Congenital vaccinia	—	
Variola virus (Chapter 27)	Abortion	Congenital variola		
Mumps virus	Abortion	—	Possible association with endocardial fibroelastosis	
Influenza virus	Possible abortion	—	—	—
Malaria (Chapter 27)		Hepatosplenomegaly, jaundice, anemia, fever, poor feeding, vomiting		

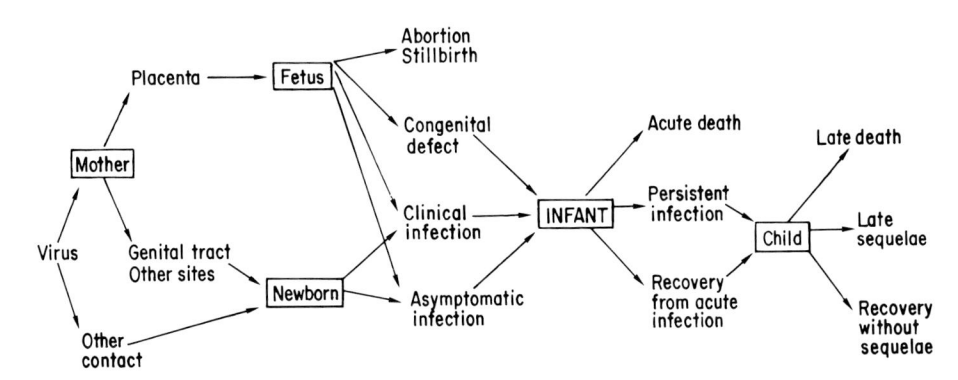

Fig. 28-1. Pathogenesis of viral infections in the fetus and newborn. (From Overall, J.C., Jr.: Viral infections of the fetus and neonate. In Feigin, R.D., and Cherry, J.D., editors: Textbook of pediatric infectious diseases, Philadelphia, 1981, W.B. Saunders Co.)

the blood-brain barrier in adults, although it may cross the placenta and invade the fetus.

The usual sequence of events is maternal viral infection, viremia, infection of placenta, and spread to fetus. Viral agents also may be transmitted to the newborn at the time of delivery or in the postpartum period. Both the type-2 strain of herpes simplex virus and CMV are examples of viruses that frequently are isolated from the genital tract during pregnancy, often in the absence of any signs of maternal disease, and may be transmitted directly to the infant at the time of delivery, particularly if there is premature rupture of the membranes. Enterovirus infections, particularly with Coxsackie and, as recognized more recently, ECHO viruses, have been associated with severe disseminated infections in the neonate. Both have occurred in infants born to mothers with clinical illness around the time of delivery and were presumably transmitted at delivery or in the postpartum period (p. 679). A similar situation applies for hepatitis B where viral antigen has been found in amniotic fluid, vaginal secretions, and maternal blood. Varicella-zoster virus may be acquired congenitally by an infant born to a mother with an active varicella infection, or the contact may occur after delivery when the mother is still in the contagious phase of the disease. Since it is often difficult to determine if transplacental transmission occurred prior to delivery, temporary separation of the infant and the mother may be warranted in those situations where the maternal disease is still contagious and infection poses a potentially serious threat to the neonate.

The fetus may manifest a variety of outcomes of the host-parasite interaction, such as congenital rubella, varicella, and CMV infection (Fig. 28-1). Alternatively, the fetus may manifest no overt evidence of infection, as is the usual case with congenital toxoplasmosis. Unfortunately the host-parasite interaction that results in subclinical or inapparent infection may be associated with persistence of the agent and in some circumstances with late sequelae, including hearing loss, mental retardation, and even more serious degenerative disease of the CNS. Such long-range effects from asymptomatic congenital infection are now recognized in infants with CMV, rubella, and toxoplasma infections. Finally, fetal death, abortion, or stillbirth is associated with maternal infections that occur during the first trimester of pregnancy. Although an organism may be isolated from the products of conception in some circumstances, this is not always the case. In this latter situation fetal death also could be the result of maternal illness possibly associated with fever, toxins, metabolic alterations, or vascular changes. The fetus thus is one part of a parasite-mother-fetus relationship. The nature of the infection, the degree of resistance of the mother, and the stage of development of the fetus are all determinants of the outcome of the interaction.

FREQUENCY OF INFECTIONS

A number of factors can influence the frequency of maternal infection and thus are determinants of involvement of the fetus. Most congenital infections occur during primary infection in the mother. In the case of CMV severe disease occurs in the fetus during primary maternal infections. However, subsequent infants born to the same mother may acquire CMV during a reactivation of recurrence of the viral infection. In contrast, congenital rubella syndrome does not occur in infants born to immune mothers. Transplacental hepatitis B is also more likely to occur during a primary maternal infection, as are toxoplasmosis and the rare occurrences of congenital chickenpox, measles, smallpox, or enterovirus infections. On the other hand, organisms such as herpes simplex virus, CMV, and hepatitis B, which may be acquired at the time of delivery, are commonly present as chronic or reactivated latent infections in the mother.

A major factor that influences the outcome of an infection in utero is the gestational age of the fetus at the time of exposure. In the congenital rubella syndrome as many as 85% of infants born to mothers who had rubella during the second month of pregnancy have malformations. This decreases to 14% to 25% if the exposure occurred during the third month and to 6% to 17% with infection in the fourth month. A similar effect of gestational age also is observed in CMV and varicella-zoster virus infections, although this is less well documented because of the asymptomatic nature of most CMV infections and the infrequent occurrence of varicella during pregnancy. In contrast, a third-trimester maternal infection with *Toxoplasma* organisms has a greater probability of being transmitted to the fetus, but the infection frequently results in milder or subclinical infection in the infant. However, maternal toxoplasma infection during the first or second trimester is less frequently transmitted to the fetus but is more likely to result in serious clinical manifestations when the fetus in involved. Similarly the transplacental transmission of hepatitis B also appears to be more frequent when acute maternal disease occurs in the third trimester.

A number of social and environmental factors also influence the incidence of maternal infection and therefore the frequency of fetal and neonatal disease. The development of virus vaccines has had a major impact during recent years; smallpox has been eradicated, and the use of the vaccinia virus vaccine has been discontinued; rubella vaccines have eliminated major rubella epidemics and significantly decreased the occurrence of rubella in women of childbearing age. The other viral vaccines—measles, mumps, and poliomyelitis—almost have eliminated the risk of these diseases during pregnancy. The question remains, however, whether waning immunity in an adult population immunized as infants

Table 28-2. Approximate frequency of viral and protozoal infections in the mother during pregnancy and in the newborn

Infectious agent	Mother (number per 1,000 pregnancies)	Neonate (number per 1,000 live births)
Cytomegalovirus		
During pregnancy, congenital	10-70	6-34
At delivery, natal	30-130	20-70
Rubella virus		
1964 Epidemic	20-40	3-7
Interepidemic, prevaccine	0.1-2	0.1-0.7
After vaccine	0.03-0.7	0.03-0.2
Hepatitis B virus	1-160	0-61
Herpes simplex virus	1-10	0.03-0.3
Toxoplasma gondii	1-10	0.03-1

may predispose them to the occurrence of these former childhood diseases during the childbearing years.

Ethnic and socioeconomic factors also exert an influence. Mothers of oriental extraction have a significantly higher rate of chronic HB_sAg and HB_eAg carriage. This results in a higher frequency of natal and postnatal hepatitis B infection in their offspring. CMV infection appears to be more common in lower socioeconomic groups, and social factors such as drug abuse and sexual promiscuity contribute to the incidence of hepatitis, CMV, and genital herpes.

Finally, the frequency of *recognized* infection is dependent on the method of indentification of involved infants. Since most congenital CMV, rubella, toxoplasmic, and hepatitis B infections are asymptomatic in the neonatal period, clinical case-finding methods alone clearly will underestimate the true frequency of infection. Epidemiologic observations (e.g., rubella or enterovirus epidemic in the community), clinical or laboratory information from the mother (e.g., viral illness with a rash or presence of HB_sAg in the serum), or screening tests in the newborn (e.g., elevated quantitative IgM in cord blood serum) often have been used to select a group of neonates at high risk of congenital or neonatal infection. The performance of additional laboratory tests in these high-risk neonates to identify potential specific causative agents has led in many instances to the demonstration of infection rates much higher than previously suspected.

The data reported in Table 28-2 have been obtained by a variety of methods, and some are based on relatively small population samples. Nevertheless they still provide an estimate of the relative frequency of the various infections.

Cytomegalovirus infection

CMV infection is diagnosed by means of virus isolation from urine specimens and cervical swabs in pregnant women or by the demonstration of specific anti-CMV IgM in the cord blood serum of the neonate. Surveys indicate that 10 to 40 per 1,000 women excrete virus in the urine during pregnancy and that 30 to 60 per 1,000 are excreters at the time of delivery. Isolation from cervical swabs is more common; the virus is recovered from 10 to 70 per 1,000 women during pregnancy and up to 130 per 1,000 at delivery. The rate of recovery from both the urine and the cervix increases during pregnancy. It is not possible, however, to estimate the frequency of clinical disease during pregnancy, since CMV infection is usually asymptomatic.

Congenital infection of the neonate has been documented to occur in 6 to 34 per 1,000 live births, as evidenced by the isolation of virus from urine specimens obtained from newborns in the first 24 hours of life. Specific IgM antibody against CMV has been demonstrated in cord blood serum in 6 per 1,000 live births. The newborn also may acquire CMV infection at the time of birth from the mother who has virus present in her cervical secretions, presumably by aspiration of the infected secretions. The rate of perinatal infection has been estimated to be about 20 per 1,000 live births. On the other hand, approximately 50% of infants born to a mother with known CMV genital tract infection acquire a natal infection, and, since up to 130 per 1,000 women in lower socioeconomic groups may excrete the virus at the time of delivery, the actual frequency of perinatal CMV infection may be as high as 60 to 70 per 1,000 in some populations.

Rubella

The use of the rubella vaccine is modifying the epidemiologic patterns of this disease in the United States, and the data available from periods before development of the vaccine may not be applicable in the future. As a guideline, however, earlier information indicates that the frequency of serologically proved clinical rubella among 30,000 pregnant women in the Collaborative Perinatal Research Study was approximately 1 per 1,000 during nonepidemic years but rose to 22 per 1,000 during the 1964 rubella epidemic. The total figure for rubella during pregnancy, however, is likely to be at least twice as high, since as many as half to two thirds of maternal rubella infections are subclinical or are not diagnosed as rubella. An incidence of congenital rubella of 0.7 per 1,000 live births was demonstrated in a study screening cord blood sera for the presence of rubella-specific IgM antibody. During the 1964 epidemic there were an estimated 20,000 babies born with congenital rubella syndrome in the United States, or approximately 5 per 1,000 live births. The current frequency of congenital rubella infection clearly has been modified by the use of the rubella vaccine. In contrast to the experience during 1964, only 23 to 77 cases of congenital rubella syndrome were reported annually in the United States from 1970 to 1979. It is estimated that the frequency of malformations in infants is highest when the maternal infection occurs early in pregnancy. After the first trimester maternal rubella may result in fetal loss or in infants with neurologic sequelae, but the precise frequency is not known.

Hepatitis B virus

In neonates hepatitis B virus is currently the major concern. Hepatitis A does not appear to be transmitted across the placenta and therefore is not a problem. Although evidence suggests that non–A, non–B hepatitis may be transmitted from mother to child, particularly during an acute infection in the third trimester of pregnancy, adequate data are not available to define the magnitude of the problem at the present. Hepatitis B virus (serum hepatitis) is associated with acute symptomatic or asymptomatic infections, chronic infections, or an asymptomatic carrier state. The serum from an infected individual may contain pleomorphic spherical particles 20 to 22 nm in diameter, filamentous forms that are also 20 to 22 nm in diameter, and Dane particles (42 nm in diameter), which are thought to be the complete virion. The presence of the hepatitis virus or viral antigens can be detected in the serum of infected individuals by a variety of immunologic methods. HB_sAg is the surface antigen of the virus. HB_cAg is a virus-specific antigen that is thought to be the internal component of the Dane particle. Patients who have recovered from hepatitis B usually have antibody directed either against the surface and/or core antigen. Another hepatitis B virus antigen, the e antigen, has been described. Although HB_eAg has not been fully characterized, it is found in the sera of some HB_sAg-positive individuals, and its presence in maternal sera has been associated with transmission of hepatitis B to the neonate. Antibody also may develop against the e antigen, and the presence of anti-HB_e in serum of the mother is correlated with lack of transmission of the infection to her offspring. The most commonly used tests to identify HB_sAg in the serum are radioimmunoassay and counterimmunoelectrophoresis.

During pregnancy the hepatitis B virus may produce acute clinical disease in the mother, or the antigen may be present in the serum of mothers who are chronic asymptomatic carriers (HB_sAg positive). The frequency of occurrence of HB_sAg in the serum of pregnant women is highly variable and is influenced by the socioeconomic status, ethnic origin, and geographic location of the population surveyed. In the United States 0.1% to 0.3% of the general population are carriers. The prevalence may increase in multiply transfused patients (3.8%), drug addicts (4.2%), and Asians, particularly Chinese (2.5% to 15%).

The frequency of HB_sAg in the neonate is even more variable and is dependent on the population studied. Vertical transmission of infection from mother to fetus or infant may occur by the following routes: (1) transplacental, either during pregnancy or at the time of delivery secondary to leaks in the placenta, (2) during delivery by exposure to amniotic fluid, vaginal secretions, or maternal blood containing HB_sAg, and (3) after birth by fecal-oral spread or ingestion of breast milk. HB_sAg has been demonstrated in the cord blood at delivery, in breast milk of maternal carriers, and in the gastric contents of infants born to carrier mothers.

Differences in the time of exposure, the route of inoculation, and the size of the viral inoculum may explain the wide variation in the time of onset of antigenemia in the infected neonate. An onset of antigenemia prior to 2 months of age suggests an exposure in utero. An onset from 2 to 5 months is compatible with infection at the time of delivery, whereas infants who contract the infection postnatally may become HB_sAg positive after 6 months. In mothers known to be HB_sAg carriers at the time of delivery, antigen has been shown to be present in cord sera in from none to 43% of the newborns. The presence of antigen in the cord blood does not necessarily indicate infection, and such infants may clear HB_sAg and never develop any further evidence of either antigen or antibody. Most series from populations in the United States or Western Europe, however, indicate a very low rate of vertical transmission. In one study of 18 children born to European HB_sAg carrier mothers, none of the infants developed clinical evidence of hepatitis, none became chronic carriers, and the three who became transiently HB_sAg positive did so after 6 months of age. Importantly, none of the mothers were HB_eAg positive. In contrast, a study of Chinese women showed that 40% of 158 infants born to HB_sAg carriers developed HB_sAg or anti-Hb_s in their sera during infancy, and 22% became chronic carriers. A different situation exists, however, when a woman develops acute hepatitis during pregnancy. Unlike CMV and rubella, maternal hepatitis B infection has not been associated with an increased incidence of abortion, stillbirth, congenital malformations, or intrauterine growth retardation. Also unlike rubella, the risk of infection of the fetus when maternal infection occurs in the first two trimesters is low but increases during the third trimester, as evidenced by the presence of HB$_s$Ag in the neonates' serum. Schweitzer and associates reported the occurrence of neonatal infection in only 1 of 10 babies born to mothers who had hepatitis in the first two trimesters but in 16 of 21 (76%) when the illness occurred in the third trimester or during the first 2 months after delivery.

Infants born to mothers with hepatitis may follow one of five courses, which are discussed under clinical manifestations. Of those infants who are infected either at the time of delivery or during the early neonatal period, most show no signs of acute illness but may remain chronic carriers for long periods. Liver function studies, however, may be abnormal in some of these infants, and liver biopsies may show evidence of mild unresolved hepatitis. A small number of infants who acquire hepatitis transplacentally or around the time of delivery may develop acute icteric hepatitis, usually followed by recovery and development of antibody. The long-term outcome of asymptomatic infants with persistent antigenemia is not known at the current time. A few infants will have clinical and/or biochemical evidence of chronic liver disease. Death from fulminant hepatitis B virus infection in the neonate or young infant is rare but has occurred, particularly in successive children born to the same chronic carrier mother.

Toxoplasmosis

Maternal infection with the parasite *Toxoplasma gondii* is usually asymptomatic. Only 15% of French women with serologic evidence of toxoplasmosis during pregnancy manifested clinical disease, usually a mild febrile illness with cervical adenopathy. Among 23,617 pregnant women analyzed by the Collaborative Perinatal Research Study in the United States, 6.4 per 1,000 developed an infection with *Toxoplasma* organisms, as evidenced by a rise in their antibody titer against this organism.

Not all infants born to a mother with evidence of toxoplasmosis during pregnancy become infected. One to three infants per 1,000 live births have IgM antibody directed against this organism, indicating intrauterine infection. The incidence of fetal infection increases throughout pregnancy, but the most severe involvement results from maternal infection occurring during the first and second trimesters. In 180 pregnancies with acquired maternal toxoplasmosis 61% had no evidence of fetal infection, 3% resulted in abortion or stillbirth, and 36% produced an infant with serologic or parasitologic evidence of congenital toxoplasmosis. Of the 64 infants with congenital toxoplasmosis, 11% had severe, 17% had mild, and 72% had subclinical disease in the neonatal period.

Herpes simplex

Infection of the newborn with herpes simplex virus occurs primarily at delivery when the infant passes through the infected genital tract of the mother. There have been, however, several case reports of presumed transplacental transmission of the virus with the birth of a congenitally infected infant. In addition, transmission of the virus to the neonate from extragenital sites in the mother and even from nonmaternal sources has been documented. Since infected infants may have high titers of virus present in lesions or oral secretions, precautions should be taken to prevent spread within the nursery. Approximately 70% of the cases of neonatal herpes infection are caused by the genital, or type 2, strain of herpes simplex virus and the remainder by the oral, or type 1, strain.

Since the virus may be transmitted to the newborn from a variety of sources, it is difficult to provide a true estimate of the frequency. Nahmias and associates have suggested that maternal herpes simplex infection occurs at an incidence of 1 to 10 per 1,000 pregnancies and that the neonatal infection may be seen in 0.1 to 0.5 per 1,000 live births. However, the reported annual incidence of neonatal herpes in the United States (approximately 120 cases) suggests a lower frequency of about 0.03 per 1,000, or about 1 per 30,000 deliveries. Genital herpes infections are more common in lower socioeconomic groups. The frequency of neonatal herpes also is influenced by the time during pregnancy when the maternal infection occurs. The greatest risk of neonatal infection is when the mother has a primary herpetic infection during the last 3 weeks of pregnancy. The presence of clinically recognizable genital herpes at the time of delivery should be considered an indication for cesarean section to prevent acquisition of the virus by the infant during the birth process.

Coxsackie and other viral infections

Serologic evidence of Coxsackie B virus (types 1 to 6) infection during pregnancy has been demonstrated in 9% of a small series of 198 women in the Collaborative Perinatal Research Study. Disseminated Coxsackie B infection of the neonate is rare, but milder forms of disease and asymptomatic infections with Coxsackie viruses as well as a spectrum of disease from mild to severe with ECHO viruses may be more common than has been recognized (p. 680). Maternal mumps, varicella-zoster, and rubella were considerably less frequent among women in the Collaborative Study, and disease in the neonate was a rare event.

Malaria

As a result of the influx of refugees from Southeast Asia, congenital malaria, an extremely rare disease in the United States, is now being seen with increased frequency. In 1980 seven cases were reported. Congenital malaria should be included in the differential diagnosis of systemic infection in infants born to mothers who may have malaria (Chapter 27).

Summary of frequency

Approximately 5% of the 30,000 pregnancies in the Collaborative Study were complicated by at least one definitive or presumed viral infection, excluding the common cold. Most women might be expected to have at least one upper respiratory or gastrointestinal tract infection during any 9-month period. Since the overwhelming majority of viral infections during pregnancy are limited to the respiratory or gastrointestinal tract, these are not likely to represent a threat to the fetus. However, it may not be possible to identify many mild or subclinical viral infections in the mother or newborn. Some of these asymptomatic maternal illnesses still may be associated with infection of the fetus. The role that newly identified viral agents such as the coronaviruses, which cause respiratory tract infections, and the parvoviruses and rotaviruses, which cause gastrointestinal tract infections, may play in causing fetal and neonatal disease is at present unknown (Chapter 27). The precise contribution of viruses and protozoa to abortion, stillbirth, congenital malformation, neonatal infections, and long-term sequelae also remains incompletely defined. In most cases the cause of fetal loss and congenital malformation cannot be determined. With the exception of CMV, herpes simplex, influenza, hepatitis, and toxoplasmosis, the agents listed in Table 28-1 are either rare or are being eliminated because of vaccines. On the basis of current knowledge, then, one would conclude that viruses and protozoa do not play a major role in neonatal morbidity or mortality. Nevertheless the seriousness of many neonatal viral and protozoal infections, together with the future development of antiviral chemotherapy, necessitates that those concerned with the care of newborns be cognizant of the clinical manifestations of these infections.

CLINICAL MANIFESTATIONS
Differential diagnosis

Viral and protozoal infections in the newborn often may have similar clinical findings. It should be reemphasized, however, that the majority of viral and toxoplasmic infections of the neonate are asymptomatic: over 90% of

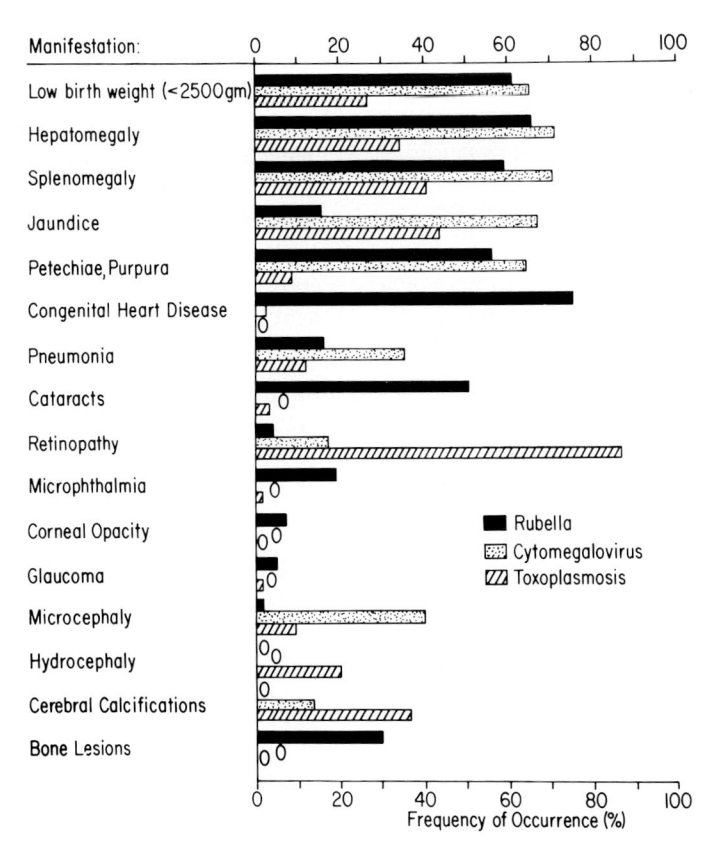

Fig. 28-2. Manifestations of symptomatic congenital rubella and CMV infections and toxoplasmosis in the neonate. (From Overall, J.C., Jr.: Viral infections of the fetus and neonate. In Feigin, R.D., and Cherry, J.D., editors: Textbook of pediatric infectious diseases, Philadelphia, 1981, W.B. Saunders Co.)

CMV, approximately two thirds of rubella and toxoplasmosis, and most hepatitis B infections. In contrast, less than 2% of neonatal herpes infections are asymptomatic. In attempting to establish an etiologic diagnosis in symptomatic infants, however, certain clinical features may provide helpful clues. The manifestations of congenital rubella and CMV infections that appear in the first months of life in symptomatic infants are summarized in Fig. 28-2. The features of congenital toxoplasmosis included in this figure represent those signs and symptoms occurring in symptomatic infants before the diagnosis or during the acute stage of the disease in the first year of life. The diagnosis of congenital toxoplasmosis, however, was made in 80% of these infants by 4 months of age. Low birth weight, hepatomegaly, splenomegaly, jaundice, and pneumonia may be seen with relatively similar frequency in all three infections. The presence of congenital heart disease, bone lesions, cataracts, microphthalmia, corneal opacity, or glaucoma is highly suggestive of rubella, whereas microcephaly, hydrocephalus, and cerebral calcifications are rarely seen. In contrast, pneumonia and microcephaly are relatively more common in CMV infection, whereas congenital heart disease, bone lesions, and externally visible eye findings are rare. The prominent features of toxoplasmosis include chorioretinitis, hydrocephalus, and cerebral calcifications, whereas congenital heart disease, nonretinal eye findings, and bone lesions are seldom seen. Thus infants with early to midgestation in utero infections commonly are seen at birth with congenital abnormalities, intrauterine growth retardation, and other manifestations of disease. In contrast, neonates who are exposed late in gestation or near the time of delivery usually are asymptomatic initially but subsequently develop signs and symptoms days, weeks, months, or even years later.

In contrast to the findings in congenital rubella, CMV, and toxoplasmic infections, disease caused by herpes simplex virus or the enteroviruses may be seen as a fulminant systemic illness that resembles neonatal bacterial sepsis (Fig. 28-3). Failure to isolate bacteria from blood, spinal fluid, or urine cultures should suggest the possibility of a viral cause, particularly herpes simplex virus or an enterovirus. Vesicular skin lesions, chorioretinits, keratoconjunctivitis, and encephalitis are characteristic of herpes, whereas aseptic meningitis and hepatitis are prominent in enterovirus infections. Although there are

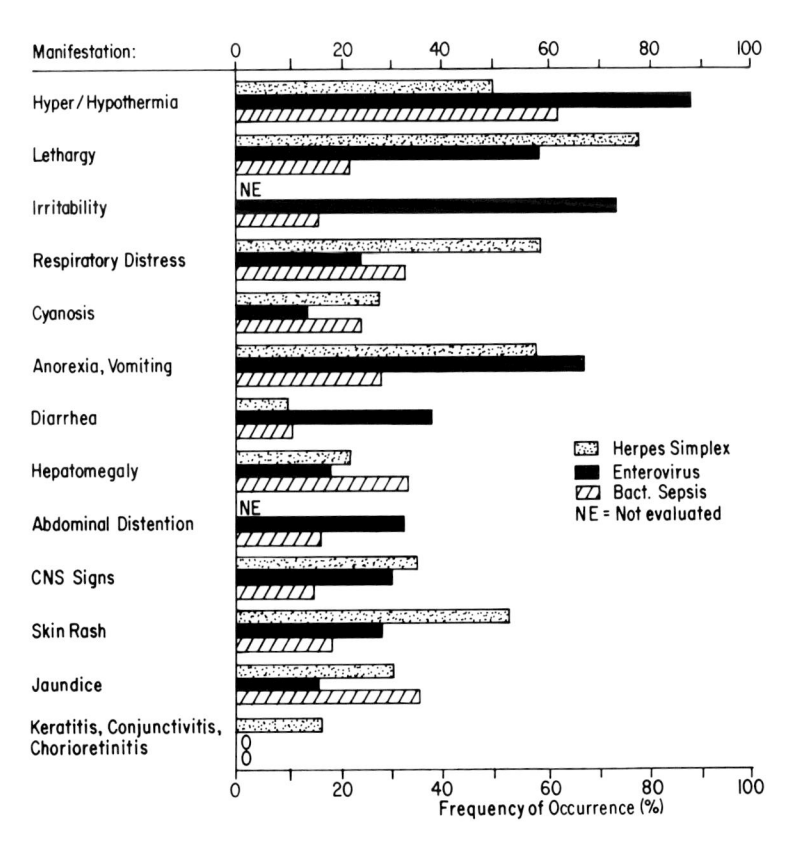

Fig. 28-3. Manifestations of herpes simplex and enterovirus infections and bacterial sepsis in the neonate. (From Overall, J.C., Jr.: Viral infections of the fetus and neonate. In Feigin, R.D., and Cherry, J.D., editors: Textbook of pediatric infectious diseases, Philadelphia, 1981, W.B. Saunders Co.)

certain clinical features which may be associated with each of these specific causative agents, the overlap in manifestations may result in the inability to make a diagnosis on clinical grounds alone. Under these circumstances the laboratory assumes a major role in establishing a definitive diagnosis.

Congenital cytomegalovirus infection

The classic congenital CMV infection, or cytomegalic inclusion disease, has been considered a symptomatic systemic illness in the neonate that frequently results in microcephaly and psychomotor retardation. Milder forms of infections, however, are much more common, and it is now evident that over 90% of neonatal CMV infections are asymptomatic.

The manifestations of the symptomatic form of congenital CMV infection in the neonate are summarized in Fig. 28-2. Evidence of intrauterine growth retardation was noted among the low birth weight infants; 7 of 13 in one series were small for their gestational age. Hepatosplenomegaly and icterus are the most consistent findings in the neonatal period. Hepatomegaly is usually the result of neonatal hepatitis and is accompanied by direct-reacting hyperbilirubinemia and elevation of alkaline phosphatase and serum transaminase enzyme values. Liver involvement is indicated by isolation of the virus from biopsy specimens and histologic evidence of hepatitis, cholangitis, fatty metamorphosis, and interstitial fibrosis. Extramedullary hematopoiesis is responsible for the splenomegaly and hepatomegaly in infants with no evidence of hepatitis. Hepatosplenomegaly and icterus often may persist for many months without the development of severe chronic liver disease. Petechiae and purpura are the result of thrombocytopenia, which usually resolves spontaneously in a few weeks or months. Major bleeding as a complication of the thrombocytopenia has been reported only rarely. Indirect hyperbilirubinemia, reticulocytosis, and/or normoblastemia suggests hemolytic anemia, which usually resolves spontaneously in several months. Pneumonia is the result of the direct viral involvement of the lung, as indicated by isolation of virus and demonstration of typical cytomegalic inclusion cells in autopsy specimens of lung tissue. The chorioretinitis observed in cytomegalic inclusion disease is quite similar to that seen in toxoplasmosis. Involvement of the CNS by the virus results in the most severe sequelae of the disease. Microcephaly may not be present at birth but may become apparent at a year of age or later because of the retarded growth rate in the brain as compared with somatic tissues. Sixty-six percent of the 42 patients had evidence of microcephaly when monitored beyond the neonatal period (Fig. 28-2). It is likely that this figure would be higher if longer follow-up analyses were available. Classically the cerebral calcifications in cytomegalic inclusion disease occur in a periventricular location, whereas those in toxoplasmosis exhibit a diffuse pattern, but there may be considerable overlap between the two. The presence of microcephaly, cerebral calcifications, or abnormal neurologic signs in the early weeks of life is associated with a high frequency of death or severe mental retardation. Of the 42 patients who were monitored for 9 months to 9 years, 17% died, 62% had neurologic sequelae (mental retardation, seizures, spasticity, visual loss, or combinations of these), and only 21% had no evidence of CNS dysfunction. It is important to observe these infants until at least school age to determine that sequelae are not present.

The vast majority of infants with congenital CMV infection have clinically inapparent disease in the neonatal period. Although the potential long-term effects of the asymptomatic congenital infection have not been completely defined, infants identified at birth by a positive urine culture in the first 24 hours of life or by the presence of CMV IgM antibody in cord blood serum are currently being studied. The evidence indicates that an IQ of less than 90 may be observed in 39% of these patients, compared with 28% of control subjects. Hearing loss occurs in 36% of patients, in contrast to 9% of control subjects. In one series school failure was predicted in 36% of patients but in only 14% of the control subjects. These findings indicate that the inapparent congenital infection may result in significant hearing loss and contribute to impaired intellectual functioning and poor school performance. More recently CMV has been shown to cause hospital-acquired infection in newborn intensive care unit infants. The illness is seen primarily in preterm infants 4 to 6 weeks of age who received multiple blood transfusions. The usual presentation is an acute septic illness in an infant who had been progressing satisfactorily. Hepatosplenomegaly, gray pallor, deterioration of respiratory status, and atypical lymphocytosis are commonly observed. In one series 4 of 29 involved infants died. It is not known whether infants who recover will suffer any long-term sequelae. The occurrence of CMV infection in 38% of infants receiving blood from a CMV antibody–positive donor in one study suggests that blood transfusions for newborns should use only CMV antibody–negative donors.

Congenital rubella

Although newborns may be seen initially with the classic syndrome, as many as two thirds of proved cases of congenital rubella may be asymptomatic in the neonatal period. The clinical features of symptomatic congenital rubella present in the neonatal period (early onset), based on the combined experience from several institutions, are illustrated in Fig. 28-2. Although thrombocytopenic purpura is a frequent manifestation of congenital rubella, the material included from one series that was selected on the basis of purpura is a relatively higher frequency of this clinical finding. The rates of occurrence of purpura in most series range from 15% to 50%. Thrombocytopenia is almost always present in association with the purpura and usually resolves spontaneously in the first month of life. Neonatal thrombocytopenic purpura is a poor prognostic sign, since it usually occurs in severely affected infants with multiple malformations. As high as 35% of these patients with purpura may die during the first year, in contrast to a mortality during the first 18 months of only 13% of all children with congenital rubella. Although the thrombocytopenia may be profound, death from hemorrhage is rare. The low birth weight of infants with rubella syndrome is probably the result of intrauterine growth retardation; even when born prematurely, the infant is often small for his estimated gestational age. Direct involvement of the liver by rubella virus results in neonatal hepatitis, as evidenced by hepatomegaly, a predominantly direct-reacting hyperbilirubinemia, and elevations of alkaline phosphatase and serum transaminase enzyme values. Pathologic studies usually have demonstrated hepatocellular disease with necrosis, giant cell formation, bile stasis, and fibrosis, but extrahepatic biliary obstruction also has been demonstrated. Congenital heart disease usually is detectable in the neonatal period, although specific lesions may not be defined until later in life when appropriate catheterization studies are performed. Interstitial pneumonia with cough, tachypnea, and breathlessness as the primary manifestations of congenital rubella has been reported. Six of seven patients in one series with this syndrome died in the first year of life as a result of their pulmonary disease. The histopathology of the lung is characterized by acute to subacute to chronic interstitial pneumonitis. Isolation of rubella virus from lung specimens indicates active viral infection in this organ. Although cataracts are the most characteristic ocular lesion in rubella syndrome, they may not be visualized until after the neonatal period. Retinitis is described as widespread, mottled or blotchy, black pigmentary deposits that are quite variable in size and location; it has little or no effect on retinal function. The frequency of occurrence of retinitis in the combined data from six series of children monitored for several years was 36%. Bone lesions are another typical finding in congenital rubella in the neonatal period. We have observed one newborn in whom the only manifestation of rubella infection was the presence of bone lesions. Roentgenographic studies reveal small linear areas of radiolucency and increased bone density in a longitudinal axis of the metaphyseal area in the long bones of the upper and lower extremities. Absence of periosteal reaction is helpful in differentiating the lesions from those seen in congenital syphilis. The abnormality results from disturbances in laying down and calcification of osteoid and usually resolves by 2 to 3 months of age.

Manifestations of CNS involvement such as lethargy, irritability, tone disturbances, and bulging fontanel are often present in the neonatal period. One or more seizures occurred in 27 of a group of 100 infants with congenital rubella syndrome or a history of maternal rubella; however, the majority of these occurred after the neonatal period. Elevation of protein levels was present in most spinal fluid specimens obtained in the neonatal period; pleocytosis was less frequent. Rubella virus is frequently present in the CNS as evidenced by the isolation of virus from 25 to 99 spinal fluid specimens obtained during the first 3 months of life. The extent of impairment in infants at 18 months of age is not readily predictable on the basis of clinical symptomatology or virus isolation in the first few weeks of life. Severe involvement is more frequent, however, in infants with seizures and with high levels of protein in the cerebrospinal fluid during the neonatal period.

Infants with maternal or laboratory evidence of congenital infection with rubella virus who do not demonstrate any sign of clinical illness in the neonatal period still may go on to develop hearing loss, mental retardation, or other abnormalities later in life. This is especially true in those infants whose mothers had rubella after the first trimester. The most important delayed manifestations of congenital rubella are hearing loss (87% of the 426 infants referred to the New York City Rubella Project in whom hearing was tested), congenital heart disease (46%), mental retardation (39%), and cataract or glaucoma (34%). Abnormal hearing may not become apparent until school age. In one series of patients with congenital rubella several children had normal hearing when tested at 2 years of age, yet significant hearing loss was demonstrated at 7 years. The hearing loss may be profound and contribute significantly to the impaired speech development and the learning disabilities of these children. The most common congenital heart lesions are patent ductus arteriosus (69%), pulmonary artery stenosis (49%), pulmonary valvular stenosis (39%), aortic valvular stenosis (6%), aortic arch anomalies (6%), and ventricular septal defect (5%). Children may have more than one cardiac defect. When mental retardation is present, it is unfortunately frequently severe (67% of the children with retardation in the New York City Rubella Project). Psychiatric disorders, including reactive behavior disorder, cerebral dysfunction, and infantile autism, also have been observed. Diabetes mellitus has been observed in 15% to 20% of adults with congenital rubella. Onset is usually in the second and third decade of life. Other late manifestations of the congenital rubella syndrome include chronic lymphocytic thyroiditis, thymic hypoplasia, abnormal dermatoglyphics, chromosomal abnormalities, pancreatic insufficiency, and progressive panencephalitis. As one might expect, severity of the long-term sequelae appears to correlate with the number of defects observed in early life.

Hepatitis B

The clinical syndrome of neonatal hepatitis is infrequently associated with a specific causative agent. Relatively few data are available concerning hepatitis A (infectious hepatitis) and non–A, non–B hepatitis in the newborn. Hepatitis B virus may cross the placenta or be acquired at the time of delivery or during the neonatal period. The fetus or newborn infant exposed to hepatitis B virus may follow one of several course: (1) asymptomatic transient hepatitis B antigenemia, followed by the production of anti-HB$_s$, (2) asymptomatic persistent antigenemia, variably associated with mild and fluctuating elevations of liver enzymes, (3) symptomatic hepatitis with recovery and clearance of the antigen, (4) symptomatic hepatitis that becomes chronic persistent or chronic active with continued presence of hepatitis B antigenemia, and (5) acute fulminant hepatitis with death. The majority of infants have asymptomatic transient hepatitis B antigenemia. It should be noted, however, that infants born to mothers who had hepatitis during the pregnancy often have a low birth weight, although no other stigmata have been recognized. Any infant born to a mother with hepatitis (HB Ag positive) should be tested for the presence of HB Ag in the cord blood and at intervals for at least 12 months. The identification of HB$_s$Ag in the cord blood, however, does not necessarily indicate infection, since such infants may clear the antigen from their blood and never develop subsequent antigenemia or antibody. If the infant develops evidence of infection (becomes HB$_s$Ag positive), careful observation with determination of HB$_s$Ag and anti-HB$_s$ antibody as well as tests of liver chemistries should be repeated at periodic intervals.

A small number of infants who acquire hepatitis B in utero or around the time of delivery may develop the clinical signs of acute hepatitis with alterations in liver chemistries. These infants usually follow a benign course, recover, and develop antibody. In contrast, neonates who acquire an antigenemia but are asymptomatic in the newborn period commonly become chronic carriers. Such carriers may manifest continuing biochemical, histologic, and virologic evidence of chronic liver involvement. Liver biopsies from infants who fall into this classification show histologic changes compatible with continuing unresolved hepatitis and the presence of virus particles in the nuclei of hepatocytes. Most also have elevations of transaminase activity, which may be characterized by one of three courses: (1) extremely high levels that fluctuate markedly, (2) moderate elevations that are reasonably stable, or (3) slight elevations that are also relatively stable for long periods. The ultimate outcome of chronic hepatitis B in these children is unknown, as are the factors that determine which pattern of hepatitis B will occur in an involved infant.

Congenital toxoplasmosis

Over 70% of infants born with congenital toxoplasmosis do not manifest signs of clinical illness in the neonatal period. The most common findings during the first few months of life in the 152 infants with symptomatic infection with Eichenwald's series are illustrated in Fig. 28-2. These infants fall into two major groups: (1) infants with generalized disease in whom the primary manifestations of low birth weight, hepatosplenomegaly, icterus, and anemia are observed in the first several weeks of life, and (2) infants with primarily neurologic disease in whom the major findings are abnormal spinal fluid, convulsions, intracranial calcifications, and hydrocephalus or microcephaly. These latter findings, with the exception of the abnormal spinal fluid, are not seen until after 1 month of age in the majority of infants. Chorioretinitis, the most common lesion in congenital toxoplasmosis, occurs in both groups of infants but usually is not apparent in the neonatal period. Postmortem examination of infants who died in the neonatal period reveals multiple foci of necrosis with encysted forms of the *Toxoplasma* parasite in myocardium, renal glomeruli and tubules, the adrenal gland, and the brain. The enlarged liver and spleen are the result of marked extramedullary hematopoiesis; parasites are rarely seen. The overall mortality in Eichenwald's series was 12%; 90% of the survivors developed serious neurologic sequelae, such as mental retardation, convulsions, spasticity, palsies, severely impaired vision, hydrocephalus or microcephaly, and deafness.

The infants with asymptomatic, or silent, congenital toxoplasmosis are diagnosed by the demonstration of a seroconversion or a significant rise in antitoxoplasmic antibodies in the mother during pregnancy or the presence of specific antitoxoplasmic IgM antibodies in the cord blood serum or in serum obtained from the neonate soon after birth. These infants usually have abnormal spinal fluid with lymphocytosis and elevated protein levels in the neonatal period. In one study of 13 newborns diagnosed because of routine screening tests or during the evaluation of nonspecific findings, 11 (85%) developed chorioretinitis and 5 (39%) neurologic sequelae. The onset of eye disease occurred as early as 1 month to as late as 9.3 years. Neurologic defects included microcephaly, seizures, severe psychomotor retardation, mild cerebellar dysfunction, and delay in development. In another group of 11 children who were asymptomatic as neonates but who were diagnosed because of the onset of symptoms later in life, 10 out of 11 (91%) had chorioretinitis, and 8 out of 11 (73%) had neurologic sequelae. Sixteen of the children in these two groups had skull films, and 5 (31%) had intracranial calcifications. All had neurologic sequelae.

These data indicate that a majority of infants with subclinical congenital toxoplasmosis in the neonatal period develop clinical manifestations of their disease later in life.

Neonatal herpes simplex

Unlike most other viruses associated with significant disease in the neonatal period, herpes simplex virus rarely causes an intrauterine infection. More commonly herpetic infections of the neonate are acquired during the birth process; this is supported by the usual incubation period of 6 to 11 days between birth and onset of disease. Infected patients have been recognized, however, at birth and at 3 weeks after birth. Three patterns of disease have been described: (1) disseminated infection with or without CNS involvement occurring in two thirds of involved infants, (2) infection localized to the CNS, skin, eye, or oral cavity present in one third, and (3) asymptomatic infection present in less than 1%. The most common presentation is the disseminated form with involvement of multiple organ systems, resulting in a clinical picture resembling that of sepsis or generalized enterovirus infection (Fig. 28-3). Distinguishing features that should suggest the possibility of neonatal herpes include vesicular skin rash, keratoconjunctivitis, mouth ulcers, and encephalitis. In the recent National Institutes of Health (NIH) collaborative study 50% of infants with neonatal herpes were premature. Importantly, signs and symptoms of acute herpetic disease did not occur until after discharge from the nursery in two thirds of the cases. Skin vesicles were the presenting features in 71% of infants, evidence of CNS or other target-organ involvement was present in 18%, and the remaining 11% had both skin vesicles and disseminated disease. Seventy percent of infants that were initially seen with skin lesions progressed to CNS or disseminated disease, indicating that treatment should not be delayed because the disease appears to be localized. The prognosis in untreated neonatal herpes is very poor. In the review of 298 cases by Nahmias and associates 72% succumbed to the infection, and another 16% developed serious neurologic sequelae. In contrast, those infants with only localized involvement without CNS or systemic disease have a better prognosis.

Several cases of congenital herpes simplex virus infection have been reported, but these are much less common than infections acquired at birth. These infants have a vesicular rash present at birth or within the first day or two of life, diffuse brain damage, microcephaly, and intracranial calcifications. Less commonly observed features include chorioretinitis, retinal dysplasia, cataracts, and microphthalmia.

The source of infection may not be readily ascertained, and the absence of recognizable genital lesions in the mother does not rule out the consideration of herpesvirus infection in the neonate. In the NIH study 70% of the maternal infections were asymptomatic. Furthermore in approximately 30% of infected infants the oral strains are responsible. Since there now is evidence indicating that herpes simplex virus has been acquired postnatally from an infected mother, usually with a type-1 oral herpetic lesion, from hospital personnel, from family members, or by nosocomial transmission from other neonates, isolation precautions should be applied to a newborn with known or suspected herpesvirus infection.

Congenital malaria

Infants born to mothers with malaria may become infected, particularly if there is maternal parasitemia during delivery. Congenital infection can occur with all four human species of malaria. These infants usually are seen during the first month of life with signs of sepsis, including poor feeding, lethargy, fever, hepatosplenomegaly, anemia, jaundice, vomiting, diarrhea, pallor, and cyanosis. The adult presentation of fever and paroxysms of chills and sweats usually is not observed. The diagnosis should be considered in infants of mothers with a history of malaria exposure, particularly in recent Asian immigrants (Chapter 27).

DIAGNOSIS
Maternal history and physical examination

A history of illness in the mother during pregnancy may be helpful in suggesting the likely causative agent in a neonate suspected of having an intrauterine or perinatal viral infection. For example, illness associated with a rash or history of exposure to such an illness may suggest rubella, whereas a mild febrile episode with cervical adenopathy might implicate *Toxoplasma* organisms. Some rubella and the majority of CMV and toxoplasmic infections are not clinically apparent. Genital herpes often results in painful ulcerations on the vulva or cervical lesions that can be recognized on physical examination. Although most enterovirus infections do not result in a sufficiently distinctive clinical picture to permit diagnosis, pleurodynia is one recognized syndrome that may be caused by the Coxsackie B group of viruses. The season of the year in which the mother was ill may be helpful, since enterovirus infections usually occur during the late summer through fall; often there is a recognized outbreak in the community. Maternal mumps, varicella-zoster, and measles may be diagnosed clinically.

Isolation of a pathogen

The most direct method of establishing the diagnosis of an infection in the neonatal period is the isolation of the agent from an appropriate site in the infected mother or infant. The best methods for isolation of CMV are from freshly voided clean-catch urine specimens and, in the mother, from a cervical swab. Virus excretion in the urine of congenitally infected infants may continue for several years after birth. The best site for obtaining rubella virus in the infant is the throat, although the virus has been recovered from spinal fluid and less frequently from the urine. Virus has been recovered from the throats of approximately 80% of infected infants from birth to 1 month of age, 60% from 1 to 4 months, 30% from 5 to 8 months, 10% from 9 months to 1 year, and 3% from 1 to 2 years. Rubella virus has been isolated from cataractous lens tissue of children as old as 31 months. This persistence of virus excretion makes the infant with congenital infection a possible source of transmission. There are reports of rubella and of CMV infection in family members and nursing personnel caring for infected infants. Although precautions should be taken with regard to exposure of pregnant women to these infants, the actual risk of infection has not been defined.

French workers have reported that *Toxoplasma* organisms can be isolated from placental tissue in 95% and from cord blood in 43% of infants with serologically confirmed congenital toxoplasmosis. Most laboratories, however, do not have the facilities or the expertise required for the mouse-inoculation techniques necessary for successful isolation of this organism.

The diagnosis of genital herpes simplex infection in the mother can be documented by the demonstration of cells with intranuclear inclusions or multinucleated giant cells on a Giemsa-stained smear of the base of a vesicle or ulcer or on a Papanicolaou smear. Herpes simplex virus can be cultured from a swab of the ulcerative lesions in the mother or from new vesicular lesions, throat swabs, urine, and often spinal fluid in the infant if there is disseminated disease. In infants with isolated involvement of the CNS, brain biopsy may be required for diagnosis. Frequently the cytopathic effect typical of herpes simplex virus can be observed in tissue culture as early as 24 to 48 hours after inoculation.

Each of the aforementioned three viral agents is fairly labile and may be lost by freezing and thawing; thus specimens should be transferred promptly to the laboratory and cultured fresh. Transport of specimens from a long distance to the virus diagnostic laboratory is not likely to result in successful isolation of these agents unless special precautions are used in handling. In this situation diagnosis should be sought by serologic methods.

Enteroviruses can be isolated from stool specimens, throat swab material, and sometimes spinal fluid if there is evidence of CNS infection. These agents are relatively stable; specimens may be stored in an ordinary refrigerator at 4° C for short periods and shipped to the diagnostic laboratory in a tightly sealed vial in dry ice. Although vaccinia and varicella viruses can be recovered from skin vesicles, the diagnosis usually can be made clinically from the appearance of the lesions. In any suspected fetal or neonatal infection, isolation of the pathogen can be attempted with autopsy tissue, especially if it is performed soon after death. Isolation of a virus from spinal fluid, urine, or a skin vesicle is strong evidence of a causative association. However, one should interpret cautiously the isolation, particularly of enteroviruses, from throat swabs or stool specimens. Virus isolation data must be considered in association with the clinical picture and the results of antibody assays in both mother and infant.

Serologic studies

Serum samples may be submitted to state health laboratories for the TORCH (*Toxoplasma*, other, rubella, cytomegalovirus, and herpes simplex) screen. Most laboratories use passive hemagglutination or immunofluorescence techniques for antibody against *Toxoplasma* organisms, hemagglutination inhibition for rubella, and complement-fixing or passive hemagglutination for CMV and herpes simplex. Serologic confirmation of a maternal viral or protozoal illness requires serum specimens that bracket the illness. The presence of a high antibody titer against one of the TORCH agents in a single serum specimen obtained from the mother after delivery of an abnormal infant may provide suggestive evidence that the infant is infected with that agent. The major value of the maternal serum obtained at delivery, however, is to provide an opportunity for comparison with antibody titers in the cord blood serum or in serum obtained from the infant. Except for early stages of infection, antibodies to the TORCH agents are predominantly IgG and are passed transplacentally from mother to fetus. Thus any antibodies present in maternal blood will be found at approximately the same titer in the infant. The half-life of passively transferred antibody is between 3 and 4 weeks. A serum sample obtained from the infant at 3 to 4 months of age should show a significant drop if the antibody present in the newborn period was passively transferred from the mother. The titer should remain the same or become elevated if the infant was infected and has begun to produce his own humoral antibody response. After 6 months any antibody present is likely to have been produced by the infant in response to an infection. Thus even serum specimens obtained from older infants can be used in establishing the cause of congenital viral infection.

A quantitatively elevated level of IgM in cord blood serum has been used as a screening test in an attempt to identify infants who have had intrauterine infection. Since IgM antibody is not passed transplacentally from mother to fetus in the absence of a placental leak, any specific IgM antibody in the cord blood is of fetal and not maternal origin. Although it has been shown that significantly more infants with elevated cord IgM levels than infants with normal levels have had intrauterine infection, not all infants with such infections have an elevated IgM level. The quantitative IgM level has been elevated in approximately 75% of the serum samples submitted to the Centers for Disease Control (CDC) in Atlanta from symptomatic infants in whom a diagnosis of one of the TORCH agents was subsequently made. In the majority of infants with elevated cord IgM levels identified by routine screening it has not been possible to identify a specific intrauterine infection (CMV, rubella, *Toxoplasma* organisms, syphilis, or others) with currently available techniques. Although assay for quantitative level of IgM in the cord serum is not an ideal screening test because of the high frequency of false positive results, an elevated level does indicate that further evaluation should be undertaken.

Tests for specific IgM antibody using fluorescent antibody or ultracentrifugation techniques have been developed for CMV, rubella virus, *Toxoplasma* organisms, and herpes simplex virus. The CMV IgM test on cord blood serum has been positive in 90% of infants excreting the virus in their urine in the first 24 hours of life and in over 99% of those who show symptoms in the neonatal period. The presence of rubella IgM in cord blood also appears to correlate with symptoms of disease in the neonatal period and therefore long-term sequelae. In contrast, specific IgM has been absent in 75% of cord serum from infants who were eventually shown to have congenital toxoplasmosis, presumably either because the infection occurred so early in gestation that IgM was no longer present in fetal serum or because of inhibition of the fetal humoral response by the transplacental passage of specific maternal IgG. Although specific IgM has been shown to be present in the serum of infants with neonatal herpes simplex infection, it does not appear until after 7 to 10 days of illness have elapsed; thus the value of this test in making an early diagnosis is reduced. In the future it seems likely that the specific IgM antibody test will become the most practical and rapid diagnostic test for congenital CMV, rubella, and toxoplasmic infections. Serum samples from selected infants (those with clinical manifestations suggestive of an intrauterine infection plus an elevated quantitative IgM level) may be submitted to the CDC through state health laboratories for specific IgM antibody tests. For the present virus isolation appears to be the best means for diagnosis of neonatal herpes simplex infection. For the enterovirus group (Coxsackie and ECHO viruses) both virus isolation, depending on the site from which it was recovered, and serologic data are important for definitive diagnosis.

TREATMENT AND PREVENTION

For the majority of viral infections, whether congenital or acquired around the time of delivery, no effective therapy is available. The progression of disease in infants who were asymptomatic at birth, however, suggests that, when and if effective antiviral agents are developed, it may be possible to ameliorate the course of the disease.

Cytomegalovirus and rubella

There is no known effective antiviral therapy for either CMV or rubella. Rubella vaccine has reduced the incidence of congenital rubella, but a CMV vaccine is still being developed.

Herpes simplex virus

Vidarabine (adenine arabinoside or ara-A) has been shown to be of benefit in adults with herpes encephalitis. The results of the recent NIH collaborative study of neonatal herpes indicate that arabinosyladenine significantly reduced mortality from 74% in the placebo control group to 38% in the treated infants. Therapy was most effective against localized disease, and the best prognosis occurred in neonates with superficial involvement of skin, eye, or mouth. The dosage is 15 mg/kg/day, administered intravenously over 12 hours for 10 days at a concentration of 0.7 mg/ml or less in a standard intravenous solution. It is possible that higher doses may be more effective, but adequate data on benefits and toxicity are not available at this time. Treatment should be started early, and the diagnosis should be confirmed by virus isolation.

Toxoplasmosis

Although definitive data are not available and a controlled randomized study is yet to be carried out, present evidence suggests that treatment may decrease the incidence of adverse sequelae. Therapy would appear to be appropriate for a symptomatic newborn and for an asymptomatic infant with proven infection, i.e., a rising titer of antibody or a positive IgM *Toxoplasma* organism fluorescent antibody test on the infant's blood. Therapy consists of pyrimethamine, 1 mg/kg/day, orally, and then 0.5 mg/kg/day for 21 to 30 days, along with sulfadiazine, 25 mg/kg/day, orally for 21 to 30 days. Folinic acid, 2 to 6 mg, also should be given three times a week to prevent anemia. The treatment may be repeated when there is evidence of ongoing disease after a course of therapy.

Malaria

Infants with congenital malaria should be treated, although experience with this disease in the United States is limited. Chloroquine is the drug of choice for all four human strains unless the infection is caused by chloroquine-resistant *Plasmodium falciparum* (Chapter 27).

Hepatitis B

Although vidarabine and human interferon have been used in adults with chronic active hepatitis, there are no data that support the use of these antiviral agents in neonates. On the other hand, there is increasing evidence that γ-globulin may prevent the development of hepatitis B in infants born to infected mothers. Hepatitis B immune globulin (HBIG) is preferable to regular γ-globulin preparations because of higher antibody titers to hepatitis B. Candidates for HBIG administration include infants born to mothers infected with acute hepatitis B in the third trimester, babies of mothers who are chronic carriers with HB_eAg in their serum, and infants of mothers who delivered a previously infected child. Two different regimens have been used or recommended: (1) 0.5 to 1 ml at birth followed by the same dose at 3 months of age, and (2) 0.5 ml/kg at birth and then 0.16 ml/kg every month for 6 months. In a controlled study using this latter regimen 5 of 20 untreated infants became HB Ag positive, compared with none out of 21 who received HBIG.

Lowell A. Glasgow
James C. Overall, Jr.

BIBLIOGRAPHY
General

Blattner, R.J., Williamson, A.P., and Heys, F.M.: Role of viruses in the etiology of congenital malformations, Prog. Med. Virol. **15**:1, 1973.

Charles D., and Finland, M., editors: Obstetric and perinatal infections, Philadelphia, 1973, Lea & Febiger.

Cherry, J.D., Soriano, F., and Jahn, C.L.: Search for perinatal viral infection; a prospective clinical, virological, and serological study, Am. J. Dis. Child. **116**:245, 1968.

Eichenwald, H.F., McCracken, G.H., Jr., and Kindberg, S.J.: Virus infections of the newborn, Prog. Med. Virol. **9**:35, 1967.

Elliott, K., and Knight, J., editors: Symposium on Intrauterine Infections, Amsterdam, 1973, Elsevier/North Holland Biomedical Press.

Kibrick, S.: Viral infections of the fetus and newborn. In Perspectives in virology, vol. 2, Minneapolis, 1961, Burgess Publishing Co.

Krugman, S., and Gershon, A.A., editors: Infections of the fetus and the newborn infant, New York, 1975, Alan R. Liss, Inc.

Mims, C.A.: Pathogenesis of viral infections of the fetus, Prog. Med. Virol. **10**:194, 1968.

Monif, G.R.G.: Viral infections of the human fetus, London, 1969, Macmillan Press, Ltd.

Nahmias, A.J.: The TORCH complex, Hosp. Pract. **9**:65, 1974.

Overall, J.C., Jr., and Glasgow, L.A.: Virus infections of the fetus and newborn infant, J. Pediatr. **77**:315, 1970.

Sanders, D.H., and Cramblett, H.G.: Viral infections in hospitalized neonates, Am. J. Dis. Child. **116**:251, 1968.

Sever, J.L.: Perinatal infections affecting the developing fetus and newborn. In The prevention of mental retardation through control of infectious disease, Washington, D.C., 1966, U.S. Department of Health, Education, and Welfare.

Sever, J.L., Larsen, J.W., and Grossman, J.H.: Handbook of perinatal infections, Boston, 1979, Little, Brown & Co.

Sever, J.L., and White, L.R.: Intrauterine viral infections, Ann. Rev. Med. **19**:471, 1968.

CMV infection

Ballard, R.A.: Acquired cytomegalovirus infection in preterm infants, Am. J. Dis. Child. **133**:482, 1979.

Benson, J.W.T., Bodden, S.J., and Tobin, J.O'H.: Cytomegalovirus and blood transfusion in neonates, Arch. Dis. Child. **54**:538, 1979.

Hanshaw, J.B.: Congenital cytomegalovirus infection; laboratory methods of detection, J. Pediatr. **75**:1179, 1969.

Hanshaw, J.B., and others: CNS sequelae of congenital cytomegalovirus infection. In Krugman, S., and Gershon, A.A., editors: Infections of the fetus and the newborn infant, New York, 1975, Alan R. Liss, Inc.

Kuman, M.L., Nankervis, G.A., and Gold, E.: Inapparent congenital cytomegalovirus infection; a followup study, N. Engl. J. Med. **288**:1370, 1973.

McCracken, G.H., Jr., and others: Congenital cytomegalic inclusion disease; a longitudinal study of 20 patients, Am. J. Dis. Child. **117**:522, 1969.

Medearis, D.N., Jr.: Observations concerning human cytomegalovirus infection and disease, Bull. Johns Hopkins Hosp. **114**:181, 1964.

Reynolds, D.W., and others: Maternal cytomegalovirus excretion and perinatal infection, N. Engl. J. Med. **289**:1, 1973.

Reynolds, D.W., and others: Inapparent congenital cytomegalovirus infection with elevated cord IgM levels; causal relation with auditory and mental deficiency, N. Engl. J. Med. **290**:291, 1974.

Weller, G.H., and Hanshaw, J.B.: Virologic and clinical observations on cytomegalic inclusion disease, N. Engl. J. Med. **266**:1233, 1962.

Rubella

Cooper, L.Z.: Congenital rubella in the United States. In Krugman, S., and Gershon, A.A., editors: Infections of the fetus and the newborn infant, New York, 1975, Alan R. Liss, Inc.

Cooper, L.Z., and others: neonatal thrombocytopenic purpura and other manifestations of rubella contracted in utero, Am. J. Dis. Child. **110**:416, 1965.

Desmond, M.M., and others: Congenital rubella encephalitis, J. Pediatr. **71**:311, 1967.

Dudgeon, J.A.: Congenital rubella in the United Kingdom of Great Britain. In Krugman, S., and Gershon, A.A., editors: Infections of the fetus and the newborn infant, New York, 1975, Alan R. Liss, Inc.

Hardy, J.B., and others: Adverse fetal outcome following maternal rubella after the first trimester of pregnancy, J.A.M.A. **207**:2414, 1969.

Horstmann, D.M., and others: Maternal rubella and the rubella syndrome in infants, Am. J. Dis. Child. **110**:408, 1965.

Korones, S.B., and others: Congenital rubella syndrome; new clinical aspects with recovery of virus from affected infants, J. Pediatr. **67**:166, 1965.

Lindquist, J.M., and others: Congenital rubella syndrome as a systemic infection, Br. Med. J. **2**:1401, 1965.

Modlin, J.F., and Brandling-Bennet, A.D.: Surveillance of the congenital rubella syndrome, 1969-73, J. Infect. Dis. **130**:316, 1974.

National Communicable Disease Center: Rubella surveillance, Washington, D.C., June 1969, U.S. Department of Health, Education, and Welfare.

Phelan, P., and Campbell, P.: Pulmonary complications of rubella embryopathy, J. Pediatr. **75**:202, 1969.

Rudolph, A.J., Singleton, E.B., and Rosenberg, H.S.: Osseous manifestations of the congenital rubella syndrome, Am. J. Dis. Child. **110**:428, 1965.

Sever, J.L., Nelson, K.B., and Gilkeson, M.R.: Rubella epidemic, 1964; effect on 6000 pregnancies, Am. J. Dis. Child. **118**:123, 1969.

Weller, T.H., Alford, C.A., Jr., and Neva, F.A.: Changing epidemiologic concepts of rubella, with particular reference to unique characteristics of the congenital infection, Yale J. Biol. Med. **37**:455, 1965.

Hepatitis B

Keyes, T.F., and others: Maternal and neonatal Australia antigen, Calif. Med. **115**:1, 1971.

Kohler, P.F., and others: Prevention of chronic neonatal hepatitis B virus infection with antibody to hepatitis B surface antigen, N. Engl. J. Med. **291**:1378, 1974.

Krugman, S.: Viral hepatitis; recent developments and prospects for prevention, J. Pediatr. **87**:1067, 1975.

Papaevangelou, G., and Hoofnagle, J.H.: Transmission of hepatitis B virus infection by asymptomatic chronic HB$_s$Ag carrier mothers, Pediatrics **63**:602, 1979.

Papaevangelou, G., Hoofnagle, J.H., and Kremastinou, T.: Transplacental transmission of hepatitis B virus by symptom-free chronic carrier mothers, Lancet **2**:746, 1974.

Reesink, H.W., and others: Prevention of chronic HB$_s$Ag-positive mothers by hepatitis B immunoglobulin, Lancet **2**:436, 1979.

Schweitzer, I.L., and others: Factors influencing neonatal infection by hepatitis B virus, Gastroenterology **65**:277, 1973.

Schweitzer, I.L., and others: Viral hepatitis in neonates and infants, Am. J. Med. **55**:762, 1973.

Toxoplasmosis

Alford, C.A., Jr., Stagno, S., and Reynolds, D.W.: Toxoplasmosis; silent congenital infection. In Krugman, S., and Gershon, A.A., editors: Infections of the fetus and the newborn infant, New York, 1975, Alan R. Liss, Inc.

Desmonts, G., and Couvreur, J: Congenital toxoplasmosis; a prospective study of 378 pregnancies, N. Engl. J. Med. **290**:110, 1974.

Desmonts, G., and Couvreur, J.: Toxoplasmosis; epidemiologic and serologic aspects of perinatal infection. In Krugman, S., and Gershon, A.A., editors: Infections of the fetus and the newborn infant, New York, 1975, Alan R. Liss, Inc.

Eichenwald, H.F.: A study of congenital toxoplasmosis. In Siim, J.C., editor: Proceedings of the Conference on Clinical Aspects and Diagnostic Problems of Toxoplasmosis in Pediatrics, Baltimore, 1956, Williams & Wilkins Co.

Feldman, H.A.: Toxoplasmosis, Pediatrics **22**:559, 1958.

Miller, M.J., Seaman, E., and Remington, J.S.: The clinical spectrum of congenital toxoplasmosis; problems in recognition, J. Pediatr. **70**:714, 1967.

Remington, J.: Toxoplasmosis. In Charles, D., and Finland, M., editors: Obstetric and perinatal infections, Philadelphia, 1973, Lea & Febiger.

Sever, J.L.: Perinatal infections affecting the developing fetus and newborn. In The prevention of mental retardation through control of infectious disease, Washington, D.C., 1966, U.S. Department of Health, Education, and Welfare.

Wilson, C.B., and others: Development of Adverse Sequelae in children born with subclinical congenital *Toxoplasma* infection, Pediatrics **66**:767, 1980.

Herpes simplex

Brunell, P.A.: Prevention and treatment of neonatal herpes, Pediatrics **66**:806, 1980.

Dowdle, W.R., and others: Association of antigenic type of herpesvirus hominis with site of viral recovery, J. Immunol. **99**:974, 1967.

Music, S.I., Fine, E.M., and Togo, Y.: Zoster-like disease in the newborn due to herpes simplex virus, N. Engl. J. Med. **284**:24, 1971.

Nahmias, A.J., Josey, W.E., and Naib, Z.M.: Neonatal herpes simplex infection; role of genital infection in mother as the source of virus in the newborn, J.A.M.A. **199**:164, 1967.

Nahmias, A.J., and others: Newborn infection with herpesvirus hominis types 1 and 2, J. Pediatr. **75**:1194, 1969.

Nahmias, A.J., and others: Herpes simplex virus infection of the fetus and newborn. In Krugman, S., and Gershon, A.A., editors: Infections of the fetus and the newborn infant, New York, 1975, Alan R. Liss, Inc.

South, M.A., and Others: Congenital malformations of the central nervous system associated with genital (type 2) herpesvirus, J. Pediatr. **75**:13, 1969.

Whitley, R.J., and others: The natural history of herpes simplex virus infection of mother and newborn, Pediatrics. **66**:489, 1980.

Whitley, R.J., and others: Vidarabine therapy of neonatal herpes simplex virus infection, Pediatrics. **66**:495, 1980.

Diagnosis

Alford, C.A., and others: Subclinical central nervous system disease of neonates; a prospective study of infants born with increased levels of IgM, J. Pediatr. **75**:1167, 1969.

Hanshaw, J.B., Steinfield, H.J., and White, C.J.: Fluorescent antibody tests for cytomegalovirus macroglobulin, N. Engl. J. Med. **279**:566, 1968.

McCracken, G.H., Jr., and others: Serum immunoglobulin levels in newborn infants. II. Survey of cord and followup sera from 123 infants with congenital rubella, J. Pediatr. **74**:383, 1969.

CHAPTER 29 # The blood and hematopoietic system

HEMATOPOIESIS IN THE EMBRYO AND FETUS

To understand the marked differences in blood counts between newborns and premature infants compared with adult values, one must understand the development of the formed elements of the blood in utero. On about day 14 of gestation, mesenchyme in the blood islands of the yolk sac begins to differentiate into primitive megaloblastic-looking blood cells, and peripheral cells become the endothelium of blood vessels. This intravascular phase of hematopoiesis lasts for about 2 months and is followed by the hepatic phase. During this 3- to 4-month period the liver produces large amounts of erythroblasts, megakaryocytes, and granulocytes. Spleen and thymus begin to produce blood cells at this time, followed shortly by lymph node activity resulting in detectable monocytes and lymphocytes by the fifth month. By the last trimester, bone marrow is the major site of production, although the liver continues to make some blood cells as late as the first postnatal week. Cellularity is maximal from the thirtieth week, so a newborn can increase blood production only by expanding the volume of marrow.

The blood cells in utero

By the sixteenth week of gestation the primitive nucleated erythroblasts in the blood are almost entirely replaced by definitive mature red blood cells. The erythrocytes present in the blood at this stage are considerably larger than those present at the time of birth, and the hemoglobin concentration of the blood and the red blood cell count are significantly lower than the normal postnatal levels (Fig. 29-1). A gradual increase in the red blood cell count occurs throughout the fetal period together with a decreasing size of the red blood cells. Reticulocytosis is prominent in the early fetus, and at 10 weeks of gestation as many as 80% of the red blood cells may be reticulocytes. By 30 weeks the reticulocyte count reaches a minimum of about 4%.

Leukocytes are present only in small numbers during the first half of gestation. Granulocyte counts are less than 50% of adult values before the twenty-sixth week and increase prominently in the last 2 to 3 months of fetal life (Fig. 29-1). Lymphocyte counts reach approximately two thirds of the values at term by about 20 weeks of gestation, then increase gradually.

Small numbers of megakaryocytes have been observed as early as the yolk sac stage of hematopoiesis. Platelets are present in the blood by 11 weeks of gestation, and by 30 weeks the platelet count approaches normal adult values.

NORMAL HEMATOLOGIC VALUES IN THE NEWBORN

The concentration of hemoglobin in cord blood at birth averages approximately 17 gm/dl; a wide range of values of between 14 and 20 gm/dl generally is accepted as normal. Hematocrit values of cord blood average about 55%, with a normal range of 43% to 63%. The red blood cell count is correspondingly elevated, with a mean of approximately $5.5 \times 10^6/mm^3$. These values may be modified by a number of factors that must be taken into consideration if a meaningful interpretation of hematologic data in the newborn is to be made.

An important determinant is the duration of gestation. During the final weeks of intrauterine life the hemoglobin concentration of blood undergoes a rapid increase (Fig. 29-1), with average increments of 1 to 3 gm/dl occurring between the thirty-eighth and fortieth weeks. This magnitude of change will be reflected in a correspondingly reduced hemoglobin concentration at birth in prematurely born as compared with full-term infants. In

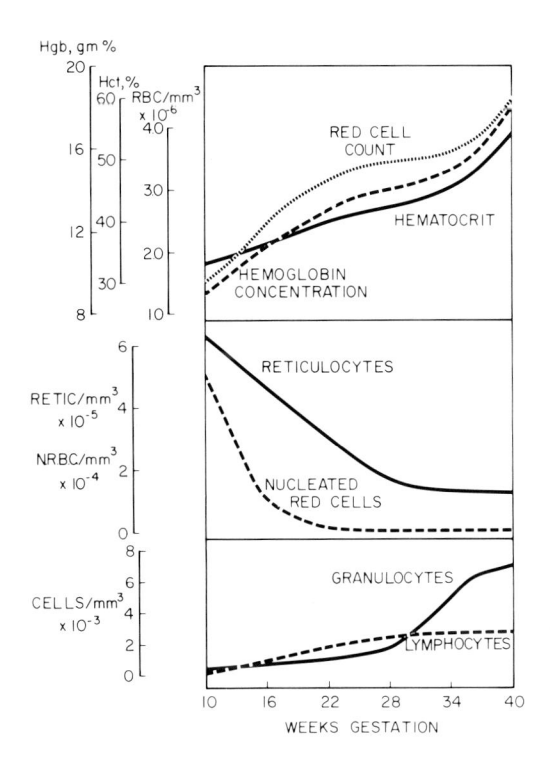

Fig. 29-1. Hematologic changes during prenatal development.

a study of premature infants having birth weights of less than 1,200 gm, a mean hemoglobin concentration of 15.6 gm/dl was found, as compared with 17.1 gm/dl in full-term infants.

The length of time allowed to elapse before the cord is clamped at delivery can have a considerable effect on the blood volume and total circulating red blood cell mass of the newborn. The placental vessels contain approximately 100 ml of blood at term, and transfusion of a major fraction of the blood contained in the placenta can occur under conditions that promote emptying of the placental vessels at delivery. Placing the infant below the level of the placenta and delaying clamping the cord for several minutes after birth can increase the blood volume of the infant by as much as 40% to 60%. Usher found that newborns with delayed clamping of the cord had mean blood volumes of 126 ml/kg as compared with 78 ml/kg in infants whose cords were clamped immediately at birth. In both groups of infants the average hematocrit value was the same at birth, but after 48 hours mean hematocrit values of 65% were obtained in the group with delayed clamping of the cord and 48% in the infants in whom placental transfusion was prevented. Increased hemoglobin and hematocrit values can be demonstrated for at least 3 or 4 days in infants with delayed cord clamping.

The effect of transfusion of placental blood into the infant at birth may result in even greater increases in the blood volume in the premature infant. The quantity of blood in the placenta undergoes little change in the last 2 to 3 months of gestation, during which time the blood volume of the infant increases considerably. The preterm infant can thus receive a proportionately larger fraction of blood volume by the addition of placental blood.

It remains unclear whether the addition of the placental blood to the circulation is advantageous to the infant. Although the rapid increase in blood volume that occurs might impose significant stress on the heart and pulmonary vasculature, it has been reported that a decreased incidence of neonatal respiratory distress may occur in infants in whom clamping the cord is delayed. Furthermore, infants having a larger circulating red blood cell mass at birth will gain an increased storage supply of iron resulting from breakdown of the additional hemoglobin; however, this may contribute to hyperbilirubinemia in the first week of life. This supplementary iron can be used at a later time for hemoglobin production and will help to prevent iron deficiency if dietary intake is inadequate to supply the iron requirements for rapid growth during later infancy.

During the first week of life, hematocrit and hemoglobin values obtained from capillary blood may be markedly higher than venous samples due to peripheral venous stasis. This may allow significant anemia to be undiagnosed. Warming the infant's heel may decrease the difference between capillary and venous values. Sick infants should always have venipuncture hematocrits, since acidosis and hypotension increase peripheral stasis.

An additional modifying factor that occurs within the first few hours following delivery is a shift in the distribution of fluid to produce a decrease in the circulating plasma volume and a corresponding increase in the red blood cell concentration in the blood. An elevation in the hemoglobin value of approximately 2 gm/100 ml above cord blood values persists until the end of the first week of life (Fig. 29-2).

Reticulocyte counts in cord blood of normal infants average 4% to 5%, and in most cord blood samples nucleated red blood cell precursors are also present. These findings are accompanied by elevated erythropoietin levels and erythroid hyperplasia in the bone marrow and are interpreted to represent compensatory red blood cell production resulting, in part, from the decreased oxygen saturation of the fetal blood, which ranges from approximately 30% saturation in the umbilical artery to 65% in the umbilical vein. An additional contributing factor is the high oxygen affinity of the fetal blood because of the predominance of fetal hemoglobin in the red blood cells; the result of this increase is an impairment of oxygen release to the tissue. In infants with intrauterine growth

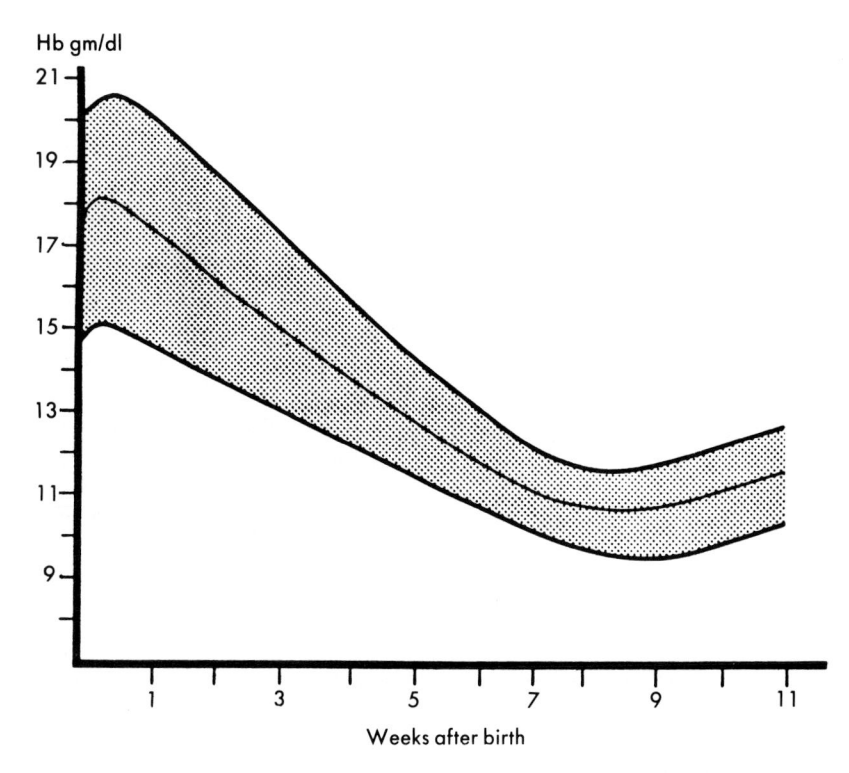

Fig. 29-2. Normal hemotocrit values in full term infants ± S.D.

retardation, hypoxia in utero appears to occur to a more severe extent, and these infants frequently demonstrate higher than normal levels of erythropoietin and a greater degree of erythrocytosis.

The erythrocytes of the newborn are considerably larger than those of adults, reflected in an increase in the mean cellular diameter and mean corpuscular volume indices (Table 29-1). The red blood cells have increased hemoglobin content, but the mean corpuscular hemoglobin concentration (MCHC) is within the normal range established for erythrocytes of adults.

A number of physiologic and metabolic characteristics of erythrocytes of newborns also differ from those of red blood cells of older children and adults. Permeability of the fetal red blood cell membrane to sodium and potassium is increased, and glucose utilization and adenosine triphosphate (ATP) production by the erythrocytes are correspondingly elevated. The latter changes appear in part to represent compensatory activities that serve to maintain normal concentrations of intracellular cations by means of an augmented rate of energy-dependent ion transport.

Red blood cell survival is shortened to a mild or moderate degree in the full-term infant as compared with the normal adult erythrocyte survival time of 100 to 120 days. In the premature infant, shortening of the red blood cell life span is even greater, although considerable variability has been reported. The reduced life span of the erythrocytes of the infant may be related to the relatively larger size of the fetal erythrocyte, which, together with greater cell rigidity, renders the erythrocytes less compliant and deformable within the small blood vessels and may cause them to be more susceptible to intravascular damage. In addition, the increased permeability of the red blood cell membrane to sodium and

Table 29-1. Normal hematologic values in cord blood of the full-term newborn

Hemoglobin concentration	14.0-20.0 gm/dl
Red blood cell count	4,200,000-5,800,000/mm^3
Hematocrit	43-63%
Mean cell diameter	8.0-8.3 μm
Mean corpuscular volume (MCV)	100-120 μm^3
Mean corpuscular hemoglobin (MCH)	32-40 pg
Mean corpuscular hemoglobin concentration (MCHC)	30-34%
Reticulocyte count	3-7%
Nucleated red blood cell count	200-600/mm^3
White blood cell count	10,000-30,000/mm^3
Granulocytes	40-80%
Lymphocytes	20-40%
Monocytes	3-10%
Platelet count	150,000-350,000/mm^3
Serum iron concentration	125-225 μg/dl
Total iron-binding capacity	150-350 μg/dl

potassium predisposes the red blood cells to the development of adverse osmotic changes within the cells, adding further risk of premature cell destruction, particularly within the spleen and other reticuloendothelial organs.

An increase in the activity of a number of glycolytic red blood cell enzymes also has been demonstrated in the blood of newborns. However, these changes may reflect the presence of a larger percentage of young red blood cells rather than a specific characteristic of the cells. Other enzymes, including carbonic anhydrase and NADH-dependent methemoglobin reductase, exhibit reduced activity in the red blood cells of the newborn. The decrease in the latter enzyme is a major factor in accounting for the elevated levels of methemoglobin in the blood of newborns, particularly in premature infants, as well as the predisposition of young infants to form methemoglobin more readily in the presence of precipitating factors.

From 70% to 90% of the hemoglobin in the blood of the fetus and newborn is fetal hemoglobin. This hemoglobin type continues to predominate through the first weeks of postnatal life, after which it gradually becomes replaced by adult hemoglobin. A functional difference between fetal and adult hemoglobin results from the ability of the latter to interact with low-molecular weight phosphorylated compounds in the cell to produce altered oxygen-binding properties of the hemoglobin. When adult hemoglobin combines with these substances, which include 2,3-diphosphoglycerate (2,3-DPG), ATP, and related compounds, a marked decrease in oxygen affinity occurs. Fetal hemoglobin, on the other hand, undergoes virtually no participation in this type of interaction. The result of this difference in the behavior of adult and fetal hemoglobins is a leftward shift of the oxygen dissociation curve of fetal blood as compared with the blood of adults, representing a relatively greater oxygen affinity of the fetal blood. This property may be of considerable benefit to the fetus in utero by facilitating placental oxygen exchange from maternal blood to the fetal erythrocytes. However, because of the high oxygen affinity of the fetal hemoglobin, release of oxygen to the tissues is impeded, which may be disadvantageous to the newborn, particularly if anemia is present.

The leukocyte count at birth averages approximately 20,000/mm^3, with a wide normal range from 9,000 to 30,000. Approximately 70% of the white blood cells consists of neutrophils, which often include band forms, and occasionally a small number of metamyelocytes and myelocytes. The white count usually drops with bacterial infection, and rare blast forms may appear in the blood smear. After the first week of life the differential count shifts to a predominance of lymphocytes, which persists until 4 or 5 years of age. Phagocytic activity of the neutrophils may be less than normal, but the difference appears to be related to opsonization factors in the serum of the infant rather than to an intrinsic defect of the leukocytes.

Platelet counts of full-term infants range from 150,000 to 300,000/mm^3, which are usually considered to be normal values for adults. Some reports have indicated slightly lower values in some premature infants. In any infant, however, a platelet count of less than 100,000/mm^3 should be considered abnormal.

The bone marrow findings of the newborn reflect the extremely active production of blood cells, particularly erythrocytes, which is characteristic of this period of life. The bone marrow at birth is highly cellular and occupies virtually the entire medullary cavity of all of the bones. Consequently, diagnostic bone marrow aspiration in young infants can be performed in long bone areas, such as the tibias, whereas in the older child and adult these bones contain primarily fatty tissue. Erythroid precursors comprise approximately 40% of the cellular elements present in aspirated bone marrow specimens.

HEMATOLOGIC CHANGES IN THE NEONATE AND INFANT

Within hours after birth of a normal infant the low oxygen saturation of the blood increases to reach approximately 95% saturation. The striking changes in erythropoiesis that occur in the first weeks of life are largely attributable to the improved oxygenation of the blood and tissues of the infant. Erythropoietin levels, which are elevated at birth, rapidly fall to undetectable levels. In the bone marrow, erythropoietic activity becomes suppressed, with red blood cell precursors comprising less than 10% of the nucleated elements by the end of the first week of postnatal life. The reticulocytosis, which is characteristic at birth, also decreases rapidly to reach less than 1% by 5 to 7 days. Nucleated red blood cell precursors disappear even more rapidly and after 2 to 4 days are usually no longer demonstrable in the blood of normal infants.

The postnatal suppression of erythropoiesis, combined with the expansion of the blood volume of the infant caused by rapid growth, produces a progressive decline in the hemoglobin concentration of the infant, beginning near the end of the first week of life and reaching its low point after 2 to 3 months. This physiologic anemia of infancy may result in a hemoglobin concentration of as low as 9.0 gm/dl (11.0 ± 2.0) in a normal full-term infant. These changes do not represent any abnormality or nutritional deficiency in the infant, and the hematologic events at this stage are not affected by the administration of iron or other hematinic agents. With the resumption of active erythropoiesis following the second to third months, if irons supplies are adequate, the hemoglobin concentration of the infant gradually increases to reach a mean level of 12.5 gm/dl, which persists throughout early childhood.

In premature infants, particularly those with birth weights of less than 1,500 gm, the physiologic decrease in hemoglobin concentration develops earlier than in full-term infants and reaches a lower ultimate level. Minimum values are achieved by 4 to 7 weeks, and hemoglobin concentrations of 7 to 8 mg/dl may occur in apparently healthy infants. Resumption of active erythropoiesis in the premature infant is also initiated earlier in postnatal life than in the full-term infant.

The supply of available iron stores in the full-term infant is usually sufficient to sustain normal red blood cell production for approximately the first 6 months of life, even without additional exogenous iron. Thereafter the iron needs related to growth require an intake of approximately 1 mg/kg daily if anemia is to be prevented. In the infant whose iron reserve at birth is diminished, the need for additional iron intake develops earlier. Included in this group are premature infants and infants with blood loss during the fetal or neonatal periods.

Although the iron needs of the normal full-term infant during the first year of life can usually be met by adequate dietary intake, some of these infants develop iron deficiency. It has therefore been recommended that iron supplementation be included in the diet of all infants throughout the first year of life. Iron-enriched cereals and milk formulas generally provide the most convenient and reliable means for providing this supplementary iron. In the premature infant dietary iron is virtually never adequate, and iron supplementation is mandatory to prevent the development of anemia. In these infants it is desirable to introduce iron-enriched milk formula or other iron-containing preparations into the diet during the early weeks of life. Although exogenous iron is not incorporated into hemoglobin to a significant extent in young infants, orally administered iron is nevertheless absorbed and stored by the infant and can be used for hemoglobin synthesis at a later time when the need for additional iron develops.

ANEMIA IN THE NEWBORN PERIOD
Anemia caused by hemorrhage
Fetal-maternal transfusion

Transplacental transfusion of fetal blood into the circulation of the mother has been known for many years to be the basis for maternal antibody formation against fetal erythrocytes in the pathogenesis of isoimmune hemolytic disease. It was first suggested by Weiner that fetal blood loss by this mechanism could occur to an extent sufficient enough to produce anemia at birth. An anemic infant subsequently studied by Chown showed substantial evidence of fetal-maternal hemorrhage; blood from the mother was found to contain an elevated percentage of fetal hemoglobin, and large numbers of erythrocytes were present, having antigenic properties characteristic of the infant's cells but not of those of the mother. The changes in the maternal blood gradually disappeared over a period of several weeks following the delivery. In a survey by Cohen and associates of over 600 pregnancies, fetal erythrocytes were detected in maternal blood in approximately 50% of the cases. In about 1% of the pregnancies the transplacental hemorrhage appeared to be of sufficient magnitude to produce anemia in the infant.

Clinical manifestations. In a majority of patients the bleeding appears to occur at a slow rate over a prolonged period of time before delivery. The degree of anemia in the newborn can vary widely, ranging from mild to very severe. Jaundice is characteristically absent, the Coombs antiglobulin test is negative, and the liver and spleen are not enlarged; these findings allow this condition to be readily distinguished from the anemia of isoimmune hemolytic disease. Pallor and tachycardia are present to a degree related to the severity of the anemia. The infant otherwise is usually active and in no apparent distress. The anemia is accompanied by polychromatophilia of the erythrocytes, by elevated reticulocyte counts, and often by increased numbers of nucleated red blood cells. If the anemia is severe and is the result of chronic long-term hemorrhage, the hematologic findings characteristic of severe iron-deficiency anemia will be present, including hypochromia and microcytosis of the erythrocytes, decreased serum iron levels, and an absence of stainable iron in aspirated bone marrow.

If the fetal-maternal transfusion occurs acutely at the time of labor or delivery, the findings in the infant will reflect the rapid reduction in the blood volume (p. 255). Loss of more than 40 ml of blood can be sufficient to produce findings of hypovolemic shock. The infant may appear weak and pale, with tachycardia and labored respirations. Anemia can usually be demonstrated; but if insufficient time has elapsed for compensatory hemodilution to occur, the hemoglobin concentration may not be significantly depressed. Acute blood loss usually can be confirmed, however, by a decreased umbilical venous pressure. The presumptive diagnosis of severe acute blood loss should be considered in any pale neonate in distress when the liver or spleen is not enlarged, and appropriate measures should be undertaken immediately to confirm or disprove this possibility.

Laboratory manifestations. Loss of fetal blood into the maternal circulation can be established by demonstrating the presence of fetal erythrocytes in the mother's blood. The most widely applicable technique is the slide elution procedure of Kleihauer and Betke. In this procedure, which is performed rapidly and easily, unstained blood

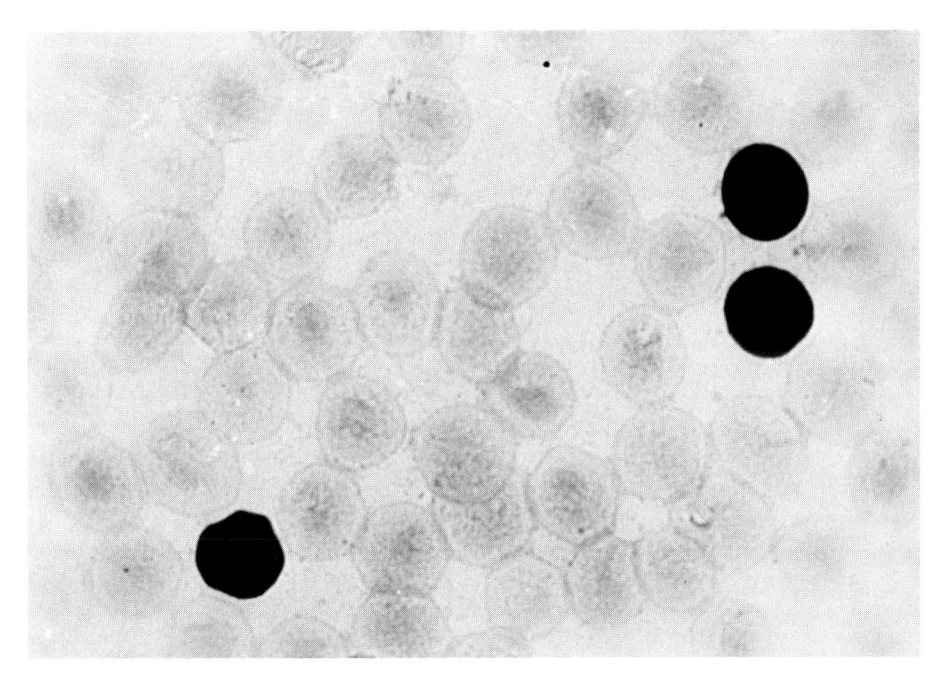

Fig. 29-3. Fetal erythrocytes in maternal blood following a transplacental hemorrhage. The slide was stained following elution of adult hemoglobin by the Kleihauer-Betke procedure. The fetal cells are darkly stained, whereas those of the mother are barely visible.

smears are fixed and then incubated in an acidic buffer that causes adult hemoglobin to be eluted from the erythrocytes. Fetal hemoglobin resists elution under these conditions and remains within the intact red blood cells. After staining, the fetal hemoglobin-containing erythrocytes become visible as darkly stained cells, while the erythrocytes of maternal origin, which contain principally adult hemoglobin, appear as clear, ghostlike cells (Fig. 29-3). The presence of even small numbers of fetal cells in maternal blood is readily ascertained by this procedure, and by determination of the percentage of fetal cells present an estimate of the quantity of blood transfused can be made. If major blood group incompatibility exists between the mother and infant, transfused fetal erythrocytes may be rapidly removed from the maternal circulation and may not be detectable in blood smears from the mother. Under these conditions the mother may develop fever or a shaking chill, representing a transfusion reaction to the infusion of incompatible blood. Buffy coat smears of the maternal blood may demonstrate erythrophagocytosis when blood group incompatibility exists and may be helpful in establishing a diagnosis when the slide elution test for fetal cells is negative.

Treatment. Treatment of the infant depends on both the severity of the anemia and whether the blood loss occurred acutely or chronically. In the infant with a mild degree of anemia, particularly when there is evidence that the blood loss was not acute, no immediate therapy is usually necessary if the infant is vigorous and in no distress. If tachycardia or marked pallor is present, a transfusion of packed red blood cells is indicated. In the severely affected infant with findings of iron deficiency caused by prolonged hemorrhage, incipient heart failure may be present, and transfusion may impose a risk of vascular overload. Under these conditions a partial exchange transfusion using packed red blood cells is preferable. When transfusions are done in these infants, it is rarely necessary to increase the hemoglobin concentration to more than 11 to 12 gm/dl to achieve complete relief of symptoms of anemia. Iron therapy is essential in subsequent care because of depletion of the iron stores, which is invariably present. Adequate iron supplementation in these infants can be achieved by the regular use of an iron-enriched milk formula or by oral administration of an iron preparation sufficient to provide 2 to 3 mg of elemental iron per kilogram daily. The iron supplementation should be started in early infancy and continued throughout the first year of life to ensure that the iron needs for growth of the infant are fully met.

In the neonate with findings of hypovolemic shock at birth because of acute bleeding into the maternal circulation shortly before delivery, rapid diagnosis and prompt institution of therapy are essential to prevent irreversible changes. Therapy is directed toward rapid restoration of the infant's blood volume and should be started immediately after the condition is recognized. Fresh type O, Rh-negative blood, 10 to 20 ml/kg, should be injected rapidly through an umbilical catheter. When blood is not readily available, albumin solutions, plasma, or dextran may be given in the initial infusion, to be followed by whole blood as soon as it becomes available. The response to blood replacement in these infants is usually dramatic. Tachycardia and tachypnea rapidly subside, and tone and activity improve promptly. Subsequent additional transfusions with packed red blood cells are indicated if signs of distress persist or if the hemoglobin concentration falls to less than 8 to 9 gm/dl after fluid equilibration in the plasma has taken place. Orally administered iron should be given to these infants and continued throughout the first year.

Blood loss in utero from one twin to another

incidence and etiology. Newborn monovular twins frequently exhibit large differences in their hemoglobin concentrations at birth, with anemia being present in one twin and polycythemia in the other. In approximately 70% of monovular twin pregnancies the placentas are monochorial and almost invariably contain vascular communications between the fetal circulations (p. 213). When a significant degree of arteriovenous anastomosis exists between the placental circulation of one twin and the other, the opportunity exists for the twin on the arterial limb of the communication to infuse blood into the circulation of the other. A study of 130 monochorial twin pregnancies indicated an incidence of at least 15% significant blood loss from one twin to the other. A high mortality of the affected twins occurred, often with death in utero early in the pregnancy. Of 38 of these infants born alive, only 13 survived, suggesting that this complication may be a major factor to account for the higher mortality of monochorial as compared with dichorial twin pregnancies.

Clinical manifestations. In the donor twin, anemia may vary from mild to severe. Red blood cell hypochromia and microcytosis are often present as a reflection of iron deficiency caused by the prolonged blood loss. Elevated reticulocyte counts and large numbers of nucleated red blood cells represent a compensatory increase of erythrocyte production. The anemia is often accompanied by oligohydramnios and hypotension. If blood loss has been extensive, the infant may exhibit pallor, weakness, and tachycardia.

The polycythemic infant presents a ruddy appearance and often is larger than the anemic twin. The infant may show evidence of hypertension, which can be associated with heart failure and pulmonary edema. Hyperviscosity of the blood results from the increased red blood cell mass and can predispose these infants to venous thrombosis of hemorrhage. Hyperbilirubinemia may accompany breakdown of the increased numbers of red blood cells.

Treatment. The donor twin may require supportive transfusions if symptomatic anemia is present. With severe anemia a partial exchange transfusion with packed red blood cells minimizes the risk of circulatory overload. If the infant is asymptomatic and the anemia is not severe, orally administered iron will usually be all that is required.

In the polycythemic twin, phlebotomy is indicated if complications arise as a result of hyperviscosity of the blood or from circulatory overload. The hemoglobin concentration can be reduced most effectively by performing a partial exchange transfusion using plasma to replace the blood that is removed. Phototherapy may be useful in minimizing the risk of dangerous hyperbilirubinemia in these infants. Serial determinations of the serum bilirubin level should be performed, and exchange transfusion should be considered if there is hyperbilirubinemia (p. 766).

Obstetric hemorrhage

Incidence. Anemia in newborns caused by acute obstetric hemorrhage occurs at a rate of approximately 1 per 1,000 live births. This complication may result from obstetric accidents in otherwise normal pregnancies or be predisposed by abnormalities of the umbilical cord, umbilical vessels, or placenta.

Etiology. Rupture of the normal umbilical cord has been documented as a cause of neonatal hemorrhage primarily following precipitous, often unattended deliveries. Although this now occurs uncommonly, it should be considered when an anemic infant with a history of an uncontrolled delivery is encountered. When the cord is abnormally short or is entangled with the infant, it may become torn in the course of even a normal delivery. Varices or aneurysms of the umbilical vessels may produce areas of focal weakness that predispose the infant to rupture of the cord. When the placental insertion of the umbilical cord is abnormal (p. 211), giving rise to anomalous aberrant vessels lying free on the placental surface or to a diffuse velamentous insertion, the unprotected vessels become easily subjected to laceration during the delivery with the risk of considerable blood loss by the infant. A not infrequent anomaly is multilobularity of the placenta, in which one or more accessory lobules exist apart from the main body of the placenta. The lobules are joined by fragile communicating vessels that become easily disrupted during labor and delivery, accompanied by hemorrhage.

In placenta previa and abruptio placentae, hemorrhage from the placental surface can result in blood loss from the infant as well as from the mother. In these disorders the incidence of stillbirths is high, and surviving infants frequently are severely anemic at birth. Acute blood loss following accidental incision of the placenta at cesarean section is also not uncommon, particularly in placenta previa. Tearing or separation of the placenta during delivery of the infant through the uterine incision may also lead to significant blood loss.

Clinical manifestations. In anemia developing as a result of obstetric hemorrhage, the findings in the infant at birth are attributable to acute blood loss, and following severe hemorrhage may include pallor, tachycardia, irregular respirations, decreased tone, and a weak cry. The central venous pressure will often be reduced. The hemoglobin concentration immediately after delivery may not reflect the true magnitude of blood loss; but usually 6 to 12 hours later, after hemodilution has occurred, the anemia will be fully apparent.

Treatment. Therapy is directed toward rapid expansion of the blood volume with transfusions of fresh whole blood whenever possible, as described in the preceding sections. Dietary supplementation with orally administered iron should be started early and in adequate amounts to prevent later development of iron deficiency.

Postnatal hemorrhage

Hemorrhage in the first days of life as a cause of anemia most often results from birth trauma. When a congenital or acquired disorder of hemostasis is present in the infant, postpartum hemorrhage is not uncommon, even in the absence of unusual trauma at delivery. Postnatal bleeding may be apparent or occult and in either case may result in gradual or rapidly progressive anemia. The sudden onset of shock in a previously well infant sometimes may be the first indication of occult hemorrhage. In any infant who develops anemia beyond the first day of life, without jaundice or other evidence of hemolysis, every attempt should be made to ascertain or exclude the presence of internal bleeding. In premature infants, in cases of multiple births, and following breech or traumatic deliveries the risk of postnatal hemorrhage is increased.

Hemorrhage into the scalp associated with a caput succedaneum occurs commonly (p. 218) but usually subsides within a few days, producing no untoward effect. Occasionally a substantial quantity of blood may be lost into the scalp, resulting in anemia of sufficient severity to require supportive transfusions of packed red blood cells. Subperiosteal hemorrhages (cephalhematomas) occur with or without fracture of the skull (p. 218). The hemorrhage is often gradual and may continue for 1 to 3 days, after which it usually subsides spontaneously. Massive blood loss requiring tranfusion occurs in rare instances. A more frequent complication in these infants is the development of jaundice following degradation of the extravasated blood. The bilirubin level may become sufficiently elevated to produce kernicterus if the hemorrhage has been extensive.

Intracranial hemorrhage may result as a complication of birth trauma, and intraventricular hemorrhage is particularly prevalent in premature infants (p. 367). Subarachnoid or subdural hemorrhage may be of sufficient severity to produce anemia, for which small transfusions of packed red blood cells should be given.

Hemorrhage into the liver, spleen, adrenals, or kidneys, following rupture or laceration of these organs, may also produce anemia in the perinatal period. Predisposing factors include traumatic or breech delivery, prematurity, disorders of hemostasis, and conditions that produce swelling or distension of the abdominal organs. The liver is most commonly affected. Hemorrhage may be mild and limited to subcapsular bleeding or may result from rupture of the parenchyma and capsule of the liver, with massive blood loss into the peritoneal cavity. With progressive subcapsular hepatic hemorrhage the infant may appear well until rupture of the capsule ensues, followed by rapid development of hemoperitoneum and hypovolemic shock (p. 232). Splenic rupture in the newborn period occurs uncommonly but may follow a traumatic delivery (p. 233). In a majority of the reported examples of this complication, splenic distension associated with splenomegaly caused by isoimmune hemolytic disease was present. Retroperitoneal hemorrhage involving the adrenals, or less commonly the kidneys, usually follows a traumatic delivery and may produce anemia (p. 233). Findings attributable to blood loss often develop soon after birth and are accompanied by an enlarging flank mass. In some infants the adrenal hemorrhage may be manifested as unexplained jaundice together with a mass in the flank in an otherwise healthy-appearing infant. The diagnosis can often be established by the finding of a radiolucent suprarenal mass and downward and lateral displacement of the kidney on an excretory urogram. These findings may be similar to those of congenital neuroblastoma. Arteriography through the umbilical artery will usually show increased vascularity in neuroblastoma, whereas an avascular lesion is seen in adrenal hemorrhage.

Anemia due to hemorrhagic disorders
Development of hemostasis in the newborn

In spite of modern blood component therapy, hemorrhage is a direct cause of death in many premature and full-term infants. It may occur as specific organ-related bleeding, such as intracranial or pulmonary hemorrhage, or as part of a generalized bleeding diathesis, such as

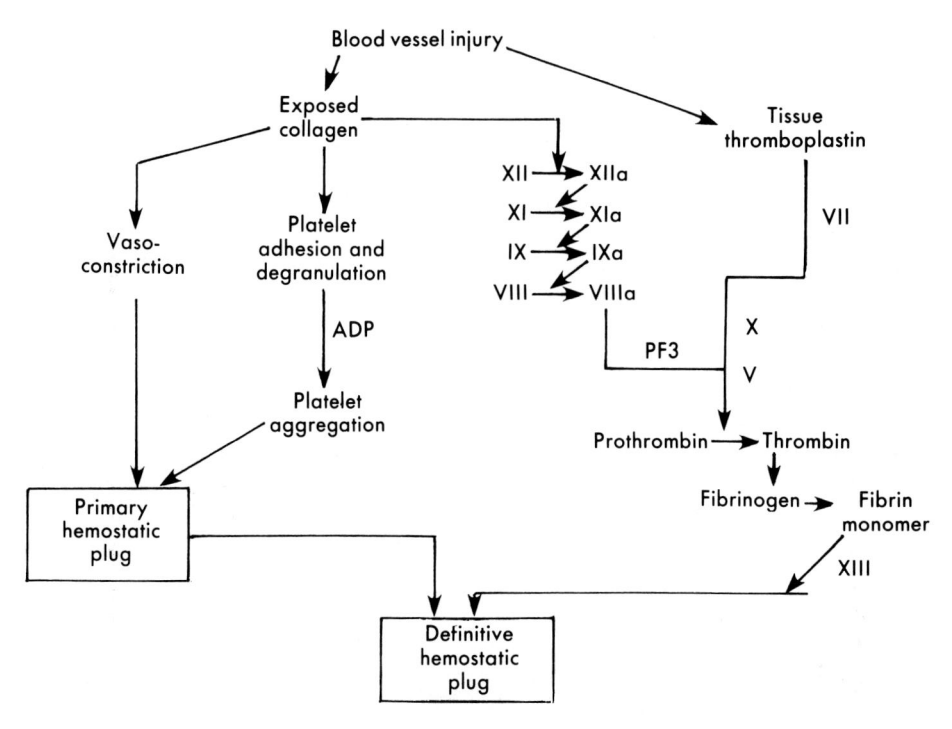

Fig. 29-4. Intravascular clotting cascade. Components of normal hemostasis.

disseminated intravascular coagulation (DIC). Normal hemostatic mechanisms are still incompletely understood in the fetus and newborn, but some knowledge of these values is essential for proper treatment of bleeding neonates.

Normal hemostasis requires the interaction of three separate components: (1) the endothelial lining of the blood vessel, (2) platelet release, and (3) the intravascular clotting cascade (Fig. 29-4). Although an abnormality in one of these arms may be tolerated with minimum bleeding, changes in more than one arm usually cause significant bleeding. For example, an infant with a platelet count of 20,000/mm^3 due to isoimmune thrombocytopenia is usually asymptomatic, but if the same infant develops bacterial sepsis with DIC, fatal bleeding may occur.

When a vessel wall is injured, it immediately contracts while the exposed collagen activates the clotting cascade and causes platelet adhesion and degranulation to occur with ADP release. The resulting platelet aggregate plugs the vessel temporarily until it can react with fibrin polymer to form the definitive clot. Except for small premature infants who have increased vascular fragility, vessel integrity and platelet number are normal in newborns, and therefore the bleeding time is normal. A mild, transient platelet function deficit is present in newborns, which produces slight decrease in platelet factor 3 release and aggregation with epinephrine, ADP, collagen, and thrombin.

There is no placental transfer of clotting factors, which are slightly decreased in full-term infants and moderately decreased in premature infants (Table 29-2). The vitamin K–dependent factors (prothrombin and factors VII, IX, and X) are significantly decreased and may drop low enough to cause clinical bleeding if vitamin K is not administered during the first day of life. Antihemophilic factor (VIII) is normal at birth. Factor VIII antigen is normal or even above normal, with a mean of 182% on the first day of life. There may be low-grade consumption during delivery, which decreases the level of circulating procoagulant without changing the level of antigen.

Although fibrinolytic activity (as measured by the euglobulin lysis time) is increased in all newborns, fibrin split products are not increased, possibly due to rapid liver clearance. As discussed previously, most of the clotting factors are decreased in the newborn, but the whole-blood clotting time is shortened. This paradox can be explained by decreased levels of circulating anticoagulants, particularly antithrombin III, an α_2-globulin. Small for date and postmature infants have partial thromboplastin times (PTT), prothrombin times, and thrombin times that are slightly more prolonged than those of full-term infants. The fibrinogen, factor V, and factor VIII

Table 29-2. Hemostatic function

Hemostatic factor or component	Premature infant	Full-term infant	Age adult level is attained
Vascular and platelet function			
Vasoconstriction	Present	Present	At birth
Capillary fragility	Increased	Normal	At birth
Bleeding time	Normal	Normal	At birth
Platelet count	Normal	Normal	At birth
Platelet function	↓↓ Aggregative ability	↓ Aggregative ability ↓ Clot retraction ↓ Platelet factor 3 availability	Not established
Coagulation			
Whole blood clotting time	Decreased	↓ Or normal	At birth
Partial thromboplastin time (PTT) (adult normal, 35-45 seconds)	70-145 seconds	45-70 seconds	2-9 months
Prothrombin time (PT) (adult normal, 12-14 seconds)	12-21 seconds	13-20 seconds	3-4 days
Thrombin time (TT) (adult normal, 8-10 seconds)	11-17 seconds	10-16 seconds	Few days
Thrombotest (II, VII, IX, X)	30%-50%	40%-68%	2-12 months
XII (Hageman factor)	10%-50%	25%-60%	9-14 days
IX (PTA)	5%-20%	15%-70%	1-2 months
IX (PTC)	10%-25%	20%-60%	3-9 months
VIII (AHF)	20%-80%	70%-150%	At birth
VII (proconvertin)	20%-45%	20%-70%	2-12 months
X (Stuart-Prower factor)	10%-45%	20%-55%	2-12 months
V (proaccelerin)	50%-85%	80%-200%	At birth
II (prothrombin)	20%-80%	26%-65%	2-12 months
I (fibrinogen) (gm/dl)	150%-300%	150%-300%	2-4 days
XIII (fibrin-stabilizing factor)	100%	100%	At birth
Fibrin split products (μg/ml)	0-10	0-7	
Antithrombin III	48%	55%	

Modified from Bleyer, W.A., Hakami, N., and Shepard, T.H.: J. Pediatr. **79**:838, 1971.

levels are normal. Their platelet counts are also slightly low, averaging 130,000/mm^3.

Congenital coagulation disorders

Hemophilia is by far the most common inherited coagulation disorder to cause bleeding in the neonatal period. Since both classic hemophilia and Christmas disease are X-linked, they occur almost exclusively in males. Fifty percent of infants with severe hemophilia develop bleeding in the first week of life, from either birth trauma, routine heel sticks, or circumcision. A positive family history occurs in two thirds of cases and helps confirm the clinical diagnosis. Laboratory findings show a prolonged PTT with a normal prothrombin time. However, since the PTT is prolonged in normal newborns also, a factor VIII or IX assay must be run. A very low level of factor VIII combined with a normal level of factor VIII–related antigen confirms the diagnosis of classic hemophilia. The assay should be performed on the mother at the same time to confirm that she is a carrier, since most mothers of hemophiliacs are shown to be carriers when careful studies are done. Resorption of blood from skin or other hemorrhagic sites may occasionally produce hyperbilirubinemia in a neonate. If specific treatment of bleeding is required, cryoprecipitate should be used rather than commercial factor VIII concentrates, since newborns are more susceptible to the markedly increased risk of hepatitis associated with concentrates. Fresh frozen plasma in a dosage of 10 ml/kg should be given for infants with Christmas disease.

Factor XIII (fibrin-stabilizing factor) deficiency is rare but causes delayed bleeding at several days of age. The most common bleeding site is the umbilical stump, which may not start bleeding until 2 or 3 days of age. The disorder is autosomal recessive and therefore occurs in both sexes. Routine clotting studies are all normal, and diagnosis requires special factor assays using solubility of a euglobulin clot in 6M urea. Fresh frozen plasma is the only treatment.

Vitamin K deficiency is much less common in newborns now that nurseries give vitamin K injections to all infants in the first 24 hours of life (K$_1$ oxide, 0.5 to 1.0 mg parenterally). Neonates lack vitamin K stores and need additional amounts at birth. Because of their immature livers, premature infants are particularly prone to hemorrhagic diseases. Inadvertent failure to administer vitamin K is the most common cause of this disorder, but maternal therapy with hydantoin anticonvulsants or coumadin or parenteral alimentation of the infant without adequate vitamin K supplementation may cause the need for additional vitamin. Prolonged use of broad-spectrum antibiotics also may lower the amount of vitamin K synthesized by gut flora and result in deficiency. Babies with this disorder tend to look normal except for bleeding on the second to fourth day of life with gastrointestinal, cutaneous, or central nervous system hemorrhage. Studies show a prolonged prothrombin time and PTT with normal platelet counts and fibrinogen levels. Intravenous vitamin K is usually sufficient therapy, and plasma is rarely required.

Platelet disorders

The causes of thrombocytopenia in newborns can be grouped into 3 types of disorders: (1) immune, (2) congenital problems where thrombocytopenia may be only one of a group of abnormalities, and (3) infection. Thrombocytopenia is generally defined as less than 150,000 platelets/mm^3 in any age patient. Although the count is most accurately done by phase-contrast microscopy, examination of a carefully made blood film is the simplest way to estimate platelet count. Normally, five platelets should be present on an oil-immersion field.

Bleeding due to decreased platelets classically causes petechiae plus epistaxis, melena, and central nervous system bleeding. The level of platelets at which bleeding signs occur is extremely variable. Petechiae rarely occur until platelets drop below 60,000/mm^3, and spontaneous hemorrhage is unlikely with counts above 30,000/mm^3. The presence of additional problems such as sepsis or hypervolemia frequently triggers or worsens clinical bleeding in a patient who is already thrombocytopenic.

In neonatal immune thrombocytopenia, IgG platelet antibodies cross the placenta and coat the platelet, causing its rapid removal from the circulation, usually by the spleen or occasionally by the liver, thus shortening the platelet life span to a few hours. Harrington and associates have shown by in vitro techniques that the IgG is adsorbed to the platelet membrane and affects autologous as well as homologous platelets. As few as 50 to 100 antibody molecules can sensitize a platelet for destruction, corresponding to only a 1% saturation of antigenic sites on the membrane. Techniques for measuring platelet antibodies are many and varied and are available only in research laboratories. The best techniques currently in use are indirect and depend on antibody-induced injury of the platelet membrane to trigger a reaction, e.g., the platelet factor 3 release method uses release of PF3 to stimulate clotting in a partially activated plasma system. ^{14}C-labeled serotonin release is measured in another assay.

Active, or autoimmune, neonatal thrombocytopenia is a possible complication when the mother has circulating platelet antibodies due to an autoimmune disease such as lupus erythematosus or idiopathic thrombocytopenic purpura (ITP). This disorder is best diagnosed by maternal history and platelet count. When the maternal platelet count is normal, the infant is rarely affected unless the mother has been splenectomized. However, when the maternal count is low, 50%-90% of infants are affected.

Passive, or isoimmune, thrombocytopenia is analogous to erythroblastosis and can occur alone or in conjunction with red cell sensitization. The incidence of this disorder is about 3 per 10,000 live births. The mother produces an antiplatelet antibody on stimulation by fetal platelets, which cross the placenta. The antibody is most commonly directed against the Pl^{a1} antigen, since only 3% of the population is negative for this antigen, and therefore a Pl^{a1}-negative mother has a high probability of sensitization.

The major therapeutic dilemma in immune thrombocytopenia is deciding which mothers are at risk for a thrombocytopenic infant. In autoimmune thrombocytopenia, bleeding is likely if maternal platelets are low. Isoimmune disorders are rarely detected until after an affected child has been born. Since the disorder may occur with subsequent pregnancies, later babies should all be considered to have a high risk for thrombocytopenia. When an infant has a low platelet count, the most risky period is delivery itself. For this reason, caesarean section is recommended for all infants judged at high risk. If the mother's platelet count is less than 60,000/mm^3 to 100,000/mm^3, she should be given platelet transfusions prior to surgery.

Once the infant is born without problems, he has a very low risk of significant bleeding and rarely needs treatment. The parents can be reassured that the disorder is self-limited and will clear when the maternal IgG is metabolized, usually in 4 to 8 weeks. If an infant has more than minor skin bleeding after delivery, the only effective treatment is platelet transfusions. The mother is the ideal platelet donor, since she is Pl^{a1} negative, but she has circulating antibodies that are difficult to remove, even by washing the platelets. If bleeding persists in spite of platelet transfusions, exchange transfusion with fresh whole blood will eliminate much of the antibody while also raising the infant's platelet count. Babies with significant bleeding into an enclosed space, such as intracranially, may develop delayed jaundice as the blood is resorbed. Fig. 29-5 shows the typical response to transfused platelets in an infant with isoimmune thrombocytopenia. There are several rare but interesting causes of neonatal thrombocytopenia due to decreased platelet production as shown by megakaryocytic hypoplasia in bone marrow aspirate or biopsy specimens.

Isolated congenital hypoplastic thrombocytopenia is seen in babies who are otherwise healthy but have unremitting thrombocytopenia. Most such cases described in the literature are probably due to other causes, such as congenital viral infections.

Infants with thrombocytopenia–absent radii syndrome (TAR) have megakaryocytic hypoplasia associated with limb deformities varying from bilateral absent radii to phocomelia. They may also have minor renal or skeletal abnormalities. Fig. 29-6 shows an infant with this disorder. In addition to severe thrombocytopenia, these babies have a characteristic leukocytosis during the first few weeks of life with a marked shift to the left in the differential count, frequently including 1% to 5% circulating blasts. The leukocytosis usually resolves after several months, but severe thrombocytopenia persists for years. If the children survive the first few months of life, their bleeding symptoms usually improve because the platelet count rises to above 10,000/mm^3 by age 4 or 5 years. However, mortality from intracerebral bleeding in the neonatal period is significant. These infants are almost always mentally normal and manage well with good orthopedic and psychosocial support. Probably incomplete forms of the syndrome exist where a child has the blood abnormalities of TAR, but less severe orthope-

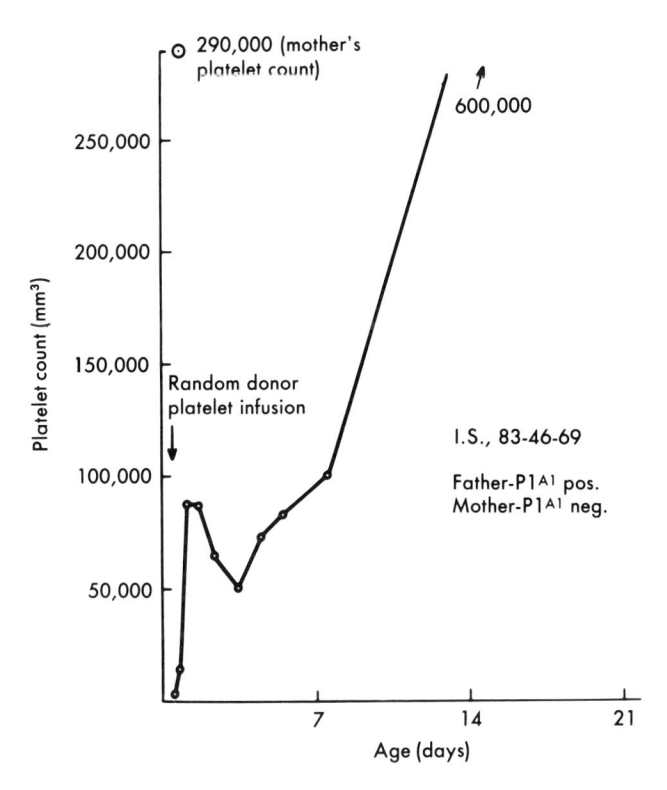

Fig. 29-5. Neonatal response to random donor platelet transfusions in isoimmune disease with low titers of circulating antibody. Survival curves probably represent combined effects of antibody dilution and increasing endogenous platelet survival.

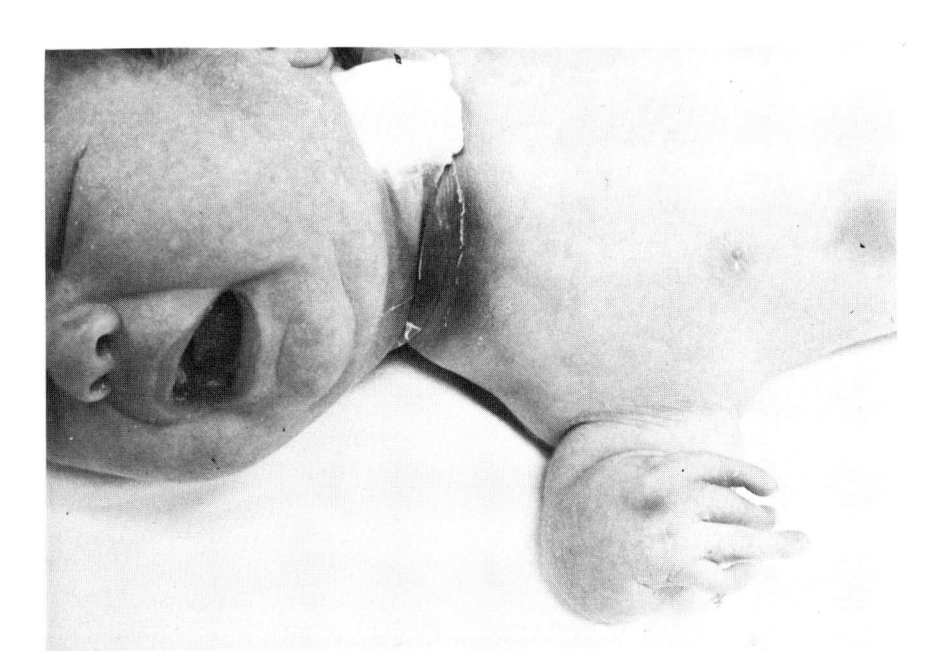

Fig. 29-6. Hand anomalies and skin hemorrhage in a newborn with thrombocytopenia–absent radius syndrome.

dic deformities. In this situation the leukocyte abnormalities are a useful marker.

Several other uncommon disorders may cause neonatal thrombocytopenia, including the sex-linked Wiskott-Aldrich syndrome, Schwachman's syndrome (neutropenia and pancreatic insufficiency), and trisomy 13 or trisomy 18.

Bacterial or viral infections are probably the most common causes of neonatal thrombocytopenia. This may occur as part of disseminated intravascular coagulation or as an isolated event. Each of the TORCH infections can cause severe thrombocytopenia, and every infant with unidentified thrombocytopenia should have a TORCH titer run. The mechanism is usually viral or bacterial adherence to the platelet membrane, causing it to be destroyed in the spleen. An element of bone marrow suppression frequently is also present and contributes to the thrombocytopenia.

Disseminated intravascular coagulation (DIC)

Despite numerous publications on DIC, treatment of this disorder remains difficult and controversial. DIC occurs when the balance between circulating procoagulants, proteases, endothelial lining, and blood flow is upset, either locally or systemically, producing apparent consumption of intrinsic clotting factors. The primary defect also can be an alteration in the fibrinogen molecule itself. It is important to remember, however, that DIC is a *syndrome* that occurs secondary to a variety of primary events, an outline of which follows*:

A. Hypoxia-acidosis
 1. Hyaline membrane disease
 2. Asphyxia
B. Infectious diseases
 1. Disseminated viral diseases
 2. Bacterial septicemia
 3. Protozoal infections—toxoplasmosis
C. Obstetric conditions
 1. Abruptio placentae
 2. Dead twin fetus
 3. Chorioangioma
 4. Eclampsia and preeclampsia
 5. Infants who are small for gestational age or who are postmature
D. Miscellaneous diseases and conditions
 1. Severe erythroblastosis fetalis (Rh isoimmunization)
 2. Necrotizing enterocolitis
 3. Shock

This complication typically is recognized in a very sick neonate who suddenly develops generalized bleeding with oozing from puncture sites, catheter insertions, and endotracheal tubes. Because diagnosis may be difficult in newborns who normally have prolonged clotting studies, all sick neonates should have clotting studies performed on admission as a baseline of comparison should bleeding develop later.

The diagnosis of DIC is based on laboratory findings of thrombocytopenia, increased PTT and prothrombin time, and decreased fibrinogen levels.

A. Minimal criteria for DIC
 1. Thrombocytopenia
 2. ↑ PTT
 3. ↑ Prothrombin time
 4. Hypofibrinogenemia
B. Helpful confirmative tests
 1. ↑ Thrombin time (not corrected by protamine)
 2. ↑ Fibrin split products
 3. ↓ Levels of factors V and VIII

If additional tests are available, prolonged thrombin time, fibrin split products, and decreased levels of factors V and VIII will confirm the diagnosis. Once successful therapy is initiated, the intrinsic clotting factors usually increase first, and it may take 5 to 10 days for platelets to revert to normal levels.

The most important issue in therapy of DIC is whether the triggering event (e.g., septicemia, asphyxia) is treatable and reversible. If it is not, the infant will probably die regardless of how vigorously the blood abnormalities are treated.

Most centers now feel that supportive care with blood components is the best treatment of DIC, having the least chance of causing further stress to an already sick infant. Fresh frozen plasma, 10 cc/kg, provides all intrinsic clotting factors and can be repeated every 12 to 24 hours if bleeding persists. If platelets are less that 20,000 to 40,000/mm^3, one or two platelet packs should also be given. Since one unit of platelets also contains fibrinogen and factor VII, platelets alone frequently are adequate treatment of a bleeding episode and are particularly useful when one does not want to push large intravascular volumes into a small infant. For the rare infant whose bleeding persists despite these measures, exchange transfusion with fresh, heparinized blood will provide clotting factors and platelets while also eliminating some of the circulating fibrin split production.

Heparinization has been effective in reversing DIC in some situations in adults and has occasionally been recommended for children. There has never been any objective evidence that heparin reverses DIC in children, however, and heparinization of small infants frequently triggers even more bleeding in an infant who is already critically ill. In addition, heparin has a prolonged half-life in neonates, and it is very difficult to monitor heparinization accurately, since all clotting tests are prolonged in normal newborns.

*From Corrigan, J.J., Jr.: Am. J. Pediatr. Hematol./Oncol. 1:245, 1979. ©1979, Masson Publishing USA, Inc., New York.

Table 29-3. Laboratory evaluation of the bleeding infant

	Platelet count	Prothrombin time	PTT	Fibrinogen	Factor VIII
Well infant					
Thrombocytopenia	↓	N	N	N	N
Vitamin K deficiency	N	↑	↑	N	N
Classic hemophilia	N	N	↑	N	↓↓
Sick infant					
DIC	↓	↑	↑	↓↓	↓
Liver disease	N-↓	↑	↑	Sl↓	N-↑
Infection	N-↓	N	N-↑	↑	↑

Evaluation of a bleeding newborn

In the evaluation of a neonate with bleeding, first determine whether the bleeding is localized or generalized. Localized bleeding, such as subperiosteal or intraventricular or intrapulmonary hemorrhage, is almost always a local phenomenon and not due to a generalized coagulopathy, but the latter two are frequently triggered by asphyxia and may ultimately progress to DIC.

Table 29-3 illustrates the laboratory evaluation of a bleeding infant. Because infection, either viral or bacterial, is the most common cause of neonatal bleeding, all such infants should have a thorough search for infection, including TORCH titers and careful bacterial cultures. A good screening series of clotting tests includes a platelet count, prothrombin time, PTT, and fibrinogen level. If thrombocytopenia is the only abnormality in an otherwise vigorous infant, specific causes such as platelet antibodies, congenital megakaryocytic hypoplasia with TAR, or Schwachman's or Wiskott-Aldrich syndrome must be suspected. If platelets are normal, but PTT and prothrombin time are prolonged, the child probably has had inadequate vitamin K; an intravenous dose of 1 mg can be given as a diagnostic trial. Healthy males with a prolonged PTT probably have hemophilia; a specific assay for antihemophilic factor or Christmas factor will confirm the diagnosis.

An infant who suddenly becomes ill with generalized bleeding usually has bleeding either from thrombocytopenia plus vasculitis or from thrombocytopenia associated with a full-blown DIC syndrome. Occasionally, liver disease can be confused with DIC, but this is very uncommon in neonates. Liver disease must be severe to decrease production of factors II, VII, IX and X enough to prolong the PTT. Fibrinogen levels never get below 60 to 80 mg/dl without consumption, since a small amount of fibrinogen is made by extrahepatic sources such as vascular endothelium. Therefore a fibrinogen level of less than 50 mg/dl is due either to DIC or, rarely, to congenital hypofibrinogenemia.

Laboratory assessment of hemostasis

It is possible, with the use of a limited number of screening tests, to identify the underlying pathologic process and thus initiate appropriate evaluation of specific testing procedures in virtually any hemostatic disorder. The *partial thromboplastin time* (PTT) is a readily available and reliable screening test for assessing a well-circumscribed group of plasma coagulation factors. Prolongation of the PTT occurs with deficiency of all coagulation factors with the exception of VII and XIII. Deficiencies in the extrinsic pathway (factors I, II, V, VII, and X) are evaluated by the *prothrombin time* (PT). The *euglobulin lysis time* screens for deficiencies in fibrinolysis. Rapid screening assays for factor XIII (urea solubility) and fibrinogen are readily available in any comprehensive neonatology center. The *platelet count* is a specific indicator of platelet numbers, and the *bleeding time* offers insight into the vascular component of hemostasis as well as platelet function.

Congenital anemias due to erythrocyte underproduction

Congenital hypoplastic anemia (CHA)

Congenital hypoplastic anemia has been described under a variety of names, including chronic aregenerative anemia, erythrogenesis imperfecta, pure red cell aplasia, and Diamond-Blackfan anemia. It was initially described as a distinct entity in 1938. There is an equal sex distribution and no clear-cut genetic pattern of inheritance in the majority of cases, although both full- and half-siblings have been affected. Gradual onset of severe anemia occurs in the first months of life, with 72% of patients presenting by the age of 4 months. Reticulocytopenia in the peripheral blood reflects the marked diminution of erythrocyte precursors in the bone marrow (erythroblastopenia). Total white count, absolute neutrophil count, and platelet count are all normal.

Several features characteristic of fetal erythrocytes persist throughout life in these patients, including macrocytosis (MCV usually greater than 100 μm³), elevated levels of hemoglobin F, heterogeneously distributed among the red cell population, and expression of the "i" antigen on the surface of erythrocytes. These features are often helpful in distinguishing CHA from transient erythroblastopenia of childhood (TEC), in which the MCV is usually less than 90 μm³ at presentation and in remission. This disorder may also present in the first months of life but requires no specific therapy and has no long-term consequences.

Levels of erythropoietin are elevated in CHA. The mechanism of suppression of erythropoiesis is not known. Immunologic factors are suspected, since both serum and lymphocytes have been found to inhibit bone marrow erythroid colony growth in vitro. It is probable that multiple mechanisms are active, and CHA does not have a single pathogenesis underlying all cases of the disorder. Neither nutritional factors nor lack of stimulating hormones appears to contribute to lack of erythrocyte production, however.

Several constitutional anomalies, including triphalangeal thumbs, have been reported in association with CHA. Peripheral blood lymphocyte and bone marrow chromosomes are normal, in contrast to Fanconi's anemia, which usually presents beyond the neonatal period and involves multiple cell lines. Several patients with CHA have developed acute leukemia in adolescence or young adulthood. Short stature is a consistent finding but is not usually evident at birth, with only about 20% of patients small for gestational age. Short stature does not appear to be solely a feature of corticosteroid therapy but may be aggravated by chronic use of drugs.

Infants present with gradually increasing pallor, poor feeding, and listlessness. Physical examination is usually unremarkable except for pallor unless the child is in congestive heart failure, in which case hepatomegaly with or without splenomegaly and flow murmurs suggestive of cardiovascular decompensation may be present. These findings reverse with transfusion. Evaluation includes complete blood count with reticulocyte count, red cell indices, and bone marrow examination.

Prior to the availability of corticosteroids, therapy was only supportive, with monthly red cell transfusions required to maintain adequate oxygenation. Use of washed packed red cells is advisable to minimize sensitization and transfusion reactions. Complications for chronically transfusion-dependent patients include development of hepatitis, production of antibodies to minor red cell antigens, hypersplenism, and iron overload, with liver and heart failure and death in the second to third decade of life.

The majority of patients respond to corticosteroid therapy with improvement or normalization of the hemoglobin and independence of transfusion therapy. The response to steroids appears to be greatest when treatment is instituted early. Patients started on steroids 6 months or more into their illness have a lower response rate. A proportion of patients fail to respond to steroids and remain transfusion dependent. After initial daily prednisone, erythroid activity may be preserved by every-other-day or other intermittent schedules for steroid therapy to minimize the complications of long-term daily steroid use. Some patients remit with the onset of puberty and become independent of transfusion or steroid therapy, but this is an erratic occurrence. Therapy is begun with the equivalent of 2 mg prednisone/kg body weight, but occasionally higher doses are needed to obtain a response. If the disease is steroid responsive, reticulocytosis is commonly seen within 1 to 2 weeks, but occasionally a longer period is required, and 6 to 8 weeks should be completed before concluding that the process is not responsive. Androgens have no place in the management of CHA. The mechanism of action of corticosteroid therapy is unclear, but the observation of its efficacy serves to underscore the possible immune etiology of CHA.

Most patients survive at least into young adulthood. Causes of death include transfusional hemosiderosis and septicemia following splenectomy performed for hypersplenism in chronically transfused patients. Steroid-responsive patients have a far better survival rate but experience the consequences of long-term steroid therapy and have markedly short stature.

For the nonresponders, red cell transfusion support, including iron chelation therapy for control of hemosiderosis, is the major alternative approach. Unchecked, hemosiderosis invariably leads to hypersplenism, skin pigmentation, impaired sexual maturation, pancreatic insufficiency, bone age retardation, and cardiomyopathy. Chelation can be carried out with parenterally administered desferrioxamine. From infancy to preschool age graded daily doses ranging from 100 to 500 mg may be administered via intramuscular or subcutaneous injection. In the older patient iron chelation is readily administered via perfusion pump in a daily dose range of 500 to 1,000 mg. The role of vitamin C as a chelation enhancer is questionable. It does, in fact, facilitate iron absorption and thus is best avoided. Although sufficient chelation does not occur until iron stores are approximately 10 times normal, it is nonetheless advisable to initiate therapy early in high transfusion regimen patients. However, attention must be paid to the possible occurrence of allergic reactions and cataract formation. Splenectomy has no proven therapeutic benefit other than its value in patients who develop hypersplenism. Another major risk of prolonged transfusion support is the development of red cell antibodies. For steroid-dependent or severely anemic, steroid-unresponsive patients with an HLA identical, mixed leukocyte culture (MLC) nonreactive donor, marrow transplantation should be considered.

Anemias of endocrine insufficiency

The normochromic, normocytic anemias of adrenal insufficiency, hypothyroidism, and pituitary insufficiency are usually mild, i.e., hemoglobin levels rarely fall below 8 gm/dl. However, in hypoadrenalism the severity of the anemia may be obscured by a contracted plasma volume. Therapy is directed at correction of the underlying deficiency. Although macrocytosis is occasionally noted in this group of disorders, it probably reflects the large red cell size characteristic of the newborn. True megaloblastic changes occur only in the presence of associated folate or vitamin B_{12} deficiency. A modest increase in icterus may also be present as a result of early (intramarrow) red cell senescence.

Osteopetrosis

Osteopetrosis (Albers-Schönberg disease) is an autosomal recessive disease characterized by defective osteoclast (and perhaps monocyte) production function that leads to thickened and brittle cortical bone formation, frequent fractures, growth retardation, and diminution in marrow space. The net effect is a compromise of erythroid as well as granulocyte and megakaryocyte development. Hematopoietic adjustment usually occurs via extramedullary hematopoiesis. The resultant normochromic, normocytic anemia is frequently accompanied by immature or nucleated red cells in the peripheral circulation. The combination of repeated transfusions and extramedullary blood formation ultimately leads to hypersplenism. Although variations in severity are typical, the early onset form is usually fatal. Until recently, therapy was essentially supportive. For patients with HLA identical, MLC nonreactive donors, it is possible to restore marrow function following allogeneic transplantation of both hematopoietic and the osteoclast progenitors.

Constitutional pancytopenia

The Fanconi variant of constitutional aplastic anemia is characterized by moderate to severe pancytopenia in association with one or more congenital defects, including hyperpigmentation, absent or hypoplastic thumbs, combination absent radii and thumbs (in contrast to absent radii with thumbs in the radial-platelet hypoplasia syndrome), decreased numbers of carpal bones, microphthalmia, hyperreflexia, microcephaly, short stature, decreased bone age, strabismus, developmental abnormalities of the ears, double ureters, and ectopic and/or horseshoe kidneys.

The phenotypic expression of this disorder may precede the hematologic manifestation by a few months to as many as 15 years. Approximately 10% of these patients never develop hematologic disease.

Chromosomal abnormalities, uniformly seen in this disorder, include increased frequency of breakage, endoreduplications, and defective chromatid exchanges. The precise relationship between the chromosomal abnormalities and the hematologic manifestations is unclear, although the defective DNA repair mechanism (abnormal chromatic exchanges) suggests that the hematologic manifestations, i.e., both the aplasia and subsequent leukemia, are secondarily induced. Elevated fetal hemoglobin levels, not uniformly distributed throughout the red cell mass, and the presence of the i antigen are commonly seen in this disorder. The leukemic transformation occurs in about 7% of these patients and is almost exclusively of the acute monocytic or monomyelocytic variety.

In the majority of cases androgen therapy effectively increases erythroid production and to a lesser extent granulocyte and platelet production. One such example is oxymetholone administered orally in a dosage of 1 to 3 mg/kg/day. Once a response is identified, the dosage should be reduced to the minimum amount capable of maintaining a sustained response. Corticosteroids, other than their ability to diminish testosterone-induced skeletal maturation, offer no additional therapeutic advantage. For the androgen-nonresponsive patient, red cell transfusion support accompanied by iron chelation therapy is the only major alternative. However, marrow transplantation from a genotypically normal HLA identical, MLC nonreactive sibling is an appropriate consideration. Androgen therapy must be carefully monitored because of potential hepatotoxicity and the risk of late-occurring hepatic carcinoma. The familial variant of constitutional aplastic anemia, so-called because of the lack of skeletal and chromosomal abnormalities, is otherwise identical in hematologic expression and therapeutic responsiveness.

Acquired anemias due to erythrocyte underproduction

Transient erythroblastopenia of childhood (TEC)

Transient erythroblastopenia of childhood is frequently confused with congenital erythroid hypoplasia (CEH). Unlike CEH, however, most cases occur between 6 months and 4 years of age and usually follow viral infections. It rarely lasts longer than 4 months and usually disappears without any sequelae. When TEC occurs in prematurely born patients, the anemia may be so pro-

Table 29-4. Comparison of congenital erythroid hypoplasia and transient erythroblastopenia

	Congenital	Transient
Onset	Essentially all under 6 months of age	Most between 6 months and 4 years of age
Etiology	Variable inheritance	Viral, idiopathic
Skeletal defects	Present in approximately one third of patients	None
Chromosomal defects	Rare, unrelated	None
Male:female	1:1	1:1
Hematologic findings		
MCV	$>95\ \mu m^3$	$<90\ \mu m^3$
Pure red cell aplasia	Present	Present
Hgb F	Usually increased	Consistent with age
i antigen	Usually present	Absent
Therapy	Corticosteroid response in >85% of cases	None necessary
Prognosis	Spontaneous remission in 10%-15% of cases; hemosiderosis in long-term red cell transfused patients	Complete recovery in 6-8 weeks

found as to require red cell transfusion, but the marrow myeloid to erythroid ratio rarely exceeds 10:1. In its rare recurrent form, TEC probably represents a variant of CEH. The distinguishing characteristics of CEH and TEC are noted in Table 29-4.

Aplastic crises of hemolytic disease

Transient red cell hypoplasia often accompanies certain hemolytic disorders, notably sickle cell disease and hereditary spherocytosis, and less commonly enzyme-induced hemolytic disorders. Viral infections, on occasion, have been implicated in the etiology of aplastic crises in these disorders, and there are presumptive data to suggest a possible causal relationship with a "conditioned" folate deficiency, i.e., excessive demands imposed by rapid growth and accelerated marrow turnover time. Typical findings in the aplastic crises of hemolytic disease include listlessness, rapid onset of pallor, and increased icterus. The pertinent hematologic findings include anemia with reticulocytopenia. Associated granulocytopenia and thrombocytopenia are uncommon but may occur as a consequence of severe folate depletion.

Idiopathic acquired aplastic anemia

Although acquired aplastic anemia has a peak incidence between 3 and 7 years of age, it may occur at any age, including infancy. A variety of etiologic factors have been incriminated, and it may in fact be the forerunner of acute leukemia. The distinguishing features between congenital and acquired aplastic anemia are noted in Table 29-5. Both groups of disorders are characterized by varying degrees of pancytopenia, but only rarely is the acquired from responsive to either corticosteroid or androgen therapy. Indeed, those patients who are rapidly responsive to corticosteroid therapy may very likely be preleukemic. The treatment of choice, wherever possible, is marrow transplantation. Over 70% of patients so treated maintain successful remission and experience long-term, indefinite disease-free states. In the absence of a compatible donor, blood product support is the only alternative and should be carried out in accordance with the guidelines presented in other sections of this chapter.

Folic acid and vitamin B_{12}

Serum folate levels in the newborn are two or three times higher than those obtained in normal adults. However, within 3 or 4 weeks of birth they frequently fall into the "deficiency range" in temporal association with the "physiologic" hemoglobin decline (Fig. 29-7). In the small premature infant (<1,500 gm) the serum folate decrement results in a 10% to 30% incidence of "folate deficiency," i.e., 0.5 ng/μl. Administration of supplemental folate usually repairs the deficit but does not slow the rate of hemoglobin decline despite the disappearance of formaminoglutamic acid secretion, an end-stage metabolite of folate deficiency seen in such patients. Nonetheless, folate requirements for small premature infants are excessive and are not met by the amounts present in otherwise modified cow's milk preparations. Accordingly, supplemental folate (1 to 2 mg/week) should be administered to all premature infants to prevent the occurrence of "conditioned" deficiencies as a result of infection or chronic hemolysis.

The pattern of serum vitamin B_{12} levels parallels that of folate, but there are essentially no data comparing hemoglobin response to vitamin B_{12} supplementation. On the other hand, known deficiency states have been described and include maternally induced deficiency, malabsorption defects, and juvenile pernicious anemia. As in folate deficiency, the hematologic sine qua non is megaloblastic maturation with reticulocytopenia.

Most of the folate and vitamin B_{12} data were obtained

Table 29-5. Comparison of constitutional (familial, Fanconi's) and acquired aplastic anemia

	Constitutional	Acquired
Onset	0.5 to 15 years of age	Any age but more frequent after 5 years
Etiology	Autosomal recessive (Fanconi's) Autosomal recessive or incomplete dominant (familial)	Drugs, chemicals, radiation, viral, PHN* idiopathic, preleukemia
Skeletal defects	Present in Fanconi's type; absent in familial type	Absent
Chromosomal defects	Present in Fanconi's type; absent in familial type	Absent
Male:female	2:1	1:1
Hematologic findings		
Pancytopenia†	Present‡	Present‡
Hgb F	Usually increased	Occasionally increased
i antigen	Usually present	Occasionally present
Therapy	Response to androgens in >85% of cases; consider marrow transplant in nonresponders with HL-A identical, MLC nonreactive donors	Response to androgens in <10% of cases; consider marrow transplant in all severe cases
Prognosis	Guarded, with risk of terminal leukemia or hepatic carcinoma	Poor in severe cases unable to be transplanted; occasional spontaneous remission

*Paroxysmal nocturnal hemoglobinuria: sugar water and Ham tests positive.
†Congenital amegakaryocytic thrombocytopenia is probably an early manifestation of constitutional aplastic anemia.
‡Severe pancytopenia: absolute granulocyte count <500/mm³, platelet count <20,000/mm³, reticulocyte count <1.0%.

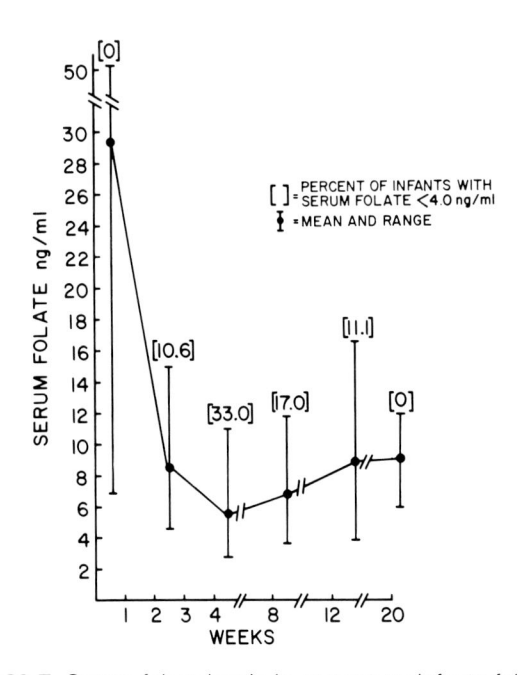

Fig. 29-7. Serum folate levels in premature infants fall dramatically during the first month of life. By 4 weeks, 33% of infants have "deficiency" values below 4 ng/ml. Although supplementation has not been shown to alter the hemoglobin decline in these patients, most of the data were obtained prior to knowledge of the effects of vitamin E deficiency on red cell survival.

without the awareness of tocopherol and glutathione peroxidase studies. It is thus reasonable to conclude that repeat studies of these interrelationships using multivariant analyses will help clarify the roles of folate and vitamin B_{12} in early infant nutrition.

Anemias due to red cell destruction

Accelerated red cell destruction due to intrinsic or acquired abnormalities of erythrocytes is common in the perinatal period. Isoimmune hemolytic disease is unique to this age group. Certain clinical features are prominent in hemolytic disease of the newborn and are affected by physiologic factors characteristic of the neonatal period.

Catabolism of hemoglobin is increased in all hemolytic states. The newborn liver is significantly less able to conjugate bilirubin than the mature liver, and hyperbilirubinemia is predominantly unconjugated, or indirect reacting. One gram of hemoglobin yields approximately 35 mg bilirubin.

Hematopoiesis occurs in the spleen and liver normally during the third trimester and may be pronounced in hemolytic states. Extramedullary hematopoiesis occurs more readily in this period, and hepatosplenomegaly due to myeloid metaplasia is often a prominent feature of hemolytic states.

Immature erythroid and myeloid precursors are released more readily from the bone marrow and other sites of hematopoiesis in the newborn period than later in life. Thus circulating marrow elements are frequently found in peripheral blood, a finding termed *erythroblastosis*. Young myeloid cells may also circulate when hematopoiesis is particularly brisk.

The blood-brain barrier of newborn infants is unusually permeable to bilirubin in the plasma that is not bound to plasma proteins, particularly albumin. This makes infants susceptible to the development of kernicterus, or bilirubin staining of the brain, which does not occur with higher levels of bilirubin in older children and adults. The damage to nervous tissue is irreversible. It is seen at relatively low concentrations of bilirubin in premature infants because of low serum albumin and proportionately greater unbound bilirubin. Drugs and hydrogen ions may displace bilirubin and predispose to development of kernicterus in certain circumstances. Prevention of kernicterus is the major concern in treatment of hyperbilirubinemia due to hemolytic disease of the newborn.

The major causes of hemolytic disease in the newborn period include immune destruction of red cells due to passively transferred maternal antibody, intrinsic defects in the red cell, and infection.

Isoimmune hemolytic disease

Maternal IgG, or 7S antibody, passes across the placenta. If the antibodies are directed against antigens present on fetal erythrocytes, they bind to the red cell membrane and may cause the target cells to be removed by tissue macrophages. IgM, or 19S antibody, does not cross the placenta and does not cause hemolysis in the fetus. Hemolysis is extravascular. Free hemoglobin is not found in the serum except in rare cases of severe hemolysis. This reflects the fact that the antibodies act by altering the red cell membrane to enhance clearance of the cells and not primarily by fixing complement. Complement components are low even in term infants, and most IgG antibodies fix complement less efficiently than IgM antibodies. The major sites of destruction are the liver and spleen. The efficiency of clearance relates to the amount of antigen on the membrane, the amount of antibody bound to the antigens, the biologic activity of the antibody, and the maturity of macrophage function, particularly splenic function.

Red cell antigens are glycoproteins whose expression is genetically determined. Persons who are type O produce antibodies to blood group antigens A and B, termed *naturally occurring antibodies*. Their production appears to be incited by bacterial glycoproteins that are antigenically similar to the A and B substances. Type A persons produce anti-B, and type B persons produce anti-A. Most of these naturally occurring antibodies are IgM and do not cross the placenta. If a fraction of the antibodies is IgG, they may be passively transferred and may cause hemolysis if the infant carries the red cell antigen. Thus ABO hemolysis is frequently not due to maternal sensitization but to passive transfer of antibody directed at cross-reacting antigens. In contrast, Rh and minor blood groups do not react with such antibodies, and hemolysis induced by antibodies is due to maternal sensitization to fetal antigens.

ABO incompatibility

Individuals who lack the A and B factors normally demonstrate antibodies against the factors that are absent. Type O persons produce anti-A and anti-B antibodies, primarily 19S globulins. Frequently, some of the anti-A activity in type O and type B individuals can be demonstrated in the 7S fraction of serum. If this antibody crosses the placenta of an infant whose red cells bear the A substance, the infant may develop hemolysis. Thus hemolytic disease due to anti-A may occur following a first pregnancy in an unsensitized mother, and subsequent pregnancies are not likely to produce severely affected infants. ABO hemolytic disease may also occur due to antibody production in a sensitized mother. Blood group substance A_1 appears to be the most strongly antigenic of the major blood group antigens and is associated with the largest number of cases of clinically apparent hemolysis. Expression of the A and B substances is relatively poorly developed in the fetus and newborn. The antigen density is lower than later in life and probably accounts for the relatively mild hemolysis accompanying many cases of ABO incompatibility. Approximately 39% of infants of type O mothers are either type A (31%) or type B (9%). The cord blood Coombs test is positive in approximately 33% of these pregnancies, but a relatively small percentage require intervention for control of hyperbilirubinemia or anemia. The spectrum of disease is extremely broad. The incidence and severity may be greater in black than in white infants.

The naturally occurring anti-A IgG is a univalent or "incomplete" antibody that agglutinates type A cells well in 20% albumin but poorly in saline. Thus it may be difficult to demonstrate Coombs positivity unless appropriate steps are taken. Hemolysis due to anti-A and anti-B antibodies is characterized by the presence of spherocytes on the baby's blood smear. Spherocyte formation is thought to result from removal of a portion of the red cell membrane in the spleen, with release of cells containing reduced surface area and somewhat reduced cell volume.

RH incompatibility

The antigens in the Rh system are determined by three closely linked genes that segregate as alleles. The antigens are termed C, c, D, d, E, and e. The d antigen is inferred but has not been demonstrated. Several rare variants have also been identified and have been associated with isoimmune hemolytic disease, including C^w, C^x, and D^u. Individuals are defined as Rh positive if their red cells express the D antigen and may be either homozygous (D/D) or heterozygous (D/d) for the D antigen. Rh-negative individuals are homozygous d/d. The D antigen is highly antigenic and is expressed on the red cell membrane as early as the eleventh week of fetal life. These facts are probably responsible for the severity of Rh hemolytic anemia, which is associated with hemolysis early in fetal life and high titers of antibodies. The incidence of hemolytic disease of the newborn due to Rh antibodies varies with racial groups. Approximately 85% of Caucasians are Rh positive, as are 93% of blacks and 99% of Orientals. Rh incompatibility occurs only if the mother is Rh negative. Hemolytic disease is approximately three times as common in Caucasians as in blacks and is rare in Chinese.

Fetal cells may enter the maternal circulation at any time during a pregnancy, but fetomaternal transfusion is most common with trauma related to delivery or amniocentesis. Fetal cells can be demonstrated in the maternal circulation of up to 50% of patients following delivery, but the volume of bleeding is rarely more than about 0.2 ml. Approximately 1.0 ml of blood appears to be necessary to sensitize the mother to the antigens of the fetal cells. If the mother has naturally occurring antibodies to one of the major blood group antigens (A or B) present on fetal cells, the fetal cells may be destroyed before the mother has a chance to become sensitized to other antigens (such as D) present on the same cell. This is thought to account for the fact that Rh sensitization is less frequent in pregnancies in which ABO incompatibility also exists. Because most transplacental bleeding occurs around the time of delivery, Rh-negative mothers rarely become sensitized to Rh-positive fetal cells prior to term in the first pregnancy unless they have had previous transfusion with Rh positive blood. The probability of sensitization increases with each Rh-positive infant, and subsequent pregnancies are more likely to be affected, but fewer than 10% of Rh-negative women who bear Rh-positive infants are eventually sensitized.

Immunization to the D antigen incites production of both 19S and 7S globulins. The 7S globulins are capable of transplacental transfer and coat fetal cells bearing the D antigen. These cells are then destroyed in the fetal liver and spleen, with resulting anemia and compensatory increase in erythropoiesis. The severity of the disorder varies from minimal hemolysis without clinical manifestations to uncompensated anemia with erythroblastosis and hydrops fetalis. Successive Rh-positive pregnancies in sensitized women incite increasing titers of antibodies, and the clinical severity tends to increase with each affected pregnancy. This is not the case in ABO incompatibility, even when the mother is sensitized to major blood group antigens. The titer of maternal antibody cannot be used as a reliable guide to the severity of disease in the infant, but a high or rising anti D titer in a sensitized Rh-negative woman suggests significant hemolytic disease in the infant and may be used as an indication for amniocentesis to confirm the diagnosis and assess severity of hemolysis.

Jaundice is usually minimal or absent at birth because bilirubin is rapidly transported across the placenta and metabolized and excreted by the mother. With active hemolysis, however, jaundice is apparent within the first 12 to 24 hours of postnatal life and increases rapidly. The most severely affected infants have hydrops fetalis, marked pallor, edema, ascites, pleural effusion, and congestive heart failure. The placentas are often also edematous and pale. In the most severe forms, disseminated intravascular coagulation may accompany brisk hemolysis, much like severe hemolytic transfusion reactions. Anemia at birth is most commonly associated with Rh incompatibility but may be seen in isoimmune hemolytic disease due to other blood group incompatibilities.

The incidence of Rh hemolytic disease has been greatly diminished by the prophylactic use of anti-D immune globulin following delivery, abortion, or amniocentesis in unsensitized Rh-negative women. High-titer anti-D serum is obtained from sensitized Rh-negative women or men deliberately immunized with Rh-positive cells. Administration of the gammaglobulin fraction of this serum within 72 hours of delivery results in clearance of circulating Rh-positive cells and prevents immune recognition of the foreign antigen by the mother. This procedure is not completely effective because transplacental bleeding may occur prior to delivery, and sensitization may antedate administration of the immune globulin. Extensive fetal-maternal transfusion results in more circulating Rh-positive cells than can be cleared with the standard dosage of immune globulin, and sensitization may occur unless the dosage is substantially increased in this situation. However, the vast majority of instances of sensitization of Rh-negative women occur because of failure to administer anti-D globulin following abortion or delivery of an Rh-positive infant.

Because the severity of Rh hemolytic disease tends to become progressively greater with each affected pregnancy, management extends into the prenatal period. The majority of stillborn infants with hydrops fetalis are delivered at 37 weeks' gestation or later. Thus early delivery of severely affected children may facilitate hematologic management if the lung function has matured sufficiently to permit extrauterine survival. Intrauterine transfusion may be given to support the infant until delivery is feasible.

Spectrophotometric assessment of bilirubin in amniotic fluid is used to determine the need for intervention (intrauterine transfusion or early delivery) in affected infants. If the maternal anti-D titer is greater than 1:16 and rising in a woman who has delivered a previous stillborn infant or an infant requiring exchange transfusion for Rh incompatibility, amniocentesis is performed and the optical density rise at 450 μm is determined according to the method of Liley. The result is interpreted according to the zone into which the measurement falls related to gestational age of the fetus. Over 95% of severely affected infants can be identified by serial examination of amniotic fluid spectrophotometry, which facilitates selection of infants for intrauterine transfusion and early delivery. Amniocentesis should be performed at about 21 weeks' gestation and repeated every 7 to 21 days, depending on the initial reading, in pregnancies at risk.

Intrauterine transfusion is feasible because red cells are absorbed intact from the peritoneal cavity. The cells enter the subdiaphragmatic lymphatics and are transported into the right lymphatic duct and into the circulation over 7 or 8 days. Infusion of excessive volumes of red cells results in increased intraperitoneal pressure with occlusion of the umbilical vein, so it is important that the volume be limited. Inadvertent trauma to the heart and major arteries is associated with mortality, but many fetal organs have been punctured without apparent adverse effects. Washed, packed O negative red cells should be used for intrauterine transfusion. Fatal and nonfatal lymphocyte engraftment has been reported, mandating the use of red cells that are at least white-cell poor, and preferably irradiated, to prevent lymphocyte engraftment and graft-versus-host disease.

Other minor blood group incompatibilities

Sensitization to any of the minor blood group antigens can be associated with isoimmune hemolytic disease. These include Kell, Duffy, Lewis, Kidd, M, S, and others. The less antigenic components of the Rh system, C, c, E, and e, can also be associated with hemolytic disease of the newborn. The spectrum varies from subclinical evidence of sensitization to active hemolysis with hyperbilirubinemia requiring exchange transfusion. Hydrops fetalis with intrauterine or perinatal death has been reported with anti-Kell hemolytic disease.

Diagnosis of isoimmune hemolytic disease of the newborn. Jaundice in the first few days of life is the most frequent feature leading to diagnosis of isoimmune hemolysis. The bilirubin in cord blood rarely exceeds 5 mg/dl even in the most severe cases but begins to accumulate within the first 24 hours in most cases. The bilirubin is predominantly unconjugated because of the immaturity of the liver enzymes responsible for glucuronidation.

Anemia is rarely present at birth except in hemolytic disease due to Rh incompatibility but develops as hemolysis increases. Hepatomegaly and splenomegaly may be present due to extramedullary hematopoiesis, reticuloendothelial hyperplasia associated with extravascular hemolysis, and occasionally to congestive heart failure with severe anemia.

The blood smear shows evidence of active erythropoiesis, with polychromasia, reticulocytosis, and nucleated red blood cells. In severe cases, less mature erythroid precursors and sometimes myeloid precursors are found in the peripheral blood. Macrocytosis reflects the increase in young cells as well as the normally elevated red cell volume in the newborn period. Densely stained microspherocytes are often prominent in ABO incompatibility and are associated with increased osmotic fragility of the red cells (Fig. 29-8). Spherocytes are also seen in minor blood group incompatibilities but not in Rh hemolytic disease. If the rate of red cell production equals the rate of destruction, anemia may be absent despite active hemolysis. When active hemolytic disease is present at birth, the suppression of erythropoiesis, which normally occurs within the first 24 hours of birth due to decreased erythropoietin production, is not seen.

Blood group incompatibility between mother and infant and the presence of antibody bound to the infant's erythrocytes must be demonstrated to establish a definitive diagnosis of isoimmune hemolytic disease. The direct Coombs antiglobulin test for detection of bound antibody is the most useful test but may be negative in mild cases of hemolysis if small amounts of antibody are present on the cell. In ABO disease the albumin Coombs test is more sensitive than the test performed in saline because the antibodies are often univalent ("incomplete"). An indirect Coombs test on the mother's serum may detect free antibodies when these cannot be identified on the infant's cells. Occasionally in Rh hemolytic disease the antibody may mask the D antigen, and the cells may falsely type as Rh negative. This occurs in a setting of severe hemolytic disease in an infant whose Rh-negative mother has a positive indirect Coombs test and has previously borne affected infants, but its occurrence should not obscure the diagnosis.

Management. Management is directed at prevention of the complications of hyperbilirubinemia and anemia. Hyperbilirubinemia is associated with neurologic damage due to binding of unconjugated bilirubin that is not bound to serum albumin to the brain stem and basal ganglia. Unconjugated bilirubin complexes with phospholipids in membranes and binds at lipid-water interphases. Binding to albumin is rapid and reversible, and an equilibrium is rapidly established in plasma and extracellular fluid. Beyond the neonatal period the blood-brain barrier is less permeable to penetration of unconjugated bilirubin, and most pathologic conditions associated with

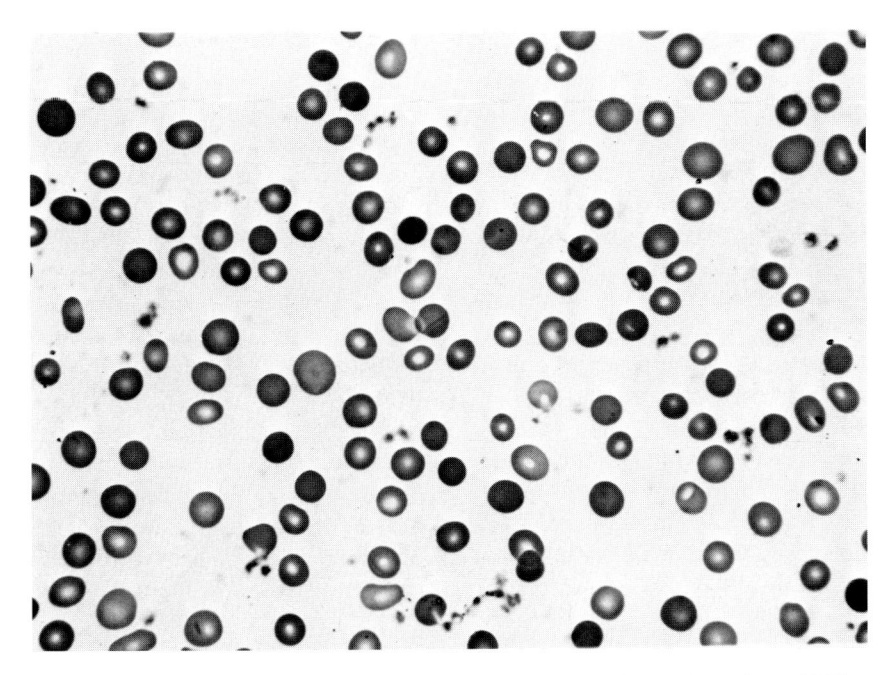

Fig. 29-8. Microspherocytes in ABO incompatability. (Wright's stain; ×800.)

jaundice are accompanied by an increase in direct-reacting bilirubin. Thus the neurologic sequelae of hyperbilirubinemia are rarely seen except in this age group.

The first clinical sign of kernicterus is lethargy. Hypotonia and poor feeding are other early signs associated with loss of the sucking reflex. The hypotonia is replaced by hypertonia within the first few weeks, and most infants become opisthotonic and spastic. Long-term consequences are high-frequency nerve deafness, athetoid movements, mental retardation, and dysplasia of dental enamel. Frequently there is a transient period of clinical improvement that may lead to the impression that damage has not occurred. Kernicterus is never present at birth because of transplacental passage of bilirubin and should be regarded as a preventable disorder. Clinical manifestations in infants with hemolytic disease usually appear between the second and sixth day of life. Kernicterus rarely occurs at bilirubin levels below 20 mg/dl in full-term, otherwise healthy infants. Prematurity and low serum albumin levels also predispose to the development of kernicterus at lower bilirubin levels, as do acidosis and certain drugs by displacing bilirubin from albumin-binding sites. Nomograms have been constructed that facilitate decision making in jaundiced infants by taking into account infant age, the birth weight, and the level of bilirubin at which observation, phototherapy, and exchange transfusion are indicated.

Phototherapy. Exposure of free or bound bilirubin to blue light (wavelengths 400 to 500 nm) causes a change in configuration from the normal Z form to a photobilirubin, termed the E form. Photobilirubin does not form an insoluble acid, is nontoxic to nervous tissue, and is excreted in the bile without conjugation. The Z configuration is more stable, however, and the E form is transformed back to the Z form in the dark. These changes take place both in vivo and in vitro. Light exposure of the skin lowers plasma bilirubin through this conversion, and increased excretion of the photobilirubin may prevent the development of high, toxic levels. No serious short-term consequences of phototherapy are known, although deposition of pigments may darken the skin, and biochemical evidence of riboflavin deficiency has been demonstrated. There is concern about possible long-term side effects of phototherapy based largely on the possible carcinogenic hazard of radiation exposure. In vitro tests of mutagenicity have confirmed the theoretical hazards, but the clinical significance is as yet unknown. Continuous exposure to light is less mutagenic than intermittent exposure and is preferred. The infant's eyes must be protected from direct light exposure, and shielding the Isolette may decrease the exposure of nursery personnel.

Exhange transfusion. Exchange transfusion has two goals in hemolytic disease of the newborn: removal of sensitized, damaged erythrocytes, which contribute to the rate of hemolysis, and removal of unconjugated bilirubin, which may cause neurologic damage. Exchange of twice the total blood volume (calculated as 80 ml/kg body weight) will replace 85% of the infant's red cells and a substantial portion of plasma containing both antibody and bilirubin. Both antibody and bilirubin are distributed throughout the extracellular fluid, however, and reenter the plasma following exchange transfusion. In addition, tissue-bound bilirubin may also reenter the circulation, and rebound elevations in bilirubin following exchange transfusion are common. The first exchange transfusion serves to remove sensitized erythrocytes and correct anemia. Subsequent exchange transfusions are directed primarily at removal of bilirubin, much of which is released from tissue-binding sites.

Several considerations arise in the selection of blood for exchange transfusion. The erythrocytes should not express the antigen against which the maternal antibody is directed and should be compatible with both the mother's and baby's blood. If type O blood is used in a type A or type B patient, it should have a low titer of anti-A or anti-B. Optimally the blood should be freshly drawn and less than 2 days old if possible. Blood stored for longer periods may contain elevated levels of potassium due to hemolysis, and the erythrocytes are depleted of ATP and 2,3-DPG, which renders them less capable of delivering oxygen to the tissues. Neutropenia and thrombocytopenia may accompany multiple exchange transfusions, and clotting factors may be depleted if plasma components or old blood is used. There have been several instances of fatal generalized intravascular sickling in infants who have received exchange transfusion with blood from donors with sickle cell trait (Hb AS) or sickle-C disease (Hb SC). These donors were not anemic and were unaware of their hemoglobinopathies, so it is wise to be sure that the sickle preparation is negative in blood intended for exchange transfusion. Graft-versus-host disease has been described in infants, particularly prematures, receiving exchange transfusion with fresh blood containing viable lymphocytes. This is not a common clinical problem, although transient mild skin rashes, diarrhea, or liver function abnormalities may be unrecognized manifestations of graft-versus-host disease. This has been associated with deaths in infants receiving intrauterine transfusions, and such blood should be completely free from lymphocytes or irradiated to prevent graft-versus-host disease.

The hazards of exchange transfusion include introduction of infectious agents, either from umbilical vein catheterization or contamination of blood or intravenous infusion solutions, arrhythmias due to hypocalcemia when blood anticoagulated with acid-citrate-dextrose is used, congestive heart failure or shock, if careful attention to maintenance of intravascular volume is not paid, and thrombosis of the inferior vena cava related to the placement of the catheter. The procedure should be performed under rigidly aseptic conditions, with continuous cardiac and respiratory monitoring, and the infant must be kept warm. Slow infusion of 1 ml of 10% calcium gluconate after each 100 ml of citrated blood is given will prevent arrhythmias and excessive bleeding. The bilirubin and hematocrit levels should be determined immediately after transfusion and again within 2 hours after equilibration has occurred.

Delayed manifestation. Anemia occurring late following isoimmune hemolytic disease is not necessarily related to the severity of the acute process. Infants with mild hemolytic disease may experience an abrupt increase in the rate of red cell destruction after 1 week of age. This may be due to improved splenic function and more effective clearance of sensitized cells. If the liver enzymes responsible for bilirubin metabolism have also matured, jaundice may not accompany the drop in hemoglobin. Infants who have had exchange transfusions continue to have detectable passively transferred maternal antibody. As their production of erythrocytes bearing the offending antigen increases, hemolysis may accelerate. Infants who are not anemic in the first 48 hours of life normally cease producing erythropoietin and red cells. Anemia developing in the next few weeks may not incite erythropoiesis, since the bone marrow is relatively less sensitive to stimulation during this period. Thus ongoing hemolysis may lead to anemia after the first week of life, which is not compensated by increased red cell production. Infants with mild hemolysis must be followed more closely than other infants to detect the occasional infant who develops severe and even life-threatening anemia.

Since the hemolysis is extravascular, iron is stored in the reticuloendothelial cells of the liver and spleen and is available for reuse. Even infants who have had exchange transfusion should not be depleted of iron stores. Infants who have particularly active bone marrow with ongoing hemolysis or early anemia should receive folic acid supplementation to prevent the development of megaloblastic anemia.

A small number of infants with isoimmune hemolytic disease develop persistent jaundice with an elevation in the conjugated, direct-reacting component. This may be associated with abnormalities of liver enzymes and was formerly termed the *inspissated bile syndrome*. Its pathogenesis is uncertain, and in most instances the laboratory abnormalities disappear by 3 to 6 months of age.

Prognosis. The prognosis for infants with isoimmune hemolytic disease is related to the degree of hyperbilirubinemia. Although the levels of bilirubin that are associated with major anatomic abnormalities and gross functional defects are well known, it is less clear whether lower levels of bilirubin elevations are associated with more subtle intellectual or neurologic impairment. These possibilities are under active investigation, and the criteria for therapeutic intervention may be revised as more information becomes available.

QUANTITATIVE DISORDERS OF GLOBIN CHAIN SYNTHESIS

All hemoglobin molecules are constructed of four heme groups and four globin chains. The different varieties of hemoglobins vary in their globin chain components. Embryonic hemoglobins produced in the first trimester include Gower 1, composed of four ϵ-chains (ϵ_4), Gower 2 ($\alpha_2\epsilon_2$), and Portland ($\zeta_2\gamma_2$). Beyond early embryonic life all hemoglobins contain two α-chains and vary only in their non-α-globin chains. Hemoglobin F, the major fetal hemoglobin, contains two α- and two γ-chains ($\alpha_2\gamma_2$). The major adult hemoglobin, Hb A, contains two α- and two β-chains ($\alpha_2\beta_2$). A minor constituent of adult hemoglobin is Hb A_2 ($\alpha_2\delta_2$). Newer techniques of molecular biology have yielded much information about the genetics of the hemoglobinopathies and of normal hemoglobin synthesis (Fig. 29-9).

The α-globin chains are carried on chromosome 16 and are duplicated in most populations. Thus most persons have two haploid sets of α-genes, or a total of four gene copies. The non-α-genes are carried on chromosome 11 (Fig. 29-10). The δ- and β-genes are closely linked. There are two γ-genes on the same chromosome that are similar in structure, but one gene produces more glutamine ($^G\gamma$) and the other contains more alanine ($^A\gamma$). Although there is a small amount of β-chain production beginning late in the first trimester, which permits prenatal diagnosis of hemoglobinopathies, γ-chain production predominates. After birth, γ-chain production ceases and is replaced by β-chain production. This is termed the *fetal-to-adult "switch,"* and the mechanisms that control it are not well understood. Similar processes occur in sheep and other mammals, permitting study of animal models that may illuminate control mechanisms active in humans.

Fetal hemoglobin resists elution from cells with mild acid solutions, which forms the basis of the acid elution or Kleihauer-Betke stain for detection of cells bearing Hb F. It also resists alkali denaturation and migrates differently from Hb A, Hb A_2, Hb S, and Hb C. Hb A_2 and other adult hemoglobins interact with the anion 2,3-DPG, which decreases the oxygen affinity of hemoglobin and improves delivery of oxygen to the tissues. Hb F exhibits minimal interaction with 2,3-DPG and has a higher oxygen affinity than Hb A under physiologic conditions within the red cell. This higher oxygen affinity facilitates the transport of oxygen across the placenta at the cost of somewhat less effective oxygen delivery.

Small amounts of β-chain production can be detected as early as 10 weeks, permitting intrauterine diagnosis of hemoglobinopathies affecting the β-chain. To date, the greatest experience is with techniques that require demonstration of the rates of production of globin chains by fetal reticulocytes and thus require fetal blood sampling. This is performed with a fetoscope, and blood is drawn directly from fetal placental vessels. The quantities of blood required are small, but contamination with maternal blood can make confident diagnosis of hemoglobinopathies difficult. Newer techniques of examination of DNA using restriction endonucleases may permit intra-

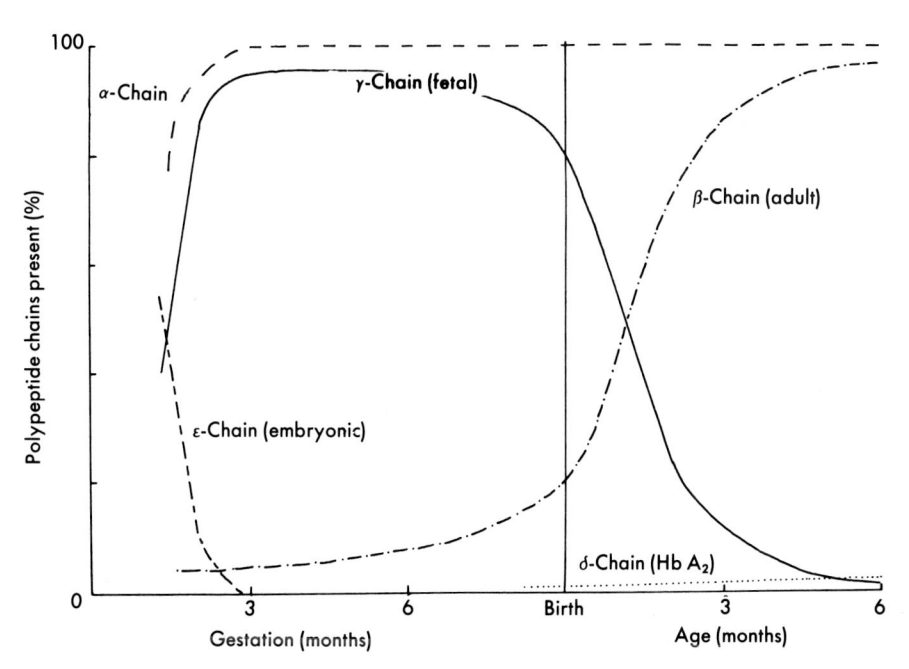

Fig. 29-9. Development of human hemoglobin chains. (From Huens, E.R., and others: Cold Spring Harbor Symp. Quant. Biol. **29**:327, 1964. Copyright 1964.)

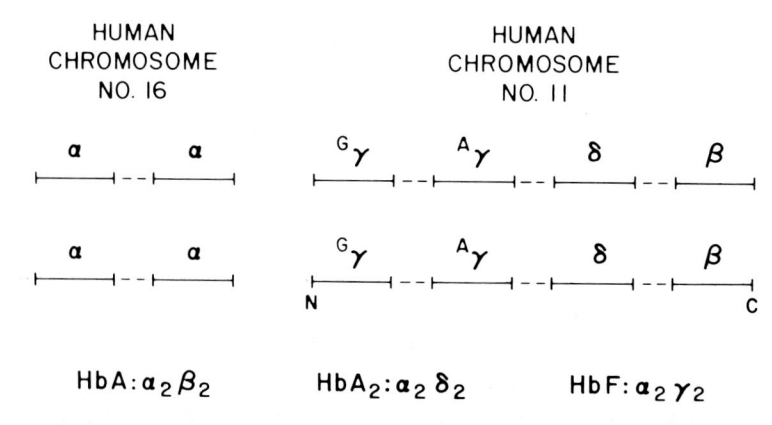

Fig. 29-10. Number and chromosomal arrangement of nonembryonic human globin genes. (From Forget, B.G., and others: Structure of the human globin genes. In Maniatis, T., Axel, R., and Fox, C.F., editors: Eukaryotic gene regulation: ICN-UCLA Symposia on Molecular and Cellular Biology, vol. 14, New York, 1979, Academic Press, Inc.)

uterine diagnosis using cells that do not synthesize hemoglobin, allowing use of amniotic fluid fibroblasts.

There are two major classes of disorders of hemoglobins: the thalassemias, which represent disorders of the quantity of globin chain production, and hemoglobinopathies, which represent disorders of globin chain structure. Because the hemoglobins vary at different stages of fetal development, the clinical expression of these disorders varies from severe and lethal in utero to no significant disease in the newborn period. Abnormalities of α-chains are expressed throughout prenatal and postnatal life, abnormal γ-chains are present only in the fetal and neonatal period, and abnormal β-chains are rarely associated with disease states before 3 to 6 months of age.

Thalassemias

The thalassemias are designated according to the globin chain that is underproduced. α-Thalassemia is associated with an excess of non-α-chain production (γ, β, and δ) over α-chains. β-Thalassemia is associated with an excess of α- over non-α-chains, with the β-chain production the major abnormality.

α-Thalassemias comprise a diverse group of disorders. α-Genes usually number four in each cell. The α-thalassemias result from deletion of various numbers of these genes. One absent gene results in a state designated the *silent carrier*; affected persons are detected only by sophisticated studies done in the process of evaluating families. Deletion of two genes results in microcytosis, usually without anemia. Deletion of three genes results in a microcytic anemia with Hb Bart's (γ_4) detectable in cord blood because of the excess of γ-chains. Deletion of all four genes results in hydrops fetalis. Infants are usually stillborn or die shortly after birth. This degree of severity is seen in Chinese and some other Asian populations. In these populations only about 1% of people are Rh negative, and Rh hemolytic disease is rare. α-Thalassemia is a more common cause of hydrops fetalis than Rh hemolytic disease in these areas.

Some racial groups, particularly blacks, normally have only two α-genes. The rate of α-chain production is normal, and chain synthesis is balanced. α-Thalassemias occur only with further deletions.

Infants with homozygous α-thalassemia are delivered severely anemic with all of the clinical features of hydrops fetalis. The erythrocytes are hypochromic and have inclusions due to precipitated globin chains demonstrable on supravital staining. Reticulocytosis and erythroblastosis are evident on smear. Hemoglobin electrophoresis demonstrates predominantly Bart's (γ_4), with smaller amounts of hemoglobins H (β_4) and Portland ($\zeta_2\gamma_2$).

The unstable abnormal hemoglobins precipitate within the cells, which leads to intramedullary hemolysis with ineffective erythropoiesis. In addition, the major hemoglobin, Bart's, has such a high oxygen affinity that it does not deliver oxygen effectively, and there is severe tissue hypoxia with growth failure. Hb Portland has normal oxygen-carrying capacity, which may explain why some affected infants survive into the third trimester.

In areas with large Asian populations, α-thalassemia is the major cause of nonimmune hydrops fetalis. Other causes of nonimmune hydrops include severe anemia due to blood loss or hemolysis (e.g., pyruvate kinase deficiency), major cardiovascular anomalies, congenital nephrosis, renal vein thrombosis, intrauterine infections, certain chromosomal anomalies, placental malformations, and maternal diabetes and toxemia. Ultrasonography has proved useful in the intrauterine evaluation of hydrops of any cause.

β-Thalassemia, or Cooley's anemia, consists of a group of related disorders in which β-chain production is diminished or absent. In contrast to the α-thalassemias, the genetic material that codes for the β-chain is present in most kindreds with β-thalassemias. β-Chain production is diminished because of abnormal control processes, abnormal messenger RNAs, or disorders of later processing of the chain. If β-chain production is completely absent, patients are severely anemic and are dependent on transfusions for life. Because γ-chain production is normal, however, these patients do not present with anemia until 3 to 6 months of age. If there is some β-chain production, patients may experience a marked but compensated anemia and may avoid chronic transfusion. One variant, δβ-thalassemia, results from the deletion of both the δ- and β-genes, which are adjacent on chromosome 11. These patients continue to produce γ-chains and express a condition termed *hereditary persistence of fetal hemoglobin*.

The anemia of β-thalassemia is due both to ineffective erythropoiesis, with premature destruction of erythrocytes due to precipitated α-chains in the cells, and decreased production of hemoglobin. Hepatosplenomegaly, with extramedullary hematopoiesis, is a prominent feature of the disorder. The medullary cavity of bones is greatly expanded by exuberant attempts to raise the hemoglobin level, and pathologic fractures may occur. All these features resolve with aggressive transfusion therapy to suppress erythropoiesis and maintain a normal hemoglobin level. Patients usually die of transfusional iron overload in the second and third decades of life. β-Thalassemias are most common in persons of Mediterranean background.

Abnormalities of globin chain structure

A number of abnormalities of γ-chain structure have been detected in the course of cord blood screening for other disorders. None has been associated with anemia or clinical disease and is not detectable past early infancy.

β-Chain abnormalities account for the majority of the known variant hemoglobins. Many are hemoglobins of abnormal (usually increased) oxygen affinity, known as M hemoglobins. The major disorders of clinical significance in the United States are sickle cell disease and hemoglobin C disease. Because of the low levels of β-chain production, these rarely cause any clinical problems in the newborn period. Prenatal diagnosis is possible at about 14 weeks' gestation.

Hemoglobin C disease alone is not associated with significant morbidity or mortality in childhood. Sickle cell disease and SC disease are accompanied by sickling phenomena that may be life threatening, and early diagnosis is advisable to permit management decisions that should prevent much of the early mortality of sickle cell disease. About 12% of infants born with sickle cell disease die by age 2. Of these, the majority die of infection, most between 6 months and 2 years. Several infants have been reported who have died of generalized intravascular sickling in the neonatal period and have not had abnormally high levels of sickle hemoglobin. At least two infants have died from exchange transfusion performed with blood containing sickle hemoglobin (sickle cell trait, and SC disease).

Cord blood screening is done in many institutions to identify affected infants. Because of the high levels of Hb F at birth, it may be difficult to accurately quantitate the hemoglobins. However, identification of Hb S with or without Hb A and Hb C permits identification of infants at risk for significant hemoglobinopathies and defines a group of infants who should have a quantitative electrophoresis repeated at 3 to 6 months. Because of the low levels of the S, the hemoglobin solubility tests (Sickledex) are not usually suitable for screening in the newborn period. The metabisulfite tests for sickling may or may not demonstrate abnormalities on cord blood.

Methemoglobinemia

Methemoglobin is an otherwise normal hemoglobin in which the iron is oxidized and unable to carry oxygen. Normally iron is present in the reduced ferrous state. Oxidation to the ferric state occurs at a slow rate under normal conditions, but methemoglobin is reduced by an enzyme designated NADH-dependent diaphorase. Several other pathways exist but are not responsible for significant regeneration of ferrous iron. Activity of this enzyme is substantially reduced in normal full-term infants and is very low in premature infants; it rises to adult levels in erythrocytes by 4 months of age. In some populations, including Navajo Indians, congenital deficiency of this enzyme persists past early infancy. In newborns, methomoglobinemia is usually associated with oxidant stresses that increase the levels of methemoglobin. In congenital diaphorase deficiency, methemoglobinemia may be present continually without unusual oxidant or drug exposure.

When greater than 10% of hemoglobin is present as methemoglobin, the skin becomes dusky, and the blood develops a brown color that is not altered by direct exposure of the patient or the blood to high concentrations of oxygen. A variety of drugs and chemicals precipitate acute episodes of methemoglobinemia in newborns, including phenacetin, certain sulfonamides, aniline and its derivatives, and nitrites, which may contaminate well water and are present in some folk medications ("sweet spirits of nitre"). Infant food prepared from soil-grown vegetables, such as carrots, containing high levels of nitrates from fertilizer have caused clinically significant methemoglobinemia. In many cases the source of the oxidant causing methemoglobinemia is never identified and may include municipal water sources. Most of these infants have been bottle-fed on formulas prepared with tap water. In addition to the reduced level of diaphorase, the γ-chain of Hb F interacts with oxidants in such a way as to make Hb F more susceptible to methemoglobin formation than Hb A. In congenital diaphorase deficiency, significant neonatal methemoglobinemia may be present in heterozygotes as well as homozygotes for this autosomal recessive disorder.

The usual symptoms related to methemoglobinemia are tachypnea and tachycardia, and the major clinical finding is cyanosis at rest. The severity of illness is related to the levels of methemoglobinemia. Since methemoglobin cannot carry oxygen, these patients are functionally anemic. If the condition develops rapidly and methemoglobin levels are 30% or greater, infants may be dyspneic and irritable. Clinically apparent cyanosis implies methemoglobin levels of 10% or greater, but levels as high as 60% to 70% have been described in severely affected infants and may be fatal. A simple screening test for the presence of methemoglobin is performed by placing a drop of the infant's blood and that of a normal control on filter paper, which is waved gently in air for 30 seconds to oxygenate the hemoglobin. Control venous blood should turn red, whereas blood containing elevated levels of methemoglobin remains brown. A spectrophotometric procedure will confirm the diagnosis and quantitate the abnormal hemoglobin.

Once the diagnosis is established, a cause must be sought. Environmental sources of toxins should be reviewed and should include drugs, source of food and water, and topical agents, such as diaper marking dyes, which may be absorbed. If no source is sought, assay of the infant's erythrocytes for NADH-reductase levels and electrophoresis for detection of one of the abnormal M hemoglobins is indicated. The M hemoglobins are due to single amino acid substitutions that enable the globin chains to form stable complexes with ferric rather than ferrous ions. These hemoglobins are resistant to reduction by the usual intraerythrocyte enzymes. Most M hemoglobins are due to β-chain mutations and are not evident in the newborn period. A few are due to α-chain substitutions and may manifest neonatal methemoglobinemia. The major problems in differential diagnosis are congenital cardiac conditions such as tetralogy of Fallot and severe respiratory disease, but diagnostic clinical features are usually apparent.

Treatment of methemoglobinemia due to NADH-reductase deficiency or to oxidant exposure is administration of methylene blue at a dosage of 1 to 2 mg/kg intravenously. Methemoglobin levels fall within 1 or 2 hours. Failure of response suggests an abnormal hemoglobin. Recurrence without reexposure to toxins suggests enzyme deficiency. Ascorbic acid in doses of 300 to 400 mg orally per day may also be effective and may be sufficient in mild cases. Excessive administration of methylene blue may damage erythrocytes and produce a hemolytic anemia and should be avoided.

Unstable hemoglobins

Congenital Heinz body hemolytic anemias are a group of disorders associated with structurally abnormal hemoglobins that precipitate within the cell. Both α- and β-chain mutants have been described. Some are electrophoretically identical to Hb A, and other techniques must be used to establish the existence of an abnormal hemoglobin. All patients are heterozygotes, and almost a third appear to represent spontaneous mutations. These are uncommon genes, and the probability of homozygosity is very low. The spleen selectively removes the precipitated Heinz bodies, so the abnormal hemoglobin comprises only 10% to 30% of the total hemoglobin, with the remainder consisting primarily of Hb A. Following splenectomy, the number of Heinz bodies and the proportion of abnormal hemoglobin increase. The peripheral smear may demonstrate slight hypochromia, microcytosis, and basophilic stippling but may be entirely normal. To establish the diagnosis, demonstration of Heinz bodies on a supravital preparation is particularly useful. Incubation of the blood for 24 to 48 hours increases the yield, especially in patients whose spleens are intact. Heating red cell hemolysates to 50° for 1 hour produces a visible precipitate.

Since only about 25% of patients with unstable hemoglobins have α-chain mutations, most are not apparent in the immediate neonatal period. Those who do demonstrate the disorder early may have mild hyperbilirubinemia or significant hemolysis, depending on the variant. Anemia is rarely severe enough to require transfusion. Patients should receive folic acid supplementation, avoid oxidant drugs (which may aggravate Heinz body formation), and may require splenectomy if hemolysis is severe.

Congenital deficiencies of red cell enzymes

Normal erythrocytes differ metabolically from adult erythrocytes in a number of ways. Some of these differences reflect the fact that the red cell life span of fetal cells is approximately half that of adult erythrocytes. Many appear to be intrinsic differences between fetal and adult red cells. For instance, neonatal erythrocytes have elevated levels of glucose phosphate isomerase, phosphoglycerate kinase, enolase, and glyceraldehyde-3-phosphate, but lower levels of phosphofructokinase. They are deficient in several enzymes that protect against oxidant damage, including NADH-dependent methemoglobin reductase (diaphorase), catalase, and glutathione peroxidase. These may predispose the infant's red cells to Heinz body formation, methemoglobinemia, and hemolysis with relatively mild oxidant stresses. When hereditary enzyme deficiency is superimposed on the ordinary metabolic alterations of fetal red cells, significant hemolysis is often more of a problem than it is later in life.

Glucose-6-phosphate dehydrogenase

The gene for G6PD is carried on the X chromosome. Over 100 variants have been identified. Most are distinguishable electrophoretically from the "normal" A enzyme, but relatively few are associated with disease. The enzyme is unstable, and intracellular levels of G6PD do not decline to the region that would make the red cell susceptible to oxidant damage before 120 days, and thus do not limit the red cell life span. Unstable variants decline in activity at a greater rate. Mature erythrocytes are anucleate and cannot replenish the supply of enzyme by new synthesis. The rate of decay of enzyme activity determines the severity of the disease. Older cells are more susceptible to hemolysis with oxidant damage than young cells, which have higher levels of G6PD.

Because this is an X-linked disorder, males are most commonly affected. Studies of this enzyme resulted in promulgation of the *Lyon hypothesis*, which holds that the X chromosome is randomly inactivated in individual cells in females. Thus, rather than having a uniform population of cells with enzyme levels and electrophoretic patterns reflecting both the normal and abnormal enzyme, heterozygous females have two populations of cells. In one population the normal enzyme is expressed and no abnormal enzyme is identifiable, and in another population only the abnormal enzyme can be found. Some heterozygous females may have significant G6PD deficiency if a large proportion of their cells express only the abnormal enzyme. Populations with a high frequency of abnormal G6PD enzymes include blacks, Southern Europeans, Sephardic Jews, Chinese, Southeast Asians, and Arabs.

Drug-induced hemolysis is the most characteristic manifestation of relatively mild G6PD deficiency. This is the form most often seen in blacks, with a gene frequency of 14% in American blacks. The red cell survival is normal under ordinary conditions, but acute hemolysis develops with infection or exposure to certain drugs. The concomitant events of infection and drug exposure may result in markedly more severe hemolysis than occurs with either alone, which is particularly relevant for administration of aspirin, which does not appear to cause hemolysis without infection but does so with active infection. The role of infection may relate in part to generation of hydrogen peroxide by phagocytic cells ingesting microorganisms.

Congenital nonspherocytic hemolytic anemia occurs with more severe enzyme deficiencies, such as the Mediterranean variant. Affected individuals have a population of older red cells that are unable to metabolize the oxidants generated by normal events and thus develop Heinz bodies and are destroyed prematurely. These persons have an additional population of younger red cells susceptible to hemolysis with oxidant stresses such as infection or drugs and may hemolyze much of their red cell volume with fatal consequences. *Favism* is the term applied to acute hemolysis with ingestion of fava beans in persons with severe G6PD deficiency. Infants with G6PD deficiency may develop acute, severe hemolysis with maternal ingestion of fava beans or oxidant drugs either while the infant is in utero or via breast milk.

The clinical severity of the disorder is determined by the nature of the abnormal enzyme, the maturity of the infant, and the degree and extent of oxygen and/or drug therapy. Many instances of hyperbilirubinemia with hemolysis (fall in hemoglobin and reticulocytosis) associated with neonatal G6PD deficiency may occur without obvious precipitating factors. This may be sufficient to cause kernicterus and require exchange transfusion.

The smear demonstrates some fragmentation and poikilocytosis due to removal of cytoplasm and membrane in the spleen. Heinz bodies can be demonstrated by supravital staining with cresyl violet. Several screening tests for G6PD deficiency are easily performed, but the degree of reticulocytosis affects the result. Since young red cells have higher levels of G6PD, the test should be performed again after recovery when the reticulocyte count is low if a normal result is obtained during an acute hemolytic reaction. An alternative approach is to test only the denser cells by differential centrifugation, since these are the older fraction of red cells and more likely to be deficient in G6PD.

Drug-induced hemolysis occurs with glutathione synthetase deficiency, glutathione reductase deficiency, and glutathione peroxidase deficiency. The inability to detoxify oxidants is the same as it is in G6PD deficiency. These are uncommon disorders and are associated with reduced levels of glutathione and formation of Heinz bodies with exposure to acetylphenylhydrazine. G6PD levels are normal. Specific enzymatic assays are required to establish the diagnosis. These disorders may be associated with neonatal hyperbilirubinemia.

Pyruvate kinase

Pyruvate kinase (PK) is carried on an autosomal chromosome, and its deficiency is the most commonly encountered enzymopathy of the glycolytic pathway

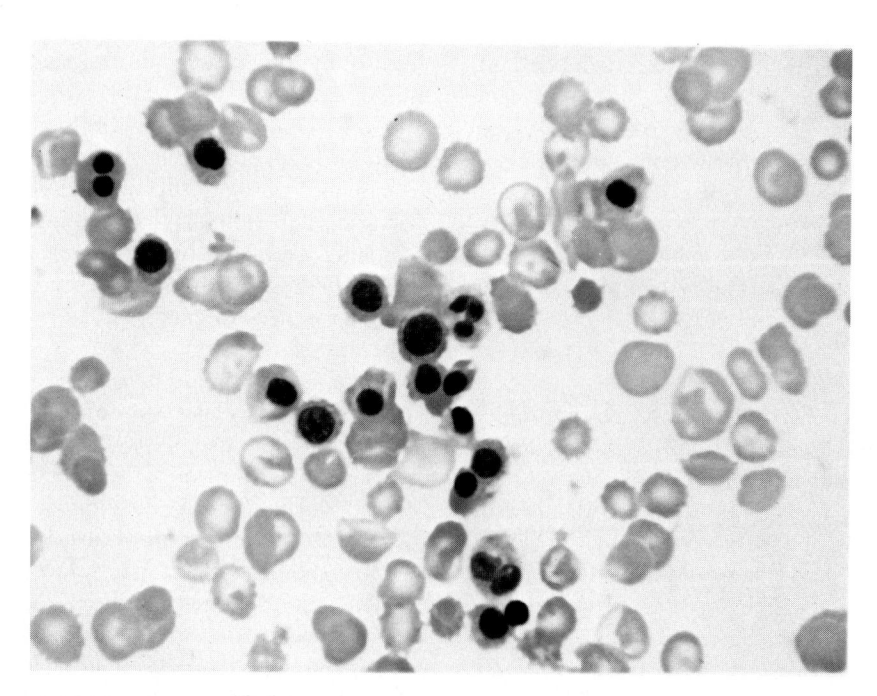

Fig. 29-11. Cord blood smear from an infant with severe pyruvate kinase deficiency and erythroblastosis fetalis. (Wright's stain; ×800.)

associated with anemia. It catalyzes the conversion of phosphoenolpyruvate to pyruvate, with generation of ATP. Intracellular levels of ATP are diminished, and the sodium-potassium pump in the red cell membrane does not function well, particularly with incubation. Potassium loss exceeds sodium gain initially, and the cells lose water and become crenated (desiccytes). These cells are poorly deformable and are removed on passage through liver and spleen. There is some evidence that reticulocytes may be selectively destroyed in the bone marrow, liver, and spleen. The reason for this is not clear but may relate to the higher rate of glycolysis seen in reticulocytes. The spleens of these patients are full of reticulocytes, and tagged mature PK-deficient red cells may have a normal survival time.

Several abnormalities have been described. In some families the level of enzyme activity is diminished. In others the enzyme is kinetically abnormal, and in still others the enzyme is unstable and decreases with red cell age. Since it is autosomally determined, two abnormal enzymes may coexist in the same cell. Carriers for mutant enzymes do not demonstrate hemolysis. The disorder may be difficult to diagnose even with quantitative assays of PK activity, especially if the enzyme has abnormal kinetics and the assay is performed with high levels of phosphoenolpyruvate. The buildup of products prior to this reaction, especially 2,3-DPG, may aid in making the diagnosis.

Certain population groups have a relatively high incidence of PK deficiency, notably Northern Europeans and Amish groups. Persistent jaundice and the presence of a nonspherocytic hemolytic anemia should suggest the diagnosis of PK deficiency. Although there are morphologic abnormalities of the cells observed in wet preparations with a phase contrast microscope, the Wright-stained smear is unremarkable except for polychromasia consistent with the degree of reticulocytosis (Fig. 29-11). Despite significant anemia, patients are rarely symptomatic, which is probably due in part to the elevated levels of 2,3-DPG, which lower oxygen affinity and improve tissue oxygen delivery.

The clinical course is highly variable. Hyperbilirubinemia in the newborn period is common, and persistent jaundice and transfusion requirement are not unusual. Patients are described who have a fully compensated hemolytic anemia with persistent hyperbilirubinemia but no anemia. More commonly, the hemolytic rate is significant, and patients are splenectomized early in life with variable response. Most patients derive some benefit from splenectomy, with a rise in hemoglobin and reduction or elimination of transfusion requirement. Occasional patients do not benefit at all from splenectomy. Bilirubin gallstones are frequent, and aplastic crises with infection may result in rapid development of severe anemia. Folic acid supplementation is required, but iron is reused, and dietary supplementation should not be given. This is especially true if significant numbers of transfusions have been required.

Disorders of the red cell membrane

The red cell membrane has been extensively studied and many of the functional components characterized at a molecular level. It is an ideal system for the study of membranes because it is easy to purify and the cells can be obtained in large quantity by noninvasive techniques. The membrane consists of a lipid bilayer with intrinsic proteins traversing the lipids and a complex protein lattice that underlies and inserts into the lipid. The red cell shape is dictated by the protein lattice, which must also be sufficiently deformable to permit the cell to traverse the capillary beds of all tissues and to escape destruction in the spleen. Several disorders of red cell shape have been associated with congenital hemolytic anemias. Most present in the newborn period with hyperbilirubinemia and varying degrees of hemolysis.

Hereditary spherocytosis

This disorder is an autosomal dominant disease in which the abnormality of shape leads to entrapment of the cells in splenic sinusoids and hemolysis. The cells are dense with a high mean corpuscular hemoglobin concentration and a reduced membrane area. The cell has a more spherical shape than normal as a consequence of the reduced surface-to-volume ratio. The red cell membranes are inherently unstable, which leads to loss of membrane and spherocytosis; the cause of the instability is unknown. Two metabolic lesions are described. The first is an abnormality in the activity of a membrane protein kinase that phosphorylates the protein spectrin, a major component of the fibrillary lattice that maintains the shape of the erythrocyte. This has been variable in cases of hereditary spherocytosis, and its relationship to the pathogenesis of the disease is not known. The second defect is an increased permeability to sodium. It is likely that this is an epiphenomenon, since membrane instability and spherocytosis are not found in hereditary stomatocytosis, in which the permeability defect is much greater.

Hereditary spherocytosis affects about 1 in 5,000 infants and is most common in Northern Europeans. About 25% of cases are sporadic. Neonatal jaundice is very common and may require exchange transfusion. The diagnosis may be difficult in the newborn period for several reasons. ABO incompatibility is also associated with spherocytosis, although there is usually more variability in the size and shape of the red cells in isoimmune hemolytic disease. The MCHC is elevated in hereditary spherocytosis but not in ABO incompatibility. In the neonatal period, osmotic fragility is normally less marked than in adult cells, so the osmotic fragility test in neonates with spherocytosis may fall into the "normal" range for adults. All spherocytes are osmotically fragile, so the osmotic fragility test is not specific for hereditary spherocytosis. Family studies may be useful to establish a diagnosis of neonatal hemolysis due to hereditary spherocytosis if other test results are equivocal.

Beyond the newborn period, most patients develop a chronic hemolytic anemia whose severity varies from fully compensated (reticulocytosis without anemia) to severe (requiring periodic transfusions). Gallstones eventually develop in many patients with chronic hemolytic anemias. Splenectomy is usually recommended in hereditary spherocytosis, since it eliminates the hemolysis, although the erythrocyte abnormalities remain. Because of the hazards of postsplenectomy infection, splenectomy should be delayed until at least age 5 unless the anemia is marked. Whether the long-term hazards of gallstones exceed those of postsplenectomy infection is not clear.

Hereditary elliptocytosis

Although more common than hereditary spherocytosis, in the majority of cases this disorder is not associated with disease. Normal persons may have up to 15% elliptocytes on smear; greater than 25% is required to make the diagnosis. In the 10% of patients in whom this condition is more than a morphologic curiosity, hemolysis may be severe. The osmotic fragility and sodium leak are similar to those of hereditary spherocytosis cells in cases with hemolysis, and splenectomy is useful. This may be a cause of neonatal jaundice, and the smear is usually strikingly abnormal (Fig. 29-12). It is an autosomal dominant, so family studies may help confirm the diagnosis.

Hereditary stomatocytosis

In this disorder the red cells are swollen and cup shaped and there is an extreme defect in cation permeability. The cells tend to accumulate sodium in excess of potassium loss and gain volume. There is a marked increase in the activity of the sodium-potassium pump in response to the increase in intracellular sodium, with consequent increase in requirement for energy in the form of ATP. In the hypoglycemic, stagnant environment of the spleen, these cells are unable to fulfill their energy needs and are destroyed. Splenectomy reduces the rate of hemolysis but may not eliminate it. These cells are also abnormally rigid and poorly deformable, which contributes to their rapid rate of destruction. In one instance, biochemical correction of the permeability defect, with reduction of the energy requirement and intracellular water, also corrected the abnormality in deformability, which suggests that this is a secondary defect.

As with other defects in the membrane, hereditary stomatocytosis may be accompanied by hyperbilirubinemia in the newborn period and may be severe enough to require exchange transfusion.

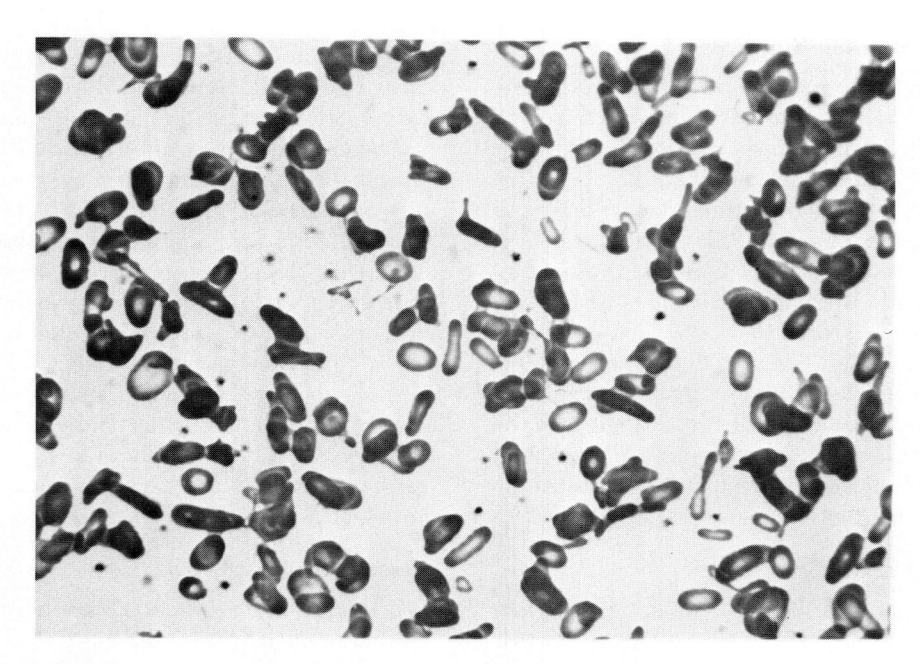

Fig. 29-12. Peripheral blood smear at age 1 week from an infant with hereditary elliptocytosis. (Wright's stain; ×800.)

Acanthocytes and acanthocytosis

Acanthocytes are erythrocytes with multiple projections from the surface due to an excess of membrane per unit cell volume—the obverse of spherocytosis. In most instances they reflect abnormalities of plasma lipids. The lipids of the red cell membrane exchange with those free in serum. Spur cells and acanthocytes are morphologically identical but have differences in their lipid profiles, with an excess of cholesterol-to-phospholipid ratio in both. The associated conditions include liver disease, particularly with biliary obstruction, abetalipoproteinemia, and deficiency of lecithin: cholesterol acyltransferase. The latter two conditions are inborn metabolic errors that are familial and rare. Acanthocytes may be seen transiently in the newborn period without associated disease or significant hemolysis, which may reflect liver immaturity. Often there is no cogent explanation of the phenomenon.

Vitamin E

Vitamin E (tocopherol) is a fat-soluble antioxidant found abundantly in nature in combination with unsaturated fatty acids. It is, in effect, the antirancidity vitamin. Although it occurs in a number of isomeric forms, the dextrorotary form of α-tocopherol is biologically the most effective cogener.

In the immediate newborn period, serum tocopherol values range from 0.3 to 0.7 mg/dl, or one-third to one-half that of maternal levels. Maintenance of normal levels depends exclusively on adequate dietary sources and effective absorption. The first unequivocal description of anemia secondary to vitamin E deficiency was identified in 1965 and was followed in rapid succession by a number of additional reports. In these studies the infants were either fed fat-rich formulas stripped of tocopherol or were too young to absorb tocopherol in quantities sufficient to provide adequate antioxidant protection. Also included were premature infants further stressed by such prooxidant agents as trivalent iron. In the small premature infant, i.e., less than 1,500 gm birth weight, a relatively greater polyunsaturated fatty acid content is present in the erythrocyte membrane than that identified in the full-term infant or adult. Thus any combination of excessive polyunsaturated fatty acid intake (more than 35% of the fat content), inadequate tocopherol intake, or oxidative stress, i.e., iron administration, may result in an absolute or "conditioned" vitamin E deficiency and lead, in turn, to significant hemolysis (Figs. 29-13 and 29-14).

The characteristic hematologic findings include anemia with reticulocytosis and occasionally thrombocytosis, the latter very likely due to a nonspecific increase in marrow activity. A less common event is peripheral edema, presumably the result of oxidative damage to vascular endothelium. In the full-blown disorder, appreciable losses of red cell membrane phosphatidyl ethanolamine

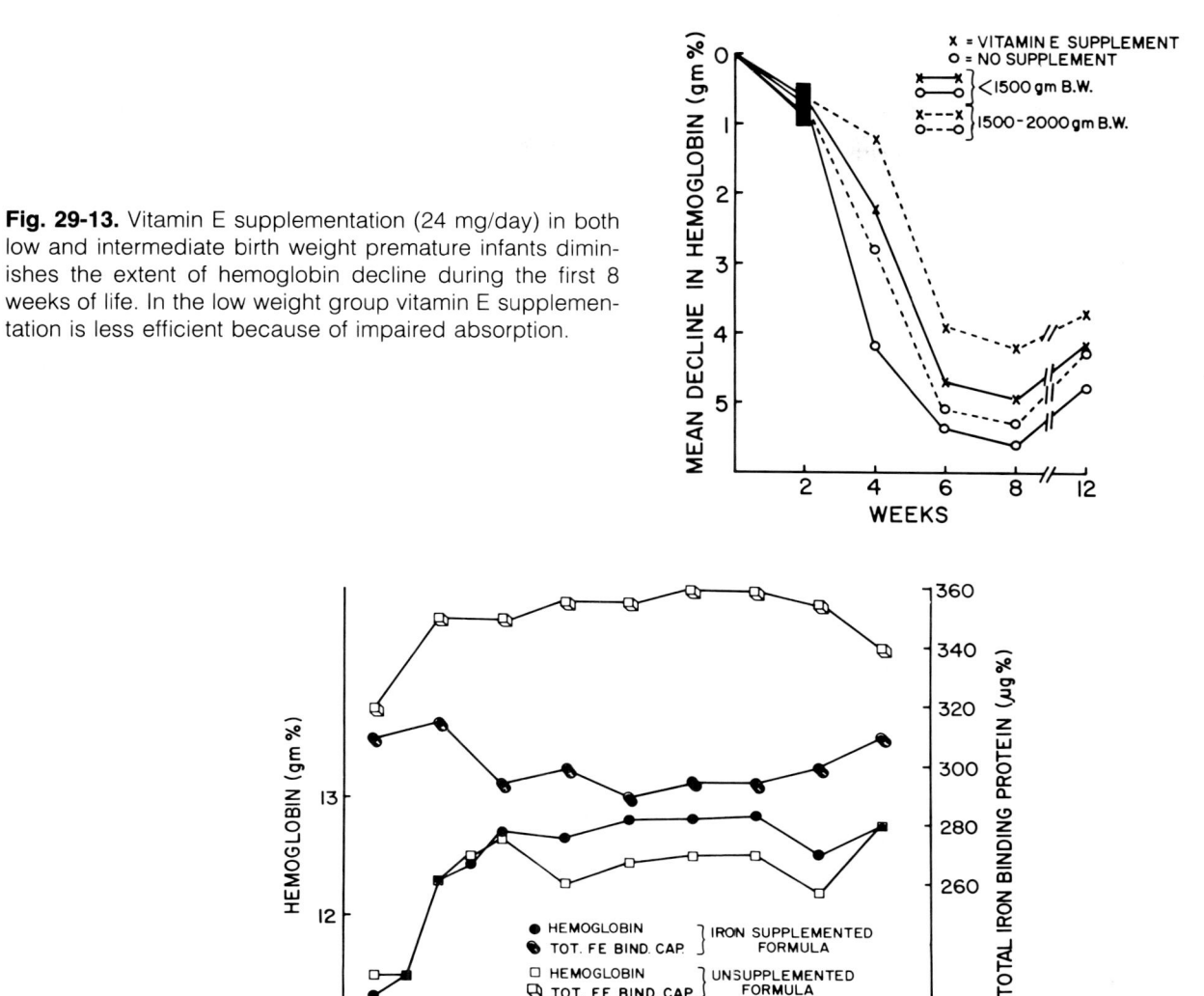

Fig. 29-13. Vitamin E supplementation (24 mg/day) in both low and intermediate birth weight premature infants diminishes the extent of hemoglobin decline during the first 8 weeks of life. In the low weight group vitamin E supplementation is less efficient because of impaired absorption.

Fig. 29-14. Although the hemoglobin differences between term infants fed iron-supplemented and unsupplemented formulas are not significant, evidence for iron deficiency is well demonstrated by the higher levels of unsaturated iron-binding protein in the supplemented group.

occur in temporal association with demonstrable increases in red cell fragility in dilute hydrogen peroxide solutions.

Glutathione peroxidase functions in concert with tocopherol in maintenance of erythrocyte lipid stability. It is synthesized solely in the presence of trace quantities of selenium, which is present in variable distribution in soil. Its content in cow's milk is approximately 14 ng/dl, or half that of human milk. Thus any infant fed solely cow's milk preparations for extended periods of time is at risk for the development of selenium depletion and, accordingly, glutathione peroxidase deficiency. The risk of such an occurrence is almost exclusive to the small premature infant.

It has recently been shown that vitamin E deficiency in the small premature infant can be aborted by the early parenteral administration of tocopherol (25 mg intramuscularly for 5 days) in association with low-fat formulas (15% of the total fat as polyunsaturated fatty acids). With this regimen it is also possible to provide early iron pro-

Fig. 29-15. Serum tocopherol values of 0.5 mg/dl or less do not necessarily imply "deficiency." However, in the absence of PUFA:tocopherol ratio determinations, any small premature infant with a serum tocopherol level below 0.5 mg/dl may be considered suspect.

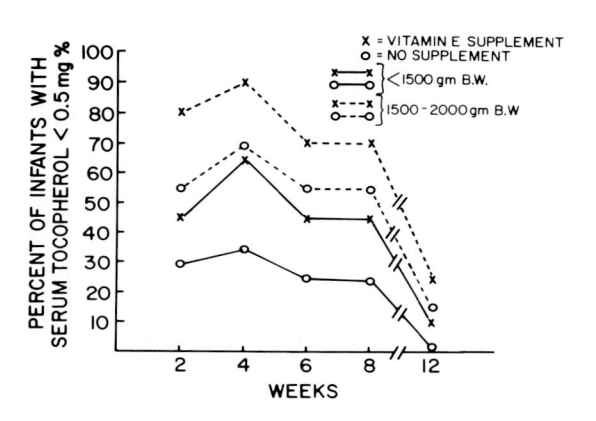

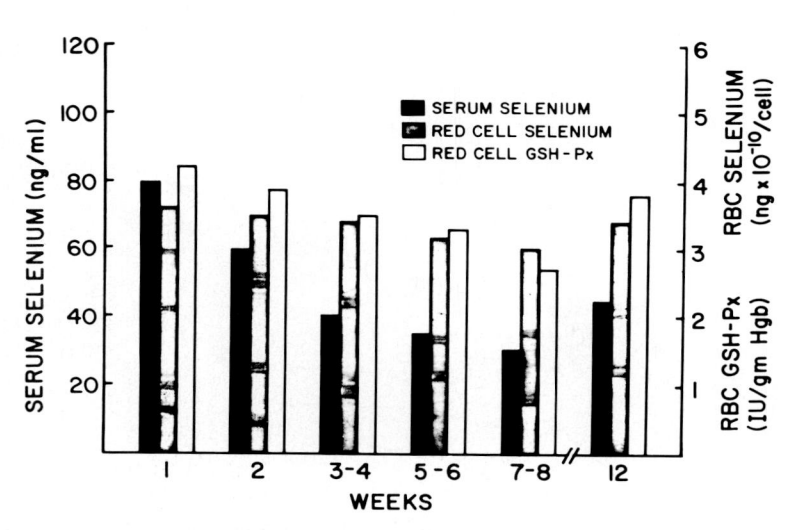

Fig. 29-16. The decline in serum selenium levels precedes the fall in red cell selenium and glutathione peroxidase activity. Normal adult serum selenium levels range from 120 to 200 ng/ml.

phylaxis to diminish the risk of developing the hematologic sequelae of iron deficiency during the ensuing rapid growth period. In animal studies of induced selenium deficiency, tocopherol has, to varying degrees, diminished the extent of oxidative-induced membrane damage. Whether the high-dose, parenteral tocopherol regimen functions in a similar manner in the selenium-deficient patient awaits verification. For the older premature infant whose ability to absorb tocopherol is essentially unimpaired, a similar formula enriched solely with 13 IU of tocopherol/L is sufficient to maintain tocopherol adequacy (serum tocopherol levels > 1.0 mg/dl and thus protect against increased membrane peroxidation (Fig. 29-15). In these infants, early iron administration is not essential and can, in fact, be withheld for 6 to 8 weeks or until such time as additional foodstuffs (with additional selenium) are added. The hematologic and biochemical patterns relating to tocopherol and selenium during prematurity are noted in Fig. 29-16.

It is readily apparent that iron supplementation is an obvious requisite for the rapidly growing premature infant. Similar recommendations apply to term infants, particularly those fed modified cow's milk preparation. Term infants, as a rule, generally do not exhibit blatant hematologic manifestations of iron deficiency if fed a properly supervised diet. However, laboratory manifestations of subclinical iron deficiency probably occur in most cow's milk-fed infants. Hemoglobin values during the first 18 months of life in non-iron-supplemented and iron-supplemented term infants are essentially similar, but consistently elevated iron-binding protein values are noted in the non-iron-supplemented group (Fig. 29-17). It is therefore reasonable to conclude that many non-iron-supplemented infants function on marginal iron

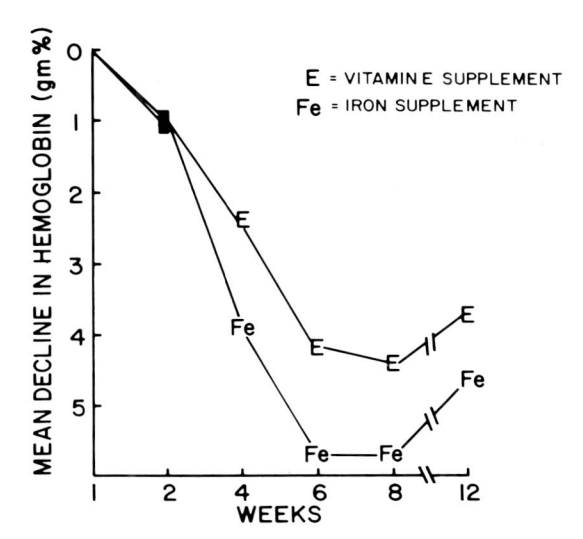

Fig. 29-17. The administration of iron (3 mg/kg/day) to low birth weight (1,500 gm) premature infants intensifies hemoglobin losses during the first 6 to 10 weeks. Conversely, vitamin E supplementation protects against excessive hemoglobin loss (see Fig. 29-13.)

reserves. Because of the greater bioavailability of iron in breast-fed as compared with cow's milk–fed infants who receive essentially equivalent quantities of iron, iron supplementation for breast-fed infants is probably unnecessary until 6 months of age.

POLYCYTHEMIA

Among the known causes of neonatal polycythemia are twin-twin transfusion, maternal-fetal transfusion, and excessive delays in cord clamping. Neonatal polycythemia on occasion has been associated with events relating to placental insufficiency, i.e., toxemia, placenta previa, postmaturity, and infants small for gestational age. It has also been identified in congenital adrenal hyperplasia, thyrotoxicosis, and in infants of diabetic mothers. In the endocrine-related disorders, hypocalcemia and hypoglycemia are common sequelae but may also occur in the absence of endocrine dysfunction, solely on the basis of polycythemia-induced thrombotic episodes. It has also been described in Down's syndrome with elevated erythropoietic levels and in the hyperplastic visceromegaly syndrome (Beckwith-Wiedemann). With rare exceptions, cases of erythrocytosis due to high oxygen affinity hemoglobinopathies are the results of β-chain defects and thus not manifest at birth. The characteristic findings in neonatal polycythemia include varying degrees of plethora, listlessness, and icterus. As the severity increases, additional findings include respiratory distress with modest cyanosis, seizures, and diffuse thrombotic disease. In every situation an etiologic search should include a careful appraisal of the maternal endocrine status, investigation of maternal and infant blood types, chromosomal analyses in an opposite-sex transfusion, fetal hemoglobin levels, IgM/IgA titers, and assessment of any antecedent maternal event such as toxemia or placenta previa. In twin-twin transfusions there is an increased likelihood of identifying a seriously anemic donor twin.

Virtually all symptoms relate to the increase in blood viscosity, and thus the decision to interrupt a polycythemic event must be based on knowledge of both pathophysiology and the ongoing clinical status. For example, a hematocrit level of 60% is associated with a viscosity three to five times greater than a 40% hematocrit level. The hyperviscosity induced by the markedly increased erythroid mass is often further exaggerated by a poorly deformable red cell. The net effect is extensive impairment of the microcirculatory dynamics and an intensification of the hypoxic stimulus to red cell production. Accordingly, therapy should always be directed to those who are obviously symptomatic, or empirically, those whose hematocrit values exceed 70%. All other infants should be observed frequently and treated at the first sign of changes in symptomatology. Therapy should be designed to reduce red cell mass without loss of blood volume. Simple phlebotomy is thus inappropriate because of the risk of producing a hypovolemic state. Plasma transfusions are equally ill advised because such therapy implies a secondary or relative polycythemia, which rarely if ever occurs in this age group and can only be verified by radioisotope labeling studies. The most effective approach is partial exchange transfusion with fresh frozen plasma designed to reduce the hematocrit to an acceptable level of 55% or less. The following formula is a useful guide:

$$\text{Volume of exchange (ml)} = \text{Blood volume} \times \frac{\text{Observed-desired hematocrit}}{\text{Observed hematocrit}}$$

This procedure can be performed using aliquots equivalent to 10% of the estimated blood volume. Repeat hematocrits are obtained at the conclusion of the exchange transfusion procedure and at six hourly intervals during the ensuing 24 hours. Thrombocytopenia, due either to marrow overcrowding or peripheral destruction, occasionally accompanies severe polycythemia but rarely causes problems. It is therefore unnecessary to compromise volume with additional platelet infusions, particularly in light of knowledge that the platelet count usually reverts to normal within 24 to 48 hours following exchange transfusion. In twin-twin polycythemic states the symptomatic or severely anemic donor sibling (hemoglobin less than 7.0 gm/dl) should be treated in accordance with guidelines set forth for the treatment of acute blood loss. However, blood removed during the exchange transfusion, because of admixing and lack of sterility, must never be used for reinfusion into the donor twin. In the anemic but otherwise asymptomatic twin, treatment solely with oral iron is sufficient.

BLOOD COMPONENT REPLACEMENT THERAPY
Red cell transfusion

Knowledge of the blood volume variations in the neonate is a prerequisite to effective replacement therapy. In the term infant the range in blood volume is 80 to 95 ml/kg. In the premature infant the blood volume per unit weight is larger, i.e., 90 to 110 ml/kg, and somewhat more variable. Treatment of acute blood loss in the neonate thus presupposes knowledge not only of the gestationally related differences but also of the reliability of measurable parameters. The most effective indicator is the central venous pressure. Blood pressure, pulse, or hemoglobin/hematocrit determinations are not reliable indicators of acute blood loss. As a reference guide, however, a systolic blood pressure below 50 mm Hg or a pulse rate greater than 170 per minute is strongly suggestive of blood loss in excess of 20% of the estimated blood volume. Hemoglobin and/or hematocrit determinations are virtually useless because of the variability in plasma restoration time, which may take as long as 20 or as few as 6 hours following an acute hemorrhagic event. Once the blood volume is restored, as indicated by a normal central venous pressure, the hemoglobin and/or hematocrit values may then be used as corroborative follow-up information. However, it is inadvisable to use levels obtained from capillary blood because of errors concomitant on peripheral pooling or stasis. In the premature infant the disparity between peripheral and central hemoglobin/hematocrit determinations often results in a lack of conformity that may last for 3 or 4 weeks. In the term infant the discrepancy rarely persists beyond 5 to 7 days. An outline of the various events leading to neonatal blood loss follows.

A. Prenatal external losses
 1. Fetal-maternal transfusion
 2. Twin-twin transfusion
B. Prenatal/perinatal/postnatal internal losses
 1. Cephalhematoma
 2. Caput succedaneum
 3. Intracerebral
 4. Retroperitoneal
 5. Hepatic rupture
 6. Splenic rupture
C. Obstetric external losses
 1. Placenta previa
 2. Abruptio placentae
 3. Placental tear at cesarean section
 4. Umbilical cord rupture
    a. Varices
    b. Torsion
 5. Placental vessel rupture
    a. Defective communication
    b. Abnormal insertion

Acute blood loss should be treated with "fresh" whole blood, i.e., not older than 72 hours of age, to replace coagulation factor losses, maintain a sufficient oxygen transport mechanism, and obviate hyperkalemia. If whole blood is not immediately available, plasma, plasma expanders, or saline may be used until an appropriately cross-matched sample is obtained. In dire emergencies, i.e., when immediate blood support is dictated, low-titered O negative blood may be administered in advance of an appropriately cross-matched sample. An alternative is the use of type-specific red cells admixed to a prearranged hematocrit with fresh frozen plasma or preferably platelet-rich plasma, particularly if there is an associated thrombocytopenia. It is also appropriate to irradiate the blood (500 rad) to prevent the possible occurrence of graft-versus-host disease in a potentially immunoincompetent recipient.

Only rarely are red cell transfusions necessary for the treatment of chronic blood loss. Identification of this type of event should presuppose chronic intrauterine blood loss, as in protracted fetal-maternal hemorrhage. In such infants the usual symptom is pallor. Other clinical manifestations of lesser frequency include congestive heart failure and/or hepatomegaly. Apart from a low hemoglobin value at birth, i.e., less than 12 gm/dl, altered red cell morphology (hypochromia, microcytosis, anisocytosis, poikilocytosis), variable degrees of normoblastosis, and a low serum iron level with an elevated total iron-binding capacity, there are relatively few additional findings. The venous pressure is usually normal or moderately elevated, and on occasion one may note peripheral edema. For the most part these infants are vigorous, and even pallor often goes undetected. Jaundice in excess of the "physiologic levels" is an uncommon event and, when seen, should alert the practitioner to the possibility of hemolytic disease. The diagnosis of fetal-maternal hemorrhage can be made with certainty by demonstrating the presence of fetal red cells in the maternal circulation. A variety of different tests are available in this regard and include differential agglutination, fluorescent antibody, and acid elution (Kleihauer-Betke) techniques. The latter is a simple and reliable method for use in essentially all instances of suspected fetal-maternal blood loss, except for the rare example of a maternal hemoglobin abnormality characterized by increased levels of fetal hemoglobin (as in hereditary persistence of fetal hemoglobin, thalassemia, or sickle cell disease). In effect, for any nonisoimmunized, metabolically intact, anemic infant in whom overt blood loss is suspected but not identified, the possibility of fetal-maternal blood loss should be investigated and include an examination of the placenta for tears or malformations. Because most of these infants are essentially asymptomatic at birth, it is appropriate to treat solely with oral iron (3 mg of elemental iron/kg/day) administered for at least 3 months to correct the hemoglobin defect as well as replenish iron stores. However, if the clinical course suggests the need for transfusion support, red cells rather than whole blood should be administered because only a red cell deficit exists. For example, a 1.8-kg infant on day 3 is noted to be pale and otherwise asymptomatic. The central venous pressure is normal, and the hemoglobin is 8 gm/dl. On day 9, without a change in hemoglobin value, the patient experiences several apneic spells and is noted to have increasing hepatomegaly. All indications suggest prior fetal-maternal blood loss. It is decided to repair the hemoglobin value to 14 gm/dl using packed red cells, which generally have a hematocrit range of 65% to 75% (hemoglobin concentration 20 to 25 gm/dl). To calculate the transfusion requirements, the following formula is used:

$$\text{Cell volume (ml)} = \frac{\text{Patient weight (kg)} \times \text{Blood volume (ml/kg} \times \text{desired observed hemoglobin)}}{\text{Hemoglobin (gm/dl) of packed cells}}$$

$$= \frac{1.8 \times 100 \times (14 - 8)}{25}$$

$$= 43 \text{ ml}$$

For this patient the blood volume is estimated at 100 ml/kg, and the hemoglobin concentration of the packed cells is actually determined. To compensate for possible blood volume lability, the transfusion is administered slowly, i.e., 20 ml per hour.

Platelet transfusion

The treatment of thrombocytopenic bleeding is best performed with single-donor units and, preferably, type-specific support if multiple transfusions are anticipated. Donors should be carefully screened to preclude the administration of antiaggregating agents such as aspirin and indomethacin. For the treatment of bleeding secondary to isoimmune thrombocytopenia, the optimum platelet source is the mother. However, unrelated single-donor platelet support will suffice because of the relatively short-lived process. Irrespective of the events leading to the peripheral destruction of platelets, the goal in treating thrombocytopenic bleeding is maintenance of a platelet count in excess of 30,000/mm^3. Rarely does bleeding occur or persist above this level. A two-unit plasma exchange technique offers the most efficient platelet yield, has the advantage of returning plasma and red cells to the donor, provides approximately 70% of the estimated platelet mass, and is free from the clumping effect that occurs with platelets separated from sedimented whole blood and stored at 4° C. A variety of automated collecting processes are currently operative, and the reader is urged to develop a familiarity with the local or regional collection program. The keynote in platelet support, irrespective of the collection system, is freshly obtained samples, i.e., less than 24 hours old. Platelets more than 48 hours old rarely will produce an incremental response. As a general guide, each collection unit, or 50 ml, contains from 5 to 8 × 10^{10} platelets. One can thus estimate the number of units or fractions thereof needed to raise the platelet number in excess of 30,000/mm^3 merely by calculating the total circulating volume relative to the estimated platelet number per unit. This standard 50-ml size can also be concentrated to as little as a 10-ml volume but at the risk of a 30% to 50% loss in platelet viability. For example, a bleeding thrombocytopenic neonate with a blood volume of 300 ml has a platelet count of 10,000/mm^3 (1 × 10^4/mm^3). The total platelet volume is 1 × 10^7/ml × 300, or 0.3 × 10^{10}. A half unit (25 ml) contains 2.5 × 10^{10} platelets, or, assuming a viability of 70%, 1.7 × 10^{10} platelets. The anticipated net effect should be a sixfold increase in platelet volume, i.e., a rise in platelet count to 70,000/mm^3.

Granulocyte transfusion

Granulocyte transfusion therapy appears to be the most effective when used in the treatment of gram-negative infections in association with an absolute granulocyte count below 500/mm^3. There are no data to support the use of granulocyte transfusions in patients with gram-positive infections or viral, fungal, or parasitic disorders. Ideally, such transfusions should be administered no less than once a day until the infection is either eradicated or until the granulocyte count exceeds 500/mm^3. The administration unitage is not as precise for granulocytes as it is for platelets, and one rarely observes a granulocyte response per se primarily because of the brief life span of granulocytes within the vascular space. Depending in part on the type of processing equipment, a general guide to granulocyte transfusion is the likelihood that 4 to 8 L of processed blood will yield approximately 5 × 10^9 granulocytes/mm^3. Febrile reactions commonly occur with repeated granulocyte transfusions and can be controlled with concomitant steroid and antihistamine administration. As with red cell and platelet transfusions, it is also advisable to irradiate granulocytes prior to infusion in small (immunoincompetent) infants to prevent lymphocyte engraftment.

DISORDERS OF PHAGOCYTIC CELLS

Polymorphonuclear leukocytes, monocytes, and tissue macrophages are all derived from the bone marrow. A stem cell common to other marrow elements is the ultimate precursor. Myelopoiesis, or production of neutrophils and monocytes, takes place in the liver, spleen, and bone marrow but apparently does not occur in the yolk sac, which is the site of erythropoiesis in the first trimester. Monocytes leave the marrow and mature into fixed tissue macrophages in other organs, including the liver, spleen, and lungs. Under normal conditions in neonates and adults a reserve of mature neutrophils is present in the marrow that exceeds the circulating pool by a factor of 10. These mature cells are released under conditions of stress or infection. In addition, intravascular neutrophils are free in the circulation and adhere to vessel walls in "circulating" and "marginal" pools that exist in equilibrium. Neutrophils form the first line of defense against bacterial infection and are able to migrate into areas of infection, ingest organisms, and kill them rapidly. Monocytes form the second line of defense, arriving in the inflammatory infiltrate much less rapidly then neutrophils. Monocytes are important for defense against fungal infections as well as against bacteria. Phagocytes are also major factors in wound healing, being needed for removal of necrotic material as well as for prevention of infection. In addition, tissue macrophages are the major site of destruction of sensitized or damaged erythrocytes in hemolytic disease, regardless of the nature of the red cell abnormality.

Phagocytic cells interact in complex fashion with humoral factors, which regulate the recognition of foreign material and the formation of inflammatory exudates. The major humoral factors are immunoglobulins and components of the complement and coagulation systems. IgG, 7S globulin, crosses the placenta and provides the neonate with passive protection against some organisms. The amount of protection varies with the gestational age of the infant (since much of the IgG is acquired in the last month of pregnancy) and with the immune status of the mother. Complement components are synthesized by the infant, with much of the contribution coming from the liver, including the macrophages therein. Low levels of some components, particularly in the alternate or properdin pathway, even in healthy full-term infants, may contribute to increased susceptibility to infection. Activated complement factors and some coagulation factors are potent "chemoattractants," or stimulators of migration toward a gradient. The factors, although beyond the scope of this section, contribute heavily to normal function of phagocytic cells.

Neutrophil kinetics

The absolute neutrophil count tends to be markedly elevated at birth and in the first few days of life. Since lymphocytosis is a normal finding at this age, the total white count may be quite high. The high neutrophil count is related to several factors. The rate of marrow *production* is high because of an elevated level of a hormone, termed *colony-stimulating factor*, which increases the rates of division and maturation of marrow precursors. The rate of *release* from the marrow is increased at the time of delivery, perhaps because of the stress of delivery, with release of epinephrine and endogenous cortisol. In addition, the rate of *demargination* of the intravascular pool is increased by the same factors that accelerate release. By 1 week of age the absolute neutrophil count has reached the levels normally seen later in childhood. Because of the lymphocytosis that is normal at this age, the percentage of neutrophils may be lower than in older children, but the absolute numbers should be the same.

Neutropenia

An absolute neutrophil count less than 1,500/mm^3 constitutes neutropenia. Some persons, particularly black males, normally run somewhat lower counts, but this is rarely detected in the neonatal period.

Neutropenia due to an increase in the rate of destruction of cells is associated with a number of processes. Exhaustion of marrow stores, which is rarely seen outside the newborn period, has been associated with severe infection. Necrotizing enterocolitis may cause massive emigration of neutrophils into the gastrointestinal tract and deplete the marrow reserves. Neutropenia associated with necrotizing enterocolitis has a particularly poor prognosis. Neutrophil transfusion may be of potential benefit in these children. They require very small volumes, which can be obtained in the course of preparation of platelet packs or neutrophil transfusions for other patients. Staphylococcal septicemia is also associated with neutropenia due to exhaustion of stores. Depletion of reserves with repeated exchange transfusion has also been described but has not been associated with infectious complications.

Immune neutropenia may be due to maternal antibody production, analogous to isoimmune hemolytic disease or thrombocytopenia. This is usually transient, and the neutrophil count begins to rise within 2 weeks. If the child does not contract an infection, it is a benign and self-limited process. Drug-induced neutropenia may occur in infants, possibly from transplacentally acquired drugs. These include sulfonamides, semisynthetic penicillins, propylthiouracil, methimazole, and gold salts. Congenital autoimmune neutropenia has been described in several patients, and the specificity of the antibodies is known in some cases. These infants tend to have severe neutropenia or agranulocytosis and have significant infections. These antibodies do not tend to disappear, and the patients remain chronically neutropenic.

Neutropenia due to impaired production of neutrophils has a variable prognosis, which depends on the severity of the neutropenia. If the neutrophil count is greater than 500, patients usually have minor infectious problems but not serious or life-threatening septicemia. There are a variety of ill-defined patterns, with variable degrees of monocytosis in the peripheral blood, eosinophilia, and bone marrow morphologies. At present, no good system for classifying these patients and no rational basis for selecting therapy except for antimicrobial coverage appropriate for the organisms causing infection exist. Certain groups of patients are more easily defined by their clinical patterns.

Cyclic neutropenia appears to be due to disordered regulation of myelopoiesis. It is a hereditary condition with dominant transmission. Patients have repeated episodes of fevers, mouth sores, and ulceration of other mucosal surfaces. The majority of patients cycle at 21-day intervals, with a marked monocytosis accompanying the periods of agranulocytosis. The bone marrow morphology varies with the time of the cycle. Most patients have recurrent infections, but severe deep tissue infections are relatively uncommon, probably because the most profound neutropenia lasts only 4 or 5 days, and organisms are killed in the periods of normal numbers of neutrophils. Macrophages are normal. This may present in the newborn period, but repeated determination of blood counts and several months of close follow-up are required to make the diagnosis unless there is a family history.

Bone marrow dysfunction with pancreatic insufficiency, or Schwachman-Diamond syndrome, includes patients whose significant problems are variable. Some are most affected by malnutrition and dwarfism, whereas others are incapacitated primarily by recurrent infections. The sweat test is normal in these patients, but the picture of pancreatic insufficiency with recurrent pulmonary infections may closely mimic cystic fibrosis. Hypoplastic anemia and thrombocytopenia are also present, but neutropenia is usually the most significant component of the marrow dysfunction. Treatment includes pancreatic enzyme replacement and aggressive treatment of infections, but the management is generally unsatisfactory. The symptoms are usually present after a month of age and are not recognized in the neonatal period.

Infantile genetic agranulocytosis, or Kostmann's syndrome, is a severe form of hereditary neutropenia with apparently autosomal recessive inheritance. Children usually have infections and associated agranulocytosis in the newborn period. Marked degrees of monocytosis are characteristics of this disease and may afford at least some protection against bacterial infection. Skin and respiratory tract infections are difficult to control, and most patients die of infection in childhood. Subtle chromosomal abnormalities have been detected in some cases, and several patients who have survived the first decade have developed myeloid leukemias. The marrow precursors seem to grow normally in culture, and there have been no inhibitors of proliferation indentified. The nature of the defect in this devastating condition remains undefined.

Reticular dysgenesis is the ultimate immunologic deficiency state. Patients have severe combined immune deficiency, without T or B lymphocyte function, and agranulocytosis. Presentation is early in infancy, with rapid death from overwhelming infection the rule unless a compatible donor for bone marrow transplantation can be found. As in other defects in lymphocyte function, it is important to suspect the diagnosis early to facilitate therapy and counseling. Blood products that might contain viable lymphocytes should be irradiated to prevent the establishment of potentially lethal graft-versus-host disease.

Phagocyte function in the newborn

See also Chapter 26.

The increased susceptibility of the newborn to infection has prompted study of the function of neonatal neutrophils and monocytes. Chemotaxis of neutrophils is normal or only minimally depressed in normal term and preterm infants but may be abnormally low in conditions of serious illness or stress. Migration into skin windows in vivo and formation of acute inflammatory exudates is equivalent to that seen in older children. Chemotaxis by monocytes, however, has been found to be abnormal in several studies, and monocyte migration into skin windows is significantly delayed. The membranes of these cells are less deformable than in older children. The impairment of monocyte migration may be biologically significant and render the infant more susceptible to fungal infections, as well as delaying the clearance of established bacterial infection.

Phagocytosis by neutrophils from full-term and preterm neonates is normal but may be depressed with stress. Monocyte phagocytosis is also normal in most studies, although there is some variability depending on the system used.

Oxidative metabolism, which has major importance in effective killing of many bacteria and fungi, is increased in neonatal neutrophils. Glucose oxidation and hydrogen peroxide production are increased in unstimulated cells compared with those of older individuals. Intracellular bacterial killing is slightly impaired with some test organisms but not with others.

The *spleen* has several roles in host defenses. It is a reservoir for functioning lymphocytes, and it acts as a filter for removal of blood-borne organisms. The phagocytic or filter function can be assessed in several ways.

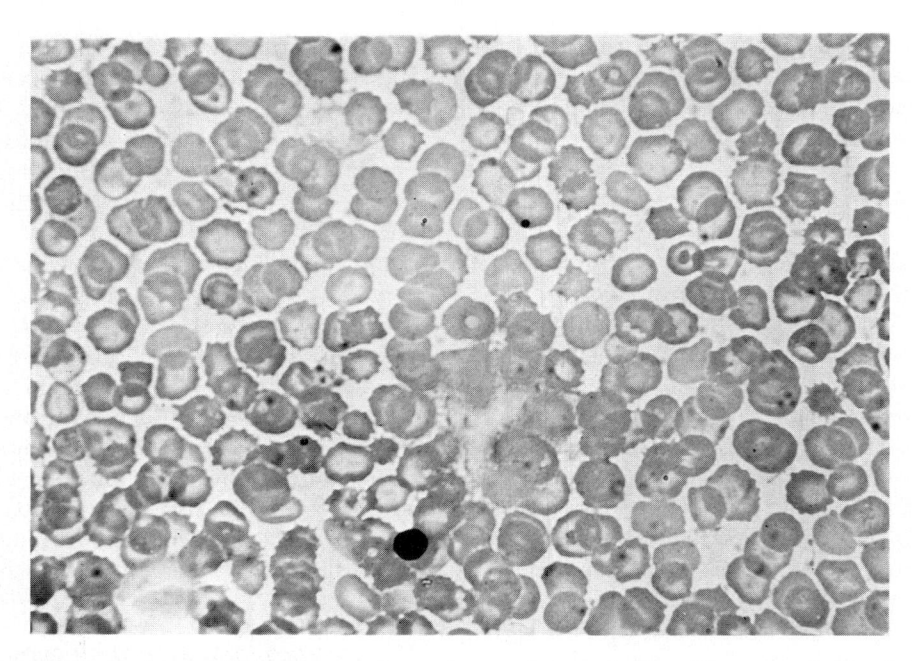

Fig. 29-18. Peripheral blood smear at age 1 week from an infant with congenital asplenia and cyanotic congenital heart disease (Ivemark's syndrome), showing nucleated red cells, acanthocytes, and multiple Howell-Jolly bodies. (Wright's stain; ×800.)

Radionuclide scanning reflects the phagocytic functions but is not a sensitive tool. The spleen normally removes intraerythrocytic particulate matter, such as Heinz bodies and Howell-Jolly bodies, and "polishes" the surface of erythrocytes by removing "pits," which can be seen under phase contrast (Fig. 29-18). Through these techniques, splenic function can be shown to be abnormal in fetal humans and rats and can be shown to mature with advancing gestational and postnatal age. Until the final month of gestation the percentage of red cells having surface pits is three to six times the normal values in children over 1 year of age. It is about twice normal at term birth and reaches normal levels before 1 month of age. The immaturity of splenic macrophages may contribute to the higher incidence of bloodstream infections in neonates and may reflect the defect in monocyte function, since the macrophages ultimately derive from monocytes.

Disorders of phagocyte function

Defects in neutrophil chemotaxis are not common in the newborn period. Several defects have been identified that have been associated with major infectious problems. These include an abnormal neutrophil contractile protein, actin, with both impaired chemotaxis and phagocytosis. A disorder of neutrophil release from the marrow, termed the *lazy leukocyte syndrome*, is characterized by severe neutropenia with bone marrow myeloid hyperplasia. The marrow neutrophils have been found to have markedly impaired motility. Several infants have been described with impaired chemotaxis, recurrent infections, and delayed separation of the umbilical cord. The umbilical cords of these infants did not separate until at least 5 weeks of age, and three of four related children died of infection in infancy. A girl with mental retardation, hypotonia, and defective complement-mediated ingestion and chemotaxis died of septicemia at age 10 after life-long severe infectious problems beginning with omphalitis in the newborn period. There are two major syndromes associated with defective killing of ingested organisms: chronic granulomatous disease and Chediak-Higashi syndrome.

Chronic granulomatous disease

In this condition the phagocytic cells are all unable to use oxygen for intracellular killing. About 86% of patients are male, and X-linked inheritance is the major mode of transmission. There are sporadic cases of autosomal recessive inheritance or spontaneous mutations. Neutrophils and monocytes possess a membrane-bound oxidase that generates a reactive radical (superoxide) from molecular oxygen. This in turn is converted to hydrogen peroxide, which is active in bacterial killing. Patients with chronic granulomatous disease do not produce superoxide or hydrogen peroxide, and their cells are unable to kill organisms that produce catalase. Catalase detoxifies hydrogen peroxide, which is produced by the organisms themselves as a metabolic product. *Staphylococcus aureus, E. coli, Serratia marcescens, Aspergillus, Candida albicans,* and several other organisms are major causes of infections in these patients. Chemotaxis and ingestion are normal, and the organisms survive inside the cells with establishment of granulomata. Skin infections, pneumonia, liver abscesses, fistula formation, and bacteremia are frequent complications. The spectrum of the disease is wide, with some patients dying of infections in the neonatal period and others relatively mildly affected. The molecular basis of the metabolic defects are not yet known.

Chediak-Higashi syndrome

Partial oculocutaneous albinism, massive granules in many cells, and defective bacterial killing due to delayed degranulation of neutrophils and monocytes are the characteristic features of this autosomal recessive disorder. These patients have several associated defects, including a chemotactic defect and increased levels of oxidative metabolism. Microtubule formation is abnormal, and intracellular levels of cyclic guanosine monophosphate (GMP) are low. Pharmacologic measures that elevate cyclic GMP improve microtubule assembly as well as neutrophil migration and bacterial killing. However, most of these patients are relatively well until they develop hepatosplenomegaly, lymphadenopathy, and pancytopenia with high fevers. This accelerated, or lymphoma-like, phase leads to rapid death from bleeding and infection associated with agranulocytosis and thrombocytopenia. Neonatal manifestations of infection are uncommon, but the disorder can be diagnosed from the morphologic appearance of the granules in the peripheral blood smear and the partial albinism.

Congenital asplenia

Congenital asplenia or polysplenia is found as an isolated anomaly or in association with other congenital defects. Asplenia with dextrocardia and cyanotic congenital heart disease is termed *Ivemark's syndrome*. Polysplenia is associated with splenic dysfunction and should be treated as functional asplenia, although it is not as major an immunologic impairment. Diagnosis is suspected in the presence of anomalies known to be associated with asplenia and may be confirmed by splenic scan. Howell-Jolly bodies are not infrequently present in normal newborns but are seen in greater numbers in asplenia. It is important to identify these patients early because they are susceptible to development of overwhelming infection with a variety of organisms, including gram-negative organisms and pneumococcus. Administration of prophylactic antibiotics should be seriously considered, and children should be managed like other young children who are splenectomized early in life.

SOLID TUMORS IN THE NEWBORN

Although infrequent, a number of different solid tumors occur in infancy. Because most arise as abdominal masses, a thorough abdominal examination should be a part of all newborn evaluations. Included among the more common abdominal tumors are neuroblastoma, nephroblastoma (Wilms' tumor), rhabdomyosarcoma, hepatoblastoma, and teratoma. Rarely, cases of transplacental passage of tumor from mother to infant have been reported. Most of these incidents have dealt with malignant melanoma in which the placenta was extensively replaced by tumor. Transplacental passage of Hodgkin's disease, lymphosarcoma, and bronchogenic carcinoma also have been reported. In addition, several cases of choriocarcinoma of the placenta with transfer to the mother of the malignant trophoblast have been identified. Retinoblastoma, another relatively common tumor in the noenate, is covered in the section on ophthalmology.

Congenital mesoblastic nephroma and Wilms' tumor

For many years congenital mesoblastic nephroma was thought to be a variant of Wilms' tumor. In 1967 Bolande emphasized the benign nature of this tumor, which may grow to be very large but will not metastasize. Pathologically the tumor consists of mesenchymal elements without the tubular differentiation commonly seen in Wilms' tumor. Ultrasonography or computed tomography performed at birth or shortly thereafter will reveal a large, hard abdominal mass that is part of the kidney. Excisional surgery is curative, since the tumor is benign, and radiotherapy and/or chemotherapy should not be given, especially since these treatments are relatively toxic in small infants.

Wilms' tumor also occurs in the neonate and should be treated in accordance with the degree of involvement, as outlined in the National Wilms' Tumor Study Programs. Vincristine, actinomycin D, and doxorubicin (Adriamycin) have been used with impressive success in these patients, but the dosage must be modified to account for excessive toxicity in the small neonate. Radiotherapy is also a highly effective modality. The sarcomatous variant of Wilms' tumor, albeit exceedingly rare, is highly resistant to both radiotherapy and chemotherapy.

Neuroblastoma

The incidence of clinical tumor is less than 1 per 10,000 live births. However, autopsy series of newborns dying from a variety of causes have shown that 1 in 40 have neuroblastoma in situ on serial sectioning of adrenal glands. Whether this phenomenon is due to maturation of the tumor or to specific immunologically mediated suppression is a moot point. The tumor arises from neural crest tissue and therefore can occur anywhere along the sympathetic chain. In the neonate the adrenal is a primary site in approximately 70% of the cases, and the tumor is evident as an abdominal mass. Ten percent of the tumors arise from the posterior mediastinum. The liver is the most commonly occurring metastatic site, although virtually any area may be involved. On occasion the liver may be so huge as to mimic hydrops fetalis, an impression further intensified by the occurrence of anemia secondary to marrow replacement. Skin metastases appear as bluish subcutaneous nodules and are frequently referred to as "blueberry muffin spots." Orbital metastases, although rare, may produce a disfiguring proptosis. With progression of the disease severe cachexia is the major sequela.

Once neuroblastoma is suspected, timed urine samples should be obtained for quantitative catecholamine assays. If all metabolites are assayed, the test will confirm the diagnosis in over 95% of patients. Evaluation should also include abdominal films in search of calcific-like densities, intravenous pyelogram, skeletal roentgenograms and bone scans, bone marrow aspiration and biopsy, liver-spleen scan, computerized tomography, and ultrasonography. As a single test, ultrasonography is probably the most reliable imaging procedure.

If the tumor is completely resectable, surgery is the most effective therapeutic endeavor. In stage IVS disease (localized abdominal primary tumor with metastases limited to liver, bone marrow, and/or skin), cure is possible with removal of the primary tumor only. Most centers elect merely to observe young infants with localized disease, since urinary catecholamines offer a reliable way to monitor tumor activity. A short course of radiation therapy (up to 500 rad) or a single dose of cyclophosphamide (up to 300 mg/kg) may be sufficient to diminish massive liver involvement in stage IVS patients. For unresectable tumors, increased urinary catecholamine levels will confirm the diagnosis and eliminate the need to obtain biopsy tissue. Although there has never been conclusive proof that radiotherapy or chemotherapy alone alters survival in neuroblastoma, there is clearly a role for these modalities in infants with disseminated or bulky disease. These tumors are very radiosensitive, and small amounts of radiotherapy (1,000 to 2,500 rad) will usually relieve acute symptoms caused by tumor compression of vital structures. Cyclophosphamide is the most effective single agent and is usually given in combination with vincristine, DTIC (dimethyl-triazeno-imidazole-carboxamide), and doxorubicin. Experimental approaches now under investigation include immunotherapy, whole-body irradiation, and bone marrow allografting. In spite of the poor prognosis for children with disseminated disease, neonates with neuroblastoma have an overall survival of 60% to 70%, and the physician should therefore be vigorous in diagnosing and treating these infants promptly.

Rhabdomyosarcoma

Rhabdomyosarcoma, a tumor of striated muscle cells, has a peak incidence at the toddler and teenage ranges but is also seen in newborns. Although head and neck sites are the most common overall, neonates tend to develop abdominal or pelvic tumors, which are usually evident as a mass in the abdomen or pelvis. Symptoms may develop due to ureteral or urethral compression or bowel obstruction. The botryoid sarcoma variant may cause a large nodular mass to protrude from the bladder or vagina.

There are four pathologic types of rhabdomyosarcoma: embryonal, alveolar, botryoid, and pleomorphic. The prognosis is best for the embryonal and worst for the pleomorphic type. The botryoid type is a variant of the embryonal type in which the tumor grows in cystic formations beneath a mucosal surface such as the bladder lining.

Because this tumor is highly infiltrative, complete excisional surgery is often difficult. It is important to coordinate therapy between surgeons, radiotherapists, and oncologists, since early radiotherapy and chemotherapy may eliminate the need for radical ablative surgery. Results of the first Intergroup Rhabdomyosarcoma Study showed that pelvic and extremity primaries have a high incidence of lymph node spread at diagnosis, but the prognosis is excellent if all gross tumor can be removed at operation.

The most effective drugs for this tumor are vincristine, cyclophosphamide, actinomycin D, and doxorubicin. Most oncologists use intensive chemotherapy with three or more of these drugs given for a period of 15 to 18 months.

Hepatoblastoma

Hepatic tumors are rare in children. When they occur, they are usually seen in small infants. There is a high incidence of associated anomalies, including hemihypertrophy, renal abnormalities, Meckel's diverticulum, and absent adrenal gland. Hemihypertrophy also occurs with increased frequency in patients with Wilms' tumor. Rarely does hepatoblastoma cause jaundice or other abnormalities of liver function. The presenting signs include an enlarging abdominal mass, weight loss, and cachexia. Painful pressure on the celiac nerve axis is frequent. Alpha-fetoprotein levels are usually elevated and serve as a reliable tumor marker if serially obtained. It is important to note, however, that alpha-fetoprotein values tend to be elevated in the normal neonate and thus

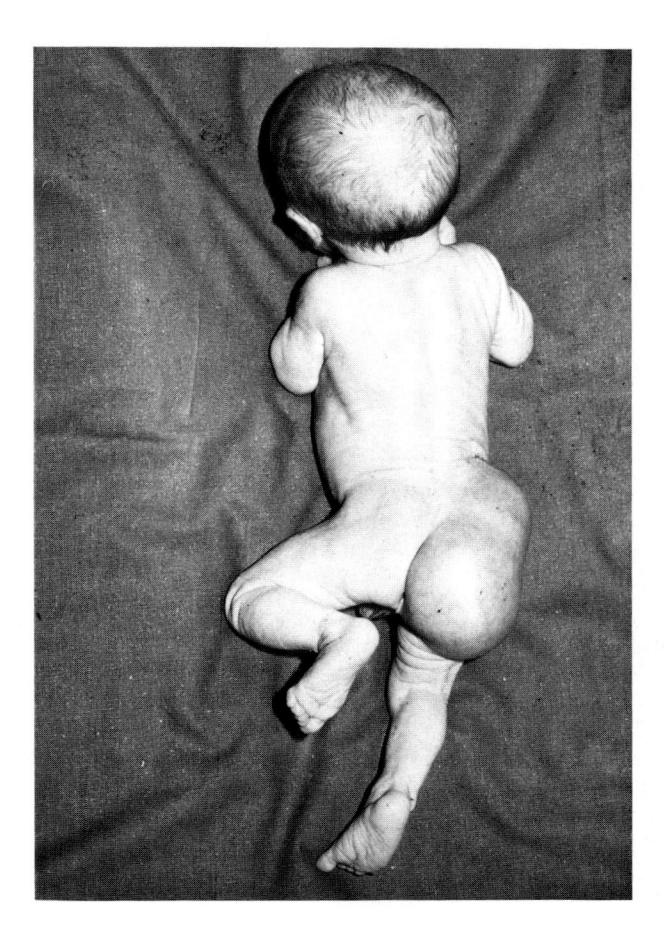

Fig. 29-19. Three-month-old infant with a slowly inlarging right buttock mass. Excision of the tumor showed sacrococcygeal teratoma.

cannot be relied on as a single determination. Complete resection offers the best chance for cure. If the tumor has not metastasized to lungs or bone and is localized to one lobe of the liver, the long-term survival after surgery is about 60%. Combination chemotherapy is an effective adjunct, whereas radiation therapy has essentially no role.

Teratoma

Sacrococcygeal teratomas (Fig. 29-19) are the most common solid tumors of the neonatal period and must be differentiated from myelomeningoceles, pilonidal cysts, hemangiomas, and chordomas. It is important that these tumors be diagnosed early, since they may undergo malignant degeneration rapidly, within a few weeks up to 6 months. Often these seemingly benign tumors have associated areas of malignant change. Accordingly, the pathologist must search carefully during histopathologic processing. In the neonate, 5% to 10% of these tumors have associated malignant areas, and in older infants the incidence increases to 50% to 60%.

There is extraordinary variation in the size of the buttocks or perianal area in such patients. A careful rectal examination, however, invariably reveals a mass because the tumor originates from an area near the anterior surface of the sacrum and within reach of digital examination. On lateral radiographic evaluation the rectum is displaced forward, and calcific-like densities may be visualized occasionally. Complete excision is the major therapeutic modality, since malignant teratomas do not respond well to either radiotherapy or multiagent chemotherapy.

Samuel Gross
Susan B. Shurin
Elizabeth M. Gordon

BIBLIOGRAPHY
Hematopoiesis in the embryo and fetus

Oski, F.A., and Naiman, J.L.: Hematologic problems in the newborn, Philadelphia, 1972, W.B. Saunders Co.

Schulman, I.: Characteristics of the blood in foetal life: oxygen supply to the human foetus, Oxford, 1959, Blackwell Scientific Publications Ltd.

Thomas, D.B., and Yaffey, J.M.: Human foetal haemopoiesis. I. The cellular composition of the foetal blood, Br. J. Haematol. 8:290, 1962.

Walker, J., and Turnbull, E.P.N.: Haemoglobin and red cells in the human foetus and their relation to the oxygen content of the blood in the vessels of the umbilical cord, Lancet 2:312, 1953.

Normal hematologic values in the newborn

Gairdner, D., Marks, J., and Roscoe, J.D.: Blood formation in infancy: normal erythropoiesis, Arch. Dis. Child. **27**:214, 1952.

Humbert, J.R., and others: Polycythemia in small for gestational age infants, J. Pediatr. **75**:812, 1969.

Iron nutrition in infancy, Sixty-second Ross Conference on Pediatric Research, Chicago, 1970, Ross Laboratories.

Linderkamp, O., and others: Capillary-venous hematocrit differences in newborn infants, Eur. J. Pediatr. **127**:9, 1977.

Maurer, H.S., Behrman, R.E., and Honig, G.R.: Dependence of the oxygen affinity of blood on the presence of foetal or adult haemoglobin, Nature **227**:338, 1970.

Monroe, B.L., and others: The neonatal blood count in health and disease. I. Reference values for neutrophilic cells, J. Pediatr. **95**:89, 1979.

O'Brien, R.T., and Pearson, H.A.: Physiologic anemia of the newborn infant, J. Pediatr. **79**:132, 1971.

Oski, F., and Naiman, J.L.: Hematologic problems in the newborn, Philadelphia, 1966, W.B. Saunders Co.

Oski, F.A., and Smith, C.: Red cell metabolism in the premature infant. III. Apparent inappropriate glucose consumption for cell age, Pediatrics **41**:473, 1968.

Schulman, I.: The anemia of prematurity, J. Pediatr. **54**:663, 1959.

Usher, R., Shephard, M., and Lind, J.: The blood volume of the newborn infant and placental transfusion, Acta Paediatr. Scand. **52**:497, 1963.

Van der elst, C.W., Malan, A.F., and Heese, H. de V.: Haematocrit values and blood viscosity in the newborn infant, S. Afr. Med. J. **53**:494, 1978.

Xanthou, M.: Leukocyte blood picture in healthy full term and premature babies during neonatal life, Arch. Dis. Child. **43**:242, 1970.

Yac, A.C., and Lind, J.: Placental transfusion, Am. J. Dis. Child. **127**:128, 1974.

Anemia due to hemorrhagic disorders

Aballi, A.J., Puapondh, Y., and Desposito, F.: Platelet counts in thriving premature infants, Pediatrics **42**:685, 1968.

Anthony, B., and Krivit, W.: Neonatal thrombocytopenic purpura, Pediatrics **30**:766, 1962.

Barnard, D.R., and Hathaway, W.E.: Neonatal thrombosis, Am. J. Pediatr. Hem./Onc. **1**:235, 1979.

Bleyer, W.A., Hakami, N., and Shepard, T.H.: The development of hemostasis in the human fetus and newborn infant, J. Pediatr. **79**:838, 1971.

Corrigan, J.J.: Heparin therapy in bacterial septicemia, J. Pediatr. **91**:695, 1977.

Corrigan, J.J.: Activation of coagulation and disseminated intravascular coagulation in the newborn, Am. J. Pediatr. Hem./Onc. **1**:245, 1979.

Corrigan, J.J., Sell, E.J., and Page, C.: Hageman factor and disseminated intravascular coagulation (DIC) in newborns and rabbits, Pediatr. Res. **11**:916, 1977.

Glader, B.E., and Buchanan, G.R.: The bleeding neonate, Pediatrics **58**:548, 1976.

Hall, J.G., and others: Thrombocytopenia with absent radius, Medicine **48**:411, 1969.

Hathaway, W.E.: The bleeding newborn, Semin. Hematol. **12**:175, 1975.

Maak, B., Scheidt, B., and Frenzel, J.: Factor VIII activity and factor VIII related antigen in newborns, Eur. J. Pediatr. **128**:283, 1978.

McIntosh, S., and others: Neonatal isoimmune purpura: response to platelet infusions, J. Pediatr. **82**:1020, 1973.

Merskey, C.: Defibrination syndrome or . . . ? Blood **41**:599, 1973.

Perlman, M., and Divilansky, A.: Blood coagulation status of small-for-dates and postmature infants, Arch Dis. Child. **50**:424, 1975.

Sell, E.J., and Corrigan, J.J.: Platelet counts, fibrinogen concentrations, and factor V and factor VIII levels in healthy infants according to gestational age, J. Pediatr. **82**:1028, 1973.

Stuart, M.J.: Platelet function in the neonate, Am. J. Pediatr. Hem./Onc. **1**:227, 1979.

Zipursky, A., and others: Clinical and laboratory diagnosis of hemostatic disorders in newborn infants, Am. J. Pediatr. Hem./Onc. **1**:217, 1979.

Anemias due to erythrocyte underproduction—congenital and acquired

Adamson, J.W., and others: Erythrocytosis associated with hemoglobin Rainier: oxygen equilibria and marrow regulation, Clin. Invest. **48**:1376, 1969.

Altman, K.I., and Miller, G.: A disturbance of tryptophan metabolites in congenital hypoplastic anemia, Nature **172**:868, 1953.

Bergstedt, J.: Monozygotic twins, one with high erythrocyte values and jaundice, the other with anemia neonatorum and no jaundice, Acta Pediatr. **46**:201, 1957.

Coccia, P.F., and others: Successful bone-marrow transplantation for infantile malignant osteopetrosis, N. Engl. J. Med. **302**:701, 1980.

Cohen, F., Zeulzer, W.W., and Evans, M.M.: Identification of blood group antigens and minor cell populations by the fluorescent antibody method, Blood **15**:884, 1960.

Dent, C.E., and others: Studies in osteopetrosis, Arch. Dis. Child. **40**:7, 1965.

Diamond, L.K., and Blackfan, K.D.: Hypoplastic anemia, Am. J. Dis. Child. **54**:464, 1938.

Diamond, L.K., and others: Congenital (erythroid) hypoplastic anemia, Am. J. Dis. Child. **102**:403, 1961.

Diamond, L.K., and others: Congenital hypoplastic anemia, Adv. Pediatr. **22**:349, 1976.

Fanconi, G.: Familaire infantile perniziosaartige Anamie (pernizioses Blutbild und Konstitution), Jb. Kinderheilk. **117**:257, 1927.

Fanconi, G.: Familial constitutional panmyelocytopathy, Fanconi's anemia. I. Clinical aspects, Semin. Hematol. **4**:233, 1967.

Garriga, S., and Crosby, W.H.: The incidence of leukemia in families of patients with hypoplasia of the marrow, Blood **14**:1008, 1959.

Grieg, H.B., and others: The familial crisis in hereditary spherocytosis: report of five cases, S. Afr. J. Med. Sci. **23**:17, 1958.

Gross, S., and Guilford, M.V.: Vitamin E and lipid relationships in premature infants, J. Nutr. **100**:1099, 1970.

Gross, S., and Melhorn, D.K.: Vitamin E, red cell lipids and red cell stability in prematurity, Ann. N.Y. Acad. Sci. **203**:141, 1972.

Gross, S., and Newman, A.J.: Turner's syndrome with congenital erythroid hypoplasia, Lancet **1**:449, 1967.

Gross, S., and others: Hematological studies of erythropoietic porphyria: a new case with severe hemolysis, chronic thrombocytopenia and folic acid deficiency, Blood **23**:762, 1964.

Gtaeber, J.E., Williams, M.L., and Oski, F.A.: The use of intramuscular vitamin E in the premature infant, J. Pediatr. **90**:282, 1977.

Hadjimarkos, D.M.: Selenium content of human milk: possible effect on dental caries, J. Pediatr. **63**:273, 1963.

Hakami, N., and others: Neonatal megaloblastic anemia due to inherited transcobalamin. II. Deficiency in two siblings, N. Engl. J. Med. **285**:1163, 1971.

Hammond, D., and others: Production, utilization and excretion of erythropoietin. I, Chronic anemias; II, Aplastic crisis; III, Erythropoietic effect of normal plasma, Ann. N.Y. Acad. Sci. **149**:516, 1968.

Hassan, H., and others: Syndrome in premature infants associated with low plasma vitamin E levels and high polyunsaturated fatty acid diet, Am. J. Clin. Nutr. **19**:147, 1966.

Hirst, E., and Robertson, T.I.: The syndrome of thymoma and erythroblastopenic anemia, Medicine (Baltimore) **46**:225, 1967.

Humbert, J.R., and others: Polycythemia in small for gestational age infants, J. Pediatr. **75**:812, 1969.

Jones, R.A., and Silver, S.: The detection of minor erythrocyte population by mixed agglutinates, Blood **13**:763, 1958.

Kleihauer, E., Braun, H., and Betke, K.: Demonstration von fetalem Hamoglobin in den Erythrocyten eines Blutauusstrichs, Klin. Wochenschr. **35**:637, 1957.

Lampkin, B., and others: Megaloblastic anemia of infancy secondary to maternal pernicious anemia, N. Engl. J. Med. **274**:1168, 1966.

Lowe, C.F., and others: Iron balance and requirements in infancy. Committee on Nutrition, American Academy of Pediatrics, Pediatrics **43**:134, 1969.

Melhorn, D.K., and Gross, S.: Vitamin E dependent anemia in the premature infant. I. Relationships between gestational age and absorption of vitamin E. J. Pediatr. **79**:569, 1971.

Melhorn, D.K., and Gross, S.: Vitamin E dependent anemia in the premature infant. II. Effects of large doses of medicinal iron, J. Pediatr. **79**:581, 1971.

Michael, A.F., Jr., and Mauer, A.M.: Maternal-fetal transfusion as a cause of plethora in the neonatal period, Pediatrics **28**:458, 1961.

Mott, M.G., and others: Congenital (erythroid) hypoplastic anemia: modified expression in males, Arch. Dis. Child. **44**:757, 1969.

Muth, O.H., and others: Effect of selenium on white muscle disease, Science **128**:1090, 1958.

Naiman, J.L., and Schlackman, N.: Transient thrombocytopenia in the neonatal polycythemia syndrome, Proc. Soc. Pediatr. Res. **5**:241, 1971.

Naveh, D., and others: Neonatal polycythemia and elevated plasma erythropoietin (ESF) in Down's syndrome, Proc. Am. Soc. Hematol. **38**:142, 1971.

Newman, A.J., and Gross, S.: Capillary and venous hematocrit in the newborn, Clin. Pediatr. (Phila) **6**:8, 1967.

Nixon, A.D., and Buchanan, J.G.: Haemolytic anemia due to pyruvate kinase deficiency, N.Z. Med. J. **66**:859, 1967.

Oski, F.A., and Naiman, J.L.: Hematological problems in the newborn, ed. 2, Philadelphia, 1972, W.B. Saunders Co.

Oski, F.A., and Barness, L.A.: Vitamin E deficiency. Cause of anemia in infants? J.A.M.A. **193**:47, 1965.

Price, J.M., and others: Excretion of urinary tryptophan metabolites by patients with congenital hypoplastic anemia (Diamond-Blackfan syndrome), J. Lab. Clin. Med. **75**:316, 1970.

Rotruck, J.A., and others: Selenium: biochemical role as a component of glutathione peroxidase, Science **179**:588, 1973.

Sacks, M.O.: Occurrence of anemia and polycythemia in phenotypically dissimilar single ovum human twins, Pediatrics **24**:604, 1959.

Schmid, W.: Familial constitutional panmyelocytopathy, Fanconi's anemia. II. Discussion of the cytogenetic findings in Fanconi's anemia, Semin. Hematol. **4**:241, 1967.

Shojania, A.M., and Gross, S.: Folic acid deficiency and prematurity, J. Pediatr. **64**:323, 1964.

Shahidi, N.T., and Diamond, L.K.: Testosterone-induced remission in aplastic anemia, A.M.A. J. Dis. Child. **98**:293, 1959.

Shearer, T.R., and Hadjimarkos, D.M.: Geographic distribution of selenium in human milk, Arch. Environ. Health **30**:230, 1975.

Singer, K., and others: Aplastic crisis in sickle cell anemia: a study of its mechanism and its relationship to other types of hemolytic crisis, J. Lab. Clin. Med. **35**:721, 1950.

Sisson, T.R.C., and others: The blood volume of infants, J. Pediatr. **55**:163, 1959.

Sjolin, S., and Wranne, L.: Treatment of congenital hypoplastic anaemia with prednisone, Scand. J. Haematol. **7**:63, 1970.

Tartaglia, A.P., and others: Chromosome abnormality and hypocalcemia in congenital erythroid hypoplasia, Am. J. Med. **41**:990, 1966.

Thomes, E.D., and others: Aplastic anemia treated by marrow transplantation, Lancet **1**:284, 1972.

Tillman, W., Prindull, G., and Schroter, W.: Severe anemia due to transient pure red cell aplasia in early childhood, Eur. J. Pediatr. **123**:51, 1976.

Usher, R., and others: The blood volume of the newborn infant and placental transfusion, Acta Pediatr. **52**:497, 1963.

Wang, W.C., and others: Differentiation of transient erythroblastopenia of childhood from congenital hypoplastic anemia, J. Pediatr. **88**:784, 1976.

Zaizov, R., and others: Familial aplastic anaemia without congenital

Hemolytic anemias caused by intrinsic abnormalities of the erythrocyte membrane

Cutting, H.O., and others: Autosomal dominant hemolytic anemia characterized by ovalocytosis: a family study of seven involved members, Am. J. Med. **39**:21, 1965.

Jacob, H.S.: Hereditary spherocytosis: a disease of the red cell membrane, Semin. Hematol. **2**:139, 1965.

Mentzer, W.C., Lubin, B.H., and Emmons, S.: Correction of the permeability defect in hereditary stomatocytosis by dimethyl adipimidate, N. Engl. J. Med. **294**:1200, 1976.

Truccoo, J.I., and Brown, A.K.: Neonatal manifestations of hereditary spherocytosis, Am. J. Dis. Child. **113**:263, 1967.

Valentine, W.N.: The molecular lesion of hereditary spherocytosis (HS): a continuing enigma, Blood **49**:241, 1977.

Isoimmune hemolytic disease

Bowman, J.M.: Rh erythroblastosis fetalis 1975, Semin. Hematol. **12**:189, 1975.

Bowman, J.M.: Suppression of Rh isoimmunization, Obstet. Gynecol. **52**:385, 1978.

Broderson, R.: Bilirubin transport in the newborn infant, reviewed with relation to kernicterus, J. Pediatr. **96**:349, 1980.

Cockington, R.A.: A guide to the use of phototherapy in the management of neonatal hyperbilirubinemia, J. Pediatr. **95**:281, 1979.

Cohen, F., and others: Mechanisms of isoimmunization. I. The transplacental passage of fetal erythrocytes in hemospecific pregnancies, Blood **23**:621, 1964.

Desjardins, L., and others: The spectrum of ABO hemolytic disease of the newborn infant, J. Pediatr. **95**:447, 1979.

Dunn, P.M.: Obstructive jaundice and haemolytic disease of the newborn, Arch. Dis. Child. **38**:54, 1963.

Etches, P.C., and others: Nonimmune hydrops fetalis: report of 22 cases including three siblings, Pediatrics **64**:326, 1979.

Gromisch, D.S., and others: Light (phototherapy) induced riboflavin deficiency in the neonate, J. Pediatr. **90**:118, 1977.

Grundbacher, F.J.: ABO hemolytic disease of the newborn: a family study with emphasis on the strength of the A antigen, Pediatrics **35**:916, 1965.

Hardyment, A.F., and others: Follow up of intrauterine transfused surviving children, Am. J. Obstet. Gynecol. **133**:235, 1979.

Hutchinson, A.A., and others: Nonimmunologic hydrops fetalis: a review of 61 cases, Obstet. Gynecol. **59**:347, 1982.

Komazawa, M., and Oski, F.A.: Biochemical characteristics of "young" and "old" erythrocytes of the newborn infant, J. Pediatr. **87**:102, 1975.

Miyazaki, S., and others: Coombs positive hemolytic anemia in congenital rubella, J. Pediatr. **94**:759, 1979.

Pearson, H.W.: Life-span of the fetal red blood cell, J. Pediatr. **70**:166, 1967.

Peevy, K.J., and Wiseman, H.J.: ABO hemolytic disease of the newborn: evaluation of management and identification of racial and antigenic factors, Pediatrics **61**:574, 1978.

Pochedly, C.: Etiology of late anemia of hemolytic disease of the newborn, Clin. Med. **78**:30, 1971.

Scanlon, J.W., and Muirhead, D.M.: Hydrops fetalis due to anti-Kell isoimmune disease: survival with optimal long-term outcome, J. Pediatr. **88:**484, 1976.

Sisson, T.R.C., and others: Phototherapy of jaundice in newborn infants. I. ABO blood group incompatibility, J. Pediatr. **79:**904, 1971.

Valaes, T., and Hyte, M.: Effect of exchange transfusion on bilirubin binding, Pediatrics **59:**881, 1977.

Van Praagh, R.: Diagnosis of kernicterus in the neonatal period, Pediatrics **28:**870, 1961.

Whang-Peng, J., and others: The transplacental passage of fetal leukocytes into the maternal blood, Proc. Soc. Exp. Biol. Med. **142:**50, 1973.

Quantitative disorders of globin chain synthesis

Alter, B.P.: Prenatal diagnosis of hemoglobinopathies and other hematologic diseases, J. Pediatr. **95:**501, 1979.

Asakura, T., and others: A rapid test for sickle hemoglobin, J.A.M.A. **233:**156, 1975.

Fisch, R.O., and others: Methemoglobinemia in a hospital nursery, a search for causative factors, J.A.M.A. **185:**760, 1963.

Forget, B.G.: Molecular genetics of humen hemoglobin synthesis, Ann. Int. Med. **91:**605, 1979.

Hegyi, T., and others: Sickle cell anemia in the newborn, Pediatrics **60:**213, 1977.

Huntsman, R.G., Metters, J.S., and Yawson, G.I.: The diagnosis of sickle cell disease in the newborn infant, J. Pediatr. **80:**279, 1972.

Kan, Y.W., Allen, A., and Lowenstein, L.: Hydrops fetalis with alpha thalassemia, N. Engl. J. Med. **276:**18, 1967.

Minnich, V., and others: Alpha, beta, and gamma polypeptide chains during the neonatal period with description of a fetal form of hemoglobin Da-St. Louis, Blood **19:**137, 1962.

Necheles, T.F., and Allen, D.M.: Heinz-body anemias, N. Engl. J. Med. **280:**203, 1969.

Powars, D., Schroeder, W.A., and White, L.: Rapid diagnosis of sickle cell disease at birth by microcolumn chromatography, Pediatrics **55:**630, 1975.

Weatherall, D.J.: The thalassemia syndromes, Oxford, 1965, Blackwell Scientific Publications, Ltd.

White, J.M., and Dacie, J.V.: The unstable hemoglobin: molecular and clinical features, Prog. Hematol. **7:**69, 1971.

Congenital deficiencies of red cell enzymes

Beutler, E.: Glucose-6-phosphate dehydrogenase and nonspherocytic congenital hemolytic anemia, Semin. Hematol. **2:**91, 1965.

Beutler, E.: Abnormalities of the hexose monophosphate shunt, Semin. Hematol. **8:**311, 1971.

Jaffe, E.R.: Hereditary hemolytic disorders and enzymatic deficiencies of human erythrocytes, Blood **35:**116, 1970.

Hibbard, B.Z., and others: Severe methemoglobinemia in an infant **93:**816, 1978.

Lopez, R., and Cooperman, J.M.: Glucose-6-phosphate dehydrogenase deficiency and hyperbilirubinemia in the newborn, Am. J. Dis. Child. **122:**66, 1971.

Mentzer, W.C., and Collier, E.: Hydrops fetalis associated with erythrocyte G-6-PD deficiency and maternal ingestion of fava beans and ascorbic acid, J. Pediatr. **86:**565, 1975.

Necheles, T.F., Boles, T.A., and Allen, D.M.: Erythrocyte glutathione-peroxidase deficiency and hemolytic disease of the newborn infant, J. Pediatr. **72:**319, 1968.

Valentine, W.N.: Deficiencies associated with Embden-Meyerhof pathway and other metabolic pathways, Semin. Hematol. **8:**348, 1971.

Disorders of phagocytic cells

Hutter, J.J., Hathaway, W.E., and Wayne, E.R.: Hematologic abnormalities in severe neonatal necrotizing enterocolitis, J. Pediatr. **88:**1026, 1976.

Lalezari, P., and others: Chronic autoimmune neutropenia due to anti-NA2 antibody, N. Engl. J. Med. **293:**744, 1975.

Weetman, R.M., and Boxer, L.A.: Childhood neutropenia, Pediatr. Clin. North Am. **27:**361, 1980.

Zipursky, A., and others: The hematology of bacterial infections in premature infants, Pediatrics **57:**839, 1976.

Neutrophil function disorders

Blume, R.S., and Wolff, S.M.: The Chédiak-Higashi syndrome: studies in four patients and a review of the literature, Medicine **51:**247, 1972.

Gotoff, S.P.: Neonatal immunity, J. Pediatr. **85:**149, 1974.

Hayward, A.R., and others: Delayed separation of the umbilical cord, widespread infections, and defective neutrophil mobility, Lancet **1:**1099, 1976.

Stoerner, J.W., and others: Polymorphonuclear leukocyte function in newborn infants, J. Pediatr. **93:**862, 1978.

Weston, W.L., and others: Monocyte-macrophage function in the newborn, Am. J. Dis. Child. **131:**1241, 1977.

Splenic function

Freedman, R.M., and others: Development of splenic reticuloendothelial function in neonates, J. Pediatr. **96:**466, 1980.

Majeski, J.A., and Upshur, J.K.: Asplenia syndrome: a study of congenital anomalies in 16 cases, J.A.M.A. **240:**1508, 1978.

Ozsoylu, S., Hosain, F., and McIntyre, P.A.: Functional development of phagocytic activity of the spleen, J. Pediatr. **90:**560, 1977.

Waldman, J., and others: Sepsis and congenital asplenia, J. Pediatr. **90:**555, 1977.

Nonhematologic malignant neoplasms in the newborn

Bolande, R.P., Brough, A.J., and Izant, R.J.: Congenital mesoblastic nephroma of infancy: a report of eight cases and the relationship to Wilms' tumor, Pediatrics **40:**272, 1967.

Evans, A.E.: Treatment of neuroblastoma, Cancer **30:**1595, 1972.

Kinnear, E., Wilson, L., and Draper, G.: Neuroblastoma: its history and prognosis: a study of 487 cases, Br. Med. J. **3:**301, 1976.

Lemire, R.J., Graham, C.S., and Beckwith, J.B.: Skin-covered sacrococcygeal masses in infants and children, J. Pediatr. **79:**948, 1971.

Maurer, M.: Solid tumors in children, N. Engl. J. Med. **299:**1345, 1978.

Pochedly, C.: Neuroblastoma, Acton, Mass., 1976, Publishing Sciences Group, Inc.

Schwartz, A.D.: Congenital malignant disorders. In Schaffer, A.J., and Avery, M.E., editors: Diseases of the newborn, Philadelphia, 1977, W.B. Saunders Co.

Sutow, W.W., Vietti, T.J., And Fernbach, D.J.: Clinical pediatric oncology, ed. 2, St. Louis, 1977, The C.V. Mosby Co.

CHAPTER 30 Jaundice and liver disease

The yellow discoloration of the skin and other organs caused by accumulation of bilirubin and designated as *jaundice*, or *icterus*, is generally considered a sign of a serious clinical pathologic condition in the older child and adult. The challenge of neonatal jaundice is to distinguish normal physiology from pathosis and the benign situation from the threatening one.

CLASSIFICATION OF NEONATAL JAUNDICE

Two types of bilirubin must be recognized for clinical purposes: unconjugated (indirect reacting) and conjugated (direct reacting). Hyperbilirubinemia, characterized by the retention of unconjugated bilirubin, is by far the most common type of hyperbilirubinemia in the neonate; unconjugated bilirubin is the type of pigment found in "physiologic jaundice" and in pathologic states in which there is increased production, decreased hepatic conjugation, or decreased hepatic uptake of bilirubin. Conjugated hyperbilirubinemia is far less common in the neonate and most often denotes a serious derangement of hepatic function, particularly interference with excretion of bilirubin from the liver into bile or obstruction of the flow of bile in the biliary tree. Jaundice and hepatic disease in the newborn period, as in the older child and adult, can best be classified according to the type of bilirubin retained (conjugated or unconjugated).

Unconjugated hyperbilirubinemia in the human, regardless of age, is defined as an elevation of the indirect-reacting serum bilirubin concentration to greater than 1.0 or 1.5 mg/dl, depending on the standard used in calibration of the van den Bergh reaction. Nearly all adults and older children will have indirect-reacting bilirubin concentrations in serum of less than 0.8 mg/dl. *Conjugated hyperbilirubinemia* is defined as an elevation of the direct-reacting fraction in the van den Bergh reaction to greater than 1.5 or 2 mg/dl, or when this fraction accounts for more than 10% of the total serum bilirubin concentration. The latter portion of the definition is added to guard against overinterpretation of direct reactions in newborns with markedly elevated indirect-reacting bilirubin concentrations, because up to 10% of the *unconjugated* pigment will behave as *direct-reacting* pigment in the van den Bergh reaction. Clinical situations in which the direct-reacting serum bilirubin concentration is equal or close to the total bilirubin concentration are extremely rare, especially in the newborn period. In the usual clinical situation the elevated direct-reacting fraction accounts for 20% to 70% of the total pigment. This "mixed" hyperbilirubinemia should be considered primarily in the classification of conjugated hyperbilirubinemia, since the significant pathosis will usually relate to interference with hepatic cell excretion and bile transport rather than to abnormalities of increased bilirubin production or deficient hepatic bilirubin uptake or conjugation.

Classification of hyperbilirubinemia as conjugated or unconjugated requires performance of a determination of serum bilirubin concentration that distinguishes between direct- and indirect-reacting pigments. The prototype of all such methods is the van den Bergh test, a modification of the Ehrlich diazo reaction. More recent modifications permit determinations using as little as 50 µL of serum from a jaundiced neonate. The technique currently recommended because of its precision and sensitivity is that of Jendrassik and Grof, which is used in the automated techniques available in most hospital laboratories. Direct spectrophotometric techniques that fail to distinguish direct- from indirect-reacting pigment are not recommended but may serve as backup in emergency situations.

PART ONE
Unconjugated hyperbilirubinemia
PHYSIOLOGY
Bilirubin synthesis

The pathways of bilirubin synthesis, transport, and metabolism are summarized in Fig. 30-1. In the normal adult bilirubin is derived primarily from the degradation of heme contained in the circulating erythrocyte when senescence of the red cell results in its lysis in the reticuloendothelial cells of the body. Erythrocyte precursors and nonhemoglobin heme proteins (mainly cytochromes) normally contribute about 15% of the bilirubin excreted into bile. In the newborn total bilirubin production probably is increased severalfold as a result of a shortened circulating erythrocyte life span (reduced to 70 to 90 days as compared with 120 days in the adult), increased heme degradation from the very large pool of hematopoietic tissue that ceases to function shortly after birth, and possibly increased turnover of cytochromes. In addition to increased synthesis of bilirubin, the load of bilirubin presented to the liver is increased as a result of enhanced absorption of unconjugated bilirubin by the intestinal mucosa with return of bilirubin to the liver by way of the enterohepatic circulation. In the newborn enhanced intestinal reabsorption may result from starvation, from the absence of intestinal bacteria necessary for the conversion of bilirubin to colorless urobilinogens and pigmented stercobilins, from the large bilirubin pool that exists in meconium, and from slow intestinal motility.

The pathway by which hemoglobin, an iron-porphyrin complex bound to a globin, is converted to bilirubin in the reticuloendothelial cell is not fully known. Reticuloendothelial cells contain a microsomal enzyme, heme oxygenase, that is capable of oxidizing the alpha-methene bridge carbon of the heme molecule after loss of iron and globin to form the green pigment, biliverdin. The single carbon atom lost from the heme molecule is converted quantitatively to carbon monoxide. The carbon monoxide thus formed is excreted by the lung unchanged. Although there are other potential endogenous and exogenous sources of carbon monoxide, quantitative estimation of its excretion or synthesis offers a reasonably accurate assessment of the rate of heme degradation from all sources and of bilirubin synthesis. It is believed that nonhemoglobin heme undergoes the same degradative process. Biliverdin, a water-soluble pigment, is rapidly reduced by the enzyme biliverdin reductase and by nonenzymatic reducing agents in the reticuloendothelial cell to form bilirubin. The degradation of 1 gm of hemoglobin forms 34 mg of bilirubin.

Bilirubin transport in plasma

The unconjugated bilirubin released into the circulation by the reticuloendothelial cell is rapidly bound to albumin, since this nonpolar pigment is almost totally insoluble in water at pH 7.4. Recent studies indicate that the solubility of bilirubin is less than 0.01 mg/dl. Each molecule of adult human albumin is capable of binding at least two molecules of bilirubin; the first molecule is more tightly bound than the second. Additional binding sites with weaker affinities also may exist but are probably of little clinical importance. Newborns have been found to have a lower plasma-binding capacity for bilirubin because of reduced albumin concentrations and reduced molar binding capacities as compared with the adult or older child. This may be of importance in determining and evaluating the risk of the newborn for bilirubin encephalopathy (kernicterus).

Hepatic uptake of bilirubin

The hepatocyte is the only cell in the body capable of removing significant quantities of unconjugated bilirubin from the circulation and converting it by conjugation with other substances into a form from which either the liver cell or the kidney can excrete the pigment into bile or urine. Bilirubin enters the liver cell by a process of carrier-mediated diffusion, with ligandin (Y protein) of the liver cell cytoplasm as the major intracellular bilirubin-binding protein. Another intracellular protein, Z, also binds bilirubin but with a lower affinity. Bilirubin dissociates from circulating albumin before its entry into the liver cell. Ligandin also binds corticosteroids and exogenous substances, including sulfobromophthalein (BSP). The balance between hepatic cell uptake and excretion of bilirubin and the rate of bilirubin production determines the serum unconjugated bilirubin concentration under normal circumstances.

Conjugation of bilirubin

Bilirubin excretion into bile requires conversion of the nonpolar unconjugated bilirubin into a more polar, more water-soluble substance. In the human this is accomplished almost entirely by conjugation of each molecule of bilirubin with two molecules of glucuronic acid by a two-step conjugation process. (Phototherapy achieves the same result, i.e., conversion of bilirubin to a more polar water-soluble substance.) In the normal adult this process accounts for the disposal of approximately 95% of all bilirubin. The remaining portion is converted to water-soluble substances by conjugation with substances other than glucuronic acid or by oxidation, hydroxylation, or reduction.

Bilirubin is presumed to be transported by ligandin to the endoplasmic reticulum, the site of the first of the two

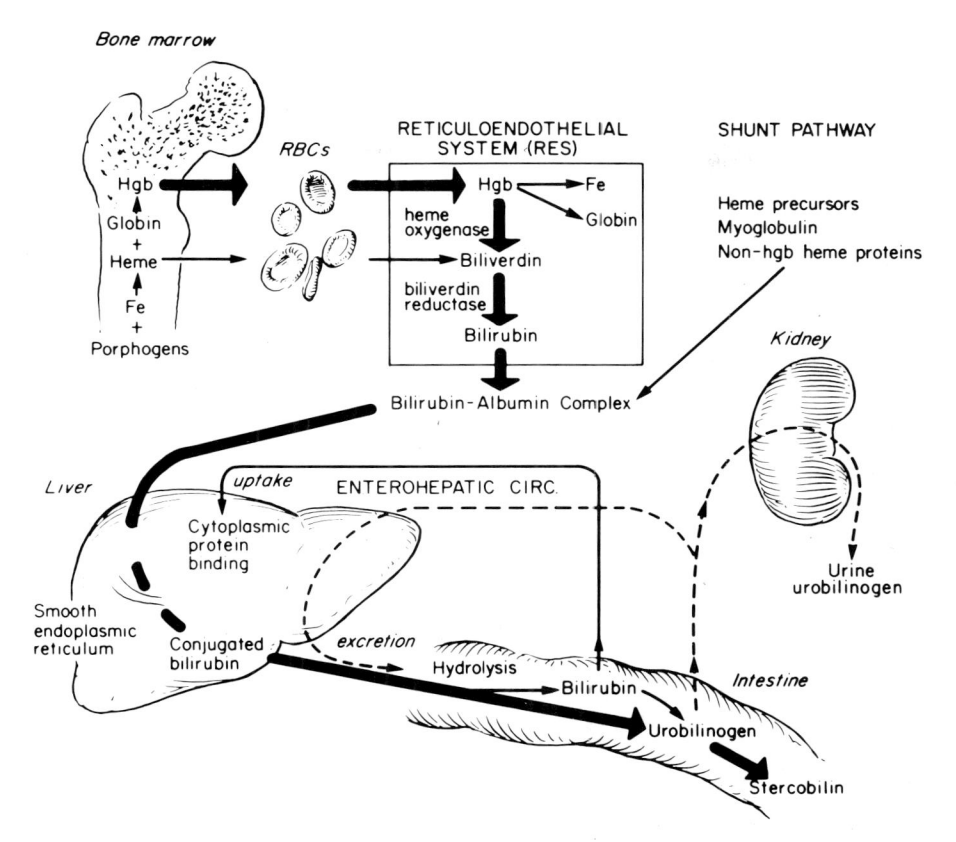

Fig. 30-1. The pathways of bilirubin synthesis, transport, and metabolism. (From Assali, N.S.: Pathophysiology of gestation, New York, 1972, Academic Press, Inc.)

conjugating enzymes, UDP glucuronyl transferase. This enzyme catalyzes the transfer of one glucuronic acid molecule from the activated UDP glucuronic acid to one of the two propionic side groups on one of the central pyrrole rings of bilirubin to form bilirubin monoglucuronide. UDP glucuronic acid is synthesized by the soluble cytoplasmic enzyme uridine diphosphoglucose dehydrogenase from uridine diphosphoglucose, which in turn had been synthesized from free glucose. The total capacity of UDP glucuronyl transferase to form the monoglucuronide of bilirubin has been estimated to be a hundredfold greater than the normal load of bilirubin presented to the liver for disposal. Thus only with reduction in enzyme activity to less than 1% of normal would unconjugated bilirubin retention result.

Although bilirubin monoglucuronide is water soluble and capable of being excreted into bile without further alteration, approximately two thirds of the total bilirubin excreted into bile in adult human is found to be in the form of a diglucuronide. The enzyme responsible for this second step of conjugation reaction is UDP-glucuronate glucuronyl transferase (transglucuronidase) and is located in the canalicular portion of the hepatocyte plasma cell membrane. The substrate for this transglucuronidation is bilirubin monoglucuronide itself. The enzyme transfers one molecule of glucuronic acid from one molecule of bilirubin monoglucuronide to another, resulting in formation of one molecule of bilirubin diglucuronide, which is then excreted from the cell, and one molecule of unconjugated bilirubin, which is then returned to the endoplasmic reticulum for subsequent reconjugation.

Both bilirubin monoglucuronide and bilirubin diglucuronide will be measured in the van den Bergh reaction as direct-reacting pigment, since both are relatively water soluble. In circumstances in which increased loads of bilirubin are delivered to the liver, resulting in retention of conjugated bilirubin, as in severe chronic hemolysis, the pigment retained is bilirubin monoglucuronide.

At least two additional carbohydrate conjugates of bilirubin also can be formed: conjugates with glucose and xylose and possibly other carbohydrates, sulfates, and taurine. These nonglucuronide conjugates account for no more than 10% of the total bilirubin conjugates excreted in bile in humans.

Bilirubin excretion

The transfer of bilirubin from hepatocyte into bile can occur after nonpolar bilirubin IX$_\alpha$ has been converted to a more polar, water-soluble compound, usually by the process of two-step conjugation in the liver just described. The excretory process itself appears to be an energy-dependent concentrative process in which bile bilirubin concentrations are approximately a hundredfold greater than hepatocyte cytoplasmic bilirubin concentrations. The physiology of hepatic bilirubin excretion is discussed further in the section on conjugated hyperbilirubinemia of the newborn.

Enteric bilirubin absorption

Bilirubin monoglucuronides and diglucuronides are relatively unstable conjugates and readily hydrolyzed to unconjugated bilirubin both nonenzymatically under the influence of mild alkaline conditions, as noted in the duodenum and jejunum, and enzymatically by the enteric mucosal enzyme, β-glucuronidase. Unconjugated bilirubin then may be reabsorbed across the intestinal mucosa to return to the liver via the portal circulation. Although quantitative estimates of the disposal of bilirubin have been performed only for adult humans, these data indicate that approximately 25% of the total bilirubin excreted into the intestine is reabsorbed as unconjugated bilirubin. Approximately 10% of the total is excreted in stool as unaltered bilirubin, whereas the remaining pigment is converted to urobilinoids, the majority of which is excreted in stool, and a small portion of which is reabsorbed in the colon and subsequently excreted by both the liver and the kidney.

PHYSIOLOGIC JAUNDICE OF THE NEWBORN

Unconjugated hyperbilirubinemia of the newborn regardless of cause can be understood only in the context of physiologic jaundice of the newborn, since this is the visible demonstration of developmental limitations of bilirubin metabolism and transport in the newborn period. All other abnormal situations are superimposed on these developmental processes.

In the full-term human neonate physiologic jaundice is characterized by a progressive rise in serum unconjugated bilirubin concentrations from approximately 2 mg/dl in cord blood to a mean peak of 6 mg/dl between 60 and 72 hours of age, followed by a rapid decline to approximately 2 mg/dl by the fifth day of life (Fig. 30-2). This early period of physiologic jaundice has been designated *phase I physiologic jaundice*. During the period from the fifth to tenth day of life serum bilirubin concentrations decline very slowly, reaching the normal adult value of 1 mg/dl or less by the end of that period. This later period of minimal, slowly declining hyperbilirubinemia has been designated *phase II physiologic jaundice*. Based on studies in the newborn rhesus monkey, an animal with a similar pattern of neonatal physiologic jaundice, phase I results from the combination of a sixfold increase in the load of bilirubin presented to the

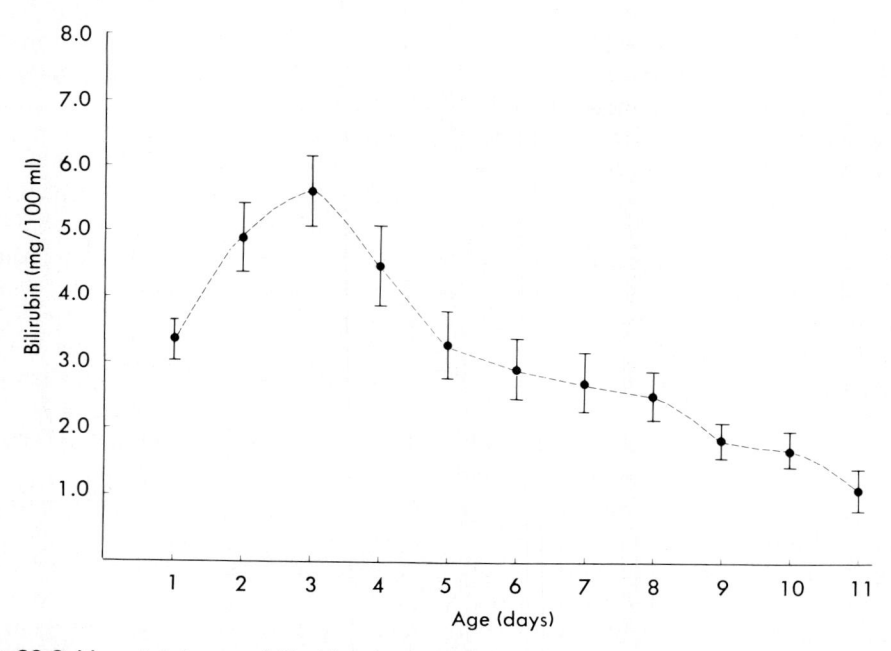

Fig. 30-2. Mean total serum bilirubin concentrations in 22 full-term normal infants during the first 11 days of life.

liver and a marked deficiency in hepatic bilirubin glucuronyl transferase activity. The presence of either of these factors alone would not result in retention of unconjugated bilirubin. Hepatic uptake and excretion of bilirubin are also deficient during this period but are not rate-limiting steps in transport of bilirubin from plasma into bile. The very large increase in bilirubin load appears to result primarily from increased enteric reabsorption of unconjugated bilirubin. Increased de novo synthesis of bilirubin both from circulating and precursor erythrocytes and from nonhemoglobin heme degradation possibly also may contribute to this load. In the newborn monkey the markedly increased load persists for 3 to 6 weeks; similar data are not yet available for the human neonate. Deficient conjugation of bilirubin may result from insufficient enzyme synthesis, inhibition of enzymatic activity by naturally occurring substances, deficient synthesis of the glucuronide donor uridine diphosphoglucuronic acid (UDPGA), or a combination of these factors. Phase II physiologic jaundice appears to result from an imbalance in which hepatic uptake of bilirubin is diminished while the increased bilirubin load presented to the liver persists. Developmental deficiency of ligandin may contribute to deficient uptake of bilirubin.

Despite the development of physiologic jaundice of some degree in nearly every newborn, only approximately half of all full-term newborns are visibly jaundiced during the first 3 days of life. This is because serum bilirubin concentrations of less than 5 mg/dl usually are not reflected in cutaneous icterus in the newborn, unlike the situation in the older child and adult in whom jaundice will be noticeable in the sclerae and skin at serum bilirubin concentrations as low as 2 mg/dl. Variations in duration of hyperbilirubinemia and in skin color and perfusion may account for these differences. Since routine daily serum bilirubin determinations are not usually performed on full-term or even premature newborns, careful scrutiny of the nursery population several times a day by experienced personnel is essential to detect significant hyperbilirubinemia requiring further investigation. Lack of knowledge and the inherently complex developmental nature of physiologic jaundice prevent one from defining it simply by a serum bilirubin concentration above a specific level. For practical reasons having to do with risks of bilirubin encephalopathy and the likelihood of finding a superimposed explanation for the hyperbilirubinemia, a serum concentration exceeding 5 mg/dl during the first 24 hours of life should alert the physician to the need for further investigation.

Physiologic jaundice in the premature infant

Physiologic jaundice in the premature infant is more severe than in the full-term infant, with mean peak concentrations reaching 10 to 12 mg/dl by the fifth day of life. This delay in reaching the maximum concentration as compared with the full-term infant reflects the delay, primarily, in the maturation of hepatic glucuronyl transferase activity in the premature infant. Since mean peak unconjugated bilirubin concentrations of 10 to 12 mg/dl may be associated with bilirubin encephalopathy in certain low birth weight infants, all degrees of visible jaundice in premature infants should be monitored closely and investigated fully. Normal serum bilirubin concentrations in premature infants may not be reached in many cases until the end of the first month of life.

Physiologic jaundice in the postmature infant

Nearly all postmature infants and approximately half of all small-for date infants may be expected to have little or no physiologic jaundice, with serum bilirubin concentrations often less than 2.5 mg/dl. The mechanism for this acceleration of hepatic maturation is unknown. Similarly infants of mothers treated with phenobarbital, a drug known to stimulate hepatic glucuronyl transferase activity, and those of heroin users have less than the anticipated severity of physiologic jaundice. Other drugs, less well investigated, also may have similar effects.

Conjugated hyperbilirubinemia may occur in combination with physiologic jaundice when excretory mechanisms are unable to cope with the quantity of bilirubin presented to and conjugated by the liver. Severe uptake or conjugating deficiency, however, may mask excretory defects for a brief period by preventing sufficient conjugated pigment from reaching the excretory transport step and thus preventing retention and regurgitation of conjugated pigment despite a defect in hepatic excretion.

Bilirubin transport in the fetus

In the fetus synthesized unconjugated bilirubin is transferred rapidly across the placenta into the maternal circulation for excretion by the maternal liver. Small amounts of bilirubin apparently are excreted by the fetal liver into a sluggish bile flow, since meconium accumulates significant amounts of bilirubin during the course of gestation. Unconjugated bilirubin also may be transferred from the maternal circulation *into* the fetus. In those rare situations in which a pregnant woman has significant unconjugated hyperbilirubinemia, a similar degree of hyperbilirubinemia would be anticipated in cord blood. Conjugated pigment is not transferred in either direction across the placenta. Therefore conjugated hyperbilirubinemia in the mother, as in hepatitis or recurrent jaundice of pregnancy, will not be reflected in the cord blood. In recent years it has been recognized that severe hemolytic disease in the fetus results in small but significant increases in amniotic fluid unconjugated bilirubin concentrations. It is not known how bilirubin enters the amniotic fluid pool, but suggestions have ranged from transfer directly across the placenta from the maternal circulation, to transudation of pigment across the amniotic membranes or cord vessels, to secretion of bilirubin in the pulmonary fluids flowing from the fetal lung into the fetal pharynx and oral cavity and then into the amniotic fluid. The measurement of bilirubin concentrations in amniotic fluid by the optical density (ΔOD) technique has markedly improved management of the erythroblastotic infant (Chapter 5).

Genetic and ethnic influences on physiologic jaundice

The severity of physiologic jaundice differs greatly between oriental and other ethnic populations. Mean maximal serum unconjugated bilirubin concentrations in Chinese, Japanese, Korean, and American Indian full-term newborns are between 10 and 14 mg/dl, approximately double those of the nonoriental populations. The incidence of bilirubin toxicity as defined by autopsy-proved kernicterus also is increased significantly in oriental neonates. There is no evidence for increased hemolysis in oriental newborns to account for these dramatic differences. Glucose-6-phosphate dehydrogenase (G6PD) deficiency is far more common in Orientals than in whites; however, it does not relate directly to the increased severity of neonatal jaundice.

Certain geographic isolates also demonstrate a markedly increased incidence of unconjugated hyperbilirubinemia of the newborn without associated hemolysis. The most dramatic of these are from certain islands off the coast of Greece, especially the islands of Lesbos and Rhodes. As in the oriental populations, the incidence of G6PD deficiency in these populations also is markedly increased compared with the world incidence and with the remainder of the Greek population, but this does not directly account for most of those infants with increased serum bilirubin concentrations. The incidence of kernicterus also is much greater in the newborns from these Greek islands than in those of the mainland population.

It has been suggested that the increased incidence of neonatal unconjugated hyperbilirubinemia in oriental and other geographically identifiable populations may result either from environmental influences, such as the maternal ingestion of certain ethnically characteristic herbal medications or foods, or from a genetic predisposition to slower maturation of hepatic bilirubin metabolism. Oriental groups living in the United States appear to have the same severity of neonatal jaundice as those in the Orient, suggesting that geographic factors alone are not determinant. The question of drugs and foods, as well as that of genetic factors, remains to be investigated.

Hemolysis, ecchymoses, and other factors that increase bilirubin synthesis in the newborn are particularly likely to produce severe hyperbilirubinemia in these high-risk populations.

PATHOLOGIC STATES OF UNCONJUGATED HYPERBILIRUBINEMIA

Superimposed on the physiologic limitations that result in physiologic jaundice are several specific disorders that may further increase serum unconjugated bilirubin concentrations, prolong unconjugated hyperbilirubinemia beyond the normal period of physiologic jaundice, or both. Most disorders causing exaggerated unconjugated hyperbilirubinemia can be classified in a functional manner according to the step in the pathway most severely affected, that is, (1) bilirubin production, (2) hepatic uptake, or (3) hepatic conjugation. The level of the serum bilirubin concentration does not in itself indicate whether the cause is physiologic or pathologic. Moderate hemolytic disease in one infant with very poor hepatic uptake and conjugation of bilirubin may result in a very rapid rise in the serum bilirubin concentration to 20 mg/dl, whereas the same degree of hemolysis in an infant with much greater hepatic bilirubin uptake and conjugating capacity may result in a slowly rising serum bilirubin concentration that reaches only 6 mg/dl in the same period. Since the balance between bilirubin load and hepatic bilirubin transport processes is so delicate, a small increase in bilirubin production may result in a very marked rise in the serum concentration. Thus it is often very difficult to distinguish between severe physiologic limitations and minor pathologic states.

Increased bilirubin production

Although increased bilirubin production could result from pathologic states in which nonhemoglobin heme (such as cytochromes) and erythrocyte hemoglobin precursor heme degradation is increased because of specific disease states, such disorders in fact have not been identified in the newborn period. Destruction of circulating erythrocytes is the largest single category of disorders leading to exaggerated unconjugated hyperbilirubinemia in the newborn period. These disorders are listed in the outline later in this section and are discussed in more detail in Chapter 29.

Rh erythroblastosis

This was at one time the leading cause of bilirubin encephalopathy and a frequent and serious clinical problem (p. 34). With the introduction of antiRh(D) antisera for prophylactic treatment of all unsensitized Rh-negative mothers following delivery of an Rh-positive infant or performance of an abortion, the incidence of Rh disease has been greatly reduced. Mothers sensitized before the development of immune serum prophylaxis and those without access to preventive treatment still continue to deliver affected infants. Jaundice is only one of many problems affecting the infant with Rh erythroblastosis.

Destruction of erythrocytes and production of large amounts of bilirubin begin in utero, but nearly all erythroblastotic infants are not icteric at birth, because serum bilirubin concentrations are kept below 5 mg/dl by transfer of unconjugated bilirubin across the placenta. Jaundice may appear, however, within 30 minutes after delivery. Classically the serum bilirubin is all indirect-reacting, although small amounts of conjugated bilirubin have been noted. In recent years, with survival of some very severely affected fetuses, particularly those receiving intrauterine transfusions (p. 34), moderate to marked *conjugated* hyperbilirubinemia has been seen in cord blood or during the first days of life. Total cord bilirubin concentrations may be as high as 40 mg/dl, with as much as 80% direct-reacting bilirubin, since conjugated bilirubin is not transported across the placenta. The reason for the development of direct-reacting bilirubin in sera is unknown, but it has been suggested that hepatic conjugation may mature more rapidly than usual as a result of chronic exposure to bilirubin in utero, whereas excretory function lags behind. In severe erythroblastosis, hepatic excretory function also may be adversely affected by development of hepatic swelling secondary to heart failure and by congestion caused by severe extramedullary hematopoiesis in liver, anemia, and poor hepatic perfusion and oxygenation.

CONDITIONS ASSOCIATED WITH INCREASED ERYTHROCYTE DESTRUCTION

A. Isoimmunization
   1. Rh incompatibility
   2. ABO incompatibility
   3. Other blood group incompatibilities
B. Erythrocyte biochemical defects
   1. G6PD deficiency
   2. Pyruvate kinase deficiency
   3. Hexokinase deficiency
   4. Congenital erythropoietic porphyria
C. Structural abnormalities of erythrocytes
   1. Hereditary spherocytosis
   2. Hereditary elliptocytosis
   3. Infantile pyknocytosis
   4. Others
D. Infection
   1. Bacterial (such as syphilis)
   2. Viral (such as rubella)
   3. Protozoal (such as toxoplasmosis)
E. Sequestered blood
   1. Subdural hematoma/cephalohematoma
   2. Ecchymoses
   3. Hemangiomas

The risk of kernicterus in states of severe hemolysis, as in Rh erythroblastosis, may be greater than in nonhemolytic hyperbilirubinemia of the same degree. This is suggested both by the increased incidence of brain damage in association with Rh hemolytic disease and by studies suggesting disproportionately decreased albumin binding of bilirubin in association with hemolytic disease.

ABO hemolytic disease

See p. 726.

Infants with group A or B erythrocytes may have increased hyperbilirubinemia, hemolysis, and positive Coombs' tests because of transfer of maternal anti-A or anti-B antibody into the fetal circulation. Although similar to Rh disease, the disorder may occur in the firstborn without prior sensitization of the mother and is generally milder and of shorter duration; however, it may also cause severe hemolysis, jaundice, and kernicterus.

Other causes of increased bilirubin production

These include erythrocyte enzyme deficiencies (G6PD deficiency and others), infection, sequestered blood, and structural abnormalities of erythrocytes. The clinical manifestations may be extremely subtle with little or no detectable decrease in hematocrit levels, elevation or reticulocyte count, or clearly definable abnormality of the erythrocyte on microscopic examination of the peripheral smear. A relatively small decrease in erythrocyte life span may enhance bilirubin production sufficiently to raise serum bilirubin concentrations to dangerous levels. No currently available clinical laboratory tool will assist in defining the contribution to hyperbilirubinemia of increased hemolysis of such small degree. Ultimately measurement of carbon monoxide production rates may permit quantitative assessments of heme degradation.

Glucose-6-phosphate dehydrogenase deficiency

See p. 735.

This deficiency is characterized by marked genetic heterogeneity, such that the majority of infants with the deficiency will not demonstrate exaggerated neonatal jaundice. In the American black population G6PD deficiency is a relatively mild disorder, and exaggerated jaundice in the newborn is unusual and occurs generally only in association with exposure to certain known inciting agents, such as naphthalene or high-dose synthetic vitamin K (K_3). Mediterranean and oriental types of G6PD deficiency are more often readily apparent, with exaggerated jaundice more common and an associated high incidence of kernicterus. In the more severe form of the disease jaundice may not become apparent until the second or third day of life and may then persist into the second and even third weeks, in association with obvious hemolysis. Those infants developing hemolysis later in the newborn period either may have relatively less hyperbilirubinemia, reflecting their maturing hepatic bilirubin metabolism, or may have significant elevations of direct-reacting bilirubin in sera, indicating that hepatic uptake and conjugation of bilirubin have matured relatively more rapidly than the excretory pathway, resulting in retention of conjugated bilirubin.

Severe neonatal jaundice may be associated with *erythrocyte pyruvate kinase deficiency, 2,3-diphosphoglycerate mutase deficiency, 6-phosphogluconic dehydrogenase deficiency*, and probably many other enzymatic defects yet to be defined. Although extremely rare, the recessively inherited *congenital erythropoietic porphyria* may be present with mixed hyperbilirubinemia, splenomegaly, and anemia at birth and may be suspected by the pink reddish brown urine that fluoresces readily under ultraviolet light.

As in the case of the red blood cell enzyme defects, structural defects of erythrocytes may or may not cause exaggerated neonatal jaundice. *Hereditary spherocytosis* (p. 737) is associated with neonatal jaundice in approximately half the cases and must be differentiated from ABO incompatibility, since the latter disorder also is characterized by increased numbers of spherocytes in the peripheral smear. Coombs' testing and examination of the parents and other family members for evidence of spherocytes help distinguish the two disorders. Since the disease is inherited as an autosomal dominant trait in most cases, the diagnosis may be suspected more strongly when one parent has either splenomegaly or a history of splenectomy. In some patients, however, differentiation cannot be made, and only continued examination of the peripheral smear beyond the newborn period will determine whether hereditary spherocytosis is the correct diagnosis. *Hereditary elliptocytosis* rarely causes hemolysis in the newborn (p. 737). A transient abnormality of erythrocyte morphology associated with hemolysis and neonatal jaundice is the disorder known as *infantile pyknocytosis*. Small, irregular, dense red blood cells with spiny projections are seen in the peripheral smear and account for more than 5% of the total red cell population. Anemia and hemolysis persist throughout the first month of life and often into the second or third month. Jaundice is most severe during the first 2 weeks of life. This disorder was recognized with greater frequency some years ago and now has become quite rare. In vitro studies of erythrocytes and plasma from these infants suggested that the abnormality resided in an extracorpuscular factor. The changing incidence of this disorder suggests that it may be a manifestation of an unknown exogenous toxic factor.

All the aforementioned disorders that may cause exaggerated hemolysis will result in more severe hyperbilirubinemia in the premature infant than in the full-term infant. Although more severe neonatal jaundice is characteristic of the premature infant, efforts should be made to detect abnormalities of erythrocytes in all jaundiced low birth weight infants. Since G6PD deficiency is by far the most common enzymatic defect, all infants with severe hyperbilirubinemia should have determinations of G6PD enzyme levels on preexchange transfusion blood specimens. Smears of the peripheral blood always should be examined as part of the evaluation of all infants with serum total bilirubin concentrations greater than 12 mg/dl.

Exaggerated *unconjugated* hyperbilirubinemia often is cited as a sign of bacterial sepsis; the mechanism is thought to be related to increased red cell destruction. However, the frequency of this association is unknown. More clearly related to bacterial sepsis, especially with *Escherichia coli*, *Proteus* organisms and pneumococci, is the development of conjugated hyperbilirubinemia; this is believed to be a result of inhibition of hepatic excretion of bilirubin by bacterial toxins (p. 653).

Hepatic uptake deficiency

Defective hepatic uptake of bilirubin has been suggested as one of the possible contributing causes of chronic unconjugated hyperbilirubinemia in adults (Gilbert's syndrome). Aside from animal studies which suggest that physiologic jaundice of the newborn may result from defective bilirubin uptake, there are no data to suggest that exaggerated hyperbilirubinemia of the newborn results from specific defects in hepatic bilirubin uptake.

Deficient conjugation of bilirubin
Inherited defects

Two genetically and functionally distinct disorders associated with inherited lifelong deficiency of hepatic glucuronyl transferase activity have been described.

Crigler-Najjar syndrome. This is the rarer and more severe of these chronic nonhemolytic unconjugated hyperbilirubinemias and has been designated type I glucuronyl transferase deficiency. Only approximately 100 infants with type I glucuronyl transferase deficiency have been reported.

Clinical manifestations. Inherited as an autosomal recessive trait, in the homozygous form severe unconjugated hyperbilirubinemia develops during the first 3 days of life and progresses in an unremitting fashion to reach serum concentrations of 25 to 35 mg/dl during the first month of life. Kernicterus occurs commonly during the early neonatal period, although recently there have been some survivors without neurologic sequelae. Stools are pale yellow, and examination of bile obtained either at surgery or by duodenal intubation reveals extremely low bilirubin concentrations (less than 10 mg/dl) and the total absence of bilirubin glucuronide. Bilirubin glucuronide formation measured in vitro with liver obtained by biopsy is absent. Formation of most nonbilirubin glucuronides is either severely reduced or absent. With either direct hepatic enzymatic assay or indirect measurement of glucuronide formation both parents are found to have partial defects (approximately 50% of normal), but serum bilirubin concentrations will be normal. During the first week of life the recognition of this disorder may be difficult because of confusion with other types of exaggerated unconjugated hyperbilirubinemia. Persistence of unconjugated hyperbilirubinemia at concentrations exceeding 20 mg/dl beyond the first week of life in the absence of obvious hemolysis should alert one to consider this syndrome. In the nursing newborn the much more common disorder of breast milk jaundice also must be considered (p. 762), but management of breast-feeding, as outlined later, will rapidly differentiate the two.

The diagnosis may be strongly suggested by the persistence of unconjugated hyperbilirubinemia, but it can be established only by direct measurement of hepatic glucuronyl transferase activity. Open surgical biopsy to obtain a specimen of liver should be avoided, since anesthesia and physiologic alterations associated with surgery may precipitate kernicterus. The diagnosis can be strongly supported by identifying partial defects in conjugation in both parents in the absence of jaundice. Duodenal intubation in which bile is obtained that contains little bilirubin is strong circumstantial evidence of the diagnosis, but dilutional effects may be confusing. Direct collection of bile from the gallbladder or common duct with concentrations below 10 mg/dl would be diagnostic, but the surgical intervention necessary is an unwarranted risk. Differentiation from type II glucuronyl transferase deficiency may be achieved by the failure of type I patients to respond to a week of phenobarbital administration with a marked decline in serum bilirubin concentration. This failure to respond to phenobarbital suggests that the basic defect in the type I disorder is the synthesis of a structurally defective enzyme.

Treatment. The management of these infants requires maintenance of serum bilirubin concentrations below 20 mg/dl during at least the first 2 to 4 weeks of life. Under certain circumstances serum bilirubin concentrations should be kept even lower (p. 767). The risk of kernicterus persists into adult life, but the serum bilirubin concentrations required to produce brain injury beyond the newborn period are considerably higher, perhaps above 35 mg/dl. Exchange transfusion may be the preferred method for reducing the serum bilirubin concentration in these infants, but repeated frequent exchange transfusions are required. For this reason most of these infants have been placed under phototherapy (p. 768) either after one or more exchange transfusions or before exchange. Phototherapy generally has been continued throughout the early years of life in the hope that his will prevent the development of kernicterus. Most recent patients indeed have survived without apparent brain damage. Whether this is because of the use of phototherapy or related to improved general newborn care is not known. In the older infants and children phototherapy has been used mainly at night, during sleep periods, permitting the children to have normal activities during the daytime. Despite attempts to expose the older children to phototherapy of the highest intensities and longest durations possible, increasingly poorer responses of the serum bilirubin concentration to phototherapy have been observed with aging. This may result from increased skin thickness or a changing distribution of the bilirubin pool. Prompt management of all intercurrent infections, febrile episodes, and other types of illness may help prevent later development of kernicterus. Kernicterus may develop at *any age* if serum bilirubin concentrations increase to 45 to 55 mg/dl. Despite vigorous efforts to reduce serum bilirubin concentrations, *all* type I patients have developed severe kernicterus at or before achieving young adulthood, even when neurologically normal throughout childhood.

Glucuronyl transferase deficiency type II. This disorder may be manifested in a manner very similar to that of the type I syndrome, or it may be a much less severe disorder, even without neonatal manifestations.

Clinical manifestations. In those infants in whom the disorder becomes apparent during the newborn period, unconjugated hyperbilirubinemia generally will appear during the first 3 days of life with serum bilirubin concentrations that may be either in a range compatible with physiologic jaundice (less than 12 mg/dl) or exaggerated. Characteristically, however, bilirubin concentrations will remain more elevated than expected (greater than 3 mg/dl) into the third week of life and persist thereafter at concentrations that range from minimal elevations of greater than 1.5 mg/dl to as high as 22 mg/dl. There may be uncertainty for some period as to whether chronic hyperbilirubinemia has developed. Although kernicterus has been reported in two patients with type II syndrome, its occurrence is unusual. Evidence of hemolytic disease is absent (although it may occur coincidentally), stool color is normal, and the infants are otherwise healthy.

Since this disorder is inherited as an autosomal dominant trait with marked variability of penetrance, one of the parents will be either minimally to severely icteric or at least demonstrate a defect in bilirubin conjugation when tested for this function. Other members of the family also may either appear icteric or have detectable low-grade unconjugated hyperbilirubinemia. Screening of the parents and other close relatives for hyperbilirubinemia is a useful method for supporting the diagnosis when it is suspected. A definitive diagnosis can be made only by direct or indirect testing of the infant and the parents for the capacity to form glucuronides of bilirubin or other suitable substances (such as menthol or salicylamide). Bilirubin glucuronide formation can be tested in vitro by performance of a percutaneous liver biopsy. Administration of substances conjugated as glucuronides in liver and excreted in urine, such as menthol or salicylamide, obviates the need for liver biopsy but is unfortunately less specific and accurate. Regardless of the method used, the levels of conjugation are extemely low and indistinguishable from those found in the type I syndrome. Once a deficiency in conjugation is established, it is necessary to distinguish between types I and II. Although examination of gallbladder bile will demonstrate that type I cases have extremely low bilirubin concentrations and type II cases have nearly normal concentrations (50 to 100 mg/dl), this would necessitate surgical exploration, a dangerous procedure for any severely jaundiced infant. Genetic studies may indicate that only one parent and family members from that parent's lineage are affected, suggesting that the infant has type II syndrome, but such studies are not always possible or definitive. Since jaundiced infants and adults with the type II syndrome respond readily to administration of phenobarbital, with a sharp decline in serum bilirubin concentrations to 2 to 3 mg/dl within 7 to 10 days, whereas individuals with type I syndrome demonstrate no change in serum bilirubin concentration, the response to phenobarbital may be used as a simple clinical tool to differentiate the two. A dosage of 5mg/kg/day given once a day is sufficient for infants and young children. Adults usually will respond to administration of only 60 mg/day.

Treatment. The response to phenobarbital administration may be used not only as a diagnostic test but also, when chronically administered, for long-term reduction of bilirubin concentrations for cosmetic and psychosocial reasons. At the serum bilirubin concentrations observed in type II patients there should be no long-term risk of kernicterus, unless there is coincidental hemolytic disease.

Pregnancy in the patient with either type I conjugating defect or more severe forms of type II syndrome may present a special hazard to both the mother and fetus. During pregnancy serum bilirubin concentrations my rise, and bilirubin binding by albumin may be altered, thus increasing the risk to the mother of neurologic manifestations of severe unconjugated hyperbilirubinemia. Unconjugated bilirubin crosses the placenta in both directions. With severe unconjugated hyperbilirubinemia in the mother markedly elevated unconjugated bilirubin concentrations may be anticipated in the fetus, raising the possibility of congenital kernicterus, which has not yet been observed.

Acquired defects

Late-onset breast milk jaundice. A small cohort of breast-fed infants develop a syndrome characterized by the relatively late onset of exaggerated unconjugated hyperbilirubinemia at a time when jaundice would normally be abating. The estimated incidence is 1 per 200 breast-fed infants. A normal pattern of physiologic jaundice is observed during the first 3 days of life, following which the serum bilirubin concentrations rise to reach maximum unconjugated bilirubin concentrations of 10 to 27 mg/dl by the tenth to fifteenth day of life in the absence of hemolysis and other evidence of illness. Weight gain and bowel function are characteristically normal. Often the infants are not noted by the parents or other caregivers to be abnormal in any way. Interruption of nursing and substitution with artificial feeding or nursing by another woman for 2 to 4 days result in a prompt decline of the serum bilirubin concentration to approximately half the original level. Resumption of nursing by the mother results in a small but significant increase in serum indirect bilirubin concentrations of 1 to 3 mg/dl in most infants or arrest of the decline in bilirubin concentrations in others. Failure to respond in this manner indicates that the infant's jaundice is unrelated to breast-feeding, and other causes should be sought. It should be emphasized that interruption of nursing is *not* recommended as a routine procedure in all jaundiced breast-fed infants but should be reserved for those infants whose serum bilirubin concentrations approach levels considered dangerous for development of kernicterus (p. 764). Since this syndrome is most commonly seen in full-term otherwise normal infants, serum bilirubin levels that remain below 20 mg/dl in these infants may be considered to be safe during the first 4 weeks of life, and nursing need not be interrupted. The rare inherited defects in hepatic bilirubin metabolism (type II especially) may occur in breast-fed infants, leading to the erroneous diagnosis of breast-feeding jaundice. It will become clear, however, that a chonic disorder exists when, after termination of nursing weeks or even months later, unconjugated hyperbilirubinemia persists. Since persistence of low-grade unconjugated hyperbilirubinemia poses no threat to the newborn or older infant, delay in recognition of the defect poses no hazard. The breast-feeding jaundice syndrome may be anticipated when there is a history of *prolonged* unconjugated hyperbilirubinemia in other breast-fed infants of the mother, since approximately 70% of the nursed infants of these women may be expected to have the syndrome. Similarly in the artificially fed infants of these same mothers prolonged, severe jaundice is rare.

This syndrome was attributed in earlier studies to the presence of an isomerically abnormal progesterone metabolite, pregnane-3α, 20β-diol, in milk. This steroid metabolite had been shown to be a competitive inhibitor of glucuronyl transferase in vitro. More recent studies have indicated that the milk associated with this syndrome also contains high concentrations of nonesterified long-chain fatty acids. This led to the suggestion that certain of these fatty acids act as inhibitors of hepatic glucuronyl transferase, resulting in retention of unconjugated bilirubin. This mechanism has not been demonstrated in vivo, however. Although the presence of both pregnane-3α, 20β-diol and increased amounts of nonesterified fatty acids in these human milks has been amply confirmed, the role of these agents in pathophysiology of this syndrome remains uncertain. Milk from these mothers enhances reabsorption of bilirubin.

Early-onset breast milk jaundice. The relationship between accentuated unconjugated hyperbilirubinemia in the first week of life and breast-feeding has not been fully established. This entity frequently is claimed to be seen by many clinicians but has never been adequately documented. In some hospital nurseries it is said to be the single most frequent cause of neonatal jaundice in full-term newborn infants. It is clear that this is not a universal finding, however. Two prospective studies failed to show any significant differences between serum bilirubin concentrations of breast- and bottle-fed infants during the first 3 days of life. The possible difference in the incidence of this entity between hospitals may be related to differences in breast-feeding practices. In many hospital settings breast-feeding mothers are not encouraged to nurse their infants with sufficient frequency (at least every 2 hours in the early days of lactation) to permit rapid and effective development of lactation. Poor advice and inappropriate supplementation with water and/or formula also may serve to inhibit lactation. Starvation or reduced caloric intake is known to produce elevated unconjugated serum bilirubin levels in many animal species, including humans. The mechanism by which starvation may induce unconjugated hyperbilirubinemia in the neonate has not been studied.

Since it is clear that not all jaundice in the breast-fed neonate is a result of breast-feeding, the clinician is faced with the difficult dilemma of whether breast-feeding should be interrupted when the serum bilirubin concentration is rising or markedly elevated. There is unfortunately no firm clinical experience or studies on which to base a recommendation. Breast-feeding should not be interrupted routinely but only when serum bilirubin concentrations are at or near potentially toxic levels.

Transient familial neonatal hyperbilirubinemia. This is a rare syndrome in which every infant of certain mothers may be expected to develop severe unconjugated hyperbilirubinemia during the first 48 hours of life, with bilirubin concentrations usually reaching 20 mg/dl or greater. Many of these infants develop kernicterus unless exchange transfusions are performed. Hemolysis is absent, and the infants are otherwise healthy. The sera of these infants and their mothers are found to contain high concentrations of an unidentified inhibitor of glucuronyl transferase when tested in vitro. The inhibitor is present in maternal sera during the second and third trimesters of pregnancy and in both maternal and newborn sera at the time of delivery. Although sera from normal pregnant women and newborns also inhibit glucuronyl transferase activity to a small degree, sera from these mothers and infants are 4 to 10 times as inhibitory. The serum inhibitory effect gradually declines after delivery to become normal by approximately 14 days post partum. Coincident with the decrease in inhibition, there is a gradual decline in serum bilirubin concentrations in the newborn.

Pyloric stenosis. This disorder is associated with the development of unconjugated hyperbilirubinemia in 10% to 25% of the infants at the time vomiting begins, usually during the second or third week of life (p. 499). There is no relationship between the development of jaundice and the degree of dehydration or electrolyte imbalance. Hepatic glucuronyl transferase activity is markedly depressed in the jaundiced infants but not in anicteric infants with pyloric stenosis. The mechanism of diminished glucuronyl tranferase activity is unknown but may relate to the presence of an inhibitory substance elaborated in the intestinal tract. *Duodenal and jejunal obstruction* also is associated with exaggerated unconjugated hyperbilirubinemia. Surgical relief of the obstructive enteropathy results in return of serum bilirubin concentrations to normal within 2 to 3 days. *Lower intestinal obstruction*, as in Hirschsprung's disease, also may result in unconjugated hyperbilirubinemia, although usually of milder degree than with upper intestinal tract disease. In this situation as well as in upper intestinal tract obstructions hyperbilirubinemia may result from increased reabsorption of unconjugated bilirubin from the intestine as a result of enteric stasis, which may lead to increased hydrolysis of bilirubin glucuronide to unconjugated bilirubin and enhanced reabsorption by intestinal mucosa.

Drugs administered to newborns must be considered as potential agents that may exaggerate unconjugated hyperbilirubinemia not only by initiating hemolysis in certain metabolic defects of erythrocytes (G6PD deficiency) but also by inhibition of hepatic glucuronyl transferase activity. Many drugs that have been used in neonatal therapy (such as streptomycin and chloramphenicol) are capable of inhibiting the enzyme in vitro, but only novobiocin has ever been demonstrated to actually produce unconjugated hyperbilirubinemia. Novobiocin is a noncompetitive inhibitor of glucuronyl transferase. The use of any new drug in the neonate should alert the staff to the need to observe for increased jaundice.

Exaggerated neonatal jaundice with undefined mechanisms

Maternal diabetes is associated with an increased incidence of exaggerated and prolonged unconjugated hyperbilirubinemia in the offspring (Chapter 3). This is unrelated to the severity and duration of the maternal diabetes. Exaggerated jaundice often is attributed to the prematurity of the infant of the diabetic mother. However, even when one compares infants of identical gestational age, there is an increased incidence, duration, and severity of jaundice in the infant of the diabetic mother. The mechanism is unexplained. Early feeding (before 12 hours of age) may reduce the severity of the hyperbilirubinemia.

Hypothyroidism in the newborn is another disorder in which exaggerated unconjugated hyperbilirubinemia has been observed (p. 890). Approximately 10% of the hypothyroid infants may by expected to have prolonged and exaggerated jaundice. Treatment with thyroid hormone will promptly alleviate the hyperbilirubinemia. Congenital hypothyroidism often is difficult to diagnose in the newborn, and persistence of unconjugated hyperbilirubinemia should suggest the possibility of thyroid insufficiency.

BILIRUBIN TOXICITY
Kernicterus

See p. 760.

The recognition that unconjugated bilirubin has the capability of entering the brain cell under certain circumstances and causing the death of those cells is the reason for the urgency of carefully observing every jaundiced newborn (and certain newborns without apparent clinical jaundice) and treating neonatal jaundice.

Pathology

The staining and necrosis of neurons results in *bilirubin encephalopathy*. The areas of the brain most commonly affected are the basal ganglia, hippocampal cortex, and subthalamic nuclei. The cerebral cortex generally is spared. Only unconjugated bilirubin enters neurons. Although the diagnosis of kernicterus at autopsy has always relied on the grossly yellow staining of brain tissue and the accompanying neuronal necrosis, recent animal studies have suggested that significant functional impairment of brain function may result from hyperbilirubinemia even when there is no obvious yellow staining or histologic evidence of cell damage. This suggests that very small quantities of bilirubin may be cytotoxic.

Approximately half of all infants with kernicterus observed at autopsy have extraneural lesions of bilirubin toxicity. These include necrosis of renal tubular cells, intestinal mucosa, and pancreatic cells in association with intracellular crystals of bilirubin. Gastrointestinal (GI) hemorrhage may accompany these lesions.

Clinical manifestations

In the classic presentation of bilirubin encephalopathy, the newborn progressively develops lethargy, rigidity, opisthotonos, high-pitched cry, fever, and convulsions over a period of up to 24 hours (p. 760). This is followed by death in approximately half the infants so affected. Premature infants with autopsy-proved kernicterus generally have none of these characteristic clinical findings. Survivors of neonatal manifestations of bilirubin encephalopathy often demonstrate choreoathetoid cerebral palsy, high-frequency deafness, and less often mental retardation during later infancy and childhood. These sequelae of kernicterus also may develop in infants who never manifest clinical signs of bilirubin encephalopathy during the newborn period. In addition, some infants may have sequelae of subclinical bilirubin encephalopathy characterized only by the later development of mild disorders of motor function or abnormal cognitive function or both, collectively called minimal brain dysfunction. Premature infants are particularly susceptible to this type of subtle bilirubin-related brain damage.

Pathogenesis

The pathogenesis of bilirubin encephalopathy is complex and poorly understood. Although certain sequelae (such as choreoathetoid cerebral palsy) are specific, most sequelae are not and could as well be the result of hypoxic, vascular, or infectious injury. Furthermore both clinical and laboratory studies have indicated that certain neonatal risk factors, which in themselves produce brain damage, also increase the likelihood that kernicterus will develop in the presence of mild to moderate unconjugated hyperbilirubinemia. Leading among these factors is hypoxia. The relationship between brain hypoxia and kernicterus is so close that some investigators have suggested that kernicterus will not develop in the absence of some degree of central nervous system (CNS) hypoxia. The theory of this relationship may be particularly valid

Table 30-1. Recommended maximum total serum bilirubin concentrations (mg/dl)*

Birth weight category (gm)†	Uncomplicated course	Complicated course‡
Less than 1,000	10	10§
1,000-1,249	13	10
1,250-1,499	15	13
1,500-1,999	17	15
2,000-2,499	18	17
2,500 and up	20	18

*Direct-reacting bilirubin concentrations are not subtracted unless they amount to more than 50% of the total serum bilirubin concentration; applicable during the first 28 days of life.
†Equivalent gestational age categories may be used in lieu of birth weight for small for gestational age infants.
‡Complications include perinatal asphyxia and acidosis, postnatal hypoxia and acidosis, significant and persistent hypothermia, hypoalbuminemia, hemolysis, and hypoglycemia.
§Septicemia or meningitis: all infants with proven or highly suspected bacterial infection should be treated as <1,000–gm infants regardless of birth weight.

for those clinical situations in which kernicterus develops at relatively low serum bilirubin concentrations (5 to 15 mg/dl), as in the very immature premature infant. Other factors that enhance the development of kernicterus are hypoglycemia, acidosis, bacterial infection (sepsis and meningitis), hypothermia, moderate to severe hemolysis, administration of certain drugs (sulfonamides), hypoalbuminemia, and deficient albumin binding of bilirubin. The mechanism (or mechanisms) by which each of these pathologic states enhances the development of kernicterus is, in part, speculative. Nevertheless the recognition of the importance of these factors has led to their inclusion in virtually every schema for establishing criteria for treatment of neonatal hyperbilirubinemia (see section on management and Table 30-1).

In the pathogenesis of kernicterus unconjugated bilirubin moves from the plasma pool into the neuron. This movement results either from (1) a reduction in the quantity or quality of binding of bilirubin by the circulating albumin, or (2) a major alteration in a membrane function of the brain cell that normally excludes bilirubin from entry (the so-called blood-brain barrier). In most clinical situations both factors are operative. The human albumin molecule is capable of binding at least two molecules of bilirubin; the first molecule is more tightly bound than the second. Additional classes of binding sites, if operative in vivo, have much lower affinities than the first two. At a molar ratio of 1, each gram of human albumin binds 8.4 mg of bilirubin. Thus, at an average serum albumin concentration of 3.5 gm/dl, the first binding site should be capable of binding 29.4 mg of bilirubin per 100 ml serum. The second binding site should be capable of binding an additional 29.4 mg/dl for a total binding capacity of 58.8 mg/dl. Various techniques are available to measure albumin binding of bilirubin, but their application and interpretation in clinical management are not generally accepted. The dye-binding methods (2-[4-hydroxybenzeneazo] benzoic acid [HBABA] and Direct-Yellow-7 [DY7]) are based on the measurement of reserve binding sites on the albumin molecule and should be capable of indicating impending risk; the column chromatographic methods (Sephadex G-25), the salicylate displacement spectrophotometric method (saturation index), the red cell uptake method, and the oxidation technique (peroxidase method) all should be capable of detecting either small amounts of unbound bilirubin ("free" bilirubin) or "loosely bound" bilirubin. In general, there is an increased risk of developing kernicterus when there is either an increase in "loose" or "free" bilirubin in the circulation or when binding capacity approaches dangerously close to saturation; however, present data are insufficient to permit a recommendation as to the use of either a single method or combination of methods or numerical standards for the application of any of these methods. The critical point at which the risk of kernicterus is probably significantly increased is when the first binding site on albumin is saturated.

Some of the factors implicated as increasing the risk of kernicterus in the newborn may operate by direct alteration of albumin binding of bilirubin. Thus acidosis, of even mild degree, the sulfonamide drugs, and possibly sodium benzoate (a preservative in certain drugs) may diminish the binding of bilirubin by albumin; hemolysis may interfere with binding by release of heme pigments into the circulation that may compete with bilirubin for albumin-binding sites; hypoglycemia, hypothermia, and sepsis may act similarly by increasing free fatty acid concentrations in plasma. Free fatty acids may interfere with binding either by direct competitive displacement of bilirubin, by binding to nonbilirubin binding sites on albumin to produce conformational changes of the albumin molecule with consequent weakening of bilirubin binding, or by complex formation with bilirubin to form a freely circulating pigment not bound to albumin. The increased risk of kernicterus in the newborn and particularly in the premature infant, as compared with the adult, and the demonstration of significantly reduced binding capacity for bilirubin by albumin in the newborn have led to the additional suggestion that a fetal type of albumin, with reduced binding affinity, may exist. Kernicterus has been reported to occur in adults with type I glucuronyl transferase deficiency but only when serum bilirubin concentrations have reached 45 to 55 mg/dl. This contrasts with the situation in the full-term newborn in which an increased incidence of kernicterus may be anticipated at concentration above 20 mg/dl and even at concentrations exceeding 16 mg/dl. Even lower serum bilirubin concentrations have been associated with kernicterus in the small and sick premature infant.

Many mechanisms have been proposed to explain both the entrance of bilirubin into the neuron and the resultant damage to cellular metabolism. Unconjugated bilirubin is a lipid-soluble substance with almost no aqueous solubility. Passage into the lipid moieties of cell membranes and from there into lipids of subcellular organelles (mitochondria) to block critical steps in transport or energy metabolism is possible. Binding to specific proteins in cell membranes or within the cell is also possible. Although it appears to the pathologist that kernicterus is an irreversible form of brain damage, transient or reversible states of bilirubin intoxication have been suggested by clinical observations of increasing lethargy with increasing bilirubin concentrations and awakening after exchange transfusion. These reversible states remain to be confirmed, but the suggestion of a significant, otherwise unexplained change in the neurobehavioral status of a jaundiced newborn should be considered sufficient basis for institution of immediate exchange transfusion regardless of serum bilirubin concentration or the values of binding studies.

MANAGEMENT OF UNCONJUGATED HYPERBILIRUBINEMIA
Diagnostic clinical and laboratory studies

After performance of appropriate diagnostic tests to establish the cause of the unconjugated hyperbilirubinemia, the clinician is faced with two major decisions: when to institute therapy and which technique (or techniques) to use. Diagnostic studies to determine the presence of hemolytic diseases should be undertaken in full-term infants who become clinically icteric during the first 24 hours of life or whose bilirubin concentrations exceed 12 mg/dl thereafter. All hospitals should routinely determine the maternal blood group and Rh type at the time of onset of labor and infant blood group, Rh type, and direct Coombs' test immediately after delivery. Additional tests should include hemoglobin or hematocrit determinations, smear of peripheral blood for erythrocyte morphology, and reticulocyte count. In the presence of significant icterus with a potential ABO incompatibility (type O mother and type A, B, or AB infant), the direct Coombs test should be repeated at least once when originally negative, since initial false negatives have been seen. If evidence of hemolysis develops or if the infant requires either simple or exchange transfusion, blood should be sent for determination of erythrocyte G6PD activity. A careful history from the parents may reveal familial patterns of neonatal hyperbilirubinemia or anemia or ethnic patterns associated with severe neonatal jaundice. Observation of the parents for jaundice and even determination of serum bilirubin concentrations in them also may be useful in the diagnosis of familial types of hemolytic disease or inherited hepatic dysfunction. Patterns of feeding (time of onset, breastfeeding) also may be of importance. More extensive studies for rarer forms of hemolytic disease and enzyme assays for glucuronyl transferase activity may be deferred until the chronicity of the disease has been established; this is usually after the first month of life. Studies for hepatocellular disease (such as hepatitis and obstructive biliary disease), including serum glutamic-oxaloacetic transaminase (SGOT) and serum glutamic-pyruvic transaminase (SGPT), alkaline phosphatase, and cholesterol, need to be performed only when there is a significant elevation of the direct-reacting bilirubin. A careful physical examination with special attention to liver and spleen size, skin appearance, and neurobehavioral status should be performed frequently in the evaluation of a jaundiced infant. Skin color cannot be relied on for estimation of serum bilirubin concentrations, and it is essential that serum bilirubin determinations be performed on every infant at the time jaundice is first observed and as frequently thereafter as needed to establish the pattern of increase. Recent development of reflectance photometers permits more precise measurement of bilirubin levels than is possible by visual inspection, but cutaneous determinations should be used only for screening purposes. Precise serum bilirubin methods should be used in confirmation. In most patients a repeat determination in 4 to 8 hours will be necessary the first day jaundice is noted and at least daily thereafter until a clear pattern of decline is observed. In some patients serum bilirubin concentrations may be monitored on an ambulatory basis, eliminating the need for prolonged hospitalization only for the purpose of obtaining serum bilirubin concentrations. In most cases a hematocrit value should be determined simultaneously with each bilirubin determination. Direct-reacting bilirubin concentrations should be determined at the time of the first bilirubin estimation and at least once a day thereafter.

The method of management chosen for an individual infant will determine in part the serum bilirubin concentration at which therapy is instituted. It is essential therefore that every newborn nursery and neonatal intensive care unit have an established policy regarding the methods to be used and criteria for initiation of therapy.

Exchange transfusion

Exchange transfusion is the standard mode of therapy for treatment of hyperbilirubinemia to prevent kernicterus and for correction of anemia in erythroblastosis fetalis (p. 742). With this technique approximately 85% of the circulating red blood cells will be replaced when the equivalent of two infant blood volumes (160 ml/kg body weight) is used in aliquots not to exceed 10% of the total blood volume. Serum bilirubin concentrations usually will be reduced by 50%. Although it is a relatively safe procedure in experienced hands, it carries a mortality risk of 0.1% to 1% and a significant morbidity and is time consuming and expensive. The procedure usually takes 1 to 2 hours to complete. Slower exchanges theoretically should increase the quantity of bilirubin removed by permitting equilibration of pigment from tissue, but the differences are too small to justify the increased risk of prolonging the duration of manipulation. The indications for exchange transfusion should be individualized to some extent and might be based on a variety of criteria that includes serum bilirubin concentrations, albumin concentrations, and measurements of albumin binding of bilirubin. Since the two latter techniques still require evaluation, the recommendations contained in Table 30-1 use only the serum bilirubin concentration, birth weight (or gestational age equivalent), and adjustments for increased risk factors. These criteria are proposed largely on the basis of clinical observations and represent the concensus judgment of a number of neonatologists participating in a controlled clinical trial of phototherapy under the auspices of the National Institute of Child Health and Human Development. No infant is permitted to have a serum unconjugated bilirubin concentration in excess of 20 mg/dl during the first 28 days of life, and direct-reacting bilirubin is not subtracted from the total unless the direct-reacting portion exceeds 50% of the total bilirubin. Although direct-reacting bilirubin does not enter the CNS and does not in itself cause kernicterus, it is not known whether direct-reacting bilirubin can partially displace unconjugated bilirubin from albumin-binding sites to increase the risk of kernicterus. The same criteria are used on the first day of life as on subsequent days, but in the face of rapidly rising serum bilirubin concentrations, as may be seen in Rh erythroblastosis or other types of erythroblastosis, the decision to perform the exchange should anticipate the rise (from the previous serum bilirubin concentrations, the hemoglobin, and the reticulocyte count) so that the exchange is under way by the time the critical level is reached. In the severely affected, hydropic or nonhydropic erythroblastotic infant, clinical judgment rather than laboratory data should be used to decide whether the infant requires immediate exchange transfusion after delivery. In this situation a partial exchange transfusion using packed red blood cells coupled with reduction in blood volume if venous pressure is elevated and with measures to ensure adequate ventilation and correction of acidosis and shock often will be life saving. In most exchange transfusions fresh whole or reconstituted acid citrate dextrose (ACD) or citrate phosphate dextrose (CPD) anticoagulated blood should be used. If blood older than 5 days *must* be used, the pH should be checked and sodium bicarbonate added to correct the pH to 7.1; correction to pH 7.4 may result in later excessive rebound alkalosis as the citrate is metabolized. Use of heparinized blood avoids any additional osmolar loads and may obviate the need to administer calcium or correct for acidosis but may result in hypoglycemia and markedly increased free fatty acid concentrations.

The administration of salt-poor albumin (1 gm/kg) to infants 1 to 2 hours before exchange transfusion to increase the efficiency of bilirubin removal by shifting more tissue-bound bilirubin into the circulation has been advocated and shown to increase the bilirubin removed by 40%. Since the total amount of bilirubin removed during an exchange transfusion is only a small portion of the total body pool of bilirubin, this increase may not significantly alter subsequent bilirubin concentrations or the need for additional exchange transfusions. Although probably benign, the transient increase in serum bilirubin concentration after albumin administration theoretically could increase the risk of kernicterus rather than reduce it if there are local phenomena at the brain level that alter albumin binding of bilirubin.

The potential complications of exchange transfusion are listed in Table 30-2. Preparations for emergency situations should be made before initiation of the procedure.

Table 30-2. Complications of exchange transfusion

System	Specific problem
Vascular	Embolization (air thrombus)
	Thrombosis of portal vein
	Necrotizing enterocolitis (?)
	Perforation of vessel
	Uncontrollable hemorrhage
Cardiac	Arrhythmias (mechanical or chemical)
	Cardiac arrest
	Heart failure caused by volume overload
Electrolyte	Hyperkalemia
	Hypernatremia
	Hypocalcemia
	Acute hypercalcemia
	Acidosis
	Alkalosis
Coagulation	Hemorrhagic disorder caused by overheparinization
	Thrombocytopenia
	Microembolization with intravascular hemolysis
Infectious	Bacteremia
	Hepatitis B
	Cytomegalovirus
Immunologic	Transfusion mismatch reaction
Miscellaneous	Mechanical injury to donor cells
	Hypothermia

Adapted from Odell, G.B., and others: Pediatr. Clin. North Am. **9**:605, 1962.

Table 30-3. Guidelines for use of phototherapy in newborn period*

Birth weight category (gm)	Indication for phototherapy
Less than 1,500	Start during first 24 hours of life regardless of serum bilirubin concentration
1,500-1,999	Without hemolysis at 10 mg/dl; with hemolysis at 8 mg/dl
2,000-2,499	Without hemolysis at 12 mg/dl; with hemolysis at 10 mg/dl
2,500 and over	Without hemolysis in healthy infant, withhold use of phototherapy; with hemolysis, or in presence of factors that contraindicate use of exchange transfusion, at 15 mg/dl

*Phototherapy to be continued until serum bilirubin concentration has stabilized at or fallen to less than half of exchange transfusion indication level shown in Table 30-1.

Phototherapy

Despite the unquestioned ability of phototherapy to reduce serum bilirubin concentrations in most infants, continued uncertainty regarding the effectiveness of phototherapy in preventing kernicterus and the potential long-term side effects has led to controversy about its application as a routine clinical procedure. A national collaborative study is underway at the present to evaluate both the efficacy and safety of phototherapy. When the final results of this study are known, more rational recommendations on its use will then be possible.

At our medical center phototherapy is being used prophylactically for all infants with birth weights less than 1,500 gm, therapeutically for all low birth weight infants more than 1,500 gm, and only for those full-term infants with prolonged hyperbilirubinemia after at least one exchange transfusion (Table 30-3). In the very low birth weight infants prophylactic phototherapy is being used because of the excessive morbidity and mortality observed during exchange transfusions. In the full-term, otherwise well infant with hyperbilirubinemia exchange transfusion is well tolerated with almost no mortality risk. Furthermore institution of phototherapy in this group may actually prolong hospitalization, since in the majority of full-term infants serum bilirubin concentrations already may have begun to fall by the time hyperbilirubinemia is recognized and phototherapy initiated.

Two independent mechanisms have been proposed to explain the action of phototherapy in reducing serum bilirubin concentrations in newborn infants. The first and the major pathway is photoisomerization of unconjugated bilirubin IXα. Chemical structure of unconjugated bilirubin IXα is usually in the 5Z, 15Z configuration. In this form the −COOH group of each carboxymethyl side chain interacts via three hydrogen bonds with the C=O and N−H group of the pyrrole rings in the opposite half molecule. As a result, the ionization of the two −COOH groups is inhibited, and therefore the molecule is nonpolar and water-insoluble. Unconjugated bilirubin undergoes Z to E isomerization when illuminated. With tetrapyrrolic bilirubin IXα either one or both of the bridge double bonds could undergo isomerization, yielding 5E, 15Z; 5Z, 15E; and 5E, 15E isomers. The E configuration spatially precludes hydrogen bonding of the molecule, which therefore becomes free to ionize and renders the E isomer more polar than the Z isomer.

At least two pairs of photoisomers have been identified. The first pair, photobilirubin IA and IB, is presumably the two possible E, Z isomers. The second pair, photobilirubin IIA and IIB, is most likely two rotamers of the 5E, 15E isomer. Both pairs presumably are formed rapidly in the skin, subcutaneous tissue, and their capillaries. Being more polar, these isomers partition into the plasma, continuously shifting the equilibrium to promote more isomer formation. These isomers are rapidly taken by the liver and transported into bile. Isomers I, destabilized by bile acids, rapidly revert to native unconjugated bilirubin IXα. The isomers II remain mostly intact and are the major polar photoproducts found in bile. This photoisomerization pathway may be responsible for over 80% of the augmented bilirubin catabolism during the phototherapy.

The second pathway involves a variety of oxidation reactions with bilirubin, resulting from an autosensitized reaction involving singlet oxygen. The products formed by these reactions are multiple but include biliverdin, dipyrroles, and monopyrroles. Many of these products are colorless, nonreactive in the van den Bergh test, and presumably excreted by the liver and kidney without need for conjugation. Compared with the first pathway, this second mechanism appears to play a minor role in photocatabolism of unconjugated bilirubin in vivo.

In applying phototherapy, banks of eight or ten fluorescent lamps are placed approximately 12 to 16 inches above an unclothed infant lying in an open bassinet or an incubator. A shield of the correct type of Plexiglas should be placed between the lamps and the infant to absorb the small amount of ultraviolet light emitted by most fluorescent lamps and to guard against injury from lamp explosion. For phototherapy various kinds of fluorescent light lamps have been used, including daylight, cool white, blue, and special blue types. Bilirubin absorbs light maximally in the blue range (from 420 to 500 nm), with peak absorption for albumin-bound bilirubin at 460 nm and for unbound bilirubin at 440 nm. Daylight and cool white lamps have a spectral peak between 550 and 600 nm and thus are less effective than special blue lamps, which have a narrow spectral range and peak between 420 and 480 nm.

Effective phototherapy must provide irradiance well

above the levels that have been determined to be minimally effective in producing bilirubin degradation, while not exceeding levels beyond which no significant increases in response are evident. A standard phototherapy unit with eight new daylight lamps operating under optimal conditions would provide clinically significant minimal effective levels for phototherapy (approximately 4 muW/cm^2/nm). According to the current knowledge a saturation point for bilirubin degradation appears to correspond to the energy output provided by a standard phototherapy unit with four daylight and four special blue lamps (approximately 0.9 μW/cm^2/nm). Increasing the distance from the lamp to the skin surface of the infant will result in a diminution of light energy by a factor equal to the square of the increase in distance. Thus doubling the distance from 12 to 24 inches will reduce the light energy reaching the infant to one fourth the original energy. The greater the surface area exposed, the greater the effectiveness of phototherapy will be. Skin pigmentation does not reduce the effectiveness of phototherapy. With time in use, fluorescent lamps reduce the energy output to a degree that varies from one type of lamp to another. A meter for monitoring lamp energy output should be used routinely during treatment. Commercially available photometers have been found to measure the same amount of irradiance with some variations. This is because of variations in peak absorptions and absorption band widths of the individual meters. For this reason comparative data have to be established when a new meter is introduced to the service.

The effect of high-intensity light exposure on the eyes of newborn human infants is uncertain, but animal studies indicate that retinal degeneration may occur after several days of continuous exposure. It is essential therefore that the eyes of all newborns exposed to phototherapy be covered with sufficient layers of opaque material to ensure against the possibility of damage. There is an increased insensible and intestinal water loss during phototherapy, which must be compensated for by an increase of about 25% in the fluid volume offered to treated infants. In addition, stools are slightly looser and more frequent. Phototherapy does not retard growth.

The *bronze baby syndrome* is associated with phototherapy. In this disorder the serum, urine, and skin become brown-black (bronze) several hours or more after an infant is placed under the phototherapy lamps. In nearly all patients direct-reacting hyperbilirubinemia has been noted either before light exposure or after the syndrome has developed. In most patients some evidence of hepatocellular disease has been suggested from chemical or histologic determinations. Increased hemolysis was suggested in one patient. In the only patient to die, kernicterus was observed at autopsy in association with the bronze baby syndrome. All other patients have recovered without apparent sequelae. The nature of the bronze pigment is unknown, and its development following high-intensity light exposure may represent an inborn error of metabolism, a preexisting hepatic excretory defect leading to retention of a pigment that would otherwise have been eliminated in bile, or a pigment derived from red blood cell destruction. Since it is not clear at this time whether this is a benign cosmetic response to phototherapy, a sign of impending liver or subclinical liver disease, or a true toxicity to phototherapy, it is essential that direct-reacting bilirubin concentrations be determined before instituting phototherapy. If significant elevation of direct-reacting pigment is found, phototherapy should not be used.

Congenital erythropoietic porphyria is another syndrome in which phototherapy is contraindicated, since it may lead to death. This rare disorder is characterized by hemolysis, splenomegaly, and pink to red urine that fluoresces orange under ultraviolet light. Exposure to visible light of moderate to high intensity and of wavelengths between 400 and 500 nm (blue) will produce severe bullous lesions on the exposed skin and may produce hemolysis. Mixed hyperbilirubinemia with a significant direct-reacting fraction also may be seen in this disease.

It also has been suggested that phototherapy may alter albumin binding of bilirubin by photooxidative damage of albumin; this has not been confirmed in vivo. Other possible dangers of phototherapy include overheating of the infant, electrical shock from poorly grounded or defective equipment, and unproved long-term effects on endocrine and sexual maturation and DNA metabolism.

Pharmacologic management

Phenobarbital is one of a large group of drugs that stimulate protein synthesis in general and hepatic glucuronyl transferase and hepatic ligandin synthesis specifically. DDT, ethanol, heroin, and certain antihistamines act similarly. After the demonstration that phenobarbital administration to a child with type II glucuronyl transferase deficiency reduced serum bilirubin concentrations, phenobarbital administration to pregnant mothers and their offspring was shown to reduce by approximately 50% peak serum bilirubin concentrations caused by physiologic jaundice. Studies in newborn rhesus monkeys have demonstrated that the major effect of this therapy is to increase hepatic glucuronyl transferase activity and the conjugation of bilirubin. It also may enhance hepatic uptake of bilirubin in the newborn. The administration of phenobarbital to newborns at the time jaundice is first observed or even immediately after delivery is much less effective than its administration to the mother during pregnancy for at least 2 weeks before delivery. The drug also is much less effective in premature infants. As a prophylactic measure, it would be necessary therefore to administer phenobarbital to large numbers of pregnant women for prolonged times during pregnancy, since the time of delivery could not be predicted with certainty. Even then the group of infants most susceptible to the toxic effects of hyperbilirubinemia—the premature—would receive little or no beneficial effect. The drug is potentially addicting, may lead to excessive sedation of the newborn, and has other potent metabolic effects in addition to those on bilirubin metabolism. For these reasons the use of phenobarbital has not achieved wide application but has been reserved largely for very specific high-risk populations. For example, in the unexplained severe hyperbilirubinemia of the newborns from the Greek coastal islands the frequency of kernicterus has been significantly reduced by general administration of phenobarbital to pregnant women during the last trimester. A dosage of 60 mg/day is sufficient for maternal administration and 5 mg/kg/day for neonatal treatment. Phenobarbital also is useful in the differentiation between types I and II glucuronyl transferase deficiency (p. 761). Combining phenobarbital treatment with phototherapy has no advantage, the effect being no greater than that of phototherapy alone.

Enteric reabsorption of unconjugated bilirubin may be a major source of increased bilirubin in the newborn period. Frequent milk feeding (cow or human) prevents the rise of serum bilirubin and enhances the bilirubin-reducing effect of phototherapy. Oral administration of nonabsorbable substances that bind bilirubin in the intestinal lumen and presumably reduce enteric absorption of bilirubin may reduce peak serum bilirubin concentrations in physiologic jaundice by about 50%. *Activated charcoal* has been used but is effective only when administered during the first 12 hours of life. *Agar* also has been shown to be effective. Further study of this type of therapy is needed before recommendations can be made regarding clinical application.

Lawrence M. Gartner
Kwang-Sun Lee

BIBLIOGRAPHY
Physiology

Arias, I.M.: Formation of bile pigment. In Arias, I.M., editor: Handbook of physiology; alimentary canal, vol. 5, section 6, Washington, D.C., 1968, American Physiological Society.

Berk, P.D., and others: Comparison of plasma bilirubin turnover and carbon monoxide production in man, J. Lab. Clin. Med. **83:**29, 1974.

Bonnet, R., Davies, J.E., and Hursthouse, M.B.: The structure of bilirubin, Nature **262:**326, 1976.

Elder, G., Gray, C.H., and Nicholson, D.C.: Bile pigment fate in gastrointestinal tract, Semin. Hematol. **9:**71, 1972.

Fleischner, G.M., and Arias, I.M.: Structure and function of ligandin and Z protein in the liver; a progressive report. In Popper, H., and Schaffner, F., editors: Progress in liver disease, vol. 5, New York, 1976, Grune & Stratton, Inc.

Gartner, L.M., Lane, D.L., and Cornelius, C.E.: Bilirubin transport by liver in adult *Macaca mulatta*, Am. J. Physiol. **220:**1528, 1971.

Jansen, P.L.M., and others: Enzymatic conversion of bilirubin monoglucuronide to diglucuronide by rat liver plasma membranes, J. Biol. Chem. **252:**2710, 1977.

Lee, K.S., and Gartner, L.M.: Spectrophotometric characteristics of bilirubin, Pediatr. Res. **10:**782, 1976.

Schmid, R.: Bilirubin metabolism: state of the art, Gastroenterology **74:**1307, 1978.

Schmid, R., and McDonagh, A.F.: The enzymatic formation of bilirubin, Ann. N.Y. Acad. Sci. **244:**533, 1975.

Physiologic jaundice of the newborn

Bernstein, R.B., and others: Bilirubin metabolism in the fetus, J. Clin. Invest. **48:**1678, 1969.

Gartner, L.M., and others: Development of bilirubin transport and metabolism in the newborn rhesus monkey, Pediatr. **90:**513, 1977.

Levi, A.J., Gatmaitan, Z., and Arias, I.M.: Deficiency of hepatic organic anion-binding protein, impaired organic anion uptake by liver and "physiologic" jaundice in newborn monkeys, N. Engl. J. Med. **283:**1136, 1970.

Maisels, M.J.: Bilirubin; on understanding and influencing its metabolism in the newborn infant, Pediatr. Clin. North Am. **19:**447, 1972.

Odell, G.B.: Neonatal jaundice, In Popper, H., and Schaffner, F., editors: Progress in liver diseases, vol. 5, New York, 1976, Grune & Stratton, Inc.

Thaler, M.M.: Neonatal hyperbilirubinemia, Semin. Hematol. **9:**107, 1972.

Vaisman, S.L., Lee, K.S., and Gartner, L.M.: Various bilirubin conjugates in pregnant and nonpregnant rats with and without phenobarbital treatment, Pediatr. Res. **10:**111, 1976.

Vest, M., Strebel, L., and Hauenstein, D.: The extent of "shunt" bilirubin and erythrocyte survival in the newborn infant measured by the administration of (^{15}N) glycine, Biochem. J. **95:**11, 1965.

Yeung, C.Y.: Neonatal hyperbilirubinemia, Chin. Trop. Geogr. Med. **25:**151, 1973.

Pathologic states of unconjugated hyperbilirubinemia

Berk, P.D., Wolkoff, A.W., and Berlin, N.I.: Inborn errors of bilirubin metabolism, Med. Clin. North Am. **59:**803, 1975.

Cornelius, C.E., and Gronwall, R.R.: A mutation in Southdown sheep affecting the hepatic uptake of BSP, indocyanine green, rose bengal, sodium cholate and phylloerythrin from blood, Fed. Proc. **24:**144, 1965.

Gartner, L.M.: The functional basis of physiologic jaundice of the newborn. In Goresky, C.A., and Fisher, M.M., editors: Jaundice, vol. 2, New York, 1975, Plenum Publishing Corp.

Garner, L.M., and Arias, I.M.: Studies of prolonged neonatal jaundice in the breast fed infant, J. Pediatr. **68:**54, 1966.

Gartner, L.M., and Hollander, M: Disorders of bilirubin metabolism. In Assali, N., editor: Pathophysiology of gestation, vol. 3, New York, 1972, Academic Press, Inc.

Jaffe, E.R.: Hereditary hemolytic disorders and enzymatic deficiencies of human erythrocytes, Blood **35:**116, 1970.

Liley, A.W.: The use of amniocentesis and fetal transfusion in erythroblastosis fetalis, Pediatrics **35:**836, 1965.

Luzzatto, L.: Genetic heterogeneity and pathophysiology of G6PD deficiency, Br. J. Haematol. **28:**151, 1974.

Meyer, U.A., and Schmid, R.: Congenital erythropoietic porphyria. In

Stanbury, J.B., Wyngaarden, J.B., and Frederickson, S.S., editors: The metabolic basis of inherited disease, ed. 4, New York, 1978, McGraw-Hill Book Co.

Odievre, M.: Breast feeding and neonatal hyperbilirubinemia. In Berenberg, S.R., editor: Liver diseases of infancy and childhood, The Hague, 1976, Martinus Nijhoff Medical Division.

Orzalezi, M., and others: ABO system incompatibility: relationship between direct Coombs test positivity and neonatal jaundice, Pediatrics **51**:288, 1973.

Oski, F.: Oxytocin and neonatal hyperbilirubinemia, Am. J. Dis. Child. **129**:1139, 1975.

Smith, D.W., and others: Congenital hypothyroidism; signs and symptoms in the newborn period, J. Pediatr. **87**:958, 1975.

Taylor, P.M., and others: Hyperbilirubinemia in infants of diabetic mothers, Biol. Neonate **5**:289, 1963.

Winfield, C.R., and MacFaul, R.: Clinical study of prolonged jaundice in breast- and bottle-fed babies, Arch. Dis. Child. **53**:506, 1978.

Woolley, M.M., and others: Jaundice, hypertrophic pyloric stenosis, and hepatic glucuronyl transferase, J. Pediatr. Surg. **9**:359, 1974.

Wysowski, D.K., and others: Epidemic neonatal hyperbilirubinemia and use of a phenolic disinfectant detergent, Pediatrics **61**:165, 1978.

Bilirubin toxicity

Cashore, W.J., and others: Clinical application of neonatal bilirubin-binding determinations: current status, J. Pediatr. **93**:827, 1978.

Cowger, M.L.: Bilirubin encephalopathy. In Gaull, G., editor: Biology of brain dysfunction, vol. 2, New York, 1973, Plenum Publishing Corp.

Diamond, I.: Bilirubin binding and kernicterus. In Schulman, I., editor: Advances in pediatrics, vol. 16, Chicago, 1969, Year Book Medical Publishers, Inc.

Diamond, I., and Schmid, R.: Experimental bilirubin encephalopathy; the mode of entry of bilirubin-^{14}C into the central nervous system, J. Clin. Invest. **45**:678, 1966.

Gartner, L.M., and Lee, K.S.: Bilirubin binding, free fatty acids and a new concept for the pathogenesis of kernicterus. II. Bilirubin metabolism in the newborn, Birth Defects **12**:264, 1976.

Gartner, L.M., and others: Kernicterus; high incidence in premature infants with low serum bilirubin concentrations, Pediatrics **45**:906, 1970.

Lee, K.S., and Gartner, L.M.: Bilirubin binding by plasma proteins: a critical evaluation of methods and clinical implications, Rev. Perinatal Med. **2**:319, 1978.

Lee, K.S., Gartner, L.M., and Vaisman, S.L.: Measurement of bilirubin-albumin binding. I. Comparative analysis of four methods and four human serum albumin preparations, Pediatr. Res. **12**:301, 1978.

Lucey, J.F., and others: Kernicterus in asphyxiated newborn rhesus monkeys, Exp. Neurol. **9**:43, 1964.

Mustafa, M.G., and King, T.E.: Binding of bilirubin with lipids; a possible mechanism of its toxic reactions in mitochondria, J. Biol. Chem. **245**:1084, 1970.

Naeye, R.L.: Amniotic fluid infections, neonatal hyperbilirubinemia and psychomotor impairment, Pediatrics **62**:497, 1978.

Odell, G.B., Storey, G.N.B., and Rosenberg, L.A.: Studies in kernicterus. III. The saturation of serum proteins with bilirubin during neonatal life and its relationship to brain damage at 5 years, J. Pediatr. **76**:12, 1970.

Pearlman, M.A., and others: Absence of kernicterus in low-birth-weight infants from 1971 through 1976; comparison with findings in 1966 and 1967, Pediatrics **62**:460, 1978.

Silverman, W.A., and others: A difference in mortality rate and incidence of kernicterus among premature infants allotted to two prophylactic antibacterial regimens, Pediatrics **18**:614, 1956.

Management of unconjugated hyperbilirubinemia

Bowman, J.M.: Neonatal management. In Queenan, J.T., and others, editors: Modern management of the Rh problem, ed. 2, New York, 1977, Harper & Row Publishers, Inc.

Clark, C.F., and others: The "bronze baby" syndrome: postmortem data, J. Pediatr. **88**:461, 1976.

Committee on Phototherapy in the Newborn: Final report of the Committee on Phototherapy in the Newborn, Washington, D.C., 1974, Division of Medical Sciences, National Research Council, National Academy of Sciences.

Lee, K.S., and others: Unconjugated hyperbilirubinemia in very low birth weight infants, Clin. Perinatol. **4**:305, 1977.

McDonagh, A.F., Palma, L.A., and Lightener, D.A.: Blue light and bilirubin excretion, Science **208**:145, 1980.

Moller, J.: Agar ingestion and serum bilirubin values in newborn infants, Acta Obstet. Gynecol. Scand. **53**:61, 1974.

Panagopoulos, G., Valaes, T., and Doxiadis, S.A.: Morbidity and mortality related to exchange transfusions, J. Pediatr. **74**:247, 1969.

Wurtman, R.J.: Effects of light on metabolic processes. In Bergsma, D., editor: Bilirubin metabolism in the newborn, Birth Defects **6**:60, 1970.

Vaisman, S.L., and Gartner, L.M.: Pharmacologic treatment of neonatal hyperbilirubinemia, Clin. Perinatol. **2**:37, 1975.

PART TWO

Conjugated hyperbilirubinemia

Jaundice in the neonatal period may be associated with a rise in the direct-reacting fraction of serum bilirubin. This is indicative of a defect or insufficiency in bile secretion or biliary flow or both and therefore is commonly accompanied by a rise in serum levels of other constituents of bile, such as bile salts and phospholipids. It frequently is referred to as obstructive jaundice, although the term is inaccurate, since it implies mechanical blockage, which is present in only the minority of cases. The designation *cholestasis* may more precisely describe this group of disorders. Conjugated hyperbilirubinemia may result from primary defects either in the hepatocellular phase of bile excretion or in canalicular or ductal function or from loss of patency of these structures.

PATHOPHYSIOLOGY

The *hepatocellular phase* involves the transport of conjugated bilirubin across the hepatic cell membrane. This passage occurs at a specific site in the hepatocyte referred to as the biliary pole. Structurally the cytoplasm at this pole is distinguished by a paucity of mitochondria and ribosomes and by the presence of a network of microfilaments, visible with the electron microscope and demonstrated to represent the contractile protein actin. The role of this protein in bile excretion is unknown. The cell membrane at the biliary pole is differentiated to form microvilli and becomes one facet in the usually multifaceted bile canaliculus formed by two, sometimes three, adjacent hepatocytes (Figs. 30-3 and 30-4). The junction

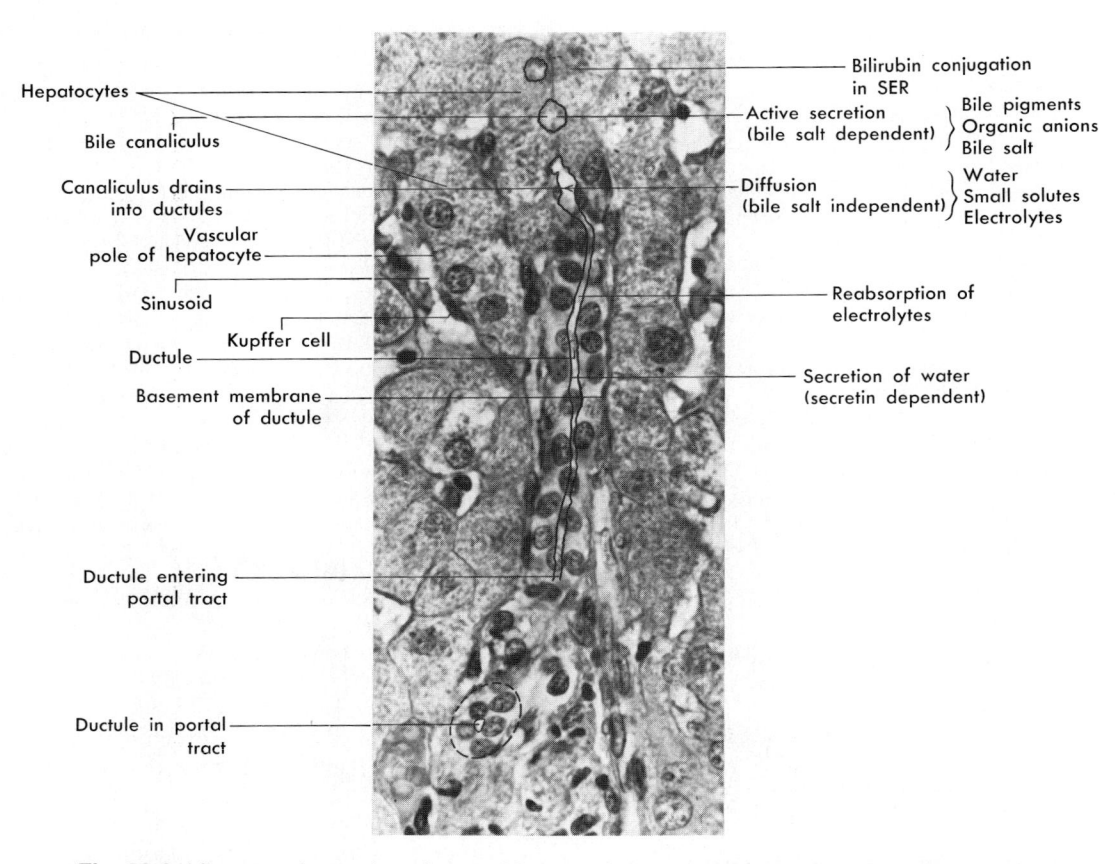

Fig. 30-3. Microscopic section of normal liver depicting transition between bile canaliculus and bile ductule entering portal tract. Anatomic structures are identified to left of illustration, and corresponding physiologic events are listed on right.

between hepatocytes bordering the bile canaliculus is called the "tight junction" and under normal circumstances forms an efficient barrier preventing the contents of the bile canaliculus from reaching the perisinusoidal space of Disse or the vascular compartments. The bile canaliculus, the smallest of the conduits for bile, is therefore an integral part of the hepatocyte. It follows that injury to the hepatocyte may result in impairment of the cellular phase of bile excretion and breakdown of the tight junctions, leading to the clinical and laboratory findings of obstructive jaundice. If cellular damage is extensive, hyperbilirubinemia may be associated with other laboratory abnormalities that reflect impairment of other hepatocellular functions. On the other hand, injury may be limited to the processes responsible for bile transport at the biliary pole, thus resulting in the isolated laboratory finding of conjugated hyperbilirubinemia. A liver biopsy taken in the early stages of one of the diseases caused by hepatocellular defect in bile secretion characteristically would show bile pigment granules in hepatocytes and bile in canaliculi: thus *intracellular* and *intracanalicular* cholestasis. Bile pigment granules are not seen in normal hepatocytes, and the lumens of bile canaliculi are not clearly visualized in routine histologic preparations of normal liver tissue (Fig. 30-4). When examined with the electron microscope, the canalicular lumen is normally small and contains no bile. It is partially obliterated by the projecting microvilli (Fig. 30-3). On rare occasions liver biopsies from patients with conjugated hyperbilirubinemia fail to show any abnormalities when examined with the light microscope.

The *ductal phase* of bile excretion includes those events which take place in the biliary system distal to the bile canaliculus (Fig. 30-3). The intrahepatic component comprises the bile ductules (the initial portion of which is frequently referred to as the canal of Hering); the interlobular (portal) bile ducts, always associated with a vein and an arteriole; and the right and left hepatic ducts, which in some individuals may partially extend beyond the liver capsule. The extrahepatic component includes the common hepatic duct, the cystic duct, the gallbladder, and the common bile duct (choledochus). Most diseases affecting the *extrahepatic* bile ducts are associated with segmental or diffuse luminal obliteration and are

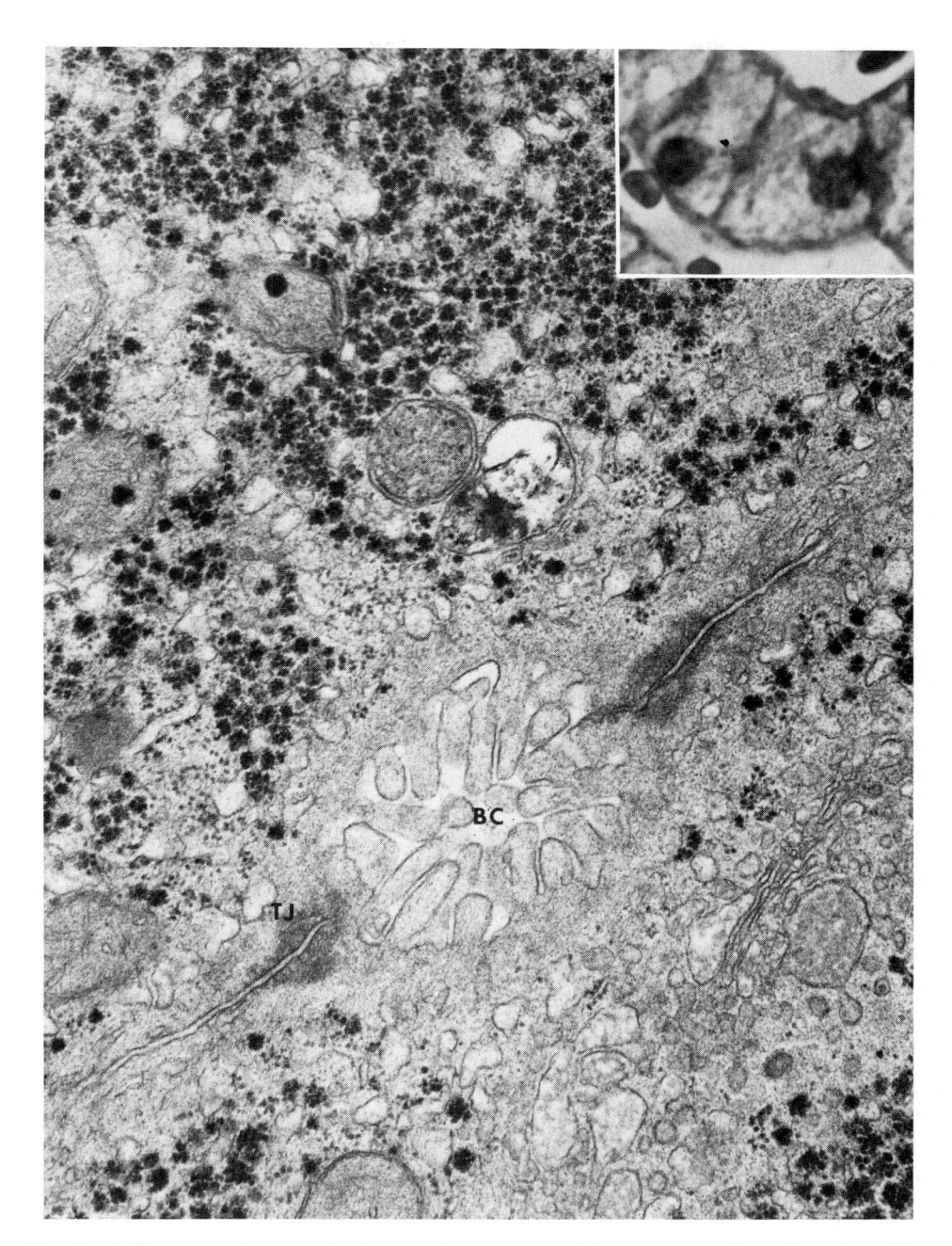

Fig. 30-4. Electron micrograph of two adjacent normal hepatocytes. Note the microvillar surface of the bile canaliculus *(BC)*. Tight junctions *(TJ)* border the canaliculus. Insert illustrates a high-power view of two adjacent hepatocytes as seen in the light microscope. In such preparations bile canaliculi appear as poorly defined condensations of the cell membrane. (Courtesy Dr. L. Biempica, Albert Einstein College of Medicine.) (Epon-embedded; ×6,000.)

expressions primarily of mechanical disturbance in bile flow. Diseases involving the *intrahepatic* ducts are complex and probably result both from mechanical obstruction to the flow of bile and from abnormalities of the biochemical pathways involved in the process of bile secretion (such as bile salt synthesis and transport). A characteristic tissue response to mechanical obstruction of a major bile duct is dilatation and proliferation of the proximal portions of the intrahepatic biliary system, including the ductules and canals of Hering, structures that are outside the confines of the portal tracts. The stimulus responsible for this proliferation is unknown. A constant accompaniment to bile duct proliferation is an increase in connective tissue, which leads eventually to cirrhosis. Although bile secretory defects initially may be either cellular or ductal, any long-standing abnormality in the flow of bile leads to hepatic parenchymal cell damage.

The accompanying outline lists diseases that may be seen as conjugated hyperbilirubinemia in the neonatal period. They are divided into those primarily caused by a defect in the hepatocellular phase of bile secretion and those caused by ductal disturbances. In most of these disorders direct-reacting bilirubin accounts for 50% to 90% of total serum bilirubin. A small amount of indirect-reacting bilirubin is always present, reflecting mild hemolysis, defective uptake and excretion, or hydrolysis of conjugated bilirubin. Early in the onset of conjugated hyperbilirubinemia in the neonate the direct-reacting portion may account for only 10% to 25% of the total serum bilirubin. As hepatic conjugation and uptake of bilirubin mature, the indirect-reacting portion usually decreases, whereas the direct portion increases.

DISEASES THAT MAY BE SEEN AS CONJUGATED HYPERBILIRUBINEMIA IN THE NEONATAL PERIOD

A. Hepatocellular disturbances in bilirubin excretion
  1. Primary hepatitis
     a. Neonatal idiopathic hepatitis (giant cell hepatitis)
     b. Hepatitis caused by identified infectious agents
        (1) Hepatitis B (HB$_s$AG)
        (2) Rubella
        (3) Cytomegalovirus
        (4) *Toxoplasma* organisms
        (5) Coxsackie virus
        (6) Syphilis
        (7) Herpes simplex, varicella-zoster
        (8) *Listeria* organisms
        (9) Tubercle bacillus
  2. "Toxic hepatitis"
     a. Systemic infectious diseases
        (1) *E. coli* (sepsis or urinary tract)
        (2) Pneumococci
        (3) *Proteus* organisms
        (4) *Salmonella* organisms
        (5) Idiopathic diarrhea
     b. Intestinal obstruction
     c. Parenteral alimentation
     d. Ischemic necrosis
  3. Hematologic disorders
     a. Erythroblastosis fetalis (severe forms)
     b. Congenital erythropoietic porphyria
  4. Metabolic and heredofamilial disorders
     a. Alpha$_1$-antitrypsin deficiency
     b. Galactosemia
     c. Tyrosinemia
     d. Fructosemia
     e. Glycogen storage disease type IV
     f. Lipid storage diseases
        (1) Niemann-Pick disease
        (2) Gaucher's disease
        (3) Wolman's disease
     g. Cerebrohepatorenal syndrome (Zellweger's syndrome)
     h. Trisomy E
     i. Fibrocystic disease
     j. Familial idiopathic cholestasis: Byler's disease
B. Ductal disturbances in bilirubin excretion
  1. Extrahepatic biliary atresia
     a. Without associated malformations
     b. Associated with trisomy E
     c. Associated with polysplenia-heterotaxia syndrome
  2. Intrahepatic biliary atresia (paucity of intrahepatic ducts)
  3. Intrahepatic atresia associated with lymphedema
  4. Extrahepatic stenosis and choledochal cyst
  5. Bile plug syndrome
  6. Fibrocystic disease
  7. Tumors of the liver and biliary tract
  8. Periductal lymphadenopathy

SPECIFIC DISORDERS
Biliary atresia and neonatal hepatitis

Biliary atresia and idiopathic neonatal hepatitis occur with approximately similar frequency and together account for about 90% of all cases of neonatal conjugated hyperbilirubinemia. *Biliary atresia* includes a group of diseases in which there is luminal obliteration or apparent absence of all or segments of the biliary duct system. Involvement may be limited to the major extrahepatic bile ducts or, much more rarely, may involve intrahepatic branches located in portal tracts. The latter situation usually is designated as paucity of intrahepatic bile ducts, or intrahepatic biliary atresia. In rare instances atresia of the major bile ducts coexists with absence or paucity of intrahepatic bile ducts. *Idiopathic neonatal hepatitis*, as used here, includes those infants with prolonged conjugated hyperbilirubinemia without apparent stigmata of generalized viral illness, evidence of an identifiable infectious agent, or etiologically specific metabolic abnormality. On liver biopsy this group is characterized by extensive transformation of hepatocytes into multinucleated giant cells and is therefore sometimes referred to as neonatal giant cell hepatitis. Necrosis and inflammation are probably always present but are transient, and therefore their absence at any given time does not exclude the diagnosis.

Differentiation between these two groups of diseases may be extremely difficult in the early stages; however, an early accurate diagnosis is essential for the choice of proper clinical management. Extrahepatic biliary atresia, the most frequent form of atresia, requires early surgical intervention. Unrelieved by surgery, the defect inevitably leads to death from biliary cirrhosis in the first 3 years of life. Those rare infants with both extrahepatic atresia and paucity of intrahepatic ducts have a significantly longer life expectancy (see under prognosis). The prognosis in neonatal hepatitis is uncertain. A significant number either expire from hepatic insufficiency or progress to chronic liver disease, whereas some recover without sequelae.

Etiology and pathogenesis

The cause of biliary atresia and of neonatal hepatitis remains undetermined. The long-held view that biliary atresia represents a congenital developmental anomaly is now thought untenable. In the majority of cases biliary atresia and neonatal hepatitis occur as isolated abnormalities, and both are considered representative of acquired conditions, probably caused by the same or similar factors. Viral agents are strongly suspected.

Recent serologic studies indicate that a high proportion (68%) of infants with biliary atresia have antibodies to Reovirus type 3, whereas less than 7% of age-matched controls have these antibodies. These findings suggest that biliary atresia may be etiologically related to perinatal infection with Reovirus type 3. In fact, a hepatobiliary disease bearing strong resemblance to human biliary atresia can be experimentally induced in very young mice by infection with Reovirus type 3.

In support of the acquired nature of biliary atresia is the absence of reported cases in stillborn fetuses and the rare association with other malformations. Similarly clinical evidence of total obstruction to the flow of bile (such as acholic stools or colorless meconium) is not detected in the early stages of jaundice. The onset of conjugated hyperbilirubinemia and acholic stools is frequently delayed until 2 weeks of life or even later. Microscopic changes observed in the extrahepatic biliary system or "fibrous cords" removed during the Kasai procedure (see under treatment) strongly suggest a sequence of changes reflecting an injury progressing from epithelial necrosis and inflammation to fibrosis and scarring (see Fig. 30-6). Clinical pathologic observations over a long period indicate that some patients fulfill all known criteria for neonatal hepatitis, including surgical demonstration of patent biliary ducts in the early stages of jaundice, and then go on to develop extrahepatic biliary atresia. Landing has proposed the concept of "infantile obstructive cholangiopathy" to include neonatal hepatitis, biliary atresia, and choledochal cyst. According to his theory injury may occur either in utero or in the perinatal period, but the consequences of such injury and therefore clinically manifested disease are delayed until sometime after birth. Injury, regardless of its nature, affects primarily structures involved in bile secretion. It is likely that in all patients with neonatal hepatitis or any of the forms of biliary atresia both hepatocytes and the biliary epithelium are involved. Clinical manifestations and outcome may depend on the severity and dominance of lesions in a specific location. Thus primary damage to hepatocytes may result in clinical manifestations of neonatal hepatitis, whereas injury to portal radicles of the biliary duct system may result in paucity of intrahepatic ducts, and injury to major bile ducts and gallbladder may result in extrahepatic atresia. Choledochal cyst may represent the mildest form of extrahepatic atresia, in which injury involves only a short segment of the bile duct and results in dilatation or cyst formation of the proximal portion.

Associated conditions

Most patients with neonatal hepatitis and biliary atresia represent isolated cases without familial incidence or associated anomalies. Rare familial occurrences of both neonatal hepatitis and biliary atresia have been reported, however. Furthermore both neonatal hepatitis and biliary atresia occur more frequently in patients with trisomy E (trisomy 18) than in the general population. Biliary atresia has been observed in 50% of reported patients with the polysplenia-heterotaxia syndrome. This syndrome is characterized by situs inversus of abdominal organs, intestinal malrotation, multiple spleens, centrally placed liver, and a variety of cardiac, pulmonary, and vascular malformations. The inferior vena cava is frequently absent and renders these patients unsuitable for liver transplantation when they have inoperable biliary atresia. Familial occurence of intrahepatic paucity of bile ducts (intrahepatic biliary atresia) has been described in association with other abnormalities. One familial syndrome includes cholestasis, paucity of intrahepatic bile ducts, and lymphedema of the lower extremities. Most patients in this group are from families of Norwegian extraction. Another syndrome includes cholestasis, paucity of intrahepatic bile ducts, unusual facies, vertebral malformations, cardiac murmurs, and retarded mental, physical, and sexual development (Alagille syndrome).

Clinical and laboratory manifestations

Early clinical manifestations of both biliary atresia and neonatal hepatitis may be limited to jaundice. In a small

Table 30-4. Clinical and biochemical findings in neonatal hepatitis and biliary atresia

	Neonatal hepatitis	Biliary atresia
Hepatomegaly	+	+
Splenomegaly	±	− (+ Late)
SGOT	+ (Rarely may be high)	+ (Usually not over 300)
SGPT		
Alkaline phosphatase	+	+
Bilirubin	5-40 mg/dl	5-20 mg/dl
Hemolytic anemia and reticulocytosis	+ (Most cases)	+ (Occasionally)

proportion of patients, especially among those who later develop neonatal hepatitis, jaundice may be apparent at birth, documented by increased concentrations of conjugated bilirubin in umbilical cord blood. No case of extrahepatic biliary atresia has ever been described in which elevation of *direct-reacting* bilirubin was found in the cord blood. In most patients with either hepatitis or atresia jaundice becomes apparent between the second and sixth weeks of life. The dark yellow staining of diapers from the presence of bilirubin in the urine often prompts the parents to seek medical advice. Jaundice is frequently first noted by the physician during a "well baby" visit. Hepatomegaly may be present in both neonatal hepatitis and biliary atresia. Splenomegaly is more frequently present in neonatal hepatitis, but this is not a constant finding. Its presence in biliary atresia usually signifies cirrhosis. Total obstruction to the flow of bile is reflected by acholic stools and may be observed in both neonatal hepatitis and biliary atresia. It is always transient and incomplete in neonatal hepatitis, but its duration is variable and may extend beyond the crucial period during which an accurate diagnosis must be established if surgical correction is needed. A summary of clinical and biochemical findings in biliary atresia and neonatal hepatitis is presented in Table 30-4. Routine clinical and laboratory findings usually will not distinguish between extrahepatic biliary atresia and neonatal hepatitis. A routine series of diagnostic laboratory tests is suggested, however, to establish the severity of hepatic involvement and to screen for possible causes (see outline that follows). In patients with intrahepatic paucity of bile ducts early clinical manifestations and laboratory findings are identical to those observed in patients with extrahepatic biliary atresia. Later in the first year of life, however, intrahepatic paucity of bile ducts is characterized by rising serum cholesterol concentrations well beyond those observed in other forms of infantile liver disease. Levels over 1,000 mg/dl may be seen as early as the third month of life. Cutaneous xanthomata are prominent in the later stages of this disease, usually after 1 year of age. The failure of routine laboratory tests to distinguish between neonatal hepatitis and biliary atresia has led to continued search for other distinguishing biochemical characteristics. Lipoprotein X is found in the sera of all patients with significant cholestasis, and therefore a qualitative analysis is not helpful in the differential diagnosis. Following treatment with cholestyramine, however, there may be a decrease in the level of lipoprotein X in patients with neonatal hepatitis and an increase in patients with atresia. Alpha-fetoproteins are frequently present in the sera of patients with neonatal hepatitis but may be absent in patients with biliary atresia.

RECOMMENDED LABORATORY TESTS FOR EVALUATION OF NEONATAL CONJUGATED HYPERBILIRUBINEMIA

A. Liver function tests
   1. Total and direct-reacting serum bilirubin, total serum protein, and serum protein electrophoresis
   2. SGOT, SGPT, alkaline phosphatase (and 5'-nucleotidase if alkaline phosphatase elevated), gamma glutamyl transpeptidase (GGTP)
   3. Cholesterol
   4. Serum and urine bile acid concentrations if available
   5. Alpha$_1$-antitrypsin
   6. ^{131}I-labeled rose bengal excretion test
   7. Alpha-fetoprotein and lipoprotein X(?)
B. Hematologic tests
   1. Complete blood count, smear, and reticulocyte count
   2. Direct Coombs' test and erythrocyte G6PD
   3. Platelet count
   4. Prothrombin time and partial thromboplastin time
C. Tests for infectious diseases
   1. Cord blood IgM
   2. VDRL, FTA-ABS, complement fixation titers for rubella, cytomegalovirus, and herpesvirus, and Sabin's dye titer for toxoplasmosis
   3. HB$_s$AG (Australia antigen) in both infant and mother
   4. Viral cultures from nose, pharynx, blood, stool, urine, and cerebrospinal fluid
D. Urine tests
   1. Routine urinalysis, including protein and reducing substances
   2. Urine culture
   3. Bilirubin and urobilinogen
   4. Amino acid screening
E. Liver biopsy
   1. Light microscopy
   2. Specific enzyme assay (if indicated)
F. Radiologic/ultrasound studies as indicated
G. Additional specific diagnostic studies for metabolic disorders to be performed as indicated or suspected

The single most helpful diagnostic tool in differential diagnosis between biliary atresia and neonatal hepatitis is the ^{131}I-labeled rose bengal excretion test. This test should be performed in infants with acholic or light-colored stools. For 2 days preceding and 3 days following

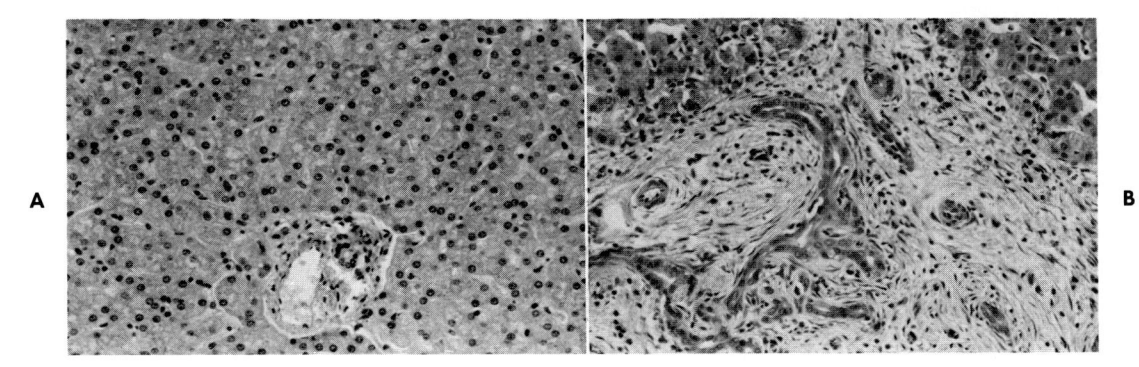

Fig. 30-5. A, Portal tract of normal infant, containing large, thin-walled vein and single cross section of bile duct. **B,** Portal tract from infant with biliary atresia. Note marked enlargement of tract from fibrosis that surrounds multiple elongated bile ducts. (Both micrographs ×60.)

administration of ^{131}I-labeled rose bengal, 2 drops of Lugol's solution should be given daily to block the thyroid uptake of ^{131}I. The ^{131}I-labeled rose bengal should be administered intravenously in a dosage of 1μCi diluted in 1 ml saline per kg of body weight. The stools should be collected for the following 72 hours. To avoid errors in interpretation, it is essential to avoid urine contamination of stool. Simultaneous serial scanning of the abdomen should be performed during the 72 hours following ^{131}I-labeled rose bengal administration. Rose bengal is excreted into the biliary system unchanged by the hepatocyte. Under normal conditions 90% of the injected dye is recovered in the stools at the end of 72 hours. Although excretion may be very low in neonatal hepatitis, levels below 5% at the end of 72 hours indicate complete mechanical obstruction. In some infants with extrahepatic atresia, excretion may be as low as 0.1% of the administered dose. Abdominal scanning techniques using the gamma camera have been suggested to avoid the need for stool collection. If significant radioactivity is detected within the intestine, excretion may be assumed to have exceeded 10%. The fine distinction between those infants having excretions of less than 5% and those with between 5% and 10% is probably not possible without 72-hour stool collection and accurate counting of the low-level radioactivity in it. The abdominal scanning technique during rose bengal studies also may reveal the presence of a choledochal cyst.

Liver biopsy

Histopathologic examination of the liver is an integral part of the evaluation of any patient with persistent conjugated hyperbilirubinemia. It is best performed and analyzed after all other pertinent laboratory data have been gathered. A percutaneous liver biopsy usually yields adequate tissue for microscopic and, if desired, electron-microscopic and virologic studies. In experienced hands it is a safe procedure, and in the majority of patients (90% to 95%) it establishes or confirms the correct diagnosis, sparing the infant with neonatal hepatitis an unnecessary surgical procedure. Before the biopsy, however, it must be ascertained that the prothrombin time is within 3 to 5 seconds of normal and that the platelet count is greater than 100,000. A prolonged prothrombin time may be corrected in some patients by administration of vitamin K. In some situations in which a biopsy is urgently required, fresh-frozen plasma may be administered before and 6 hours after percutaneous biopsy. Postoperatively infants must be observed closely for vital signs or clinical changes that indicate significant bleeding, bile peritonitis, or pneumothorax, the rare but significant complications of the procedure. In the final analysis the rose bengal test and a percutaneous liver biopsy are the only reliable means available without surgical exploration to distinguish between neonatal hepatitis and extrahepatic biliary obstruction.

Interpretation of liver biopsy

Biliary atresia. The most critical information to be derived from the liver biopsy is the determination of the presence or absence of changes indicative of mechanical blockage in the major bile ducts. It has been shown in patients and in animal experiments that, soon after obstruction of the common bile duct, ducts and ductules in portal tracts and in the periportal zones begin to proliferate. This phenomenon involves most, if not all, portal tracts and is present even at the periphery of the liver far removed from the site of obstruction. At least three portal tracts should be available for examination. In biliary atresia all tracts will show some degree of proliferation (Fig. 30-5). Minimal and rare proliferation of bile ductules, frequently limited to just one portal tract in a needle biopsy, may be seen in neonatal giant cell hepatitis and probably reflects a localized or incomplete block caused by bile inspissation. In early stages of biliary atre-

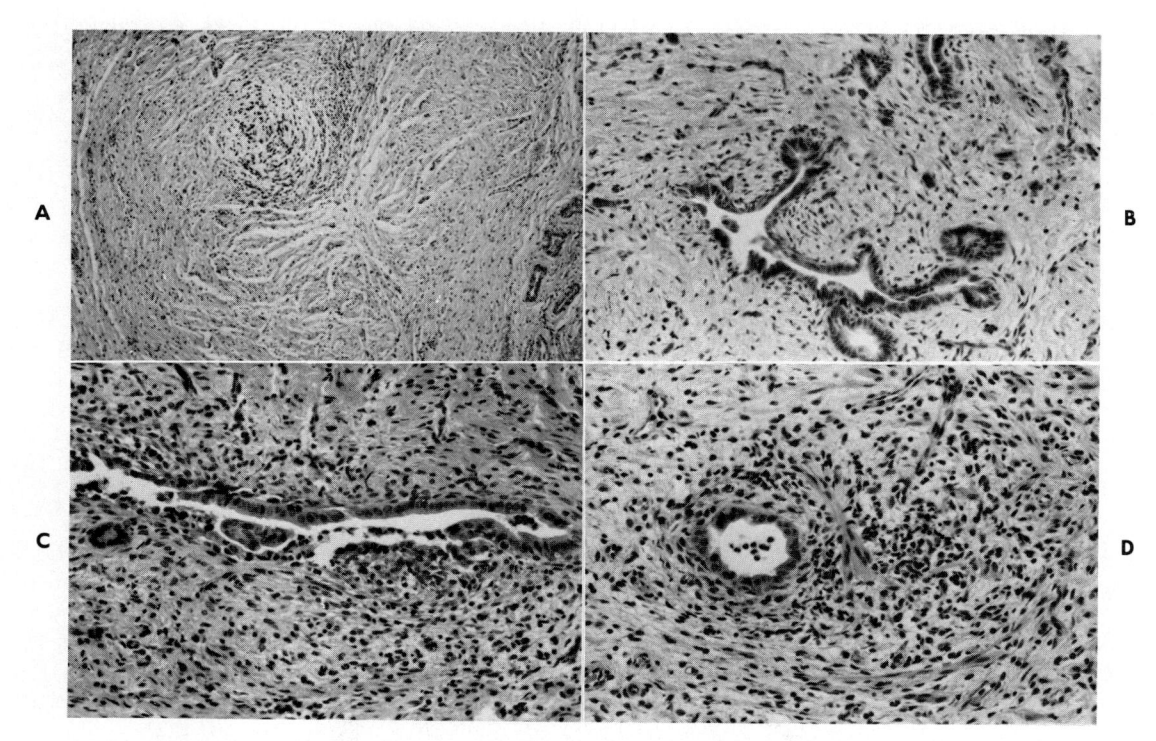

Fig. 30-6. Microscopic preparations of "fibrous remnant" of extrahepatic biliary system resected during Kasai procedure for biliary atresia. **A,** Most distal portion of specimen, showing complete obliteration of lumen by fibrous tissue. **B** to **D,** More proximal segments illustrating a spectrum of changes that includes necrosis of lining epithelium, acute and chronic inflammation, mural fibrosis with distortion of lumen, and great variation in size of ductlike structures. (All micrographs ×60.)

sia ductular proliferation may be present without fibrosis, which will regularly develop later. Ducts frequently appear distorted (Fig. 30-6) because of a discrepancy between the rate of proliferation of biliary epithelium and that of the surrounding fibrous tissue. In percutaneous needle biopsies proliferated ducts are usually empty but on occasion may contain bile. In later stages of biliary atresia identifiable bile ducts in portal tracts may be absent, a condition referred to as secondary intrahepatic biliary atresia. Extensive paucity (atresia) of portal bile ducts, whether primary or secondary, is associated with a clinical syndrome resembling that observed in primary biliary cirrhosis, or sclerosing cholangitis, with hypercholesterolemia, xanthomata, and pruritus. Other changes in portal tracts include occasional inflammatory exudate, dilatation of lymphatic channels, and tortuous thick-walled arterioles. The liver parenchyma in biliary atresia shows intracanalicular and intracellular cholestasis with the intracanalicular component predominating (Fig. 30-7). In one third of all patients with biliary atresia there is giant cell transformation of hepatocytes. In most cases this transformation is limited to the centrilobular areas and is not accompanied by necrosis and inflammation. Extramedullary hematopoiesis also may be present.

Neonatal hepatitis. This disorder is characterized by marked irregularity in the size of hepatocytes and numerous giant cells (Figs. 30-8 and 30-9). Giant cells may contain from 4 to 100 nuclei. The cytoplasm of these giant cells is usually foamy and contains bile pigment. Intracanalicular cholestasis is less prominent than in biliary atresia. In fact bile canaliculi appear reduced in number when giant cells are abundant. Necrosis and inflammation are usually present. Kupffer cells are swollen and contain iron, bile pigment, and lipofuscin, probably representing phagocytosed debris of destroyed liver cells. Extramedullary hematopoiesis is almost always present. Although all these findings also may be seen in some cases of biliary atresia, it is the absence of portal bile duct proliferation that distinguishes neonatal hepatitis from biliary atresia (Figs. 30-5 and 30-8).

Treatment of neonatal hepatitis

Clinical management of neonatal hepatitis consists of supportive measures, since no specific therapy is known. Many infants have transient but significant obstruction to

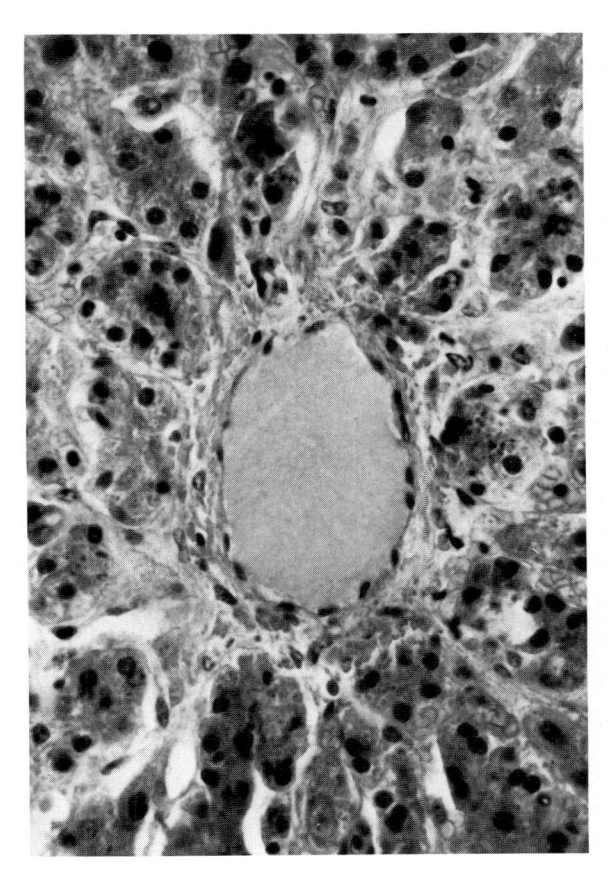

Fig. 30-7. Extrahepatic biliary atresia. Central vein surrounding hepatocytes. Intracanalicular bile plugs are present. In addition, hepatocytes contain intracytoplasmic bile pigment granules. (Paraffin embedding and hematoxylin-eosin staining.)

the flow of bile and often require replacement of fat-soluble vitamins, particularly D and K. Subclinical rickets is common in these infants and may contribute to the increase in serum levels of alkaline phosphatase. Persistence of acholic or very pale stools without significant lowering of direct-reacting serum bilirubin concentrations after 1 month should be viewed as an indication for repeat clinical study, including liver biopsy. This practice will permit detection of patients who sclerose their bile ducts after an initial phase of hepatitis and who are therefore suitable candidates for exploratory laparotomy and corrective surgery. On rare occasions patients with neonatal hepatitis and complete obstruction, as evidenced by acholic stools, may recover rapidly after operative cholangiography that shows normal extrahepatic ducts. This phenomenon is probably a result of "flushing out" of inspissated bile in the extrahepatic biliary system, with consequent relief of obstruction.

Fluctuations in stool color should alert the clinician to the possibility of the existence of a choledochal cyst. This can usually be diagnosed with ultrasound and treated surgically.

There are no early reliable criteria on which the prognosis of a particular patient can be based.

Treatment of biliary atresia

When the clinical evaluation indicates complete biliary obstruction or proves inconclusive, the patient should undergo an exploratory laparotomy. On entry of the abdomen after initial scrutiny of the biliary system an operative cholangiogram should be performed to confirm and characterize the extrahepatic lesion and define its extent. Operative examination of these infants should be performed only by surgeons prepared to proceed with corrective procedures if necessary. Reoperation after an exploratory laparotomy increases the technical difficulties and delays the institution of corrective measures.

Reconstitution of normal biliary drainage by direct anastomosis of existing bile ducts to the GI tract is possible in only a very small proportion of patients with biliary atresia (estimated at 5% to 10%). These include the rare cases of choledochal cyst and occlusion of a short segment of the common bile duct by a valve, membrane, or fibrosis. In most patients with biliary atresia there are

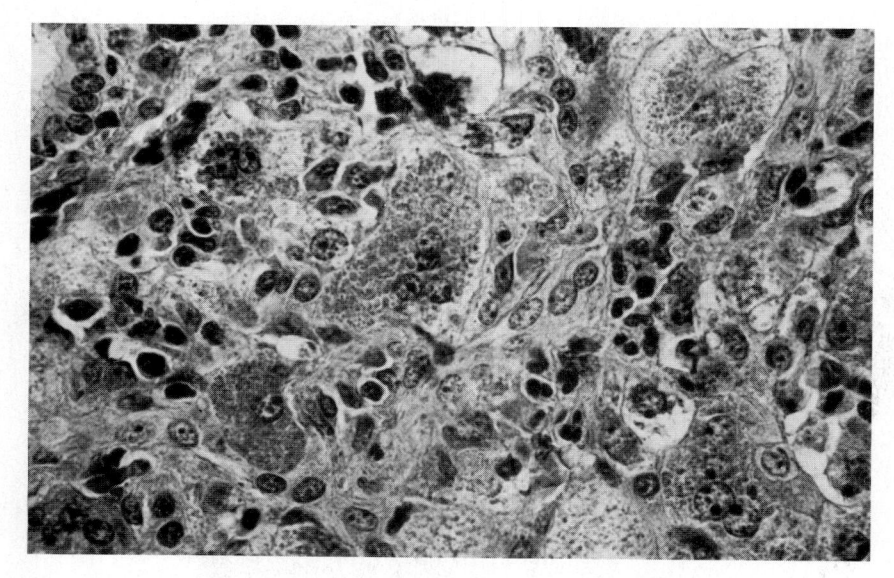

Fig. 30-8. Neonatal hepatitis. Note the marked cellular irregularity obliterating the normal orderly plate arrangement. Intracanalicular bile is present. Small cells in sinusoids represent Kupffer cells and elements of extramedullary hematopoiesis. (Paraffin embedding and hematoxylin-eosin staining; ×60.)

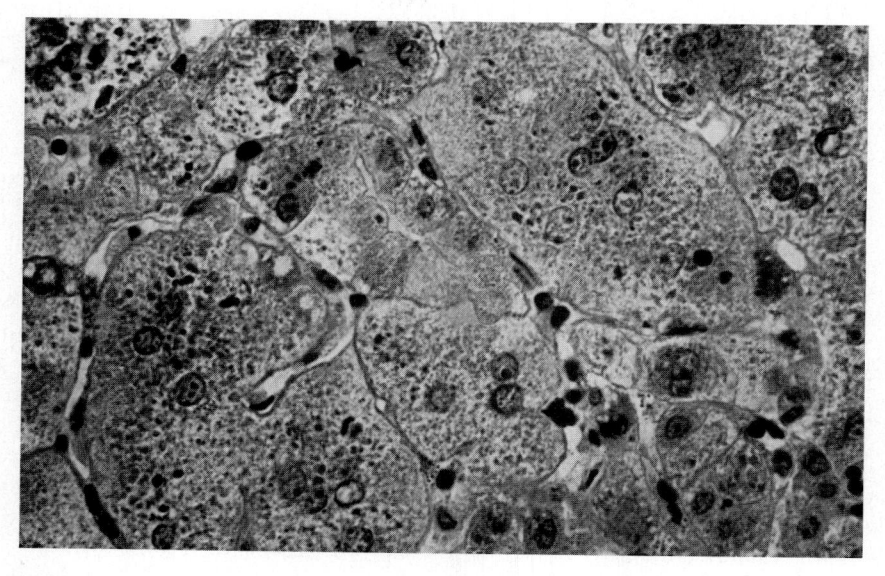

Fig. 30-9. High-power view of transformed giant hepatocytes. Most of the intracytoplasmic granules represent bile pigment. (Paraffin embedding and hematoxylin-eosin staining; ×200.)

no grossly visible ducts proximal to the atretic segment; in the past all these patients were considered inoperable. Untreated patients, although jaundiced, often appear clinically well in the first few months of life but deteriorate rapidly following development of cirrhosis with clinical manifestations of portal hypertension, ascites, hypersplenism, infection, and hemorrhage.

In 1968 Kasai and associates described an operative procedure in which the transected fibrous tissue of the porta hepatis is anastomosed to a Roux-en-Y loop of small intestine (portoenterostomy). Reconstitution of bile flow depends on the presence in the porta hepatis of bile duct–like structures that, although very small (100 to 800μm), are patent and confluent (Fig. 30-6). If the gallbladder and the cystic duct are patent and drain bile from intrahepatic ducts, a portocholecystostomy can be performed.

The optimal time for operation is not well established, but most centers report no success after the age of 4 months or at a time when cirrhosis is advanced. Mild hepatic fibrosis may undergo regression after reestablishment of bile drainage. Operative success is judged by the onset of bile drainage, which usually occurs between 1 and 4 days after surgery. The most frequent complication is that of ascending cholangitis, which may result in sclerosis and occlusion of the existing bile ducts. Recent modifications in technique have reduced the frequency of complications. Despite establishment of biliary drainage in approximately 40% to 60% of cases, the majority of these infants proceed to advanced cirrhosis and death.

Prognosis

At present relatively few long-term survivors or cures have been reported, but the number of patients alive and apparently well with no evidence of jaundice 2 years following operation is increasing. In a disease with mortality approaching 100% even a small salvage rate must be considered significant. Liver transplantation has been done in patients with biliary atresia or neonatal hepatitis that has progressed to cirrhosis. Few infants achieve normal liver function, and survival beyond 2 years is exceptional. The longest known survivor of transplantation at present is 7 years old.

Bile plug syndrome

Mechanical obstruction of a major bile duct may be caused by precipitated bile and mucus within the lumen (p. 482). The cause is obscure, although in a few patients it may be associated with cystic fibrosis. Clinical and pathologic findings are identical to those observed in biliary atresia and choledochal cyst. Diagnosis is made at surgery, and the bile plug usually can be removed. The condition is not known to recur.

Hepatitis caused by known infectious agents

In a small proportion of infants with neonatal hepatitis a specific infectious agent may be identified either by direct isolation and culture or by serologic tests that detect specific antibodies (p. 696). In some patients viral antigen may be demonstrated with liver biopsy, using fluorescein-tagged antibodies. Among infectious agents reported in association with neonatal hepatitis are bacteria such as *Treponema pallidum* and *Listeria* organisms and viruses such as rubella virus, Coxsackie virus, the herpesviruses (herpes simplex and varicella-zoster), cytomegalovirus, and adenovirus. The protozoon *Toxoplasma gondii* also has been reported. Fetal infection may take place in utero either by transplacental spread or by an ascending infection of the amniotic fluid, usually after rupture of membranes. In some cases infection may occur during delivery by aspiration of vaginal contents. Clinically patients in this group may appear sick and fail to thrive and also may have evidence of CNS and other organ involvement (p. 702). In many patients there are stigmata of generalized infection. Laboratory findings are similar to those seen in idiopathic neonatal hepatitis, but stools are not acholic, and therefore biliary atresia usually is not suspected.

Liver biopsy may be helpful in the diagnosis, especially in infections with the herpes viruses. These DNA viruses replicate in the nucleus, resulting in intranuclear inclusion bodies that can be seen with the light microscope. Cytomegalic inclusion disease is characterized by marked enlargement of hepatocytes and biliary epithelium caused by large intranuclear as well as intracytoplasmic inclusions. In some cases, however, the virus has been isolated from patients in whom liver biopsy results were typical of neonatal giant cell hepatitis with no evidence of inclusions.

Hepatitis B surface antigen (HB_sAg) may be transmitted from mother to infant, probably by aspiration of vaginal contents or blood during delivery (p. 696). With few exceptions infants born to HB_sAG-positive mothers show no antigenemia in cord blood or in the first month of life. Repeated serologic tests indicate that HB_sAg appears in the serum of these infants between 5 and 7 weeks of life and reaches a peak at 10 weeks. Antigenemia in the newborn may be associated with liver injury, and both may persist for many months or possibly years. It is necessary therefore to closely observe all infants of HB_sAg-positive mothers for many years for clinical and laboratory evidence of chronic liver disease. Severe and even fulminant neonatal hepatitis associated with HB_sAg has been described in infants of chronic carriers and after neonatal transfusions. The prophylactic use of hyperimmune serum for infants born to HB_sAg-positive mothers is strongly recommended by some investigators. Such therapy should be initiated as soon as possible.

Neonatal liver injury in metabolic disorders

Several metabolic disorders result in hepatocellular injury and give rise to a clinical pathologic syndrome that may resemble neonatal hepatitis or biliary atresia. The most commonly observed conditions are α-1-antitrypsin deficiency, galactosemia, tyrosinemia, and cystic fibrosis.

α-1-*Antitrypsin deficiency* in the homozygous state (PiZZ) may be manifested by neonatal liver injury. It is estimated that only 10% to 20% of all individuals with this abnormality will have liver disease. The majority of PiZZ individuals never develop clinical evidence of liver disease but may develop pulmonary emphysema as adults. Patients with α$_1$-antitrypsin deficiency may show all the signs and symptoms of neonatal hepatitis or biliary atresia, including acholic stools. Liver biopsy also may show changes consistent with either one of the aforementioned conditions; bile duct proliferation may be so pronounced that exploratory laparotomy is performed. In some patients hepatocytes, particularly in the periportal zone, contain intracytoplasmic inclusions that give a positive reaction with periodic acid–Schiff (PAS) stain. When frozen liver sections are incubated with fluorescein-tagged antibodies against α$_1$-antitrypsin, they bind with these inclusions, thus identifying them as α$_1$-antitrypsin. Similar identification of the intracytoplasmic inclusions can be carried out in paraffin-embedded tissue using the immunoperoxidase (PAP) technique. In many infants neonatal cholestasis may regress before the age of 6 months and reappear in later childhood or adolescence when the patient becomes cirrhotic. The pathogenesis of liver disease associated with this anomaly is not understood.

In *galactosemia* and *tyrosinemia* the infants fail to thrive and appear sick (pp. 817 and 831). Liver biopsy shows marked fatty accumulation in hepatocytes associated with fibrosis that may be quite extensive even in the first weeks of life. If there is no restriction of intake of foods containing galactose or tyrosine, cirrhosis develops and may lead to death in early infancy.

Cystic fibrosis may be associated with neonatal liver injury that clinically mimics neonatal hepatitis or biliary atresia. Injury is apparently caused by inspissation of mucus and bile in bile ducts. Such inspissation in a major extrahepatic duct may be responsible for the bile plug syndrome described previously. When smaller ducts are partially or completely obstructed by the inspissated material, a localized proliferation of bile ducts and associated fibrosis may develop and lead to a condition known as focal biliary cirrhosis. In some infants the dominant histologic abnormality consists of intracanalicular bile stasis and giant cell transformation of hepatocytes.

Liver injury associated with parenteral alimentation

Intravenous parenteral alimentation is being used with increasing frequency in many institutions (p. 310). Following prolonged use (several weeks or longer) many infants show evidence of conjugated hyperbilirubinemia, which may persist for some time after cessation of this mode of feeding. Liver biopsy shows evidence of hepatocellular injury with swelling of hepatocytes, necrosis, cholestasis, and occasional giant cell transformation. There is no information available as to the specific cause or eventual outcome of this abnormality.

Other causes of conjugated hyperbilirubinemia

Sepsis occasionally is associated with conjugated hyperbilirubinemia in the neonatal period. In some patients generalized bacterial infection may induce hemolysis, whereas in other cases hemolysis cannot be demonstrated, and toxic phenomena may induce functional cholestasis. Postmortem examinations of neonates with severe sepsis have shown central bile stasis, focal hepatocellular necrosis, and giant cell transformation in some patients. In others no hepatic pathosis can be demonstrated. Severe urinary tract infection, particularly with coliform bacilli, is associated with this syndrome; in this case generalized septicemia is not an essential feature, and cholestasis may be caused by massive endotoxin release. Antibiotic treatment is followed by prompt relief of hyperbilirubinemia.

Isolated cases of conjugated hyperbilirubinemia have been described in association with storage diseases, such as *Niemann-Pick disease* and *Gaucher's disease*, and with a familial disorder characterized by extreme *fatty liver*. Bland focal hepatic ischemic necrosis, typically with little or no inflammatory response, has been described in patients with *hypoplastic left-heart syndrome*, severe internal *hemorrhage*, and rarely in association with *umbilical vein catheterization*.

Conjugated hyperbilirubinemia associated with *cerebrohepatorenal syndrome*, *glycogenosis (type IV)*, and *familial recurrent cholestasis*, including *Byler's disease*, usually occurs beyond the neonatal period. *Indian childhood cirrhosis* and *congenital hepatic fibrosis* (with or without infantile polycystic disease of kidneys) rarely are seen with significant conjugated hyperbilirubinemia in the neonatal period. Additional rare causes of conjugated hyperbilirubinemia include tumors, such as *metastatic neuroblastoma* and primary *hepatoblastoma*. In these cases development of jaundice is usually delayed until after 2 months of age. Tumors and enlarged periductal lymph nodes also may obstruct the extrahepatic biliary ducts.

Rachel Morecki
Lawrence M. Gartner
Kwang-Sun Lee

BIBLIOGRAPHY

Pathophysiology

Andres, J.M., and others: Developmental hepatology and mechanisms of liver dysfunction, part I, J. Pediatr. **90**:686, 1977.

French, S.W., and Davies, P.L.: Ultrastructural localization of actin-like filaments in rat hepatocytes, Gastroenterology **68**:765, 1975.

Phillips, M.J., and others: Microfilament dysfunction as a possible cause of intrahepatic cholestasis, Gastroenterology **69**;48, 1975.

Popper, H., and Schaffner, F.: Pathophysiology of cholestasis, Hum. Pathol. **1**:1, 1970.

Biliary atresia and neonatal hepatitis

Aagenaes, O.: Hereditary recurrent cholestasis with lymphoedema; two families, Acta Paediatr. Scand. **63**:465, 1974.

Aagenaes, O., van der Hagen, C.B., and Refsum, S.: Hereditary recurrent intrahepatic cholestasis from birth, Arch. Dis. Child. **43**:646, 1968.

Aagenaes, O., and other others: Neonatal cholestasis in alpha-1-antitrypsin deficient children, Acta Paediatr. Scand. **61**:632, 1972.

Alagille, D.: Clinical aspects of neonatal hepatitis, Am. J. Dis. Child. **123**:287, 1972.

Alagille, D., and others: Hepatic ductular hypoplasia associated with characteristic facies, vertebral malformations, retarded physical, mental and sexual development and cardiac murmur, J. Pediatr. **86**:63, 1975.

Alpert, L.I., Strauss, L., and Hirschhorn, K.: Neonatal hepatitis and biliary atresia associated with trisomy 17-18 syndrome, N. Engl. J. Med. **280**:16, 1969.

Altman, R.P., Chandra, R., and Lilly, G.R.: Ongoing cirrhosis after porticoenterostomy in infants—biliary atresia, J. Pediatr. Surg. **10**:685, 1975.

Ballow, M., and others: Progressive familial intrahepatic cholestasis, Pediatrics **51**:998, 1973.

Bangaru, B., and others: Comparative studies of biliary atresia in the human newborn and Reovirus 3 induced cholangitis in weanling mice, Lab. Invest. **43**:456, 1980.

Brent, R.L., and others: Persistent jaundice in infancy, J. Pediatr. **61**:111, 1962.

Brough, A.J., and Bernstein, J.: Conjugated hyperbilirubinemia in early infancy: a reassessment of liver biopsy, Hum. Pathol. **5**:507, 1974.

Campbell, D.P., Poley, J.R., and Alauporic, P.: Determination of serum lipoprotein X for the early differentiation between neonatal hepatitis and biliary atresia, J. Surg. Res. **18**;385, 1975.

Chandra, R.S.: Biliary atresia and other structural anomalies in the congenital polysplenia syndrome, J. Pediatr. **85**:649, 1974.

Craig, J.M., and Landing, B.H.: Form of hepatitis in neonatal period simulating biliary atresia, Arch. Surg. **54**:321, 1952.

Danks, D.M., and Bodian, M.: A genetic study of neonatal obstructive jaundice, Arch. Dis. Child. **38**:378, 1963.

Danks, D.M., and others: Extrahepatic biliary atresia; the frequency of potentially operable cases, Am. J. Dis. Child. **128**;684, 1974.

Danks, D.M., and others: Prognosis of babies with neonatal hepatitis, Arch. Dis. Child. **52**:368, 1977.

Gellis, S.S.: Biliary atresia, Pediatrics **55**:8, 1975.

Greco, M.A., and Finegold, M.J.: Familial giant cell hepatitis; report of two cases and review of the literature, Arch. Pathol. **95**:240, 1973.

Haas, J.: Bile duct and liver pathology in biliary atresia, World J. Surg. **2**:561, 1978.

Haas, L.: Intrahepatic cholestasis in the newborn, Arch. Dis. Child. **43**:438, 1968.

Hitch, D.C., Shikes, R.H., and Lilly, G.R.: Determinants of survival after Kasai's operation for biliary atresia using actuarial analysis, J. Pediatr. Surg. **14**:310, 1979.

Javitt, N.B., and others: Cholestatic syndromes in infancy; diagnostic value of serum bile acid pattern and cholestyramine administration, Pediatr. Res. **7**:119, 1973.

Kasai, M., Watanabe, I., and Ohi, R.: Follow-up studies of long-term survivors after hepatic portoenterostomy for "non-correctable" biliary atresia, J. Pediatr. Surg. **10**:173, 1975.

Kasai, M., and others: Surgical treatment of biliary atresia, J. Pediatr. Surg. **3**:665, 1968.

Kasai, M. and others: Technique and results of operative management of biliary atresia, World J. Surg. **2**:571, 1978.

Kattamis, C.A., Demetrios, D., and Matsaniotis, N.S.: Australia antigen and neonatal hepatitis syndrome, Pediatrics **54**:1257, 1974.

Kobayashi, A., and Ohbe, Y.: Choledochal cyst in infancy and childhood; analysis of 16 cases, Arch. Dis. Child. **52**:121, 1977.

Kobayashi, A., and others: Bone disease in infants and children with hepatobiliary disease, Arch. Dis. Child. **49**:641, 1974.

Landing, B.H.: Considerations of the pathogenesis of neonatal hepatitis, biliary atresia and choledochal cyst; the concept of infantile obstructive cholangiopathy, Prog. Pediatr. Surg. **6**:113, 1974.

Lawson, E.E., and Boggs, J.D.: Long-term follow-up of neonatal hepatitis; safety and value of surgical exploration, Pediatrics **53**:650, 1974.

Morecki, R., Glaser, J., and Horwitz, M.: Etiology of biliary atresia: the role of Reovirus type 3 infection. In Proceedings of the International Workshop on Biliary Atresia, New York, 1981, Marcel Dekker. (In press.)

Mowat, A.P., Pscharopoulos, H.T., and Williams, R.: Extrahepatic biliary atresia versus neonatal hepatitis; a review of 137 prospectively investigated infants, Arch. Dis. Child. **51**:763, 1976.

Odievre, M.: Long term results of surgical treatment of biliary atresia, World J. Surg. **2**:589, 1978.

Sharp, H.L., and Krivit, W.: Hereditary lymphedema and obstructive jaundice, J. Pediatr. **78**:491, 1971.

Sharp, H.L., and others: Cholestyramine therapy in patients with a paucity of intrahepatic bile ducts, J. Pediatr. **71**:723, 1967.

Smetana, H.F., and others: Neonatal jaundice; a critical review of persistent obstructive jaundice in infancy, Arch. Pathol. **80**:553, 1965.

Stiehl, A., Thaler, M., and Admirand, W.H.: Effects of phenobarbital on bile salt metabolism in cholestasis due to intrahepatic bile duct hypoplasia, Pediatrics **51**:992, 1971.

Strauss, L., Valderrama, E., and Alpert, L.I.: Biliary tract anomalies; the relationship of biliary atresia to neonatal hepatitis; Fourth Conference on the Clinical Delineation of Birth Defects, Birth Defects **82**:135, 1972.

Valman, H.B., France, N.E., and Wallis, P.G.: Prolonged neonatal jaundice in cystic fibrosis, Arch. Dis. Child. **46**:805, 1971.

Zeltzer, P.M., and others: Differentiation between neonatal hepatitis and biliary atresia by measuring serum-alpha-fetoprotein, Lancet **1**:373, 1974.

Hepatitis caused by known infectious agents

Allen, L., and Murphy, W.R.: Listeriosis, South. Med. J. **51**:1454, 1958.

Beckett, R.S., and Flynn, F.J.J.: Toxoplasmosis; report of two new cases with classification and demonstration of organisms in the human placenta, N. Engl. J. Med. **249**:345, 1953.

Chiba, S , and others: Primary cytomegalovirus infection and liver involvement in early infancy, Tohoku J. Exp. Med. **117**:143, 1975.

Desmonts, G., and Couvreur, J.: Congenital toxoplasmosis; a prospective study of 378 pregnancies, N. Engl. J. Med. **290**:1110, 1974.

Dupuy, J.M., Frommel, D., and Alagille, D.: Severe viral hepatitis type B in infancy, Lancet **1**:191, 1975.

Dupuy, J.M., and others: Hepatitis in children; study of 80 cases of B-type acute and chronic hepatitis, J. Pediatr. **92**:17, 1978.

Escobedo, M.B., and others: The frequency of jaundice in neonatal bacterial infections, Clin. Pediatr. **13**:656, 1974.

Hamilton, J.R., and Sass-Kortsak, A.: Jaundice associated with severe bacterial infection in young infants, J. Pediatr. **63**:121, 1963.

Kattamis, C.A., and others: Australia antigen and neonatal hepatitis syndrome, Pediatrics **54**:1257, 1974.

Nahmias, A.J., and others: The TORCH complex—perinatal infections associated with toxoplasma, rubella, cytomegalo- and herpes simplex viruses, Pediatr. Res. **5**:405, 1971.

Newman, C.G.H.: Perinatal varicella, Lancet **2**:1159, 1965.

Pugh, R.C.B., Newns, G.H., and Dudgeon, J.A.: Hepatic necrosis in disseminated herpes simplex, Arch. Dis. Child. **29**;60, 1954.

Rotthauwe, H.W.: Viral hepatitis in infancy and childhood, Clin. Gastroenterol. **3**:437, 1974.

Schweitzer, I.L., and others: Hepatitis and hepatitis associated antigen in 56 mother-infant pairs, J.A.M.A. **220**:1092, 1972.

Scott, R.B., Wilkins, W., and Kessler, A.: Viral hepatitis in early infancy; report of three fatal cases in siblings simulating biliary atresia, Pediatrics **13**:447, 1954.

Strauss, L., and Bernstein, J.: Neonatal hepatitis in congenital rubella, Arch. Pathol. **86**:317, 1968.

Zuckerman, A.J.: Viral infections of liver in childhood, Postgrad. Med. J. **50**:338, 1974.

Bile plug syndrome

Bernstein, J., Brayland, R., and Brough, J.: Bile plug syndrome; a correctable cause of obstructive jaundice in infants, Pediatrics **43**:273, 1969.

Liver injury associated with parenteral alimentation

Bernstein, J., and others: Conjugated hyperbilirubinemia in infancy associated with parenteral alimentation, J. Pediatr. **90**:361, 1977.

Tovloukian, R., and Seashore, J.H.: Hepatic secretory obstruction with total parenteral nutrition in the infant, J. Pediatr. Surg. **10**;353, 1974.

Metabolic disorders and other causes

Aagenaes, O., and others: Pathology and pathogenesis of liver disease in alpha-1-antitrypsin deficient individuals, Postgrad. Med. J. **50**;365, 1974.

Alagille, D., and others: Hepatic ductular hypoplasia associated with characteristic facies, vertebral malformations, retarded physical, mental, and sexual development, and cardiac murmur, J. Pediatr. **86**:63, 1975.

Bennett, C.E.: Congenital galactosemia, U.S. Armed Forces Med. J. **9**:112, 1958.

Cottrall, K., Cook, J.L., and Mowat, A.P.: Neonatal hepatitis syndrome and alpha-1-antitrypsin deficiency; an epidemiologic study in Southeast England, Postgrad. Med. J. **50**:376, 1974.

Crocker, A.C., and Farber, S.: Niemann-Pick disease; a review of 18 patients, Medicine **37**:1, 1958.

Dunn, P.M.: Obstructive jaundice and haemolytic disease of the newborn, Arch. Dis. Child. **38**:54, 1963.

Genz, J., Jagenburg, R., and Zetterström, R.: Tyrosinemia, J. Pediatr. **66**:670, 1965.

Hardwick, D., and Dimmick, J.: Metabolic cirrhoses of infancy and early childhood, Perspect. Pediatr. Pathol. **3**:103, 1976.

Lieberman, E., and others: Polycystic disease of kidneys and liver; clinical radiologic and pathologic correlation, Medicine **50**:277, 1971.

McAdams, A.J., Hug, G., and Boue, K.E.: Glycogen storage disease, type I to X; criteria for morphologic diagnosis, Hum. Pathol. **5**:463, 1974.

Nayak, N.C., and Ramalingaswami, V.: Childhood cirrhosis. In Becker, F.F., editor: The liver; normal and abnormal functions. B. The biochemistry of disease, series no. 5, New York, 1975, Marcel Dekker, Inc.

Odievre, M., and others: Alpha-1 antitrypsin deficiency in liver disease in children; phenotypes, manifestations and prognosis, Pediatrics **57**;226, 1976.

Oppenheimer, E.H., and Esterly, J.R.: Hepatic changes in young infants with cystic fibrosis; possible relation to focal biliary cirrhosis, J. Pediatr. **86**:683, 1975.

Porter, C.A., and others: α_1-Antitrypsin deficiency and neonatal hepatitis, Br. Med. J. **3**:435, 1972.

Ragazzini, F., Bartolozzi, G., and Ciampolini, M.: Neonatal cholestasis. In Gentilini, P., and others, editors: Intrahepatic cholestasis, New York, 1975, Raven Press.

Sass-Kortsak, A.: Management of young infants presenting with direct-reacting hyperbilirubinemia, Pediatr. Clin. North Am. **21**:777, 1974.

Sveger, T.: Liver disease and alpha-1 antitrypsin deficiency detected by screening of 200,000 infants, N. Engl. J. Med. **294**:1316, 1976.

Townsend, E.H., Jr., Mason, H.H., and Strong, P.S.: Galactosemia and its relation to Laennec's cirrhosis; review of literature and presentation of six additional cases, Pediatrics **7**:760, 1951.

Walker, W., and Mathis, R.K.: Hepatomegaly; an approach to differential diagnosis, Pediatr. Clin. North Am. **22**:929, 1975.

CHAPTER 31 The kidney and urinary tract

RENAL FUNCTION AND ITS MORPHOLOGIC CORRELATES

During intrauterine life the function of the nephric system is minimal; homeostasis of the fetus is dependent on the placenta, as evidenced by the absence at birth of abnormalities in fluid and electrolyte balance in newborns with bilateral renal agenesis. Formation and excretion of urine are essential, however, for the maintenance of an adequate amount of amniotic fluid. Moreover urine formation plays a role in the embryogenesis of the urinary system.

At birth the kidneys have a combined weight of about 25 gm, compared with 40 gm at 3 months of age and 300 gm in the adult. They often demonstrate persistence of a fetal lobular structure and, because of the laxity of the abdominal wall, are readily palpable. Because of the centrifugal growth of this organ, the medullary and juxtamedullary areas are thicker than the cortical area. The kidney of the full-term newborn contains its full complement of nephrons (800,000 to 1,000,000 per kidney). According to Potter and Thierstein formation of new glomeruli ceases when the length of the fetus reaches 46 to 49 cm and his weight reaches 2,100 to 2,500 gm. At birth the surface area of the glomerular capillaries and the length of the tubule are about one tenth those of the adult.

The most important distinctive physiologic feature of the newborn kidney is its relatively low level of function. Measurements performed some 30 years ago have established that the glomerular filtration rate (GFR) of the newborn is lower than that of the adult, even when corrections are made for body weight or surface area. More recent studies carried out in full-term or premature neonates have confirmed the initial finding and enabled us to establish a pattern of postnatal development of renal function. For unknown reasons the conceptual age of 34 weeks was found to represent a crucial point in the maturation of renal function in humans. A substantial and sudden increase in GFR appears to occur at this age regardless of whether development occurs in the intrauterine or extrauterine environment. However, for infants of the same conceptual age the rate of glomerular filtration is substantially higher in those born prematurely than in those who depended on the placenta for the maintenance of body homeostasis (Fig. 31-1). The low levels of glomerular filtration explain in part why the newborn is unable to dispose rapidly and efficiently of excess water and solute. This limitation is of no consequence under normal circumstances because the process of growth is associated with a high degree of anabolism of substances such as nitrogen, potassium, sodium, calcium, phosphorus, and water. Another characteristic of the newborn kidney is the more advanced maturation of the juxtamedullary nephrons. These nephrons, which are endowed with long loops of Henle, have a great capacity to reabsorb sodium and water and are principally responsible for the concentration of urine. The fact that the newborn is unable to reach levels of urine osmolality in excess of 700 mOsm/L, compared with 1,300 mOsm/L in the older child, is only in small part the result of morphologic immaturity. The main reason is the limited availability of urea, which constitutes about half the total osmolality of the renal medullary interstitium in the mature kidney. The almost complete anabolism of protein, which is characteristic of the healthy newborn, results in relatively little urea for excretion. Within 2 or 3 months, if protein is provided in sufficient amounts, the kidney reaches a concentrating ability which approaches that of the mature organ.

Another peculiarity of the kidney during early extra-

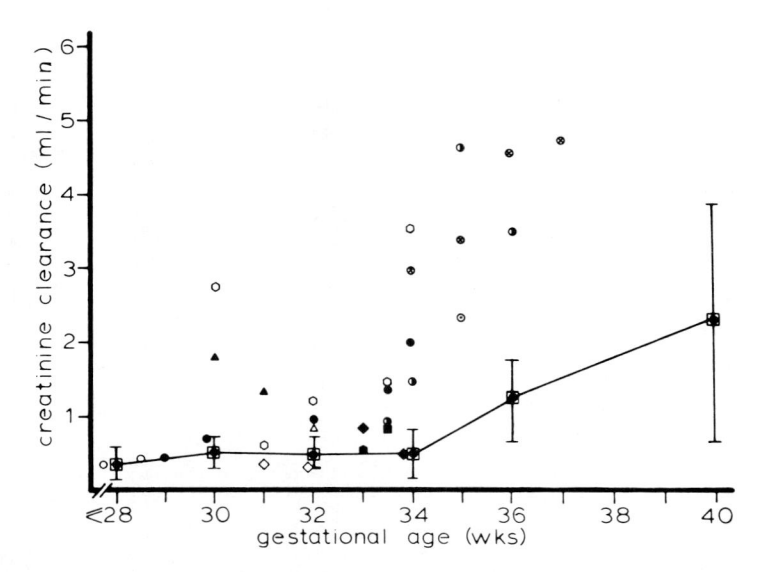

Fig. 31-1. Relationship between creatinine clearance and conceptional age (gestational plus postnatal ages). The line connects values of infants studied at birth, whereas the mass plot represents values obtained in infants studied at later dates. Measurements done in one infant at various ages are marked with the same symbol.

uterine life is the high degree of both anatomic and functional heterogeneity of its nephrons, related principally to the difference between relatively mature inner and immature outer cortex. For example, an elevenfold difference in tubular length has been found among the nephrons of the same kidney, resulting in a variable range of transport capacity of different nephrons. The glomeruli, on the other hand, show a much smaller degree of variation. Morphologic studies also show that the ratio between glomerular diameter and tubular volume is higher in the infant than later in life. This characteristic has been considered to result in a functional imbalance between the capacity to filter and the capacity to reabsorb or secrete and to explain why the newborn excretes in the urine a higher fraction of the filtered load of substances such as amino acids, phosphate, and bicarbonate. Recent studies indicate that in the newborn the glomerular capillary surface area might be smaller than suggested by measurements of glomerular diameter and that functional glomerulotubular balance is maintained for some substances such as sodium and glucose but not for others, such as bicarbonate.

The concentration of bicarbonate in blood is controlled by its renal threshold. This mechanism allows bicarbonate to remain in the blood only as long as its concentration is below a certain level. Above this level (the renal threshold) filtered bicarbonate is incompletely reabsorbed, and thus some is excreted in the urine. If the threshold is low, as it is in the newborn, the concentration of bicarbonate in serum, and therefore, the buffering capacity of the blood, is maintained at a low level.

This is a factor contributing to the tendency to develop acidosis in the newborn period, especially in premature and low birth weight infants (Fig. 31-1). Also responsible for this phenomenon are an increased production of organic acids and, because of the inability of the kidney to establish a steep gradient of H^+ during the first few days of life, failure to excrete strongly acidic urine. The low phosphate intake that is prevalent at this early age contributes to a low rate of excretion of titratable acid. Thus, if phosphate is added to the diet, a significant increase in urinary titratable acid ensues. Finally, ammoniogenesis also is diminished during the first few weeks of life, even under conditions of stress such as administration of ammonium or calcium chloride. The response of the kidney to acid loading becomes comparable to that of the adult by the end of the first month of life.

In summary, the immature kidney is characterized by a generally low functional capacity. The low rate of glomerular filtration limits the ability of the kidney to dispose rapidly of a fluid or solute load. The even greater limitations in tubular reabsorption may result in inappropriate loss in urine of substances present in the glomerular filtrate such as certain amino acids and bicarbonate. Although none of these limitations has a detrimental effect in a healthy neonate, they restrict the ability of the newborn to respond to stress.

REACTION OF THE IMMATURE KIDNEY TO INJURY

The tissue reaction of the newborn to suppuration, ischemic necrosis, and hemorrhage incorporates a greater proliferative or regenerative component than that in the adult. After injury epithelial cells undergo dedifferentiation and apparent multiplication to form distinctive glomerular and tubular forms that mimic a fetal appearance. Such epithelial patterns incorporate both regressive transformation and failure of differentiation. Although commonly seen in dysplastic kidneys, they do not in themselves signify a developmental anomaly, nor do they constitute evidence of an underlying congenital abnormality in an otherwise diseased kidney. These epithelial abnormalities, both glomerular and tubular, often coexist with involutional changes. For example, glomerular hyalinization, sometimes referred to as *congenital glomerulosclerosis*, is a process common enough to be regarded as normal. Ten percent of glomeruli will show histologic evidence of glomerulosclerosis and obsolescence, although we do not understand either the pathogenesis or the significance of the finding. Such changes are found in increased numbers as a consequence of renal necrosis, ischemic damage, and urinary tract obstruction. There is also increased severity of glomerulosclerosis in premature infants and in those with congenital heart disease.

Glomerulosclerosis frequently is accompanied by focal glomerular cyst formation; variable tubular atrophy and tubular cyst formation also may be present. In autosomal trisomy D and E syndromes, sclerotic glomeruli, incorporating both primitive and cystic changes, often are found in the peripheral cortex. Tiny cystic glomeruli are found in the peripheral cortex as subcapsular microcysts in many syndromes of multiple congenital malformations. The cysts are rarely of functional consequence and should not be confused with polycystic disease. It is not known if they are truly abnormalities of renal development and morphogenesis or if they are acquired changes of formed nephrons secondary to undefined metabolic, nephrotoxic influences. Cyst formation seems to be a common response of the fetal or neonatal kidney to severe forms of injury. Congenital urinary tract obstruction may be associated with cystic tubular dilatation, an uncommon effect of obstruction in later life.

An important aspect of the reaction of immature kidneys to injury is the effect on subsequent renal growth. Parenchymal disease beginning very early in life may lead to very small, end-stage kidneys, probably because subsequent growth and development are impaired by extensive epithelial damage, fibrosis, and vascular changes. In localized or unilateral diseases, on the other hand, the uninvolved parenchyma is capable of considerable compensatory hypertrophy and functional adaptation. This may relate to the great capacity of the immature fetal kidney for proliferation. All changes, even in full-term newborns, take place in the existing nephrons, and no new ones are formed.

INVESTIGATION FOR RENAL DISEASE

Clinical evaluation of the kidneys must include assessment of both morphologic status and functional capacity.

Morphologic evaluation

Gross morphologic characteristics can be investigated by a variety of roentgenographic and radioisotopic methods. A plain film of the abdomen often delineates the edge of the kidney, providing information concerning renal size and shape. In the neonate a small kidney almost always reflects a developmental abnormality rather than the effects of acquired disease. An irregular contour may be indicative of scarring following vascular obstruction or infection. This should be differentiated from fetal lobulation, which often persists into extrauterine life.

Ultrasonography (echography, sonography) is a method based on the property of tissues of varied density to produce echoes when sound waves of high frequency are directed toward them. This technique allows identification of an abnormal abdominal mass, such as a hydronephrotic kidney, or of the absence of a normal structure, as in unilateral renal agenesis. It also can distinguish cystic from solid formation. The noninvasive nature of this technique and the fact that it allows identification of structural anomalies regardless of the functional status make it very suitable for the investigation of the urinary tract in the newborn (Chapter 8).

Radioisotopic methods such as the renal scan and the renogram have the advantage of requiring much lower irradiation than the usual roentgenographic technique. The renal scan is of value in locating anomalous kidneys, determining kidney size, and demonstrating renal and other abdominal masses and changes in renal vascular perfusion. In the infant the renogram is used mainly in the investigation of urinary tract obstruction.

Excretory urography is still a widely used and valuable method of roentgenographic investigation of the kidney (p. 1077). The usual dose of 50% diatrizoate (Hypaque) sodium given to a child is 1 ml/kg, but in infants a dose of 3 ml/kg (up to a total of 20 ml) is used. For evaluation of a mass in the neonate as much as 5 ml/kg may be given. Since 50% diatrizoate has an osmolarity of 1,000 mOsm/L and a sodium concentration of 50 mEq/L, the material should be used with caution in dehydrated infants and in those with cardiac failure or renal insufficiency. Films taken shortly after the injection of contrast material reveal a "bodygram" effect from opacification of the vascular space. As a consequence, organs or other masses that are highly vascular are opaque, whereas avascular structures such as cysts are translucent and surrounded by a dark shadow. Since the renal parenchyma is visualized during the same phase, the resulting nephrogram can be used for measurement of kidney size and cortical thickness. Subsequent films permit visualization of the entire urinary tract and serve to define the status of the calyceal system, pelves, ureters, and bladder.

Voiding cystourethrography should be considered an essential part of the roentgenologic examination whenever obstructive uropathy is suspected or urinary tract infection has been documented. A 12% to 15% solution of a water-soluble contrast medium is instilled into the bladder through a catheter lubricated with an antibiotic ointment (a no. 5 feeding tube is adequate for the newborn). The catheter is removed when complete filling of the bladder is evidenced by leakage around the tube. Fluoroscopic observation of the urethra during voiding and of the bladder and lower ureters toward the end of voiding is essential.

Aortography and selective renal angiography are used in the differential diagnosis of abdominal masses, although their role is controversial. The inferior venacavogram may be of great help in the diagnosis of renal vein thrombosis. However, at least 30% of normal newborns fill the azygos and the hemiazygos septa during this procedure, and this finding therefore should not be considered diagnostic of obstruction. The diagnosis of Wilms' tumor usually can be confirmed by an intravenous urogram; although most of these tumors have a distinctive vascular pattern, some are avascular, and an angiogram may not help in the differentiation from an abscess. Angiography is of value in the diagnosis of vascular anomalies, such as segmental hypoplasia and arterial obstruction.

The microscopic morphologic characteristics of the kidney can be investigated by examining tissue obtained by *needle biopsy*. This procedure is used in the diagnosis of parenchymal renal disease; in expert hands the associated risks are minimal. Although indications for performing a renal biopsy in the newborn are limited, it is an extremely valuable procedure in appropriate patients.

Functional evaluation

Examination of a *freshly voided specimen of urine* provides immediate, invaluable information regarding the condition of the kidney. Although the neonate excretes a higher fraction of filtered protein in urine than does the older child, the concentration usually does not exceed 5 to 10 mg/dl of urine; as a consequence, protein is not detected by conventional methods of testing, such as Albustix or 10% sulfosalicylic acid. In the past the claim that the urine of the newborn contains significant amounts of protein was based on testing with trichloroacetic acid, which gave false positive results by reacting with urates.

Microscopic examination of the sediment obtained by centrifugation of a 10-ml aliquot of urine for 5 minutes should reveal less than 2 or 3 white blood cells (WBC) per high-power field and usually no red blood cells (RBC) and no casts or bacteria. Abnormal numbers of leukocytes are usually interpreted as indicative of infection. It should be realized, however, that leukocyturia occurs in many noninfectious conditions as well, including obstructive uropathy and a number of types of glomerulonephritis. More than a few cellular casts in the urinary sediment suggest renal parenchymal disease; RBC casts are the hallmark of glomerulonephritis.

The *Addis count* provides quantitative information on the rate of excretion in the urine of cells, casts, and protein. In addition, it can serve as a test of concentrating ability if appropriate restriction of fluid intake is imposed before and during the collection period. Since an accurately timed collection is essential for this determination, the test is difficult to perform in the infant. Moreover data from which the normal range can be established are extremely limited; up to 100,000 WBCs and 75,000 RBCs are considered normal. Detection of casts is unusual in the absence of disease. The amount of protein should not exceed 5 to 10 mg/12 hours. After an overnight thirst older children normally have a concentrated urine of at least 900 mOsm/L. After the first few days of life an osmolality of 700 or more is expected in infants' urine.

Since the elimination from the blood of certain substances, such as *urea* and *creatinine*, depends on the rate of glomerular filtration, their *plasma concentrations* serve as indicators of the level of renal function. However, the relationship between their concentrations in plasma and GFR is described by a hyperbola, so that until renal function is severely impaired, the increase in plasma urea and creatinine concentrations is relatively small, and their concentrations still may fall within the normal range. Furthermore the concentration of these substances in healthy infants is much lower than it is in older children. A creatinine concentration of 0.6 mg/dl, for instance, which is well within what is generally accepted to be the normal range for older children and adults, might represent a 100% increase over normal in a newborn and signify therefore a 50% reduction in GFR. Technical difficulties in accurately measuring creatinine in concentrations below 0.5 mg/dl further complicate interpretation of the results. Finally, the concentration of urea in plasma is markedly affected by the intake and rate of anabolism of protein.

A better estimate of the functional capacity of the kidney is given by measurement of GFR by one of a variety of *clearance methods*. The renal clearance is the amount of plasma that would need to be totally cleared of a particular substance by the kidney per unit of time to account for its rate of excretion in urine. The mathematic expression is $C = (U \times V)/P$, in which C is renal clearance, U is concentration in urine of the substance under study, V is volume of urine per unit of time, and P is the concentration in plasma of the substance under study. Conventionally clearances are expressed as milliliters per minute per 1.73 m² of body surface area. If a substance is freely filterable through the glomerular membrane, is physiologically inert, and is neither reabsorbed nor secreted, its clearance is equal to GFR. Inulin, a polymer of fructose, is such a substance. Its clearance remains the best determinant of GFR. However, since a continuous infusion of inulin must be given to maintain an adequate blood concentration during the test, and since the measurement of inulin involves a tedious chemical procedure, the clearance of inulin is not measured routinely. Nevertheless with this method GFR has been shown to be 25 to 30 ml/minute/1.73 m² during the first few days of life and 50 ml/minute/1.73 m² by the end of the first month. It must be emphasized, however, that individual variation and variability related to the method make interpretation of isolated results difficult unless they are clearly abnormal.

To obviate the need for continuous infusion, the clearance of some substances normally present in blood may be used to estimate GFR. The most commonly used are urea and creatinine. The advantage of the urea clearance is the high concentration of urea in blood and urine and the ease of its chemical determination. The disadvantage is the dependence of its excretion on the rate of urine flow, since urea is variably reabsorbed during passage through the nephron. At moderate rates of urine flow (2 to 6 ml/minute/1.73 m²) approximately 60% of the filtered urea is excreted in the urine, and thus the clearance of urea represents approximately 60% of the actual GFR. The main advantage of the creatinine clearance is its independence of rate of urine flow. However, the low concentration of creatinine in the plasma of infants and young children makes the laboratory method difficult and inaccurate. Since creatinine is excreted by tubular secretion as well as by glomerular filtration, its clearance may overestimate true GFR. Nevertheless the clearance of creatinine remains the best and most widely used method for measurement of GFR under usual clinical circumstances.

Recent progress in the mathematic analysis of multicompartmental models has made the calculation of GFR possible from the plasma disappearance curve of a substance injected intravenously as a single bolus. Substances excreted by glomerular filtration that can be labeled with isotopes, such as ^{125}I-iothalamate sodium and ^{51}Cr-labeled EDTA, as well as compounds that can be measured accurately by chemical methods, such as inulin, can be employed. This method obviates the need for the continuous infusion and timed urine collections that are so difficult to obtain in infants and small children. The amount of radioactivity provided by a single procedure is negligible. It appears, however, that the method overestimates the true GFR by approximately 30% during the first 2 weeks of life.

Many clinical situations require assessment of *renal acidifying mechanisms*. This is done by a determination of urinary pH and rates of excretion of titratable acid and ammonium during spontaneous metabolic acidosis or after administration of ammonium chloride and by performance of a bicarbonate titration. After the first few days of life healthy infants are able to achieve a urinary pH as low as 5. In the presence of acidemia higher values cannot be considered normal.

PRESENTING SIGNS AND SYMPTOMS

It is characteristic of the seriously ill newborn to have nonspecific signs of disease, such as fever, irritability, poor feeding, and failure to thrive. In such infants disease of the kidneys and urinary tract must be considered in the differential diagnosis. Certain signs that point directly toward urinary tract disease are discussed in this section.

Disorders of micturition

Ninety-two percent of healthy infants pass urine within the first 24 hours after birth and 99% by 48 hours. Often the first micturition takes place in the delivery room and goes unnoticed. If a newborn does not urinate within 72 hours, serious consideration should be given to the possibility of bilateral renal agenesis (p. 793), urinary tract obstruction (p. 797), or a renovascular accident (p. 791). Of these possibilities, the most important to diagnose is obstructive uropathy, since it is amenable to surgical correction. Perinatal asphyxia has been implicated recently as a cause of urinary retention in the newborn. Abnormalities in the volume of urine passed by the newborn each 24 hours are practically impossible to assess unless special attention is directed to the urinary system. The frequency of micturition varies from 2 to 6 times during the first and second days of life and from 5 to 25 times during the subsequent 24 hours. The daily urinary volume is 30 to 60 ml during the first and second days, 100 to 300 ml during the following week, and 30 to 50 ml/kg/24 hours subsequently.

Oliguria (urinary output below 15 to 20 ml/kg/24 hours) most often is a consequence of dehydration. Oliguria or anuria also can result from hypoxia, malformation, renovascular accident, or urinary tract obstruction. Oliguria of prerenal origin, as in association with diarrheal disease, maternal diabetes, or respiratory distress syndrome (RDS), usually can be identified by the high solute content of the urine, whereas in oliguria of true renal insufficiency urinary osmolality is low. Urinary retention can mimic anuria of renal origin. This retention can result from asphyxia, neurologic abnormalities such as meningitis or disturbances in the innervation of the bladder (for example, meningomyelocele), or from obstruction secondary to phimosis, posterior urethral valves, balanoposthitis, or vulvovaginitis. Palpation of the urinary bladder and, if necessary, bladder catheterization establish the diagnosis. *Polyuria* is most often the result of a defect in concentrating capacity, secondary to medullary abnormalities in renal dysplasia (p. 794), to renal hypoplasia (p. 794), or to nephronophthsis or medullary cystic disease (p. 796). It also is seen in association with lack of antidiuretic hormone or nephrogenic diabetes insipidus (p. 803).

Table 31-1. Proteinuria in the newborn

Gestational age (weeks)	Number	Amount of protein (mg/m²/hour) Mean	Range
<28	5	0.86	0.2-1.3
30	12	2.08	0-9.4
32	15	2.32	0-5.2
34	15	2.48	0-13.1
36	17	1.27	0-4.6
40	26	1.29	0-6.1

Proteinuria

Small amounts of protein ordinarily pass through the semipermeable glomerular basement membrane. Although the concentration of these proteins in the proximal tubular fluid probably does not exceed 1 to 2 mg/dl, it can account for a significant loss of protein through the uninary tract. Under normal circumstances more than 95% of this protein is reabsorbed in the proximal tubule. The remainder of the nephron also is able to reabsorb protein, allowing only very small amounts to appear in the final urine. The protein content of the normal urine may be as high as 10 to 25 mg/24 hours in children; de Luna and Hullet reported a mean urinary excretion in newborns of 45 mg/24 hours. However, no more than 10% of full-term and 20% of premature babies have proteinuria in excess of 25 mg/24 hours. The average rates of protein excretion in newborns of various gestational ages are shown in Table 31-1. The usual semiquantitative methods of measurement do not detect concentrations of protein below 5 to 10 mg/dl; as a consequence, significant amounts of protein can pass unnoticed under conditions of diuresis.

Protein excretion in 12- to 24-hour urine collections should be determined whenever renal disease is suspected. Documentation of proteinuria is only the first step in the diagnosis of kidney disease, however, since nearly any form of injury, whether glomerular or tubular, can result in an increase in the excretion of protein. Furthermore nonrenal disorders such as cardiac insufficiency, venous obstruction, pulmonary edema, and fever may be accompanied by transient proteinuria.

Hematuria

Blood can enter the urine at any point of the urinary system from the kidney to the urethra. In the normal newborn the excretion of RBCs in urine does not exceed 100 per minute, or 75,000 per 12 hours. Red urine usually indicates hematuria, but it also may be caused by the presence of bile pigments, porphyrins, urate, or hemoglobin. The differential diagnosis between hemoglobinuria and hematuria is easy to make if the urine is examined soon after collection. After standing, RBCs may hemolyze, especially in hypotonic urine, and no longer appear as formed elements. When hematuria is diagnosed, its origin must be determined. Extraurinary sources must be excluded. The next step is to determine if the RBCs originate from the upper or the lower urinary tract. Examination of a freshly voided urine specimen to detect the presence or red cell or other types of casts is extremely helpful, the presence of casts being pathognomonic of parenchymal renal disease. Hematuria in the newborn may result from perinatal asphyxia, a renovascular accident (p. 791), cortical and medullary necrosis (p. 807), neoplasia (p. 808), obstructive uropathy (p. 797), infection (p. 804), nephritis (p. 799), or coagulopathy (p. 808).

Pyuria

Pyuria is the presence of an abnormal number of WBCs in the urine. We do not expect to detect more than 2 to 3 WBCs per high-power field in a centrifuged specimen of urine. Littlewood found that bag specimens of well-mixed, uncentrifuged urine obtained from 600 newborns on the sixth or seventh day of life contained 5 or less WBCs per mm³ in 98% of boys but in only 56% of girls. The percentage in girls increased to 94% when a clean-catch technique was used, suggesting perineal contamination of the bag specimens. The most common cause of pyuria is urinary tract infection (p. 804). Increased rates of excretion of WBCs also can accompany nephritis (p. 799) and nephrosis (p. 800) and can be indicative of any type of inflammatory process within the urinary tract.

Edema

Accumulation of fluid in the interstitial space is a common manifestation of renal disease. It can be the consequence of a decrease in the colloid osmotic pressure of the plasma proteins, as in the nephrotic syndrome, or of a marked decrease in GFR, as in the various nephritides and congenital malformations. Almost invariably the pathophysiologic mechanism is complex, involving, in addition to physical factors, hypersecretion of aldosterone, and possibly inhibition of a natriuretic hormone. At an early stage the retention of fluid can be detected only by repeated accurate measurements of weight. Later swelling becomes obvious. It is generally stated that the edema of renal disease involves primarily the face and is soft, whitish, and painless. None of the characteristics, however, is specific.

Ascites is the intraabdominal accumulation of fluid (p. 532). It can occur in the nephrotic syndrome, in which case the fluid has the character of an exudate with a protein content that usually does not exceed 500 mg/dl. A more common, although still unusual, cause of ascites in the newborn is obstruction of the lower urinary tract, particularly in association with posterior urethral valves. The ascitic fluid represents urine that has leaked through a ruptured pelvis or calyx. The differential diagnosis includes chylous ascites, ascites caused by syphilis, hepatobiliary obstruction, ruptured intraabdominal cyst, meconium peritonitis, and bile ascites.

Edema occasionally is found in premature babies during the first few days of life and results from shifts of fluid between body water compartments. *Late edema* develops among some newborns with birth weights below 1,300 gm and a young gestational age. The accumulation of fluid corresponds to 35 to 36 weeks of gestation. No other gross abnormalities are found in these babies, and the edema usually is transitory. There are no significant differences in external water and electrolyte balances. A difference is observed, however, in the distribution of fluids between various body compartments, with the extracellular compartment being larger than normal in the edematous babies. The cause of this condition remains obscure, although some of these cases have been shown to be associated with vitamin E deficiency and anemia (p. 712). Unusual causes of edema in the newborn include primary lymphedema (Milroy's disease), congenital lymphedema with gonadal dysgenesis, the syndrome of inappropriate antidiuretic hormone secretion, hyperaldosteronism, congenital analbuminemia, severe protein deficiency, protein-losing gastroenteropathy, scleredema, syphilis, erythroblastosis fetalis, and hereditary angioneurotic edema. The differential diagnosis also includes maternal diabetes.

Abdominal masses

Examination of the abdomen by palpation usually can be performed easily during the first 48 hours of extrauterine life because of the laxity of the abdominal muscles. The kidneys of the newborn are in a lower position than they are later in life, the right usually being lower than the left. The technique of examination described by Mussels and associates led to the suspicion of renal

Table 31-2. Renal anomalies found in 56 of 10,000 newborn infants

Findings	Infants (number)	Percent of total
Horseshoe kidney	16	29
Renal agenesis, unilateral	15	27
Left	10	
Right	5	
Pelvic kidney	9	17
Left	5	
Right	4	
Hypoplastic kidney, unilateral	3	6
Renal agenesis, bilateral	2	4
Polycystic kidney	2	3
Multicystic kidney	2	3
Crossed renal ectopia	2	3
Double kidney, unilateral	2	3
Double collecting system, unilateral	1	2
Enlarged kidneys, bilateral	1	2
Wilms' tumor	1	2

anomalies in 77 of 10,000 infants; 56 of these anomalies were confirmed by intravenous pyelography (Table 31-2). Conditions accounting for an apparently large kidney are hydronephrosis (p. 798), tumor (p. 808), thrombosis of the renal vein (p. 801), and cystic disease (p. 794). The possibility of an adrenal hemorrhage also should be kept in mind. A smooth mass is more likely to be the result of hydronephrosis or renal vein thrombosis, whereas an irregular surface suggests malformation or cystic disease. Ultrasonogram, renal scintiscan, or intravenous pyelogram often is helpful in the differential diagnosis. A renal venacavogram may be necessary when renal vein thrombosis is suspected.

RENAL INSUFFICIENCY AND RENAL FAILURE

Inadequacy of renal function may be a consequence of developmental anomalies, may arise from prerenal factors such as dehydration and shock, or may be the result of acquired disease of the kidneys. The following are causes of acute renal failure in the newborn:

A. Prerenal
 1. Hypoxemia
 2. Hypokalemia
 3. Hypotension
 4. Cardiac failure
 5. Hemorrhage
 6. Sepsis
 7. Asphyxia
B. Renal
 1. Vascular accidents
 2. Nephrotoxins
 3. Pyelonephritis
 4. Nephritis

5. Hypoplasia/dysplasia
6. Renal agenesis
C. Postrenal
1. Neurogenic bladder
2. "Asphyxiated bladder"
3. Obstructive uropathy

Clinical manifestations

Renal insufficiency often is suspected on the basis of oliguria or anuria, or it may be detected from biochemical examination of the blood. Urinary output less than 15 to 20 ml/kg/24 hours in the newborn (beyond the first few days of life) is oliguria. It is vital to determine if the cause of oliguria or anuria is *prenatal* (caused by inadequacy of the blood supply to the kidney), *postrenal* (urine is formed but not voided because of obstructive uropathy or a neurogenic bladder), or *true renal failure* (malfunction of the kidneys caused by intrinsic renal disease). This differentiation is readily made in many instances, but at times it can be rather difficult. The variables that are of help in the differential diagnosis between prerenal and true renal failure are listed in Table 31-3.

Transient renal impairment with oliguria and azotemia has been observed in asphyxiated infants. GFR and urinary output often are diminished, and sodium excretion is increased in newborns with RDS. Acute renal failure is also an important complication of cardiac surgery in young infants, with attendant hypotension and hypoperfusion, and it may be of sufficient severity to affect the outcome. Functional studies have shown depressed GFR and urea clearance, diminished excretion of creatinine, and impaired dilution and acidification. Increased numbers of cells and casts are found in the urinary sediment. Tubular necrosis in postmortem material is, however, uncommon, and there has been poor correlation between clinical and pathologic findings. The observations suggest that functional impairment results from poor cortical perfusion and that tubular injury is a reflection of cortical ischemia rather than the cause of functional impairment.

Extensive roentgenologic or urologic investigation may be required to demonstrate the cause of postrenal failure. In prerenal failure, if insufficiency of the vascular volume is suspected, the response to administration of fluid may be helpful; isotonic saline in a dose of 15 to 20 ml/kg or on rare occasions mannitol (0.5 gm/kg in a 20% solution) can be given intravenously in 20 to 30 minutes. A prompt increase in urinary output suggests that additional fluids may be needed. If there is no response, care must be taken to avoid administration of excessive amounts of fluids to "force" a diuresis.

Treatment

Treatment of renal insufficiency in the neonate is similar to treatment in the older child. Consideration must be given to maintenance of the balance of water, electrolytes, and hydrogen ions and to provision of optimal nutrition. Acute renal insufficiency is treated by providing a fluid intake equal to insensible water loss (25 to 40 ml/kg/24 hours) plus urinary output. In the anuric or severely oliguric patient solute requiring urinary excretion is not given. In addition to withholding potassium, it may be necessary to reduce dangerously high plasma levels. When the concentration in plasma exceeds 5 mEq/L, polystyrene sodium sulfonate (Kayexalate), a Na^+/K^+ exchange resin, can be given (by enema or by mouth) in a starting dose of 0.5 to 1.5 gm/kg. This is repeated as needed. Moderate or severe degrees of acidemia are treated by administration of sodium bicarbonate. Peritoneal dialysis may be indicated in the infant with total renal failure lasting more than 7 to 10 days or when severe metabolic disturbances cannot be managed with medical treatment alone.

In infants with chronic renal insufficiency adequate nutrition requires special attention. Mild to moderate degrees of renal insufficiency usually can be managed with proprietary formulas, such as PM 60-40 or SMA, as the sole source of nutrition. The usual dose of supplemental vitamins should be given. With lesser degrees of function other specific therapy may be required. Normal levels of pH and bicarbonate in the blood should be maintained by administration of sodium bicarbonate. This dosage is adjusted according to the patient, starting with 1 to 2 mEq/kg/day and increasing as needed. Concentrations of calcium and inorganic phosphate in the blood should be measured frequently. Young infants fed low-phosphate diets usually do not develop hyperphosphatemia until they reach advanced stages of renal failure. In such patients phosphate-binding gels (such as aluminum hydroxide gel [Amphojel]) can be administered, although they are usually poorly tolerated. A dosage of 50 to 150 mg/kg/day given orally is customary. If the plasma calcium level falls significantly below normal, supplemental oral calcium (such as calcium gluconate [Calglucon]) is given in a dosage of 10 to 20 mg (of elemental calcium) per kg per day. If these measures are not successful in maintaining normal blood levels of calcium,

Table 31-3. Differential diagnosis between prerenal and renal failure in newborns

	Prerenal	Renal
Urine sodium (mEq/L)	< 10	> 25
Fractional excretion of sodium (%)	< 1.5	> 3.5
Urine/plasma osmolarity	> 1.5	< 1.1
Urine/plasma creatinine	> 30	< 10
Urine/plasma urea	> 30	< 10

pharmacologic doses of vitamin D should be prescribed, starting with a dosage of 10,000 units/day. Recently oral dihydrotachysterol (DHT), an analog of vitamin D, and 1,25-dihydroxycholecalciferol (calcitriol), which are active in the absence of the kidneys, have been used successfully. Care must be taken to avoid too vigorous therapy and induction of hypercalcemia. The serum calcium × phosphate product should not be allowed to exceed 70.

In infants with severe uremia vomiting may be a most troublesome symptom. Treatment with one of the phenothiazine drugs may be helpful. Hypertension in infants (p. 617) is treated as in older children. Every effort should be made to maintain normal blood pressure. Treatment is usually initiated with a diuretic, such as hydrochlorothiazide (1 to 2 mg/kg/day), to which hydralazine hydrochloride (1 to 2 mg/kg/day in four divided doses), propranolol (0.5 to 1 mg/kg/day in 2 to 4 divided doses), or methyldopa (2 to 5 mg/kg/day) has been added. If these drugs are unsuccessful, guanethidine sulfate can be used (0.2 to 0.3 mg/kg/day as a single dose). Diazoxide, 5 mg/kg intravenously, is indicated whenever prompt decrease in diastolic pressure is required.

Infants who cannot be maintained in a satisfactory metabolic state by dietary and medical therapy alone are candidates for dialysis. Peritoneal dialysis can be used for short periods but may be inadvisable if prolonged treatment is anticipated. Hemodialysis, although technically difficult, has been done in infants, and candidates for such therapy should be referred to appropriate centers. Renal transplantation has not been successful in the neonate; but as experience is gained and technical problems are solved, it is likely to become available for even the smallest infants.

MALFORMATIONS
Renal maldevelopment

Clinical manifestations of renal maldevelopment in the newborn provide few clues to specific anatomic or etiologic diagnoses. Renal enlargement at times is detectable on abdominal palpation and occasionally causes abdominal distension. An inability to palpate the kidney may be an indication of renal agenesis or hypoplasia. Oliguria is less apparent than anuria, and abnormalities of micturition may be undetected. Unusual delay or difficulty in passing urine is reason for evaluating the renal status of the baby. Less specific clinical abnormalities include poor feeding, fussiness, vomiting, dehydration, and persistent respiratory difficulty. A high degree of suspicion is required to establish the diagnosis within the first few days of life, and clinical examination should include urinalysis, blood chemical determinations, ultrasonography, and excretory urography. Urologic examination may be necessary to evaluate abnormalities of the lower urinary tract. Therapy tends to be supportive rather than curative. Certain lesions are lethal because of irremediable parenchymal malformation or because of severe urinary tract obstruction, which often is associated with renal dysplasia. The infant mortality for all genitourinary malformations is approximately 10 per 100,000 live births, with 90% in the first month. Less severe degrees of malformation lead to partial functional impairment with few differentiating features. The objectives of prompt clinical recognition are to arrest and prevent continuing deterioration, especially by identifying those cases amenable to surgical intervention.

Abnormalities of renal development considered in this section include agenesis (the lack of renal embryogenesis), dysplasia (an altered embryogenesis and abnormal differentiation of metanephric structures), and polycystic disease (a diffuse cystic alteration of the kidney without evidence of other maldevelopment). In renal agenesis one or both kidneys are lacking. The diagnosis of dysplasia rests on the finding of abnormally differentiated metanephric structures. Such abnormalities may affect all or part of a kidney, and examples of dysplasia encompass both extremely small, rudimentary kidneys and greatly enlarged kidneys. Some types are markedly cystic, but they must be differentiated from polycystic disease, even though the kidneys may be diffusely or totally affected. Polycystic disease differs clinically and morphologically from cystic dysplasia.

Bilateral renal agenesis, the complete absence of both kidneys, is a common malformation, occurring in approximately 1 of 10,000 deliveries. This condition is characterized by certain external features, including an abnormal facies with a wizened look, known as Potter's facies (Fig. 31-2). The ears are low set, often with folded helices, the chin is small, and the nose seems to be turned down at the tip. A skin crease characteristically curves around the inner canthus of the eye and runs laterally over the cheek. The legs commonly are bowed and the feet clubbed. These abnormalities and vernix nodules (amnion nodosum) on the placental membranes have been attributed to oligohydramnios (p. 47), a state common to several malformations in which fetal urination is absent or markedly diminished. The presence of oligohydramnios, in addition to the failure to detect kidneys and bladder by ultrasonography, can help in the antenatal diagnosis of Potter's syndrome.

Most cases are sporadic; a few familial instances have been noted, suggesting a genetic origin. The existence of an extra Y chromosome may be one of the predisposing factors. Chromosomal studies have shown normal karyotypes. Males are affected considerably more often than females. Infants with bilateral renal agenesis commonly are born prematurely, with evidence of intrauterine growth retardation. Breech deliveries are therefore com-

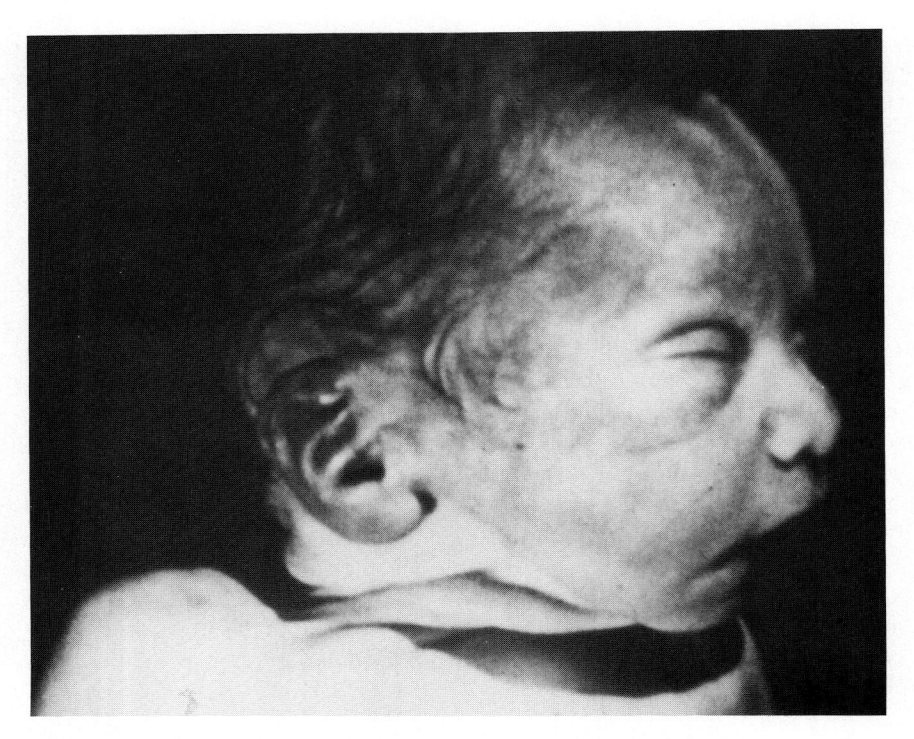

Fig. 31-2. Potter's facies. Characteristic are epicanthal folds, hypertelorism, low-set ears, mongoloid slant of the eyes, crease below the lower lip, and receded chin.

mon. A large number of affected infants, perhaps 40%, are stillborn, and most of the others die shortly after birth. A major postnatal problem is severe respiratory distress secondary to pulmonary hypoplasia with pneumothorax (p. 453). The lung may weigh as little as half the expected amount and often appears histologically to be underdeveloped. Occasionally infants surviving for several days appear to have died of renal failure.

Other frequently associated internal abnormalities include anal, duodenal, and esophageal atresia, colonic agenesis, and Meckel's diverticulum. The internal genitalia derived from the paramesonephric duct are usually defective or lacking (vas deferens and seminal vesicle in the male and the uterus and upper vagina in the female). The absence of one umbilical artery often is observed. Malformations of the caudal region of the fetus have been described with some frequency, and sirenomelic monsters characteristically have renal agenesis. Unilateral agenesis is a problem in newborns only in the event of injury to the other kidney.

Renal dysplasia, a condition of abnormal metanephric differentiation, is also a relatively frequent renal problem in the newborn. Severe bilateral dysplasia, like agenesis, is associated with oligohydramnios, Potter's facies, and death from respiratory distress or renal insufficiency within the first few days of life. Morphologic studies reveal two common anatomic forms of dysplasia: (1) aplastic kidneys, which are extremely small, sometimes barely recognizable buttons of tissue, and (2) multicystic kidneys, which are enlarged and grossly cystic. The two conditions are structurally similar, except for the cysts, and form the two ends of a spectrum of parenchymal malformation. The essential anatomic features are structural disorganization and histologic evidence of altered metanephric differentiation. The latter takes the form of metaplastic cartilage and abnormal ductal and nephronic elements. Cysts arise as terminal dilatations of collecting tubules (Fig. 31-3). Since cyst formation is variable, the two conditions cannot always be sharply separated. Multicystic dysplasia is the most common form of cystic renal disease in the newborn, and bilateral multicystic dysplasia in our experience has been more common than polycystic disease. The condition is only rarely familial; it does occasionally occur in association with chromosome abnormalities such as trisomy D and trisomy E.

Renal dysplasia must be differentiated from *hypoplasia*, in which the parenchyma is deficient although normally formed. Simple renal hypoplasia without evidence of parenchymal maldevelopment is seldom severe enough to cause renal insufficiency during the neonatal period. The abnormality was reported to occur in the fetal alcohol syndrome. Oligonephronic hypoplasia,

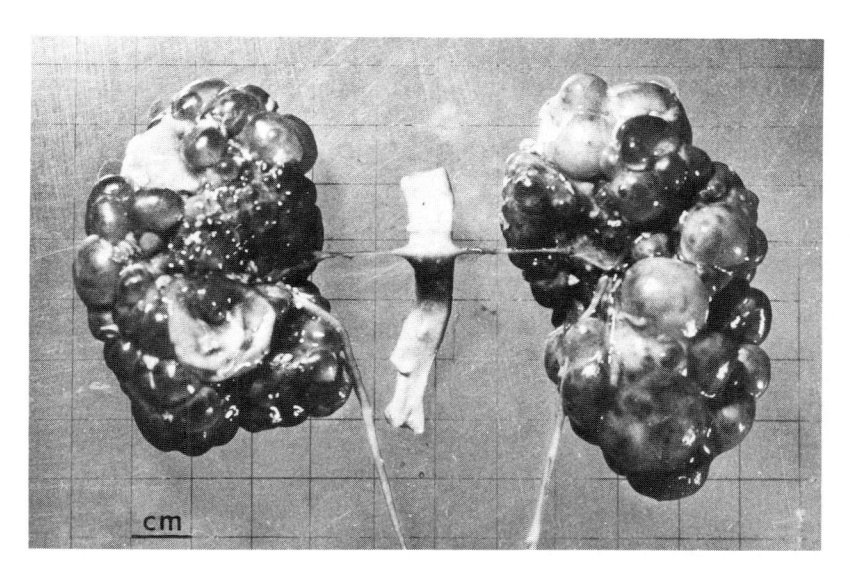

Fig. 31-3. Bilateral multicystic dysplasia in a newborn. The kidneys are enlarged and irregularly cystic, and the usual reniform configuration is barely apparent. Both ureters are atretic, and the renal arteries are extremely small. This condition is a cause of total renal nonfunction.

which also becomes clinically apparent in older children, is characterized by a decreased number but markedly increased size of nephrons.

Renal dysplasia commonly is associated with other anomalies of the urinary tract, with a frequency approximating 90%. Our experience has shown multicystic kidneys to be associated invariably with ureteral atresia and pyelocalyceal occlusion. The state of the ureter in renal aplasia has been more variable, partly because of the difficulty in drawing a sharp line between aplasia and less severe degrees of malformation. Consequently descriptions of ureteral stenosis, ectopy, and dilatation are not uncommon in reports of renal aplasia. With bilateral aplastic or multicystic kidneys abnormalities of the lower urinary tract, such as small bladders and constricted or occluded urethras, may reflect the lack of urine production. Malformations of other systems, particularly cardiovascular and gastrointestinal, are common. The frequency of renal involvement in newborns with multiple malformations is high.

Both aplastic and multicystic kidneys can be unilateral. Unilateral aplasia is asymptomatic, and its disclosure in newborns is usually an incidental finding in the study of another condition. The differential diagnosis of unilateral nonvisualization includes agenesis and severe hypoplasia. Unilateral multicystic kidney, on the other hand, frequently appears as a flank mass, more often on the left side and more often in males. Enlargement is usually moderate, although cystic kidneys can weigh several hundred grams and cause fetal dystocia. Ultrasonography may be diagnostic. Excretory urography usually fails to visualize the kidney, but high-dose urography ("total body opacification") may show selective concentration of contrast medium and partial opacification of the abnormal kidney. Endoscopic examination may reveal absence of ureteral orifice or nonpatency of the ureter. Although the lesion seems to be relatively innocuous with only rare reports of associated hypertension, most of these kidneys are removed, perhaps unnecessarily. The risk of a malignant nephroblastoma, often cited to justify surgery, is very remote. The prognosis in very young infants is uncertain, mainly because the contralateral kidney is hypoplastic or hydronephrotic in at least one third of patients. A careful assessment is mandatory, therefore, to identify abnormalities correctable by reconstructive surgery. The lesion of multicystic dysplasia is not, however, a progressive disease to which the other kidney will eventually succumb. The contralateral kidney often is hypertrophied and seems to be unduly susceptible to infection and lithiasis in older individuals.

An uncommon form of severe cystic dysplasia has been observed in newborns also suffering from cerebral malformation with encephalocele, eye anomalies, cleft palate, congenital heart disease, and polydactyly (an assortment of congenital abnormalities known as *Meckel's syndrome*). The clinical manifestations are nonspecific, and the severity of renal involvement is highly variable. The lesion superficially resembles polycystic disease in that the kidneys are enlarged and spongy, they retain a reniform configuration, and the pelves and ureters are patent. Gross examination, however, does reveal a lack of medullary differentiation and demarcation. Histologic

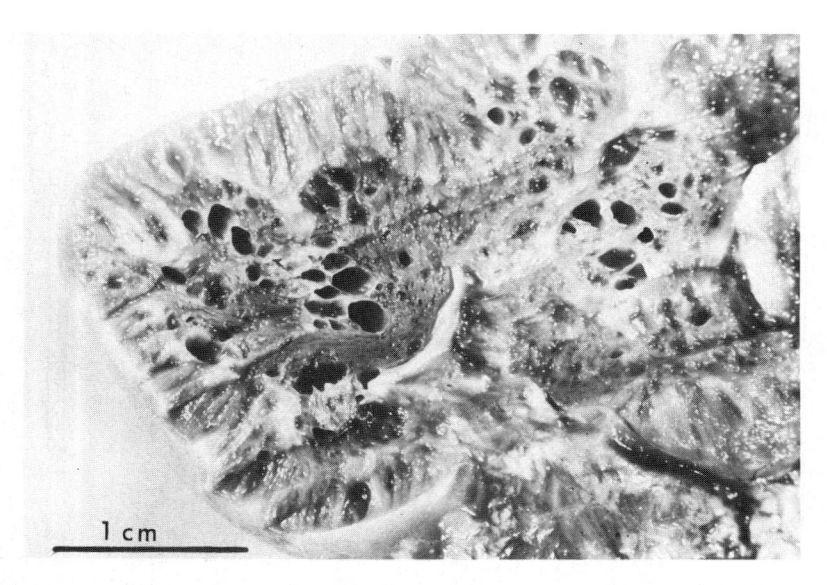

Fig. 31-4. Infantile polycystic disease in a newborn, showing the preservation of lobar structure and cortical-medullary differentiation. The cortex is thickened and spongy, and the medullary pyramids contain grossly apparent cysts; the latter are sometimes visible radiographically. (From Elkin, M., and Bernstein, J.: Clin. Radiol. **20:**68, 1969.)

examination discloses large numbers of cystic collecting tubules with little metanephric differentiation. Infants with less severe degrees of parenchymal maldevelopment with patent urinary tracts retain limited capacity to function; they have different clinical and pathologic implications because they can excrete urine and concentrate contrast media to some degree. Cortical dysplasia with variable functional impairment has been observed in association with *Jeune's syndrome* and *Zellweger's cerebrohepatorenal syndrome*. Trifling cortical cystic lesions in syndromes of multiple malformations are without functional significance for the newborn.

Cystic dysplasia must be differentiated from *polycystic disease*, which occurs in autosomal dominant and autosomal recessive forms. Autosomal recessive disease is by far the more common in newborns and has long been known as *infantile* polycystic disease (IPCD). Autosomal dominant disease, the typical *adult* polycystic disease (APCD), recently has been recognized to account for symptomatic neonatal disease with severe renal enlargement. Either type can appear sporadically or can affect multiple siblings. The clinical features on occasion may suffice to differentiate the two, and renal biopsies are often decisive, but a carefully taken family history commonly provides the best clue of all.

IPCD appears in newborns as bilaterally, often asymmetrically enlarged, diffusely spongy kidneys. There is dilatation of collecting tubules with relatively little fibrosis. IPCD is differentiated from cystic dysplasia by the preservation of renal shape and landmarks and by the absence of dysplastic microscopic elements (Fig. 31-4). Microdissection also has shown that the principal site of dilatation is in the collecting tubules. Portions of nephrons, including glomeruli, are variably dilated, and medullary collecting ducts are characteristically ectatic. In about a third of the patients polycystic changes are also present in the liver and only rarely in other organs.

Many affected infants are stillborn, and the majority of those born alive die within the first few days of life. The condition can be diagnosed clinically in infants with Potter's facies, abdominal enlargement, and a history of oligohydramnios. Abdominal distension at times has been severe enough to cause fetal dystocia. Respiratory distress and congestive heart failure are common. Electrocardiograms show left ventricular hypertrophy and left ventricular strain. Other infants have less severe renal insufficiency and survive the neonatal period. Again, ultrasonographic examination should be diagnostic. Excretory urography discloses delayed concentration of dye, a mottled nephrogram, and retention of contrast medium in small cysts (Fig. 31-5). Urograms in infants with better preservation of renal function show medullary ductal ectasia, the characteristic roentgenographic picture of IPCD.

Variation in clinical expression and in anatomic findings probably is related to the natural history and progression of a single disease. However, it also has been suggested that IPCD consists of several age-related, genetically different entities with somewhat differing morphologic characteristics and clinical expression.

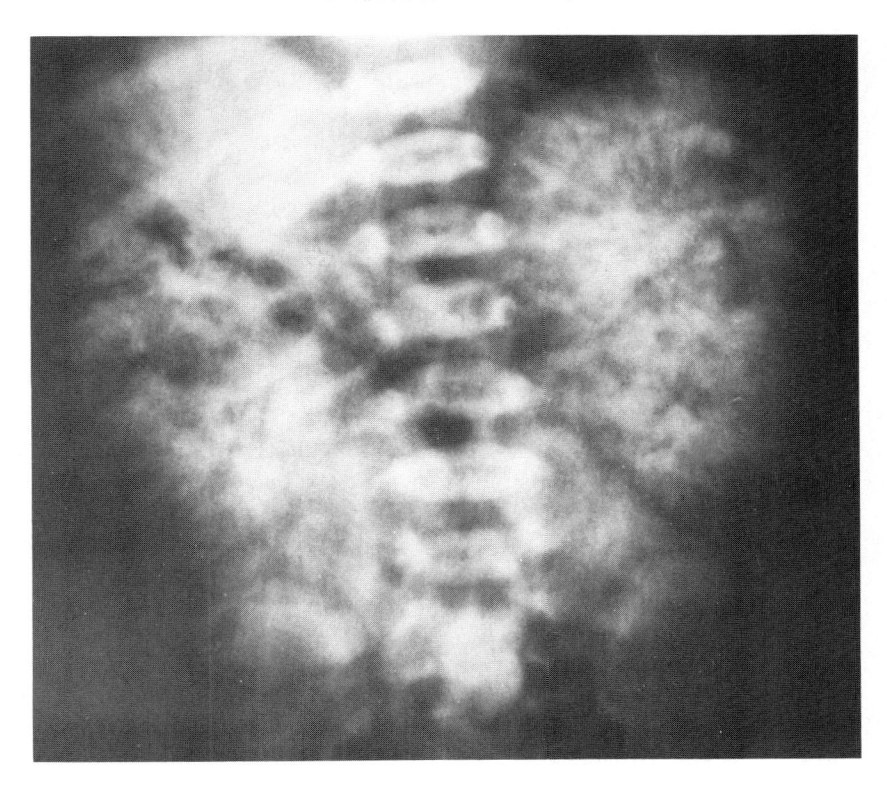

Fig. 31-5. Radiologic presentation of infantile polycystic disease. The irregular renal contour is caused by the presence of cysts.

Infants surviving the neonatal period often suffer from gradually increasing renal insufficiency. Hypertension usually appears. Older children also develop hepatic fibrosis and portal hypertension as part of the clinical spectrum of IPCD.

Adult polycystic disease recently has been recognized to cause serious renal disease in newborns. The roentgenographic pattern is irregular; some babies with APCD *seem* to have had mild medullary ductal ectasia. The cysts reside in nephrons, and cortical involvement may be very patchy. Severe neonatal involvement is, however, diffuse, and morphologic studies of renal biopsies show severe glomerular dilatation. Glomerular cysts cannot be regarded as synonymous with or pathognomonic of APCD, since they do occur in many other conditions, but symptomatic neonatal disease with glomerular cysts carries a presumptive diagnosis of APCD. Urographic studies of the parents of such babies have revealed typical APCD. There is a suggestion that the disease may stabilize in infants surviving the neonatal period, to progress in a more typical fashion during later childhood and early adulthood. Treatment of both forms of polycystic disease is supportive, with measures to avoid the lethal complications of hypertension.

Urinary tract obstruction

Obstruction of the urinary tract produces dilatation above the site of the lesion, and a retrograde rise in hydrostatic pressure may result in hydronephrosis and impairment of renal structure and function. Severe cases of obstruction are first seen in infancy, whereas milder ones are detected later in childhood. The presenting symptoms (such as failure to thrive, respiratory distress, abdominal distension, and vomiting) often are not specific, although a distended bladder or a hydronephrotic kidney, when palpated, is the clue to diagnosis. Ultrasonography usually will provide confirmatory evidence.

Urinary obstruction in early fetal life is a cause of renal parenchymal maldevelopment. An example is the condition known as ectopic ureterocele, encountered mostly in females. The kidney and ureter are duplicated, and one of the ureters, generally the one that drains the upper pole of the duplex kidney, opens ectopically in the trigone or bladder neck, commonly terminating in an intravesical cyst. The obstructed segment of kidney is usually dysplastic and the normally draining segment usually is normally developed.

On excretory urography the diagnosis is suggested by the duplication of the collecting system and a poorly visualized upper pole of the kidney. Visualization of only the

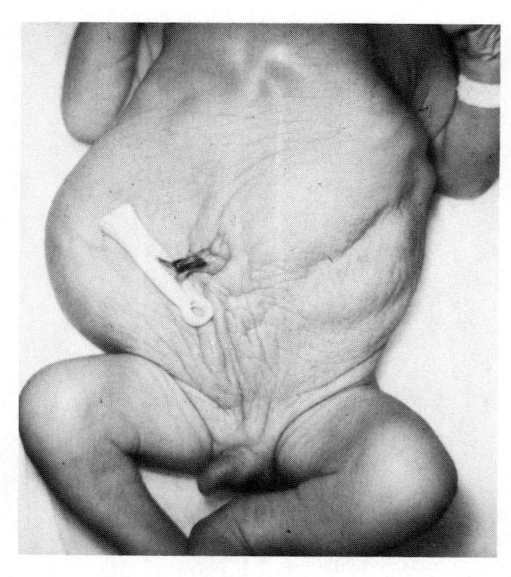

Fig. 31-6. Prune-belly syndrome. Note the distended, flabby abdomen wrinkled like a prune.

lower pole reveals the "drooping lily" sign, with little or no evidence of function in the upper pole. Cystography, when done with a minimum of contrast material, discloses a filling defect in the bladder, corresponding to the ureterocele. The diagnosis can be confirmed by cystoscopy. Treatment consists of heminephrectomy, ureterectomy, excision or uncapping of the ureterocele, and often reimplantation of the refluxing ipsilateral ureter.

Obstruction at the ureteropelvic junction occasionally causes giant hydronephrosis, which may be evident in the first month of life. Severe hydronephrosis often is associated with dysplastic parenchymal changes. On occasion the kidney associated with ureteral or ureteropelvic occlusion is normally formed and merely hydronephrotic. In such instances we have theorized that the obstructive ureteral lesion was acquired relatively late in gestation, perhaps shortly before birth, since many of these specimens are only moderately hydronephrotic despite a complete ureteral obstruction, suggesting a course of short duration. Corrective surgery may preserve adequate renal function in the children with mild hydronephrosis, although the roentgenologic appearance of the collecting system scarcely improves with time.

Lower urinary tract obstruction is more common in the newborn and occurs almost exclusively in males. The most frequent cause is valvular obstruction of the posterior urethra; other obstructive lesions with similar effects of varying severity are urethral atresia, cysts of the verumontanum, and urethral diverticula. Clinical findings of outlet obstruction early in life relate to urinary retention. Fetal ascites also has been described. Mild degrees of obstruction may go undetected for years, and severe obstruction results in vesical dilatation, hydroureter, and hydronephrosis. Respiratory distress, abdominal distension, vomiting, and poor feeding are frequent complaints. Urethral obstruction occasionally is associated with aplasia or absence of the abdominal musculature, the "prune-belly" syndrome (Fig. 31-6).

Bilateral flank masses and a midline suprapubic mass in male infants are evidence of bladder neck or urethral obstruction, despite a common clinical inclination to think first of cystic kidneys. Poor urinary stream, dribbling, and other abnormalities in micturition are apparent early in life. There may be complete obstruction, with failure to pass urine at birth. Roentgenographic studies show the obstruction usually as a dilated prostatic urethra ending abruptly at cusplike valves. The bladder is heavily trabeculated, there is evidence of secondary hypertrophy, and ureteral reflux is common. Infection is frequent, particularly after instrumentation. Obstructing valves are most often exaggerations of two mucosal folds that are normally continuous with the lower end of the verumontanum. Supraverumontanal folds and mucosal diaphragms are less common. Obstruction results not just from coaptation of the folds but also from a narrow, stenotic orifice between them. Ureteral dilatation and tortuosity need not be symmetric, and hydronephrosis is often only moderate. Infants with an obstruction severe enough to be apparent in the newborn period frequently have associated renal parenchymal maldevelopment, presumably resulting from the effect of obstruction on the developing kidney in utero. Renal dysplasia is much less often associated with milder degrees of obstruction apparent later in life. The most severe cases of posterior urethral valves and the highest mortality related to this malformation are encountered in the neonatal period. A case where there is evidence of bladder outflow obstruction should be considered an emergency, and immediate steps should be taken to establish the cause. The medical and surgical management should be thoroughly integrated. Any surgical procedure beyond catheterization of the bladder should await correction of fluid and electrolyte abnormalities. Some of these babies may need peritoneal dialysis before surgery. Removing the urethral obstruction is only part of the treatment. Ureteral dilatation and tortuosity are secondary causes of obstruction, frequently requiring draining of the upper urinary tract. Infection must be treated vigorously to prevent continuing renal damage, but the impairment imposed by parenchymal malformation cannot be reversed.

The condition known as the *prune-belly syndrome*, or *congenital absence of the abdominal musculature*, is first seen as a distended, flabby abdomen, which is creased like a prune (Fig. 31-6). Female infants comprise less than 5% of cases. The condition is rarely familial, and no cytogenetic abnormality has been detected. Failure of testicular descent is characteristic. Other congenital malformations, such as pulmonary hypoplasia, intestinal malrotation, and imperforate anus, also may be present. The ureters are dilated and tortuous, and the kidneys are hydronephrotic and often dysplastic, suggesting that a generalized developmental defect of abdominal parietes and mesenchyma is responsible for the entire syndrome. The bladder is large, dilated, and hypertrophied, indicating that infravesical obstruction also might be a causative factor. Aplasia or agenesis of the abdominal musculature has been seen in association with urethral atresia, urethral diverticulum, and posterior urethral valves. The bladder, however, is not trabeculated, despite its large capacity, and complete emptying often can be observed radiographically. The posterior urethra, also characteristically dilated, tapers at the membranous urethra, but evidence of increased resistance is lacking. Prognosis is related to the degree of obstruction, the extent of associated renal dysplasia, and the control of infection. Reconstructive surgery has been of limited help, and vigorous antibacterial therapy may be the main factor in prolonging survival. Drainage of the upper tract may be necessary to control infection and prevent continuing damage to kidneys that are frequently dysplastic. When there is associated urethral atresia, the prognosis is poor.

The Ochoa syndrome also is characterized by lower urinary tract obstruction in association with a peculiar facies. The condition probably is transmitted as an autosomal dominant trait.

Other abnormalities of the newborn, such as *exstrophy of the bladder, epispadias,* and *neurogenic bladder* (p. 386) caused by meningomyelocele, are problems in urologic management and require careful control of infection.

Vesicoureteral reflux

The prevalence of vesicoureteral reflux (VUR) among healthy newborns is unknown but appears to be low. None was detected in one series of 26 full-term and 66 premature newborns. A review of the literature revealed a rate of 0.4% among 1,015 normal infants and children. However, the number increases sharply in newborns with urinary tract infection. Among 160 newborns subjected to roentgenologic investigation because of bacteriuria, 61 were found to have VUR, 46 to a moderate or severe degree. In 77% of the 41 children monitored the reflux disappeared spontaneously, in the majority of them during the first year of life. The long-term prognosis of infants with VUR depends on the severity of the abnormality and the association with pyelonephritis. Renal scarring, hypoplasia of the kidney, and hypertension commonly are encountered among children with severe grades of reflux. There is a good likelihood that segmental hypoplasia (Ask-Upmark kidney) is a form of reflux nephropathy. Based on current knowledge a voiding cystourethrogram is indicated in any newborn with bacteriuria associated with fever or persisting beyond 1 week of age. Because of a high familial incidence of VUR, there are some who advocate screening in siblings of children with a history of reflux. The treatment of VUR may be medical (prophylaxis of urinary tract infection) in the mild and moderate degrees of reflux and must be surgical in severe forms.

NEPHRITIS

Acute glomerulonephritis is common in the neonatal period. Its principal cause today is congenital syphilis, a disease of resurgent clinical importance. Congenital luetic nephritis may result in the nephrotic syndrome in newborns and young infants. Other infants may have the clinical findings of hemorrhagic nephritis with hematuria, cylindruria, and moderate azotemia, accompanied by mild to moderate proteinuria. Pathologic studies have shown a proliferative glomerulonephritis with extramembranous deposits of immunoglobulin and complement. Mesangial proliferation may be minimal, despite immune deposits corresponding to a membranous nephropathy. The glomerular lesion frequently is accompanied by prominent cortical infiltrates of plasmacytes and lymphocytes, which may be strong clues to the diagnosis in renal biopsies. The clinical diagnosis usually rests on demonstrating other stigmata of syphilis and positive serologic tests (p. 674). Antibiotic therapy is ordinarily effective in treating the lesion and in reversing the nephrotic syndrome. A proliferative glomerulonephritis with subendothelial deposits of immunoglobulin has been described in congenital toxoplasmosis. It too has been associated with the nephrotic syndrome. Congenital systemic infection with cytomegalovirus, herpesvirus, or rubella virus may cause an interstitial nephritis with tubular lesions. These abnormalities usually have been postmortem findings of little clinical importance. Glomerular necrosis has been described in cytomegalic inclusion disease.

Chronic glomerulonephritis has been described in several necropsy studies. The patients were severely ill newborns, and in at least one report a rapidly progressing anemia suggested a hemolytic-uremic syndrome. Studies of renal function have been lacking, however, and it is presumed that the infants suffered from renal insufficiency. Some infants have been edematous, and the lesion has been associated with the nephrotic syndrome. The glomeruli were diminished by sclerosis and hyalinization, and severe epithelial proliferation and crescent formation were present in those which remained. Tubular atrophy and cast formation, intersti-

Fig. 31-7. Congenital nephrotic syndrome. Microscopic examination discloses sclerotic and proliferative changes in the glomeruli. The collecting tubules, particularly those near the corticomedullary junction, are dilated to microcystic proportions. (PAS stain; ×40.)

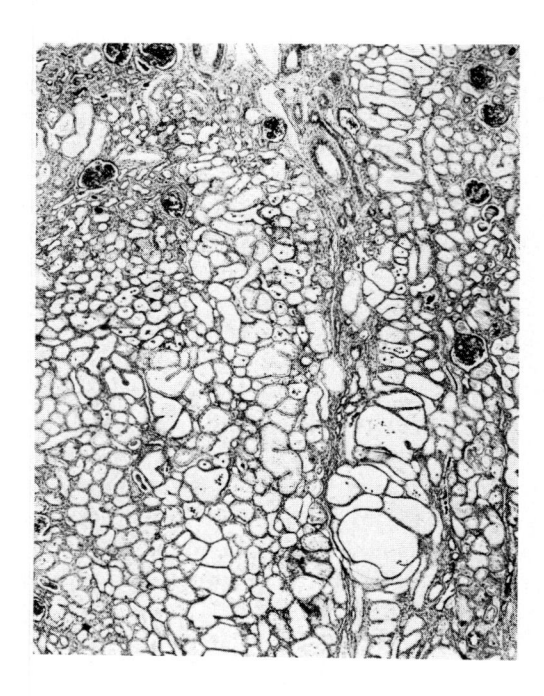

tial inflammation, fibrosis, and vascular sclerosis complete the picture. The lesion must be differentiated from *congenital glomerulosclerosis*, a process of glomerular involution and hyalinization that takes place in many and perhaps all newborns. Some cases reported as chronic glomerulonephritis may have been examples of severe diffuse mesangial sclerosis, as described in the section on congenital nephrotic syndrome. The number of sclerotic glomeruli found incidentally in newborns dying of other diseases, without renal symptoms, has been as high as 20%, although a figure of 5% to 10% is most commonly accepted. These glomerular changes may be associated with slight focal tubular atrophy; more extensive changes reflect some other disease.

THE NEPHROTIC SYNDROME

The characteristic features of the nephrotic syndrome—proteinuria, hypoproteinemia, hyperlipidemia, and edema—rarely are encountered during neonatal life. When present, they are usually the expression of the congenital nephrotic syndrome, a familial disease with an autosomal recessive type of inheritance.

Congenital nephrotic syndrome
Clinical manifestations

The majority of the cases of congenital nephrotic syndrome have been reported in Finland, where at least 130 families have been identified. Some 24 families, comprising 40 children, have been reported from the United States, and many other questionable cases have been described. The onset of the disease occurs during intrauterine life, as evidenced by large and abnormal placentas, qualitative similarity between protein content of the amniotic fluid and fetal urine, delivery of small for gestational age and premature babies in about 90% of the cases, faulty intrauterine calcification of the bones, erythroblastosis, and polycythemia (probably reflecting intrauterine anoxia). About 95% of the cases become manifest during the first 8 weeks of life, with most of the children showing proteinuria from the very first day. Pallor, mottling of the skin, cyanosis, and respiratory distress are accompanying symptoms. Protein electrophoresis shows low levels of albumin and IgG and high levels of α-globulin, mostly α_1-macroglobulin.

Prenatal diagnosis is possible because the concentration of α-fetoprotein is elevated in amniotic fluid and maternal serum.

Pathology

The characteristic lesion of the Finnish type of congenital nephrotic syndrome is the so-called microcystic kidney, which has been seen in approximately a third to a fourth of reported cases (Fig. 31-7). The cysts lie within dilated tubules near the corticomedullary junctions, but there is no evidence that they represent a primary abnormality in renal tubular development. Although initially the glomeruli may be only minimally altered, except for ultrastructural evidence of fusion of the foot processes, they undergo progressive sclerosis. Immunofluorescent studies generally have been negative. Another type of lesion found in early infantile nephrotic syndrome is diffuse mesangial sclerosis; the glomeruli are small and compact, containing increased matrix with few patent capillary loops and eventually undergoing complete sclerosis. In some patients the glomerular lesions are similar to those seen in later childhood and include minimal change, segmental glomerulosclerosis, and membranous nephropathy. Such patients respond to therapy much like older children do.

Etiology

The cause of the congenital nephrotic syndrome is unknown. Toxic factors such as mercury and phenol, infectious agents such as *Escherichia coli* and *Toxoplasma* organisms, and drugs such as corticosteroids have been considered but never documented. An immunologic process has been incriminated in the pathogenesis. Skin transplanted from infants born with this disease to their mothers undergoes accelerated rejection, suggesting intrauterine sensitization to the fetus. However, this could be the consequence of fetal-maternal transfusion resulting from placental damage. In nine patients with the congenital nephrotic syndrome γ-globulin and complement were demonstrated by immunofluorescent techniques in renal tissue obtained by biopsy or autopsy. These results have been challenged by Hoyer and associates and by Rapola and Savilahti.

Treatment

The condition is resistant to all forms of therapy. Approximately 75% of the patients succumb, most to infection, during the first 6 months of life. Isolated children have been reported with longer survival times. Recent attempts have been made to perform dialysis and transplants in these children.

Other forms of the nephrotic syndrome

Congenital syphilis, congenital toxoplasmosis, renal vein thrombosis, and cytomegalic inclusion disease are associated with a nephrotic syndrome in early life. A heterogeneous group of patients has been included under the name *atypical familial nephrosis*.

Congenital syphilis accounts for an increasing number of newborns with the nephrotic syndrome. The clinical presentation and the morphologic changes in the kidney are described on p. 674. Important differences from congenital nephrosis, which must be considered in the differential diagnosis, are the high levels of IgG in the serum (in contrast to the low levels encountered in congenital nephrosis) and the good response to antibiotic therapy. Congenital syphilis also must be differentiated from *congenital toxoplasmosis*, in which serum immunoglobulin values may be normal.

Renal vein thrombosis in the nephrotic syndrome occurs principally as a complication of membranous glomerulonephritis. Primary renal vein thrombosis (p. 806) does not lead to severe proteinuria and the nephrotic syndrome.

Cytomegalovirus infection occasionally has been associated with a nephrotic syndrome. None of the patients manifested symptoms of cytomegalic inclusion disease, such as jaundice, petechiae, or central nervous system disturbance.

Atypical familial nephrotic syndrome includes children with the nephrotic syndrome who are within the age range of congenital nephrosis but show a benign course and children who have the onset of the disease later in life but show changes characteristic of the congenital type of nephrosis. No such case has been described in Finland. Many children with this syndrome are offspring of related parents; some of them are identical twins; and in all families more than one sibling has shown signs of the disease.

ANOMALIES OF RENAL TUBULAR FUNCTION

Dysfunction of the renal tubule can result from a primary defect in the transport ability of the renal tubular membrane or can be secondary to a systemic disorder or disease. Primary defects include conditions such as renal glucosuria, renal tubular acidosis (RTA), renal phosphaturia, and the renal aminoacidurias. The latter group includes, among others, cystinosis, glycogen storage disease, Wilson's disease, galactosemia, heavy metal poisoning, hyperglobulinemia, and idiopathic and secondary hypercalcemia. The causes of the majority of these anomalies of renal tubular transport are unknown; some are inherited, a few are self-limited, many are inconsequential, some have a serious impact on growth and development, and some are amenable to therapy. This is a heterogeneous group of conditions which have as their common denominator one or more disturbances in the function of the renal tubule.

Cystinuria, Hartnup disease, familial iminoglycinuria, hereditary glycinuria, glucoglycinuria, and congenital lysinuria, although present from birth, usually become symptomatic beyond the newborn period. The same is true for tubular disorders, such as hereditary hypophosphatemia (familial vitamin D–resistant rickets), pseudohypoparathyroidism, and most forms of the Fanconi syndrome, including cystinosis (p. 802). The availability of screening tests for these anomalies makes possible their early recognition and treatment. Only some of the major syndromes particularly pertinent to the newborn period are discussed here.

Renal glucosuria

Glucose does not appear in the urine unless its concentration in blood reaches a level that is about twice normal. In patients with renal glucosuria the renal threshold for this substance is diminished, and glucose is excreted in the urine at normal or slightly elevated blood concentrations. Depending on the level of the threshold, glucose is found in the urine either consistently or only after a load, such as following a meal rich in carbohydrates. Two forms of renal glucosuria are described. In one of them (type A) the defect involves a depression in both the threshold and the maximal capacity to reabsorb glucose (T_mG). The other variety (type B) is characterized by a low threshold and a normal T_mG. Since the blood level at which T_mG is observed is far removed from the threshold, the magnitude of the glucosuria relates little to the level of the T_mG. No evidence exists regarding a defect in the intestinal transport of glucose in patients with renal glucosuria, although such an association has been documented in the familial glucose-galactose malabsorption syndrome.

The defect in renal glucosuria is present from birth and may account for otherwise unexplained episodes of hypoglycemia. The inheritance in the majority of patients is autosomal dominant, although an autosomal recessive mode of transmission also has been described. Results of examination of the renal tubular structures by light microscopy are normal; alterations in the mitochondria have been found on electron micrographs. No therapy is necessary other than recognition of the condition, avoidance of confusion with diabetes mellitus, and provision of a normal intake of carbohydrates.

The aminoacidurias

The amino acids normally present in the glomerular filtrate are actively reabsorbed, almost quantitatively, in the proximal tubule. The moiety that escapes reabsorption can be detected in the urine by paper or column chromatography. The excretory pattern varies with age, both quantitatively and qualitatively. In normal full-term infants ranging in age from 16 days to 4 months there is a relatively high fractional excretion of threonine, serine, proline, glycine, and alanine, suggesting immaturity of only certain transport mechanisms.

An abnormal excretion of amino acids in urine can result from (1) an increase in the filtered load that exceeds the reabsorptive capacity of the tubule, (2) competition of two or more amino acids for the same transport site, or (3) a selective or generalized defect of the transport system. Characteristically in the renal aminoacidurias plasma concentrations are normal. Five specific sites for the transport of amino acids have been described. The first system carries dibasic amino acids (lysine, arginine, and ornithine) and is defective in a condition known as *hyperdibasic aminoaciduria*. In *cystinuria*, in addition to these amino acids, excessive amounts of cystine are excreted. The second transport mechanism is responsible for reabsorption of the acidic amino acids (glutamic and aspartic acids). No human defect in the renal transport of glutamic acid has been identified, but a few patients with aspartyl-glycosaminuria have been described. The third pathway transports imino acids (proline and hydroxyproline) and glycine and is defective in *familial iminoglycinuria*. The remainder of the neutral amino acids share a common transport site, as evidenced by the fact that they are all excreted in excess in *Hartnup disease*. Studies of patients with β-alaninemia have served to define the fifth transport system, that for the β-amino compounds, such as β-alanine, β-isobutyric acid, and taurine.

A number of conditions are characterized by the excretion in the urine of abnormal amounts of most, if not all, amino acids. Yet in another group the impairment in proximal tubular reabsorption extends to other substances, such as glucose, phosphate, and bicarbonate (Fanconi's syndrome). In most cases the diagnosis of aminoaciduria cannot be made safely before 4 months of age, because in early postnatal life the excretion of amino acids is high. Nevertheless their existence can be suspected, particularly when the disease is present in family members. In some instances a prenatal diagnosis can be made by amniocentesis. Many of these abnormalities are inherited as autosomal recessive traits, and a few are X linked.

Cystinosis

Cystinosis, inherited as an autosomal recessive trait, is characterized by accumulation of cystine in the lysosomal fraction of the cells. Plasma cystine levels are normal. The symptoms result from involvement of several organ systems. The infantile form, which is the most severe, has been detected as early as the first month of life by the presence of aminoaciduria in apparently normal siblings of affected children. Thirst, vomiting, diarrhea, dehydration, unexplained fever, and failure to thrive usually become evident much later in infancy. If the child does not die of infection, acidosis, or hypokalemia, renal insufficiency ultimately occurs.

A reliable method of making a positive diagnosis is the determination of the cystine content of peripheral leukocytes, which is markedly elevated (up to 100 times normal). Treatment is symptomatic. Observation of patients who have undergone renal transplantation indicates deposition of cystine in the renal interstitium and not in the tubular cells, as is characteristic of cystinosis.

Oculocerebrorenal dystrophy (Lowe's syndrome)

Lowe's syndrome is characterized by multiple tubular dysfunctions, mental retardation, and severe congenital ocular anomalies. The condition is transmitted by a sex-linked recessive gene; all but four of the affected subjects reported were males. The female cases probably represent a different entity. The time of onset varies from the first few months to late childhood. Cataracts, frequently coexisting with glaucoma, are prominent features. The involvement of the nervous system is manifested by severe mental retardation, muscular hypotonia, and tendinous areflexia. Cryptorchidism is common. The renal disorder is characterized by proteinuria, aminoaciduria, and sometimes glucosuria. Therapy is symptomatic. Prognosis depends on the severity of the mental retardation.

Pseudohypoaldosteronism

Pseudohypoaldosteronism results from unresponsiveness of the renal tubule to aldosterone. The consequence is abnormal loss of sodium, hyponatremia, hyperkalemia, and metabolic acidosis. Plasma renin activity and aldosterone concentration are high. The mode of inheritance is sex linked. The symptoms (anorexia, vomiting, failure to thrive) appear 2 to 3 weeks after birth. Differentiation from the salt-losing form of adrenal hyperplasia is made by appropriate investigation of steroid metabolism (p. 915). In pseudohypoaldosteronism the excretion of 17-ketosteroids and 17-hydroxysteroids is normal, whereas the excretion of aldosterone is very high. Treatment is urgent and consists of administration of large quantities of sodium chloride. The need for salt supplementation seems to diminish with age.

Nephrogenic diabetes insipidus

Nephrogenic diabetes insipidus is characterized by insensitivity of the renal tubule to vasopressin. Most of the homozygotes are male, suggesting a sex-linked mode of inheritance. However, asymptomatic females have been reported. Symptoms appear shortly after birth; dehydration, unexplained fever, and failure to thrive are prominent. Polyuria and polydipsia usually are detected later. A significant delay in psychomotor development often occurs, apparently caused by chronic dehydration.

The pathogenesis is unknown. Differential diagnosis should include antidiuretic hormone lack, diabetes insipidus, bilateral renal hypoplasia, hydronephrosis, medullary cystic disease, or oligomeganephronia. Laboratory tests reveal hyperelectrolytemia with dilute urine. Vasopressin is ineffective. A water-deprivation test should be avoided.

The prognosis is good if the diagnosis is made early in life. Therapy consists of administration of sufficient fluids to maintain normal hydration. In infants the need for water can be minimized by giving a solute-poor milk. Thiazide diuretics have been shown to be effective in decreasing urinary volume and improving concentrating ability, although their mechanism of action remains unclear. Indomethacin, an inhibitor of prostaglandin synthesis, was reported to improve the concentrating ability and act synergistically with chlorothiazide.

Renal tubular acidosis

RTA is a defect in the reabsorption of bicarbonate or secretion of hydrogen ion that is not related to a decrease in GFR. RTA has three forms: the *proximal* type, resulting from the inability of the kidney to maintain a normal threshold for bicarbonate; the *distal* type, resulting from the inability of the kidney to establish an adequate gradient of secretion of hydrogen; and a *mixed* form that has been described recently.

Proximal renal tubular acidosis

Proximal RTA can appear as an isolated defect or coexist with other proximal tubular anomalies, as in the Fanconi syndrome (p. 802) or oculocerebrorenal syndrome (p. 802). The primary form is characterized clinically by failure to thrive and chemically by hyperchloremic acidosis. The great majority of patients are male. A transient form of proximal RTA also has been observed in newborns who have acute infections. This is self-limited but can account for transitory, "unexplained" metabolic acidosis.

Clinical manifestations. The diagnosis is made by demonstration of a low renal threshold for bicarbonate and a normal renal acidifying capacity. The former is determined by a study of bicarbonate reabsorption during continuous infusion of increasing amounts of bicarbonate. There is normal variation in threshold with age; the infant has a bicarbonate threshold of 20 to 22 mmol/L, whereas in the adult the threshold is 24 to 26 mmol. The threshold in the premature infant appears to be lower, perhaps 18 to 20 mmol/L. The ability of the kidney to acidify the urine is tested by administration of an acid load (ammonium chloride) and a test of the pH of the urine. Although during the first few days of life the newborn may not be able to lower urinary pH below 6.5 or 6.0, beyond this period urinary pH should reach a value of at least 5.0.

Etiology. The nature of the defect is unknown. Children with primary proximal RTA do not have a defect in urinary concentration and do not show evidence of rickets, urolithiasis, or nephrocalcinosis.

Treatment. Therapy consists of administration of sodium citrate or bicarbonate, usually in amounts exceeding 5 mEq/kg/day. The solution should be administered at frequent intervals, since it will leak into the urine shortly after being administered when bicarbonate concentration in blood exceeds the threshold. The condition is self-limited; most patients with primary RTA recover by 2 to 3 years of age.

Distal renal tubular acidosis

Distal RTA is a persistent defect in urinary acidification that usually occurs in isolated cases but may be inherited as an autosomal dominant trait.

Clinical manifestations. The condition affects females predominantly and tends to become overt after the age of 2 years. However, the onset often can be traced to the first months of life by a history of vomiting, anorexia, polyuria, dehydration, and failure to thrive. Beyond infancy, polyuria, growth retardation, nephrocalcinosis, and interstitial nephritis are the prevailing features. Rickets or osteomalacia, commonly encountered in adults with distal RTA, occurs rarely in children.

Etiology. The nature of the defect that prevents the kidney from establishing an adequate gradient of hydrogen ion between peritubular blood and tubular fluid is not known. Evidence that the defect is intrinsic to the renal tubular epithelium is provided by the normal behavior of the transplanted kidney in 15 patients with distal RTA.

Diagnosis. The diagnosis is made by observation of a urinary pH consistently above 6.5 or 7.0, despite spontaneous or induced metabolic acidosis.

Treatment. Therapy consists of administration of sodium bicarbonate, usually in amounts of 1 to 3 mEq/kg/day. The dose may need to be higher in the newborn. Some patients may require supplemental potassium as well. The dose is adjusted to maintain blood pH and bicarbonate within normal limits to ensure a maximal opportunity for normal growth. In addition, therapy is directed toward prevention of nephrocalcinosis; the dose should be sufficient to keep the excretion of calcium in urine below 2 mg/kg/24 hours.

Prognosis. Although primary distal RTA is a permanent defect, when it is correctly treated, the prognosis for growth and prevention of renal insufficiency is good.

INFECTION OF THE URINARY TRACT

See also Chapter 27.

Asymptomatic bacteriuria has been found in less than 1% of apparently healthy full-term infants; there may be a slight male preponderance. By contrast, studies in premature infants have demonstrated bacteriuria, confirmed by suprapubic puncture, in 2% to 5%.

Diagnostic methods

A variety of methods are available for collection of urine from the newborn for urinalysis and bacteriologic examination. Measures must be taken to avoid cellular and bacterial contamination. The simplest method involves careful cleansing of the external genitalia with soap and water, thorough rinsing to ensure removal of all soap residue, and application of a *sterile plastic bag;* Lincoln and Winberg also have suggested irrigation of the preputial folds of male infants. After application of the bag the baby is checked every 10 to 15 minutes so that the bag can be removed shortly after urination has occurred. If a stool is passed, or if the bag has been in place for more than 1 hour, the bag is removed, the baby is cleansed again, and a fresh bag is affixed.

Catheterization of the bladder is difficult to perform in the neonate because of the normally occurring phimosis of the male and the obscure position of the urethral orifice in the female. If a "bag" specimen is inadequate, a urine specimen should be obtained by suprapubic puncture of the bladder rather than by bladder catheterization.

Suprapubic aspiration of urine from the bladder is easily performed with 24- or 25-gauge, 1-inch needle. The needle is directed perpendicular to the skin, in the midline, 1 inch above the symphysis. In 10% to 15% of attempts no specimen will be obtained because insufficient urine is present in the bladder. Minimal degrees of hematuria are observed transiently in some infants and should be of no concern. This method may be contraindicated for infants with thrombocytopenia, coagulation disorders, or other conditions associated with a bleeding diathesis.

There are insufficient data on what level of bacterial concentration in a clear-voided, or "bag," urine represents the statistical dividing line between contamination and true bacteriuria in infants. Most workers have viewed counts in excess of 10^4 organisms per ml with suspicion, requiring that repeated examinations consistently demonstrate equal or greater numbers of the same organism to confirm the diagnosis. We have had the experience, however, of meeting these criteria only to find sterile urine from a suprapubic aspirate. Initial screening therefore should be performed on bag urine; those with bacterial counts in excess of 10^4 per ml should be repeated, and those found again to be in excess of 10^4 should be examined by suprapubic aspiration. Examination of urine collected by the bag technique will reveal no bacterial growth or less than 10^4 organisms per ml in 70% to 90% of cases, thus excluding these infants from further consideration. Infants with bacterial counts above 10^4 are candidates for repeat examination, although with this method even counts above 10^5 most often prove to be caused by contamination. It is assumed that any bacterial growth in urine obtained by suprapubic aspiration represents true bacteriuria, thus obviating the need for quantitation. Nevertheless, since most infected urine contains bacteria in excess of 10^5 or even 10^6 per ml, quantitation of bacteria in suprapubic aspirates can be helpful in that concentrations below 10^4 or 10^3 must be viewed as possibly representing contamination, despite the technique of collection. The great majority of cultures from infected infants reveal one organism; mixed cultures therefore are also suggestive of contamination.

In the infant about to be treated with antibiotics urine

should be collected by suprapubic aspiration rather than by bag technique, since the former technique yields the most reliable results; once antibiotic therapy is initiated, there is no further opportunity to distinguish between true and false positive reactions. If the clinical circumstances permit repeated examination of the urine before institution of antibiotic therapy, the simpler bag technique is acceptable, since positive reactions then can be confirmed or refuted by examination of a suprapubic aspirate.

Unfortunately it is difficult to determine what amount of leukocyturia is normal in the newborn. Houston found 76% of uninfected infants and children to have 0 to 10 leukocytes per mm^3 of urine, with another 20% falling within the range of 11 to 50. Lincoln and Winberg concluded on the basis of a survey of 500 newborns that normal males should have less than 25 and normal females less than 50 WBCs per mm^3 in clean-catch urine specimens. In contrast, Littlewood found less than 5 leukocytes per mm^3 in clean-catch urine specimens in 97% of male and 94% of female infants. However, Gower and associates reported that the presence of even more than 10 WBCs per mm^3 in suprapubic aspirates usually was not associated with a positive culture. There is a strong association between pyuria and bacteriuria in infants. Nevertheless most infants with pyuria do not have bacteriuria; conversely, significant bacteriuria can occur in the absence of pyuria. Therefore the final diagnosis of urinary tract infection in the neonate lies in the demonstration of bacteriuria.

Etiology

The spectrum of organisms that has been cultured from the urine of infants is similar to that from the urine of older children with urinary tract infection. *E. coli* predominates, but *Aerobacter*, *Klebsiella*, *Pseudomonas*, and *Proteus* organisms, coliform bacteria, and enterococci are encountered more frequently in infants than in older children (p. 668).

Pathogenesis

The majority of urinary tract infections in older infants and children represent ascending infections, that is, entry of organisms through the urethra, migration into the bladder, and then in certain instances extension to the kidneys. Information concerning the route of entry in neonates is not available. Infants found on routine screening to have significant bacteriuria may well have a simple cystitis, which represents a pathogenesis similar to that observed in older subjects. Although proof is lacking, at least some if not all instances of pyelonephritis that occur in the newborn in the absence of urologic malformation represent cases of blood-borne infection, with organisms lodging in the kidney during the course of bacteremia. Many infants with pyelonephritis, diagnosed during life or after death, do have associated septicemia. It is difficult to determine, however, whether the septicemia preceded or occurred as a consequence of the pyelonephritis.

In the majority of neonates with urinary tract infection urologic-radiologic examination reveals structurally normal kidneys and collecting systems. This finding is in striking contrast to infants diagnosed as having urinary tract infection during the remainder of the first year of life in whom the prevalence of urologic malformation has been reported to be as high as 50% to 80%.

Pathology

Postmortem studies of acute pyelonephritis have shown pus-containing tubules and ductules, interstitial edema progressing to fibrosis, and interstitial cellular infiltrates. Proliferative glomerular changes, seen occasionally, have been regarded as reactive. The lesion seems to be capable of complete resolution, unless suppuration and fibrosis supervene. Chronic and recurrent pyelonephritis, commonly associated with hydronephrosis, is accompanied by fibrosis, tubular atrophy, and glomerulosclerosis. Changes once regarded as localized nephronic malformations predisposing the infant to infection may be secondary sclerotic vascular changes; they are common and often are associated with hypertension.

Clinical manifestations

The majority of infants with urinary tract infection are asymptomatic; however, even in the sick infant there may be little clinical evidence to suggest infection of the urinary tract. The low incidence of asymptomatic bacteriuria in healthy full-term infants suggests that routine screening in this age group is not a profitable undertaking. In contrast, the infant with any evidence of illness is an excellent candidate for otherwise silent urinary tract infection; accordingly he should be examined appropriately. Screening of apparently healthy premature infants has detected significant bacteriuria in 2% to 5%, with some reports showing the incidence to be considerably higher than this. Repeated screening of premature infants during their stay in the nursery is worthwhile. Pyelonephritis has been reported to occur three to four times more commonly in male than in female infants.

Neonates with pyelonephritis may exhibit relatively little evidence of serious infection, or they may appear as toxic, septic, desperately ill infants. A syndrome of pyelonephritis, hepatomeagaly, hemolytic anemia, and jaundice (direct- and indirect-reacting bilirubin) has been described in several reports. Other features include poor feeding, lethargy, irritability, occasional vomiting and diarrhea, and azotemia. Hemolysis may be severe enough to require transfusion. The pathogenesis of this syndrome is unknown. The organisms most commonly cultured are the low-numbered serotypes of *E. coli*, especially 04:H5. As in presumptive septicemia (p. 650), treatment is urgent and cannot await the results of cultures. The response to antibiotic therapy usually is prompt, with a return of the blood urea to normal, resolution of hepatomegaly, clearing of jaundice, and cessation of hemolysis.

Treatment

See p. 654 for discussion of specific antibiotic therapy. Treatment should be followed by urologic investigation, including intravenous urogram and voiding cystourethrogram. Of utmost importance is the long-term follow-up monitoring, with repeated examination of the urine for possible recurrence of infection.

VASCULAR DISORDERS OF THE KIDNEY

Circulatory disturbances of the kidney include arterial obstruction, venous thrombosis, cortical necrosis, medullary necrosis, and tubular necrosis. These lesions constitute the most common group of acquired renal diseases in the newborn. All of them are believed to be related to obstruction or diversion of renal blood flow, and the ensuing renal necrosis relates in part to the extent, type, and location of the circulatory abnormality. The degree of renal injury is, however, quite variable; renal vein thrombosis, for example, is associated with complete cortical infarction in one case and inconsequential alteration in another. The clinical triad of renal enlargement, hematuria, and azotemia applies to almost the entire group of disorders of the kidney. The clinical identification of a specific condition or anatomic lesion is seldom possible. In general, therapy tends to be conservative and consists principally of maintaining adequate hydration. Anticoagulation appears not to have been helpful. Peritoneal dialysis has been used with some success in newborns.

Arterial obstruction

This lesion is usually acute and most often the result of thromboembolism. The embolus may originate from a thrombus arising in the ductus arteriosus. Thrombosis developing as a complication of umbilical artery catheterization has become more common in recent years. The renal arteries can be obstructed by an embolus or by a large thrombus occluding the aortic lumen. The ensuing renal infarction may be unilateral or bilateral and total or segmental, depending on the number and distribution of emboli. Embolic lesions also appear in the extremities, gastrointestinal tract, and head. Renal infarction results in an enlarged kidney and either oliguria and hematuria or anuria. There may be vomiting and abdominal tenderness. Infants also develop severe, acute hypertension and may be seen in congestive heart failure without obvious cause. Serum creatinine and blood urea nitrogen levels are elevated. Plasma renin activity is usually in excess of 100 mg/ml/hour, and renal scans indicate a diminution of the renal blood flow. Angiography may be needed to confirm the location of the vascular obstruction. An important consequence of unilateral or segmental arterial occlusion is subsequent renal atrophy with chronic hypertension. Segmental hypoplasia should be considered in the differential diagnosis. Hypertension may be transient and thus manageable by medical means, but it also can be severe and persistent, necessitating a nephrectomy. Hydralazine, 0.1 to 0.15 mg/kg, or diazoxide, 3 to 5 mg/kg, given intravenously, has been used successfully to control hypertension. The reason for surgery should be the persistence of the hypertension rather than the extent of the infarction, since the capacity of the kidney to recover functionally is impossible to predict in the early stages of the disease (p. 617).

Thrombosis of the renal veins

This lesion has been more common than arterial occlusion, although its frequency may have declined in recent years as the result of better fluid management and rehydration of distressed infants.

Clinical manifestations

Approximately half of over 300 reported cases have been in infants under 2 months of age. The most important factor in its pathogenesis appears to be dehydration, a mechanism that can account for cases of both antenatal and postnatal thrombosis. Other factors in newborns include relative polycythemia, relatively low renal blood flow and blood pressure, anoxia, and birth injury. Babies born to diabetic mothers seem to be particularly susceptible, perhaps as the result of glucosuria, polyuria, and dehydration or as the result of extravascular fluid shifts, hypovolemia, and effective dehydration. The intrauterine origin of the lesion has been amply demonstrated. We have observed organizing venous thrombi in a newborn with anencephaly, another condition that may be associated with polyuria and intrauterine dehydration. Renal vein thrombosis also is a complication of diarrhea of the newborn.

The vascular lesion occurs with or without renal infarction. Venous infarction can result in considerable renal enlargement and anuria or oligohematuria. Thrombocytopenia and depletion of clotting factors are frequent findings, suggesting intravascular consumption, but disseminated coagulation has not been clearly demonstrated. Vomiting, lethargy, anorexia, fever, shock, and associated findings may be related to the initiating causes as much as to the renal lesion. Excretory urography usually discloses nonopacification or slight, diffuse opacification. A venogram may demonstrate vena caval thrombosis. As a later phenomenon, the thrombi, undergoing calcification, occasionally are visible radiographically as radially oriented markings. The thrombi involve the smaller, intrarenal veins; thus surgical thrombectomy is unlikely to be beneficial.

Treatment

The lesion can be unilateral or bilateral, the former occurring more frequently. Prompt nephrectomy has been advocated in the past in the treatment of unilateral disease to prevent rapid progression and death. However, medical therapy developed in relation to bilateral venous thrombosis now has been extended to unilateral involvement. Such measures include rehydration and possible anticoagulation. The results of this approach are as good as those obtained with surgery.

Prognosis

Survival probably depends on the severity of the morbid state that precipitates the renal lesion and on the presence or absence of renal infarction, which cannot be reconstituted by either form of therapy. Heparin therapy for anticoagulation is potentially dangerous because of bleeding, and its effectiveness has not been established. The late hazards of medical management are renal atrophy, tubular dysfunction, and occasional hypertension.

Cortical and medullary necrosis

These two lesions overlap clinically and often coexist pathologically. The frequency of the lesions seems to be increasing relative to renal vein thrombosis, perhaps

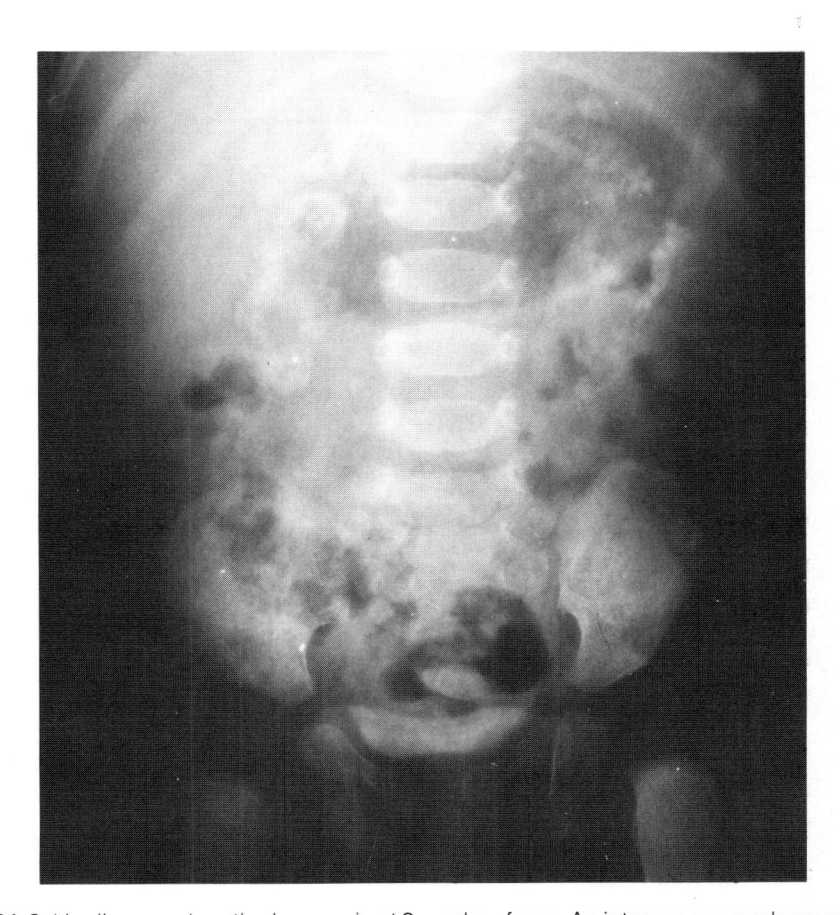

Fig. 31-8. Healing renal cortical necrosis at 9 weeks of age. An intravenous pyelogram at 10 minutes showing a faint nephrogram and faint opacification of the left renal pelvis and bladder. Bilateral renal cortical and adrenal calcification are evident. (From Leonidas, J. C., Berdon, W. E., and Gribetz, D.: J. Pediatr. **79:**623, 1971.)

because of longer survival of severely ill newborns in intensive care nurseries.

Clinical manifestations

The clinical findings are nonspecific and include renal enlargement, anuria or oliguria, and hematuria. Both cortical and medullary necrosis in newborns have been associated with severe anemia and asphyxia. Blood loss in anemic shock has been attributed to twin-twin transfusion, fetal-maternal transfusion, uteroplacental hemorrhage, and severe hemolytic disease. Asphyxial shock commonly is associated with maternal toxemia, and advanced cortical necrosis has been seen in stillborn infants. It has been argued that in hemorrhagic and asphyxial shock renal cortical perfusion is diminished to the point of ischemic tissue necrosis, a mechanism similar to that producing tubular necrosis. Some infants also have thrombocytopenia, and small arteriolar, glomerular, and venular thrombi in the kidney have been interpreted as evidence of disseminated intravascular coagulation. Few patients with documented disseminated intravascular coagulation have had renal cortical necrosis, however, and the local vascular changes may be secondary to severely altered renal circulation. Cortical necrosis also occurs in association with sepsis, diarrhea, and dehydration. Medullary necrosis in infants with congenital heart disease has been related to the toxicity of large doses of angiographic contrast medium, and medullary necrosis in infants with severe hyperbilirubinemia and kernicterus seems to be secondary to the direct toxic effects of unconjugated bilirubin concentrated in the renal medulla.

Pathology

Both cortical necrosis and medullary necrosis are usually bilateral, but involvement may be patchy or focal. The lesion is a bland, coagulative, ischemic necrosis. Medullary necrosis is commonly hemorrhagic and accompanied by variable cortical involvement. Both conditions are accompanied by focal necrosis in other organs: the liver, adrenal gland, intestines, and the brain. Necrotic cortical tissue undergoes calcification, producing within weeks a characteristic pattern of bilateral, symmetric cortical calcification. There may be poor renal visualization by excretory urography because of cortical damage and impaired function. Medullary necrosis may be recognized radiographically by a deformed pyelocalyceal system with evidence of papillary necrosis and cavitation (Fig. 31-8).

Treatment

The clinical differentiation of these two conditions from renal vein thrombosis may be very difficult, but in all three the clinical management is similar, consisting of careful control of fluids, judicious use of anticoagulation, and treatment of renal failure. Indications for surgical intervention are not clearly defined, even in cases with caval thrombosis.

Prognosis

The prognosis is related to the underlying causes as well as to the severity of the renal lesion. As the result of improved supportive care and improved handling of renal failure, relatively long survival times have been described. Prolonged survival may be complicated by severe hypertension. Sparing of juxtamedullary nephrons through collateral circulation in the inner cortex may account for relatively good tubular function despite severe glomerular insufficiency in surviving infants. Percutaneous renal biopsy may be of value in judging the severity of cortical damage.

TUMORS OF THE KIDNEY

Renal tumors in the newborn are uncommon, although they constitute the largest group of malignant neoplasms in childhood. The majority of neonatal renal tumors are leiomyomatous masses, sometimes referred to as *hamartomas* or *congenital mesoblastic nephromas*. Wilms' tumors, when they do occur, may be well differentiated and consist of cystic and tubular structures. Other renal neoplasms, including renal cell carcinoma, lymphoma, and teratoma, are medical rarities in the newborn. In general, renal tumors occurring early in infancy offer a considerably better outlook than do those in later childhood. The difference is in large measure a result of the relative frequency of mesoblastic nephroma and of well-differentiated Wilms' variants, which carry a good prognosis. Sarcomatous tumors have a poorer prognosis, even in young children. Only a few mesoblastic nephromas, perhaps 1% to 2%, have shown aggressive behavior, and the occurrence of true malignancy with distant metastases has been denied. Cystic Wilms' tumors and nephroblastomas with tubular differentiation also are rarely malignant. However, typical Wilms' tumors in the newborn may pursue the usual malignant course.

Clinical manifestations

In newborns, as in older infants, the initial finding is usually that of abdominal swelling or a palpable mass, often detected by the parents. There may be a history of vomiting and fever, and laboratory examination may disclose hematuria and an elevated erythrocyte sedimentation rate. Older infants frequently have hypertension; it does occur in newborns, but its incidence is unknown.

Wilms' tumors have been associated with several nonrenal malformations, among them congenital aniridia and hemihypertrophy, which also has been associated with adrenal and hepatic tumors, visceral hemangiomas, and pigmented nevi. Aniridia occurs as part of a syndrome that includes cataracts, microcephaly, mental retardation, growth retardation, misshapen ears, and cryptorchidism. A syndrome that encompasses male pseudohermaphroditism with occasional agonadism, glomerulonephritis with nephrotic syndrome, and renal failure and hypertension also has included Wilms' tumor. The Beckwith-Wiedemann syndrome of omphalocele and visceromegaly also is associated with subsequent development of Wilms' tumor (p. 858). The external malformations are seen at birth; the tumors develop later. These syndromes, despite their infrequency, should alert physicians to the risk of subsequent malignancy in affected patients.

Pathology

Congenital mesoblastic nephromas are morphologically distinctive, differing grossly and microscopically from typical nephroblastomas. The tumors are usually solitary, unencapsulated, and firm or rubbery. The cut surface has a whorled appearance, resembling uterine leiomyoma, and cysts are variably present. Histopathologic examination shows the tumor to be composed of sheets and intertwined bands of spindle, fibrous, and muscular cells, among which are nests and clusters of atypical and distorted glomeruli and tubules. The contained nephronic elements may be either (1) initially normal parenchyma entrapped within the expanding tumor, or (2) renal elements differentiating out of the metanephric mesenchyma that constitutes the tumor. Foci of rhabdomyomatous differentiation, angiomatous differentiation, cartilaginous differentiation, and hematopoietic infiltration may be seen. Cysts frequently are lined by epithelial cells that appear to have differentiated out of the adjacent stroma. Mitotic activity usually is meager. Increased mitotic activity and cellular atypia may be clues to the rare case that recurs or metastasizes; criteria of aggressive behavior have not been clearly established.

Differentiated Wilms' tumors contain masses of cysts, tubules, and even glomeruli, with little intervening undifferentiated stroma. The degree of epithelial differentiation along the tubules may be variable, but an embryonal appearance usually predominates. More typical nephroblastomas consist of undifferentiated mesenchyma, with only focal muscular and epithelial differentiation. Nephroblastomas usually are discrete, compressing the adjacent kidney tissue into a relatively fibrous capsule. True encapsulation is lacking, however, and the tumor invades the adjacent kidney, renal veins, and contiguous organs. Metastases are principally hematogeneous: lungs, liver, bones, and the opposite kidney.

The multilocular cystic nephroma is a benign renal tumor that consists of large cysts separated by fibrous septa. The solid portions of the tumor are usually poorly cellular, but cellular forms that are intermediates between obviously benign types and cystic Wilms' tumors do exist. These tumors thus are regarded as part of the spectrum of neoplasms arising from metanephric blastema, a spectrum that includes the multilocular cystic nephroma, the well-differentiated tubular nephroblastoma, and the typical Wilms' tumor. There is also some gradation between multilocular cysts and mesoblastic nephromas, and precise differentiation at times may be difficult.

An interesting condition is the occurrence within the renal cortex of small nodules of undifferentiated tissue that resemble nephroblastoma. Such nodules are commonly seen in trisomy E, and they have been reported in syndromes of fetal gigantism and hemihypertrophy. The nodules are usually bilateral and present in the outer cortex. When small and grossly inapparent, they have been referred to as *nodular blastema*. When the cortex is distorted by large masses of blastematous tissue, the condition is referred to as *nephroblastomatosis*. These two abnormalities, which are developmental in origin, are believed to be related to nephroblastoma. They are frequently found in kidneys resected because of Wilms' tumor, and Wilms' tumors on a few occasions have been reported to coexist with bilateral nephroblastomatosis. Therefore they may provide a link between the malformations and the subsequent development of Wilms' tumor in the syndromes previously noted.

Diagnosis

The differential diagnosis of abdominal masses in the newborn includes neuroblastomas, retroperitoneal tumors and cysts, splenomegaly, hepatic tumors, ovarian cysts and tumors, intestinal duplications, and several renal abnormalities. Radiography and sonography are important in localizing the lesion to the kidney, in excluding hydronephrosis and polycystic disease, and in identifying ectopic, fused, and solitary kidneys. Excretory urography commonly shows flattening and distortion of the pyelocalyceal system, a finding common to all intrarenal masses. Excretion of contrast medium, however, may be so impaired by infiltrating tumor or by secondary vascular obstruction that the roentgenograms show only a nonfunctioning renal mass. Arteriography may be of additional help in identifying and localizing the tumor, but the characteristically abnormal vasculature is common to mesoblastic nephroma, Wilms' tumor, and multilocular cyst. The leiomyomatous and cystic tumors tend to be less vascular. During the nephrographic phase of the arteriogram the denser renal tissue is seen to be displaced by the tumor. Occasional Wilms' tumors are avascular, perhaps because of hemorrhagic or cystic degeneration, and differentiation from cystic lesions may then be difficult. Renal angiography is also of value in defining the extent of neoplastic involvement and in evaluating the contralateral kidney before surgery.

Bilaterality in nephroblastomas (all ages) occurs in approximately 4% of patients; its frequency in newborns is obscured by other developmental abnormalities, particularly nephroblastomatosis. Wilms' tumors also may coexist with other renal abnormalities, including cystic disease, duplication, fusion, and ectopia, thus complicating radiologic interpretation. Wilms' tumors also have occurred with greater than expected frequency in horseshoe-shaped and solitary kidneys.

Treatment

Definitive therapy should be instituted promptly after the diagnosis has been confirmed. The presence of a localized intrarenal mass necessitates surgical exploration. Primary treatment is nephrectomy, and the benign mesenchymal tumors require no additional postoperative therapy. The greatest danger lies in overtreatment with secondary damage, especially from irradiation.

Prognosis

The prognosis in neonatal renal tumors is good; this estimate takes into account the benign variants of early infancy. The survival of all infants younger than 1 year may be 70% to 80%. Infants of this age with typical Wilms' tumor, however, may have no better a prognosis than do older children. Clinical staging is of help in determining outcome; tumors confined to the kidney have an excellent prognosis, but progressively poorer results can be anticipated with tumors that extend into the renal fossa and vessels.

Adrian Spitzer
Jay Bernstein
Chester M. Edelmann, Jr.

BIBLIOGRAPHY
Renal function and its morphologic correlates

Arant, B.S., Jr.: Developmental patterns of renal functional maturation compared in the human neonate, J. Pediatr. 92:705, 1978.

Brodehl, J., and Gellisen, K.: Endogenous renal transport of free amino acids in infancy and childhood, Pediatrics 42:395, 1968.

Dean, R.F.A., and McCance, R.A.: Inulin, diodone, creatinine and urea clearances in newborn infants, J. Physiol. 106:431, 1947.

Edelmann, C.M., Jr., Barnett, H.L., and Troupkou, V.: Renal concentrating mechanism in newborn infants; effects of dietary protein and water content, role of urea and responsiveness to antidiuretic hormone, J. Clin. Invest. 39:1062, 1960.

Fawer, C.L., Torrado, A., and Guignard, J.P.: Maturation of renal function in full-term and premature neonates, Helv. Paediatr. Acta 34:11, 1979.

Fetterman, G.H., and others: The growth and maturation of human glomeruli and proximal convolutions from term to adulthood; studies by microdissection, Pediatrics 35:601, 1965.

Guignard, J.P., and others: Glomerular filtration rate in the first 3 weeks of life, J. Pediatr. 87:269, 1972.

Hatemi, N., and McCance, R.A.: Renal aspects of acid base control in the newly born. III. Response to acidifying drugs, Acta Paediatr. Scand. 50:603, 1961.

McCance, R.A.: The maintenance of stability in the newly born. I. Chemical exchange, Arch. Dis. Child. 34:459, 1959.

McCance, R.A., and von Finck, M.A.: The titratable acidity, pH, ammonia and phosphates in the urines of very young infants, Arch. Dis. Child. 22:200, 1947.

McCance, R.A., and Widdowson, E.M.: Renal function before birth, Proc. R. Soc. Lond. 141:488, 1953.

Potter, E.L., and Thierstein, S.T.: Glomerular development in the kidney as an index of fetal maturity, J. Pediatr. 22:695, 1943.

Schwartz, G.J., and others: Late metabolic acidosis: a reassessment of the definition, J. Pediatr. 95:102, 1979.

Reaction of the immature kidney to injury

Bernstein, J.: Developmental abnormalities of the renal parenchyma; renal hypoplasia and dysplasia. In Sommers, S.C., editor: Pathology annual 1968, New York, 1968, Appleton-Century-Crofts.

Bernstein, J., and Meyer, R.: Congenital abnormalities of the urinary system. II. Renal cortical and medullary necrosis, J. Pediatr. 59:657, 1961.

Emery, J.L., and Macdonald, M.S.: Involuting and scarred glomeruli in the kidneys of infants, Am. J. Pathol. 36:713, 1960.

Kanasawa, M., and others: Dwarfed kidneys in children; the classification, etiology, and significance of bilateral small kidneys in 11 children, Am. J. Dis. Child. 109:130, 1965.

Malt, R.A.: Compensatory growth of the kidney, N. Engl. J. Med. 280:1446, 1969.

Osathanondh, V., and Potter, E.L.: Pathogenesis of polycystic kidneys; type 4 due to urethral obstruction, Arch. Pathol. 77:502, 1964.

Investigation for renal disease

Dunbar, J.S., and Nogrady, B.: Excretory urography in the first year of life, Radiol. Clin. North Am. 10:367, 1972.

Fawer, C.L., Torrado, A., and Guignard, J.P.: Single injection clearance in the neonate, Biol. Neonate 35:321, 1979.

Frank, J.L., Potter, B.M., and Shkolnika, A.: Neonatal ultrasonography. In Rosenfeld, A.T., editor: Genitourinary ultrasonography, New York, 1979, Churchill-Livingstone.

Goldman, H.S., and Freeman, L.M.: Radiographic and radioisotopic methods of evaluation of the kidneys and urinary tract, Pediatr. Clin. North Am. 18:409, 1971.

Kassirer, J.P.: Clinical evaluation of kidney function; glomerular function, N. Engl. J. Med. 285:385, 1971.

Lang, E.K.: Contribution of arteriography in the assessment of renal lesions encountered in the neonatal period and infancy, Radiology 110:429, 1974.

Stonestreet, B.S., Bell, E.F., and Oh, W.: Validity of endogenous creatinine clearance in low birth weights infants, Pediatr. Res. 13:1012, 1979.

Disorders of micturition

Ivey, H.H.: The asphyxiated bladder as a cause of delayed micturition in the newborn, J. Urol. 120:498, 1978.

Lattimer, J.K., Uson, A.C., and Melicow, M.M.: Urologic emergencies in newborn infants, Pediatrics 29:310, 1962.

Lawson, J.S., and Hewstone, A.S.: Microscopic appearance of urine in newborn period, Arch. Dis. Child. 39:287, 1964.

Moore, E.S., and Galvez, M.B.: Delayed micturition in the newborn period, J. Pediatr. 80:867, 1972.

Sherry, S.N., and Kramer, I.: The time of passage of the first stool and first urine by the newborn infant, J. Pediatr. 46:158, 1955.

Proteinuria

deLuna, M.B., and Hullet, W.H.: Urinary protein excretion in healthy infants, children and adults, Proc. Am. Soc. Nephrol. **16:**16, 1967.

Peterson, P.A., Evrin, P., and Berggard, I.: Differentiation of glomerular, tubular, and normal proteinuria; determinations of urinary excretion of beta-2-macroglobulin, albumin, and total protein, J. Clin. Invest. **48:**1189, 1969.

Hematuria

Angella, J.J., Prieto, E.N., and Fogel, B.J.: Hemoglobinuria associated with hemolytic disease for the newborn infant, J. Pediatr. **71:**530, 1967.

Emanuel, B., and Aronson, N.: Neonatal hematuria, Am. J. Dis. Child. **128:**204, 1974.

Pyuria

Gruikshand, G., and Edmond, E.: "Clean catch" urines in the newborn; bacteriology and cell excretion patterns in first week of life, Br. Med. J. **4:**705, 1967.

Lincoln, K., and Winberg, J.: Studies of urinary tract infection in infancy and childhood. III. Quantitative estimation of cellular excretion in unselected neonates, Acta Paediatr. Scand. **53:**447, 1964.

Littlewood, J.M.: White cells and bacteria in voided urine of healthy newborns, Arch. Dis. Child. **46:**167, 1971.

Edema

Cywes, S., Wynne, J.M., and Louw, J.H.: Urinary ascites in newborn; with a report of two cases, J. Pediatr. Surg. **3:**350, 1968.

Fisher, D.A.: Obscure and unusual edema, Pediatrics **37:**506, 1966.

Kagan, B.M., and Felix, N.S.: Edema of infancy, Pediatr. Clin. North Am. **2:**391, 1955.

MacLaurin, J.C.: Changes in body water distribution during the first 2 weeks of life, Arch. Dis. Child. **41:**286, 1966.

Wu, P.Y.K., and others: "Late edema" in low birth weight infants, Pediatrics **41:**67, 1968.

Abdominal masses

Longio, L.A., and Martin, L.W.: Abdominal masses in the newborn infant, Pediatrics **21:**596, 1958.

Mussels, M., Gaudry, C.L., and Bason, W.M.: Renal anomalies in the newborn found by deep palpation, Pediatrics **47:**97, 1971.

Renal insufficiency and renal failure

Barratt, T.M.: Renal failure in the first year of life, Br. Med. Bull. **27:**115, 1971.

Chesney, R.W., and others: Acute renal failure; an important complication of cardiac surgery in infants, J. Pediatr. **87:**381, 1975.

Dobrin, R.S., Larsen, C.D., and Holliday, M.A.: The critically ill child; acute renal failure, Pediatrics **48:**286, 1971.

Fine, R.N., and others: Hemodialysis in infants under 1 year of age for acute poisoning, Am. J. Dis. Child. **116:**657, 1968.

Holliday, M.A., Potter, D.E., and Dobrin, R.S.: Treatment of renal failure in children, Pediatr. Clin. North Am. **18:**613, 1971.

Mathew, O.P., and others: Neonatal renal failure: usefulness of diagnostic indices, Pediatrics **65:**57, 1980.

Norman, M.E., and Asadi, F.K.: A prospective study of acute renal failure in newborn infants, Pediatrics **63:**475, 1974.

Malformations

Bain, A.D., and Scott, J.S.: Renal agenesis and severe urinary dysplasia; a review of 50 cases with particular reference to associated anomalies, Br. Med. J. **1:**841, 1960.

Bernstein, J.: Developmental abnormalities of the renal parenchyma; renal hypoplasia and dysplasia. In Sommers, S.C., editor: Pathology annual 1968, New York, 1968, Appleton-Century-Crofts.

Bernstein, J.: Heritable cystic disorders of the kidney; the mythology of polycystic disease, Pediatr. Clin. North Am. **18:**435, 1971.

Bernstein, J., Brough, A.J., and McAdams, A.J.: The renal lesion in syndromes of multiple congenital malformations; cerebrohepatorenal syndrome; Jeune asphyxiating thoracic dystrophy; tuberous sclerosis; Meckel syndrome. In Bergsma, D., editor: Birth defects, vol. 10, Baltimore, 1974, Williams & Wilkins Co.

Buchta, R.M., and others: Familial bilateral renal agenesis and hereditary renal dysplasia, Z. Kinderheilkd. **115:**111, 1973.

Burke, E.C., Shin, M.H., and Kelalis, P.P.: Prune-belly syndrome; clinical findings and survival, Am. J. Dis. Child. **117:**668, 1969.

Cain, D.R., and others: Familial renal agenesis and total dysplasia, Am. J. Dis. Child. **128:**377, 1974.

Davidson, W.M., and Ross, G.I.M.: Bilateral absence of the kidneys and related congenital anomalies, J. Pathol. **68:**459, 1954.

Elejalde, B.R.: Genetic and diagnostic considerations in these families with abnormalities of facial expression and congenital urinary obstruction; the Ochoa syndrome, Am. J. Med. Genet. **3:**97, 1979.

Elkin, M., and Bernstein, J.: Cystic diseases of the kidney, radiological and pathological considerations, Clin. Radiol. **20:**65, 1969.

Javadpour, N., and others: Hypertension in a child caused by a multicystic kidney, J. Urol. **104:**918, 1970.

Johannessen, J.V., Haneberg, B., and Moe, P.J.: Bilateral multicystic dysplasia of the kidneys, Beitr. Pathol. **148:**290, 1973.

Kaye, C., and Lewy, P.R.: Congenital appearance of adult-type (autosomal dominant) polycystic kidney disease; report of a case, J. Pediatr. **84:**807, 1974.

Kyaw, M.M.: Roentgenologic triad of congenital multicystic kidney, Am. J. Roentgenol. Radium Ther. Nucl. Med. **119:**710, 1973.

Leonidas, J.C., Strauss, L., and Krasna, I.H.: Roentgen diagnosis of multicystic renal dysplasia in infancy by high dose urography, J. Urol. **108:**963, 1972.

Lieberman, E., and others: Infantile polycystic disease of the kidneys and liver; clinical, pathological and radiological correlations and comparison with congenital hepatic fibrosis, Medicine **50:**277, 1971.

Lundin, P.M., and Olow, I.: Polycystic kidneys in newborns, infants, and children; a clinical pathological study, Acta Paediatr. **50:**185, 1961.

Machin, G.A.: Urinary tract malformations in the XYY male, Clin. Genet. **14:**370, 1972.

Newman, L., and others: Unilateral total renal dysplasia in children, Am. J. Roentgenol. Radium Ther. Nucl. Med. **116:**778, 1972.

North, A.F., Jr., Eldredge, D.M., and Tapley, W.B.: Abdominal distention at birth due to ascites associated with obstructive uropathy, Am. J. Dis. child. **111:**613, 1966.

Passarage, E., and Sutherland, J.M.: Potter's syndrome; chromosome analysis of three cases with Potter's syndrome or related syndromes, Am. J. Dis. Child. **109:**80, 1965.

Potter, E.L.: Bilateral absence of ureters and kidneys; a report of 50 cases, Obstet. Gynecol. **25:**3, 1965.

Qazi, Q., and others: Renal anomalies in fetal alcohol syndrome, Pediatrics **63:**886, 1979.

Risdon, R.A.: Renal dysplasia. I. A clinico-pathological study of 76 cases, J. Clin. Pathol. **24:**57, 1971.

Risdon, R.A.: Renal dysplasia, II. A necropsy study of 41 cases, J. Clin. Pathol. **24:**65, 1971.

Risdon, R.A., Young, L.W., and Chrispin, A.R.: Renal hypoplasia and dysplasia; a radiological and pathological correlation, Pediatr. Radiol. **3:**213, 1975.

Ross, D.G., and Travers, H.: Infantile presentation of adult-type polycystic disease in a large kindred, J. Pediatr. **87:**760, 1975.

Vesicoureteral reflux

Acton, C.M., and Drew, J.H.: Vesicoureteral reflux in the neonatal period. In Hodson, J., and Kincaid-Smith, P., editors: Reflux nephropathy, New York, 1979, Masson Publishing USA, Inc.

Blaufox, M.D., and others: Radionuclide scintigraphy for detection of vesico-ureteral reflux in children, J. Pediatr. **79**:239, 1971.

Drew, J.H., and Acton, C.M.: Radiological findings in newborn infants with urinary infection, Arch. Dis. Child. **51**:620, 1976.

Iannaccone, G., and Panzironi, P.E.: Ureteral reflux in normal infants, Acta Radiol. **44**:451, 1955.

Johnston, J.H., and Mix, L.W.: The Ask-Upmark kidney: a form of ascending pyelonephritis? Br. J. Urol. **48:393, 1976.**

Peters, P.C., Johnson, D.E., and Jackson, J.H.: The incidence of vesicoureteral reflux in the premature child, J. Urol. **97**:159, 1967.

Rolleston, G.L., Shannon, F.T., and Utley, W.L.F.: Relationship of infantile vesicoureteric reflux to renal damage, Br. Med. J. **1**:460, 1970.

Rolleston, G.L., Shannon, F.T., and Utley, W.L.F.: Follow-up of vesico-ureteric reflux in the newborn, Kidney Int. (Suppl.) **8**:S59, 1975.

Nephritis

Claireaux, A.E., and Pearson, M.G.: Chronic nephritis in a newborn infant, Arch. Dis. Child. **30**:366, 1955.

Collins, R.D.: Chronic glomerulonephritis in a newborn child, Am. J. Dis. Child. **87**:478, 1954.

Kaplan, B.S., and others: The glomerulopathy of congenital syphilis; an immune deposit disease, J. Pediatr. **81**:1154, 1972.

Shahin, M.D., Papadopoulou, Z.L., and Jenis, E.H.: Congenital nephrotic syndrome associated with congenital toxoplasmosis, J. Pediatr. **85**:366, 1974.

Taitz, L.S., Isaacson, C., and Stein, H.: Acute nephritis associated with congenital syphilis, Br. Med. J. **2**:152, 1961.

Wiggelinkhuizen, J., and others: Congenital syphilis and glomerulonephritis with evidence for immune pathogenesis, Arch. Dis. Child. **48**:375, 1973.

Yuceoglu, A.M., and others: The glomerulopathy of congenital syphilis; a curable immune-deposit disease, J.A.M.A. **229**:1085, 1974.

Nephrotic syndrome

Aula, P., and others: Prenatal diagnosis in congenital nephrosis in 23 high-risk families, Am. J. Dis. Child. **132**:984, 1978.

Habib, R., and Bois, E.: Hétérogéité des syndromes néphrotiques á début précoce du nourrisson (syndrome néphrotique "infantile"); étude anatomo-clinique et génétique de 37 observations, Helv. Paediatr. Acta **28**:91, 1973.

Hallman, N., Norio, R., and Rapola, J.: Congenital nephrotic syndrome, Nephron **11**:101, 1973.

Hoyer, J.R., and others: The nephrotic syndrome of infancy: clinical, morphologic, and immunologic studies of four infants, Pediatrics **40**:233, 1967.

Kaplan, B.S., Bureau, M.A., and Drummond, K.N.: The nephrotic syndrome in the first year of life; is a pathologic classification possible? J. Pediatr. **85**:615, 1974.

Kouvalainen, K.: Immunological studies on the congenital nephrotic syndrome, Am. J. Dis. Child. **104**:554, 1962.

McDonald, R., Wiggelinkhuizen, J., and Kaschula, R.O.C.: The nephrotic syndrome in very young infants, Am. J. Dis. Child. **122**:507, 1971.

Medearis, D.N.: Cytomegalic inclusion disease; an analysis of the clinical features based on the literature and six additional cases, Pediatrics **19**:467, 1957.

Norio, R.: Heredity in the congenital nephrotic syndrome; a genetic study of 57 Finnish families with a review of reported cases, Ann. Paediatr. Fenn. **12** (Suppl. 27):1, 1966.

Papaioannou, A.C., Asrow, G.G., and Schuckmell, N.H.: Nephrotic syndrome in early infancy as a manifestation of congenital syphilis, Pediatrics **27**:636, 1961.

Rapola, J., and Savilahti, E.: Immunofluorescent and morphological studies in congenital nephrotic syndrome, Acta Paediatr. Scand. **60**:253, 1971.

Walker, C.H.M., and others: Hemodialysis in infantile nephrotic syndrome, Am. J. Dis. Child. **106**:479, 1963.

Wiggelinkhuizen, J., and others: Alpha fetoprotein in the antenatal diagnosis of the congenital nephrotic syndrome, J. Pediatr. **89**:452, 1976.

Renal glucosuria

Elsas, L.J., and others: Renal and intestinal hexose transport in familial glucose-galactose malabsorption, J. Clin. Invest. **49**:576, 1970.

Monasterio, G., and others: Renal diabetes as a congenital tubular dysplasia, Am. J. Med. **37**:44, 1964.

Aminoacidurias

Brodehl, J., and Gellissen, K.: Endogenous renal transport of free amino acids in infancy and childhood, Pediatrics **42**:395, 1968.

Chisolm, J.J., Jr., and Harrison, H.E.: Aminoaciduria, Pediatr. Clin. North Am. **7**:333, 1960.

Chisolm, J.J., Jr., and Harrison, H.E.: Aminoaciduria in vitamin D deficiency states, in premature infants and older infants with rickets, J. Pediatr. **60**:206, 1962.

Pruzansky, W.: Cystinuria and cystine urolithiasis in childhood, Acta Paediatr. Scand. **55**:97, 1966.

Rosenberg, L.E., Durant, J.L., and Elsas, L.J.: Familial iminoglycinuria; an inborn error of renal tubular transport, N. Engl. J. Med. **278**:1407, 1968.

Whelan, D.T., and Scriver, G.R.: Hyperdibasic aminoaciduria; an inherited disorder of amino acid transport, Pediatr. Res. **2**:525, 1968.

Cystinosis

Cramhall, J.C., and others: Cystinosis; plasma cystine and cysteine concentrations and the effect of D-penicillamine and dietary treatment, Am. J. Med. **44**:330, 1968.

Seegmiller, J.E., and others: Cystinosis, Ann. Int. Med. **68**:883, 1968.

Serp, M., and others: Dietary treatment of cystinosis, Acta Paediatr. Scand. **57**:409, 1968.

States, B., and others: Prenatal diagnosis of cystinosis, J. Pediatr. **87**:558, 1975.

Worthen, H.G.: Growth failure due to diseases of the proximal tubule, J. Pediatr. **57**:14, 1960.

Pseudohypoaldosteronism

Cheek, D.B., and Perry, J.N.: A salt wasting syndrome in infancy, Arch. Dis. Child. **33**:252, 1958.

Donnell, G.N., Litman, N., and Roldan, M.: Pseudohypoadrenalcorticism; renal sodium loss, hyponatremia, and hyperkalemia due to renal tubular insensitivity to mineralocorticoid, Am. J. Dis. Child. **97**:813, 1959.

Nephrogenic diabetes insipidus

Blachar, Y., and others: The effect of inhibition of prostaglandin synthesis on free water and osmolar clearances in patients with hereditary nephrogenic diabetes insipidus, Int. J. Pediatr. Nephrol. **1**:48, 1980.

Friss-Hansen, P., Skadhauge, E., and Zetterstrom, R.: Fluid and electrolyte metabolism in nephrogenic diabetes insipidus, Acta Paediatr. Scand. (Suppl.) 146:57, 1957.

Gautier, P.E., and Sympkiss, M.: The management of nephrogenic diabetes insipidus in early life, Acta Paediatr. Scand. 46:354, 1957.

Schotland, M.G., Grumbach, M.M., and Strauss, J.: The effect of chlorothiazides in nephrogenic diabetes insipidus, Pediatrics 31:741, 1963.

Renal tubular acidosis

Morris, R.C.: Renal tubular acidosis; mechanisms, classification and implications, N. Engl. J. Med. 281:1405, 1969.

Rodriguez-Soriano, J., and Edelmann, C.M., Jr.: Renal tubular acidosis, Ann. Rev. Med. 20:363, 1969.

Rodriguez-Soriano, J., Vallo, A., and Garcia-Fuentes, M.: Distal renal tubular acidosis in infancy; a bicarbonate wasting state, J. Pediatr. 86:524, 1975.

Infection of the urinary tract

Edelmann, C.M., Jr., Ogwo, J., and Fine, B.P.: The prevalence of bacteriuria in full-term and premature newborn infants, J. Pediatr. 82:125, 1973.

Gower, P.E., and others: Urinary infection in two selected neonatal populations, Arch. Dis. Child. 45:259, 1970.

Houston, I.B.: Pus cell and bacterial counts in the diagnosis of urinary tract infections in childhood, Arch. Dis. Child. 38:600, 1963.

Lincoln, K., and Winberg, J.: Studies of urinary tract infections in infancy and childhood. II. Quantitative estimation of bacteriuria in unselected neonates with special reference to the occurrence of asymptomatic infections, Acta Paediatr. Scand. 53:307, 1964.

Lincoln, K., and Winberg, J.: Studies of urinary tract infections in infancy and childhood. III. Quantitative estimation of cellular excretion in unselected neonates, Acta Paediatr. Scand. 53:447, 1964.

Littlewood, J.M.: White cells and bacteria in voided urine of healthy newborns Arch. Dis. Child. 46:167, 1971.

Littlewood, J.M.: Sixty-six infants with urinary tract infection in first year of life, Arch. Dis. Child. 47:218, 1972.

Newman, C.G.H., O'Neill, P., and Parker, A.: Pyuria in infancy and the role of suprapubic aspiration of urine in diagnosis of infections of the urinary tract, Br. Med. J. 2:277, 1967.

Seeler, R.A., and Hahn, K.: Jaundice in urinary tract infection in infancy, Am. J. Dis. Child. 118:553, 1969.

Vascular disorders of the kidney

Adelman, R.D., and others: Nonsurgical management of renovascular hypertension in the neonate, Pediatrics 62:71, 1978.

Arneil, G.C., and others: Renal venous thrombosis, Clin. Nephrol. 1:119, 1973.

Bauer, S.B., and others: Neonatal hypertension; a complication of umbilical-artery catheterization, N. Engl. J. Med. 293:1032, 1975.

Belman, A.B., and King, L.R.: The pathology and treatment of renal vein thrombosis in the newborn, J. Urol. 107:852, 1972.

Belman, A.B., and others: Nonoperative treatment of unilateral renal vein thrombosis in the newborn, J.A.M.A. 211:1165, 1970.

Bernstein, J., and Meyer, R.: Congenital abnormalities of the urinary system. II. Renal cortical and medullary necrosis, J. Pediatr. 59:657, 1961.

Brough, A.J., and Zuelzer, W.W.: Renal vascular disease, Pediatr. Clin. North Am. 11:533, 1964.

Chesney, R.W., and others: Acute renal failure; an important complication of cardiac surgery in infants, J. Pediatr. 87:381, 1975.

Demarquez, J.L., and others: Thrombose de la veine renale chez le nouveau-ne; traitement par l'urokinase, Arch. Fr. Pediatr. 32:281, 1972.

Dimmick, J.E., Hardwick, D.F., and Ho-Yuen, B.: A case of renal necrosis and fibrosis in the immediate newborn period; association with the twin-to-twin transfusion syndrome, Am. J. Dis. Child. 122:345, 1971.

Ford, K.T., Teplick, S.K., and Clark, R.E.: Renal artery embolism causing neonatal hypertension; a complication of umbilical artery catheterization, Radiology 113:169, 1974.

Groshong, T.D., and others: Renal function following cortical necrosis in childhood, J. Pediatr. 79:267, 1971.

Gruskin, A.B., and others: Effects of angiography on renal function and histology in infants and piglets, J. Pediatr. 76:42, 1970.

Halvorsen, J.F., and Moe, P.J.: Renal vein thrombosis in neonates; report of three cases treated with nephrectomy, Acta Paediatr. Scand. 64:373, 1975.

Leonidas, J.C., Berdon, W.E., and Gribetz, D.: Bilateral renal cortical necrosis in the newborn infant; roentgenographic diagnosis, J. Pediatr. 79:623, 1971.

McDonald, P., and others: Some radiologic observations in renal vein thrombosis, Am. J. Roentgenol. Radium Ther. Nucl. Med. 120:368, 1974.

Mauer, S.M., and others: Bilateral renal vein thrombosis in infancy; report of a survivor following surgical intervention, J. Pediatr. 78:509, 1971.

Siegel, S.R., Fisher, D.A., and Oh, W.: Renal function and serum aldosterone levels in infants with respiratory distress syndrome, J. Pediatr. 83:854, 1973.

Stark, H., and Geiger, R.: Renal tubular dysfunction following vascular accidents of the kidneys in the newborn period, J. Pediatr. 83:933, 1973.

Svenningsen, N.W., and Aronson, A.S.: Postnatal development of renal concentration capacity as estimated by DDAVP-test in normal and asphyxiated neonates, Biol. Neonate 25:230, 1974.

Takeuchi, A., and Benirschke, K.: Renal venous thrombosis of the newborn and its relation to maternal diabetes, Biol. Neonate 3:237, 1961.

Torrado, A., and others: Hypoxaemia and renal function in newborns with respiratory distress syndrome (RDS), Helv. Paediatr. Acta 29:399, 1974.

Tumors of the kidney

Berdon, W.E., Wigger, H.J., and Baker, D.H.: Fetal renal hematoma, a benign tumor to be distinguished from Wilms' tumor; report of 3 cases, Am. J. Roentgenol. Radium Ther. Nucl. Med. 118:18, 1973.

Bolande, R.P.: Congenital and infantile neoplasia of the kidney, Lancet 2:1497, 1974.

Bolande, R.P., Brough, A.J., and Izant, R.J., Jr.: Congenital mesoblastic nephroma of infancy; a report of eight cases and the relationship of Wilms' tumor, Pediatrics 40:272, 1967.

Bove, K.E., Koffler, H., and McAdams, A.J.: Nodular renal blastema, definition and possible significance, Cancer 24:323, 1969.

Brown, J.M.: Cystic partially differentiated nephroblastoma, J. Pathol. 115:175, 1975.

Drash, A., and others: A syndrome of male pseudohermaphroditis, Wilms' tumor, hypertension, and degenerative renal disease, J. Pediatr. 76:585, 1970.

Favara, B.E., Johnson, W., and Ito, J.: Renal tumors in the neonatal period, Cancer 22:845, 1968.

Fowler, M.: Differentiated nephroblastoma; solid, cystic, or mixed, J. Pathol. 105:215, 1971.

Joshi, V.V., and others: Congenital mesoblastic nephroma of infancy; report of a case with unusual clinical behavior, Am. J. Clin. Pathol. 60:811, 1973.

Liban, E., and Kozenitzky, I.L.: Metanephric hamartomas and nephroblastomatosis in siblings, Cancer 25:885, 1970.

Mankad, V.N., Gray, G.F., Jr., and Miller, D.R.: Bilateral nephroblastomatosis and Klippel Trenaunay syndrome, Cancer 33:1462, 1974.

Miller, R.W., Fraumeni, J.F., Jr., and Manning, M.D.: Association of Wilms' tumor with aniridia, hemihypertrophy and other congenital malformations, N. Engl. J. Med. 270:922, 1964.

Perlman, M., Levin, M., and Wittels, B.: Syndrome of fetal gigantism, renal hamartomas, and nephroblastomatosis with Wilms' tumor, Cancer 35:1212, 1975.

Poole, C.A., and Viamonte, M., Jr.: Unusual renal masses in pediatric age group, Am. J. Roentgenol. 109:368, 1970.

Walker, D., and Richard, G.A.: Fetal hamartoma of the kidney; recurrence and death of patient, J. Urol. 110:352, 1973.

CHAPTER 32 Inborn errors of metabolism

This chapter limits itself to those diseases which have clinical manifestations in the neonatal period and to those for which therapy has been advised even though clinical manifestations are lacking.

In the recognition of inborn errors of metabolism in the newborn period the most important clue is the history of a sibling affected by a metabolic disorder. There are few specific signs of these diseases. Most affected infants are products of normal pregnancies and are clinically normal at birth. At varying intervals after birth they may develop lethargy, poor feeding, and persistent vomiting, generally with some evidence of depression of central nervous system function. Seizures may occur. Frequently myoclonic, the seizures also may be major and either generalized or focal. Although some affected infants have normal or increased muscle tone, the majority show rather profound hypotonia. The tachypnea and hyperventilation of metabolic acidosis may be noted. In a number of diverse disorders prolonged and unusually severe neonatal jaundice has been observed.

The initial laboratory evaluation of an infant suspected of having metabolic disease should include (1) complete blood count, including leukocyte differential and platelet counts (2) urinalysis with tests for glucose, reducing substance, ketones, and acids reactive with 2,4-dinitrophenylhydrazine, (3) measurement of arterial (or arterialized capillary) pH, P_{CO_2}, and P_{O_2} (or oxygen saturation), and (4) measurement of plasma glucose, sodium, potassium, chloride, bicarbonate, calcium, magnesium, and ammonia.

If the results obtained in this evaluation are normal and the infant shows clear-cut neurologic deterioration, quantitative analysis of amino acids in cerebrospinal fluid should be obtained.

All these initial steps, with the possible exception of quantitative amino acid analysis, can be carried out rapidly, leading to a rational approach to further investigation and to management. Other necessary components in the overall assessment of the suspect infant include quantitative analysis of plasma amino acids, quantitative analysis of amino acids and organic acids in urine, and skin biopsy for establishment of fibroblast cultures for subsequent biochemical analysis (such cultures also can be established from material obtained at autopsy).

If a diagnosis is established in a surviving infant, there are four general approaches to management:

1. If efficacy of any therapeutic measure has not been demonstrated, one may elect to employ no specific management.
2. One may restrict the intake of the metabolite that accumulates in the disorder. This approach is effective in classic phenylketonuria but may not be generally applicable. For example, in some disorders it is possible that adequate levels of the normal product of the blocked reaction are dependent in part on stimulation of residual enzyme activity by high levels of the precursor metabolite.
3. One may increase the intake of the normal metabolite that is not produced because of the metabolic error. This approach has produced chemical remission in orotic aciduria. It requires that the administered metabolite be absorbed and transported effectively to the site of need.
4. One may administer large amounts of the cofactor(s) that participates in the blocked reaction (megavitamin therapy). This form of management has been dramatically effective in some cases—generally, although not always, in disorders involving vitamin metabolism.

It is frequently necessary in practice to institute man-

Table 32-1. Some vitamins employed in megavitamin therapy

Vitamin	Recommended allowance (mg/day)	100 × (mg/day)	1,000 × (mg/day)	Toxicity
Pyridoxine	0.3	30	300	None
Thiamine	0.3	30	300	None
Riboflavin	0.4	40	400	None
Niacinamide	6	600	6,000	None (short term)
Cobalamin*	0.0005	0.05	0.5	None
Folic acid	0.03	3	30	Loss of seizure control
Ascorbic acid	35	3,500	35,000	None
Biotin†	0.035	3.5	35	None
Pantothenic acid	2	200	2,000	None

*Recommended megavitamin dose: hydroxocobalamin 2 mg/day IM.
†Recommended megavitamin dose: biotin 10 to 40 mg/day PO.

agement of a seriously ill infant before the results of specific tests are known. In such circumstances general principles of management are as follows: specimens for the studies previously outlined must be collected as a first priority, both for patient management and for future genetic counseling. Catabolic stress should be minimized by providing the infant with 30 gm of glucose/kg/day (120 kcal/kg/day) for the first few days of management. Megavitamin therapy may be therapeutically effective (Table 32-1). Exchange transfusion or peritoneal dialysis may ameliorate the condition sufficiently to allow definitive diagnosis and management.

NEONATAL SCREENING TESTS

Screening tests for inherited diseases are widely employed in neonatal nurseries. The specific disorders are discussed in detail later in the chapter.

The general usefulness of any given test is a function of its sensitivity and specificity on the one hand, and the possibility of effective intervention on the other. Given current obstetric practice, the former consideration means that the disease must be expressed sufficiently on the third day of life to allow its detection, and that the test employed must be positive in virtually 100% of affected infants and negative in virtually 100% of nonaffected infants. Effectiveness of intervention is to some extent a matter of judgment. All would agree that congenital hypothyroidism detected by screening can be effectively treated. Many would not agree that sickle cell disease can be more effectively treated because it is detected by neonatal screening, but the issue becomes more complex when genetic counseling is included as a major component of the total process of intervention.

Since neonatal screening is generally government funded, an element of practicality is added: a screening program should be cost effective, i.e., should result in a lowering in the cost to government of medical care for its citizens. Hence a disease for which screening is employed should be common enough and disabling enough to have a reasonably large associated cost to society, and this cost should be significantly lowered by detection and treatment in the neonatal period.

Another practical consideration involves both the type of sample to be used for screening and the laboratory techniques to be employed. What has evolved as most effective is collection of whole blood obtained by heelstick on filter paper strips and transport of the dried strips to central laboratories, where automated methods of testing can be used at relatively little cost.

The following diseases are generally included in neonatal screening programs in the United States:

1. Congenital hypothyroidism affects roughly 1 in 5,000 infants, can be efficiently detected in dried blood spots, and can be effectively treated at low cost with great reduction in morbidity. (See Chapter 33, part three.)
2. Phenylketonuria affects 1 in 16,000 infants, can be efficiently detected, and can be treated effectively at a cost that is high but much lower in both human and monetary terms than the cost of not screening for and treating the disease.
3. Galactosemia affects 1 in 50,000 to 100,000 infants. The screening assay for galactose in blood (Paigen) is relatively efficient, but the disease is so severe in many neonates that the result of the screening test may be reported too late. Treatment of the disease is very effective and not costly.
4. Maple syrup urine disease affects approximately 1 in 200,000 infants. The screening test is quite reliable but may not be reported in time to prevent life-threatening illness in some affected infants. Treatment is very costly, its success dependent in significant part on the severity of the chemical defect.
5. Homocystinuria affects approximately 1 in 100,000 infants. The screening test currently used mea-

sures the level of methionine in whole blood: it is not very sensitive, although relatively specific under current feeding practices. Pyridoxine-responsive homocystinuria is effectively treated at low cost. If treatment requires a diet with altered amino acid composition, the cost of treatment rises significantly, and effectiveness is somewhat less predictable.

It is obvious from this discussion that large-scale neonatal screening for phenylketonuria and congenital hypothyroidism is easily justified, that a reliable cribside test for galactosemia would be preferable to large-scale screening, and that large-scale neonatal screening for maple syrup urine disease and homocystinuria has limited usefulness. Screening programs are in a state of evolution, and tests will be added or deleted as their merits dictate.

DISORDERS OF AMINO ACID METABOLISM
Disorders of the metabolism of phenylalanine and tyrosine
Phenylketonuria

Clinically there are two forms of phenylketonuria. The first, classic phenylketonuria, is the result of a deficiency of phenylalanine hydroxylase and responds both chemically and clinically to a diet restricted in phenylalanine. The second form, sometimes called (inappropriately) malignant hyperphenylalaninemia, is the result of defective metabolism of the coenzyme for phenylalanine hydroxylase, tetrahydrobiopterin. In this form of the disorder dietary restriction of phenylalanine results in lowering of plasma phenylalanine without affecting the neurologic consequences of the disease.

Etiology and pathogenesis. It has been repeatedly demonstrated that phenylalanine hydroxylase activity is absent or nearly so in classic phenylketonuria. The pathogenesis of the clinical disease is unclear but is without doubt related to accumulation in tissues and body fluids of unmetabolized phenylalanine, since restriction of dietary phenylalanine is therapeutically effective.

In the normal growing infant dietary phenylalanine is in part used for protein synthesis and in part hydroxylated to form tyrosine (Fig. 32-1). In the latter reaction tetrahydrobiopterin, the cofactor, is oxidized to dihydrobiopterin. Tetrahydrobiopterin then is regenerated in a NADPH-dependent reaction catalyzed by dihydrobiopterin reductase. Tetrahydrobiopterin is synthesized de novo in a series of reactions currently under investigation. Although neither phenylalanine nor tyrosine can be synthesized de novo, phenylalanine can spare the dietary requirement for phenylalanine. This irreversibility is also significant for the interpretation of laboratory data. Defects in metabolism of tyrosine have no direct effect on the level of phenylalanine in plasma; individuals with

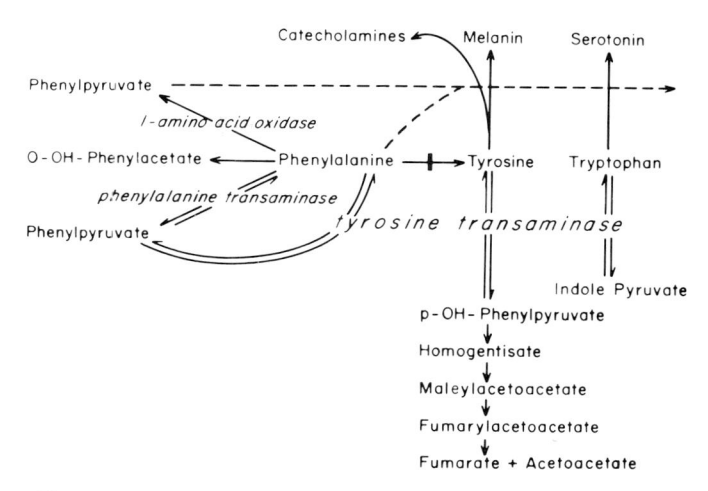

Fig. 32-1. Schematic representation of the metabolism of phenylalanine, tyrosine, and tryptophan. Solid crossbar indicates the metabolic block demonstrated in phenylketonuria, whereas broken crossbars indicate postulated secondary metabolic blocks.

hereditary tyrosinosis characteristically exhibit normal plasma levels of phenylalanine. Therefore an elevation of plasma phenylalanine occurring under normal dietary conditions indicates an impairment in phenylalanine hydroxylation. The degradation of tyrosine is initiated in the liver by tyrosine transaminase, an enzyme that also catalyzes the transamination of phenylalanine and tryptophan. In the experimental animal any of these three aromatic amino acids is capable of inducing increased activity of tyrosine transaminase.

In a quantitative sense the metabolic pathway of phenylalanine and tyrosine evolves during the latter part of gestation. As a result, premature infants are likely to show elevations in both phenylalanine and tyrosine in plasma. Full-term infants do so less frequently. This condition commonly is called *transient tyrosinemia*. The elevations in both phenylalanine and tyrosine can be extreme, more than 20 times normal, and indeed may not be without risk of neurologic sequelae. In this regard it should be noted that identification of transient tyrosinemia occurred during an era when infants commonly received formulas that contained four times as much protein per ounce as human milk does. One recent study of a small group of premature infants showed no elevations above normal in plasma phenylalanine and tyrosine when dietary intake simulated that provided by human milk. The quantitative aspects of phenylalanine metabolism are thus relatively simple, but the physiologic ramifications of impairments in the pathway also involve considerations of both the neurochemical metabolism of phenylalanine and the interrelationships of the metabolism of the three aromatic amino acids: phenylalanine, tyrosine, and tryptophan. Phenylalanine and tyrosine are

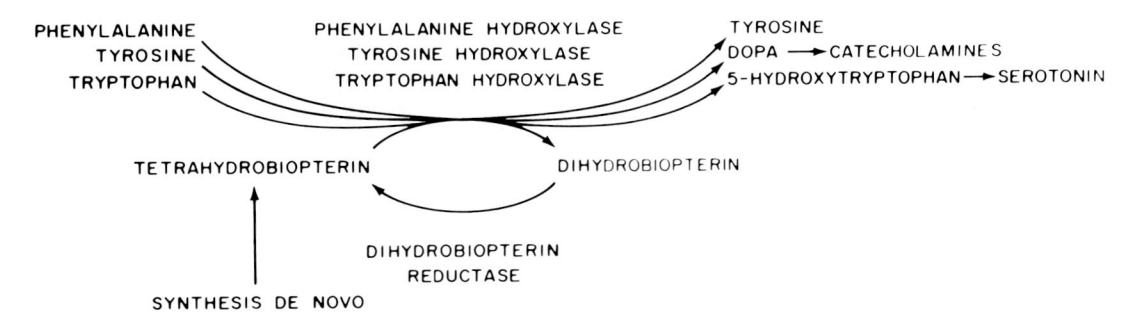

Fig. 32-2. Biopterin metabolism and its relationship to the synthesis of neurotransmitters.

precursors of epinephrine, norepinephrine, dopamine, and octopamine, and tryptophan is a precursor of serotonin (Fig. 32-2). Because the aromatic amino acids have analogous structures and share enzymatic pathways, it can be expected that great excesses in tissue levels of one, for example, phenylalanine, can impair the conversion of the others, for example, tyrosine and tryptophan, into neurally active compounds. Furthermore the hydroxylations of phenylalanine to form tyrosine, of tyrosine to form dopa, and of tryptophan to form 5-hydroxytryptophan all require tetrahydrobiopterin. In the two inborn errors of biopterin metabolism now defined—the first a deficiency of dihydrobiopterin reductase, the second a failure in de novo synthesis of tetrahydrobiopterin—hyperphenylalaninemia occurs together with reduced amounts of neurotransmitters whose synthesis is dependent on the availability of tetrahydrobiopterin.

It is a simplifying and attractive hypothesis, as yet unproven, that the neurologic disorder in phenylketonuria of whatever cause occurs as a result of impaired or disordered synthesis of neurotransmitters. In the classic disease phenylalanine accumulations in excess of 20 times normal interfere with the normal metabolism of tyrosine and tryptophan. In the variant disorder deficiency of tetrahydrobiopterin interferes with normal metabolism of all three aromatic amino acids, although not with the degradative pathways for tyrosine and tryptophan.

Clinical manifestations. There are no reliable clinical manifestations of phenylketonuria in the neonatal period. Feeding difficulties, choking spells, and vomiting occur in some patients. Hypertrophic pyloric stenosis has been diagnosed in a number of patients, and the association may well be more than coincidental. Since the definition of phenylketonuria caused by defective cofactor metabolism it has become apparent that clinical difficulties in the neonatal period are more likely to occur in this form of the disease than in classic phenylketonuria. In any case neonatal neurologic development in phenylketonuria cannot be distinguished from normal.

Diagnosis. Although urinary phenylpyruvic acid is the hallmark of phenylketonuria, its appearance cannot be relied on in the neonatal period. The classic criterion for the diagnosis of phenylketonuria in the neonatal period is plasma phenylalanine of 20 mg/dl or more associated with low or normal plasma tyrosine, both values obtained while the infant is receiving normal feedings. Berry has suggested that 15 mg/dl is more clinically relevant than 20 mg/dl in predicting risk for cerebral injury in classic phenylketonuria, which accounts for at least 95% of affected subjects. The number of patients known to have cofactor-related disease is too small to allow a definition of the range of values for plasma phenylalanine associated with this condition, which is at least as clinically dangerous as classic phenylketonuria.

It has been proposed that the response of plasma phenylalanine to test doses of tetrahydrobiopterin be used to define cofactor-related disease in hyperphenylalaninemic infants. Lack of response indicates absence of phenylalanine hydroxylase, whereas a fall in plasma phenylalanine indicates either defective de novo synthesis or defective regeneration of tetrahydrobiopterin. Unfortunately it is possible that, in the presence of deficient but not absent phenylalanine hydroxylase, a great excess of tetrahydrobiopterin could stimulate hydroxylation of phenylalanine, thus lowering plasma phenylalanine. Quantitation of pterins (metabolites of the biopterin pathway) also has been proposed as a means of defining the presence or absence of cofactor-related disease. At this writing these techniques are becoming widely available in the United States.

Treatment of classic phenylketonuria. The evidence regarding diet therapy in phenylketonuria strongly indicates that restriction of phenylalanine intake is beneficial and also that overrestriction of dietary phenylalanine is detrimental to the health of these infants. The objective of therapy as currently practiced is to reduce plasma phenylalanine to a level that allows normal intellectual development while giving amounts of dietary phenylalanine adequate enough to ensure against phenylalanine deficiency. The usual requirement for phenylalanine in the neonatal period is 60 to 80 mg/kg/day. Infants diagnosed as having treatable hyperphenylalaninemia therefore are given a low-phenylalanine formula (3 mg phenylalanine per ounce of prepared formula) together with enough cow's milk (50 mg phenylalanine per ounce of prepared formula) to provide 70 mg phenylalanine/kg/day. Plasma phenylalanine is monitored and dietary phenylalanine adjusted to achieve an appropriate level of phenylalanine in plasma. Adequate growth cannot be achieved unless plasma phenylalanine is allowed to remain several milligrams per deciliter above the normal fasting level. Our clinic strives to maintain the plasma phenylalanine level at 8 to 10 mg/dl with consistently negative reactions to urinary ferric chloride tests. Solid food is added at appropriate intervals, according to a diet plan such as that offered by a manufacturer of low phenylalanine formula.

The hazards of a treatment program for phenylketonuria cannot be overemphasized. Points of particular concern are given in the following sections.

Accuracy of diagnosis. The criteria previously given are appropriate for a single point in time only. Apparent phenylalanine tolerance, as manifested by plasma phenylalanine levels, may change markedly with time. Borderline patients not selected for treatment should be observed closely. Those subjected to treatment should be assessed periodically for accuracy of diagnosis. For this purpose a trial of unlimited phenylalanine intake is preferred over an abrupt test of phenylalanine tolerance.

Overtreatment: phenylalanine deficiency. Rouse has documented the hazards of prolonged inappropriate restriction of phenylalanine in the diet of infants not having phenylketonuria. Hackney and co-workers suggested that disappointing results in dietary treatment may in part be the result of unrecognized phenylalanine deficiency. In young infants both phenylalanine requirement and phenylalanine intake may fluctuate widely over short periods of time under ideal conditions. Stress, such as infection, accentuates such fluctuations. It is therefore necessary to monitor plasma phenylalanine at very frequent intervals. The following schedule is suggested:

0 to 6 months	Twice weekly
6 months to 1 year	Once weekly
1 year to 18 months	Twice monthly
18 months until cessation of therapy	Once monthly

The analyses must be promptly performed and the results immediately applied to management.

Growth. Many appropriately treated patients do not grow normally. The distinction between impairment of growth caused by phenylalanine deficiency and that caused by the effects of a largely synthetic diet is sometimes difficult to make.

Treatment for cofactor-related phenylketonuria. For variant phenylketonuria in which tetrahydrobiopterin metabolism is defective, it would seem appropriate to treat with tetrahydrobiopterin. Such therapy may indeed lower plasma phenylalanine, obviating the need for a phenylalanine-restricted diet. However, because neither the cofactor nor any of its metabolites has been shown to cross the blood-brain barrier, cofactor therapy is unlikely to prevent brain damage. For this reason treatment with L-dopa, 5-hydroxytryptophan, and carbidopa has ben recommended in addition to management of plasma phenylalanine. Clinical efficacy has been reasonably well demonstrated in older infants so treated.

Treatment of hyperphenylalaninemia. Infants whose serum phenylalanine is greater than 10 mg/dl but less than 20 mg/dl are best managed initially by restricting dietary protein to 2 gm/kg/day. Serum phenylalanine generally falls to concentrations less than 10 mg/dl with this management. Should it fail to do so, it is best to use a regimen of specific phenylalanine restriction as in classic phenylketonuria.

Genetics. Classic phenylketonuria is inherited as an autosomal recessive disease. There is at present no test that allows reliably accurate discrimination between heterozygous and normal individuals. There is as yet insufficient information concerning the cofactor-related disease to allow a definite statement regarding its pattern of inheritance. The limited available data are consistent with autosomal recessive transmission.

Tyrosinosis

Tyrosinosis is a rare disorder in which plasma and urinary tyrosine are greatly increased. The only known clinical abnormality that is consistently present is the Richner-Hanhart syndrome (keratoconjunctivitis palmoplantaris). Conjunctival irritation has been noted in the neonatal period. In one case impairment in the transamination of tyrosine was demonstrated (Fig. 32-1).

Acute tyrosinosis, chronic tyrosinemia, hypermethioninemia

These terms are applied to a heterogeneous group of disorders in which it now seems likely that no primary defect in tyrosine or methionine metabolism exists. The clinical manifestations are predominantly those of acute and chronic liver disease, renal tubular dysfunction, and impairment of central nervous system development.

Etiology and pathogenesis. A number of infants seen within the first year of life, primarily with manifestations of severe hepatic dysfunction, have been shown to have striking elevations of plasma tyrosine and/or methionine. Enzymatic defects in the metabolic pathways for the affected amino acids have been clearly documented in these infants. However, in some instances the condition has proved to be self-limited and the clinical course compatible with neonatal hepatitis. On the other hand, some of these infants have shown only partial recovery, with persistence of low-grade liver disease and disorders of renal tubular function, associated with chronic elevation of plasma tyrosine. Familial incidence compatible with autosomal recessive inheritance has been documented in the latter group. Cases of chronic disease have been reported in which acute disease was never present. Since hereditary fructose intolerance, galactosemia, and fructose-1,6-diphosphatase deficiency all have been shown to produce the clinical and laboratory findings of acute tyrosinosis, it is entirely possible that a genotype having no primary effect on the metabolism of tyrosine can produce the manifestations of acute tyrosinosis and chronic tyrosinemia.

Clinical manifestations. The manifestations of this syndrome in the neonatal period are largely those of acute hepatic dysfunction. Listlessness, vomiting, diarrhea, abdominal enlargement with hepatomegaly, splenomegaly, and the development of ascites are prominent clinical features. Bleeding disorders are common, and coma may evolve in the course of this disorder. Mortality is high in the neonatal period.

It is readily apparent that these manifestations are similar to those of hereditary fructose intolerance, galactosemia, and neonatal septicemia, all of which enter into the differential diagnosis of this condition.

Laboratory manifestations. Moderate to striking elevations of plasma tyrosine or methionine or both are present. In acute tyrosinosis, tyrosyluria is a constant finding. Hyperphenylalaninemia and elevation of other plasma amino acids may be seen. Hypoglycemia, hypophosphatemia, and galactosuria have been noted. The results of the usual tests of hepatic function are grossly abnormal. Anemia, thrombocytopenia, and leukopenia are common.

Treatment. Some patients with acute tyrosinosis have responded favorably to a diet restricted in tyrosine and phenylalanine. Plasma levels of tyrosine predictably have fallen under this treatment, but clinical response has been less uniform. It seems likely that the amount and type of carbohydrate in the diet are as important as the amino acid composition, but studies to date do not allow a clear recommendation as to carbohydrate feeding. Given the mortality associated with the condition, it is probably wise both to employ low-phenylalanine, low-tyrosine feedings and to alter the carbohydrate source for affected infants (for example, from sucrose to lactose or from lactose to sucrose).

Prognosis. The disorder may be fatal early, enter a chronic phase, or remit completely; the result probably is dependent on both cause and management.

Genetics. As indicated earlier, a genetic basis for some forms of this disorder has been clearly established.

Alcaptonuria

Alcaptonuria, a disorder of the oxidation of homogentisic acid (Fig. 32-1), leads to the excretion of large amounts of homogentisic acid in the urine. The only manifestation of the disorder in the neonatal period is the darkening of diapers on standing. This reaction is the basis for the diagnostic test in which sodium hydroxide is added to freshly voided urine or dropped onto a freshly wet diaper. The production of a blackish brown stain is almost immediate and is virtually diagnostic of alcaptonuria. Plasma tyrosine and phenylalanine are normal in alcaptonuria.

Although a low-phenylalanine, low-tyrosine diet has been recommended in this condition to prevent the deposition of melanin-like by-products in joint cartilage, there is little justification for the imposition of such an abnormal diet in children with this disorder.

Alcaptonuria is inherited as an autosomal recessive disease.

Homocystinuria

Homocystinuria is a disorder of the metabolism of sulfur-containing amino acids that is associated with a progressive clinical syndrome involving the eye, the integument, the bones and connective tissues, the blood vessels and the central nervous system.

Etiology and pathogenesis. The fundamental defect in homocystinuria is marked reduction in the activity of cystathionine synthetase. This defect leads to the accumulation of homocystine in blood and urine and generally of methionine in the blood. The synthesis of cystine also is impaired. It is generally believed that homocystine and/or the products of its altered metabolism are responsible for the slowly evolving clinical syndrome. Although the results of therapy support this view, the pathogenesis of the disease is by no means clear. Mechanisms have been proposed whereby homocystine, homocysteine, and homocysteic acid could alter the tertiary structure of connective tissue proteins, damage vascular endothelium, alter platelet function, and otherwise inappropriately activate the clotting mechanism. A number of these mechanisms are quite attractive intellectually, but as yet none are proven.

Clinical manifestations. Infants with homocystinuria are normal at birth and remain so throughout the neonatal period. The clinical manifestations are progressive. Most characteristic is ectopia lentis, which commonly appears between 2½ and 3⅓ years of age. Many affected individuals develop constitutional features of Marfan's syndrome, malar flush, and livedo reticularis of the lower extremities. Roughly half the patients have intellectual deficits. Thrombotic episodes involving both small and large arteries and veins are a constant threat to the older homocystinuric individual.

The characteristic laboratory manifestation of homocystinuria is the presence of homocystine in the urine. This substance can be readily detected by the cyanide-nitroprusside test for compounds containing —S—S— or —S—H groups. Confirmation of the diagnosis is best obtained by column chromatography of amino acids from plasma or urine. The amount of free homocystine in homocystinuric plasma is relatively small. Since homocystine reacts readily with plasma protein, the diagnosis can be missed if plasma samples are allowed to stand for long periods prior to analysis. Rarely homocystine appears in the blood and urine of subjects who have other metabolic disorders. It is therefore worthwhile to exclude both cystathioninuria with secondary homocystinuria and defective cobalamin metabolism giving rise to both homocystinuria and methylmalonic aciduria.

Treatment. The goal of management in homocystinuria is the normalization of plasma homocystine, methionine, and cystine. In about half the affected subjects this goal can be approached effectively by the administration of large doses of pyridoxine, a cofactor for cystathionine synthetase. Effective dosages have ranged from 25 to 1,000 mg/day in older subjects, the wide range reflecting both genetic heterogeneity and in all likelihood the presence of unrecognized folate depletion in some of the treated subjects. For those whose response to megavitamin therapy is less than ideal, a diet low in methionine and enriched in cystine should be employed. With this scheme of management reasonable control of plasma homocystine can be achieved with lowering of plasma methionine. Plasma cystine has proved more refractory to therapy. In any case the available, albeit limited, evidence suggests clinical efficacy.

Genetics. Homocystinuria is inherited as an autosomal recessive disease.

Nonketotic hyperglycinemia

Nonketotic hyperglycinemia is a familial disorder of glycine metabolism in which profound dysfunction of the nervous system is noted shortly after birth. A large percentage of affected infants die within the first 2 weeks of life, and most of the remainder exhibit severe motor and mental retardation.

Etiology and pathogenesis. Of the many pathways of glycine metabolism noted in Fig. 32-3, only glycine cleavage is known to be affected in nonketotic hyperglycinemia, and this appears to be the primary phenomenon in the pathogenesis of this disorder. The mechanism through which the profound clinical effects of the disease are produced is unclear. Extreme elevation in plasma glycine, seen in infants undergoing total parenteral nutrition, has no apparent clinical effect. No forceful argument can be made at this time that abnormalities in gluconeogenesis and methyl group metabolism, occurring as secondary effects of the defect in glycine cleavage, are clinically significant. On the other hand, Perry has pointed out that the clinical manifestations of hyperglycemia correlate with the concentration of glycine in cerebrospinal fluid, not with concentration in plasma, and that such elevations of glycine in cerebrospinal fluid are seen only in nonketotic hyperglycinemia. The hypothesis that glycine excess in the central nervous system produces the clinical disease by altering neurotransmission gained some support from the observation that two affected infants showed clinical improvement when treated with strychnine, an antagonist to glycine in neurotransmission. Other patients so treated have shown no clinical response.

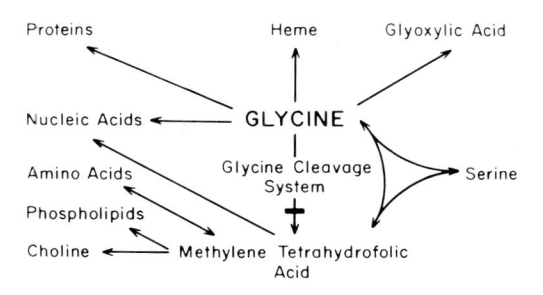

Fig. 32-3. Schematic representation of the metabolism of glycine. Crossbar indicates the metabolic block in nonketotic hyperglycinemia.

Clinical manifestations. Almost all patients with this disorder show serious abnormalities within the first few days of life. Poor feeding, lethargy, and hypotonia progressing to coma and apnea have been noted regularly. Seizures, both myoclonic and generalized, are common. Physical examination reveals lack of responsiveness, hypotonia, and diminished Moro and deep tendon reflexes.

In severely affected infants who survive the first 2 weeks of life, a waxing and waning course evolves in which prolonged periods of muscle spasm alternate with brief periods of relaxation. Seizures, typically myoclonic, occur both singly and in bursts. Poor feeding occurs for protracted periods, and motor and mental development is profoundly retarded.

Laboratory manifestations. The essential laboratory finding in nonketotic hyperglycinemia is striking elevation of glycine in cerebrospinal fluid. Plasma and urinary glycine levels are almost always elevated, but the abnormality in blood and urine is much less specific than that in cerebrospinal fluid. Arterial Pco$_2$ may be increased and Po$_2$ decreased as a result of respiratory depression.

Treatment. Aside from the previously noted reports of the efficacy of strychnine therapy in two patients, no effective management of nonketotic hyperglycinemia has been achieved. Dietary therapy and the use of sodium benzoate, methionine, and alanine have been attempted without clinical success.

Genetics. Nonketotic hyperglycinemia is inherited as an autosomal recessive disease.

Histidinemia

Histidinemia is a disorder of the catabolism of histidine caused by lack of histidase activity. It is characterized by the excretion of imidazolepyruvic acid, which gives positive reactions to ferric chloride and 2,4-dinitrophenylhydrazine tests on urine samples, similar to the reactions obtained in phenylketonuria. Plasma histidine is generally four to ten times normal.

Even though there may be considerable genetic heterogeneity in histidinemia, there is no clear evidence at present that it is a harmful condition. There are no neonatal manifestations other than the laboratory findings just noted. Although dietary therapy has been proposed for affected neonates, it cannot be recommended at this time.

DISORDERS OF THE UREA CYCLE

Disorders of the urea cycle severe enough to cause clinical disease in the neonate have as their hallmarks profound encephalopathy and striking elevation of blood ammonia. In the past it was thought that all infants exhibiting these signs were lethally affected. Developments over the past decade now indicate that some potentially lethal inborn errors of the urea cycle can be treated simply and effectively and that lethal hyperammonemic encephalopathy can occur both as a secondary phenomenon early in the course of treatable disorders of the propionate pathway and also as a self-limited phenomenon in infants who have no definable inborn disorder of metabolism. These discoveries clearly mandate an aggressive approach to the management of hyperammonemic encephalopathy in the neonate.

Etiology and pathogenesis

Urea accounts for two thirds of the total urinary nitrogen excreted by the neonate and thus is clearly the major excretory product in nitrogen metabolism. From a quantitative standpoint urea is produced by the liver alone. Its synthesis occurs in five reactions (Fig. 32-4), the first two of which are mitochondrial and energy requiring. The last three reactions occur in the cytosol (Fig. 32-5). Functionally the smooth flow of nitrogen into urea also requires integrity of the hepatic circulation, of transmembrane transport systems, and of general mitochondrial function. Although urea is an end product in that it is not metabolized by mammals, it is a dynamic metabolite functionally. A substantial fraction of the total urea pool is broken down by intestinal microorganisms. The nitrogen, liberated as ammonia, returns to the liver via the portal circulation, where it is either incorporated into amino acids or reincorporated into urea. That human metabolism is oriented toward ammonia fixation is reflected in the normal values for the concentration of ammonia in peripheral blood—25 μmol/L, compared with 500 μmol/L for blood urea nitrogen. Nitrogen destined for excretion in peripheral tissues is transported to the liver predominantly as glutamine and alanine. Chemical hyperammonemia of mild degree can occur in a variety of stressful conditions, but severe hyperammonemia of clinical significance is indicative of a profound disruption in hepatic function, be it circulatory or caused by hepatocellular destruction or deficient activity of one or more of the urea cycle enzymes. Chemically these disorders can be defined as hepatic inability to clear the blood of preformed ammonia and of glutamine.

Clinical manifestations

In the neonate severe hyperammonemia is manifested by a progressive illness beginning with poor feeding, with the evolution of hyperpnea, seizures that may be generalized or focal, waxing and waning consciousness, and ultimately coma and death. Muscle tone may be increased early, or there may be alternating hypertonia and hypotonia. Ultimately there is profound hypotonia. Primitive reflexes are progressively lost. A number of affected infants (including some with inherited defects in the urea cycle) have had pulmonary hemorrhage without apparent primary respiratory disease. Clinical hyperammonemia also has developed within the context of neonatal respiratory distress syndrome (RDS).

Specific entities
Idiopathic, self-limited, neonatal hyperammonemia

This entity has only recently been described. Affected infants generally but not always have been prematurely born. Some have shown signs of fetal distress, and some have had RDS. Signs of encephalopathy—poor feeding, disturbed respiratory pattern, and seizures—generally have appeared within the first 24 to 48 hours of life. Plasma ammonia values have ranged from 170 to 3,000 μmol/dl. When measured, plasma glutamine has been increased as well. Analyses of urea cycle enzymes and of urinary organic acids have been unrevealing. Exchange transfusion has been recommended as preferable to peritoneal dialysis in the management of hyperammonemia.

I concur with this recommendation with regard to this specific entity. Depression of central nervous system function often has been severe enough to necessitate ventilatory assistance. Nonetheless not all survivors have shown long-term neurologic deficits.

Reye's syndrome (encephalopathy and fatty degeneration of the viscera)

Reye's syndrome has been reported to occur in the neonate. However, fatty metamorphosis of viscera and encephalopathy are common findings in diverse inborn errors of metabolism causing lethal disease in neonates. An acute, acquired disease of this type, superimposed on a normal metabolic substrate, has not been demonstrated in the neonate.

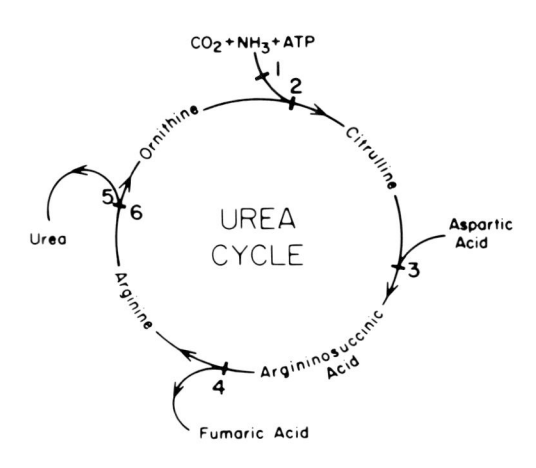

Carbamylphosphate synthetase deficiency (Figs. 32-4 and 32-5)

Several patients with deficiency of carbamylphosphate synthetase and apparently adequate activity of other urea cycle enzymes have been reported. One of these had a complex disorder without documented hyperammonemia, whereas another had clinical and chemical ammonia intoxication within the neonatal period. The latter patient had, in addition, hyperglycinemia, intermittent neutropenia, and ketoacidosis but no definable disorder of organic acid metabolism. Since a sibling had a similar clinical illness, it is presumed that the disorder was inherited. Other neonates with clinical diseases consistent with hyperammonemia have shown deficiencies of hepatic carbamylphosphate synthetase.

Fig. 32-4. Numbers denote enzymes whose function is impaired in the various errors of urea synthesis: *1*, carbamyl phosphate synthetase; *2*, ornithine carbamyl transferase; *3*, argininosuccinic acid synthetase; *4*, argininosuccinic acid lyase; *5*, arginase, primary defect; and *6*, arginase, secondary defect caused by elevated levels of lysine.

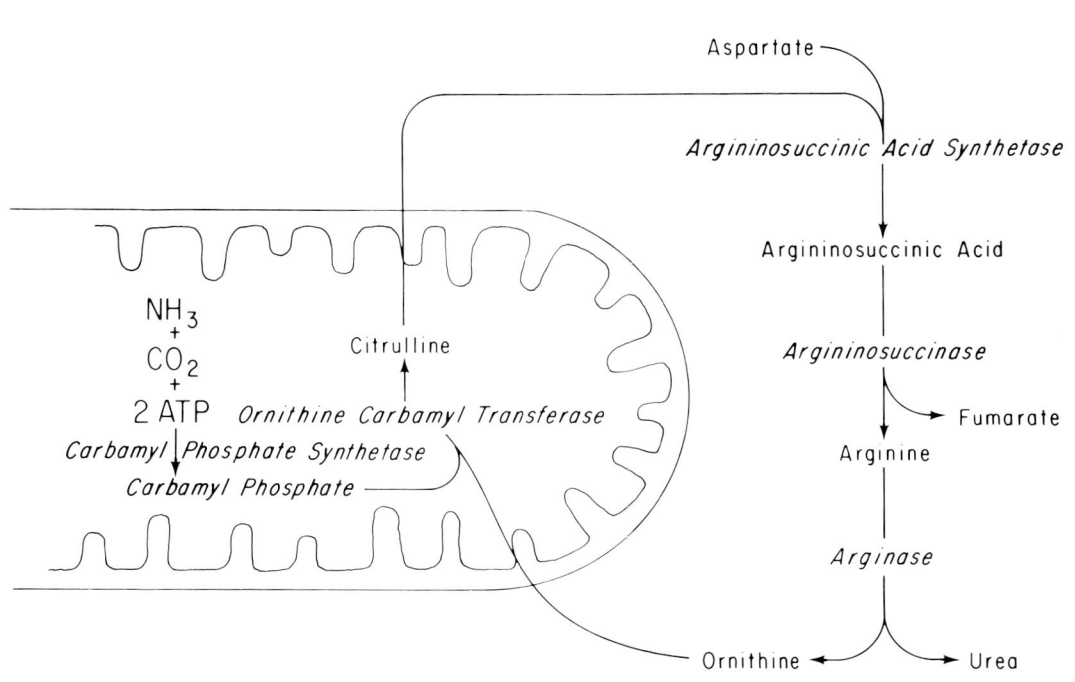

Fig. 32-5. The urea cycle, an intramitochondrial and extramitochondrial process.

Sex-linked hyperammonemia: ornithine carbamyltransferase deficiency (Fig. 32-4)

Ornithine carbamyltransferase deficiency is unique among these disorders in that it shows sex-linked inheritance. The majority of patients recognized thus far have been females, with reduced but not absent enzyme activity. Mother-to-daughter transmission has been demonstrated. Affected males have shown either a variant enzyme or absence of enzyme activity. Absence of enzyme activity is lethal within the first week of life in affected males, if untreated.

Surviving patients with ornithine carbamyltransferase deficiency generally show elevations in plasma and urinary glutamine and alanine. Most have excreted large amounts of orotic acid, apparently synthesized in response to diminished use of carbamylphosphate for citrulline synthesis. Diagnosis is made by enzyme assay of liver tissue.

Argininosuccinicaciduria (Fig. 32-4)

Unique among these disorders is the peculiarly friable hair seen even within the neonatal period in infants with argininosuccinicaciduria. Inheritance in argininosuccinicaciduria is of the autosomal recessive type. Definitive diagnosis may be established by finding large amounts of argininosuccinic acid in the urine or by enzyme assay.

Arginase deficiency (Fig. 32-4)

Arginase deficiency has only recently been recognized. There has been no known instance of neonatal presentation. Diagnosis is made by enzyme assay.

Lysine intolerance with hyperammonemia (Fig. 32-4)

A single instance of lysine intolerance with hyperammonemia has been recorded, without neonatal manifestations. It is postulated that in this disease an impairment in lysine catabolism results in elevated tissue levels of lysine and that the elevated tissue lysine competitively inhibits the hydrolysis of arginine by arginase.

N-Acetylglutamate synthetase deficiency

In broken mitochondrial preparations in vitro, N-acetylglutamate is required in catalytic amounts for carbamylphosphate synthesis. Whole mitochondria do not have this requirement, presumably because sufficient quantities of the compound are synthesized within the organelle.

Deficiency of the synthetase has been reported in a single infant whose sibling had died in the neonatal period with findings at autopsy suggestive of hyperammonemia. In the surviving infant, therapy with carbamylglutamate was reported to be effective.

Management. The management of hyperammonemia involves reduction in the load of metabolic nitrogen destined for excretion as both a short-term and long-term goal and removal of free ammonia and its precursors from the body as a short-term goal. Initial management of the sick neonate includes therefore sterilization of the intestine with colistin or neomycin (short term), cessation of protein feedings (short term), provision of high carbohydrate intake (100 to 120 kcal/kg/day) by continuous intravenous infusion, and exchange transfusion or peritoneal dialysis (short term). During the initial phase of management citrullinemia and argininosuccinicacidemia must be ruled out. The presence of either disease is an indication for the immediate initiation of therapy with arginine in dosages of 2 to 4 mmol/kg/day. When a stable clinical state is achieved, protein feedings can be resumed. It is advisable to administer 0.25 to 0.5 gm/kg/day of a high-quality protein with a total caloric intake of 120 kcal/kg/day. The protein can be increased slowly (no more often than every fourth day) to achieve the best attainable balance between neurologic state and growth. In all primary disorders of the urea cycle except arginase deficiency arginine can be considered an essential amino acid, and sufficient arginine should be administered to maintain normal plasma arginine concentrations. In citrullinemia and argininosuccinicaciduria additional arginine is likely to be beneficial in that it provides a source of ornithine to be used in the synthesis of citrulline and argininosuccinic acid, which are obligatory end products of nitrogen metabolism in these conditions.

The results of long-term management are determined in large part by the degree to which nitrogen elimination is impaired. If the impairment is extremely severe, the aforementioned long-term management will not suffice. For such cases formulas containing either crystalline amino acids or mixtures of amino acids and keto acid analogs of amino acids have been employed successfully. Because the catabolic stress associated with minor infections has led to lethal hyperammonemia in most patients so treated, long-term usefulness of this form of management is questionable at this time.

DISORDERS OF ORGANIC ACID METABOLISM

This large group of diseases, each of which is rare, accounts for a small but significant fraction of neonatal clinical illness. In each of these disorders the metabolism of one or more organic acids is disturbed, leading to accumulation of affected acids in the body. Because they are strong acids, their urinary excretion places a heavy burden on the renal acidification mechanism. The accumulated acids have, in addition, a variety of effects on chemical physiology, some of which are clinically devastating. Manifestations vary from patient to patient and are dependent on the nature and severity of the defect, dietary intake, the presence or absence of intercurrent infection, and so forth. Hyperpnea caused by metabolic acidosis is the most common manifestation, but feeding difficulties, vomiting, and depression of central nervous system function, with or without seizures, are also prominent. Chemically, in addition to metabolic acidosis, there may be hypoglycemia, hyperammonemia, and disturbances in serum electrolytes (hypocalcemia, hypokalemia), all of which are poorly understood. In the clinical application of readily available laboratory tests the most valuable sign of organic acidosis is an increase in the undetermined anion fraction in plasma. When defined as serum Na − (serum Cl + serum bicarbonate), this value is normally 10 to 15 mEq/L. Slight increases occur in dehydration because of decreased glomerular filtration, but values greater than 17 mEq/L in well-hydrated infants and greater than 20 mEq/L under any circumstances are highly suspicious. It must be recognized, however, that hypoxemia and poor perfusion of tissues can give rise to organic acidosis without an underlying enzymatic defect. In such cases the predominant acid accumulated is lactic acid, although a number of others may be present in both blood and urine.

Maple syrup urine disease

Maple syrup urine disease, or branched-chain aminoaciduria, is the result of an impairment in the decarboxylation of the keto acid derivatives of the three branched-chain amino acids: leucine, isoleucine, and valine (Fig. 32-6). Profound depression of the central nervous system and death early in life occur in the vast majority of untreated patients.

Etiology and pathogenesis

The transamination of the branched-chain amino acids occurs normally in maple syrup urine disease, but the keto acids produced by transamination are not oxidized normally. Since the transamination reaction is freely reversible, accumulation of these keto acids leads to a corresponding increase in the levels of the branched-chain amino acids. The clinical manifestations of the disease are correlated with elevations in plasma leucine and α-ketoisocaproic acid, but not with accumulations of isoleucine, valine, and their keto acid analogs. The metabolic acidosis observed in this disease is only in part explained by the excretory load of these specific organic acids. The mechanism by which the profound disturbance of the central nervous system is produced remains unknown. On postmortem examination the brains of affected infants exhibit defective myelinization and spongy degeneration of the white matter. Although hypoglycemia and excessive glycogen deposition in the liver have been noted in these patients, the central nervous system manifestations cannot be explained solely on the basis of hypoglycemia.

Clinical manifestations

Affected infants appear normal at birth. Onset of clinical manifestations generally occurs very early; most patients exhibit profound illness within a week. Initially there may be rapid, shallow respirations, soon followed by profound alteration in consciousness. The infant appears apathetic and characteristically develops alternating hypertonia and hypotonia, accompanied by brief tonic seizures. The odor of maple syrup usually is detected at the time of clinical illness but occasionally has not been noted in fatally affected infants. The untreated disease is rapidly progressive, and death occurs within the neonatal period generally from respiratory failure, with or without complicating bronchopneumonia.

Laboratory manifestations

The presence of α-keto organic acids in the urine, as detected by the 2,4-dinitrophenylhydrazine text, is characteristic of the untreated disease and strongly suggests the diagnosis in infants whose clinical presentation is compatible with the disorder. The diagnosis is confirmed by finding striking elevations of leucine, isoleucine, and valine in plasma. These amino acids also are excreted in the urine in abnormal amounts. Alloisoleucine, an enantiomer of isoleucine, is also present in plasma. This amino acid was identified erroneously as methionine in early descriptions of the disorder.

Metabolic acidosis is probably characteristic of the untreated disease, although most reports do not emphasize this aspect of maple syrup urine disease. Hypoglycemia usually occurs.

Treatment

Restriction of dietary leucine, isoleucine, and valine has been employed with some degree of success. Dietary treatment requires frequent monitoring of plasma leucine, isoleucine, and valine to provide sufficient amounts of these essential amino acids for growth and development while avoiding the severely deleterious effects of excessive administration. Crises with central nervous system dysfunction and metabolic acidosis are associated not only with dietary indiscretion but also with infections and other forms of stress. Dietary therapy must be continued for life.

Crises have been treated successfully by peritoneal dialysis. This therapy also has been suggested for neonates who have become severely affected prior to the institution of dietary therapy.

A thiamine-responsive form of the disease has been described.

Prognosis

Even with early institution of therapy the prognosis for both life and normal intellectual development is guard-

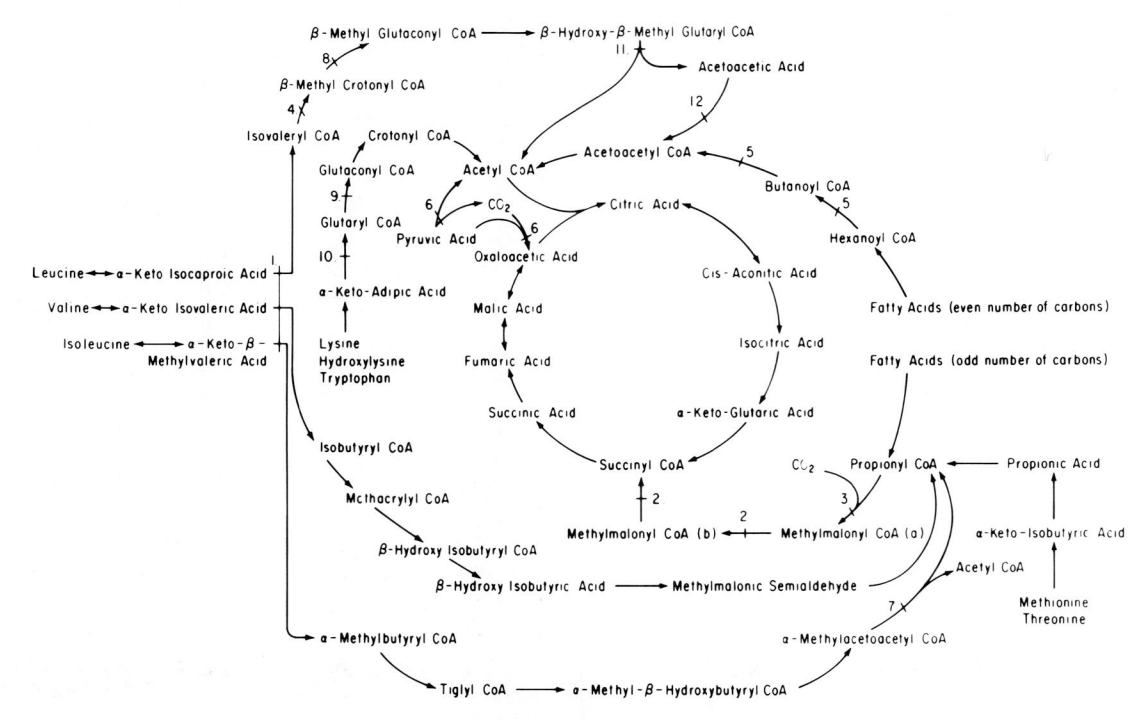

826 Behrman's neonatal-perinatal medicine: diseases of the fetus and infant

Fig. 32-6. Some pathways of organic acid metabolism. Inborn errors are numbered as follows: *1*, maple syrup urine disease; *2*, methylmalonic acidemia; *3*, propionic acidemia; *4*, isovaleric acidemia; *5*, hexanoic-butanoic acidemia; *6*, lactic acidosis; *7*, β-ketothiolase deficiency; *8*, β-methyl crotonylglycinuria; *9*, glutaric aciduria type I; *10*, α-keto adipic aciduria; *11*, 3-hydroxy-3-methylglutaric aciduria; *12*, succinyl-CoA: 3-ketoacid CoA-transferase deficiency.

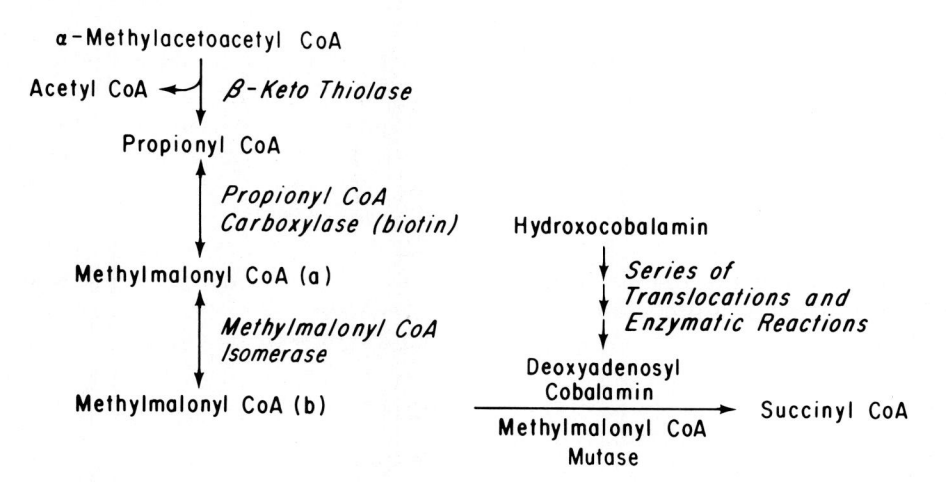

Fig. 32-7. Propionate pathway. Inborn errors of every process indicated have been described.

ed. An intermittent form of the disease has been reported in which typical crises occur in children who are otherwise clinically normal. The metabolic defect appears to be similar to but less severe than that found in the classic form of the disease. The relation of the intermittent variety to clinical disease in the neonate has not been elucidated.

Genetics

The disease shows autosomal recessive inheritance.

Disorders of propionate pathway

Disorders of the propionate pathway—β-ketothiolase deficiency, propionic acidemia, and methylmalonic acidemia—all give rise to the ketotic hyperglycinemia syndrome: protein intolerance with ketonuria, ketoacidosis, hypoglycemia, hyperammonemia, hyperglycinemia, neutropenia, thrombocytopenia, and anemia. Manifestations generally are noted during the neonatal period.

Genetically determined enzymatic defects have been described for each of the processes involved in the pathway from α-methyl acetoacetyl CoA to succinyl CoA (Figs. 32-6 and 32-7). The most distal defect, β-ketothiolase deficiency, involves primarily the degradation of isoleucine. The other enzyme defects also impair the catabolism of methionine, valine, possibly threonine, cholesterol, and fatty acids with odd numbers of carbon atoms.

Intestinal microorganisms contribute significantly to the load of compounds that are metabolized in the propionate pathway. The pathway is thus a major one whose disruption can be expected to be profoundly deleterious. However, the mechanism by which each of the components of the ketotic hyperglycinemia syndrome is produced remains unknown.

Of great practical importance is that deficiencies in propionyl CoA carboxylase activity in some cases are caused by defective metabolism of the cofactor biotin and are responsive to biotin therapy (Fig. 32-7). Similarly methylmalonic acidemia may be caused by a number of defects in cobalamin metabolism (Fig. 32-7). Such defects may respond to cobalamin therapy.

Clinical manifestations

Although slowly developing clinical disease occurs in association with these enzymatic defects, clinical presentation in the neonatal period is more common. Lethargy, poor feeding, vomiting, and hyperpnea are likely to progress to frank coma, the clinical disease being exacerbated by protein feedings. Seizures are uncommon.

Laboratory manifestations

Laboratory findings in the neonatal period are disturbingly protean. A striking but frequently overlooked clue to the diagnosis is ketonuria. Even in the presence of ketonuria there may be no acidosis but rather hyperammonemia of such degree as to suggest a primary defect in urea cycle function. In a number of affected infants ketoacidosis has been profound, occurring at times together with grossly elevated blood ammonia (greater than 300 μmol/L). The combination of neonatal ketoacidosis and extreme hyperammonemia is virtually diagnostic of a defect in the propionate pathway. Neutropenia, thrombocytopenia, and anemia are only intermittently present, as is hyperglycinemia. Hypoglycemia is very common, particularly during exacerbations of ketoacidosis. The diagnosis is forwarded by determination of the specific pattern of organic acids in blood and/or urine and definitively made by demonstration of the specific enzymatic defect.

Treatment

Initial management is directed toward (1) correction of hypoglycemia if present, (2) management of hyperammonemia (see section on defects of the urea cycle), and (3) management of metabolic acidosis. Sterilization of the intestine is beneficial in that it reduces the absorption of intermediates in the pathway produced by intestinal microorganisms. Glucose infusions sufficient to supply total caloric need are also helpful in that they retard the breakdown of protein. Large doses of sodium bicarbonate may be required initially (20 mEq/kg/day). Once appropriate samples of blood and urine have been collected, it is advisable to employ megavitamin therapy: biotin, 10 mg/day orally, and hydroxycobalamin, 2 mg/day intramuscularly. Once stabilization has been achieved, oral feedings can be instituted employing a diet high in carbohydrates and low in protein (0.5 gm/kg/day). Protein intake then can be liberalized gradually to achieve the best possible clinical state. Throughout the course of the illness, but particularly during crises, careful attention must be paid to the hematologic abnormalities. Severe infection is a serious risk during episodes of neutropenia, and transfusion of whole blood and of platelet concentrates may be required for management of anemia and thrombocytopenia.

Prognosis

Defects in the propionate pathway may be lethal in spite of optimal management, but a number of infants, critically ill at diagnosis, have responded well to treatment. Intellectual and motor development is likely to be delayed but not necessarily profoundly so.

Genetics

Autosomal recessive inheritance is indicated in each of the disorders of the propionate pathway.

Congenital lactic acidosis

Lactic acidosis is most commonly encountered as the result of hypoxemia and/or poor perfusion of tissues. It also can be seen as a complication of a number of metabolic disorders in which the known primary defect does not involve lactate metabolism (hereditary fructose intolerance, fructose-1,6-diphosphatase deficiency, and glycogenosis type I). In a third group of patients lactic acidosis is so dominant a characteristic of the illness as to assume primary importance in nomenclature: hence the term *congenital lactic acidosis*.

Etiology and pathogenesis

The metabolism of lactate is essentially that of pyruvate, with which both lactate and alanine are in equilibrium. Quantitatively pyruvate is catabolized through pyruvate dehydrogenase (with thiamine pyrophosphate and lipoic acid as cofactors) and the citric acid cycle. This pathway seems normally to predominate under conditions of glucose excess. Alternatively pyruvate can be carboxylated to form oxaloacetate in a reaction catalyzed by pyruvate carboxylase, a biotin-requiring enzyme. Oxaloacetate can be used catalytically in the tricarboxylic acid cycle and quantitatively for the synthesis of glucose via phosphoenolpyruvate and reverse glycolysis. The latter sequence of reactions seems to be most active when glucose is in limited supply. The flow of pyruvate through one or the other pathway, however, is dependent on the integrity of other systems. If the function of the electron transport chain is impaired, as, for example, by anoxia, the action of pyruvate dehydrogenase is slowed. Furthermore, because both pyruvate dehydrogenase and pyruvate carboxylase are mitochondrial enzymes, structural and functional integrity of mitochondria is necessary for their proper functions. In fact, then, lactic acidosis could be accounted for in any number of ways, and indeed infants with lactic acidosis as the predominant manifestation of congenital metabolic disease are a heterogeneous group. Only in the past decade has a systematic effort been made to examine the activities of the pyruvate dehydrogenase complex and of pyruvate carboxylase in these infants. The electron transport chain has been studied in only one or two patients. Thus no systematic classification of defects is possible. In general it can be said: (1) most infants with congenital lactic acidosis tolerate excess glucose well (not to be expected with pyruvate dehydrogenase deficiency); (2) most are normoglycemic or nearly so (not to be expected with pyruvate carboxylase deficiency); (3) brain damage in most tends to be severe; (4) some have neuropathologic findings of subacute necrotizing encephalomyelitis and, because of the resemblance of these anatomic findings to those of experimental thiamine deficiency, are thought to have defects of pyruvate dehydrogenase; and (5) some have ketoacidosis, suggesting that the tricarboxylic acid cycle is deprived of oxaloacetate because of pyruvate carboxylase deficiency.

Clinical manifestations

The majority of infants with congenital lactic acidosis are undoubtedly acidotic from birth. In many instances the acidosis is manifest only by mild hyperpnea and poor feeding and is not recognized until some weeks later when intercurrent infection precipitates a severe acidotic crisis. As a group, these infants are profoundly hypotonic and inattentive. They do not follow, and many show optic atrophy early. Although physically normal at birth, they tend to become obese early. Seizures are relatively common and tend to be myoclonic in type. When generalized seizures occur, there is a strong likelihood of hypoglycemia. Tetany has been reported and is thought to be secondary to the formation of calcium lactate complexes in plasma. Development tends to be extremely retarded. Befitting the heterogeneous nature of the disorder, some infants have been hypertonic, and some have shown spontaneous improvement.

Laboratory manifestations

The undetermined anion fraction of plasma electrolytes is increased, with the increase largely accounted for by lactate. Oxygen saturation and Po_2 are normal, and Pco_2 is decreased. Pyruvate and alanine are increased in plasma, and urine contains excessive lactate, pyruvate, and alanine. Blood glucose is generally normal, but hypoglycemia has been noted in some cases. When profound depression of the central nervous system occurs, Po_2 may fall and Pco_2 rise as a result of hypoventilation. Thus the infant, who is cyanotic and comatose when first examined, may have either decreased oxygenation with secondary lactic acidosis or intrinsic lactic acidosis with secondary hypoventilation. In the former case establishment of adequate oxygenation results in relatively prompt ameliorization of the lactic acidosis.

Treatment

Initial management is directed toward correction of the metabolic acidosis. Adequate oxygenation of tissues must be ensured. Intravenous sodium bicarbonate generally is required, sometimes in dosages as high as 20 mEq/kg/day. Because of the need for such large amounts of sodium in therapy, edema and hypernatremia are constant threats, requiring careful attention to sodium and water balance with judicious use of diuretics. After appropriate specimens have been obtained for diagnostic purposes, megavitamin therapy is indicated.

Biotin, 10 mg/day, and thiamine, 50 to 200 mg/day, generally are employed (dosages used have been variable). Lipoic acid, pathothenic acid, and niacin also have been used. For most patients it can be expected that diet therapy will have little influence on the clinical course of the disease. In a few patients glucose administration has been associated with increased lactate in plasma, suggesting that pyruvate dehydrogenase is specifically affected and that a high fat, low carbohydrate diet may be beneficial. However, transfusion with citrated blood also has precipitated acidotic crises in some patients, suggesting that these individuals have deficiencies in activity of both pyruvate dehydrogenase and α-ketoglutarate dehydrogenase, which is closely related to pyruvate dehydrogenase and a key enzyme in the citric acid cycle. For such individuals glycolysis may be an important source of energy. Thus carbohydrate restriction probably is not indicated and may be deleterious. Patients with presumed pyruvate carboxylase deficiency may have impaired production of oxaloacetic acid. It is possible that supplementation of the diet of such patients with aspartic acid, which can be transaminated to oxaloacetic acid, would increase their ability to use both carbohydrates and fats as sources of energy.

If stabilization of the infant on feedings can be achieved, oral sodium bicarbonate therapy is likely to be required. The dose needed to maintain acid-base homeostasis varies both from individual and from day to day. To avoid alkalosis, I have employed a regimen in which the pH of freshly voided urine is monitored and bicarbonate supplements administered only when urine pH falls below 7.

Prognosis

The outlook for infants with congenital lactic acidosis undoubtedly depends primarily on the nature of the enzyme defect and its responsiveness to cofactor therapy. Severe developmental retardation, with or without death in early infancy, is most likely, but a few patients have done relatively well.

Genetics

Congenital lactic acidosis has been reported in siblings. Because of the heterogeneous nature of the disorder and the small number of cases, no definitive statement regarding inheritance is possible.

Isovaleric acidemia (sweaty feet syndrome)

Isovaleric acidemia is similar clinically to disorders of the propionate pathway.

Etiology and pathogenesis

An enzymatic defect in the catabolic pathway for leucine is responsible for this disease and generally gives rise to metabolic acidosis, depression of the central nervous system, and pancytopenia early in life. Although all these manifestations are common in the presence of accumulations of short-chain fatty acids, the pathogenetic mechanisms are unclear.

Clinical manifestations

Clinically normal at birth, the affected infant characteristically develops tachypnea within the neonatal period. In reported cases the odor of sweaty feet generally has been noted early. Seizures and central nervous system depression with respiratory impairment are not unusual, and serious infection, presumably caused by anemia and neutropenia, frequently has complicated the neonatal course of the illness.

Laboratory manifestations

Metabolic acidosis with an increase in the undetermined anion fraction is a constant finding. Ketosis is found during acidotic crises. Depression of erythrocytes, neutrophils, and platelets is common.

Treatment

As in other organic acidoses, large doses of sodium bicarbonate and even peritoneal dialysis may be required to achieve initial stabilization. Vigorous supportive therapy, including antibiotics and transfusion, also may be required. By analogy with methylmalonic acidemia, sterilization of the intestine is likely to be beneficial. Long-term management entails a high-calorie diet low in protein (perhaps specifically restricted as to leucine) and supplemental sodium bicarbonate as indicated. There is evidence that glycine supplementation, by increasing the formation of isovaleryl glycine, also may be of benefit.

Prognosis

Mortality in the neonatal period has been high in the past, as a result of both depression of central nervous system function and complications associated with pancytopenia. In survivors some degree of developmental retardation can be anticipated.

Genetics

The disease shows autosomal recessive inheritance.

Other disorders of organic acid metabolism
β-Methyl crotonylglycinuria

A number of instances of this entity have bee described. Manifestations have included metabolic ac dosis, amyotonia syndrome, and mucocutaneous can diasis. At this point it would appear that most affec individuals suffer from a defect in biotin metaboli leading to deficient activity of a number of bi requiring enzymes. In most reported patients therapeutic response to biotin, 10 mg/day, has dramatic.

In most instances the disorder has shown autosomal recessive inheritance.

α-Ketoadipic aciduria

This disorder is apparently rare but has been reported to produce intermittent metabolic acidosis in the neonatal period. Levels of plasma and urinary α-aminoadipic acid are increased, as might be expected, and increase further when a lysine load is administered. Specific therapy has not been reported. The mode of inheritance is unknown.

3-OH,3-Methylglutaric aciduria

This recently described defect in leucine catabolism can give rise to both metabolic acidosis and profound hypoglycemia in the neonatal period. Plasma amino acids (including leucine) are normal.

D-Glyceric aciduria

A single infant, with clinical manifestations similar to those of nonketotic hyperglycinemia, was found to have elevated D-glyceric acid in urine and blood. The elevations were not sufficient to cause metabolic acidosis. Serum glycine was increased, but the concentration of glycine in cerebrospinal fluid was not reported.

Glutaric aciduria type I

This rare disorder probably causes no clinically recognizable disease in the neonate but gives rise in later months to a progressive movement disorder characterized by delayed motor development, dystonia, and choreoathetosis.

Glutaric aciduria type II

Several infants, all of whom died within the neonatal period, were found to excrete in urine large amounts of glutaric acid along with other organic acids, particularly [...] acid. The nature of the disease is unclear, but it [...] appear to involve more than an isolated defect in [...] abolism of glutaric acid.

butanoic aciduria (sweaty feet syndrome)

[...]ents, of whom three were siblings, were [...] this disorder, whose postulated cause is [...] green acyl dehydrogenase that initiates [...] hexanoyl CoA and butanoyl CoA. Clini[...] was lethal in all four infants, who had [...]al acidosis and septicemia. More [...]zen urine from one of the patients [...] infant suffered from isovaleric aci[...]roducts of which are easily con[...] butanoic acids in the chromato[...] earlier study.

Succincyl CoA: 3-keto acid CoA-transferase deficiency

At least two infants are known to have been affected by this disorder. Ketoacidosis was evident early in both infants, one of whom died at 6 months and the other at 21 months. Genetic transmission seems assured on the basis of family histories.

DISORDERS OF MONOSACCHARIDE METABOLISM
Neonatal diabetes mellitus

Carbohydrate intolerance to an extent requiring insulin therapy has been noted with some frequency in the neonatal period. The disorder may be temporary or permanent.

Etiology and pathogenesis

The cause of diabetes mellitus, when it occurs in the neonate, is unknown. No consistent abnormalities of pancreatic tissue have been noted in autopsy material from infants with this disorder. Plasma insulin levels have not shown a consistent pattern in the few subjects in whom measurements have been made.

There is some association between the development of diabetes mellitus in the neonatal period and postmaturity and low birth weight, neonatal hypoglycemia, and steroid therapy early in the neonatal period.

Clinical manifestations

The age of patients at detection of this disorder has varied from 4 to 44 days. The most prominent manifestations have been weight loss and dehydration in association with polyuria. Characteristically the affected infant maintains a good oral intake and does not become comatose. The vast majority probably have some degree of metabolic acidosis, but severe ketonuria is not the rule.

Laboratory manifestations

In the excellent review of this disorder by Gentz and Cornblath blood sugar was noted to range from 245 to 2,300 mg/dl in affected infants. Hypernatremia was common, and ketonuria was variable, but metabolic acidosis was detected in most subjects whose acid-base status was evaluated.

Treatment

All patients with this disorder require careful attention to fluid and electrolyte balance. The dose of insulin required to achieve carbohydrate homeostasis varies markedly from patient to patient and from day to day in individual patients. Except for the severely ill infant, insulin therapy should be gradually instituted. Initially one-fourth unit of regular insulin per kilogram of body weight should be administered and the blood sugar monitored for 12 hours to assess the insulin sensitivity of the patient. It is not always possible to establish a regimen of management that employs a single injection of insulin each day. For many patients coverage with regular insulin on the basis of degree of glycosuria is optimal management for the first several months of life. Dietary allowances of protein and carbohydrate should be liberal. Since the risk of insulin-induced hypoglycemia with secondary brain damage is high in the early months of life, it is best not to attempt to achieve aglycosuria.

Prognosis

Gentz and Cornblath found that 30 of 50 patients with neonatal diabetes had temporary disorders requiring treatment for a mean period of 65 days. For those neonates with permanent diabetes there is no indication that prognosis is worse than it is for individuals who develop diabetes later in life.

Genetics

There is a relatively high incidence of diabetes mellitus in the families of affected infants but no clearly defined inheritance pattern for the disorder.

DISORDERS OF GALACTOSE METABOLISM
Galactokinase deficiency

Deficient activity of galactokinase results in disordered metabolism of galactose and the development of cataracts.

Etiology and pathogenesis

The initial step in the metabolism of dietary galactose is the phosphorylation of galactose, a reaction catalyzed by galactokinase. When this reaction is impaired, ingested galactose is either excreted in the urine or metabolized by unusual pathways. Marked reduction in activity of galactokinase thus results in postprandial galactosuria and in the production of galactitol by enzymatic reduction of galactose. There is substantial evidence to suggest that galactitol, acting as a nondiffusible osmotic agent within the lens, causes swelling of the lens fibers and ultimately distortion of the architecture of the lens. In addition, the reduction of galactose to galactitol drains the lens of compounds that are able to act as hydrogen donors in the stabilization of sulfhydryl-containing proteins. The instability of affected proteins, coupled with the osmotic effects of galactose, finally leads to cataract formation.

Clinical manifestations

In individuals homozygous for galactokinase deficiency cataract formation occurs early in life and has been noted within the neonatal period. Cataract formation in the third and fourth decades of life has been reported in individuals apparently heterozygous for this disorder. Dysfunction of liver and kidney are not seen in galactokinase deficiency, nor is hypoglycemia produced by galactose ingestion. Pseudotumor cerebri, however, has been reported to occur early in the course.

Laboratory manifestations

The diagnosis is established by demonstration of reduction of activity of galactokinase in red blood cells. Measurement of galactose in blood and urine in the postprandial state can be employed as a screening procedure. Increased urinary galactitol is a more constant finding in this disorder than is either galactosuria or galactosemia.

Treatment

Elimination of galactose from the diet is the treatment of choice. Resorption of cataracts has been reported in some individuals so treated. It appears that galactose restriction should be lifelong in this disorder.

Prognosis

The prognosis for general health is excellent, the only morbidity associated with this condition being visual impairment caused by cataracts.

Galactosemia

Galactosemia is a hereditary disorder of the metabolism of galactose-1-phosphate that is analogous to hereditary fructose intolerance, in which manifestations of renal disease and liver dysfunction follow the ingestion of galactose. Cataracts and some degree of mental retardation are also features of galactosemia.

Etiology and pathogenesis

The biochemical lesion in galactosemia is lack of activity of galactose-1-phosphate uridylyltransferase. This impairment of function leads to the accumulation within cells of galactose-1-phosphate; galactose accumulates both intracellularly and extracellularly. Cataract formation presumably occurs by the mechanism proposed for the development of cataracts in patients with galactokinase deficiency. The disorders of hepatic and renal function appear to be well correlated with the intracellular levels of galactose-1-phosphate. As in the case of hereditary fructose intolerance, hypoglycemia occurs promptly on the administration of galactose, and renal function can be shown to be impaired during the course of a galactose tolerance test. Although galactose-1-phosphate is known to inhibit phosphoglucomutase in vitro, the precise mechanism by which hypoglycemia occurs is not completely understood. The cerebral, renal, and hepatic lesions of galactosemia have not been satisfactorily explained.

Clinical manifestations

Infants with galactosemia are physically normal at birth, although their birth weights may be somewhat lower than those of unaffected siblings. Clinical manifestations may be fulminant, with death occurring within the first few days of life or delayed until some weeks after birth. Vomiting and diarrhea, hepatosplenomegaly, and jaundice, frequently associated with anemia, are the cardinal manifestations. Renal tubular acidosis may occur. Cataracts are usually but not invariably present in the neonatal period. The clinical manifestations that occur early within the neonatal period are strikingly similar to those of neonatal septicemia, and in a number of instances the coexistence of these two entities has been demonstrated. In those infants whose disease has a more insidious onset, clinical manifestations may be predominantly those of failure to thrive associated with hepatomegaly. The major clinical risk to life is progressive liver dysfunction complicated by cirrhosis.

Laboratory manifestations

The diagnosis of galactosemia is made by finding absence or near absence of activity of galactose-1-phosphate uridylyltransferase in red blood cell hemolysates. Some genetic variants of the disorder have been described in which the activity of the enzyme is reduced or unusually unstable. Therefore in some instances it may be necessary to obtain clarification of the diagnosis by measurement of red blood cell galactose-1-phosphate. The normal value for red blood cell galactose-1-phosphate is less than 1 mg/gm of hemoglobin. Untreated galactosemia is always accompanied by marked elevation in red blood cell galactose-1-phosphate. This determination is also useful in monitoring dietary therapy; most clinics restrict galactose to the extent necessary to maintain red blood cell galactose-1-phosphate at 4 mg/gm of hemoglobin or less.

Measurement of blood and urinary galactose has some value in screening but cannot be depended on to exclude the diagnosis of galactosemia in an infant who is so ill as to have little intake of galactose.

The galactose tolerance test has no place in the diagnosis of neonatal galactosemia. It is potentially dangerous and offers no advantage over the assay of red blood cell galactose-1-phosphate uridylyltransferase and galactose-1-phosphate.

Treatment

Prompt and progressive improvement follows the elimination of galactose from the affected infant's diet. Non-lactose-containing formulas, such as Nutramigen and Prosobee, may be used for this purpose. The very ill neonate may require vigorous supportive therapy, including transfusion and antibiotics for infection, in addition to elimination of dietary galactose. The appropriate duration of dietary treatment is not exactly known. It appears that the risk of severe liver and renal damage and of cataracts is limited to infancy and that tolerance for dietary galactose increases with age.

If the diagnosis of galactosemia is suspected in a very ill neonate, the proper course of action is to institute a galactose-free diet, obtaining blood for enzymatic evaluation whenever this is feasible. The elimination of galactose from the diet does not invalidate the enzyme assay, irrespective of the duration of elimination of dietary galactose.

Prognosis

The mortality of individuals with galactosemia symptomatic in the neonatal period is approximately 20%. This is thought to be related to delay in the institution of therapy but may be related in part to concomitant severe bacterial infection. For patients successfully treated in the neonatal period the prognosis for general health is good. Appropriate treatment generally is associated with complete resolution of the hepatic and renal lesions and occasionally even of cataracts. Cataract formation does not progress after the institution of therapy.

Statistically there is an inverse relationship between the age at onset of therapy and intellectual achievement. However, some galactosemic infants recognized at birth and treated promptly have shown inadequate intellectual development when compared with their siblings. Furthermore there is a high incidence of behavioral and learning disorders in the population of galactosemic infants, whether treated or untreated.

Genetics

Galactosemia is inherited as an autosomal recessive disease. Since there is considerable heterogeneity within the population of galactosemic individuals, enzymatic evaluation of the parents of the galactosemic infant is advisable.

Uridine-diphospho-galactose 4-epimerase deficiency

Both the catabolism of galactose and its synthesis from glucose are dependent in large part on the interconversion of uridine-diphospho-glucose and uridine-diphospho-galactose, which is catalyzed by an epimerase.

Deficiency of the epimerase in erythrocytes, but not in liver, has been noted several times. Affected subjects show no clinical disease. One infant with deficiency of the enzyme in liver as well as erythrocytes had typical clinical galactosemia. Presumed to be unable either to synthesize or catabolize galactose, the infant was treated with galactose restriction, not galactose elimination, and responded well to this management.

DISORDERS OF FRUCTOSE METABOLISM
Deficiency of fructose kinase: essential fructosuria

Essential fructosuria, an asymptomatic disorder that results in fructosuria after the ingestion of fructose by affected subjects, is caused by an inborn deficiency in the enzymatic phosphorylation of fructose. It has no apparent clinical significance.

Hereditary fructose intolerance

Hereditary fructose intolerance is a serious disorder of carbohydrate metabolism; the ingestion of fructose produces hypoglycemia, abdominal pain, vomiting, and severe liver and kidney dysfunction.

Etiology and pathogenesis

In hereditary fructose intolerance there is a marked decrease in the activity of fructose-1-phosphate aldolase and usually a reduction in the activity of fructose-1,6-diphosphate aldolase. Since the two enzymatic activities are closely related chemically, it appears possible that the disorder is related to an abnormality in a single protein. In affected subjects the ratio of fructose-1-phosphate aldolase to fructose-1,6-diphosphate aldolase is almost always found to be greater that 2, whereas the normal ratio of these activities is less than 2.

In response to fructose ingestion or infusion, patients exhibit a variable rise in blood fructose and a prompt and striking fall in blood glucose. Plasma inorganic phosphate falls, whereas plasma magnesium rises somewhat. Serum glutamic oxaloacetic transaminase (SGOT) and serum glutamic pyruvic transaminase (SGPT) also rise on the ingestion of fructose, and there is a marked increase in the excretion of amino acids. The exact mechanism responsible for these findings is not entirely understood, although generally it is considered to be related to the impairment in the metabolism of phosphorylated hexose. In vitro fructose-1-phosphate exhibits glycogenolysis. Clinically the hypoglycemia of hereditary fructose intolerance does not respond to glucagon.

Clinical manifestations

Affected infants are normal at birth. Clinical manifestations occur only when the infants receive formulas containing fructose or sucrose. When such formulas are fed, vomiting, sometimes accompanied by diarrhea, promptly develops. There may be postprandial seizures. With continued ingestion of fructose evidence of liver dysfunction appears, with hepatomegaly, jaundice of the obstructive type, and bleeding. At the same time renal function is impaired, with a substantial number of patients developing renal tubular acidosis. If fructose is not eliminated from the diet, progressive deterioration and death may occur within the neonatal period.

Affected infants who survive the early months of life frequently develop a striking aversion to sweets.

Laboratory manifestations

Definitive evidence of this disorder is reduction in the level of activity of fructose-1-phosphate aldolase, together with elevation of the ratio of fructose-1-phosphate aldolase to fructose-1,6-diphosphate aldolase in liver tissue obtained by biopsy. An alternative method of diagnosis requiring less elaborate laboratory facilities is provided by the fructose tolerance test. Fructose, 0.5 gm/kg body weight, is injected intravenously over a few minutes. In the presence of hereditary fructose intolerance there is a striking reduction in blood glucose and plasma phosphate levels. If the question of hereditary fructose intolerance arises in the neonate, fructose should be eliminated from the diet as a therapeutic trial. Definitive tests may be delayed for a year or two if the fructose-free diet proves effective.

Elevations of plasma tyrosine and methionine have been noted in an infant with hereditary fructose intolerance.

In addition to evidence of impaired renal acidification, urinary abnormalities in hereditary fructose intolerance include generalized aminoaciduria, tyrosyluria, intermittent fructosuria, and occasionally galactosuria.

Treatment

The acute manifestations of fructose intolerance are ameliorated by the infusion of glucose. Definitive management is the elimination of fructose from the diet. Supportive measures may be necessary for acutely ill infants. In the management of these patients it is good to remember that orally administered medications sweetened with sucrose or fructose are contraindicated.

Prognosis

For those patients who survive early infancy, the prognosis is excellent. The vast majority of affected adults show no clinical disease but retain a rigid aversion to dietary fructose. Interestingly dental caries is virtually absent in persons with hereditary fructose intolerance.

Genetics

In general, family histories of hereditary fructose intolerance are compatible with autosomal recessive transmission. However, the disorder appears to have shown dominant inheritance in several families.

Fructose-1,6-diphosphatase deficiency

Fructose-1,6-diphosphatase catalyzes a critical step in the reversal of the glycolytic pathway. Deficiency of the enzyme is associated not only with hypoglycemia but also with overproduction of pyruvic and lactic acids and alanine.

Clinical manifestations

Limited information on the neonatal presentation suggests that hyperpnea, poor feeding, vomiting, and depression of the central nervous system predominate as manifestations. The liver is characteristically enlarged.

Laboratory manifestations

In addition to lactic acidosis and hypoglycemia, there is characteristically ketosis. The liver shows fatty infiltration and, in addition, may have increased glycogen. Fructose-1,6-diphosphatase activity in the liver is markedly reduced or absent.

Treatment

Correction of lactic acidosis should be carried out vigorously with sodium bicarbonate and with sufficient glucose to both correct the hypoglycemia and suppress gluconeogenesis. Long-term management with a low-protein, fructose-free diet has been advised. In older children with deficiency of fructose-1,6-diphosphatase, folic acid therapy has been reported to increase the activity of the enzyme and ameliorate symptoms.

Prognosis

For infants with neonatal disease the prognosis is guarded.

Genetics

Autosomal recessive inheritance is probable.

GLYCOGENOSES

Glycogenoses (Table 32-2 and Fig. 32-8) can be made somewhat less bewildering if the disorders are divided into three groups that reflect the associated clinical diseases: (1) disorders that directly affect glucose homeostasis (types I, III, VI, and VIII), (2) disorders that affect primarily general hepatic function without directly involving glucose homeostasis (type IV), and (3) disorders that primarily affect neuromuscular function (types

Table 32-2. Glycogenoses

Cori type	Eponym	Deficient enzyme	Affected tissue
I	von Gierke	Glucose-6-phosphatase	Liver, platelets Kidney Gastrointestinal tract
II	Pompe	Acid maltase	All tissues
III	Forbes	Debrancher	Liver, RBC, WBC Muscle variably
IV	Andersen	Brancher	All tissues
V	McArdle	Muscle phosphorylase	Muscle
VI	Hers	Liver phosphorylase	Liver, WBC
VII	Tarui	Muscle phosphofructokinase	Muscle, ?RBC
VIII	Hug and Schubert	Phosphorylase kinase	Liver, WBC, all other tissues

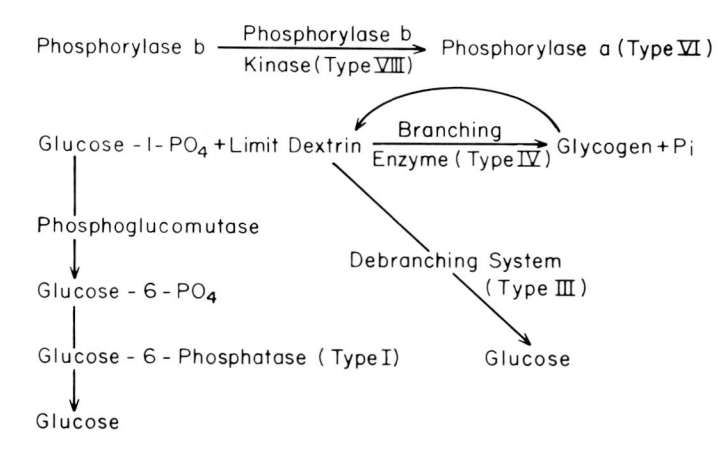

Fig. 32-8. Reactions impaired in the principal types of hepatomegalic glycogenosis. The Cori classification of the disease produced is indicated parenthetically.

II and V). For the physician caring for newborn infants a further simplification can be made by considering those disorders which can be expected to have clinical manifestations during the neonatal period. All the disorders that affect glucose homeostasis fall into this category at least in theory. Of the disorders that primarily affect neuromuscular function, only type II has neonatal manifestations. Since this disease is a disorder of lysosomal function, it is discussed in the section on lysosomal disorders. In the second group, which contains only type IV, there is no neonatal manifestation; the disease is manifested by hepatomegaly at several months of age, followed by progressive cirrhosis, hepatic dysfunction, and death within the first few years of life.

Disorders affecting glucose homeostasis
Etiology and pathogenesis

During fetal life glycogen storage is greatly predominant over glycogenolysis. As a result, fetuses having glycogenoses affecting glucose homeostasis can be expected to be normal, or nearly so, at the end of gestation. Abnormality can be anticipated only when glycogenolysis is required for fuel homeostasis. Although such a requirement may occur during gestation, it certainly occurs during the stress of labor, delivery, and the adaptation to extrauterine life. In the normal infant the energy needs associated with this stress are met in part by glucose released from stored glycogen and in part by the release of free fatty acids from adipose tissue. Surprisingly most infants with inborn errors in the release of glucose from glycogen do not manifest illness during the neonatal period. Too few affected infants have been studied in the neonatal period to allow a proven explanation, but some tentative conclusions can be drawn from the physiology of these disorders in later life. First, the disorders of the breakdown of glycogen itself, debrancher deficiency and defects in the phosphorylase cascade, tend to be clinically mild. Hypoglycemia is generally of modest degree and, if severe, accompanied by ketosis. Gluconeogenesis proceeds normally. Thus a metabolic fuel is generally available. Second, patients with severe clinical disease, a minority of the total, almost always have type I glycogenosis, deficiency of glucose-6-phosphatase. This disease is more frequently manifested in the neonatal period, has high rates of mortality and morbidity, and is potentially treatable.

In type I glycogenosis the degradation of glycogen proceeds normally, but the resultant glucose-1-phosphate cannot be converted to free glucose. The accumulation of phosphorylated glucose results in increased glycolysis with the production of excessive amounts of lactate. For reasons that are as yet unclear, the release of free fatty acids and the production of ketone bodies are suppressed. Because gluconeogenesis proceeds through phosphorylated intermediates, it too is lacking. Blood glucose tends to fall to very low levels without a concomitant rise in free fatty acids. Plasma lactate can rise rapidly, producing severe metabolic acidosis. Lactate becomes the major circulating fuel, apparently used effectively by some affected infants but not by others.

The excess of glucose-6-phosphate in type I disease also leads to excessive synthesis of lipids, occasionally associated with xanthomatosis. Hyperuricemia also occurs, in part because of the effect of lactate on uric acid excretion but also because of an increase in uric acid synthesis.

Clinical manifestations

As indicated previously, the affected infant is likely to be physically normal at birth. In disorders other than type I glycogenosis progressive enlargement of the liver with or without hypoglycemia and ketosis is the likely course of the illness. In type I disease early neonatal hypoglycemia is common, with associated hyperpnea caused by lactic acidosis. These can occur prior to enlargement of the liver. Hypoglycemic seizures may be prominent, or the infant may be depressed, waking only for feedings.

Laboratory manifestations

Blood glucose concentration is variable but in type I disease tends to fall precipitously in the after-absorptive state, with lactate in plasma rising concomitantly. Ketonuria sometimes is noted and generally is indicative of a disorder other than type I. The most important single laboratory test in the evaluation of this group of patients is measurement of the response of blood glucose and lactate to the intravenous administration of glucagon (100 µg/kg). This test should be performed 2 hours after feeding, with measurement of blood glucose and lactate made 30 minutes, 15 minutes, and immediately before the administration of the hormone and at 15-minute intervals for an hour thereafter. Failure to respond to glucagon with a rise in blood glucose of 4 mmol/L (72 mg/dl) can be considered diagnostic of glycogenosis. Coupled with this diagnostic result, a sharp rise in plasma lactate in response to glucagon is diagnostic of type I glycogenosis.

Inferences can be made by analyses of erythrocytes, leukocytes, and platelets for both amount and structure of glycogen and for the various enzymatic activities, but refinement of diagnosis is best accomplished by enzymatic analysis of liver tissue obtained by percutaneous biopsy. Although general liver function is not seriously affected in these infants, defects of coagulation should be looked for and corrected, if present, before biopsy. Platelet dysfunction has been noted in type I glycogenosis.

A variant of type I, called type Ib, has been shown to be caused not by deficiency of glucose-6-phosphatase but by failure of function of the translocater that permits entry of glucose-6-phosphate into microsomes where the enzyme is localized. Subjects affected by type Ib have neutropenia in addition to the other manifestations of type I disease.

Treatment

Treatment is directed toward prevention of hypoglycemia by frequent feedings and toward minimization of glycogen accumulation by employing only glucose and its polymers as the carbohydrate in the diet. It may be necessary to give feedings every 2 hours during the day and night. Alternatively continuous intragastric feedings can be employed at night, with frequent normally administered feedings during the day. This regimen has achieved notable success in the management of type I glycogenosis. Acidotic crises in type I glycogenosis may be quite severe, requiring both sufficient glucose to suppress glycogenolysis and massive doses of sodium bicarbonate. During more quiescent periods small oral doses of bicarbonate suffice to control the lactic acidosis. Hyperuricemia may require allopurinol therapy. Hyperlipidemia with xanthomatosis has been reported to respond to substitution of medium-chain triglycerides for the ordinary fat in the diet.

Prognosis

For patients with disorders other than type I the prognosis is quite good; most show mild disease in infancy with progressive improvement in later childhood. Although the prognosis for patients with type I disease has greatly improved with the introduction of continuous nocturnal intragastric feedings, the outlook must remain guarded. Sudden death from an overwhelming crisis is not unusual. Irreversible cerebral damage may occur before the disorder is recognized. Retardation of growth, persistent hypotonia, and delay in sexual maturation remain problems.

DISORDERS OF LIPID METABOLISM
Hyperlipoproteinemia

In recent years evidence has accumulated that links premature atherosclerotic cardiovascular disease with inborn errors of lipid metabolism (Table 32-3). Although xanthomatosis may appear in the neonatal period in these diseases, the life-threatening cardiovascular manifestations do not appear for years to decades after birth. In some instances even the abnormalities of plasma lipids, which appear to be genetically determined, are not manifested during childhood. The demonstration that dietary manipulation, with or without the addition of drugs such as cholestyramine and clofibrate, can cause the plasma lipids of some diseased subjects to return to normal or near normal levels has led to an interest in the prevention of the clinical manifestations of these disorders by similar therapy instituted early in infancy.

Type I hyperlipoproteinemia

Type I hyperlipoproteinemia, a rare disorder, is the result of the failure of release of lipoprotein lipase activity in response to the ingestion of fat. This failure leads to the accumulation in plasma of a large number of chylomicrons, giving the plasma a "cream of tomato soup" appearance. The hyperlipoproteinemia is accompanied by hypercholesterolemia and in many cases the development of xanthomata. Although this disease is not a lysosomal storage disorder, hepatosplenomegaly with infiltration by foam cells is common in early childhood. Affected individuals develop episodes of abdominal pain that sometimes are associated with evidence of pancreatitis. Premature cardiovascular disease of the atherosclerotic type apparently is not a feature of this disorder.

The lactescence of plasma develops quite soon after the dietary intake of fat is established, and xanthomata have been reported within the neonatal period. Elimination of fat from the diet causes prompt remission in the hyperlipidemia.

A diet containing adequate amounts of essential fatty acids and medium-chain triglycerides rather than the usual dietary fat may be of benefit to patients with this disorder. No systematic trial of this management has been made, nor is any likely considering the rarity of the condition. Type I hyperlipoproteinemia is inherited as an autosomal recessive disease, and heterozygous individuals have no abnormality detectable by present methods.

Type II hyperlipoproteinemia

Type II hyperlipoproteinemia, or familial hypercholesterolemia, is a genetic disorder that has clinical manifestations in both heterozygous and homozygous individuals. Although the pathogenesis of type II hyperlipoproteinemia has not been completely elucidated, it is known that there is a failure of the normal feedback inhibition of cholesterol synthesis in affected individuals.

Clinical manifestations in the neonatal period are not common, but xanthomata have been noted at birth. Hypercholesterolemia is present in cord blood in a large number of affected subjects. Individuals homozygous for this disease characteristically exhibit plasma cholesterol levels in excess of 500 mg/dl, whereas heterozygous individuals have elevated levels but to a lesser degree. Hypertriglyceridemia, although present, is not striking, and fasting plasma is clear.

Homozygous subjects have an extremely high mortal-

Table 32-3. Hyperlipidemia

Frederickson type	Plasma triglycerides	Cholesterol	Xanthomata	Synonym
I	Increased (milky plasma)	Increased	Present	Familial hyperchylomicronemia
II	Slightly increased (clear plasma)	Increased	Present	Familial hypercholesterolemia
III	Normal	Normal	Absent	"Floating beta" disorder
IV	Normal	Normal	Absent	Familial endogenous hyperlipemia
V	Normal	Normal	Absent	Familial endogenous and exogenous hyperlipemia

ity from atherosclerotic cardiovascular disease in the first 3 decades of life. The prognosis for the heterozygous state is somewhat better, although these individuals are subject to premature atherosclerotic cardiovascular disease. The management of homozygous subjects has been attempted by both surgical and medical techniques. Portacaval anastamosis, ileal bypass, and repeated plasmapheresis, with and without the use of cholestyramine, clofibrate, and nicotinic acid, have been employed with varying success. There is no clear treatment of choice. For heterozygous individuals control of cholesterol intake and the use of a sequestering agent such as cholestyramine have been advised. Neither efficacy nor safety of treatment in early life has been established.

The other types of hyperlipoproteinemia have neither clinical manifestations nor detectable laboratory abnormalities in the neonatal period.

Congenital lipodystrophy

Congenital lipodystrophy is a rare disorder, characterized by the absence of fat deposits in skin and viscera.

Etiology and pathogenesis

Concepts concerning the pathogenesis of congenital lipodystrophy have undergone considerable change in recent years. It now seems likely that the effect of insulin on the adipocyte is inhibited, leading both to failure of activation of lipoprotein lipase and to impairment of fat storage. In some older subjects with lipodystrophy, antibodies to insulin receptors have been demonstrated. In other patients the inhibition may be mediated through some as yet unidentified hormonal molecule, perhaps secreted by the hypothalamus. In any case serum insulin levels are consistently elevated, and insulin resistance can be demonstrated.

Clinical manifestations

Affected infants are long and thin at birth, already exhibiting an absence of subcutaneous fat. The face is typically wrinkled. Hepatomegaly, which is always present in later life, is not a prominent finding in neonates. No disability has been attributed to the disorder in early life. The fully developed clinical picture of lipodystrophy—insulin-resistant diabetes mellitus, acanthosis nigricans, hepatomegaly, and hyperchylomicronemia—evolves over the first decade of life.

Laboratory manifestations

There may be no laboratory abnormality in the affected neonate, with hyperlipidemia and glucose intolerance developing only with time. Hypoglycemia has been noted early in the course of one patient.

Treatment

There is no specific treatment for this disorder, although the hyperlipidemia generally responds to a low-fat diet.

Prognosis

The prognosis for life and general health is good during the early years. The disorder is disfiguring and in about half the patients is associated with mental deficiency. Acanthosis nigricans is characteristic of later stages, as is diabetes mellitus with its accompanying microangiopathy. Fatty infiltration of the liver, accompanied by fibrosis, is invariably present in the fully developed disorder, and liver dysfunction may result.

Genetics

Current evidence strongly suggests autosomal recessive inheritance.

DISORDERS OF LYSOSOMAL FUNCTION

Over the past 2 decades investigations employing electron microscopy and the cytochemistry of subcellular particles have resulted in both the discovery and simultaneous explanation of a large number of "new" storage diseases and also the reexamination of the older, largely clinical descriptions of storage diseases. The process is by no means complete but at this writing has produced a much more orderly and systematic classification of storage diseases, which are now so numerous as to bewilder all but the specialist. This review attempts to put these disorders into perspective and to single out for brief discussion those which can be recognized clinically in the neonatal period.

Etiology and pathogenesis

An increasing number of storage diseases are being classified as disorders of lysosomal function. The lysosome is an intracellular organelle whose role is the isolation of molecules from the cytosol and the degradation of these molecules. Under the electron microscope the lysosome is seen as a cytoplasmic membrane enclosing various cellular constituents. It is characterized by its high acid phosphatase activity.

Hers suggested the following criteria for disorders of lysosomal function: (1) the disease is characterized by storage of material within lysosomes; (2) the stored material can be degraded by a mixture of normal lysosomal enzymes; and (3) an enzymatic activity necessary for this degradation is absent from affected tissues.

Subsequent studies have expanded the original concept: if several hydrolytic enzymes share a common protein subunit, a genetic defect in the synthesis of that subunit can impair the activities of all the enzymes sharing the subunit. The inborn defect may involve a hydrolytic enzyme whose function is necessary not only for the degradation of molecules but also for the modification of other hydrolytic enzymes so that they can be accumulated within the lysosome. The defect may involve a function subsequent to degradation, that is, physiologically appropriate disposal of the products of degradation. Lysosomal storage also may occur as a secondary phenomenon when there is excessive production of a substance normally accumulated by lysosomes. Storage disorder also may be induced by drugs.

It is beyond the scope of this chapter to review all the lysosomal disorders that can be diagnosed at or before birth by appropriate chemical analysis. This discussion concerns only those diseases which can be expected to produce clinical manifestations during the early weeks of life. It must be borne in mind that all the storage diseases are progressive; clinical manifestations appear when accumulated material has grossly distorted morphologic characteristics or function or both. Factors such as the normal rate of turnover of the stored material, the degree of deficiency of the enzymes involved, and the degree of awareness of the observer determine the time of initial manifestation or recognition. Not only the pathogenesis of storage diseases but also their treatment have been the subject of intense investigation. A number of schemes for enzyme replacement have been developed. Some of these are promising, although none to my knowledge is unequivocally effective. The question of therapy should be investigated thoroughly at the time any of these diseases is diagnosed.

Amino acid storage disease

Cystine storage disease, more commonly referred to as the de Toni–Fanconi syndrome, probably does not produce clinical disease within the first month of life, although it may be diagnosed in the neonatal period by appropriate laboratory studies. An infant having evidence of gross renal tubular dysfunction in this period should be investigated for primary renal tubular disease, galactosemia, hereditary fructose intolerance, and glucose-6-phosphatase deficiency.

Polysaccharide storage disease

Glycogen storage disease type II

Pompe's disease, or type II glycogen storage disease, has been observed to produce clinical abnormalities from birth, although this observation is not necessary for the diagnosis.

Etiology and pathogenesis. Pompe's disease is the prototype for diseases of lysosomal function. The causative biochemical lesion is absence of activity of a lysosomal hydrolytic enzyme, acid maltase (acid α-glucosidase). The cytoplasmic enzymes of glycogen synthesis and degradation—those responsible for the maintenance of glucose homeostasis—are present in normal amounts and function normally. However, two factors prevent hydrolysis of glycogen engulfed by lysosomes. The first is the absence of the hydrolytic enzyme that normally accomplishes the function. The second is that the glycogenolytic enzymes of cytoplasm cannot catalyze this hydrolysis in the hostile lysosomal environment. For reasons as yet obscure the devastating effects of the disease occur in the neuromuscular system, even though lysosomal accumulation of glycogen can be demonstrated in many other tissues, including liver and kidney. Mechanical distortion of cellular architecture has been incriminated in the malfunction of nerve and muscle.

Clinical features. Clinical manifestations can appear at any time during the first few months of life. The single most constant finding is profound muscular hypotonia, with diminution of reflexes but without loss of muscle mass. The muscles are firm to the touch. Cardiac failure as a result of myocardial involvement in the disease is very common as the initial complaint. Cardiomegaly is massive, and no murmur suggesting a congenital malformation is present. Hepatomegaly, when present, probably is related to congestive heart failure. Alertness is unaffected. The initial response to cardiotonic measures is generally good, but the overall course of the disease is one of relentless progression. Death is usually the result of respiratory failure, with or without complicating bronchopneumonia.

Laboratory studies. Results of all tests of hepatic glycogen release are normal, as is the structure of the glycogen stored by these patients. The electrocardiogram characteristically shows very large QRS deflections, a shortened PR interval, and a leftward axis. The electromyogram shows typical and virtually diagnostic myotonic discharges. Nerve conduction is slowed.

Confirmation of the diagnosis may be made by demonstration of typical lysosomal inclusions of glycogen in white blood cells, liver, or muscle. Enzymatic confirmation also may be obtained using these tissues, although some patients with Pompe's disease with normal levels of acid maltase in white blood cells have been reported.

Treatment. Attempts have been made to treat such patients by infusing an appropriate enzyme mixture obtained from cultures of *Aspergillus niger*. Beneficial effects have been noted in serial electron micrographs of material obtained by liver biopsy, but no substantive clinical benefit has been shown. Therapy at this time is only supportive.

Prognosis. In general, patients with cardiac involvement as a primary manifestation die within the first year of life, whereas those whose clinical disease does not involve the myocardium may survive for several years.

Genetics. Evidence suggests an autosomal recessive inheritance, although there is a preponderance of males among the reported patients.

Neutral lipidoses
Wolman's disease

Wolman's disease is a disorder of the storage of cholesterol and triglycerides, involving viscera much more than the central nervous system and leading to death within the first few months of life.

Etiology and pathogenesis. The absence of an acid lipase activity (E600-resistant acid esterase) leads to the accumulation of cholesterol and triglycerides within intracellular membranous cytoplasmic bodies throughout the body. The liver, spleen, adrenal glands, and gastrointestinal tract are most prominently involved. The nervous system shows definable but less striking abnormalities.

Clinical manifestations. Infants with Wolman's disease show failure to thrive from birth. Vomiting and diarrhea are prominent manifestations, as is progressive abdominal distention with hepatosplenomegaly of massive proportions. The infants show progressive inanition, with maintenance of apparently normal alertness until very late in the course of the disease.

Laboratory manifestations. The most important diagnostic sign is the presence of enlarged calcified adrenal glands on the abdominal roentgenogram. Vacuolated leukocytes are prominent in peripheral blood smears, and foam cells in the bone marrow are characteristic. The diagnosis is established by the demonstration of abnormal accumulation of triglycerides and cholesterol in biopsy tissue; the liver is the preferred organ for biopsy. Confirmation by assay of acid lipase activity is useful and may become an essential diagnostic technique.

Treatment. Although several agents known to influence cholesterol metabolism have been used to treat this disorder, no success has been reported. Because of the involvement of the adrenal cortex, replacement therapy with adrenal steroids may be indicated. Such therapy has not altered the course of the disease.

Prognosis. The prognosis is uniformly poor, and death usually occurs within the first 6 months.

Genetics. Analysis of the few reported cases indicates autosomal recessive inheritance.

Mucopolysaccharidoses

It is likely that the classic mucopolysaccharidoses (Hurler's, Hunter's, Sanfilippo's, Morquio's, Scheie's, and Maroteaux-Lamy syndromes) cannot be detected clinically in the neonatal period. "Congenital" cases reported in previous years now are generally thought to be examples of more profound lysosomal dysfunction, currently classified as mucolipidoses. To the original six mucopolysaccharidoses, there has been added a seventh with which neonatal clinical disease has been associated.

β-Glucuronidase deficiency (mucopolysaccharidosis VII)

Only a few patients with this disease have been described, and there is apparently considerable genetic heterogeneity among them. Some have had clinical disease in the neonatal period.

Etiology and pathogenesis. As its name implies, the disease is caused by deficiency of lysosomal β-glucuronidase. It must be presumed that the defect is more profound in those affected subjects who are clinically abnormal at birth.

Clinical manifestations. The affected infant may exhibit the Hurler syndrome at birth: hepatosplenomegaly, dysostosis multiplex, and hernias. Corneal clouding has not been noted early and may not always occur. Motor and mental development is variably affected.

Laboratory manifestations. Roentgenologic changes of dysostosis are present early. Inclusions are present in granulocytes. Excretion of mucopolysaccharides in urine is increased, although not dramatically so. The diagnosis is made by demonstration of the specific enzyme defect in leukocytes or fibroblasts. Treatment is supportive, but enzyme replacement should be considered. Autosomal recessive inheritance has been demonstrated.

Complex lipidoses
Farber's disease

Farber's disease is an infantile disorder of ceramide storage that is characterized by the accumulation of this material in granulomatous lesions, which involve the skin, subcutaneous tissues, joints, larynx, liver, and central nervous system. It is generally lethal within the first 2 years of life.

Etiology and pathogenesis. The biochemical basis of Farber's disease is, in all likelihood, deficiency of acid ceramidase. Ceramide accumulates in foam cells in many tissues in this disorder, and these foam cells accumulate within granulomas, which appear to evolve into the hyaline fibrotic masses characteristic of the disease. The inflammatory character of Farber's disease is unique among the storage diseases.

Clinical manifestations. Painful swelling of multiple joints, hoarseness, and stridor may appear at any time during the first few weeks of life. Palpable nodules develop in skin and subcutaneous tissue, particularly over the joints. Hepatomegaly and deterioration of central nervous system function, with the evolution of retinal cherry-red spots, form the remainder of the fully developed disease.

Laboratory manifestations. Roentgenographic examination reveals generalized demineralization of bone, destruction of normal joint relationships, erosion of bones at the articular surfaces, and soft tissue calcification. Routine laboratory studies are not helpful in diagnosis, although occasional lipid-laden cells may be found in the bone marrow. Microscopic examination of a nodule obtained by biopsy is the best means currently available to confirm the clinical diagnosis, although it may well be supplanted in the near future by assay of acid ceramidase.

Treatment. Although antiinflammatory agents may provide some symptomatic relief, there is no truly effective therapy for this condition.

Prognosis. The prognosis is uniformly poor; death characteristically occurs within the first 2 years.

Genetics. The disease has occurred in siblings and in both males and females and thus is likely to show autosomal recessive inheritance.

Gaucher's disease: malignant infantile form

The malignant form of Gaucher's disease is caused by the widespread storage of glucosyl cerebroside in brain, liver, spleen, and other tissues. It is a progressive disorder, with severe central nervous system dysfunction and death generally occurring within the first year of life.

Etiology and pathogenesis. The fundamental biochemical lesion in malignant infantile Gaucher's disease is marked reduction in the activity of glucosyl cerebrosidase. The consequent accumulation of glucosyl cerebroside is considered to be responsible for the clinical findings, although the pathogenetic mechanisms have not been elucidated. There is some degree of neuronal loss on pathologic examination of the brain.

Clinical manifestations. The clinical features of the disease can develop at any time within the first few years of life. Feeding difficulties, vomiting, hepatosplenomegaly, and muscular hypertonia are found in various combinations. Cough and respiratory difficulty are also common. Deterioration of central nervous system function is characteristic, with the evolution of a vegetative state. Retinal cherry-red spots do not develop.

Laboratory manifestations. The serum acid phosphatase is elevated to a striking degree. Absolute confirmation of the diagnosis requires demonstration of the enzymatic deficiency in leukocytes or tissue obtained by biopsy. Microscopic examination of bone marrow and of other tissue generally reveals cellular characteristics specific enough to establish the diagnosis.

Treatment. Treatment is supportive.

Genetics. Gaucher's disease is inherited as an autosomal recessive disorder.

Gaucher's disease: chronic nonneuronopathic form

Although the chronic nonneuronopathic form of Gaucher's disease seldom is recognized in the early months and years of life, it seems likely that the visceral manifestations noted in malignant Gaucher's disease in early life are in fact present at similar ages in the nonneuronopathic disease. The striking differences are the normal neural function and much better prognosis of the nonneuronopathic disease.

Ganglioside storage disease
Tay-Sachs disease

Tay-Sachs disease is a progressive infantile disease of neurologic function, characterized by regression of development, blindness, spasticity, and ultimate fatality. It exhibits no characteristic clinical manifestations outside the nervous system.

Etiology and pathogenesis. Tay-Sachs disease is a result of a deficiency of activity of hexosaminidase A, which is necessary for the degradation of ganglioside GM_2. Although the accumulation of ganglioside GM_2 probably is generalized in a chemical sense, clinically significant accumulation is limited to the nervous system and predominantly to the gray matter of the central nervous system. The precise mechanism by which clinical disease occurs is unknown. Infants dying very early have shrunken brains showing enlarged lateral ventricles and gliosis; those dying late in the disease have enlarged brains with small ventricles, the result of progressive storage of ganglioside.

Clinical manifestations. The onset of clinical manifestations is generally within the first 8 months of life, but onset prior to 3 months of age is unusual. There is gradual deterioration of cortical function. The most characteristic clinical manifestation is hyperacusis, a striking extensor response to sharp sounds. Lack of normal awareness, poor muscle tone, and spasticity also are noted frequently. The retinal cherry-red spots that eventually develop in nearly all patients with Tay-Sachs disease are not present in the neonatal period. Seizures, which may be myoclonic, focal, or generalized, have occurred in the neonatal period but are unusual early in the course of the disease.

Laboratory manifestations. The absence of hexosaminidase A activity in any of several tissues, including white blood cells, liver, and skin fibroblasts, is diagnostic of Tay-Sachs disease. Reduction in the activity of fructose-1-phosphate aldolase in the red blood cells has been documented, but the measurement of this activity cannot be considered a substitute for the assay of hexosaminidase A.

Therapy. No specific therapy is available.

Prognosis. The course is relentlessly progressive, and death generally occurs 13 to 30 months after the onset of clinical manifestations.

Genetics. Tay-Sachs disease shows autosomal recessive inheritance. The disease occurs predominantly in Ashkenazi Jews.

Neimann-Pick disease type A

Infantile Neimann-Pick disease is a progressive disease associated with the storage of sphingomyelin in the nervous system and viscera.

Etiology and pathogenesis. Severe deficiency of sphingomyelinase in all tissues leads to the intracellular accumulation of sphingomyelin within membranous cytoplasmic bodies. The predominant clinical effects are in the nervous system.

Clinical manifestations. Neimann-Pick disease usually is recognized after the neonatal period. Persistent neonatal jaundice and hepatosplenomegaly have been noted retrospectively in a number of patients. The retinal cherry-red spots develop quite early in many cases but are not reliably present within the neonatal period. Neurologic deterioration usually occurs after the neonatal period.

Laboratory manifestations. Vacuolated leukocytes may be observed in blood smears, and Niemann-Pick cells (lipid-laden macrophages) can be seen in the bone marrow. The level of plasma acid phosphatase occasionally is elevated. Specific diagnosis depends on the demonstration of sphingomyelin accumulation and of markedly reduced activity of sphingomyelinase in tissue obtained by biopsy or in tissue cultures of skin fibroblasts or bone marrow. The enzymatic defect also has been demonstrated in peripheral leukocytes.

Therapy. No specific therapy is available.

Prognosis. The disorder exhibits autosomal recessive inheritance. A preponderance of reported cases have occurred in Jews, but no racial or ethnic group appears to be spared.

Niemann-Pick disease type B

Type B Niemann-Pick disease is different from type A disease only in that the nervous system is spared in type B disease. Visceral manifestations are similar in the two disorders, but the prognosis is better in type B disease; the course resembles that of chronic Gaucher's disease.

Mucolipidoses

The term *mucolipidoses* describes diseases combining elements of mucopolysaccharidosis, e.g., dysostosis multiplex, and elements of lipidosis, e.g., macular cherry-red spots. The diseases so classified include a number of entities that are clinically evident early in life. The excretion of mucopolysaccharide in the urine generally is not increased. However, in a number of these diseases smaller urinary polysaccharides containing excess sialic acid (*N*-acetyl neuraminic acid) have been found in abnormal amounts. Thus a subgroup, the sialidoses, has evolved in which it would appear that deficient neuraminidase activities are causative.

Generalized gangliosidosis

Generalized gangliosidosis is a disorder combining the morphologic features of Hurler's syndrome with a clinical course similar to that of the infantile cerebral lipidoses.

Etiology and pathogenesis. Ganglioside GM_1 is the major storage material, but there is also storage of mucopolysaccharides. Assays of lysosomal enzymes have revealed marked deficiencies of activity of β-galactosidases A, B, C, and D.

Clinical manifestations. It seems likely that cases reported as neonatal or congenital Hurler's syndrome represent instances of generalized gangliosidosis or other mucolipidoses. Hurler's facies, hepatosplenomegaly, and skeletal abnormalities may be seen at birth or very shortly thereafter. Developmental retardation is manifested very early, and there is profound failure to thrive. Macular cherry-red spots appear in approximately 50% of cases.

Laboratory manifestations. The excretion of mucopolysaccharides in the urine is normal. However, 10% to 80% of leukocytes contain Reilly bodies, and bone marrow examination reveals finely vacuolated histiocytic cells. Similar evidence of storage is seen in biopsy material from various tissues, particularly the liver. Definitive diagnosis requires demonstration of marked deficiency in β-galactosidases A, B, and C.

Treatment. There is no specific treatment.

Prognosis. The prognosis is uniformly poor. Death usually occurs prior to 2 years of age as a result of pulmonary complications.

Genetics. Autosomal recessive inheritance occurs.

I-cell diseases (mucolipidosis II)

I-cell disease is a disorder of lysosomal function characterized by rapid accumulation of heterogeneous material within lysosomes, onset of clinical disease during fetal life, and rapid progression of disease postnatally.

Etiology and pathogenesis. I-cell disease currently is considered to be a sialidosis because of the accumulation of sialic acid–rich macromolecules among the stored material. The lysosomes themselves are deficient in a number of hydrolytic activities. The enzymes affected are in fact synthesized but are not concentrated within lysosomes and exhibit different electrophoretic mobilities from those observed in studies of normal lysosomal hydrolases. The discovery of neuraminidase deficiency in I-cell disease suggests the possibility that this deficiency results both in the storage of sialic acid–rich substances and also in failure of a posttranslational modification of other hydrolases that is necessary for their localization within lysosomes.

Clinical manifestations. Affected infants have low birth weights and subsequent growth failure. These infants are quiet from birth and show severe developmental retardation early in life. The skin may be somewhat thickened and tight. There is no hepatosplenomegaly, and the corneas are clear. Although Hurlerlike bony abnormalities are not recognizable clinically, careful examination of roentgenograms will reveal their presence.

Laboratory manifestations. The usual tests of mucopolysacchariduria give normal results, but thin-layer chromatography reveals excessive excretion of smaller saccharides containing sialic acid. No inclusions are seen in leukocytes. The diagnosis is established by finding typical inclusions within cultured fibroblasts.

Treatment. No specific treatment is known for I-cell disease. The prognosis is poor.

Mannosidosis

Mannosidosis is a recently described storage disease in which hepatosplenomegaly, skeletal changes, central nervous system dysfunction, and marmoration of skin may appear within weeks after birth.

The absence of acid α-mannosidase has been demonstrated. Vacuolated lymphocytes and polymorphonuclear inclusions are seen in the bone marrow.

There is no specific treatment, and the prognosis is poor.

Mucolipidosis IV

Mucolipidosis IV is relatively slowly progressive but is of interest in that corneal clouding without dysostosis or organomegaly is apparent within the first few weeks of life.

Nephrosialidosis

Nephrosialidosis is quite rare, and reported cases may not represent a homogeneous entity. In any case clinical manifestations are present at or shortly after birth. These include hepatosplenomegaly, inguinal hernias and ascites. Dysostosis develops during the early months of life. Massive proteinuria occurs and presumably is responsible for the ascites and subsequently for the evolution of anasarca.

Uncategorized storage disorders: stiff skin syndrome

Four patients have been described who have stiff skin and limitation of joint mobility; clinical manifestations have been noted in the newborn period. Histologic changes in the skin suggest mucopolysaccharide storage.

John F. Nicholson

BIBLIOGRAPHY
General

Cornblath, M., and Schwartz, R.: Disorders of carbohydrate metabolism in infancy, ed. 2, Philadelphia, 1978, W.B. Saunders Co.

Danks, D.M.: Management of newborn babies in whom serious metabolic illness is anticipated, Arch. Dis. Child. **49:**576, 1974.

Mamunes, P.: Neonatal screening tests, Pediatr. Clin. North Am. **27:**733, 1981.

Novogroder, M.: Neonatal screening for hypothyroidism, Pediatr. Clin. North Am. **27:**881, 1981.

Scriver, C.R., and Rosenberg, L.E.: Amino acid metabolism and its disorders, Philadelphia, 1973, W.B. Saunders Co.

Stanbury, J.B., Wyngaarden, J.B., and Frederickson, D.S., editors: The metabolic basis of inherited disease, ed. 4, New York, 1978, McGraw-Hill Book Co.

Phenylketonuria

Berlow, S.: Progress in phenylketonuria: defects in the metabolism of biopterin, Pediatrics **65:**837, 1980.

Berry, H.K.: The diagnosis of phenylketonuria: a commentary, Am. J. Dis. Child. **135:**211, 1981.

Hackney, I.M., Davidson, W., and Linsao, L.: Phenylketonuria; mental development, behavior, and termination of low phenylalanine diet, J. Pediatr. **72:**646, 1968.

Kang, E.S., Sollee, N.D., and Gerald, P.S.: Results of treatment and termination of the diet in phenylketonuria (PKU), Pediatrics **46:**881, 1970.

Kennedy, J.L., and others: The early treatment of phenylketonuria, Am. J. Dis. Child. **113:**16, 1967.

Mamunes, P., and others: Intellectual deficits after transient tyrosinemia in the term neonate, Pediatrics **57:**675, 1976.

Rouse, B.M.: Phenylalanine deficiency syndrome, J. Pediatr. **69:**246, 1966.

Snyderman, S.E., and others: The phenylalanine requirement of the normal infant, J. Nutr. **56:**253, 1953.

Tyrosinosis, acute tyrosinosis, and chronic tyrosinemia

Bakker, H.D., and others: Fructose-1,6-diphosphatase deficiency: another enzyme defect which can present itself with the clinical features of "tyrosinosis," Clin. Chim. Acta **55**:41, 1974.

Gaull, G.E., and others: Biochemical observations on so-called hereditary tyrosinosis, Pediatr. Res. **4**:337, 1970.

Grant, D.B., Alexander, F.W., and Seakins, J.W.T.: Abnormal tyrosine metabolism in hereditary fructose intolerance, Acta Paediatr. Scand. **59**:432, 1970.

Sandberg, H.O.: Bilateral keratopathy and tyrosinosis, Acta Ophthalmol. **53**:760, 1975.

Scriver, C.R., Larochelle, J., and Silverberg, M.: Hereditary tyrosinemia and tyrosyluria in a French Canadian geographic isolate, Am. J. Dis. Child. **113**:41, 1967.

Yu, J.S., Walker-Smith, J.A., and Burnard, E.D.: Neonatal hepatitis in premature infants simulating hereditary tyrosinosis, Arch. Dis. Child. **46**:306, 1971.

Nonketotic hyperglycinemia

Arneson, D., and others: Strychnine therapy in nonketotic hyperglycinemia, Pediatrics **63**:369, 1979.

Perry, T.L., and others: Studies of the glycine cleavage enzyme system in brain from infants with glycine encephalopathy, Pediatr. Res. **11**:1192, 1977.

Homocystinuria

Hagberg, B., and Iambraeces, L.: Some aspects of the diagnosis and treatment of homocystinuria, Dev. Med. Child. Neurol. **10**:470, 1968.

Histidinemia

Neville, G.R., and others: Histidinaemia—study of relation between clinical and biochemical findings in seven subjects, Arch. Dis. Child. **47**:190, 1972.

Thalhammer, O., Schreibenreiter, S., and Pantlitschko, M.: Histidinemia; detection by routine newborn screening and biochemical observations on three unrelated cases, Z. Kinderheilkd. **109**:279, 1971.

Disorders of the urea cycle

Bachman, C., and others: N-Acetylglutamate synthetase deficiency: a disorder of ammonia detoxification, N. Engl. J. Med. **304**:543, 1981.

Ballard, R.A., and others: Transient hyperammonemia of the preterm infant, N. Engl. J. Med. **299**:9230, 1978.

Brusilow, S.W., Valle, D.L., and Batshaw, M.: New pathways of nitrogen excretion in inborn errors of urea synthesis, Lancet **2**:452, 1979.

Packman, S., and others: Severe hyperammonemia in a newborn infant with methylmalonyl-CoA mutase deficiency, J. Pediatr. **92**:759, 1978.

Snyderman, S.E., and others: The therapy of hyperammonemia due to ornithine transcarbamylase deficiency in a male neonate, Pediatrics **56**:65, 1975.

Terheggen, H.G., and others: Familial hyperargininemia, Arch. Dis. Child. **50**:57, 1975.

van der Zee, S.P.M., and others: Citrullinemia with rapidly fatal neonatal course, Arch. Dis. Child. **46**:847, 1971.

Disorders of organic acid metabolism

Bakkaren, J.A.J.M., and others: Organic aciduria in hypoxic premature newborns simulating an inborn error of metabolism, Eur. J. Pediatr. **127**:41, 1977.

Mantovani, J.F., and others: Presentation with pseudotumor cerebri and CT abnormalities, J. Pediatr. **96**:279, 1980.

Maple syrup urine disease

Goodman, S.I., and others: The treatment of maple syrup urine disease, J. Pediatr. **75**:485, 1969.

Sallan, S.E., and Cottom, D.: Peritoneal dialysis in maple syrup urine disease, Lancet **2**:1423, 1969.

Scriver, C.R., and others: Thiamine-responsive maple-syrup-urine disease, Lancet **2**:310, 1971.

Snyderman, S.E.: The therapy of maple syrup urine disease, Am. J. Dis. Child. **113**:68, 1967.

Defects in the propionate pathway

Brandt, I.K., and others: Propionic acidemia (ketotic hyperglycinemia): dietary treatment resulting in normal growth and development, Pediatrics **53**:391, 1974.

Hsia, Y.E., Lilljeqvist, A.C., and Rosenberg, L.E.: Vitamin B12-dependent methylmalonicaciduria: amino acid toxicity, long chain ketonuria, and protective effect of vitamin B12, Pediatrics **46**:497, 1970.

Keating, J.P., and others: Hyperglycinemia with ketosis due to a defect in isoleucine metabolism: a preliminary report, Pediatrics **50**:890, 1972.

Nyhan, W.L., and others: Response to dietary therapy in B12 unresponsive to methylmalonic acidemia, Pediatrics **57**:539, 1973.

Congenital lactic acidosis

Brunette, M.G., and others: Thiamine responsive lactic acidosis in a patient with deficient low-Km pyruvate carboxylase activity in liver, Pediatrics **50**:702, 1972.

Farrell, D.F., and others: Absence of pyruvate decarboxylase activity in man; a cause of congenital lactic acidosis, Science **187**:1082, 1975.

Gautier, E.: Lactic acidosis in infancy, Helv. Med. Acta **35**:423, 1970.

Green, H.L., Schubert, W.K., and Hug, G.: Chronic lactic acidosis of infancy, J. Pediatr. **76**:753, 1970.

Hartmann, A.F., Sr., and others: Lactate metabolism; studies of a child with a serious congenital deviation, J. Pediatr. **61**:165, 1962.

Lie, S.O., and others: Fatal congenital lactic acidosis in two siblings. I. Clinical and pathological findings, Acta Paediatr. Scand. **60**:129, 1971.

Robinson, B.H., and Sherwood, W.G.: Pyruvate dehydrogenase phosphatase deficiency: a cause of congenital chronic lactic acidosis in infancy, Pediatr. Res. **9**:935, 1975.

Saudubray, J.M., and others: Neonatal congenital lactic acidosis with pyruvate carboxylase deficiency in two siblings, Acta Paediatr. Scand. **65**:717, 1976.

von Biervliet, J.P., and others: Hereditary mitochondrial myopathy with lactic acidemia, a DeToni-Fanconi-Debre syndrome, and a defective respiratory chain in voluntary striated muscles, Pediatr. Res. **11**:1088, 1977.

Isovaleric acidemia

Kelleher, J.F., Jr., and others: The pancytopenia of isovaleric acidemia, Pediatrics **65**:1023, 1980.

Krieger, I., and Tanaka, K.: Therapeutic effects of glycine in isovaleric acidemia, Pediatr. Res. **10**:25, 1976.

Levy, H.L., and others: Isovaleric acidemia; results of family study and dietary treatment, Pediatrics **52**:83, 1973.

Newman, C.G.H., and others: Neonatal death associated with isovaleric acidemia, Lancet **2**:439, 1967.

Other disorders of organic acid metabolism

Brandt, N.J., and others: Glutaric aciduria in chorio-athetosis, Clin. Genet. 13:77, 1978.

Cowan, M.J., and others: Multiple biotin-dependent carboxylase deficiencies associated with defects in T-cell and B-cell immunity, Lancet 2:115, 1979.

Gregersen, N., and others: Glutaric aciduria; clinical and laboratory findings in two brothers, J. Pediatr. 90:740, 1977.

Przyrembel, H., and others: Alpha-ketoadipic aciduria, a new inborn error of lysine metabolism; biochemical studies, Clin. Chim. Acta 58:257, 1975.

Przyrembel, H., and others: Glutaric aciduria type II; report on a previously undescribed metabolic disorder, Clin. Chim. Acta 66:227, 1976.

Schutgens, R.B.H., and others: Lethal hypoglycemia in a child with a deficiency of 3-hydroxy-3-methyl glutaryl coenzyme-A-lyase, J. Pediatr. 94:89, 1979.

Stokke, O., and others: Beta-methylcrotonyl-CoA carboxylase deficiency: a new metabolic error in leucine degradation, Pediatrics 49:726, 1972.

Tildon, J.T., and Cornblath, M.: Succinyl-CoA: 3-CoA: 3-ketoacid CoA-transferase deficiency, J. Clin. Invest. 51:493, 1972.

Neonatal diabetes mellitus

Gentz, J.C.H., and Cornblath, M.: Transient diabetes in the newborn, Adv. Pediatr. 16:345, 1969.

Disorders of galactose metabolism

Holton, J.B., and others: Galactosemia: a new severe variant due to uridine diphosphate galactose-4-epimerase deficiency, Arch. Dis. Child. 56:885, 1981.

Huttenlocher, P., Hillman, R., and Hsia, Y.: Pseudotumor cerebri in galactosemia, J. Pediatr. 76:902, 1970.

Glycogenoses

Perlman, M., Aker, M., and Slonim, A.E.: Successful treatment of severe type I glycogen storage disease with neonatal presentation by nocturnal intragastric feeding, J. Pediatr. 94:772, 1979.

Spencer-Peet, J., and others. Hepatic glycogen storage disease, Q. J. Med 40:95, 1971.

Disorders of lipid metabolism

Seip, M.: Generalized lipodystrophy, Ergeb. Inn. Med. Kinderheilkd. 31:59, 1971.

Disorders of lysosomal storage

Berman, E.R., and others: Congenital corneal clouding with abnormal systemic storage bodies; a new variant of mucolipidosis, J. Pediatr. 84:519, 1974.

Clement, D.H., and Godman, G.C.: Glycogen disease resembling mongolism, cretinism, and amyotonia congenita, J. Pediatr. 36:11, 1950.

Dean, M.F., and others: Enzyme replacement therapy by fibroblast transplantation; long-term biochemical study in three cases of Hunter's syndrome, J. Clin. Invest. 63:138, 1979.

Esterly, N.B., and McKusick, V.A.: Stiff skin syndrome, Pediatrics 47:360, 1971.

Hers, H.G.: Inborn lysosomal diseases, Gastroenterology 448:625, 1965.

Hirshhorn, R., and Weissmann, G.: Genetic disorders of lysosomes, Prog. Med. Genet. 1:49, 1976.

Humbel, R., and Collart, N.: Oligosaccharides in urine of patients with glycoprotein storage disease. I. Rapid detection by thin-layer chromatography, Clin. Chim. Acta 60:143, 1975.

Kelly, T.E., and Graetz, G.: Isolated acid neuraminidase deficiency: a distinct lysosomal storage disease, Am. J. Med. Genet. 1:31, 1977.

Kjellman, B., and others: Mannosidosis: a clinical and histopathologic study, J. Pediatr. 75:366, 1969.

Leroy, J.G., and others: I-cell disease: a clinical picture, J. Pediatr. 79:360, 1971.

Moser, H.W., and others: Farber's lipogranulomatosis, Am. J. Med. 47:869, 1969.

Rosenstein, B.: Glycogen storage disease of the heart in a newborn infant, J. Pediatr. 65:126, 1964.

Schneider, J.A., Wong, J., and Seegmiller, J.E.: The early diagnosis of cystinosis, J. Pediatr. 74:1114, 1969.

Sly, W.S., and others: Beta glucuronidase deficiency; report of clinical, radiologic and biochemical features of a new mucopolysaccharidosis, J. Pediatr. 82:249, 1973.

Spranger, J., Gehler, J., and Cantz, M.: Mucolipidosis I—a sialidosis, Am. J. Med. Genet. 1:21, 1977.

Spranger, J.W., and Wiedeman, H.R.: The genetic mucolipidoses; diagnosis and differential diagnosis, Humangenetik 9:113, 1970.

Thomas, G.H., and others: Increased levels of sialic acid associated with a sialidase deficiency in I-cell disease (mucolipidosis II) fibroblasts, Biochem. Biophys. Res. Commun. 71:188, 1976.

von Bassewitz, D.B., and others: Vacuolated lymphocytes in type II glycogenosis, Eur. J. Pediat. 127:1, 1977.

Wolman, M., and others: Primary familial xanthomatosis with involvement and calcification of the adrenals, Pediatrics 28:742, 1961.

CHAPTER 33 **Metabolic and endocrine disorders**

PART ONE

Carbohydrate metabolism in the fetus and neonate

Emerging from an intrauterine environment, where nutritional needs are continuously provided by the maternal circulation and regulated by placental exchange, the newborn must effect major physiologic and metabolic changes over a short period to adjust to intermittent enteral feeding. During intrauterine life, readjustments in maternal metabolism are required to provide for the progressively increasing demands of the growing fetus. The fetus prepares for extrauterine survival by increasing energy stores and developing enzymatic processes for rapid mobilization of stored energy. As carbohydrate stores become depleted postnatally, the neonate must develop the capacity for hepatic glucose production from other sources. However, abnormalities in the maternal or placental environment may modify the postnatal development of glucose homeostasis.

METABOLIC ADJUSTMENTS DURING PREGNANCY

When food is withheld from a pregnant woman, the use of endogenous fuel occurs more rapidly than in a nonpregnant state, since the mother must supply not only her own needs but also those of the growing fetus. The following biochemical differences are found between gravid and nongravid women following an overnight fast: (1) plasma glucose values are lower, and hypoglycemia may supervene if fasting is prolonged; (2) plasma amino acids are lower, and aminoaciduria is present; (3) muscle catabolism and activation of gluconeogenesis occur more rapidly; (4) maternal lipolysis is increased with elevated values for free fatty acids and ketones; (5) plasma insulin concentration may be lower during the first trimester, but during late pregnancy, insulin is increased even though blood sugar is lower.

In addition to alterations during fasting, maternal metabolism is significantly changed during alimentation. The response to exogenous glucose in late pregnancy is accompanied by an excessive outpouring of insulin. However, the hypoglycemic action of exogenous insulin is significantly diminished. Thus pregnancy is characterized by augmentation of insulin release concomitant with increased peripheral resistance. Since more insulin is needed during late pregnancy for maintenance of carbohydrate homeostasis, the inability to provide compensatory hyperinsulinism results in gestational diabetes (Chapter 3). The rapid reversibility of glucose intolerance in gestational diabetes suggests that the fetoplacental unit exerts this critical stress.

The placenta may exert its influence on maternal metabolism in two ways: (1) it may play a role in the extraction and degradation of maternal hormones, such as insulin, and (2) it is a site of production of hormones, such as human placental lactogen, estrogens, and progesterone, that may affect carbohydrate metabolism. Human placental lactogen is similar to growth hormone and exerts a significant antiinsulin action; it also increases lipolysis. Human placental lactogen secretion is increased with progressive human placental lactogen fetoplacental growth, and at the end of pregnancy its concentration is 750 times that of growth hormone. Although it is difficult to assign relative importance to individual hormones, in concert they effect an enhanced turnover of fat in adipose tissue, cause pancreatic hyperplasia, and increase the amount of insulin required for glucose disposition.

Serum cortisol, which exerts peripheral insulin antagonism, also is increased during pregnancy. However, most of the increase is attributable to biologically inactive protein-bound hormone, which is elevated under the influence of estrogen. Serum growth hormone concentration is not increased during pregnancy and may be decreased. Plasma glucagon concentration, after an overnight fast, is the same in pregnant women during late gestation as in normal controls and is therefore not responsible for the increased insulin resistance.

During periods of food ingestion, mechanisms exist that selectively favor maternal repletion and anabolism. For example, a larger proportion of the ingested glucose is converted to triglyceride, and there is greater suppression of glucagon following exogenous glucose ingestion; thus a more conducive intrahepatic setting for glycogen deposition is provided.

PLACENTAL TRANSPORT OF NUTRIENTS AND HORMONES

Maternal glucose crosses the placenta to the fetus by facilitated diffusion (Fig. 33-1). Glucose concentration in amniotic fluid decreases with increasing gestational age; fetal urine is probably the major source of this glucose, and, as maturation of kidney tubules results in greater glucose reabsorption, less appears in amniotic fluid. Recent evidence suggests that the placenta is capable of producing lactate and that lactate is then provided to the fetus in sufficient quantities to account for 25% of fetal oxidative metabolism. Amino acids are actively transported to the fetus against a transplacental gradient with maintenance of amino acids at levels 1.1 to 4.3 times those in maternal plasma. There is more rapid transport of L-amino acids than D-isomers. Transplacental passage of esterified and free fatty acids is limited in the human; however, ketone bodies readily cross the placenta. In contrast, there is an effective physiologic barrier to the transport of insulin, glucagon, growth hormone, and placental lactogen in the human placenta. There is dissociation of fetal and maternal levels, and equilibrium across the placenta does not occur with any of these hormones. However, all the lipid-soluble steroid hormones are transported freely across the placenta.

FETAL GLUCOSE METABOLISM
(see also Chapter 7)
Energy source and stores

The rate of glucose uptake by the fetus via the umbilical circulation is related to the maternal blood glucose level. The concentration of glucose in fetal blood is approximately one third lower than that in maternal blood. Glucose is the major source of energy throughout fetal life; however, in sheep, amino acids and lactate also provide a significant amount of the fuel for fetal oxygen consumption during late gestation. Fetal hepatic glycogen stores have been identified by the ninth week of

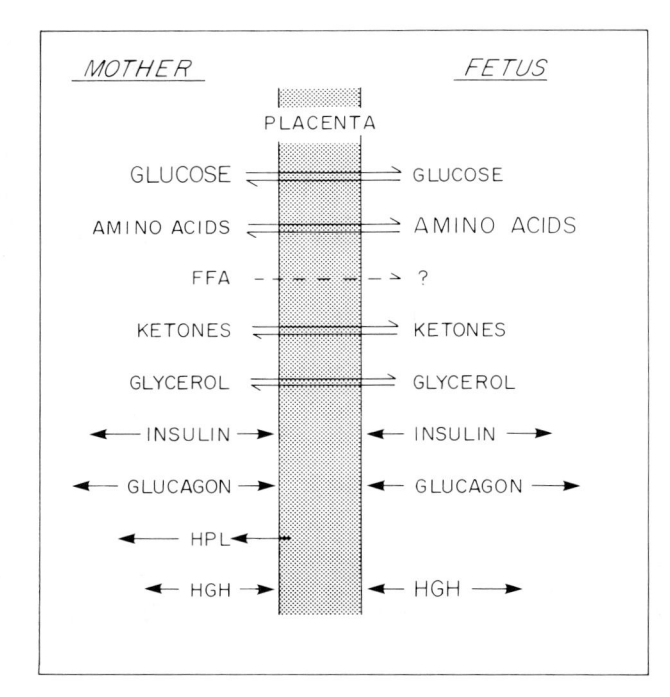

Fig. 33-1. Placental permeability and the relationship between maternal and fetal fuels and hormones. (From Freinkel, N., and Metzger, B.E. In Pregnancy metabolism, Diabetes and the Fetus, CIBA Foundation Symposium no. 63, Amsterdam, 1979, Excerpta Medica.

gestation and at term are three times (150 mg/gm liver) those of a well-fed adult; skeletal muscle glycogen is three to five times that of adults, and cardiac muscle glycogen is 10 times the adult value. Another source of stored energy resides in fetal adipose tissue triglycerides that accumulate in the last trimester. This accumulation of adipose tissue is predominantly a result of synthesis from glucose, since there is limited transfer of free fatty acids from the mother.

During hypoxia the fetus may meet metabolic requirements primarily by glucose production from glycogenolysis and glycolysis. In chronic sheep preparations, total maternal starvation causes a prompt fall in maternal and fetal blood glucose levels for the first 48 hours, but a stable plateau is reached subsequently; the fetus then increases amino acid catabolism, which accounts for most of the fetal oxygen consumption. The human fetus has the potential to replace substrate glucose with β-OH-butyrate for energy during periods of maternal starvation and glucose deprivation.

Fetal hormones

In the human, proinsulin separated from human fetal pancreatic extracts comprises 0.1% to 1.6% of the total insulin values irrespective of the age of the fetus, a proportion similar to that in the adult. Immunoreactive insulin has been demonstrated in both plasma and pancreatic tissue as early as 8 weeks' gestation; the source appears to be the fetal pancreas, since the placenta is impermeable to insulin. At 13 to 18 weeks of gestation, fetal insulin response to sustained maternal hyperglycemia is negliglible. At term, however, the fetus is capable of a significant response to prolonged hyperglycemia, although to a lesser degree than are adults. Since the fetus is continuously receiving glucose from the mother, there is minimal requirement for insulin response. With repeated episodes of hyperglycemia, as in maternal diabetes, greater insulin response is seen, indicating that β-cell sensitivity is being induced or enhanced. That insulin may modify the growth rate in utero has been shown by the positive correlation between fetal plasma insulin concentration and fetal weight.

Human growth hormone has been measured as early as 9 weeks of gestation and increases rapidly between the eleventh and sixteenth weeks. Since the transplacental transfer of human growth hormone is negligible, the fetal pituitary appears to be its source in the fetus. At term, fetal plasma human growth hormone levels are higher than those of maternal plasma. Unlike those of adults, fetal human growth hormone levels are not suppressed during hyperglycemia and actually show a paradoxical rise.

The pancreatic α-cells are detectable at approximately 8 to 11 weeks' gestation and constitute 30% of the islet cells at term. Circulating glucagon has been found in fetal plasma as early as the fifteenth week. Fetal pancreatic and circulating glucagon must be of fetal origin, since maternal glucagon does not cross the placenta. Peak concentrations of glucagon in the pancreas are reached at 24 to 26 weeks of gestation and are approximately two or three times higher than those of adult human pancreas. Similar to those of human growth hormone, glucagon levels fail to diminish during constant glucose infusion. Although the physiologic function of fetal glucagon is unknown, its effect on fetal carbohydrate metabolism is probably minimal. Cortisol is synthesized in a cooperative effort between mother and fetus, involving the fetal zone of the adrenal cortex and progesterone secreted by the placenta as substrate. The fetal adrenal gland can also synthesize cortisol from acetate.

Fetal enzymes

Metabolism in the fetus in large part reflects its dependence on maternally derived substrates. Glucose for energy is continually provided and need not be synthesized. The fetus actively incorporates amino acid into protein and synthesizes triglycerides from glucose. The human fetal liver has the enzymatic capacity for gluconeogenesis and glycogenolysis as early as the third month of gestation. However, if maternal glucose provision is adequate and placental transfer normal, there is no requirement for fetal gluconeogenesis. Nevertheless, during early human fetal life the absolute levels of gluconeogenic enzymes are 10% to 70% of adult values. This does not necessarily mean that these enzymes are rate limiting under these conditions, since early fetal liver may produce glucose from pyruvate. In contrast to its potential role as a provider of glucose, under normal states of maternal nutrition fetal hepatic glycogen content actually increases linearly at this early gestational age. Because of fetal dependence on glucose metabolism, one would also expect high activity of important glycolytic enzymes. Indeed, hexokinase and pyruvate kinase are high in fetal rat tissues and decrease at birth. As the rat fetus approaches term, there is a marked increase in glycogen synthetase and phosphorylase with a predominance of synthetase, thus facilitating deposition of hepatic glycogen.

NEONATAL GLUCOSE METABOLISM

The newborn must supply its own substrate to meet the energy requirements for maintenance of body temperature, respiration, muscular activity, and regulation of blood glucose. The concentration of glucose in umbilical venous blood approximates 70% to 80% of that in the mother and is higher than in the umbilical arterial blood. During the first 4 to 6 hours of postnatal life, glucose values fall, stabilizing between 50 and 60 mg/dl. By the third day, glucose values equilibrate at 60 to 70 mg/dl in full-sized neonates and at lower levels in low birth weight infants. Blood glucose values remain lower in low birth weight than in full-sized infants throughout the first month of life. Intense lipid mobilization begins within a few minutes after birth and is reflected by a rapid rise in glycerol and free fatty acid. The respiratory quotient declines from levels approaching 1.0 to levels of 0.7 by the third postnatal day, suggesting a changeover from a predominantly carbohydrate to a predominantly fat metabolism at a time when liver glycogen and blood glucose are decreasing. Furthermore, a progressive rise in blood ketones occurs within a few hours after birth and reaches a peak in 2 to 3 days, indicating increased oxidation of free fatty acids. Lipolysis is probably initiated by activation of the autonomic nervous system secondary to cold stimulation of the skin at the time of birth or to clamping of the cord.

Blood glucose concentration is normally maintained at a relatively constant level by a fine balance between hepatic glucose output and peripheral glucose uptake. The latter is influenced by factors such as body temperature, muscular activity, and insulin concentration. Normal neonates have a low capacity for removal of a rapidly injected glucose load, as demonstrated by glucose disappearance rates between 1.0% and 1.3% during the first

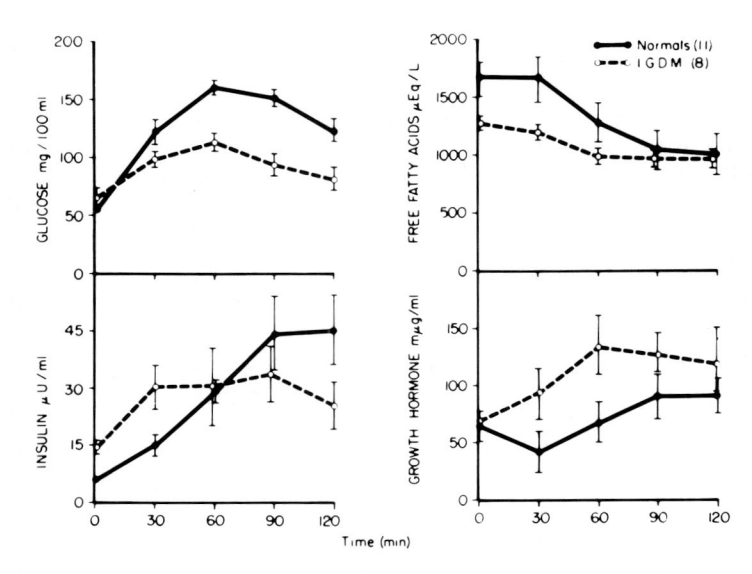

Fig. 33-2. Blood glucose, plasma insulin, free fatty acids, and growth hormone values (mean ± S.E.) at fasting and following 2 gm/kg glucose administered orally in 11 normal newborns and 8 infants of gestational diabetic mothers. (From Pildes, R.S., and others: Pediatrics **44**:76, 1969.)

24 hours of life. By 5 to 7 days of age, however, glucose disappearance rates are significantly higher than during the first 24 hours of life.

Several groups have begun to study glucose kinetics in infants using the Steele steady state infusion technique with stable isotope tracers. Glucose production is higher in the newborn than in the adult. Kalhan and associates, using glucose-1-^{13}C in normal term infants at 2 to 4 hours of age and prior to feeding, measure glucose production of 4.4 ± 0.4 (mean ± S.D.) mg/kg/minute. Adult values are approximately half those reported in normal neonates.

Hepatic glucose output depends on (1) adequate glycogen stores, (2) sufficient supplies of endogenous gluconeogenic precursors, (3) a normally functioning hepatic gluconeogenetic and glycogenolytic system, and (4) a normal endocrine system for modulating these processes. At birth the neonate has glycogen stores that are greater than those in the adult. However, because of a twofold greater basal glucose utilization, these stores are rapidly depleted and begin to decline within 2 to 3 hours after birth, remain low for several days, and then gradually rise to adult levels. Muscle and cardiac carbohydrate levels fall more slowly. During asphyxia, energy requirements are met by anaerobic glycolysis, an inefficient mechanism that results in a limited amount of energy and rapid depletion of glycogen stores. In premature infants there is marked reduction of both total carbohydrate and fat content, and depletion of liver carbohydrate occurs within 12 hours after birth. Endogenous gluconeogenic substrate availability probably is not a limiting factor, since the concentration of plasma amino acids is increased at birth as a consequence of active placental transport. Similarly, other gluconeogenic precursors, such as lactate, pyruvate, and glycerol, also are increased.

The fall in blood glucose that normally occurs after birth is accompanied by an elevated level of human growth hormone, a relatively low concentration of immunoreactive insulin, and an increase in plasma glucagon. The neonate shows an attenuated but significant insulin response to a variety of stimuli. Following oral administration of glucose the insulin response in the normal neonate is similar to that in adults with chemical diabetes, that is, a lag in insulin response and a delayed peak (Fig. 33-2). The premature infant has a minimal and variable insulin response, but the values are markedly increased by intravenous administration of glucose plus amino acids. The physiologic role of human growth hormone has not been defined; human growth hormone values are high during the first 48 to 72 hours and gradually decline but are still elevated at 8 weeks of age. In addition, the newborn shows a paradoxical rise in human growth hormone following glucose infusion. Plasma glucagon values at birth are similar to or slightly higher than maternal levels. A surge in glucagon release is seen within hours after birth, which is probably mediated via adrenergic mechanisms and not as a response to hypoglycemia. Glucagon and human growth hormone are not suppressed during hypoglycemia. In healthy newborns, intravenous and oral alanine feedings raise plasma glucagon and glucose levels. The adrenal medulla secretes little epineph-

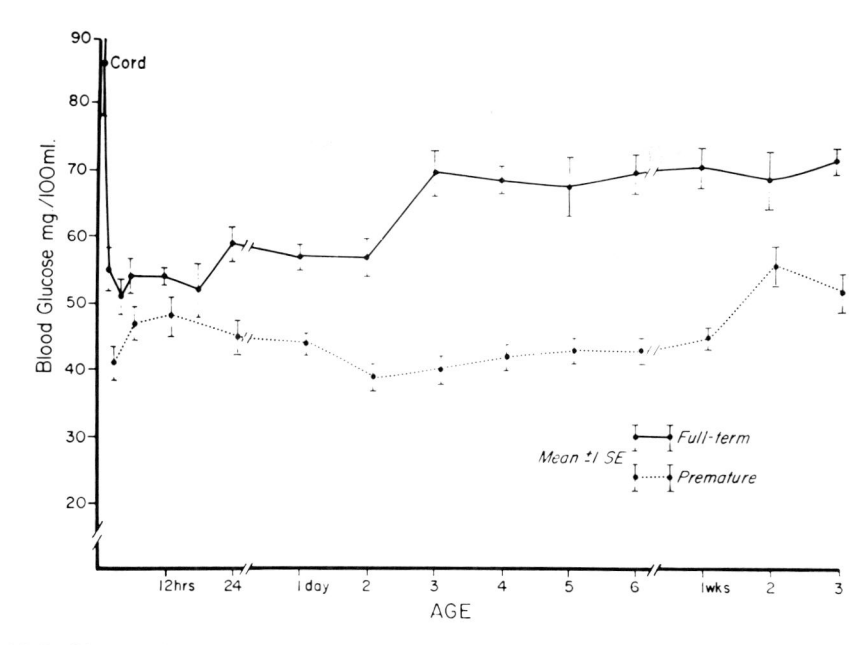

Fig. 33-3. Glucose levels in 179 infants more than 2.5 kg and in 104 low birth weight infants (< 2.5 kg) during the neonatal period. (Reprinted, by permission, From Cornblath, M., and Reisner, S.H.: N. Engl. J. Med. **273:**278, 1965.)

rine at birth and is not a significant regulator of neonatal blood glucose concentration. Nevertheless, hypoglycemia stimulates epinephrine secretion, probably through increased activity of the sympathetic plexus mediated by the splanchnic nerve. The newborn adrenal cortex rapidly establishes independent cortisol production controlled by pituitary adrenocorticotropic hormone (ACTH).

Adaptation to prolonged starvation in adult humans is facilitated by the ability of the brain to derive much of its energy through oxidation of ketone bodies; this decreases the need for gluconeogenesis and spares muscle protein. Enzymes involved in ketone body utilization pathways are present in brain tissue of human fetuses and in newborns. That ketone bodies are used by the brains of infants and children has been shown by measurements of arteriovenous differences across the brain.

THE CLINICAL PROBLEM OF HYPOGLYCEMIA

Ideally, hypoglycemia should be defined as a state of tissue glucose insufficiency (notably the central nervous system). At present there are no means of determining tissue glucose insufficiency except for the variable and inconsistent symptoms attributable to low glucose levels. Since the significance of low glucose concentration without symptoms is not well understood, symptoms cannot be used as sole criteria in determining tissue glucose insufficiency. Because of these problems, we prefer to use a definition of hypoglycemia based on the statistical distribution of whole blood glucose values in large surveys of low birth weight (less than 2.5 kg) and full-sized neonates (2.5 kg or more) as proposed by Cornblath and Schwartz (Fig. 33-3). The values represent two standard deviations below the mean for a particular population. Because most laboratories no longer use whole blood for glucose determinations, the original definitions have been converted to plasma values. Thus hypoglycemia in the first 72 hours is defined as two plasma glucose levels less than 25 mg/dl in low-birth-weight neonates and less than 35 mg/dl in full-sized neonates. After 72 hours, hypoglycemia in full-sized neonates is defined as plasma glucose levels less than 45 mg/dl. Changing practices in maternal and neonatal care over the past 10 years may have altered these definitions. However, we have not seen symptomatic infants with glucose values above the ranges defined who have had alleviation of their symptoms with glucose infusions.

Clinical manifestations

These are nonspecific, but the episodic nature and the frequent clustering of symptoms and signs are highly suggestive (see following list). Convulsions, a dramatic and serious manifestation, have been noted in 20% to 25% of neonates with hypoglycemia. Cardiac arrest at 6 hours of age, associated with a blood glucose value of 8 mg/dl, was the presenting symptom in one of our infants who subsequently proved to have human growth hormone deficiency. Often the symptoms are insidious and consist of somnolence, lethargy, and refusal to feed.

CLINICAL SIGNS COMMONLY ASSOCIATED WITH NEONATAL HYPOGLYCEMIA

Tremors or jitteriness
Irritability
Apneic spells
Cyanotic spells
Convulsions
Limpness
Lethargy
Hypothermia
High-pitched or weak cry
Refusal to feed
Eye-rolling
Cardiac failure
Cardiac arrest
Sweating

A variety of clinical entities may cause symptoms similar to those of hypoglycemia. Moreover, hypoglycemia may also be present as an additional contributing factor to a primary disease.

Laboratory manifestations

Factors that are frequently overlooked in the interpretation of a glucose concentration are the type of sample and the method of analysis. Whole blood includes red cells, which, because of their lower water content, have a glucose concentration lower than that of plasma. Plasma glucose values are higher than those of blood by about 14%; the percent difference may be greater at very low (less than 30 mg/dl) values because of a greater probability of laboratory error. Whole blood glucose also varies in accordance with the hematocrit value; in addition, neonatal red blood cells contain high concentrations of glycolytic intermediates such as reduced glutathione. Thus whole blood must be deproteinized with zinc hydroxide before analysis. Capillary blood samples should be collected from a warm heel and taken to the laboratory on ice, since the rate of in vitro glycolysis is increased in neonatal red blood cells; the blood glucose level may be lowered by 18 mg/dl/hour if the sample is allowed to stand at room temperature.

A large number of enzymatic and chemical methods are currently used for glucose determinations. Those which employ reducing methods may give falsely elevated glucose values, since non-glucose-reducing substances may range up to 60 mg/dl in newborn blood. True sugar method can be used, since galactose and fructose levels are minimal in normal infants. However, enzymatic procedures using glucose oxidase or glucose-6-phosphate dehydrogenase, which specifically measure glucose, are preferable.

The need for a rapid, simple method of blood sugar determination has led to the development of enzyme test strips (Dextrostix). Accuracy of this method depends on placing a large drop of blood so that it completely covers the strip for exactly 1 minute and washing it with a controlled stream of water. The test strips, if allowed to stand for prolonged periods because of infrequent use, may give erroneously low values. Modification of the technique using plasma and the development of the reflectance meter (Ames Co.) have improved the results; these techniques are reliable when used by experienced personnel, but enough error exists to require that all abnormal or borderline values be confirmed with standard laboratory methods.

Differential diagnosis

Hypoglycemia may be caused by a wide variety of pathologic conditions and is a common finding in many hereditary disorders of carbohydrate and amino acid metabolism, as shown in the following outline. Discussion of individual entities is limited to disorders of carbohydrate metabolism that occur in the neonatal period.

A. Asymptomatic (transient)
B. Symptomatic (transient, idiopathic)
C. Specific etiology
   1. Hyperinsulinism
      a. Maternal diabetes
      b. Erythroblastosis
      c. Beckwith-Wiedemann syndrome
      d. Infant giants
      e. β-Cell nesidioblastosis-adenoma spectrum
      f. Functional β-cell hyperplasia
      g. Leucine sensitivity
      h. Maternal drugs
   2. Endocrine disorders
      a. Panhypopituitarism
      b. Isolated growth hormone deficiency
      c. Cortisol deficiency
         (1) ACTH unresponsiveness
         (2) Isolated glucocorticoid deficiency
         (3) Maternal steroid therapy
         (4) Adrenal hemorrhage
         (5) Adrenogenital syndrome
      d. Hypothyroidism
      e. Glucagon deficiency
   3. Hereditary defects in metabolism
      a. Carbohydrate metabolism
         (1) Galactosemia
         (2) Glycogen storage disease type 1
         (3) Fructose intolerance
      b. Amino acid metabolism
         (1) Maple syrup urine disease
         (2) Propionicacidemia
         (3) Methylmalonic acidemia
         (4) Hereditary tyrosinemia

D. Associated with other neonatal problems
  1. Iatrogenic
     a. Following abrupt cessation of intravenous fluids
     b. Following exchange transfusion
     c. Hypothermia
     d. Malpositioned umbilical artery catheter
  2. Miscellaneous
     a. Neonatal infection
     b. Cardiac malformation
     c. Hypothermia
     d. Hyperviscosity
     e. Chronic diarrhea
     f. Antiinsulin antibodies
     g. Central nervous system abnormalities

Asymptomatic transient neonatal hypoglycemia

Asymptomatic hypoglycemia may be seen frequently before onset of feedings, especially in premature or small for gestational age infants. The true incidence of asymptomatic hypoglycemia is impossible to ascertain, since its presence has usually been determined by chance sampling. Gutberlet and Cornblath have suggested that this be considered as early transitional or adaptive hypoglycemia following the withdrawal of substrate supplied from the mother. Infants in this category are not necessarily small for gestational age (SGA), but appropriate for gestational age and large for gestational age babies have similar problems. There is no sex predilection; perinatal hypoxia, prematurity, maternal toxemia and diabetes, twinning, and delayed feedings may contribute to the hypoglycemia. If symptoms are present, they may be due to the underlying disease, especially if they are not alleviated by glucose. Hypoglycemia is of short duration and rarely recurs. The infants may respond spontaneously to oral feedings or to relatively low concentrations of constant glucose infusions. Extensive long-term follow up data are not available, but current data indicate that the prognosis is more favorable than in patients with symptomatic hypoglycemia. Nevertheless, hypoglycemia should be treated until normoglycemia is established.

Symptomatic transient idiopathic neonatal hypoglycemia
Incidence and etiology

The incidence of idiopathic transient symptomatic neonatal hypoglycemia varies between 1.3 and 3 per 1,000 live births. Twice as many male as female infants are affected. Among low birth weight infants, 5.7% may be affected; the incidence rises to 15% in low birth weight infants who are symptomatic and below the fiftieth percentile for gestational age. The smaller of twins who weighs less than 2.0 kg and is discordant by 25% in weight when compared with the larger twin has a 70% chance of developing symptomatic hypoglycemia (Fig. 33-4).

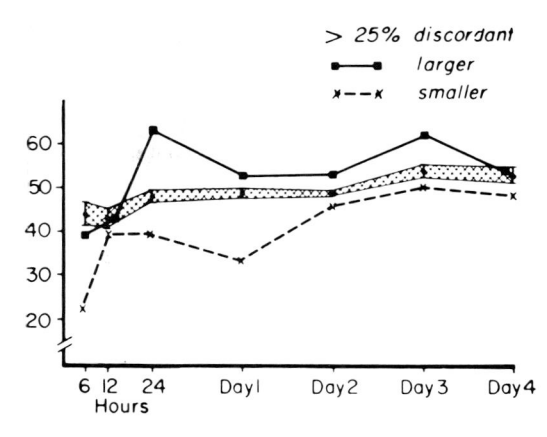

Fig. 33-4. Mean blood glucose values in twins whose birth weights were discordant by more than 25%. Mean ± S.D. of 100 pairs of twins is shown by crosshatch. (From Pildes, R.S., and others: Pediatrics **40**:69, 1967.)

Clinical and laboratory manifestations

The infants may be born preterm, at term, or postterm, although preterm infants predominate. Intrauterine growth retardation, manifested by a birth weight below the tenth percentile for gestational age on the Lubchenco intrauterine growth curve, is present in about 75% of the infants (Fig. 33-5). Postterm neonates need not be below the tenth percentile; instead, intrauterine growth retardation is exhibited by a disproportionately low weight-length ratio and clinical signs of dysmaturity. In general, weight is affected to a greater degree than length and head circumference; however, the latter two are below the tenth percentile in a significant number of infants. Decreased head circumference also may indicate microcephaly, which in some patients may be the primary etiologic factor causing hypoglycemia.

Maternal age is not a significant factor, but toxemia is found in a high proportion of mothers. There is no correlation between hypoglycemia and duration of labor, premature rupture of membranes, or the type of analgesia or anesthesia. Birth hypoxia is frequently present.

Symptoms begin within the first 24 hours in about 40% of the infants and after 72 hours in 14%. Associated laboratory features include polycythemia, a frequent observation in intrauterine malnutrition, and hypocalcemia (less than 7.0 mg/dl), which has been found in 20% of the infants and is probably related to prematurity, toxemia, or birth anoxia rather than to intrauterine malnutrition. Cardiomegaly was demonstrated on roentgenogram in 12 and cardiac failure in 4 of 76 infants in one study. The

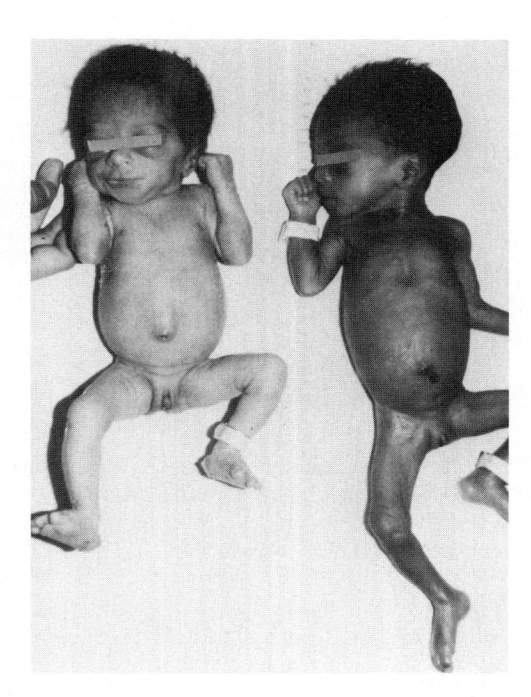

Fig. 33-5. SGA infant, 40 weeks' gestation and 1,100 gm at birth, compared with an AGA infant of 32 weeks' gestation. The SGA infant had asymptomatic hypoglycemia.

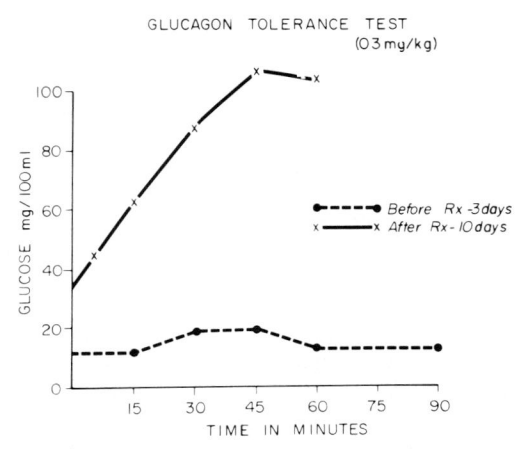

Fig. 33-6. Whole blood glucose values following glucagon tolerance test in SGA hypoglycemic neonate shown in Fig. 33-5, before and after treatment with hydrocortisone.

cause of cardiomegaly is unknown, but cardiac congenital anomalies need not be present, and cardiomegaly recedes after carbohydrate homeostasis is established. Polycythemia is a frequent finding in SGA infants and may be a factor in the pathogenesis of cardiomegaly. However, cardiomegaly and congestive failure also have been found in hypoglycemic infants with normal hematocrit values.

Pathogenesis

The association of hypoglycemia with intrauterine growth retardation has led to many studies of carbohydrate homeostasis in SGA infants. Hypoglycemia is not uniformly present in SGA infants, and factors other than intrauterine growth retardation may be necessary to precipitate hypoglycemia in some SGA infants (see following outline). Since SGA infants have experienced nutritional restriction during gestation, it seems reasonable to expect reduced amounts of hepatic glycogen and total body fat. Supportive evidence includes low hepatic carbohydrate levels at postmortem of SGA infants as compared with appropriate for gestational age (AGA) full-term infants and stillbirths. Normoglycemic SGA infants may show adequate glucagon response to exogenous glucose, but hypoglycemic SGA infants have a reduced glycemic response with rapid improvement following therapy (Fig. 33-6). A relative decrease in liver glycogen available per unit of brain weight may be inferred from the disproportionately increased brain-liver weight ratio in SGA infants. Decreased gluconeogenesis has been suggested because of increased blood levels of alanine and lactate in SGA as compared with AGA infants. In hypoglycemic SGA newborns, levels of gluconeogenic amino acids entering at pyruvate, such as proline, glycine, and valine, are significantly higher than in normoglycemic SGA infants. Decreased gluconeogenesis is also indicated by the poor glycemic response to intravenous and oral alanine of SGA neonates compared with that of normal neonates. Administration of hydrocortisone results in a hyperglycemic response to alanine, which may have been facilitated by lowering plasma insulin levels or by increasing gluconeogenesis from alanine.

Glucose utilization following intravenous glucose administration, particularly in full-term SGA hypoglycemic newborns, may be significantly increased as compared with that in normal controls (Fig. 33-7). Insulin values, appropriately depressed in SGA infants, may be elevated in some hypoglycemic SGA neonates. This suggests that β-cell function usually adapts itself to intrauterine starvation but that the adaptation may not be universal in all hypoglycemic SGA infants. The importance of glucagon in the etiology of hypoglycemia is unknown. Human growth hormone secretion appears normal, deficient secretion of catecholamines has been implicated, and a low cortisol production rate has been reported. Finally, the finding of hypoglycemia in microcephalic neonates suggests a defective central nervous system mechanism for glucose homeostasis in some infants.

Following is an outline of the pathogenesis of transient neonatal hypoglycemia:

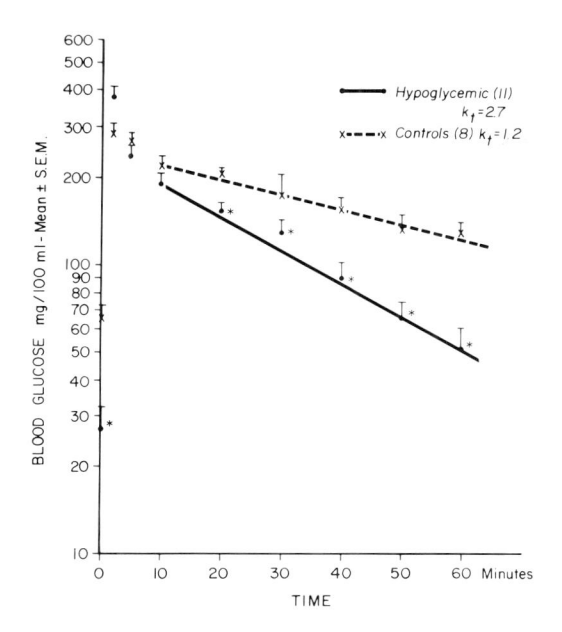

Fig. 33-7. Glucose disappearance rates (k_t) in 8 normal controls and 11 full-term SGA hypoglycemic neonates. (From Pildes, R.S., and others: Pediatrics **52**:75, 1973.)

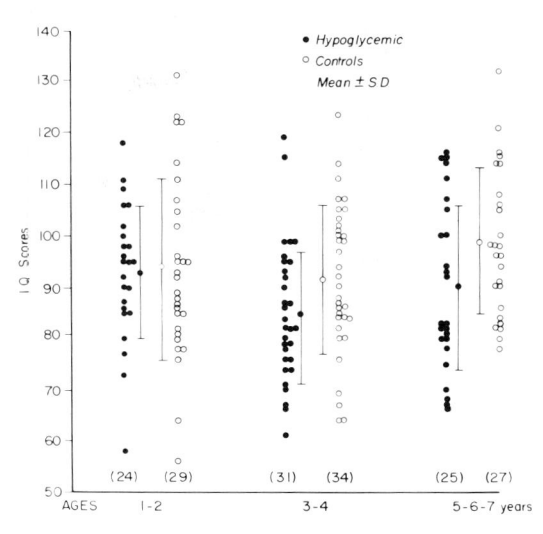

Fig. 33-8. Individual IQ scores in hypoglycemic neonates compared with those of equally high-risk but normoglycemic controls. (From Pildes, R.S., and others: Pediatrics **54**:5, 1974.)

A. Inadequate production of glucose
   1. Decreased glycogen and fat stores
   2. Defective gluconeogenesis
   3. Decreased glucose-sparing substrates such as:
      a. Ketones
      b. Glycerol
B. Excessive utilization
   1. Increased peripheral glucose disappearance in some infants
   2. Inadequate counterinsulin hormones
   3. Increased needs
      a. Increased oxygen consumption in SGA infants
      b. Anoxia
      c. Large brain-liver ratio

Pathology

Evidence that neuronal glucose deprivation specifically damages nerve cells is difficult to substantiate, since hypoxia, acidosis, and other underlying factors commonly coexist with severe hypoglycemia. Adult rhesus monkeys subjected to gross insulin hypoglycemia had evidence of damage to the neocortex. In newborn rat pups made hypoglycemic with insulin once per day for 18 days, there was generalized diminution of brain weight, cellularity, and protein content. Widespread neuronal damage has been described in three of six infants who had prolonged hypoglycemia and died in the first week of life.

Prognosis

Untreated hypoglycemia may result in severe neurologic deficit or death. In a long-term prospective follow-up of a group of 39 treated hypoglycemic infants and 41 matched normoglycemic high-risk control neonates, mean height and weight were similar in the two groups at 5 to 7 years of age. However, head circumference, which had been significantly smaller at birth in the hypoglycemic newborns, remained smaller. Abnormal neurologic development could not be ascribed solely to hypoglycemia, except in 2 of 30 infants who had repeated evaluations. Convulsions in the neonatal period were associated with increased neurologic abnormalities and with recurrent nonhypoglycemic seizures. A greater number of hypoglycemic neonates had IQ scores below 86 than did the controls (Fig. 33-8), although the mean IQ scores were not significantly different. Thus, although treatment resulted in less severe damage than had been expected from previous reports, these studies suggest that treatment of symptomatic infants should be even more aggressive to improve the prognosis.

The hypoglycemia is usually self-limited, but recurrences may be common during the first few days as intravenous fluids infiltrate or are too rapidly discontinued before oral feedings are well tolerated. Recurrent hypoglycemic episodes also occur during the first few months of life in 10% to 15% of the infants. In children with ketotic hypoglycemia, retrospective studies show an increased incidence of neonatal hypoglycemia.

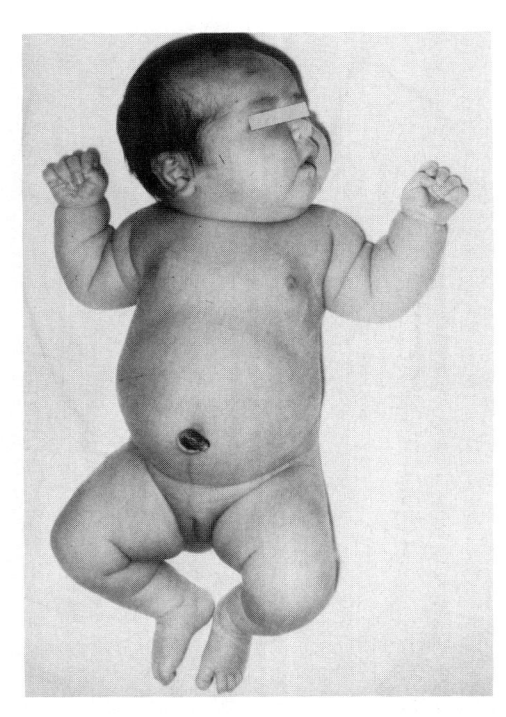

Fig. 33-9. Infant of gestational diabetic mother born at 40 weeks' gestation. Birth weight, 4.7 kg; postnatal age, 1 week.

Infant of the diabetic mother (see also Chapter 3)
Clinical and laboratory manifestation

Infants of diabetic mothers may be LGA but physiologically immature (Fig. 33-9). They need not be large; diabetic mothers with severe vascular disease may give birth to SGA infants. In our nursery, most infants of diabetic mothers are AGA, and the incidence of LGA infants approximates 30%. Typically, the infant has a round, cherubic face and appears plethoric. The excessive weight is due to increased body fat and enlargement of viscera, primarily liver, adrenals, and heart. The umbilical cord and placenta are also enlarged. Skeletal length is increased in proportion to weight, but the brain appears disproportionately small because it does not increase in size abnormally. The development of ossification centers does not correspond to weight and length but rather to gestational age (or even less than the infant's gestational age). There is considerable reduction in total and extracellular water. Skinfold thickness and adipose cell diameter correlate significantly with maternal blood glucose during the third trimester. Recently maternal glycohemoglobin concentration (Hb A_{1c}) has also been shown to be a predictor of birth weight and skinfold thickness in infants of diabetic mothers. During the first days of life the infants are generally tremulous and hyperexcitable, although hypotonia, lethargy, and poor sucking also may occur. Clinical problems in the neonate are extremely variable. In retrospective studies, respiratory distress syndrome (RDS) was found in greater frequency in infants of diabetic mothers than in infants of comparable gestational age regardless of mode of delivery until 38.5 weeks of gestation. In our nursery the incidence of respiratory distress in infants of both gestational and insulin-dependent diabetic mothers is 30% to 40%, but RDS is rare; "wet lung" syndrome or transient tachypnea is the primary cause of respiratory distress (p. 447). Increased cardiothymic shadow is found in approximately 35% and congestive heart failure, judged by tachypnea, tachycardia, and hepatomegaly in 5% to 17% of the infants (Fig. 33-10). Poor control of maternal diabetes may be responsible for the differences in incidence of congestive failure in various centers. Electrocardiograms may be abnormal and show marked right ventricular hypertrophy, combined ventricular hypertrophy, and, rarely, left ventricular hypertrophy. Echocardiographic studies have emphasized the presence of a wide spectrum of hypertrophic cardiomyopathy. Disproportionate septal hypertrophy and abnormal ventricular wall thickening, at times resulting in obstruction of the left ventricle outflow tracts, have been reported. The findings may be indistinguishable from those of hypertrophic subaortic stenosis, but the natural history appears to be benign. Digitalis is contraindicated if heart failure is due to hypertrophic cardiomyopathy; propranolol may be used to reduce ventricular contractility.

Immediately after birth, blood glucose levels fall precipitously to levels lower than those in normal infants (Fig. 33-11). A nadir is reached between 1 and 3 hours of age; by 4 to 6 hours spontaneous recovery usually begins. Blood glucose levels below 30 mg/dl occur in 40% to 50% of infants of diabetic mothers, but the infants are usually asymptomatic; symptomatic hypoglycemia occurs in a small percentage of these infants. The frequency of this complication is greater in infants born to insulin-dependent mothers, in infants whose mothers are poorly controlled during pregnancy, and in those whose mothers receive large doses of intravenous glucose during labor or at the time of delivery. Some centers are beginning to report that infants of insulin-dependent diabetic mothers are having less neonatal complications than those of gestational diabetic mothers, presumably because the gestational diabetic is not diagnosed until late in pregnancy, whereas the insulin-dependent diabetic is closely followed during her pregnancy. Hypocalcemia is prevalent in infants of diabetic mothers, even when gestational age and perinatal complications are taken into consideration. Since symptoms of hypocalcemia are similar to those of hypoglycemia, the former must be taken into consideration when therapy for hypoglycemia is ineffective. In general, hypoglycemia is seen during the first hours after birth; hypocalcemia occurs between 24 and 36 hours of

Metabolic and endocrine disorders   855

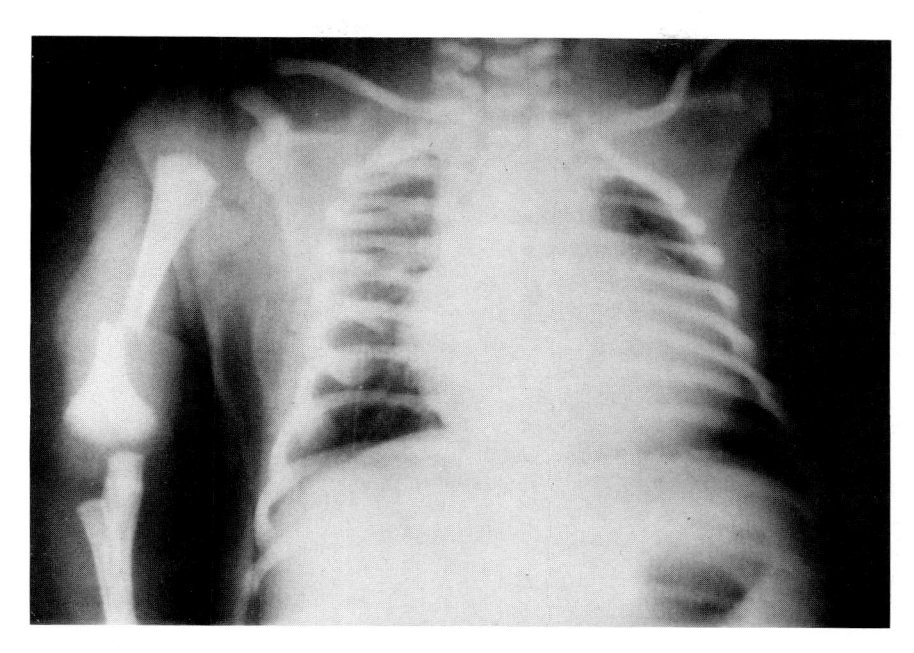

Fig. 33-10. Chest roentgenogram of a vaginally delivered full-term infant of a diabetic mother weighing 4.7 kg. The infant had cardiomegaly, hepatomegaly, congested lung fields, and fractures of the right humerus and left clavicle.

Fig. 33-11. Serial changes in the concentration of glucose in the blood of infants immediately following delivery. Mothers with gestational diabetes had abnormal intravenous glucose tolerance tests during pregnancy but received no insulin. (Reprinted, by permission of the New England Journal of Medicine from McCann, M.L., and others: N. Engl. J. Med. **275:**1, 1966.)

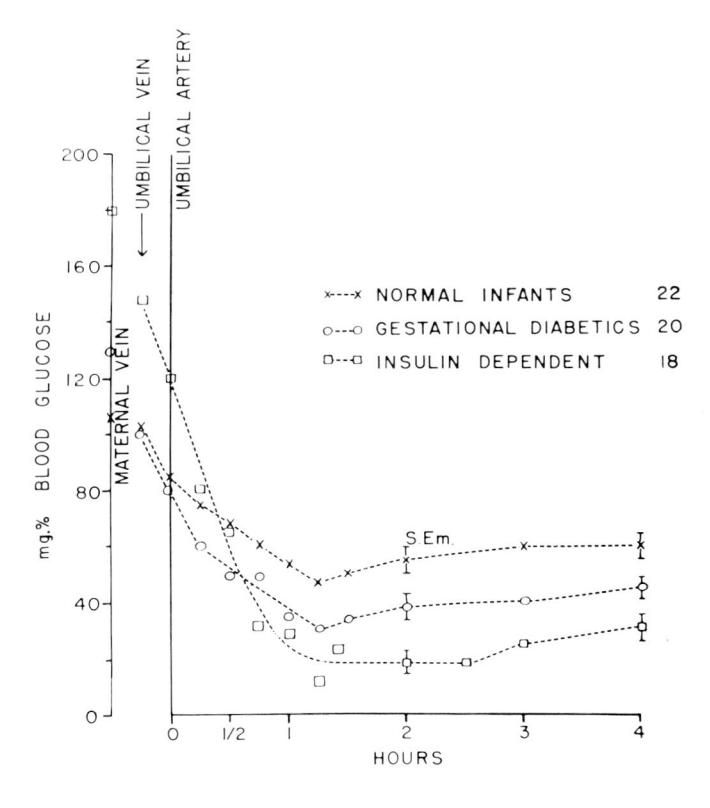

Table 33-1. Collaborative perinatal project: frequency of major malformations in children of diabetic pregnancies

System	%	Diabetic-nondiabetic ratio*
CNS	2.29	3.4
Musculoskeletal	5.29	1.5
Sensory	0.35	1.5
Cardiovascular	2.47	5.6
Respiratory	1.94	2.7
Genitourinary	3.35	3.6
Alimentary	3.53	1.8

*Nondiabetics: $n = 47,408$; diabetics: $n = 567$.
From Chung, C.S., and Myrianthopoulos, N.C.: Effect of maternal diabetes on congenital malformations. In Bergsma, D., editor: Factors affecting risks of congenital malformations, Florida: Symposia Specialists for The National Foundation–March of Dimes, BD:OAS **XI** (10):23, 1975.

age. In many infants, however, jitteriness remains and cannot be explained either by hypocalcemia or hypoglycemia. Other problems include nonhemolytic hyperbilirubinemia, polycythemia, neonatal small left colon syndrome, and, rarely, renal vein thrombosis. Of 42 consecutively followed infants of diabetic mothers in our nursery, only one had a renal vein thrombosis (2.4%). The infants usually have unilateral or bilateral flank masses and hematuria. Management consists of adequate hydration as long as renal function is maintained and fluid restriction if renal failure supervenes. The use of heparin is of questionable benefit. Removal of the kidney is not indicated unless hypertension occurs during follow-up. Neonatal small left colon syndrome presents with failure to pass meconium, abdominal distension, and bile-stained vomitus. Contrast enemas show a markedly diminished caliber of the left colon from the splenic flexure. The syndrome is transient, and immature ganglion cells may be present in the intermyenteric plexus.

Congenital anomalies are two to four times more frequent among infants of diabetic mothers than among normal controls and more commonly affect multiple organ systems; cardiovascular, central nervous system, and genitourinary malformations predominate (Table 33-1). The types of anomalies do not appear to be specific, with the possible exception of the caudal regression syndrome (Fig. 33-12). Anomalies are no more frequent in the offspring of diabetic fathers and prediabetic mothers than among those of nondiabetics. This is consistent with the hypothesis that anomalies may be the result of metabolic disturbances.

Electroencephalograms and sleep-pattern studies suggest physiologic immaturity of the brain. However, peripheral nerve conduction velocities are generally consistent with gestational age, indicating normal myelinization.

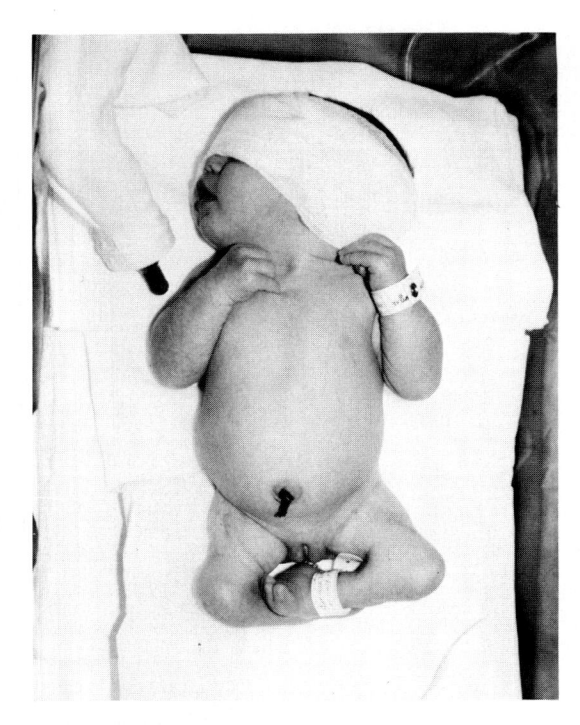

Fig. 33-12. Infant of diabetic mother with caudal regression syndrome (sacral agenesis).

Pathogenesis

No single physiologic or biochemical event can explain the diverse clinical manifestations. Pedersen has suggested the following pathogenetic sequence: maternal hyperglycemia causes fetal hyperglycemia and hypertrophy of the fetal pancreatic islets, leading to fetal hyperinsulinism. An expanded Pedersen hypothesis has been proposed as a result of metabolic changes found in even the mildest of gestational diabetics. These include increased levels of glucose, selected amino acids, lipids, and ketones ("mixed nutrients"). Thus a surfeit of "mixed nutrients" is available to the fetus as long as vascular complications are not present. In addition, the β-cells may be more sensitive to the insulinogenic action of amino acids. The combination of hyperinsulinism and increased mixed nutrients causes increased hepatic glucose uptake and glycogen synthesis, accelerated lipogenesis and augmented protein synthesis, thus leading to the characteristic macrosomia of these infants. Pathologic correlates include hypertrophy and hyperplasia of the pancreatic islets with a disproportionate increase in the percentage of β-cells. In addition, there is myocardial hypertrophy, an increased amount of cytoplasm in the liver cells, and extramedullary hematopoiesis. The separation of the placenta suddenly interrupts glucose infusion into the neonate without affecting insulin concentration proportionately; this causes hypoglycemia during the first hours after birth. The hyperinsulinemia has been difficult to document in infants of diabetic mothers because of placental transfer of maternal antiinsulin antibodies, which interfere with the radioimmunoassay of insulin. However, hyperinsulinism has been substantiated from measurements of immunoreactive insulin from infants of gestational diabetic mothers and from infants whose mothers have had few or no insulin antibodies. In addition, oral glucose tolerance tests in infants of gestational diabetic mothers and in normal newborns have demonstrated a significantly higher fasting plasma insulin level in the infants of gestational diabetic mothers despite similar glucose levels; infants of gestational diabetic mothers responded with a prompt elevation of plasma insulin and assimilated the glucose load more rapidly. Measurement of C-peptide, which is released by the β-cells in amounts equimolar with insulin, has confirmed the presence of hyperinsulinism in infants of insulin-dependent mothers. C-Peptide levels were increased in cord blood of infants of diabetic mothers as compared with normal controls and were directly related to the severity of maternal diabetes. Higher cord levels of C-peptide were significantly associated with neonatal hypoglycemia and macrosomia, whereas no correlation was found with RDS. Cord levels of C-peptide in infants of diabetic mothers were also elevated at less than 34 weeks' gestation. In addition, infants of diabetic mothers show a prompt C-peptide increase within 2 minutes following an intravenous bolus of glucose in contrast to the delayed response of normal newborns. Further supports for hyperinsulinemia are the findings of increased glucose disappearance rates of endogenous and exogenous intravenous glucose and the enhanced plasma insulin response following arginine administration as compared with that in normal newborns. Hepatic glucose production rates in infants of diabetic mothers are significantly lower than in control infants, providing additional evidence for suppression of hepatic glucose output during hyperinsulinemic states. Plasma free fatty acid and D-β-hydroxybutyrate levels during the first 60 minutes of postnatal life are lower in infants of diabetic mothers than in normal controls, another manifestation of the hyperinsulinemia. However, plasma glycerol levels increase. The lower free fatty acid levels, despite increased glycerol levels, have been explained by an increased rate of reesterification of free fatty acid with α-glycerophosphate derived from glycogen within adipose tissue.

Although hyperinsulinism is probably the principal cause of hypoglycemia, deficient catecholamine and glucagon responses also have been demonstrated and may contribute to hypoglycemia by facilitating insulin action. However, cortisol and human growth hormone levels are similar in infants of diabetic mothers and in normal infants; thus these hormonal responses are appropriate and adequate. Insulin appears to be the important growth factor in fetal development. This may be due to direct action on cell proliferation or indirectly through stimulation of amino acid and glucose uptake into fetal tissues. On the other hand, there is delay of pulmonary functional maturity, which may reflect insulin-induced alterations in lung growth and substrate flow. In rabbit fetal lung cultures the addition of insulin abolished the stimulatory effect of cortisol on lecithin synthesis. Insulin delayed the appearance of lamellar bodies in type II cells and increased glycogen content of the alveolar lining cells (p. 408).

Treatment

Meticulous diabetes control during pregnancy leads to improved survival among infants of diabetic mothers. Prevention of ketoacidosis and recognition and treatment of toxemia and urinary tract infection are particularly important. Attempts should be made to maintain fasting plasma glucose values below 100 mg/dl, and postprandial blood sugar values should be kept below 150 mg/dl. Despite these precautions, 10% of intrauterine deaths defy explanation; moreover, some mothers appear predisposed to recurrent stillbirths.

To determine the optimum time of interrupting the pregnancy, the possibility of extrauterine survival must be weighed against that of intrauterine death (Chapter 3). Hospitalization of diabetic patients, other than gestational diabetic patients, is recommended after 34 weeks of gestation. Bed rest, 24-hour urinary estriol determinations as an indication of fetal well-being, weekly oxytocin challenge tests to determine fetal response to the stress of labor, and amniotic fluid lecithin/sphingomyelin ratios to evaluate pulmonary maturity are indicated. Many fetuses can be carried to term, thus preventing the complications of prematurity. Vaginal delivery is preferred, but obstetric factors may justify termination of pregnancy by cesarean section. During labor the rate of glucose infusion should not exceed 200 ml per hour of a 5% dextrose solution in order to prevent a precipitous fall in neonatal blood glucose.

Ideally, delivery should take place in a hospital having a special care nursery where the newborn can be carefully monitored. Glucose values are checked hourly during the first 6 hours of age or until definite recovery is established. Feedings can be started as soon as the infant is stable, usually within 2 to 4 hours after birth, and continued at 3-hour intervals. The first feeding is human milk, 20 cal/oz formula, or 5% dextrose water. If nipple feedings are not tolerated, continuous nasogastric milk infusions can be administered. Treatment is then directed at individual clinical problems.

Prognosis

Perinatal mortality has improved in all series as a result of early identification and good control of diabetes, coupled with delayed delivery to prevent low birth weight. Detection of excessive size and fetal monitoring during labor should lead to prevention of birth trauma and fetal asphyxia. Postneonatal mortality is higher than in normal controls, primarily because of an increased proportion of infants of diabetic mothers with congenital anomalies who survive the newborn period.

Physical growth during childhood and adolescence has been studied by several investigators. Children of diabetic mothers whose birth weight index was greater than or equal to 1.5 had greater weight/height indices at follow-up examination 1 to 19 years later. Macrosomia at birth may be associated with increased number or size of fat cells and predisposes the infant to subsequent obesity. Thus the tendency to obesity in the infant of the diabetic mother is probably secondary to birth weight and not necessarily due to persistently abnormal metabolism.

The incidence of subsequent overt diabetes varies between 0.5% and 1.0% in most studies, but rates of 7% and 11% have also been reported by White and Laron, respectively. These rates are related to genetic factors and not due to fetal life during maternal diabetes. The risk of subsequent diabetes for the infant of a diabetic mother is no greater than that for the infant of a diabetic father. In all series the rate is 10 to 30 times higher than in the normal population. Abnormal glucose tolerance tests have been observed in 12% to 14% of children studied.

Neurologic and developmental outcome of the infant of the diabetic mother vary considerably. The determinants of poor outcome are poor control, early onset of diabetes and vascular complications, low birth weight and prematurity, and perinatal complications. Maternal acetonuria has been associated with delayed psychomotor development. Psychomotor development was followed in 749 infants of diabetic mothers for 1 to 26 years by Yssing in Denmark. Major cerebral handicaps were seen in 18% of the patients, and cerebral palsy and epilepsy were three to five times more common than in the normal population. SGA infants appear to have a greater incidence of borderline to low IQ values. Haworth and associates noted 30% mental subnormality in 37 infants of diabetic mothers at 4½ years of age, which was not related to the presence of hypoglycemia. More recent studies of 57 infants of diabetic mothers, whose mothers had strict control of their diabetes, reveal normal physical and mental development at 5 years of age. Thus improved perinatal outcome should also be associated with improved quality of survival.

Erythroblastosis fetalis

Hypoglycemia is a significant complication of severe erythroblastosis fetalis (p. 727). The incidence varies from 17.8% of infants with cord hemoglobin concentrations below 10 gm/dl to 1.9% of those with higher cord hemoglobin values and 31% of infants after exchange transfusions. Although the condition is often asymptomatic, the diagnosis of symptomatic hypoglycemia may be overlooked because the symptoms are ascribed to the primary disease. Hyperinsulinemia has been demonstrated before and during exchange transfusion. Histologically the total numbers of α- and β-cells are proportionally increased because of hyperplasia of the pancreatic islets; this, in turn, leads to increased total extractable pancreatic insulin and elevated insulin concentration in cord blood. Plasma and urine insulin values are elevated, and plasma free fatty acid levels are decreased. The α-cell proliferation results in a significant decrease in plasma glucagon following an intravenous bolus of glucose. It is not known how the hemolytic disease influences the development of the endocrine pancreas. Inhibition of insulin activity in vitro by hemolysates, such as glutathione reductase, suggests that products of hemolysis may inactivate circulating insulin, thus stimulating compensatory islet cell hyperplasia. Hypoglycemia, as a late sequela, has been reported in two siblings, ages 7 and 25 months, who had severe erythroblastosis as neonates; this suggests that the disturbance in carbohydrate metabolism may persist for some years.

Beckwith-Wiedemann syndrome (hyperplastic fetal visceromegaly)

The most frequent features of this syndrome are macroglossia, omphalocele, and visceromegaly (Fig. 33-13). Of the numerous additional anomalies recorded, those occurring most consistently include facial nevus flammeus, abnormal ear lobe grooves, microcephaly, visceromegaly, renal medullary dysplasia, cytomegaly of the adrenal cortex, and hyperplasia of many organs. Somatic overgrowth may be asymmetrical, resulting in hemihypertrophy; advanced physical development may be striking. These patients along with those having incomplete forms of Beckwith-Wiedemann syndrome are also at higher risk of developing intraabdominal neoplasia, particularly nephroblastoma.

Symptomatic hypoglycemia occurs in one third to one half of all patients; symptoms usually start within the first 24 hours after birth but may be delayed up to the third day. The hypoglycemia may be severe, difficult to control, and may persist for several months. It is likely that many of the fatalities in patients who have been diag-

mia and hypocalcemia also have been observed. Pathologically, islet cell hyperplasia has been demonstrated. Basal hyperinsulinemia and hyperresponsiveness of insulin secretion to glucose and tolbutamide have been demonstrated.

The syndrome is found in siblings, although in some affected individuals only minor anomalies are present. An autosomal dominant mode of inheritance with incomplete penetrance and variable expressivity has been postulated, although the syndrome also has been considered autosomal recessive. Patients are cytogenetically normal.

Severe hypoglycemia also has been observed in infants of extremely high birth weights who do not have the congenital anomalies noted in the Beckwith-Wiedemann syndrome. These infants have been referred to as *infant giants;* their birth weights range from 3.8 to 5.3 kg. Pancreatic hyperplasia has been described in some of these infants.

β-Cell nesidioblastosis-adenoma spectrum

Although rare, these entities must be considered in any neonate with persistent symptomatic hypoglycemia in whom no immediately apparent cause can be found. The neonates are usually AGA or LGA, lack any positive physical findings, have a noncontributory maternal history, and have severe hypoglycemia resistant to conventional medical management.

There is a relatively high blood insulin level in the presence of hypoglycemia, and fluctuating insulin and glucose levels are not directly related to glucose intake. Normal peripheral insulin values, however, have been reported. Insulin levels in the insulinoma tumor tissue in adults are strikingly high and consist primarily of proinsulin. Tolerance tests may be difficult to perform because of the inability to fast the patient even for short periods of time. Metabolic studies performed during continuous glucose infusions followed by abrupt cessation of infusate may prove useful but are dangerous. Definitive therapy for infants with hypoglycemia in the nesidioblastosis-adenoma spectrum is early subtotal pancreatectomy. These infants have a high incidence of neurologic damage, which is probably a reflection of poor preoperative glucose control. In most instances preoperative medical therapy consisting of various combinations of glucose infusion, corticosteroid, epinephrine, diazoxide, glucagon, and phenytoin fails to control the hypoglycemia. Recently continuous somatostatin infusion with the addition of glucagon to correct the somatostatin-induced hypoglucagonemia has been successfully used for temporary preoperative medical therapy.

β-Cell nesidioblastosis can be differentiated from islet cell adenoma or from functional islet cell hyperplasia only at the time of surgery. If an islet cell tumor is not

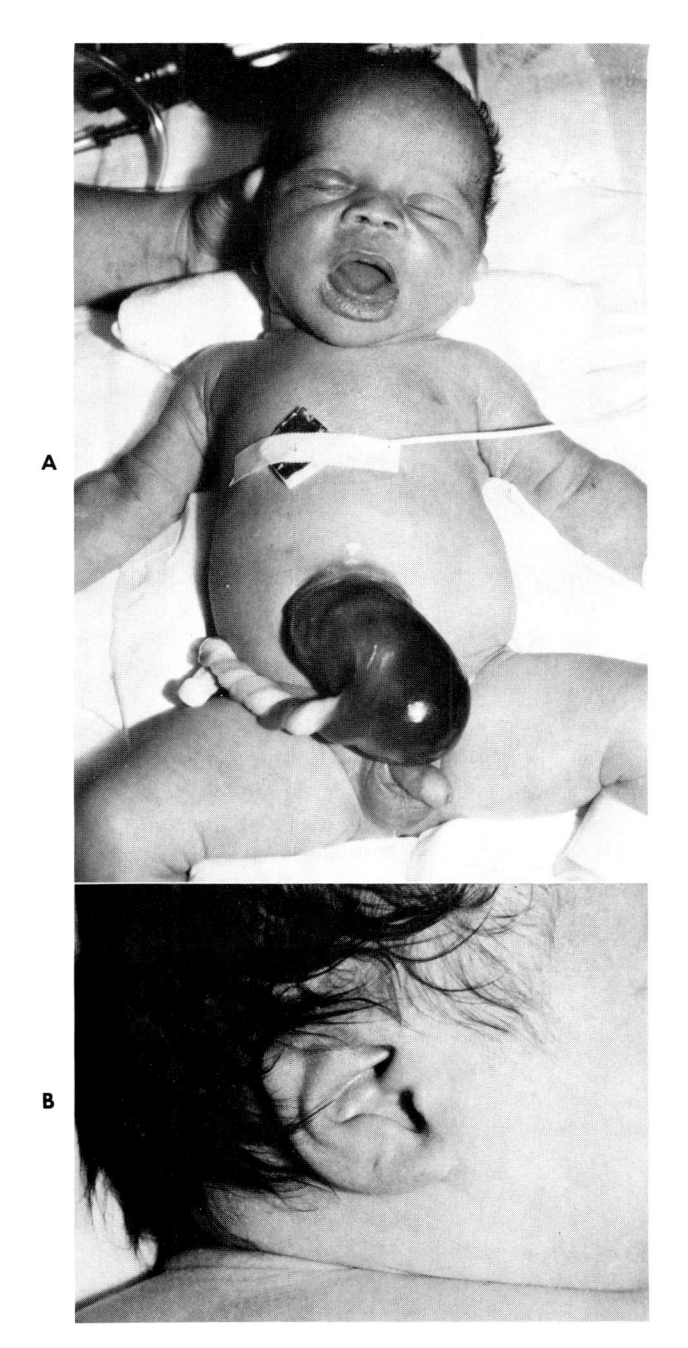

Fig. 33-13. Newborn infant weighing 3.8 kg with Beckwith-Wiedemann syndrome showing **(A)** macroglossia and omphalocele and **(B)** vertical earlobe grooves.

nosed retrospectively were due to the unrecognized hypoglycemia. Intelligence is normal in many patients, although mild to moderate retardation was a regular feature in Beckwith's original series. Mental retardation may be due, in part, to undetected hypoglycemia in the neonatal period or during infancy. Neonatal polycythe-

found, at least 80% to 95% of the pancreas is excised, since the adenoma may not be visible at laparotomy. The pancreatic tissue should be stained with an insulin-specific stain.

Nesidioblastosis is not simple β-cell hyperplasia, but rather involves all islet cell types and is characterized by disorganization and proliferation of islet cells. It is differentiated from localized adenoma, in which the pathologic finding of "nesidioblastosis" is confined to the tumor. Familial nesidioblastosis suggestive of autosomal recessive inheritance has been reported. There have also been reports linking nesidioblastosis with some cases of sudden infant death.

Leucine-induced hypoglycemia

Patients with leucine sensitivity have hyperresponsiveness to the amino acid L-leucine. Leucine sensitivity may be seen with various disorders associated with increased insulin release. Symptoms may be present from birth or appear later in the first year of life. Classically, symptoms occur within 30 minutes of a high-protein meal but may occur after a prolonged fast. Symptoms may be mild at first but increase in severity and result in permanent neurologic impairment if unrecognized and untreated. To make the diagnosis, a significant fall in blood glucose (50%) should occur within 20 to 45 minutes following oral administration of L-leucine. Similar results, however, may be obtained in 70% of patients with insulinomas, since nonspecific increased insulin release may be induced by leucine. Therapy consists of a low-leucine diet and postprandial and bedtime carbohydrate supplements. Prompt recognition and treatment may prevent psychomotor retardation. The hypoglycemia tends to improve spontaneously by 4 to 6 years of age.

Maternal drugs

The antidiabetic drugs tolbutamide and chlorpropamide cross the placenta and produce pancreatic β-cell hyperplasia and increased insulin release. Tolbutamide has a markedly prolonged half-life in the neonate and has been found in higher concentrations in the newborn after delivery than in maternal blood. Protracted hypoglycemia may occur when maternal glucose supply is interrupted. Exchange transfusion has been required in one infant whose mother received chlorpropamide and in whom hypoglycemia was unresponsive to all conventional methods of management.

Benzothiadiazide diuretics may also cause postneonatal hypoglycemia either by stimulation of fetal β-cells or secondary to elevation of maternal glucose levels.

Oral β-sympathomimetic tocolytic drugs have caused sustained hypoglycemia and elevated cord blood insulin levels in infants delivered within 2 days of termination of tocolytic therapy (Chapter 11, part two).

Hypoglycemia and pituitary deficiency

Neonatal hypoglycemia associated with anterior pituitary hypofunction may represent a series of separate syndromes with defects ranging from no structural abnormalities in the brain to anencephaly. Although considered rare, the true incidence is unknown, since the disorder is usually unrecognized because of the absence of characteristic physical findings.

Clinical and laboratory manifestations

Symptoms of hypoglycemia may begin during the first hours of postnatal life and are marked by their severity. They include sudden and profound limpness, convulsions, apnea, cardiovascular collapse, and cardiac arrest. The infants are of normal length and weight, born at term or post term. Males predominate in a ratio of 2:1, but five of the six neonates in our series were male. Physical examination is often unrevealing; some male infants have a small phallus, poorly developed scrotum, and/or small undescended testes (Fig. 33-14). In a few patients, facial abnormalities consisting of cleft lip and palate, poorly developed nasal septum, and hypotelorism have been described. Although the infants are of normal size at birth, growth retardation and delayed bone age may be found by 6 to 8 weeks of age.

Tolerance tests and other studies are sometimes difficult to perform because the severity and persistence of symptoms require immediate glucose therapy and frequently steroids. However, determinations of glucose, insulin, and human growth hormone during continuous glucose infusions may be helpful. Normal neonates show an increased, albeit attenuated, insulin response and an elevated basal human growth hormone level that are not suppressed by hyperglycemia. Low human growth hormone and insulin values that do not rise during hyperglycemia suggest pituitary hypofunction. Cord blood human growth hormone levels in normal newborns are markedly elevated but in congenital hypopituitarism are in the normal adult range. Further studies with an intravenous bolus of glucose, glucagon, arginine, or L-dopa provide confirmatory evidence. Because tolbutamide or insulin may provoke severe hypoglycemia, these tests are not indicated. Specific growth hormone deficiency, without other associated endocrine abnormalities, has been described. However, repeated careful evaluation by radioimmunoassay techniques may reveal associated endocrine hypoadrenalism and hypothyroidism. In patients with pituitary "aplasia," thyrotropin (thyroid-stimulating hormone, TSH), thyroxine (T_4), and prolactin were low and did not show a significant increase after

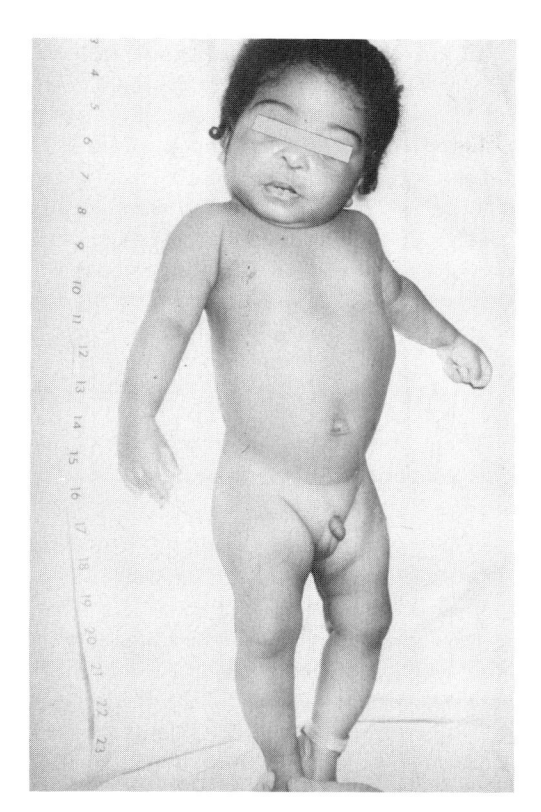

Fig. 33-14. Thirteen-month-old infant with pituitary hypofunction showing repaired cleft lip, delayed growth (59 cm), and small phallus and scrotum.

stimulation by thyroid-releasing hormone (TRH). Others have shown a rise in thyroid-stimulating hormone following stimulation with thyroid-releasing hormone, suggesting a primary hypothalamic defect. Other evidence for deficient hypothalamic releasing hormones includes increased prolactin levels and poor luteinizing hormone (LH) response following stimulation with releasing hormones. The adrenals respond to ACTH stimulation, but a deficiency of ACTH may be demonstrated by the use of metyrapone. Although thyroid function studies may be normal at first, abnormalities can be seen later in infancy.

Pathology

At postmortem examination the pituitary gland may be hypoplastic or aplastic, the thyroid and adrenal glands small, and the cellular architecture of the adrenals disorganized, with atrophy or absence of the fetal cortex. In three infants, multiple congenital anomalies of the central nervous system, including holoprosencephaly and arrhinencephaly, were found. A pneumoencephalogram of another infant demonstrated absence of the septum pellucidum and massa intermedia. In one of our infants with cleft lip and palate the pneumoencephalogram was normal. Hypoplasia or aplasia of the adenohypophysis without cerebral or facial anomalies also may occur. Different expressions of the same syndrome may occur, depending on the extent of pituitary hypoplasia or other central nervous system anomalies or both.

Pathogenesis

The underlying pathogenetic mechanisms remain unclear, although aplasia of the anterior pituitary was found in siblings of three patients and in two patients with familial history of consanguinity. This is consistent with a possible autosomal recessive inheritance. A familial history could not be obtained in any of our six patients; the infant with cleft lip and palate, however, has seven normal siblings. Whether the disorder is due to failure of the pituitary to form or degeneration of the pituitary is unknown. It is also possible that abnormalities of the hypothalamus with a deficiency of hypophysiotropic releasing hormones are responsible for the multiple endocrinopathies observed in these infants. The pathophysiologic relationships among pituitary hypoplasia, the central nervous system anomalies, and the other pituitary hypofunctions are unknown.

Treatment

Therapy consists of replacement with human growth hormone (1 to 2 mg intramuscularly three times weekly), thyroid hormone if hypothyroidism is documented, and physiologic doses of hydrocortisone (5 mg twice daily) for proven hypoadrenalism. Although human growth hormone administration does not always improve physical growth, hypoglycemia is corrected. Bone age may remain retarded, and continuous evaluation of thyroid function should be undertaken even if this was normal at the outset. Testosterone cream (5%) applied topically twice a day or testosterone enanthate (25 or 50 mg) given in three monthly injections has been used to increase the size of the corpora of the penis.

Prognosis

Many patients die in early infancy, and others may have severe physical and mental retardation. It is therefore imperative that early recognition and prompt therapy be instituted.

Cortisol deficiency

ACTH unresponsiveness is a hereditary disorder in which the adrenal glands fail to produce adequate cortisol, but aldosterone secretion is normal and ACTH levels are elevated. Feeding problems, failure to thrive, and regurgitation occur in the neonatal period; hypoglycemia, convulsions, and shock or death may occur in infancy or early childhood. The syndrome is characterized by hyperpigmentation, normal serum electrolyte concentrations, and an unusually severe untoward response to illness or stress. There is often a history of affected siblings, and an autosomal recessive mode of inheritance has been suggested. The pathogenesis of this syndrome is poorly understood. Differentiation of the zones of adrenal cortex in utero require ACTH, except for the zona glomerulosa, which is primarily under renin-angiotensin control. Histologic examination of the adrenal glands of patients with ACTH unresponsiveness has revealed an intact zona glomerulosa and atrophy of the fasciculata and reticularis zones. Migeon and associates have postulated an abnormlity at the site (or sites) of ACTH action or cortisol biosynthesis.

Familial isolated glucocorticoid deficiency also has been described in a family of five siblings; in two of the infants, glucocorticoid production was normal initially and deficient at a later age. This suggests that in some families there may be a degenerative process in the adrenal gland.

Maternal steroid therapy resulting in neonatal subclinical adrenal insufficiency was reported in an infant having Cushingoid facies, transient hypoglycemia, and poor response at 20 hours to intravenous corticotropin.

Adrenal hemorrhage is discussed in Chapter 17.

Adrenogenital syndrome is discussed in Chapter 33, part three.

Hypothyroidism

See Chapter 33, part three.

Congenital glucagon deficiency

Two male infants have been reported with glucagon deficiency; the disorder became evident on the second to third day of postnatal life with repeated convulsive movements, hypotonia, weak cry, and poor suck. In both infants the diagnosis was based on a low basal glucagon concentration and a strong hyperglycemic response to glucagon. In one of the infants there was a lack of response to glucagon. In one there was a lack of response to hypoglycemia and alanine infusion. Both parents of this infant were closely related and had partly deficient glucagon secretion; two siblings of this infant died before 5 months of age with probable hypoglycemia. Thus an autosomal recessive inherited disorder is suggested.

Galactosemia

See p. 831.

Infants with hereditary galactose intolerance are usually normal at birth. Evidence that the fetus is susceptible to the untoward effects of galactose in utero has been demonstrated by the presence of cataracts as early as 7 days after birth in some neonates. Postnatal exposure to milk results in vomiting and diarrhea, poor weight gain, and prolonged jaundice. The liver is enlarged, smooth, firm, and not tender. Hypoglycemia is not a consistent finding. If the condition is untreated, lamellar or zonular cataracts develop and there is a progressive mental retardation and cirrhosis. A milder course has been described in some infants, with failure to thrive as the most constant feature. The cause of the hypoglycemia is unknown, but it may be inhibition of phosphoglucomutase by galactose, which results in decreased hepatic output of glucose.

Glycogen storage disease type I (Von Gierke's disease)

Of the many liver glycogen storage diseases, type I glucose-6-phosphatase deficiency is the most likely to present in the neonatal period (p. 838). The genetic defect is autosomal recessive; the heterozygote cannot be detected biochemically, and amniotic fluid analysis is not helpful in predicting the disease. In the most severe form the syndrome may manifest itself in the first days or weeks after birth with profound hypoglycemia (blood glucose level less than 10 mg/dl) and acidosis. The infant appears ill and agitated and has deep, rapid respirations. Recurrent acidosis is the most common cause of readmission to the hospital. Hypoglycemia, although profound, may be asymptomatic. The only physical stigma of glycogen storage disease type I in the neonate is moderate hepatomegaly. The relatively normal appearance shortly after birth suggests that the disease is well controlled in utero. This could be expected, since the fetus is receiving therapeutic total parenteral nutrition from the mother. However, with time the characteristic physical findings appear: short stature, fat doll-like facies, and a protuberant abdomen occupied by an enlarged, firm smooth liver that may reach the iliac crest. Splenomegaly and cardiomegaly are absent. Easy bruising and bleeding tendencies, especially nasal and gastrointestinal, frequently occur.

Laboratory findings following an overnight fast show hypoglycemia, elevated lactate and pyruvate levels, metabolic acidosis, hyperlipidemia, ketonuria and ketonemia, and elevated uric acid concentrations. Serum electrolyte levels may be falsely low because of lipid displacement. Bleeding time is prolonged, and there is reduced platelet adhesion and defective collagen and epinephrine-induced aggregation, suggesting an intrinsic defect in platelet release. The diagnosis may be inferred from the absence of glucose rise and elevated lactate and pyruvate levels during glucagon and galactose tolerance tests. Absence of glucose-6-phosphatase enzymatic activity in liver biopsies provides confirmatory evidence.

Therapy consists primarily of frequent high-carbohydrate feedings, oral sodium bicarbonate for prevention of acidosis, early recognition of infection, and treatment of hyperuricemia and bleeding episodes. Long-term benefits of portacaval shunts remain doubtful. In a recent report a newborn with with lactic acidosis and hypoglycemia 24 hours after birth was treated with continuous nocturnal intragastric feeding of 5% glucose solution initiated on the twelfth day. During her first 2 years of follow-up she demonstrated normal growth and development. Continuous overnight intragastric infusion with glucose (0.5 gm/kg/hour) or Vivonex also has been helpful in controlling symptoms and improving growth in older children.

Prognosis in early infancy is guarded, but survival beyond adolescence is often associated with improvement of symptoms. Growth retardation continues, but mental retardation is not a constant feature despite profound hypoglycemia; the brain of patients with glycogen storage disease may be capable of using alternate substrates, such as ketone bodies.

Fructose intolerance

Hereditary fructose intolerance may occur in the neonatal period if the susceptible infant is fed a sucrose-containing formula or is given table sugar, fruits, or fruit juices. Symptoms include vomiting, failure to thrive, excessive sweating, and unconsciousness or convulsions. Hypoglucosemia is frequent, as are fructosemia and fructosuria following ingestion of fructose.

Hereditary defects in amino acid metabolism

See Chapter 32.

Hypoglycemia associated with other neonatal problems

Iatrogenic causes

Reactive hypoglycemia may follow abrupt cessation of hypertonic glucose infusions or exchange transfusions. Acid-citrate-dextrose and citrate-phosphate-dextrose blood contains a significant quantity of glucose, which may stimulate insulin release and cause subsequent hypoglycemia 2 to 3 hours after exchange transfusion is discontinued. Heparinized blood does not contain glucose and may cause hypoglycemia during the exchange. On the other hand, heparin may elevate free fatty acid levels, which secondarily causes hypoglycemia after the exchange. Marked variability of blood glucose values also may occur as a result of changing rates of glucose infusions. Refractory hypoglycemia has been associated with an umbilical artery catheter positioned near the origin of the vessels supplying the pancreas (T11 to L1). Direct glucose infusion into the vessels of the pancreas resulted in a reactive hyperinsulinemic response and hypoglycemia.

Infection

Hypoglycemia, both symptomatic and asymptomatic, has been described in neonatal sepsis caused primarily by gram-negative bacilli. Glucose disappearance rates were significantly faster in the infected, as compared with healthy, neonates; hyperinsulinism could not be demonstrated.

Congenital cardiac malformations

The mean blood glucose concentration in neonates and older children with congenital cyanotic heart disease may be lower than in healthy controls. Glucose disappearance rates and fasting insulin and growth hormone values are normal, but glucose values following glucagon administration are lower than in healthy children. Although the mechanism is unknown, chronic hypoxia leading to decreased glycogen stores may be a contributing factor. Hypoglycemia may also lead to cardiomegaly and congestive heart failure in the absence of congenital malformations.

Hypothermia

The occurrence of hypothermia secondary to hypoglycemia has been well documented and is a useful clinical sign. Studies in adults using 2-deoxy-D-glucose suggest that hypoglycemia, directly or secondarily, may affect a central thermoregulatory center in the hypothalamus that is sensitive to glucose. Hypoglycemia also may be secondary to hypothermia. The normal core temperature in the neonate is from 36.5° to 37.5° C. If body temperature falls, heat production is increased several times the basal level, resulting in a more rapid depletion of energy stores. Hypoglycemia has been reported in neonates with severe cold injury after prolonged exposure to cold with rectal temperatures below 32° C.

Hyperviscosity

An increased rate of glucose disposal without hyperinsulinemia is part of the syndrome of hyperviscosity and responds to partial exchange transfusion (Chapter 29).

Acute and chronic diarrhea

Hypoglycemia occurs in children with acute diarrheal disease due to typhoid, cholera, shigellosis, chronic malnutrition, and kwashiorkor. We have seen four infants, 4 to 8 weeks of age, with hypoglycemia associated with severe diarrhea and secondary malnutrition; in two infants glucagon tolerance tests did not show a rise in blood glucose, suggesting that hepatic glycogen stores had been depleted.

DIAGNOSTIC EVALUATION OF NEONATAL HYPOGLYCEMIA

A detailed history and a meticulous physical examination are of utmost importance to avoid numerous provocative stimulatory studies. In most instances of neonatal hypoglycemia the underlying disease process is obvious, and further studies are not necessary. Important maternal historical factors include family history of diabetes, blood group incompatibility, toxemia, hypertension, drug intake, familial history of hypoglycemia, or unexplained stillbirth and infant deaths. Physical examination will determine if the infant is SGA or LGA, is postmature, has erythroblastosis, or is an infant of a prediabetic or diabetic mother. Further diagnostic studies are not required unless hypoglycemia is persistent. Macrosomia, abnormal umbilicus, and protuberant tongue are diagnostic features of the Beckwith-Wiedemann syndrome. The presence of chubby, doll-like facies and hepatomegaly without a maternal diabetic history may indicate glycogen storage disease. Cataracts, jaundice, failure to thrive, hepatomegaly, and reducing substances in the urine suggest galactosemia. Abnormalities of the genitalia are associated with pituitary deficiency. Similarly, cleft lip or palate or other facial anomalies may be associated with central nervous system abnormalities and pituitary hypoplasia; roentgenograms in infants with pituitary hypofunction may reveal delayed bone age. The absence of any positive family history association with a normal-appearing, AGA neonate is highly suggestive of an insulinoma. In neonates, hypoglycemia is usually associated with the fasting state; therefore a history of symptoms shortly after milk intake suggests leucine sensitivity or galactosemia.

In older infants and children a 24- to 36-hour fast is recommended for assessment of the various parameters involved in carbohydrate homeostasis. The time required for the development of hypoglycemia in a normal neonate, however, is significantly less, and a prolonged fast may have serious consequences. We have seen one infant with human growth hormone deficiency become limp, bradycardiac, and apneic and have a blood glucose level of 9 mg/dl after a 6-hour fast. Initial baseline laboratory determinations when the diagnosis is not readily apparent should include glucose, insulin, human growth hormone, cortisol, and, if glycogen disease is a consideration, lactate, pyruvate, ketones, pH, and buffer base. Samples should be drawn at least 3 to 4 hours after a feeding or at the time of hyoglycemia. Provocative tolerance tests depend on the results of these studies coupled with the physical findings. Not all tolerance tests are indicated; moreover, it is frequently difficult to obtain sufficient blood for a variety of studies. Selectivity is therefore essential. Glucagon tolerance tests after a 6- to 8-hour fast, for example, are indicated if glycogen storage disease is considered. Glucagon tolerance tests, however, are not of value for pituitary hypofunction or hyperinsulinism. Studies of thyroid and adrenal function are necessary when human growth hormone deficiency has been established or a clinical picture consistent with hypothyroidism or congenital adrenal hyperplasia is present. If hypoglycemia is intractable, biochemical determinations can be done during continuous glucose infusion followed by abrupt cessation of the infusate over a 90- to 120-minute period. It is mandatory that an intravenous line be kept open and a constant vigil maintained by the physician of any infant undergoing prolonged starvation or tolerance tests that are likely to produce hypoglycemia.

TREATMENT OF NEONATAL HYPOGLYCEMIA

The management of neonatal hypoglycemia requires identification of the high-risk infant, implementation of oral feedings within the first 3 to 4 hours after birth, and minimization of caloric expenditures by maintenance of a neutral core temperature. In addition, careful monitoring for clinical symptoms and blood glucose determinations are essential. If routine assessment is made by use of Dextrostix, abnormal or borderline values should be checked in the laboratory. In asymptomatic high-risk infants, glucose concentrations should be measured before the first feeding and at least 3 hours after a subsequent feeding. Formula can be given at 2- to 3-hour intervals. In general, however, oral feeding should not be used as a therapeutic regimen but as an adjunct to intravenous fluids. Oral glucose is ineffective in treatment of hypoglycemia and, in high concentrations, may cause gastric irritation.

Intravenous glucose

Following a diagnosis of hypoglycemia, intravenous therapy should be initiated promptly. Asymptomatic infants respond within 10 to 20 minutes to 10% glucose solution infused at a rate of 8 mg/kg/minute. For immediate correction a minibolus of 200 mg/kg of 10% glucose can be injected over 1 minute followed by continuous glucose infusion of 8 mg/kg/minute (Fig. 33-15). Glucose values should be monitored hourly until stable, and the amount of glucose in the infusate should be decreased gradually by 2 mg/kg/minute as glucose values become stabilized. We treat all hypoglycemic infants regardless of presence or absence of symptoms as if they were at risk for developing brain damage.

Infusion of hypertonic solutions into a peripheral vein is preferable to infusion through an umbilical vessel. However, in emergency situations or when peripheral

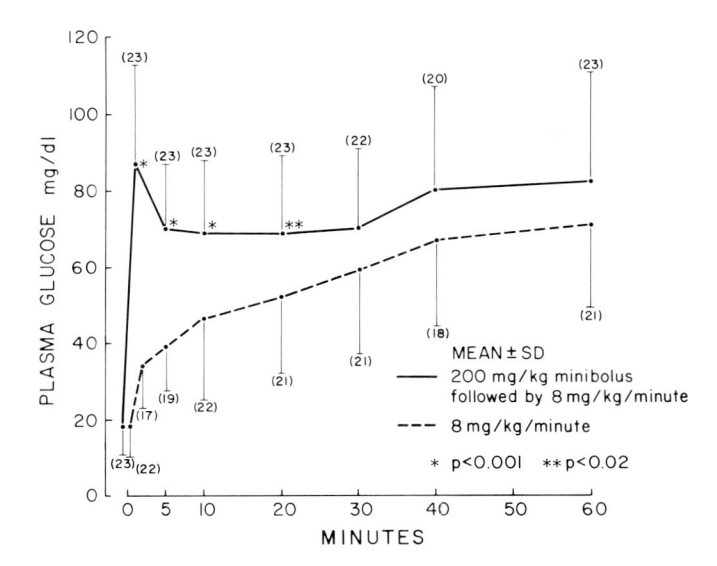

Fig. 33-15. Treatment of 23 hypoglycemic neonates with 200 mg/kg glucose minibolus followed by 8 mg/kg/minute constant glucose infusion, compared with treatment of 22 hypoglycemic neonates with only 8 mg/kg/minute constant glucose infusion. (From Lilien, L.D., and others. J. Pediatr. **97**:295, 1980.)

veins are unavailable, a properly placed umbilical artery or venous line may be used. To prevent reactive hypoglycemia, glucose should be infused by pump and immediately restarted if the infusion infiltrates. In infants with intractable hypoglycemia, glucose should be infused simultaneously in two peripheral intravenous sites to ensure uninterrupted glucose infusion in cases of infiltration. Increases in glucose infusion, i.e., greater than 12 to 14 mg/kg/minute, may produce risk of fluid overload, venous thrombosis, or slough at the intravenous site. Therefore, if increased rates of 12 to 14 mg/kg/minute are needed to maintain euglycemia, hydrocortisone is started. Infants who do not respond to hydrocortisone may need additional or alternative therapy, depending on the etiology of hypoglycemia.

Steroids

Hydrocortisone, 10 mg/kg/day given in two doses intravenously, intramuscularly, or orally, has been shown to reduce peripheral glucose utilization, to increase the effects of exogenous glucagon, and to enhance gluconeogenesis. Hydrocortisone is started if plasma glucose values are not above 40 mg/dl shortly after intravenous glucose therapy or if hypoglycemia recurs. Prednisone (2 mg/kg/day) may also be used. Intravenous fluids are tapered first; hydrocortisone is continued until the infant is stable for 48 hours after intravenous fluids have been discontinued. Steroids are usually necessary for 5 to 7 days.

Epinephrine

A trial dose of epinephrine 1:1,000 (0.01 ml/kg), a maintenance dose of epinephrine 1:200 in 25% glycerine solution (0.01 to 0.005 ml/kg/6 hours [Sus-Phrine]) administered subcutaneously, or ephedrine sulphate (0.5 mg/kg/3 hours) orally has been recommended for infants with hyperinsulinism and has been used particularly in infants of diabetic mothers. Epinephrine mobilizes stored fuels from the liver by glycogenolysis, stimulates gluconeogenesis, stimulates lipolysis in adipose tissue, and exerts an effect on the endocrine pancreas by suppressing insulin and augmenting glucagon secretion. However, epinephrine may have adverse effects by raising lactate levels in the blood.

Diazoxide

This drug (10 to 15 mg/kg/day divided tid) given intravenously or orally suppresses pancreatic insulin release and may be effective in protracted hypoglycemia due to hyperinsulinism. Failure to respond to diazoxide should not be used as an argument that an infant is not suffering from hyperinsulinemic hypoglycemia. Side effects include generalized hirsutism, hyperglycemia, ketosis, sodium retention, and hypotension. To prevent the hypotensive side effects, intravenous diazoxide should be given slowly to allow for adequate serum protein binding. The drug has not been investigated widely and should not be used except when all other medical management is ineffective.

Glucagon

Glucagon (0.3 mg/kg intravenously or intramuscularly) has no place in the treatment of neonatal hypoglycemia except possibly in asymptomatic infants of diabetic mothers during the first 4 hours of age or as specific therapy for glucagon deficiency (for maintenance therapy in glucagon deficiency, zinc protamine glucagon, 0.1 to 0.5 mg/kg/12 hours intramuscularly). Glucagon raises blood sugar through glycogenolysis and gluconeogenesis. It is therefore not effective in SGA neonates who may have depletion of glycogen stores and defective gluconeogenesis. Since glucagon may also stimulate insulin release and thus lead to rebound hypoglycemia, it should be accompanied by continuous glucose infusion.

Human growth hormone

Human growth hormone (1 to 2 mg/day intramuscularly three times per week) is supplied through the National Pituitary Foundation for hypoglycemia due to pituitary hypofunction.

Somatostatin

Somatostatin (3.5 to 48 μg/kg/hour by continuous intravenous infusion) suppresses insulin as well as glucagon secretion. Stomatostatin may cause a bleeding diathesis. It has been of benefit for preoperative control along with glucagon in some infants with suspected nesidioblastosis-adenoma syndrome.

Pancreatectomy

Removal of 80% to 95% of the pancreas is recommended in rare persistent cases of hyperinsulinemic hypoglycemia where all other measures have failed. Surgery should be performed within 2 to 3 weeks of onset of hypoglycemia and failure of medical therapy, since severe brain damage is a common finding at follow-up.

HYPERGLYCEMIA

The definition of hyperglycemia, just as of hypoglycemia, is based on statistical studies of whole blood glucose values in a large population of neonates. When whole blood glucose values are converted to plasma glucose values, the upper limit of normal is 145 mg/dl. Neonatal mortality is significantly higher in hyperglycemic than in euglycemic premature infants. In a study of 75 consecutively studied premature infants during the first 5 days of postnatal age, neonatal mortality was 59% in hyperglycemic and 12% in euglycemic infants. Increased morbidity may be caused by osmotic diuresis and ventricular hemorrhage secondary to hyperosmolarity. Eighteen milligrams of glucose will increase plasma osmolarity by 1 mOsm.

Hyperglycemia is frequently reported in premature infants who are given intravenous glucose infusion (Fig.

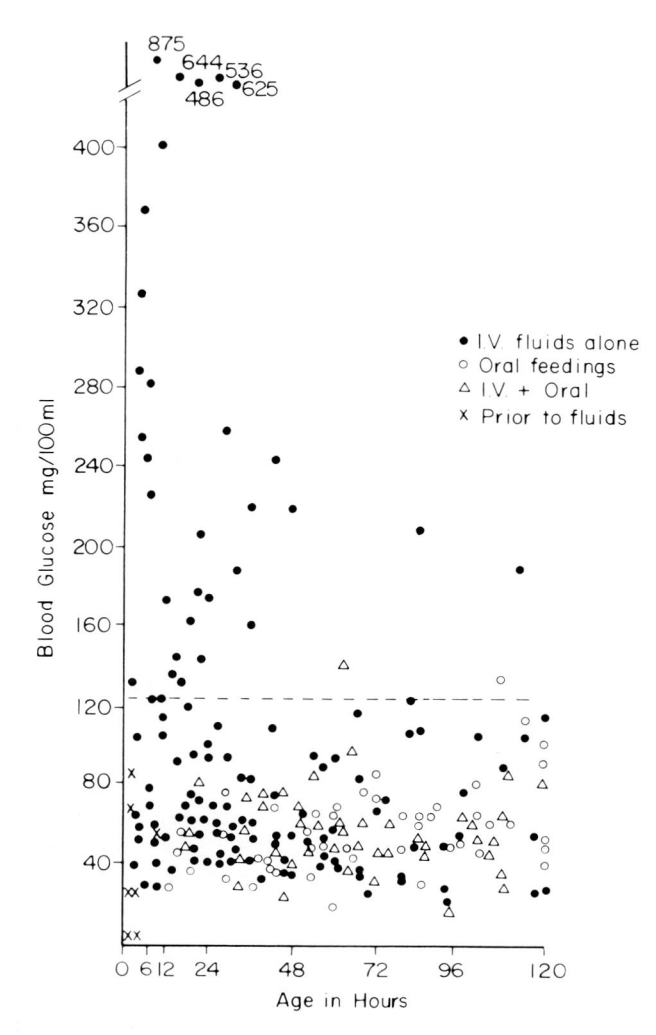

Fig. 33-16. Blood glucose values in infants <2,000 gms during the first 5 days of postnatal life. Hyperglycemia was common in infants who were given glucose infusions (rate 3 to 7 mg/kg/minute). (From Zarif, M., Pildes, R.S., and Vidyasagar, D.: Diabetes **25**:428, 1976.)

33-16). In one study hyperglycemia was found in 56% of infants who weighed less than 1,100 gm who received glucose infusion rates greater than 6.6 mg/kg/minute. In our nursery, hyperglycemia was seen in 47% of infants who weighed less than 1,500 gm who received a mean glucose infusion of 4.3 mg/kg/minute.

Premature infants most likely to develop hyperglycemia are usually of very low birth weight, have low Apgar scores, show respiratory distress, and may be septic. The most significant factor associated with hyperglycemia in our studies has been stress.

In low birth weight infants the association of hyperglycemia with a significant rise in serum insulin has been postulated to be the result of either persistent endogenous glucose production or diminished peripheral glucose utilization. In small premature infants, new glucose production is not suppressed by a continuous infusion of exogenous glucose. Thus relative insulin deficiency may be present despite high insulin values.

The use of xanthines in premature infants with apnea and the maternal use of diazoxide have also been associated with neonatal hyperglycemia.

We have observed a premature infant who had mild tachypnea and persistent hyperglycemia on the first day of life whose blood culture revealed group B *Streptococcus* organisms. Others have reported a premature infant with two separate episodes of hyperglycemia, each associated with symptomatic *Escherichia coli* sepsis. Insulin levels in this infant were abnormally low at times when the serum glucose level was elevated, indicating inadequate insulin response.

Infants at risk of hyperglycemia need frequent monitoring of plasma glucose. Since many of those very sick infants require transport to tertiary centers, Dextrostix or plasma glucose concentration assessments should be performed prior to transport; glucose infusion should not exceed 4 mg/kg/minute. When hyperglycemia is present in a small premature infant, constant monitoring of plasma glucose levels and reduction of glucose concentration in intravenous fluids are necessary; insulin may be indicated, as is correction of fluid and electrolyte losses from osmotic diuresis.

Hyperglycemia is also seen in neonates with diabetes mellitus (p. 830). Although permanent diabetes mellitus has been reported in several neonates, the more common manifestation of this syndrome is transient. Infants with transient diabetes mellitus are usually less than 6 weeks of age; they frequently are SGA and on occasion have had an antecedent history of transient neonatal hypoglycemia. Presenting symptoms are failure to thrive, dehydration, and fever. Infection or underlying central nervous system lesions are present in one third of the infants. Blood glucose levels range from 250 to 2,300 mg/dl, and minimal ketones are present in the urine. Insulin values are low and do not increase following an intravenous bolus of glucose. With recovery of the patient, insulin values increase and return to normal. Treatment usually consists of adequate hydration. Exogenous insulin may be given if hyperglycemia persists, but the requirements are usually low, since these infants are quite sensitive to insulin. Complete recovery is the rule, and permanent diabetes mellitus has not been seen in long-term follow-ups. However, 10% of these infants may be mentally retarded. This may be due to an underlying central nervous system hemorrhage or may be secondary to overzealous treatment with insulin with resultant hypoglycemia.

Rosita S. Pildes
Lawrence D. Lilien

BIBLIOGRAPHY

Adam, P.A.J.: Control of glucose metabolism in the human fetus and newborn infant, Adv. Metab. Disord. 5:183, 1971.

Adam, P.A.J., and others: Oxidation of glucose and D-β-OH-butyrate by the early human fetal brain, Acta Paediatr. Scand. 64:17, 1975.

Anderson, J.M., Milner, R.D.G., and Stritch, S.J.: Effects of neonatal hypoglycemia on the nervous system: a pathological study, J. Neurol. Neurosurg. Psychiatry 30:295, 1967.

Barrett, C.T., and Oliver, T.K., Jr.: Hypoglycemia and hyperinsulinism in infants with erythroblastosis, N. Engl. J. Med. 278:1260, 1968.

Beckwith, J.B.: Extreme cytomegaly of the adrenal fetal cortex, omphalocele, hyperplasia of the kidneys and pancreas and Leydig-cell hyperplasia: another syndrome? Paper presented to the Western Society for Pediatric Research, Los Angeles, 1963.

Belman, A.B.: Renal vein thrombosis in infants and childhood: a contemporary survey, Clin. Pediatr. 15:1033, 1976.

Benedetti-Massi, F., and others: Blood glucose and plasma insulin and glucagon response during intravenous glucose tolerance test in newborn infants affected by erythroblastosis fetalis, Acta Paediatr. Scand. 64:113, 1975.

Bennett, P.H., Webner, C., and Miller, M.: Congenital anomalies and the diabetic and prediabetic pregnancy. In Pregnancy metabolism, diabetes and the fetus, CIBA Foundation Symposium no. 63, Amsterdam, 1979, Excerpta Medica, p. 207.

Benzing, G., and others: Simultaneous hypoglycemia and acute congestive heart failure, Circulation 40:209, 1969.

Bier, D.M., and others: Glucose production rate in infancy and childhood, Pediatr. Res. 10:405, 1976.

Block, M.B., and others C-peptide immunoreactivity (CPR); a new method for studying infants of insulin-treated mothers, Pediatrics 53:923, 1974.

Bloom, S.R., and Johnston, D.I.: Failure of glucagon release in infants of diabetic mothers, Br. Med. J. 4:453, 1972.

Bloomgarden, Z.T., and others: Treatment of intractable neonatal hypoglycemia with somatostatin plus glucagon, J. Pediatr. 96:148, 1980.

Blum, D., and others: Studies of hypoglycemia in small-for-date newborns, Arch. Dis. Child. 44:304, 1969.

Brazy, J.E., and Pupkin, M.J.: Effects of maternal isoxsuprine administration on preterm infants, J. Pediatr. 94:444, 1979.

Breitweser, J.A., and others: Cardiac septal hypertrophy in hyperinsulinemic infants, J. Pediatr. 96:535, 1980.

Buist, N.R.M., and others: Congenital islet cell adenoma causing hypoglycemia in a newborn, Pediatrics 47:605, 1971.

Burd, L.I., and others: Placental production and foetal utilization of lactate and pyruvate, Nature 254:710, 1975.

Burstein, R.L., Papile, L., and Greenberg, R.E.: Mechanisms of hyperglycemia in small premature infants (abstr.), Pediatr. Res. 14:568, 1980.

Christiansen, R.O., and Johnson, J.D.: Studies of insulin secretion in infantile hypoglycemia, Pediatr. Res. 8:157, 1975.

Chung, G.S., and Myrianthopoulos, N.C.: Factors affecting risks of congenital malformations, Birth Defects 11(10):23, 1975.

Churchill, J.A., Berendes, H.W., and Nemore, J.: Neuropsychological deficits in children of diabetic mothers: a report from the collaborative study of cerebral palsy, Am. J. Obstet. Gynecol. 105:257, 1969.

Cochrane, W.A., and others: Familial hypoglycemia induced by amino acids, J. Clin. Invest. 35:411, 1956.

Cornblath, M., Parker, M.L., and Reisner, S.H.: Secretion and metabolism of growth hormone in premature and full-term infants, J. Clin. Endocrinol. Metab. 25:209, 1965.

Cornblath, M., and Schwartz, R.: Carbohydrate metabolism in the neonate, ed. 2, Philadelphia, 1976, W.B. Saunders Co.

Cowett, R.M., and others: Glucose disposal of low birth weight infants: steady state hyperglycemia produced by constant intravenous glucose infusion, Pediatrics **63**:389, 1979.

Cowett, R.M., and others: Kinetic studies with ^{13}C-U-glucose in pregnant women and their offspring (abstr.), Pediatr. Res. **13**:357, 1979.

Daniel, R.R., and others: Carbohydrate metabolism in pregnancy. XI. Response of plasma glucagon during normal pregnancy and in gestational diabetes, Diabetes **23**:771, 1974.

Davidson, D.C., Blackwood, M.J., and Fox, E.G.: Neonatal hypoglycemia with congenital malformation of pancreatic islets, Arch. Dis. Child. **49**:151, 1974.

Davis, W.S., and Campbell, J.B.: Neonatal small left colon syndrome, Am. J. Dis. Child. **129**:1024, 1975.

Driscoll, S.G., and Steinke, J.: Pancreatic insulin content in severe erythroblastosis fetalis, Pediatrics **39**:448, 1967.

Epstein, M., Nicholls, E., and Stubblefield, P.G.: Neonatal hypoglycemia after beta-sympathomimetic tocolytic therapy, J. Pediatr. **94**:449, 1979.

Falorni, A., and others: Glucose metabolism and insulin secretion in the newborn infant, Diabetes **23**:172, 1973.

Farquhar, J.W.: Prognosis for babies born to diabetic mothers in Edinburgh, Arch. Dis. Child. **44**:36, 1969.

Fiser, R.H., and others: Insulin-glucagon substrate interrelationships in the neonatal sheep, Am. J. Obstet. Gynecol. **120**:944, 1974.

Freinkel, N., and Metzger, B.E.: Pregnancy as a tissue culture experience: the critical implications of maternal metabolism for fetal development. In Pregnancy metabolism, diabetes and the fetus, CIBA Foundation Symposium No. 63, Amsterdam, 1979, Excerpta Medica, p. 3.

Gács, G., Kun, E., and Berend, K.: Hypoglycemia in infants and children with cyanotic congenital heart disease, Acta Paediatr. Acad. Sci. Hung. **4**:105, 1973.

Garces, L.Y., Drash, A., and Kenny, F.M.: Islet cell tumor in the neonate, Pediatrics **41**:789, 1968.

Gentz, J.C.H., Persson, B.E.H., and Zetterstrom, R.: On the diagnosis of sympotomatic neonatal hypoglycemia, Acta Paediatr. Scand. **58**:449, 1969.

Gentz, J.C.H., and others: Intravenous glucose tolerance, plasma insulin, free fatty acids and hydroxybutyrate in underweight newborn infants, Acta Paediatr. Scand. **58**:481, 1969.

Grajwer, L.A., Lilien, L.D., and Pildes, R.S.: Neonatal subclinical adrenal insufficiency—result of maternal steroid therapy, J.A.M.A. **238**:1279, 1977.

Grasso, S., and others: Insulin secretion in the premature infant: response to glucose and amino acids, Diabetes **22**:349, 1973.

Gross, I., and Smith, G.J.: Insulin delays the morphological maturation of fetal rat lung in vitro, Pediatr. Res. **11**:515, 1977.

Hakanson, D.O., and Sunderji, S.G.: HbA$_{1c}$ and newborn skinfold thickness: reflection of maternal diabetic control (abstr.), Pediatr. Res. **14**:573, 1980.

Haworth, J.C., Dilling, L.A., and Van Woert, M.: Blood glucose determination in infants and children: the reflectance meter-enzyme test strip system, Am. J. Dis. Child. **123**:469, 1972.

Haworth, J.C., Dilling, L.A., and Vidyasagar, D.: Hypoglycemia in infants of diabetic mothers: effect of epinephrine therapy, J. Pediatr. **82**:94, 1973.

Haworth, J.C., McRae, K.N., and Dilling, L.A.: Prognosis of infants of diabetic mothers in relation to neonatal hypoglycemia, Dev. Med. Child. Neurol. **18**:471, 1975.

Haymond, M.W., Karl, I.E., and Pagliara, A.S.: Increased gluconeogenic substrates in the small-for-gestational age infant, N. Engl. J. Med. **291**:322, 1974.

Hazeltine, F.G.: Hypoglycemia and Rh erythroblastosis fetalis, Pediatrics **39**:696, 1967.

Hintz, R.L., Menking, M., and Sotos, J.F.: Holoprosencephaly with endocrine dysgenesis, J. Pediatr. **72**:81, 1968.

Hirschborn, N., and others: Hypoglycemia in children with acute diarrhea, Lancet **1**:128, 1966.

Humbart, J.R., and Gotlin, R.W.: Growth hormone levels in normoglycemia and hypoglycemia infants born small for gestational age, Pediatrics **48**:190, 1971.

James, T., Blessa, M., and Boggs, T.R.: Recurrent hyperglycemia associated with sepsis in a neonate, Am. J. Dis. Child. **133**:645, 1979.

Johnson, J.D., and others: Hypoplasia of the anterior pituitary and neonatal hypoglycemia, J. Pediatr. **82**:634, 1973.

Kalhan, S.C., Savin, S.M., and Adam, P.A.J.: Measurement of glucose turnover in the human newborn with glucose-1-^{13}C, J. Clin. Endocrinol. Metab. **43**:704, 1976.

Kalhan, S.C., Savin, S.M., and Adam, P.A.J.: Attenuated glucose production rate in newborn infants of insulin-dependent diabetic mothers, N. Engl. J. Med. **296**:375, 1977.

Kaye, R., and others: Catecholamine excretion in spontaneously occurring asymptomatic neonatal hypoglycemia, Pediatr. Res. **4**:295, 1970.

Kenny, F.M., and Precyasombat, C.: Cortisol production rate. VI. Hypoglycemia in the neonatal and postnatal period and in association with dwarfism, J. Pediatr. **70**:65, 1967.

King, K.C., and others: Human maternal and fetal insulin response to arginine, N. Engl. J. Med. **285**:603, 1971.

King, K.C., and others: Insulin response to arginine in normal newborns and infants of diabetic mothers, Diabetes **23**:816, 1974.

Kitson, H.F., and others: Somatostatin treatment of insulin excess due to β-cell adenoma in a neonate, J. Pediatr. **96**:145, 1980.

Koivisto, M., Blanco-Sequiros, M., and Krause, N.: Neonatal symptomatic and asymptomatic hypoglycemia: a follow-up study of 151 children, Dev. Med. Child. Neurol. **14**:603, 1972.

Kollee, L.A., and others: Persistent neonatal hypoglycaemia due to glucagon deficiency, Arch. Dis. Child. **53**:422, 1978.

Kornhauser, D., Adam, P.A.J., and Schwartz, R.: Glucose production and utilization in the newborn puppy, Pediatr. Res. **4**:120, 1970.

LeDune, M.A.: Intravenous glucose tolerance and plasma insulin studies in small-for-dates infants, Arch. Dis. Child. **47**:111, 1971.

LeDune, M.A.: Response to glucagon in small-for-dates hypoglycemic and non-hypoglycemic newborn infants, Arch. Dis. Child. **47**:754, 1972.

Light, I.J., Keenan, W.J., and Sutherland, J.M.: Maternal intravenous glucose administration as a cause of hypoglycemia in the infant of the diabetic mother, Am. J. Obstet. Gynecol. **113**:345, 1972.

Lilien, L.D., Grajwer, L.A., and Pildes, R.S.: Treatment of neonatal hypoglycemia with continuous intravenous glucose infusions, J. Pediatr. **91**:779, 1977.

Lilien, L.D., and others: Hyperglycemia in stressed small premature neonates, J. Pediatr. **94**:454, 1979.

Lilien, L.D., and others: Treatment of neonatal hypoglycemia with minibolus and intravenous glucose infusion, J. Pediatr. **97**:295, 1980.

Lovinger, R.D., Kaplan, S.L., and Grumbach, M.M.: Congenital hypopituitarism associated with neonatal hypoglycemia and microphallus: four cases secondary to hypothalmic hormone deficiencies, J. Pediatr. **87**:1171, 1975.

Lubchenco, L.O., and Bard, H.: Incidence of hypoglycemia in newborn infants classified by birth weight and gestational age, Pediatrics **47**:831, 1971.

Mann, T.P., and Elliot, R.I.K.: Neonatal cold injury due to accidental exposure to cold, Lancet **1**:229, 1957.

McCann, M.L., and others: Effects of fructose on hypoglucosemia in infants of diabetic mothers, N. Engl. J. Med. **275**:1, 1966.

Mestyan, J., Schultz, K., and Horvath, M.: Comparative glycemic responses to alanine in normal term and small for gestational age infants, J. Pediatr. **85**:276, 1974.

Mestyan, J., and others: Hyperaminoacidemia due to accumulation of gluconeogenic amino acid precursors in hypoglycemic small-for-gestational age infants, J. Pediatr. 87:409, 1975.

Metzger, B.E., and others: Effects of gestational diabetes on diurnal profiles of plasma glucose, lipids and individual amino acids, Diabetes Care 3:402, 1980.

Migeon, C.J., and others: The syndrome of congenital adrenocortical unresponsiveness to ACTH: report of six cases, Pediatr. Res. 2:501, 1968.

Milsap, R.L., and Auld, P.A.M.: Neonatal hyperglycemia following maternal diazoxide administration, J.A.M.A. 243:144, 1980.

Moncrieff, M.W., Hill, D.S., and Arthur, L.J.H.: Congenital absence of pituitary gland and adrenal hypoplasia, Arch. Dis. Child. 47:251, 1972.

Naeye, R.L.: Infants of diabetic mothers: a quantitative morphologic study, Pediatrics 35:980, 1965.

Nagel, J.W., and others: Refractory hypoglycemia associated with a malpositioned umbilical artery catheter, Pediatrics 64:315, 1979.

Nakagawa, S., and others: A new type of hypoglycemia in a newborn infant, Diabetologia 9:367, 1973.

Nejad, S.A., and Senior, B.: A familial syndrome of isolated aplasia of the anterior pituitary, J. Pediatr. 84:79, 1974.

Nitzan, M., and Groffman, H.: Hepatic gluconeogenesis and lipogenesis in experimental intrauterine growth retardation in the rat, Am. J. Obstet. Gynecol. 109:623, 1971.

Obenshain, S.S., and others: Human fetal insulin response to sustained maternal hyperglycemia, N. Engl. J. Med. 283:566, 1970.

Pagliara, A.S., and others: Hypoglycemia in infancy and childhood, J. Pediatr. 85:365, 1973.

Pedersen, J.: The pregnant diabetic and her newborn: problems and management, ed. 2, Baltimore, 1977, The Williams & Wilkins Co.

Perlman, M., Aker, M., and Slonim, A.E.: Successful treatment of severe type 1 glucogen storage disease with neonatal presentation by nocturnal intragastric feeding, J. Pediatr. 94:772, 1979.

Persson, B.: Carboyhdrate and lipid metabolism in the newborn infant, Acta Anaesthesiol. Scand. 55:50, 1974.

Persson, B., Gentz, J., and Kellum, M.: Metabolic observations in infants of strictly controlled diabetic mothers, Acta Paediatr. Scand. 62:465, 1973.

Persson, B., Settergren, G., and Dahlquist, G.: Cerebral arteriovenous differences of acetoacetate and D-β-hydroxybutrate in children, Acta Paediatr. Scand. 61:273, 1972.

Persson, B., and Tunell, R.: Influence of environmental temperature and acidosis on lipid mobilization in the human infant during the first two hours after birth, Acta Paediatr. Scand. 60:385, 1971.

Pildes, R.S.: Insulin in normal and pathological pregnancies and its effects on the fetus and newborn, Pediatr. Adolesc. Endocrinol. 5:213, 1979.

Pildes, R.S., Patel, D.A., and Nitzan, M.: Glucose disappearance rate in symptomatic neonatal hypoglycemia, Pediatrics 75:91, 1973.

Pildes, R.S., and others: The incidence of neonatal hypoglycemia: a completed survey, J. Pediatr. 70:76, 1967.

Pildes, R.S., and others: Plasma insulin response during oral glucose tolerance tests in newborns of normal and gestational diabetic mothers, Pediatrics 44:76, 1969.

Pildes, R.S., and others: A prospective controlled study of neonatal hypoglycemia, Pediatrics 54:5, 1974.

Pollak, A., and others: Glucose disposal in low-birth-weight infants during steady-state hyperglycemia: effects of exogenous insulin administration, Pediatrics 61:546, 1978.

Räihä, N.C.R., and Lindros, K.O.: Development of some enzymes involved in gluconeogenesis in human liver, Ann. Med. Exp. Biol. Fenn. 47:146, 1969.

Raivio, K.O., and Osterlund, K.: Hypoglycemia and hyperinsulinemia associated with erythroblastosis fetalis, Pediatrics 43:217, 1969.

Rastogi, G.K., Letarte, J., and Fraser, T.R.: Proinsulin content of pancreas in human fetus of healthy mothers, Lancet 1:7, 1970.

Reid, M.M., and others: Cardiomegaly in association with neonatal hypoglycemia, Acta Paediatr. Scand. 60:295, 1970.

Robert, M.F., and others: Association between maternal diabetes and the respiratory distress syndrome in the newborn, N. Engl. J. Med. 294:357, 1976.

Sann, L., and others: Effect of intravenous hydrocortisone administration on glucose homeostasis in small for gestational age infants, Acta Paediatr. Scand. 68:113, 1979.

Schwartz, S.S., and others: Familial nesidioblastosis: severe neonatal hypoglycemia in two families, J. Pediatr. 95:44, 1979.

Schiff, D., and Lowy, C.: Hypoglycemia and excretion of insulin in urine in hemolytic disease of the newborn, Pediatr. Res. 4:280, 1970.

Schiff, D., Stern, L., and Leduc, J.: Chemical thermogenesis in newborn infants: catecholamine excretion and the plasma non-esterified fatty acid response to cold exposure, Pediatrics 37:577, 1966.

Schiff, D., and others: Metabolic effects of exchange transfusions, J. Pediatr. 78:603, 1971.

Schiff, D., and others: Metabolic aspects of the Beckwith-Wiedemann syndrome, J. Pediatr. 82:258, 1973.

Senior, B., and others: Benzothiadiazides and neonatal hypoglycemia, Lancet 2:377, 1976.

Senterre, J., and Karlberg, P.: Respiratory quotient and metabolic rate in normal full term and small for date newborn infants, Acta Paediatr. Scand. 59:653, 1970.

Shah, M.P.K., and Farquhar, J.W.: Children of diabetic mothers—subsequent weight. In Camerini-Davalos, R.A., and Cole, H.A., editors: Early diabetes in early life, New York, 1975, Academic Press, Inc.

Shelley, H.J., and Neligan, G.A.: Neonatal hypoglycemia, Br. Med. Bull. 22:34, 1966.

Simmons, M.A., and others: Fetal metabolic response to maternal starvation, Pediatr. Res. 8:830, 1974.

Smith, B.T., and others: Insulin antagonism of cortisol action on lecithin synthesis by cultured fetal lung cells, J. Pediatr. 87:953, 1975.

Snyder, R.D., and Robinson, A.: Leucine-induced hypoglycemia, Am. J. Dis. Child. 113:566, 1967.

Sokoloff, L.: Metabolism of ketone bodies by the brain, Annu. Rev. Med. 24:271, 1973.

Soltész, G., Mestyán, J., and Schultz, K.: Glucose disappearance rate and changes in plasma nutrients after intravenously injected glucose in normoglycemic and hypoglycemic underweight newborns, Biol. Neonate 21:184, 1972.

Sosenko, I.R., and others: The infant of the diabetic mother—correlation of increased cord C-peptide levels with macrosomia and hypoglycemia, N. Engl. J. Med. 301:859, 1979.

Sotelo-Avila, C., Gonzalez-Crussi, F., and Fowler, J.W.: Complete and incomplete forms of Beckwith-Wiedemann syndrome: their oncogenic potential, J. Pediatr. 96:47, 1980.

Sperling, M.A., DeLamater, P.V., and Phelps, D.: Spontaneous and amino-acid stimulated glucagon secretion in the immediate postnatal period, J. Clin. Invest. 53:1159, 1974.

Stern, L., Ramos, A.D., and Leduc, J.: Urinary catecholamine excretion in infants of diabetic mothers, Pediatrics 42:598, 1968.

Tsang, R.C., and others: Parathyroid function in infants of diabetic mothers, Pediatrics 86:399, 1975.

van Assche, F.A., and others: The endocrine pancreas in erythroblastosis fetalis, Biol. Neonate 15:176, 1970.

Vidnes, J., and Oyasaeter, S.: Glucagon deficiency causing severe neonatal hypoglycemia in a patient with normal insulin secretion, Pediatr. Res. 11:943, 1977.

White, P.: Pregnancy and diabetes, Med. Clin. North Am. 49:1015, 1965.

Widness, J.A., and others: Glycohemoglobin (HbA_{1c}): a predictor of birth weight in infants of diabetic mothers, J. Pediatr. **92**:8, 1978.

Williams, P.R., and others: Effects of oral alanine feeding on blood glucose, plasma glucagon and insulin concentrations in small-for-gestational age infants, N. Engl. J. Med. **292**:612, 1975.

Yakovac, W.C., Baker, L., and Hummeler, K.: Beta cell nesidioblastosis in idiopathic hypoglycemia of infancy, J. Pediatr. **79**:226, 1971.

Yen, S.S.C.: Endocrine regulation of metabolic homeostasis during pregnancy, Clin. Obstet. Gynecol. **16**:130, 1973.

Yeung, C.Y., Lee, V.W.Y., and Yeung, C.M.: Glucose disappearance rates in neonatal infection, J. Pediatr. **82**:486, 1973.

Yssing, M.: Long-term prognosis of children born to mothers diabetic when pregnant. In Camerini-Davalos, R.A., and Cole, H.A., editors: Early diabetes in early life, New York, 1975, Academic Press Inc.

Zarif, M., Pildes, R.S., and Vidyasagar, D.: Insulin and growth hormone responses in neonatal hyperglycemia, Diabetes **25**:428, 1976.

Zucker, P., and Simon, G.: Prolonged symptomatic neonatal hypoglycemia associated with chlorpropamide therapy, Pediatrics **42**:824, 1968.

PART TWO

Disorders of calcium and magnesium metabolism

CALCIUM PHYSIOLOGY

Recent developments in the understanding of normal calcium physiology have provided a basis for reexamining the pathophysiologic considerations in disordered neonatal calcium homeostasis. Current research has confirmed the complex interrelationships of calcium (Ca) with phosphate (P), magnesium (Mg), and acid-base status, and with the three major Ca regulatory hormones: parathyroid hormone, vitamin D, and calcitonin (Table 33-2).

Ca in blood circulates as three important fractions: (1) protein bound, (2) complexed, and (3) ionized. Complexed Ca (complexed with bicarbonate, phosphate, or citrate) and ionized Ca are also termed ultrafiltrable Ca (or non-protein-bound Ca). Ionized Ca is the only physiologically active fraction of blood Ca. Total Ca levels in blood might be reduced as the result of low plasma protein; however, if the ionized Ca remains normal, there may be no physiologic changes. On the other hand, total Ca levels may be unchanged when chelating agents are used, such as the citrate in acid-citrated blood; in this instance ionized Ca is lowered, with potentially significant physiologic effects. There are problems in the use of the McClean-Hastings nomogram for prediction of ionized Ca from the total Ca and protein values. Whenever possible, direct measurement of the ionized Ca with an ion electrode would be preferable. In general, however, total and ionized Ca do correlate over a wide range of Ca values in the newborn, although the predictability of ionized Ca from total Ca alone is poor. The same considerations apply to the use of electrocardiographic determinations of the QT or Q_0T interval; although there is a correlation with ionized Ca, the predictability is as low as that for total Ca.

Table 33-2. Biochemical and hormonal effects on calcium and phosphate levels

Factors	Usual effect on serum Ca	Usual effect on serum P
Biochemical		
Ca	Increase	—
P	Decrease	Increase
Mg	Increase	—
Alkalosis	Decrease	—
Hormonal		
Parathyroid hormone	Increase	Decrease
Vitamin D	Increase	Increase
Calcitonin	Decrease	Decrease

Calcium balance

During pregnancy there is rapid transfer of Ca from mother to fetus via an active placental pump. In the last trimester of pregnancy there is a net transfer of Ca of 100 to 150 mg/kg of fetal body weight. Radiocalcium balance studies in the pregnant rat have shown that about 30% of the total fetal bone is derived from the maternal skeleton; the remainder is from maternal dietary sources. Ionized Ca levels in the blood of mammalian fetuses are high and nearly always greater than that of the mother. At birth there is an abrupt termination of the maternal to fetal Ca supply. To maintain serum Ca homeostasis at this time, it is estimated that an increase of 16% to 20% of Ca flux from fetal bone to extracellular space would be required, unless sufficient exogenous intake of Ca could be achieved. Since dietary Ca in the first few days of life is significantly less than the amount normally received through maternal to fetal transfer, a fall in serum Ca would be expected to occur. However, if normal physiologic processes are operative, compensatory mechanisms would be activated to restore Ca equilibrium immediately. In sick neonates even greater deprivation of Ca is common because of the conventional withholding of milk feeding and the substitution of Ca-free intravenous feeding. In premature infants, infants with birth asphyxia, and infants of diabetic mothers, serum Ca levels are generally correlated with the amount of oral Ca intake.

Phosphate

Active placental P transport occurs in utero from mother to fetus, with fetal serum P levels being significantly greater than maternal values. At birth endogenous breakdown of tissue glycogen occurs with release of P into the extracellular space, further increasing the P load of the infant. Neonatal renal excretion of P is poor because of decreased glomerular filtration rate or decreased parathyroid hormone production (decreased parathyroid hormone increases the renal tubular reabsorption of P). Decreased responsiveness of the renal tubules to parathyroid hormone has been proposed as a reason for decreased P excretion in the human, although the kidneys of fetal sheep are responsive to the action of parathyroid hormone. Excess P with hyperphosphatemia is a well-known cause of hypocalcemia. Hypocalcemia occurs because of deposition of Ca in bone and soft tissue, blunting of parathyroid hormone activity at the bone site, and through the augmentation of calcitonin action at the bone site. Excessive endogenous P loading has been proposed as a factor in the cause of early neonatal hypocalcemia (see further). This type of hypocalcemia is generally associated with hyperphosphatemia, which is not derived from exogenous sources, since milk intake is minimal at this age. In late neonatal hypocalcemia, excessive exogenous dietary P is an important factor causing hypocalcemia. The use of cow's milk types of formula (evaporated milks) and the early introduction of cereals to infants (which generally have a high P content) may lead to hypocalcemia. Most proprietary formulas have P contents higher than that of breast milk (though less than that of evaporated milk) and tend to cause some degree of hyperphosphatemia but have negligible effects on serum Ca.

Acid-base

Acute changes in acid-base status directly affect Ca homeostasis. Decreases in pH increase ionized Ca, and increases in pH decrease ionized Ca. In adults the decrease in ionized Ca in acute alkalosis stimulates the activity of the parathyroid glands. Chronic changes in acid-base status also may affect Ca balance. In chronic acidosis there is mobilization of Ca from bone to the extracellular space, and in chronic alkalosis the reverse occurs. Several reports have documented the clinical association of early neonatal hypocalcemia in sick infants with the amount of bicarbonate administered for the correction of acidosis. It is not clear, however, whether the bicarbonate correction of acidosis adversely affects serum Ca or whether the severity of the illness adversely affects serum Ca. In later infancy, when metabolic acidosis of diarrheal dehydration has been corrected by alkali administration, postacidotic hypocalcemic tetany can result. Ca metabolism in the neonatal period can also affect acid-base status. In the rapidly growing premature infant, deposition of Ca into bone releases hydrogen ions into the extracellular space and is a possible contributing cause of the late metabolic acidosis of prematurity (p. 322).

Parathyroid hormone

The parathyroid glands are the most important organs in the control of Ca homeostasis. Parathyroid hormone increases serum Ca primarily by increasing bone resorption of Ca (an action that requires vitamin D), by decreasing renal excretion of Ca, and by increasing intestinal absorption of Ca (through its effect on the production of the final metabolite of vitamin D, 1α,25-dihydroxycholecalciferol). Concurrently, its phosphaturic action removes the P released into the circulation by its bone action, minimizing the possible adverse effect of hyperphosphatemia on Ca homeostasis.

Parathyroid hormone production is regulated by the ionized Ca that reaches the parathyroid glands. Decreases in ionized Ca stimulate, and increases suppress, the production of parathyroid hormone, providing a sensitive feedback mechanism for the control of Ca homeostasis. Acute decreases in Mg also stimulate, and increases suppress, parathyroid hormone production. More recently, many other factors have been identified that stimulate parathyroid hormone production, such as epinephrine and β-adrenergic agents and decreases in strontium. The parathyroid hormone that is secreted from the parathyroid glands has a molecular weight of 9,500 and contains the biologically active N-terminal group. Fragments circulating in the blood include a 7,500 molecular weight moiety (biologically inactive, containing the inactive C-terminal) and 4,500 molecular weight and smaller fragments, some of which have biologic activity. Radioimmunoassays currently available for the assay of parathyroid hormone concentrations vary in their ability to recognize the N- or C-terminal of the hormone.

Human fetal parathyroid glands are functionally active as early as 12 weeks of gestation, as demonstrated by their ability to resorb bone. In sheep the fetal parathyroid glands can respond to appropriate acute hypocalcemic challenges in spite of probable suppression of function by the high ionized Ca levels in utero. Parathyroid hormone probably does not cross the placental barrier in either direction. However, *maternal hyperparathyroidism* has been shown to adversely affect the parathyroid function of the fetus. The sequence is probably as follows: maternal hyperparathyroidism results in maternal hypercalcemia, which leads to fetal hypercalcemia and suppression of the fetal parathyroids. Conversely, *maternal hypoparathyroidism* has resulted in fetal and neonatal hyperparathyroidism. The suggested sequence is as follows: maternal hypoparathyroidism, if untreated, leads to maternal hypocalcemia, fetal hypocalcemia, and secondary fetal and neonatal hyperparathyroidism.

After birth, decreases in serum Ca are precipitated by the abrupt termination of Ca supply and the imposition of an endogenous P load from tissue breakdown that cannot be excreted by the kidneys. Normally the parathyroid glands should respond by appropriate increases in production of parathyroid hormone, which would act appropriately on target organs to increase and normalize serum Ca concentrations. It was previously proposed that the target organs in the neonate might not be responsive to parathyroid hormone. Recent studies, however, indicate that the neonate shows an appropriate calcemic response when challenged with parathyroid hormone. On the other hand, the ability of the neonatal parathyroids to produce parathyroid hormone may be diminished in some infants. In normal full-term infants, when serum Ca levels fall slightly after birth, parathyroid hormone levels increase appropriately. However, in premature infants and infants of diabetic mothers there is no significant increase in parathyroid hormone level in response to marked decreases in serum Ca. The reason for the state of functional hypoparathyroidism in these infants is unclear but may be related to the high levels of ionized Ca in utero, which could have suppressed the fetal parathyroids. With time, all infants apparently increase their serum parathyroid hormone concentrations, even to hyperparathyroid levels, presumably in response to the hypocalcemic stress.

Vitamin D

The sequence for vitamin D metabolism in the body is as follows: vitamin D_3 (cholecalciferol) is either ingested and absorbed in the jejunum and duodenum or synthesized from precursors in the skin under ultraviolet irradiation; transport of vitamin D_3 to the liver results in the first 25-hydroxylation step to 25-hydroxycholecalciferol (25-hydroxy-D); the latter metabolite is the major circulating vitamin D metabolite in the body (in adults, 25-hydroxy-D levels range from 10 to 65 ng/ml); it is transported to the kidney for 1α-hydroxylation to $1\alpha,25$-dihydroxycholecalciferol; this last metabolite is the most

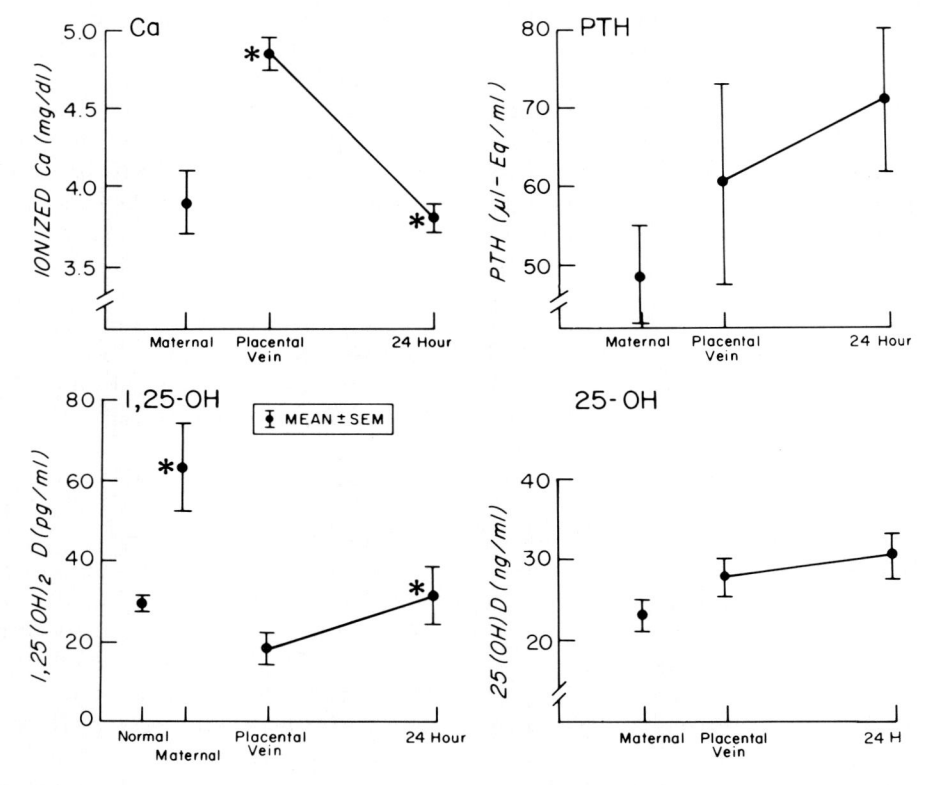

Fig. 33-17. Calcium and 1,25-dihydroxycholecalciferol in normal full-term infants. Placental vein ionized calcium levels are higher than maternal values and fall after birth. Serum 1,25-dihydroxycholecalciferol values in mothers are significantly higher than values in normal adults and placental vein. Placental vein 1,25-dihydroxycholecalciferol concentrations are lower than those in adults at birth but revert to normal values at 24 hours. Serum parathyroid hormone and 25-hydroxy vitamin D concentrations in this study were not significantly changed after birth. (Reprinted, by permission of the New England Journal of Medicine, from Steichen, J.J., and others: N. Engl. J. Med. **302**:315, 1980.)

active of the vitamin D metabolites and is the final metabolite, which acts on the target organs for vitamin D metabolism. The main factors increasing the rate of conversion of 25-hydroxycholecalciferol to 1α,25-dihydroxycholecalciferol are hypocalcemia, parathyroid hormone (possibly through its hypophosphatemic effect) and hypophosphatemia. Hypocalcemia might affect vitamin D metabolism also through stimulation of parathyroid hormone production and, subsequently, 1α,25-dihydroxycholecalciferol production.

Vitamin D metabolites act on the intestine to absorb Ca and P; on the bone, in concert with parathyroid hormone, to mobilize Ca and P from bone; and on the kidney to conserve Ca and P. Thus vitamin D sufficiency is necessary for maintenance of normal Ca and P homeostasis. In rats, vitamin D and 25-hydroxycholecalciferol cross the placenta from mother to fetus. Limited quantities of 1α,25-dihydroxycholecalciferol appear to cross the monkey placenta. During human pregnancy, maternal serum 1α,25-dihydroxycholecalcified concentrations are elevated, but fetal concentrations are low. The importance of vitamin D metabolites in utero is uncertain. However, certain immigrants to the United Kingdom who are vitamin D deficient have offspring who are more prone to late neonatal hypocalcemia. It has been suggested that vitamin D deficiency may lead to maternal hyperparathyroidism and fetal hypoparathyroidism, but it is also possible that decreased vitamin D in the mother leads to mild vitamin D deficiency in the infant and increased susceptibility to hypocalcemia. In premature infants there may be decreased 25-hydroxycholecalciferol levels. This may be due to decreased placental transfer, malabsorption of vitamin D, or decreased hepatic hydroxylation or increased turnover of the metabolite. Theoretically, decreased vitamin D levels would adversely affect serum Ca levels. In term infants, serum 1α,25-dihydroxycholecalciferol concentrations are low at birth but increase to normal ranges by 24 hours of life, possibly reflecting the need for optimal intestinal calcium and phosphorus absorption (Fig. 33-17).

Adequate bone mineralization in infancy requires adequate vitamin D and mineral supplies. It is generally believed that 200 IU of vitamin D each day with 100 mg/kg/day of Ca would satisfy the usual needs. The requirements of these substances in small premature infants who currently are surviving the immediate postpartum period is unclear. Clinical reports of undermineralization of bone in such infants receiving standard proprietary formulas can be documented by photon absorptiometry (Fig. 33-18). Supplementation of such formulas with calcium (to achieve an intake of 250 mg/kg/day) and phosphate (125 mg/kg/day) appears to improve bone mineralization (Fig. 33-19).

Calcitonin

Calcitonin is produced mainly by the C-cells of the thyroid gland, which are embryologically derived from neural crest tissue. Calcitonin is a 32–amino acid mole-

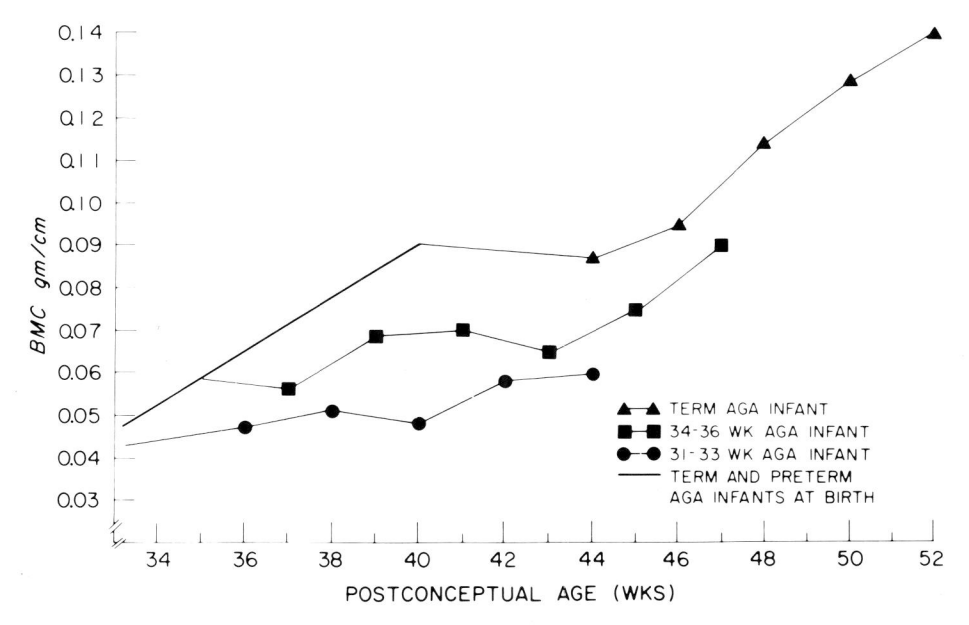

Fig. 33-18. Postnatal bone mineralization in preterm infants on standard proprietary formulas is significantly decreased compared with intrauterine bone mineralization rates. *BMC*, Bone mineral content. (Adapted from data in Minton, S., Steichen, J.J., and Tsang, R.C.: J. Pediatr. **95**:1037, 1979.)

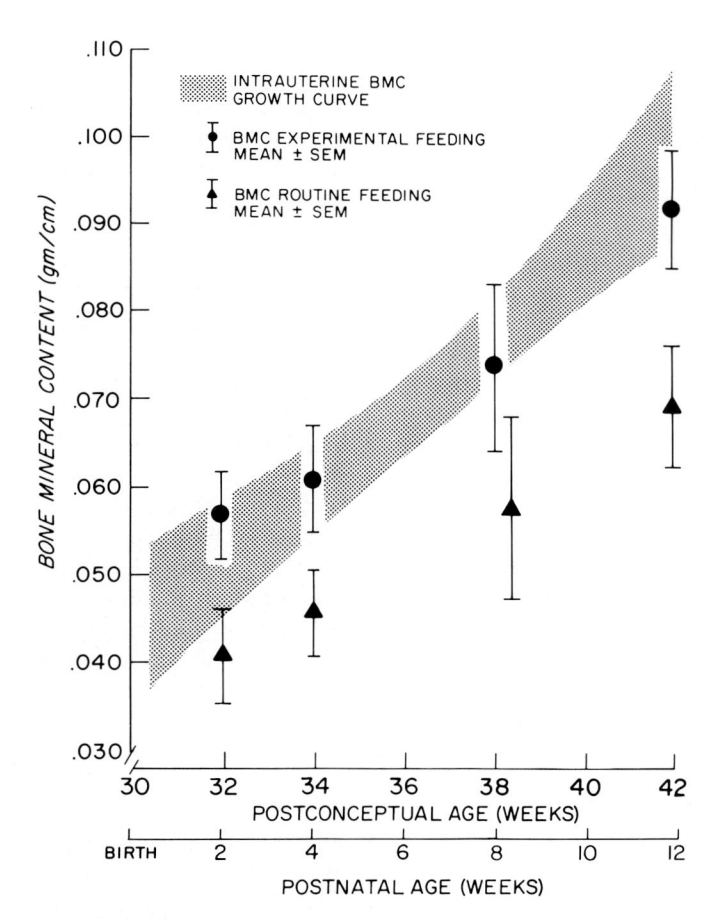

Fig. 33-19. In premature (28 to 32 week) infants fed an experimental formula fortified with calcium (1,260 mg/L) and phosphate (630 mg/L) postnatal bone mineralization is greater than that of premature infants fed standard proprietary formula and approximates the bone mineralization achieved in utero. Similar results are seen in 32 to 35 week gestation infants. (From Steichen, J.J., Gratton, T.L., and Tsang, R.C.:J. Pediatr. **96:**528, 1980.)

cule that acts at the bone site to antagonize the effect of parathyroid hormone by decreasing the amount of Ca and P being released from the bone; at the kidney site calcitonin has both calciuric and phosphaturic effects. Thus the overall effect of calcitonin is to decrease serum Ca and P. Factors that increase the production of calcitonin include increases in circulating calcium and magnesium and increases in the gastrointestinal (GI) hormones: gastrin, glucagon, and pancreozymin. These hormones are released secondary to food in the GI tract; for example, glycine and gastric distension stimulate gastrin release, intraduodenal glucose stimulates enteroglucagon, and intraduodenal fat stimulates pancreozymin. Thus it is suggested that this GI-thyroid–C-cell system serves to prevent marked increases in serum Ca during food ingestion. In utero, calcitonin-secreting C-cells are functionally active. In ovine, porcine, and bovine fetuses given Ca infusions, appropriate increases in calcitonin secretion are produced. Calcitonin activity at the bone site is also present in fetal life. High levels of serum calcitonin occur in fetal animals and newborn humans. After birth, in newborns there is a further increase in serum calcitonin levels. The physiologic importance of this increase in serum calcitonin is unclear. On theoretical grounds, calcitonin would be advantageous for infants in protecting the skeleton from excessive bone resorption; however, this could lead to decreases in serum Ca and serum P. It is uncertain whether calcitonin is a cause of neonatal hypocalcemia; excess calcitonin, however, would not explain the hyperphosphatemia associated with hypocalcemia.

CLINICAL CONDITIONS OF CALCIUM DISTURBANCE
Hypocalcemia
"Early" neonatal hypocalcemia

Neonatal hypocalcemia that occurs in the first few days of life is the most common type of neonatal hypocalcemia. Definitions vary as to the level of serum Ca required for the diagnosis of hypocalcemia, but most authors agree that when serum Ca falls below 7 mg/dl, the infant should be considered hypocalcemic. At 7 mg/dl, ionized Ca levels are low, and body mechanisms for conservation of Ca are activated. In early neonatal hypocalcemia, serum Ca values fall to their lowest levels at 24 to 48 hours of age. In general, one third of premature infants 37 weeks' gestational age or less, one half of infants of insulin-dependent diabetic mothers, and 30% of infants with birth asphyxia (1-minute Apgar score of 6 or less) have hypocalcemia.

With the advent of ionized Ca determinations in clinical laboratories, the definition of neonatal hypocalcemia should be revised to include conditions where the level of ionized Ca in serum falls below 3 to 3.5 mg/dl. Normal ranges in different laboratories vary mainly because of variations in currently available specific ion electrodes (reported adult normal values have ranged from 3.5 to 4.5 mg/dl or 4 to 5 mg/dl).

Prematurity. Serum Ca values after birth, in the first few days of life, correlate directly with gestational age (Fig. 33-20). Thus less mature infants have a greater probability of developing hypocalcemia. Hypocalcemia in premature infants is related in part to decreased Ca intake from decreased milk intake, increased endogenous P loading, and transient functional hypoparathyroidism. Birth asphyxia in some infants compounds the problems. Other etiologic factors that have been suggested as causes of hypocalcemia include the correction of acidosis with alkali and decreased circulating vitamin D metabolites. Gestational age rather than birth weight

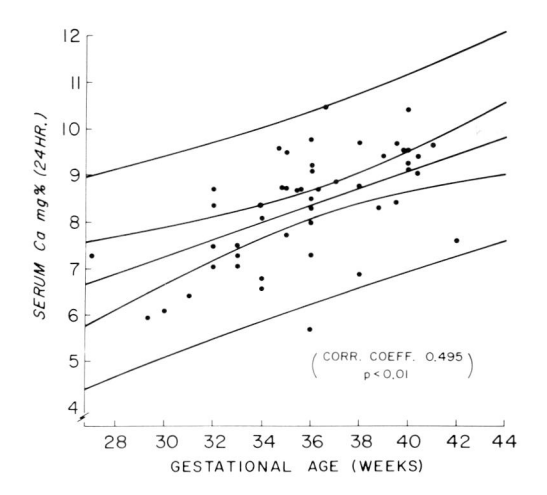

Fig. 33-20. Serum Ca in relation to gestational age at 24 hours of age. (From Tsang, R.C., and others: J. Pediatr. **82**:423, 1973.)

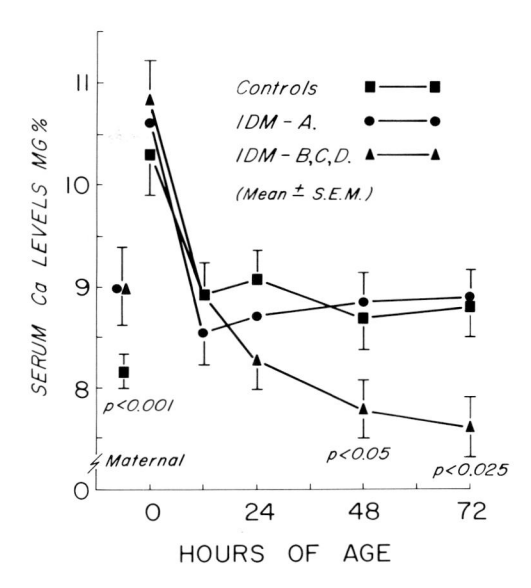

Fig. 33-21. Serum Ca levels in infants of class B, C, and D diabetic mothers and infants of class A diabetic mothers compared with levels in control infants matched for sex, gestational age, and presence or absence of birth asphyxia. (From Tsang, R.C., and others: J. Pediatr. **80**:384, 1972.)

itself appears to be an important determinant of neonatal Ca homeostasis. Thus SGA infants do not develop hypocalcemia unless they are also gestationally premature or have birth asphyxia (see further).

Neonatal hypocalcemia is associated with hyperphosphatemia and generally occurs at an age (24-48 hours) when blood pH's (which are generally low in the first few hours after birth in these infants) have reverted to normal. In nearly all instances, hypocalcemia is temporary and shows a gradual reversion toward normal after 1 to 3 days. Factors that contribute to the restoration include improvement in Ca intake when milk feeding increases, increased excretion of P, and restoration of parathyroid function. Ca supplementation may hasten the restorative process.

Infants of diabetic mothers. Infants of diabetic mothers are often delivered prematurely and often have birth asphyxia. Since prematurity and birth asphyxia are significantly associated with hypocalcemia, decreased serum Ca in infants of diabetic mothers relates in part to these two complications. In addition, maternal diabetes itself exerts a separate effect on serum Ca (Fig. 33-21). In carefully controlled studies comparing infants of diabetic mothers with infants of nondiabetic mothers, matched for gestational age and presence or absence of birth asphyxia, serum Ca is significantly lower in infants of diabetic mothers. The degree of hypocalcemia also varies directly with the severity of maternal diabetes, classified by White's criteria (p. 23). Other factors that adversely affect serum Ca in infants of diabetic mothers are the limitation of food and Ca intake because of illness (for example, respiratory distress and poor feeding), endogenous P loading from increased tissue glycogen breakdown, and impaired parathyroid hormone production.

Neonatal hypocalcemia in infants of diabetic mothers is generally associated with hyperphosphatemia and hypomagnesemia. Hypocalcemia lasts for only a few days with spontaneous resolution hastened by factors outlined in the discussion of hypocalcemia of prematurity.

Birth asphyxia. Many infants with birth asphyxia are gestationally immature and thus may have decreased serum Ca. However, matched controlled observations have demonstrated that birth asphyxia and gestational immaturity are two separate factors influencing the incidence of hypocalcemia in the immediate neonatal period (Fig. 33-22). In birth asphyxia the factors of decreased Ca intake and increased endogenous P loading appear important, although the role of the parathyroids has not been clarified. The hypocalcemia of birth asphyxia often occurs in association with hypomagnesemia and hyperphosphatemia and is generally of a transitory nature.

"Late" neonatal hypocalcemia

Hypocalcemia occurring in neonates beyond the first 2 to 4 days of life is termed "late" neonatal hypocalcemia. The term is often reserved for infants with cow's milk–induced hypocalcemia, who constitute, in some geographic areas, the largest group of infants with late hypocalcemia.

Calcium deficiency. Any intestinal malabsorption syndrome, such as celiac disease or shortened bowel syndromes, can lead to malabsorption of Ca, since Ca absorption is carried out primarily in the small intestine.

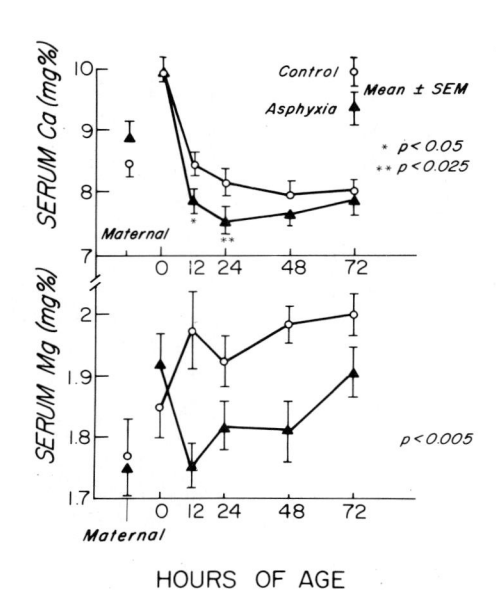

Fig. 33-22. Serum Ca and Mg levels in infants with birth asphyxia compared with levels in control infants matched for sex and gestational age. Serum Mg levels in infants with birth asphyxia were significantly lower from 12 to 72 hours of age. (From Tsang, R.C., and others: J. Pediatr. **84:**428, 1974.)

Concomitant malabsorption of vitamin D or Mg will further disrupt Ca balance.

Phosphate loading. In areas of the world where modified cow's milk with high P content (for example, evaporated milk) is given to neonates, hypocalcemia is commonly observed. The markedly reduced number of infants in the United States currently seen with this disorder may be related to the introduction of proprietary formulas with P contents lower than that in cow's milk and the continuation of breast milk feeding (low P content). P-induced hypocalcemia commonly occurs at the end of a week of relatively high P feeding. In immigrants to the United Kingdom, maternal vitamin D deficiency recently has been proposed as an additional etiologic factor in this condition. The parathyroid glands become hyperplastic in response to P-induced hypocalcemia in an attempt to correct the hypocalcemia. Early introduction of cereals to infants carries with it the potential risk of hypocalcemia because of the generally high P content of commercial cereals.

Hypomagnesemia. Hypomagnesemia, particularly from intestinal Mg malabsorption, has generally presented with hypocalcemia. Hypocalcemia will not be corrected unless the Mg disturbance is first rectified (see further).

Acid-base disturbances. Infants with acidosis secondary to diarrhea who receive alkali therapy to correct their acidosis may develop "postacidotic" tetany with decreases in total and ultrafiltrable Ca. Infants with chronic respiratory disease who become alkalotic because of hyperventilation with mechanical respirators or overcorrection with alkali infusions also may develop decreases in ionized Ca and signs of hypocalcemia.

Parathyroid disorders. The term *transient congenital idiopathic hypoparathyroidism* is applied to a group of infants who resemble infants with early neonatal hypocalcemia. Biochemically, there is hypocalcemia, hyperphosphatemia, and target organ responsiveness to parathyroid hormone. The diagnosis, however, may be delayed beyond the first few days of life, and the disease lasts for a few days to a few weeks, resolving either spontaneously or with short courses of vitamin D. This condition may simply represent an extension of early neonatal hypocalcemia that was not recognized in the immediate neonatal period. True *congenital hypoparathyroidism* can occur as a sex-linked condition, in association with ring chromosomes (16 or 18), or as part of DiGeorge's syndrome (congenital absence of the thymus and parathyroids). In the last condition, hypocalcemia is associated with thymic-dependent immunologic deficiencies (p. 646). *Secondary hypoparathyroidism* may occur in offspring of mothers with hyperparathyroidism. The condition is generally transient, lasting for a few days to a few weeks, and supportive therapy with Ca and vitamin D generally suffices. In some instances protracted neonatal hypocalcemia has suggested that a maternal Ca disorder was present. *Pseudohypoparathyroidism*, or target organ unresponsiveness to parathyroid hormone, is a disease of later childhood and generally is not detected in the neonatal period.

Disordered vitamin D metabolism. *Dietary deficiency of vitamin D* is less common in the western world. Rapidly growing small premature infants who do not receive supplemental vitamin D, other than that contained in their limited intake of milk, have developed radiologic signs of rickets. In infants with vitamin D deficiency, there is defective intestinal absorption of Ca and P and development of hypocalcemia and hypophosphatemia. In *neonatal liver disease*, including neonatal hepatitis and biliary atresia, disordered hepatic 25-hydroxylation of vitamin D may lead to hypocalcemia, hypophosphatemia, and rickets (p. 774). In normal subjects there appears to be active enterohepatic circulation of 25-hydroxycholecalciferol. In liver disease, decreased bile salt secretion may result in decreased absorption of 25-hydroxycholecalciferol, further compounding the disturbance in vitamin D metabolism. In the kidneys of infants with *vitamin D–dependency rickets*, there may be a congenital metabolic block in the conversion of 25-hydroxycholecalciferol to the final 1α,25-dihydroxycholecalciferol. Reduction in the available amount of the final active vitamin D metabolite results in hypocalcemia and rickets. In all these conditions, parathyroid hyperplasia may develop in an attempt to correct the hypocalcemia associated with disordered vitamin D metabolism. Hyperparathyroidism may worsen the bone picture by increasing bone resorption, although this serves to partially rectify the hypocalcemia. In addition, the hyperparathyroidism results in hyperphosphaturia and aminoaciduria.

Clinical and laboratory manifestations

The classic description of neonatal hypocalcemic tetany—high-pitched cry, Chvostek's sign (facial muscle twitching when stimulated), and Trousseau's sign (for example, carpal spasm after constriction of the upper arm)—is useful in the older infant but is of little diagnostic value in the first few days of life. In the early neonatal period the main clinical signs are jitteriness (increased neuromuscular irritability and activity), twitching (jerky movements of one or more extremities), and generalized convulsions. However, in many neonates with jitteriness, serum Ca (total or ionized) may be normal. This is particularly evident in SGA infants who may be normocalcemic, normomagnesemic, and normoglycemic and yet have hypertonicity and increased neuromuscular activity.

Serum Ca, P, Mg, and protein determinations should be obtained and followed serially when hypocalcemia is suspected. Ionized Ca determinations are very helpful if available; care should be exercised in obtaining the blood sample, since changes in blood pH will affect ionized Ca values. The sample should be a free-flowing blood sample, anaerobically obtained and sealed in capillary tubes before immediate analysis. Blood parathyroid hormone levels provide an index of the activity of the parathyroid glands, although, in general, serial levels of parathyroid hormone in relation to changes in serum Ca afford a better idea of the actual functional activity of the parathyroids. Blood 25-hydroxy-D and 1,25-dihydroxycholecalciferol determinations, if available, provide an index of vitamin D metabolism. Electrocardiographic determination of the QT_c or Q_0T_c interval may be useful. A corrected QT interval (QT_c, corrected for heart rate) greater than 0.40 second and a corrected Q_0T (or Q_0T_c, origin of Q to origin of T) greater than 0.20 second suggest hypocalcemia, although neither measurement predicts the ionized Ca value. Electrocardiographic monitoring may be used to gauge the response to Ca salt therapy. Chest roentgenograms for the thymic silhouette are important in considering associated immunologic abnormalities. Efforts to diagnose the other biochemical or hormonal causes of hypocalcemia may be necessary when these conditions are suspected.

Treatment

Treatment of symptomatic hypocalcemia is the administration of Ca salts. Acute intravenous administration of 10% Ca gluconate, 2 ml/kg body weight (18 mg elemental Ca/kg), should be given into a peripheral vein over a period of 10 minutes with either electrocardiographic or heart rate monitoring. The infusion should be discontinued if bradycardia occurs. When this dose of Ca salts is given to an adult or older child, there is parathyroid suppression, so that usually this amount should not be exceeded. Continued follow-up intravenous supplementation of Ca at the rate of 75 mg elemental Ca/kg/day generally is sufficient to achieve normocalcemia. When normocalcemia is achieved, stepwise reduction of intravenous Ca (37 mg/kg each day, 18 mg/kg for the last day) may help to prevent rebound hypocalcemia. Complications of intravenous Ca therapy include extravasation of Ca into soft tissue with Ca deposition or sloughing of skin, and inadvertent rapid infusion with resultant bradycardia. Particular care should be exercised when the Ca infusion is given into an umbilical venous catheter tip close to the heart. Intraarterial infusions are inadvisable because of potential vascular complications. Alternatively, where infants can tolerate oral fluids, oral administration of Ca gluconate in the same dosage is useful after initial acute correction. The only complication is an increased frequency of bowel movements, especially when the recommended dosage is exceeded.

In asymptomatic hypocalcemia, opinions vary as to the intensity of therapy required. In most instances, hypocalcemia resolves itself spontaneously. Whenever possible, Ca gluconate should be given orally and is generally successful, obviating intravenous therapy with its attendant complications.

In hypocalcemic conditions secondary to other disorders, therapy for the primary disease is important. In P-induced hypocalcemia, use of a low-P formula (such as Similac PM 60/40) and avoidance of cereals are indicated. The use of aluminum hydroxide gel (Amphojel) to decrease P absorption is effective, but the long-range effects are unknown. Hypomagnesemia generally requires therapy before hypocalcemia can be successfully treated. When hypocalcemia is persistent, the use of vitamin D or one of its metabolites may be helpful, since vitamin D raises serum Ca levels primarily by increasing intestinal absorption of Ca. Dosages of vitamin D are approximately 400 IU for vitamin D deficiency (2,000 to 10,000 IU initially), 2,000 to 10,000 IU for hepatic disease, 10,000 IU to 100,000 for true hypoparathyroidism, and 5,000 to 50,000 IU for vitamin D–dependency rickets. Repeated therapeutic doses of parathyroid extract are inadvisable because of the possibility of antibody production and refractoriness to therapy.

Hypercalcemia

Hypercalcemia is present when total Ca in serum is above 10.5 to 11 mg/dl or ionized Ca is above 4.5 to 5 mg/dl. Clinical signs include hypotonia, weakness, lethargy, weight loss or poor weight gain, constipation, vomiting, poor feeding, convulsions, polyuria, and polydipsia.

Parathyroid disorders

Primary hyperparathyroidism. Congenital primary hyperparathyroidism is a rare disorder of diffuse clear cell parathyroid hyperplasia. Adenomas of the parathyroid are not seen in the neonatal period, although they may develop in later childhood. Familial patterns are occasionally reported and are compatible with recessive inheritance. The condition may not be clinically apparent and may be discovered only at autopsy. Alternatively, clinical signs may be present at birth or delayed for 30 months. Laboratory findings include hypercalcemia up to 25 mg/dl, hypophosphatemia, hyperphosphatasia, hypercalciuria, and phosphaturia; aminoaciduria and albuminuria are seen occasionally. Radiography of the long bones may show diffuse demineralization, subperiosteal resorption in the phalanges, and occasionally osteitis fibrosa and spontaneous fractures. Nephrocalcinosis is rarely seen by radiography but is often detectable histologically. The prognosis for patients with untreated primary hyperparathyroidism is grave, with progressive deterioration and death. Definitive treatment is surgical with subtotal parathyroidectomy; success depends on early diagnosis before severe clinical problems occur.

Secondary hyperparathyroidism. *Congenital hyperparathyroidism* secondary to maternal hypoparathyroidism is a rare cause of hypercalcemia in the newborn. The condition is related to poor control of maternal Ca metabolism during pregnancy. Maternal hypocalcemia is thought to lead to fetal hypocalcemia and consequent chronic stimulation of the fetal parathyroid glands. Infants present with the clinical, biochemical, or skeletal features of hyperparathyroidism. The condition is transient with a relatively good prognosis for the infants, provided supportive measures are instituted.

Vitamin D disturbances

Idiopathic hypercalcemia syndrome. A severe form of this syndrome was originally described by Fanconi in infants with failure to thrive, hypercalcemia, hypercalciuria, azotemia, renal acidosis, and osteosclerosis. These infants have a characteristic elfin facies and may have severe mental retardation. A systolic heart murmur is often heard, and supravalvular aortic stenosis may be present. Lightwood and Payne described a more benign form of hypercalcemia. The infants suffer from failure to thrive, vomiting, and constipation. Hypercalcemia and azotemia are present, but mental retardation and osteosclerosis are not observed. In general this latter form of hypercalcemia is easily reversible, and the prognosis is good, except in rare instances where the infants die during the acute phase of extreme hypercalcemia.

The pathogenesis of idiopathic hypercalcemia is not known. Vitamin D has been strongly implicated because of the epidemiologic association of hypercalcemia and excessive vitamin D fortification of milk in Great Britain. An increased incidence of infantile hypercalcemia occurred at a time when infants were often receiving 4,000 units of vitamin D per day from fortified commercial milk, infant cereals, and vitamin D supplements. Alternatively, both neonatal and infantile hypersensitivity to vitamin D and the prolonged persistence of vitamin D metabolites in the body have been suggested as etiologic factors. Intrauterine sensitization of the fetus to vitamin D also has been proposed but is unproved. Maternal rabbits given very large doses of vitamin D give birth to offspring with generalized vascular lesions, some of which are suggestive of supravalvular aortic stenosis. In clinical practice, concern has been expressed that large doses of vitamin D administered to pregnant hypoparathyroid women may lead to the syndrome of severe idiopathic hypercalcemia; however, no detrimental effects have been seen in these infants, provided the mothers remain normocalcemic during pregnancy. This suggests that, if there are detrimental effects on the fetus from maternal vitamin D excess, maternal or fetal hypercalcemia rather than vitamin D might be the toxic agent. Finally, hypercalcemia even of long duration may not necessarily be harmful, as demonstrated by a condition described as *benign familial hypercalcemia*, where family members with hypercalcemia of long duration demonstrate no other biochemical, osseous, or parathyroid abnormalities.

Subcutaneous fat necrosis. Small areas of subcutaneous fat necrosis are frequently seen in newborns over areas of increased pressure and are usually of little clinical significance (p. 217). Occasionally, however, extensive areas of fat are necrotic, particularly over the back and limbs, in infants born of difficult deliveries, in hypothermic infants, or large infants of diabetic mothers. Fat necrosis usually appears during the first few days of life, and hypercalcemia follows in the next week or weeks. The clinical signs are similar to those of the benign form of idiopathic hypercalcemia and usually begin around 2 months of age with vomiting and failure to thrive, although in severe instances, renal calculi, renal insufficiency, and convulsions can be seen. Proposed pathogenetic mechanisms include abnormalities in fat metabolism, abnormal regulation of Ca physiology secondary to sudden release of large amounts of Ca from the subcutaneous fat, or abnormal sensitivity to vitamin D.

Miscellaneous causes

Iatrogenic hypercalcemia. Increased serum Ca levels may be seen as a result of overtreatment of hypocalcemia. After exchange transfusions with citrated blood and intermittent intravenous supplementation of Ca, measurements of total Ca in the infant's blood may be deceptively high, although ionized fractions may be low because of citrate complexing effects.

Paraneoplastic syndrome. In older children and adults hypercalcemia may be associated with malignancies. Hypercalcemia may be secondary to nephroblastoma in young infants.

Clinical and laboratory manifestations

The history affords the greatest information for the diagnosis and treatment of hypercalcemia. A close questioning of the mother is important to establish any history of excessive vitamin D intakes during pregnancy or in the neonatal period, especially in regard to vitamin D–fortified foods (milks, cereals) and supplements. A history of familial or maternal Ca-P disease should be investigated. The history of a difficult labor may alert the physician to the presence of fat necrosis. The onset of clinical signs in the immediate neonatal period or later gives some idea as to the severity and possible pathogenetic mechanisms involved. The clinical signs of hypercalcemia are usually nonspecific, except for fat necrosis and elfin facies. Plasma protein should be measured to rule out increases in total Ca from dysproteinemic states. Ionized Ca determinations are important in some cases. Plasma P determinations are useful in parathyroid disturbances (decreased) but are of less value in other disorders. Determination of the percent of renal tubular reabsorption of P may help in distinguishing parathyroid disorders (decreased, less than 85%) from nonparathyroid conditions. The mother's Ca-P status should be determined. Measurement of parathyroid hormone levels, especially in conjunction with tests stimulating parathyroid hormone release (such as disodium ethylene diamine tetraacetate, EDTA, stimulation tests), will be helpful in differentiating hypercalcemia from parathyroid or nonparathyroid causes. Plasma 25-hydroxy-D determinations may be useful in instances where vitamin D excess is suspected. ECG may show shortening of the QT interval. Bone radiographs will identify demineralization or osteolytic lesions (parathyroid overactivity) or osteosclerotic lesions (vitamin D excess) consistent with the etiology of the hypercalcemia.

Treatment

Therapy of hypercalcemia includes restriction of dietary Ca, discontinuation of vitamin D intake (through the use of breast milk or vitamin D–free formulas or cow's milk), and avoidance of sunlight. In acute hypercalcemia cortiocosteroids may be useful (prednisone, 2 mg/kg body weight daily) in decreasing intestinal Ca absorption. Furosemide diuretics are effective as calciuretic agents, provided water and electrolyte balance are maintained. Alternative modes of therapy include the intravenous use of EDTA or calcitonin. The potential side effects of these drugs, especially for long-term therapy in the infant, are unknown.

MAGNESIUM PHYSIOLOGY

Mg metabolism is intimately related to Ca homeostasis. Hypomagnesemia leads to hypocalcemia primarily because hypomagnesemia results in hypoparathyrodism and, less commonly, because hypomagnesemia can lead to target organ unresponsiveness to parathyroid hormone. In contradistinction to Ca, which is primarily an extracellular cation, Mg is an intracellular cation. Tissue Mg depletion may not be associated with clinically evident decreases in Mg concentration in the blood. Factors that affect plasma Mg concentrations include P, parathyroid hormone, and vitamin D. Increased plasma P can lead to decreases in plasma Mg as well as Ca. Parathyroid hormone can act to increase serum Mg concentrations. Excessive vitamin D may lead to hypomagnesemia, possibly because of increased intestinal absorption of Ca; increased Ca absorption results in competitive Mg malabsorption. Alternatively, excessive vitamin D may lead to redistribution of Mg in the body fluids. Calcitonin may act to decrease serum Mg levels.

CLINICAL CONDITIONS OF MAGNESIUM DISTURBANCE
Hypomagnesemia

Hypomagnesemia occurs when serum Mg levels fall below 1.5 mg/dl, although clinical signs usually do not develop until serum Mg levels fall below 1.2 mg/dl. Neonatal hypomagnesemia can result from decreased Mg supply, increased Mg loss, or disordered Mg homeostasis.

Decreased magnesium supply

Sporadic primary intestinal Mg malabsorption has been reported in rare instances in infancy, requiring apparent lifelong supplementation with Mg salts. Similarly, surgical procedures that reduce small-intestinal

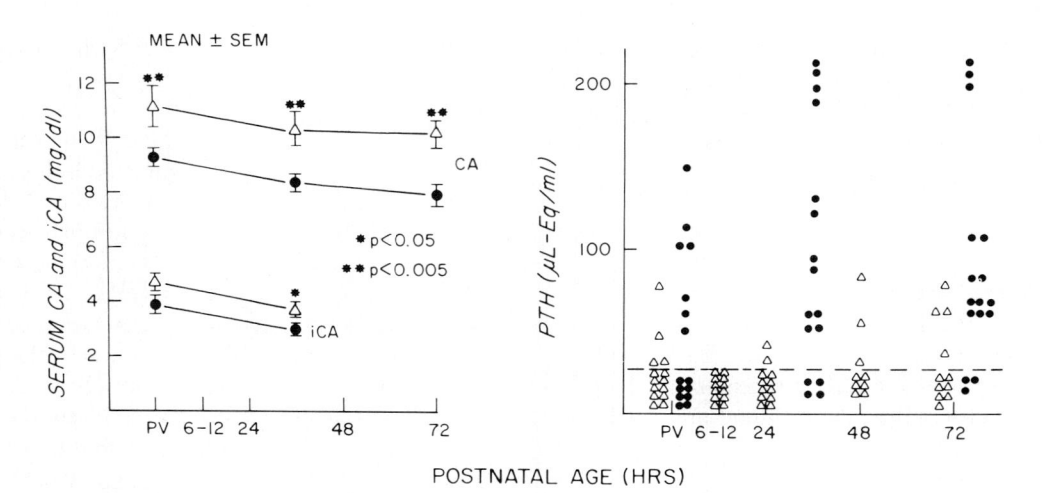

Fig. 33-23. Maternal hypermagnesemia is reflected in neonatal hypermagnesemia. Neonatal hypermagnesemia results in suppression of parathyroid hormone, but elevation of serum total and ionized Ca. △, Hypermagnesemic infants; ●, controls. (From Donovan, E.F., and others: J. Pediatr. **96**:305, 1980.)

length can lead to Mg deprivation. Infants with intrauterine growth retardation and infants born of mothers with hypomagnesemia may represent conditions where the maternal supply or placental transfer of Mg may be deficient.

Increased magnesium loss

The increased loss of Mg caused by repeated exchange blood transfusions with acid citrated blood of low Mg content may lead to hypomagnesemia.

Disordered homeostasis

Neonatal hypoparathyroidism may be associated with hypomagnesemia. Hypoparathyroidism may be sporadic, familial, or related to maternal hyperparathyroidism. In these instances, hypomagnesemia may be detected in the neonatal period or might not be diagnosed until later childhood. Treatment of hypomagnesemia generally facilitates the management of hypocalcemia.

Transient hypomagnesemia may occur in infants of diabetic mothers. The incidence of hypomagnesemia increases with the severity of maternal diabetes. In these infants, hypomagnesemia is associated with decreased parathyroid function. It is uncertain whether the hypomagnesemia is a factor causing the functional hypoparathyroidism or whether the hypoparathyroidism results in hypomagnesemia. Another possible cause for the hypomagnesemia in infants of diabetic mothers is maternal hypomagnesemia. Clinically, there is little correlation between hypomagnesemia in these infants and signs of neuromuscular irritability.

Conflicting studies have been published regarding the effect of birth asphyxia on neonatal Mg homeostasis. One study suggested that serum Mg levels might be high in infants with birth asphyxia. Recent studies of the hypocalcemia of birth asphyxia have demonstrated the association of decreased serum Mg and increased serum P with the hypocalcemia. The differences in results may reflect differences in gestational ages of the infants studied, since there is an inverse relation between gestational age and neonatal serum Mg levels.

Hyperphosphatemia, in addition to causing hypocalcemia, can also lead to hypomagnesemia. Thus cow's milk feeding has the potential for causing hypomagnesemia in infants.

Hypermagnesemia

The upper limit of normal for serum Mg levels in infancy is 2.8 mg/dl. The most important cause of neonatal hypermagnesia is maternal hypermagnesemia from magnesium sulfate therapy for toxemia of pregnancy. Neonatal neuromuscular depression (curare-like effect) may occur with hypermagnesemia, and respiratory failure (CNS depression) can occur in extreme cases. It may be difficult to separate the effects of the hypermagnesemia from the effects of birth asphyxia itself, since birth asphyxia may occur in infants of toxemic mothers who do not receive Mg therapy. Apgar scores after birth do not correlate with the serum Mg concentrations, but neuromuscular depression may correlate with the duration of Mg therapy given to the mother. Neonatal parathyroid function is suppressed by hypermagnesemia. However, serum Ca concentrations appear to be increased in hypermagnesemic infants, possibly related to direct effects of Mg facilitating the release of Ca from bone (Fig. 33-23).

Formerly, another cause of neonatal hypermagnesemia was the use of magnesium sulfate enemas, prescribed for the therapy of respiratory distress syndrome; this therapy is not efficacious and is dangerous.

Clinical and laboratory manifestations

Hypomagnesemia should be considered in any high-risk infant just described and in any infant with hypocalcemia who does not respond clinically or biochemically to Ca or vitamin D therapy. It may occur with the signs of neuromuscular hyperexcitability, muscle twitching, and tonic, clonic, generalized, or focal seizures. Electrocardiographic changes of T wave inversion and ST depression may occur. Total body Mg depletion may be confirmed by the use of a test measuring the excretion of an intravenous Mg load of 6 mg elemental Mg per kilogram of body weight; Mg-depleted subjects will excrete less than 60% of the infused Mg.

Hypermagnesemia should be suspected in depressed infants born of mothers who have received magnesium sulfate therapy. Depending on the severity of the hypermagnesemia, the signs may include neuromuscular depression, hypotension (usually at Mg levels above 4 to 6 mg/dl in adults), difficulty in urination (above 5 mg/dl), CNS depression (above 6 to 8 mg/dl), respiratory depression, and coma (above 12 to 17 mg/dl). Electrocardiographic signs include tachycardia or bradycardia and increased atrioventricular and ventricular contraction time.

Treatment

Hypomagnesemia should not be treated with Ca or vitamin D, which may cause further decrease in serum Mg. Therapy with Mg salt is the treatment of choice. The average amount of magnesium sulfate required in the neonate is 0.25 ml/kg of body weight of a 50% solution (100 mg of elemental Mg/ml) given intramuscularly. Electroencephalographic monitoring during intravenous Mg salt therapy is unlikely to show dramatic changes in electroencephalographic patterns. The dose of Mg can be repeated in conjunction with twice-daily monitoring of serum Mg levels during the first few days. Maintenance 50% magnesium sulfate (0.25 ml/kg) may be given orally daily. Four to five times higher doses may be required in malabsorptive states, although diarrhea may ensue with these doses.

In hypermagnesemic conditions, supportive therapy is usually sufficient, since the Mg excess is gradually removed through urinary excretion. Adequate hydration is important to ensure adequate urinary flow. In hypermagnesemia associated with neuromuscular depression, diuretic therapy might be attempted, since in adults organic mercurials and ethacrynic acid diuretics increase Mg excretion; this mode of therapy, however, is unproved in the neonate. Exchange blood transfusions may be useful in severe depression by removing the excess Mg from the infant's blood.

Reginald C. Tsang
Jean J. Steichen

BIBLIOGRAPHY
Calcium and magnesium physiology

Anast, C., and others: Evidence for parathyroid failure in magnesium deficiency, Scinece 177:606, 1972.

Avioli, L.V., and Haddad, J.G.: Vitamin D: current concepts, Metabolism 22:507, 1973.

Comar, C.L.: Radiocalcium studies in pregnancy, Ann. N.Y. Acad. Sci. 64:281, 1956.

Foster, G.V., Byfield, P.G.H., and Gudmundsson, T.V.: Calcitonin, J. Clin. Endocrinol. Metab. 1:93, 1972.

Garel, J.M., Care, A.D., and Barlet, J.P.: A radioimmunoassay for ovine calcitonin: an evaluation of calcitonin secretion during gestation, lactation and foetal life, J. Endocrinol. 62:497, 1974.

Garel, J.M., and Dumont, C.: Distribution and inactivation of labelled parathyroid hormone in rat fetus, Horm. Metab. Res. 4:217, 1972.

Garel, J.M., and Tarlet, M.P.: The effects of calcitonin and parathormone on plasma magnesium levels before and after birth in the rat, J. Endocrinol. 61:1, 1974.

Haddad, J.G., Jr., Bousseau, V., and Avioli, L.V.: Placental transfer of vitamin D_3 and 25-hydroxycholecalciferol in the rat, J. Lab. Clin. Med. 77:908, 1971.

Littledike, E.T., Arnaud, C.D., and Whipp, S.C.: Calcitonin secretion in ovine, porcine, and bovine fetuses, Proc. Soc. Exp. Biol. Med. 139:428, 1972.

Miller, E.R., and others: Mineral balance studies with the baby pig: effects of dietary vitamin D_2 level upon calcium, phosphorus and magnesium balance, J. Nutr. 85:255, 1965.

Minton, S.D., Steichen, J.J., and Tsang, R.C.: Bone mineralization in term and preterm appropriate for gestational age infants, J. Pediatr. 95:1037, 1979.

Omdahl, J.L., and DeLuca, H.F.: Regulation of vitamin D metabolism and function, Physiol. Rev. 53:327, 1973.

Parsons, J.A., and Potts, J.T.: Physiology and chemistry of parathyroid hormone, J. Clin. Endocrinol. Metab. 1:33, 1973.

Ramberg, C.F., Jr., and others: Kinetic analysis of calcium transport across the placenta, J. Appl. Physiol. 35:682, 1973.

Richardson, J.A., and Welt, L.G.: The hypomagnesemia of vitamin D administration, Proc. Soc. Exp. Biol. Med. 118:512, 1965.

Schedewie, H., and others: Placental crossover and fetal tissue distribution of 1,25(OH) vitamin D in rhesus monkey (abstr.), Pediatr. Res. 14:580, 1980.

Scothorne, R.J.: Functional capacity of fetal parathyroid glands with reference to their clinical use as homografts, Ann. N.Y. Acad. Sci. 120:669, 1964.

Shami, Y., and Radde, I.C.: The effect of the Ca/Mg concentration on placental (Ca/Mg)-ATPase activity, Biochim. Biophys. Acta 255:665, 1972.

Smith, F.G., Jr., and others: Fetal response to parathyroid hormone in sheep, J. Appl. Physiol. 27:276, 1969.

Smith, F.G., Jr., and others: Parathyroid hormone in foetal and adult sheep: the effect of hypocalcemia, J. Endocrinol. 53:339, 1972.

Steichen, J.J., Gratton, T.L., and Tsang, R.C.: Osteopenia of prematurity: the cause and possible treatment, J. Pediatr. 96:528, 1980.

Steichen, J.J. and others: Elevated serum $1,25(OH)_2$ vitamin D concentrations in rickets of prematurity, J. Pediatr. 99:293, 1981.

Steichen, J.J., and others: Vitamin D homeostasis in the perinatal period: 1,25-dihydroxy vitamin D in maternal, cord and neonatal blood, N. Engl. J. Med. 302:315, 1980.

Swaminathan, R., and others: The relationship between food, gastrointestinal hormones and calcitonin secretion, J. Endocrinol. **59**:217, 1973.

Hypocalcemia

Bergman, L., Kjellmer, I., and Selstam, U.: Calcitonin and parathyroid hormone: relation to early neonatal hypocalcemia in infants of diabetic mothers, Biol. Neonate **24**:1, 1974.

Brown, D.R., Tsang, R.C., and Chen, I.-W.: Oral calcium supplementation in premature and asphyxiated neonates, J. Pediatr. **89**:973, 1976.

Colletti, R.B., and others: Detection of hypocalcemia in susceptible neonates, N. Engl. J. Med. **290**:931, 1974.

Fanconi, A., and Prader, A.: Transient congenital idiopathic hypoparathyroidism, Helv. Paediatr. Acta **22**:342, 1967.

Hillman, L.S., and Haddad, J.G.: Perinatal vitamin D metabolism. II. Serial 25-hydroxy-vitamin D concentrations in sera of term and premature infants, J. Pediatr. **86**:928, 1975.

Linarelli, L.G., Bobik, J., and Bobik, C.: Newborn urinary cyclic AMP and developmental responsiveness to parathyroid hormone, Pediatrics **50**:14, 1972.

Scriver, C.R.: Commentary: vitamin D dependency, Pediatrics **45**:361, 1976.

Tsang, R.C., and Brown, D.R.: Calcium and magnesium in premature infants and infants of diabetic mothers. In Seelig, M.S., editor: Nutritional imbalances in infant and adult disease, New York, 1977, Spectrum Press.

Tsang, R.C., and others: Hypocalcemia in infants of diabetic mothers: studies in Ca, P, and Mg metabolism and in parathormone responsiveness, J. Pediatr. **80**:384, 1972.

Tsang, R.C., and others: Neonatal parathyroid function: role of gestational and postnatal age, J. Pediatr. **83**:728, 1973.

Tsang, R.C., and others: Possible pathogenic factors in neonatal hypocalcemia of prematurity, J. Pediatr. **82**:423, 1973.

Tsang, R.C., and others: Neonatal hypocalcemia in birth asphyxia, J. Pediatr. **84**:428, 1974.

Tsang, R.C., and others: Parathyroid function in infants of diabetic mothers, J. Pediatr. **86**:399, 1975.

Tsang, R.C., and others: Studies in calcium metabolism in infants with intrauterine growth retardation, J. Pediatr. **86**:936, 1975.

Hypercalcemia

Fanconi, G., and others: Chronische Hypercalcamie kombiniert mit osteosklerose Hyperazotamie, Minderwuchs und kongenitalen Missbildungen, Helv. Paediatr. Acta **7**:314, 1952.

Fellers, F.X., and Schwartz, R.: Etiology of the severe form of idiopathic hypercalcemia of infancy, N. Enlg. J. Med. **259**:1050, 1958.

Foley, T.P., and others: Familial benign hypercalcemia, J. Pediatr. **81**:1060, 1972.

Fraser, D.: The relation between infantile hypercalcemia and vitamin D—public health implications in North America, Pediatrics **40**:1050, 1967.

Friedman, W.F., and Mills, L.F.: The relationship between vitamin D and the craniofacial and dental anomalies of the supravalvular aortic stenosis syndrome, Pediatrics **43**:12, 1969.

Gerloczy, F., and Farkas, K.: Hyperparathyroidism in a newborn: mother with chronic hypoparathyroidism, Acta Med. Acad. Sci. Hung. **4**:73, 1953.

Goldbloom, R.B., Gillis, D.A., and Prasad, M.: Hereditary parathyroid hyperplasia: a surgical emergency of early infancy, Pediatrics **49**:514, 1972.

Grantmyer, E.B.: Roentgenographic features of "primary hyperparathyroidism in infancy," J. Can. Assoc. Radiol. **24**:257, 1973.

Hillman, D.A., and others: Neonatal familial primary hyperparathyroidism, N. Engl. J. Med. **270**:483, 1964.

Juif, J.-G., and others: L'hypercalcemie associée á un nephroblastome: syndrome paraneoplasique chez le jeune enfant, Arch. Fr. Pediatr. **31**:553, 1974.

Kaplan, E.: The parathyroid gland in infancy, Arch. Pathol. **34**:1042, 1942.

Landing, B.H., and Kamoshita, S.: Congenital hyperparathyroidism secondary to maternal hypoparathyroidism, J. Pediatr. **77**:842, 1970.

Lightwood, R., and Payne, W.W.: Discussion of British Paediatric Association: proceedings of twenty-third general meeting, Arch. Dis. Child. **27**:297, 1952.

Michael, A.F., Hong, R., and West, C.: Hypercalcemia in infancy associated with subcutaneous fat necrosis and calcifications, Am. J. Dis. Child. **104**:235, 1962.

Najjar, S.S., Aftimos, S.F., and Kurani, R.F.: Furosemide therapy for hypercalcemia in infants, J. Pediatr. **81**:1171, 1972.

Pratt, E.L., Geren, B.B., and Neuhasure, E.B.D.: Hypercalcemia and idiopathic hyperplasia of the parathyroid glands in an infant, J. Pediatr. **30**:388, 1947.

Seelig, M.S.: Vitamin D and cardiovascular, renal and brain damage in infancy and childhood, Ann. N.Y. Acad. Sci. **147**:537, 1969.

Tsang, R.C., and others: Parathyroid function tests with EDTA in infancy and childhood, J. Pediatr. **88**:250, 1976.

Magnesium disturbances

Anast, C.S.: Serum magnesium levels in the newborn, Pediatrics **33**:969, 1964.

Dancis, J., Springer, D., and Cohlan, S.A.: Fetal homeostasis in maternal malnutrition. II. Magnesium deprivation, Pediatr. Res. **55**:131, 1971.

Donovan, E.F., and others: Neonatal hypermagnesemia: effect on parathyroid hormone and calcium homeostasis, J. Pediatr. **96**:305, 1980.

Harris, I., and Wilkinson, A.W.: Magnesium depletion in children, Lancet **2**:735, 1971.

Jukarainen, E.: Plasma magnesium levels during the first five days of life, Acata Paediatr. Scand. **222**(suppl.):1, 1971.

Lipsitz, P.J.: The clinical and biochemical effects of excess magnesium in the newborn, Pediatrics **47**:501, 1971.

Paunier, L., and others: Primary hypomagnesemia with secondary hypocalcemia in an infant, Pediatrics **41**:355, 1968.

Skyberg, D., and others: Neonatal hypomagnesemia with selective malabsorption of magnesium: a clinical entity, Scand. J. Clin. Invest. **21**:355, 1968.

Stone, S.R., and Pritchard, J.A.: Effect of maternally administered magnesium sulfate on the neonate, Obstet. Gynecol. **35**:574, 1970.

Suh, S.M., and others: Pathogenesis of hypocalcemia in primary hypomagnesemia: normal end-organ responsiveness to parathyroid hormone and impaired parathyroid gland function, J. Clin. Invest. **52**:153, 1973.

Tsang, R.C.: Neonatal magnesium disturbances: a review, Am. J. Dis. Child. **124**:282, 1972.

Tsang, R.C., and others: Hypomagnesemia in infants of diabetic mothers: perinatal studies, J. Pediatr. **89**:115, 1976.

PART THREE
Thyroid disorders

Thyroid disorders of neonates must be considered in the light of many physiologic factors that influence the fetal and neonatal thyroid function. These include embryogenesis of thyroid, action of thyroid hormones, synthesis and transport of these hormones, regulatory mechanisms of thyroid function, fetal-maternal relationships, and the dynamic alteration of thyroid function with birth.

EMBRYOGENESIS OF THYROID

The major portion of human thyroid originates from the median anlage, which arises from the pharyngeal floor and is identifiable in the 17-day-old embryo. Initially, the median anlage is in close contact with the endothelial tubes of the embryonic heart. Following the descent of the heart the rapidly growing median thyroid is progressively pulled caudally until it reaches its definitive level in front of the second to sixth tracheal ring. The pharyngeal region contracts to become a narrow stalk, the thyroglossal duct, which subsequently atrophies. The descent of the heart may influence the downward movement of thyroid because of its topographic contact. Usually the median anlage grows caudally so that no lumen is left in the tract of its descent. Ectopic thyroid and persistent thyroglossal duct or cyst are the results of abnormalities of the thyroid descent. The lateral parts of the descending median anlage expand to form the thyroid lobes and the isthmus.

The second anlage of the thyroid is composed of a pair of ultimobranchial bodies arising from caudal extension of the fourth pharyngeal pouch. This anlage is initially connected to the pharynx by the ductus pharyngobranchialis IV (late seventh week). Subsequently the pharyngeal connection is lost and the ductal lumen becomes obliterated. The ultimobranchial bodies are incorporated into the expanding lateral lobes of the median anlage. The contribution of ultimobranchial bodies to the ultimate thyroid tissue is small, and its differentiation appears to require the influence of the median anlage. There is evidence to suggest that the cells arising from ultimobranchial bodies are identifiable as parafollicular cells or C-cells in mammals and that these cells are the source of thyrocalcitonin.

By the latter part of the tenth week the histiogenesis of the thyroid is virtually complete, although the follicles do not contain colloid. A single layer of epithelial cells surrounds the follicular lumen. Thyroxine has been detected in the serum of a 78-day-old fetus. Thus the fetal thyroid contributes to the fetal requirement of thyroidal hormones by the beginning of the second trimester. The pituitary regulatory mechanism of the fetal thyroid may begin to operate at this stage, as evidenced by the detection of TSH in the fetal blood.

PHYSIOLOGIC ACTION OF THYROID HORMONES

The principal functions of the thyroid are to synthesize, store, and release the thyroid hormones, thyroxine (T_4) and triiodothyronine (T_3), into the circulation. T_3 has one less iodine atom than T_4 and is more potent than T_4 in its physiologic action; this is caused by its greater speed of action rather than a qualitative difference in its metabolic effects. Therefore physiologic action of these two hormones need not be considered separately.

One of the principal actions of T_4 is to stimulate the rate of cellular oxidation in a large variety of tissues, leading to increased oxygen consumption, liberation of carbon dioxide, and production of heat. Changes in the basal metabolic rate (BMR) in hypothyroidism and hyperthyroidism are well known. This action of T_4 may be mediated through increased microsomal protein synthesis. Clinically, the calorigenic action of T_4 affects the circulation by increasing the heart rate, stroke volume and cardiac output. The pulse pressure is widened mainly by a decrease in the diastolic pressure and by some elevation in the systolic pressure. Circulation time is shortened. In hypothyroidism the ECG may show decreased voltage of all complexes, prolongation of the PR interval, and depression or inversion of the T wave. The effect on the ECG, however, may be secondary to myxedema of the myocardium.

T_4 affects protein metabolism. There is a negative nitrogen balance in hyperthyroidism, unless the patient is protected by adequate caloric intake to cover the increased energy requirement. In severe hypothyroidism, deposition of a mucoprotein containing hyaluronic acid occurs in extracellular myxedematous fluid.

T_4 influences the incorporation of creatine into the phosphocreatine cycle. In hypothyroidism there is an excessive storage of creatine, and in hyperthyroidism the urinary excretion of creatine is increased. However, the total excretion of creatine and creatinine is not affected by T_4. Thus T_4 changes the urinary creatine to creatinine ratio; creatine accounts for 10% to 30% in the normal child, 0% to 10% in hypothyroidism, and 25% to 65% in hyperthyroidism.

The effect of T_4 on lipid metabolism is seen in the elevated serum cholesterol level in hypothyroidism, except in infants. The total neutral fats, fatty acids, and phospholipids of the serum also are increased in hypothyroidism.

T_4 also affects the metabolism of carbohydrates, calcium, vitamins, and water and the liver function. The rate of glucose absorption and use is increased by T_4. In hypothyroidism, hypercalcemia may occur, the serum carotene level may be high, and the glucuronic acid conjugation mechanism of the liver may be impaired. Retention of water in the extracellular compartment occurs in hypothyroidism, producing the myxedematous fluid. In hyperthyroidism, on the other hand, increased calcium excretion in the urine and feces may lead to demineralization of the bones.

Another principal action of T_4 and T_3 is their effect on growth and development. Thyroidectomy in neonatal monkeys results in defective growth and development of the brain, and in untreated cretinism, mental retardation often ensues. The degree of mental retardation in cretinism is related to the severity and duration of the hypothyroid state of the infant whose brain is growing. The brain is more susceptible to lack of the thyroid hormones during its rapid growth and development, whereas defective growth and permanent damage do not occur if hypothyroidism begins after morphologic maturation of the brain is completed.

Other aspects of growth and development also require thyroid hormones. When hypothyroidism occurs in childhood, dental eruption, linear growth, and skeletal maturation are retarded. The retardation of skeletal maturation results in immature skeletal proportions and immature facial contours and contributes to the characteristic body configuration of hypothyroidism, which is different from that seen in stunted growth caused by isolated growth hormone deficiency. Ossification of cartilage is also disturbed in hypothyroidism. This produces the characteristic picture of epiphyseal dysgenesis in roentgenograms of the ossifying epiphyseal centers.

T_4 also affects the peripheral nerves. In hypothyroidism the relaxation phase of the ankle and knee jerk reflexes is prolonged. In hyperthyroidism, sympathetic and autonomic response may be exaggerated.

In addition to the classic thyroid hormones, T_4 and T_3, a calcium-lowering principle is found in the thyroid gland, thyrocalcitonin or calcitonin. Although thyrocalcitonin has hypocalcemic and hypophosphatemic actions when administered to humans, its physiologic role is not yet understood. Thyroidectomy does not lead to hypercalcemia.

SYNTHESIS, RELEASE, TRANSPORT, AND UTILIZATION OF THYROID HORMONES

The biologically active thyroid hormones, L-thyroxine (T_4) and 3,5,3'-triiodothyronine (T_3), are iodinated amino acids. Their synthesis occurs exclusively within the follicular cells. Iodine is supplied to the body mainly through dietary intake. However, it can be absorbed readily from the skin and lungs. Thus application of iodine-containing ointment or lotion to the skin can result in misleadingly high protein-bound iodine (PBI) levels. Although some organic iodine compounds, including T_4 and T_3, can be absorbed unchanged from the gastrointestinal tract, most are reduced and absorbed as ionic iodide. Generally, one fourth to one third of ingested iodide is taken up by the thyroid, which constitutes the basis for ^{131}I uptake studies. This iodide-trapping mechanism involves an active transport process, an iodide pump that is dependent on oxidative phosphorylation. The iodide pump is present both at the basal and apical surfaces of follicular cells, the former serving to concentrate iodide into the cells from the extracellular space and the latter serving to pump iodide into the follicular lumen as a secondary reservoir. The mechanism is capable of maintaining the intrathyroidal iodide concentration some 20-fold to 100-fold higher than that of serum. In one type of goitrous cretinism there is a defect in this iodide transport mechanism.

Immediately on entering the follicular cells, iodide is oxidized to an active form for iodination of thyroglobulin, probably by a peroxidase enzyme system. Thyroglobulin, a glycoprotein, is synthesized by the ribosomes of the follicular cells and is then secreted into the follicular lumen. Almost all of the iodine taken up by the thyroid is rapidly incorporated into the 3-position and the 5-position of the many tyrosyl residues of thyroglobulin to form monoiodotyrosine (MIT) and diiodotyrosine (DIT). Once iodide is organically bound to the tyrosyl residues, it can no longer be released readily from the thyroid. Defects in the iodide organification can be seen in two types of goitrous cretinism.

Synthesis of T_3 requires coupling between MIT and DIT molecules, accompanied by elimination of an alanine residue. T_4 is formed by coupling between two molecules of DIT. These reactions occur within the structure of thyroglobulin and involve oxidative processes. Several patients with goitrous hypothyroidism caused by a coupling defect have been described.

Secretion of T_4 and T_3 into the circulation requires liberation of these moieties from the peptide bonds. Thyroglobulin molecules pass from the lumen of the follicles into the follicular cells where proteolysis takes place. Congenital hypothyroidism may occur as a result of abnormal proteolysis of thyroglobulin. Of the approximately 125 tyrosyl residues in the thyroglobulin, only 10 or so form iodothyronines, whereas another 20 consist of MIT and DIT. Following proteolysis of thyroglobulin, the freed MIT and DIT are deiodinated by the iodotyrosine deionidase, and the liberated iodide is reused by the thyroid for iodination. A defective deiodination mechanism of free iodotyrosines results in depletion of iodine as these iodine-containing molecules are released into the circulation and wastage of these compounds as they are subsequently excreted into the urine. This results in goitrous cretinism.

T_4 and T_3 secreted into the circulation are transported by loosely attaching, through noncovalent bonds, to the plasma proteins. Three proteins play a role in the transport system. Over 75% of T_4 is normally bound to thyroxine-binding globulin (TBG). The second carrier protein is the T_4-binding prealbumin (TBPA); only about 15% of T_4 is bound to TBPA. The third protein is the serum albumin, which usually carries less than 10% of the circulating T_4. Whereas T_4 binds with all three proteins, T_3 binds only with TBG and albumin, and its intensity of binding is considerably less than that of T_4. The protein-bound thyroid hormones are biologically inactive and are in equilibrium with active non-protein-bound hormones. Although quantitatively insignificant, the non-protein-bound thyroxine or free thyroxine (FT_4) concentration more accurately indicates the metabolic status of the individual, since only FT_4 can enter the cells and exert its effect. If the capacity of TBG is increased, a rise in the concentration of total hormone will follow, and the concentration of free hormone will be maintained at the normal level.

The exact mechanism by which free T_4 exerts its biologic effect is not known. Recent studies suggest that a significant proportion of T_4 undergoes peripheral deiodination to produce T_3. There is a growing body of evidence to suggest that T_3, derived mainly from peripheral conversion of T_4, is the principal functional thyroid hormone. Catabolism of iodothyronines involves further deiodination, deamination, decarboxylation, and conjugation.

REGULATORY MECHANISM OF THYROID FUNCTION

The major control mechanism of thyroid function is the hypothalamic-pituitary-thyroid axis. The basophilic cells of the anterior pituitary gland produce and store TSH, which is a glycoprotein capable of rapidly increasing the intrathyroidal cyclic adenosine monophosphate (cyclic AMP). It causes increased uptake of iodine by the thyroid, accelerates virtually all steps of iodothyronine synthesis and release, and increases the size and vascularity of the thyroid gland. It has been suggested that these changes may be mediated by the increase in cyclic AMP. The secretion and the plasma level of TSH are inversely related to the levels of free (non-protein-bound) thyroid hormones. The inhibitory feedback action of free iodothyronines involves a direct action of these hormones on the pituitary gland without involving the hypothalamus. Thus the secretion of TSH is directly regulated through an intrinsic mechanism of the pituitary gland that is sensitive to the levels of free iodothyronines. However, the hypothalamus does influence TSH secretion. The hypothalamus secretes TRH, which stimulates the release of TSH by the pituitary gland. TRH is a tripeptide, L-pyroglutamyl-L-histidyl-L-proline-amide. Although the precise anatomic locations of TRH biosynthesis are not known, TRH synthetase is found in the median eminence and ventral and dorsal hypothalamus. When TRH is infused, it rapidly stimulates the release of TSH into the circulation, and the plasma TSH reaches a peak value in 20 to 30 minutes. The plasma half-life of TRH is extremely short and probably does not exceed 4 minutes. Exposure to cold environment increases TRH synthetase activity. TRH synthetase activity is reduced in hypothyroid animals and is increased in hyperthyroid animals. The hypothalamus may regulate the set point of feedback control as a thermostat through TRH, with iodothyronines playing a positive feedback role in TRH synthesis. This control probably operates in neonates whose circulating TSH becomes rapidly elevated after parturition. Administration of TRH stimulates the secretion of prolactin and HGH in addition to the release of TSH. In the majority of children with idiopathic hypopituitarism, TSH release after TRH administration is normal, indicating an impaired TRH secretion rather than a primary TSH deficiency. TRH-mediated TSH release can be augmented by administration of theophylline or estradiol and may be blunted by administration of L-dopa or glucocorticoids. However, clinically significant hypothyroidism rarely, if ever, occurs following prolonged administration of large amounts of glucocorticoids or ACTH.

In addition to the hypothalamic-pituitary regulation, the thyroid is responsive to an intrinsic autoregulatory mechanism, the intrathyroidal iodide, which compensates for the fluctuation in dietary iodine intake.

COMMONLY USED CHEMICAL THYROID FUNCTION TESTS
Protein-bound iodine

In the PBI test, serum or plasma proteins are precipitated, organic iodine is converted to iodide, and the total iodide is quantitated. Usually, T_4 accounts for 80% to 90% of the PBI. Since this test measures the total iodide, it is influenced not only by the T_4 levels but also by the levels of inorganic iodine, organic iodine (including MIT and DIT), and iodothyronine-binding proteins. Administration of T_3 results in a fall of PBI; it suppresses the endogenous T_4 secretion, and it contributes little to the serum iodine, since it is administered in small quantities because of its much greater biologic activity compared with T_4. The availability of T_4-binding sites on TBG also affects the PBI. Phenytoin (Dilantin) competes with T_4 at the TBG-binding sites, while phenytoin and salicylates displace T_4 from the TBPA-binding sites. Thus these drugs are capable of depressing the PBI value.

T_4-column

The most commonly used procedure employs an anion-exchange resin to separate the protein-bound T_4

from other organic and inorganic iodine in serum or plasma. The eluted fraction containing T_4 obtained from this chromatographic step is subjected to quantitative iodide determination. This iodide content is referred to as thyroxine-iodine (T_4-I). The T_4-I measured by this method is approximately 10% to 25% less than the PBI value. The difference between PBI and T_4-I values is often increased in goitrous cretinism due to inborn errors of T_4 synthesis, hyperthyroidism, and thyroiditis because of the release of hormonally inactive iodoproteins into the circulation. Although iodotyrosines and most of the inorganic and organic iodines do not interfere with T_4-I determination, organic iodine is not completely eliminated. Nevertheless, this method is superior in its specificity to that of PBI. Changes in the T_4-binding capacity of the plasma proteins affect T_4-I measured by this method as in the PBI. Inorganic iodine, which crosses the placental barrier, administered in a large dose can falsely elevate T_4-I through nonspecific iodination of plasma proteins. Iodine contamination also occurs from iodinated dyes used as x-ray contrast media. Iophenoxic acid (Teridax), formerly used for gallbladder series, has been shown to cross the placenta and interfere with T_4 determination for many years.

T_4 by competitive protein binding (Murphy-Pattee test)

The Murphy-Pattee method of assessing T_4-I does not depend on iodine determination. The method involves reacting a crude extract of the patient's T_4 with standardized human TBG saturated with radioactive T_4. The T_4 in the extract competitively displaces the radioactive T_4 from TBG in proportional amounts. The bound and the newly freed radioactive T_4 are separated, and the radioactivity in each fraction is measured. Comparison of these measurements against a standard curve permits the patient's T_4 level to be expressed in terms of µg of T_4-I per deciliter. The value obtained by the Murphy-Pattee method is identical to that obtained by the T_4-column assay in the absence of an interfering substance. The nature of the competitive protein-binding assay eliminates interference by exogenous iodinated substances. However, interference by changes in T_4-binding capacity of the plasma proteins, including the competitive displacement of endogenous T_4 from the binding proteins by phenytoin, salicylates, and T_3, affect the Murphy-Pattee test. The normal values in the neonatal period range from 8.2 to 16.6 µg T_4 per deciliter.

T_4 determination by radioimmunoassay

Development of a radioimmunoassay for T_4 has largely replaced the use of PBI and T_4-I as routine thyroid function tests. The T_4-binding antiserum is produced by immunizing rabbits against thyroglobulin. Unextracted serum is incubated with the antiserum in the presence of radioactive T_4 (^{125}I-T_4). This incubation is carried out in a solution containing 8-anilino-1-naphthalene-sulfonic acid (ANS), which displaces T_4 from TBG and makes both the unlabeled and radioactive T_4 available for reaction with T_4-binding antiserum. T_4, freed from TBG and TBPA in the specimen, competes with the ^{125}I-T_4 for the binding sites on the antiserum in proportion to its total amounts. The ^{125}I-T_4 bound to the antiserum is then separated from the free ^{125}I-$T_4$4, and comparison of ^{125}I-T_4 in these two fractions against a standard curve permits the patient's T_4 level to be expressed in micrograms per deciliter. Although the principles involved in T_4 determination by radioimmunoassay are similar to those of the Murphy-Pattee method, radioimmunoassay procedure does not require an initial extraction step and leads to a greater precision. Furthermore, this procedure requires only a very small quantity of blood (< 50 µl). These advantages have been exploited for screening neonates for possible hypothyroidism. Furthermore, T_4 by radioimmunoassay is affected by fewer interfering factors than either T_4 by column or competitive protein binding (CPB). However, as in T_4 by CPB, radioactivity in the samples can interfere with the assay. Other interfering factors include D-isomer of T_4, hyperbilirubinemia, and marked changes in TBG. Normal adult values of serum T_4 by radioimmunoassay are slightly higher than those by the CPB method (8.33 ± 2.42 S.D. for T_4 by radioimmunoassay, and 7.51 ± 1.90 S.D. for T_4 by CPB, in micrograms per deciliter).

Free thyroxine

The four methods just described largely measure the biologically inactive protein-bound T_4. In contrast, the minute amounts of free T_4 (FT_4) in the serum cannot be determined by conventional analytic technique. The method of estimating the FT_4 depends on the fact that the level of FT_4 is governed by an equilibrium between the levels of binding proteins, protein-bound T_4, and FT_4, following the law of mass action. FT_4 does not depend on the T_4-binding capacity as such, since a change in such capacity will soon be compensated by a concordant change in the amount of T_4 released from the thyroid. To estimate the FT_4, serum is equilibrated with a tracer dose of radioactive T_4, which apportions itself between free and bound forms in the same ratio as that of the endogenous hormone. The dialyzable fraction of the labeled serum contains the radioactive FT_4 in amounts proportional to the endogenous FT_4. The concentration of FT_4 in the serum is calculated as the product of the total T_4-I and the dialyzable fraction. In normal adult serum, FT_4 averages about 2 mμg/dl, although normal values vary from laboratory to laboratory because of different techniques used.

T_3 by radioimmunoassay

Development of T_3-binding antiserum by immunization of rabbits against T_3–bovine-serum–albumin conjugate allows application of radioimmunoassay principles to the measurements of total serum T_3 levels. The method is very similar to that of T_4 by radioimmunoassay, except that ^{125}I-T_3 is used. The published normal adult levels of total serum T_3 range from about 100 to 200 mμg/dl and are significantly lower in the cord blood.

Free T_3 (FT_3) concentration in serum or plasma also can be estimated by adopting a method similar to that used in FT_4 determination. FT_3 concentration is usually expressed in picograms per deciliter (pg/dl).

TSH by radioimmunoassay

Serum concentration of TSH can be measured by application of the radioimmunoassay principles. Unknown serum is mixed with ^{125}I-TSH, buffer, and rabbit antiserum to human TSH. TSH bound to the antibody is then separated from the unbound TSH. The ^{125}I-TSH measurements in these two fractions are compared with a curve obtained by use of a reference standard human TSH in various concentrations. The patient's serum TSH is expressed in units per milliliter of the reference standard. In general, the euthyroid values in adults are less than 3 μU to 10 μU/ml. TSH is elevated in primary hypothyroidism. There also is a surge of TSH release at parturition that reaches a peak within 2 hours after birth. TSH in the cord serum is usually less than 20 μU/ml, and concentrations of greater than 60 μU/ml are suggestive of congenital hypothyroidism. Thus TSH assay of the cord serum can provide a means for screening such infants. Because of the limitation in the sensitivity of the assay, it is difficult to distinguish euthyroid individuals from those with TSH deficiency or thyrotoxicosis by TSH by radioimmunoassay alone.

Assessment of thyroxine-binding protein saturation

T_3-resin uptake

A tracer dose of radioactive T_3, which competes for binding sites with the endogenous hormones, is added to the serum. When the specimen is passed through resin, the unbound radioactive T_3 is absorbed on the resin and can be measured by a radioassay. The amount of radioactive T_3 taken up by the resin is inversely proportional to the unsaturated T_4-binding capacity of the plasma proteins.

T_3-resin uptake is often expressed as a T_3-resin uptake ratio (T_3U ratio), which is a ratio between the T_3-resin uptake of the patient's serum and the T_3-resin uptake of a pool of normal serum. The normal value is about 1.0.

TBG test

Since the major portion of plasma T_4 is bound to TBG, measurement of the binding capacity of TBG gives a good approximation of T_4-binding protein capacity. In this method the serum is equilibrated with a large excess of radioactive T_4. By relating the proportion of radioactive T_4 in the TBG area to the T_4-I, it is possible to estimate the TBG values in terms of micrograms of T_4-binding capacity per deciliter of serum. The binding capacity of TBG is increased by estrogens and therefore in pregnancy and neonates. It may be increased in acute hepatitis and in a genetic disorder (p. 774). It is decreased by administration of androgens or glucocorticoids. In the nephrotic syndrome, chronic hepatic disease, and a sex-linked genetic disorder it also is decreased. Phenytoin competes with the T_4-binding sites of TBG and gives a falsely low value. In all these circumstances T_3-resin uptake is inversely related to the TBG test. T_3-resin uptake is increased by administration of salicylates, since this drug competes with T_4 at the TBPA-binding sites. More recently, a radioimmunoassay method for measurement of TBG has been developed. This method allows TBG concentration to be assessed directly in milligrams per deciliter.

THYROID FUNCTION: FETAL-MATERNAL RELATIONSHIP

T_4 is detectable in the fetal serum by the twelfth week of gestation. Thereafter, both the total T_4-I and FT_4 increase linearly in relation to the gestational age. The mean cord concentration of T_4 by radioimmunoassay between 20 and 30 weeks of gestation is 5.5 ± 1.6 (S.D.) μg/dl. At term the T_4-I reaches a level of 12.6 ± 4.0 (S.D.) μg/dl in the umbilical cord serum, which is 10% to 20% lower than the corresponding value in maternal serum and is also about 15% lower than the T_4 measured by radioimmunoassay. The FT_4 in the cord blood is equal to or higher than that in the maternal blood. Fetal T_4 metabolism differs markedly from that of postnatal life. In the fetus, T_4 is metabolized predominantly to reverse T_3 (RT_3), 3,3′,5′-triiodothyronine, rather than to T_3. The RT_3 has minimum metabolic activity compared to T_3. Thus serum concentrations and production rates of RT_3 are much higher in the fetus, whereas concentrations of both T_3 and FT_3 in the fetal circulation are lower than in adults. The T_3 and FT_3 levels in the cord blood have been shown to be 30% to 50% of the maternal concentrations at term. TSH is also present in the 12-week-old fetus and rapidly rises thereafter, paralleling the increas-

Table 33-3. Representative serum values of total and free thyroid hormones, TBG, and TSH in cord blood and early neonatal period compared with adult and maternal values*

References	Source of serum or age of infant	Number of subjects	T₄ (µg/dl)	FT₄ (mµg/dl)	T₃ (mµg/dl)	FT₃ (pg/dl)	TBG (mg/dl)	TSH (µU/ml)
Abuid, Stinson, and Larsen	Cord blood	7-8	12.0 ± 1.6	1.85 ± 0.22	49 ± 6	150 ± 20		
	15 minutes	5-6	13.3 ± 2.5		79 ± 13			
	90 minutes	7	14.1 ± 1.9		191 ± 16			
	24 hours	3-4	22.3 ± 1.6		262 ± 41			
	48 hours	3-4	21.9 ± 1.3		191 ± 37			
	Mothers at term	7-8	12.8 ± 1.4	1.40 ± 0.16	145 ± 12	310 ± 40		
Erenberg, Phelps, Lam, and Fisher	Cord blood	26	11.9 ± 0.41	2.9 ± 0.12	50.5 ± 3.6	146 ± 12	5.4 ± 0.47	
	60 minutes	8-12			293	863		
	24 hours	10-21	16.2		419	1260		
	36-48 hours	9		7.0				
	60-72 hours	7-19		6.0	220	620		
	5 days	6	12.6					
	Pregnant women	17	14.3 ± 0.66	2.7 ± 0.15	173.0 ± 8.4	398 ± 30	8.7 ± 0.58	
	Adults	40	8.3 ± 0.38	2.4 ± 0.12	122.0 ± 5.3	378 ± 27	3.5 ± 0.67	
Abuid, Klein, Foley, and Larsen	Cord blood	27-30	10.9 ± 0.3	2.23 ± 0.12	48 ± 3	130 ± 10		8.5 ± 0.7
	3 days	23-26	17.2 ± 0.5	4.87 ± 0.33	125 ± 8	410 ± 20		7.3 ± 1.0
	6 weeks	15	10.3 ± 0.4	2.07 ± 0.08	163 ± 6	400 ± 20		<2.5
	Mothers at term	8	12.8 ± 1.4	1.40 ± 0.16	145 ± 12	310 ± 40		
	Adults	11	8.8 ± 0.5	1.92 ± 0.10	112 ± 5	290 ± 20		

*T₄, T₃, TBG, and TSH were measured by RIA methods, and FT₄ and FT₃ by assessment of the dialyzable fractions. All values are the mean or mean ± standard error of the mean.

Table 33-4. Normal range for T_4, T_3, T_3 resin uptake, TBG, and TSH in infancy and childhood*

Age	Total T_4 (μg/dl) Mean	Range†	Total T_3 (ng/dl) Mean	Range†	T_3 resin uptake (%) Mean	Range†	TBG (mg/dl) Mean	Range†	TSH (μU/ml) Mean	Range†
Cord blood	10.2	7.4-13.0	45	15-75	0.90	0.75-1.05	5.6	—	9.0	<2.5-17.4
1 to 3 days	17.2	11.8-22.6	124	32-216	1.15	0.90-1.40	5.0	—	8.0	<2.5-13.3
1 to 2 weeks	13.2	9.8-16.6	250	—	1.00	0.85-1.15	—	—	—	—
2 to 4 weeks	11.0	7.0-15.0	160	160-240	0.95	0.80-1.15	—	—	4.0	0.6-10.0
1 to 4 months	10.3	7.2-14.4	163	117-209	0.90	0.75-1.05	—	—	<2.5	<2.5
4 to 12 months	11.0	7.8-16.5	176	110-280	0.98	0.88-1.12	4.4	3.1-5.6	2.1	0.6-6.3
1 to 5 years	10.5	7.3-15.0	168	105-269	0.99	0.88-1.12	4.2	2.9-5.4	2.0	0.6-6.3
5 to 10 years	9.3	6.4-13.3	150	94-241	1.00	0.88-1.12	3.8	2.5-5.0	2.0	0.6-6.3
10 to 15 years	8.1	5.6-11.7	113	83-213	1.01	0.88-1.12	3.3	2.1-4.6	1.9	0.6-6.3
Adult	8.4	4.3-12.5	125	70-204	1.01	0.85-1.14	3.5	2.1-5.5	1.8	0.2-7.6

*T_4, T_3, TSH, and TBG are measured by radioimmnoassay; T_4 results measured by competitive protein binding are 15% lower.
†Range equals ±2 S.D. from mean value.
From LaFranchi, S.H.: Pediatr. Clin. North Am. **26**:33, 1979.

ing levels of FT_4. It does not correlate with levels of fetal T_4-I or the maternal FT_4. The TSH level is higher in the fetus than in the mother, and at term the fetal value is more than twice that found in the mother. This suggests that fetal TSH regulates fetal thyroid function.

T_4-binding proteins also can be detected in the 12-week-old fetus. During early fetal life, T_4 seems to be bound mainly to the TBPA and albumin. The fetal concentration of TBG increases rapidly and by midgestation reaches a level close to that in a full-term infant. During early gestation the rise of fetal TBG parallels the increase in T_4-I, and the proportion of T_4 bound to TBG similarly increases during this period. The binding capacity of TBG in premature and full-term infants is close to one and one-half times that of the normal adult but is lower than that of the mother. The high level of TBG in the neonate is caused by a transplacental transfer of estrogens from the mother and, to a large extent, accounts for the high PBI or T_4-I values in these infants. The level of TBPA is low in both newborn and maternal sera. The TBPA probably plays a minor role after midgestation.

Shortly after birth a transient but marked hyperactivity occurs in the thyroid function of neonates (Tables 33-3 and 33-4). Within the first minutes of life a dramatic release of TSH occurs, reaching a peak level of approximately 100 μU/ml at 30 minutes of age. This hypersecretion of TSH persists with decreasing intensity over the following 24 to 72 hours. There is evidence that this acute rise of TSH may be stimulated, at least in part, by the drop in body temperature of the fetus with birth. In response to the postnatal TSH surge, the levels of PBI, T_4-I, FT_4, T_3, FT_3, and T_3-resin uptake increase progressively during the first hours of extrauterine life, reaching a peak by about 48 hours of age. The increase in serum T_3 and FT_3 is more marked than that of T_4 and FT_4 during this period. Thus neonates experience a physiologic hyperthyroid state during the first several days of life. Absence of such chemical hyperthyroid state constitutes strong evidence for congenital hypothyroidism. The levels of these thyroid hormones remain elevated during the first 2 weeks of life and gradually fall thereafter, reaching high normal adult values by 4 to 6 weeks of age. True adult levels are not reached until puberty (Table 33-4). The serum TBG levels remain essentially unchanged during the first 5 days of life.

Iodine kinetics in infants and children are also different from those in the adult. The thyroid weighs about 2 gm at birth, which is about one tenth of the adult weight. The 24-hour ^{131}I uptake by the thyroid is similar to that of the adult after the first month of age. Thus the concentration of ^{131}I per gram of thyroid tissue in the infant is greater than that in the adult. The thyroid of the infant is more susceptible to damage by radiation. The T_4 turnover rate is also higher in infants and children than in the adult. This accounts for the greater thyroid hormone requirement in children per unit of body weight.

In considering the fetal-maternal relationship, the placenta is of major importance. TSH does not cross the placental barrier. The placenta is almost completely impermeable to T_4 during the early stage of pregnancy, and at term the T_4 transport across the placenta is slow and limited. Thus the fetus during the first trimester either does not require T_4 for its growth and development or is totally dependent on small amounts of maternal T_4. During the later stages of gestation, the fetus is largely dependent on its own T_4 production. Iodides cross the placenta readily. Iodides or iodine, when given in a large quantity, produces a transient inhibition of T_4 synthesis by diminishing the iodination process, probably through its effect on thyroidal autoregulation. Thus, in rare instances, iodine given to the mother in large amounts has produced goiter in the offspring.

Other clinically important compounds that can affect the fetal thyroid function by crossing the placenta from mother to fetus are the antithyroid compounds (goitrogens) and the long-acting thyroid stimulator (LATS). The former include perchlorates and thionamide compounds such as thiourea, thiouracil, propylthiouracil, methimazole, and carbimazole. Transplacental transfer of these drugs can result in fetal goiter with or without hypothyroidism. LATS, a substance with certain characteristics of globulin, is produced in Graves' disease and stimulates the thyroid function in a manner similar to that of TSH. Transfer of LATS across the placenta into the fetus can result in neonatal thyrotoxicosis.

The amniotic fluid contains a high level of RT_3, reflecting the high production rate by the fetus by 15 weeks of gestation. However, it is not known whether the fetal thyroid status can be assessed by determining the level of RT_3 in the amniotic fluid. The T_4, T_3, and TSH levels in amniotic fluid do not correlate well with the fetal thyroid state.

In human milk, T_4 is present in insignificant amounts. The concentrations of T_3 and RT_3 in human milk vary considerably from specimen to specimen. However, it is suggested that the T_3 concentration in breast milk is insufficient to prevent the detrimental effects of hypothyroidism, although it may alleviate the symptoms in certain cases.

CONGENITAL HYPOTHYROIDISM (CRETINISM)

Congenital hypothyroidism, or cretinism, is a deficiency of the thyroid believed to have been present at or before birth. Cretinism must be diagnosed promptly because delay in treatment can lead to irreversible brain damage. Yet the overt signs of hypothyroidism are rarely present at birth, and abnormalities of thyroid function may be overlooked during the neonatal period. The dynamic changes in thyroid function following birth, the elevated levels of TBG in neonates, and the sudden deprivation of maternal T_4, however inefficient its transplacental transfer may be, all contribute to the difficulty in establishing a diagnosis.

Etiology and pathogenesis

The etiologic classification of congenital hypothyroidism is shown in the following outline. The term *sporadic cretinism* applies to all forms of primary congenital hypothyroidism, except those caused by dietary iodine deficiency and those caused by inborn errors of hormone synthesis or metabolism.

A. Primary hypothyroidism
   1. Defective embryogenesis of thyroid
      a. Agenesis (athyreosis)
      b. Dysgenesis
         (1) Thyroid remnant in normal location
         (2) Maldescent or ectopic thyroid gland
   2. Inborn error of hormone synthesis or metabolism (familial cretinism)
      a. Iodide-trapping defect
      b. Iodide organification defect
         (1) Without deafness
         (2) With deafness (Pendred's syndrome)
      c. Coupling defect of iodotyrosines
      d. Deiodination defect
         (1) Generalized
         (2) Limited to thyroid gland
         (3) Limited to peripheral tissues
      e. Defect of thyroglobulin
      f. Goiter with calcification
      g. Peripheral tissue unresponsiveness to thyroid hormone
      h. Unresponsiveness of thyroid to TSH
   3. Goitrous cretinism caused by maternal ingestion of goitrogens
   4. Iodine deficiency (endemic goiter)
B. Secondary hypothyroidism
   1. TSH deficiency
   2. TRH deficiency

In contrast to the clear-cut preponderance of thyroid disorders in females over males during childhood and adult life, there is no sex difference in the incidence of congenital hypothyroidism. The relative incidence of each type of cretinism varies widely in different geographic locations.

In the nongoitrous regions, *defective embryogenesis* of the thyroid accounts for 70% to 85% of all cretinism. Failure in the anatomic development of the thyroid gland may be complete or partial. Residual thyroid tissue in the normal position or in ectopic areas is detected in 60% to 80% of infants and children with hypothyroid. Ectopic thyroid is usually composed of a remnant of undescended thyroid tissue (cryptothyroid) and is situated in the midline. The undescended thyroid is located in the base of the tongue in about half the cases, between the tongue and the hyoid bone in about one fourth, and between the hyoid bone and normal location in the remaining cases. The ectopic tissue is often capable of undergoing compensatory hypertrophy when the hormone production becomes inadequate and may be found as a midline mass. The cause of defective embryogenesis of the thyroid is unknown. Dysgenesis of the thyroid can occasionally be a familial condition. Destruction of the fetal thyroid by maternal thyroid antibodies acquired transplacentally has been suggested as a possible etiologic factor in some instances of sporadic athyreotic cretinism. Genetically determined *errors of T_4 synthesis or metabolism* involve deficiency of one or more enzymes necessary at various stages of the biosynthetic and metabolic pathways. Impaired hormonal secretion results in hypersecretion of TSH, usually leading to compensatory hyperplasia of the thyroid. Hence familial cretinism is often referred to as goitrous cretinism. Hypothyroidism or goiter or both may or may not be present in the newborn and infant, depending on the degree and time of onset of hormonal deficiency. Family members of a goitrous cretin often are found to have less severe defects manifested by goiter without associated hypothyroidism. The exact enzyme defect in some goitrous cretins, including those assumed to result from defects in the coupling mechanism and thyroglobulin synthesis, is still unknown. Cretins caused by a *defect in the trapping of iodide* can be confused with infants with athyreosis because of the lack of administered radioiodine to concentrate in the neck. However, a goiter is present in these patients, and the saliva fails to concentrate radioiodine. The iodine-trapping defect is an autosomal recessive trait.

There are two types of *defects in the organification of iodide:* one in which iodide peroxidase is deficient and another in which an iodide transferase is lacking. The former is generally associated with more severe hypothyroidism. The latter is called *Pendred's syndrome* and is associated with congenital deafness and usually a small euthyroid goiter. Both types of iodide organification defects are transmitted as an autosomal recessive trait.

The mode of transmission of other inborn errors of thyroid hormone synthesis or metabolism has not been clearly established, although autosomal recessive inheritance has been suggested for most entities.

In the *coupling defect* of iodotyrosines, T_4 and T_3 are decreased, and MIT and DIT are increased in both the serum and thyroid gland. In patients with deiodination defects there is a rapid turnover of thyroid iodine and wastage of iodotyrosines into the urine. The defect may be generalized, or it may be limited to intrathyroid or peripheral deiodination.

A *defect in thyroglobulin synthesis* was postulated in patients who had abnormal iodoproteins in their sera. Other unusual types of familial cretinism include a large kindred with goiter characterized by extensive intrathyroid calcification. The transmission pattern in this family suggests an autosomal dominant trait. A family with possible inability of the peripheral tissue to respond to T_4 also has been reported. The affected members of this family had deaf-mutism, goiter, delayed bone maturation, and elevated levels of PBI.

Unresponsiveness of the thyroid to TSH have been reported in two boys who had congenital hypothyroidism without a goiter. The serum TSH was elevated in these individuals, and TSH stimulation test gave no response. A coupling abnormality between the TSH receptor and the TSH receptor–adenylate cyclase system was suggested as the pathogenetic process.

Maternal *ingestion of antithyroid drugs*, especially the thiocarbamides and potassium perchlorate, can cause neonatal goitrous hypothyroidism. Although the correlation between the dosage of drug and the incidence of neonatal goiter is poor, prolonged administration of large doses of these drugs increases the risk of goitrous cretinism. Administration of inorganic iodides to the mother in large amounts, usually for treatment of various respiratory disorders, can also produce a large congenital goiter filled with colloid (Fig. 33-24). Radioiodine treatment given to pregnant women during the second trimester has resulted in hypothyroidism in the offspring. The hypothyroidism was not obvious at birth in most instances.

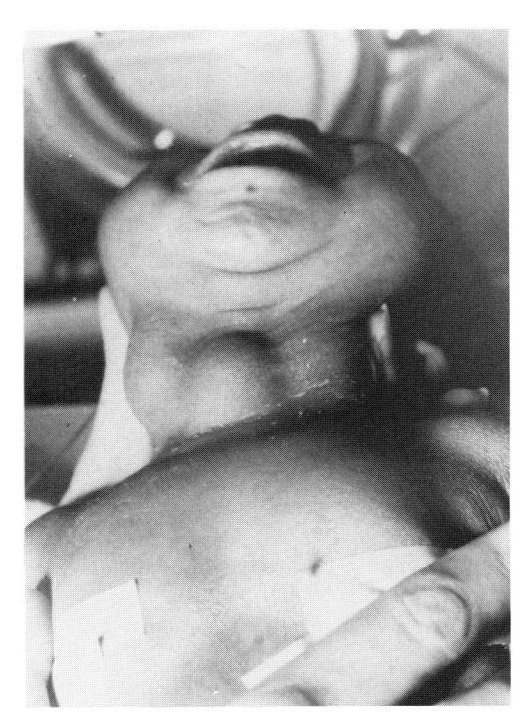

Fig. 33-24. Iodine-induced goiter in a neonate. The lateral bulging of the neck is caused by enlarged lateral lobes of the thyroid.

Endemic goiter occurs in large land areas where dietary iodine is deficient. However, the incidence of goiter in neonates is relatively low in these areas, and many individuals living in the same environment do not develop goiter. These observations suggest that there may be other factors superimposed on iodine deficiency.

Secondary hypothyroidism has been considered to be extremely rare in neonates. However, an increasing number of such infants have been discovered in recent years through neonatal thyroid screening programs. The majority of these patients have TRH deficiency resulting in low serum levels of T_4 and TSH, but they do respond to TRH infusion by a sharp rise in circulating TSH. TSH deficiency is rare in neonates. Pituitary aplasia, when

Table 33-5. Incidence of various neonatal hypothyroidism and TBG deficiency

	Primary hypothyroid			Secondary hypothyroid	Transient hypothyroid	TBG deficiency
Aplastic or hypoplastic gland (63%)	1 in 4,254	Normal or enlarged gland (14%)	Ectopic thyroid tissue (23%)	1 in 68,200	1 in 37,370	1 in 8,913

present, is usually associated with anencephaly or other severe malformations of the brain. These patients rarely survive beyond the neonatal period.

Neonatal screening for hypothyroidism and incidence of congenital hypothyroidism

The availability of highly sensitive and specific radioimmunoassay systems for T_4 and TSH led to the development of screening programs for neonatal hypothyroidism. During the past few years a number of states in the United States and provinces in Canada have mandated such screening through legislation, and screening programs have been established in Europe and Japan.

Most, if not all, programs in the United States use the filter paper spot technique. Capillary blood specimens from a heel stick are obtained at 2 to 5 days of life. The filter paper designed for this purpose bears printed circles. Blood samples are placed in these circular areas so as to fill and saturate the areas. Initially T_4 is measured from these specimens. Specimens that fall in the lowest, approximately third, percentile are subsequently subjected to TSH determinations. This method has the following advantages: (1) it can be easily incorporated into the existing metabolic-genetic screening programs (e.g., phenylketonuria screening); (2) it provides for a comprehensive screening capable of identifying infants with primary hypothyroidism and those at risk for secondary hypothyroid and TBG deficiency; (3) the selectivity is high, since the acute physiologic increase of T_4 at 2 to 5 days of life is lacking in hypothyroid infants; (4) it will detect most of the cases of compensated hypothyroidism; (5) it has the lowest recall rate of 1% to 2%; and (6) it appears to be capable of detecting nearly all infants with congenital hypothyroidism.

From various mass screening programs in North America, the overall incidence of congenital hypothyroidism appears to be one in 3,684 births (a total of 1,046,362 infants screened by various methods). Significantly, only 2.9% of 277 hypothyroid infants were suspected on the basis of clinical evidence prior to the reporting of the screening results. The incidence of various types of neonatal hypothyroidism and TBG deficiency as tabulated from the screening programs is shown in Table 33-5. A preliminary estimate of the incidence of goitrous hypothyroidism is one in 30,824 neonates. Most of the infants with transient hypothyroidism were born of mothers who received goitrogens during pregnancy. However, several infants were found to have idiopathic transient hypothyroidism with an elevated TSH.

Widespread use of screening programs has lead to an increased frequency of diagnosing thyroid-binding globulin deficiency. This X-linked trait occurs as frequently as one in 10,000 births. The T_4 and TSH concentration will be low, with the T_3 resin uptake elevated. The diagnosis can be confirmed by a very low thyroid-binding globulin concentration measured by a specific radioimmunoassay. It is important to identify these infants, since they have normal free T_4 levels and should not be treated with thyroid hormone.

Premature infants frequently have low levels of T_4 and free T_4 when compared with the normal range for full-term infants. Serious illness is also associated with low T_4 values. With gestations less than 30 weeks, low thyroid-binding globulin (TBG) may be present, but after 30 weeks TBG has reached the level present at term and therefore does not account for the low levels of T_4. In one study 25% of preterm infants had low T_4 and TSH levels. TBG was normal and TSH not elevated. TRH administration produced a rise in TSH and T_4, suggesting that the defect was in the hypothalamus (tertiary hypothyroidism). By 6 months of age all infants had T_4 levels in the normal range, thus documenting the transient nature of the defect. Developmental attainment at 1 year of age was equal to a matched control group that did not have low T_4 levels. Data on further development of these infants are not yet available.

Clinical manifestations

Even in the athyreotic cretins the classic clinical features of cretinism are usually absent at birth and appear only gradually after about 6 weeks. In patients with a functional remnant of thyroid tissue and in patients with some types of familial cretinism, the clinical manifestations may be delayed several months or years, depending on the functional state of the thyroid. Nevertheless, signs of hypothyroidism can be detected by careful observation within the first few weeks of life in more severe forms of cretinism. The early manifestations include lethargy, inactivity, hypotonia, large anterior and posterior fontanels, feeding difficulty, respiratory

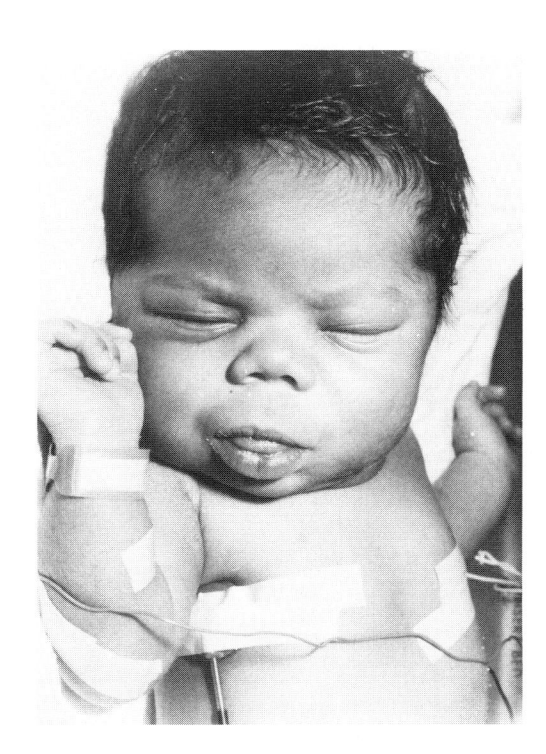

Fig. 33-25. Typical facial features of cretinism.

distress, pallor, perioral cyanosis, mottled skin, poor or hoarse cry, constipation, and hypothermia. The feeding difficulty is often first noted by the mother or a nurse as the infant readily falls asleep after sucking for a short period, necessitating repeated stimulation and thus requiring a prolonged period to complete the feeding. The respiratory distress is caused by myxedema of the airway and is characterized by noisy breathing, nasal stuffiness, and intermittent cyanosis, especially in the perioral area. These respiratory symptoms may lead one to suspect congenital anomalies of the airway or congenital heart disease. After the first 2 weeks of life, prolonged physiologic jaundice may be an indication of hypothyroidism. The jaundice may appear to be further prolonged when carotenemia is superimposed after feeding a diet high in carotene.

The classic features of cretinism usually occur after about 6 weeks of life (Fig. 33-25). These include the typical facies, characterized by depressed nasal bridge, relatively narrow forehead, and puffy eyelids, thick, dry, and cold skin, coarse hair, which may appear long and abundant, and large tongue; abdominal distension; umbilical hernia; hyporeflexia; bradycardia; hypotension with widened pulse pressure; anemia; and widely patent cranial sutures.

Lingual thyroid occasionally can be seen in infants and children as a discrete round mass at the base of the tongue, especially when it is hypertrophied from endogenous TSH stimulation (Fig. 33-26). The base of the tongue must be firmly depressed to visualize this mass.

In some instances, sublingual thyroid is palpable as a round midline mass deep under the mandible.

Neonatal goiters may be extremely large, asymmetrical, and grotesque and may be confused with a hygroma or other type of mass (see Fig. 33-24). Alternatively, the goiter may be quite small and escape notice on a cursory examination.

The onset of symptoms in infants with secondary hypothyroidism tends to be gradual, as some T_4 production occurs. However, signs of other pituitary hormone deficiencies and/or signs of congenital midbrain defects are commonly present. These include neonatal hypoglycemia, small penis, hypospadias, undescended testes, wandering nystagmus, or cleft lip or palate.

Laboratory manifestations

There is no single test by which a diagnosis of cretinism can be established. When the diagnosis is suspected, several appropriate thyroid function tests should be employed. It is advisable to assess both the T_4 level and the saturation of T_4-binding proteins. Elevated levels of serum TSH may be a reliable indication of cretinism. However, the TSH level in the cord blood is normally higher than the adult value, and there is a physiologic TSH surge during the first 48 hours of life (p. 885). The results of these tests must be interpreted in combination and in light of the infant's age and the clinical evidence for hypothyroidism. Many acute and chronic nonthyroidal illnesses, including the respiratory distress syndrome, affect some thyroid function tests but do not

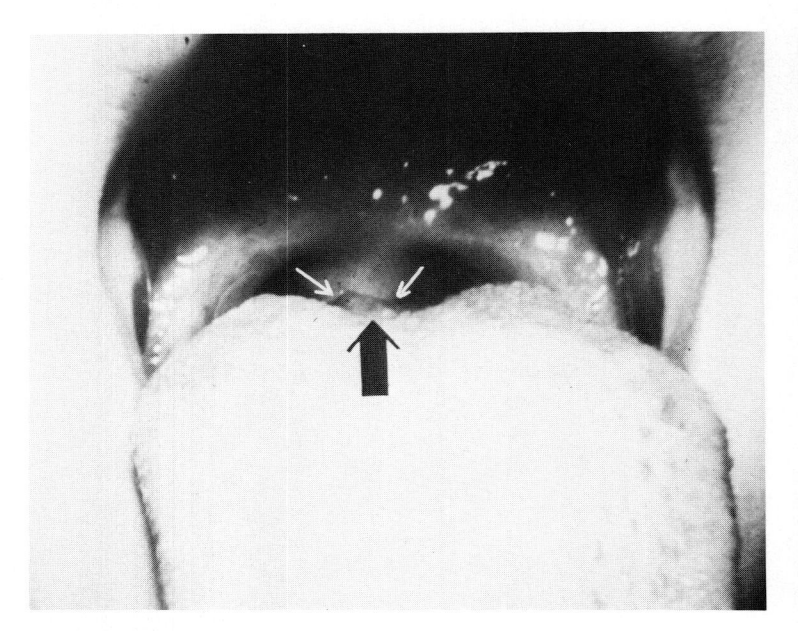

Fig. 33-26. Visualization of a lingual thyroid.

produce hypothyroidism. The typical laboratory findings are low serum T_4, FT_4, and T_3, elevated RT_3, and normal TSH. In certain types of hypothyroidism, such as iodine-deficient cretinism, preferential synthesis of T_3 may occur. Therefore normal or high T_3 alone does not exclude hypothyroidism any more than normal T_4 does.

Severe hyponatremia in association with inappropriate antidiuretic hormone secretion is known to occur in elderly individuals with hypothyroidism. This syndrome has been reported in at least one infant with congenital hypothyroidism.

Retardation of bone maturation is present in about half of the cretins at birth. Thus the assessment of bone age is particularly useful in the newborn. However, roentgenographic examination of the hand and wrist, which is most commonly used in estimating bone age, is almost totally useless during the neonatal period, since the first ossification center, the hamate, does not appear in the normal infant until 3 to 4 months of age. Retardation of bone maturation in neonates is best assessed by x-ray examination of the knee and the foot. The ossification centers of the calcaneus and talus appear at about the twenty-sixth to twenty-eighth week of gestation, and the distal femur at about the thirty-fourth to thirty-sixth week of intrauterine life. The absence of the distal femoral epiphyses in a newborn weighing 3,000 gm or more or the absence of the distal femoral and proximal tibial epiphyses in an infant weighing 2,500 to 3,000 gm at birth suggests intrauterine thyroid hormone deficiency.

Ossification of the cartilages of the epiphyses is also disturbed in hypothyroidism. Normally, ossification begins from the center of the cartilage and extends peripherally in an orderly manner. In hypothyroidism, calcification of epiphyseal centers starts from multiple irregular foci scattered in the developing cartilage. The irregular calcification pattern appears in the roentgenogram as stippled or fragmented ossification centers and is referred to as *epiphyseal dysgenesis* (Fig. 33-27). This finding is highly characteristic of hypothyroidism and provides a strong clue for the diagnosis. A roentgenographic examination of the knee and the foot is useful in detecting epiphyseal dysgenesis during the neonatal period. Abnormal changes occur in the epiphyseal cartilage secondary to thyroid hormone deficiency before calcification so that even after the hypothyroidism is treated, the characteristic pattern of calcification, epiphyseal dysgenesis, may appear in all centers that normally would have calcified during the period of deficiency.

A goiter and tracheal compression by an enlarged thyroid also may be visualized by roentgenographic examination of the neck.

An estimate of visceral myxedema may be made by detecting a low voltage of all complexes in the ECG and EEG. A roentgenogram of the chest also may reveal the presence of cardiomegaly, reflecting myxedema of the heart.

Measurements of the serum cholesterol levels and the BMR are not reliable diagnostic aids in the assessment of thyroid function during the neonatal period. Tests that utilize in vivo administration of radioiodine or technetium 99 (technetium shares with iodide the same active transport mechanism into the thyroid) are unnecessary for the diagnosis of many cretins. However, a radioiodine uptake test can be used to confirm the presence of an agenetic or dysgenetic thyroid. The thyroid 24-hour

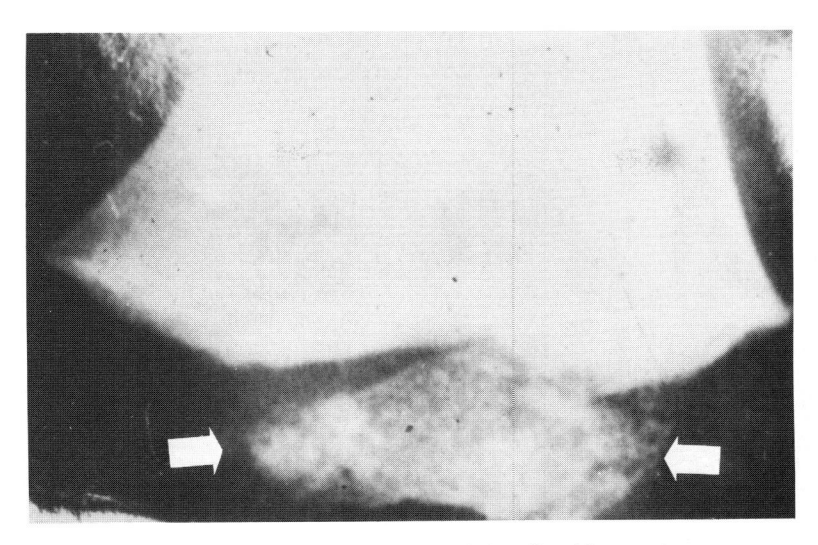

Fig. 33-27. Epiphyseal dysgenesis of the distal femoral center.

uptake of radioiodine is variable during the first several weeks and may exceed 90% during the first week of life. A 24-hour uptake of less than 2% is highly suggestive of thyroid agenesis, and if the uptake is less than 10%, presence of a dysgenetic thyroid can be suspected. An ectopic thyroid is usually not detected by the radioiodine uptake test because of the relatively small aperture of the counter used for such a study. In neonates, radioiodine should be administered through a nasogastric tube, and the tube should then be flushed with water to prevent any loss of the tracer. To detect an undescended thyroid, a scintillation scan of the pharyngeal area and the neck may be obtained after administration of radioiodine.

The presence of defective iodine-trapping mechanism can be suspected in goitrous cretins when the thyroid fails to concentrate radioiodine within 2 to 4 hours after oral administration of the tracer. The defect can be demonstrated by comparing the radioiodine concentrations in simultaneously obtained samples of the saliva and plasma 1 to 2 hours after the administration of the tracer. In the normal individual the salivary concentration is about tenfold greater than that in the plasma, whereas the salivary glands of patients with defective iodine trapping fail to concentrate radioiodine.

In patients with an iodide organification defect, the iodide taken up by the thyroid is readily released from the gland. When the thyroid uptake of radioiodine is measured at 2, 4, 6, and 24 hours after oral administration of radioiodine in these patients, the uptake may be normal or elevated during the earlier hours. However, the uptake rapidly declines within 24 hours. In normal individuals, on the other hand, the thyroid uptake of radioiodine gradually increases during the first 4 to 6 hours and remains at a plateau level of 15% to 30% of the administered dose at the end of 24 hours. When rapid organification of inorganic iodide fails to take place in the thyroid, an anion such as perchlorate can competitively inhibit the iodine accumulation, and there is a net loss of iodide from the gland. This property of perchlorate is utilized in the perchlorate discharge test. This test involves measuring the 2-hour thyroid uptake of radioiodine and then administering sodium or potassium perchlorate orally in amounts of 10 mg/kg of body weight. One to 2 hours thereafter, the thyroid uptake is remeasured. If the uptake decreases by more than 10% to 15% of the initial value, the presence of a defect in normal organification of iodide is suggested.

Differentiation among other types of familial cretinism is more difficult and often technically impossible to achieve during infancy. The studies required for the differential diagnosis usually involve administration of radioactive substances in doses greater than considered safe for infants. Thus, in most instances, patients should be treated for a few years and a definitive study undertaken at a later date. However, secretion of abnormal iodoproteins into the circulation, as would occur in the coupling defect of iodotyrosines, can be suspected when there is a greater than normal discrepancy between the PBI level and the T_4-I or T_4 value (p. 883).

The diagnosis of cretinism caused by maternal ingestion of goitrogens is usually established from the history and is confirmed by its self-limiting course. The reactions to the perchlorate discharge test are positive in both iodine-induced goiter and following administration of antithyroid drugs.

In cretinism caused by iodine deficiency, the radioiodine uptake is elevated.

Secondary hypothyroidism may be suspected in infants with both low T_4 and TSH. The TRH infusion test may be employed to distinguish hypothalamic TRH deficiency from pituitary TSH deficiency. Serum TSH levels increase in normal children and in patients with TRH deficiency within 10 minutes after intravenous administration of TRH, peaking at 20 to 45 minutes and returning to baseline levels by 2 hours.

Differential diagnosis

Errors of diagnosis of cretinism usually result from a failure to suspect the condition or from diagnosing other disorders as hypothyroidism. These errors commonly arise from basing the diagnosis on a few suggestive clinical features and misinterpreting the laboratory data.

During the early neonatal period, respiratory difficulty, pallor, and cyanosis in cretinism must be differentiated from other common causes of respiratory distress and from congenital heart disease. Lethargy, inactivity, hypotonia, and feeding difficulty may be mistaken for manifestations of sepsis or brain damage from a variety of causes. The prolonged jaundice in cretinism must not be confused with icterus caused by hemolytic anemia, septicemia, or hepatic disease. The coarse facial features, macroglossia, and dry skin of cretinism can mislead one to suspect Hurler's syndrome, chondrodystrophy, or mongolism. In rare instances hypothyroidism has been found in patients with mongolism. A large goiter must not be confused with a hygroma, cyst, or tumor of the neck. A lingual thyroid, when visible or obstructing the airway, has been mistaken for a tumor of the pharyngeal area. Although epiphyseal dysgenesis may resemble osteochondritis deformans in its roentgenographic appearance, the latter does not occur during the neonatal period.

Treatment

All hypothyroid infants, with or without goiter, should be rendered euthyroid as promptly as possible by substitution therapy. Neonates with a euthyroid goiter should be regarded as being in a state of impending hypothyroidism and, in most instances, should be treated. Desiccated thyroid, sodium-L-thyroxine, or triiodothyronine can be used for treatment. Desiccated thyroid has the advantages of being inexpensive and maintaining the T_4 value within the normal range when the patient is rendered euthyroid. Desiccated thyroid has an estimated plasma half-life of 6.9 days in the adult; its latent period, the interval between administration of the drug and the onset of its effect, is longer than that of T_3. One drawback in using desiccated thyroid for replacement has been reported recently. Daily doses of desiccated thyroid sufficient to maintain a clinical euthyroid state and normal serum T_4 and TSH levels produced serum T_3 levels higher than the normal range in most children and adolescents. Such elevation of T_3 was not induced by appropriate doses of sodium-L-thyroxine. The authors suggest that sodium-L-thyroxine is the drug of choice for treatment of hypothyroidism. Sodium-L-thyroxine is better standardized for its potency than desiccated thyroid but will result in slightly elevated T_4 value. Sixty-five milligrams (1 grain) of desiccated thyroid is the equivalent of 100 µg of L-thyroxine and 35 µg of T_3.

In the treatment of infants with severe myxedema, possible complications should be kept in mind. Cardiac insufficiency from overtaxing the myxedematous heart by too rapid a mobilization of the myxedema fluid into the circulation is well known in the adult. This complication is prevented by administering a small dose of thyroid hormone at first and gradually increasing the dosage. The infant, however, generally tolerates a rapid restoration to the euthyroid state better than the adult, and some authors have advocated a prompt restoration of T_4 to a normal value. It is my opinion that thyroid hormone should be increased judiciously when evidence of severe myxedema, particularly of the heart, is present. Aspiration of food is another complication of cretins; it may occur after therapy has been started, when the infants begin to feed more vigorously. It results from an impairment in swallowing, caused by myxedema of the pharyngeal area, compounded by increased appetite as the euthyroid state is restored. Therefore, when myxedema is severe, the infant should be fed carefully and slowly by an expert nurse during the early phase of treatment.

There are different views on the exact mode of treatment of severe cretinism. Initially the patient may be given orally 8 mg of desiccated thyroid per day; after 1 week the dosage is increased to 16 mg; at 2 weeks, to 32 mg; at 3 weeks, to 48 mg; at 4 weeks, to 65 mg; and thereafter this dosage is maintained during the first 2 years of life. This or a similar schedule of treatment has been used successfully by a large number of physicians over a period of many years. Alternatively, because of the more rapid action and shorter half-life of T_3, others prefer to use this drug in treatment of infants with hypothyroidism. The patient is started on 5 µg of T_3 per day administered orally; after 7 days the dosage is increased to 10 µg; thereafter it is increased by 5 µg every 4 to 5 days until it reaches 25 µg/day; then T_3 is discontinued, and the patient is placed on the maintenance dosage of desiccated thyroid of 65 mg/day or 9 µg/kg/day of sodium-L-thyroxine. The dosage should be adjusted so that a clinical euthyroid state and normal or high normal serum T_4 levels can be maintained. The initially elevated serum TSH levels in primary hypothyroidism may not suppress to the normal range for many months despite an adequate replacement therapy. Therefore TSH levels should not be used as the sole criterion for evaluating the adequacy of treatment.

Restoration of milder hypothyroidism to a euthyroid state can be accomplished more rapidly. Patients with a euthyroid goiter may be placed on a maintenance dosage of thyroid hormone immediately.

Until hypothyroidism is corrected, the infant should be kept under careful observation, and cardiovascular function should be monitored. Clinical observation should be supplemented by following the growth curve, the maturation of the bones, and the T_4 levels. All cretins, except those caused by maternal ingestion of goitrogens and by iodine deficiency, require lifetime substitution therapy.

Goitrous cretinism caused by maternal ingestion of goitrogens is a self-limiting condition. The blocking effect of antithyroid drugs usually disappears several days after birth. Therefore, if the goiter is small and the patient is euthyroid, no treatment is required. If the patient is hypothyroid, however, or if the goiter is large, it is safer to treat the infant for several weeks or months. The antithyroid agents are secreted in breast milk. Shrinkage of the goiter may be hastened by substitution therapy, and the treatment can be withdrawn after the thyroid returns to normal size. Occasionally, the goiter may be huge, and asphyxia may occur in the neonate from a goiter that encircles the trachea. This complication is most commonly seen in iodide-induced goiter and constitutes a medical emergency.

Endemic cretins should be given substitution therapy for an indefinite period, unless iodine prophylaxis can be ensured in the specific geographic location.

Prognosis

Shortly after adequate substitution therapy is instituted, all clinical manifestations of hypothyroidism will disappear, and accelerated linear growth will occur if growth was retarded before the treatment. After a period of "catch-up" growth, an optimal rate of growth will be maintained. Goiter or hypertrophied ectopic thyroid will gradually shrink in size when the patient is properly treated. The coarse hair is gradually lost and is replaced by finer, normal hair over a period of several months. The marked acceleration in bone maturation (catch-up) occurs after a latent period of a few months, and thereafter the osseous development should parallel the chronologic age. When hypothyroidism is treated with a slightly excessive dosage of thyroid hormones for a prolonged period, the bone maturation may gradually exceed the chronologic age, even though the patient may fail to show overt signs of hyperthyroidism or have clearly elevated levels of T_4. With substitution therapy, epiphyseal dysgenesis will appear in centers that failed to calcify while the patient was hypothyroid, and then the calcification will coalesce to form a normal epiphysis.

Although the prognosis for physical recovery is good, the prognosis for normal mental and neurologic performance is uncertain and less favorable. The eventual IQ of severe cretins is inversely related to the duration of thyroid hormone deficiency. Irreversible brain damage can occur from fetal hypothyroidism as well as from postnatal hormone deficiency. Therefore the prognosis for mental development of a cretin should be guarded, even if the treatment is initiated soon after birth. It is my impression that the mental ability of neonates with marked delay in the bone maturation is likely to be worse than that in those with mild or no retardation in bone age. Mental and neurologic competence of cretins is also related to the severity of hypothyroidism. However, even mild cretins, treated promptly after birth, may have impairment of arithmetic ability, speech, or fine motor coordination in later life.

GOITERS

The majority of neonatal goiters result from maternal ingestion of goitrogens. Prominent goiter only occasionally is the manifestation of familial goitrous cretinism. Most euthyroid goiters of newborns are brought about by compensatory hypertrophy of the thyroid and thus are potentially indicative of impending hypothyroidism. Therefore these goiters should be treated appropriately.

Congenital neoplasms of the thyroid rarely occur. They include Hürthle cell tumor and adenocarcinoma. I have also encountered a teratoma of the thyroid in a newborn that was suggested by calcification within the thyroid. Neoplasm can be suspected when a nodular goiter is present. Radioiodine scintiscan reveals a cold nodular area corresponding to the location of the neoplasm where uptake of radioiodine is lacking. A diagnosis of neoplasm should be confirmed by a biopsy.

THYROTOXICOSIS
Etiology and pathogenesis

Neonatal thyrotoxicosis was previously believed to occur by transplacental transfer of LATS or other thyroid-stimulating immunoglobulins from the mother. Approximately 50% of patients are born to mothers known to have Graves' disease either prior to or during the pregnancy. However, neonatal thyrotoxicosis may occur in infants without detectable thyroid-stimulating immunoglobulins, and mothers with detectable LATS may give birth to normal infants. Family studies, observation on twins, and age-specific incidence rates suggest that this disease occurs at random in a genetically preselected population. Thus the pathogenesis of congenital Graves' disease has proved elusive.

Clinical manifestations

When neonatal thyrotoxicosis occurs in the infant born to a mother with untreated active Graves' disease, the clinical manifestations of hyperthyroidism may become apparent within the first 24 hours of life. Infants may be born prematurely from such a mother. Irritability, excessive movement, tremor, flushing of the cheeks, sweating, increased appetite, weight loss or lack of weight gain, supraventricular tachycardia, goiter, and exophthalmos may be observed. Although a goiter is inevitably present in neonatal thyrotoxicosis, its size varies considerably; it may be small and escape notice on a cursory examination, or it may be large enough to cause tracheal compression. Furthermore, the goiter may increase in size during the early neonatal period. Exophthalmos is usually mild when present. Hepatosplenomegaly, thrombocytopenia, and hypoprothrombinemia have been reported in isolated instances. In severe neonatal thyrotoxicosis, hyperthermia, arrhythmias, and cardiac failure may occur; and, if the condition is untreated, death may ensue.

The course of the syndrome, in a classic form, is self-limited because of the gradual depletion of transplacentally acquired LATS. The signs and symptoms subside spontaneously after 3 to 12 weeks, depending on the severity of the disease, which in turn is probably related to the titer of LATS in the plasma of the neonate. Goiter, however, may persist for some time after all signs of hyperthyroidism disappear. The thyroid gradually returns to normal size. It has been emphasized recently that, in other forms, neonatal thyrotoxicosis may not be a transient disorder and may persist for months or years.

In the infant born to a mother who received antithyroid medications for treatment of Graves' disease during the latter part of pregnancy, the onset of clinical manifestations may be modified by transplacental acquisition of the antithyroid agent as well as LATS. At birth the infant may be euthyroid or even hypothyroid, and the presence of a goiter may be the only abnormal feature. Since the plasma half-life of antithyroid agents is short, the typical manifestations of neonatal thyrotoxicosis may appear several days after birth. If the infant is born in a hypothyroid state, a period of euthyroidism may follow within a few days, and thyrotoxicosis may not occur until 5 to 7 days after birth.

Diagnosis and differential diagnosis

A maternal history of Graves' disease before or during pregnancy is important in the diagnosis of neonatal thyrotoxicosis. Information concerning the treatment of maternal hyperthyroidism also must be obtained. The infant should be examined repeatedly for signs of thyrotoxicosis, and the neck should be palpated carefully to detect a goiter. Determination of FT_4 should be obtained, together with an assessment of T_4-binding protein saturation. The data should be interpreted in relation to the clinical features and age of the neonate. The determination of radioiodine uptake by the thyroid has little value during the neonatal period. LATS can be determined by a bioassay in sera of the mother, umbilical cord, and infant. A high titer of LATS will strongly support the diagnosis of neonatal thyrotoxicosis. Serial determinations of LATS in the neonate are also helpful.

In the euthyroid or hypothyroid neonate born to a mother who received antithyroid medication during the latter part of pregnancy, it is virtually impossible to predict whether thyrotoxicosis will ensue. Therefore serial examinations of the infant must be undertaken during the first 10 days of life.

Although neonatal thyrotoxicosis can be confused with various neurologic disorders, congenital heart disease, or sepsis, a positive maternal history of Graves' disease and the presence of a goiter should readily alert one to the correct diagnosis. In normal neonates and infants the thyroid gland is rarely palpable. Therefore, in general, a palpable thyroid in these individuals should be regarded as a goiter.

Treatment

The treatment of thyrotoxicosis in a neonate is similar to that in an older child and involves the use of antithyroid drugs. Care should be exercised not to induce hypothyroidism with excessive medication. Iodine (Lugol's Solution), propylthiouracil, or methimazole is commonly used. Lugol's Solution can be given in doses of 1 drop three times daily. Although iodine rapidly inhibits the release of T_4 from the thyroid, its effect tends to disappear after several weeks. Propylthiouracil is given orally in amounts of 10 mg/kg/day in three divided doses at 8-hour intervals. Methimazole is given in amounts of 1 mg/kg/day in three divided doses. Circulating T_4 has a half-life of 6.9 days, and therefore little or no clinical response to antithyroid drugs can be expected during the first few days of therapy. After 1 to 3 months of therapy the dosage of antithyroid drug should be reduced or its administration discontinued to determine whether the disease has a self-limited course.

Most signs and symptoms, including the cardiovascular manifestations, of hyperthyroidism are closely related to increased adrenergic response. Antiadrenergic agents, therefore, can alleviate many of the untoward manifestations of thyrotoxicosis. In contrast to antithyroid drugs, these agents can rapidly diminish the severity of thyrotoxicity, and their effects are evident within a few hours. Thus reserpine or propranolol hydrochloride, together with iodine or propylthiouracil, may be used in the treatment of severe neonatal thyrotoxicosis. Propranolol hydrochloride is given orally in a dosage of 2 mg/kg/day in two or more divided doses. Digitalization may be necessary in neonates with cardiac failure. Under these circumstances reserpine may be contraindicated or must be used with extreme caution. A large goiter compressing the trachea and resulting in asphyxia must be treated surgically by splitting the isthmus.

The euthyroid or hypothyroid infant born to a mother who received antithyroid medications during the pregnancy should be managed as described in the section on congenital hypothyroidism, since these neonates may or may not be kept under close observation. If the infant has already received thyroid hormone, it should be discontinued as soon as thyrotoxic manifestations occur, and appropriate management of hyperthyroidism must be initiated. A mother who is receiving an antithyroid medication should not be allowed to breast-feed the infant, since these agents are secreted into the milk.

Prognosis

Neonatal thyrotoxicosis carries a mortality of about 15% if it is not recognized and treated properly. However, in many instances the syndrome has a self-limited duration and no sequelae have been recognized. A goiter may resolve slowly over a period of several months. Premature closure of all cranial sutures occasionally occurs. It is advisable to obtain a roentgenogram of the skull at 6 to 12 months of age.

FAMILIAL ABNORMALITIES OF THYROXINE-BINDING GLOBULIN

Genetic disorders resulting in either increased or decreased levels of thyroxine-binding globulin (TBG) have been reported. Affected individuals are healthy and asymptomatic, since a change in the level of TBG does not lead to an alteration of the FT_4 level. The disorders are usually discovered fortuitously by studying the T_4, which reveals unexpectedly high or low values. The only clinical significance of these conditions, therefore, lies in the fact that abnormal T_4 levels may lead to erroneous diagnosis.

Decreased TBG

In several families, affected males had no detectable TBG. Moreover, there was no male-to-male transmission of the trait. A female member in one of these families had no detectable TBG and a sex chromosome constitution of XO. Thus, in these families, the trait appeared to be transmitted as an X-linked gene. In another family, however, a deficiency of TBG was found in three males and three females of two generations. The mode of transmission in this family suggested an autosomal dominant trait.

Increased TBG

Studies in two families with increased TBG suggest that the trait was inherited as an autosomal dominant gene. In another family, affected males transmitted the trait to female but not to male offspring, suggesting that the trait was X linked.

The conflicting reports on the mode of inheritance of both the decreased and the increased TBG traits are difficult to reconcile at present. Since the TBG levels were estimated from its binding capacity of T_4, the reported increased TBG may merely reflect an elevated binding capacity of the protein without a quantitative increase in the amount of circulating TBG. Thus the level of TBG may be controlled by more than one gene, one of which could be a regulator gene.

Akira Morishima

BIBLIOGRAPHY

Abuid, J., and others: Total and free triiodothyronine and thyroxine in early infancy, J. Clin. Endocrinol. Metab. **39**:263, 1974.

Abuid, J., Stinson, D.A., and Larsen, P.R.: Serum triiodothyronine and thyroxine in the neonate and the acute increases in these hormones following delivery, J. Clin. Invest. **52**:1195, 1973.

Anderson, H.J.: Hypothyroidism: nongoitrous hypothyroidism. In Gardner, L.I., editor: Endocrine and genetic diseases of childhood, Philadelphia, 1969, W.B. Saunders Co.

Bongiovanni, A.M., and others: Sporadic goiter of the newborn, J. Clin. Endocrinol. Metab. **16**:146, 1956.

Braverman, L.E., Ingbar, S.H., and Sterling, K.: Conversion of thyroxine (T_4) to triiodothyronine (T_3) in athyreotic human subjects, J. Clin. Invest. **49**:855, 1970.

Chopra, I.J.: A radioimmunoassay for measurement of thyroxine in unextracted serum, J. Clin. Endocrinol. Metab. **34**:938, 1972.

Chopra, I.J., and Crandall, B.F.: Thyroid hormones and thyrotropin in amniotic fluid, N. Engl. J. Med. **293**:740, 1975.

Codaccioni, J.L., and others: Congenital hypothyroidism associated with thyrotropin unresponsiveness and thyroid cell membrane alterations, J. Clin. Endocrinol. Metab. **50**:932, 1980.

Cuestas, P.A., and Engel, R.R.: Thyroid function in preterm infants with respiratory distress syndrome, J. Pediatr. **94**:643, 1979.

Czernichow, P., and others: Thyroid function studies in paired maternal-cord sera and sequential observations of thyrotropic hormone release during the first 72 hours of life, Pediatr. Res. **5**:53, 1971.

Delange, F., and others: Transient hypothyroidism in the newborn infant, J. Pediatr. **92**:974, 1978.

Erenberg, A., and others: Total and free thyroid hormone concentrations in the neonatal period, Pediatrics **53**:211, 1974.

Fisher, D.A.: Thyroid development and disorders of thyroid function in the newborn, N. Engl. J. Med. **304**:702, 1981.

Fisher, D.A., Oddie, T.H., and Burroughs, J.C.: Thyroidal radioiodine uptake rate measurement in infants, Am. J. Dis. Child. **103**:738, 1962.

Fisher, D.A., and Odell, W.D.: Acute release of thyrotropin in the newborn, J. Clin. Invest. **48**:1670, 1969.

Fisher, D.A., and Burrow, G.N., editors: Perinatal thyroid physiology and disease, Kroc Foundation Symposia Series, no. 3, New York, 1975, Raven Press.

Fisher, D.A., and others: Screening for congenital hypothyroidism: results of screening one million North American infants, J. Pediatr. **94**:700, 1979.

Florsheim, W.H., and others: Familial elevation of serum thyroxine-binding capacity, J. Clin. Endocrinol. Metab. **22**:735, 1962.

French, F.S., and Van Wyk, J.J.: Fetal hypothyroidism, J. Pediatr. **64**:589, 1964.

Gorodzinsky, P., and others: Cord serum thyroxine and thyrotropin values between 20 and 30 weeks' gestation, J. Pediatr. **94**:971, 1979.

Greene, H.G., and others: Cretinism associated with maternal sodium iodide I[131] therapy during pregnancy, Am. J. Dis. Child. **122**:247, 1971.

Greenberg, A.H., and others: Observations on the maturation of thyroid function in early fetal life, J. Clin. Invest. **49**:1790, 1970.

Grumbach, M.M., and Werner, S.C.: Transfer of thyroid hormone across the human placenta at term, J. Clin. Endocrinol. Metab. **16**:1392, 1956.

Hadeed, A.J., and others: Significance of transient postnatal hypothyroxinemia in premature infants with and without respiratory distress syndrome, J. Pediatr. **68**:494, 1981.

Heidemann, P., and Stubbe, P.: Serum 3,5,3'-triiodothyronine, thyroxine, and thyrotropin in hypothyroid infant with congenital goiter and the response to iodine, J. Clin. Endocrinol. Metab. **47**:189, 1978.

Hirsch, P.F., Voekel, E.F., and Munson, P.L.: Thyrocalcitonin: hypocalcemic hypophosphatemic principle of the thyroid gland, Science **146**:412, 1964.

Klein, A.H., Agustin, A.V., and Foley, T.P., Jr.: Successful laboratory screening for congenital hypothyroidism, Lancet **2**:77, 1974.

LaFranchi, S.H.: Hypothyroidism, Pediatr. Clin. North Am. **26**:33, 1979.

Larsen, P.R., and Broskin, K.: Thyroxine (T$_4$) immunoassay using filter paper blood samples for screening of neonates for hypothyroidism, Pediatr. Res. **9**:604, 1975.

Larsen, P.R., and others: Immunoassay of thyroxine in unextracted human serum, J. Clin. Endocrinol. Metab. **37**:177, 1973.

Little, G., and others: "Cryptothyroidism": the major cause of sporadic "athyreotic" cretinism, J. Clin. Endocrinol. Metab. **25**:1529, 1965.

Marrow, W.J.: Hurthle cell tumor of the thyroid gland in an infant, Arch. Pathol. **40**:387, 1945.

Marshall, J.S., Levy, R.P., and Steinberg, A.G.: Human thyroxine-binding globulin deficiency: a genetic study, N. Engl. J. Med. **274**:1469, 1966.

McKenzie, J.M.: Neonatal Graves' disease, J. Clin. Endocrinol. Metab. **24**:660, 1964.

Odell, W.D., Wilber, J.F., and Paul, W.E.: Radioimmunoassay of thyrotropin in human serum, J. Clin. Endocrinol. Metab. **25**:1179, 1965.

Oppenheimer, J.H., and Surks, M.I.: The peripheral action of the thyroid hormones, Med. Clin. North Am. **59**:1055, 1975.

Parker, R.H., and Beierwaltes, W.H.: Thyroid antibodies during pregnancy and in the newborn, J. Clin. Endocrinol. Metab. **21**:792, 1961.

Patel, Y.C., Burger, H.G., and Hudson, B.: Radioimmunoassay of serum thyrotropin: sensitivity and specificity, J. Clin. Endocrinol. Metab. **33**:768, 1971.

Penny, R., and Frasier, S.D.: Elevated serum concentrations of triiodothyronine in hypothyroid patients, Am. J. Dis. Child. **134**:16, 1980.

Perry, R.D., Hodgman, J.E., and Starr, P.: Maternal, cord, and serial venous blood: protein-bound iodine, thyroid-binding globulin, thyroid-binding albumin, and prealbumin values in premature infants, Pediatrics **35**:759, 1965.

Robles-Valdes, C., Mayans, J.A.R., and Lomeli, J.I.A.: Severe hyponatremia in congenital hypothyroidism, J. Pediatr. **94**:631, 1979.

Rogers, W.M.: Normal and anomalous development of the thyroid: normal development. In Werner, S.C., and Ingbar, S.H., editors: The thyroid, ed. 3, section 22, New York, 1971, Harper & Row, Publishers.

Schultz, R.M., Glassman, M.S., and MacGillivary, M.H.: Elevated threshold of thyrotropin suppression in congenital hypothyroidism, Am. J. Dis. Child. **123**:19, 1980.

Smith, C.S., and Howard, N.J.: Propranolol in treatment of neonatal thyrotoxicosis, J. Pediatr. **83**:1046, 1973.

Sokoloff, L., and others: Mechanisms of stimulation of protein synthesis by thyroid hormones in vitro, Proc. Natl. Acad. Sci. U.S.A. **60**:652, 1968.

Stanbury, J.B., and others: Congenital hypothyroidism with impaired thyroid response to thyrotropin, N. Engl. J. Med. **279**:1132, 1968.

Stanbury, J.B., Wyngaarden, J.B., and Fredrickson, D.S.: The metabolic basis of inherited disease, ed. 2, New York, 1966, McGraw-Hill Book Co., Inc.

Sunshine, P., Kusumoto, H., and Kriss, J.P.: Survival time of circulating long-acting thyroid stimulator in neonatal thyrotoxicosis: implications for diagnosis and therapy of the disorder, Pediatrics **36**:869, 1965.

Varma, S.K., and others: Thyroxine, triiodothyronine, and reverse triiodothyronine concentrations in human milk, J. Pediatr. **93**:803, 1978.

Wayne, E.J., Koutras, D.A., and Alexander, W.D.: Clinical aspects of iodine metabolism, Oxford, 1964, Blackwell Scientific Publications Ltd.

Weinstein, I.B., and Kitchin, F.D.: Genetic factors in thyroid disease. In Werner, S.C., and Ingbar, S.H., editors: The thyroid, ed. 3, section 26, New York, 1971, Harper & Row, Publishers.

Wilber, J.F.: Thyrotropin releasing hormone: secretion and action, Ann. Rev. Int. Med. **34**:353, 1973.

PART FOUR

Abnormalities of sexual differentiation

Genetic sex is determined at fertilization, but the actual differentiation begins at 6 weeks of gestation and is largely completed by 14 weeks. This chapter reviews normal and abnormal sexual differentiation, diagnostic categories for various disorders, and practical information for the recognition, diagnosis, and management of neonates with intersex problems. The term *intersex problem* is defined as a discrepancy in the genetic, gonadal, or genital makeup of an individual. The term *hermaphrodite* is often used interchangeably but is more restrictive. Male pseudohermaphrodites have testes with incomplete masculinization; female pseudohermaphrodites have ovaries with some virilization of the genitalia; and true hermaphrodites have both ovarian and testicular tissue.

FETAL SEX DIFFERENTIATION: EMBRYOLOGY AND ENDOCRINOLOGY
Gonadal development

The gonads of both sexes develop from the indifferent gonad, first seen at 5 weeks of gestation as the genital ridge, located on the medial aspect of the mesonephros. The primordial germ cells are seen as early as 4½ days of gestation. They migrate from the entoderm of the allantois and yolk sac and reach the genital ridge at 26 or 27 days and later.

Testicular differentiation

Differentiation of the testis begins at 6 weeks of gestation when the cells of the primitive gonad interact to form the epithelial or primary sex cords and intervening connective tissue. The cord cells, thought to be of epithelial origin, become the primitive Sertoli cells, and the primordial germ cells become incorporated into the cords and develop into spermatogonia. In the seventh and eighth weeks the cords in the cortex loop to form the seminiferous cords, and in the hilum they anastomose to form the rete cords or rete testis. From 8 weeks on the seminiferous cords become coiled and thickened and contain eight to ten layers of Sertoli cells, whereas the spermatogonia remain located near the basement membrane of the cords. The seminiferous cords and rete testis become lumenized in the second half of gestation.

The fetal testis is characterized by the appearance of Leydig cells, in the interstitium between the seminiferous cords, beginning at approximately 8 to 8½ weeks, and these may be mesenchymal in origin. The Leydig cells increase strikingly in number during the third month, occupy half the volume of the testis by the middle of the fourth month, and then show a significant fall in numbers; some Leydig cells are present postnatally but disappear within a few months due to a physiologic lack of gonadotropin stimulation.

As the fetus elongates, the testis descends and occupies a more caudal position. In the sixth and seventh months the cremasteric muscle differentiates in the caudal testicular ligament to form the testicular gubernaculum, which penetrates the inguinal canal and is anchored to the connective tissue of the scrotum. The testis descends behind the peritoneum and reaches the scrotum by the eighth or ninth month; the inguinal canal closes after testicular descent is complete.

Ovarian differentiation

Differentiation of the ovary begins gradually at 6½ to 8 weeks of gestation. The cord cells become the primitive granulosa cells, which are analogous to the Sertoli cells. The primary sex cords show little development in the medulla or hilum, and epithelioid interstitial cells (analogous to Leydig cells) are not seen. In the cortex, however, the primordial germ cells, now called oogonia, undergo intensive mitotic division during the third month to form a thick zone of mostly oogonia interspersed with a few primitive granulosa cells. Primitive granulosa cells begin to organize around the oocytes to form primordial follicles.

The late fetal ovary (15 to 18 weeks onward) is characterized by the development of primary follicles, which surround follicular cells to form a basement membrane, and each follicle becomes surrounded by connective tissue. At 18 to 22 weeks about 7 million oogonia and oocytes are present, but by birth only 2 million are present, with half of these undergoing degeneration and atresia; only about 400,000 oocytes will persist into reproductive life, of which only approximately 400 are ovulated during the woman's reproductive period.

Development of the genital ducts

The internal genital ducts develop from separate anlagen, the mesonephric or wolffian ducts in the male and the paramesonephric or müllerian ducts in the female (Fig. 33-28). The wolffian ducts are formed in 26- to 32-day-old embryos; the müllerian ducts arise at 44 to 48 days and develop in close association with the wolffian ducts, which serve as a guide to the caudal progression of the müllerian ducts. In the absence of wolffian ducts, the müllerian ducts will not develop.

In the male fetus the müllerian ducts begin to undergo regression at 8 weeks, shortly after the ipsilateral testicular seminiferous cords have differentiated and preceding the appearance of Leydig cells, and regression is completed by 9½ to 10 weeks. Differentiation of the wolffian ducts is testosterone dependent and begins at about 8½ weeks. The wolffian ducts differentiate into the epididymis and vas deferens, and beginning at 10½ weeks the seminal vesicles and their ejaculatory ducts develop at the caudal end from lateral outpouchings. The wolffian ducts project into the urogenital sinus just lateral to the termination of the fused müllerian ducts.

The female genital ducts differentiate later than the male genital ducts. In the absence of ipsilateral testes, the müllerian ducts form the fallopian tubes, uterus, and upper portion of the vagina beginning in the third month of gestation. The wolffian ducts, in the absence of *local* testosterone produced by an ipsilateral testis, rapidly disappear, and by 13 weeks degeneration of these ducts is complete (Fig. 33-28). The fallopian tubes later descend with the ovaries and are included in a fold of peritoneum called the broad ligament. At birth the position of the uterus is vertical, and uterine development is disproportionate in that the uterine cervix is twice as large as the fundus and remains so until puberty. Mater-

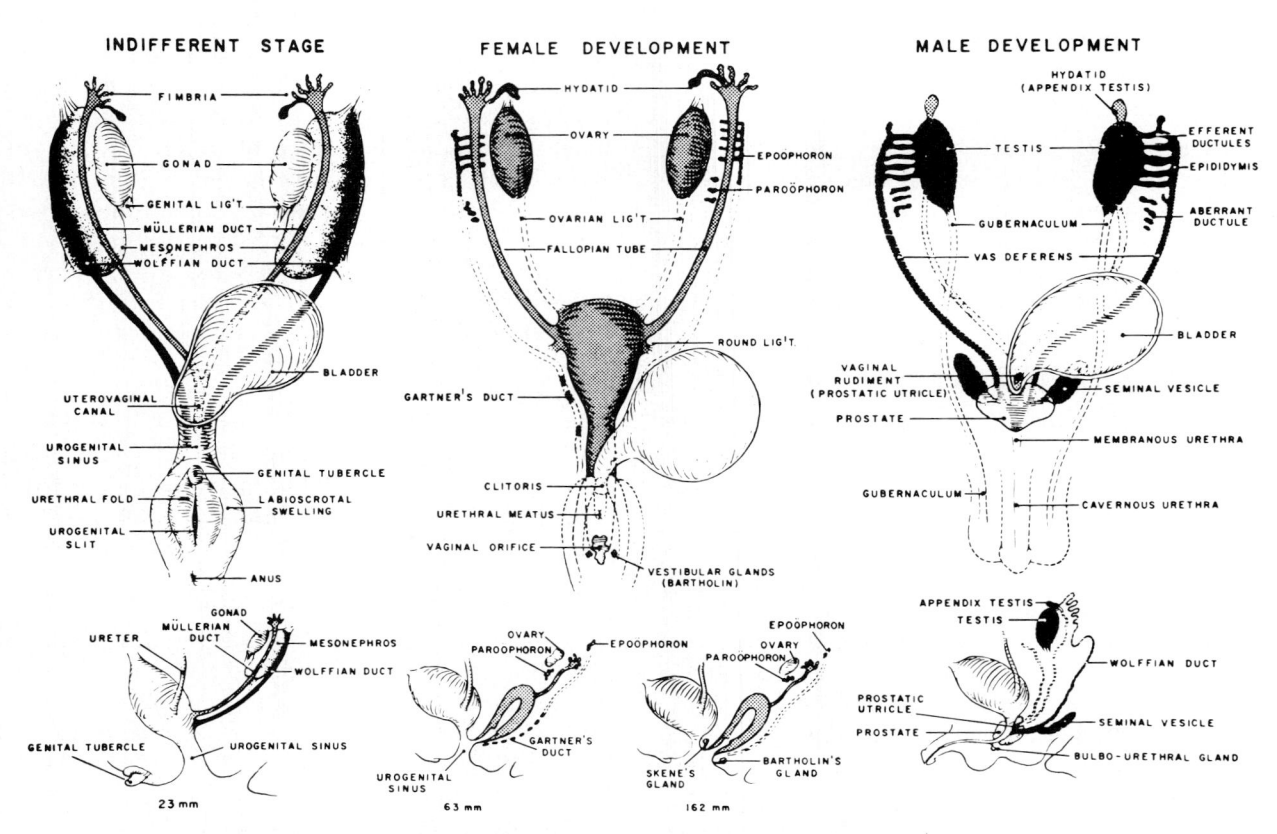

Fig. 33-28. Internal genital duct differentiation. *Left,* Wolffian and müllerian ducts in a 7½-week-old fetus at the indifferent stage. *Center,* Female fetus beyond 13 weeks. *Right,* Male fetus beyond 14 weeks. (From Grumbach, M.M., and Van Wyk, J.J.: Disorders of sexual differentiation. In Williams, R.H., editor: Textbook of endocrinology, Philadelphia, 1974, W.B. Saunders Co.)

nal estrogens probably stimulate uterine growth in utero, so its size at birth is larger than at several months of age; endometrial hyperplasia occasionally may result in transient neonatal uterine bleeding.

The development of the vagina depends on the caudal müllerian ducts having made contact with the entodermal epithelium of the urogenital sinus. At this junction a multilayered solid epithelial cord known as the vaginal plate is formed; it disintegrates beyond 4 months to form the vaginal lumen. It is not clear whether the lower portion of the vagina is derived from the urogenital sinus and the upper portion is of müllerian origin, or whether the vagina is entirely of urogenital sinus origin. The origin of the hymen is also unclear, but it is thought to be derived from the mesenchyme that separated the vagina from the urogenital sinus.

Development of the external genitalia

The male and female embryos share common genital primordia that inherently will develop along female lines unless systemic androgens, specifically dihydrotestosterone (DHT), induce male differentiation.

The indifferent stage of the external genitalia lasts until the ninth week when, in the presence of *systemic* androgens, masculinization begins with the lengthening of the anogenital distance. The urogenital and labioscrotal folds begin to fuse in the midline, beginning caudally and progressing anteriorly. The urethra develops with fusion of the urogenital folds to form both the membranous urethra in the perineum and the penile urethra along the ventral surface of the phallus. Midline fusion of the labioscrotal folds forms the scrotal raphe, whereas the penile raphe represents the fused portions of the urogenital folds. These processes are complete in the 14-week fetus.

In the female fetus at 9 weeks the anogenital distance does not increase, and the urogenital folds and labioscrotal swellings do not fuse. The labioscrotal swellings develop predominantly in their caudal portions, but less so than in male fetuses, and remain unfused as they transform into the labia majora. The urogenital folds develop into the labia minora. The epithelium of the vaginal vestibule between the labia minora and the hymen is entodermal, being derived from the urogenital sinus,

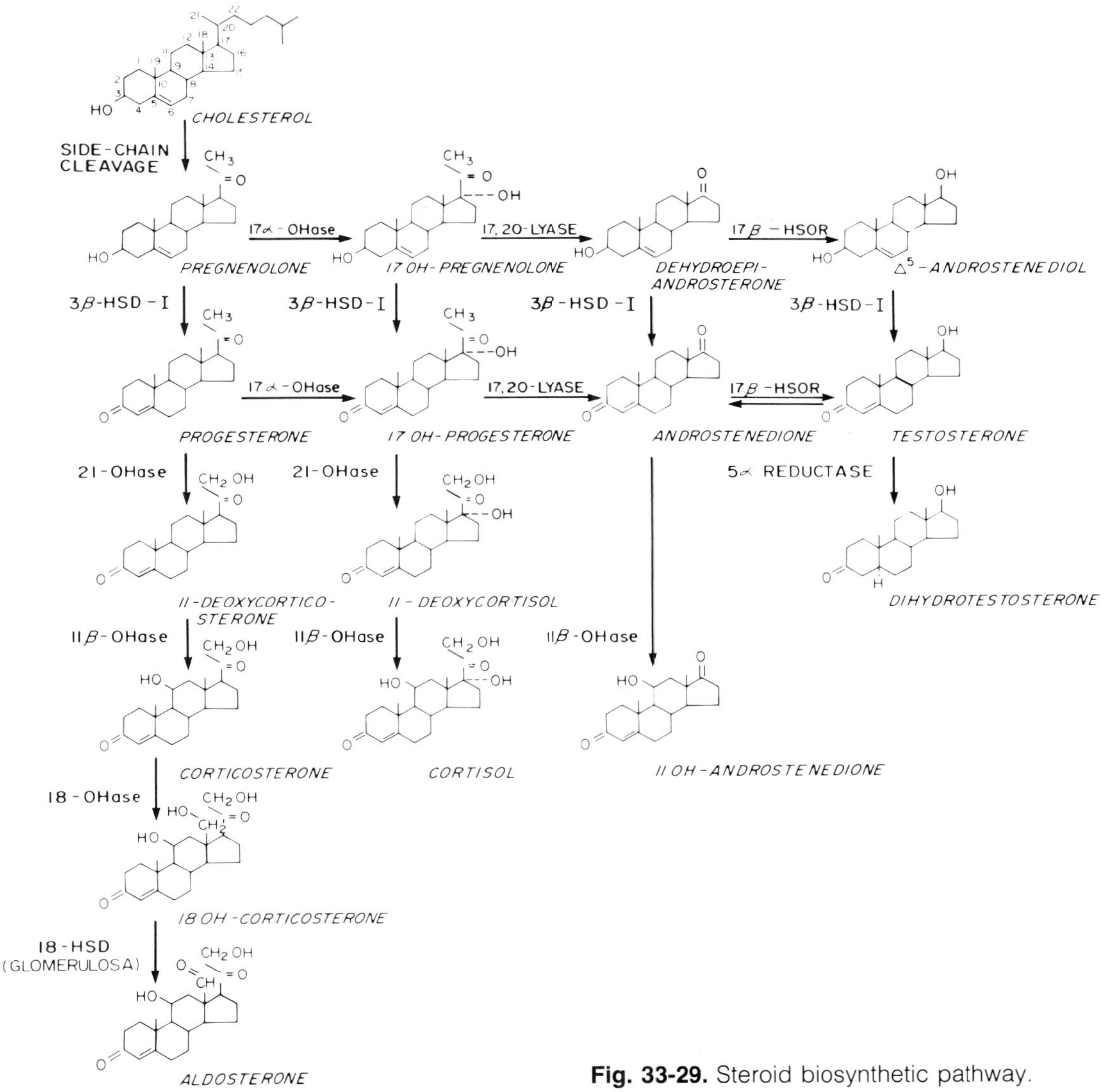

Fig. 33-29. Steroid biosynthetic pathway.

whereas the epithelium between the labia minora and majora is ectodermal in origin.

Fetal gonadal endocrine function

Müllerian-inhibiting factor (MIF) is a protein secreted by the seminiferous tubules, most probably by the Sertoli cells, beginning around 7½ weeks, as judged by the onset of müllerian duct regression. It is thought to be secreted locally, since it induces only ipsilateral müllerian duct regression. Levels of MIF activity in the human fetal testis decline by late pregnancy and are low at birth; continued MIF activity may be maintained in the infantile testis to 9 months of age or beyond. Whether MIF is necessary for testicular descent or other developmental functions is not known.

The major hormone produced by the fetal testis is testosterone. It is synthesized by the Leydig cells beginning at 8½ weeks, and testicular production achieves peak serum testosterone levels at 12 to 18 weeks. In the second half of gestation, males show a gradual decline, and females a rise, in serum testosterone levels, so that by the third trimester males have similar or only slightly higher levels than females. Fetal serum dihydrotestosterone (DHT) levels have not been measured, but other steroids, including androstenedione, dehydroepiandrosterone, 17-hydroxyprogesterone, and progesterone, are produced by the fetal testis (Fig. 33-29).

The major stimulus for testicular secretion of testosterone during the period of genital differentiation is believed to be placental human chorionic gonadotropin (HCG), whereas fetal pituitary luteinizing hormone (LH) is believed to be the principal stimulus during the second

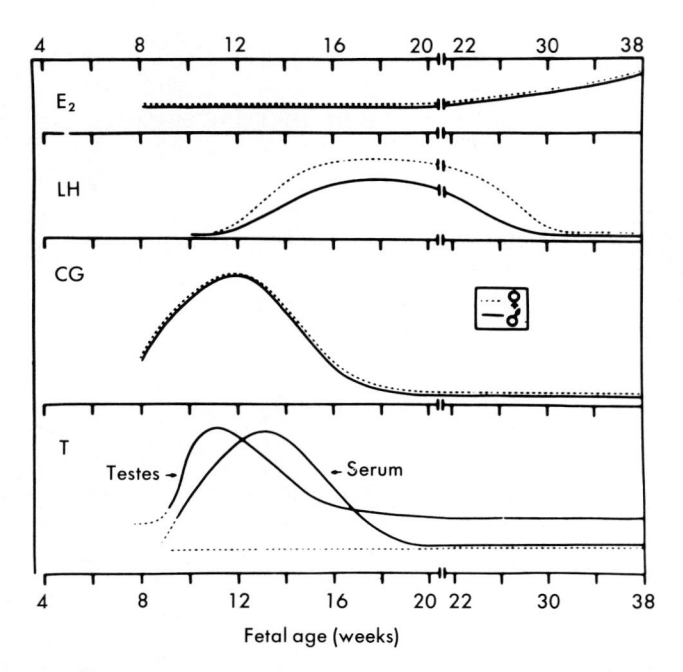

Fig. 33-30. Serum levels of estradiol (E$_2$), LH, HCG (CG), and serum and testicular concentrations of testosterone (T) throughout fetal life. (From Reyes, F.I., Winter, J.D.S., and Faiman, C.: Gonadotropin-gonadal interrelationships in the fetus. In New, M.I., and Fiser, R.J., Jr., editors: Diabetes and other endocrine disorders during pregnancy and in the newborn, Progress in Clinical and Biological Research, vol. 10, New York, 1976, Alan R. Liss.)

half of gestation, when growth of the penis and other genitalia occurs (Fig. 33-30). Fetal serum HCG levels are estimated to be 15 to 150 times lower than maternal levels, suggesting that only a small fraction of placental HCG reaches the fetus. Nonetheless, the fetal testes are able to bind and respond to HCG with production of testosterone. Fetal serum LH levels correlate with the subsequent maintenance and decline in serum testosterone.

The fetal ovary, like the testis, develops some capacity for steroid biosynthesis starting at 8 weeks gestation in that it becomes capable of converting testosterone or androstenedione to estrone and estradiol. Whether the fetal ovaries actually produce estrogens or other hormones has never been demonstrated; most estrogen present in the fetus is produced by the placenta. Amniotic fluid levels of estradiol at 12 to 16 weeks are, however, slightly higher in females, which raises a possibility of ovarian synthesis of estrogen. Estradiol synthesis is believed to be mediated by follicle-stimulating hormone (FSH) and may play some local role in ovarian differentiation.

CONTROL OF FETAL SEX DIFFERENTIATION
Gonadal differentiation: H-Y antigen

Gonadal differentiation is predominantly controlled by the Y chromosome; in its presence the bipotential gonad will differentiate into a testis, and in its absence ovarian differentiation will occur. The number of X chromosomes has no bearing on the differentiation of the early gonad. This control appears to be exerted during the sixth and seventh weeks of gestation, when the primordial germ cells interact with the somatic (epithelial and mesenchymal) cells of the gonadal blastema to form either seminiferous cords or irregular groups of cells that will lead to follicular formation. The differentiation of Y-chromosomal gonadal cells into seminiferous cords is attributed to the presence of a specific cell surface membrane protein, the H-Y (histocompatibility-Y) antigen, which is regulated by the H-Y gene, located on the short arm of the Y chromosome. In gonadal cells lacking a Y chromosome the H-Y antigen is absent, and these cells undergo early ovarian differentiation.

The concept of the H-Y antigen explains many of the disorders of gonadal differentiation. The finding of testicular tissue in the absence of a Y chromosome can be explained by translocation of the H-Y gene to an X or an autosomal chromosome. The absence of testicular tissue in an XY individual can be explained by a selective loss or mutation of the H-Y gene, the lack of a normal receptor for the H-Y antigen, or the loss or mutation of a gene that may regulate the H-Y gene. These latter two functions are postulated to be linked to the X chromosome. As helpful as these concepts are, however, it still remains to be definitely proven that it is the H-Y antigen, and not another closely related genetic product, that is the testis determinant.

In the absence of testicular differentiation, the indifferent gonad will undergo early ovarian development, regardless of the chromosomal makeup of its component cells. Early ovarian differentiation does not require two X chromosomes and thus may also be seen in 45,XO fetuses, since the second X chromosome in somatic cells (including the somatic cells in the gonad) is normally inactivated. The exception to this rule occurs with oocytes, in which both X chromosomes must be active for normal development to occur. Since the differentiation of oocytes is needed for later ovarian development, only ovaries associated with two or more X chromosomes will subsequently develop normally. In 45,XO fetuses, late ovarian development fails to occur, and the primordial follicles and germ cells degenerate rapidly. The resultant gonad appears as an elongated whitish streak that microscopically shows whorls of fibrous tissue (appearing like ovarian stroma) lacking in germ cells or epithelial (endocrine) elements. This streak gonad is characteristic for the gonadal dysgenesis syndromes. Y-chromosomal fetuses who fail to undergo testicular differentiation are believed to undergo the same early ovarian differentiation and late degeneration as occurs in the 45,XO fetus. They also have streak gonads postnatally and are categorized as having gonadal dysgenesis, but they carry a high risk for development of gonadal tumors, unlike gonadal dysgenesis patients with X chromosome abnormalities. This may be due to the persistence of residual XY germ cells that did not degenerate.

Spermatogonia that lose the Y chromosome are nonviable, suggesting that genes on the Y chromosome are necessary for spermatogenesis. The X chromosome is normally inactivated in the spermatocyte, but the presence of a second X chromosome, e.g., 47,XXY syndrome, will result in meiotic failure, loss of germ cells, and infertility.

Control of genital differentiation

The inherent tendency of the fetus is to develop along female lines. In the absence of testes, female sex differentiation occurs regardless of whether an ovary, streak gonad, or no gonad is present; a male fetus castrated early also undergoes female sex differentiation.

Male sex differentiation requires bilateral testes, which produce MIF and testosterone. MIF acts locally to cause regression of the ipsilateral müllerian duct only. If only one testis is present, müllerian duct development will take place on the contralateral side. The entire length of the müllerian duct is not sensitive to MIF at the same time, so its regression takes place sequentially, starting either at its cranial end or at the section adjacent to the caudal end of the testis. Testosterone does not cause müllerian duct regression.

Testosterone secreted by the fetal testis acts locally to stimulate differentiation of the ipsilateral wolffian duct and additionally serves as a prohormone in the masculinization of the external genitalia. If one testis is present, the contralateral wolffian duct will degenerate, indicating that systemic testosterone is not adequate for stimulation of wolffian differentiation. Thus testosterone derived from maternal sources or from the fetal adrenals, as in congenital adrenal hyperplasia, will not induce wolffian development.

The external genitalia and urogenital sinus undergo male differentiation as a result of the action of DHT, which is produced peripherally within these tissues from the single-step conversion of testosterone by the 5α-reductase enzyme. DHT in turn must bind to the androgen receptor to induce cell differentiation. Testosterone itself serves only as a prohormone and does not induce external genital male differentiation. The source of the systemic testosterone does not matter, so androgens derived from maternal sources or from the fetal adrenals in congenital adrenal hyperplasia may also induce masculinization of the external genitalia, if metabolized to DHT. The absence of one testis is usually associated with incomplete masculinization of the external genitalia, suggesting that two testes are generally required to provide adequate systemic levels of testosterone and consequently adequate DHT. If 5α-reductase activity is deficient, DHT will not be produced, and the external genitalia will follow their inherent tendency and differentiate along female lines, with only slight masculinization occurring, since this enzyme deficiency is typically not complete. A distal blind vaginal pouch also develops. The period in which DHT may induce changes is limited to before 14 weeks of gestational age; any deficiency of male differentiation, such as incomplete labioscrotal fusion, cannot be corrected beyond this time. Hypospadias thus may reflect an error in differentiation, for whatever reason, that occurred between 9 and 14 weeks of gestation.

Cells that are stimulated by androgens to undergo differentiation are referred to as target cells; these include not only the cells of the wolffian duct or the external genitalia and urogenital sinus but also the cells of the bone marrow, liver, kidney, and other tissues. Target cells in both male and female fetuses normally have the potential to respond if androgens are present.

The effect of androgens on target cells is mediated by a specific protein receptor located in the cytosol and a specific acceptor, presumably a nonhistone protein, located in the nucleus. Testosterone enters target cells by passive diffusion and either remains unmetabolized or is reduced via the 5α-reductase enzyme to DHT. Testosterone or DHT then binds to the androgen receptor, and this receptor-steroid complex is translocated to the nucleus where it interacts with a specific acceptor. This interaction results in transcription of certain genes with consequent production of new mRNA and synthesis of new proteins, resulting in differentiation of the target cells (Fig. 33-31, A). Androgen receptors have been identified in many tissues from various species and in fetuses as early as 8 weeks of gestational age. They are present equally in the target cells of both sexes.

A deficiency of androgen-receptor binding results in partial to complete androgen insensitivity (Fig. 33-31, B). In terms of fetal sex differentiation, androgen-mediated events of wolffian duct differentiation, masculinization of the external genitalia, and growth of genital structures would be impaired or completely fail to occur, depending on the extent of receptor deficiency. XY patients with complete androgen insensitivity (commonly referred to as testicular feminization syndrome) have bilateral testes and absence of müllerian ducts with fail-

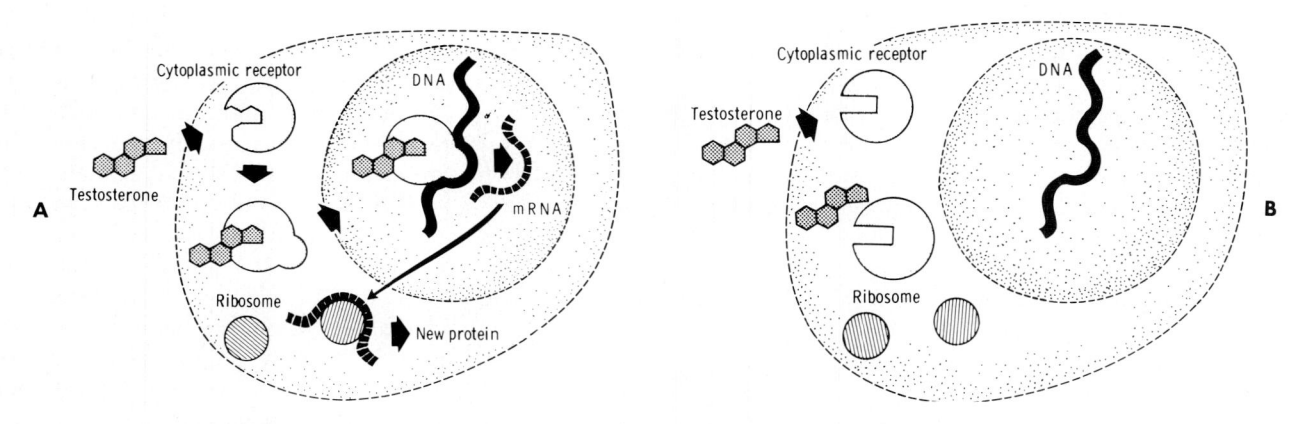

Fig. 33-31. A, Role of the androgen receptor in mediating testosterone (or DHT) action within the target cell. **B,** Consequence of loss of specific binding of testosterone (or DHT) by the androgen receptor. Testosterone freely diffuses into the target cell, but in the absence of receptor binding the formation of the receptor-steroid complex is impaired or absent, resulting in failure to stimulate target cell differentiation. The target cell thus behaves as though androgens were absent, or in a female manner. (From Imperato-McGinley, J., and Peterson, R.E.: Am. J. Med. **61**:251, 1976.)

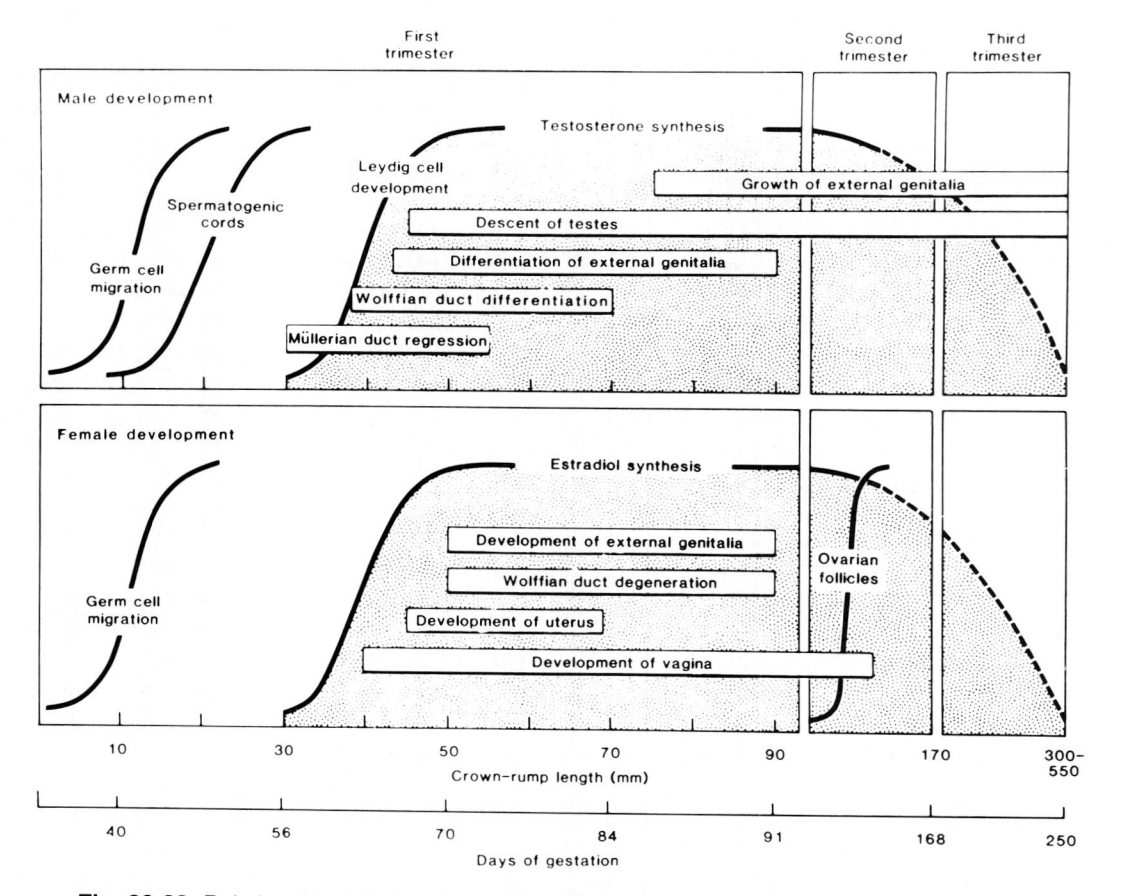

Fig. 33-32. Relationship between gonadal and genital differentiation and development in male *(top)* and female *(bottom)* fetuses from 5 weeks of gestational age to term. (The curve showing estradiol synthesis by the female ovary should be ignored, since there is no evidence for significant estradiol secretion by the human fetal ovary; estradiol also is not considered to be of any importance in fetal sex differentiation.) (From Wilson, J.D., George, F.W., and Griffin, J.E.: Science **211**:1278, 1981. Copyright 1981 by the American Association for the Advancement of Science.)

ure of formation of wolffian ducts, complete lack of masculinization of the external genitalia, and a distal vaginal pouch, giving them a normal phenotypic female appearance. Patients with partial androgen insensitivity have partial wolffian duct development and partial masculinization of the external genitalia (one example is the pedigree originally described by Reifenstein). The receptor deficiency may be so slight as to result only in a micropenis or infertility. The gene responsible for formation of the cytosolic androgen receptor is X linked. Androgen insensitivity also may be due to an abnormality beyond the androgen receptor step, such as a deficiency in the nuclear acceptor or in the events related to transcription of mRNA or new protein formation.

In summary, fetal sex differentiation occurs between 6 and 14 weeks of gestational age, with growth of the genitalia occurring thereafter (Fig. 33-32). The inherent development of the fetus is along female lines. The only abnormalities seen in female sex differentiation are the abnormalities of ovarian development, e.g., 45,XO Turner's syndrome, and in the exposure of the female fetus to abnormally elevated levels of androgens that lead to masculinization of the external genitalia, e.g., congenital adrenal hyperplasia. Male sex differentiation is more complicated and requires the H-Y gene, the H-Y antigen and its receptor, bilateral testes producing MIF and testosterone, and 5α-reductase activity and intact androgen receptor function in the target cells. There are thus many more disorders associated with abnormal male sex differentiation than female sex differentiation. These disorders are classified in the following outline.

A. Disorders of gonadal development
  1. True hermaphroditism
  2. Gonadal dysgenesis
     a. X chromosome abnormalities (Turner's syndrome)
     b. XX gonadal dysgenesis
     c. Y chromosome abnormalities (including mixed gonadal dysgenesis)
     d. XY gonadal dysgenesis
  3. Disorders of testicular development
     a. Dysgenetic testes (renal disease, Wilms' tumor)
     b. Testicular regression syndromes
        (1) Early (XY gonadal agenesis)
        (2) Late (congenital anorchia)
     c. Rudimentary or small testes
     d. Seminiferous tubule dysgenesis (Klinefelter's and XX male syndromes)
B. Disorders of testicular function
  1. Abnormalities of gonadotropin stimulation
  2. Abnormalities of müllerian-inhibiting factor
  3. Testosterone biosynthetic defects
C. Disorders of androgen-dependent target cells
  1. 5α-Reductase deficiency
  2. Androgen insensitivity syndromes
     a. Complete (testicular feminization syndrome)
     b. Partial (incomplete testicular feminization)
D. Female pseudohermaphroditism
  1. Congenital adrenal hyperplasia
     a. 21-Hydroxylase deficiency
        (1) Simple virilizing form
        (2) Salt-losing form
     b. 11β-Hydroxylase deficiency
     c. 3β-Hydroxysteroid dehydrogenase deficiency
  2. Maternally-derived androgenic substances
     a. Virilizing ovarian or adrenal tumors
     b. Androgen, progestin, or estrogen therapy
  3. Idiopathic
E. Other disorders of sexual development
  1. Hypospadias, micropenis, cryptorchidism
  2. Müllerian aplasia, vaginal agenesis

DISORDERS OF GONADAL DEVELOPMENT
True hermaphroditism

True hermaphroditism is defined as the coexistence in an individual of ovarian and testicular tissue in either the same gonad or opposite gonads. The ovarian tissue must contain ovarian follicles or corpora albicantia, since fibrous stroma alone does not necessarily connote ovarian tissue; for testicular tissue to be definitely diagnosed, it must contain seminiferous tubules or spermatozoa. Several chromosome karyotypes are seen in true hermaphroditism: three fifths of the cases are 46,XX, one fifth are 46,XY or 45,XO/46,XY, and one fifth show mosaicism or chimerism, being 46,XX/46,XY or 46,XX/47,XXY. The most frequently occurring gonadal combinations are an ovary and testis, or an ovary and ovotestis. The ovotestis accounts for 41% of all gonads in this condition, with the ovary and testis accounting for 32% and 22%, respectively; occasional patients may have a unilateral streak gonad or a tumor.

The internal genital ducts generally reflect the gonadal constitution. On the side of an ovary a fallopian tube is almost always seen, and on the side of the testis the vas deferens and epididymis are almost always present, with a few cases having a fallopian tube as well. On the side of an ovotestis a vas is seen 35% of the time, and a fallopian tube, often closed at the fimbrial end, is seen 65% of the time; rarely both a vas and a tube are present. A uterus is described in about 83% of patients, but it is usually hypoplastic, unicornuate, or otherwise maldeveloped.

The external genitalia are usually ambiguous, although a number of cases have been reported with normal male or female appearance. The urethra most commonly opens on the perineum as a urogenital sinus, giving an appearance of perineal hypospadias. The phallus is usually larger than a normal clitoris and often has chordee; it often is of sufficient size to give the genitalia a more masculine appearance (Fig. 33-33). Unilateral or bilateral gonads are palpable in 61% of patients, more frequently on the right side; about 60% are ovotestes and much of the remainder are testes, but rarely an ovary may

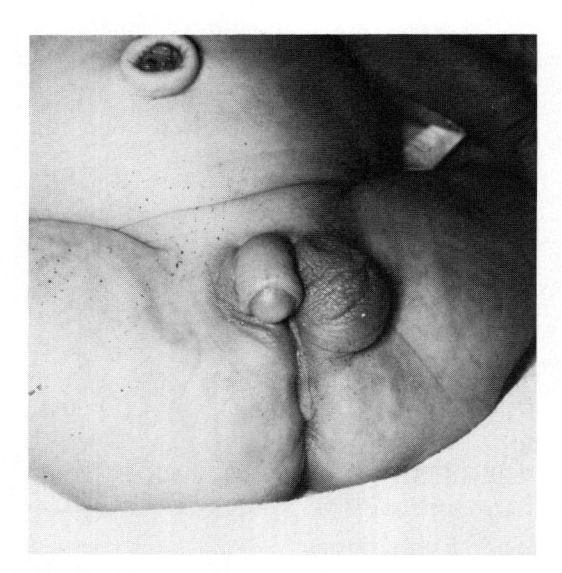

Fig. 33-33. True hermaphrodite with scrotal testis and abdominal ovotestis. The genital ambiguity is not specific for this disorder.

descend. The ovotestis is more likely to descend if it contains a greater proportion of testicular tissue. Histologically the ovarian portion of the ovotestis is usually normal, with the predominant abnormality being a reduction in the number of primordial follicles. The testicular portion, however, is abnormal in more than 90%; germ cells may be present, but complete spermatogenesis has not been observed.

The testosterone response to HCG stimulation in three patients has been low or low-normal. Fertility has been rarely reported; self-impregnation has not been documented. Gonadal tumors occur in 1.9% to 2.6% and have a greater frequency in Y-chromatin–positive patients. Renal abnormalities have been noted in 4.6% of 150 cases reviewed.

The incidence of true hermaphroditism is unknown. Most cases occur sporadically, but several affected families have been reported. There are three possible causes of true hermaphroditism: (1) chimerism or mosaicism involving the second X and the Y chromosome, (2) translocation of the H-Y gene locus to an X chromosome or an autosome, or conversely, possible translocation of an ovarian gene locus from the X to the Y chromosome or an autosome, and (3) the possibility of an autosomal gene mutation that causes sex reversal. Chimerism refers to the presence of two cell lines that originate from different zygotes, whereas in mosaicism the different cell lines originate from a common zygote by nondisjunction.

Most cases of true hermaphroditism are potentially recognizable in the neonatal period because of ambiguous genitalia. If a gonad is an ovotestis, one pole may feel firmer, the other softer. The majority will have a palpable uterus. Approximately 70% of cases will be X-chromatin positive on buccal smear; in these individuals it is necessary to rule out female pseudohermaphroditism, particularly congenital adrenal hyperplasia. The definitive diagnosis requires a gonadal biopsy, but this is preferably delayed beyond the neonatal period until the infant weighs at least 9 kg, since there is no urgency in making the diagnosis. The assignment of sex of rearing should be based on the size of the phallus and the likelihood of satisfactorily correcting the external genital abnormalities to give a normal male or female appearance by early childhood. The chances for fertility are extremely poor as a male and only a little better as a female, so this should not be a factor in deciding the sex of rearing, although the presence of a normal uterus would be an argument for female assignment. The chromosome karyotype also should not be a factor. A decision as to sex of rearing should not be delayed until a gonadal biopsy is done because the gonadal findings should not have any bearing.

Gonadal dysgenesis

Turner, in 1938, described a series of phenotypic females who had a triad of somatic features consisting of infantilism (short stature, delayed bone age, and absence of secondary sexual development), webbing of the skin of the neck, and deformity of the elbow (cubitus valgus). Other investigators subsequently noted similar patients to have gonadal dysgenesis (manifested as bilateral streak gonads) with elevated gonadotropins; other somatic abnormalities were also frequently associated. In 1959 the cause of this form of gonadal dysgenesis was found to be a loss of the second X chromosome, i.e., a 45,XO chromosome karyotype. Variant forms of this syndrome were also recognized in which patients had only partial deletions of the second X chromosome or X chromosome mosaicism such as XO/XX.

The eponym *Turner's syndrome* came to be used synonymously with the diagnosis of gonadal dysgenesis, which was unfortunate, since other forms of described gonadal dysgenesis had very different causes and often totally lacked the somatic abnormalities described by Turner. They did have in common the presence of bilateral streak gonads and a female phenotype. The somatic abnormalities described by Turner appear to be controlled by genes located on the X chromosome, and thus they usually occur simultaneously in those cases of gonadal dysgenesis due to an abnormality of the second X chromosome. However, some patients with Y chromosome abnormalities and gonadal dysgenesis also have Turner's somatic stigmata, since the presence of an abnormal Y chromosome often leads to the development of mosaicism with 45,XO cell lines. It is the presence of these 45,XO cells that results in some Y chromosome cases having an appearance of Turner's syndrome, yet the cause and the complications of their gonadal dysgenesis are very different from those due to abnormalities of the X chromosome.

The streak gonad found in all forms of gonadal dysgenesis is an elongated, whitish streak of tissue consisting of whorls of connective tissue, suggestive of ovarian stroma, that contain no germinal elements or endocrine or other epithelial elements. Affected patients have normal müllerian duct development, absence of wolffian ducts, and phenotypically female external genitalia. Secondary sexual development fails to occur at puberty without therapeutic intervention, and these individuals are hypergonadotropic. Turner's syndrome patients are not at increased risk for mental retardation. A portion of neonates with Turner's syndrome have somatic abnormalities that permit their identification in the nursery. The most diagnostic features are lymphedema on the dorsa of the hands or feet, loose posterior neck folds (often with a low nuchal hairline), horseshoe kidney or other renal abnormalities, and coarctation of the aorta (this occurs in males 2.3 times more frequently than in females). Other features often present in the neonatal period include intrauterine growth retardation and neurosensory hearing loss; the genitalia are usually normal.

Patients with X chromosome mosaicism or partial deletion of the second X chromosome as a group have fewer somatic and gonadal manifestations than are seen in 45,XO Turner's syndrome. In cases of mosaicism it is thought that the relative proportion of XX to XO cells may determine the extent to which normal development of gonadal and somatic tissues may occur. Turner's syndrome patients having only a partial deletion of the X chromosome also manifest a modified phenotype, depending on the portion of the X chromosome deleted. The combined incidence of 45,XO and mosaic Turner's syndrome is approximately 1 in 2,000 female neonates.

The cause of monosomy X is unknown. The mean maternal and paternal ages are not raised, so nondisjunction is not thought to be important; a postfertilization abnormality is thought to be most likely. The incidence of the 45,XO karyotype in spontaneous abortuses is very high, generally estimated to be 10%. The mean incidence of living 45,XO newborns, however, is only approximately 1 in 5,000 female births, suggesting that about 99% of XO fetuses abort. The reasons for this high mortality are unclear because few XO fetuses have been examined, and many of these were macerated. The ovaries in the 45,XO fetus do develop normally in the first few months in utero but then are presumed to undergo accelerated degeneration.

An infant or child suspected of having Turner's syndrome may be screened with a buccal smear, recognizing that false negative and false positive results may occur. (In the first few days of life, 46,XX female neonates normally may have a reduced percentage of sex-chromatin–positive nuclei of as low as 4%.) Patients with mosaicism of the X chromosome will usually have fewer than 20% sex-chromatin–positive cells; patients with only partial deletions of the X chromosome may have a normal buccal smear, but the sex chromatin body may be abnormally sized. A definitive diagnosis requires a chromosome karyotype. There is a high rate of failure in the culture of 45,XO cells, so repeated attempts may be necessary. Banding techniques should be used, and 20 or more cells should be assessed for the possibility of mosaicism. At times, multiple tissues need to be karyotyped before mosaicism may be identified. Serum FSH is abnormally elevated in infancy and again beyond age 10 to 12 years but is normal in childhood.

Patients with *XX gonadal dysgenesis* have bilateral streak gonads with intact müllerian duct structures and female external genitalia. They differ from patients with Turner's syndrome in that they usually have normal stature, absence of Turner's stigmata, no abnormality of the X chromosome, and their condition may frequently be familial. Isolated instances of clitoromegaly have been described, due to testosterone production by either hilar cells or luteinized gonadal stromal cells in a streak gonad; only patients who have clitoromegaly are likely to be recognized in infancy.

Several variants of *gonadal dysgenesis due to abnormalities of the Y chromosome* have been described. A small number of patients have been reported with abnormal gonadal or statural development and a partial deletion of the Y chromosome without chromosomal mosaicism. These cases have provided some insight as to the possible location of the gene loci for testicular development.

An abnormal or partially deleted Y chromosome will frequently result in chromosome mosaicism, usually XO/XY or XO/XYY. Gonadal and somatic development in these cases is determined by the relative prevalence of the XO and the XY cell lines and whether the Y chromosome has retained or lost the H-Y locus. Affected patients present a wide range of gonadal and somatic phenotypes. At one end of the spectrum they appear identical with 45,XO Turner's syndrome patients, who have bilateral streak gonads and müllerian structures, female external genitalia, short stature, and the somatic abnormalities of Turner's syndrome. However, they also have a 15% to 20% risk of gonadal tumor development and are at increased risk of unwanted virilization. At the other end of the spectrum are a few XO/XY phenotypic males with almost normal male external genitalia, bilateral testes and wolffian duct development, absence of müllerian structures, normal stature, and absence of Turner's stigmata. Whether they have an increased risk of gonadal tumor formation is unknown.

Individuals toward the middle of the spectrum are most frequently seen having ambiguous genitalia, varying degrees of testicular development (testicular development might be dysgenetic or normal, and unilateral or bilateral), persistence of müllerian structures, and variable presence of short stature or Turner's stigmata. They are also at high risk for gonadal tumor development and often have a gonadal tumor obscuring the original gonadal architecture. A subset of this group is the syndrome of mixed gonadal dysgenesis.

Mixed gonadal dysgenesis is a term first used to describe individuals with a unilateral functioning testis and a contralateral streak or absent gonad. All have some degree of virilization of the external genitalia, ranging from clitoromegaly or partial labial fusion to almost normal male external genitalia; slightly more than half have a urogenital sinus. All patients have some müllerian development, consisting of an upper vagina, uterus, and a fallopian tube usually on the side having a streak or absent gonad. An epididymis or vas deferens may be present on the testicular side in half the cases, and the testis is most frequently located in the inguinal canal. Variably normal to diminished or absent testosterone responses have been reported with HCG stimulation, and gonadotropins have been normal or elevated. Gonadal tumors occur in 22%, affecting either the testis or the streak gonad; a gonadal tumor has not been described in a scrotal testis.

Management of these patients involves appropriate sex assignment in the newborn period and prophylactic removal of dysgenetic gonads later in infancy or early childhood because of the increased risk of tumor formation. The cause of mixed gonadal dysgenesis is thought to be an abnormality of the Y chromosome. Its main significance is the observation that the unilateral testis affects wolffian and müllerian duct development only on the side having a testis.

The syndrome of *XY gonadal dysgenesis* is characterized by a normal XY karyotype with the presence of bilateral streak gonads, intact müllerian structures, and a female phenotype with absence of the somatic abnormalities of Turner's syndrome. Most cases occur sporadically, but family aggregates have been reported, some involving two or three generations, compatible with either X-linked recessive or autosomal dominant male-limited inheritance. XY gonadal dysgenesis is genetically heterogeneous in that some individuals are H-Y antigen negative, and others are H-Y antigen positive. In the latter, it is postulated that the receptor for the H-Y antigen must be abnormally formed or absent.

Clinical recognition of 46,XY gonadal dysgenesis is possible in the newborn period in infants with clitoromegaly; occasional neonates have presented with edema of the feet, and there appears to be a significant association with camptomelic dwarfism. There is a very high risk for the development of gonadal tumors in XY gonadal dysgenesis, approximately 5% in the first decade of life (occurring as early as 3 years of age) and overall about 30%.

Prophylactic removal of the streak or dysgenetic gonads is indicated in infancy. The sex of rearing should be female. The syndrome of XY gonadal dysgenesis has often been categorized with XX gonadal dysgenesis under the general term of XY and XX pure gonadal dysgenesis ("pure" because the Turner's somatic stigmata are usually absent). This seems inappropriate. The cause of the XY form appears to be related to abnormalities of the H-Y antigen or its receptors, whereas the XX form appears to be due to an autosomal mutation that affects ovarian development. The importance of XY gonadal dysgenesis is that it proves Jost's hypothesis that early castration or failure of testicular development will result in a female genital phenotype, regardless of chromosome constitution.

Disorders of testicular development

Male pseudohermaphroditism comprises male infants who have testes with incomplete development of internal genital ducts or external genitalia. This designation includes patients with disorders of testicular development, disorders of testicular function, and disorders of androgen-dependent target cells.

Dysgenetic testes

Dysgenetic testes are defined by the following characteristics: (1) their failure to induce regression of the ipsilateral müllerian duct structures, (2) their association with incomplete masculinization of the genitalia, (3) their variably abnormal testicular histology, and (4) their increased predisposition to develop tumors originating from the germinal structures. The testes may be of normal or small size and are usually cryptorchid. The chromosome karyotype commonly is 46,XY, but other karyotypes are seen. This disorder is to be differentiated from mixed gonadal dysgenesis and the persistent müllerian duct syndrome; dysgenetic testicular tissue is also seen in true hermaphroditism.

Many male pseudohermaphrodites, including many with dysgenetic testes, have been reported with the *occurrence of degenerative renal disease or Wilms' tumor* arising within the first 3 years of life. The nature of the pseudohermaphroditism has not been well characterized in most cases and probably is quite variable. Many cases have not been karyotyped: one was XX/XY and others are 46,XY. Although many reported patients had ambiguous genitalia or occasionally female genitalia secondary to XY gonadal dysgenesis, some patients have had male-appearing genitalia with either a small penis or with cryptorchidism or anorchia. Many with ambiguous genitalia have had müllerian duct structures. The testes seldom have been studied histologically, being either absent or cryptorchid. It is hypothesized that there is a basic embryogenic abnormality affecting the urogenital or mesonephric structures. Infants with dysgenetic male pseudohermaphroditism should be examined for aniridia and development of abdominal masses and should have their renal status assessed to exclude Wilms' tumor or degenerative renal disease.

Testicular regression syndromes

Early regression with genital ambiguity (XY gonadal agenesis). At least 15 patients with a presumed or demonstrated XY chromosome karyotype have been reported with complete absence of testes (including absence of gonadal streaks), virtually complete absence of both müllerian and wolffian duct derivatives, and female to partially masculinized genitalia. Their gonadal and genital features may be explained as being caused by very early regression of the developing fetal testes, between approximately 8 and 10 weeks. Testicular failure must have occurred after the initial production of MIF by Sertoli cells but before the Leydig cells could produce sufficient testosterone for a reasonable period of time.

Other XY individuals have been documented to have complete absence of testes with quite well-developed wolffian structures but incomplete masculinization of external genitalia. Presumably testicular regression occurred slightly later than in those cases completely lacking internal genital ducts.

Late regression: congenital anorchia (vanishing testes syndrome). More than 100 cases have been reported of cryptorchid 46,XY males who on exploration were found to have bilateral anorchia, but with normal development of wolffian structures, absence of müllerian structures, and normal male external genitalia. The vas deferens ends blindly, often without an epididymis, either in the inguinal canal or upper scrotum, retroperitoneally near the usual location of the internal inguinal ring, or in the iliac fossa. Neonates and infants with anorchia should show a failure of any rise in testosterone during either endogenous LH or exogenous HCG stimulation; serum LH and FSH levels should be abnormally elevated beyond 1 to 2 weeks of age for several months. In the 46,XY individual with a male phenotype these findings are pathognomonic, and surgical exploration is unnecessary. In patients with monorchia, endocrine testing is not helpful in ruling out an abdominal gonad, and surgical exploration is indicated. The cause of congenital anorchia is not established, but the most likely explanation for at least a portion of cases, including those occurring shortly after birth, is vascular occlusion or trauma due to testicular hemorrhage, torsion of the testis, breech delivery, or similar events. Infections, teratogens, or hereditary factors may play a role. The possibility that bilateral congenital anorchia is related to early testicular regression has been raised.

Rudimentary or small testes

A few 46,XY patients have been described with abnormally small testes associated with either a micropenis or ambiguous genitalia, or hypogonadism in adulthood. They have male internal genital ducts and lack any müllerian structures. It is not certain what constitutes a small testis in neonates. Testes with a longest diameter of 1 cm or more are probably normal, and a measurement of 0.5 or 0.6 cm is considered abnormally small, but whether 0.8 cm represents a low or normal measurement is not known. It is unclear whether rudimentary or small testes represent a distinct entity or if they represent an attenuated form of testicular regression or, alternatively, a different form of dysgenetic testes. The differential diagnosis includes pituitary gonadotropin deficiency in patients with a micropenis, and in patients with ambiguous genitalia, mixed gonadal dysgenesis. The sex of rearing is dictated principally by penile size and the likelihood of adequately correcting the ambiguous genitalia.

Seminiferous tubule dysgenesis (Klinefelter's, or 47,XXY, syndrome and its variants)

The major clinical manifestations of classic Klinefelter's syndrome (47,XXY) develop with onset of puberty, and most patients are recognized at this time or beyond. The constant features are a male phenotype and small testes, associated with azoospermia (93%) and histologic evidence of impaired spermatogenesis (100%). Infants with 47,XXY Klinefelter's syndrome only occasionally have features that might permit their recognition. Testes may be small, firm, or soft in affected neonates. Cryptorchidism and hypospadias occur infrequently; a few infants have been born with a very small penis. In 63 infants detected at seven centers, major congenital abnormalities occurred in 18%, including cleft palate, inguinal hernia, and cryptorchidism each occurring in four patients and other abnormalities occurring singly. Minor abnormalities occurred in 26%, including clinodactyly in 19%. Mental, motor, speech, and emotional development is frequently impaired. Testicular histology in the first year of life has varied from normal to extensively abnormal, with decreased to absent spermatogonia. Gonadotropin and testosterone studies have not been published in neonates or infants. Patients with Klinefelter's syndrome may be predisposed to the development of germ cell tumors, particularly those of extragonadal origin, which have occurred as early as a few months of age.

The incidence of the 47,XXY karyotype in a total of 111,402 live newborn males screened in 10 chromatin and chromosome surveys is 1:994; if the Klinefelter variants are added, the incidence of all Klinefelter's syndrome patients is 1:779. Increased maternal age is associated with an additional X chromosome in both male and female offspring, although this effect is not so marked as that seen for autosomal trisomies.

Among the variant forms of Klinefelter's syndrome, patients with 48,XXXY and 49,XXXXY karyotypes are more likely to be recognized early in life. All have somatic abnormalities and mental retardation, and many have a hypoplastic penis; of those with the 49,XXXXY karyotypes, all also have cryptorchidism and 14% have cardiac defects. Patients with 48,XXYY and 46,XY/47,XXY karyotypes are unlikely to be recognized in infancy, as are most XX males, but about 10% to 20% of XX males do have ambiguous genitalia.

DISORDERS OF TESTICULAR FUNCTION
Abnormalities of gonadotropin stimulation: deficiency of fetal pituitary LH secretion

Fetal pituitary LH normally stimulates the fetal testis in the second half of gestation when levels of placentally derived HCG have become low. During this period the genital structures have long completed their differentiation and only undergo growth, which in part is believed to be testosterone mediated. Male 46,XY neonates lacking LH thus do not have ambiguous genitalia or even hypospadias but may show either cryptorchidism, often with a small, "un-lived-in" scrotum, or a small penis (Fig. 33-34); some may have a micropenis at birth. Since FSH deficiency usually accompanies a lack of LH, the testes also tend to be small.

Gonadotropin deficiency may be due to pituitary aplasia or hypopituitarism associated with other pituitary hormone deficiencies. If growth hormone deficiency coexists, there is a stronger likelihood for a small or micropenis and for hypoglycemia to occur in the neonatal period. The combination of hypoglycemia with a micropenis should suggest hypopituitarism; TSH and ACTH deficiencies often accompany the growth hormone and gonadotropin deficiencies in these patients.

Persistent müllerian duct syndrome

More than 80 cases have been described at surgery or autopsy of phenotypic males having bilateral fallopian tubes and a uterus associated with normal wolffian structures, male external genitalia, and, when determined, a 46,XY karyotype. The müllerian structures may be hypoplastic or partially rudimentary. These individuals usually have cryptorchidism or an inguinal hernia, and in those with unilateral cryptorchidism the hernia is often on the contralateral side. The vas deferens is frequently continuous with, or embedded in, the posterior wall of the uterus, and malignant gonadal tumors have been reported. The cause of this syndrome is considered to be either a deficiency of MIF, synthesis of an abnormal MIF, an MIF receptor defect, or a defect in timing of its secretion.

Testosterone biosynthetic defects

Five enzymatic steps are involved in the biosynthesis of testosterone from cholesterol. The first three steps are also necessary for the biosynthesis of cortisol, and defects involving their enzymes include cholesterol side-chain cleavage enzyme-complex (20,22-desmolase) deficiency, 3β-hydroxysteroid dehydrogenase deficiency, and 17α-hydroxylase deficiency. Patients having any of these three disorders will have cortisol deficiency and decreased or absent androgen and estrogen synthesis. They are classified as having congenital adrenal hyperplasia but differ from the more common 21-hydroxylase forms in that the male, or 46,XY, patients have ambiguous genitalia and thus are usually recognized at birth, whereas the female, or 46,XX, patients have female or only slightly virilized genitalia and thus may not be recognized until they have developed adrenal insufficiency. These three disorders are discussed in the section on congenital adrenal hyperplasia.

Defects involving the remaining two testosterone bio-

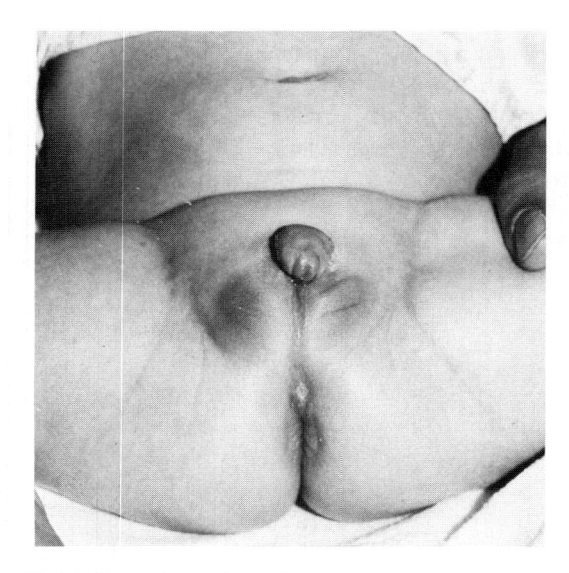

Fig. 33-34. Gonadotropin deficiency with undescended testes, compact scrotum, and small penis.

synthetic enzymes, which are not needed for cortisol synthesis, include 17,20-desmolase deficiency and 17β-hydroxysteroid oxidoreductase deficiency. The enzyme *17,20-desmolase (or 17,20-lyase)*, present in adrenal and gonadal tissue, is necessary for the production of the C_{19} steroids, dehydroepiandrosterone (DHA) and androstenedione, which serve as precursors for both androgens and estrogens. In the neonatal period, 46,XY patients with this enzyme deficiency may have ambiguous genitalia or, if the deficiency is complete, inguinal gonads in otherwise female-appearing genitalia. Some may have no clinically recognizable abnormality and do not come to medical attention until puberty. Similarly affected 46,XX patients would be expected to be normal in infancy. The XY patients should show low levels of testosterone, DHAS, and androstenedione and abnormally increased levels of 17-hydroxyprogesterone and 17-hydroxypregnenolone in the first months of life, when normal male infants would have increased levels, or after HCG stimulation.

The decision as to sex of rearing of the affected 46,XY neonate can be made in the first days of life without knowledge of the biochemical findings. It should be based on the size of the penis and the potential for successfully correcting the external genitalia along the lines of the intended sex of rearing.

The enzyme *17β-hydroxysteroid oxidoreductase (17-ketosteroid reductase)* is necessary primarily for conversion of androstenedione to testosterone, and of estrone to estradiol. It is present in both gonadal and in peripheral tissues but only to a very small extent in adrenocortical tissue. Its deficiency is associated primarily with diminished testosterone synthesis, resulting in failure of male differentiation in utero. The 46,XY patients with this enzyme deficiency have had a normal or slightly masculinized female genital appearance. Müllerian structures are absent, and many patients have an epididymis and vas deferens bilaterally. Testes may be descended.

Neonates and infants should show a low or low-normal serum level of testosterone and a markedly elevated level of androstenedione during periods of endogenous LH or exogenous HCG stimulation. Modest elevations of 17α-hydroxyprogesterone, a precursor of androstenedione, may occur. Serum LH levels should be elevated beyond the first 1 or 2 weeks.

DISORDERS OF ANDROGEN-DEPENDENT TARGET CELLS: 5α-REDUCTASE DEFICIENCY

Patients with 5α-reductase enzyme deficiency are unable to transform testosterone to DHT and thus have reduced or negligible production of DHT. The consequence in males is that differentiation in utero of the external genitalia (urogenital sinus, urogenital folds, and genital tubercle) fails to occur. Affected males thus have normally developed testes and male internal ducts and absent müllerian duct structures but female-appearing

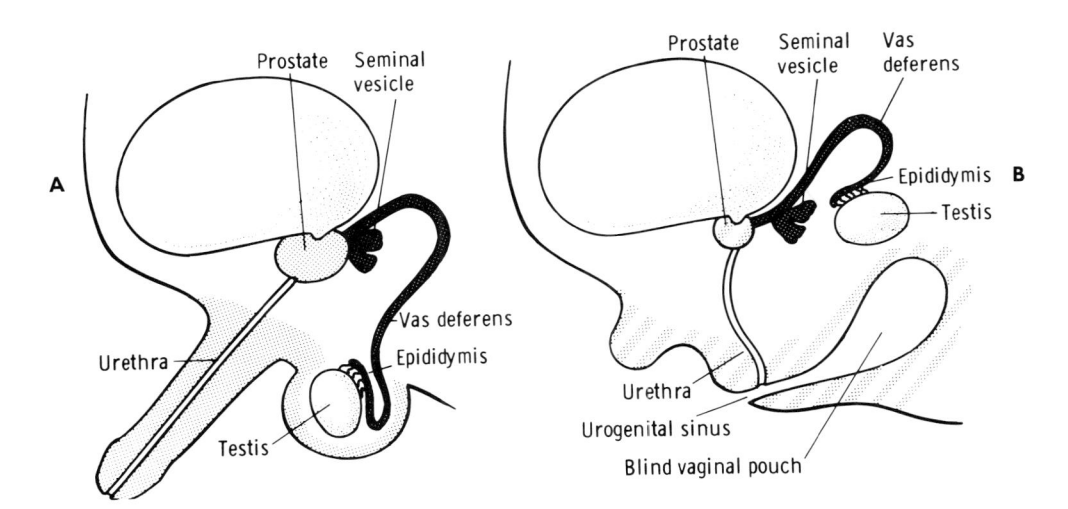

Fig. 33-35. A, Male differentiation of the external genitalia and urogenital sinus structures is DHT-stimulated (light stippled area), whereas wolffian duct differentiation is testosterone-stimulated (dark stippled area). **B,** 5α-Reductase deficiency results in impaired male differentiation of DHT-responsive tissues. The external genitalia appear female, and the vesicovaginal septum develops to create a distal blind vaginal pouch (in this diagram) opening into a urogenital sinus. Wolffian duct differentiation is normal. (From Imperato-McGinley, J., and Peterson, R.E., Am. J. Med. **61:**251, 1976.)

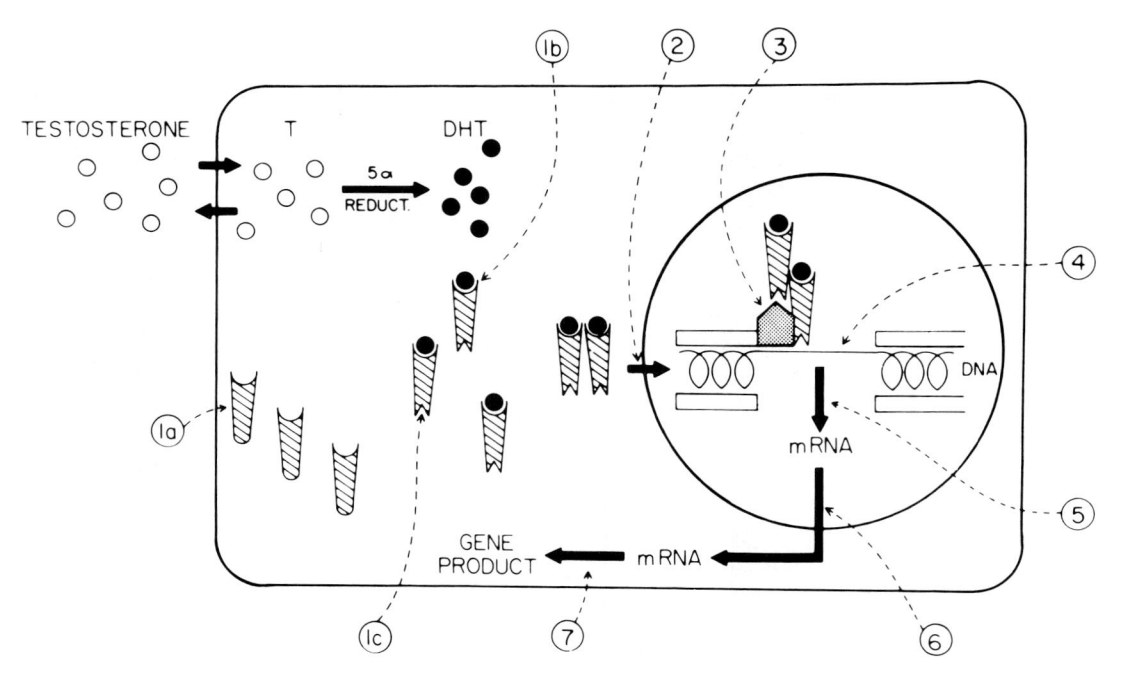

Fig. 33-36. Androgen-dependent target cell showing steroid hormone action. Numbers refer to sites where mutations might result in androgen insensitivity. *1*, Mutations affecting cytosol androgen-receptor protein, including *a*, absent protein, *b*, abnormality of androgen (DHT in this diagram) binding site, *c*, abnormality of acceptor binding site; *2*, defective translocation of androgen-receptor complex to nucleus; *3*, abnormalities of nuclear acceptor site; *4*, abnormal regulatory molecules; *5*, abnormal transcription of nuclear mRNA; *6*, abnormal mRNA processing; *7*, abnormal translation in synthesis of new protein. (From Fichman, K.R., Migeon, B.R., and Migeon, C.J.: Genetic disorders of male sexual development. In Harris, H., and Hirschhorn, K., editors: Advances in human genetics, vol. 10, New York, 1980, Plenum Press.)

external genitalia. In the cases reported to date, the external genitalia have been partially virilized, presumably because the enzyme deficiency has never been total. At birth all patients have been potentially recognizable: all have had clitoromegaly and, with rare exception, a single perineal orifice (giving an appearance of perineal hypospadias) that proved to be a urogenital sinus opening. Some cases have had posterior labial fusion, and most have had a small, distal vaginal pouch (Fig. 33-35). Among the reported cases, most were reared as females. At puberty, noncastrated individuals show striking virilization, except that certain secondary sexual characteristics do not appear. There is no published experience yet as to the biochemical findings in affected neonates or infants in the first year of life. Based on the findings in adults, it is reasonable to expect that under gonadotropin stimulation serum testosterone (T) will be elevated, and DHT will be low, causing the T:DHT ratio to be abnormally elevated. The T:DHT ratio may be elevated in patients with androgen insensitivity, but they have normal serum levels of DHT. The inheritance of 5α-reductase deficiency is autosomal recessive. Affected 46,XX females have no genital abnormalities. Determination of the sex of rearing is particularly difficult in this disorder because there is some prospect for fertility, but the penile length achieved has been very small (not more than half of normal adult size). There is no experience to show whether early intervention with DHT therapy can provide an adequate penile length either during childhood or by adulthood. Phallic length should be used to decide on the sex of rearing in the neonate or young infant.

Syndromes of androgen insensitivity
Complete androgen insensitivity (testicular feminization syndrome)

The androgen insensitivity syndrome refers to those disorders in which peripheral tissues are partially or completely incapable of responding to stimulation by any androgen (Fig. 33-36). Androgen-mediated events, such as masculine differentiation in utero or virilization during puberty, fail to occur or are impaired to a variable extent, depending on the completeness of the defect. The classic example of this syndrome is *complete androgen insensi-*

tivity, also called *testicular feminization*. Affected individuals have a 46,XY karyotype with bilateral testes and no müllerian structures but with failure of wolffian duct development and complete absence of any masculinization of the external genitalia. They have normal female-appearing external genitalia with a distal vaginal pouch. The testes are of normal size and may be intraabdominal or descended into the inguinal canal or labia majora. More than half the patients have an inguinal hernia. At puberty these patients undergo normal female breast development and labial growth and acquire a female habitus. Gender identity remains female in adulthood. Occurrence of the syndrome is familial in 30% of cases, and inheritance is X-linked recessive. Spontaneous mutation is thought to account for the sporadic cases. There is an increased risk of gonadal malignancy occurring after the first two decades. Patients with complete androgen insensitivity come to early medical attention either because of a history of an affected relative or because of an inguinal hernia or labial mass. This syndrome can be simply screened for in the neonate by establishing the absence of a uterine cervix via rectal examination. In addition, basal testosterone levels should be elevated in the male range in the first 36 hours of life and at 30 to 60 days and slightly beyond.

The sex of rearing of these individuals should be unequivocally female. Their testes ideally should be left in the abdomen until the latter part of the second decade so that they may feminize normally at puberty.

Partial androgen insensitivity (incomplete testicular feminization)

This syndrome includes those disorders in which peripheral tissues are partially unable to respond to androgen stimulation. Affected individuals are 46,XY and have bilateral testes and no müllerian structures, but they differ from patients with complete androgen insensitivity in that they have some masculinization of their external genitalia. The extent of masculinization, which should be evident at birth, may range from clitoromegaly or posterior labial fusion to phenotypically normal male-appearing genitalia. A significant portion of recognized cases have perineal, perineoscrotal, or penile hypospadias. Wolffian duct development also occurs but is often incomplete, and the external genital appearance may not necessarily correlate with the extent of wolffian duct development.

Androgen insensitivity has been demonstrated in several patients when administration of exogenous testosterone or DHT failed to induce either retention of nitrogen or phosphorus or suppression of serum LH levels. However, in other instances androgen administration, usually in higher dose, was able to induce either nitrogen retention or LH suppression. These observations are compatible with the partial nature of the disorder.

Neonates with partial androgen insensitivity usually come to medical attention because of ambiguous genitalia or because of a positive family history. Diagnosis is based on finding a 46,XY karyotype, absence of müllerian structures, normal to increased levels of testosterone and DHT during the periods of gonadotropin stimulation, and elevated LH levels between 1 and 2 weeks and about 6 to 12 months of age. The differential diagnosis includes disorders of testosterone biosynthesis and 5α-reductase deficiency; patients with true hermaphroditism, mixed gonadal dysgenesis, or maternal exposure to progestins may have similar features. Definitive diagnosis requires demonstration of a deficient metabolic response to androgen stimulation or a deficiency in the cytoplasmic androgen receptor protein. These studies are usually done only in research centers, so most patients are not definitively diagnosed.

Determination of the sex of rearing in the neonate or young infant should be based on penile size.

FEMALE PSEUDOHERMAPHRODITISM

Female pseudohermaphroditism comprises female infants who have ovaries with a variable degree of genital virilization. Congenital adrenal hyperplasia (CAH) is a major cause of masculinization that must always be considered in the neonatal period. All forms of CAH are described here, even though the less frequent enzymatic defects may lead to ambiguity of external genitalia in male infants.

Congenital adrenal hyperplasia

Congenital adrenal hyperplasia comprises five different inherited enzyme disorders, which have in common deficient cortisol synthesis with consequent hypersecretion of ACTH and adrenocortical hyperplasia. The affected enzymes are those involved in the pathway leading from cholesterol to cortisol: the cholesterol side-chain cleavage enzyme complex (or 20,22-desmolase), 3β-hydroxysteroid dehydrogenase, 17α-hydroxylase, 21-hydroxylase, and 11β-hydroxylase. Except for 17α-hydroxylase, these enzymes are also necessary for mineralocorticoid (aldosterone) biosynthesis (see Fig. 33-29). The first three enzymes are also present in gonadal tissue, and their deficiency results in deficient testosterone synthesis and abnormal male sex differentiation; female neonates with 3β-hydroxysteroid dehydrogenase deficiency may be modestly virilized. Estrogen synthesis is also impaired in these three enzyme deficiencies, but this is not of clinical significance until puberty. The 21- and 11β-hydroxylases are found predominantly in the adrenal cortex and minimally in gonadal tissue; their deficiency results in excess formation of precursor ste-

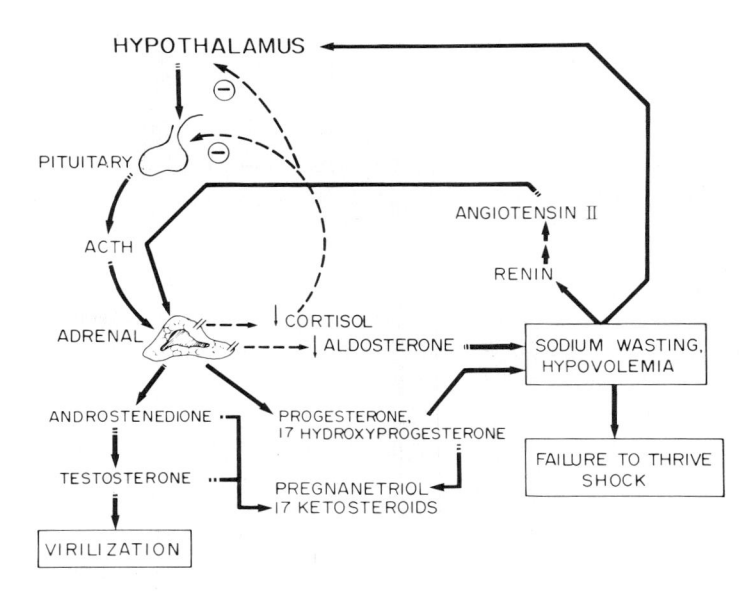

Fig. 33-37. Pathophysiology of 21-hydroxylase deficiency. In the simple virilizing form, cortisol biosynthesis is deficient (aldosterone biosynthesis is not deficient). This results in increased secretion of ACTH, which stimulates increased adrenal production of progesterone and 17-hydroxyprogesterone (salt-losing steroids) and of androgens that induce masculinization. During periods of stress the cortisol deficiency may become clinically apparent. Affected patients otherwise thrive because the steroid deficiency usually can be compensated for. In the salt-losing form diagrammed above, aldosterone biosynthesis also is deficient and leads to sodium wasting and failure to thrive. This, coupled with a more severe cortisol deficiency, will lead to adrenal crisis, usually in the neonatal period.

roids, which are metabolized to result in increased androgen synthesis. Affected females are usually abnormally virilized in utero and thus recognizable at birth, whereas affected males have no recognizable genital abnormalities at birth; if untreated, both sexes virilize during infancy and childhood.

These five enzyme deficiencies are clinically important because of the adrenal insufficiency that is associated. This is life threatening and needs to be recognized and managed early. Affected neonates with abnormal sexual differentiation may be identified at birth, before symptoms of adrenal insufficiency appear; others with normal sexual development are recognized when an adrenal crisis occurs.

21-Hydroxylase deficiency

21-Hydroxylase enzyme deficiency is by far the most common cause of congenital adrenal hyperplasia (CAH), accounting for 90% to 95% of all cases. Two forms are seen: a simple virilizing form in which the enzyme deficiency is partial, and a salt-losing form in which the enzyme deficiency is more complete. Both forms are characterized by abnormal virilization. In the simple virilizing form the partial enzyme block can be compensated for, so adrenal insufficiency tends not to occur except in stressful circumstances. In the salt-losing form adrenal insufficiency occurs under basal conditions and tends to manifest in the neonatal period as an adrenal crisis.

Partial 21-hydroxylase deficiency (simple virilizing form). The 21-hydroxylase enzyme is necessary for the conversion of 17-hydroxyprogesterone to 11-deoxycortisol (compound S) and of progesterone to 11-deoxycorticosterone (DOC). Partial deficiency of this enzyme results in an impairment of cortisol and aldosterone biosynthesis, which is compensated for by increased secretion of ACTH and angiotensin. This causes overproduction of the steroids before the enzyme block and a secondary increased secretion of adrenal androgens, which are converted in peripheral tissues to testosterone and DHT where they cause abnormal virilization (Fig. 33-37).

Affected fetuses produce increased amounts of androgens from the first trimester. In the female fetus this leads to varying degrees of male differentiation of the external genitalia and urogenital sinus, but the internal genital ducts develop normally along female lines without any wolffian duct development. At birth the spectrum of masculinization in females ranges from mild clitoromegaly, usually with some posterior labial fusion, to occasionally complete male differentiation with the urethra opening at the tip of a male-sized phallus; the latter may have a normal male appearance except that the

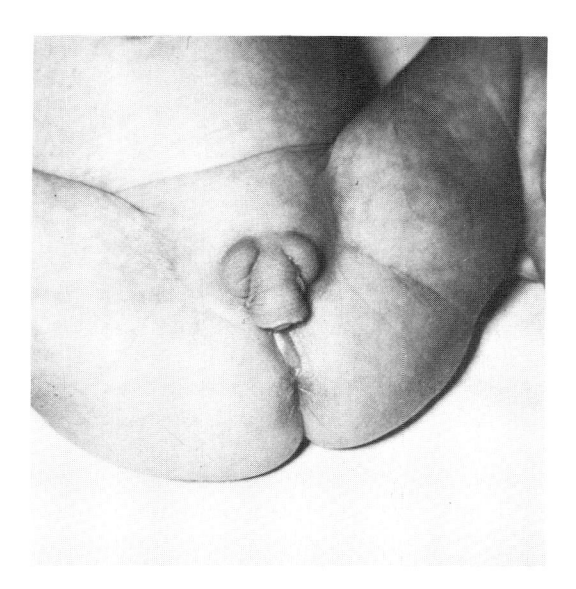

Fig. 33-38. Genitalia of female infant with 21-hydroxylase deficiency congenital adrenal hyperplasia.

gonads are impalpable. In the male the increased secretion of fetal adrenal androgens is of little significance in relation to the fetal production of testicular androgens. The external genitalia are usually normal at birth (very rarely an affected male has had hypospadias); there may be slight enlargement of the penis, but this is rarely recognizable as such. Female and male neonates may have increased pigmentation of the genitalia or areolae. The extent of male differentiation in female fetuses tends to reflect the severity of the enzyme defect, so females with the simple virilizing form tend to show less extensive male differentiation than the salt losers (Fig. 33-38).

Untreated simple virilizers continue to produce excessive androgens postnatally, resulting in accelerated growth and skeletal maturation and the appearance of androgen-induced sexual changes. Patients with mild CAH generally do not develop symptoms of adrenal insufficiency unless exposed to major stress or significant salt depletion (reduced salt intake, vomiting, excessive sweating). A few simple virilizers and salt losers have come to medical attention because of recurrent hypoglycemic episodes or seizures, usually occurring during common infections. Associated congenital anomalies, such as renal abnormalities, are occasionally seen in CAH, although their incidence is not greater than occurs in the general population.

Severe or complete 21-hydroxylase deficiency (salt-losing form). Severe deficiency of the 21-hydroxylase enzyme results in significant impairment of cortisol and aldosterone synthesis, which cannot be compensated for by the increased levels of ACTH and angiotensin. The development of cortisol and aldosterone deficiency, usually in the first weeks of life, results in an acute adrenal crisis and sodium wasting. This characterizes the salt-losing form of CAH and distinguishes it from the simple virilizing form (see Fig. 33-37).

The precursor steroids, 17-hydroxyprogesterone and progesterone, and 16α-hydroxyprogesterone, a metabolite of progesterone, are produced in increased amounts and have adverse effects of their own, since they function as salt-losing hormones. They may act directly on the renal tubules to cause sodium wasting, but more likely they act competitively to inhibit aldosterone action at the distal tubule, since they do not cause sodium wasting in the absence of mineralocorticoids. Their presence in a setting of diminished levels of mineralocorticoids has the effect of increasing the severity of the hypoaldosteronism by causing an additional amount of sodium wasting by the kidney. The production of C_{19} androgens also tends to be greater in the salt-losing form because of the more intense ACTH and angiotensin stimulation. Female salt losers collectively show more complete masculinization of the external genitalia than simple virilizers, some being incorrectly designated as male at birth (Fig. 33-38). Male salt losers may have a larger penile size at birth but not so much as to be clinically noticeable; they generally come to medical attention when they develop adrenal insufficiency.

Symptoms or signs of adrenal insufficiency are not present at birth and rarely occur before the end of the first week of life. Approximately half of salt losers have an adrenal crisis between 6 and 14 days of age, only a small number have an earlier crisis, and more than three fourths will have had their first crisis by 1 month of age. Less severely affected individuals may present in the following months, usually in association with a stressful condition causing decreased salt intake or increased salt losses, and a few escape having any crisis. The early symptoms and signs are nonspecific and include lethargy, poor appetite, regurgitation of feedings, failure to gain weight, or weight loss. Hyperkalemia, hyponatremia, and metabolic acidosis may be seen early. The regurgitation of feedings may progress to projectile vomiting. Severe symptoms and signs may occur rapidly, including dehydration, hypotension, muscle weakness, obtundation, a gray or cyanotic appearance, cold and clammy skin, hyperkalemic cardiac conduction abnormalities, and hyponatremic or hypoglycemic seizures. The differential diagnosis in the male infant without ambiguity includes sepsis, pyloric stenosis, or congenital heart disease. Patients with pyloric stenosis are differentiated by the presence of metabolic alkalosis.

The development of an acute adrenal crisis is in part due to hypoaldosteronism, which results in renal sodium wasting with depletion of total body sodium, and impaired ability to secrete potassium and hydrogen ions in the distal tubule. The decreased total body sodium results in hypovolemia and hyponatremia. Hypovolemia causes decreased tissue perfusion, which accounts for many of the early symptoms just described and eventually results in hypotension and shock.

Hypocortisolemia represents the other major component of adrenal insufficiency and results in impairment of cardiovascular, metabolic, and other systemic functions. Among the cardiovascular effects associated with glucocorticoid deficiency are decreased stroke volume and cardiac output, decreased blood pressure, and decreased vascular tone or reactivity. Depletion of renin substrate occurs in the presence of cortisol deficiency and impairs the renin-angiotensin axis, leading to circulatory failure. Norepinephrine raises the peripheral blood pressure only in the presence of cortisol, suggesting that cortisol exerts a permissive action. There is also impaired ability to concentrate the urine due to reduced responsiveness of the renal collecting tubules to vasopressin.

Cortisol deficiency is associated with an inability to maintain normal hepatic glycogen stores, which during a period of starvation may lead to hypoglycemia. Fat becomes the primary source of energy, which may lead to lipid depletion. Cortisol is normally important for mobilizing increased glucose production by the liver, both by inducing gluconeogenic enzymes and by its permissive effect on epinephrine- and glucagon-induced glycogenolysis. Cortisol also induces protein breakdown and increased formation of amino acids, which may serve as substrate for gluconeogenesis. Cortisol deficiency is associated with impaired muscle activity, a normochromic, normocytic anemia, and eosinophilia.

The mechanism for the delay in adrenal crisis is that the newborn normally has a very low aldosterone secretion rate in the first few days or first week of life (9 to 41 μg/24 hours with a mean of 23 μg/24 hours at age 3 hours to 7 days), which rises dramatically (25 to 138 μg/24 hours with a mean of 72 μg/24 hours at 8 days to 12 months). Plasma aldosterone concentrations nonetheless are high in the first week, attributed to a low metabolic clearance rate because of neonatal hepatic immaturity. With maturation of the liver, an increased amount of aldosterone must be secreted to maintain adequate plasma levels. The salt loser is thus spared in the first few days of life but is unable to subsequently meet increased aldosterone secretory requirements. A second reason for the delay is that it typically takes several days of complete glucocorticoid withdrawal for a crisis to develop and longer if some cortisol is present.

Biochemical findings

Blood. The serum level of cortisol and the cortisol production rate are normal in the untreated simple virilizing form of CAH and can be increased further in response to ACTH administration, although often not to the extent seen in normal individuals. In the salt-losing form of CAH, serum cortisol levels tend to be low-normal or low, and the cortisol production rate is low. An inadequate rise of each of these parameters is seen in response to ACTH administration. ACTH levels in the untreated patients of both forms of CAH are elevated, but more in the salt losers.

The aldosterone production rate in the simple virilizer is also corrected and actually is elevated, although hyperaldosterone-induced effects (hypokalemia, metabolic alkalosis, hypertension) are not seen. This elevation is thought to be secondary to the presence of increased levels of the salt-losing steroids, 17-hydroxyprogesterone and progesterone, which antagonize mineralocorticoid action at the distal tubules. Plasma renin activity is also elevated, which supports this explanation. In the salt loser the aldosterone production rate under conditions of normal sodium replacement ranges from low up to normal in patients with mild salt losing. Unlike the simple virilizing form, however, no increase in aldosterone production is seen in response to sodium restriction or ACTH administration.

Of the steroids preceding the enzyme block, 17-hydroxyprogesterone is the most strikingly elevated. Its serum levels are increased 20 to 300 times above the upper limit of normal, to levels of 40 to 600 ng/ml and occasionally higher, whereas serum progesterone levels are increased six to 75 times.

Two principal routes of metabolism of 17-hydroxyprogesterone are by 11β-hydroxylation to form 21-deoxycortisol, and by side-chain cleavage to form the C_{19} androgens. Serum 21-deoxycortisol levels are markedly elevated, ranging from 18 to 169 ng/ml (normal is less than 1 ng/ml). The biochemical effects of 21-deoxycortisol, if any, are unknown, but in the routine laboratory assays for cortisol, 21-deoxycortisol may cross-react significantly and cause the cortisol measurements to appear higher than they actually are.

The major C_{19} androgen produced is androstenedione, which is principally derived from the side-chain cleavage of 17-hydroxyprogesterone. Serum levels of androstenedione range from 2.2 to 55 ng/ml (upper normal in children under 7 years is 0.42 ng/ml). Of the other C_{19} adrenal steroids secreted, serum levels of DHA are usually elevated, whereas serum levels of the sulfate and glucuronide esters of androstenedione or DHA are elevated in some but normal in others. The adrenal C_{19} steroids have little biologic effect of their own but can serve as prohormones for testosterone synthesis. Approximately 15% of the androstenedione produced is metabolized in peripheral tissues (particularly liver, muscle, and skin) to testosterone, with the adrenal synthesizing very little testosterone directly. Serum testosterone levels in affected children range between 1.1 and 6 ng/ml (normal is less than 0.4 ng/ml), and the serum androstenedione to testosterone ratios range between 2:1 and 7:1. In female and in male patients about two thirds and one third of the testosterone produced, respectively, is derived from adrenal-synthesized androstenedione; the remaining portions reflect that amount under normal circumstances.

Urine. The steroids produced by the adrenal are ultimately metabolized to physiologically inactive forms and are made more water soluble for excretion in the urine or kidneys, adrenals, and connective tissue also metabolize these steroids. Several steroid metabolites are excreted in the meconium and feces of newborns, but more than 90% of steroid excretion is found in the urine at all ages, chiefly as glucuronide or sulfate conjugates or in hydroxylated forms.

The 24-hour urine steroid pattern in 21-hydroxylase deficiency classically shows significant elevations of pregnanetriol and the 17-ketosteroids. Urine levels of pregnanetriol in these infants are 0.2 to 10 mg/24 hours in the neonatal period (normally barely detectable or less than 0.1 mg/24 hours). Some infants may have initially normal pregnanetriol levels. Urinary free 17-hydroxyprogesterone has recently been found by Wong and associates to be superior to pregnanetriol, particularly in neonates, for the diagnosis of 21-hydroxylase deficiency. Urinary 17-ketosteroids range between 2 and 40 mg/24 hours in infants as compared with normal levels in the first 3 to 4 weeks of life of up to 2.5 mg/24 hours. The urinary 17-hydroxycorticosteroids, which reflect cortisol metabolism, are normal or low; urinary free cortisol presumably behaves similarly.

Pathology. The bilateral adrenal glands are characteristically hyperplastic and enlarged; the hyperplasia is initially diffuse, and the surface is convoluted or cerebriform. Microscopically the effects of excessive ACTH stimulation are seen. Most of the adrenal cortex is composed of eosinophilic compact cells with finely granular cytoplasm containing fine lipid droplets, which extend from the medulla toward the outer cortex. The zona glomerulosa, from which mineralocorticoids are produced, is less well described but is stated to be two to four times wider in the simple virilizing form of CAH but is either normal or absent in the salt-losing form.

Differential diagnosis. 11β-Hydroxylase deficiency is frequently misdiagnosed as 21-hydroxylase deficiency and needs to be ruled out by measurement of 11-deoxycortisol. The differential diagnosis of adrenal insufficiency includes ACTH deficiency or hypopituitarism, congenital adrenal hypoplasia or aplasia, hereditary ACTH unresponsiveness, other inherited enzyme deficiencies in cortisol or aldosterone synthesis, pseudohypoaldosteronism, adrenal hemorrhage, Wolman's disease, adrenoleukodystrophy (neonatal or childhood forms), and adrenal suppression following pharmacologic glucocorticoid therapy given to the mother during pregnancy or to the infant. Hyponatremia also may occur with inadequate sodium intake or excessive losses, in water overload, inappropriate ADH, congestive heart failure, cirrhosis, nephrotic syndrome, potassium depletion, or with diuretic therapy.

Treatment. Cortisol replacement, equivalent to the amount secreted daily in normal individuals (12 mg/m²/24 hours), is the treatment of choice. It suppresses the increased output of ACTH and thereby causes the ACTH-stimulated adrenocortical activity to be decreased. Any existing aldosterone secretion is maintained by endogenous angiotensin stimulation, and the reduction in 17-hydroxyprogesterone and progesterone results in a diminished salt-losing tendency. Adrenal androgen secretion is also decreased so that abnormal virilization no longer occurs. Patients with the salt-losing form require replacement sodium and mineralocorticoid therapy in addition to cortisol.

Cortisol replacement may be given intramuscularly or orally, but allowance must be made for differences in the potency, absorption, and duration of action of the different preparations available. Cortisone acetate is the intramuscular preparation used; it has a duration of action of 3 days. Its physiologic replacement dosage averages 16mg/m²/24 hours or 45 to 50 mg/m² every 3 days. The phosphate and succinate esters of hydrocortisone are generally limited to intravenous usage because they have a short duration of action of about 8 hours. Hydrocortisone is the oral preparation of choice. Because of its short half-life and its partial inactivation by gastric acidity, the maintenance hydrocortisone dosage approaches twice physiologic production, or 20 to 25 mg/m²/day (range of 16 to 30 mg/m²/day) given in three divided doses. Prednisone, prednisolone, and dexamethasone are not used in infants and growing children because they are so much more potent and difficult to adjust and are more likely to cause growth suppression. At the initiation of therapy and *during periods of stress or illness two to three times the maintenance dose should be given*. The levels of 17-hydroxyprogesterone and other abnormally elevated steroids should fall toward normal within several days.

A salt-losing adrenal crisis is treated with saline-glucose infusion, hydrocortisone, and DOCA (desoxycorticosterone acetate), 1 to 2 mg intramuscularly once daily (twice-daily doses may be needed initially). Acidosis should be corrected by the addition of bicarbonate; hyperkalemia may result in cardiac toxicity, and hypoglycemia rarely may occur. Hydrocortisone can be withheld until diagnostic tests are completed but should be administered if blood pressure and other functions are not correctible with DOCA and fluid-electrolyte replacement. Overtreatment with DOCA or saline solutions can result in hypernatremia, hypertension, metabolic alkalosis, or fluid retention with cardiac or pulmonary failure. Sodium replacement is essential for mineralocorticoid therapy to be effective, and dehydration must be corrected to permit normal glomerular filtration.

The cardiac toxicity of hyperkalemia is made worse by hypocalemia, hyponatremia, metabolic acidosis, or rapid elevations of potassium. The latter may occur with the administration of potassium-containing antiboiotics or use of stored blood for transfusion, or by tissue destruction or hemolysis; hypovolemia may cause impaired renal tubular secretion of potassium. The treatment of choice of hyperkalemia due to adrenal insufficiency is mineralocorticoid replacement. Mineralocorticoids cannot act in the face of inadequate sodium for exchange with potassium at the renal tubule, so adequate sodium replacement is important. If cardiac toxicity is severe, the most rapidly effective therapeutic measure is intravenous calcium infusion (given as 10% calcium gluconate, 0.4 ml/kg); administered slowly, it will result in a shift of potassium into cells and should be considered for severe hyperkalemia.

Maintenance mineralocorticoid replacement therapy in infants is provided either parenterally or orally. Two 125-mg DOCA pellets implanted in a subcutaneous pocket located infrascapularly will last 9 to 10 months or occasionally slightly longer; DOC pivalate, 25 mg intramuscularly once monthly may be given instead. Alternatively, oral therapy with 9α-fludrocortisone acetate (Florinef), 0.05 to 0.1 mg daily and occasionally 0.15 mg daily, is given; DOCA, 1 mg intramuscularly, may be substituted on days when oral therapy cannot be given. Salt supplementation (1 to 3 gm daily) is sometimes given in the first 3 to 6 months because the renal tubules are less able to conserve sodium. The level of plasma renin activity serves as a guide to the need for added salt.

Sex of rearing. The sex of rearing should be female in all 46,XX CAH patients, regardless of the extent of masculinization of their genitalia. This is based on the observation that they have normal ovaries and müllerian structures and have the potential to lead normal, fertile lives as females. Surgical correction of the masculinized external genitalia in female patients is done when a reasonable body size has been achieved, usually toward the end of the first year and preferably no later than 18 months of age. Patients maintained under good control with steroid replacement therapy should show normal growth and development.

Genetics, detection of heterozygotes, fetal and newborn screening. The 21-hydroxylase deficiency is one of the most common autosomal recessive disorders, having an estimated incidence of one per 5,000 to 10,000 births. Obligate heterozygotes (parents of affected children) have a significantly greater than normal rise of serum 17-hydroxyprogesterone, 17-hydroxyprogesterone plus progesterone, or 21-deoxycortisol within 30 to 360 minutes of intravenous ACTH stimulation. These studies demonstrate the existence in the heterozygote of a partial biochemical defect that manifests only under conditions of maximum ACTH stimulation. The exact nature of the enzyme defect is not known. One hypothesis suggests that separate 21-hydroxylases are involved in aldosterone and cortisol biosynthesis and that in simple virilizers only the latter is defective, whereas in salt losers both enzymes are abnormal. Against this is the finding in many non–salt losers that aldosterone biosynthesis is partially deficient.

The prenatal diagnosis of CAH has been made by finding abnormally elevated levels of amniotic fluid 17-hydroxyprogesterone. In the few cases reported, 17-hydroxyprogesterone was markedly elevated as early as 14 weeks of gestational age, with levels being higher through 30 to 34 weeks and perhaps longer. The experience is too limited to know the reliability of this method. HLA genotyping of cultured amniotic fluid cells in conjunction with measurement of amniotic fluid 17-hydroxyprogesterone has also been successfully used to diagnose and rule out CAH in different fetuses. Screening of newborns for CAH is technically feasible by measurement of 17-hydroxyprogesterone in either cord blood or on blood collected on filter paper at several days of age.

11β-Hydroxylase deficiency

Deficiency of 11β-hydroxylase results in impaired synthesis of cortisol and aldosterone, increased formation of 11-deoxycorticosterone (DOC), which has significant mineralocorticoid activity of its own, and increased androgen synthesis, which occurs as a result of the increased levels of precursor steroids. Although it is the second most common form of congenital adrenal hyperplasia, it accounts for only 3% to 5% of the total CAH cases. It was first recognized in 1951 and 1952 by Wilkins and associates, who reported a group of patients who had virilizing CAH with hypertension that remitted when adrenal activity was suppressed by small doses of cortisone. These authors speculated correctly that the hypertension was secondary to excessive secretion of DOC.

The clinical picture of 11β-hydroxylase deficiency is heterogenous in that not all patients develop hypertension, and the relative severities of their virilization, hypertension, and biochemical findings do not always correlate. Hypertension is present in 60% to 80% of patients. Hypokalemia is inconsistently present, and serum sodium levels are upper normal to minimally elevated. Females are usually born with some masculinization of external genitalia, but some have no genital abnormalities at birth. Males are normal at birth, but both sexes may have hyperpigmentation of the genitalia and areolae. Postnatal virilization affects both sexes; some males have developed gynecomastia in infancy or childhood.

The characteristic biochemical abnormality seen is an elevated serum level of 11-deoxycortisol (compound S), with reported levels ranging between 80 and 400 ng/ml (normal is 7.8 ± 5.3 ng/ml). Serum DOC levels also have been elevated in the few patients measured, ranging between 10 and 180 ng/ml (normal is 0.06 ng/ml). Urinary tetrahydro-11-deoxycortisol (THS) levels are characteristically elevated. Serum levels of 17-hydroxyprogesterone and androstenedione are also increased and may cause diagnostic confusion with 21-hydroxylase deficiency.

11β-Hydroxylase deficiency should be considered in XX neonates with masculinization of the external genitalia and in any patients beyond the neonatal period with abnormal virilization; it should also be considered in all hypertensive patients. The diagnosis is based on finding elevated serum levels of 11-deoxycortisol and DOC and increased urinary levels of THS and in demonstrating their suppressibility with cortisol replacement therapy. The differential diagnosis includes 21-hydroxylase deficiency and, beyond the neonatal period, a virilizing adrenal or ovarian tumor.

Treatment is with cortisol replacement therapy, as outlined for 21-hydroxylase deficiency. The sex of rearing should agree with the gonadal sex, since these individuals can develop and function perfectly normally and be fertile. It is most likely that 11β-hydroxylase is autosomal recessive, based on examination of pedigrees, and prenatal diagnosis has been successfully accomplished with measurement of THS levels in amniotic fluid and maternal urine.

3β-Hydroxysteroid dehydrogenase deficiency

Deficiency of 3β-hydroxysteroid dehydrogenase (HSD) results in adrenal insufficiency with sodium wasting and ambiguous genitalia in both sexes. The first patients documented to have this deficiency were described by Bongiovanni in 1961 and 1962, and to date at least 22 patients have been reported. About three fourths of the patients have shown signs of the disorder between ages 1 week and 3 months with symptoms of adrenal insufficiency, e.g., failure to thrive, dehydration, or sodium wasting. The genitalia of the female patients varied from normal to mildly masculinized, whereas most of the males have had marked genital ambiguity. Biochemically there is impaired synthesis of cortisol, aldosterone, and testosterone, which may be compensated for in milder cases, and there is an accumulation of the precursor 3β-hydroxy-Δ^5-steroids, 17-hydroxypregnenolone, and pregnenolone; DHA, DHAS, and androstenediol have been elevated in some, but not all, patients studied.

3β-HSD deficiency should be considered in XY males with ambiguous genitalia, XX females with clitoromegaly or posterior labial fusion, and in patients with adrenal insufficiency or failure to thrive. The differential diagnosis includes 21-hydroxylase deficiency and a virilizing adrenal or ovarian tumor. Treatment for this disorder is the same as for 21-hydroxylase deficiency.

Cholesterol side-chain cleavage enzyme (20,22-desmolase) deficiency (congenital lipoid adrenal hyperplasia)

Deficiency of the cholesterol side-chain cleavage enzyme complex (SCC deficiency) results in impaired synthesis of all adrenal and gonadal steroids. The clinical course for most cases has been the development of severe adrenal insufficiency, in some cases occurring in the first days of life but in milder cases beginning beyond several weeks of age. Sodium wasting has often been quite marked. Many patients have died within the first several months of life. The XX female patients have had normal female external genitalia; in the XY male patients the external genitalia have appeared female or ambiguous, and a blind vaginal pouch has frequently been present.

The adrenal glands are enlarged with a characteristically enormous accumulation of lipid, giving the name *congenital lipoid adrenal hyperplasia*. Biochemically there is a decreased to absent production of all adrenal steroids, depending on the severity of the defect, and an accumulation of cholesterol and its esters in the adrenal. Serum cholesterol levels have not been elevated; in one case the urinary cholesterol level was elevated to 0.8 and 0.9 mg/24 hours (normal is 0.11 to 0.35 mg/24 hours).

SCC deficiency should be considered in cases of adrenal insufficiency and in XY males with ambiguous genitalia. The diagnosis is based on demonstrating a deficiency of the glucocorticoids, mineralocorticoids, and androgens, an increase in urinary cholesterol, and the presence of bilateral adrenal hyperplasia via ultrasound or CT scan. In XX females with adrenal insufficiency and no genital abnormalities, the differentiation of SCC deficiency from congenital adrenal hypoplasia is very difficult and depends on demonstrating the presence or absence of the adrenal glands. The inheritance of SCC deficiency is probably autosomal recessive.

Treatment includes cortisol, salt, and mineralocorticoid replacement therapy, as outlined for 21-hydroxylase deficiency. This needs to be given aggressively in infancy to reduce the high mortality risk. The sex of rearing in males should be based on phallic size and the chances for achieving normal-appearing genitalia by early childhood.

17α-Hydroxylase deficiency

Deficiency of 17α-hydroxylase results in impaired synthesis of cortisol, androgens, and estrogens. The resultant increased ACTH secretion causes increased formation of the precursor steroid, progesterone, the steroids in the mineralocorticoid pathway except aldosterone, and adrenocortical hyperplasia. Clinically this results in hypokalemic alkalosis, borderline hypernatremia, and hypertension; whether these findings are present in affected neonates or infants is not known because no data are available. Adrenal insufficiency does not occur because of the mineralocorticoid and glucocorticoid properties of DOC and corticosterone. XX female patients have normal genitalia at birth, but XY male patients have phenotypically female to poorly masculinized external genitalia, often with a distal vagina or prostatic utricle, and variable testicular descent. The internal gland ducts are appropriate for the gonadal sex, although wolffian duct development may be incomplete.

The serum levels and production rates of cortisol are low to low-normal, whereas those for DOC and corticosterone are markedly elevated; serum levels of progesterone are also elevated but occasionally have been normal. The serum level and production rate of aldosterone and the level of plasma renin activity are low due to the increased DOC. Cortisol replacement therapy corrects these abnormalities, and in most patients aldosterone secretion returns to normal, although in several cases it has remained abnormally low. Serum levels of testosterone are low and show a poor rise following HCG stimulation, and serum levels of LH and FSH are elevated. Urinary 17-hydroxycorticosteroids and 17-ketosteroids are low to low-normal, whereas the tetrahydro-derivatives of DOC and corticosterone are characteristically elevated; pregnanediol ranges from normal to elevated. Cortisol replacement is given as described for 21-hydroxylase deficiency, but mineralocorticoid therapy is not necessary unless aldosterone secretion fails to return to normal.

The sex of rearing of XY patients should be female, unless the genitalia are sufficiently male sized at birth and surgically correctible. The inheritance is believed to be autosomal recessive.

Maternally derived androgenic substances

Masculinization of the female fetus occasionally occurs from exposure to androgens or certain other agents derived from the maternal circulation. The extent of masculinization is related to the compound, dosage, duration of exposure, and timing of exposure. Exposure at 8 to 12 weeks' gestation may result in midline fusion of the labioscrotal folds, opening of the vagina and urethra into a common urogenital sinus, and in more severe cases development of a prostate and possibly seminal vesicles. Exposure beyond 12 to 14 weeks can only result in clitoromegaly and hypertrophy of the labia majora but no midline fusion or development of a urogenital sinus. Maternally derived androgens usually do not stimulate wolffian duct development, and the müllerian duct structures and bilateral ovaries develop normally.

Androgen-secreting tumors of the ovary occur rarely in pregnant women, and only one case of virilizing adrenal tumor has been reported. Among the reasons why a considerable portion of female fetuses do not undergo masculinization is that the placenta aromatizes most maternal androgens before they cross over to the fetus, and the high maternal (versus fetal) levels of sex-steroid binding globulin favors concentration of these androgens on the maternal side.

Maternal ingestion of synthetic progestins or androgens may cause abnormal masculinization of the female fetus. In the male fetus, progestin exposure from 8 to 12 weeks' gestation may increase the risk of hypospadias. These substances have been given to pregnant women because of habitual or threatened abortions, as pregnancy-test drugs, as a postcoital "morning-after" pill, as an oral contraceptive, or occasionally for other medical problems such as endometriosis, breast cancer, or alopecia. Since these medications have often been given for only part of the pregnancy, the extent of clitoral enlargement, urethral displacement, and labioscrotal fusion is often discordant, unlike the other causes of female pseudohermaphroditism. The mother may rarely show mild androgenization. Advanced skeletal maturation occurs in the offspring exposed to the more androgenic substances.

Paradoxical masculinization of female fetuses has also occurred in a very small number of pregnancies in which diethylstilbestrol was administered. In contrast, males exposed to diethylstilbesetrol in utero have had an increased incidence of cryptorchidism and hypoplastic testes. The affected female offspring had clitoromegaly, with midline labioscrotal fusion and formation of a urogenital sinus occurring in those exposed between 8 and 12 weeks' gestation. Inhibition of 3β-hydroxysteroid dehydrogenase with secondarily increased adrenal androgen production is one postulated mechanism. Although diethylstilbestrol has been contraindicated in the treatment of pregnancy complications since 1971, it is still used as a postcoital contraceptive and for certain medical problems. Females exposed prenatally to diethylstilbestrol have an increased incidence of structural abnormalities of the vagina, cervix, and uterine cavity, increased pregnancy wastage (possibly related to the structural abnormalities), and an increased incidence of clear cell adenocarcinoma of the genital tract. The exposed female offspring need to have periodic screening for the development of clear cell adenocarcinoma beginning at age 14 years, or sooner if vaginal bleeding or discharge occurs.

The masculinization of females that occurs with androgen or other drug exposure in utero does not progress postnatally. Biochemical studies show normal levels of androgens or their metabolites and of 17-hydroxyprogesterone. Surgical correction of midline labioscrotal fusion or of major clitoromegaly should be done by age 18 months; mild clitoromegaly need not be corrected, since the clitoris will become less prominent with an increase in general body size.

Idiopathic female pseudohermaphroditism

Female pseudohermaphroditism unrelated to adrenal disorders or maternal drug ingestion is often associated with other congenital malformations, particularly imperforate anus, renal agenesis, duplication or hydronephrosis of the kidneys, or other abnormalities of the lower intestinal or genitourinary tract. The ovaries are usually normal, but there may be absence or malformation of the müllerian structures. The cause of this form of female pseudohermaphroditism is unknown. Idiopathic clitoral hypertrophy, with or without labioscrotal fusion, sometimes occurs without any evidence for androgen or other drug exposure and without other associated congenital abnormalities.

OTHER DISORDERS OF SEXUAL DEVELOPMENT
Hypospadias

Hypospadias is a developmental abnormality in which the urethral meatus lies proximal to the tip of the glans penis, either on the ventral surface of the penis or on the perineum. It is the second most common genital abnormality (after cryptorchidism) in male newborns, with an incidence in different series reported to be 0.3%, 0.61%, or 0.82%. It occurs less frequently in blacks (0.39%) than in whites (0.61%). The types of hypospadias seen comprise approximately 87% glandular or coronal, 10% penile, and 3% penoscrotal and perineal, although higher proportions of the latter type have been reported.

Other anomalies frequently accompany the hypospadias. Chordee (ventral curvature of the penis) is usually caused by fibrous tissue growth in the area of failed urethral development. Its location (glandular or midshaft) and severity are easier to assess in the erect penis. The prepuce in the hypospadic penis is usually deficient ventrally and thus appears hooded. Other genital anomalies include meatal stenosis, hydrocele, cryptorchidism in 8% to 10%, and inguinal hernia in 8% of patients. More severe forms of hypospadias are often associated with incompletely translocated labioscrotal folds or a shawl scrotum and with a prostatic utricle. Urinary tract abnormalities are seen in 9% to 28% of cases of hypospadias, with renal ectopia and horseshoe kidneys having a higher than normal prevalence. The incidence of urinary tract abnormalities appear to be similar for all grades of severity of hypospadias. Ultrasound examination of the kidneys and ureters should be considered.

Male relatives of affected infants are at increased risk for having hypospadias. About 7% to 8% of hypospadic patients have a brother or father with hypospadias, and second- and third-degree relatives are affected at rates of 2.3% and 1.0%, respectively. Index cases with more severe degrees of hypospadias have a higher incidence of hypospadic first-degree relatives, reaching 16.7% in individuals with perineoscrotal hypospadias. This familial tendency is thought to be due to a polygenic mode of inheritance.

Mild hypospadias (glandular to penile) occurring alone, without other genital abnormalities or dysmorphic features, is very unlikely to have an associated endocrinopathy, intersex problem, or chromosomal abnormality. Severe hypospadias (penoscrotal or perineal) occurring alone, however, is associated with approximately a 15% risk of such problems occurring. The addition of other genital abnormalities (cryptorchidism or abnormally small penis) increases the risk of occurrence of an intersex problem or endocrinopathy to 35% in mild, or 79% in severe, hypospadias. Hypospadias occurs with increased incidence in certain rare syndromes, many of which carry a very poor prognosis. The cause of hypospadias in at least some cases is due to a partial deficiency in either testosterone production, conversion of testosterone to dihydrotestosterone (5α-reductase deficiency), or in the function of the cytoplasmic androgen receptor protein (partial androgen insensitivity). In 4% to 9% of cases maternal exposure to progestins at 5 to about 14 weeks of gestation has been a cause of hypospadias.

The evaluation of hypospadias in the newborn should include a history for possible maternal drug exposure and a family history of hypospadias, endocrine, or intersex problems; a physical examination to evaluate the hypospadias, identify somatic or other genital abnormalities, and exclude the presence of a uterus or gross abnormality of the kidneys; and an assessment of penile length to be certain that rearing the infant as a male is appropriate. Additional studies are not necessary in infants with mild hypospadias without other abnormalities. Studies should be considered in hypospadic infants at greater risk for an endocrine or intersex problem.

The immediate concerns in the evaluation of neonatal hypospadias relate to withholding circumcision, selection of sex of rearing, identification of possible male or female pseudohermaphrodites, and recognition of syn-

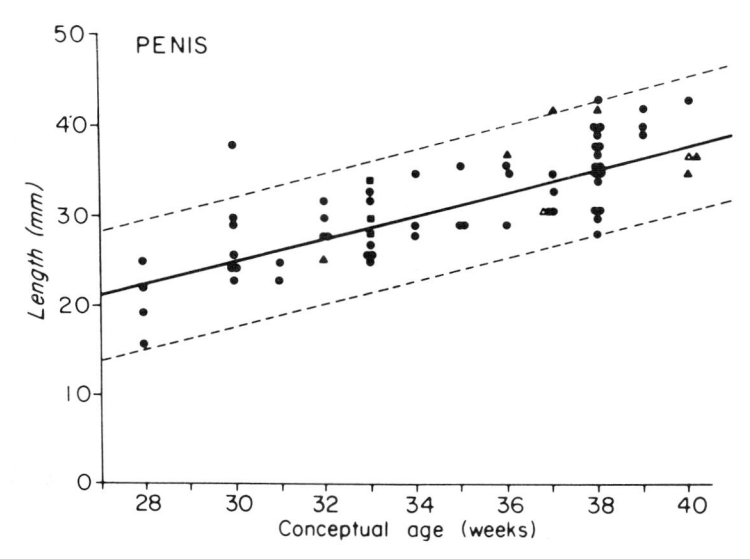

Fig. 33-39. Stretched penile lengths (mean ±2 S.D.) in 63 normal premature and full-term male infants (●), two small-for-gestational-age infants (△), seven large-for-gestational age infants (▲), and four twins (■). (From Feldman, K.W., and Smith, D.W.: J. Pediatr. **86**:395, 1975.)

dromes that may have a poor prognosis. If penile length is found to be abnormally small, assuming that correction has been made for some loss of length due to chordee, female sex of rearing should be considered. If both gonads are impalpable, the possibility must be seriously considered that the infant has female pseudohermaphroditism, e.g., congenital adrenal hyperplasia.

Surgical repair of hypospadias is generally done beyond infancy, ideally at 3 to 5 years of age, with the goal being completion of repair before entering school. Surgical correction of chordee is sometimes done separately at 1 or 2 years of age. It is important for the boy to be able to stand to urinate before he begins school and that his genital appearance be close to normal so that he may develop a normal body image. Multistage operations are usually required for more severe forms of hypospadias, and complication rates may be 10% to 25%. Education of the family and preparation of the patient for these procedures are very important.

Micropenis

A micropenis is arbitrarily defined as a penis with a normally formed urethra that opens at the tip of the glans in which either (1) the stretched length is more than 2.5 standard deviations below the mean for age or (2) the penile corpora cavernosa are absent or severely deficient in size, resulting in an abnormally thin penis, regardless of penile length. The fully stretched penile length should be measured with the ruler pressed against the pubic ramus, depressing the suprapubic fat pad completely.

The cause of most cases of micropenis is endocrinologic and reflects a deficiency of those factors needed for normal penile growth to occur beyond 14 weeks of gestation. The major causes include hypogonadotropic hypogonadism (30%), primary hypogonadism (25%), partial androgen insensitivity (2%), and idiopathic or undiagnosed (43%). Growth hormone deficiency may accompany hypogonadotropic hypogonadism, although it is unknown whether growth hormone alone (without LH deficiency) can cause micropenis. Other congenital malformations and chromosome abnormalities are frequently associated. The diagnostic evaluation of micropenis includes measurement of serum testosterone and LH and FSH levels. An HCG stimulation test should be done if testosterone elevation is not seen, and this may increase penile size if a testosterone rise is elicited. A chromosome karyotype may need to be determined.

The selection of sex of rearing is based principally on penile size, since there is a rough correlation of penile size in infancy with its final size in adulthood. The sex of rearing should be female if the stretched penile length is less than 1.5 cm or if the penile corpora cavernosa are severely deficient or absent, and male if the stretched length is 2.0 cm or more and if penile diameter is adequate. The length criteria should be adjusted for the premature neonate (Fig. 33-39). The administration of a course of testosterone therapy to assess penile responsiveness is not useful, since virtually all patients, including those with partial androgen insensitivity, will show some increase in penile size. This test does not predict whether a patient can achieve a normal penile length in adulthood. The treatment of micropenis in patients reared as male is with intermittent, brief courses of testosterone enanthate given intramuscularly. Surgical correction of a micropenis is generally not recommended. If female sex of rearing is selected, genital reconstructive surgery should be done before 18 months of age.

Cryptorchidism

Cryptorchidism refers to those conditions in which one or both testes have failed to descend completely into the scrotum; it is the most common genital abnormality found in newborns.

The incidence of cryptorchidism in full-term males is estimated to be 2.7% and in premature males about 21%, increasing with earlier gestational age. It is also more frequently bilateral with earlier gestational age (bilateral 27% to 39% of the time at term and 68% of the time in preterm infants). Postnatal testicular descent into the scrotum is achieved by 6 weeks in 50% of cryptorchid full-term newborns and by 3 months in 90% of cryptorchid prematures; an additional 25% of cryptorchid full-term males have testicular descent during the remainder of the first year of life into a high scrotal position. At 1 year of age the overall incidence of cryptorchidism is 0.78%, with 75% of full-term and 90% of premature cryptorchid newborns having attained a scrotal position.

The cause of cryptorchidism in most individuals is unknown. In conditions of abnormal abdominal wall development, such as bladder exstrophy, gastroschisis, omphalocele, and prune-belly syndrome, bilateral cryptorchidism is almost invariable. Cryptorchidism, usually bilateral, occurs in syndromes having abnormal hypothalamic-pituitary-gonadal function.

Torsion of the testis occurs more frequently in cryptorchidism, particularly in the neonatal and infancy periods, and occasionally in utero. It may be difficult to diagnose, so destruction of the testis often results. If a scrotal testis is involved, the clinical presentation includes a scrotal mass, which is either nontender or only mildly so, with reddish to bluish discoloration of the scrotal skin. The patient is usually otherwise well, and the mildness of symptoms often delays diagnosis. Torsion of the impalpable cryptorchid testis is much more difficult to identify early because pain and irritability may be intermittent; some neonates have had an abdominal mass.

Hypospadias occurs in about 3% of bilaterally cryptorchid patients. Patients having either unilateral or bilateral cryptorchidism and hypospadias are at an overall 53% risk for having an intersex problem, the risk being higher for bilateral involvement and for a more caudal location of the urethral meatus.

A congenital inguinal hernia is associated with cryptorchidism in 65% to 90% of cases. It results when the processus vaginalis fails to close and is considered significant if large enough to permit abdominal contents to enter, in which case repair may be necessary in early infancy.

The generally accepted approach in the management of true cryptorchidism is to plan for orchiopexy sometime between 2 and 5 years of age. A more aggressive approach is to first give a course of low-dose HCG treatment (e.g., 500 units IM twice weekly for 2 to 6 weeks) at some time after 2 to 4 months of age.

Müllerian aplasia, vaginal agenesis

Congenital absence of the vagina in the 46,XX female with otherwise normal external genitalia is a developmental abnormality thought to result from failure of the müllerian ducts to make contact with the posterior portion of the urogenital sinus. Aplasia of the müllerian ducts occurs from a caudal to cephalic direction, so that complete absence of the uterus is always accompanied by absence of the vagina. Ovarian development usually proceeds normally, but hypoplasia or absence of ovaries is occasionally seen. Urinary tract abnormalities are seen in many, and there is increased frequency of skeletal abnormalities. Patients may be identified on physical examination at birth by absence of a vagina, and those with an intact uterus may have hydrometra at birth.

About 5% to 10% of patients have partial absence of the vagina with agenesis of only the lower one-third. The fallopian tubes, uterus, and upper portion of the vagina are entirely normal. This is presumably a result of failure of urogenital sinus epithelium to invade the vagina at 4 to 5 months of gestation, and renal abnormalities may again be present.

RECOGNITION AND EVALUATION OF INTERSEX PROBLEMS
Recognition

Most intersex patients have some abnormality of their external genitalia and are thus potentially identifiable at birth. The genitalia do not need to appear "ambiguous" to qualify for a diagnostic evaluation. An intersex problem is likely to be present if an individual has either (1) two or more abnormalities of the external genital structures or (2) presence of one of certain single genital abnormalities. Not all patients with abnormal genitalia will be found to have an identifiable intersex problem. Possibly a teratogenic event, a partial hormone deficiency not detectable by ordinary testing, or a timing defect occurring at a critical period in development resulted in abnormal genital differentiation.

CHARACTERISTICS OF AMBIGUOUS GENITALIA

A. Abnormality of any two of the following
1. Size of phallus
2. Location of urethral meatus
3. Fusion of labioscrotal folds
4. Location or size of gonads

B. Presence of any one of the following abnormalities
1. With male-appearing genitalia
   a. Impalpable gonads (e.g., congenital adrenal hyperplasia, anorchia)
   b. Small gonads* (e.g., Klinefelter's syndrome, dysgenetic or rudimentary testes)
   c. Micropenis† (e.g., growth hormone, LH or testosterone deficiencies; partial androgen insensitivity; idiopathic)
   d. Inguinal mass (e.g., persistent müllerian duct syndrome)
2. With female-appearing genitalia
   a. Posterior labial fusion (e.g., congenital adrenal hyperplasia, maternal androgens, testosterone deficiency, partial androgen insensitivity)
   b. Clitoromegaly‡ (e.g., congenital adrenal hyperplasia, maternal androgens, gonadal dysgenesis, testosterone deficiency, partial androgen insensitivity, infiltration by tumor)
   c. Palpable gonads (e.g., true hermaphroditism, complete androgen insensitivity, male pseudohermaphroditism)
   d. Inguinal mass (e.g., true hermaphroditism, complete androgen insensitivity, male pseudohermaphroditism)

Some intersex patients have no abnormality of the external genitalia but may be recognizable by the presence of abnormal somatic features, e.g., lymphedema of the dorsa of the feet or hands, loose posterior neck folds, horseshoe kidney, coarctation of the aorta, or other somatic stigmata in Turner's syndrome, camptomelic dwarfism (bowing and angulation of the lower limbs, flat facies, shortened vertebrae) in XY gonadal dysgenesis, or hyperpigmentation in congenital adrenal hyperplasia. Finally, some intersex patients appear phenotypically normal at birth, e.g., many cases of gonadal dysgenesis, persistent müllerian duct syndrome, and complete androgen insensitivity syndrome, and may not come to medical attention until an older age.

---

*A gonad is abnormally small if the longest diameter is less than approximately 0.8 cm.
†Length of the penis is determined of the maximally stretched penis, with the ruler depressing the suprapubic fat pad above the pubic symphysis and measurement made from the base of the penis to the tip of the glans, ignoring excess foreskin. Normal measurements at various ages are published (Fig. 33-39). A micropenis is defined as being below −2.5 S.D. of the mean for age.
‡A clitoris is abnormally enlarged if its breadth is more than 6 mm or if it protrudes from between the labia majora when the legs are together.

A neonate suspected of having an intersex problem should have the pronouncement of his sex deferred. The parents of the neonate instead should be told something along the following lines: "The genitalia are unfinished in their development, and we will need a few days to perform some studies to determine which sex this baby was intended to be reared as." Most of the diagnostic evaluation can be performed within 2 or 3 days, at which time the sex of rearing can almost always be determined, often without a definitive diagnosis being known.

Clinical evaluation

The evaluation of the neonate suspected of having an intersex problem is outlined below. The history, physical examination, and buccal smear for chromatin bodies are done at the outset, and a 10- to 15-ml blood sample is obtained for measurement of steroid hormones, ideally within the first 24 or 36 hours of age, when testosterone levels are physiologically increased if testicular tissue is present (Fig. 33-40). Basal blood samples are diagnostically useful at certain specified ages. A 24-hour urine collection is not necessary if the radioimmunoassays for serum steroids are available. Endoscopy of the urovaginal orifices is done prior to retrograde genitography; endoscopy is important to ascertain where the radiopaque contrast material is injected. The gonadal biopsy is necessary only in certain disorders and is preferably deferred until the infant is bigger.

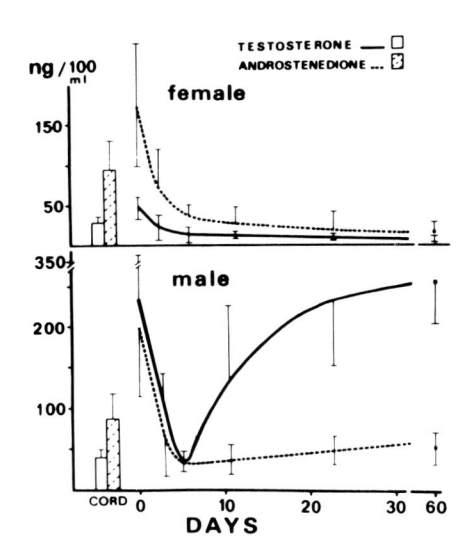

Fig. 33-40. Pattern of testosterone and androstenedione plasma levels during the first month of life in normal neonates. The curves join the mean values (±1 .S.D.) between the different age groups. (From Forest, M.G., and Cathiard, A.M.: J. Clin. Endocrinol. Metab. **41**:977, 1975. © 1975, The Endocrine Society.)

OUTLINE OF DIAGNOSTIC EVALUATION OF INTERSEX PROBLEMS*

History: maternal androgens, drugs, teratogens; affected relatives; sibs died in infancy; consanguinity

Physical: gonads, rectal, genitalia, hyperpigmentation, Turner's stigmata, dysmorphic features

Chromosomes: buccal smear for X and Y chromatin; chromosome karyotype

Anatomic: endoscopy, retrograde genitogram; (?) ultrasound

Biochemical: obtain 10 to 15 ml of blood in first 24 to 36 hours of life (see below for other optimal ages)

If patient is:	Obtain serum levels (at appropriate ages) of:
XX with müllerian ducts	17-OHP, Cpd S, and T; also 17-hydroxypregnenolone in mild virilization
XX without müllerian ducts	T, LH, FSH, estradiol
XY with müllerian ducts	T, LH, FSH
XY without müllerian ducts	T, LH, FSH, dihydrotestosterone; if T is low and testes are normal size, measure androstenedione, 17-OHP, 17-hydroxypregnenolone, urinary cholesterol

Gonadal biopsy (generally deferred until older age): limited to certain diagnoses: true hermaphroditism, gonadal dysgenesis with a Y chromosome, dysgenetic testes, rudimentary testes, persistent müllerian duct syndrome, Leydig cell agenesis, deficient LH receptor, and XX male

Ages when hormone levels in basal blood samples are diagnostically useful:

1. 17-OHP, Cpd S, 17-hydroxypregnenolone, progesterone, or urinary cholesterol, to diagnose congenital adrenal hyperplasia—any age, including cord blood
2. Testosterone, dihydrotestosterone—first 24 to 36 hours of life or at 1 to 2 weeks to 4 to 6 months of age (peak levels occur at 30 to 60 days in term neonates, later in premature neonates)
3. Androstenedione or 17-OHP to diagnose testosterone biosynthetic defect—same ages as for testosterone
4. LH, FSH, or estradiol—1 to 2 weeks to 4 to 6 months of age; FSH may remain increased in normal female neonates up to approximately 2 years of age
5. HCG stimulation testing is necessary to evaluate for the presence of testes between 2 days and 2 weeks of age and beyond 4 to 6 months of age.

The presence of abnormal genitalia raises one of the following questions: (1) if the infant is 46,XX, why are the genitalia excessively masculinized; and (2) if the infant is 46,XY, why is masculinization of the genitalia incomplete or severely deficient? Assessment of the genetic, gonadal, and biochemical status should provide a satisfactory answer. The genetic status can be known within 1 day

*Cpd S, Compound S or 11-deoxycortisol; FSH, follicle-stimulating hormone; HCG, human chorionic gonadotropin; LH, luteinizing hormone; 17-OHP, 17α-hydroxyprogesterone; T, testosterone.

with reasonable certainty by assessing for both the X and Y chromatin on the buccal smear. 46,XX neonates may normally show a lowered percentage of X chromatin, to as low as 4%, in the first several days of life. The karyotype is the definitive analysis, and some laboratories can provide results within 4 or 5 working days.

The gonadal status can be inferred in the neonatal period from knowledge of the following:

1. *Gonadal descent and size.* For practical purposes, only a gonad containing testicular tissue, i.e., a testis or ovotestis, can descend to a position where it is palpable (an ovary virtually never descends); a small gonad may be rudimentary or dysgenetic.
2. *Müllerian duct structures.* Presence of a uterine cervix indicates either one or both gonads did not produce MIF; the presence of bilateral fallopian tubes indicates both gonads failed to produce MIF.
3. *Chromosomes.* Bilateral ovaries can be present only if no Y and two X chromosomes are present. Testes, dysgenetic testes, ovotestes, streak gonads, or no gonads may occur with any karyotype.

The biochemical studies will further clarify the gonadal status or may provide a definitive diagnosis in many patients.

1. Elevated levels of testosterone occur physiologically in the neonatal period at specified time periods in the presence of functioning testes (Fig. 33-40) or may occur abnormally at any time from adrenal secretion of androgens in congenital adrenal hyperplasia; decreased levels of testosterone occur if Leydig cells are deficient or absent, if LH activity is impaired, or if there is a testosterone biosynthetic defect; levels of DHT should follow a pattern similar to those of testosterone.
2. An elevated cord or peripheral blood level of 17-hydroxyprogesterone, 11-deoxycortisol (compound S), or 17-hydroxypregnenolone is diagnostic of 21- or 11β-hydroxylase or 3β-hydroxysteroid dehydrogenase deficiencies, respectively, and would imply that any increased levels of testosterone were adrenal and not testicular in origin in a 46,XX patient.
3. Levels of estradiol in female infants with bilateral ovaries overlap but may be higher (up to 75 pg/ml) than in male infants with testes (up to 35 pg/ml) in the first several months.
4. An elevated level of FSH connotes dysgenetic or absent testicular or ovarian tissue (FSH elevation may not occur until several months of age in some).
5. An elevated level of LH in males beyond 1 to 2 weeks of age indicates impaired testosterone synthesis.

The actual process used to arrive at a final diagnosis is charted in flow diagrams for XY and XX patients, respectively (Figs. 33-41 and 33-42). The appearance of the external genitalia is almost never characteristic for a specific diagnosis and is not diagnostically useful. Since the assay for the androgen receptor is not yet available in

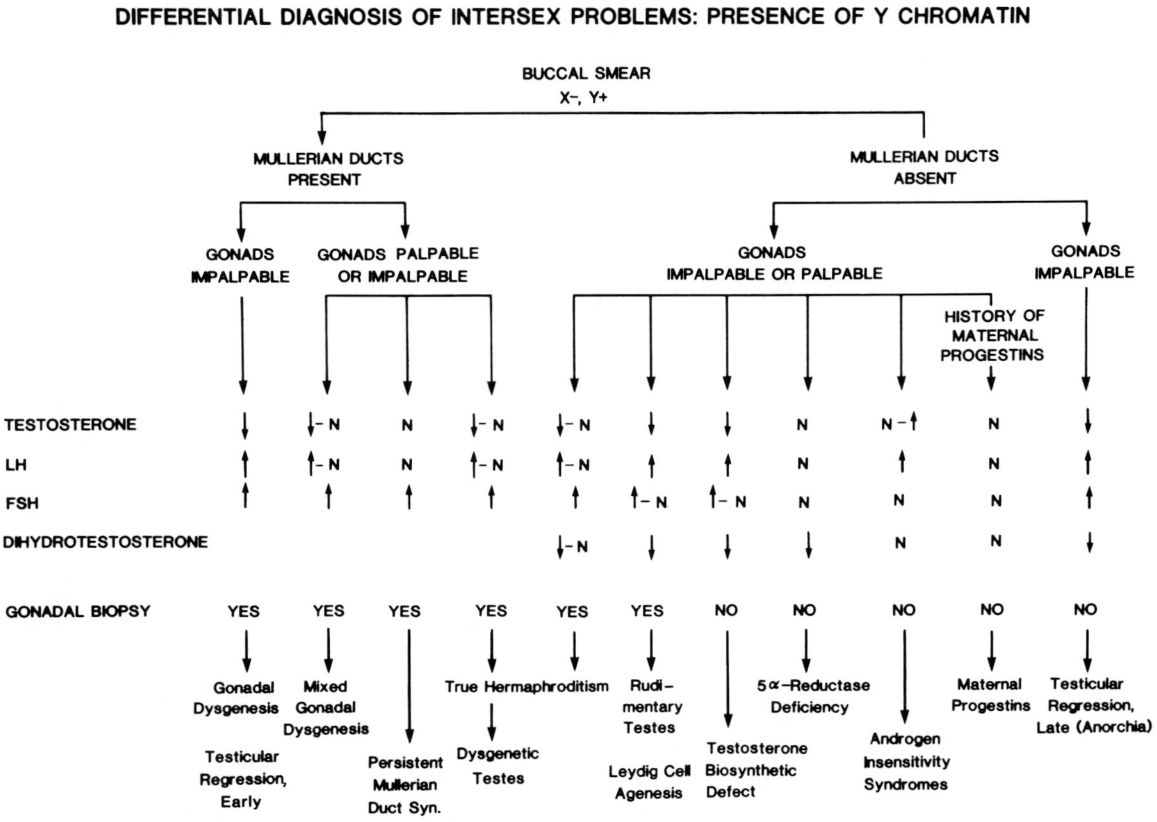

DIFFERENTIAL DIAGNOSIS OF INTERSEX PROBLEMS: PRESENCE OF Y CHROMATIN

	|	|	|	|	|	|	|	|	|	|
TESTOSTERONE	↓	↓-N	N	↓-N	↓-N	↓	↓	N	N-↑	N	↓
LH	↑	↑-N	N	↑-N	↑-N	↑	↑	N	N	N	↑
FSH	↑	↑	↑	↑	↑	↑-N	↑-N	N	N	N	N
DIHYDROTESTOSTERONE					↓-N	↓	↓	↓	N	N	↓
GONADAL BIOPSY	YES	YES	YES	YES	YES	YES	NO	NO	NO	NO	NO

Branches (left to right):
- Müllerian Ducts Present, Gonads Impalpable → Gonadal Dysgenesis; Testicular Regression, Early
- Müllerian Ducts Present, Gonads Palpable or Impalpable → Mixed Gonadal Dysgenesis
- Müllerian Ducts Present → Persistent Müllerian Duct Syn.
- Müllerian Ducts Present → True Hermaphroditism; Dysgenetic Testes
- Müllerian Ducts Absent, Gonads Impalpable or Palpable → Rudimentary Testes; Leydig Cell Agenesis
- → Testosterone Biosynthetic Defect
- → 5α-Reductase Deficiency
- → Androgen Insensitivity Syndromes
- History of Maternal Progestins → Maternal Progestins
- Gonads Impalpable → Testicular Regression, Late (Anorchia)

Fig. 33-41. Flow diagram for the diagnosis of XY intersex disorders: presence of Y chromatin. True hermaphrodites may also present with absence of müllerian ducts. *Nl*, Normal range; ↓, decreased; ↑, increased.

commercial laboratories, the diagnosis of the androgen insensitivity syndromes is made by deduction. In some cases of XY, or male, pseudohermaphroditism it may not be possible to distinguish between two or three diagnoses because of overlapping features and unavailability of certain tests.

Sex assignment

The selection of sex of rearing of the intersex neonate is usually made when the chromatin and müllerian duct status is known, or it occasionally may need to be deferred until the biochemical results are returned. The decision is best made in consultation with appropriate specialists. If bilateral ovaries are deduced to be present, the neonate should be reared as female; if bilateral ovaries are not present, the sex of rearing is determined by the length of the penis. It is best to make this decision as early as possible. Infants who were incorrectly sex-assigned at birth may successfully undergo sex reassignment up to 18 months to 2 years of age, but beyond this time it is felt that gender identity is sufficiently fixed and should not be altered.

The reason for rearing all neonates with bilateral ovaries as female, despite many having well-masculinized external genitalia, is that these patients are capable of normal female hormone secretion and are potentially fertile; their genitalia can be reconstructed to a normal female phenotype with only one or two surgical procedures. As males they would require life-long hormonal therapy and would be infertile; hypospadias repair and hysterectomy would be necessary.

If bilateral ovaries are absent, the principal criterion for male sex of rearing is whether one may expect a patient to achieve a normal penile size in both childhood and adulthood. As yet there is no evidence to show that a neonate having an abnormally small penis, e.g., a length of 4 S.D. below the mean, can be treated so that his penile length will reach a normal size in adulthood, i.e, within 2 S.D. of the mean. A trial of testosterone or dihydrotestosterone therapy in infancy to determine if the penis will grow is not recommended, since it does not predict whether a normal penile size can be attained in adulthood. If penile length is severely diminished, it is safer for that patient to be reared as a female.

DIFFERENTIAL DIAGNOSIS OF INTERSEX PROBLEMS: ABSENCE OF Y CHROMATIN

	± Somatic Malformations	History of Maternal Androgens	21 OHase	11β OHase	3β HSDase	True Hermaphroditism	XX Male
17-HYDROXYPROGESTERONE	N	N	↑↑	↑	±↑	N	N
11-DEOXYCORTISOL (CPD S)	N	N	N	↑↑	N	N	N
17-HYDROXYPREGNENOLONE	N	N	↑	±↑	↑↑	N	N
TESTOSTERONE	N	N	↑	↑	±↑	F–M	M
LH	N	N				N–↑	N–↑
FSH	N	N				↑	↑
ESTRADIOL						M–F	M
GONADAL BIOPSY	NO	NO	NO	NO	NO	YES	YES
	Idiopathic	Maternal Androgens	\multicolumn{3}{c	}{Congenital Adrenal Hyperplasia}	True Hermaphroditism	XX Male

Buccal Smear X+, Y−
- Mullerian Ducts Present → Gonads Impalpable
- Mullerian Ducts Absent → Gonads Impalpable or Palpable; Gonads Palpable

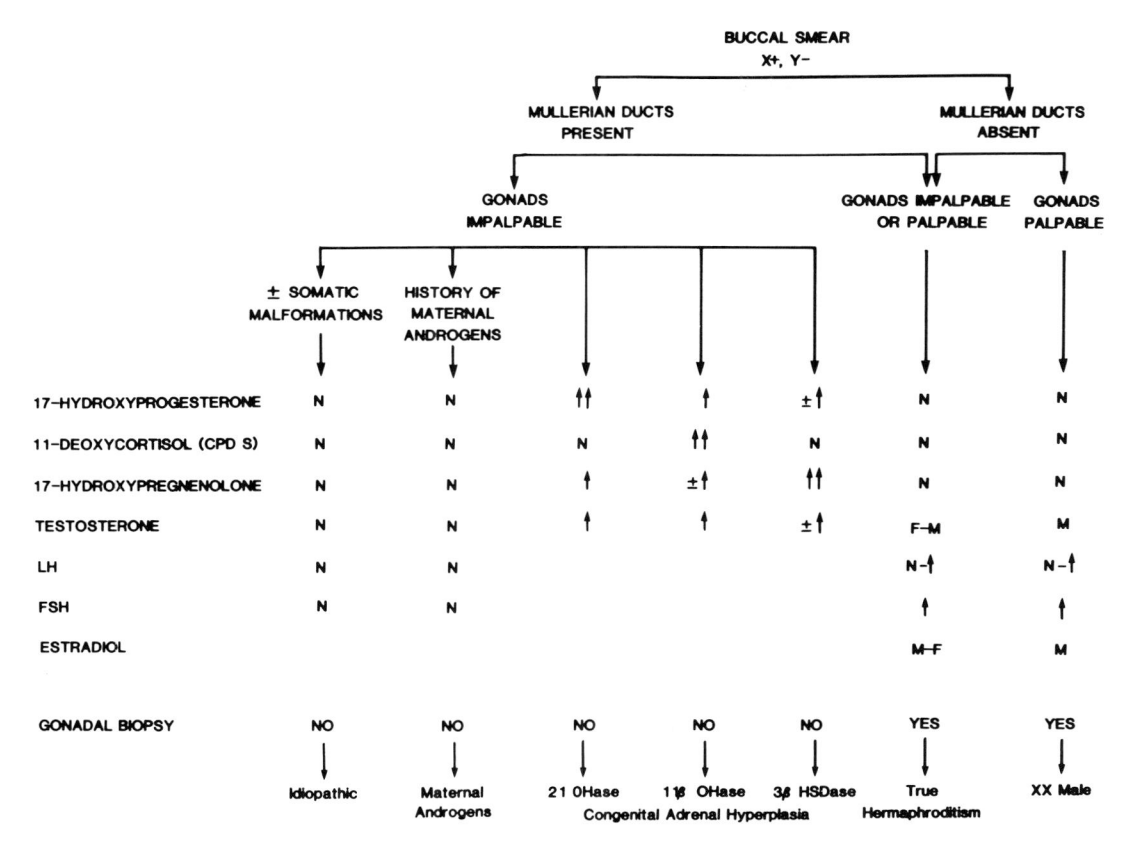

Fig. 33-42. Flow diagram for the diagnosis of XX intersex disorders: absence of Y chromatin. *F*, Female range; *M*, male range; *Nl*, normal range; ↓, decreased; ↑, increased.

CRITERIA FOR SELECTION OF SEX OF REARING FOR INTERSEX NEONATES OR INFANTS

A. Female sex of rearing if:
  1. Bilateral ovaries are present, regardless of degree of masculinization of genitalia.
  or
  2. Stretched penile length is less than 1.5 cm.
B. Male sex of rearing if:
  1. Ovaries are absent.
  and
  2. Stretched penile length is greater than 2 cm.
C. Modifying factors:
  1. If stretched penile length is borderline (1.5 to 2.0 cm in a term neonate), female sex of rearing is recommended if the patient has:
    a. Partial androgen insensitivity
    b. Severe mental retardation or major medical problems requiring other extensive medical or surgical interventions
    c. A prospect for shortened adult height, e.g., gonadal dysgenesis
    or
    d. Difficult surgical repair of genitalia
  2. If penile chordee is present, allow for an increase in penile length that will occur when the chordee is corrected.
  3. In premature neonates the stretched penile lengths are normally shorter (Fig. 33-39).

In summary, the underlying aims in selecting the more appropriate sex of rearing are (1) that the genitalia be correctable to a normal size and function by early childhood, so that the child may grow up with a normal body image and gender identity; (2) that the genitalia be normal in size and function in adulthood to permit normal penile-vaginal intercourse; and (3) if the first two goals are feasible, that fertility should be retained.

Management

The most immediate concern in a neonate with abnormal genitalia is whether congenital adrenal hyperplasia is present. One may expect the onset of adrenal insufficiency to occur between 4 and 14 days in 50% of affected patients and later in the rest, but not earlier. The specific treatment is described in the section on congenital adrenal hyperplasia.

Infants reared as male with a small penis should be treated with testosterone, administered intramuscularly, to increase penile size into the normal range for age. The bone age needs to be monitored. Topical testosterone therapy is not recommended. If testes are undescended after age 6 months, a course of LH-releasing hormone (LHRH) or HCG treatment may bring on testicular descent, particularly in bilateral undescent. Nonresponders should have an orchiopexy done by age 4 years. Dysgenetic testes should be removed, and prosthetic testes may be placed in the scrotum.

Surgical correction of the ambiguous genitalia in patients reared as female is best done by age 18 months and is usually done when the infant has attained a reasonable size, e.g., a body weight of 9 kg. Clitoral reduction is preferably done by resection of the corpora cavernosa and suturing the glans to the pubis; clitoral recession or amputation is not recommended. There is debate as to whether vaginal orifice exteriorization should be done in infancy. Construction of a vagina in a patient lacking a vagina is deferred until adulthood when she plans to be sexually active. Wolffian duct structures do not need to be removed.

Surgical correction of ambiguous genitalia in the male should be completed before the boy enters school so that he will have a normal genital appearance and be able to stand to urinate. Circumcision of the penis should not be done before hypospadias repair. Plastic surgical attempts to increase penile size are not recommended, since no method is available that can provide a reasonably normal appearing and functional penis. Only androgen therapy is of benefit. Male patients having a vagina that enters a urogenital sinus may have urinary incontinence if the vagina acts as a reservoir, in which case the vagina should be excised. Müllerian duct structures do not necessarily need to be removed because the wolffian ducts may be embedded in its walls and thus unintentionally removed, although occasional cases of uterine cancer have been reported.

The gonads should be removed either (1) if their hormonal production will lead to inappropriate virilization or feminization in patients reared as female or male, respectively, or (2) if they are at increased risk for tumor development. The increased levels of testosterone produced by the testes in the first half year of life are generally not a major problem, and afterward the testes are relatively inactive hormonally until puberty. Ovarian sex steroid production is not clinically important until puberty. Gonadal tissue destined to secrete sex hormones inappropriate for the sex of rearing is removed at some time prior to the onset of puberty.

Patients with streak or dysgenetic gonads having a Y chromosome are at markedly increased risk for tumor development, occurring as early as 3 to 5 years of age.

Gonadectomy should be performed in the first few years of life, particularly in individuals with a Y gonadal streak. In complete androgen insensitivity syndrome it is considered safe to leave the testes in situ until 15 to 18 years of age. Intersex patients lacking a Y chromosome and testicular tissue do not appear to be at increased risk for gonadal tumor development.

Patients with hypogonadism will require testosterone or estrogen-progesterone replacement therapy at puberty. The sex steroids are not necessary for normal growth prior to puberty.

Genetic counseling should be provided to the family when the diagnosis is known. Heterozygote detection is available for 21-hydroxylase deficiency, and prenatal diagnosis has been reported for 21- and 11β-hydroxylase deficiencies and is possible for complete androgen insensitivity syndrome. Many families benefit by the involvement of a social worker or psychologist who may assist the family in understanding confusing medical issues and in dealing with their emotions. As the patient grows up he will need to gradually learn the facts of his disorder.

Female patients exposed to increased androgens in utero may show an increase in their level of activity, tomboyishness, greater preference for pursuing career interests, decreased interest in maternal roles, and more male friends. Boys exposed to decreased levels of androgens or increased levels of progesterone in utero may show less typically masculine behavior. Some patients will have learning disability or behavioral or psychologic problems that may be related to their underlying disorder, e.g., Klinefelter's syndrome, or to abnormalities of body image or gender identity, for which psychologic counseling may be of benefit. The prognosis for most well-managed patients, however, is that they can expect to grow up with a normal body image and gender identity, attain appropriate scholastic and job-related goals, lead a normal social life, become married if they wish, and have normal sexual relations. Since many patients will be infertile, they should expect to have their children by adoption.

Robert K. Danish

BIBLIOGRAPHY
Fetal sexual differentiation

Forest, M.G., and others: Concentration of 14 steroid hormones in human amniotic fluid of midpregnancy, J. Clin. Endocrinol. Metab. **51**:816, 1980.

Gordon, J.W., and Ruddle, F.H.: Mammalian gonadal determination and gametogenesis, Science **211**:1265, 1981.

Haseltine F.P., and Ohno, S.: Mechanisms of gonadal differentiation, Science **211**:1272, 1981.

Imperato-McGinley, J., and Peterson, R.E.: Male pseudohermaphroditism: the complexities of male phenotypic development, Am. J. Med. **61**:251, 1976.

Jirasek, J.E.: Morphogenesis of the genital system in the human, Birth Defects Orig. Art. Ser. **13**(2):13, 1977.

Josso, N., Picard, J.-Y., and Tran, D.: The antimüllerian hormone, Recent Prog. Horm. Res. **33**:117, 1977.

Kaplan, S.L., Grumbach. M.M., and Aubert, M.L.: The ontogenesis of pituitary hormones and hypothalamic factors in the human fetus: maturation of central nervous system regulation of anterior pituitary function, Recent Prog. Horm. Res. **32**:161, 1976.

O'Rahilly, R.: The development of the vagina in the human, Birth Defects Orig. Art. Ser. **13**(2):123, 1977.

Reyes, F.I., Winter, J.S.D., and Faiman, C.: Gonadotropin-gonadal interrelationships in the fetus. In New, M.I., and Fiser, R.H., Jr., editors: Diabetes and other endocrine disorders during pregnancy and in the newborn, Progress in Clinical and Biological Research, vol. 10, New York, 1976, Alan R. Liss.

Tapanainen, J., and others: Age-related changes in endogenous steroids of human fetal testis during early and midpregnancy, J. Clin. Endocrinol. Metab. **52**:98, 1981.

Wachtel, S.S., and Ohno, S.: The immunogenetics of sexual development. In Steinberg, A.G., and others, editors: Progress in medical genetics, vol. 3, Philadelphia, 1979, W.B. Saunders Co.

Wilson, J.D.: Sexual differentiation, Annu. Rev. Physiol. **40**:279, 1978.

Wilson, J.D., George, F.W., and Griffin, J.E.: The hormonal control of sexual development, Science **211**:1278, 1981.

Disorders of gonadal development

Aynsley-Green, A., and others: Congenital bilateral anorchia in childhood: a clinical, endocrine and therapeutic evaluation of twenty-one cases, Clin. Endocrinol. **5**:381, 1976.

Barakat, A.Y., and others: Pseudohermaphroditism, nephron disorder and Wilms' tumor: a unifying concept, Pediatrics **54**:366, 1974.

Bloomgarden, Z.T., and others: Genetic and endocrine findings in a 48,XXYY male, J. Clin. Endocrinol. Metab. **50**:740, 1980.

Bove, K.E.: Gonadal dysgenesis in a newborn with XO karyotype, Am. J. Dis. Child. **120**:363, 1970.

Brosnan, P.G., and others: A new familial syndrome of 46,XY gonadal dysgenesis with anomalies of ectodermal and mesodermal structures, J. Pediatr. **97**:586, 1980.

Brown, D.M., Markland, C., and Dehner, L.P.: Leydig cell hypoplasia: a cause of male pseudohermaphroditism, J. Clin. Endocrinol. Metab. **46**:1, 1978.

Campbell, W.A., and Price, W.H.: Congenital hypothyroidism in Klinefelter's syndrome, J. Med. Genet. **16**:439, 1979.

Conte, F.A., and Grumbach, M.M.: Pathogenesis, classification, diagnosis, and treatment of anomalies of sex. In De Groot, L.J., editor: Endocrinology, vol. 3, New York, 1979, Grune & Stratton, Inc.

Conte, F.A., Grumbach, M.M., and Kaplan, S.L.: A diphasic pattern of gonadotropin secretion in patients with the syndrome of gonadal dysgenesis, J. Clin. Endocrinol. Metab. **40**:670, 1975.

Edlow, J.B., and others: Neonatal Klinefelter's syndrome, Am. J. Dis. Child. **118**:788, 1969.

Edman, C.D., and others: Embryonic testicular regression: a clinical spectrum of XY agonadal individuals, Obstet. Gynecol. **49**:208, 1977.

Fichman, K.R., Migeon, B.R., and Migeon, C.J.: Genetic disorders of male sexual differentiation. In Harris, H., and Hirschhorn, K., editors: Advances in human genetics, vol. 10, New York, 1980, Plenum Press.

German, J., and others: Genetically determined sex-reversal in 46,XY humans, Science **202**:53, 1978.

Gordon, R.R., and O'Neill, E.M.: Turner's infantile phenotype, Br. Med. J. **1**:483, 1969.

Haddad, H.M., and Wilkins, L.: Congenital anomalies associated with gonadal aplasia: review of 55 cases, Pediatrics **23**:885, 1959.

Harris, J.S., and Heller, R.H.: The detection of Klinefelter's syndrome at birth, Clin. Pediatr. **13**:581, 1974.

Hoefnagel, D., and others: Camptomelic dwarfism associated with XY-gonadal dysgenesis and chromosome anomalies, Clin. Genet. **13**:489, 1978.

Hsueh, W.A., Hsu, T.H., and Federman, D.D.: Endocrine features of Klinefelter's syndrome, Medicine **57**:447, 1978.

Jacobs, P.A.: The incidence and etiology of sex chromosome abnormalities in man, Birth Defects Orig. Art. Ser. **15**(1):3, 1979.

Josso, N., and Briard, M.-L.: Embryonic testicular regression syndrome: variable phenotypic expression in siblings, J. Pediatr. **97**:200, 1980.

Karsh, R.B., and others: Congenital heart disease in 49,XXXXY syndrome, Pediatrics **56**:462, 1975.

Koo, G.C., and others: Mapping the locus of the H-Y gene on the human Y chromosome, Science **198**:940, 1977.

Litvak, A.S., and others: The association of significant renal anomalies with Turner's syndrome, J. Urol. **120**:671, 1978.

Murken, J.-D., and others: Klinefelter's syndrome in a fetus, Lancet **2**:171, 1974.

Najjar, S.S., Takla, R.J., and Nassar, V.H.: The syndrome of rudimentary testes: occurrence in five siblings, J. Pediatr. **84**:119, 1974.

Nielsen, J., and others: Klinefelter's syndrome and trisomy 18 in a newborn boy, Clin. Genet. **13**:259, 1978.

Rajfer, J., and others: Dysgenetic male pseudohermaphroditism, J. Urol. **119**:525, 1978.

Robinson, A.: Neonatal deaths and sex-chromosome anomalies, Lancet **1**:1223, 1974.

Robinson, A., and others: Summary of clinical findings: profiles of children with 47,XXY, 47,XXX and 47,XYY karyotypes, Birth Defects Orig. Art. Ser. **15**(1):261, 1979.

Roe, T.F., and Alfi, O.S.: Ambiguous genitalia in XX male children: report of two infants, Pediatrics **60**:55, 1977.

Rosenthal, A.: Cardiovascular malformations in Klinefelter's syndrome: report of three cases, J. Pediatr. **80**:471, 1972.

Rushton, D.I., and others: The fetal manifestations of the 45,XO karyotype, J. Obstet. Gynaecol. Br. Commonw. **76**:266, 1969.

Ruvalcaba, R.H.A., Gogue, H.P., and Kelley, V.C.: Discordance of congenital bilateral anorchia in uniovular twins: 17 years of observation on growth and development, Pediatrics **67**:276, 1981.

Shapiro, L.R., and others: Deceleration of intellectual development in a XXXXY child, Am. J. Dis. Child. **122**:163, 1971.

Simpson, J.L.: Gonadal dysgenesis. In Simpson, J.L.: Disorders of sexual differentiation: etiology and clinical delineation, New York, 1976, Academic Press, Inc.

Simpson, J.L.: True hermaphroditism: etiology and phenotypic considerations, Birth Defects Orig. Art. Ser. **14**:(6C):9, 1978.

Szpunar, J., and Rybak, M.: Middle ear disease in Turner's syndrome, Arch. Otolaryngol. **87**:34, 1968.

Warburton, D., and others: Monosomy X: a chromosomal anomaly associated with young maternal age, Lancet **1**:167, 1980.

Weiss, L.: Additional evidence of gradual loss of germ cells in the pathogenesis of streak ovaries in Turner's syndrome, J. Med. Genet. **8**:540, 1971.

Winters, S.J., and others: H-Y antigen mosaicism in the gonad of a 46,XX true hermaphrodite, N. Engl. J. Med. **300**:745, 1979.

Wolf, U.: XY gonadal dysgenesis and the H-Y antigen: report on 12 cases, Hum. Genet. **47**:269, 1979.

Zah, W., Kalderon, A.E., and Tucci, J.R.: Mixed gonadal dysgenesis: a case report and review of the world literature, Acta Endocrinol. **197**(Suppl.):1, 1975.

Disorders of testicular function and androgen-dependent target cells

Amrhein, J.A., and others: Androgen insensitivity in man: evidence for genetic heterogeneity, Proc. Natl. Acad. Sci. USA **73**:891, 1976.

Amrhein, J.A., and others: Partial androgen insensitivity: the Reifenstein syndrome revisited, N. Engl. J. Med. **297**:350, 1977.

Danish, R.K., and others: Micropenis. II. Hypogonadotropic hypogonadism, Johns Hopkins Med. J. **146:**177, 1980.

Goebelsmann, U., and others: Male pseudohermaphroditism consistent with 17,20-desmolase deficiency, Gynecol. Invest. **7:**138, 1976.

Griffin, J.E., and Wilson, J.D.: The syndromes of androgen resistance, N. Engl. J. Med. **302:**198, 1980.

Imperato-McGinley, J., and others: Androgens and the evolution of male-gender identity among male pseudohermaphrodites with 5α-reductase deficiency, N. Engl. J. Med. **300:**1233, 1979.

Imperato-McGinley, J., and others: Male pseudohermaphroditism secondary to 17β-hydroxysteroid dehydrogenase deficiency: gender role change with puberty, J. Clin. Endocrinol. Metab. **49:**391, 1979.

Keenan, B.S., and others: Syndrome of androgen insensitivity in man: absence of 5α-dihydrotestosterone binding protein in skin fibroblasts, J. Clin. Endocrinol. Metab. **38:**1143, 1974.

Keenan, B.S., and others: Male pseudohermaphroditism with partial androgen insensitivity, Pediatrics **59:**224, 1977.

Lovinger, R., Kaplan, S., and Grumbach, M.: Congenital hypopituitarism associated with neonatal hypoglycemia and microphallus: four cases secondary to hypothalamic hormone deficiencies, J. Pediatr. **87:**1171, 1975.

Meyer, W.J., III, Migeon, B.R., and Migeon, C.J.: Locus on human X chromosome for dihydrotestosterone receptor and androgen insensitivity, Proc. Natl. Acad. Sci. U.S.A. **72:**1469, 1975.

Saenger, P., and others: Prepubertal diagnosis of 5α-reductase deficiency, J. Clin. Endocrinol. Metab. **46:**627, 1978.

Virdis, R., and others: Endocrine studies in a pubertal male pseudohermaphrodite with 17-ketosteroid reductase deficiency, Acta Endocrinol. **87:**212, 1978.

Weiss, E.B., and others: Persistent müllerian duct syndrome in male identical twins, Pediatrics **61:**797, 1978.

Female pseudohermaphroditism and congenital adrenal hyperplasia

Barnes, A.B., and others: Fertility and outcome of pregnancy in women exposed in utero to diethylstilbestrol, N. Engl. J. Med. **302:**609, 1980.

Bongiovanni, A.M.: Urinary steroidal pattern of infants with congenital adrenal hyperplasia due to 3-beta-hydroxysteroid dehydrogenase deficiency, J. Steroid Biochem. **13:**809, 1980.

Brook, C.G.D., and others: Experience with long-term therapy in congenital adrenal hyperplasia, J. Pediatr. **85:**12, 1974.

Bongiovanni, A.M.: Androgens, estrogens, and the fetus. In New, M.I., and Fiser, R.H., Jr., editors: Diabetes and other endocrine disorders during pregnancy and in the newborn, Progress in Clinical and Biological Research, vol. 10, New York, 1976, Alan R. Liss.

Bongiovanni, A.M.: Congenital adrenal hyperplasia and related conditions. In Stanbury, J.B., Wyngaarden, J.B., and Fredrickson, D.S., editors: The metabolic basis of inherited disease, ed. 4, New York, 1978, McGraw-Hill Book Co., Inc.

Cavallo, A., and others: The use of plasma androstenedione in monitoring therapy of patients with congenital adrenal hyperplasia, J. Pediatr. **95:**33, 1979.

dePeretti, E., and others: Endocrine studies in two children with male pseudohermaphroditism due to 3β-hydroxysteroid (3β-HSD) dehydrogenase defect. In Genazzani, A.R., Thijssen, J.H.H., and Siiteri, P.K., editors: Adrenal androgens, New York, 1980, Raven Press.

Finkelstein, M., and Shaefer, J.M.: Inborn errors of steroid biosynthesis, Physiol. Rev. **59:**353, 1979.

Gutai, J.P., Lee, P.A., Johnsonbaugh, R.E.: Detection of the heterozygous state in siblings of patients with congenital adrenal hyperplasia due to 21-hydroxylase deficiency, J. Pediatr. **94:**770, 1979.

Haymond, M.W., and Weldon, V.V.: Female pseudohermaphroditism secondary to a maternal virilizing tumor: case report and review of the literature, J. Pediatr. **82:**682, 1973.

Hensleigh, P.A., Carter, R.P., and Grotjan, H.E., Jr.: Fetal protection against masculinization with hyperreaction luteinalis and virilization, J. Clin. Endocrinol. Metab. **40:**816, 1975.

Holcombe, J.H., Keenan, B.S., and Clayton, G.W.: Plasma 17α-hydroxyprogesterone and aldosterone concentrations in infants and children with congenital adrenal hyperplasia—the role of salt-losing hormones in salt wasting, J. Pediatr. **98:**573, 1981.

Holcombe, J.H., and others: Neonatal salt loss in the hypertensive form of congenital adrenal hyperplasia, Pediatrics **65:**777, 1980.

Hughes, I.A., and Laurence, K.M.: Antenatal diagnosis of congenital adrenal hyperplasia, Lancet **2:**7, 1979.

Jones, H.W., and Verkauf, B.S.: Surgical treatment in congenital adrenal hyperplasia: age at operation and other prognostic factors, Obstet. Gynecol. **36:**1, 1970.

Kai, H., and others: Female pseudohermaphroditism caused by maternal congenital adrenal hyperplasia, J. Pediatr. **95:**418, 1979.

Klouda, P.T., Harris, R., and Price, D.A.: Linkage and association between HLA and 21-hydroxylase deficiency, J. Med. Genet. **17:**337, 1980.

Koizumi, S., and others: Cholesterol side-chain cleavage enzyme activity and cytochrome P-450 content in adrenal mitochondria of a patient with congenital lipoid adrenal hyperplasia (Prader disease), Clin. Chim. Acta **77:**301, 1977.

Koshimizu, T.: Plasma renin activity and aldosterone concentration in normal subjects and patients with salt-losing type of congenital adrenal hyperplasia during infancy, Clin. Endocrinol. **10:**515, 1979.

Kowarski, A., and others: Aldosterone secretion rate in congenital adrenal hyperplasia: a discussion of the theories on the pathogenesis of the salt-losing form of the syndrome, J. Clin. Invest. **44:**1505, 1965.

Lee, P.A., and others, editors: Congenital adrenal hyperplasia, Baltimore, 1977, University Park Press.

Lorenzen, F., and others: Studies of the C-21 and C-19 steroids and HLA genotyping in siblings and parents of patients with congenital adrenal hyperplasia due to 21-hydroxylase deficiency, J. Clin. Endocrinol. Metab. **50:**572, 1980.

McKenna, T.J., and others: Pregnenolone, 17-OH-pregnenolone, and testosterone in plasma of patients with congenital adrenal hyperplasia, J. Clin. Endocrinol. Metab. **42:**918, 1976.

Migeon, C.J.: Diagnosis and treatment of adrenogenital disorders. In DeGroot, L.J., editor: Endocrinology, vol. 3, New York, 1979, Grune & Stratton, Inc.

Migeon, C.J., and Kenny, F.M.: Cortisol production rate. V. Congenital virilizing adrenal hyperplasia, J. Pediatr. **69:**779, 1966.

Park, I.J., Jones, H.W., Jr., and Melhem, R.E.: Nonadrenal familial female hermaphroditism, Am. J. Obstet. Gynecol. **112:**930, 1972.

Park, I.J., and others: Special female hermaphroditism associated with multiple disorders, Obstet. Gynecol. **39:**100, 1972.

Pollack, M.S., and others: Prenatal diagnosis of congenital adrenal hyperplasia (21-hydroxylase deficiency) by HLA typing, Lancet **1:**1107, 1979.

Rosenberg, B., Hendren, W.H., and Crawford, J.D.: Posterior urethrovaginal communication in apparent males with congenital adrenocortical hyperplasia, N. Engl. J. Med. **280:**131, 1969.

Rösler, A., and others: Prenatal diagnosis of 11β-hydroxylase deficiency congenital adrenal hyperplasia, J. Clin. Endocrinol. Metab. **49:**546, 1979.

Rovner, D.R., and others: 17α-Hydroxylase deficiency: a combination of hydroxylation defect and reversible blockade in aldosterone biosynthesis, Acta Endocrinol. **90:**490, 1979.

Shackleton, C.H.L.: Congenital adrenal hyperplasia caused by defect in steroid 21-hydroxylase: establishment of definitive urinary steroid

excretion pattern during first weeks of life, Clin. Chim. Acta 67:287, 1976.
Sotiropoulos, A., and others: Long-term assessment of genital reconstruction in female pseudohermaphrodites, J. Urol. 115:599, 1976.
Taylor, N.F., Clymo, A.B., and Shackleton, C.H.L.: Steroid excretion by an infant with 3β-hydroxysteroid dehydrogenase deficiency during conventional replacement therapy and following corticotrophin stimulation, J. Endocrinol. 80:62P, 1979.
Verhoeven, A.T.M., and others: Virilization in pregnancy coexisting with an (ovarian) mucinous cystadenoma: a case report and review of virilizing ovarian tumors in pregnancy, Obstet. Gynecol. Surv. 28:597, 1973.
Waldhäusl, W., and others: Combined 17α- and 18-hydroxylase deficiency associated with complete male pseudohermaphroditism and hypoaldosteronism, J. Clin. Endocrinol. Metab. 46:236, 1978.
Wong, E.T., and others: Urinary 17α-hydroxyprogesterone in diagnosis and management of congenital adrenal hyperplasia, J. Clin. Endocrinol. Metab. 49:377, 1979.

Hypospadias, micropenis, cryptorchidism, and müllerian aplasia

Aarskog, D.: Maternal progestins as a possible cause of hypospadias, N. Engl. J. Med. 300:75, 1979.
Auldist, A.W., and Ferguson, R.S.: Torsion of the testis in the newborn, Aust. N.Z. J. Surg. 45:14, 1975.
Buyse, M., and Feingold, M.: Syndromes associated with abnormal external genitalia. In Vallet, H.L., and Porter, I.H., editors: Genetic mechanisms of sexual development, New York, 1979, Academic Press, Inc.
Cryptorchidism and gonadotrophin therapy (editorial), Lancet 1:1344, 1978.
Danish, R.K., and others: Micropenis. II. Hypogonadotropic hypogonadism, Johns Hopkins Med. J. 146:177, 1980.
Duncan, P.A., and others: The MURCS association: müllerian duct aplasia, renal aplasia, and cervicothoracic somite dysplasia, J. Pediatr. 95:399, 1979.
Fonkalsrud, E.W., and Mengel, W., editors: The undescended testis, Chicago, 1980, Year Book Medical Publishers, Inc.
Gendrel, D., Roger, M., and Job, J.-C.: Plasma gonadotropin and testosterone values in infants with cryptorchidism, J. Pediatr. 97:217, 1980.
Hadziselimovic, F., Herzog, B., and Seguchi, H.: Surgical correction of cryptorchism at 2 years: electron microscopic and morphometric investigations, J. Pediatr. Surg. 10:19, 1975.
Lee, P.A., and others: Micropenis. I. Criteria, etiologies and classification, Johns Hopkins Med. J. 146:156, 1980.
Lee, P.A., and others: Micropenis. III. Primary hypogonadism, partial androgen insensitivity syndrome, and idiopathic disorders, Johns Hopkins Med. J. 147:175, 1980.
Levitt, S.B., and others: The impalpable testis: a rational approach to management, J. Urol. 120:515, 1978.
Lutzker, L.G., Kogan, S.J., and Levitt, S.B.: Is routine intravenous urography indicated in patients with hypospadias? Pediatrics 59:630, 1977.
Mengel, W., and others: Studies on cryptorchidism: a comparison of histological findings in the germinative epithelium before and after the second year of life, J. Pediatr. Surg. 9:445, 1974.
Rajfer, J., and Walsh, P.C.: The incidence of intersexuality in patients with hypospadias and cryptorchidism, J. Urol. 116:769, 1976.
Robinow, M., and Shaw, A.: The McKusick-Kaufman syndrome: recessively inherited vaginal atresia, hydrometrocolpos, uterovaginal duplications, anorectal anomalies, postaxial polydactyly, and congenital heart disease, J. Pediatr. 94:776, 1979.
Russell, L.J., Weaver, D.D., and Bull, M.J.: The axial mesodermal dysplasia spectrum, Pediatrics 67:176, 1981.
Shapiro, S.R., and Bodai, B.I.: Current concepts of the undescended testis, Surg. Gynecol. Obstet. 147:617, 1978.
Svensson, J., and Snochowski, M.: Androgen receptor levels in preputial skin from boys with hypospadias, J. Clin. Endocrinol. Metab. 49:340, 1979.
Waaler, P.E., and Maurseth, K.: Cryptorchidism: is routine intravenous pyelography indicated? Arch. Dis. Child. 51:324, 1976.

Diagnosis and management of intersex problems

Chaussain, J.L., and others: Longitudinal study of plasma testosterone in male pseudohermaphrodites during early infancy, J. Clin. Endocrinol. Metab. 49:305, 1979.
Fauré, C., Fortier-Beaulieu, M., and Josso, N.: Genitography in intersex conditions concerning 86 cases, Ann. Radiol. 12:259, 1969.
Feldman, K.W., and Smith, D.W.: Fetal phallic growth and penile standards for newborn male infants, J. Pediatr. 86:395, 1975.
Fonkalsrud, E.W., Kaplan, S., and Lippe, B.: Experience with reduction clitoroplasty for clitoral hypertrophy, Ann. Surg. 186:221, 1977.
Forest, M.G., and Cathiard, A.M.: Pattern of plasma testosterone and Δ^4-androstenedione in normal newborns: evidence for testicular activity at birth, J. Clin. Endocrinol. Metab. 41:977, 1975.
Gendrel, D., and others: Simultaneous postnatal rise of plasma LH and testosterone in male infants, J. Pediatr. 97:600, 1980.
Guthrie, R.D., Smith, D.W., and Graham, C.B.: Testosterone treatment for micropenis during early childhood, J. Pediatr. 83:247, 1973.
Jones, H.W., Jr.: Problems of sex differentiation—surgical correction, Birth Defects Orig. Art. Ser. 14(6C):63, 1978.
Lippe, B.M., and Sample, W.F.: Pelvic ultrasonography in pediatric and adolescent endocrine disorders, J. Pediatr. 92:897, 1978.
Manuel, M., Katayama, K.P., and Jones, H.W., Jr.: The age of occurrence of gonadal tumors in intersex patients with a Y chromosome, Am. J. Obstet. Gynecol. 124:293, 1976.
Money, J., Hampson, J.G., and Hampson, J.L.: Hermaphroditism: recommendations concerning assignment of sex, change of sex, and psychologic management, Bull. Johns Hopkins Hosp. 97:284, 1955.
Pang, S., and others: Dihydrotestosterone and its relationship to testosterone in infancy and childhood, J. Clin. Endocrinol. Metab. 48:821, 1979.
Riley, W.J., and Rosenbloom, A.L.: Clitoral size in infancy, J. Pediatr. 96:918, 1980.
Simpson, J.L., and Photopulos, G.: The relationship of neoplasia to disorders of abnormal sexual differentiation, Birth Defects Orig. Art. Ser. 12(1):15, 1976.
Winter, J.S.D., and others: Pituitary-gonadal relations in infancy. 2. Patterns of serum gonadal steroid concentrations in man from birth to two years of age, J. Clin. Endocrinol. Metab. 42:679, 1976.

PART FIVE

Infants of addicted mothers

There has been a steady increase in the abuse of narcotic drugs over the last decade. In 1975 (according to NIDA figures) there were approximately 570,000 to 724,000 narcotic addicts in the United States, of whom about 24% were in treatment (methadone maintenance or detoxification program). In New York City alone there were about 250,000 addicts, with about 48% addicts in treatment. It has been estimated that 20% to 40% of these addicts are polydrug abusers, consuming additional quantities of alcohol, psychoactive drugs, barbiturates, and other drugs, thereby compounding the drug addiction problem even further. Women comprise 30% of addicts, and 75% are of childbearing age. As a result, an increasing number of babies are born exhibiting the withdrawal syndromes secondary to maternal drug abuse.

HEROIN
Pathology and pathogenesis

Heroin (diacetylmorphine) readily crosses the placenta. It is deacetylated in the liver to monoacetylmorphine and then to morphine. Once in the fetus, heroin is distributed widely and variably throughout the fetal tissues and body compartments. There appear to be significant differences in its distribution between immature infants and adults. Studies of pregnant animals given morphine have shown the concentration in fetal brain was two to three times that in the maternal brain, and similar differences in distribution are likely for heroin.

Fifty percent of infants born to heroin-addicted women are of low birth weight, and 50% of these are small for gestational age (SGA). Postmortem studies of placentas of heroin-addicted mothers have demonstrated that the increased incidence of prematurity may be due to a high rate of chorioamnionitis or other maternal infection. In addition, autopsies of SGA infants born to narcotic-addicted mothers reveal their organs to be small and consisting of diminished numbers of cells that are of normal size. These autopsy results differ from those obtained from malnourished infants born to nonaddicted mothers, whose organs show a decrease in both number and size of their cells. Therefore it has been postulated that maternal undernutrition is not the only factor responsible for the antenatal growth retardation observed in infants of narcotic addicts; heroin may have a direct growth-inhibiting effect on the fetus.

The incidence of congenital anomalies in infants born to addicted mothers is not higher than in the general population. An increased rate of stillbirths has, however, been reported in those mothers in whom heroin was withdrawn during pregnancy.

Clinical manifestations

Heroin withdrawal symptoms and signs occur in 50% to 75% of infants born to addicted mothers and usually begin within the first 24 to 48 hours of life. The incidence of withdrawal depends on several factors: (1) the dosage of heroin (less than 6 mg/day is associated with no or mild withdrawal symptoms), (2) the duration of maternal addiction (less than 1 year, 55%; greater than 1 year, 73% incidence of withdrawal), and (3) the time of last maternal dose (there is a higher incidence of withdrawal if heroin is taken within 24 hours of birth). The withdrawal syndrome may consist of a combination of any of the following: irritability, jitteriness, coarse tremors, high-pitched cry, fist-sucking, sneezing, yawning, tachypnea, poor feeding, regurgitation, vomiting, diarrhea, sweating, hypothermia or hyperthermia, hypertonia, hyperreflexia, myoclonus, and, less commonly, seizures. In addition, an abnormal sleep cycle with absence of quiet sleep and disturbance of active sleep has been described in these infants. Sucking studies have shown a decrease in both the rate and intensity of sucking.

Infants born to heroin addicts have a low incidence of hyperbilirubinemia and respiratory distress syndrome (RDS). The decreased incidence of hyperbilirubinemia probably is due to induction of the glucuronyl transferase enzyme system by heroin. The low incidence of RDS may be due to a direct effect of heroin on lung maturation with an accelerated production of surfactant, as suggested by animal studies.

Treatment

Therapy for the withdrawal syndrome is recommended in the following situations: (1) severe irritability and tremors that interfere with feeding and sleep, (2) vomiting and diarrhea, (3) seizures, (4) hyperthermia or hypothermia, and (5) severe tachypnea interfering with feedings. Other causes of these symptoms should be excluded before initiating treatment.

Many neonatal units use a withdrawal evaluation scoring system to decide on the necessity of treatment and its efficacy. Treatment should include one of the following drugs: phenobarbital, paregoric, or diazepam singly or in combination (Table 33-6). The choice of medication varies in individual nurseries. The initial dose of phenobarbital or diazepam should be a high mg/kg loading dose followed by a lower maintenance dosage to allow an adequate plasma level and rapid clinical response. While maintenance therapy is being given, plasma drug level monitoring is desirable to prevent toxicity. Once a clinical response has been achieved, the medication should be tapered gradually (every other day) and discontinued. The duration of treatment in neonatal heroin withdrawal may vary from 4 days to 6 weeks.

Prognosis

With appropriate management in the neonatal period the mortality of heroin-addicted infants does not exceed 3% to 4%; in the late 1950s the reported mortality was 34%, with most infants dying of severe dehydration and shock secondary to diarrhea and vomiting. The follow-up of surviving infants often is incomplete because many addicted mothers will not bring their infants for appointments or because the infants have been placed in foster care. Wilson and associates have reported on 22 children

Table 33-6. Dosage schedule

Drug	Dosage
Phenobarbital*	5-20 mg/kg loading dose IM, then 4-6 mg/kg/day maintenance, q12h PO
Paregoric	4-6 drops every 4-6 hours PO; if no improvement, increase dosage by 2 drops until clinical improvement is apparent
Diazepam (Valium)	0.3-0.5 mg/kg/day (0.9-1.5 mg/kg/day); initial dose IM and then PO q8h
Methadone	0.1-0.5 mg/kg/day every 4-12 hours PO

*Phenobarbital plasma levels should be evaluated frequently to prevent toxicity.

born to heroin addicts at 3 to 6 years of age. They demonstrated deficiencies in both height and weight. In addition, 14% had head circumferences less than 3% on the growth chart. Their overall intellectual functioning was not significantly different from that of normal controls, but they exhibited significant difficulties in the general processes of perception and cognition. They also scored significantly lower than controls in tasks requiring attention, concentration, and short-term memory. These children appeared more aggressive, compulsive, and active than their matched controls, often having an uncontrollable temper.

METHADONE

Methadone, a synthetic opiate, has been the therapy of choice for heroin addiction since its introduction for this purpose by Dole and Nyswander in 1965. It blocks the euphoric effects of heroin, thus reducing the craving for the drug. Methadone is metabolized by the liver into two major metabolites and at least five additional metabolites via N-demethylation, aromatic ring hydroxylation, and degradation of both side chains. The metabolites are excreted in the urine, feces, and bile. Methadone itself crosses the placenta. The maternal-to-cord plasma ratio of methadone is 2.7:1, and the maternal-to-neonatal plasma methadone ratio at about 1 hour of life is 2.2:1, indicating placental limitation of transport of methadone, rapid tissue binding, or both.

Incidence

An increasing number of infants have been born to methadone-maintained mothers. These mothers seem to have better prenatal care and a somewhat better lifestyle than those taking heroin. However, there is a high incidence of multiple drug abuse, including alcohol, barbiturates, tranquilizers, and other psychoactive drugs; additionally, these mothers are often heavy smokers. The incidence of methadone withdrawal in the infants varies from 70% to 90%, according to most published reports.

Clinical manifestations

Infants born to methadone-maintained mothers are of higher birth weights than infants of heroin addicts and subsequently have a lower incidence of intrauterine growth retardation. According to Kandall the birth weights of these infants correlate with the first trimester dose of methadone; the higher the methadone dose (at dosage greater than 40 mg/day), the heavier the infant at birth. The mechanism for this is not known. No increase in the incidence of congenital anomalies has been reported in children born to methadone-maintained mothers.

Thrombocytosis and increased platelet-aggregating activity have been reported in infants born to mothers receiving methadone maintenance and/or involved in other polydrug abuse. This phenomenon of unknown etiology occurred after the first week of life and persisted for over 16 weeks. In addition, abnormal thyroid function (increased T_3 and T_4 levels) has been described in newborn infants of methadone-treated mothers.

The signs and symptoms of withdrawal in the infant are more severe and prolonged than the withdrawal symptoms seen in infants of heroin-addicted mothers. The clinical manifestations are similar to those described for heroin withdrawal. The incidence of seizures is higher in the infants of methadone-maintained mothers (10% to 20%). When seizures are present, they usually occur between the seventh and tenth days of life. The infants have the same disturbances in their sleep cycles as infants of heroin-addicted mothers (no quiet sleep and abnormal REM sleep).

The incidence and severity of withdrawal syndromes in infants of methadone-maintained mothers depend on the maternal and fetal metabolism and excretion of the drug. The higher the level of methadone in maternal plasma and the more rapid the neonatal metabolism and excretion, the higher the incidence of moderate to severe symptoms and signs of withdrawal. The lower the maternal level of methadone and the slower the metabolism and excretion of methadone in the neonate, the less chance the infant has of developing manifestations of drug withdrawal. The time of onset of methadone withdrawal symptoms depends on the time of the last maternal dose. For example, in one study, when the last maternal dose was within 20 hours of delivery, the onset of withdrawal usually occurred between 24 and 52 hours of life; when the maternal dose of methadone was taken more than 20 hours before delivery, the onset of symptoms occurred before 24 hours of life. In addition, the symptomatic infants did not develop the withdrawal syndrome until plasma levels fell below 0.06 µg/ml.

A syndrome of late-onset withdrawal has been described in some infants born to methadone-maintained mothers. This occurs at 2 to 4 weeks of age either with or without previously occurring withdrawal manifestations.

The symptoms are similar to those of early withdrawal and often are accompanied by a voracious appetite but poor weight gain. The symptoms may continue for several weeks and require continuing treatment. This late withdrawal syndrome may be the result of the strong tissue binding of methadone and resultant slow excretion, or of the discontinuation of other drugs taken by the mother that are no longer transferred to the infant after delivery.

Treatment

Therapy for methadone withdrawal includes the same drugs used for heroin withdrawal: phenobarbital, paregoric, and methadone (Table 33-6). The duration of treatment is usually longer than for infants of heroin-addicted mothers (5 days to 4 months).

Prognosis

The few follow-up studies of these infants that are available reveal a higher incidence of hyperactivity, learning and behavior disorders, and poor social adjustment. An increased incidence of sudden infant death has been reported in infants born to methadone-maintained mothers.

ALCOHOL

Alcohol crosses the placenta readily and rapidly reaches the fetus. In studies of mothers receiving alcohol for suppression of labor, blood levels of alcohol in the mother and her fetus were similar. After birth, blood alcohol levels are higher in the neonate and are eliminated more slowly than in the mother. Acute alcohol withdrawal has been well documented in the adult, but only a few case reports are available in the pediatric literature, although acute withdrawal has been reported in neonates born to mothers receiving alcohol suppression for premature labor. The syndrome consists of the following: an odor of alcohol on the breath for several hours after birth, a 72-hour phase of hyperactivity, tremors and seizures followed by a 48-hour phase of lethargy, and finally a return to normal activity and responsiveness.

Recently, much attention has been focused on the effects of chronic in utero alcohol exposure of infants born to mothers who are moderate to heavy alcohol consumers. Chronic alcohol exposure during pregnancy may result in a multitude of symptoms, varying from mild to severe and consisting of an increased rate of spontaneous abortions and stillbirths, congenital abnormalities, and/or mental retardation. The severity and frequency of these effects are related to dosage, pattern of alcohol consumption, time of gestation, and individual susceptibility. The risk of congenital anomalies from chronic in utero alcohol exposure, compared with a population that has only occasional or no alcohol intake, is 10% if the mothers consume more than 1 or 2 oz of absolute alcohol per day, 19% if they consume more than 2 oz of absolute alcohol, and 40% if they consume more than 5 oz of absolute alcohol per day during pregnancy.

The *fetal alcohol syndrome* and *alcohol-related birth defects* consist of the following:

1. Central nervous system: microcephaly, withdrawal symptoms, including irritability and tremors, apnea and seizures, abdominal distension, and opisthotonos. The irritability seen in these infants may persist for several months to years with mild to moderate mental retardation.
2. Growth deficiency of perinatal onset, continuing postnatally.
3. Facial characteristics: short palpebral fissures, hypoplastic philtrum, thinned upper vermilion, and retrognathia.
4. A variety of anomalies, including cardiac abnormalities (ventricular septal defect, tetralogy of Fallot), joint defects, limitation of motion of elbow and phalangeal joints, hip dysplasia, anomalies of external genitalia, hypoplasia of labia or hypospadias, and skin hemangiomas.

The frequency of expression of major and minor components of the fetal alcohol syndrome has been reported as 1 or 2 in 1,000 live births. The frequency of a partial expression is 3 to 5 in 1,000 live births.

Birth weight appears to be reduced if absolute alcohol intake exceeds 1 oz per day prior to pregnancy and during the third trimester of pregnancy. This growth retardation continues through childhood. Studies evaluating human growth hormone, luteinizing hormone, FSH, PTH, testosterone, and thyroxine, as well as bone age, have shown these all to be within the normal limits.

Follow-up of infants and children born to mothers who were chronic alcoholics has revealed an average IQ of 67. There was no correlation between dysmorphogenesis and the intelligence score. The low IQ is thought to reflect central nervous system damage secondary to alcohol and/or its metabolites.

Treatment

The treatment of acute alcohol withdrawal includes the same drugs that are used in the narcotic abstinence syndrome. Prevention of fetal alcohol syndrome or alcohol-related birth defects should center around appropriate management and follow-up of the mother's alcohol intake before and after pregnancy. The recommendation of the National Institute for Alcohol Abuse is not to consume more than an absolute maximum of two drinks per day during pregnancy, that is, 1⅓ oz of absolute alcohol, to prevent any alcohol-associated birth defects or long-term consequences.

PHENOBARBITAL

Phenobarbital is commonly used in the treatment of seizure disorders and for sedation. It also is a commonly abused drug among patients of all socioeconomic classes. Phenobarbital crosses the placenta readily and is distributed rapidly throughout the fetus, with the greatest concentrations in the liver and brain. Infants of phenobarbital-addicted mothers are usually full term and of appropriate weight for gestational age. Their Apgar scores usually are good. The incidence of phenobarbital withdrawal symptoms is not known. When they do occur, symptoms begin at a median age of 7 days (range, 2 to 14 days) and may last for 2 to 4 months. Desmond and associates described two stages of phenobarbital withdrawal: an acute stage consisting of irritability, constant crying, sleeplessness, hiccups, and mouthing movements, followed by a subacute stage during which there is a voracious appetite, frequent regurgitation and gagging, episodic irritability, hyperacusis, sweating, and a disturbed sleep pattern. The second stage may last from 2 to 4 months. The late onset of phenobarbital withdrawal probably is due to its slow metabolism and excretion by the newborn. Treatment consists of swaddling, frequent feedings, and protection from noxious external stimuli. If there is no improvement with these methods, the infant should be given phenobarbital and then slowly withdrawn from this drug after control of symptoms.

MISCELLANEOUS DRUGS

Recently several cases have been reported of a neonatal withdrawal syndrome from pentazocine, a nonnarcotic analgesic that previously was thought to be nonaddictive. Infants born to chronic users of pentazocine have commenced withdrawal symptoms at about 24 hours of age. The symptoms of withdrawal include hypertonia, hyperactivity, tremors, and vomiting. Treatment with phenobarbital for 14 to 17 days has been effective.

Other drugs that may cause withdrawal symptoms include codeine, propoxyphene, and diazepam. No reports are available concerning withdrawal from chlordiazepoxide (Librium) and meprobamate, but a fourfold increase in the incidence of malformation has been reported in infants born to mothers taking these drugs during early pregnancy. There are no reported cases of amphetamine withdrawal in the newborn. Pregnancy rarely continues to term in heavy methamphetamine users, possibly because of malnutrition or the direct effects of amphetamine on the fetus. Similarly, there are no available reports on the condition of infants born to cocaine users. Because these women tend to be multiple drug abusers, it is difficult to identify any specific effects on their neonates due to cocaine alone.

URINARY DRUG-SCREENING METHODS

There are several methods for urinary identification of morphine, methadone, amphetamines, phenothiazines, barbiturates, and sedatives. The methods include fluorometry, ultraviolet spectrophotometry, thin-layer chromatography, gas-liquid chromatography, mass spectrophotometry, and immunoassay system. Gas-liquid chromatography and mass spectrophotometry are the most accurate of these and also the most complicated and time consuming. The other methods, which are less accurate but technically easier and less time consuming, are more appropriate for a screening program. The sensitivity of the screening methods is such that a minimum of 1 to 5 μg/ml of these drugs is detectable. The most commonly used method is thin-layer chromatography with various extractions procedures and chromogenic sprays. The immunoassay system, employing a bacterial antigen-antibody lysosome system, is the simplest and most rapid system available at present but will detect only morphine, methadone, cocaine derivatives, amphetamines, and barbiturates. For a more complete qualitative drug analysis, thin-layer chromatography and mass spectrophotometry can be used. Alcohol is best detected using an autoanalyzer and the enzyme alcohol dehydrogenase. It is sensitive to 0.1 mg of alcohol per deciliter in the blood.

Tove S. Rosen

BIBLIOGRAPHY
Heroin

Cohen, S.: Narcotism: dimensions of the problems in recent developments in chemotherapy of narcotic addiction, Ann. N.Y. Acad. Sci. **311**:4, 1978.

Ingall, D., and Zuckenstatter, M.: Diagnosis and treatment of the passively addicted newborn, Hosp. Pract., 1970.

Kahn, E.J., Neumann, L.L., and Polk, G.A.: The course of heroin withdrawal syndrome in newborn infants treated with phenobarbital and chlorpromazine, J. Pediatr. **75**:495, 1969.

Naeye, R.L., and others: Fetal complications of maternal heroin addiction: abnormal growth, infections and episodes of stress, J. Pediatr. **83**:1055, 1973.

Nathenson, G., and others: The effect of maternal heroin addiction on neonatal jaundice, J. Pediatr. **81**:899, 1972.

Ramenteria, J.L., and Nurrag, N.N.: Narcotic withdrawal in pregnancy: stillbirth incidence with a case report, Am. J. Obstet. Gynecol. **116**:1152, 1973.

Stone, M.L., and others: Narcotic addiction in pregnancy, Am. J. Obstet. Gynecol. **109**:716, 1971.

Taeusch, H.W., Jr., and others: Heroin induction of lung maturation and growth retardation in fetal rabbits, J. Pediatr. **82**:869, 1972.

Wilson, G.S., Desmond, M.M., and Verniaud, W.M.: Early development of infants of heroin-addicted mothers, Am. J. Dis. Child. **126**:457, 1973.

Wilson, G.S., and others: The development of preschool children of heroin addicted mothers: a controlled study, Pediatrics **63**:135, 1979.

Zinberg, N.E., and others: Patterns of heroin use, Ann. N.Y. Acad. Sci. **311**:10, 1978.

Methadone

Anngard, E., and others: Disposition of methadone in methadone maintenance, Clin. Pharmacol. Ther. 14:194, 1975.

Blinick, G., and others: Methadone assays in pregnant women and progeny, Am. J. Obstet. Gynecol. 121:617, 1974.

Burstein, Y., and others: Thrombocytosis and increased circulating platelet aggregates in newborn infants of polydrug users, J. Pediatr. 94:895, 1979.

Davis, M.M., Brown, B.S., and Glendinning, S.T.: Neonatal effects of heroin addiction and methadone-treated pregnancies: preliminary report on 70 live births. In Proceedings of the Fifth National Conference on Methadone Treatment, New York, 1973, National Association for Prevention of Addiction to Narcotics.

Herlinger, R.A., Kandall, S.R., and Vaughn, N.G.: Neonatal seizures associated with narcotics withdrawal, J. Pediatr. 91:638, 1977.

Kandall, S.R., and others: Birth weights and maternal narcotic use. In Senay, E., Shorty, V., and Alkane, H., editors: Development in the field of drug abuse, Proceedings of the 1974 National Association for the Prevention of Addiction to Narcotics, Cambridge, Mass., 1974, Shenkman Publishing Co.

Lipsitz, P., and Blatman, S.: Newborn infants of mothers on methadone maintenance, N.Y. State J. Med. 74:994, 1974.

Pierson, P.S., Howard, P., and Kleber, H.D.: Sudden deaths in infants born to methadone-maintained addicts, J.A.M.A. 220:1733, 1972.

Rajegowda, B.K., and others: Methadone withdrawal in newborn infants, J. Pediatr. 81:532, 1972.

Rosen, T.S., and Pippenger, C.E.: Pharmacologic observation on the neonatal withdrawal syndrome, J. Pediatr. 88:1044, 1976.

Heroin and methadone

Nathenson, G., Golden, G., and Litt, I.F.: Diazepam in the management of the neonatal narcotic withdrawal syndrome, Pediatrics 48:523, 1971.

Reddy, A.M., Harper, R.G., and Stern, G.: Observation on heroin and methadone withdrawal in the newborn, Pediatrics 48:353, 1971.

Rothstein, P., and Gould, J.B.: Born with a habit: infants of drug-addicted mothers, Pediatr. Clin. North Am. 21:307, 1974.

Schulman, C.A.: Alterations of the sleep cycle in heroin addicted and "suspect" newborns, Neuropaediatrie 1:89, 1969.

Zelson, C., Sook, J.L., and Casalino, M.: Neonatal narcotic addiction, N. Engl. J. Med. 289:1216, 1973.

Alcohol

Clarren, S.K., and Smith, D.W.: The fetal alcohol syndrome, N. Engl. J. Med. 298:1063, 1978.

Clarren, S.K., and others: Brain malformations related to prenatal exposure to ethanol, J. Pediatr. 92:64, 1978.

Green, G.H.: Infants of alcoholic mothers, Am. J. Obstet. Gynecol. 118:713, 1974.

Hanson, J.W., Streissguth, A.P., and Smith, D.W.: The effects of moderate alcohol consumption during pregnancy on fetal growth and morphogenesis, J. Pediatr. 11:219, 1977.

Jones, K.L., and others: Pattern of malformation in offspring of chronic alcoholic mothers, Lancet 1:7815, 1973.

Jones, K.L., and others: Outcome in offspring of chronic alcoholic women, Lancet 1:1076, 1974.

Nichols, M.M.: Acute alcohol withdrawal syndrome in a newborn, Am. J. Dis. Child. 113:714, 1967.

Ouelette, E.M., and others: Adverse effects on offspring of maternal alcohol abuse during pregnancy, N. Engl. J. Med. 297:528, 1977.

Peden, V.H., Sammon, J.T., and Downey, D.A.: Intravenously induced infantile intoxication with ethanol, J. Pediatr. 83:490, 1973.

Pierog, S., Chandavasur, O., and Wexler, O.: Withdrawal symptoms in infants with fetal alcohol syndrome, J. Pediatr. 90:630, 1977.

A Report to the Governor of the State of New York on Fetal Alcohol Syndrome by Task Force on FAS/ARBD, Shelia B. Blume, Chairman, New York State Division of Alcoholism and Alcohol Abuse, Nov. 1979.

Ulleland, C.N., and others: The offspring of alcoholic mothers (abstr.), Pediatrics 4:474, 1970.

Phenobarbital

Desmond, M., and others: Maternal barbiturate utilization and neonatal withdrawal symptomatology, J. Pediatr. 80:190, 1972.

Bleyer, A.W., and Marshall, R.E.: Barbiturate withdrawal syndrome in a passively addicted infant, J.A.M.A. 221:185, 1972.

Pippenger, C.E., and Rosen, T.S.: Phenobarbital plasma levels in neonates, Clin. Perinatol. 2:111, 1975.

Miscellaneous drugs

Gariott, J.C., and Spruill, F.G.: Detection of methamphetamine in a newborn infant, J. Forens. Sci. 18:434, 1973.

Goetz, R.L., and Bain, R.V.: Neonatal withdrawal symptoms associated with maternal use of pentazocine, J. Pediatr. 84:887, 1974.

Klein, R.B., Blatman, S., and Little, G.A.: Probable neonatal propoxyphene withdrawal: a case report, Pediatrics 55:882, 1975.

Kopelman, A.E.: Fetal addiction to pentazocine, Pediatrics 55:888, 1975.

Milkovich, B.A., and Van den Berg, B.J.: Effects of prenatal meprobamate and chlordiazepoxide hydrochloride on human embryonic and fetal development, N. Engl. J. Med. 291:1268, 1974.

Van Leeuwen, G., Guthrie, R., and Stange, F.: Narcotic withdrawal reaction in a newborn infant due to codeine, Pediatrics 36:635, 1965.

Urinary drug-screening methods

Dole, V.P., and others: Detection of narcotic, sedative and amphetamine drugs in urine, N.Y. State J. Med. 72:471, 1972.

Inturrisi, C.E., and Verebely, K.: A gas-liquid chromatographic method for the quantitative determination of methadone in human plasma and urine, J. Chromatogr. 65:361, 1972.

Mule, S.J.: Routine identification of drugs of abuse in human urine. I. Application of fluorometry, thin-layer chromatography and gas-liquid chromatography, J. Chromatogr. 55:255, 1971.

Rubinstein, K.E., Schneider, R.S., and Ullman, E.F.: Homogenous enzyme immunoassay: a new immunoassay technique, Biochem. Biophys. Res. Commun. 47:846, 1972.

CHAPTER 34 **The skin**

The skin of the newborn may have a variety of lesions: some innocent, temporary, and the result of a physiologic reaction, others the result of episodic disease, and still others indicative of a serious, potentially fatal underlying disorder. The definitive diagnosis of specific skin lesions requires an understanding of the physiologic characteristics and peculiarities of neonatal skin, a recognition of primary skin lesions, and knowledge of their significance.

BIOLOGY OF FETAL AND NEONATAL SKIN
Structure of the epidermis

Human skin has two distinct interdependent components: the epidermis, derived from the fetal periderm, and the dermis, which together provide a regenerating protective coat. The epidermis has marked regional variations in thickness, color, permeability, and surface chemical components. It consists of a highly ordered compact layering of keratinocytes and melanocytes. A third distinct cell type, the Langerhans cell, is also recognized.

The young keratinocytes are columnar basal cells that produce and contain a filamentous protein, keratin. They lie adjacent to the dermis, separated from it by a narrow basement membrane. The basal keratinocytes divide and migrate toward the surface. Their cellular structure is replaced by keratin, and the cells become dehydrated and flattened, forming a tough, resilient, anuclear, relatively impermeable membrane. In infants these cells of the stratum corneum are more uniform in size than those of children or adults.

Another important component of the epidermis is the melanocyte, a cell of neural crest origin capable of producing melanin, which migrates into the dermis and is first visible in the 10-week-old fetus. The melanocytes in the basal layer contain melanin at about the fourth month of fetal age. Melanin protects against ultraviolet radiation damage to vital nuclear elements. Melanin protects against ultraviolet radiation damage to vital nuclear elements. Melanin granules (melanosomes) are formed in the melanocytic cytoplasm and move via the dendritic processes toward the basal cell. As the basal keratinocyte matures, its melanin is dispersed as a fine intracellular granular dust that may be visualized in the horny layer. Melanin production is low; the newborn is not as pigmented as the older child and is more sensitive to sunlight. Yet there is no significant difference in the number of melanocytes in light, medium, or deeply pigmented skin or in infant or adult skin. The difference in color is a result of the number and size of melanosomes and the activity of individual melanocytes.

The epidermis is less adherent to the dermis in the early weeks of life, resulting in a greater propensity to blister formation in the newborn. The permeability of the stratum corneum in the newborn appears to vary with the gestational age of the infant. Nachman and Esterly assessed permeability by comparing the skin blanching response in infants of varying gestational ages to the topical application of a 10% phenylephrine (Neo-Synephrine) solution. The skin of the youngest infants (28 to 34 weeks) had the most rapid and prolonged response, whereas the skin of full-term infants in most instances failed to blanch even on the first day of life.

The appendages

The appendages derive from invaginations of epidermal germinative buds into the dermis. They include hair, sebaceous glands, apocrine glands, eccrine glands, and nails. The arrector pili muscle is attached to the hair follicle.

Lanugo (fine, soft, immature hair) frequently covers the scalp and brow in the premature infant; the scalp line may be poorly demarcated. Lanugo also may cover the face; scalp hair is usually somewhat coarser and more mature earlier in dark-haired infants. The growth phases of the hair follicle are usually synchronous at birth; 80% of the follicles are in the resting state. During the first few months of life the synchrony between hair loss and regrowth is disturbed, and hair may become coarse and thick, acquiring an adult distribution, or there may be a temporary alopecia. There are also sex differences in hair growth; boys' hair grows faster than girls' hair. In both sexes scalp hair growth is slower at the crown. The following outline shows disorders associated with abnormal amounts and morphologic characteristics of hair.

A. Disorders with hypertrichosis
  1. Generalized
     a. Congenital lipodystrophy
     b. Cornelia de Lange syndrome
     c. Craniofacial dysostosis with dental, eye, and cardiac anomalies
     d. Hypertrichosis lanuginosa universalis
     e. Hypertrichosis with gingival fibromatosis
     f. Leprechaunism
     g. Mucopolysaccharidoses
  2. Localized
     a. Congenital hemihypertrophy with hypertrichosis
     b. Hairy ears
     c. Hairy elbows syndrome
     d. Hairy nevi
     e. Ring chromosome E (low hairline)
     f. Trisomy 18 (back and forehead)
     g. Turner's syndrome (low occipital hairline)
B. Disorders with hypotrichosis*
  1. Anhidrotic (hypohidrotic) ectodermal dysplasia
  2. Atrichia with papular lesions
  3. Combined immunodeficiency syndrome with short-limbed dwarfism
  4. Congenital alopecia
  5. EEC syndrome (ectrodactyly, ectodermal dysplasia, cleft lip-palate)
  6. Goltz's syndrome
  7. Hallermann-Streiff syndrome (oculomandibulodyscephaly)
  8. Hidrotic ectodermal dysplasia
  9. Hypotrichosis, syndactyly, and retinitis pigmentosa
  10. Incontinentia pigmenti
  11. Keratosis follicularis spinulosa decalvans
  12. Ocular-dental-digital dysplasia
  13. Oral-facial-digital syndrome
  14. Progeria
  15. Rothmund-Thomson syndrome
  16. Seckel's syndrome
  17. Trisomy A
C. Disorders with hair of abnormal morphology
  1. Structural defects
     a. Arginosuccinicaciduria—monilethrix, trichorrhexis nodosa
     b. Hereditary trichodysplasia (Marie Unna hypotrichosis)—twisted hair
     c. Menkes' syndrome
     d. Monilethrix
     e. Netherton's syndrome—multiple defects
     f. Pili annulati
     g. Pili bifurcati
     h. Pili torti
     i. Pili torti and nerve deafness
     j. Trichorrhexis nodosa
     k. Trichoschisis
  2. Abnormal color, caliber, and fragility
     a. Cartilage-hair hypoplasia—small caliber
     b. Citrullinemia—fragile, atrophic bulbs
     c. Congenital trichomegaly with dwarfism, mental retardation, and retinal pigmentation—long brows and lashes
     d. Dyskeratosis congenita—sparse and fine hair
     e. Hartnup's disease—fine, fragile hair
     f. Hereditary enamel hypoplasia and kinky hair—abnormal curliness
     g. Homocystinuria—fine, fragile hair
     h. Marinesco—Sjögren's syndrome—fragile, brittle, rough hair
     i. Phenylketonuria—fine, light-colored hair
     j. Pierre Robin anomalad—fine, light-colored hair
     k. Trichorhinophalangeal syndrome—thin, sparse hair
     l. Trisomy 21—fine, light-colored, atrophic bulbs
     m. Tyrosinemia—fine, light-colored hair
     n. Woolly hair—abnormal curliness

Nails are fully formed at birth. Syndromes associated with nail defects are presented in the following outline.

SYNDROMES ASSOCIATED WITH NAIL DEFECTS*

A. Total or partial absence of nails; nail hypoplasia or dysplasia
  1. Acrodermatitis enteropathica
  2. Anhidrotic (hypohidrotic) ectodermal dysplasia
  3. Anonychia and ectrodactyly
  4. Apert's syndrome (acrocephalosyndactyly)
  5. Cartilage-hair hypoplasia
  6. Deafness and nail dystrophy (Feinmesser; Robinson)
  7. Dyskeratosis congenita
  8. Ellis–van Creveld syndrome
  9. Enamel hypoplasia and curly hair
  10. Epidermolysis bullosa
  11. Focal dermal hypoplasia (Goltz's syndrome)
  12. Glossopalatine ankylosis, microglossia, hypodontia, and anomalies of the extremities (Gorlin-Pindborg)
  13. Incontinentia pigmenti
  14. Larsen's syndrome
  15. Long-arm 21 deletion syndrome

*A supplementary listing may be found in the review by Muller.

*Data from Gorlin and Pindborg, 1964; Pardo-Costello and Pardo, 1960; Samman, 1972; Smith, 1976.

16. Nail-patella syndrome
17. Popliteal web syndrome
18. Progeria
19. Pyknodysostosis (Maroteaux-Lamy)
20. Rothmund-Thomson syndrome
21. Skin hypoplasia—nail dystrophy (Basan)
22. Trisomy 13
23. Trisomy 18
24. Turner's syndrome
B. Hypertrophic or abnormally large nails
    1. Congenital hemihypertrophy
    2. Familial hyperpigmentation with dystrophy of the nails (Touraine and Soulignac)
    3. Pachyonychia congenita
    4. Rubinstein-Taybi syndrome
    5. Otopalatodigital syndrome

The eccrine sweat glands are distributed throughout the integument. They arise from an epidermal downgrowth at about the sixth week of embryogenesis and are innervated by a sympathetic cholinergic mechanism. During the first 24 hours of life full-term infants usually do not sweat; at about the third day sweating begins on the face. Palmar sweating begins later. Sweating varies markedly with ambient and body temperature, crying, eating, and fever.

The sebaceous glands differentiate primarily from the epithelial portion of the hair follicle at about 13 to 15 weeks of life and almost immediately produce sebum in all hairy areas. The glands develop as solid outpouchings from the upper third of the hair follicle. These solid buds become filled with liquid centrally where the cells disintegrate; acini and ducts develop, opening most frequently into the canals between the hair follicle wall and hair shaft. The rapid growth and activity of sebaceous glands up to and immediately after birth is governed in part by maternal androgens and possibly also by endogenous steroid production by the fetus. Androgens are the only hormones that unequivocally have a stimulating effect on the sebaceous glands; estrogens depress their growth. In normal infants maternal androgens are responsible for the miniature puberty of the newborn, with its attendant infantile acne and transient development of secondary sexual characteristics. Shortly after birth the sebaceous glands of the normal infant begin a period of quiescence that lasts until puberty. Ectopic glands occur occasionally on the lips, buccal mucosa, esophagus, and vagina.

The apocrine glands are relatively large organs that originate from and empty into the hair follicle. Embryologically they develop somewhat later than the eccrine glands. Apocrine development is advanced by 7 or 8 fetal months, when the glands begin to produce a milky white fluid containing water, lipids, protein, reducing sugars, ferric iron, and ammonia; in the newborn the acini are well formed. The biologic function of the gland is unknown.

Structure of the dermis

The dermis has a symbiotic relation to and may exert a controlling influence on the epidermis. It is a metabolically active tissue that contains fibrous elements, amorphous ground substance, free cells, nerves, blood vessels, and lymphatic vessels. The fibrous elements are collagen and elastic tissue. Collagen makes up more than 90% of the connective tissue of the dermis. As age increases, collagen becomes progressively less soluble. The morphologic characteristics and chemical and physical properties of cutaneous elastic fibers are different from those of collagen. Histochemically stainable elastic tissue first appears in the 22-week-old fetus. Clinical changes in cutaneous elasticity in aging skin and in some diseases may be related to the spatial arrangement of elastic tissue or collagen fibers in the skin and to a qualitative change in the elastic fiber rather than to the quantity of elastin present in the dermis. The fibroblasts are the most numerous cells of the dermis. They produce collagen and the mucopolysaccharides of the ground substance. Mast cells (which produce heparin and histamine), histiocytes, macrophages, lymphocytes, neutrophils, and an occasional plasma cell and eosinophil are also present in the dermis. The major mucopolysaccharides in the ground substance of skin are hyaluronic acid and dermatan sulfate (chondroitin sulfate B).

The blood and lymphatic vessels

The vascular supply of the skin is closely related to its size and function. Therefore the physiologic requirements of skin vary considerably; skin blood flows range from 0.1 to 150 ml/dl of tissue per minute. The vascular network supplying the skin develops in early embryonic life from the mesoderm. The dermis and epidermis are served by networks of anastomosing arteries of three types: cutaneous, perforator, and segmental. The cutaneous vessels are arranged in the dermis in superficial and deep plexuses and are accompanied by an even more complex venous arrangement. Those capillary vessels found in the papillae enter them perpendicularly to the immediately overlying epidermis. This orderly arrangement of vessels in the superficial dermis becomes apparent only 17 weeks postnatally. The cutaneous vasculature derives from muscular perforator arteries that supply both muscle and skin. The perforator arteries themselves derive from the segmental (intercostal) vessels of the embryo. Direct cutaneous arteriovenous anastomoses are present in abundance, with glomerular organs probably responsible for thermoregulatory shunting. The appendages have special vascular networks.

Vasomotor tone is controlled by a delicate and complex series of nervous and pharmacologic mechanisms that involve the sympathetic nervous system, norepinephrine, acetylcholine, and histamine and also may involve serotonin, vasoactive polypeptides, corticosteroids, and prostaglandins. The nervous system control of thermoregulation also involves the hypothalamus, higher centers, sympathetic and sensory nerves, and the axon reflex.

Cutaneous innervation

The nerve networks in the dermis develop at a very early embryologic age and appear to be distributed in random fashion. The most superficial nerves have the smallest diameter and are the least myelinated. In addition to the dermal nerve network, which may show considerable regional variation, nerve fibers may serve particular regions or structures, such as hair follicles, eccrine glands, arrector pili muscles, and the subepidermal zone. The sebaceous glands are not innervated.

Cutaneous nerves serve overlapping cutaneous areas; one nerve impulse does not necessarily stimulate one spot on the cerebral cortex. Sensation is probably the product of several factors, including spatial and temporal patterns of nerve stimulation in skin and spinal cord, local chemical factors in the skin, previous experience, conditioning, the state of cortical arousal, and genetic factors relating to nerve stimulation threshold. Special neurologic structures include a dense perifollicular nerve network with exquisite tactile sensory properties and mucocutaneous end-organs highly concentrated in erogenous zones. Meissner's tactile organs are found in newborn skin as undeveloped structures that mature after birth. The Merkel-Ranvier corpuscles are important for two-point tactile discrimination on palms and fingertips; they are disc-shaped terminals that are seen during the twenty-eighth week of fetal life. After birth these receptors undergo little alteration. Vater-Pacini bodies are found around the digits, palms, and genitals; they are fully formed and numerous at birth.

The arrector pili muscles are innervated by sympathetic nerves, and norepinephrine acts as the neurotransmitter. The eccrine glands are innervated by sympathetic fibers, but acetylcholine acts as the neurotransmitter. Parasympathetic fibers may accompany the sensory nerves in the vessel walls and cause vasodilation. The axon reflex is poorly developed in the newborn; in the neonate of low birth weight, axon reflex sweating may be difficult to elicit.

NORMAL SKIN IN THE NEWBORN

The gross appearance of the skin at birth is related in part to the maturity of the infant. In the normal full-term infant the skin is soft, wrinkled, velvety, and covered with a greasy yellow-white material with a pH of 7.4; this is the vernix caseosa, a mixture of desquamating cells and sebum. Removal of the vernix is followed by desquamation of the epidermis in the majority of infants. The fetal epidermis is rich in glycogen. Glycogen, present in the basal layer at the sixth fetal month, diminishes as normal keratogenesis progresses but may reaccumulate at the site of an injury. The pH of the newborn skin surface is 5.7 on the dorsa of the arms and 6.4 in areas where the vernix accumulates, such as the groin, scalp, and forehead. Skin surface lipids in the first 2 weeks of life are low in cholesterol and high in wax esters compared with childhood values. Free fatty acids and triglycerides slowly decrease during the postnatal period and childhood.

Within a few hours of birth the skin develops an intense red color, which may remain for several hours. With fading of this erythema, bluish mottling (livedo reticularis) becomes evident, particularly when the infant is exposed to a cool environment. Localized mild edema also may be present over the pubis and the dorsa of the hands and feet, possibly an additional manifestation of an unstable peripheral circulation. Although the body surface tends to be less pigmented during the neonatal period than later in life, certain areas, such as the linea alba, the areolas, and the scrotum often are deeply pigmented as a result of high circulating levels of maternal and placental hormones. Palpable nodules of breast tissue, active secretion by mammary glands, and a hyperplastic vaginal epithelium are additional normal end-organ responses to these hormones.

The premature infant's skin may be readily distinguished from the full-term infant's skin. At birth it is more transparent and gelatinous and tends to be free of wrinkles. The premature infant may be covered with fine lanugo hair, which in the full-term infant has been lost or in some areas replaced by vellus hair. Sexual hormonal effects are less conspicuous in the premature infant; the scrotum is less rugose and pigmented, the labia majora are less prominent, nipples and areolas are less pigmented, and breast tissue is less palpable.

EPHEMERAL CUTANEOUS LESIONS

A number of benign and ephemeral lesions are commonly observed in a normal nursery population.

Milia

About 40% of infants have multiple yellow-white 1-mm cysts (milia) scattered over the cheeks, forehead, nose, and nasolabial folds. These may be few or numerous, but they frequently are distributed in clusters. Histologically milia are keratogenous cysts similar to Epstein's pearls in the oral cavity. These lesions usually disappear spontaneously within the first few weeks of life.

Pigmentary lesions

The most frequently encountered pigmented lesion is the mongolian spot, which occurs in over 70% of black, oriental, and American Indian infants and in up to 9% of white infants. Although the majority of these lesions are found in the lumbosacral area, occurrence at other sites is not uncommon. The pigmentation is macular and gray-blue, may cover an area 10 cm or larger in diameter, and results from an infiltrate of melanocytes deep in the dermis. These lesions gradually disappear during the first few years of life. With the exception of the massive garment nevus (a developmental defect) and some junctional nevi, most melanocytic nevi usually develop in the older infant or child. Lentigines, freckles, and cafe au lait spots also have their onset later in infancy or in early childhood, although occasionally the latter may be present at birth. Abnormal hyperpigmentation of the areolas and genitals may be evidence for the existence of an in utero glucocorticoid insufficiency associated with defects in the biosynthesis of hydrocortisone.

Macular hemangiomas (salmon patches)

Macular hemangiomas are present in 30% to 50% of normal newborns. They are usually found on the nape, the eyelids, and the glabella. In a prospective study of affected infants most of the facial lesions were not present at 1 year of age, but those on the neck were more persistent. Surveys of adult populations confirm the persistence of the nuchal lesions in about one fourth of the population.

Harlequin color change

Harlequin color change is a phenomenon observed in the immediate neonatal period and is more common in the low birth weight infant. When the infant is placed on his side, a sharp midline demarcation bisects the body into a pale upper half and an intensely red, dependent half. The peak frequency of attacks in one series occurred on the second, third, and fourth days, but episodes were observed during the first 3 weeks of life. These episodes are of no pathologic significance. They have been attributed to a temporary imbalance in the autonomic regulatory mechanism of the cutaneous vessels; there are no accompanying changes in respiratory rate, muscle tone, or response to external stimuli.

Erythema toxicum

This benign and self-limited eruption usually occurs within the first 2 days of life, but lesions may appear until the fourteenth day. The incidence of affected full-term newborns in a normal nursery population varies from 30% to 70%. The disorder is less common with decreasing birth weight and gestational age. These lesions may vary considerably in character and number; they may be firm, shotty, 1 to 3 mm in diameter, pale yellow to white papules or pustules on an erythematous base, erythematous macules (up to 3 cm), or splotchy erythema. There are no related systemic symptoms, and their cause is unknown. A microscopic examination of a Wright- or Giemsa-stained smear of these lesions demonstrates numerous eosinophils; Gram stains are negative for bacteria, and cultures are sterile. No treatment is necessary.

Transient neonatal pustular melanosis

This distinctive eruption consists of two types of lesions: small superficial vesicopustules with little or no surrounding erythema (Fig. 34-1, A) and pigmented macules often encircled by a collarette of fine scale (Fig. 34-1, B). Both types of lesions may be present at birth, but the macules are observed more frequently. The lesions may be profuse or sparse and occur on any body surface, including the palms, soles, and scalp. Sites of predilection are the forehead, submental area and anterior neck, lower back, and pretibial areas. When intact

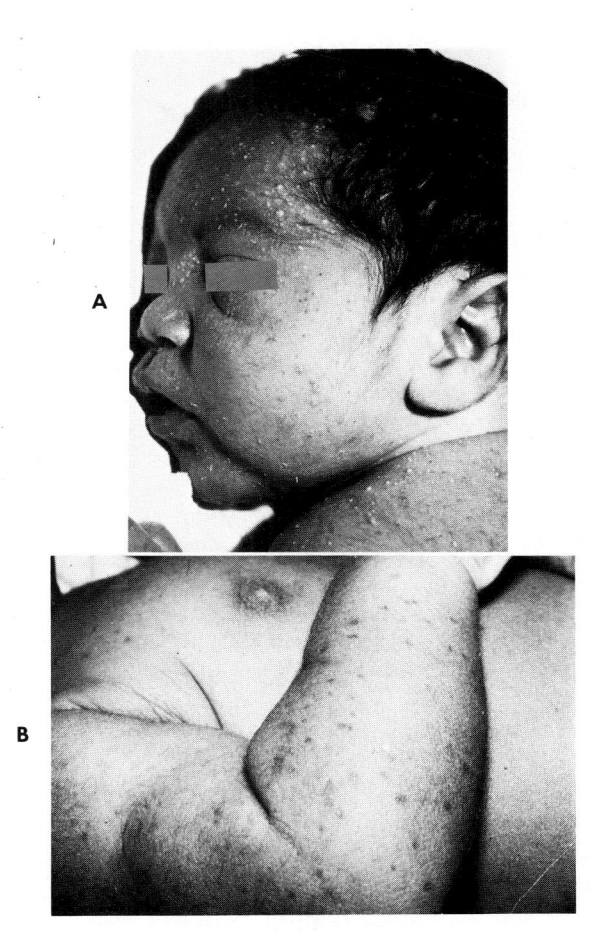

Fig. 34-1. Transient neonatal pustular melanosis. **A,** Superficial pustules on the face and shoulders of a 1-day-old infant. Some have ruptured, leaving a collarette of scale. **B,** Pigmented macules on the arm and chest of a newborn.

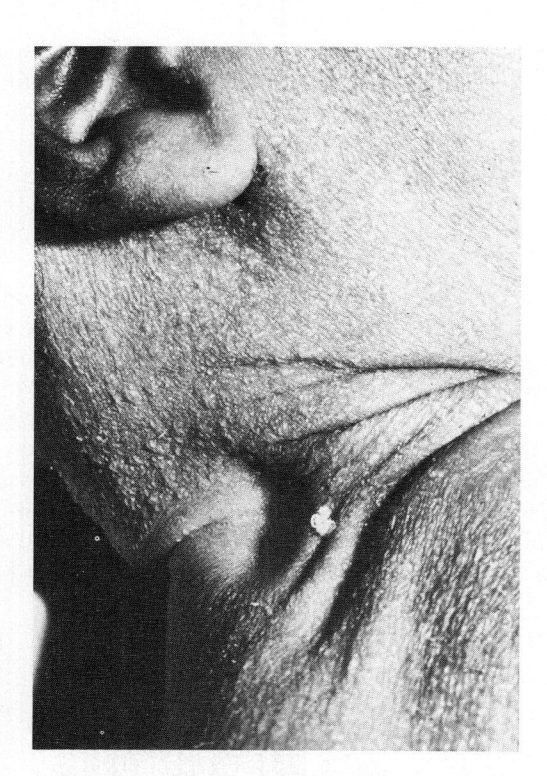

Fig. 34-2. Miliaria crystallina on the neck.

pustules rupture, a pigmented macule is often discernible central to the collarette of scale, which represents the margin of the unroofed pustule. Presumably the macules result from postinflammatory hyperpigmentation, and those present at birth may be the sequelae of in utero pustular lesions. Pustular melanosis may be confused with erythema toxicum or a staphylococcal pyoderma. Bacterial cultures and Gram stains of smears prepared from intact pustules are devoid of organisms; Wright stains of intralesional contents demonstrate cellular debris, polymorphonuclear leukocytes, and a few or no eosinophils, in contrast to erythema toxicum. Although the pustules disappear in 48 hours, the macules may persist for up to 3 months. Neither type of lesion requires therapy, and, although the cause is unknown, parents may be reassured that the disorder is benign and transient.

Miliaria

Miliaria are lesions resulting from sweat retention. They are of two types: superficial thin-walled vesicles without inflammation (miliaria crystallina) and small, erythematous, grouped papules (miliaria rubra). Lesions occur in the intertriginous areas and over the face and scalp (Fig. 34-2). During the first week of life these lesions may be exacerbated by a warm and humid environment. Miliaria is often confused with erythema toxicum; rapid resolution of the lesions differentiates them from pyoderma. No treatment is indicated.

Acne neonatorum

Acne neonatorum is an uncommon but distressing facial eruption (most often of male infants) that has its onset during the first few weeks of life. The condition resembles acne in the adolescent patient; comedones, papules, pustules, and rarely nodules may be present. The duration of acne neonatorum may vary, but usually it clears spontaneously during the latter portion of the first year of life. Although elevation of urinary 17-ketosteroid levels has been reported in affected infants, this has not been a consistent finding. Conservative treatment with mild topical preparations to produce drying and peeling should suffice. Occasionally the infant may be left with pitted scarring.

THE SCALY BABY

There are three causes of excessive scaling in the newborn. Physiologic epidermal desquamation of the normal newborn and the desquamation seen in dysmature infants are not of long-term significance. However, ichthyosis, the third cause, is a chronic inherited disease.

Physiologic desquamation and dysmaturity

The newborn with accentuated physiologic desquamation usually has a gestational age of between 40 and 42 weeks; peak shedding occurs about the eighth day of life. These infants are otherwise normal in physical appearance and behavior. In contrast, the dysmature infant (p. 64) has several distinctive characteristics. The dysmature infant's body is lean with thin extremities and little subcutaneous fat; weight is low in relation to length. The skin is parchmentlike, scaly, and stained with meconium, as are the nails and umbilical cord; the hair is abundant, and the nails are abnormally long. In both the normal infant with accentuated physiologic scaling and the dysmature infant, desquamation is a transient phenomenon, and the integument continues to serve its intended protective function. However, the infant with ichthyosis may have serious difficulty early in life because of impaired barrier function and the subsequent risks of secondary infection.

Ichthyosis

Of the four major types of ichthyosis, three may be apparent during the first month of life: X-linked ichthyosis, lamellar ichthyosis (nonbullous congenital ichthyosiform erythroderma), and epidermolytic hyperkeratosis (bullous congenital ichthyosiform erythroderma). The diagnosis depends on an analysis of the morphologic features, the histologic pattern, and pedigree information. The fourth type, ichthyosis vulgaris, is the most common and benign form and rarely has its onset before the third month of life. In addition to the aforementioned terms, two descriptive terms are applied to severely scaling newborns: the *harlequin fetus* and the *collodion baby*.

Harlequin fetus

The harlequin fetus represents the most severe form of ichthyosis. It is the result of autosomal recessive inheritance and may be an extreme form of lamellar ichthyosis. However, an abnormal cross β–fibrous protein has been demonstrated by x-ray diffraction analysis in the epidermis of one harlequin fetus. Normal α–fibrous protein has been found in all other types of ichthyosis, including lamellar ichthyosis. The skin of the harlequin fetus is hard, thick, and gray or yellow, with deep crevices running both transversely and vertically. The fissures are most prominent over areas of movement. Rigidity of the skin about the eyes results in marked ectropion, although the globe is usually normal. The ears and nose are underdeveloped, flattened, and distorted, and the lips are everted and gaping, thus producing a "fish mouth" deformity. The nails and hair may be hypoplastic or absent. Extreme inelasticity of the skin is associated with flexion deformity of all joints. The hands and feet are ischemic, hard, and waxy in appearance, with poorly developed distal digits. These infants usually do not survive after the first week or two of life.

Collodion baby

The collodion baby syndrome (lamellar exfoliation of the newborn) is less severe and more common than the harlequin fetus and may represent a phenotypic expression of several genotypes. This disorder usually eventuates in lamellar ichthyosis (recessive type), but collodion membranes also have been observed in patients with X-linked ichthyosis. Rarely, shedding of the collodion-like membrane may reveal a normal underlying integument. A significant number of these babies are premature. The infant is covered with a cellophane-like membrane, which, by its tautness, may distort the facial features and the digits. Less commonly only a part of the integument is involved. The membrane is shiny and brownish yellow, resembling an envelope of collodion or oiled parchment, and may be perforated by hair. Fissuring and peeling begin shortly after birth, and large sheets may desquamate, revealing erythema of variable intensity. Once the membrane has fissured, no respiratory difficulties are encountered. Complete shedding of the collodion membrane may take several months. Pedigree information and histopathologic examination of a skin biopsy are additional aids in the delineation of the specific type of ichthyosis.

X-linked ichthyosis

The patient with X-linked ichthyosis, if affected at birth, may have collodion membranes or only hyperkeratosis. In several studies 17% to 36% of the subjects had manifestations of the disease at birth, and 84% to 94% were affected by 3 months of age. The scales are characteristically large, thick, and dark and are prominent over the neck, anterior trunk, and extensor extremities. Sparing of palms and soles and partial sparing of the flexures are helpful diagnostic features. Usually the axillae or the antecubital fossae or both are involved early in life. Systemic manifestations are generally absent, and complications are rare. Skin biopsy is helpful (although the histologic pattern resembles that of lamellar ichthyosis), showing hyperkeratosis, a well-developed granular layer, hypertrophic epidermis, and a perivascular lymphocytic infiltrate. This form of ichthyosis is present only in males and not in heterozygous females. The cutaneous abnormality has been linked with a steroid sulfatase enzyme deficiency in the somatic tissues of affected males. Deep corneal opacities also have been described as a relatively reliable genetic marker in older boys and men with the disorder, whereas female carriers have this finding inconsistently.

Lamellar ichthyosis (nonbullous congenital ichthyosiform erythroderma)

A brilliant and generalized erythema often characterizes the scaly infant with lamellar ichthyosis. Affected babies are commonly of low birth weight. Hyperkeratosis is universal, involving the flexural areas as well as other body surfaces (Fig. 34-3), but scaling in the neonatal period is less prominent than later in childhood. The palms and soles may show only increased skin markings or may be considerably thickened. Ectropion, often severe later in life, is not usually a problem during the neonatal period. Maceration of the skin in intertriginous areas may serve as an entry point for bacterial organisms. Lamellar ichthyosis has a recessive mode of inheritance. Since it also can occur as the cutaneous feature of several rare syndromes, affected infants must be throughly evaluated, particularly for central nervous system (CNS) abnormalities.

Epidermolytic hyperkeratosis (bullous congenital ichthyosiform erythroderma)

The infant with epidermolytic hyperkeratosis has recurrent bullous lesions, as well as erythema, dryness, and peeling. During the neonatal period bullae may occur over widespread areas, resulting in extensive

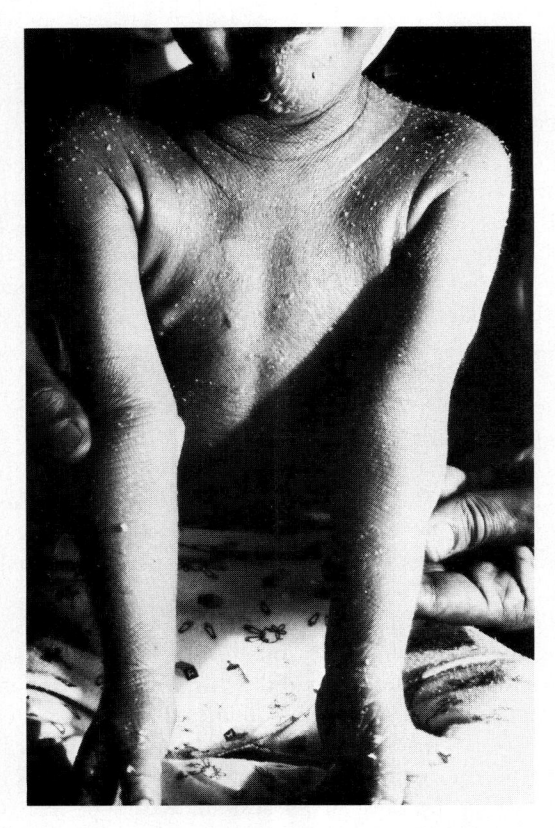

Fig. 34-3. Lamellar ichthyosis. Note generalized scaling including the flexural areas.

denudation with secondary infection, sepsis, and death. These skin lesions may be confused with those of staphylococcal scalded skin syndrome or epidermolysis bullosa. Antibiotics may be required during the first months of life. The bullous lesions become less prominent as the infant grows older and disappear completely in adulthood. The histopathologic picture in epidermolytic hyperkeratosis is diagnostic and consists of vacuolization of the epidermis, abnormally large, clumped keratin granules, hyperkeratosis, and an increased granular layer. An accurate family history is also critical, since this disorder is inherited as an autosomal dominant trait.

VESICOBULLOUS ERUPTIONS

Blistering eruptions in the neonatal period may be caused by infections, congenital diseases, or infiltrative processes or may be of unknown origin. The proper management of such infants depends on knowledge of the cause of the disease or, when this is not possible, on an understanding of the pathogenesis of the type of blister encountered. The latter is often dependent on determining at what level within the skin the blister has occurred.

Blister sites may be either epidermal or subepidermal. In the epidermis the blister can be very high (subcorneal), midepidermal, or basal. The midepidermal blister may be formed by primary separation of intercellular contacts (acantholysis), by secondary edematous disruption of intercellular contacts (spongiosis), or by intracellular injury, as seen in viral infections. The diagnosis of a blistering disease usually requires a family history, an immediate past history of the infant and mother, laboratory studies relative to finding an infectious agent, evaluation of the infant's general state of health, consideration of the morphologic characteristics of the eruption, and a biopsy of the involved skin. The biopsy should be obtained from a fresh, typical, small lesion and should include some normal surrounding skin. Treatment of erosive lesions with steroids and antibiotics should be tempered by awareness that knowledge of the metabolism and toxicity of these substances in the neonate is incomplete and that increased permeability of the skin may result in excessive absorption.

BACTERIAL AND YEAST INFECTIONS

The colonization of the newborn's skin begins at birth. The organisms acquired at birth are similar to those found on adult skin. *Staphylococcus epidermidis* (coagulase negative) predominates, but diphtheroids, streptococci, and coliform bacteria also are found. The newborn skin affords an excellent culture medium for *Staphylococcus aureus;* the groin and other skin sites may become colonized before the umbilicus. *Candida albicans* is not usually found on normal skin but may be present in the oral mucosa or in the diaper area as a result of fecal contamination.

Bullous impetigo of the newborn

The lesions of impetigo usually appear after the first few days of life. This is in contrast to congenital blistering disease that may be present at birth. The blisters vary in size and may appear on any body surface. They soon rupture, leaving a red, moist, denuded area. When the epidermis is shed in large sheets, staphylococcal scalded skin syndrome should be suspected. The organism most frequently involved is *S. aureus*, group 2 phage type. Certain phage types (for example, type 71) usually are associated with these lesions. The diagnosis is made by Gram stain and culture of the blister fluid. In atypical cases skin biopsy may be helpful by showing the characteristic intraepidermal (subcorneal) bulla filled with polymorphonuclear leukocytes. Blood cultures should be obtained from affected infants. Contacts and nursery personnel should be investigated for a source of the infecting organism. The infant should be placed in isolation and observed carefully for early signs of sepsis. A high index of suspicion during examination of other infants in the nursery is the most effective means of preventing epi-

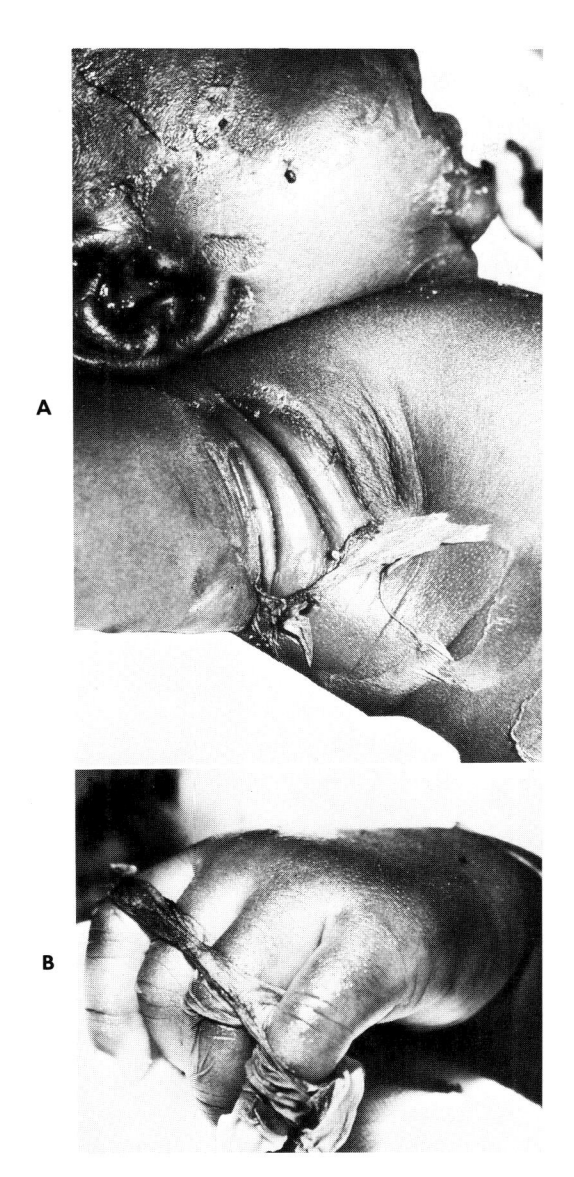

Fig. 34-4. Staphylococcal scalded skin syndrome. **A,** Extensive denudation in the axilla. **B,** Glovelike shedding of the epidermis of the hand.

demic spread of this infection (Chapter 27).

Topical therapy consists of compresses of sterile water or physiologic saline. Systemic antibiotics are indicated to cover the principal etiologic possibilities until the results of culture are available. Fluid and electrolyte replacement therapy may be required if the disease is extensive. Recovery is usually complete in several days, and there is no residual scarring.

Staphylococcal scalded skin syndrome

The scalded skin syndrome is a severe bullous eruption that has been reported at all ages. The eponym *Ritter's disease* has been used for infants up to a few weeks of age but is now obsolete.

The eruption is heralded by a bright erythema that resembles a scald. Large flaccid bullae follow and become confluent, and the skin sheds in sheets (Fig. 34-4, *A*). Frequently the entire epidermis is shed from a limb like a glove (Fig. 34-4, *B*). Conjunctivitis and ulcerations of the oral mucosa also may occur. The infant may appear toxic and sustain severe fluid losses. Some infants with a milder form of the disease display a scarlatiniform eruption without bullae or denudation.

The infecting organism in scalded skin syndrome is *S. aureus*, usually a group 2 phage type, although other phage types occasionally have been incriminated. These organisms produce an exotoxin, called exfoliatin, that is responsible for the cutaneous manifestations. Purified toxin has been demonstrated to cause scalded skin syndrome in newborn mice and more localized lesions in adult human volunteers. Histologic examination of the skin demonstrates separation at the level of the granular layer with cell death and acantholysis; there is a striking absence of inflammatory infiltrate. Since intact bullae are usually sterile, cultures should be obtained from the nasopharynx, conjunctival sac, normal skin, blood, and any other suspected site of infection. Treatment consists of prompt systemic administration of a penicillinase-resistant semisynthetic penicillin and fluid and electrolyte replacement, if necessary. A flaky desquamation occurs during the healing phase.

Viral lesions

The vesicles of variola, vaccinia, varicella, herpes zoster, and herpes simplex have similar histologic patterns (Chapter 28). The vesicle occurs in the midepidermis. There is acantholysis and marked destruction of individual cells. This results in the ballooning type of degeneration characteristic of viral vesicles. Eosinophilic mononuclear and multinucleated giant cells may be seen on a smear carefully prepared by scraping the base of a fresh vesicle and staining with Giemsa stain (the Tzanck test). These giant cells are always seen in the herpes group (varicella-zoster and simplex) and are uncommon in the pox group (variola and vaccinia). A young viral blister also may be identified according to the type of viral inclusion body found in the degenerated cells.

HEREDITARY BLISTERING DISEASES
Epidermolysis bullosa

Epidermolysis bullosa refers to a group of hereditary defects that are characterized by intraepidermal or subepidermal blisters produced by minor degrees of trauma. Epidermolysis bullosa may be grouped into two major types: those lesions which result in complete healing without scarring and those which inevitably produce

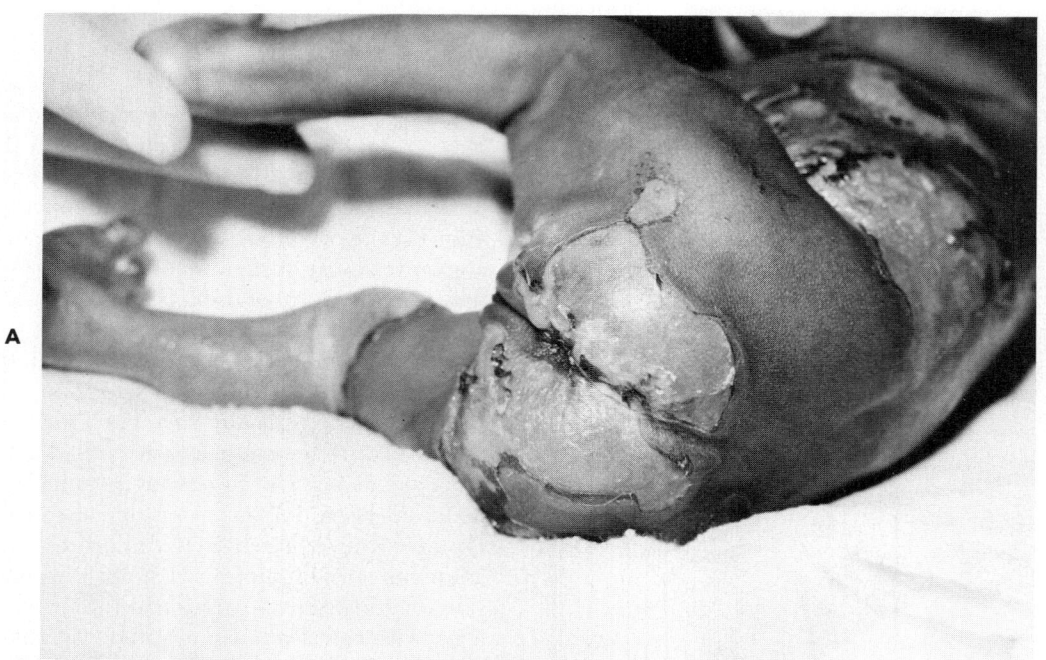

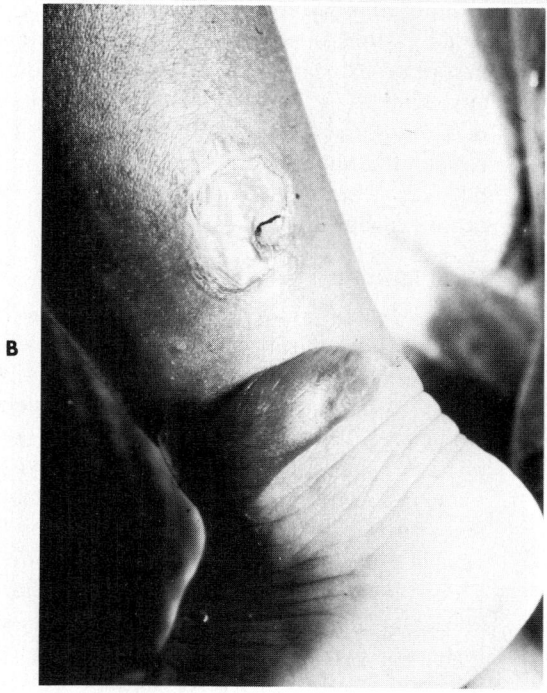

Fig. 34-5. A, Denudation secondary to blistering in an infant with epidermolysis bullosa letalis. **B,** Large intact bulla and ruptured bulla on the leg of an infant with dominant dystrophic epidermolysis bullosa.

scars. Nonscarring epidermolysis bullosa has two modes of transmission: autosomal recessive (epidermolysis bullosa letalis) and autosomal dominant (epidermolysis bullosa simplex). The term *nonscarring* refers to the manner in which an uncomplicated blister may heal. Unfortunately in the recessive form few blisters heal without complications, and scarring may result as a secondary phenomenon.

Epidermolysis bullosa letalis is usually present at birth. Sheets of epidermis loosen after minimal trauma, leaving moist erosions anywhere on the body. The nails are frequently lost. Anal and esophageal lesions also occur. Many lesions heal spontaneously, but large lesions may become infected and ulcerate. Septicemia and refractory anemia complicate the clinical course. The life span of the majority of patients is short. The blisters form between the basement membrane of the epidermis and the plasma membrane of the basal cells, lying therefore at the junction between dermis and epidermis. The cause of separation is unknown. Treatment is usually protective and palliative.

The autosomal dominant form of nonscarring epidermolysis bullosa (simplex) may be present at birth or may appear shortly thereafter in areas of trauma related to delivery (Fig. 34-5, A). The legs, feet, and scalp show erosions that heal slowly. The bullae may contain blood. Secondary infection is common. Nails usually are not involved. In contrast to the recessive form, the infants are usually in good general health. In all forms of epidermolysis bullosa, blisters may be readily elicited by gentle rubbing. Mild trauma will result in a blister within a few minutes to hours, and the resulting fresh lesions may be used for histopathologic examination. The diagnostic blister of the dominant form results from acute disintegration of basal cells. Cytolysis starts in the perinuclear region and spreads centrifugally to involve the entire basal cell. The cause is unknown. Treatment is aimed at protecting the skin from trauma, keeping lesions clean, and eradicating secondary infection.

Scarring epidermolysis bullosa (dystrophic epidermolysis bullosa) has both a recessive and a dominant form. Recessive scarring epidermolysis bullosa may occur in consanguineous families. Hemorrhagic erosions and blisters may be present at birth, especially about the feet. In contrast to the nonscarring group, milia may mark the site of healed blisters. Usually trauma precedes blister formation. The toe and finger lesions heal with fusion of digits and loss of nails, which results in a characteristic mittenlike envelope of the hands. As the fingers fuse (this usually takes several years), the hands and arms become fixed in a flexed position, and contractures develop. Repeated episodes of blistering, infection and scar formation lead to severe deformities, loss of hair, buccal mucosal scarring, dysphagia, and retarded physical and sexual development. Visceral amyloidosis, hyperglobulinemic purpura, and clotting abnormalities are associated with this severe, life-limiting disease. The electron microscopic changes in all the scarring forms are identical and diagnostic. There is a sharp separation just beneath the basement membrane (subepidermal bulla), and the normal basal layer anchoring fibrils are absent. The defect probably involves the connective tissue of the dermis immediately adjacent to the basement membrane of the epidermis. There are elevated levels of collagenase in the skin of such patients.

Treatment for scarring epidermolysis bullosa is essentially the same as that for the nonscarring forms. In selected patients surgery may be indicated for correction of flexion deformities of fused digits. Iron therapy is necessary to treat the anemia.

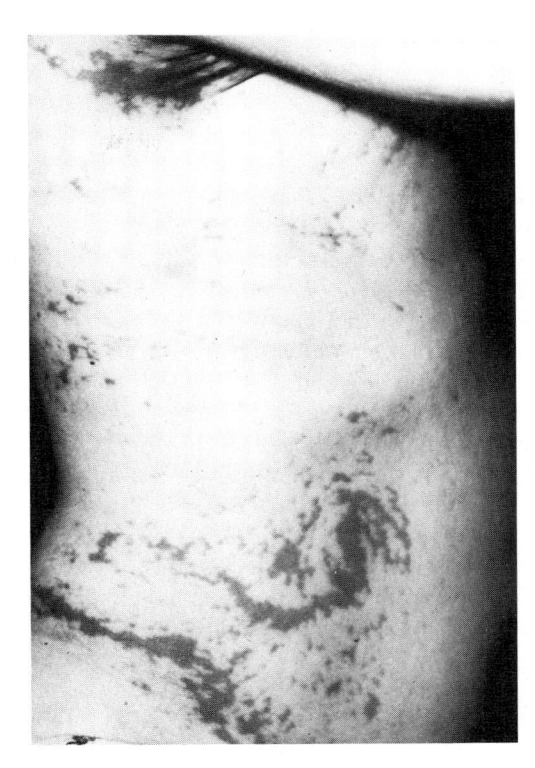

Fig. 34-6. Incontinentia pigmenti. Whorled chocolate-brown macular hyperpigmented lesions on the trunk.

The dominant form of scarring epidermolysis bullosa is less severe than the recessive type. Lesions may be present at birth, but often they appear later and are usually limited to hands, feet, and sacrum (Fig. 34-5, B). Nails may be lost, but deforming scars and contractures are infrequent. Red plaques rather than blisters may result from injury. The lesions heal with soft wrinkled scars; keloids may occur in predisposed individuals. Hypopigmentation and hyperpigmentation and milia often are found at old blister sites. The general health is usually unimpaired.

Incontinentia pigmenti

Incontinentia pigmenti is a hereditary disorder that affects the skin, skeletal system, heart, eyes, and CNS. Its mode of inheritance is probably as an X-linked dominant trait. Almost all the patients are female, but a few affected males have been reported. The cutaneous lesions are usually present at birth and have three morphologic stages. Initially there are inflammatory vesicles, which are arranged linearly and appear in crops. These are replaced by pigmented, warty excrescences, which gradually resolve and are followed by flat, pigmented patterns of whorls and lines (Fig. 34-6). These bizarre pigmented lesions represent the third and end stage, although pigmentation occasionally may accompany some of the early lesions. The blistering lesions occur on the trunk or limbs or both and vary in density from few to many. Nails and hair also may be affected. There is often a transient peripheral eosinophilia during the bullous phase of the disease. The diagnosis should be considered when inflammatory bullae arranged in lines are seen in a newborn female infant; ocular and skeletal abnormalities also may be present at this time. Faulty dentition, microcephaly, and abnormalities of the CNS can occur but may not be apparent during the neonatal period. Biopsy of a small blister demonstrates a subcorneal vesicle filled with numerous eosinophils suggestive of an inflammatory dermatitis. The differential diagnosis includes herpes simplex infection and other blistering diseases. The clinical evolution of the cutaneous process and the presence of pigment-laden macrophages in the upper dermis of end-stage lesions establishes the diagnosis. No specific therapy is required for the skin lesions; if inflammation becomes excessive during the bullous phase, treatment with compresses and topical steroids may be helpful.

OTHER BULLOUS DISEASES
Acrodermatitis enteropathica

Acrodermatitis enteropathica, a rare disorder, is inherited as an autosomal recessive trait. It is characterized by acute vesicobullous and eczematous eruptions around the mouth and genitals and on the peripheral extremities. Secondary infection with *Candida* organisms is a common complication. The onset may be as early as the third week of life, but more frequently it occurs later in infancy. Failure to thrive, hair loss, marked irritability, and paronychial lesions are additional features of the disease. Chronic, severe, and intractable diarrhea is the most serious manifestation and may be life threatening. The disease is caused by a defect in zinc metabolism, and extremely low plasma zinc levels have been documented in untreated patients; the exact nature of the defect is not known. Oral zinc sulfate has replaced diiodohydroxyquinoline as the treatment of choice and has induced dramatic remissions of the disease.

Candidiasis

See also Chapter 27.

Cutaneous candidiasis in infancy may be a mild episodic disease or a chronic disorder, or it may result in disseminated infection and death. The latter two forms often are associated with multiple endocrinopathies and/or a defect in the immune response. Candidiasis in the first 4 weeks of life is usually benign and is most often localized to the oral cavity (thrush) or the diaper area (Fig. 34-7). If maternal vaginal organisms are acquired during the birth process, the infant may manifest symptomatic mouth lesions or become an intestinal carrier. Fecal contamination is the usual source of the organism in candidal diaper dermatitis. Paronychial lesions also may occur, particularly in thumb-sucking infants. Rarely cutaneous or systemic candidiasis may be present at birth as a result of transplacental or ascending infection.

The early cutaneous lesions are vesicular with an areola of erythema; these rapidly become pustular and confluent, forming a moist erosion surrounded by satellite pustules. In the chronic mucocutaneous or granulomatous forms (rare in the neonatal period) the scalp, lips, hands, and nails may be sites of chronically scaling, heaped-up lesions. The diagnosis is aided by identification of budding yeast spores on Gram stain or of spores and pseudohyphae on a potassium hydroxide preparation. Growth of the organism is rapid on Sabouraud's or Mycosel agar.

Treatment depends on the extent of involvement. Specific topical candidicidal agents include nystatin, amphotericin B, and miconazole. Systemic administration of amphotericin B or 5-fluorocytosine should be reserved for those patients with evidence of severe disseminated disease involving more than the gastrointestinal (GI) tract and skin.

PIGMENTARY ABNORMALITIES

The melanocyte system of the newborn skin is not usually at maximal functional maturity. As a result, all babies, even black, Indian, or Chinese, may look pink or tan at birth. Within the first few weeks racial color becomes more evident because melanin production has been stimulated by exposure to light. For purposes of classification it is useful to think of pigmentary changes as diffuse or localized.

Diffuse hyperpigmentation

The intensity of pigmentation must be considered in light of the infant's genetic and racial background. Diffuse hyperpigmentation in the newborn is a very unusual occurrence. It may be caused by a gene whose main effect is on the melanocyte, by a hereditary disease that has secondary pigmentary consequences, by endocrinopathy, by a nutritional disorder, or by hepatic disease. Although in such cases hyperpigmentation may be described as diffuse, in fact it may be accentuated in certain areas, such as the face, over bony prominences, or in the flexural creases.

Localized hyperpigmentation
Flat lesions

Cafe au lait patches. These patches occasionally may be seen in the newborn period (Fig. 34-8, *A*). The lesion is flat, light brown in whites and dark brown in blacks. Single lesions are found in 19% of normal children. They have no significance. Lesions that are greater than 1.5 cm in length, more than six in number, and frequently

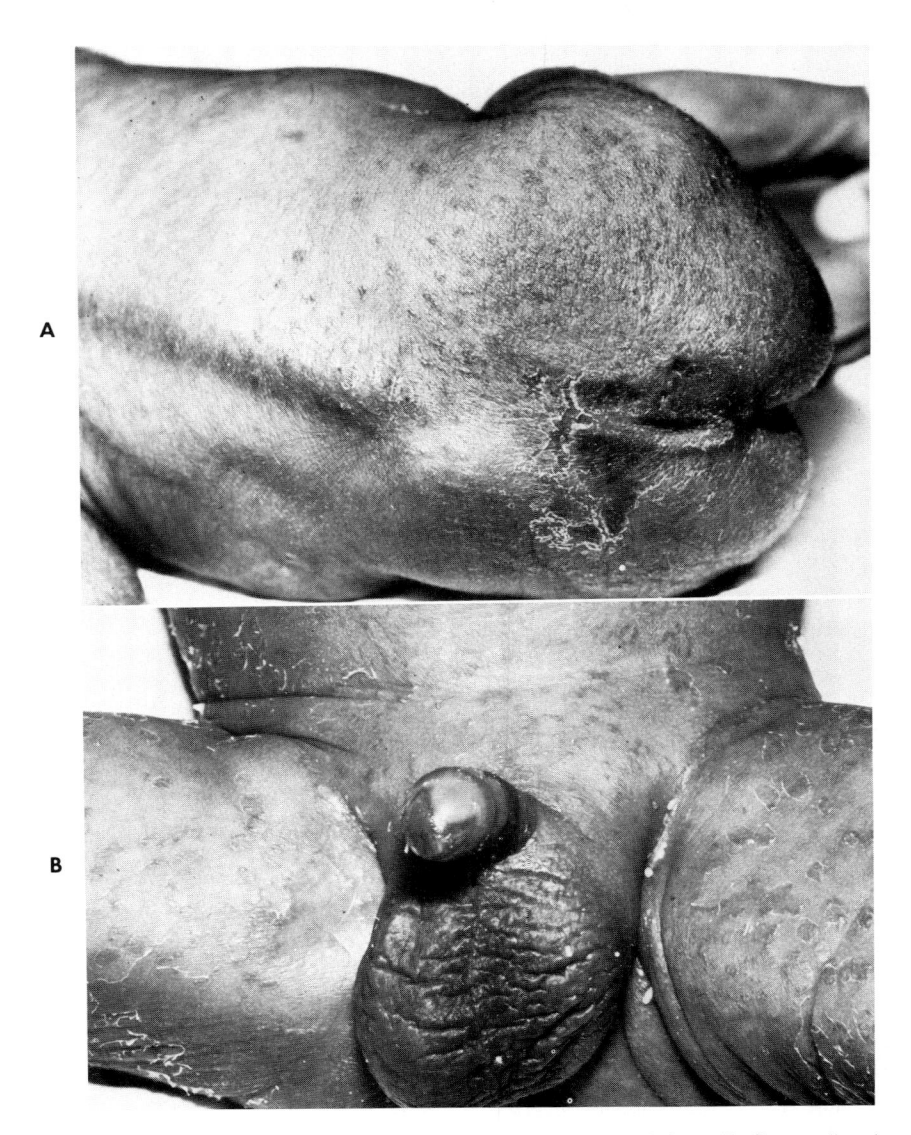

Fig. 34-7. **A,** Candidal dermatitis on the buttocks of a preterm infant. **B,** Generalized scaling, vesicopustules, and balanitis in a 10-day-old infant due to *C. albicans* infection. The mother had a candidal vaginitis during her pregnancy.

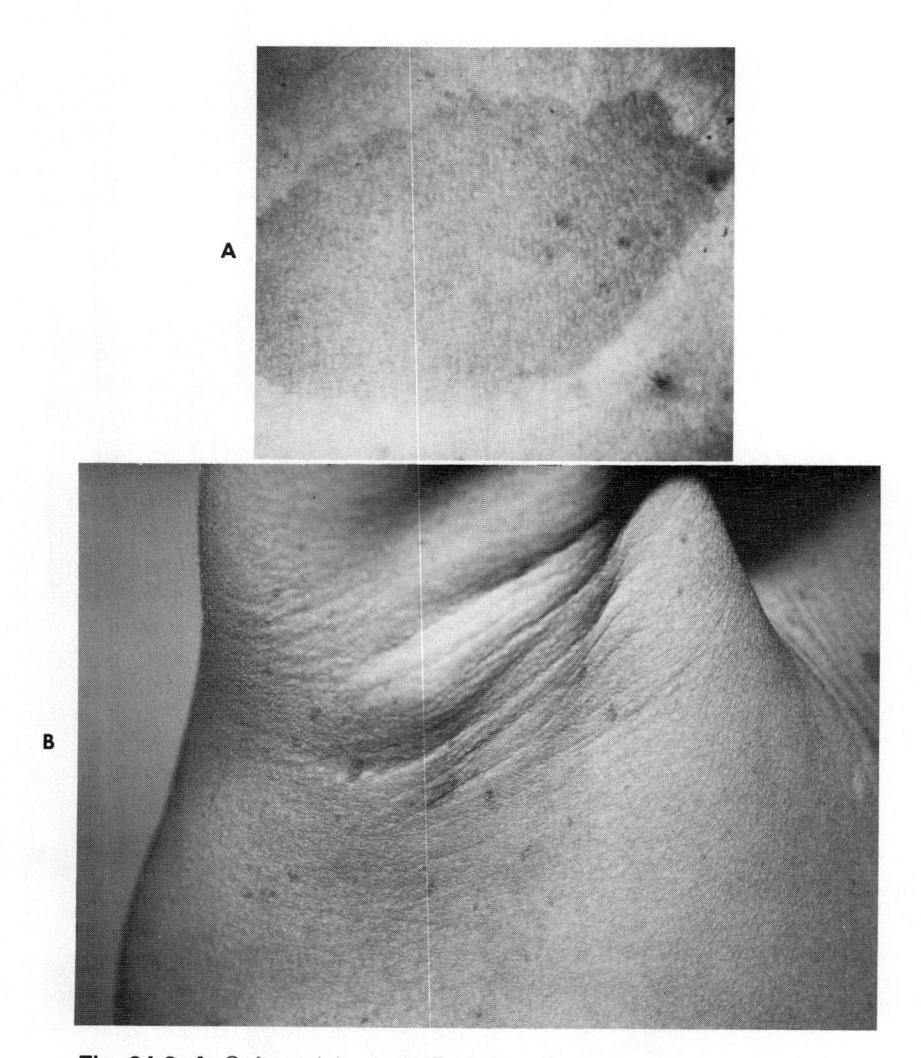

Fig. 34-8. A, Cafe au lait patch. **B,** Axillary freckling in neurofibromatosis.

accompanied by axillary freckling are diagnostic of neurofibromatosis (Fig. 34-8, *B*). The cafe au lait lesion is often the first to appear in neurofibromatosis, but the pigmented lesions may increase slowly in number so that additional genetic and histologic information is required to establish a diagnosis. Giant melanosomes may be identified in the cafe au lait spots of neurofibromatosis, and they may be found as well in the pigmentary lesions of other disorders. Patients with tuberous sclerosis also show cafe au lait spots. These are identical in appearance to those seen in neurofibromatosis but are very frequently accompanied by white macules (as discussed later).

Albright's syndrome. In Albright's syndrome the pigmented lesion is usually unilateral, elongated, and large (more than 10 cm), with a ragged, irregular ("coast of Maine") border. Macromelanosomes are less common in the melanocytes of these cafe au lait spots than in those of neurofibromatosis.

Nevocellular nevi. Approximately 1% to 2% of newborn infants have pigmented nevi of the congenital type. Small lesions (as opposed to giant pigmented nevi) are light to dark brown, often with a variegated color or speckling and an accentuated epidermal surface ridge pattern (Fig. 34-9). These lesions vary in site, size, and number but are most often solitary. Histologically many of them are characterized by the presence of nevus cells in the deeper dermis and fat and in perivascular, periappendageal, and perineural sites throughout the dermis. Although there is no clear-cut evidence that the small congenital nevus is a premalignant lesion, it is the prevailing opinion at many institutions that these lesions pose a significant enough risk to warrant removal. Should the family elect to observe rather than excise the nevus,

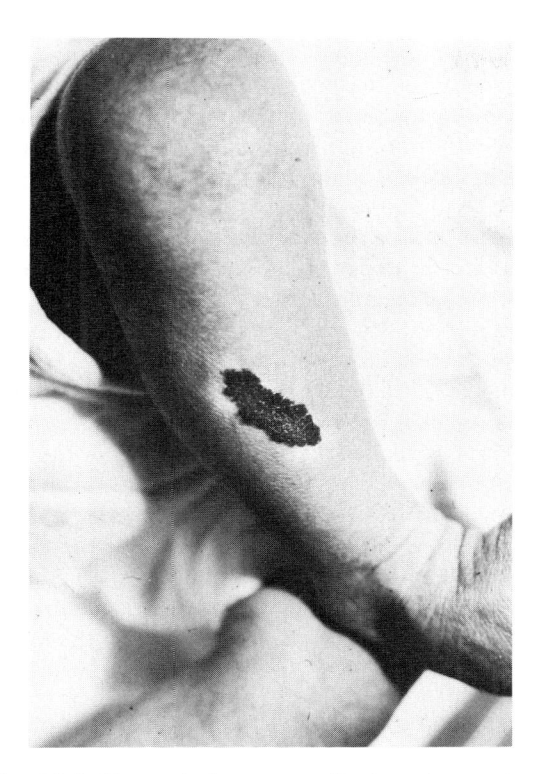

Fig. 34-9. Pigmented nevus on the leg of a newborn.

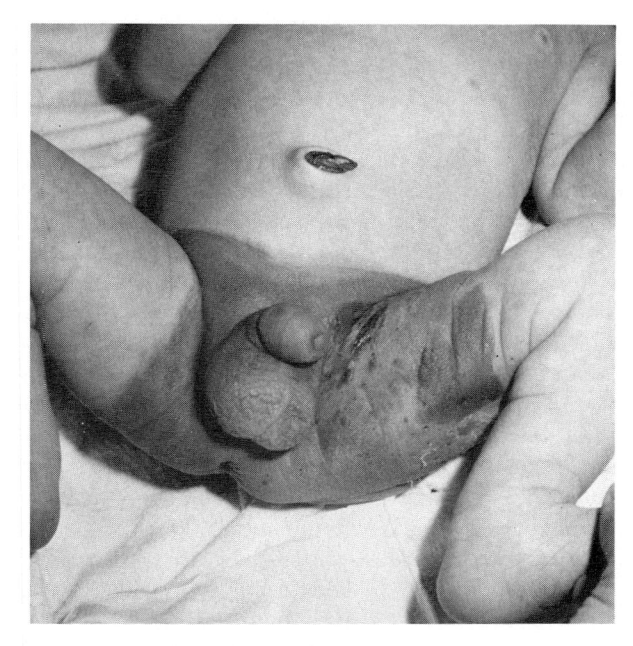

Fig. 34-10. Giant hairy nevus in the bathing trunk area.

periodic evaluation of the lesion for surface changes and associated symptoms should be carried out. Biopsy is indicated in instances where malignant change is suspected.

Peutz-Jeghers syndrome. The cutaneous lesions of the Peutz-Jeghers syndrome may be present at birth or develop soon thereafter. They consist of pigmented macules, somewhat darker than freckles, that develop around the nose and mouth. The lips and oral mucosa often are involved, as are the hands, fingertips, and nails. Macular hyperpigmentation is the only visible sign of this autosomal dominant disorder until adolescence, when the patient begins to suffer from attacks of intussusception—evidence of coexisting small bowel polyposis.

Xeroderma pigmentosum. Xeroderma pigmentosum is transmitted by an autosomal recessive gene and results in marked hypersensitivity to ultraviolet light. Soon after birth and depending on the rapidity and intensity of light exposure, the infant develops erythema, speckled hyperpigmentation, atrophy, actinic keratoses, and all known types of cutaneous malignancy. The outcome is often fatal by the second decade of life, as a result of metastatic disease. The underlying abnormality probably is caused by a deficiency in an endonuclease that is responsible for the repair of DNA damaged by ultraviolet light. Genetic heterogeneity has been demonstrated in patients with xeroderma pigmentosum who have defective excision repair of DNA. Seven complementation groups have been identified, each with a characteristic range of DNA repair rates. Patients in each of these groups differ with regard to clinical features and epidemiologic patterns. For example, neurologic involvement is usual in certain variants. Protection from ultraviolet light exposure is mandatory, since this will prevent many of the cutaneous abnormalities and tumors. Prenatal diagnosis of xeroderma pigmentosum is possible, according to Cleaver, by autoradiography to measure abnormal DNA synthesis of desquamated cells obtained from amniotic fluid.

Postinflammatory hyperpigmentation. Hyperpigmentation may result secondarily from any inflammatory process in the skin and thus may have many causes, including primary irritant dermatitis, infectious processes, panniculitis, and hereditary diseases, such as epidermolysis bullosa. The hyperpigmentation may result from an increase in melanosome production, increased melanin deposits in basal cells, increased number of keratinocytes, increase in the thickness of the stratum corneum, or deposits of melanin in dermal melanophages.

Raised lesions

The most important of the congenital pigmented nevi is the *giant hairy (garment) nevus* (Fig. 34-10). About 10% of these patients develop malignant melanoma in the lesion. These nevi are present at birth, are probably not hereditary, and may occupy 15% to 35% of the body surface, most often involving the trunk. The pigmentation is often variegated from light brown to black. The affected skin may be leathery in consistency. Almost invariably numerous pigmented nevi, other dermal nevi, and cafe au lait spots coexist elsewhere on the body. Leptomeningeal melanocytosis has been documented in some of these patients, and this latter finding may be manifested as seizures.

The melanocytic invasion may involve subcutaneous tissue, fascia, or even underlying muscle. Because of the significant incidence of malignant degeneration in these nevi and of the hideous deformity and the intense pruritus that may accompany them, it is desirable to remove these lesions surgically as soon as possible. The infant should be old enough to withstand major surgery. *Intradermal* or *compound* (involving both epidermal junction and dermis) *nevi*, circumscribed, hairy, and pigmented, may be present at birth. They occur everywhere but on the palms and soles and usually are raised, warty, and dome shaped. Histologically the melanocytic nevus cells are found localized to the upper dermis and around the appendages and contain variable amounts of pigment. Usually the diagnosis presents no problem, nor does their surgical removal.

Occasionally one may see a *blue nevus* (so called because of its Prussian-blue color), or dermal melanocytoma, at birth. They are usually 1 to 3 cm in diameter, oval, dome-shaped tumors found on the upper half of the body. They grow very slowly and have little or no known tendency to become malignant but may be difficult to differentiate clinically from vascular tumors. Excisional biopsy is diagnostic and curative of the condition.

Incontinentia pigmenti and urticaria pigmentosa (mastocytosis)

Both of these conditions, which start as blistering diseases, have hyperpigmentation as a prominent feature of the process (p. 949).

Hypopigmentation

Diffuse or localized loss of cutaneous pigment in the neonate may be caused by heredity or by a developmental disorder or may be acquired as a result of a nutritional disorder or postinflammatory changes. Decrease in cutaneous melanin may be caused by an absence or destruction of melanocytes or by a defect in one of four biologic processes: formation of melanosomes, formation of melanin, transfer of melanosomes into keratinocytes, and transport of melanosomes by keratinocytes.

Albinism (complete albinism, oculocutaneous albinism)

Albinism, which occurs in all races, has an incidence of between 1:5,000 to 1:25,000; the phenotypic picture is caused by an autosomal recessive gene. The affected infant usually has markedly reduced skin pigment, yellow or white hair, pink pupils, gray irides, photophobia, and cutaneous photosensitivity. Melanocytic nevi can be present in patients with albinism, and the nevi may or may not be pigmented. In blacks the skin may be tan; freckles can appear on exposure to light. The usual eye findings are nystagmus and a central scotoma with reduced visual acuity. Other associated abnormalities reported in albinism are small stature, mental retardation, and coagulation disorders.

The biochemical defect responsible for this disorder is a deficiency of tyrosinase, the enzyme responsible for converting tyrosine to dopa, an early step in the formation of melanin (Chapter 32). The range of tyrosinase deficiency correlates well with the spectrum of color seen in affected individuals. Structurally the melanosomes appear to be normal. Treatment is aimed at protection from ultraviolet light, since early actinic keratoses and squamous cell carcinoma are common occurrences in these patients.

Partial albinism (piebaldism)

Partial albinism is an inherited disease caused by an autosomal dominant gene. It is present at birth but may not be evident in fair-skinned infants because of a lack of contrast in skin color. The differential diagnosis may include vitiligo, achromic nevus, nevus anemicus, and the amelanotic macules of tuberous sclerosis and Addison's disease. In piebaldism the hair and skin are affected. The amelanotic areas usually involve the widow's peak and anterior scalp, forehead to the base of the nose, the chin, thorax, trunk, back, midarm, and midleg. There are normal islands of pigment within the hypomelanotic areas, and the distribution pattern is fairly constant. Examination of an amelanotic area by electron microscopy shows an absence of melanocytes or melanocytes with markedly deformed melanosomes. Repigmentation does not take place.

Phenylketonuria

Phenylketonuria, a biochemical defect, results in a variety of neurologic and cutaneous abnormalities, which include mental retardation, seizures, diffuse hypopigmentation, eczema, and photosensitivity (Chapter 32).

Chédiak-Higashi syndrome

The Chédiak-Higashi syndrome is a rare, fatal disorder transmitted by an autosomal recessive gene. Its clinical features include a diffuse to moderate reduction in cutaneous and ocular pigment, photophobia, hepatosplenomegaly, and recalcitrant, recurrent infections. The leukocytes and other cells contain large granules, and this finding has its parallel in the melanocyte, which

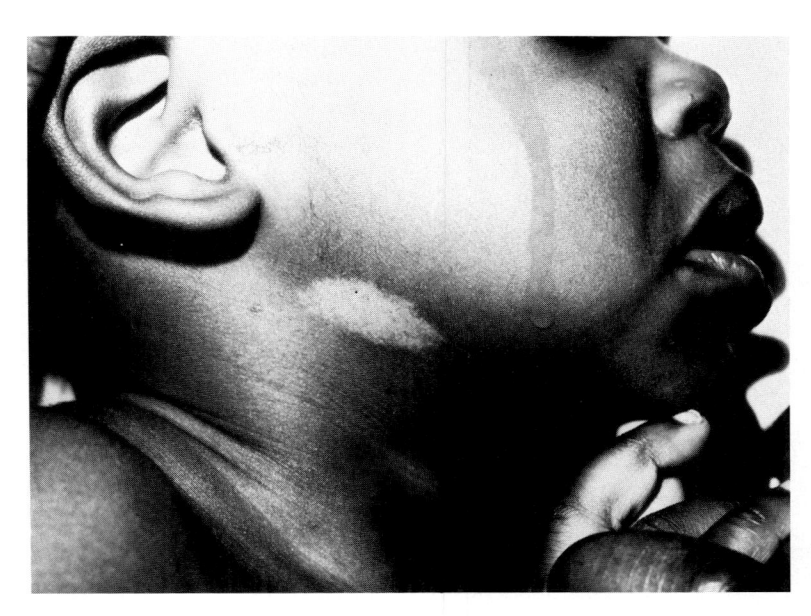

Fig. 34-11. White leaf macule in a child with tuberous sclerosis.

produces giant melanosomes. It is not known why there is a clinical pigmentary deficiency, but it appears to have little to do with true albinism. Windhorst and Padgett have speculated that the basic defect is a structural defect in the lipoprotein matrix that gives rise to the melanosome (and granulocytic lysosomes). Thus the melanin granule either is destroyed too easily or cannot be transferred to the keratinocyte (melanocytic impaction). The diagnosis may be made by the characteristic family history, physical findings, laboratory demonstration of abnormal leukocytes and melanosomes, and the usual course, which leads to death in childhood. Death results from a lymphoma-like process or infection. Hodgkin's disease recently has been reported as the fatal outcome in one patient.

Klein-Waardenburg syndrome

Klein-Waardenburg syndrome is inherited as an autosomal dominant condition; the most constant features are lateral displacement of the inner canthi of the eyes, a prominently broad nasal root, confluent eyebrows, variegation of pigment in the iris (heterochromia iridis) and fundus, congenital deafness, a white forelock, and cutaneous hypochromia. The clinical picture is quite striking, and the diagnosis usually is not difficult. Although usually limited to small areas, the hypopigmentation may be severe and extensive enough to resemble that of partial albinism.

Nevus anemicus

Nevus anemicus is a permanent pale, mottled lesion that occurs most often on the trunk. The lesions contain normal amounts of pigment. There is no decrease in the number of blood vessels in the affected area, but the vascular tone is increased because of an excess local accumulation of catecholamines. There is no effective treatment.

Nevus achromicus

Present at birth, nevus achromicus is usually a unilateral, somewhat hypopigmented, irregular-shaped, bizarre, streaky lesion. The hypopigmented area is quite uniform in color, and, in contrast to nevus anemicus, the vessels within it react normally to rubbing. The melanocytes in the affected epidermis seem to be nonfunctioning or partially functioning. Large areas of nevus achromicus may be associated with an increased incidence of mental retardation (hypomelanosis of Ito).

White spots in tuberous sclerosis

Up to 90% of infants with tuberous sclerosis have white macules that become apparent at birth or soon after (Fig. 34-11). In fair-skinned infants the hypopigmented areas may be easily demonstrated by examining the skin with a Wood's lamp. They are variable in number and may occur more frequently on the trunk and buttocks. The melanocytes within areas of macular hypopigmentation contain poorly pigmented melanosomes.

ANGIOMAS

Cutaneous hemangiomas are common developmental nevoid lesions involving the dermal and subcutaneous vasculature. They are either superficial (approximately 68%), subcutaneous (15%), or mixed (20%). The terms

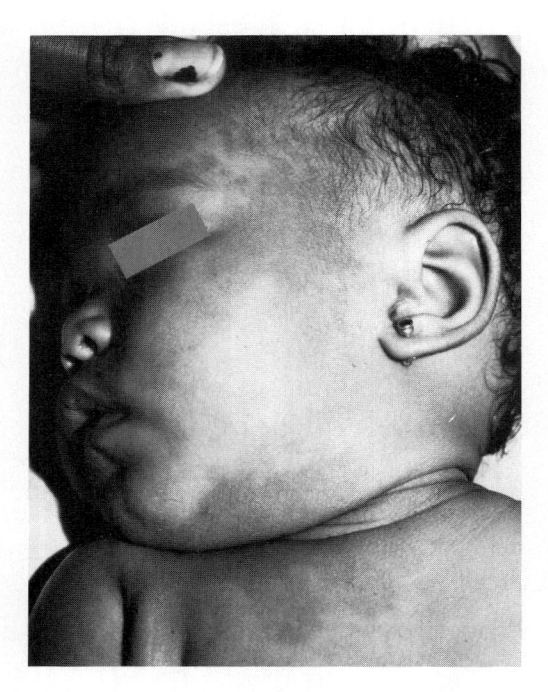

Fig. 34-12. Nevus flammeus on the upper face, chin, neck, and anterior chest. This infant had a similar lesion on the other side of the face.

capillary and *cavernous* refer to the histopathologic pattern apparent on biopsy. Capillary hemangiomas show only dilated vessels, with or without endothelial proliferation, and cavernous hemangiomas have large, dilated, blood-filled cavities with a compressed endothelial lining.

Port-wine stain, or nevus flammeus

Nevus flammeus is present at birth and should be considered a relatively permanent developmental defect. These lesions may be only a few millimeters in diameter or may cover extensive areas, occasionally involving up to half the body surface. They do not proliferate after birth; the apparent increase in size is caused by growth of the child. A nevus flammeus may be localized to any body surface, but facial lesions are probably the most common (Fig. 34-12). Port-wine nevi usually are sharply demarcated and flat, but they may have a pebbly or slightly thickened surface. Variation in color ranges from pale pink to purple. The most successful modality of treatment is the use of an opaque cosmetic cream (such as Covermark) that blends with the surrounding skin.

Most port-wine nevi occur as isolated defects and do not indicate involvement of other organs; however, occasionally the nevus flammeus may be a clue to the presence of certain vascular syndromes. The *Sturge-Weber syndrome* (encephalofacial angiomatosis) consists of a facial port-wine nevus usually in the cutaneous distribution of the trigeminal nerve, convulsions, hemiparesis contralateral to the facial lesion, and ipsilateral intracranial calcification. Ocular manifestations are frequent and include buphthalmos, glaucoma, angioma of the choroid, hemianoptic defects, and optic atrophy (Chapter 35). In a few patients the vascular defect may affect other organs. Roentgenograms of the skull of the older child show pathognomonic "tramline," double-contoured calcification in the cerebral cortex on the same side as the nevus flammeus. Electroencephalography may demonstrate unilateral depression of cortical activity, with or without spike discharges.

The prognosis depends on the extent of cerebral involvement, rapidity of progression, and response to treatment. Anticonvulsant therapy and neurosurgical procedures have been of value in some patients.

Klippel-Trenaunay-Weber syndrome

Klippel-Trenaunay-Weber syndrome is characterized by a cutaneous macular vascular nevus, venous varicosities, and overgrowth of the bony structures and soft tissues of a limb. The vascular lesions are usually apparent at birth, and boys are more frequently affected than girls. Rarely the hemangioma may be of the capillary or cavernous type, and it is often associated with arteriovenous shunts or lymphoangiomatous anomalies. Polydactyly, syndactyly, and oligodactyly have been associated findings. Complications include severe edema, phlebitis, thrombosis, and ulceration of the affected area. The prognosis depends on the extent of involvement, which should be carefully assessed by peripheral vascular studies. Surgery may be effective in preventing severe limb hypertrophy in some patients. Jobst garments are also helpful in some instances.

Macular capillary hemangiomas also occur with moderate frequency in trisomy 13, Rubenstein-Taybi syndrome (broad thumbs and toes, slanted palpebral fissures, and hypoplastic maxilla), and in the Beckwith-Wiedemann syndrome (macroglossia, omphalocele, macrosomia, and cytomegaly of the fetal adrenal gland) (p. 858).

Strawberry (nevus) hemangioma

The strawberry hemangioma is a raised, circumscribed, soft, bright red tumor that is lobulated and compressible. When a subcutaneous component is present, it consists of a bluish-red mass with less well-defined borders. If the entire nevus is deeply situated, the overlying skin may appear normal or show only a blue discoloration. The histologic pattern will depend on whether the angioma is purely capillary, cavernous, or mixed in type.

Approximately 20% to 30% of raised angiomatous nevi are present at birth (Fig. 34-13, A), and roughly 90% are

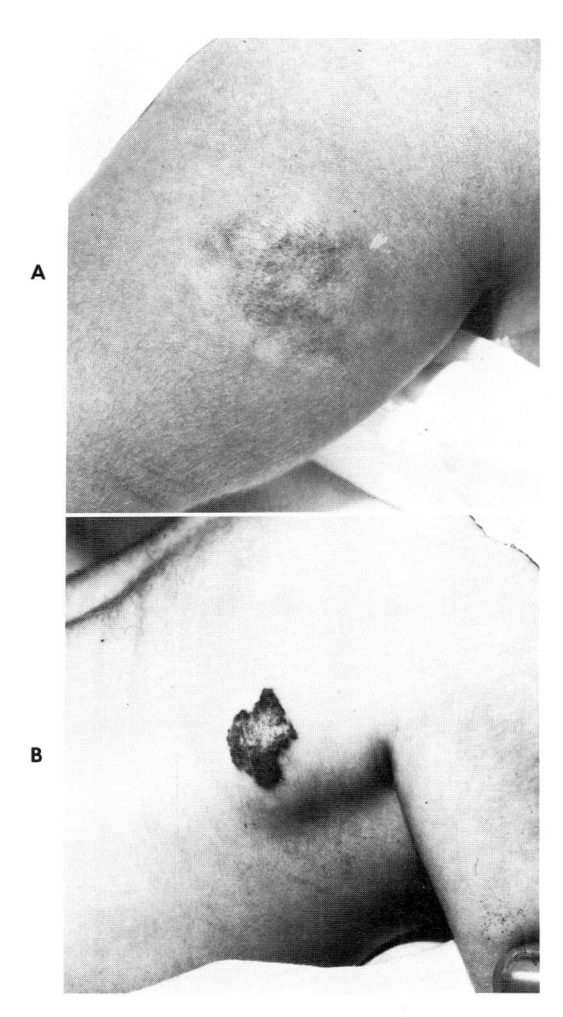

Fig. 34-13. A, Hemangioma on the thigh of a preterm infant. Areas of pallor, often an initial sign, are still present. **B,** Mixed capillary and cavernous hemangioma on the back.

evident by the second month of age. The remainder have their onset between the second and ninth month of life. Girls are affected more often than boys. The most common site is the face, and the majority of infants have a single lesion (Fig. 34-13, *B*). Virtually all these lesions show some increase in size during the first 6 months of life, often with an initial rapid growth spurt. The phase of active expansion, particularly in larger nevi, may result in ulceration, which is usually of no consequence unless complicated by secondary infection or hemorrhage.

If left untreated, most of the hemangiomas in this group will involute spontaneously. Regression may be anticipated when pale gray areas appear on the previously bright red surface of the lesion. Approximately 50% of hemangiomas disappear by 5 years of age and 70% by 7 years of age. Rapidity and completeness of resolution seem unrelated to the size of the lesion or age of appearance. In some patients there are no residual skin changes; others show variable degrees of atrophy and telangiectasia. Lesions that ulcerate tend to scar and therefore may end in a poorer cosmetic result. Profuse hemorrhage is rare unless there is an accompanying thrombocytopenia or coagulation defect. Minor degrees of hemorrhage usually can be managed by compression bandages.

The vast majority of patients with strawberry hemangiomas require no treatment other than careful follow-up monitoring to detect possible complications and to provide much needed reassurance to parents. However, under certain circumstances intervention may be indicated. Such situations include rapid growth of a lesion that compromises a vital structure or marked tissue destruction and associated symptomatic thrombocytopenia. Surgical excision is one means of approach, but an acceptable cosmetic result is not always achieved. A short intensive course of oral corticosteroids may be effective in young infants if severity of involvement warrants such therapy. Alternate-day corticosteroid therapy has been shown to be successful in some infants.

Kasabach-Merritt syndrome

The association of thrombocytopenia with hemangiomas is known as the *Kasabach-Merritt syndrome*. This phenomenon is most frequently seen in early infancy, and in one series of seven patients the median age of hospital admission was 5 weeks. Most but not all of the hemangiomas associated with thrombocytopenia are very large. Multiple coagulation defects in addition to thrombocytopenia also have been reported in association with hemangiomas. These defects include deficiency of factors II, V, and VII and hypofibrinogenemia.

In contrast to the infant with a hemangioma and normal hematologic findings, the infant with Kasabach-Merritt syndrome should be hospitalized and treated promptly. The emergence of petechiae or ecchymoses in the adjacent skin or overt bleeding is an indication for fresh blood or platelet-rich transfusions. Surgical extirpation of the lesion or a course of irradiation to the hemangioma usually results in alleviation of the thrombocytopenia. Splenectomy is not indicated. Corticosteroid therapy occasionally has been successful. A few of these infants have recovered without treatment after spontaneous involution of the hemangioma.

Miliary hemangiomatosis (diffuse neonatal hemangiomatosis)

A number of infants have been reported with multiple hemangiomas in several visceral organs. Some have had a myriad of small cutaneous lesions, most commonly in association with lesions of the GI tract, liver, CNS, and lungs. Despite supportive therapy, affected infants often die early in life from intractable high output failure, GI hemorrhage, respiratory tract obstruction, or severe neurologic deficiency caused by extensive compression of neural lesions. Corticosteroid therapy has been successful in a few instances.

Blue rubber bleb nevus syndrome

The blue rubber bleb nevus syndrome is a rare disorder consisting of multiple cavernous hemangiomas of the skin and bowel. Cutaneous lesions sometimes are present at birth, and their appearance is characteristic, as the descriptive name of this syndrome suggests. The lesions are blue to purple, rubbery, compressible protuberances that vary from a few millimeters to 3 to 4 cm in diameter. They are diffusely distributed over the body surface and may be sparse or number in the hundreds. GI lesions are common in the small bowel but also may involve the colon. Occasionally lesions in the liver, spleen, and CNS also have been noted. Severe anemia may result from recurrent episodes of GI bleeding. Neither the skin nor the bowel lesions regress spontaneously. Surgery is sometimes palliative, but it is frequently impossible to resect all the affected bowel.

Cavernous hemangiomas also have been reported as a congenital feature of Riley-Smith syndrome and Leroy's syndrome (I-cell disease). *Maffucci's syndrome* (cavernous hemangiomas and dyschondroplasia) and *Gorham's disease* (cavernous hemangiomas and disappearing bones) are not usually apparent in the neonatal period.

Lymphangiomas

Lymphangiomas are hamartomatous malformations composed of dilated lymph channels that are lined by normal lymphatic endothelium. They may be superficial or cavernous and often are associated with anomalies of the regional lymphatic vessels.

Lymphangioma circumscriptum is probably the most common type of lymphangioma and may be present at birth or appear in early childhood. Areas of predilection are the oral mucosa, the proximal limbs, and the axillary folds (Fig. 34-14). The tumor consists of clustered, small, thick-walled vesicles resembling frog spawn; it is often skin colored but may be of a blue cast because of a hemangiomatous component. Treatment is by excision; however, larger lesions may require full-thickness skin grafting. Recurrence has been noted even in full-thickness grafts.

Simple lymphangioma appears in infancy as a solitary, skin-colored, dermal or subcutaneous nodule. Following trauma it may exude serous fluid. Occasionally it has been associated with more extensive lymphatic involvement. Uncomplicated lesions may be removed by simple excision.

Cavernous lymphangioma is a diffuse, soft tissue mass consisting of large, cystic dilatations of lymphatics in the dermis, subcutaneous tissue, and intermuscular septa. Surgery is impractical in most cases.

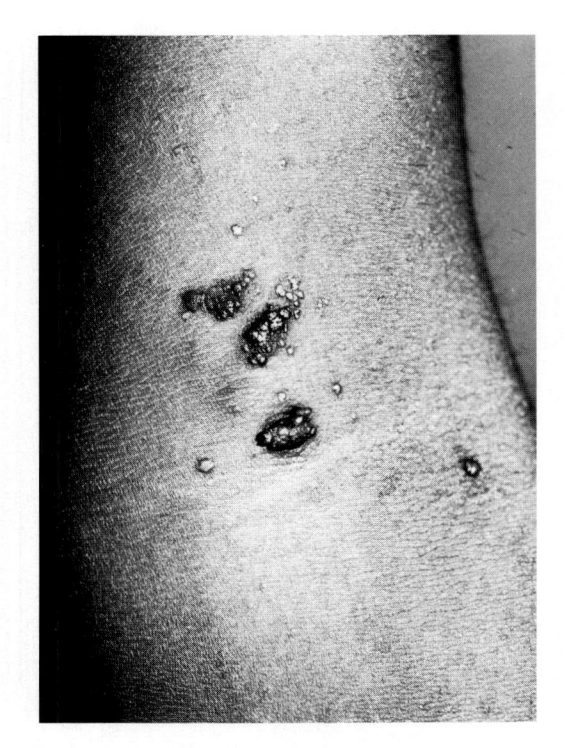

Fig. 34-14. Lymphangioma on the upper arm.

Cystic hygroma

Cystic hygroma is a benign, multilocular tumor usually found in the neck region. The tumors tend to increase in size and should be treated by surgical excision.

VERRUCOUS (EPIDERMAL OR ORGANOID) NEVI

Verrucous nevi are a group of lesions that are commonly found in the neonatal period. Most of them consist of an overgrowth of keratinocytes and may have an identifiable differentiation toward one of the appendages normally found in skin. They vary considerably in their size, clinical appearance, histologic characteristics, and evolution, depending on the topographic location of the lesion on the body. Lesions occurring in sites normally rich in sebaceous glands (such as the scalp) may look like sebaceous nevi, whereas others, found in areas where the epidermis is thick (for example, the elbow), look primarily warty in nature (Fig. 34-15).

Clinically epidermal nevi may take the following forms:
1. A string of pigmented papillomas, a few centimeters in length, found anywhere on the body.
2. Long unilateral streaks involving a limb or up to half the body (nevus unius lateris). The nails may be deformed by the process.

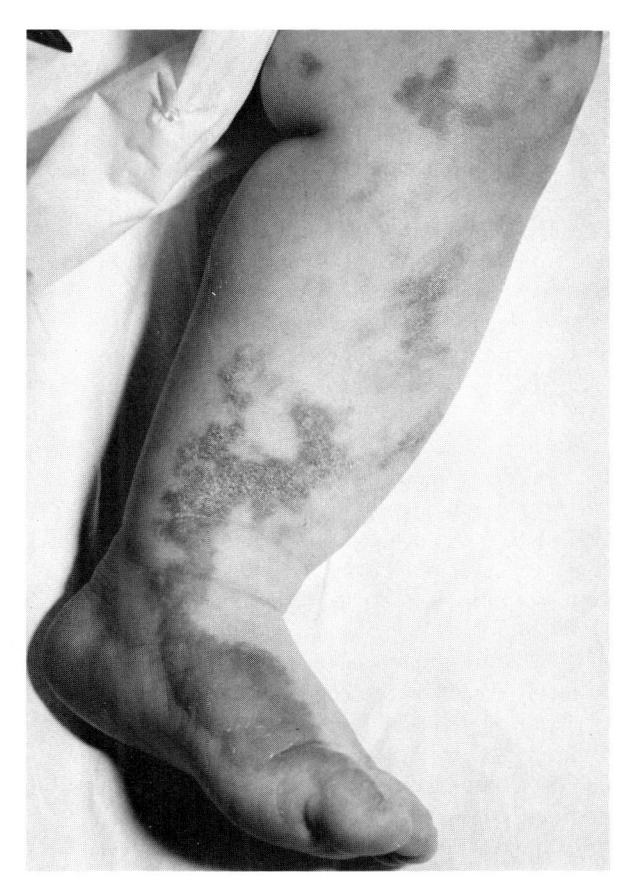

Fig. 34-15. Verrucous epidermal nevus on the leg of an infant.

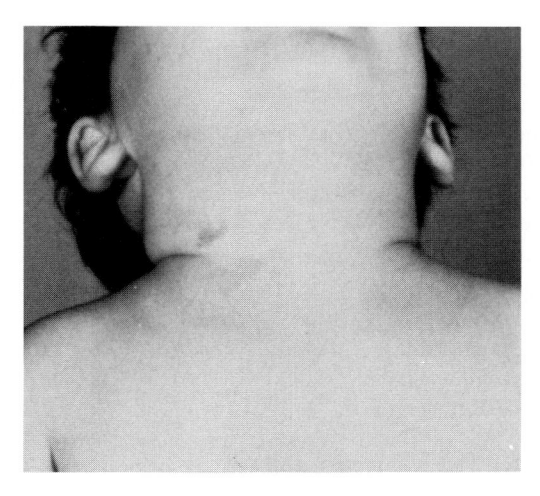

Fig. 35-16. Epidermal nevus on the right side of the neck in a child with hemihypertrophy.

3. Large, cerebriform, linear, ochre-orange lesions involving the scalp and associated with verrucous linear lesions elsewhere (including the mucous membranes). Pigmentary disorders and vascular nevi are often found in these patients.
4. A diffuse scaly eruption with a feathered, whorled, or marbled appearance.
5. Velvety hyperkeratotic areas over the extensor surfaces of hands and feet as well as in the skin folds and associated with profound mental retardation (benign congenital acanthosis nigricans).
6. A small papillomatous yellow or pink growth on the scalp, forehead, or face (simple sebaceous nevus and syringocystadenoma papilliferum). Since a significant incidence of basal cell epitheliomas occurs in these lesions, they should be studied histologically. Once the diagnosis has been established, they should be removed surgically.

The treatment of large verrucous epidermal nevi is generally unsatisfactory. The only effective treatment necessitates removal of the lesion, together with its underlying dermis. In localized lesions this may be accomplished by electrodesiccation and plastic repair; but this treatment should be delayed beyond the neonatal period, since lesions may develop over a period of years. The scars that result from surgery may be as cosmetically unsatisfactory as the original lesions, and an extension of the nevus may appear beyond the repaired area. In the older child salicylic acid (3% in cold cream) may keep the lesion soft, and water-dispersible bath oils provide some palliative relief. When the nails are involved, no treatment is effective, and aside from filing or avulsion of the affected nails, none is indicated.

The epidermal nevus syndrome

Solomon and co-workers reviewed the associated findings in 23 patients with large epidermal nevi, including all the types previously described. In more than two thirds of these patients they found associated skeletal defects, ocular and vascular anomalies, and serious CNS disease. The anomalies found included kyphoscoliosis, vertebral defects, short limbs, osseous hypertrophy, angiomas of skin and CNS, mental retardation, ocular complications, Wilms' tumor, vitamin D–resistant rickets, and convulsive disorders (Fig. 34-16). On discovering the existence of an epidermal nevus, the physician must take a careful family history and perform a thorough physical examination. Particular emphasis should be placed on the musculoskeletal and nervous systems, as well as on the eyes and skin. These infants may require baseline and periodic electroencephalographic studies, psychologic testing of intellectual development, periodic radiographic evaluation of skeletal growth, and renal studies to exclude tumor and inappropriate excretion of phosphate. Cutaneous angiomas in these patients should be removed.

ECZEMA

The term *eczema* is a source of confusion. For the purposes of this discussion eczema is a genus of skin disorder of which there are several species (for example, eczematous contact dermatitis). There are four phases of eczema, any one of which may persist as the dominant feature, depending on the age of the patient, the local physiologic characteristics of the skin involved, and the persistence of the underlying cause. The initial stage is *erythema*, which proceeds to microvesicle formation, *weeping*, or oozing. The epidermal response to the injurious process then causes a burst of rapid epidermal mitotic activity that leads to *scaling*. Finally, *lichenification* (thickening of the skin) and *pigmentary disturbances* supervene. In the young infant the first three stages predominate; lichenification is not seen.

Although the eczematous eruption itself is not difficult to recognize, it may be quite difficult to distinguish one type of eczema from another, particularly because the histologic features (spongiosis) in most of them are identical. The most common causes of eczema in the adult are least common in the newborn. Eczema is much less common in the neonatal period than in the infant older than 2 months. During the neonatal period eczema may be exogenous or endogenous. The exogenous causes include primary irritant contact dermatitis and infection. The endogenous group may be divided into those causes in which the skin's role is predominant and others in which the eruption reflects a serious systemic disease.

Primary irritancy (as opposed to allergy) is probably the most common exogenous cause of eczema in the newborn. The distribution of the eruption varies somewhat, depending on the precipitating agent. Saliva may be irritating to the face, and fecal excretions irritating to the buttocks. Detergent bubble bath, antiseptic proprietary agents, and harsh soaps containing mercury, phenol, tars, salicylic acid, or sulfur may cause an acute eczematous diaper dermatitis, which may become generalized. Precise information about what has been applied to the skin is imperative in making an accurate diagnosis.

When exogenous agents have been excluded as a cause of the eruption and the infant is otherwise quite well, several diagnoses may be entertained. One of these is *seborrheic eczema (seborrheic dermatitis)*. This condition is characterized by greasy scaling associated with patchy redness, fissuring, and occasional weeping, usually involving the scalp, ears, and perineal folds (Fig. 34-17). There is controversy as to whether seborrheic eczema is a distinct entity or whether it presages the advent of atopic dermatitis. Some infants never progress beyond the seborrheic phase of the dermatitis or develop the other features of atopic dermatitis, which in its classic form rarely is seen in the first month. *Cradle cap* is probably a minor variant of seborrheic eczema. The usual course of seborrheic eczema is one of rapid regression after 1 or 2 weeks of therapy. Occasionally a seborrheic-like process may involve the entire body, resulting in a full-blown exfoliative dermatitis (Fig. 34-18). This has been called *Leiner's disease*. Leiner's disease is associated with a defect in the function of the fifth component of complement (C5) in a few infants. Scaling also may result from staphylococcal scalded skin syndrome

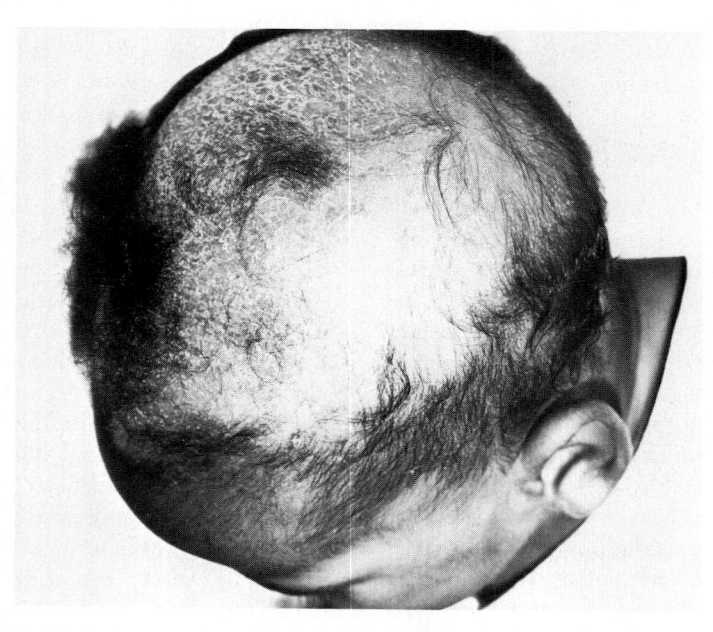

Fig. 34-17. Seborrheic dermatitis on the scalp of an infant resulting in partial alopecia.

or congenital ichthyosiform erythroderma (p. 945).

From the preceding discussion it should be clear that diaper dermatitis may have a variety of causes. Its proper management should include culture of the exudate for bacteria and yeast, the discontinuance of all ointments containing irritants, and conservative treatment for 1 or 2 weeks (see next section). If no improvement follows, a skin biopsy may be indicated.

Eczema also may be a feature of a number of systemic conditions, including histiocytosis X, Wiskott-Aldrich syndrome, ataxia-telangiectasia, X-linked agammaglobulinemia, phenylketonuria, gluten-sensitive enteropathy, and long-arm 18 deletion syndrome. Many patients with anhidrotic ectodermal dysplasia have an eczematous eruption identical to atopic dermatitis.

Topical treatment of eczema

When bacterial or fungal infection exists, appropriate antibacterial or antifungal therapy is indicated, based on the results of culture and sensitivity studies. Weeping lesions should be treated by compressing or bathing in tepid water; protective ointments (such as simple zinc oxide paste) and nonmedicated powders (such as talc) should be applied after each diaper change; soiled ointments and pastes should be removed with mineral oil. A more extensive eruption may be treated for short periods with 1% hydrocortisone cream. A scaly eruption in the scalp may be treated by frequent shampooing with a sulfur- or salicylic acid–containing shampoo. Bathing should be done in tepid water containing a water-dispersible oil. Infants with diffuse dermatitis lose heat readily and are intolerant of even mild changes in environmental temperature or humidity. Therefore humidification of the bedroom in winter and air conditioning in summer are desirable.

SUBCUTANEOUS AND INFILTRATIVE DERMATOSES
Juvenile xanthogranuloma

One fifth of infants with juvenile xanthogranuloma are affected at birth, and two thirds have onset of lesions before 6 months of age. There is no predilection for race or sex; no familial predisposition has been noted for this self-limiting disorder, which usually remains confined to the skin. The skin lesions often are restricted to the head, neck, and upper trunk and typically are reddish yellow, small papules, which may enlarge to become nodules (Fig. 34-19). Involution may leave a flat atrophic pigmented scar. Serum lipids are normal, but histologically the lesions result from an infiltrate of fat-laden histiocytes, giant cells, and mixed inflammatory cells. Ocular lesions are the most frequent complication (although rarely involvement of other organs may occur) and may result in ocular tumors, unilateral glaucoma, hyphema, uveitis, heterochromia iridis, and proptosis. Ophthalmologic consultation is required for management of the ocular lesions, but the best treatment for the skin lesions is expectant observation.

Mastocytosis

Mast cell disease may be present at birth and result in a solitary mast cell tumor, a disseminated maculopapular or nodular eruption, a bullous eruption, or a diffuse infiltration in the skin. The disseminated form may be com-

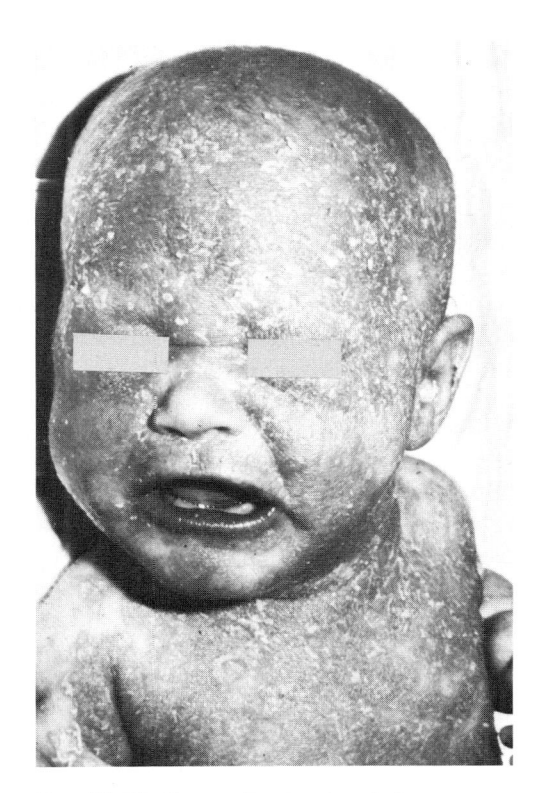

Fig. 34-18. Generalized seborrheic eczema.

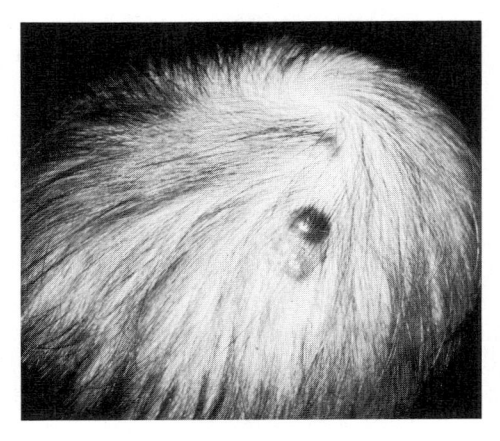

Fig. 34-19. Multiple papulonodular lesions of juvenile xanthogranuloma on the scalp.

plicated by mast cell infiltrates in internal organs. The most common form noted at birth is the firm, solitary mast cell tumor. These are generally ovoid and pink or tan and rarely exceed 6 cm in diameter. The lesions are conspicuous by their tendency to form wheals when rubbed and, in the newborn, to develop overlying blisters. Solitary lesions involute spontaneously within months to years. The maculopapular or nodular forms often become manifest in later infancy. Systemic manifestations of histamine release and residual cutaneous brown patches may be present. Treatment of disseminated forms should aim at control of the manifestations of excess histamine release, (for example, codeine, morphine and its derivatives, aspirin, and polymyxin B), and frequent monitoring for spread of the disease. Some of the distressing cutaneous symptoms, such as dermographism and pruritus, may be palliated with cyproheptadine. Hot water bathing and vigorous toweling must be avoided. The prognosis for most patients with mastocytosis, even in its disseminated cutaneous form, is good. The genetics of this condition are not clear. A few pedigrees have been reported with more than one affected family member.

Subcutaneous fat necrosis and sclerema neonatorum

Both subcutaneous fat necrosis and sclerema neonatorum occur within the first 3 months of life. Recently it has been suggested that they may be variants of the same basic disorder of fat metabolism. Sclerema neonatorum usually affects the preterm or debilitated newborn. It is manifested by diffuse hardening of the subcutaneous tissue, resulting in a tight, smooth skin that feels bound to the underlying structures. The skin is cold and stony hard. The joints become immobile and the face masklike. The affected infant also may have multiple congenital anomalies or develop sepsis, pneumonia, or severe gastroenteritis. CNS abnormalities, autonomic dysfunction, and respiratory distress frequently complicate the course of the disease. The mortality is high, but the cutaneous changes rarely last longer than 2 weeks if the infant survives. Exchange transfusion and systemic administration of steroids have been used in severely ill infants, but their efficacy has not been confirmed.

The lesions of subcutaneous fat necrosis are localized and sharply circumscribed (p. 217). They may appear as small nodules or large plaques and are found on the cheeks, buttocks, back, arms, and thighs. The affected tissue is hard, may appear reddish or violaceous, and occasionally has the texture of an orange peel. Histologically there is a granulomatous reaction in the fat, with foreign body giant cells, fibroblasts, lymphocytes, and histiocytes. Resolution of the lesion results in fibrosis. Possible precipitating causes of fat necrosis include cold exposure, trauma, asphyxia, and peripheral circulatory collapse. Usually the lesions resolve in several weeks or months without complications. Rarely calcium may be deposited in the lesion, leading to ulceration and drainage. Local drainage of calcified areas may lessen subsequent scarring.

Cold panniculitis

Cold-induced fat necrosis of the cheeks may occur in the small infant. Warm, red, indurated plaques appear a few hours to a few days following the episode of cold exposure. The lesions resolve in 2 to 3 weeks. An ice cube applied to normal skin of these patients for 2 minutes will result in formation of a nodule at the site of application. The induced nodule appears in 3 to 72 hours and parallels the course of the spontaneous lesion. The histologic picture is one of perivascular inflammation and aggregation of lipids from rupture of fat cells. Postinflammatory hyperpigmentation may mark the site of a healed nodule.

MISCELLANEOUS CONGENITAL DISEASES AFFECTING THE SKIN

A multitude of hereditary diseases affect the skin. Some of the congenital diseases that have outstanding cutaneous findings are reviewed.

Focal dermal hypoplasia (Goltz's syndrome)

Focal dermal hypoplasia is a profound mesodermal and ectodermal deficiency syndrome that appears to be inherited as an X-linked or simple dominant, mutant gene. The cutaneous lesions consist of linear streaks of atrophy, yellow-brown or red excrescences—some papillomatous and others with the appearance of partially deflated balloons—perioral and perianal papillomas, pigmentary variability, telangiectasia, sweating deficits as well as excesses, hyperkeratosis, abnormalities in the quality and density of hair, and vascular instability. There is almost complete absence of the dermis and its appendages; herniations of fat that lie just beneath the epidermis result in the characteristic yellow saclike nodules and papules. Associated with the cutaneous features are skeletal defects (spinal anomalies, microcrania, asymmetry of facial bones, absence of digits, syndactyly, phocomelia, and rib, scapular, clavicular, and pelvic anomalies), ocular anomalies (ranging from enophthalmia to minor pigmentary defects of the iris), dental anomalies, renal defects, CNS defects (mental retardation and seizures), and a variety of other soft tissue abnormalities affecting heart, stomach, rectum, and muscle.

Cutis laxa (generalized elastolysis)

There are two major forms of congenital cutis laxa: one inherited as an autosomal dominant trait and the other

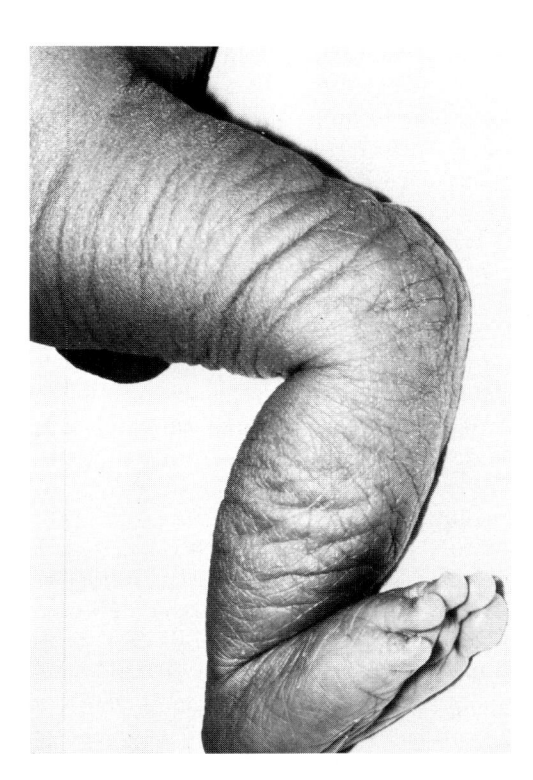

Fig. 34-20. Redundant skin on the leg of a neonate with cutis laxa and dwarfism.

inherited in an autosomal recessive manner (Fig. 34-20). In both forms of the disease affected infants have diminished resilience of the skin, which hangs in folds and results in a bloodhound appearance, at once pathetic and aged. The joints do not show hypermobility, and there is no tendency to increased bruising as in Ehlers-Danlos syndrome. Elastic tissue may be greatly diminished in the dermis and is of poor quality. The collagen has normal tensile properties. In the autosomal dominant form there are few complications, and the life span is usually normal. In the recessive type of cutis laxa, elastic fibers elsewhere in the body are defective, resulting in inguinal, diaphragmatic, and ventral hernias, rectal prolapse, diverticula of the GI and genitourinary tracts, pulmonary emphysema, and aortic aneurysms. Cardiorespiratory complications may cause death during childhood. An X-linked recessive form of cutis laxa also has been described. These patients had mild hyperextensibility of the joints and bladder diverticula in addition to lax skin.

Cutis hyperelastica (Ehlers-Danlos syndrome)

There are eight clinical forms of Ehlers-Danlos syndrome with the common features of hyperextensible skin, joint laxity, and soft tissue fragility. In addition, bleeding episodes and cardiovascular complications are characteristic of some forms of the disorder. The skin of patients with Ehlers-Danlos syndrome is hyperextensible when stretched but snaps back with normal resiliency. In contrast to cutis laxa, the skin does not hang in redundant folds, the joints are extremely hypermobile, and there is a tendency to bruise easily. Associated findings include short stature, scoliosis, periodontosis, and eye defects. Involvement of the GI tract may lead to episodes of acute blood loss. Aortic aneurysms also may develop. All forms of the disease are inherited; some are autosomal dominant traits, others are autosomal recessive, and one form is X-linked. Biochemical studies have confirmed specific enzyme defects for types IV, V, VI, and VII.

THE ECTODERMAL DYSPLASIAS
Anhidrotic (hypohidrotic) ectodermal dysplasia

Absence of sweating, hypotrichosis, and defective dentition are the most striking features of this disorder, which is usually inherited in an X-linked recessive fashion. The existence of females with the full syndrome suggests that an autosomal recessive gene may cause the same phenotype. The facies is distinctive because of frontal bossing and depression of the bridge of the nose. Eyebrows and lashes are absent or sparse. The skin around the eyes is wrinkled and frequently hyperpigmented. The skin elsewhere is thin, dry, and hypopigmented, and the cutaneous vasculature is prominent. The scalp and body hair is sparse and the ears and chin prominent. The lips are thick and everted and may show pseudorhagades. Dental anomalies range from total anodontia to hypodontia with defective teeth.

The most striking physiologic abnormality is the absence of sweating, which can be demonstrated by application to the palm of 1 drop of 5% *O*-phthalaldehyde in xylene. Absence of eccrine glands is confirmed by skin biopsy. Other glandular structures also may be absent or hypoplastic. Less constant ancillary findings include conductive hearing loss, gonadal abnormalities, stenotic lacrimal puncta, corneal dysplasia, and cataracts. Mental development is usually normal, but some degree of retardation has been seen in selected patients. Marked heat intolerance is caused by an inability to adequately regulate the body temperature by sweating. Fever occurs with increases in ambient temperature and exercise and should respond quickly to environmental cooling and rest. Some febrile reactions, however, may be caused by recurrent upper respiratory tract infections, since the respiratory mucosa also may be deficient in mucus-secreting glands. Viral respiratory tract infections in these patients tend to linger and become complicated by secondary bacterial infections in the bronchial tree. Every effort should be made to moderate extreme environmental temperatures by air conditioning. Deficient lacrimation can be palliated by the regular use of artificial tears. The nasal mucosa also must be protected by intermittent saline irrigations and application of petrolatum. It is imperative that these children have a thorough dental evaluation during the first years of life, and prostheses should be provided even for toddlers so that adequate nutrition is maintained. Reconstructive procedures can be performed later in life to improve the facial configuration. A wig may be required for patients with scant scalp hair.

The incidence of atopic diseases—asthma, allergic rhinitis, and atopic dermatitis—is increased significantly in patients with anhidrotic ectodermal dysplasia. They also have a decrease in T-cell function, which may contribute to the lingering viral respiratory tract infections from which they suffer. Atopic manifestations should be managed as they would be in otherwise normal infants and children.

Other types of ectodermal dysplasia include hidrotic ectodermal dysplasia, the EEC syndrome (ectrodactyly, ectodermal dysplasia, and cleft palate), and the Ellis–van Creveld syndrome. Isolated lack of sweat glands occurs in familial and congenital familial anhidrosis.

DIAGNOSTIC TECHNIQUES
Punch biopsy technique

Cutaneous punch biopsy may provide valuable information and is a frequently used diagnostic procedure. It is advisable to have someone hold the infant while a second person performs the procedure. Biopsy should be avoided around the eyelids and their margins, the tip and bridge of the nose, the cupid's bow of the lips, the columella of the upper lip, and the nipples. Hairy areas should be shaved. The site should be washed with soap and water; 70% alcohol is also desirable but should not be used around the eyes or genitalia. The area is infiltrated with 0.5 to 1 ml of 1% lidocaine hydrochloride without epinephrine. A sharp 3-mm punch is pressed firmly against the lesion and gently rotated until a slight give is felt. The punch is then removed. Very little effort is required to penetrate a newborn's skin. Considerable gentleness and a sharp punch are required so that the epidermis is not torn away from the dermis in performing the biopsy, particularly in the blistering diseases. It is desirable to obtain some subcutaneous fat with each biopsy. Newborn fat generally will separate quite readily. One may cut the plug away from the underlying tissue with a sharp scissors. The tissue should not be squeezed. Usually no sutures are necessary, and a simple dressing will suffice for the healing period.

The specimen should be placed in a bottle containing 10% aqueous buffered formaldehyde solution (Formalin), the cap closed, and the bottle agitated to ensure that the skin plug is immersed in the formaldehyde solution. The bottle then should be labeled as to name, date, and site of biopsy. Clinical information should be included with the specimen sent to the pathologist. It is often desirable in a general pathology laboratory to inform the pathologist that a skin biopsy from an infant is being forwarded so that special care may be taken in the processing. Tiny specimens are easily lost during the gross examination or in automated tissue-processing devices.

PRINCIPLES OF THERAPY

Treatment of the skin of the newborn requires adjustment from the adult dosage of topical medicaments. The following guidelines are useful:

1. Minor fleeting erythematous macular or papular eruptions occur at the end of the first month. Their cause is unknown, and the best treatment is patience.
2. The more severe a dermatitis, the more vulnerable is the skin, and therefore the more conservative should be the topical therapy.
3. To treat appropriately and to induce confidence in the infant's family, one should know the natural course of a skin disease and so advise the parents.
4. Systemic complications of diffuse cutaneous eruptions occur more readily in infants; they should be anticipated and treated early.
5. If lesions in different stages are present on different parts of the body surface, treat the most acute stage.
6. It is best to know and use a few topical remedies. Plain tap water is one of the safest and most helpful treatments for any acute dermatitis.

7. Pruritus is often more trying for parents than for the infant. Environmental control of temperature and humidity and mild sedation is quite helpful for uncomplicated pruritus.
8. The passage of time is the most effective treatment of small, uncomplicated cavernous hemangiomas.
9. Hexachlorophene should not be used on damaged skin, if at all.
10. Normal skin does not need extensive lubrication. If lubrication is desirable, it is better to use a cream (for example, hydrophilic ointment) than an oil.
11. Removal of a protective paste from the perineal area should be done gently with mineral oil, not by scrubbing with soap and water.
12. Lotions, pastes, talc, and ointments should not be used on weeping lesions.
13. Occlusive dressings (such as polyethylene film or Saran Wrap) should not be used in this age group.
14. Daily shampoos are not harmful if used to treat seborrheic dermatitis.
15. Exposure to sunlight should be very gradual, especially in fair-skinned infants.
16. Topical anesthetics, proteolytic enzymes, and tar ointments are rarely indicated in this age group.

Nancy B. Esterly
Lawrence M. Solomon

BIBLIOGRAPHY

Alper, J., Holmes, L.B., and Mihm, M.C., Jr.: Birthmarks with serious medical significance: nevocellular nevi sebaceous nevi, and multiple cafe au lait spots, J. Pediatr. 95:696, 1979.

Baden, H.P., Goldsmith, L.A., and Lee, L.D.: The fibrous proteins in various types of ichthyosis, J. Invest. Dermatol. 65:228, 1975.

Barman, J.M., and others: The first stage in the natural history of the human scalp hair cycle, J. Invest. Dermatol. 48:138, 1967.

Beighton, P.: The dominant and recessive forms of cutis laxa, J. Med. Genet. 9:216, 1972.

Briggaman, R.A., and Wheeler, C.E., Jr.: Epidermolysis bullosa dystrophica-recessive; a possible role of anchoring fibrils in the pathogenesis, J. Invest. Dermatol. 65:203, 1975.

Brown, A.C., and others: A congenital hair defect; trichoschisis with alternating birefringence and low sulfur content, J. Invest. Dermatol. 54:496, 1970.

Brown, S.H., Jr., Neerhout, R.C., and Fonkalsrud, E.W.: Prednisone therapy in the management of large hemangiomas in infants and children, Surgery 71:168, 1972.

Carr, A., and others: Relationship between erythema toxicum and maturity, Am. J. Dis. Child. 112:129, 1966.

Champion, R.H.: Disorders of sweat glands. In Rook, A., Wilkinson, D.S., and Ebling, F.J.G., editors: Textbook of dermatology, ed. 3, Philadelphia, 1979, F.A. Davis Co.

Cleaver, J.E.: Xeroderma pigmentosum; progress and regress, J. Invest. Dermatol. 60:374, 1973.

Davis, J., and Solomon, L.M.: T-cell dysfunction in anhidrotic ectodermal dysplasia, Acta Derm. Venereol. (Stockh.) 56:115, 1976.

Deutsch, T.A., and Esterly, N.B.: Elastic fibers in fetal dermis, J. Invest. Dermatol. 65:320, 1975.

Elias, P.M., Fritsch, P., and Epstein, E.H., Jr.: Staphylococcal scalded skin syndrome, Arch. Dermatol. 113:207, 1977.

Esterly, N.B.: The ichthyosiform dermatoses, Pediatrics 42:990, 1968.

Fost, N.C., and Esterly, N.B.: Successful treatment of juvenile hemangiomas with prednisone, J. Pediatr. 72:351, 1968.

Glimcher, M.E., Kostick, R.M., and Szabo, G.: The epidermal melanocyte system in newborn human skin; a quantitative histologic study, J. Invest. Dermatol. 61:344, 1973.

Gordon, J.: Miliary sebaceous cysts and blisters in the healthy newborn, Arch. Dis. Child. 24:286, 1949.

Gorlin, R.J., and Pindborg, J.J.: Syndromes of the head and neck, New York, 1964, McGraw-Hill Book Co.

Green, M., and Behrendt, H.: Sweating capacity of neonates, Am. J. Dis. Child. 118:725, 1969.

Griffiths, A.D.: Skin desquamation in the newborn, Biol. Neonate 10:127, 1966.

Harris, J.R., and Schick, B.: Erythema neonatorum, Am. J. Dis. Child. 92:27, 1956.

Holbrook, K.A., and Odland, G.F.: The fine structure of developing human epidermis; light, scanning, and transmission electron microscopy of the periderm, J. Invest. Dermatol. 65:16, 1975.

Holden, K.R., and Alexander, F.: Diffuse neonatal hemangiomatosis, Pediatrics 46:411, 1970.

Horsefield, G.J., and Yardley, H.J.: Sclerema neonatorum, J. Invest. Dermatol. 44:326, 1965.

Jacobs, A.H., and Walton, R.G.: The incidence of birthmarks in the neonate, Pediatrics 58:212, 1976.

Kondo, J., Sakurai, S., and Sarai, Y.: New types of exfoliation obtained from staphylococcal strains belonging to phage groups other than group II, isolated from patients with impetigo and Ritter's disease, Infect. Immun. 10:851, 1974.

Kraemer, K.H.: Xeroderma pigmentosum; a prototype disease of environmental-genetic interaction, Arch. Dermatol. 116:541, 1980.

Mackenzie, I.C.: Ordered structure of the epidermis, J. Invest. Dermatol. 65:45, 1975.

McKusick, V.A.: Heritable disorders of connective tissue, ed. 4, St. Louis, 1972, The C.V. Mosby Co.

Melish, M.E., and Glasgow, L.A.: Staphylococcal scalded skin syndrome; the expanded clinical syndrome, J. Pediatr. 78:958, 1971.

Montagna, W., and Parakkal, P.F.: The structure and function of skin, ed. 3, New York, 1974, Academic Press, Inc.

Mortenson, O., and Strougard-Andresen, P.: Harlequin color change in the newborn, Acta Obstet. Gynecol. Scand. 38:352, 1959.

Mosher, D.B., Fitzpatrick, T.B., and Ortonne, J.P.: Abnormalities of pigmentation. In Fitzpatrick, T.B., and others, editors: Dermatology in general medicine, New York, 1979, McGraw-Hill Book Co.

Muller, S.A.: Alopecia; syndromes of genetic significance, J. Invest. Dermatol. 60:475, 1973.

Nachman, R.L., and Esterly, N.B.: Increased skin permeability in preterm infants, J. Pediatr. 79:623, 1971.

Neldner, K.H., and Hambridge, K.M.: Zinc therapy of acrodermatitis enteropathica, N. Engl. J. Med. 292:879, 1975.

Pardo-Costello, V., and Pardo, O.A.: Diseases of the nails, ed. 3, Springfield, Ill., 1960, Charles C Thomas, Publisher.

Perera, P., Kurban, A.K., and Ryan, T.J.: The development of the cutaneous microvascular system in the newborn, Br. J. Dermatol. 82 (Suppl. 5):86, 1970.

Ramamurthy, R.S., and others: Transient neonatal pustular melanosis, J. Pediatr. 88:831, 1976.

Reed, W.B., Lopez, D.A., and Landing, B.: Clinical spectrum of anhidrotic ectodermal dysplasia, Arch. Dermatol. 102:134, 1970.

Reed, W.B., and others: Giant pigmented nevi, melanoma and leptomeningeal melanocytosis, Arch. Dermatol. 91:100, 1965.

Robertson, A.F., and Sotos, J.: Treatment of acrodermatitis enteropathica with zinc sulfate, Pediatrics 55:738, 1975.

Rudolph, N., and others: Congenital cutaneous candidiasis, Arch. Dermatol. 113:1101, 1977.

Sagabiel, R.W., and Odland, G.F.: Ultrastructural identification of melanocytes in early human embryos. In Riley, V., editor: Pigmentation; its genesis and biologic control, New York, 1972, Appleton-Century-Crofts.

Samman, P.D.: The nails in disease, ed. 2, London, 1972, William Heinemann Medical Books, Ltd.

Shapiro, L.G., and others: Enzymatic basis of typical X-linked ichthyosis, Lancet 2:756, 1978.

Silvers, D.N., Greenwood, R.S., and Helwig, E.B.: Cafe-au-lait spots without giant pigment granules, Arch. Dermatol. 110:87, 1974.

Simpson, J.R.: Natural history of cavernous haemangiomata, Lancet 2:1057, 1959.

Smeenk, G.: Two families with collodion babies, Br. J. Dermatol. 78:71, 1966.

Smith, D.W.: Recognizable patterns of human malformation, ed. 2, Philadelphia, 1976, W.B. Saunders Co.

Solomon, L.M., and Beerman, H.: Cold panniculitis, Arch. Dermatol. 88:897, 1963.

Somerville, D.A.: The effect of age on the normal bacterial flora of the skin, Br. J. Dermatol. 81:14, 1969.

Tromovitch, T.A., Abrams, A.A., and Jacobs, P.H.: Acne in infancy, Am. J. Dis. Child. 106:230, 1963.

Weary, P.E., Graham, G.F., and Selder, R.F., Jr.: Subcutaneous fat necrosis of the newborn, South. Med. J. 59:960, 1966.

Wessells, N.K.: Differentiation of epidermis and epidermal derivatives, N. Engl. J. Med. 277:21, 1967.

Whitehouse, D.: Diagnostic value of the cafe-au-lait spot in children, Arch. Dis. Child. 41:316, 1966.

Wilkes, T., and others: The sensitivity of the axon reflex in term and premature infants, J. Invest. Dermatol. 47:491, 1966.

Windhorst, D.B., and Padgett, B.: The Chediak-Higashi syndrome and the homologous trait in animals, J. Invest. Dermatol. 60:529, 1973.

Winkelmann, R.K.: The cutaneous innervation of the human newborn prepuce, J. Invest. Dermatol. 26:53, 1956.

Witkop, C.J., and others: Ophthalmologic, biochemical, platelet, and ultrastructural defects in various types of oculocutaneous albinism, J. Invest. Dermatol. 60:443, 1973.

CHAPTER 35 # The eye

An infant usually has contact with only one physician during the neonatal period. It is important therefore for the neonatologist or pediatrician to recognize the subtle eye findings that may help save the eye or the life of the patient. Emphasis is placed on developing the ability to recognize diseases early in their course. Blinding diseases such as congenital glaucoma, ophthalmia neonatorum, exposure of the cornea, or ocular infections will rapidly destroy useful vision unless diagnosed and treated as early as possible. Malignant orbital tumors and retinoblastomas can threaten the life of the neonate. Ocular findings may lead to a diagnosis of a general pathologic condition, such as galactosemia or rubella. A detailed examination is described for detection of occult ocular disease as well as a minimum ocular examination for all neonates. No attempt is made to make the examiner an ocular specialist, since ophthalmic consultation is frequently available if important ocular disease is suspected or discovered. Certain detailed aspects of examination and treatment are included, however, for use in localities where ophthalmic consultation may not be readily available.

The eyes are not completely developed either physiologically or anatomically at birth. They constantly change during the neonatal period. Thus a particular expected ocular reflex or response at an early age may be distinctly abnormal at a later, more mature phase. It is important to recognize the normal findings during different phases of the infant's growth to understand what is abnormal.

EXAMINATION OF THE EYE AND ORBIT

The complete ophthalmologic examination that follows requires 30 to 45 minutes; it can be shortened for the routine examination of all neonates (see following outline). A detailed examination is described for each part of the eye so that maximum information may be obtained if a subtle pathologic condition necessitates a thorough examination or if a patient's history indicates the potential for a pathologic condition in one specific segment of the eye.

MINIMAL OCULAR EXAMINATION SEQUENCE
A. History (including family history), length and possible abnormality of pregnancy, labor, and delivery
B. External examination
  1. Proportional relationship of globes and orbits to surrounding facial structures
  2. Equality of orbit, globe, and cornea to those in fellow eye
  3. Symmetry and normal contour of lids
  4. Ptosis, unilateral or bilateral
  5. Ocular motility (including fixation and following response)
  6. Pupil size, regularity, and response to light
  7. Palpation of the orbital rim and eyelids
  8. Palpation of the lacrimal sac
  9. Inspection of the lid margins and lashes
  10. Inspection of the conjunctival sac (note conjunctival and scleral color)
  11. Corneal size and clarity to the limbus
C. Internal examination
  1. Inspection of anterior chamber depth
  2. Iris, color and clarity of trabeculation
  3. Dilation of the pupils with 1% cyclopentolate (Cyclogyl) hydrochloride and 2.5% phenylephrine (Neo-Synephrine) hydrochloride
  4. Normal black pupil with direct illumination and clear red reflex through the ophthalmoscope
  5. Vitreous clarity
  6. Disc size, contour, and sharpness of detail
  7. Vessels, normal distribution and ratio
  8. Macular area pigmentation
  9. Peripheral retina

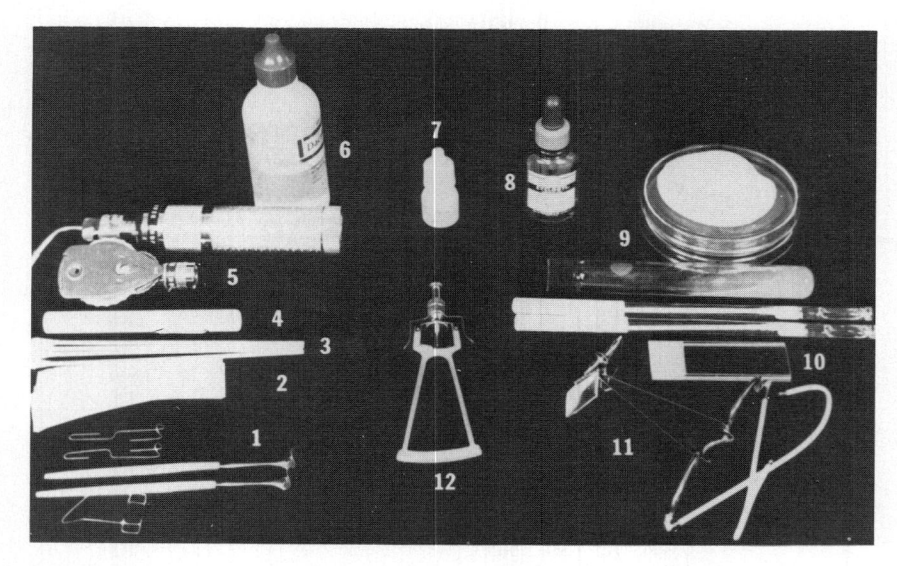

Fig. 35-1. Equipment for ocular examination: *1*, Eye speculum, paper clip retractors or Desmarres' retractors; *2*, fluorescein strips; *3*, sterile cotton-tipped applicator; *4*, penlight or otoscope; *5*, ophthalmoscope; *6*, saline or 5% dextrose irrigation; *7*, 10% phenylephrine, ophthalmic; *8*, 1% cyclopentolate, ophthalmic; *9*, culture tubes and plates, sterile swabs; *10*, glass microscope slides; *11*, loupe; and *12*, Schiøtz tonometer.

An adequate ocular examination should begin with a careful history. A family history of ocular diseases is of considerable importance. For example, a family history of retinoblastoma necessitates a thorough, periodic search of the fundus for the onset of this dominantly inherited malignant disease. Additional important information such as maternal diseases (for example, rubella), injuries, or unusual medications during the prenatal period should be noted. It is important to note the length and possible abnormalities of pregnancy, labor, and delivery; specific attention should be directed to those areas which are suggested by the pertinent history. For example, prematurity suggests the possibility of retrolental fibroplasia (RLF), and difficult delivery with obstetric forceps suggests the possibility of direct ocular trauma.

The examination should be done under comfortable circumstances. The best examining area is a surface at the height of the examiner's waist in a room where the light is bright but can be darkened easily for the intraocular examinations. A blanket should be available to swaddle the infant, and a nurse or assistant should be present to hold the infant's head or expose the eye. Irritating and forceful studies should be deferred until all general observations have been made. A great deal can be learned if the examiner takes a few moments to observe the infant while he or she is undisturbed and in a comfortable position. Observations of spontaneous general and ocular activity are considerably more reliable while the infant is being held or is nursing rather than screaming and crying (Fig. 35-1).

The general facial configuration and the external configuration of the orbit are inspected first. The orbital contents should be proportional and symmetric when compared with the overall craniofacial configuration. The lids are examined grossly and are appraised for symmetry and for both horizontal and vertical positions. The spontaneous opening and closing of the eyes are assessed. If a ptosis is present, particular attention should be paid the size of the pupils. Miosis (a small pupil) on the side of the ptosis is suggestive of Horner's syndrome. A rapid up and down movement of the lid during nursing indicates a Marcus Gunn (jaw-winking) syndrome.

The eyes should be examined for spontaneous range of motion and for conjugate movement. This is best done while the infant is undisturbed and nursing. Fixation and the ability to follow a brightly colored object, the nursing bottle, or a bright light in a dimly lit room should be noted for each eye separately and for both eyes together.

A gross estimate of vision can be obtained at this time. The pupils first should be inspected to see if they are normally round and equal in diameter. A penlight or ophthalmoscope with transilluminating head is used to shine direct light at the pupil, first in one eye and then in the other. Normally each pupil will constrict to both direct and contralateral stimulation. First, the reaction of the illuminated pupil is observed. It should constrict briskly (the response in the neonate may not be as rapid as that in an older child) and should remain constricted as long as the illumination is maintained. If it does not constrict, the contralateral pupil's reaction to the direct illumination of the first eye should be studied. If only the contralateral pupil constricts, the directly illuminated eye must have intact photoreceptors and optic nerve pathways. Failure of constriction in the directly illuminated eye in this instance may be the result of inflammation or paralysis of the iris, which prevents pupillary movement. If neither the illuminated pupil nor the contralateral pupil constricts on subsequent direct illumination), the first eye is deficient in vision and may be blind. Each eye should be tested similarly for both direct and consensual reactions.

Direct light stimulation to one eye normally should produce direct and consensual pupillary constriction. If the light is rapidly shifted to the opposite eye after pupillary constriction, both pupils should remain constricted for as long as the stimulation continues. If, however, the shift of light is followed by dilatation of the newly, directly stimulated eye, the phenomenon of pupillary escape (the Marcus Gunn pupil) has occurred. This indicates decreased vision in the eye whose pupil dilates. Rarely the pupillary reflexes will be completely normal, but the child still will not see because of intracranial abnormalities, particularly in the occipital cortex. This phenomenon is called cortical blindness.

The normal neonate frequently has small, 2-mm pupils that may show some tendency to change size symmetrically and rhythmically (hippus). The phenomenon of hippus rarely has clinical significance.

The pupillary space should be uniformly black. A white reflection of any amount is abnormal and indicates an opacity within the lens, vitreous, or retina.

Examinations that may be annoying to the infant now may be carried out. The lid margins should be inspected for regularity of contour and for the presence of the lacrimal puncta. The lacrimal puncta are seen as two minute holes in the lid margins posterior and medial to the lashes and a short distance lateral from the inner corners of the eyes. The puncta should lie next to the globe but should not be turned either in or out.

Palpation of the orbit should include examination of the orbital margin, the contents of the upper and lower lids, and the round contour of the globes. The orbital rims should be sharp in outline. In the newborn they are initially round and increase more in vertical diameter with the normal growth pattern. The area of the lacrimal sac is palpated for abnormal masses or increase in size and should be pressed against the bones of the nose and medial orbital wall. Expression of mucopurulent or purulent material from the lacrimal puncta should be noted.

To see the lash structures, the examiner should view them with magnification, as with an ocular loupe (which gives 2× to 3× magnification) or through the ophthalmoscope with the +10-diopter lens in place. Normally the lashes are directed outward in an orderly row. Abnormalities are *distichiasis*, or an additional row of lashes posterior to the gray line; *entropion*, an inward turning of the lid; and *trichiasis*, an inward turning of the lashes. Lashes that contact the cornea are dangerous. Continued irritation eventually will predispose the eye to infections of the cornea.

The lids should be separated and the conjunctival sac inspected. Lid separation may be accomplished by the use of a pediatric ocular speculum, lid retractors, or the fingers (Fig. 35-2). A useful lid retractor may be fashioned from a paper clip. The paper clip is straightened out, leaving the two bent ends. One of the ends is bent back on itself approximately ¼ inch from the tip, making a small, hook-shaped process with a rounded tip. All instruments that are introduced into the eye of course, should, be sterilized. The bulbar and palpebral conjunctiva then should be examined for the normal, moist, pinkish appearance. Redness or exudate is abnormal and often indicates infection, which can be confirmed by smear and culture. The conjunctiva of the lids overlying the tarsal plates should be examined by eversion of the lids. Eversion usually occurs quite readily when the lids are separated with fingers, particularly if the infant is attempting to squeeze the lids shut. If eversion of the lids does not occur readily, further attempts probably should not be pursued if the examiner is not an ophthalmologist, since stretching or tearing of the delicate lid structures may occur.

The normal white sclera is inspected for changes of color. Normally a bluish discoloration is present in premature infants and other small babies because of their very thin sclera. The cornea is inspected with a penlight. Magnification with a loupe or with an ophthalmoscope's +10-diopter lens in place is again employed. In premature and full-term infants during the first few days of life the cornea may be somewhat less than transparent, with a slightly hazy appearance. This is thought to be the result of corneal edema, which soon disappears. The surface of the cornea should have good luster, and the whole cornea should be absolutely transparent. A change in luster usually indicates a break or an unevenness in the anterior surface of the cornea, such as an abrasion of the cornea or corneal edema. Transparency should be complete to the extreme periphery of the cornea. Any opacity or translucency is abnormal after the first few days of life. Changes in transparency or opacification of the periphery of the cornea is associated with a local mesodermal abnormality, which may be complicated by congenital glaucoma. The horizontal diameter of the cornea should be approximately 10 mm. However, we have measured a number of apparently normal corneas that are between 9 and 10 mm in full-term infants. The average adult cornea measures 12 mm in the horizontal diameter, and this dimension is achieved during the first year of life. The corneas should be equal in size, however. An

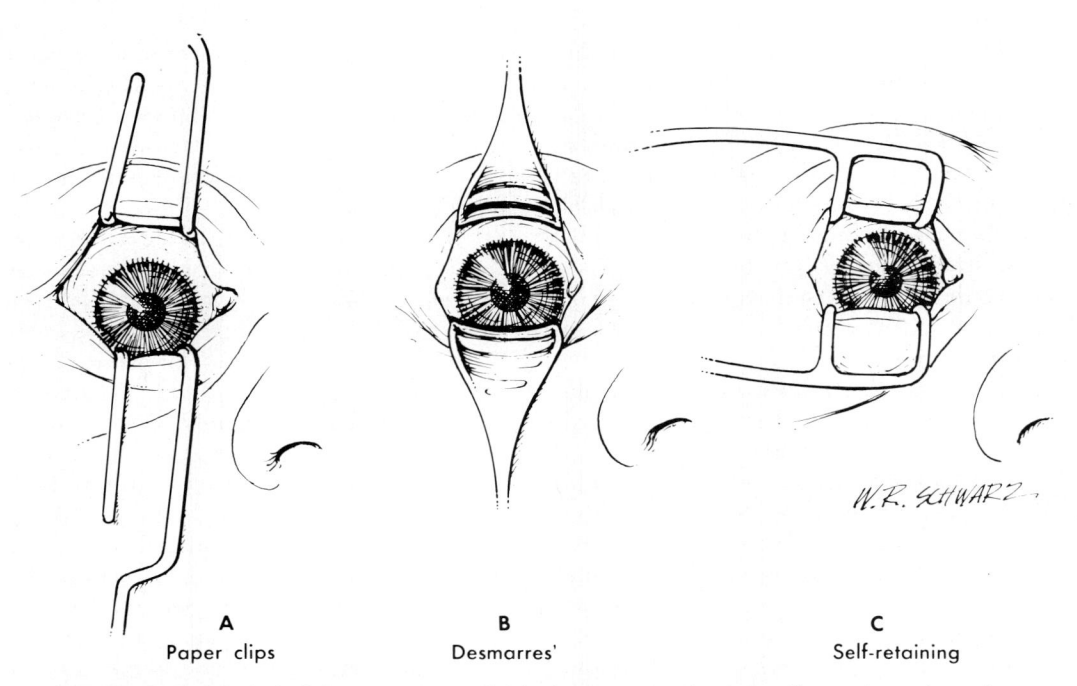

Fig. 35-2. Ophthalmic lid retractors available for eye examinations. Illustrations show the proper application and retraction. **A,** Made from ordinary paper clips; **B,** manual Desmarres' retractor; **C,** self-retaining lid retractor.

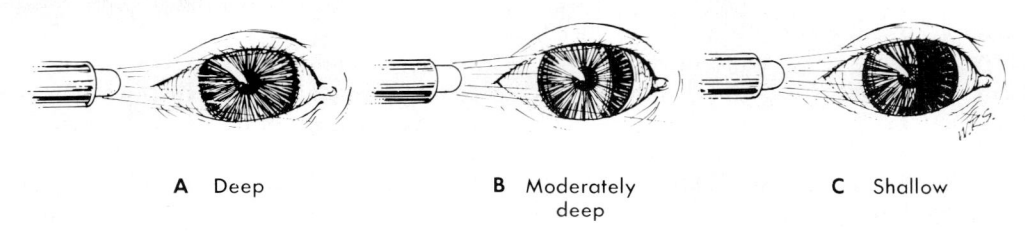

Fig. 35-3. Method of estimating the depth of the anterior chamber with a handlight. **A,** Deep anterior chamber—the iris is flat and completely illuminated by a light at right angles at the lateral canthus. **B,** If the anterior chamber is moderately shallow (less distance from the cornea to the iris), the domed shape of the iris casts a crescentlike shadow nasally; the shallower the depth, the more shadow. **C,** With an extremely shallow anterior chamber the entire nasal iris is in shadow.

accurate measurement of the cornea usually is unnecessary at this time. If congenital glaucoma is suspected because of corneal haze or enlargement or because of photophobia or tearing, an accurate measurement of corneal diameter and intraocular pressure with the infant under general anesthesia is required.

Next the anterior chamber should be inspected; it should be clear. The depth of the anterior chamber is the distance between the posterior surface of the cornea and the anterior surface of the iris. The simplest method of estimating the depth of the anterior chamber involves illuminating the iris at a right angle to the observer's line of sight; that is, the light source is directed from the temporal side in the plane of the iris (Fig. 35-3). Normally the neonate has a moderately shallow chamber. As a result of flattening of the lens and the increase in corneal diameter during the eye's growth, the anterior chamber increases in depth, and the iris flattens during the first year of life.

Normal irises are generally equal in color. Iris pigmentation is normally incomplete for the first 6 months of life; both irises develop pigmentation at the same time. The normal white infant's iris lacking pigment is blue or blue-gray for the first few weeks or months of life, whereas darkly pigmented whites and darker races may show pigmentation at birth or within the first week. *Heterochromia*, or dissimilarity in pigmentation between the two eyes, may indicate a normal hereditary pattern, congenital Horner's syndrome, or several syndromes, which are discussed later in this chapter. These may not develop until the end of the neonatal period or even later in life when full pigmentation of the iris normally occurs.

The normal lens should be clear and appear black in direct light. The red reflex through the ophthalmoscope should show no dullness or irregularities.

The fundus examination should be conducted in a dimly lit room with the infant's pupils dilated. The pupils may be safely dilated in a newborn as well as in premature infants by the use of one drop of 1% cyclopentolate and one drop of 2.5% or 10% phenylephrine. Dark irises take somewhat longer than an average of 20 minutes to dilate fully. Drops may be repeated once or twice if the pupils do not dilate well. Infants with cardiac irregularities, those with extremely flattened anterior chambers, and those with changing neurologic signs should not have their pupils dilated. In actual practice the vast majority of neonates, especially premature infants, can and should have their pupils dilated. Visualizing the fundus of the newborn eye is difficult under any circumstances and is nearly impossible with undilated pupils. The examination with the ophthalmoscope requires the use of an assistant and a small lid speculum to overcome the squeezing of the lids, the inevitable result of shining a strong light in the infant's eye.

Each eye should first be studied with the ophthalmoscope with a +10-diopter lens in place, beginning approximately 5 inches in front of the eye. Because of the sharp plane of focus of a +10-diopter lens, only one plane of depth may be studied with the ophthalmoscope at a given distance from the eye. Thus the ophthalmoscope may be used in a tomographic fashion, first to study the cornea, then the anterior chamber and iris, then the pupil and lens, and finally the anterior vitreous. Each is focused on individually as the examiner moves closer to the patient.

After the lenses in the ophthalmoscope have been changed, the posterior vitreous and the fundus can be seen and studied in detail. In eyes of near-adult anteroposterior length the fundus will be in focus with a zero or low-power lens. Most newborn eyes, especially those of premature infants, have short anteroposterior lengths, and their fundi are sharply in focus with plus diopter lenses.

The optic nerve is the largest and most readily recognized structure in the posterior pole. Its diameter with the usual ophthalmoscope should be approximately half to three fourths the diameter of the total area illuminated at one time. The optic disc is usually round and sharp in outline. It may be normally somewhat oval in its vertical diameter. Excessive elongation, especially inferiorly, may indicate a defect or coloboma of the disc. The disc appears to be larger in the myopic infant and smaller in the hyperopic infant. The optic nerve head or disc has been described as being somewhat more pale in the neonate than in the adult; however, this may be artifact caused by external pressure placed on the globe by the examiner or the assistant, which transmits pressure to blanch the small vessels of the disc. These vessels collapse, producing pallor. The retinal vessels should exit from the disc in the superior and inferior quadrants and should be smooth in outline as they curve diagonally and branch dichotomously to cover the full extent of the retina. Branches usually leave the main vessel at an angle of less than 90 degrees. The arterioles and venules of the retinal circulation should be examined for size, regularity, color, and the presence or absence of pulsation. These should be followed from the disc to the periphery as far as possible in each meridian of the clock. The macular area of the retina, which subserves precise vision and color vision, is located approximately 1½ disc diameters temporal to the disc and is identified normally by a slightly reddish brown color and by the pattern of surrounding blood vessels, which appear to converge toward it. In premature infants the normal macular coloration is usually absent, and in all neonates the foveal reflex is absent until approximately 4 months of age. The normal reddish brown pigment of the macula should be approximately ½ disc diameter in size and should show uniform regularity. Pigment mottling or stippling in the macula or elsewhere is abnormal. The examination of the retina should be continued from the macula as far toward the periphery as possible, noting the regularity of the normal pink-orange color. The far periphery of the retina, especially in the premature infant, appears pale gray and is hazy. This appearance often falsely suggests a retinal detachment. Premature and newborn infants have completely developed pigment epithelium but incompletely developed uveal pigment in the choroid. This gives a pale appearance to the fundus and offers a better view of the choroidal blood vessels, which appear as indistinct, closely packed, red, linear structures. They are broad and randomly interconnected.

Abnormalities of the fundus are located by anatomic distance from the disc, and size is related to fractions or multiples of the disc diameter. Areas of the fundus that appear to be out of focus in comparison to the rest of the surrounding fundus may indicate an elevation or tumor of the retina or underlying tumors of the choroid. Rapid rhythmic motions of the fundus while the examination is in progress may indicate the presence of nystagmus that was not obvious during external inspection.

NORMAL OCULAR FINDINGS

The eye of the newborn differs from the adult eye primarily in function, although structural differences are also present. The growth of the eye parallels that of the brain. Thus growth continues at a rapid rate for the first 3 years of life, especially during the first year. The anteroposterior dimension of the eye at birth is about 16.5 mm and grows to a maximum of approximately 24 mm in adulthood. Seventy percent of the adult eye volume is obtained by the age of 4 years. Normal values in the neonate fall within a very wide range, and possibilities of abnormality in size frequently may be substantiated only by comparison in proportion to nearby structures or by relationship to measured values in the fellow eye.

The lid apertures of the full-term infant are usually quite narrow, often being widely separated horizontally by prominent epicanthal folds. The term *telecanthus* indicates a disproportionate broadening of the medial canthal angles, a frequent finding in neonates. It is particularly noticeable in the fetal alcohol syndrome. Hypertelorism indicates a broadening of the distance between the two pupils; this is infrequent and abnormal. Measurements between the two medial canthi may vary from 18 to 22 mm. Horizontal measurement of the lid apertures varies considerably from 17 to 27 mm. These measurements should be nearly identical in the two eyes of any patient (Table 35-1).

Reflex tearing to irritants should be present shortly after birth. However, emotional tearing usually does not begin until about 3 weeks of age and is universally complete at 2 to 3 months. The latter tearing usually appears concomitantly with the onset of activity of the sebaceous glands of the skin. The newborn possesses a strong blink reflex to light and to stimulation of the lids, lashes, or cornea. The reflex response to a threatening gesture does not appear until 7 or 8 weeks of age.

The eyes should appear straight from birth for the most part. Changes in ocular position should be conjugate during the first few weeks of life. Conjugate gaze is determined by observing the light reflex from a hand light, held in front of the examiner's face to shine in an equal position on the patient's pupils. Erratic, purposeless, and independent movements of the two eyes, however, normally are observed during this period. These movements are comparable to the peripheral muscle activity seen in the extremities at the same time.

Since the macula of the newborn is structurally immature at birth, the capacity for normal acute vision is lacking. The newborn, however, has some central vision.

Retinal function is present at birth. It appears to be cortically integrated as vision, but the extent of this integration is unknown. Electroretinograms in newborns have shown an initial absence of electrical activity, especially to strong stimuli, several hours after birth. We know by the pupillary response to light and by optokinetic responses that impulses travel the visual pathways at birth and participate in visual motor function.

Optokinetics describes the reflex ocular response to a moving target. A pursuit motion occurs as the target moves across the visual field and is followed by a rapid return motion in the opposite direction to regain fixation. This is similar to what occurs while watching telephone poles or fence posts when one is traveling in a fast-moving automobile. It has been determined that, by the use of the optokinetic reflex, the infant is able to receive visual stimuli as early as 1½ hours after birth, and it has been estimated that the visual acuity of the newborn is approximately 20/700. Unfortunately most estimations of acuity rely heavily on adequate motor responses as part of the visual evaluation. Thus immature or underdeveloped motor systems may reduce or interfere with eye or head movement and decrease the accuracy of the visual analysis.

Three distinct ocular rotational reflexes may be elicited in the neonatal period. From birth and thereafter a rapid turning of the head on the shoulders produces an opposite movement of the eyes (Fig. 35-4). The *doll's eye movement* is a reflex elicited by the stretching of cervical muscles and a response by cranial oculomotor nerves and may be normal in blind or brain-damaged infants. The *vestibuloocular reflex* is elicited by holding the infant vertically and rotating the body on its long axis (Fig. 35-5). The resulting eye movement is similar to the doll's eye movement in that the eyes appear to remain stationary while the body moves; that is, longitudinal rotation to the right produces an equal and conjugate ocular rotation to the left. If there is no further rotation of the infant, the eyes return slowly to the primary position. This reflex

Table 35-1. Ocular measurements

Measurement	Full-term newborn (mm)	Premature newborn (1,000-1,300 gm) (mm)
Intermedial canthal distance	18-22	12-16
Medial canthus to lateral canthus	17-27	12-16
Anteroposterior diameter of eye at birth	16	16
Horizontal diameter of cornea	10 (average)	7.5-8 (lower limits)
	9 (lower limits)	

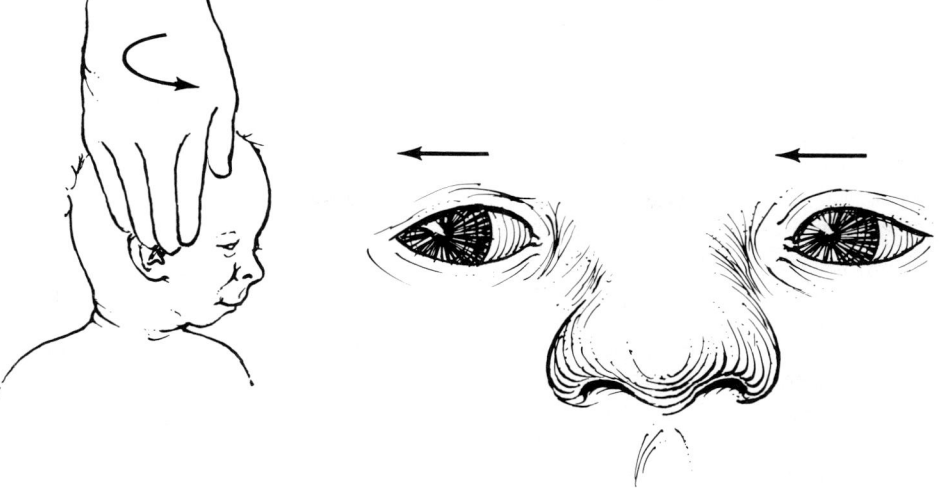

Fig. 35-4. Doll's head rotation. As the head is turned on the shoulders, a tonic neck muscle reflex produces corresponding ocular rotation in the opposite direction, as though the eyes were remaining in their original position as the head moves.

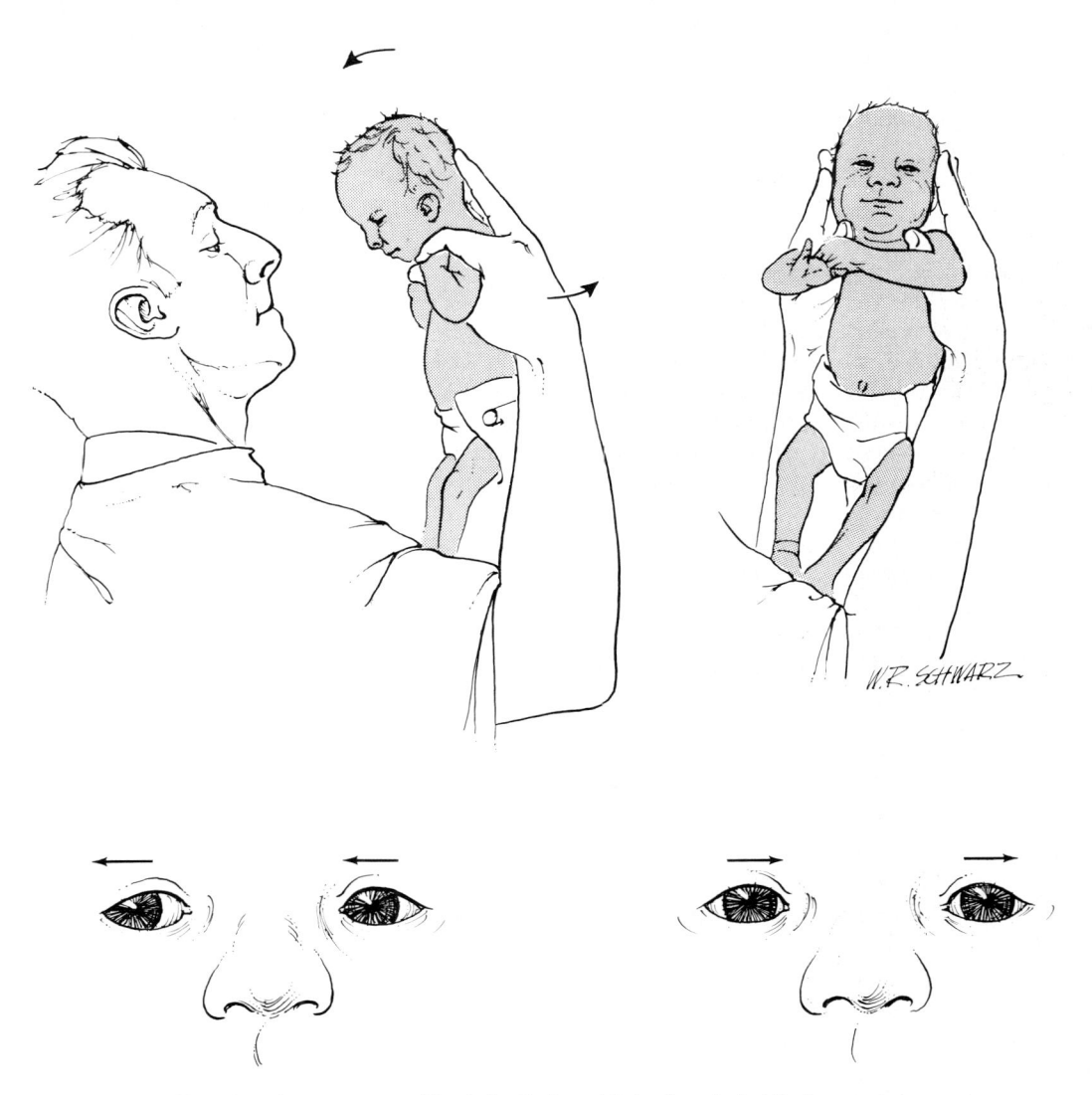

Fig. 35-5. Rotational nystagmus. The infant's head is inclined slightly forward, eyes open. With rotation, the eyes move in the opposite direction, as in doll's head rotation. When rotation stops, the recovery movement occurs in the reverse direction.

relies on functioning higher central nervous system centers and may be reduced in severely brain-damaged infants. Like the doll's eye reflex, it may be normal in blind infants.

A third rotational reflex may be elicited by holding the infant vertically, as in the vestibuloocular reflex. The infant is rotated in an arc on the long axis of the examiner. With the infant's eyes held open, the ocular rotation is first in the direction of the movement (the eyes appear to move more rapidly than the infant and in the same direction as the infant's movement). This latter ocular reflex may be a form of optokinetic nystagmus and appears to be reduced in infants with major defects of the visual system or of the central nervous system. Precise location of this reflex pathway is not known; however, it has been reduced in infants with cortical damage in whom the doll's eye and vestibuloocular reflexes were retained.

Unfortunately all such rotary or postrotary responses must rely on the evaluation of saccadic eye movements. The latter depends in part on the maturation of the motor system, which may be unpredictable in the neonate, and reduced reflex responses may be the fault of the motor system, not the visual system. Thus predictions of decreased sensory function should be made with some caution.

The macula provides central precise vision. The center of the macula is termed the *fovea;* movement of the eyes to project the object of regard onto the fovea is called fixation. The ability to maintain a somewhat unsteady gaze occurs shortly after birth, particularly if a strong light stimulus is used. However, the ability to maintain steady gaze or fixation by following an object and its movement is only weakly initiated at 5 to 6 weeks of age. At first the "following" reflex, in which the eyes pursue a moving visual stimulus, is extremely weak and occurs for only a few degrees of eye movement without any further attempt on the infant's part to locate or direct the eyes toward the target. By 3 months of age the following reflex is fully active. At this time the infant maintains fixation and pursuit movements instantaneously in both vertical and horizontal directions. At approximately 4 months central fixation is associated with the motor activity of grasping. Fusion of the two eyes with convergence ability is present at 6 months of age. The latter functions require visual acuity of approximately 20/40 to 20/60.

Visual acuity cannot be directly measured in the neonatal period. However, the amount of fixation or following ability or both that can be elicited in the infant is an accurate guide to the amount of visual function present. Central, steady fixation requires a visual acuity of at least 20/40 to 20/60. Unsteady fixation indicates an acuity of approximately 20/100. Inability to fixate on a light, even weakly, usually indicates a visual acuity of less than 20/400.

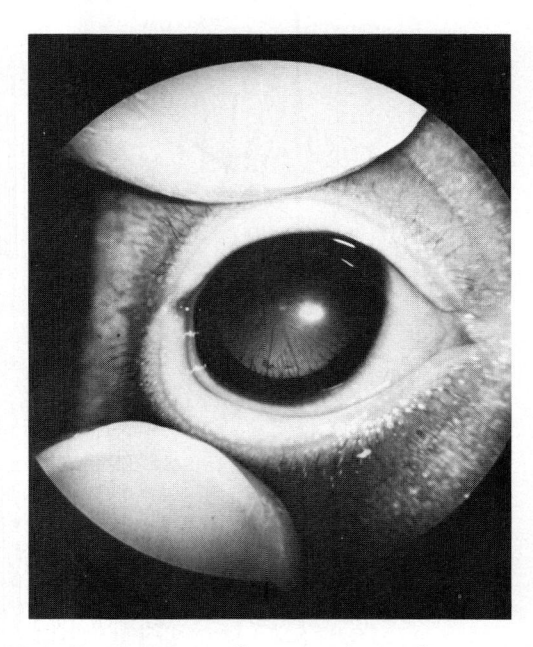

Fig. 35-6. Persistent pupillary membrane in a premature infant. Note the remnants of vascular loops of the anterior hyaloid system anterior to the lens. They will continue to atrophy during the first months of extrauterine life.

Prematurity

Prematurity imposes a number of anatomic and functional handicaps on the newborn, not the least of which involve the ocular structures. At 28 weeks' gestation the normal developmental pupillary membrane is still present and is just beginning to atrophy. The lacrimal canaliculi are growing within the lids but are not yet open. The globe is only 10 to 14 mm in diameter. At the disc Bergmeister's papilla and the hyaloid artery are beginning to atrophy. The anterior and posterior hyaloid systems surrounding the lens frequently are still present at this age. These structures begin to atrophy at the 28-week stage and continue their disappearance during the eighth month of gestation or during the premature infant's early extrauterine existence (Fig. 35-6).

The lens has been noted to have a transient period of cataractous changes in a significant number of premature infants. These have been observed during the second week after birth and persist for approximately 2 weeks. These transient opacities of the lens may be the result of a transient metabolic deficiency, possibly similar to that occurring in galactosemia. At 32 weeks' gestation the fetal nucleus of the lens is complete, but the lens may be hazy or translucent for some weeks. All the retinal layers are developed, but they are thick and gray from the equator to the periphery.

The eyelids usually are separated by this period, but the last stages of separation still may be in progress. The horizontal corneal diameter may be 7.5 to 8 mm, and the distance separating the two canthi may be 14 to 16 mm, with the horizontal lid measurement being approximately 12 to 14 mm.

THE BLIND INFANT

The pediatrician, neonatologist, or general practitioner is usually the first examiner when parents suspect that their infant is blind. This may be an infant whose eyes appear normal during external inspection. A normal ocular examination does not rule out the possibility of blindness resulting from abnormalities lying within the remaining visual pathways between the eye and the occipital cortex. Pupillary responses and doll's eye or rotational nystagmus are normal responses indicating intact subcortical reflexes. The presence of optokinetic nystagmus implies at least one intact visual cortex. Fixation, following, and reaching reflexes indicate bilaterally intact visual cortical pathways. Electroretinography and oculoencephalography (the visually evoked response) may be the only means of detecting an intact retinal function and receipt of stimulation from the retina at the cortex, respectively.

EXAMINATION OF THE BLIND INFANT

A. Subcortical reflexes
   1. Pupillary response
   2. Doll's eye movement
   3. Rotational or vestibular nystagmus
B. Visual cortical pathways
   1. Optokinetic nystagmus
   2. Fixation
   3. Following eye movements
   4. Reaching reflexes
C. Electrical responses
   1. Electroretinography
   2. Visually evoked responses (oculoencephalography)
   3. Electrooculography

REQUESTING OPHTHALMIC CONSULTATION

Routine consultation for all normal infants in the nursery is not recommended. Pathologic ocular findings in this group of neonates are sufficiently rare that ophthalmic evaluation should be requested only for those infants in whom the pediatrician's or neonatologist's ocular examination indicates the presence of an abnormality. Other indications for ophthalmic examination are if the family history indicates the presence of congenital cataracts, if retinoblastoma or congenital glaucoma has been present in family members, if intrauterine infectious disease such as rubella may have occurred in the early prenatal period, or if oxygen therapy has been administered in the neonatal period. It is recommended that the examination for retrolental fibroplasia be done at approximately 4 weeks of age. This is estimated to be the period in which the development of retrolental fibroplasia is at its most active stage.

Infants who are the products of precipitous or difficult deliveries may require a more thorough dilated indirect ophthalmoscopic examination if the neonatologist's examination indicates corneal or scleral injury or retinal hemorrhage.

Subdural hematomas and increased cerebrospinal fluid pressure, as in hydrocephalus, do not produce papilledema in neonates unless there has been premature closure of cranial sutures.

BIRTH TRAUMA

See also Chapter 17.

Eye injuries may be associated with labor and delivery and are found in increasing incidence proportional to the length of labor and difficulty of delivery. *Lid petechiae* and *hemorrhages* frequently are found in face presentations and less frequently in vertex presentations. These usually clear quite rapidly without treatment. *Subconjunctival hemorrhages* also are frequently seen and require no treatment. These findings however, should, increase the suspicion of associated intraocular injuries. Forceps deliveries, particularly when associated with improper application, may produce *lacerations of the lid or the globe*. The presence of a forceps mark or lid laceration requires a careful complete examination of the orbit for associated injuries. Forceps application also may produce *ruptures in Descemet's membrane* of the cornea. These ruptures are seen only with magnification and appear as diagonal lines in the posterior cornea. They are rapidly followed by excess hydration of the cornea, with a subsequent cloudy appearance that must be differentiated from congenital glaucoma, infections of the cornea, or diseases associated with cloudy cornea, such as the mucopolysaccharidoses. Prolonged labor or forceful delivery with forceps also may produce *bleeding into the anterior chamber*. *Retinal hemorrhages* frequently are seen after delivery. These are usually small and multiple and are scattered throughout the retina as small red dots. Notation should be made of any hemorrhage near or in the macular area, since it may be related to subnormal visual acuity and strabismus at a later date. *Retrobulbar hemorrhage* may produce protrusion or proptosis of the globe and must be differentiated from a retrobulbar tumor. Rarely the eye may be completely prolapsed, especially when the orbit is shallow; this constitutes an emergency because of exposure of the cornea and stress on the optic nerve and blood supply.

OCULAR INJURIES

Of prime importance in the treatment of ocular injuries is a full and careful evaluation of the extent of damage, with special reference to the globe itself. Ocular injuries caused by trauma in the neonatal period must be treated with the same meticulous care that is required in the adult. Because of the diminutive size of the neonate's eye, treatment usually requires microscopic evaluation and repair with the infant under general anesthesia. Lid lacerations should receive precise primary repair to minimize permanent deformity. Involvement of the lacrimal canaliculi, the lid margin, and the lacrimal gland requires special attention. Avulsion or tissue loss of the lids necessitates urgent repair to prevent exposure injuries of the cornea.

Blunt injury in the neonate may produce blood in the anterior chamber (hyphema), rupture of the globe, dislocation of the lens, vitreous hemorrhage, contusion cataract, scleral rupture, traumatic retinal detachment, retinal hemorrhages or edema, rupture of the choroid, and arterial or venous occlusion in the retina. Thermal and chemical burns may occur about the eyes and must be treated with extreme care. Treatment of these injuries requires an ophthalmologist after the usual first-aid measures of cooling and protective covering are performed. Of immediate and highest priority in the first-aid management of a chemical burn of the eye is copious irrigation with a noninjurious fluid, such as tap water, milk, or normal saline solution.

Corneal abrasions are more frequent than is realized in the infant and are suggested by a symptom of tearing in one eye. The use of eye bandages during phototherapy has increased the incidence of this complication. Diagnosis is made by staining the cornea with a fluorescein-impregnated paper strip. This is done by moistening a sterile fluorescein strip with a drop of sterile saline solution and touching its tip to the lower conjunctival fornix. The area of corneal abrasion turns light green in ordinary illumination but is best seen in a light with a cobalt blue filter. A corneal abrasion also is suggested when a small shadow cast by the irregular epithelium is seen on the iris surface. This shadow moves with movement of the examining light. Treatment required for healing in most cases is the instillation of antibiotic drops for a few days.

Lacerations may involve the conjunctiva, the cornea, or the sclera. All conjunctival lacerations should be presumed to be associated with a laceration of the globe until proved otherwise. Lacerations of the cornea or sclera require immediate evaluation and surgical repair, even when they are tiny, as in the case of a perforation from a diaper pin.

Orbital or ocular foreign bodies require specialized precise localization to determine the proper therapeutic approach. Fortunately they are rare in the neonate.

ABNORMAL FACIES

See also Chapter 38.

Eye abnormalities associated with congenital anomalies of the face, skull, or head are briefly reviewed in this section. Many abnormalities are so extensive that it is impossible to correct them totally. Treatment therefore is limited to those areas which are currently amenable to surgical correction, such as eyelid deformities, nasal and aural deficiencies, and strabismus.

Apert's syndrome

Acrocephalosyndactyly is a systemic deformity probably caused by a general mesodermal disturbance occurring about the seventh or eighth week of embryonic life. Oxycephaly, affecting primarily the anterior portion of the skull, creates high frontal bones, hypertelorism, and shallow orbits. The condition sometimes is associated with proptosis sufficient to produce corneal exposure and ulceration, exotropia, and ophthalmoplegia. The remainder of the syndrome shows syndactyly in varying degrees, skeletal deformities of the limbs, and varying degrees of mental deficiency (p. 1058).

Cornelia de Lange's syndrome

The typical facial appearance in infants with the Cornelia de Lange syndrome is a low hairline, eyebrows that are joined in the middle (synophrys), long eyelashes, and a small upturned nose. Skeletal deformities may be present, ranging from syndactyly to phocomelia. Eye disorders less frequently include hypertelorism and antimongoloid slant, strabismus, nystagmus, ptosis, high myopia, and pupillary abnormalities. Some patients with this diagnosis resemble children with the fetal alcohol syndrome.

Cretinism (congenital hypothyroidism)

Swollen eyelids, hypertelorism, and an enlarged tongue constitute an early suggestive triad (p. 890).

Crouzon's disease

Craniofacial dysostosis is a herditary abnormality (autosomal dominant) formed in part by premature union of the coronal and lambdoidal sutures, combined with hypoplasia of the maxillary area of the face. This is manifested by prominence at the superior portion of the frontal bone, hypoplasia of the superior maxilla, and shortened orbital cavities, with a prognathic jaw. Ocular defects consist of exophthalmos, exotropia, and progressive optic atrophy.

Facial clefts

Facial clefts are caused by a failure of fusion between the maxillary and lateral nasal processes during fetal development. This creates a line of cleavage between the medial end of the lower lid and the upper lid. Such colobomas may vary in extent from a very small notch to almost total absence of the entire lower lid. Atypical clefts, presumably caused by pressure of amniotic bands, may occur in any direction on the face and may produce a great variety of anomalies. All facial clefts involving colobomas of the lids that prevent lid closure, and therefore cause corneal exposure, require immediate measures to prevent damage to the exposed cornea (p. 1042).

Goldenhar's syndrome

Goldenhar's syndrome is a rare syndrome of oculoauricular dysplasia, characterized by epibulbar dermoid cysts, accessory auricular appendages, and aural fistulas. The characteristic unilateral triad also may be associated with micrognathia, macrostomia, and frequently multiple vertebral anomalies. Other ocular abnormalities less often seen include microphthalmia, microcornea, corneal ulcers, and coloboma of the upper lid. A genetic cause is uncertain.

Greig's hypertelorism

Greig's syndrome is a congenital dysostosis, which is the result of an anomaly in the development of the cranial bones. There is a gross broadening and depression of the nasal bridge, with a prominent forehead. The orbits are widely displaced and are accompanied frequently by external strabismus. Optic atrophy may occur. Proptosis is rare. Mentality is usually normal. There is maxillary hypoplasia.

Hallermann-Streiff syndrome

Oculomandibulofacial dyscephaly is characterized by hypoplasia of the mandibles, a thin, prominent nose, described as a parrot beak, and bilateral microphthalmia often associated with cataracts or microcornea or both. Glaucoma may complicate the eye findings at a later period. This syndrome may be confined to these findings or may be more severe and associated with more generalized anomalies, including atrophy of the facial skin, hypotrichosis, and marked dwarfism with dental and nasal abnormalities, which together give the infant an aged, wrinkled appearance. All cases have been sporadic in their appearance. The causative factors are unknown.

Hemifacial atrophy of Romberg

This unilateral deformity is characterized by hypoplasia of the external ear, occasional extra appendages, and an atrophic middle ear. The maxillary, malar, and palatine bones are most often smaller and flatter than normal with hemiatrophy of the mandible and absence of the zygomatic arch. The soft tissues of the face are hypoplastic and flat, and the fifth and seventh cranial nerves may be paretic. Ocular complications commonly include Horner's syndrome and an antimongoloid slant to the outer canthus. Other associated abnormalities are anophthalmia, heterochromia iridis, ptosis, oculomotor palsies, and nystagmus. The cause is unknown.

Mandibulofacial dysostosis

Also known as the *Treacher Collins* or *Franceschetti syndrome*, this anomaly is a result of inadequate differentiation of the maxillary mesoderm derived from the first branchial arch and is inherited as an irregular autosomal dominant trait. The expression of this abnormality is variable. It is characterized by an antimongoloid obliquity of the fissures, with atypical colobomas of the outer portion of the lower lids. Extraocular abnormalities are hypoplasia of the malar bone and mandible, malformations of the external ears and occasionally of the middle ear, macrostomia with a high palate and dental abnormalities, blind fistulas between the angle of the mouth and the ear, and tongue-shaped projections of the hairline onto the cheek. The Treacher Collins syndrome is differentiated from Goldenhar's syndrome by lateral lower lid colobomas in the former and ocular dermoid cysts and upper lid colobomas in the latter.

Nuclear aplasia

Facial diplegia, or Möbius syndrome, is characterized by a combination of bilateral central paresis of the sixth and seventh cranial nerves. This paresis creates a failure of lateral movements of both eyes, producing esotropia and associated bilateral facial paresis. The syndrome is inherited as an autosomal dominant trait.

Pierre Robin anomalad

The Pierre Robin anomalad is characterized by micrognathia, glossoptosis, and cleft palate. The ocular abnormalities occur in a variety of syndromes and include retinal detachment, microphthalmia, congenital glaucoma, cataracts, and high myopia (p. 1042).

Sturge-Weber syndrome

The association of capillary angiomas of the upper part of the face, the eye, and the leptomeninges forms a triad of signs also called *encephalooculofacial angiomatosis*. The capillary angioma or port-wine stain of the face (nevus flammeus) is typically unilateral and may or may not be confined to the distribution of the first or second division of the trigeminal nerve. Only those angiomas which include the forehead and the upper lid have been implicated in patients with ocular disease. The associated choroidal angioma frequently is located near the disc; it is usually indistinct and difficult to visualize without indirect ophthalmoscopy and fluorescein angiography of the fundus. If present, it may lead to macular edema and decreased visual acuity. There is no apparent hereditary pattern. Congenital glaucoma frequently occurs and, if unrecognized, can lead to irreversible blindness.

Waardenburg's syndrome

The Waardenburg syndrome is transmitted as an autosomal dominant trait and is associated with lateral displacement of the medial canthi, hyperplasia of the medial part of the eyebrows frequently coalescing in the midline, white forelock, heterochromia iridis, and nerve deafness. The fundus also may participate in the heterochromia.

Chromosomal aberrations and deletions
(see also Chapter 37)
The trisomies

Syndromes associated with trisomy of the smaller chromosomes present multiple anomalies that include both facial and ocular findings.

Trisomy 13. Trisomy D, or Patau's syndrome, is manifested by cleft palate, hair lip, polydactyly, umbilical hernia, and malformations of the heart and of the central nervous system. Ocular findings are microphthalmia, colobomas of the iris or choroid, and the occasional presence of intraocular cartilage.

Trisomy 18. Trisomy E is characterized by micrognathia, flexed fingers with the index finger overlapping the third finger, generalized hypertonicity of skeletal muscles, mental retardation, ventricular septal defect, umbilical hernia, rocker-bottom feet, and malrotation of the gut. Ocular abnormalities include corneal opacities, ptosis, strabismus, epicanthal folds, and abnormal orbital ridges. Congenital optic atrophy also has been reported.

Trisomy 21. *Down's syndrome*, or *mongolism*, is a well-recognized entity consisting of mongoloid facies, mental retardation, small obese habitus, and large tongue. The ocular abnormalities associated with this entity are epicanthus, hypertelorism, mongoloid slant of the palpebral fissures, and congenital cataracts. Brushfield's spots are found, frequently at birth, on the unusually thin, lightly colored irises of 85% of such patients. Systemic or topical therapy with atropine may result in unusual and sometimes dangerous systemic responses as well as reactions in the iris of infants with Down's syndrome.

MONGOLOID SLANT
Down's syndrome
Penta-X syndrome
Chromosome 18p− syndrome
Chromosome 18q− syndrome

ANTIMONGOLOID SLANT
Cerebral gigantism
Cornelia de Lange's syndrome
Rubinstein-Taybi syndrome
Treacher Collins syndrome
Chromosome 4p− syndrome
Chromosome 5p− syndrome (cri du chat)
Chromosome 13q− syndrome

Turner's syndrome

Infants with Turner's syndrome caused by aneuploidy of the sex chromosomes (45 chromosomes, a single X), may show ptosis, congenital cataracts, and occasionally corneal nebulae and blue scleras in the neonatal period.

Chromosomal deletions

The loss of deoxyribonucleic acid (DNA) from within a chromosome leads to a variety of syndromes, each more or less characteristic of the specific chromosome involved.

Partial deletion of the short arm of chromosomes 4 (4p−) and 5 (5p−). Infants with chromosome 4p− syndrome have low birth weights, are retarded, and may have spastic diplegia or quadriplegia. They resemble those with the syndrome of partial deletion of the short arm of chromosome 5 (5p−) because of the additional presence of microcephaly, abnormal ears, micrognathia, inguinal hernia, simian crease, and low dermal ridge count. In addition, chromosome 4p− and 5p− syndromes are characterized by antimongoloid palpebral apertures, hypertelorism, ptosis, strabismus, epicanthus, and broad nasal roots. Other features of chromosome 4p− syndrome absent in chromosome 5p− syndrome include midline scalp defect, ocular colobomas, beak-shaped nose, carplike mouth, cleft palate, preauricular or presacral dimple or sinus, hypospadias, and cryptorchidism. Chromosome 5p− syndrome is characterized by a catlike cry (cri du chat). In addition to the aforementioned features, this syndrome also is characterized by decreased tear secretion, refractive errors, tortuous retinal arterioles and venules, optic atrophy, and pupillary supersensitivity to methacholine.

Partial deletion of the long arm of chromosome 13 (13q−). Patients with this syndrome have a unique facial configuration with microcephaly, trigonocephaly, micrognathia, large malformed ears, a wide nasal bridge with hypertelorism, and protruding upper incisors. Ocular abnormalities, which may be profound, include epicanthus, microphthalmia, iris and choroidal colobomas, ptosis, cataracts, antimongoloid palpebral apertures, and retinoblastoma. Although this malignant neoplasm of the retina is inherited characteristically as an autosomal dominant trait, it has been reported in 6 of 11 patients with chromosome 13q− syndrome. Other findings include urogenital, thumb, and congenital cardiac defects.

Partial deletion of the short arm (18p−) and of the long arm (18q−) of chromosome 18. Chromosome 18p− and 18q− syndromes are characterized by mental retardation, short stature, hypertelorism, epicanthal folds, strabismus, and mongoloid or antimongoloid palpebral apertures. Patients with chromosome 18p− syndrome also have micrognathia, dental caries, moon facies, webbed neck, ptosis, flat bridge of the nose, eccentric pupils, cataract, and corneal opacities. In two cases cyclopia has occurred. Patients with chromosome 18q− syndrome also have microcephaly, midface retraction, urogenital and cardiac anomalies, optic atrophy, nystagmus, narrow palpebral apertures, myopic astigmatism, ophthalmoscopic abnormalities, oval pupils, glaucoma, and microcornea.

ABNORMAL EYELIDS
Colobomas

Colobomas of the lids are defects that may vary from a small notch of the lid borders to involvement of the entire length of the lid, either in partial or complete thickness (Fig. 35-7). Most lid colobomas are found in the medial aspect of the upper lid. When the lower lid is involved, the defect is more often in its lateral aspect.

The cause of lid colobomas is unknown; they are thought to be caused either by the localized failure of adhesion of the lid folds, resulting in a lag of growth, or by the mechanical effects of amniotic bands. Lid colobomas are very important when they prevent adequate lid closure, thus exposing the cornea. Subsequent thickening, opacification, infection, ulceration, or perforation of the unprotected cornea may occur. Surgical correction of small colobomas is accomplished by removing a **V**-shaped wedge that includes the coloboma, with subsequent primary closure of the full-thickness defect. Larger colobomatous defects require more extensive plastic repair.

LID COLOBOMAS
Isolated colobomas
Treacher Collins syndrome (lower lid)
Goldenhar's syndrome (upper lid)
Turner's syndrome (rare)

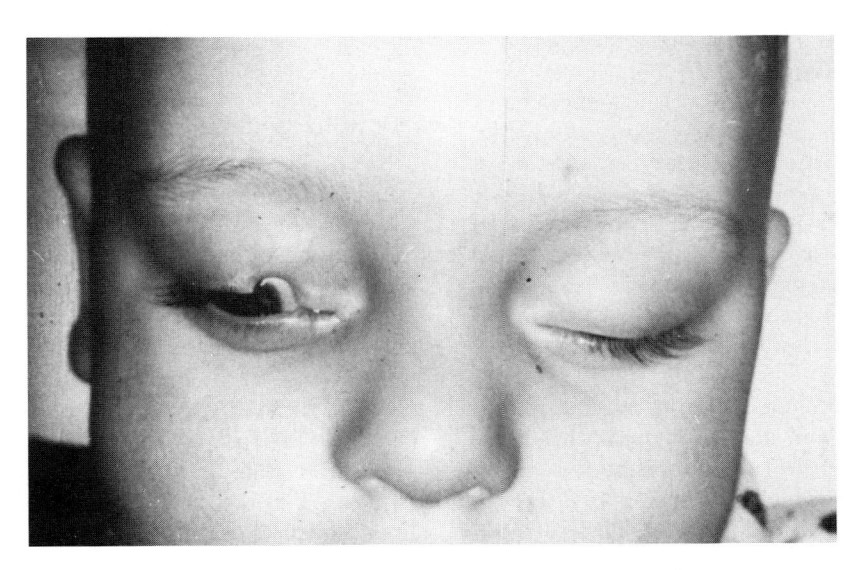

Fig. 35-7. Atypical coloboma of right upper lid.

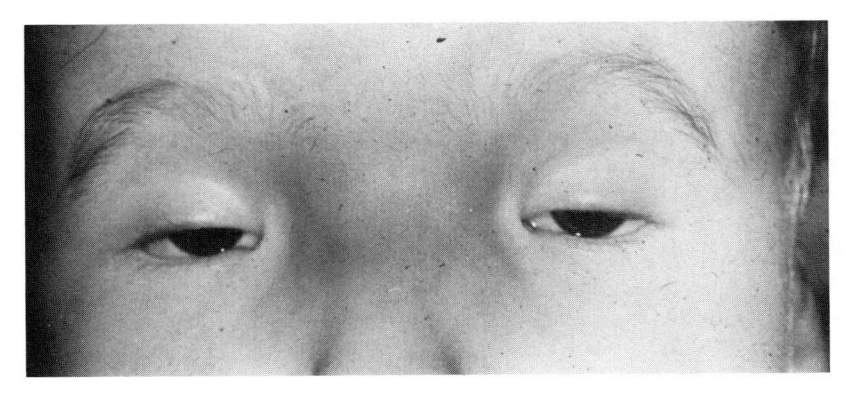

Fig. 35-8. Congenital blepharophimosis, ptosis, and epicanthus inversus (bilateral).

Congenital blepharophimosis

Blepharophimosis means eyelids that are too narrow horizontally as well as vertically (Fig. 35-8). There is usually an associated ptosis and wide epicanthus. It also is associated occasionally with microphthalmia. Lid fissure measurements usually are reduced to approximately two thirds their normal values, whereas the space between the medial canthi is considerably widened. This condition is relatively rare, and the cause is usually unknown. Autosomal dominant transmission has occurred. Treatment in the form of surgical repair is usually required; the medial and lateral canthal angles are widened where possible. Ptosis surgery may be used to strengthen the weakened upper lid levator muscle.

Epicanthus

Epicanthus is the most commonly encountered lid abnormality. A skin fold originating in the upper lid extends over the medial end of the upper lid, the medial canthus, and the caruncle and ends in the skin of the lower lid. This autosomal dominant characteristic is normally found in mongoloids. It is a frequent occurrence in many normal infants in the neonatal period and gradually disappears as the growth of the bridge of the nose obliterates the excess skin in this area. Epicanthus inversus is similar, except that the predominance of the skin fold arises in the lower lid and runs diagonally upward toward the root of the nose to overlie the medial canthus. A plastic surgical technique may be employed later in life to obliterate this extra skin fold, especially if the fold is sufficiently prominent to simulate the appearance of esotropia.

This pseudoesotropia is encountered commonly during the first year of life and decreases in appearance as the facial features mature. It is this pseudoesotropic appearance in neonates which has encouraged a "wait and it may disappear" attitude toward all esotropic-appearing infants. Whenever true esotropia is encountered, even in the neonatal period, it may represent ocular disease and deserves additional early consultation.

LID TUMORS
Hemangiomas

Hemangiomas of the lid are a relatively frequent occurrence in infancy, with an incidence of approximately 1% in full-term newborns. Approximately 20% of hemangiomas are noted at the time of birth, the remainder becoming apparent after the first several weeks or not arising until as late as the second decade of life. The incidence is greater (5%) in premature infants. In the era before the judicious use of oxygen therapy for prematurity the incidence was considerably higher, suggesting a common cause with that of retrolental fibroplasia.

Capillary hemangiomas, the most frequently encountered of the vascular tumors, may progress at a rapid rate during the first 5 to 6 months of life, producing a considerable enlargement and reddish blue discoloration of the upper or lower lid. Such tumors gradually reduce in size and may completely disappear by the second year. Treatment should initially be confined to expectant observation, since resolution is usually the rule. However, these tumors may require therapy, because of an occasionally alarming rate of growth, especially when the lesion produces gross cosmetic defects or interference with vision. Chronic obstruction of the pupillary axis will produce amblyopia.

Surgical removal is difficult and often incomplete. Roentgenograms produce radiation effects to the growth centers of the surrounding bone and possible damage to the eye. Sclerosing solutions risk damage to the periocular tissues. Carbon dioxide snow or other freezing techniques may produce cutaneous scarring. Where disproportionate growth of the hemangioma occurs, systemic corticosteroid therapy may be beneficial (although often transient) in arresting the progression or in producing some resolution.

Lymphangiomas

Lymphangiomas are slowly progressive, diffuse, soft tumors of the lids that may be present at birth or gradually may become apparent during the first several years of life. They tend to grow slowly, with cessation of growth in early adulthood. Approximately 25% of all lymphangiomas occur in the orbital or periorbital region. Of these, 80% are found in the lids. There may be sufficient vascularization to make differentiation from hemangiomas difficult except by histologic study. Because of edema and hemorrhage, these tumors tend to increase in size more dramatically than do hemangiomas. Surgical removal and repair are done when the tumor is cosmetically unacceptable. Recurrence is frequent.

Dermoid cysts

Dermoid cysts are of congenital ectodermal origin and develop in the brow, the lid, or the orbit at the closure site of an embryonic cleft. They usually occur in the lateral third of the brow or upper lid. They are soft, and the overlying skin is freely movable, whereas the cyst remains attached to the periosteum at the site of the embryonic cleft. Roentgenograms of the area are important, since these cysts frequently have connections with the cranial cavity, paranasal sinuses, or the orbit. The treatment is surgical removal if the lesion is enlarging or is cosmetically unacceptable.

Neurofibromatosis

Neurofibromatosis *(von Recklinghausen's disease)* is a congenital, autosomal dominant disease that produces tumors of proliferating Schwann cells. The presence of cafe au lait spots in the patient or parents should alert the examiner to the possibility of this disease. Lid involvement rarely occurs in the neonatal period. This disease produces a tumor, initially small and gradually enlarging, composed of wormlike tissue of the lids with overlying elephantiasis of the skin. Massive deformity of the periorbital tissue can occur. Radical excision, done for cosmetic purposes, is usually incomplete and at times is accompanied by a recurrence that is larger than the original lesion.

SPARSE EYEBROWS AND EYELASHES

The amount of upper facial hair, including the eyebrows and eyelashes, shows considerable variation in the neonate, conforming either to familial or to racial characteristics. In Eskimos and Mongols the eyebrows and eyelashes are normally less dense than in other races. The absence of eyebrows or eyelashes may occur as a congenital anomaly, usually as a part of a general alopecia. The absence of eyebrows occurs concomitantly with cryptophthalmos, where the skin is continuous over the orbits and there are no eyelids. Generalized facial hypotrichosis occurs in *ectodermal dysplasia* and the *Hallermann-Streiff syndrome* and may occur unilaterally in *congenital hemifacial atrophy of Romberg*. Cartilage-hair hypoplasia, an autosomal recessive type of short-limb dwarfism, also is characterized by sparse, thin, and lightly pigmented hair and lashes.

HYPERTRICHOSIS

Excessive hair on the lids and forehead occurs not infrequently as a dominant characteristic in males and on occasion may be extreme. Abnormalities in hair distribution may point to specific diagnoses. Simple synophrys is present in the Waardenburg syndrome as an autosomal dominant characteristic. Districhiasis is the presence of an additional row of lashes posterior to the gray line (the tarsal edge or center of the lid margin). *Districhiasis* may refer to the presence of two lashes growing from the same follicle. *Tristichiasis* is the presence of a third row of eyelashes, one or two of which are posterior to the center of the lid margin. These two conditions usually are associated with contact of the lashes with the cornea, producing corneal irritation and abrasions. Hypertrichosis involving the brows, forehead, and upper lid is seen in the *Cornelia de Lange syndrome,* a pathologic dwarfism associated with multiple congenital anomalies, also described as typus degenerativus amstelodamensis. *Hypertrichosis lanuginosa* is a condition in which the fetal lanugo persists into adult life, creating an abundant covering of hair of the eyebrows, forehead, and eyelids as well as of the remainder of the body. This anomaly also occurs as an autosomal dominant hereditary characteristic. A rare condition has been reported in which there is reduplication of the eyebrows bilaterally, the second pair occurring a short distance above the normally placed brows, with no apparent connection. The latter anomaly has been called *duplicitas supercilia*.

PTOSIS

Ptosis (droopy eyelid) is defined as an upper lid that cannot or does not rise to a normal level. In the position of primary gaze the lids normally should be elevated to a point at least midway between the pupil and the upper margin of the cornea. The examiner usually can induce momentary ocular fixation in the primary position by using a hand light in a moderately darkened room. Care must be taken not to disturb the child when evaluating for ptosis, since accurate lid position can be evaluated only in the undisturbed patient.

Ptosis is the result of dysfunction of the levator palpebrae superioris muscle, which can be variably partial or complete. Complete dysfunction is present when no elevation of the lid occurs on upward gaze. Ptosis may be present either unilaterally or bilaterally, with any gradation of function in either situation. Ptosis that is the result of absence of normal levator function will have additional signs; the normal upper lid fold may be absent, and the upper lid lashes will tend to point in a more downward position.

PTOSIS

Congenital ptosis
Congenital myasthenia gravis
Congenital Horner's syndrome
Möbius syndrome
Smith-Lemli-Opitz syndrome
Turner's syndrome (rare)
Fanconi's syndrome (infrequent)
Chromosome 4p− syndrome
Chromosome 5p− syndrome (cri du chat)
Chromosome 13q− syndrome
Trisomy 18
Transient neonatal myasthenia gravis

In the presence of a unilateral ptosis (Fig. 35-9) comparison of pupillary size with that of the opposite eye is an important factor in diagnosing Horner's syndrome. Congenital Horner's syndrome occurs as a result of birth trauma (p. 224). Subsequently the pupil remains smaller and there is less pigmentation in the iris stroma compared with the fellow pupil. Diagnosis is confirmed when one drop of 10% phenylephrine instilled into the conjunctiva produces marked elevation of an affected lid in approximately 15 to 20 minutes. Heterochromia is an associated finding if the injury to the sympathetic innervation occurred before or during the process of pigmentation of the irises and became apparent only after nor-

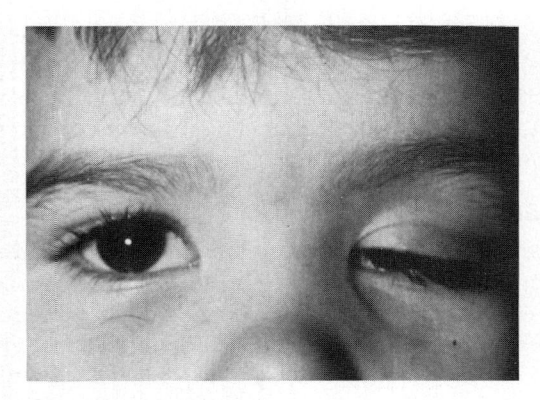

Fig. 35-9. Congenital ptosis of left upper lid.

mal pigmentation was well developed in the fellow eye.

Ptosis also may be the result of a *Marcus Gunn syndrome*. The patient with this condition shows a marked movement of the affected upper lid during nursing activity. The jaw-winking portion of the syndrome is thought to decrease or disappear in early adulthood. However, the ptosis remains. Surgical correction of the Marcus Gunn ptosis is frequently unsatisfactory because of the continued presence of the jaw-winking phenomenon, even though the ptosis may be improved by shortening the levator palpebrae muscle. The syndrome is caused by anomalous innervation of the levator palpebrae muscle (abnormal connections of the motor fibers of the pterygoid, lingual, and levator palpebrae muscles). There is a relatively toneless levator palpebrae muscle unless the jaw or tongue is additionally activated.

A temporary apparent ptosis (so-called protective ptosis) may be seen as the result of corneal or conjunctival irritation or infection and in conditions such as congenital glaucoma. These conditions always should be considered and ruled out before diagnosing other forms of ptosis, since they are the more important, and often correctable, ocular diseases.

CLOSED EYES

Eyes that have spontaneously opened at birth but then subsequently close may do so because of infection or irritation. Lid anomalies producing a failure of spontaneous lid opening at or after birth are *anophthalmia* and *cryptophthalmos*. Anophthalmia, in which there is total absence or a minute rudiment of the globe, is seen rarely. This may occur as a failure of development of the optic vesicle and is usually bilateral. Marked *microphthalmia* may simulate true anophthalmia, in which case colobomatous signs of incomplete embryonic fissure closure may be seen in either eye. The contralateral eye in this situation may be normal in size, showing only a fundus or iris coloboma inferiorly. In most patients anophthalmia is accompanied by other congenital anomalies, such as central nervous system defects and retardation. Since lid formation is not dependent on ocular formation, the lids are present with lashes and lacrimal puncta even though the globe may be absent. However, the lids remain closed and sunken without the support of the eye. The lacrimal gland is present and is capable of producing tears. Occurrence in most patients is sporadic. However, there have been some cases of familial incidence with varied types of mendelian inheritance. Treatment is only cosmetic and usually is accomplished by the use of gradually enlarging plastic molds of the conjunctival sac to stretch the lids and sac sufficiently to hold a cosmetic prosthetic shell.

In *cryptophthalmos* the eyelids fail to form their normal cleavage. Uninterrupted skin runs from the forehead to the malar area. The eyelids and eyelashes usually are absent. However, the eye can be palpated beneath the skin of the lids and may even be seen to move with the stimulation of a strong light. The anterior segment of the eye is invariably disorganized into fibrovascular tissue adherent to the subcuticular tissue of the lids. The conjunctival sac is absent. Therefore attempts to separate the lids from the ocular structures usually result in incision of the ocular tissues concomitant with the incision of the eyelids. Surgical correction therefore is not advisable in most circumstances.

THE PURULENT EYE

An eye infection is one of the most serious problems encountered in the newborn. If undiagnosed and untreated, it may rapidly proceed to loss of one or both eyes. Thus the recognition and differentiation of ophthalmia neonatorum requires vigilance and early treatment or consultation. Acute purulent conjunctivitis is a chemical or bacterial inflammation of the conjunctiva characterized by cellular infiltration and exudation.

Chemical conjunctivitis

The most common cause of ophthalmia neonatorum, referred to in some areas as the "sticky eye," is the result of instillation of 1% silver nitrate into the eye at birth. In spite of its disadvantages and occasional irritation, the *Credé prophylaxis* is statistically the most effective, least troublesome method of preventing gonococcal conjunctivitis. The rate of occurrence of chemical conjunctivitis from silver nitrate is estimated at approximately 10% of all newborns and probably is enhanced by the prolonged contact of the silver nitrate with the conjunctival sac or by excessive concentration of the silver nitrate. This is the only conjunctivitis generally present from the first day and is usually unilateral. The lids are slightly swollen, the conjunctiva is congested and edematous, and purulence is not observed. This condition clears spontaneously in 3 to 4 days if no secondary bacterial infection occurs. Ten percent sodium sulfacetamide drops four times a day may be used locally to prevent secondary infection. Secondary bacterial infection is suggested if the disease persists beyond this time or increases in severity. Cultures with sensitivity tests identify the organism and suggest appropriate treatment.

Gonorrheal conjunctivitis

Conjunctivitis caused by *Neisseria gonorrhoeae* is an acute, severe, purulent conjunctivitis with an incubation period of 2 to 5 days (p. 665). The rate of occurrence in the United States today is less than 0.03% as the result of the legal requirement of silver nitrate or penicillin instillation at birth. There have been reports of resistance to the Credé prophylaxis.

Inclusion blennorrhea

Inclusion conjunctivitis (p. 665) is another form of ophthalmia neonatorum. Differentiation from gonococcal conjunctivitis is indicated by the longer incubation period, by the primary involvement of the inferior conjunctival fornix, and by the smear. In gonococcal conjunctivitis there is involvement of both the superior and inferior fornices. The usual cultures and Gram stain are unproductive in inclusion blennorrhea. Demonstration of the typical basophilic inclusion bodies in the epithelial cells is made with Giemsa-stained smears of the conjunctival scraping of the lower lid.

Nongonococcal bacterial conjunctivitis

Ophthalmia neonatorum also may occur as the result of other common pathogens, among which are staphylococci, pneumococci, streptococci, coliform bacteria, and influenzal bacteria.

THE WATERY EYE

Epiphora (excess tearing) usually is not present until after the first 3 weeks of life, since the major portion of the lacrimal gland is not functional until that time. With the onset of emotional tearing at 3 to 4 weeks, epiphora is a frequent symptom. Although the usual causes of epiphora are blockage of the lacrimal ducts, the possibility of congenital glaucoma is the most important consideration in the differential diagnosis of this symptom. More frequent obstructions of the lacrimal drainage systems are, in order of their occurrence, obstruction of the nasolacrimal duct, obstruction at the common canaliculus, and congenital absence of the lid puncta. Stenosis of the nasolacrimal duct, which becomes more obstructed by a recurrent mild inflammation, produces excess tearing for several weeks, followed by apparent improvement and often recurrence at a later date. Congenital absence of the entire lacrimal drainage apparatus is extremely rare.

Constant epiphora is present with total obstruction of the lacrimal drainage apparatus and usually is the result of a persistent membrane at the lower end of the nasolacrimal duct. This condition creates a stagnant pooling of tears in the lacrimal sac, which contributes to chronic or recurrent *dacryocystitis*. This is heralded by a purulent exudate in the medial canthal area of the conjunctiva. Severe dacryocystitis may produce a swelling and induration of the lacrimal sac, medial and inferior to the medial canthus. Treatment of the nasolacrimal infection consists of the local instillation of antibiotic drops or ointment. If it is especially severe, systemic administration of medication and locally applied heat may be required. Repeated massage of the nasolacrimal sac at the root of the nose by the parent at home may serve to encourage the opening of the nasolacrimal duct. If the epiphora continues beyond the age of 3 to 6 months, the passage of a lacrimal probe through the nasolacrimal duct to the nose may produce an adequate opening; recurrent probings are often necessary. With obstruction of the puncta, the common canaliculus, or major obstructions in the lacrimal sac, probing is insufficient. A surgical procedure, usually accomplished later in life, is needed to bypass the tears from the conjuctival sac to the nose. Occasionally minor surgical unroofing of a congenitally closed punctum will be sufficient.

Trigeminal irritation

After the initial onset of function reflex tearing may be produced by any stimulation of the fifth cranial nerve. Therefore epiphora may occur as the result of corneal abrasion, corneal foreign body, or nasal and facial lesions that irritate the fifth cranial nerve. Chronic nasal congestion also may produce epiphora as the result of mechanical blockage of the nasolacrimal duct.

Congenital glaucoma

The presence of epiphora in the neonate always should suggest the possibility of *congenital glaucoma*, especially when epiphora is combined with photophobia. Congenital glaucoma fortunately is not very common. However, the devastating effects of the uncontrolled pressure that occurs without adequate surgical treatment are of sufficient importance to keep this disease uppermost in the mind of the examining physican. The obvious signs of enlarged corneal diameters and a cloudy cornea are not likely to be missed if these signs are present at birth. However, the onset of the glaucoma may be sufficiently delayed so that the eyes remain normal for the first weeks or months of life. The usual initial symptoms before corneal changes include epiphora, photophobia, and blepharospasm. Persistent symptoms of this nature, which are not the result of corneal abrasion or foreign body, require specific evaluation for increased intraocular pressure. Early diagnosis must be made by examination, with the infant *under general anesthesia*, for precise measurement of corneal diameters and of intraocular pressures by ocular tonometry. Congenital glaucoma is discussed in more detail in the section on the large eye (p. 987).

THE DRY EYE

Recognition of *alacrima* in the infant is important in the prevention of corneal abrasions, infections, and perforations, the inevitable results of the dry eye. During the first month the infant with alacrima of any cause may not appear to be different from the normal infant, since tear production is normally minimal during this period. The usual time of discovery is at 6 months of age or later, after the lack of tears has produced changes such as scarring or ulceration in the corneal epithelium. The tear film, with alacrima, is minimal but present. At 1 to 2 months of age early symptoms are conjunctival hyperemia and photophobia. Instead of the ample tears expected with conjunctival irritation, there is usually a sticky mucoid secretion, and the cornea shows a punctate staining with fluorescein. Treatment includes the frequent use of artificial tears such as 1% methylcellulose (as often as every 15 to 30 minutes), punctum occlusion, or tarsorrhaphy.

Congenital absence of the lacrimal secretion

Isolated congenital lack of tears, usually bilateral, is a rare anomaly. The cause is unknown but has been suggested to be either the result of hypoplasia of the lacrimal gland or the absence of innervation of the lacrimal gland structures. Treatment includes the frequent use of artificial tears and prevention of secondary infection.

Familial dysautonomia

The ocular findings in the *Riley-Day syndrome* are characteristic and may produce the initial criteria for diagnosis. There is a lack of lacrimation, corneal anesthesia, and exodeviation (divergence of the eyes). These ocular changes, plus constriction of the pupil by instillation of 0.125% of pilocarpine, may establish the diagnosis. Major systemic symptoms usually have their onset at approximately age 2 years. The abnormal swallowing mechanism, inappropriate blood pressure and respiratory control, and the ocular findings in this syndrome are the result of sympathetic and parasympathetic imbalance of an undefined type. Additional ocular findings are myopia, anisometropia (different refractive error in the two eyes), and occasionally ptosis. Tortuosity of the retinal vessels also has been noted in a majority of the patients examined for this finding. The concomitant occurrence of alacrima and corneal hypoesthesia makes the cornea particularly susceptible to corneal abrasion, infection, and ulceration. Thus corneal scarring is a frequent secondary finding in familial dysautonomia.

THE RED EYE

Conjunctival and corneal irritation from any source produces hyperemia of the conjunctiva. Probably the most frequent source of conjunctival irritation in the newborn is corneal abrasion produced by fingernails or clothing. These are of small importance and usually require little in the way of therapy except an antibiotic eyedrop and sometimes a firm patch for 1 to 2 days. However, conjunctival hyperemia also may be the initial symptom of ocular infection or congenital glaucoma; these may be devastating to the eye if left undiagnosed.

Blood in the anterior chamber of the eye, called a *hyphema*, requires ophthalmologic consultation. A hyphema occurring shortly after birth may be the result of excessive birth trauma, vascular anomalies of the iris, or the presence of blood dyscrasias. Bleeding abnormalities should be evaluated by appropriate laboratory tests. The appearance of the eye with hyphema varies with the amount of blood present in the anterior chamber. The eye may grossly show a level of red blood cells behind the cornea; there may be a diffuse, hazy red appearance; or the area of the anterior chamber may be black and opaque. Other diseases associated with anterior chamber hyphema are retinoblastoma, juvenile xanthogranuloma, and rarely retrolental fibroplasia and persistent hyperplastic primary vitreous (PHPV). A particularly severe form of secondary glaucoma occurs after hyphema in children with a sickle cell hemoglobinopathy, including sickle cell trait. Prompt screening for sickling and immediate ophthalmic consulation are indicated.

ABNORMAL ORBITS

Abnormal spatial relationships between the two orbits, creating excessively wide or excessively narrow intraorbital distances, are frequent. These abnormalities are caused by a wide variety of related cranial abnormalities involving the disproportionate growth or lack of development of the body and lesser wing of the sphenoid and ethmoid sinuses and of the maxillary processes. *Hypotelorism* (a narrowing of the intraorbital distance) is usually a secondary phenomenon associated with scaphocephaly (a boat-shaped cranium caused by premature closure of the sagittal suture). *Hypertelorism* (a widening of the intraorbital distance) is normal in the early fetus and may persist as a genetic trait. Hypertelorism may occur as an associated finding in other diseases.

HYPOTELORISM

Cebocephaly
Ocular-dental-digital dysplasia
Trisomy 13
Scaphocephaly

HYPERTELORISM

Apert's syndrome
Cerebral gigantism
Cerebrohepatorenal syndrome
Chromosome 18p− and 18q− syndromes
Crouzon's disease
Infantile hypercalcemia
Greig's hypertelorism
Median cleft face syndrome
Male Turner's syndrome
Smith-Lemli-Opitz syndrome
Chromosome 4p− syndrome
Chromosome 5p− syndrome (cri du chat)
Chromosome 13q− syndrome
Chromosome 21q− syndrome

ORBITAL TUMORS

The contents of the orbit are confined to a conical shape by its bony walls. The apex of the orbit faces posteriorly where the extraocular muscles originate and where the vascular and nerve structures enter the orbit. The bony structures of the lateral wall do not protect the orbital contents as far anteriorly as do the remaining sides of the orbit, which leaves the eye exposed to trauma more on its lateral side. At the base of the cone, anteriorly, the orbital rims form a shape circular outline in the neonate.

Tumors within the orbital cavity can most easily expand anteriorly, producing proptosis or exophthalmos. Tumors located within the cone of extraocular muscles produce a symmetric anterior displacement, whereas tumors located outside the cone of extraocular muscles displace the eye out and away from the area of origin of the tumor. Thus a tumor in the inferior portion of the orbit will displace the eye up and forward, whereas a tumor located medially will displace the eye laterally and forward. Proptosis also may occur from venous engorgement of the orbital cavity, such as that produced by a carotid-cavernous fistula. Unfortunately a cephalic bruit is often heard in the infant and is thus not pathognomonic of carotid-cavernous sinus fistulas. The diagnosis of proptosis may be confirmed if the examiner sights the eyes and lids from above, over the prominence of the eyebrows. A more anterior protrusion of the orbital contents is seen when compared with the contents of the opposite side. The proptotic eye frequently has a widened palpebral fissure.

A false diagnosis of proptosis may occur with a slight ptosis of one eye, which gives the opposite normal eye an appearance of a wider palpebral fissure. Marked enlargement of the eye, as occurs in congenital glaucoma, makes the eye appear proptotic because of the increased size of the globe. Facial abnormalities with shallow orbits, as in *Crouzon's disease*, simulate exophthalmos because of the protrusion of the normal amount of orbital structures in an abnormally shallow orbit. Since the extraocular muscles are retractors of the globe, a paralysis of all the extraocular muscles may produce proptosis of as much as 2 mm without increase in orbital contents by a tumor. If a tumor is located anterior to the equator of the globe, the tumor can extend anteriorly into the lids without producing proptosis. A diffuse extensive tumor can produce sufficient general changes to fix the eye, whereas a localized tumor produces proptosis usually without interfering with rotation of the eye.

Orbital tumors may be primary from both ectodermal and mesodermal tissues or may arise by metastasis from distant body tissues. They also may arise from the intracranial cavity or paranasal sinuses and enter the orbit by growing through bony defects in the orbital wall. Roentgenograms are valuable in the diagnosis of orbital disease. Posteroanterior, lateral, Waters', and Caldwell's projections are useful, and computed tomography is particularly helpful.

Orbital hematoma

Bleeding into the orbital contents may occur as the result of birth trauma. This bleeding produces a unilateral proptosis that tends to increase gradually in size during the first 3 or 4 hours after birth. Ecchymoses of the lids may be associated findings at birth or may occur 1 to 2 days later. Differential diagnosis includes *dermoid cysts, teratoma*, and other congenital tumors of the orbit. Treatment usually is not required, since absorption of the hematoma usually takes place over a 1- to 2-week period. It is important during this time to ensure that the cornea is not abraded and that the retinal circulation is not compromised. If examination with the direct ophthalmoscope shows compression of the arterial or venous supply at the disc, a surgical decompression of the orbit is required.

Hemangioma

Cavernous hemangioma is the most common primary orbital tumor that produces exophthalmos. In infants the hemangioma usually is not well encapsulated and frequently involves the lower lid as well as the orbit. Although observation of lid involvement assists in making the diagnosis, a biopsy frequently is required to rule out other orbital tumors. Treatment usually is deferred until after the age of 2 years, at which time spontaneous regression often occurs. The use of systemic corticosteroid therapy has been advocated when excessive growth has produced dangerous compression of the orbital structures.

Dermoid cysts

Dermoid cysts are thought to arise from a congenital nest of primitive ectoderm at the site of closure of a fetal cleft. They usually contain connective tissue, sebaceous glands, hair follicles, and smooth muscle. They often are

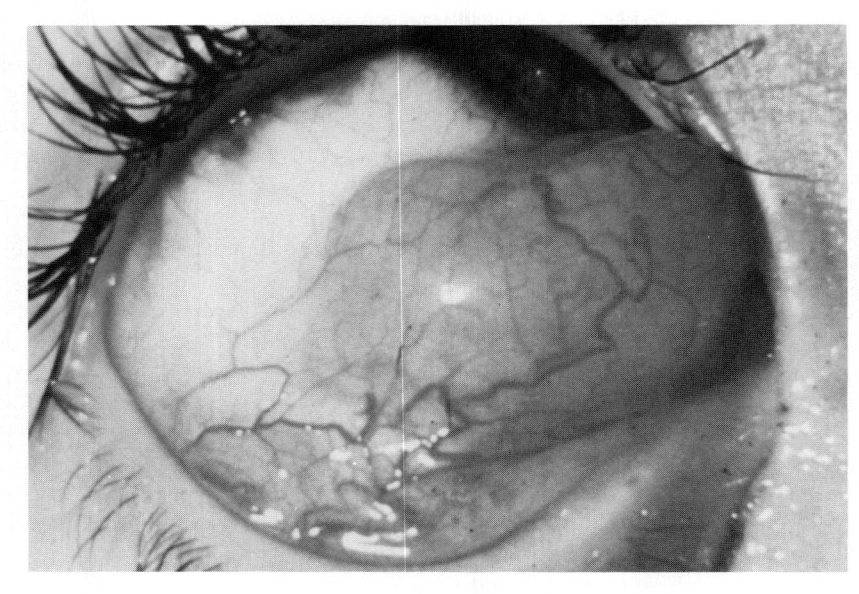

Fig. 35-10. Rhabdomyosarcoma of right orbit.

located near the orbital rim, where they are attached to bone at suture sites. Because of their location, a proptosis, combined with vertical or horizontal displacement and irregular lid swelling, is produced. Roentgenographic examination may provide evidence of teeth or show dehiscences in the bony wall where the cyst is attached. Treatment is surgical excision, which may prove difficult because of extension of the dermoid cyst through the bony suture into surrounding structures. Trauma, such as that occurring at birth, may produce a hemorrhage into the dermoid cyst. This occurs rarely, but under such circumstances differentiation from a primary hematoma of the orbit is difficult.

Teratoma

Teratoma is a primary orbital tumor composed of mesodermal and ectodermal elements. It may differentiate into a variety of tissues containing cartilage, connective tissue, skin, hair, and sebaceous glands, or endodermal epithelium. Bone is a frequent component and may be identified by orbital roentgenograms. Orbital teratomas that are present at birth produce a striking picture of massive proptosis. Treatment is early excision of the orbital contents (exenteration) both for cosmetic value and for the possible carcinomatous and sarcomatous changes that may occur within the tumor.

Rhabdomyosarcoma

Rhabdomyosarcoma is the most common malignant tumor of the orbit in children (Fig. 35-10). Although it may be found in the neonatal period, the average age of occurrence is 6 to 10 years. Rhabdomyosarcoma develops in the orbit more frequently than elsewhere in the body. It produces an exophthalmos with vertical or horizontal displacement, frequently with a palpable mass in the lid or the brow and with progressive protrusion of the eye. Diagnosis is made by biopsy. Accepted treatment has included surgical exenteration of the orbit, followed by irradiation. Recent evidence suggests that irradiation alone may be curative.

Neuroblastoma (sympathicoblastoma)

This very malignant tumor frequently originates in the adrenal gland. It may be noticed first as a unilateral or bilateral proptosis caused by metastasis to the orbit. Exophthalmos is progressive, and associated hemorrhage into the neoplastic tissue produces characteristic ecchymoses of the lid. The orbital metastasis is often the initial sign of the disease before the primary tumor is discovered. Curative treatment is not available. Exenteration of the orbit has been done in some instances to palliate the extensive exophthalmos.

Hyperthyroid exophthalmos

This rare neonatal sequela of hyperthyroidism occurs in the newborn as the result of maternal Graves' disease during the last trimester of pregnancy (p. 897). The infant is born with classic hyperthyroidism, including exophthalmos, upper lid retraction, and extraocular muscle involvement. Symptoms usually subside during the first 2 months of life.

Lymphoma

Proptosis caused by lymphomatous lesions of the orbit is rare in the neonatal period. Diagnosis is made by biopsy, and the prognosis with radiation treatment is usually good.

Orbital cellulitis

Cellulitis of the orbital tissue is rare in the neonate but is a common cause of proptosis in older children and in adults. This infection often is originally located in the paranasal sinuses and produces massive swelling of the orbital contents. The possibility of its occurrence is enhanced by a highly virulent upper respiratory tract sinus infection or a puncture wound of the orbit. The disease is characterized by rapid onset of progressive proptosis, often with redness of the lids, chemosis of the conjunctiva, and systemic signs of toxicity and hyperpyrexia. Rapid loss of vision, caused by compression of the orbital structures, can occur. Treatment includes surgical drainage of the purulent infection and systemic administration of antibiotics.

Neurofibromatosis

Neurofibromatosis *(von Recklinghausen's disease)* is also rarely seen during the neonatal period. However, plexiform neuromas of the lids and orbit have been reported in the first 3 months of life. The typical "bag of worms" tissue may produce proptosis and irregular enlargement of one or both lids. The overlying tissue becomes hypertrophic and resembles elephantiasis of the skin. Von Recklinghausen's disease also has been associated with glioma of the optic nerve, a slowly growing tumor appearing during the first 10 years of life. Invasion of the optic nerve by the glioma results in visual loss.

Letterer-Siwe disease

Letterer-Siwe disease, sometimes referred to as aleukemic reticulosis or histiocytosis, is the most severe form of lymphogranuloma. The condition usually affects children under 2 years of age and nearly always has a fatal outcome. Reticuloendothelial cells are seen to proliferate in the skin, lymph nodes, and spleen, as well as in the tissue of the orbit, producing proptosis. Hepatosplenomegaly and generalized lymphadenopathy with bone lesions and anemia are typical findings. Diagnosis is made from a biopsy of skin lesions or of lymph nodes. Palliative treatment includes corticosteroids, x-irradiation, and chemotherapy.

Congenital deformities producing proptosis

An orbital encephalocele or meningocele producing proptosis or an orbital cyst may be evident at birth or may be delayed until later years. This results from a defect in the wall between the cranial cavity and the orbit and usually is located at the suture lines. Pressure within the cranium causes herniation of brain tissue or of meninges or of both into the orbit, most often at the inner angle of the orbit at the root of the nose. Diagnosis is made by identifying the bony defect in association with the area of the orbital cyst. Clinically an encephalocele is suggested by the presence of a pulsating, fluctuant cyst that can be somewhat reduced with digital pressure or that increases with coughing or crying. Excessive manipulation of the encephalocele may produce slowing of the pulse and respiration or convulsions. Slowly progressive proptosis, with pulsation synchronous with the vascular pulse or accentuated with coughing, is diagnostic. Neurosurgical correction is difficult and has a high morbidity and mortality.

THE SMALL EYE

Microphthalmia indicates a variety of conditions in which the diameter of the neonatal eye is less than two thirds of the normal 16 mm. Pure congenital microphthalmia is a relatively rare condition with the abnormally small eye as the only clinical finding. It is associated with three features of significance: a high degree of hypermetropia, hypoplasia of the macula, and the late occurrence of glaucoma. It has been reported in both recessive and dominant transmissions. Colobomatous microphthalmia occurs when the embryonic cleft of the optic vesicle fails to close and is typically associated with other ocular anomalies such as colobomas of the iris, the ciliary body, the choroid, or the optic nerve. These may be transmitted as autosomal dominant or X-linked traits. D group deletions or trisomy also produces these abnormalities. A third group of anomalies, termed *complicated microphthalmia*, is the result of associated genetic malformations inherited as autosomal dominant, autosomal recessive, or X-linked recessive traits. It also may occur secondary to prenatal infections, such as rubella or toxoplasmosis. Microphthalmia and congenital cataract are the two most frequent clinical ocular findings in rubella infection of the embryo. Complicated micropthalmia also is associated with other ocular abnormalities, such as *Norrie's disease*.

MICROPHTHALMIA

Microphthalmia with cataract
Microphthalmia with coloboma
Hallermann-Streiff syndrome
Rubella syndrome
Trisomy 13
Ocular-dental-digital dysplasia
Trisomy 18 (infrequent)
Fanconi's syndrome (infrequent)
Congenital toxoplasmosis (infrequent)
Pierre Robin syndrome (rare)
Treacher Collins syndrome (rare)
Chromosome 13q− syndrome
Goldenhar's syndrome (rare)
Fetal alcohol syndrome

THE LARGE EYE

The presence of an abnormally enlarged eye in the neonatal period is a rare occurrence but is extremely

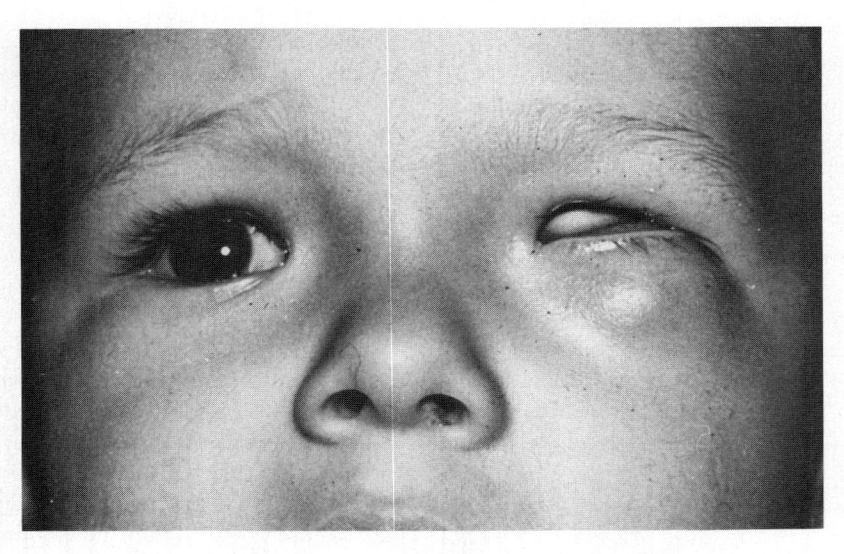

Fig. 35-11. Congenital microphthalmia with large cyst of left eye.

important to recognize. Three entities may cause an apparently enlarged eye: colobomatous microphthalmia with an associated large cyst (Fig. 35-11), congenital megalophthalmos (congenital megalocornea), and congenital glaucoma. The first results from a failure of closure of the embryonic optic vesicle. Tissue that originally was destined to become intraocular thus is located outside the eye in the orbit in a cystic structure. This may become sufficiently large that proptosis occurs, and the microphthalmic eye simulates an enlarged eye.

Megalocornea is an enlarged cornea exceeding 13 mm in diameter. The cornea is usually clear, with distinct margins and thin iris stroma. Megalocornea may represent enlargement only of the cornea, general enlargement of the anterior segment, or enlargement of the entire globe (megalophthalmos). Differentiation requires examination with the infant under anesthesia. Megalophthalmos usually is inherited as an X-linked recessive trait. It is also occasionally associated with Marfan's syndrome. The disorder is characterized by photophobia and a lack of tearing, a clear cornea, and normal ocular tensions and optic disc.

Congenital glaucoma, often transmitted as a recessive trait when it is the only abnormality, most commonly produces abnormal signs during the first year of life. Early recognition is most important to prevent progressive damage to the eye from the increased intraocular pressure (Fig. 35-12). The most frequent symptoms of congenital glaucoma are tearing, photophobia, and blepharospasm; in the neonatal period tearing may be absent from the triad. These symptoms always should suggest the possibility of congenital glaucoma, even though more common problems, such as corneal abrasion, foreign body, or ocular infection, could be present. Clouding or haziness of the cornea occurs with further advancement of the disease. This results from stretching and overhydration of the cornea. (The normal clouding of the cornea, which may be present in the newborn for the first several days of life, should be carefully observed for complete resolution.) As the disease progresses, the increased tension produces further stretching of the eye, creating increased corneal and ocular diameters. A corneal diameter of more than 12 mm should suggest glaucoma. (The normal corneal diameter is 10 to 11 mm, increasing to about 11.5 or 12 mm at 1 year of age.)

Buphthalmos (an enlarged eye caused by glaucoma) also may be secondary to a variety of diseases having obstruction of the aqueous drainage mechanism in the anterior chamber angle. The list below gives diseases associated with glaucoma.

GLAUCOMA

Isolated (congenital)
Rubella syndrome
Hallermann-Streiff syndrome
Rieger's anomaly
Lowe's syndrome
Persistent hyperplastic primary vitreous (rare)
Aniridia
Sturge-Weber syndrome
Homocystinuria (infrequent)
Marfan's syndrome (infrequent)
Weill-Marchesani syndrome (infrequent)
Neurofibromatosis (infrequent)
Ocular-dental-digital syndrome (infrequent)

Once the suspicion of glaucoma has arisen, the infant should be examined under general anesthesia by an ophthalmologist. Preanesthetic medication should consist

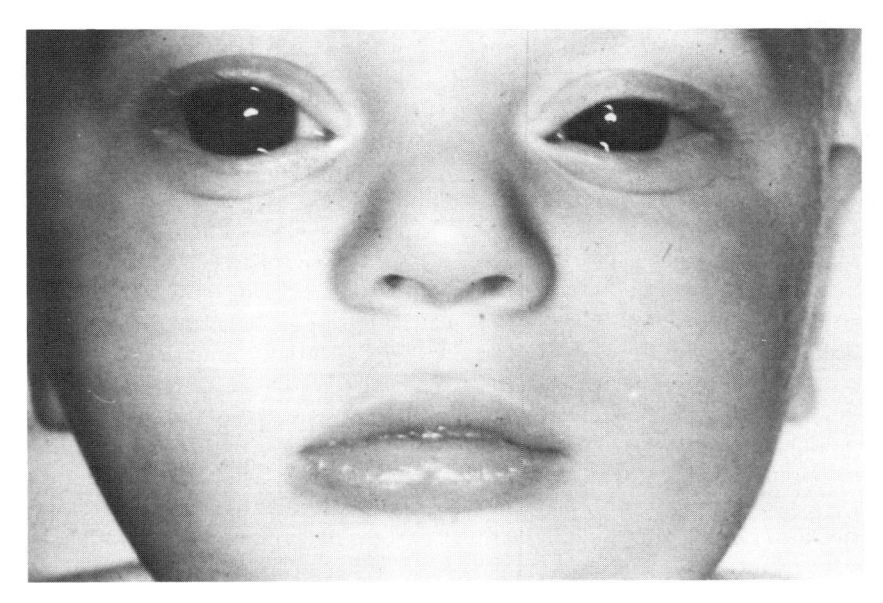

Fig. 35-12. Bilateral congenital glaucoma (buphthalmos), right eye greater than left.

only of atropine given systemically. The anesthetic agent of choice is diethyl ether. If the diagnosis is confirmed, a surgical procedure should be performed on the anterior chamber angle (goniotomy) while the infant is still under anesthesia, since medical therapy is ineffective. If the diagnosis of congenital glaucoma has been made early in its course, the percentage of successful recoveries is high; however, if there is considerable enlargement of the eye, the possibility of reducing intraocular pressure and achieving useful vision is greatly decreased.

STRABISMUS

Clinically significant strabismus is recognized less frequently in the neonatal period than in the remainder of the first decade of life. Its diagnosis is important, however, since therapy, when indicated, must begin early. Few, if any, patients with congenitally crossed eyes, for example, will spontaneously "grow out" of this problem with the passage of time. *Estropia* (crossed eyes) may occur as the result of dominant inheritance (congenital), of paralysis of the lateral rectus muscles, or of refractive errors (usually hyperopia) or may be secondary to any type of disease that reduces visual acuity in one eye. *Exotropia* (wall eyes) is seen rarely in the neonate (in congenital anomalies such as Greig's hypertelorism). The usual forms of exotropia do not appear until 1 to 2 years of age or later.

The diagnosis of strabismus can be made by the Hirschberg test, an evaluation of the pupillary light reflex on both corneas while the patient fixates binocularly on a small light source that is held before the patient's face and directed toward the pupils. The pupillary light reflex, if the patient is properly fixating with both eyes on the light source, should be positioned in the same part of the pupillary space of each eye. If the light reflex is centered in one eye and deviated to the lateral side of the pupil or cornea of the fellow eye, esotropia is present. A rough estimation of the visual acuity can be made by determining the fixation pattern of each eye while the infant's eyes fixate on a light. If one eye moves to fixate on the light centrally and steadily at all times and the other does not, the latter is certain to have poor acuity.

An alternative fixation target is the human face. This may be the most reliable target in the very early neonate and may be used for visual assessment in the same fashion as a light source.

When strabismus is present, a careful ocular examination is required to rule out the possibility of an intraocular pathologic condition. Pathologic conditions that may create esotropia are corneal opacities, cataracts, and diseases of the fundus that have reduced or destroyed macular vision, such as infections (for example, toxoplasmosis) or tumors (for example, retinoblastoma). *Fundus examination with the patient's pupils dilated is mandatory.*

Congenital esotropia may be present while the neonate is still in the nursery or may become evident during the first two weeks of life. Results of the ocular examination are otherwise normal, and visual acuity is usually equal in the two eyes. Amblyopia may develop from congenital esotropia, although it does so less frequently than in the accommodative type, which appears later in childhood.

Esotropia caused by the paralysis of the lateral rectus muscles may occur as the result of birth trauma and is diagnosed by failure of an eye to deviate laterally beyond the midline. The examination of lateral rotation is best accomplished by occlusion of one eye and observation of the opposite eye. Congenital esotropia also shows weakness of lateral gaze when both eyes are tested simultaneously but shows normal lateral rotations with one eye occluded.

Pseudostrabismus is the term given to infants who appear cross-eyed because the bridge of the nose is wide and the epicanthal folds on either side cover most of the sclera on the medial side of the cornea. True strabismus is ruled out by observation of the corneal light reflex, which is found to be symmetrically placed in both pupils.

The treatment of strabismus begins with an adequate ocular examination and a careful cycloplegic refraction. Aims in the treatment of strabismus include the prevention of strabismic amblyopia, the improvement or correction of the cosmetic appearance, and if possible the creation of binocular vision. The chances of improving amblyopia and strabismus are better the earlier therapy is begun. Treatment (drops, patching, glasses, surgery, and so on) should be completed well before the child is of school age so that the child is not handicapped by a visual or cosmetic defect.

THE CLOUDY CORNEA

The normal premature infant may have a slightly hazy cornea for the first 7 days of life, and the normal full-term infant occasionally has a similar appearance for the first 48 hours after delivery. This is thought to be caused by a temporary excess hydration of the cornea. The presence of a persistently hazy or cloudy cornea should immediately suggest congenital glaucoma. Once this has been ruled out, the following diseases are suggested.

The mucopolysaccharidoses

In the mucopolysaccharidoses various combinations of acid mucopolysaccharides are excessively deposited in the body tissues (Chapter 32). They are accumulated, as well, in the stroma of the cornea in Hurler's syndrome, Morquio's syndrome, Scheie's syndrome, and Maroteaux-Lamy syndrome. Because of progressive accumulation, corneal clouding is often minimal or invisible in the early periods of life, but it increases with age. Exact pathogenesis of this corneal clouding is not as yet known. Electron microscopic studies have shown that the stromal fibroblasts are considerably enlarged because of the presence of inclusion material in their cytoplasm. These cells may create sufficient anatomic disturbance in the stroma to produce scattering of light. The appearance in the neonatal period includes fine gray punctate opacities in the peripheral stroma, which may cause a faint and diffuse opalescence. Other ocular lesions that are associated with mucopolysaccharidoses, such as pigmentary degeneration of the retina and optic atrophy, can cause an irreversible loss of vision. Therefore the fundus should be examined through a dilated pupil in all such patients. Corneal transplantation as a method of improving visual acuity is recommended only if abnormal mental, retinal, and optic nerve functions are not associated. Differential diagnosis of ground-glass corneal opacification includes congenital glaucoma, rubella keratopathy, severe birth trauma to the cornea, and congenital hereditary corneal dystrophy. A screening diagnosis can be made by identification of the abnormal mucopolysaccharides in the urine. Intraocular pressure determinations with the infant under general anesthesia are needed to rule out congenital glaucoma. Serologic tests rule out rubella, and slit-lamp determination of stromal thickness rules out congenital hereditary corneal dystrophy.

Rubella keratopathy

Rubella embryopathy may appear at birth with a cloudy or opaque cornea that is small or of normal size without an increase in intraocular pressure (p. 983). This often has been confused with the congenital glaucoma of rubella; however, this disturbance is a local corneal defect which exhibits no progressive increase in corneal size. The opacities may vary from mild to severe and may be transient or permanent. Congenital glaucoma may be differentiated from this condition by the associated increase in intraocular pressure and by the increase in corneal diameter. True congenital glaucoma also may be one of the manifestations of rubella embryopathy.

Congenital hereditary stationary dystrophy

This rare corneal dystrophy appears at birth as a ground-glass appearance of the cornea. The corneal thickness is frequently three to four times normal and is virtually diagnostic of this disease. Intraocular pressure is occasionally mildly elevated, making the differentiation from congenital glaucoma difficult. However, progressive corneal enlargement does not occur, and the photophobia and lacrimation of isolated congenital glaucoma are not present.

THE ABNORMALLY COLORED SCLERA

The sclera of the full-term neonate is normally glistening white. The overlying conjunctiva and conjunctival vessels produce a superimposed filmy and vascular pattern. A generalized bluish discoloration of the underdeveloped sclera is normally present in premature infants. Rarely a congenital, idiopathic weakness is a small area of the sclera will produce a bulging called a *staphyloma*. The light blue color is caused by thinness of the sclera, which transmits the darker color of the underlying uveal tissue. *Osteogenesis imperfecta* may be associated with a similar bluish discoloration of the sclera in the full-term neonate because of inadequately developed scleral collagen.

DISEASES OF THE INTERNAL EYE
Aniridia, iris colobomas, and persistent pupillary membranes

Aniridia, or absence of the iris, is a rare congenital anomaly, usually bilateral, that is almost invariably associated with poor vision. A small rudimentary cuff of peripheral iris is always present grossly or microscopically. Associated findings with aniridia include severe congenital glaucoma in greater than 50% of cases, a corneal pannus, cataract, abnormal optic discs, and dislocation of the lens. Aplasia of the macula is also frequently found with aniridia and causes the nystagmus and poor visual acuity. Aniridia may result from an autosomal dominant genetic transmission or may be sporadic. The sporadic variety of aniridia is associated with Wilms' tumor in approximately 10% of cases.

Iris coloboma is one of the most common congenital abnormalities seen in the eye. Typical colobomas occur in the inferior nasal quadrant, the area of closure of the embryonic cleft (Fig. 35-13). Atypical colobomas may occur in any quadrant and rarely may be multiple. Such coloboma may vary from a small notch in the pupil to the absence of an entire segment of the iris. It usually is not associated with visual difficulties. Since typical iris colobomas are associated with an abnormal closure of the embryonic cleft, however, they also may be associated with a coloboma of the ciliary body, choroid, retina, or optic nerve. When the optic nerve or macula is involved in the coloboma, visual difficulty occurs. Thus it is always wise to look for a pathologic condition of the fundus when an iris coloboma is detected. Although iris coloboma may appear as a single ocular finding, and although it has been listed previously as a single dominant transmission, it may represent a mild or variable expression of colobomatous microphthalmia with its several modes of inheritance.

IRIS COLOBOMAS
Isolated congenital colobomas
Congenital colobomatous microphthalmia
Trisomy 13
Trisomy 18
Rieger's syndrome
Iris coloboma and anal atresia syndrome
Lowe's syndrome (infrequent)
Goldenhar's syndrome (infrequent)
Rubinstein-Taybi syndrome (infrequent)
Chromosome 13q− syndrome

Although not associated with aniridia or colobomas, *persistent pupillary membranes* may be seen in the neonate, particulary in the premature infant. These are remnants of the anterior fetal vascular coat of the lens that have failed to undergo atrophy in the seventh month of gestation. A filmy lacework of fibers radiates from the pupillary rim over the center of the lens and may persist into adulthood or, more frequently, continue to atrophy. Disappearance during the first few months of life is the rule.

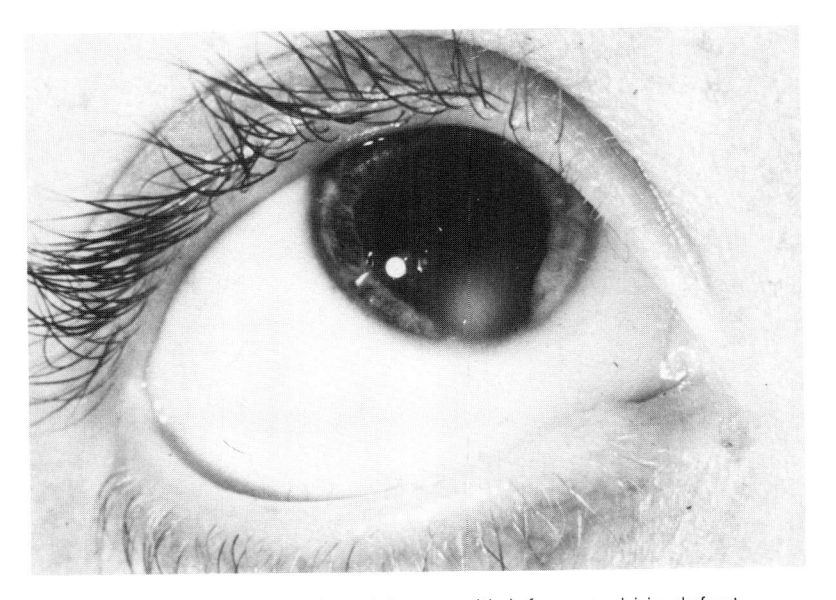

Fig. 35-13. Typical iris coloboma with inferonasal iris defect.

The unusually colored iris

Heterochromia indicates a difference in pigmentation between the two irises. Since many infants do not develop iris pigmentation until after the neonatal period, this is infrequently seen and is of little diagnostic value in this group. However, in white infants with darkly colored irises and in the darkly pigmented races some iris pigmentation is established at birth or shortly thereafter, and these neonates occasionally show abnormalities in pigmentation. Heterochromia may occur as an isolated autosomal dominant trait. Heterochromia also is associated with several syndromes; if they are present, they may be helpful in establishing the diagnosis. The hemifacial atrophy of Romberg occasionally is associated with lack of pigmentation on the side of the face that is atrophic; the Waardenburg syndrome is typically associated with heterochromia; and congenital Horner's syndrome produces heterochromia, usually after the neonatal period, as the result of failure of development of normal pigmentation in the iris on the sympathetically denervated side. Aganglionic megacolon (Hirschsprung's disease) may be associated with iris bicolor.

The white pupil

A white pupil (also called a cat's eye reflex) denotes an ocular abnormality of the lens, the vitreous, or the fundus. An understanding of the etiology of diseases associated with a white pupil is helpful in searching for genetic factors and in requesting pertinent laboratory data that may be diagnostic, as in galactosemia. Knowledge of available treatment encourages early correction before permanent visual loss occurs or before secondary complications produce irreversible ocular damage.

Examination for the white pupil

Since the infant sleeps much of the time, and since the pupils are small, the casual observation of the white pupil often is delayed until the infant becomes more alert and active. Including the observation of a red fundus reflex as a part of the normal neonatal examination of the pupil provides an early clue that an abnormality exists. This should be basic to the examination of *all* neonates. However, nothing takes the place of ophthalmoscopy through dilated pupils.

The initial examination may be made using a hand light, the light of the otoscope, or an ophthalmoscope. The pupil should be maximally dilated. With the light source held close to the eye, the pupillary reflex is evaluated for whitish discoloration; if a discoloration is present, the percentage of involvement of the pupillary area is estimated. With a +1 or +2 lens in the ophthalmoscope, a red reflex is obtained by observing the pupillary area from a position approximately 1 foot from the eye. When an extensive pathologic condition of the cornea, lens, or vitreous totally obstructs the reflection of light from the red fundus, the fundus reflex in the pupil is black. With lesser degrees of opacification or lesser amounts of diseased tissue the reflex is dull red. Irregular densities, such as those occurring in an incomplete cataract, produce a correspondingly irregular reflex (Fig. 35-14). White lesions in the fundus itself (retina and choroid) provide a white reflex rather than a black or red one. The site of the abnormality often may be localized initially by focusing through the pupil with the ophthalmoscope and the +10-diopter lens in place. Abnormalities of the lens are seen to be in focus immediately adjacent to the plane of the pupil, whereas abnormalities of the vitreous come into focus more deeply behind the pupil. In moving slightly to the side while viewing the opacity, the examiner can see that the more deeply it is placed behind the pupil, the greater the apparent relative movement of the opacity in relation to the pupil. Definitive evaluation requires ophthalmic slit-lamp examination and ophthalmoscopy with the infant under adequate sedation or gen-

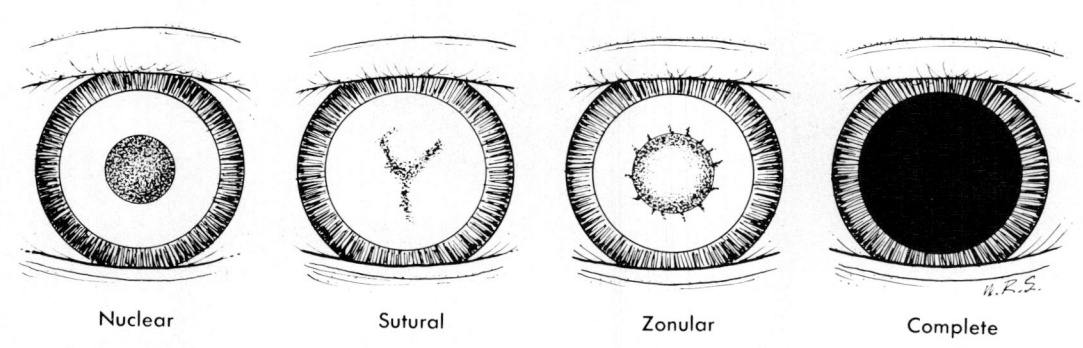

Nuclear   Sutural   Zonular   Complete

Fig. 35-14. The appearance of the red reflex with various cataracts. With the ophthalmoscope set at 0, the dilated pupil is observed with the examiner standing approximately 1 foot from the infant. The normal eye is seen to have a clear round red reflex. Lens opacities (cataracts) interrupt the red reflex, producing black opacities as shown.

eral anesthesia. The importance of this examination and its aid to diagnosis and treatment far outweigh the risks of sedation or general anesthesia.

The lens (cataracts)

A large number of morphologic types of cataracts are known, but only a brief description is presented here. The size and shape of the cataract (lens opacification) depend on the area of the lens that is being formed at the time the damage or developmental defects occur. The lens grows continuously during life, laying down new lens fibers on its external surface, much like an onion. Damage that occurs in the early fetal period produces opacifications in the very center of the lens. Such nuclear cataracts have clear layers in the periphery of the lens. Later periods of damage produce ringlike opacifications surrounded by central and peripheral clear areas (zonular cataracts). Recent damage produces peripheral opacifications near the surface of the lens (cortical cataracts). Very dense opacities cause greater visual disturbance, especially if they are located in the central anterior-to-posterior axis, whereas peripheral opacities near the equator or the lateral periphery of the lens produce little or no visual disturbance.

Etiology. Causes of cataracts may be grouped under the following headings: genetic, viral, inborn errors of metabolism, trauma, association with other eye malformations, and generalized syndromes. The following discussion begins with the most frequently encountered cataracts. The remaining causative factors are shown in Table 35-2, with evaluation as to frequency of occurrence.

Genetically determined cataracts often occur as isolated abnormalities. They are frequently present at birth but occasionally originate during childhood. The primary mode of transmission is autosomal dominant. Recessive and X-linked transmission has been recorded infrequently. The pathogenesis of genetic cataracts is not known.

The *rubella embryopathy syndrome* is composed of multiple congenital anomalies that result from maternal viremia during the first trimester of pregnancy. Cataracts are present in approximately 50% of these patients (Fig. 35-15). They may be nuclear (confined to the center of the lens) or complete (involving all layers of the lens). The rubella virus may remain dormant in lens material in the offspring for up to several years of life. Microphthalmia and anterior uveitis also may be present in the same eye. The pupil is usually small and sometimes difficult to dilate because of atrophy of the iris structures. The iris therefore transilluminates abnormally. Congenital glaucoma also occurs in 10% to 25% of patients with congenital rubella; at birth it causes an enlarged, hazy cornea. A cloudy, edematous, or white cornea, however, also may be found with normal intraocular pressure as part of the

Table 35-2. Neonatal cataracts

Type	Incidence of occurrence in the syndrome
Genetic	
Dominant	
Recessive	
X-linked recessive	
Viral	
Rubella	50% incidence
Cytomegalic inclusion disease	Infrequent
Inborn errors of metabolism	
Galactosemia	50% incidence
Galactokinase deficiency	Frequent
Lowe's syndrome	Frequent
Trauma	
Birth trauma	Infrequent
Blunt trauma	Frequent
Perforating injuries	Frequent
Battered child syndrome	Infrequent
Endocrine	
Congenital hypoparathyroidism	Frequent
Albright's hereditary osteodystrophy	Infrequent
Neurologic	
Marinesco-Sjögren syndrome	Infrequent
Smith-Lemli-Opitz syndrome	Rare
Miscellaneous	
Aniridia (sporadic or associated with Wilms' tumor	Infrequent Infrequent
Treacher Collins syndrome	Infrequent
Pierre Robin anomalad	Infrequent
Rubinstein-Taybi syndrome	Frequent
Hallermann-Streiff syndrome	
Chromosomal anomalies	
Trisomy 13	Infrequent
Trisomy 18	Infrequent
Turner's syndrome	Infrequent
Associated with other eye malformations	
Microphthalmia	Frequent
Rieger's anomaly	Infrequent

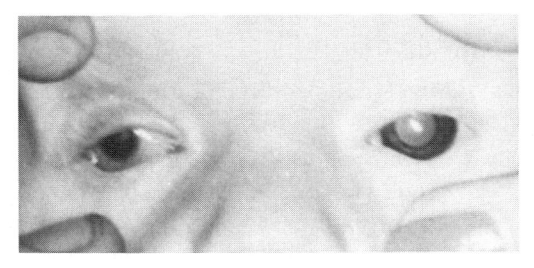

Fig. 35-15. Rubella syndrome with cataract of the left eye and microphthalmia of the right eye.

rubella embryopathy. Rubella retinopathy may be found later in life. It is a pigmentary degeneration of the retina without demonstrable effect on visual function.

Galactosemia is a hereditary inborn error of metabolism with deficiency of the enzyme galactose-1-phosphate uridyltransferase and accumulation of galactose-1-phosphate, galactose, and galactitol (p. 831). The affected neonate may be normal at birth. Subsequently cataracts may appear during the first 2 months of life. The cataracts may be zonular or may appear as the classically described drop of oil (vacuoles) in the center of the lens. The latter description results from the imbibition of water that occurs in association with accumulation of galactose and galactitol in the lens. Diagnosis is made by the finding of galactosuria or the absence of galactose-1-phosphate uridyltransferase in red blood cells. Early diagnosis and a regimen of a galactose-free diet will prevent the development or further progression of cataracts. Occasional resolution of the lens opacity also may occur if the infant receives the appropriate diet.

Treatment. All congenital cataracts require early evaluation by an ophthalmologist. Most dense cataracts need surgical treatment for prevention of amblyopia or strabismus. Some small central cataracts may be effectively treated by long-term dilatation of the pupil to expose the optically clear periphery of the lens. If dilatation is inadequate, a removal of a portion of the iris (optical iridectomy) for the same purpose may be performed surgically; however, the visual effects of lens extraction without a corrective lens will be no better than leaving the cataract in its original state. Removal of the lens (within the first few months of life if the cataract is complete), followed by contact lens application, may provide the best hope of preventing amblyopia. If the cataract affects one eye, the amblyopia treatment is less successful than when both eyes are equally affected.

Pendular nystagmus may be present in association with bilateral cataracts and may continue after surgery. This type of nystagmus is a broad to-and-fro excursion of the eyes which is approximately equal in both directions. It is usually the result, not the cause, of poor visual acuity. Treatment of bilateral dense congenital cataracts by surgical removal and subsequent correction with contact lenses may prevent the development of or may reverse pendular nystagmus.

Diseases of the vitreous and retina producing a white pupil

Diseases of the posterior portion of the eye, which may be sufficiently severe in their involvement of the vitreous or retina to produce a white reflex in the pupil, are retinoblastoma, retrolental fibroplasia, PHPV, retinal dysplasia, Norrie's disease, and incontinentia pigmenti. In addition, any lesion, such as a coloboma or medullated nerve fibers, creating a white area in the fundus may create a white pupillary reflex.

Retinoblastoma. Retinoblastoma is the most frequent malignant tumor affecting the neonatal eye. This malignancy usually produces a white pupil only when it is of sufficient size to involve a large area of the posterior segment of the eye.

Retinoblastoma occurs in approximately 1 of every 25,000 to 30,000 births, with no predilection for race or sex. The tumor arises sporadically or is inherited through an autosomal dominant mutation that exhibits approximately 80% penetrance. Most cases appear to be sporadic. The inherited variety may be gradually increasing in frequency because of a greater survival rate of patients whose retinoblastoma has been treated. Unilateral tumors are usually sporadic and may represent a somatic mutation. Bilateral retinoblastomas are usually inheritable. An affected individual who has survived the hereditary form of retinoblastoma will have about a 40% risk that each offspring will be similarly affected. An individual surviving a sporadic unilateral variety of tumor will have about a 10% chance or less that each offspring will be affected. Those surviving sporadic bilateral involvement appear to have a 40% chance that each offspring will be affected. Empirical risk figures suggest that normal parents having one affected child will have about a 6% chance that a subsequent child will be affected. However, if they have two affected children, the risk increases to 40% for each additional child.

Clinical manifestations. The tumor originates in the retina and grows anteriorly into the vitreous by direct extension or by seeding and also may grow posteriorly into the choroid. Early in its course it produces decreased vision and strabismus, and with further growth it subsequently produces a white pupil (Fig. 35-16), which is frequently detected by the parents. Any cross-eyed infant requires a fundus examination with the pupils dilated to rule out retinoblastoma. With further enlargement the tumor produces secondary glaucoma, which may be associated with pain and photophobia or symptoms identical to those of congenital glaucoma. With extension into the anterior chamber an opaque layer of white cells (hypopyon) or spontaneous bleeding (hyphema) may occur. The calcification in a retinoblastoma is most easily detected by means of ultrasound, even before it is radiologically apparent.

Diagnosis. The diagnosis of retinoblastoma is supported by finding one or more solid white masses in the fundus of the eye. Multiple tumors are present in a high percentage of patients. Small whitish opacities in the vitreous, representing an anterior seeding of the tumor, may be present. Additional confirmatory findings are the presence of calcification in the intraocular area, as shown radiologically (found in 75% of patients), and the clinical

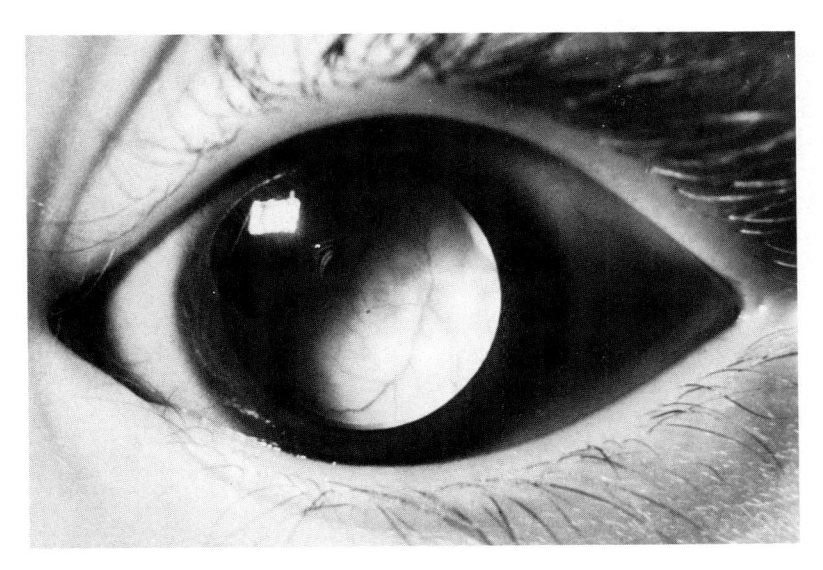

Fig. 35-16. Leukokoria, advanced retinoblastoma.

impression that the intraocular mass is solid, as shown by transillumination of the globe or by ultrasonography. Aqueous humor levels of lactic acid dehydrogenase may be elevated in comparison to serum values. The differential diagnosis may be exceedingly difficult if the tumor is advanced or atypical and may require enucleation for histologic study and positive identification. PHPV may be confused with retinoblastoma (p. 998).

Treatment. The management of retinoblastoma is determined by its size and location. Examination should be performed with the infant under anesthesia, and accurate relationships of all lesions should be plotted on retinal drawings. Reese's classification is used for grading of the severity and prognosis of the disease. This classification has five groupings. The most favorable, group I, includes small, single or multiple tumors in the posterior half of the fundus. The least favorable, group V, includes tumors involving over half the retina or seeding of the tumor into the vitreous. Intermediate groups are graded upward in severity according to increasing size and more anterior location of the tumor.

The standard treatment of retinoblastoma has been enucleation when the tumor is unilateral. Since one mode of spread of the disease is by direct extension along the optic nerve, the removal of as much optic nerve as possible in the process of enucleation is important. Recently, however, unilateral (and bilateral) tumors in groups I, II, and III have been treated by therapeutic cobalt or linear acceleration x-irradiation. With advanced bilateral disease the more involved eye is usually enucleated for histologic identification, and the remaining eye is treated with supervoltage radiation plus chemotherapeutic agents such as triethylenemelamine or cyclophosphamide (Cytoxan). Treatment modalities also include radioactive applicators for small isolated recurrent tumors in accessible locations. Photocoagulation, cryotherapy, and diathermy also have been used successfully for control of localized recurrences. Chemotherapeutic agents, such as triethylenemelamine, have been used in a palliative way, in combination with irradiation for orbital spread or distant metastases. Treatment can produce regression of the tumor, in some cases to total disappearance. In larger tumors a reduction in size occurs. The color of the tumor changes from pinkish white to grayish or glistening white. Often a regressed tumor has the appearance of cottage cheese.

Prognosis. The most significant factor in the prognosis is the stage of the disease at the time treatment is instituted. With prompt, adequate treatment, group I patients have approximately a 95% chance for 5-year survival. With advanced disease or evidence of extension beyond the globe the cure rate is markedly reduced (below 30% 5-year survival). Unfortunately radiation therapy, although it may be effective in curing the retinoblastoma, has its own complications. Children surviving treated retinoblastoma may develop new malignant disease in the irradiated tissue. The most frequent of these radiation-induced tumors is sarcoma, usually presenting in the orbit in the first 10 years after therapy; because of the location, the prognosis is exceptionally poor. Other primary malignancies also may develop.

Retrolental fibroplasia. This occurs in premature infants treated with oxygen above ambient levels (p. 437). From 1940 to 1954 the use of high oxygen concentrations in incubators was common for most premature infants in an effort to reduce brain injury from hypoxia.

During this period the incidence of retrolental fibroplasia was markedly increased. Subsequent to this time lower concentrations of oxygen have been used, and the rate of occurrence decreased. However, the treatment of respiratory distress syndrome with high oxygen concentrations, in an effort to increase the survival rate of premature infants and to decrease the morbidity from hypoxia, again has increased the occurrence rate of retrolental fibroplasia.

Pathogenesis. The pathogenesis of this disease is incompletely known, but increased arterial oxygen tensions are known to produce severe vascular constriction in the immature retinal vasculature. When an infant is returned to normal levels of oxygen, those retinal areas which would have been supplied by the vessels if they were normally developed become hypoxic. Apparently this stimulates vascular proliferation into the hypoxic area in an attempt to increase oxygenation and results in leakage, hemorrhage, and fibrous proliferation.

In an attempt to define the pathophysiology of retrolental fibroplasia, Flower produced severe cicatricial retinopathy, akin to the disease in humans, in aspirin-treated, oxygen-exposed newborn beagle puppies. In unmedicated puppies, oxygen-breathing produced retinal vasoconstriction, whereas the retinal vessels of aspirin-treated, oxygen-exposed littermates became more dilated or remained unchanged. He therefore postulated that retinal vasoconstriction was a protective rather than a pathologic response to hyperoxia. He speculated that this vasoconstrictor protective response as well as retinal vascular maturity determined the ultimate retinal response to oxygen. Prostaglandin inhibition, which influences the vascular tonus, may therefore play a role in retrolental fibroplasia. Recent studies suggest that, in addition to elevated Po_2, elevated arterial Pco_2 must be considered a potential factor in the pathogenesis of retrolental fibroplasia.

Prematurity is the most constant feature of this disease. The smaller the infant, the greater the chance for the disease to be produced. The normal retina develops relatively late in fetal development. At 3½ months' gestation only the posterior half of the retina is well differentiated. At 4 months' gestation the central retinal vessels appear at the disc and begin to vascularize the retina. By the seventh month the peripheral retina is still relatively immature, and the retinal vessels have reached only the equator of the globe. By the eighth month vascularization is complete except for the temporal periphery of the retina. Differentiation of the retina, as well as completion of the vascular supply, lags behind in the temporal retina compared with the remainder of the eye; thus the temporal retina becomes more vulnerable to the effects of high arterial oxygen concentration and is the area most likely to show the effects of retrolental fibroplasia.

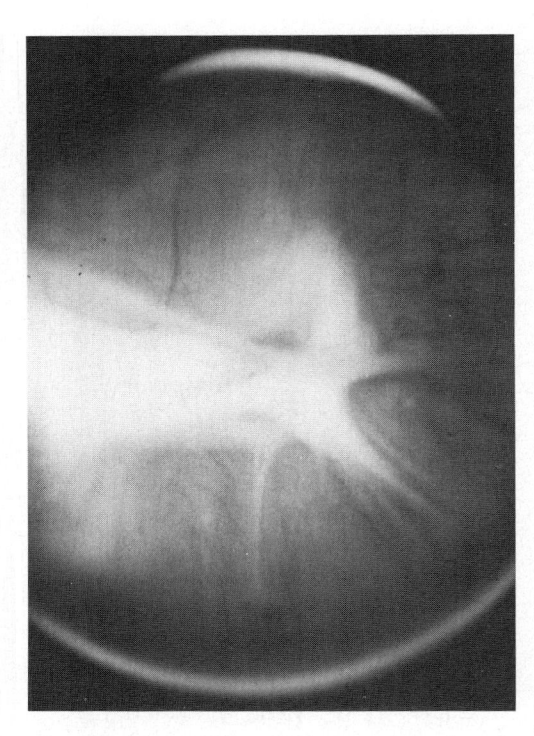

Fig. 35-17. Retrolental fibroplasia, moderately advanced, with gliotic retina drawn into upper temporal fold.

Pathology. The active stage of the disease usually begins during the first month after birth. Following the acute period of vasoconstriction, which occurs during oxygen administration, retinal vessels become dilated and tortuous. After removal of the infant from oxygen therapy the areas of incompletely formed retina develop neovascularization with tufts or arcades of newly formed, thin-walled anastomosing vessels. Small retinal hemorrhages develop from the neovascular sites and subsequently become fibrotic. Massive vitreous hemorrhage also may occur from the areas of neovascularization. The diseased, contracted vitreous produces traction and areas of retinal detachment. Further tearing of neovascular tissue occurs, with production of additional retinal and vitreous hemorrhages. With marked advancement of the disease the entire retina and its newly formed fibroblastic and neovascular tissue become detached and are pulled forward to lie just posterior to the lens, hence the name of the disease. Spontaneous regression may occur at any time during this process up to the point of fibrosis and extensive vitreous traction. There is, as yet, no way to predict accurately how often and to what extent regression will occur. In a small percentage of patients retrolental fibroplasia progresses to the severe stage, with production of a retrolental mass of fibroblastic tissue.

With cessation of the active process the eye is left with a cicatricial aftermath, which may be mild to severe, depending on the extent of the active process. Minor changes include tortuosity of the vessels and a slightly pale fundus with occasional irregular pigmentation. Myopia is common. A more advanced form shows retinal vessels that are distorted or pulled to the temporal side of the retina (Fig. 35-17). A still more advanced form shows a peripheral opaque mass in the temporal periphery, with a fold of retinal tissue extending from the optic disc to the peripheral mass. In this fold of tissue most of the major retinal blood vessels are incorporated. Where proliferation has been more marked, the retina becomes detached, and portions of or all the retina is pulled anteriorly. The most severe form is manifested by microphthalmia, a dense retrolental mass, and cataractous changes in the lens. The anterior chamber is frequently shallow, and the cornea may be cloudy as the result of secondary glaucoma. Vision is severely reduced. This latter, major form of involvement usually takes 4 to 5 months to evolve.

Clinical manifestations. Reese divides the active stage of the disease into four levels. These grades represent a semiarbitrary division of a continuation of pathologic changes.

Stage I: dilation and tortuosity of retinal vessels
Stage II: stage I plus neovascularization and some peripheral retinal clouding
Stage III: stage II plus retinal detachment in the periphery of the fundus
Stage IV: hemispheric or circumferential retinal detachment
Stage V: complete retinal detachment

A more recent classification by Kingham divides the progressive findings on a morphologic basis.

Grade I: abnormal terminal arborization of peripheral retinal vessels (much like the bristles on a broom)
Grade II: dilated terminal vessels ending in an intraretinal line of yellowish pink tissue running parallel to the ora serrata
Grade III: intraretinal line markedly thickened with new vessels that have grown into the vitreous
Grade IV: peripheral retinal detachment
Grade V: retinal detachment progressed to, or almost to, the disc

There is no method of determining which infant may develop retrolental fibroplasia when exposed to increased ambient oxygen concentrations. Vascular constriction or tortuosity or both erroneously were thought to be of some prognostic value. Arterial oxygen tension must be monitored when oxygen is administered during the neonatal period. Maintenance of a normal arterial oxygen tension (PaO$_2$) at around 60 to 80 mm Hg is critically important in managing low birth weight infants. A recent cooperative study indicates a high degree of correlation between the development of cicatricial retrolental fibroplasia and the length of time a neonate spends in a high-oxygen environment. In this study exposure to oxygen therapy for 5 weeks resulted in a very high incidence of retrolental fibroplasia. Clearly prematurity is also a major risk factor.

The probability of low birth weight infants developing retrolental fibroplasia may be affected by the interaction of numerous risk factors. Preterm infants who are the product of twin (or other multiple) pregnancies or those who have received exchange transfusions are thought to be at increased risk. Short-term exposure to high oxygen tensions may produce little or no ocular damage in some infants, whereas prolonged exposure to small increases in inspired O$_2$ levels may be likely to create undesirable retinal changes. The regularly observed wide fluctuations of PaO$_2$ in neonates with respiratory disease make routine arterial and/or transcutaneous PO$_2$ measurements mandatory (p. 430). Unfortunately the precise duration and level of elevated PaO$_2$ values that produce retinal changes are not yet known with certainty. Thus prevention of retrolental fibroplasia currently is based on the avoidance of excessively high PaO$_2$ levels and, more important, the removal of high-risk, low birth weight infants from increased oxygen environments as soon as feasible. Hittner recently reported that high doses of vitamin E may reduce the incidence and severity of retrolental fibroplasia.

Although ocular examination has no prognostic value in prevention of the disease, examination before discharge is recommended. All infants weighing less than 1,500 gm at birth and/or of less than 37 weeks' gestation are at risk and should be examined by an ophthalmologist familiar with the disease and experienced in the techniques of examination. The optimum time for examination is about 3 to 4 weeks of age. This is the approximate time when the more severe forms of retinal involvement begin to develop. Examination at an earlier age, after short-term oxygen therapy, is permissible. Vascularization of the peripheral retina to the ora serrata region is an assurance that retrolental fibroplasia will not develop at a later period. If vascularization of the peripheral retina has not progressed to the ora serrata region at the time of examination, a second evaluation with the patient's pupils dilated should be performed at approximately 6 weeks of age and at regular intervals thereafter until complete vascularization of the peripheral retina is achieved.

Therapy. Transscleral cryotherapy has been advocated as an arresting agent during the active stage of the disease. At this time there is a lack of consensus as to its effectiveness. Those advocating treatment believe that therapy must be given when there is evidence of neovascularization advancing into the vitreous. Those opposed to treatment believe there is insufficient evidence to support the advantages of therapy in a disease process that is usually self-arresting. If undertaken, therapy must by accomplished by someone who is skilled and experienced in the use of cryotherapy for this disease. The use of peripheral cryotherapy in such small eyes is complicated by the possibility of causing the destruction of large areas of ocular tissue or creating central vascular occlusion or other major problems. Photocoagulation also has been advocated, again without much verification of its clinical efficacy.

Persistent hyperplastic primary vitreous (PHPV). PHPV is a congenital anomaly that produces a white pupil at birth or shortly thereafter. This disease results from the failure of reabsorption of the embryonic hyaloid system (the primary vitreous). This embryonic system develops as a complex network of vessels growing anteriorly from the disc to surround the developing lens (the tunica vasculosa lentis). This vascular scaffolding supplies the posterior part of the eye and lens during its early formation and is replaced by the clear secondary vitreous when the eye further matures. During the fifth to eighth months of gestation the hyaloid vascular system atrophies almost completely, leaving a small, nearly transparent canal running from the disc to the posterior surface of the lens (Cloquet's canal). Failure of complete atrophy of this vascular system may leave a number of possible remnants that may be seen at birth. At the disc a small protrusion of mesodermal tissue, which extends a short distance into the vitreous, is called Bergmeister's papilla. Remnants of the hyaloid artery may be seen extending from the disc to the posterior central area of the lens. A small remnant of the tunica vasculosa lentis on the posterior central area of the lens is called a Mittendorf dot. A persistence and hyperplasia of the entire system is called PHPV.

Clinical manifestations. PHPV may appear at birth as a sheet of white tissue immediately behind the lens. It is usually most dense at the center of the lens and thins out toward the periphery. Vessels frequently are seen to radiate from its center. The retrolental mass therefore may be pinkish white. When the pupil is dilated, the ciliary processes may be seen being drawn centrally along the posterior surface of the lens toward the central mass.

PHPV is nearly always unilateral and occurs in full-term infants without history of oxygen therapy. The involved eye is usually microphthalmic. The anterior chamber is frequently shallower than in the fellow eye because fibrous contraction of the primary vitreous pulls the ciliary body centrally. In turn, the lens is forced forward. With continued organization and contraction of the primary vitreous the lens capsule may be involved, and cataract formation may occur. At this stage in development of the disease glaucoma may occur, as well as posterior chamber hemorrhages and hemorrhages into the lens. Retinal detachment occurs in the final stages, with continued vitreous traction. PHPV should be suspected in the neonate with a rapidly progressive unilateral mature cataract.

Diagnosis. Differentiation of PHPV from retrolental fibroplasia is usually possible because of the unilateral involvement and occurrence of PHPV in a full-term infant. Retrolental fibroplasia is seen bilaterally in a premature infant who has had oxygen therapy. Differentiation from retinoblastoma is aided by the presence of visible ciliary processes in the periphery of the dilated pupil and the presence of vascular elements in the central portion of the retrolental mass. Also retinoblastomas do not usually occur in microphthalmic eyes. The absence of roentgenographic evidence of calcification within the eye may be of additional value. However, because of the progressive and changing nature of PHPV, it may closely simulate retinoblastoma and may require enucleation for differentiation. A persistent embryonic iris artery or one that notches the pupil suggests the presence of PHPV, even when an opaque lens obscures its presence.

Treatment. Treatment of PHPV is ineffective in most circumstances, but experimental attempts at surgery have been made. Surgical removal of the lens and vitreous with optical correction must be attempted very early (within the first few weeks) if any degree of success is to be expected. Only very mild cases have been reported to have moderate visual success, and the prognosis for visual recovery should be extremely guarded.

Prognosis. Since the macula is poorly developed in microphthalmic eyes, even anatomically successful surgery for PHPV may not result in useful vision.

Retinal dysplasia. Retinal dysplasia is a congenital anomaly of full-term infants, is usually bilateral, and is associated with microphthalmic eyes. It may occur as part of a group of congenital anomalies, including defects of the central nervous system, cardiovascular system, and skeletal system of sufficient severity to produce early death of the infant; trisomy 13 should be considered. When the dysplasia is advanced, a white retrolental mass may be produced. Milder forms of dysplasia occur as developmental abnormalities but often are detected only by histologic techniques; results of chromosome analysis are usually normal.

Norrie's disease. This is a rare genetic disorder which is transmitted as an X-linked recessive trait. It is characterized by the presence of bilateral massive retinal detachments, resulting in a white pupil often but not always combined with deafness and mental retardation. Organization of the retinal detachment may disrupt the lens, producing cataract, or may effect the anterior chamber angle, producing congenital glaucoma. The usual result is atrophy of the globe (phthisis bulbi).

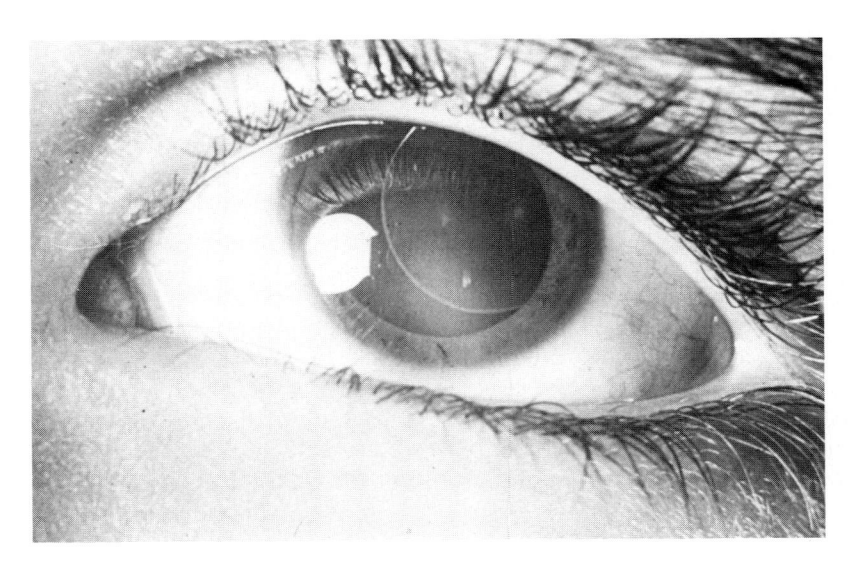

Fig. 35-18. Ectopia lentis (dislocated lens) of the left eye.

The dislocated lens

The discovery of a dislocated lens *(ectopia lentis)* in the neonatal period is helpful in the identification of systemic disease processes which are associated with this abnormality. Lens dislocation may be present in the following diseases during the neonatal period, or it may not assume its dislocated position until the first or second decade of life: homocystinuria, sulfide oxidase deficiency, hyperlysinemia, Marfan's syndrome, and Weill-Marchesani syndrome. It occurs as the result of a laxity, absence, or defect of the zonular attachments that suspend the lens from the ciliary body.

Ectopia lentis may be suggested by iridodonesis, or tremulousness of the iris, which results from the lack of normal support the lens gives to the posterior surface of the iris. Identification of an eccentric location of the lens is made by wide dilatation of the pupil and visualization of a portion of the equator of the lens in the pupillary space (Fig. 35-18). Treatment of the dislocated lens usually is not necessary during the neonatal period, unless it is complicated by cataract formation or glaucoma. The glaucoma may be caused either by complications of the cataract formation or by blockage of aqueous flow through the pupil.

The abnormal fundus

Observing the neonatal eye *through a dilated pupil* should be a routine part of the examination in every infant. With the direct ophthalmoscope the fundus appears as a flat, two-dimensional surface. However, this represents a three-dimensional organization of tissue where several successive layers are viewed simultaneously as the result of their transparency. The retinal vessels lie near the surface of the retina. Deep to the vessels, the retina is a nearly transparent layer of tissue with a sheen to its inner surface. This transparency is disturbed when abnormalities are present. It resembles a pale ghostlike sheet when it is detached. Retinal edema gives a slightly raised opalescent appearance. Infection obscures the underlying structures by a fuzzy white thickening of the retinal tissue itself.

During the neonatal period nonvascular structures of the fundus are nearly transparent because of the lack of uveal pigmentation. Therefore in all pathologic processes characterized by either a lack or an excess of pigment these defects may be only minimally suggested and may become progressively more evident as the normal uveal pigmentation becomes complete after the first 6 months of life. The choroid is the deepest layer normally visible by the ophthalmoscope. Pathologic processes that prevent its development or that destroy areas of choroid therefore will expose areas of bare sclera that will appear glistening white with the ophthalmoscope.

Hereditary abnormalities

Retinoschisis is a hereditary abnormality in which the superficial layers of the retina are split from the deeper layers and are elevated into the vitreous. This splitting creates a veil-like appearance in front of the retina. Visual function is absent in the affected tissue. Retinoschisis is a progressive, degenerative disorder, which has an X-linked recessive transmission. Macular changes and vitreous hemorrhages can occur as associated findings. Both lead to loss of vision.

Fundus albipunctatus is characterized by gray or white mottling of the fundus. This is a stationary form of retinal degeneration, transmitted as an autosomal recessive trait. Visual acuity, color vision, and visual fields are normal in patients with this disorder.

Retinitis pigmentosa is a pigmentary degeneration of the retina, which typically makes its appearance in the early teens or even later. In severe form it may rarely appear in the neonatal period. The ophthalmoscopic findings are the result of retinal pigment epithelial degeneration, with migration of the pigment to form irregular black deposits resembling bony spicules.

Leber's congenital amaurosis occasionally produces symptoms of blindness shortly after birth but usually occurs later in childhood. Typical findings are a salt-and-pepper appearance of the fundus, with a grayish cast to the retina. Electroretinography reveals severely deficient retinal function. Although autosomal recessive transmission is most common, autosomal dominance characterizes some forms of congenital amaurosis.

The diagnosis of *albinism* in the neonatal period is extremely difficult to substantiate as the result of the normal paucity of the uveal pigment during this period. The diagnosis may be suggested when pigmentation of the skin, hair, and irises fails to progress during the first several months in comparison with that of parents and siblings. Lack of pigmentation is more apparent earlier in darker races. The fundus remains quite pale and shows a prominent appearance of its choroidal vessels. Photophobia, pendular nystagmus, and abnormal transillumination of the irises are characteristic of albinism. Moderately to severely reduced vision is characteristic.

Congenital disorders

Retinal folds presumably occur as the result of overgrowth of retinal tissue in comparison with ocular size, thereby preventing total attachment of all retinal tissue to the underlying pigment epithelium and choroid. A white fold or ridge of retinal tissue may be seen running from the disc, typically inferotemporally, to the periphery. Occasionally the macular area may be involved.

Congenital grouped pigmentation is a rare finding of unknown cause in which small areas of the retina, 1 disc diameter or less in size, show hyperpigmentation. These areas typically are paired or grouped and are usually kidney shaped. They have no clinical significance but should not be confused with old inflammatory scars.

Infectious diseases

Intrauterine ocular infections occur as the result of maternal infections that cross the placental barrier (Chapters 27 and 28). Chorioretinitis occurs in patients with rubella and occasionally in patients with influenza and congenital syphilis. An irregularity of the retinal pigment develops, with what appears to be a salt-and-pepper type of distribution. Congenital cytomegalic inclusion disease may include chorioretinal lesions in any form, from large, whitish, necrotic lesions in the posterior pole to the more typical multiple, small, peripheral white areas that tend to enlarge or coalesce as the disease progresses. Congenital toxoplasmosis in its severe form may lead to large chorioretinal scars in the macular area. The chorioretinal scars appear as large white areas of exposed sclera, with prominent, darkly pigmented borders. The treatment of the eye manifestations of congenital toxoplasmosis is not established. When seen in the neonatal fundus, scar formation usually is a sign of the inactive disease. Large doses of systemically administered steroids are advocated for progressive extension of the retinal infection. Pyrimethamine (Daraprim), triple sulfa, clindamycin, sulfadiazine, and folinic acid, in combination, also have been used, although their efficacy is unproven. In addition to these intrauterine infections, postnatally acquired candidal septicemia may be associated with fluffy retinal and vitreous exudates.

Acquired fundus pathologic conditions

The retina of the premature infant is incompletely formed at birth and continues its development during the first few months of neonatal life. The periphery of the fundus from the equator to the ora serrata (the junction of the retina and the ciliary body) appears pale or grayish white, and the overlying vitreous may be somewhat hazy in appearance. These are normal findings, which gradually give way to the normal reddish pink color of the fundus as the retina progressively differentiates.

Birth trauma may produce a pathologic condition of the retina (p. 224); there may be scattered retinal hemorrhages, vitreous hemorrhage, or areas of retinal edema. (*Retrolental fibroplasia* is discussed on p. 995.) In retrolental fibroplasia a fold of retina extending from the disc to the temporal periphery, indicating marked involvement, is sometimes difficult to differentiate morphologically from a congenital retinal fold.

The abnormal macula

Best's vitelliform degeneration of the macula is an autosomal dominant disorder that rarely occurs in the neonatal period; there are cystlike changes in the macular retina, which rapidly coalesce and become yellowish. Its appearance has been likened to that of an egg yolk. This macular degeneration produces little initial reduction in visual acuity. It gradually undergoes further atrophic degeneration, with decrease in visual acuity at a much later time.

Several of the storage diseases produce an abnormal appearance of the macula, and abnormalities in the macula may be useful in detecting these disorders (Table 35-3) (Chapter 32). The abnormal appearance of the macula is produced by accumulation of the stored material in the ganglion cells of the retina. This produces a decrease in transparency of the retina except at the very center of the

Table 35-3. Neonatal macular changes

Condition	Defect
Tay-Sachs disease	Cherry-red spot
Niemann-Pick disease	Cherry-red spot
GM_1 generalized gangliosidosis	Cherry-red spot
Neuraminidase deficiency	Cherry-red spot and corneal clouding
Farber's disease	Gray macula
Best's vitelliform degeneration	Cystic macula (rare)
Toxoplasmosis	Chorioretinal scar
Coloboma	Absence of retina and choroid

macula, where no ganglion cells exist. Therefore the center of the macula retains its normal cherry-red appearance in sharp contrast to the surrounding grayish retina. Sphingolipidoses that may produce a cherry-red spot are *Tay-Sachs disease,* in which a cherry-red spot may be present shortly after birth or may develop during the first year, and *Niemann-Pick disease* (infantile), in which approximately 50% of patients develop a cherry-red spot in the macula during the neonatal period. Of the so-called mucolipidoses, *Farber's disease* has been noted to show a grayish discoloration of the macula at 6 to 8 weeks of age, and *GM_1 generalized gangliosidosis* has been found to demonstrate a cherry-red spot in the macula in approximately 30% of patients before 2 months of age. The mucopolysaccharidoses are characterized by abnormal deposition of mucopolysaccharides in the cornea, but the macula is normal. Neuraminidase deficiency (Goldberg's syndrome) appears to be a mucolipidosis with both macular cherry-red spot and mild corneal clouding.

Optic disc abnormalities

All transmissions of the visual pathways must exit the eye through the optic disc. Estimations of pallor or optic atrophy can be relied on only if careful attention is paid to preventing pressure on the orbital structures from being transmitted to the eye itself during examination of the disc. Disc margins in the neonate should be clear and distinct.

Persistence of hyaloid artery

Persistence of the central hyaloid artery is a common developmental abnormality. Its persistence in the premature infant is sufficiently frequent to be considered normal. It occurs in some 3% of full-term infants. Most frequently it is a fine thread of nearly transparent tissue, or rarely it may be patent and contain blood. It usually continues to undergo atrophic degeneration during the neonatal period and early life, with rare persistence into adulthood.

Bergmeister's papilla

The persistence of the mesodermal supporting elements of the hyaloid vascular system at the disc may leave a small protuberance of gray-white tissue extending from the disc forward into the vitreous. A small knuckle of a retinal vessel may course into this area and return to the disc before supplying the normal retina, or the papilla may be associated with one or several small, round, pearly gray cysts of remaining glial tissue. Vision usually is unimpaired.

Medullated nerve fibers

Normal myelinization of the optic nerve fibers occurs in fetal development in reverse direction to the growth of the axons themselves. Development of medullated sheaths therefore progresses from the geniculate bodies through the optic tracts, optic chiasm, and optic nerves to end normally just posterior to the optic disc. This process is usually complete at birth or within the first month of extrauterine life. Occasionally medullation of the nerve fibers proceeds through the disc and onto the retinal surface. This appears as a glistening, white, opaque area, involving the peripheral portion of the disc and extending into segments of the nearby retina. Sometimes there is no continuity between the disc and the medullated nerve fibers of the retina. The edges of the medullated areas are feathered, and the involved areas are sometimes arcuate. This process is stable after the first several months of life, and visual acuity is not often impaired, except for an enlarged area of the blind spot when measured in adults.

Conus or congenital crescent

The sharp margins of the optic disc are created by the abrupt ending of the choroid and pigment epithelium at the disc borders. On occasion one quadrant of the disc fails to have these structures extend to the immediate edge of the disc; instead they stop short in a sloping margin, which is crescent shaped. This allows the underlying sclera to be visible as a whitish crescent adjacent to the disc. This crescent is sometimes bordered by a darkly pigmented line. Two thirds of congenital crescents occur below the disc. Most eyes with congenital crescents are associated with defective vision in the form of hypermetropic astigmatism. A congenital conus should be differentiated from a myopic conus, or crescent, in that the former is present at birth, is inferiorly located, and is stationary throughout life, whereas the latter develops as the eye becomes excessively myopic and is usually temporal.

Coloboma of the disc

Coloboma of the disc is formed by a failure of adequate closure of the embryonic optic vesicle. A coloboma of the iris or choroid has a similar pathogenesis. The disc may appear enlarged and elongated, usually inferiorly or temporally. The coloboma may include the macular area. The blood vessels may be distributed normally or may be displaced to the periphery of the disc and appear to be somewhat disorganized in their initial direction from the disc. Colobomas of the disc usually are associated with defective vision.

Optic pit

Occasionally the surface of the optic disc shows a hole or pit. This pit usually is situated near the lower temporal quadrant of the disc at its border and may vary in size, shape, and depth. It is thought to be a minimal coloboma of the disc. Frequently visual defects are present with this finding. Later in life they are manifested as enlargement of the blind spot, sector field defects, or involvement of the papillomacular bundle, with production of a partial paracentral or central scotoma. In association with a pit of the optic disc, serous fluid may elevate the macula and cause reduction in visual acuity later in life.

Oblique discs

The optic nerve usually enters the posterior aspect of the eye from a slightly nasal angle. If this angle is accentuated, the nerve head or disc may be tilted obliquely, with its temporal margin considerably more posteriorly located than its nasal margin. This gives the disc an ovoid appearance, with its longest diameter in the vertical meridian. This abnormality also is frequently associated with poor visual acuity.

Hypoplasia of the optic nerve

Hypoplasia of the optic disc is a rare anomaly in which part of or all the optic nerve fibers fail to develop and reach the disc. The optic disc is smaller than normal and pale, and the retinal vessels usually are attenuated. This may occur unilaterally or bilaterally. If the condition is bilateral, the child is usually blind, or nearly so.

Congenital optic atrophy

Congenital optic atrophy is a condition of unknown cause in which the nerve fibers have been formed and subsequently have atrophied. The disc is pale and has a normal size and configuration. The child is usually blind, or vision is exceedingly poor and associated with nystagmus. The condition remains static and usually is not associated with other central nervous system disturbances.

John E. Read
Morton F. Goldberg

BIBLIOGRAPHY

Abbassi, V., Lowe, C.U., and Calcagno, P.L.: Oculo-cerebro-renal syndrome; a review, Am. J. Dis. Child. **115**:145, 1968.

Apple, D.J., and Rabb, M.F.: Clinicopathologic correlation of ocular disease, St. Louis, 1973, The C.V. Mosby Co.

Baum, J.D., and Bulpitt, C.J.: Retinal and conjunctival haemorrhage in the newborn, Arch. Dis. Child. **45**:344, 1970.

Chimonidou, E., Palimeris, G., and Velissaropoulos, P.: Retinoblastoma; some aspects concerning diagnosis, heredity, and treatment, J. Pediatr. Ophthalmol. Strabismus **16**:101, 1979.

Cogan, D.G., and Kuwabara, T.: The sphingolipidoses and the eye, Arch. Ophthalmol. **79**:437, 1968.

de Venecia, G., and Lobeck, C.C.: Successful treatment of eyelid hemangioma with prednisone, Arch. Ophthalmol. **84**:98, 1970.

Duke-Elder, S.: System of ophthalmology, vol. 3, Normal and abnormal development, part 2, Congenital deformities, St. Louis, 1964, The C.V. Mosby Co.

Egbert, P.R., and others: Visual results and ocular complications following radiotherapy for retinoblastoma, Arch. Ophthalmol. **96**:1826, 1978.

Ellsworth, R.M.: The practical management of retinoblastoma, Trans. Am. Ophthalmol. Soc. **67**:462, 1969.

Emery, J.M., and others: G_{MI}-gangliosidosis; ocular and pathological manifestations, Arch. Ophthalmol. **85**:177, 1971.

Faris, B.M., and others: The role of cryotherapy in the management of early lesions of retinoblastoma, Ann. Ophthalmol. **10**:1005, 1978.

Flower, R.W., and others: Retrolental fibroplasia: evidence for a role of the prostaglandin cascade in the pathogenesis of oxygen-induced retinopathy in the newborn beagle, Pediatr. Res. **15**:1293, 1981.

Fontaine, M.: Manifestations oculaires de la prématurité, Arch. Ophthalmol. (Paris) **31**:383, 1971.

Forbes, G.B., and Forbes, G.M.: Silver nitrate and the eyes of the newborn; Credé's contribution to preventive medicine, Am. J. Dis. Child. **121**:1, 1971.

François, E.J.: General anomalies and diseases associated with congenital cataracts. In Congenital cataracts, Springfield, Ill., 1963, Charles C Thomas, Publisher.

Fraumeni, J.F., Jr., and Glass, A.G.: Wilms' tumor and congenital aniridia, J.A.M.A. **206**:825, 1968.

Friendly, D.S.: Ocular manifestations of physical child abuse, Trans. Am. Acad. Ophthalmol. Otolaryngol. **75**:381, 1971.

Gitzelmann, R.: Hereditary galactokinase deficiency; a newly recognized cause of juvenile cataracts, Pediatr. Res. **1**:14, 1967.

Goldberg, M.F.: Waardenburg's syndrome with fundus and other anomalies, Arch. Ophthalmol. **76**:797, 1966.

Goldberg, M.F., editor: Genetic and metabolic eye disease, Boston, 1974, Little, Brown & Co.

Goldberg, M.F., Maumenee, A.E., and McKusick, V.A.: Corneal dystrophies associated with abnormalities of mucopolysaccharide metabolism, Arch. Ophthalmol. **74**:516, 1965.

Goldberg, M.F., Payne, J.W., and Brunt, P.W.: Ophthalmologic studies of familial dysautonomia; the Riley-Day syndrome, Arch. Ophthalmol. **80**:732, 1968.

Goldberg, M.F., and others: Macular cherry-red spot, corneal clouding and β-galactose deficiency; clinical, biochemical and electron microscopic study of a new autosomal recessive storage disease, Arch. Int. Med. **128**:387, 1971.

Harley, R.D., editor: Pediatric ophthalmology, Philadelphia, 1975, W.B. Saunders Co.

Hindle, N.W., and Leyton, J.: Prevention of cicatricial retrolental fibroplasia by cryotherapy, Can. J. Ophthalmol. **13**:277, 1978.

Hittner, H.M., and others: Retrolental fibroplasia: efficacy of vitamin E in a double-blind study of preterm infants, N. Engl. J. Med. **305**:1365, 1981.

Khodadoust, A.A., Mohsen, Z., and Biggs, S.L.: Optic disc in normal newborns, Am. J. Ophthalmol. **66**:502, 1968.

Kingham, J.D.: Acute retrolental fibroplasia, Arch. Ophthalmol. **95**:39, 1977.

Kingham, J.D.: Acute retrolental fibroplasia. II. Treatment of cryosurgery, Arch. Ophthalmol. **96**:2049, 1978.

Kingham, J.D.: Retrolental fibroplasia, Am. Fam. Physician **119:**125, 1979.

Kinsey, V.E., and others: PaO$_2$ levels and retrolental fibroplasia; a report of the cooperative study, Pediatrics **60:**655, 1977.

Liebman, S.D., and Gellis, S.S., editors: The pediatrician's ophthalmology, St. Louis, 1966, The C.V. Mosby Co.

McCormick, AQ.: Transient cataracts in premature infants; a new clinical entity, Can. J. Ophthalmol. **3:**202, 1968.

Newell, F.W.: Opthalmology: principles and concepts, ed. 2, St. Louis, 1969, The C.V. Mosby Co.

Parks, M.M.: Growth of the eye and development of vision. In Liebman, S.D., and Gellis, S.S., editors: The pediatrician's ophthalmology, St. Louis, 1966, The C.V. Mosby Co.

Reese, A.B.: Tumors of the eye, ed. 2, New York, 1963, Harper & Row, Publishers.

Retinopathy of Premature Conference syllabus, vols. 1 and 2, Columbus, Ohio, 1981, Ross Laboratories.

Sagerman, R.H., Cassady, R.J., and Trette, P.: Radiation therapy for rhabdomyosarcoma of the orbit, Trans. Am. Acad. Ophthalmol. Otolaryngol. **72:**849, 1968.

Scheie, H.G., and Albert, D.M.: Adler's textbook of ophthalmology, Philadelphia, 1969, W.B. Saunders Co.

Smith, D.W.: Recognizable patterns of human malformations: genetic, embryologic and clinical aspects: major problems in clinical pediatrics. vol. 3, Philadelphia, 1970, W.B. Saunders Co.

Smith, G.F., Berg, J.M., and McCreary, B.D.: de Lange syndrome. In The First Conference on the Clinical Delineation of Birth Defects. Part II. National Foundation, March of Dimes Birht Defects: Original Article Series **5:**18, 1969.

Spranger, J.W., and Wiedemann, H.R.: The genetic mucolipidoses: diagnosis and differential diagnosis, Humangenetik **9:**113, 1970.

Summitt, R.L.: Familial Goldenhar syndrome. In The First Conference on the Clinical Delineation of Bieth Defects, Part II. National Foundation, March of Dimes Birth Defects: Original Article Series **5:**106, 1969.

Symposium on Surgical and Medical Management of Congenital Anomalies of the Eye, Transactions of the New Orleans Academy of Ophthalmology, St. Louis, 1968, The C.V. Mosby Co.

Vogel, F.: Genetic prognosis in retinoblastoma. In Sorsby, A., editor: Modern trends in ophthalmology, London, 1967, Butterworth & Co. (Publishers) Ltd.

Walsh, T.J., Smith, J.L., and Shipley, T.: Neurologic blindness in infancy. In Smith, J.L., editor: Neuroophthalmology: Symposium of the University of Miami and Bascom Palmer Eye Institute, vol. 3, St. Louis, 1967, The C.V. Mosby Co.

Wilson, W.A., and Donnell, G.N.: Cataracts in galactosemia, Arch. Ophthalmol. **60:**215, 1958.

CHAPTER 36 Orthopedic problems

Significant congenital musculoskeletal abnormalities are relatively common, exceeded in frequency only by congenital abnormalities of the central nervous and cardiovascular systems. Specific limb bud abnormalities (such as congenital absence of the radius) may be associated with silent genitourinary tract abnormalities or hematologic disorders (Fanconi's syndrome). An association of other organ system anomalies always should be investigated in the neonate with skeletal abnormalities, as outlined in Chapter 38.

CLASSIFICATION OF CONGENITAL MUSCULOSKELETAL MALFORMATIONS

A classification according to parts that have been affected by certain embryologic failures recently has been proposed that places all malformations in seven categories. Only four of these categories relate to the neonate: (1) failure of formation of parts, (2) failure of differentiation (separation of parts), (3) duplications, and (4) congenital constriction bands. (See also p. 1051.)

Failure of formation of parts
Transverse limb deficiencies (congenital amputations)

These occur at any level; most commonly they are distal, involving fingertips, toes, metacarpal or metatarsal bones, or the distal aspect of the forearm or tibia. Rarely they occur above the elbow (Figs. 36-1 to 36-3). Treatment consists of early prosthetic fitting between 6 months and 1 year of age.

Longitudinal limb deficiencies

The remaining skeletal limb deficiencies are in this category. They represent absent long bones or parts of long bones (hypoplasia). The most common anomalies are congenital absence of the thumb, radius, fibula, and proximal femur. Treatment of an absent thumb is elective pollicization of the index finger to the absent thumb position (Figs. 36-4 and 36-5). The best timing varies with the surgeon; 18 months is the earliest age, but many surgeons prefer to wait until the child is 4 to 5 years old. The absent radius (congenital clubhand) is rare but produces a dislocation of the hand and wrist if not treated (Fig. 36-6). Plaster casting from the day of birth followed by surgical stabilization at 18 months of age is recommended. An absent fibula produces a shortened extremity without a normal ankle joint and requires significant surgical reconstruction. In the severe cases amputation in preschool years is recommended to achieve satisfactory ambulation (Fig. 36-7). Congenital hypoplasia of the femur (proximal femoral focal deficiency) is a dramatic and significant functional limb loss and shortening (Fig. 36-8). Early custom prosthetic fitting is required at 12 to 18 months; frequently amputation of the foot facilitates a more cosmetic prosthesis.

Failure of differentiation (nonseparation of parts)

There are multiple variations in skeletal differentiation. Only the most common and most functionally significant are presented here. *Synostosis*, or congenital bony fusion across a joint or between two long bones, occurs at the elbow, carpus, and metacarpals but most commonly in the digits (Fig. 36-9). Treatment of synostosis (division and grafting) is primarily indicated for phalangeal synostosis and is performed at 2 to 3 years of age or earlier to prevent angular digital deformity. *Syndactyly* (p. 1058) is present when the soft parts are involved without synostosis (Fig. 36-10). The anomalies of syndactyly and synostosis are most commonly seen as isolated findings but also may be associated with genetic syndromes such as Apert's syndrome. Syndactyly also is treated at 2 to 3 years of age by division and supplemental skin grafting. The feet, when involved in either syn-

Orthopedic problems **1005**

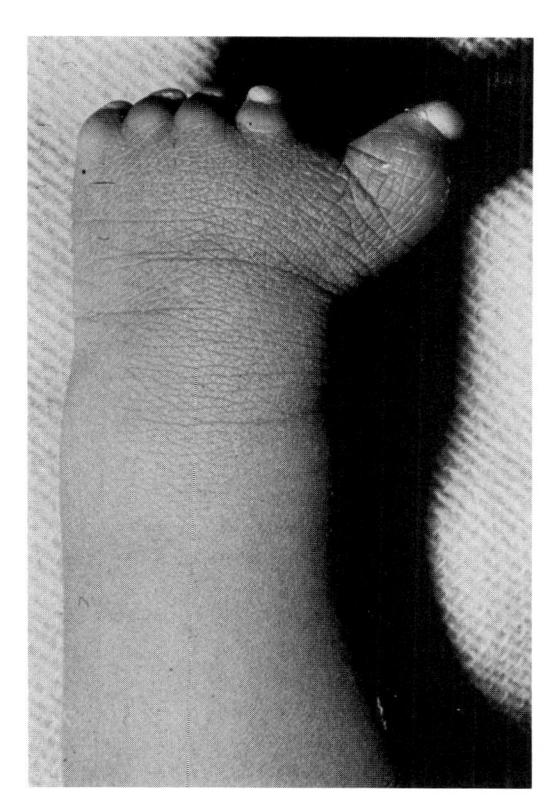

Fig. 36-1. Congenital transverse amputation of fingers at metacarpal level. Note that the thumb, wrist, and forearm are normal.

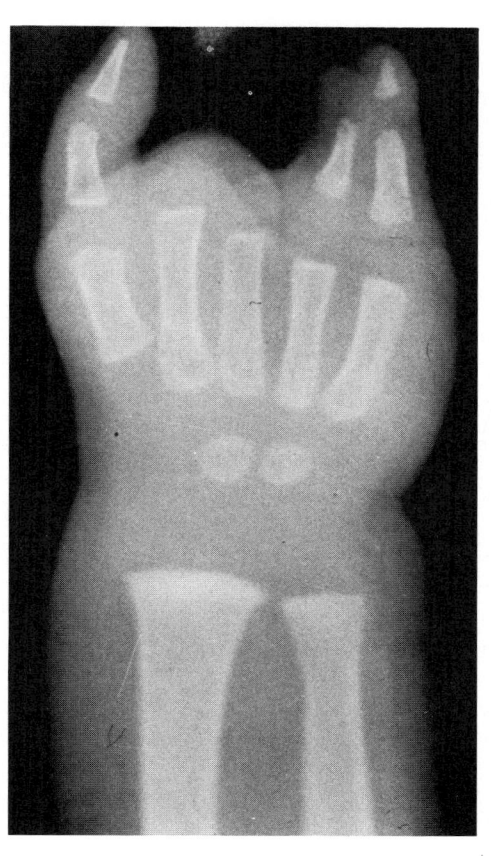

Fig. 36-2. Congenital transverse amputation of fourth and fifth fingers at proximal phalanx level, third and index fingers at metacarpal level. The thumb is normal.

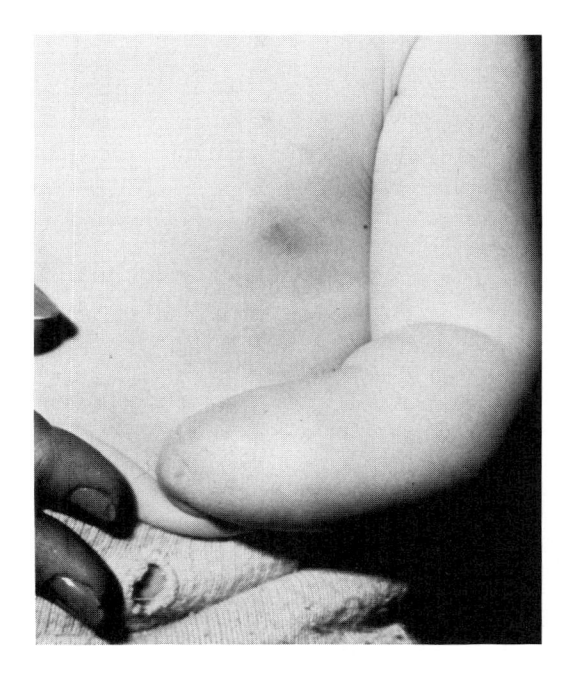

Fig. 36-3. Congenital wrist level (carpus) amputation, normal elbow and shoulder.

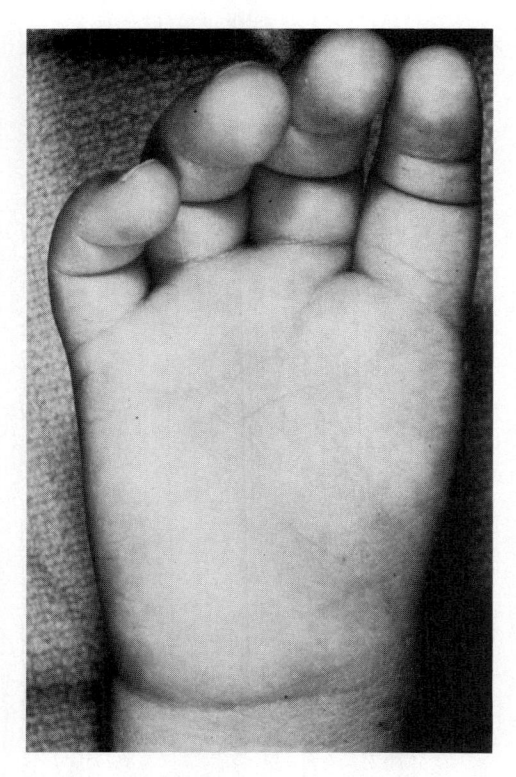

1006   Behrman's neonatal-perinatal medicine: diseases of the fetus and infant

Fig. 36-4. Absence of the thumb with a normal forearm, wrist, and adjacent fingers.

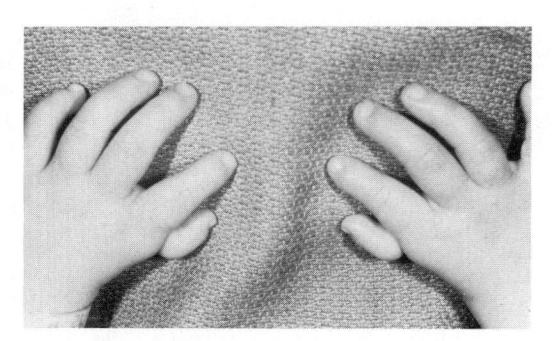

Fig. 36-5. Hypoplasia of the thumb bilaterally. Thumbs are nonfunctional and should be ablated and the bands pollicized at a later age.

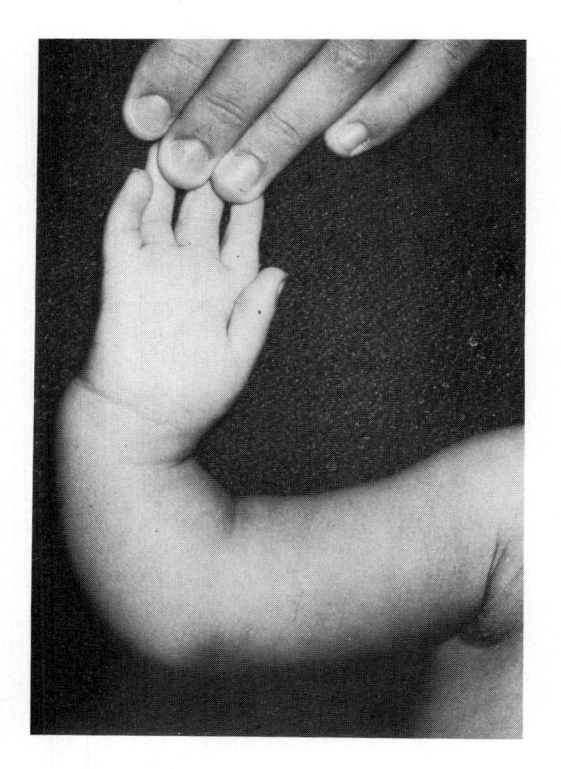

Fig. 36-6. Absent radius in a patient with normal fingers and thumb.

Fig. 36-7. Congenital absence of the tibia. This condition, despite the normal-appearing foot, should be treated by early amputation and fitting of prosthesis.

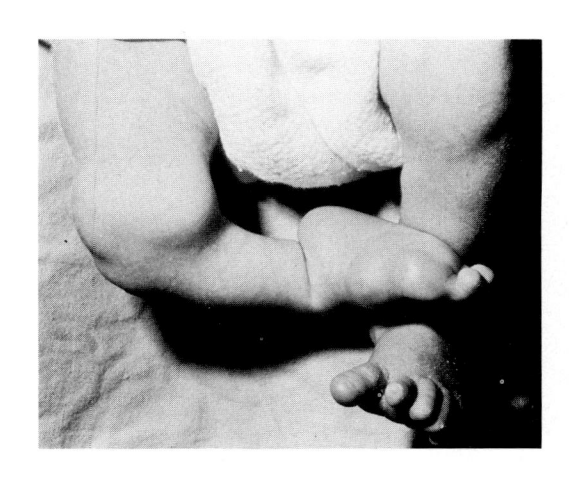

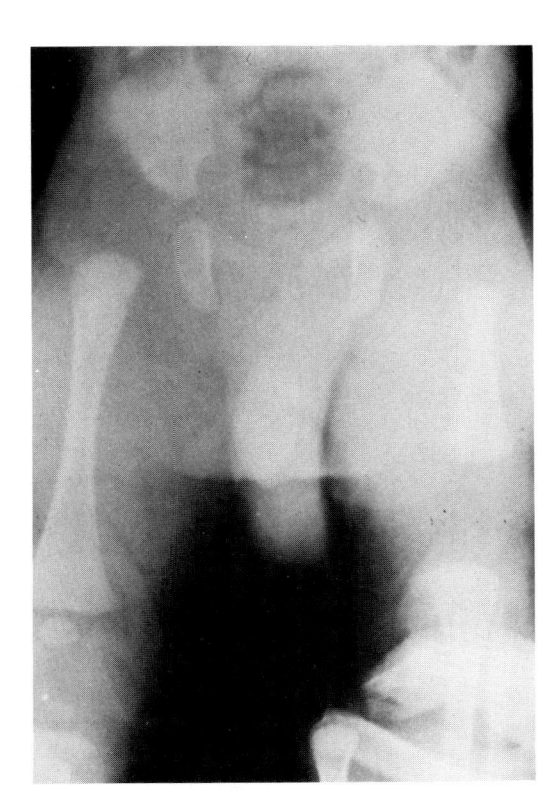

Fig. 36-8. Congenital hypoplasia of the proximal femur, sometimes known as proximal femoral focal deficiency.

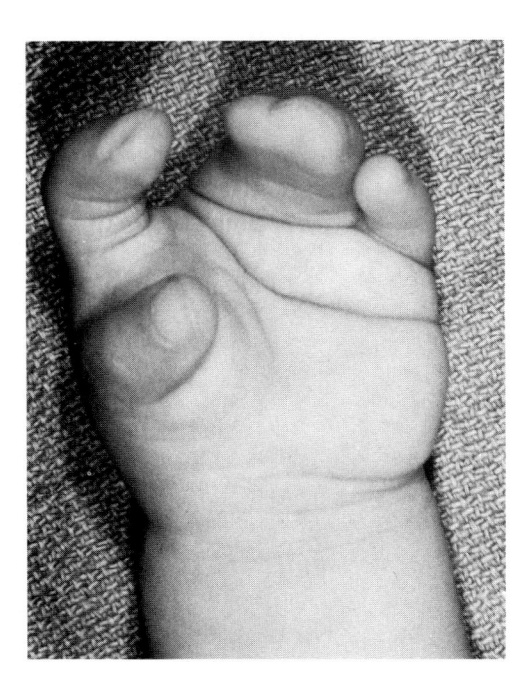

Fig. 36-9. Congenital distal synostosis of phalanges with syndactyly of third and fourth fingers.

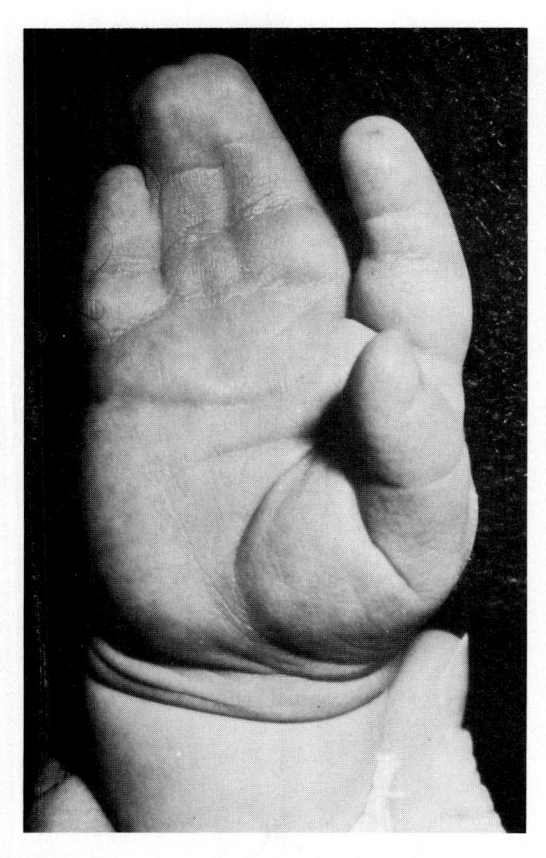

Fig. 36-10. Most commonly involved in simple syndactyly are the third and fourth fingers.

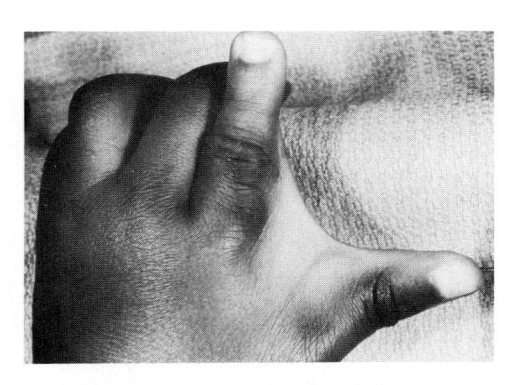

Fig. 36-11. Congenital web of thumb–index finger. Early Z-plasty and skin grafting are recommended.

ostosis or syndactyly, are treated on a more elective basis. Congenital soft tissue contracture also is a failure of differentiation. This is represented by *skin webs*, seen in the neck or thumb web space, *arthrogryposis*, *trigger digits*, and *camptodactyly* (joint contracture) (Fig. 36-11).

Duplications

Duplications probably result from a very early insult to the limb bud, so that splitting of the original embryonic part occurs. These defects may range from polydactyly to twinning or mirror bands (Fig. 36-12). The definitive treatment is elective surgical removal of the nonfunctional duplication, although on occasion the nonfunctional duplication is best retained. This procedure should be performed at 18 months; some surgeons prefer to wait until the child is 3 to 4 years old.

Congenital constriction band syndrome

Necrosis of the primordial limb bud mesenchymal tissue may produce focal scarring, which in turn produces annular constriction bands (Chapter 16) or rings (Fig. 36-13). This also may result in intrauterine gangrene and fetal amputations (Fig. 36-14). Healing of infarctions dur-

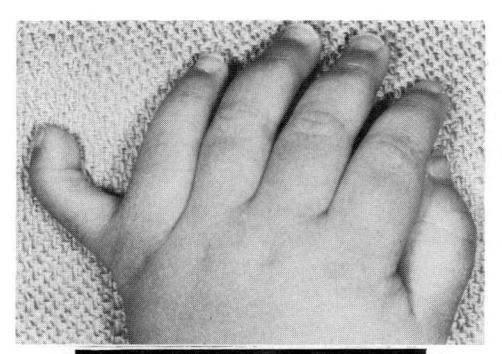

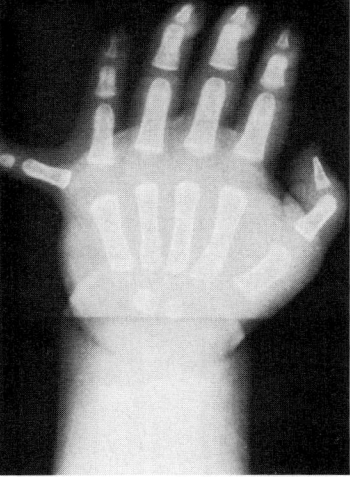

Fig. 36-12. Congenital polydactyly, the most common digit duplication, with complete bones, tendons, and nerves. Recommended treatment is early ablation by amputation.

ing the stage of separation of the parts may give the appearance of syndactyly. When the constriction band is present on the fully formed digit or extremity, release by multiple Z-plasty is indicated within the first 6 months of life to prevent edema or growth disturbance.

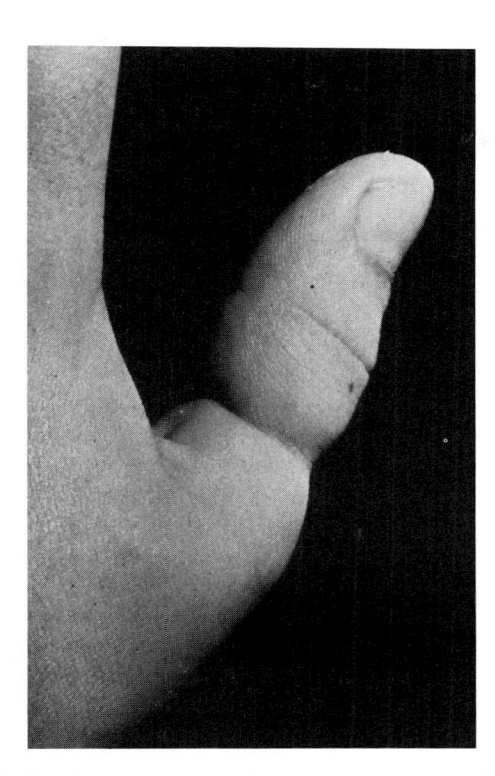

Fig. 36-13. Annular constriction ring present at base of thumb. Early Z-plasty provides successful treatment and normal growth.

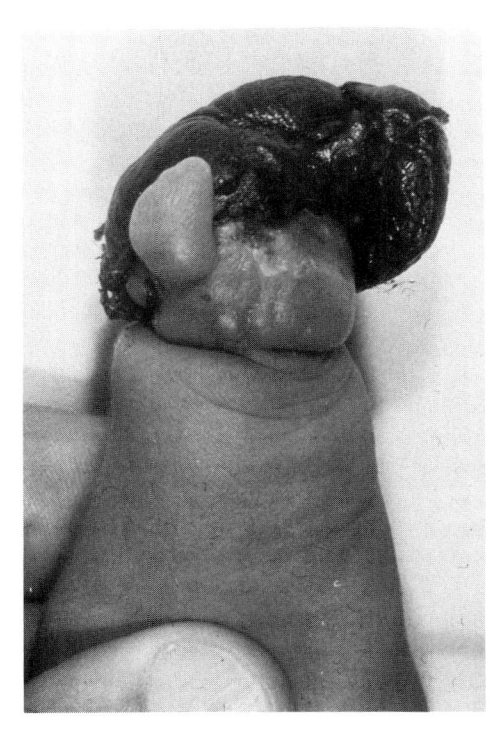

Fig. 36-14. One-week-old infant with evidence of annular band at wrist and intrauterine gangrene with fetal amputation of hand.

CONGENITAL HIP DISLOCATION

Congenital hip dislocation is one of the most challenging and important congenital abnormalities of the musculoskeletal system. It is almost as common as clubfoot and yet not as obvious at birth. Congenital hip dislocation demands a specific method of examination for its detection; unless treated early and definitively, it will lead to a painful and crippling deformity in adult life. Dislocation (luxation) refers to the femoral head being completely outside the acetabulum but still within the stretched and elongated capsule. Subluxation of the femoral head refers to the head riding on the edge of the acetabulum. The latter defect is easily reduced and is stable when the hip is flexed and abducted but is subluxated when the hip is extended and adducted. When the infant's hip is either dislocated or subluxated, the bony development of the acetabulum becomes progressively abnormal, leading to acetabular dysplasia. This discussion does not focus on the less common teratologic hip dislocation arising as part of a generalized congenital abnormality such as arthrogryposis multiplex and spina bifida.

Incidence

The left hip is affected three times more frequently than the right hip, and the condition is bilateral in only one out of every four children so affected. The disease is rare in the black population. There is considerable variation in the incidence of congenital hip dislocation in different parts of the world. In England and Sweden the frequency is estimated at approximately 1 per 1,000 live births; the incidence in northern Italy, southern France, and Japan is three times as high. The highest incidence is among the Lapps and certain American Indians and may be related to swaddling with hip extended and adducted in the first few months of life.

Etiology

Both environmental and genetic factors play a role in the causation of congenital hip dislocation. The sex ratio is approximately one male to seven females and may be related to estrogenic hormone metabolism. Primary acetabular dysplasia with poor covering of the femoral head may predispose children to congenital hip dislocation. Such dysplasia may be seen on the unaffected side in some 30% of unilateral cases of hip dislocation and is probably present but poorly recognized in many bilateral cases. Acetabular dysplasia may be found in one or both parents of affected children, and its genetic determination is probably multifactorial. Generalized joint laxity with capsular relaxation also has been demonstrated in families of some affected children. The most important environmental factor determining the incidence of congenital hip dislocation relates to the intrauterine breech posture with hips flexed and knees partially extended. There is a significantly higher incidence of congenital hip dislocation in breech presentations.

Pathology

The significant pathologic findings vary with time; initially there is only abnormal laxity of the capsule, elongation of the ligamentum teres, and a femoral head that may be small but of normal configuration. Without therapeutic intervention, growth and weight bearing stimulate further pathologic changes in the infant's hip. The femoral head becomes displaced upward and backward to lie on the ilium. The capsule elongates, extending across the acetabulum, and eventually adheres to the floor of the fossa, while the hip adductor muscles become progressively shortened. The acetabulum becomes shallow and more oblique; with persistent dislocation a secondary or false acetabulum may develop on the ilium posterior to the original fossa. The femoral head also becomes small with persistent dislocation, and its shape changes. All these changes constitute increasing obstacles to subsequent reduction of the congenitally dislocated hip.

Clinical manifestations

Apart from demonstrating definite dislocation or malformation or both, roentgenographic studies have little to offer diagnostically during the neonatal period. Diagnosis depends on clinical evaluation, which will identify more than 95% of infants with congenital hip dislocation. This evaluation, Ortolani's maneuver, is performed by placing the infant on the back with knees bent and hips flexed to 90 degrees and fully abducted. When the hip is reduced by abduction, a click is appreciated as the femoral head slides across the posterior aspect of the acetabulum and enters the socket. With adduction of the hip the femoral head redislocates out of the acetabulum with a palpable click, which can be best appreciated with the thumb on the lesser trochanter and the index finger on the greater trochanter. During this examination the infant should be relaxed and the hip adductors not tight; entry and exit clicks must be differentiated from the clicks associated with a tight iliotibial band or a gluteal tendon sliding over the greater trochanter and the knee click of a subluxating patella or a discoid meniscus.

Although Ortolani's maneuver is diagnostic for congenital hip dislocation, it has several shortcomings that limit its use during the immediate neonatal period: (1) as the hips are abducted and dislocated, the femoral head may slide so smoothly over the low rim of the acetabulum that a click is not appreciated; (2) a truly dislocated hip cannot be reduced and therefore cannot provide the characteristic exit and entrance clicks; and (3) infants with congenitally unstable hips (subluxated or subluxata-

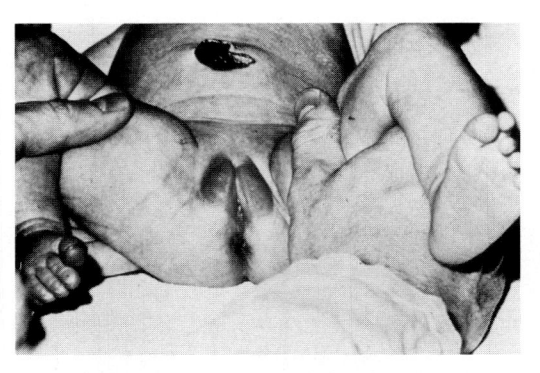

Fig. 36-15. Positioning of the hip in the newborn to perform two diagnostic tests. Ortolani's sign, or click of reduction, is elicited when abducting the hip in this manner. The "reverse" Ortolani, or Barlow, maneuver is performed by bringing the femur into adduction with flexion, causing a click of exit or dislocation.

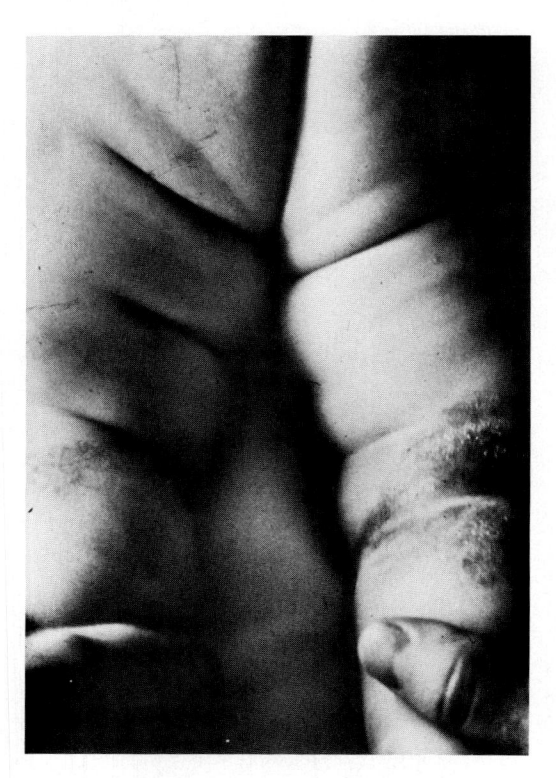

Fig. 36-16. Asymmetrical gluteal and thigh folds are not diagnostic but should alert suspicion.

ble) may escape detection only to dislocate in the future. Barlow's test, a modification of Ortolani's maneuver, therefore should be carried out on all newborns and, when combined with the latter maneuver, will detect almost all congenitally abnormal hips. In Barlow's test the infant is placed on the back with hips flexed to 90

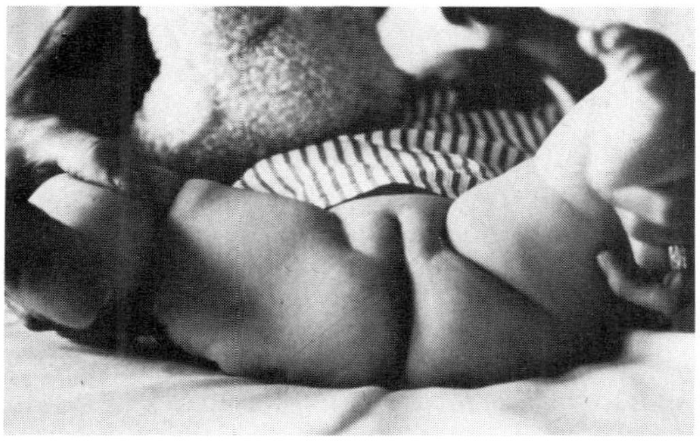

Fig. 36-17. Limitation of abduction of the thighs when hips are flexed at 90 degrees.

degrees and the knees fully flexed. The index finger of each hand is applied over the greater trochanter and the thumbs opposite the lesser trochanter in the femoral triangle. The hips are brought into midabduction, and thumb pressure is applied posteriorly over the lesser trochanter; an unstable hip will dislocate across the posterior lip of the acetabulum. With release of thumb pressure the femoral head will be reduced back into the hip socket (Fig. 36-15).

With the passage of time other physical findings appear. These findings include asymmetry of the skin folds of the thigh (Fig. 36-16), shortening of the involved extremity, limitation of passive abduction of the hip in the 90-degree flexed position (Fig. 36-17), apparent shortening of the femur as shown by differences in the knee levels with the hips flexed at right angles and the infant in the supine position (Galeazzi's sign), and piston mobility or the telescoping sign.

Treatment

Early diagnosis and appropriate therapeutic intervention are essential to avoid crippling deformity. The orthopedic treatment of congenital dislocation and subluxation of the hip varies with the age of the affected individual; only therapy that is applicable to the neonate is considered here. Initially all unstable hips, either subluxated or dislocated, should be gently reduced, which usually is not difficult at this age, and maintained in a stable position of flexion and abduction by some device, such as the Frejka pillow, orthopedic splints, or multiple diapers. The treatment of the subluxatable (dislocatable) hip is more controversial, since 75% of these hips will revert to normal during the first few weeks of life without therapeutic intervention. However, these hips also should be maintained in a stable position of flexion and abduction. Occasionally a dislocated hip is too unstable to be kept reduced by a simple device, and a plaster hip spica cast is indicated for these infants. A period of 3 to 4 months usually is required before the capsule becomes tighter and the femoral head stimulates development of the acetabulum. The hips should be periodically assessed both clinically and radiographically.

Prognosis

The crippling sequelae of congenital dislocation and subluxation of the hip can be virtually eliminated by alert diagnosis and adequate treatment in the neonatal period.

CONGENITAL KNEE DISLOCATION

Congenital knee dislocation is a rare disorder that most often is a manifestation of arthrogryposis. It consists of anterior dislocation of the knee. More commonly congenital hyperextension of the knee (genu recurvatum) occurs without dislocation and is seen in normal infants. Both conditions are more common in the female and after breech presentation, suggesting an etiologic relationship with congenital hip dislocation. The completely dislocated knee usually requires surgical correction, whereas genu recurvatum almost always spontaneously improves. Some orthopedic surgeons have advocated plaster casting for this latter abnormality.

CONGENITAL PATELLA DISLOCATION

Patella dislocation rarely occurs. The patella usually is displaced laterally, and this can occur with or without congenital dislocation of the knee. The abnormality may be bilateral. An attempt should be made to replace the patella and to apply a dressing to maintain it in the correct position. However, early reconstructive surgery frequently is indicated.

CONGENITAL SHOULDER DISLOCATION

Congenital shoulder dislocation is extremely rare. The head of the humerus may lie beneath the spine of scapula, with the arm in a position of abduction and internal rotation. This condition frequently is associated with other congenital malformations. It is often difficult to differentiate between congenital dislocation, dislocation caused by birth trauma, and subluxation secondary to obstetric paralysis. Orthopedic surgical intervention is necessary.

CONGENITAL DISLOCATION OF THE RADIUS

Congenital dislocation of the radius, a rare abnormality, usually is not detected early, because there is relatively little deformity and frequently no disability. The radial head dislocates laterally and, as a result of overgrowth, increases in length. Reconstructive surgery has little to offer, since it seldom improves function.

PSEUDARTHROSIS

Pseudarthrosis is a rare but serious abnormality that most frequently involves the tibia. The tibia, which has failed to grow normally in width, becomes angulated in its lower third, resulting in an anterior bowing of the leg before birth. It is frequently seen in children with neurofibromatosis, but the exact etiologic relationship is unknown. The thin sclerotic bone at the site of the angulation is unstable, and a pathologic fracture occurs at birth or shortly thereafter. Since the abnormal bone is avascular at this site, the fracture fails to unite, and a pseudarthrosis develops, with a resultant increase in the angular deformity. Congenital pseudarthrosis also may affect the clavicle but is often asymptomatic. Extensive orthopedic surgical manipulation is necessary for correction of pseudarthrosis.

CLUBFOOT

Clubfoot may be congenital or acquired and may accompany the oligohydramnios syndrome (p. 47). Talipes (Latin, *talus*, ankle bone, and *pes*, foot) is the generic name used to designate these foot and ankle deformities, which are conventionally described according to the position of the foot: (1) varus, or inversion; (2) valgus, or eversion; (3) equinus, or plantar flexion; and (4) calcaneus, or dorsiflexion.

Talipes equinovarus deformities are the most common and represent more than 95% of all congenital clubfeet. This abnormality occurs with a frequency of 1 per 1,000 live births; the condition is more common in males (2:1) and is bilateral in 50% of infants. All degrees of the equinovarus deformity exist, and the condition is often present in the fetus when the foot begins to form. Pathologically the muscles on the posterior and medial aspect of the leg are shortened, and the distal portions of the tibia and fibula usually show slight inward rotation (tibial torsion). In most instances the individual bones of the feet are normal at birth, and only their relationship to each other is affected.

Talipes calcaneovalgus deformities are the second most common variety of clubfoot. This is generally a mild and transient deformity involving a normal foot and is probably secondary to intrauterine malposition rather than a true developmental abnormality. Other varieties of clubfeet are extremely rare.

The therapeutic approach to children with clubfeet is similar regardless of the type. It consists of determining if the abnormality in the foot can be passively brought to the opposite position. If this maneuver proves successful, simple exercises started early in life will correct the deformity. If the foot abnormality is fixed and cannot be passively overcome, orthopedic treatment consisting of plaster cast or splintering or both is indicated. Forceful manipulation and surgery are rarely required.

Talipes varus (metatarsus primus varus) is an adduction deformity of the first metatarsal in relation to the other four metatarsals. The medial border of the forefoot is curved inward, and there is a wide space between the first and second toes. If treated early by the application of a series of corrective plaster casts, the deformity is rapidly corrected.

In *metatarsus varus* (metatarsus adductus) the forefoot, involving all five metatarsals, is adducted and inverted at the tarsometatarsal joint. The normal position of the heel and ankle readily distinguishes this condition from congenital clubfoot. Metatarsus varus usually is associated with internal tibial torsion. This deformity is quite common (2:1,000 live births) and is generally bilateral. In most patients the forefoot deformity is mild and flexible, and the prognosis is good with simple stretching and the avoidance of sleeping in the face-down position with the feet curved in. If the deformity is marked and fixed, treatment involves application of a series of plaster casts molding the foot into adduction and pronation.

Harold M. Dick

BIBLIOGRAPHY

Baker, C.J., and Rudolph, A.J.: Congenital ring constrictions and intrauterine amputations, Am. J. Dis. Child. **121**:393, 1971.

Carter, C.O., and Wilkinson, J.A.: Genetic and environmental factors in the etiology of congenital dislocation of the hip, Clin. Orthop. **33**:119, 1964.

Ferguson, A.B.: Orthopaedic surgery in infancy and childhood, ed. 4, Baltimore, 1975, Williams & Wilkins Co.

Kay, W.H.: A proposed international terminology for the classification of congenital limb deficiencies, Orthot. Prosthet. **28**:2, 33, 1970.

Palmen, K.: Preluxation of the hip joint, Acta Paediatr. Scand. **50**:129, 1961.

Salter, R.B.: Textbook of disorders and injuries of the musculoskeletal system, Baltimore, 1974, Williams & Wilkins Co.

Torpin, R.: Amniochorionic mesoblastic fibrous strings and amnionic bands, Am. J. Obstet. Gynecol. **91**:65, 1965.

von Rosen, S.: Diagnosis and treatment of congenital dislocation of the hip joint in the newborn, J. Bone Joint Surg. **44B**:284, 1962.

CHAPTER 37

Genetic disease and chromosomal abnormalities

Genetic disease and congenital malformations cause approximately 10% of deaths during the first 28 days of life and have been noted as incidental findings at autopsy in more than 20% of infants dying from other causes and in 33% of stillbirths. Children with one or more congenital anomalies make up approximately 25% of pediatric admissions to university hospitals. The National Foundation–March of Dimes of New York estimates that genetic errors afflict more than 15 million Americans with mental retardation, diabetes, complete or partial blindness, impaired hearing, defects in specific organ systems, and congenital bone, muscle, or joint disease.

Much of the neonatal morbidity and mortality of genetic disease is the result of major malformations, i.e., structural defects with potentially clinically significant consequences. The incidence of major anomalies varies according to definition and ascertainment methods but is estimated to occur in from 1% to 7% of all live births (Chapter 38). Minor malformations are detected much more frequently. In a survey of 5,000 consecutive deliveries Marden noted minor malformations in over 10% of newborns (Table 37-1). The clinical significance of minor defects lies in their frequent association with more serious anomalies. When two minor abnormalities are present, an infant's chance of having a major anomaly rises to 90%. Half of all malformations are not recognized at birth, becoming apparent as the child grows and develops.

The causes of birth defects or genetic disorders are most easily considered in terms of chromosomal abnormalities: single gene disorders with or without a known biochemical defect, multifactorial defects, environmental disorders, or those of unknown cause. Of 317 serious malformations identified among 18,355 neonates at Boston Hospital for Women, 9% were secondary to recognized chromosomal aberrations, 21% were caused by single mutant genes with mendelian inheritance, and 40% were of multifactorial origin. The remaining malformations were unclassified and probably caused in part by environmental agents. For many of the malformations encountered during the neonatal period no cause will be immediately apparent.

Table 37-1. Common minor malformations in newborns (frequency greater than 1:1,000)

Minor malformation	Percentage of newborns
Craniofacial	
Borderline micrognathia	0.32
Eye	
Inner epicanthal folds	0.42
Ear	
Lack of helical fold	3.52
Posteriorly rotated pinna	0.25
Preauricular and/or auricular skin tags	0.23
Small pinna	0.14
Auricular sinus	0.12
Skin	
Capillary hemangioma other than on face or posterior aspect of neck	1.06
Pigmented nevi	0.49
Mongoloid spots in white infants	0.21
Hand	
Simian creases	2.74
Bridged upper palmar creases	1.04
Bilateral combinations of above	0.51
Other unusual crease patterns	0.28
Clinodactyly of fifth finger	0.99
Foot	
Partial syndactyly of second and third toes	0.016
Total	12.34

Data from Marden, P.M., Smith, D.W., and McDonald, M.J.: J. Pediatr. **64**:357, 1964. Courtesy Thaddeus Kurczynski, M.D.

EVALUATION OF THE NEONATE WITH MULTIPLE MALFORMATIONS

See also Chapter 38.

An organized plan for evaluation of each neonate with multiple malformations should be developed at the time the infant is initially examined and should include a detailed pedigree and pregnancy history, physical examination, laboratory evaluation of the affected infant and parents if indicated, determination of the genetic mechanism and risk, and counseling and psychologic support for the family.

The family pedigree and pregnancy history are important sources of information in separating genetic disorders from nongenetic disease. The age, sex, and past and present health of parents, siblings, and other closely related family members should be determined. Parents may not mention stillbirths or spontaneous abortions unless specifically questioned about these events. It is also important to determine if there is consanguinity, since this increases the likelihood that an infant's disorder is caused by an autosomal recessive gene. Offspring of first-cousin marriages will have identical genes at one sixteenth of their loci. Parent-child and brother-sister matings result in children who have identical genes at 25% of their loci. Offspring of these marriages may be homozygous for a deleterious gene and therefore manifest a debilitating genetic disorder. Consanguineous marriages have the greatest effect on the incidence of recessive conditions that have a low frequency in the population. For example, if the frequency of a recessive gene in the population is 0.2, then the expected ratio of affected individuals among children of first-cousin marriages to the number of affected individuals in the general population will be 1.25:1. However, if the frequency of the recessive gene is 0.002, then this ratio will increase to 32.25:1.

The ethnic background of the infant's family and the geographic area from which they originate may be important information. Many genetic disorders occur with increased frequency among certain ethnic populations. For example, Tay-Sachs disease is noted once in every 3,600 births among Ashkenazi Jews and only once in 360,000 births in the general population. Similarly, tyrosinemia is especially common among French Canadians in the Lac St. Jean–Chicoutimi region of Quebec and extremely rare elsewhere in the world.

A history of maternal disease, notably diabetes, is associated with an increased frequency of malformations (Chapter 3) and should be specifically sought. Intrauterine growth retardation often is associated with congenital malformations. The relationship between birth weight and gestational age and the incidence of congenital malformations have been studied by Van Den Berg and Yerushalmy. These investigators have demonstrated that the severest anomalies are found in term newborns with intrauterine growth retardation, whereas the highest incidence of both minor anomalies and congenital malformations has been noted in preterm SGA infants (27%). This frequency is more than four times the incidence of anomalies seen in appropriate for gestational age preterm infants. Term infants with intrauterine growth retardation have a 9% incidence of malformations.

Polyhydramnios frequently is observed in mothers delivering infants with malformations (Chapter 6). The excessive amniotic fluid in cases with malformations often is attributed to decreased fetal swallowing; however, other factors may be important in the fluid accumulation. Malformations associated with a high frequency of polyhydramnios include Down's syndrome, trisomy 18, esophageal atresia, obstruction of the gastrointestinal tract proximal to the ileum, intrathoracic cysts, and central nervous system anomalies. Approximately 20% of infants with a history of polyhydramnios will have congenital anomalies. Thus an excess of amniotic fluid should alert the physician to search for gastrointestinal anomalies if there are no other apparent major malformations.

A detailed description of drug exposures and illnesses (especially viral syndromes) during the pregnancy should be obtained in a manner that precludes potential reinforcement of maternal guilt. Most women will recall having used several medications and having a viral syndrome at some time during pregnancy. The vast majority of illnesses will involve the upper respiratory or gastrointestinal tract and resolve spontaneously without affecting the fetus. Only rubella virus and cytomegalovirus have strong proven associations with structural malformations. It is important that a causal relationship between malformations and either drug exposure or maternal viral illnesses not be made or suggested in the process of eliciting this history. Although retrospective epidemiologic studies at times have suggested an association of an increased frequency of birth defects with many commonly used drugs (e.g., aspirin), the number of proven human teratogens is relatively small. The drug history is taken to reveal the few known teratogenic agents and to identify new teratogens. It should be clearly emphasized to both parents that the maternal drug history is most likely to be unrelated to the congenital malformations of the infant. (See Chapter 12.)

During physical examination of the infant with multiple malformations particular attention should be directed to describing and categorizing the anomalies, examining the infant's eyes, and evaluating the patterns of ridged skin (dermatoglyphics) (Chapter 38). Every infant with multiple malformations should have the eyes examined by an experienced ophthalmologist. Numerous syndromes, including those secondary to chromosomal aberrations, have eye findings that are readily detectable. With some abnormalities (for example, glaucoma or chorioretinitis) the findings are so characteristic that they may suggest specific diagnoses. The evaluation of dermatoglyphics on the palms, fingers, and soles also should be performed as part of the physical examination of these infants (p. 1052). Characteristic dermatoglyphics have been described in a number of disorders and are particularly helpful in diagnosing chromosomal syndromes.

Evaluation of the infant with multiple malformations or suspected genetic disease often includes roentgenographic studies (bone films, computed axial tomography, and intravenous pyelography), ultrasonography, cytogenetic studies, and metabolic screening or testing to diagnose inborn errors of metabolism. An orderly sequence of diagnostic testing should be based on the differential diagnosis suggested by the history and findings on physical examination. Photographs and a skeletal survey may be useful in monitoring changes in appearance or progression of roentgenographic findings suggestive of certain diagnoses.

Counseling the parents (see also p. 1060)

It should be remembered that formal genetic counseling is only one step in a long process of informing a family about their child's illness. Before delivery most parents expect their children to be normal. During the initial meeting with the physician an appraisal of the severity of the infant's problems may be overwhelming. Although many parents will accept the information and respond appropriately, some will deny that the illness is serious. In spite of the information transmitted, they may selectively remember the positive aspects of the conversation. To help counteract this denial, it is important that both parents be given the same information and, when possible, that both parents be present at all meetings. There is often a tendency for the father to want to protect the mother from the anguish that he is experiencing. When both parents continually deny the severity of the illness, it may be useful to suggest that other close family members or clergy be brought into the counseling session.

Couples may be so overwhelmed by the extent of their child's illness that they will not visit the intensive care nursery or communicate with anyone in the hospital. They may only request notification of the infant's death. This refusal to make an emotional commitment may be an attempt to protect themselves from further emotional suffering or at times reflect their inability to accept the concept of caring for an infant with a congenital defect. This approach may compound their guilt if the infant dies or may result in psychologic abandonment of a child with nonfatal disease (occasionally an infant with only a cosmetic problem). All families should be strongly encouraged to become involved with the decisions involving the care of their infants. The stimulus for continuing involvement should come from physicians, nurses, and social service personnel.

At the time of the first meeting it is inadvisable to give the parents a list of all possible diagnoses and the outcome for each disorder. If too much information is communicated, the families may be overwhelmed and confused. The extent of the illness should be described in realistic terms and be reiterated and expanded at subsequent meetings. Any decision regarding withdrawal of intensive care should be made with the family. In doing so, the parents should not be made to feel that they are responsible for letting their child die. When a child with multiple malformations dies, autopsy permission should be sought. Even when this is denied, specific arrangements must be made with the family to continue the counseling. Details of counseling for specific genetic problems are discussed after the relevant sections in this chapter.

CHROMOSOMAL ABNORMALITIES

Chromosomal abnormalities occur in approximately 1 in every 200 newborns, in 5% to 10% of perinatal deaths, and in as many as 50% of early spontaneous abortions. These disorders may be classified as numerical abnormalities of either the autosomes or sex chromosomes and structural chromosomal abnormalities that may be balanced or unbalanced. Clinically it is the autosomal trisomies and unbalanced structural chromosomal abnormalities that most often result in major developmental defects apparent during the neonatal period. Additional autosome material (e.g., trisomy) is somewhat better tolerated than deficiency of an autosome. Nevertheless, the majority of autosomal abnormalities, either duplication or deficiency, that occur in human conceptions are lost by early abortion. The amount of material that is duplicated or deficient, the particular genes within these segments, and perhaps other factors (e.g., maternal factors) influence the likelihood of live birth. Abnormalities of the sex chromosomes and balanced structural rearrangements have their greatest impact on reproductive function. The former generally are associated with gonadal dysgenesis, and the latter may result in reproductive wastage from conception of pregnancies with chromosome imbalance secondary to the parental chromosome rearrangement.

Numeric chromosomal abnormalities (aneuploidy) most often arise by *nondisjunction* (uneven distribution of chromatids or chromosomes in meiosis or mitosis) (Fig. 37-1). Nondisjunction during meiosis will result in gametes and consequently conceptions with an extra (trisomy) or missing (monosomy) chromosome. Conceptions with autosomal monosomy resulting from nondisjunction are presumably lost by abortion, prior to recognition of

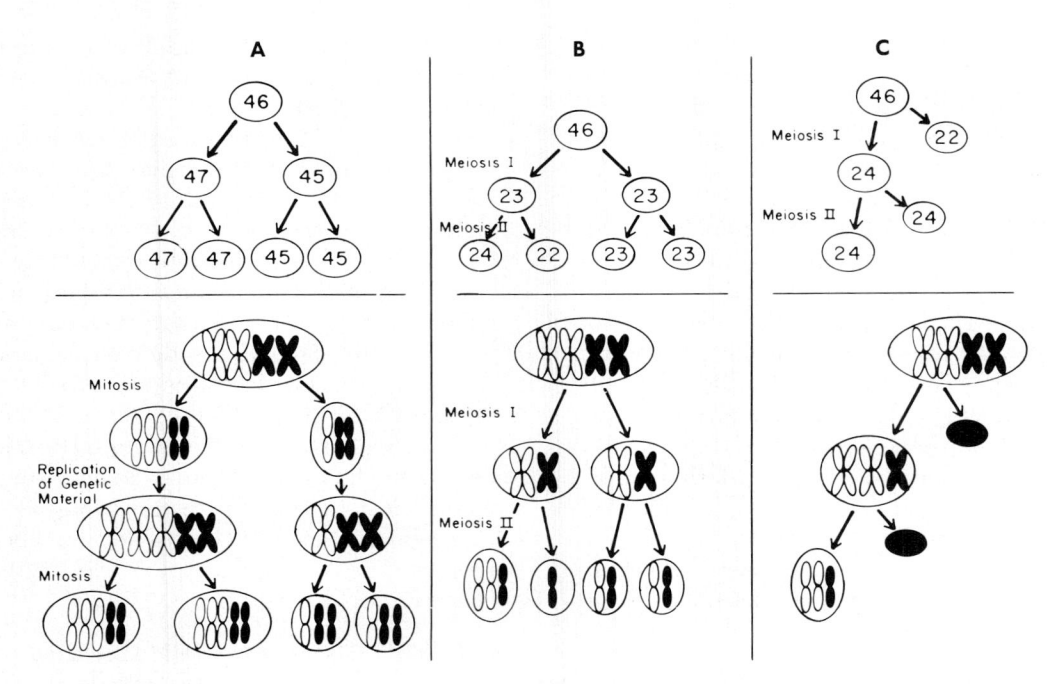

Fig. 37-1. A, Nondisjunction in mitosis demonstrating development of mosaicism with one cell line having 45 chromosomes and the other cell line having 47 chromosomes. **B,** Nondisjunction in male meiosis II resulting in spermatozoa having 22, 23, and 24 chromosomes. **C,** Nondisjunction in female meiosis I resulting in ovum with 24 chromosomes. Blackened circles represent the first and second polar bodies.

pregnancy. On the other hand, approximately 40% of the chromosomal abnormalities found in recognized early abortuses are autosomal trisomies. Nondisjunction occurring after normal gametogenesis and fertilization will result in a fetus or newborn having two or more cell lines that have differing chromosomal constitutions (mosaicism) (Fig. 37-1, A). Mosaicism is relatively more frequent in individuals with sex chromosome aneuploidy, but it also occurs with autosomal abnormalities.

Anaphase lag, a mechanism resulting in loss of a chromosome, occurs when homologous chromosomes fail to pair or segregate correctly on the spindle during cell division. The loss of one member of the chromosome pair during anaphase by this mechanism results in a monosomy and is believed to be the mechanism which accounts for a large proportion of Turner's syndrome (45,X) conceptions. X chromosome monosomy constitutes 20% of the chromosomal abnormalities in spontaneous abortion. Based on the low frequency of this abnormality in liveborn infants, it is apparent that the vast majority of Turner's syndrome conceptions are lost during early pregnancy. Anaphase lag during mitotic division following conception may give rise to mosaicism.

The autosomal trisomies (trisomy 21, 18, and 13) account for the majority of numeric chromosomal abnormalities that are diagnosed during the neonatal period. It has long been considered that nondisjunction in meiosis resulting in trisomies occurs most often during oogenesis. This is supported by the well-established association of Down's syndrome births and advancing maternal age. The identification of normal variants using banding methods, especially Q-banding (quinacrine fluorescence), permits determination of the parental origin of trisomies in a proportion of families. Such testing in informative matings indicates that the paternal origin of Down's syndrome (20% to 30% of cases) is much more frequent than previously estimated. Studies associating nondisjunction with paternal age have shown conflicting results but suggest that there may be an effect, especially after the age of 55 years. The frequency of Down's syndrome at specific paternal ages has not been defined for clinical counseling as it has for maternal age but probably does not reach the same level of clinical significance.

Causes of nondisjunction in humans, other than the association with advanced maternal age, have not been established. Familial clustering of numeric chromosomal abnormalities in isolated cases and the occurrence of children with double aneuploidies (e.g., 48,XXY, +21) suggests that there may be a genetic influence to nondisjunction in some families or individuals. Association of numeric chromosomal abnormalities with autoimmune thyroid disease, prior radiation exposure, or certain oth-

Genetic disease and chromosomal abnormalities **1017**

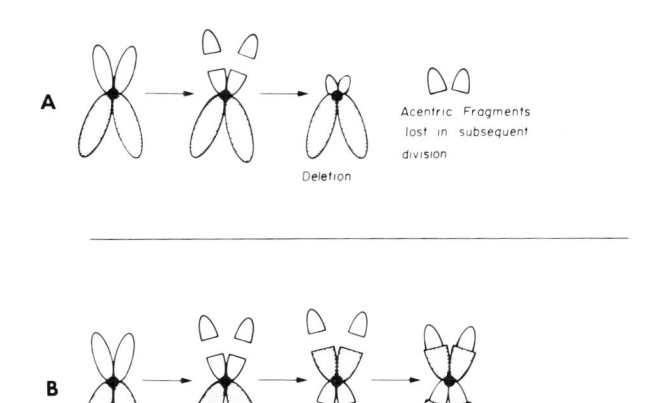

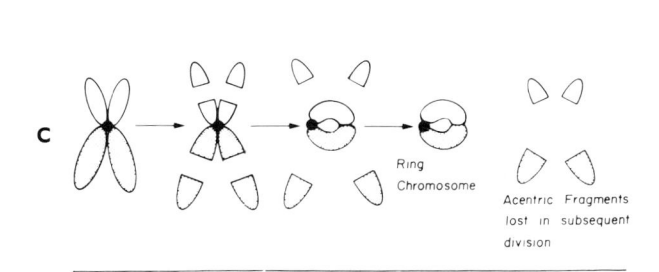

Fig. 37-2. A, Single break in the short arm of a metaphase chromosome resulting in deletion of short-arm material. **B,** Breaks in both the short arm and long arm of metaphase chromosome. Union of short arm and long arm segments adjacent to centromere results in formation of ring chromosomes.

erwise normal chromosomal variants has been suggested but not well substantiated. Because of the high frequency of spontaneous abortion and the large proportion of early abortuses who are chromosomally abnormal, studies to determine genetic or environmental factors that may cause nondisjunction must necessarily be approached through surveillance of early pregnancy wastage.

Chromosomal constitutions in which there are multiples of the haploid number ($n = 23$) of chromosomes other than diploid ($2n = 46$) are known as polyploidy (for example, triploidy, $3n = 69$, tetraploidy, $4n = 92$). Polyploidy may arise by a number of theoretic mechanisms, such as failure of segregation of chromosomes in meiosis, fertilization of an ovum by two sperm (dispermy), and failure of division and cleavage after fertilization. Triploidy and tetraploidy account for approximately 20% to 25% of the chromosomal aberrations observed in early abortuses. Of these two abnormalities, only triploidy occurs very rarely in late stillborns or live-born infants.

Structural chromosomal abnormalities result from breakage and reunion of chromosomes. These are considered balanced if all the genetic material is conserved (e.g., balanced translocations or inversions). Unequal crossing over within a rearrangement or abnormal segregation of members of pairs involved in a translocation during gametogenesis may result in an unbalanced chromosome constitution of the gamete and conception.

After a single break and loss of the chromosome fragment without a centromere (acentric fragment) the subsequent cell division will result in deletion (Fig. 37-2, A). This is most commonly exemplified by the cri du chat syndrome caused by deletion of the short arm of chromosome 5 (5p−). Two or more breaks within the same chromosome with rearrangement of material and reunion result in more complex structural abnormalities, such as ring chromosomes or inversions (Fig. 37-2, B and C). To form a ring chromosome, terminal segments of both the long arm and the short arm of the chromosome are lost as acentric fragments (Fig. 37-2, C). Inversion of material within one arm of a chromosome is known as a *paracentric inversion*. Inversions involving the centromere and the adjacent segments of each arm of the chromosome are termed *pericentric inversions*. Balanced inversions are observed quite frequently as incidental findings. For example, pericentric inversion of chromosome 9 has been observed to occur in 1% of some populations studied with seemingly no clinical consequence. To pair with an inverted homologue during meiosis, the normal chromosome must form a loop. An odd number of crossovers with the inversion loop will result in a derivative chromosome having duplication and deficiency of the terminal segments of the chromosome. In this way balanced carriers of an inversion may produce unbalanced gametes, which result in children with a chromosomal abnormality.

Abnormal separation of the centromere during cell division with separation of the replicated arms of the chromosomes, rather than separation of the chromatids, results in a structurally abnormal chromosome known as an *isochromosome* (Fig. 37-3). When examined during the metaphase of subsequent divisions, these derivative chromosomes appear as mirror images of the short arms or long arms of the original chromosome, the net effect being duplication of one set of arms and deficiency of the other. When observed clinically, isochromosomes most often involve the X chromosome and only very rarely an autosome or the Y chromosome.

Translocations result when there is breakage and exchange of material between two different chromosome pairs. Translocations are classified as balanced reciprocal when there is exchange of material between arms of two chromosomes or robertsonian when there is centric fusion (fusion at the centromere) of two acrocentric chro-

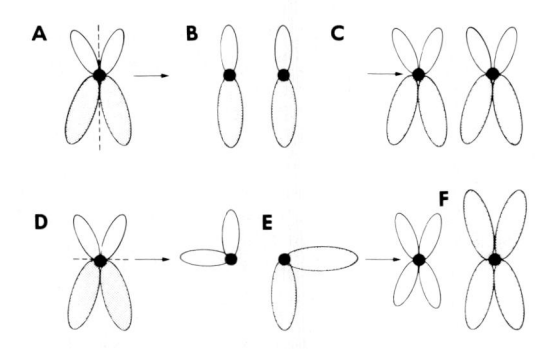

Fig. 37-3. A, Metaphase chromosome replicated for division. Dotted line depicts normal longitudinal division of centromere. **B,** Normally separated chromatids. **C,** Replicated chromosomes as seen in daughter cells during subsequent metaphase. **D,** Metaphase chromosome. Dotted line depicts abnormal division of centromere. **E,** Separated chromatids that result are "mirror image" of short arm (on left) and mirror image of long arm (on right). **F,** Replicated isochromosomes as seen in daughter cells during subsequent metaphase. The chromosome on left is an isochromosome of short arms and the chromosome on the right is an isochromosome of the long arm.

mosomes. In the latter situation there is loss of short arms, stalks, and satellites with fusion of the long arm of one acrocentric chromosome to the long arm of another. The carrier of such a translocation has only 45 chromosomes by count, that is, missing two acrocentric and having a derivative chromosome composed of the long arms of each chromosome. For example, balanced robertsonian fusion of chromosomes 13 and 14, which is the most common translocation found in humans (1:800), would be expressed karyotypically as 45,XY, −13, −14, +t (13q; 14q). The loss of repetitive DNA in the short arms of the acrocentric chromosomes does not have clinical consequences. By definition balanced translocations do not have phenotypic expression except those related to reproductive problems associated with conception of pregnancies with an unbalanced chromosome.

The occurrence of a balanced structural rearrangement of chromosomes in a newborn is most often a result of familial transmission of the rearrangement. Familial transmission of a balanced translocation or inversion can be expected in approximately 50% of normal offspring of parents who are carriers of one of these rearrangements. Abnormal phenotypic features should not be ascribed to a familial structural rearrangement or other normal variants unless it can be clearly demonstrated that there is duplication or deficiency of chromosome material in the child which is not present in the parent with the rearrangement.

Although certain mutant genes and a number of environmental agents (e.g., ionizing radiation, drugs, chemicals, and viruses) may cause breakage of chromosomes, the cause of a de novo (nonfamilial) structural abnormality cannot be determined in an individual case. A de novo structural rearrangement with duplication and/or deficiency of a chromosome segment can be considered the cause of multiple malformations in a child. As opposed to familial transmission of balanced rearrangements, the presence of a de novo structural rearrangement without apparent duplication or deficiency of chromosome segments, even by high-resolution banding techniques, should be regarded with some suspicion when the child has malformations. In such cases the possibility of duplication or deficiency of genetic material that is not within the limits of detection by currently available laboratory techniques remains a possibility.

Clinical features

A chromosomal abnormality should be considered in all stillborn or live-born infants with multiple malformations. Certain clinical findings in a neonate or child that increase the likelihood of a chromosomal abnormality being present include the following:

1. General: low birth weight, failure to thrive, short stature, developmental delay, mental retardation
2. Head: microcephaly, central nervous system malformation, dysmorphic facies, micrognathia, facial clefts, eye anomalies, malposition or malformation of the ears
3. Multisystem involvement: skeletal, cardiovascular, gastrointestinal or genitourinary malformations
4. Dermatoglyphics: abnormal or atypical patterns (p. 1052)

The striking facial resemblance and relative consistency of certain phenotypic features among infants with the same trisomy permit clinical diagnosis in a large proportion of cases. Confidence in the clinical diagnosis of tri-

Genetic disease and chromosomal abnormalities **1019**

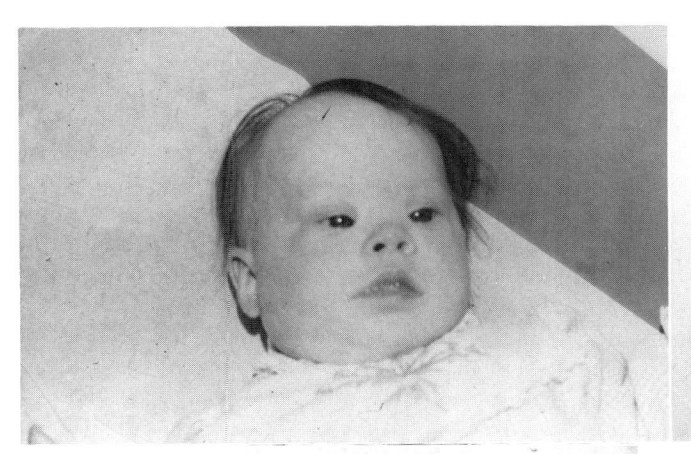

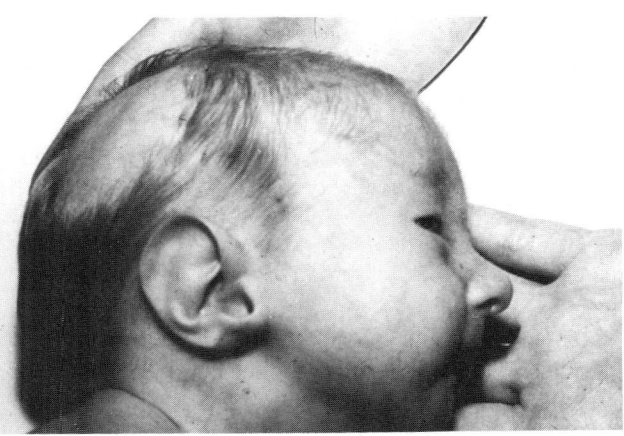

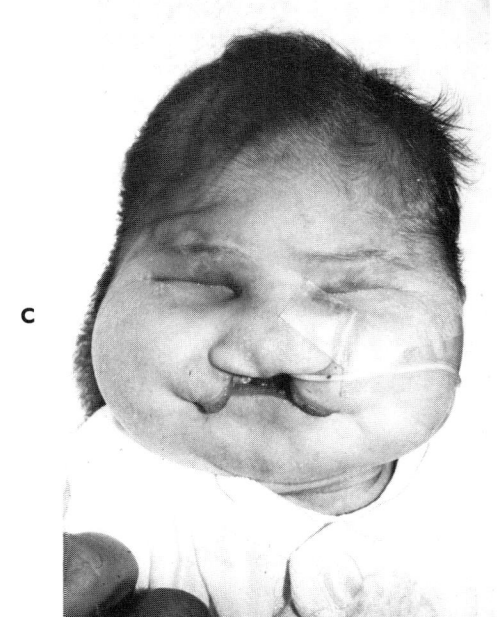

Fig. 37-4. A, Trisomy 21. Prominent features of the syndrome noted during the neonatal period are listed along with the system or organ involved. CNS: abnormal neurologic examination (hypotonia); head: mild microcephaly, flat occiput, midfacial hypoplasia; eyes: Brushfield spots, epicanthal folds, upslanting, palpebral fissures; mouth: protuberant tongue; ears: anomalous auricles; hands: simian crease, distal triradius, increased ulnar loops, short metacarpals and phalanges; fingers: dysplasia of midphalanx of fifth finger; cardiac: cardiac defects (approximately 40%); genitalia: hypogonadism; pelvis: hypoplasia, shallow acetabular angle; other: redundant skin at nape of neck, wide space between first and second toe. **B,** Trisomy 13. Prominent features of the syndrome noted during the neonatal period are listed, along with the system or organ involved. CNS: severe malformations, holoprosencephaly; head: microcephaly, sloping forehead; eyes: microphthalmia, colobomata; mouth: cleft lip/cleft palate; ears: abnormal auricles, low-set ears; hands: distal triradius, simian crease; fingers: polydactyly; chest wall: thin and/or missing ribs; cardiac: cardiac defects (over 80%); genitalia: cryptorchidism, abnormal scrotum; pelvis: hypoplasia; other: apneic spells, seizures, persistence of fetal hemoglobin, increased nuclear projection in neutrophils. **C,** Trisomy 18. Prominent features of the syndrome noted during the neonatal period are listed, along with the system or organ involved. CNS: malformations; head: narrow biparietal diameter, occipital prominence; eyes: short palpebral fissures; mouth: micrognathia, small mouth; ears: malformed auricles, low-set ears; hands: increased arches, hypoplastic nails; fingers: overlapping fingers; chest wall: short sternum; cardiac: cardiac defects (over 50%); genitalia: cryptorchidism; pelvis: small pelvis, limited hip abduction; other: growth deficiency, thrombocytopenia.

somies in the very premature infant is less likely because assessment of facial features and dysmorphic characteristics (e.g., dermatoglyphics) is more difficult. The finding of a single dysmorphic feature (e.g., transverse palmar crease or abnormal ear) in a newborn without other phenotypic features or malformations associated with a trisomy generally should be regarded as a normal variant. At times suspicious but isolated features in young children or newborns may be determined to be normal familial variations by examination of the parents or siblings.

The diagnosis of a specific chromosomal syndrome will provide the basis for searching for other malformations known to be associated with the disorder and also to formulate with the parents an approach to treatment or surgical correction of defects. In some instances diagnosis may allow reasonable prediction of the prognosis for survival and development. In cases where there is a relatively unique chromosomal disorder or one with variable phenotypic expression, caution must be exercised in predicting the prognosis.

Principal features of the three autosomal trisomies are listed in Fig. 37-4 (see also Figs. 38-1, 38-2, 38-4, 38-7, 38-21, 38-22, 38-24, 38-26, 38-28, and 38-30). Other autosomal trisomies in live-born infants are almost exclusively observed as mosaic (e.g., trisomy 8 mosaicism). It should be recognized that with mosaicism the percentage of abnormal cells observed in peripheral lymphocytes of the adult or newborn may not reflect the chromosome constitution of other tissues or organs and, more important, may not accurately reflect the fetal situation during early development. Thus, although a phenotypic syndrome may be described from review of a small number of reported cases, more variability may be expected with mosaicism than is seen in the trisomies. Clinical management and counseling in such cases must be based on phenotype rather than the relative percentage of normal and abnormal cells in peripheral lymphocyte cultures.

Structural abnormalities with duplicated or deficient chromosome segments are more reliably detected since the development of banding methods (Fig. 37-5). These methods enable identification of each member of the chromosome groups, small subsegments of the individual chromosomes, and a number of normal variants of chromosome structure. Prior to the development of chromosome banding, infants with duplicated or deficient segments often were not diagnosed, or the origin of segments involved were unidentified by conventional staining methods. As more newborns with duplication or deficiency of specific chromosome segments are diagnosed, new phenotypes are being described (such as 5p−). Caution often must be exercised in directly applying reported case history comparisons to clinical counseling of the parents. This is true not only because of the small number of similar cases which may have been reported, but particularly because many cases are relatively unique in that they involve both duplication of a segment of one chromosome and deficiency of a segment of the same or another chromosome.

With the observation of a large number of infants with a duplication or deficiency of a particular chromosome segment, phenotypic features are able to be "mapped" to specific regions or bands. In the future this experience may permit more reliable prediction of associated malformations as well as confidence in determining prognosis for survival and development. For certain types of abnormalities, such as ring chromosomes, experience only serves to underscore the variability of the phenotype.

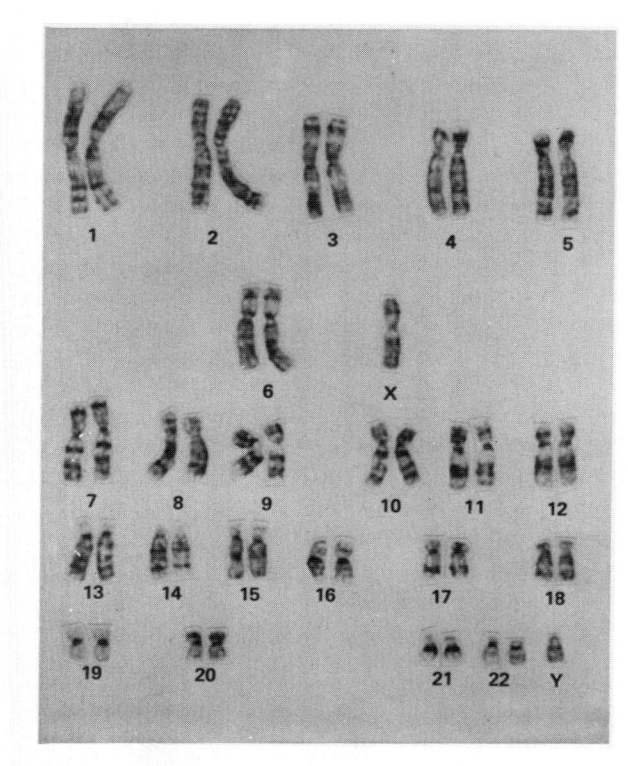

Fig. 37-5. Trypsin G-banded karyotype from normal male cell (46,XY).

Laboratory diagnosis

In most instances chromosomal diagnosis can be established by short-term (72 hours) culture of peripheral blood lymphocytes collected in heparin. The addition of a mitogen (phytohemagglutinin) to the culture medium promotes cell division, which is arrested in metaphase by an agent such as colchicine. After exposure to a hypotonic solution, used to cause swelling of the cells, the metaphases are preserved by fixative, spread on a slide, and stained for microscopic examination and photography. Pretreatment with particular chemical agents (e.g., trypsin) or stains will result in the different characteristic banding patterns. In the event that more rapid diagnosis is required, 48-hour cultures may be performed, or direct preparation of dividing cells from the bone marrow may be used. The latter procedure is particularly helpful when a lethal trisomy such as trisomy 18 or trisomy 13 is suspected in an infant, necessitating heroic life-support measures. In this situation the analysis of a limited number of cells by conventional stain, all of which are abnormal, may confirm the clinical diagnosis.

With the use of trypsin G-banding, deletions of chromosome material are readily identified. Duplicated segments may not be readily identifiable as to their chromosome of origin. In such cases the finding of a balanced parental rearrangement may provide identification of the source of the extra material. When extra material is present as a de novo event, use of several different forms of banding may identify the segment involved or narrow the possibilities.

When there is stillbirth or perinatal death of an infant suspected of having a chromosome abnormality, tissue biopsy (e.g., skin or amnion) should be obtained in the event that lymphocytes are not viable for study. Skin fibroblast chromosome analysis also may be required when recent blood transfusion renders lymphocyte chromosome analysis inaccurate. When an unusual chromosome abnormality is observed, skin biopsy provides the opportunity for permanent cell lines to be established that can be used for application of methods of chromosome study which may be developed in the future and also for research studies, such as gene mapping to specific chromosome bands. Fibroblast cultures also may be needed for confirmation or exclusion of the diagnosis of mosaicism.

Counseling the parents

Parents having a child with a chromosomal abnormality most frequently express the view that, in retrospect, they would have wished to have known the diagnosis as soon as it was suspected by the physician. Often, however, clinical diagnosis alone cannot be relied on for counseling. In most cases the parents will be aware of the malformations that the infant has. Although counseling should be individualized, it is reasonable to inform parents that these malformations suggest that the cause may be a chromosomal disorder; the normal constitution of 46 chromosomes in each cell of the body carrying all the genes also is explained at this time. The potential effect of an extra chromosome on fetal development as reflected by multisystem involvement is thus understandable. Often parents may inquire about the specific features which arouse the suspicion that there is chromosomal abnormality. If these are demonstrated to the parents, it is important to point out that many of these features in themselves are not deleterious and are often present as isolated findings in normal individuals. It should be emphasized that it is the presence of several or more of these features which suggests that a chromosomal abnormality may be present. This will help the parents understand the reasons for a chromosome study but prevent them from focusing on subtle dysmorphic features at a later time. To dispel guilt, but not to overstate the case with a complex explanation that may be irrelevant later, it is usual to explain that the presence of a chromosomal abnormality cannot be related to something the parents did or neglected to do at the time of conception or during pregnancy.

When a chromosomal abnormality is diagnosed unequivocally by the laboratory, the parents should be informed of the results. A counseling session should be arranged with both parents whenever possible. It is often useful to have a normal karyotype and the infant's karyotype available to show the parents in an effort to have them accept and understand the diagnosis. Reviewing the features of the syndrome that the child has in common with other infants having the same abnormality is also useful.

A discussion of the mechanism by which the abnormality occurs often is requested. This should be explained in terms that the parents can understand. Ultimately, for sporadic events, the parents must be told that, although we understand "how this happens," we do not understand "why this happened." When the infant has a trisomy, the parents are told that either the egg or the sperm may have contributed the extra chromosome and that in most cases it is not possible to identify the parental origin of the extra chromosome. The goal of the initial counseling session should be to promote understanding and acceptance of the diagnosis as the underlying cause of the widely dispersed malformations and problems of the infant and to alleviate parental guilt and anger.

During subsequent counseling a more detailed description of the disorder and the prognosis should be given when this is well defined. For disorders that are unique or in which the additional chromosome segment cannot be identified with confidence, giving the parents generalizations regarding chromosomal abnormalities may be subject to serious pitfalls. Rather, the child's malformations or problems should be discussed, and the prognosis for survival and development, although necessarily guarded, must be individualized or approached from a "wait and see" position.

For some parents the question of "will this happen again" comes up at this time. In a few families with recurrence of trisomy 21, mosaicism (i.e., a low-percentage

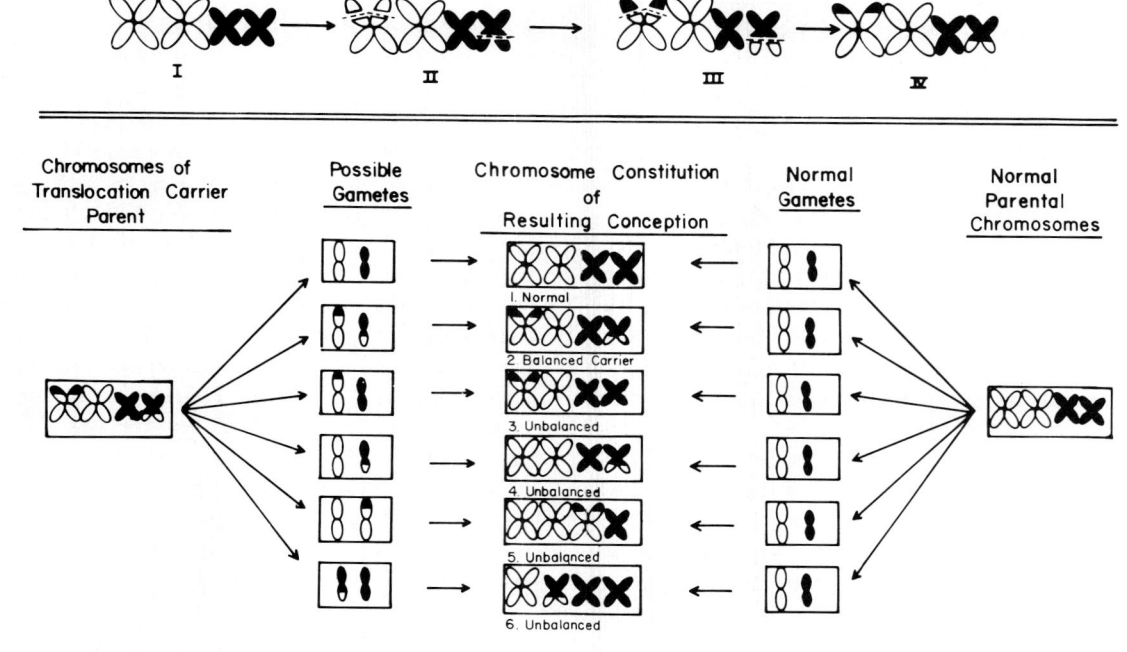

Fig. 37-6. *Upper portion; I,* Two normal chromosome pairs. *II,* Chromosome breaks occurring in one member of each chromosome pair. *III,* Exchange of broken fragments between members of each chromosome pair. *IV,* Reunion of broken fragments resulting in balanced reciprocal translocation. *Lower portion,* Possible gametic contributions from parent with balanced reciprocal translocation, and chromosome constitution of resulting conceptions after union with normal gametes from parent not carrying a translocation.

cell line with 47 +21) has been demonstrated in one parent. In such cases this provides a reasonable explanation for the occurrence of the chromosomal abnormality in the offspring and identifies the family to be at increased risk for recurrence. In the vast majority of cases parental chromosomes will be normal, and no reasonable explanation can be provided other than a sporadic occurrence of nondisjunction. In these cases the recurrence risk for trisomy 21 is estimated to be 1% to 2%. This is based on empiric data from studies of families with Down's syndrome children and is supported by experience with prenatal diagnosis. The availability of prenatal cytogenetic diagnosis for future pregnancies should be mentioned, but details regarding amniocentesis usually are reserved for a later counseling session. The knowledge that prenatal monitoring is available is often of great consolation to the parents and may also forestall premature but permanent reproductive decisions such as sterilization during this difficult adjustment period.

Empiric data establishing the risks of recurrence for trisomy 18 or trisomy 13 are not available. Based on current experience it seems reasonable to consider that this is certainly no greater than that determined for trisomy 21 and in fact may not be increased over that of the general population. Nevertheless one can expect that many of these families will elect to have prenatal cytogenetic diagnosis performed during future pregnancies for reassurance.

The guidelines for counseling a family having a child with mosaicism for autosomal trisomy are more difficult to establish. Even though mosaicism develops as a postconceptual event, it has not been determined whether this arises from a trisomic conception by anaphase lag as a secondary event or more often represents a primary error in an otherwise normal fetus. Studies of chromosomal abnormalities in abortuses suggest that the former mechanism may be more common than previously considered. Thus recurrence counseling must include the possibility that the primary abnormality was a trisomic conception.

The finding of a structural chromosomal abnormality in an infant always should be investigated by parental chromosome analysis. Balanced or unbalanced chromosome rearrangements in the child that are not inherited from either parent are considered random events. Attempts to explain isolated instances of otherwise unexplained recurrence of chromosomal abnormalities in families as being caused by gonadal mosaicism in a parent or balanced structural rearrangements below the limits of detection by current methods is somewhat speculative when counseling a family having a single child with a de novo chromosomal abnormality. Thus parents should be told that the likelihood of recurrence appears to be the same as that of the general population.

The finding of a parental balanced structural rearrangement (most often a translocation or inversion) as the cause of an unbalanced chromosome constitution in the offspring is important information for future reproduction by the parent and for other family members who may be identified as heterozygous for the same rearrangement. For translocation carriers theoretically one might predict that a sixth of pregnancies conceived would have the normal chromosome pattern, a sixth would result in balanced carrier conceptions, and the remaining two thirds of conceptions would be one of the four different unbalanced combinations (Fig. 37-6). This presumes that, after pairing in meiosis, segregation of the chromosomes involved in the translocation is random. This, however, is not necessarily the case. Diminished viability of unbalanced gametes also may be operative. Most important, the possibility of having a liveborn child with an unbalanced chromosome constitution would depend on the specific chromosome segments that might be duplicated or deficient in the offspring based on the parental karyotype. Thus prediction of the likelihood of recurrence is difficult, because empiric risk figures have only been determined for the most common translocations. For example, the risk of having a child with Down's syndrome is estimated to be 10% to 15% if a woman carries a D/G translocation of the robertsonian type involving chromosome 21 or 3% to 8% if the father is the carrier of the same translocation. On the other hand, the risk of having a child with trisomy 13 syndrome if either parent carries a 13/14 translocation appears to be quite low (less than 1%). When a translocation or inversion has resulted in a malformed live-born or late stillborn infant for whom no empiric data are available, it has been suggested that a reasonable estimate of recurrence risk is about 10% or less, or one substantial enough to justify consideration of prenatal cytogenetic diagnosis for future pregnancies.

MENDELIAN DISORDERS

Physical traits of every individual (the phenotype) are determined by multiple sets of gene pairs (alleles), with one member of each pair donated by each parent. In *recessive* traits the gene is expressed only when paired with an identical gene (homozygous state). An allele that is expressed whether homozygous or heterozygous is a *dominant* gene. Four basic patterns of inheritance have been identified: autosomal recessive, autosomal dominant, X-linked recessive, and X-linked dominant. The diagnostic criteria of each of these patterns are the following:

A. Autosomal recessive inheritance
   1. The trait appears in siblings and not in parents or other relatives.
   2. The recurrence risk is one in four for each birth.
   3. Males and females are equally affected.
B. Autosomal dominant inheritance
   1. The trait is noted both in the parents and frequently in other siblings.
   2. The trait appears in every generation.
   3. The recurrence risk is one in two for each birth.
   4. Males and females are equally affected.
C. X-linked recessive inheritance
   1. The trait is more frequently expressed in males than in females.
   2. An affected male can only transmit the defective gene to his daughter.
   3. Mothers of affected males will transmit the defective gene to half the sons and daughters. In general, only the sons will manifest the trait.
D. X-linked dominant inheritance
   1. Affected males will transmit the trait to all daughters and no sons.
   2. Affected females who are heterozygous for the defective gene will transmit the trait to half the sons and daughters.
   3. Affected females who are homozygous for the defective gene will transmit the trait to all sons and daughters.
   4. Affected females are twice as common as affected males.

There are several factors that may interfere with the ability to determine inheritance patterns. Certain phenotypes may be etiologically heterogeneous, that is, the same or similar physical characteristics may result from different genetic mechanisms. For example, Marfan's syndrome is an autosomal dominant condition whose phenotype is very similar to that observed in homocystinuria, an autosomal recessive disorder caused by a defined biochemical defect. Unless care is taken in the examination of the patient with features of Marfan's syndrome and appropriate biochemical tests are ordered, the diagnoses may be confused, and erroneous information may be given to the parents regarding the prognosis and risk of recurrence. Genetic deafness is another example of genetic heterogeneity. There are at least 16 to 18 different types of autosomal recessive deafness and numerous other autosomal dominant syndromes in which hearing may be severely impaired.

A second factor which can interfere with the ability to determine inheritance patterns is that mutations may result in multiple phenotypic abnormalities even though the primary alteration resides in a single gene. This phenomenon has been labeled *pleiotropy*. The diversity of phenotype expression from a single gene defect results in the clinical findings designated as a syndrome. Not every feature of a syndrome is detected in all individuals with the same genetic defect; environmental factors also may influence the signs or symptoms that appear. For example, voluntary or prescribed dietary restriction of a substrate when there is impaired metabolism is one approach to alleviation of symptoms or genetic treatment.

Some mutant genes are not expressed in every individual with the defect (reduced penetrance), or the expression of the trait may differ from individual to individual (variable expressivity). Both these phenomena will influence the ability to distinguish genetic from nongenetic disease and inheritance of a genetic disorder from new mutations. In more clinical terms penetrance is the percentage of individuals with the genotype who manifest the trait, and expressivity is a reflection of disease severity. Reduced penetrance and variable expressivity are more frequently observed in autosomal dominant conditions than in recessive disorders. Variation in the severity of a defect at a single locus is thought to represent heterogeneity of the mutation, the effects of modifying genes, or the influence of environmental conditions. Neurofibromatosis and cystic fibrosis are examples of inherited disorders that may demonstrate variable expressivity.

The age of the affected individual also may interfere with diagnosis of disease or determination of its inheritance pattern. Although the diagnosis of Huntington's chorea is made easily in the affected adult, manifestations of the disease are not evident in infancy or childhood. Many other inherited disorders, especially dominant diseases, become apparent only as the infant develops, and some may be detected biochemically before physical abnormalities are in evidence. Other disorders may be limited in their expression by the sex of the individual (sex-limited or sex-influenced disease). An example of a sex-limited disease is autosomal dominant precocious puberty, which occurs only in males. On the other hand, adrenogenital syndrome has been classified as a sex-influenced trait because the ratio of affected females to males is greater than 1:1. Neither of these disorders is carried on either the X or Y chromosome; however, the ability of the gene to exert its effect is influenced by the sex of the affected individual.

The Lyon hypothesis

Disorders that are carried on the X chromosome, such as hemophilia or color blindness, are rarely noted in females, even though female infants may inherit the X-linked mutant gene. The explanation for this observation is based on the random inactivation of one X chromosome in cells of the female. This theory is known as the Lyon hypothesis. One X chromosome is inactivated early in embryonic life and may be observed as a Barr body with light miscroscopy. The particular X chromosome that becomes inactivated (maternal or paternal) in any cell is randomly determined. The Lyon hypothesis explains clinical observations concerning X-linked disorders. Phenotypic females may manifest an X-linked recessive disorder when there is only a single X chromosome or there is nonrandom inactivation of one of the two X chromosomes. Nonrandom inactivation is more likely to occur in females with a structurally abnormal X chromosome and suggests that all female infants with X-linked recessive diseases should have a chromosomal analysis. The second observation explained by the Lyon hypothesis is that in a population of women carrying a defective X chromosome there will be marked variability of expression. Although most women will not manifest the abnormal trait, a small percentage of women will be affected because in a majority of their cells the abnormal X chromosome will be active as a chance phenomenon. This variability in X chromosome inactivation may make it difficult to identify female carriers of X-linked recessive disorders even when a biochemical defect or marker is available for testing (e.g., factor VIII levels for hemophilia or creatinine phosphokinase for Duchenne's muscular dystrophy). When the mother of an affected male does not have other affected sons, brothers, or uncles, the determination of new mutations from an inherited defect can be difficult. The theoretic likelihood of each possibility has been suggested for certain disorders; however, recent evidence seems to indicate that the frequency of a new mutation in the affected male is less than had been previously estimated.

Counseling the parents

For a few families with a dominant disorder it will have been clear that there was a substantial risk for an affected child. In many cases the factors previously discussed (such as variable expressivity, reduced penetrance, pleiotropy, genetic heterogeneity, and sex limitation) will result in families having interpreted for themselves some mechanism or risk other than dominant inheritance. This may give rise to the false reassurance that a particular generation of the family will be "skipped." Diagnosis of a more severely affected newborn, with subtle findings in an affected parent, and no history of the disorder in grandparents may falsely lead to the concept that the manifestations of the disease are worsening with each successive generation. Diagnosis of familial transmission of a dominant gene may require clinical or laboratory examination of parents, grandparents, or other family members suspected of having the gene. Identification of individuals with the gene can have important implications for their health as well as reproductive expectations. In some instances failure to establish inheritance of the gene suggests that the infant has a new mutation. This is particularly true for severe dominant diseases, which have diminished reproductive fitness.

An association between fresh dominant mutation and advanced paternal age has been defined. Because of the very low frequency of this type of event, prospective clinical counseling regarding this observation is not generally given. The diagnosis of a new mutation in a newborn carries a recurrence risk, which is presumably no greater than that of the general population. If familial inheritance is established or cannot be excluded, then the mode of inheritance and the 50% risk of transmission of the gene is explained to the parents. The risk then may be modified by empiric data regarding the penetrance and expression of the gene. Recently it has been observed that in infants with early onset or more severe manifestations of certain dominant disorders (e.g., myotonic dystrophy) there is more frequently maternal transmission of the gene. This interesting phenomenon remains unexplained. It has been suggested that the disease in the mother may adversely modify expression of the gene in the fetus.

A history of consanguinity suggests that the disorder in the newborn may be inherited as an autosomal recessive trait. It is important to explain to parents having a child with an autosomal recessive condition that every individual carries several deleterious recessive genes. By definition the carrier state for a recessive gene does not have clinical consequences. The birth of a child with a recessive disorder confirms that the parents are both heterozygous for the same, often rare, disorder. In addition to counseling families about future pregnancy risks (25% recurrence), it is important that they be given information regarding carrier detection of unaffected siblings and relatives who may be heterozygous for the mutant gene. For many autosomal recessive conditions biochemical testing can detect unaffected heterozygotes.

Previously affected sons, brothers, or maternal uncles may identify a disorder as X-linked recessive. Women who are carriers will transmit the gene to half their sons and daughters. With rare exceptions female heterozygotes will be unaffected because of random X chromosome inactivation. Affected males will transmit the gene to all their daughters (who will be carriers) and none of their sons. For some X-linked recessive disorders it is possible to detect unaffected female carriers using biochemical assays; however, lyonization may limit the accuracy of such testing. The possibility of a new mutation versus the probability that a woman is a carrier for an X-linked recessive disorder once she has an affected son can be calculated using formulas developed by population geneticists and the risk modified by the number of unaffected maternal male relatives. Early neonatal diagnosis of X-linked recessive disorders should be considered for males at risk. In some instances (e.g., hemophilia) this will have important implications for neonatal care. In other cases neonatal diagnosis of a disorder with delayed onset (e.g., cord blood creatinine phosphokinase for Duchenne's muscular dystrophy) may be important information to the parents for future reproduction.

MULTIFACTORIAL DEFECTS

The most common birth defects that occur as a single major malformation in an affected child have population and familial distributions that cannot be explained on the basis of a single gene or chromosomal abnormality. These are considered to occur on a continuous variability basis with an increased liability (i.e., lowered threshold in embryogenesis for the defect) because of several genes (i.e., polygenic) and also environmental factors. The combination of polygenic liability and environmental factors, which may be either maternally derived or transmitted from the maternal environment, has led to the use of the term *multifactorial* for classification of these defects.

Many of the defects in embryogenesis that are considered multifactorial also are observed as one of several or multiple malformations in infants with chromosomal disorders or single gene disorders. For example, isolated neural tube defects are considered to be multifactorial but also are observed as one of multiple malformations caused by a single gene (Meckel's syndrome, a recessive disorder) or trisomy 18, trisomy 13, triploidy, etc. Cleft lip is most often multifactorial in origin but is seen as an autosomal dominant trait when associated with lower lip pits or may be present in infants with a trisomy. Thus infants with a single obvious malformation (e.g., congenital heart defect, spina bifida, or cleft lip and palate) should be evaluated for other malformations that may indicate a chromosomal disorder, mendelian disorder, or a specific multiple malformation syndrome.

The most common multifactorial defects and their frequencies are listed in Tables 38-2 and 38-5. The relative importance of the genetic versus the environmental factors in the development of these varied defects has not been defined. Family history, epidemiologic data, and environmental exposure of the pregnancy should be ascertained and recorded for potential use in retrospective studies.

When counseling parents of a child with a multifactorial defect, it is important to point out that these are not "classically genetic" in the mendelian sense. The familial nature of the occurrence of the defects should be described (Table 37-2). The empiric data that are most applicable (e.g., geographic and ethnic) are used to determine the risk for recurrence. It is also important to

Table 37-2. Recurrence risk (percent) for the second in a sibship to be affected given that the first is born with various common congenital malformations with no other family history of such

Congenital malformation	Affected first sibling Male (%)	Affected first sibling Female (%)
Cleft lip and/or palate (England)	2.6	3.1
Talipes equinovarus (England)	1.4	1.6
Pyloric stenosis (England)	3.2	4.6
Hip dislocation (England)	4.8	3.2
Hirschsprung's disease (United States)	1.3	1.7
Atrial septal defect (England)	2.2	1.9
Ventricular septal defect (United States)	3.6	3.6
Aortic stenosis (Germany)	1.3	1.5
Anencephaly-myelomeningocele (Wales)	5.0	4.0
Anencephaly-myelomeningocele (England)	4.2	3.6

Data from Bonaiti-Pellie, C., and Smith, C.: J. Med. Genet. **11**:374, 1974; Computer Program RISKMF. Courtesy Thaddeus Kurczynski, M.D.

define the risk for other close relatives, so that the parents may suggest counseling to them, if they feel that this is appropriate. This is particularly of value when the disorder is able to be diagnosed prenatally and may be severely handicapping, as is the case with spina bifida.

ENVIRONMENTAL DISORDERS
General considerations

Congenital infections, drugs, and toxic chemicals are three classes of environmental agents accounting for approximately 7% of congenital malformations. Each is responsible for 2% to 3% of developmental defects, and radiation for less than 1%. The spectrum of congenital malformations that results will depend on the time in gestation when the embryo or fetus is exposed to the agent. Although such agents may produce detrimental effects from gametogenesis until the infant is born, periods of development during which toxic effects are most likely to occur (critical periods) have been defined.

During gametogenesis (a process that takes about 64 days in males and until the time of ovulation in females) agents that exert toxic effects probably result in death of the egg or sperm or perhaps preclinical abortion. In experimental animals LSD administration produces chromosomal breaks in meiotic cells; however, LSD has not been shown to cause malformations in humans or to increase the frequency of chromosomal disorders in offspring. As yet, preconceptual drug therapy has not been shown to have a teratogenic effect on subsequent conceptions. Several drugs, including thalidomide, methadone, and phenytoin, have been demonstrated in the semen of humans and experimental animals. In addition, two children with malformations have been reported whose fathers, but not their mothers, received thalidomide. Similarly infants with congenital malformations have been born to women whose husbands received phenytoin for epilepsy but who never took the drug themselves. The possibility that some drugs exert teratogenic effects by binding to sperm is an important area for investigation (Chapter 12).

Early embryonic development (first 3 weeks of pregnancy) begins with fertilization and ends with formation of the primitive streak. This period of development is thought to be relatively insensitive to embryotoxic influences. In some experimental animals administration of actinomycin D or cyclophosphamide during this time results in death of the embryo and structural abnormalities. Such effects may exist in human infants but have not yet been demonstrated. It is during the embryonic period (fourth to ninth week of gestation) that many adverse environmental agents exert their teratogenic effect. Such agents include drugs and toxic chemicals, radiation, and infections caused by viruses and other microorganisms. Those drugs for which a cause and effect relationship with malformations has been suggested include thalidomide, methyl mercury (Minamata disease), hydantoin, trimethadione, warfarin, aminopterin, alcohol, estrogens, and androgens (Chapter 12). Exposure to high levels of radiation during the embryonic period may produce microcephaly. Viral infections during embryonic period generally result in widespread damage to multiple organ systems (p. 692). The fetal period (ninth week of gestation until birth) may be adversely affected by numerous environmental agents; however, the outcome is usually organ damage or growth disturbance rather than malformation.

For each organ system a critical period of development may be identified during which specific malformations will result if there is interference with development. For example, myelomeningocele occurs during closure of a portion of the posterior neural tube (prior to 28 days). Cleft lip forms prior to closure of the lip at 38 days and cleft maxillary palate prior to fusion of the palatine ridges at 10 weeks. Table 37-3 lists the critical period of development for some common congenital malformations.

Radiation

Much of the information on the adverse effects of radiation comes from research on experimental animals and data accumulated on survivors of the atomic bomb at

Table 37-3. Time of development of common congenital malformations

Site of malformation	Malformation	Time of development
Face	Cleft lip	5-7 weeks
	Posterior cleft palate	8-12 weeks
Gastrointestinal tract	Esophageal atresia plus tracheoesophageal fistula	4 weeks
	Rectal atresia (with fistula)	6 weeks
	Malrotation	10 weeks
	Omphalocele	10 weeks
	Duodenal atresia	7-8 weeks
Central nervous system	Anencephaly	3-4 weeks
	Meningomyelocele	4 weeks
Cardiovascular system	Transposition of great vessels	5 weeks
	Ventricular septal defect	5-6 weeks
Genitourinary system	Agenesis of kidney	30 days
	Extroversion of bladder	4 weeks
	Bicornuate uterus	10 weeks
	Retained testis (cryptorchidism)	36-40 weeks
	Hypospadias	12 weeks
Limb	Aplasia of radius	38 days
	Syndactyly	6 weeks

Hiroshima. The central nervous system is the organ system most frequently affected. An increased incidence of microcephaly has been demonstrated in the offspring of pregnant women who were within 1,200 m of the hypocenter of the atomic bombing. Beyond this distance the frequency of microcephaly was not increased. Three factors appear to determine the extent of the radiation effect on the embryo or fetus: the dose of radiation, the time period over which this dose was administered, and the stage of gestation. The peak incidence of gross malformations occurs when the embryo is irradiated during the early organogenetic period, whereas growth retardation can result from irradiation at any stage after implantation. The preimplantation state is more sensitive to the lethal effects of radiation, and those embryos who survive irradiation at this stage rarely show malformations. A threshold or minimal dose of radiation considered to be important for induction of congenital defects in humans has not been established. For clinical counseling purposes some have suggested that less than 10 rad is a reasonable limit for reassuring patients. In general, the earlier the stage of gestation, the more sensitive is the developing organism to the effects of radiation.

The dose of natural background radiation to which every human is exposed varies from 80 mrad per year to almost 1,000 mrad per year in some parts of India and Brazil. In the United States most residents receive 100 to 400 mrad per year (40 mrad from cosmic X rays, 60 mrad from terrestrial sources, and 25 mrad from radionuclides). The human embryo and fetus are exposed to a background radiation rate of about 90 mrad for the entire gestational period. The total amount of background and fallout radiation is so low it is not thought to influence the incidence of congenital malformations.

Radionuclides administered to pregnant women for diagnostic or therapeutic purposes provide another source of radiation for the fetus. The clinical effect will depend on the type and dose of radiation and the period of gestation during which it was administered. Pathologic effects, including thyroid destruction, have been reported in the human fetus when ablative doses of radioactive iodine 131 have been given to pregnant women. If iodine 131 *must* be given, it should be used during the first 5 to 7 weeks of pregnancy before the fetal thyroid has formed. The radiation dose to the embryo or fetus should be calculated whenever radioactive material is to be administered to a pregnant woman. Once the radiation dose is calculated, rational decisions may be reached regarding the potential risk. In general, the embryo and fetus will receive much less radiation than the mother when the radioactive material does not cross the placenta in appreciable quantities. Because diagnostic roentgenograms would not be expected to exceed 10 rad, and because of concerns regarding preconceptual ovarian radiation (e.g., a possible associated increased risk of trisomic conceptions), the concept of a "safe time" in the menstrual cycle for diagnostic roentgenograms has been abandoned. Rather it seems reasonable to suggest that all unnecessary roentgenologic studies be avoided in women during the reproductive years, and whenever feasible the ovaries should be shielded.

Counseling the parents

Counseling regarding malformations potentially caused by environmental agents must be done with caution. The parental guilt generated can be overwhelming, and the medicolegal consequences should not be overlooked. Before making a firm association between the infant's defects and a particular agent, the evidence must be reviewed with care. Nevertheless, if a causal agent can be established, immunity to a viral infection or the ability to avoid a particular drug during a subsequent pregnancy provides reassurance for future reproduction.

Counseling parents during pregnancy regarding the possible effects of an environmental exposure often presents considerable difficulty. The tendency to glibly recommend abortion simply on the basis of diagnostic roentgenogram or multiple drug exposure should be avoided. It is quite clear that counseling regarding pregnancy termination should be nondirective. When proven or suspected viral or teratogenic exposure has occurred, the most reliable and up-to-date information regarding the risk should be presented to the couple along with the available options. Routine or specialized laboratory testing for viral infections must be expertly performed and interpreted. Frequently questions regarding drug exposure arise because of warnings in the lay press, an obstetrician's reluctance to offer reassurance for medicolegal reasons, or the ambivalence on the part of the patient regarding the pregnancy. For most drug exposure clear information regarding safety or possible low-level teratogenic effects has not been established. This is particularly true of new drugs or those which are likely to be used only infrequently during pregnancy. Extrapolation from animal studies or definition of risk using isolated case reports is fraught with pitfalls.

When data are not available but the drug is one that has been marketed for some time and is likely to be taken during pregnancy, counseling may be approached in a general way. Defining the population frequency of birth defects, the potential contribution of drug exposure to this, and the fact that the particular drug has not been established as a potent or possible teratogen may serve to reassure the patient. Nevertheless the inability to guarantee the safety of any specific drug for a particular pregnancy may lead to a decision on the part of the patient to terminate the pregnancy if this is an available option.

PRENATAL GENETIC DIAGNOSIS

Midtrimester prenatal diagnosis of genetic disease has developed rapidly and become widely available during the past decade. The perinatologist is in a unique position to identify families who may wish to use these services during subsequent pregnancies, either because of recurrence risk or simply for reassurance that a particular sporadic event has not recurred. Methods of prenatal diagnosis may be considered in two categories: phenotypic studies and genotypic studies. Those methods which determine the phenotype or anatomy of the fetus with regard to a particular defect or defects hold the most promise for diagnosing disorders that are multifactorial, the skeletal dysplasias, and multiple malformation syndromes for which no clear genetic cause has been defined. Methods that determine the genotype of the fetus require fetal cells for study and are used for detection of chromosomal disorders and certain mendelian diseases.

Roentgenography offers the potential for diagnosis of many of the skeletal dysplasias. The major limitation of roentgenograms for early prenatal diagnosis is the poor visualization of the fetal skeleton until beyond 20 weeks' gestation. Enhancement of visualization is achieved by amniography (injection of water-soluble contrast dye into the amniotic fluid) with maternal positioning for roentgenograms determined by fluoroscopic guidance. This procedure is useful for diagnosis of disorders having severe and characteristic skeletal findings that are detectable as early as 20 weeks of pregnancy (e.g., thrombocytopenia-absent radius [TAR] syndrome or achondrogenesis). Because of limited experience and the difficulties of visualization, inadequate or false negative testing is a concern. By outlining soft tissue, amniography provides the opportunity for diagnosis of large soft tissue masses and facilitates orientation of the fetal structures for skeletal examination. Omphalocele, sacral teratoma, encephalocele, and meningomyelocele are potentially diagnosable by this method. The diagnostic potential is limited by the ability to visualize small lesions or in the case of spina bifida those which are open but have flat surface contiguous with the fetal back. Fetal swallowing and concentration of the contrast dye in the intestinal tract are useful for diagnosis of bowel atresia or obstruction.

Ultrasound has proven to be a far more versatile method for definition of fetal anatomy than the roentgenogram (Chapter 8). The utility of ultrasound for diagnosis of birth defects first became apparent when it was recognized that consistent definition of the fetal head by 16 weeks' gestation virtually excluded the diagnosis of anencephaly. The diagnosis of early hydrocephalus, renal agenesis, polycystic kidney disease, omphalocele, encephalocele, spina bifida, and a variety of cystic or solid masses has been reported by several units. Widespread reliable diagnosis of these defects awaits further development of experience and expertise. Fetal echocardiography is promising for diagnosis of many congenital heart defects. Definition of fetal limbs and the appendicular skeleton is useful for diagnosis of reduction deformities, disorders characterized by absence of a bone (e.g., TAR) or even polydactyly. Standards for length of long bones as measured ultrasonically permit diagnosis of skeletal dysplasias characterized by shortening and/or bowing of the limbs. Defective mineralization (such as hypophosphatasia) also may be observed ultrasonically.

Direct fetal visualization is possible by percutaneous introduction of a fine-caliber endoscope, known as the fetoscope. This technique is limited by the narrow field of vision and by difficulty that may be encountered in maneuvering to a specific area of the fetal anatomy, even with ultrasonic guidance (as described later).

Amniocentesis provides a source of desquamated fetal cells, of which a proportion are viable. These cells originate from the amnion, fetal skin, and gastrointestinal and urogenital tracts. In addition to the cellular element, supernatant amniotic fluid has a number of other constituents (such as hormones and proteins) that are potentially useful for diagnosis of birth defects or genetic disease. Percutaneous amniocentesis is technically feasible as early as 14 weeks' menstrual age. The procedure may be performed on an outpatient basis; however, strict aseptic technique is required. Local anesthesia in skin may be administered prior to insertion of a spinal needle into the amniotic cavity to withdraw the fluid. The amount of fluid required varies with the study to be performed but generally ranges from a few to as much as 30 to 40 ml. The fluid that is removed rapidly reaccumulates. Patients most often return to full activity immediately after the procedure with only minimal discomfort.

The rate of successfully obtaining an adequate sample of amniotic fluid increases with advancing gestation such that generally it is recommended that the procedure be performed at 16 weeks' gestation. At this gestational age fluid usually can be obtained in 90% or more of cases by a single needle insertion. Although measurement of a constituent in supernatant fluid (e.g., alpha-fetoprotein) or direct assay of the cell pellet for enzyme activity is at times useful for diagnosis, tissue culture of the amniotic fluid cells is required in most cases. Success in establishing tissue culture of amniotic fluid cells will vary with the laboratory but can be expected in more than 95% of cases. Because of the relatively small number of viable cells collected at amniocentesis, completion of testing usually requires 2 to 3 weeks or longer.

Although regarded as safe, midtrimester amniocentesis carries important risks. Several collaborative studies have been conducted to determine the frequency of pregnancy loss attributable to this procedure. A matched control study of 1,040 patients in the United States and a similar number of patients in Canada demonstrated a fetal loss rate of 3.5% in the study group without a significant difference from control subjects. A British collaborative study showed an excess fetal loss rate among amniocentesis patients of about 1%, but the rate in control subjects was somewhat lower than expected. The reason for the differences in the findings of the British study compared with those of other studies remains unclear. Nevertheless it is generally believed that the rate of fetal loss attributable to the procedure is probably less than 0.5%. Ultrasonic placental localization is recommended prior to the procedure. A number of studies have demonstrated a reduction in the frequency of bloody fluids and particularly fetal red cells when preliminary ultrasound has been used.

Chorioamnionitis occasionally has been observed shortly after amniocentesis and inevitably results in septic abortion. The actual frequency of this complication has not been defined but is perhaps 1 or 2 in 1,000 cases. Fetal injury during midtrimester amniocentesis is almost exclusively limited to superficial scars, which may be seen as dimpling of the skin. The frequency of fetal injury varies considerably from no injuries in a number of large series to more than 1% in several smaller series. The difference in these observations is difficult to explain but may be related to experience with the procedure as well as bias of ascertainment. Interestingly, "amniocentesis injury" was reported as frequently in control newborns as in study patients in the British collaborative study. Thus it seems that the neonatal diagnosis of needle injury secondary to midtrimester amniocentesis should be made with caution. Fetomaternal bleeding occurs in about 10% of cases following midtrimester amniocentesis. Studies have shown an excess sensitization rate of 5% when Rh immunoglobulin is not administered to unsensitized Rh-negative women carrying an Rh-positive fetus who undergo early amniocentesis. This complication is avoidable by the administration of Rh immunoglobulin to these patients at the time of amniocentesis.

An increased risk of chromosomal disorders continues to be the most frequent indication of prenatal genetic diagnosis. Maternal age greater than 35 years at the time of anticipated delivery is the most common factor that enables identification of a risk which is appreciably greater than that of the general population. Although the risk for trisomy 21 increases gradually throughout the reproductive years, the rapid upswing at about age 35 years generally is taken as an indication for this testing (Table 37-4). There is a significant discrepancy between the age-related risk determined from live-born infant studies and the frequency of positive diagnosis of trisomy 21 from prenatal diagnosis experience. This may in large part be a result of the likelihood of fetal loss in these pregnancies after 16 weeks' gestation. Thus it seems most reasonable to counsel patients that their risk for having a child with a trisomy is most accurately defined from surveys of live-born children but that the chance of positive prenatal diagnosis is somewhat higher.

Others who elect to have chromosome study by amniocentesis include couples with a previous trisomic child or those in which one parent carries a balanced structural rearrangement. Sex determination when the fetus is at risk of an X-linked recessive disease is another indication for karyotyping. Although fetal sex may be determined by hormone measurement in amniotic fluid (testosterone and follicle-stimulating hormone) or nuclear sex chromatin (Barr body or Y-fluorescent bodies), the accuracy of diagnosis required is such that a standard chromosome analysis is performed.

Chromosome analysis of amniotic fluid cells may be performed for fully informed patients at no identifiable increased risk for having a child with one of these disorders. Often these couples have increased anxiety about the possibility of having a child with Down's syndrome

Table 37-4. Incidence of Down's syndrome at birth and of fetal chromosomal abnormalities at amniocentesis, by maternal age

Maternal age	Down's syndrome at birth*	Down's syndrome at second trimester Hook's study†	Down's syndrome at second trimester Golbus' study‡	Total aneuploidies at second trimester Hook's study†	Total aneuploidies at second trimester Golbus' study‡
15-19	1/1,682				
20-24	1/1,352				
25-29	1/1,133				
30	1/885				
31	1/826				
32	1/725				
33	1/592				
34	1/465				
35	1/365				
35-36					
36	1/287	0	1/143	1/104	1/66
37	1/225				
37-38					
38	1/176	1/128	1/100	1/48	1/54
39	1/139				
39-40					
40	1/109	1/149	1/45	1/75	1/35
41	1/85				
41-42					
42	1/67	1/32	1/41	1/23	1/31
43	1/53				
43-44					
44	1/41	1/18	1/18	1/14	1/10
45	1/32				
46	1/25				

From Amniocentesis for prenatal chromosomal diagnosis, Atlanta, Centers for Disease Control, U.S. Department of Health, Education, and Welfare.
*Data from Hook, E.B., and Lindsjo A.: Am. J. Hum. Genet. **30:**19, 1978.
†Data from Hook, E.B.: Birth Defects **14:**249, 1978.
‡Data from Golbus, M., and others: N. Engl. J. Med. **300:**157, 1979.

on the basis of a family member with this disorder, occupational contact with affected individuals, etc. Chromosome testing also is generally offered to patients who have amniocentesis primarily to detect other disorders (e.g., neural tube defects or inborn errors of metabolism).

The accuracy of chromosome analysis on cultured amniotic fluid cells is estimated to approach 99%. This is dependent on the ability to establish a pure culture of fetal cells without maternal cell contamination and the potential for laboratory error. Maternal cell contamination probably occurs in less than 1% of cases. When this is suspected, fetal sex confirmation by hormone measurement or comparison of parental chromosome variants with those of the amniotic cell culture by banding techniques (usually Q-banding) may clarify the origin of the cells. Polyploidy is quite frequent in amniotic cells and may be disregarded unless consistent triploidy is observed. Single aberrant cells on the basis of an in vitro phenomenon are observed from time to time and are of no apparent consequence. The diagnosis of true fetal mosaicism, however, continues to be a difficult dilemma. A consistent abnormality observed in a proportion of cells from separate cultures or in more than one patch of cells from the same culture raises the suspicion of true fetal mosaicism. Thus far, in those cases in which true fetal mosaicism has been confirmed, the abnormality has been one that also has been observed in live-born infants (e.g., trisomy 21, trisomy 13, trisomy 18, trisomy 8, or sex chromosome abnormalities). Although these observations have assisted in the clinical delineation of true fetal mosaicism from pseudomoscaicism in cultured amniotic fluid cells, this distinction is not possible in every case in which this problem arises. The finding of mosaicism or of a sex chromosome abnormality can present a significant dilemma for the parents in terms of a decision to continue or to terminate the pregnancy.

A large number of inborn errors of metabolism are diagnosable by study of cultured amniotic fluid cells (Table 37-5). The majority of these are rare autosomal recessive disorders, and a few are X-linked recessive (i.e., Hunter's syndrome, Fabry's disease, and Lesch-Nyhan

Table 37-5. Prenatal diagnosis of metabolic diseases

Disease	Diagnostic test
Lipid metabolism	
Tay-Sachs	Hexosaminidase A
Sandhoff	Hexosaminidase A and B
Gaucher	β-Glucosidase
GM$_1$ gangliosidosis	β-Galactosidase
Niemann-Pick	Sphingomyelinase
Fabry	α-Galactosidase
Metachromatic leukodystrophy	Arylsulfatase A
Krabbe	Galactosylceramide-galactosidase
Wolman	Acid esterase
Farber	Ceramidase
Familial hypercholesterolemia	Low-density lipoprotein cell–surface receptor
Mucopolysaccharidoses (MPS) and related disorders	
Hurler (MPS IH)	α-Iduronidase
Scheie (MPS IS)	α-Iduronidase
Hunter (MPS II)	Sulfoiduronate sulfatase
Sanfilippo A (MPS IIIA)	Heparan sulfate sulfamidase
Sanfilippo B (MPS IIIB)	α-N-Acetylglucosaminidase
Maroteaux-Lamy (MPS IV)	Arylsulfatase B
Mucolipidosis II (I cell disease)	Lysosomal hydrolases
Mucolipidosis III	Lysosomal hydrolases
Mucolipidosis IV	EM ultrastructure
Fucosidosis	α-Fucosidase
Mannosidosis	α-Mannosidase
Sialidosis (variant)	Neuraminidase + β-galactosidase
Amino acid metabolism	
Argininosuccinicaciduria	Argininosuccinate
Cystinosis	Cystine^{35} S uptake
Citrullinemia	Argininosuccinate synthetase
Homocystinuria	Cystathionine synthetase
Maple syrup urine disease	α-Keto acid decarboxylase
Methylmalonic acidemia	
B$_{12}$-responsive	Deoxyadenosyl-B$_{12}$ synthesis
B$_{12}$-nonresponsive	Methylmalonyl-CoA mutase
Propionic acidemia	Propionyl-CoA decarboxylase
Carbohydrate metabolism	
Glycogen storage type II	α-Glucosidase
Glycogen storage type IV	Amylo(1,4→1,6)transglucosidase
Galactosemia	Galactose-1-phosphate uridylyltransferase
Pyruvate decarboxylase deficiency	Pyruvate decarboxylase
Blood	
Hemophilia A	Factor VIII/factor VIII antigen
Sickle cell	β-Chain synthesis/restriction enzyme analysis
Homozygous β-thalassemia	β-Chain synthesis/restriction enzyme analysis
Homozygous α-thalassemia	cDNA hybridization
βδ-Thalassemia	cDNA hybridization
Chronic granulomatous disease	NBT/superoxide formation
Miscellaneous	
Combined immunodeficiency	Adenosine deaminase
Lesch-Nyhan syndrome	Hypoxanthine-guanine phosphoribosyltransferase
Menkes' syndrome	Copper uptake
Xeroderma pigmentosum	DNA repair
Hypophosphatasia	Alkaline phosphatase isoenzymes
Acute intermittent porphyria	Uroporphyrinogen I synthesis
Congenital adrenal hyperplasia (21-hydroxylase)	HLA-B linkage
Lysosomal acid phosphatase deficiency	Acid phosphatase
Congenital nephrosis	Alpha-fetoprotein

syndrome). It should be noted that cystic fibrosis, one of the more common autosomal recessive diseases in the white population, is conspicuously absent from this list. The identification of couples at risk generally is made on the basis of a previously affected child or at times by screening programs (as with Tay-Sachs disease). Occasionally identification of a couple at risk may be on the basis of carrier testing done because there is a close relative with one of these disorders. Measurement of an enzyme in supernatant fluid or uncultured cells is useful for diagnosis of only a few disorders. Most testing for inborn errors of metabolism must be conducted on cultured cells, and the number of cells required often necessitates greater delay from amniocentesis to diagnosis (4 to 6 weeks) when compared with what is required for chromosome analysis (2 to 4 weeks).

The accuracy of biochemical testing also depends on the limitations of the particular assay method used. For autosomal recessive disorders it is imperative that the affected pregnancies be clearly distinguished from those with heterozygous (maternal) carriers, since the latter group will constitute two thirds of the normal pregnancies of these parents. At times confidence in this testing is limited by the relatively small experience with the methods of prenatal diagnosis. For this reason referral of these couples or their amniotic fluid samples to centers having the greatest expertise with diagnosis of the particular disorder is recommended.

For other single gene disorders, especially many of those which are autosomal dominant, the defect is not known at the biochemical level. One approach to prenatal diagnosis is the study of a linked gene that would serve as a marker for the disease. This is only useful if there is close linkage of a marker to the gene for the disease, and this marker is detectable by amniocentesis. In addition, variability of the marker (e.g., isoenzymes) is necessary for a large proportion of matings to be informative for study. Until recently the best example of using such a system for prenatal diagnosis has been the linkage between secretor status and the gene for myotonic dystrophy. Although this is of limited use at present, rapidly accumulating information about linkages and further mapping of the human genome make this a promising direction for development of methods for prenatal diagnosis of other diseases.

Recombinant DNA technology and the linkage approach to prenatal diagnosis have recently resulted in a dramatic advance for prenatal diagnosis of hemoglobinopathies. Complementary DNA (cDNA) for hemoglobin genes was first used for prenatal diagnosis of gene deletion (e.g., homozygous α-thalassemia). This is done by extracting DNA from cultured or uncultured amniotic fluid cells, cleaving the single-stranded DNA with a restriction enzyme that is specific for a certain base sequence, and determining the presence of the gene by detecting radiolabeled cDNA on gel electrophoresis that has hybridized with the single-stranded DNA of the gene. This work led to the observation of the linkage of a mutation in the spacer segment of DNA adjacent to the gene for the β^S when cleaved by a specific restriction enzyme (HpaI). The linkage of this mutation with the β^S gene is estimated to occur in 60% to 80% of American blacks. In informative matings the presence of cDNA hybridized to β^A or β^S gene in DNA fragments of different base lengths after treatment with HpaI can determine the fetal genotype with a high degree of confidence. This technique also has been extended to the study of patients having the Mediterranean form of β-thalassemia. A linked mutation in the spacer segment has been found that is detectable by other restriction enzymes which permit prenatal diagnosis using amniotic fluid cells in a proportion of these cases. Future developments for prenatal diagnosis of other disorders by these methods will require development of cDNA for other genes and identification of closely linked markers using one of the many restriction enzymes that are available.

Measurement of alpha-fetoprotein concentration in amniotic fluid has become established as a reliable method for diagnosis of open neural tube defects and certain other disorders. This protein is the major serum protein of early fetal life and reaches peak concentration (3 to 4 mg/ml) in the fetal serum at about 14 weeks' gestation. Low-level amounts of alpha-fetoprotein are present in amniotic fluid. The concentration of alpha-fetoprotein in fetal serum declines with advancing gestational age, as does that in amniotic fluid. On the other hand, the very low concentration of alpha-fetoprotein in maternal serum (nanogram amounts) rises as pregnancy advances, with peak levels being reached at about 34 weeks' gestation.

When the fetus has an open neural tube defect, leakage of alpha-fetoprotein from the fetal blood into the amniotic fluid will cause diagnostic elevation of alpha-fetoprotein (>5 SD above the mean) in most cases. Because of the declining concentration of amniotic fluid alpha-fetoprotein during the second trimester, interpretation of this test is dependent on accurate gestational dating by ultrasound. It is now well recognized that intraamniotic fetal bleeding secondary to amniocentesis, fetal death, or a number of other defects may be associated with leakage of alpha-fetoprotein from the fetal circulation into the amniotic fluid. Other defects that have been associated with elevated amniotic fluid alpha-fetoprotein include omphalocele, sacral teratoma, cystic hygroma (most commonly associated with Turner's syndrome), and fetal nephrosis.

A practical false positive rate with measurement of

amniotic fluid alpha-fetoprotein that excludes fetal death, intraamniotic bleeding, or other serious fetal abnormalities is quite low (0.25% or less). Nevertheless, because of the problems inherent in the interpretation of a quantitative test that reflects a heterogeneous group of defects, other methods for diagnosis of neural tube defects have been sought. A number of other markers in amniotic fluid have been investigated as more specific confirmatory tests for neural tube defects. Of these, the most promising is measurement of acetylcholinesterase in amniotic fluid. Reliable anatomic definition of neural tube defects is highly desirable in establishing the diagnosis. This is possible by ultrasonographers highly experienced in evaluating fetal anatomy but is not widely available. Amniography is used by some centers in spite of the limitation in detecting flat open myeloceles or small defects.

Maternal serum alpha-fetoprotein also is increased in a large portion of pregnancies in which the fetus has a neural tube defect. Measurement of maternal serum alpha-fetoprotein serves as a useful screening test for neural tube defects. As with amniotic fluid alpha-fetoprotein, interpretation of the test is gestational-age dependent. Thus false positive or false negative results may occur on the basis of errors in gestational dating and require ultrasound confirmation of dates. Elevated maternal serum alpha-fetoprotein also is observed in a proportion of cases in which there are twins, other defects resulting in elevated amniotic fluid alpha-fetoprotein, fetal death, and fetal to maternal bleeding. As with amniotic fluid alpha-fetoprotein, elevation of concentration of alpha-fetoprotein in maternal serum is not seen with closed neural tube defects. The degree of overlap of maternal serum alpha-fetoprotein between women carrying fetuses with an open neural tube defect and those with unaffected fetuses is somewhat greater than with amniotic fluid alpha-fetoprotein measurement. At cutoff levels that detect 80% of open spina bifida and 90% of anencephaly, the false positive rate with serum alpha-fetoprotein is quite high. Often an explanation for the false positive elevation can be found by ultrasound. In the remaining cases the risk of a neural tube defect is dependent on the a priori risk of a defect, which will vary with the geographic population risk. Even in low-risk populations such as the United States the risk of a neural tube defect after two elevated maternal serum alpha-fetoprotein concentrations between 16 and 18 weeks' gestation is high enough (5%) to warrant consideration of diagnostic testing by amniocentesis.

In addition to amniocentesis, fetoscopy offers the ability to obtain fetal cells or tissue by direct biopsy. Fetal blood cells may be obtained by puncture of a vessel on the fetal surface of the placenta. Direct aspiration of fetal blood from vessels near the origin of the umbilical cord also has been successfully performed. Samples obtained by these methods are used to diagnose hemoglobinopathies by measurement of the ratios of globin chain synthesis. Families in which DNA studies are not able to be used because of the lack of a suitable linked mutation continue to require fetoscopic sampling for diagnosis. Measurement of factor VIII activity and factor VIII antigen has proven useful for diagnosis of hemophilia in male fetuses at risk. Disorders diagnosable by study of white blood cells (such as chronic granulomatous disease) or platelets also are potentially diagnosable by this technique. Histopathology on fetal skin biopsy has been used for prenatal diagnosis of icthyosis. Thus far fetoscopic blood sampling has been performed only in several hundred continuing pregnancies. From this experience it appears that the risk of abortion after this procedure is approximately 5%, and the risk of prematurity is approximately 10%.

Counseling the parents

It is important that the neonatologist recognize families who are at risk for recurrence of diagnosable defects in future pregnancies and advise the parents of the availability of testing. Complete genetic counseling should be given to all couples considering prenatal genetic diagnosis. In addition, the risks, accuracy, and limitations of the studies to be performed must be described in detail. A decision regarding prenatal genetic diagnosis is tempered by the couple's moral, ethical, and religious beliefs, in addition to their perceptions of the risks and benefits of the testing. In most instances the benefit of prenatal diagnosis will be a high degree of assurance that the fetus is not affected by a particular genetic disease. Nevertheless studies must be initiated and completed in a time sequence that will permit an abortion should there be a positive diagnosis. Clearly counseling for prenatal diagnosis and selection of reproductive options must be comprehensive but *nondirective*.

Richard A. Polin
Michael T. Mennuti

BIBLIOGRAPHY

Bergsma, D., editor: Birth defects compendium, ed. 2, The National Foundation–March of Dimes, New York, 1977, Alan R. Liss, Inc.

Berkowitz, R.L., and Coustan, D.R., editors: The handbook for drugs in pregnancy, Boston, 1981, Little, Brown & Co.

Chayen, S., editor: An assessment of the hazards of amniocentesis, Br. J. Obstet. Gynecol. **85**(Supp. 2):1, 1978.

Heinonen, O.P., Sloane, D., and Shapiro, S., editors: Birth defects and drugs in pregnancy, Littleton, Mass., 1977, Publishing Sciences Group, Inc.

McKusick, V., editor: Mendelian inheritance in man: catalogs of autosomal dominant, autosomal recessive and X-linked phenotypes, Baltimore, 1978, Johns Hopkins University Press.

NICHD National Registry for Amniocentesis Study Group: Mid-trimester amniocentesis for prenatal diagnosis: safety and accuracy, J.A.M.A. **236**:1471, 1976.

Prevention of embryonic, fetal and perinatal disease, Fogarty International Center Series on Preventitive Medicine, vol. 3, Pub. No. 76-853, Washington, D.C., Department of Health, Education, and Welfare (National Institute of Health).

Shepard, T.H., editor: Catalog of teratogenic agents, Baltimore, 1973, Johns Hopkins University Press.

Simpson, N.E., and others: Prenatal diagnosis of genetic disease in Canada: report of a collaborative study, Can. Med. Assoc. J. **115**:739, 1976.

Smith, D.W., editor: Recognizable patterns of human malformation, ed. 2, Philadelphia, 1976, W.B. Saunders Co.

Thompson, J.S., and Thompson, M.W., editors: Genetics in medicine, ed. 3, Philadelphia, 1980, W.B. Saunders Co.

U.K. Collaborative Study on Alpha-fetoprotein in Relation to Neural-tube Defects: Maternal serum-alpha-fetoprotein measurement in antenatal screening for anencephaly and spina bifida in early pregnancy, Lancet **1**:1323, 1977.

Van der Berg, B.J., and Yerushalmy, J.: The relationship of the rate of intrauterine growth of infants of low birth weight to mortality, morbidity, and congenital anomalies, J. Pediatr. **69**:531, 1966.

Warkany, J., editor: Congenital malformations, Chicago, 1971, Year Book Medical Publishers, Inc.

CHAPTER 38 Congenital malformations

Congenital malformations are a common cause of illness, long-term disability, and death in children. Their incidence varies with the age of the patient being evaluated. Although many malformations are detectable at birth, internal anomalies involving organs such as the kidneys, heart, and brain may become apparent only in succeeding years. This chapter reviews some of the significant epidemiologic and genetic aspects of congenital malformations and provides a framework for the evaluation of the dysmorphic infant. (See also Chapter 37.)

TERMINOLOGY

A number of terms used in the description of malformations require definition. A structural abnormality may be referred to as either an *anomaly* or *malformation*, both terms being synonymous. A major malformation has significant surgical and/or cosmetic consequences for the patient, whereas a minor anomaly has neither surgical nor cosmetic importance. Minor anomalies overlap with normal phenotypic variation and are arbitrarily defined as occurring in 4% or less of infants of the same racial group. A localized malformation consists of an isolated or single abnormality, such as a myelomeningocele. Multiple malformations involve more than one discrete structure or organ system.

More recently, other terms have been suggested to describe patterns of malformations. *Anomalad sequence*, or *malformation complex*, refers to a malformation together with its subsequently derived structural changes, without a particular cause being specified. An example is sirenomelia, which consists of multiple anomalies involving variable fusion of the lower extremities, abnormalities in the urogenital system, and defects of the lower intestinal tract and spine, all presumably the result of a primary disturbance in the posterior midaxis mesoderm at the primitive streak stage of development. The term *association* refers to a nonrandom occurrence of multiple malformations for which no specific or common etiology has been identified. An example is the VATER association, an acronym for a pattern of anomalies consisting of vertebral abnormalities, anal atresia, tracheoesophageal fistula with esophageal atresia, and radial and renal dysplasia. The various anomalies may occur in different combinations with no known etiology, and the patterns of malformation overlap but contrast with sirenomelia, in which the different abnormalities are structurally derived from an early localized mesodermal defect. Finally, the term *syndrome* refers to a recognized pattern of malformations with a single, specific etiology, such as the Holt-Oram syndrome, in which radial dysplasia and cardiac defects occur as a consequence of an autosomal dominant gene.

EPIDEMIOLOGY AND GENETICS
Frequency and etiology of major malformations

As indicated by the data in Tables 38-1 and 38-2, about 2% of newborn infants have a serious malformation that has surgical or cosmetic importance. This figure is a minimum estimate, since it is based on examination of newborn infants only, and additional anomalies are detected with increasing age. The largest number (86%) of congenital malformations are localized, and of this group the majority, constituting 0.58% of all newborns, are the consequence of multifactorial inheritance involving the interaction of multiple genetic and environmental factors. The most common and familiar congenital malformations fall into this category and include congenital heart disease, neural tube defects, cleft lip and/or palate, clubfoot, and congenital hip dislocation. The timing of some common developmental malformations is summarized in Table 37-3.

Approximately 20% of serious malformations are

Table 38-1. Malformations in 12,000 consecutive newborns

Type of malformation	Number of newborns	Percent of total malformations	Percent of total newborns
Localized	161	85.6	1.34
Multifactorial inheritance	70	37.2	0.58
Mendelian inheritance	41	21.8	0.34
Unknown	50	26.6	0.42
Multiple	27	14.4	0.22
Chromosomal	11	5.9	0.09
Mendelian inheritance	6	3.2	0.05
Unknown	10	5.3	0.08
Total	188	100	1.56

Data from Holmes, L.B.: N. Engl. J. Med. **192**:763, 1974.

Table 38-2. Type and etiology of major malformations in 18,155 newborns

Malformation	Number
Multifactorial inheritance	128 (0.7%)
Anencephaly-myelomeningocele-encephalocele	25
Cardiac anomalies	45
Cleft lip and/or palate	14
Clubfoot	21
Congenital hip dislocation	12
Hypospadias	8
Omphalocele	2
Bilateral renal agenesis	1
Mendelian inheritance	67 (0.4%)
Autosomal dominant disorders (excluding polydactyly)	57
Autosomal recessive disorders	9
X-linked recessive disorders	1
Chromosome abnormalities	27 (0.2%)
Down's syndrome	21
Trisomy 13	3
Other	3
Teratogenic conditions	15 (0.1%)
Infants of diabetic mothers	14
Effects of warfarin	1
Unknown	107 (0.6%)
Total number affected	344 (2%)

Data from Holmes, L.B.: N. Engl. J. Med. **195**:204, 1976.

inherited in a mendelian manner in which one locus exerts a predominant effect on the formation of a particular structure. The most common mode of mendelian inheritance for major malformations is autosomal dominant, with a minority due to autosomal recessive or, rarely, X-linked recessive genes. X-linked dominant inheritance is the least common mendelian pattern. Limb anomalies, including postaxial polydactyly, syndactyly, and brachydactyly, constitute the most prevalent major localized malformations and are frequently the result of a dominant gene. Any type of malformation, however, may be under the control of a single locus, including multiple anomalies arising in different structures or organ systems. Altogether, single major genes are responsible for 0.4% of newborns having major malformations. Inborn errors of amino acid metabolism, on the other hand, are one tenth as prevalent, occurring in 0.04% of newborns. In contrast to the amino acid disorders, relatively little is understood about the biochemical defects underlying the production of malformations by mutant genes. As a result, their specific diagnosis relies heavily on the family history and clinical evaluation.

About 0.2% of newborns have a major malformation secondary to a chromosomal disorder, and this amounts to 10% of all the major congenital malformations. It is important to note, however, that approximately 0.6% of newborns have a noteworthy chromosomal anomaly, but two thirds of these infants do not have any abnormalities detectable by physical examination at birth. Included among these early phenotypically undetectable chromosomal anomalies are common disorders of the sex chromosomes, such as 47,XXY; 47,XYY; and 47,XXX. The most prevalent malformation syndrome due to an abnormal chromosomal constitution is Down's syndrome, or trisomy 21, which occurs in about one in 1,000 births. The other common trisomies are trisomy 18 and trisomy 13, each occurring approximately once in 10,000 births. All three trisomies are more frequent with increased maternal age. Other well-known chromosomal syndromes are Kleinfelter's syndrome, due to 47,XXY, occurring in one in 1,000 male births, and Turner's syndrome, due to 45,XO present in one in 5,000 female births. Many other types of chromosomal aberrations have been identified, including translocations, inversions, ring chromosomes, and deletions. Newer techniques involving chromosome banding have made it possible to definitively identify each human chromosome and have permitted the characterization of chromosomal rearrangements not previously recognized.

Known teratogenic factors are rare causes of congenital malformations in spite of the ever-expanding list of potential teratogens in our increasingly chemical environment. As shown in Table 38-2, in studying more than 18,000 newborns, 0.1% were found to have major malformations thought to be related to teratogenic conditions. The most frequently identified were infants of diabetic mothers. Such infants appear to be at increased risk for the development of congenital heart disease, particularly transposition of the great vessels, ventricular septal defect, and coarctation of the aorta, as well as limb anomalies and sacral agenesis. The total risk of congenital anomalies is about 6% and represents a threefold increase over the normal risk. The specific factors responsible for this greater risk of malformations are not exactly clear, but labile control of the blood glucose during pregnancy does not appear to be one of them. Diabetic women with vascular complications, however, are particularly at risk of having infants with congenital malformations. (See Chapter 3.)

The relatively low risk for diabetic women may be contrasted with an apparently higher teratogenic risk in untreated maternal phenylketonuria, a relatively uncommon condition. Microcephaly, mental retardation, and various congenital anomalies have been described in the infants born to such mothers.

The occurrence of certain maternal infections during early pregnancy is well known to be associated with various congenital malformations. The most common and best understood infections are represented by the acronym TORCH, for toxoplasmosis, rubella, cytomegalic virus, and herpes hominis (Chapter 28). Herpes hominis results in a severe systemic illness in newborns that is often fatal, and survivors may have residual neurologic deficts and chorioretinitis. The other congenital infections likewise may result in an encephalopathy with various anomalies, including microcephaly, chorioretinitis, intracranial calcifications, microphthalmia, and cataracts. To a certain extent the varied clinical manifestations of these infections overlap, but a specific diagnosis can be made by the constellation of clinical findings as well as specific antibody studies.

Although many drugs may have teratogenic potential, two commonly used ones are particularly worthy of some discussion because of recent evidence suggesting a significant risk for congenital malformations. The first is chronic maternal ethanol intake, which is associated with increased perinatal mortality as well as a characteristic fetal alcohol syndrome in some cases. This pattern of malformations is characterized by growth deficiency of prenatal onset, microcephaly, short palpebral fissures, maxillary hypoplasia, and occasional other anomalies. Although originally described in alcoholic mothers, there is some suggestion that even relatively low-dose, chronic ethanol intake during pregnancy may pose a risk for the development of this syndrome (p. 936).

Maternal use of anticonvulsants, particularly phenytoin, has been implicated in the fetal hydantoin syndrome (p. 937). Characteristic features include varying combinations of growth deficiency of prenatal onset, mild mental retardation, large anterior fontanel, ocular hypertelorism, depressed nasal bridge, low-set abnormal ears, cleft lip and palate, hypoplasia of distal phalanges with nail hypoplasia, hirsutism, and other anomalies. Identical abnormalities have occurred in infants born to mothers taking barbiturates during pregnancy, and in many respects the pattern of anomalies is similar to that of the fetal alcohol syndrome. Although a number of studies of pregnancy outcome in women taking anticonvulsants, particularly but often not exclusively phenytoin, show a twofold to threefold increased risk of congenital malformations, Smith and co-workers have suggested a risk as high as 10% for major malformations and an additional risk of 30% for minor anomalies. These latter data are based on limited case studies without suitable control groups. Furthermore, the confounding effects of epilepsy per se, as well as underlying genetic predisposition to malformations, remain to be fully elucidated. Analogous confounding variables, socioenvironmental and/or genetic, also may be relevant in the fetal alcohol syndrome. These considerations point out some of the difficulties in proving a causal relationship between a potential teratogen of relatively low risk, such as phenytoin, and congenital malformations. (See Chapter 12.) Moreover, the hazards of using phenytoin in pregnant women with epilepsy must be weighed with the probable greater risk to both mother and fetus of uncontrolled seizures. It is hoped that properly designed studies in the future will provide an accurate assessment of these risks.

Somewhat less than one out of three major malformations have no known etiology, and as a group they are more frequent than severe anomalies due to either major gene or chromosome abnormalities. It is likely that, as our understanding of congenital malformations increases, specific genetic and/or environmental causes will be identified.

Malformations in aborted fetuses

Fetuses that are aborted spontaneously or therapeutically have a higher incidence of malformations than liveborn infants, and this presumably represents a natural selection process. Data on spontaneously aborted fetuses in the United States are given in Table 38-3. The common major newborn malformations, such as neural tube defects and cleft lip and palate, are also frequent in abortuses but are much more severe. Other malformations, such as cloacal exstrophy, are relatively rare in newborns

Table 38-3. Prevalence of localized malformations in spontaneously aborted fetuses and newborns (per 1,000)

Malformation	Spontaneous abortions* 2 to 8 weeks	9 to 18 weeks	≥ 19 weeks	Newborns†
Anencephaly-myelomeningocele-encephalocele	31	10	116	1.4
Cleft lip/palate	3	14.5	0	0.8
Cloacal exstrophy	0	7.3	10.6	0.1
Polydactyly	0	7.3	0	0.1

*Data from Nelson, T., Oakley, G.P., Jr., and Shepard, T.H.: Collection of human embryos and fetuses. In Hook, E.B., Javevick, D.T., and Porter, I.A., editors: Monitoring birth defects and environment: the problem of surveillance, New York, 1971, Academic Press, Inc.
†Data from Holmes, L.B.: N. Engl. J. Med. **195**:204, 1976.

but comparatively frequent in the aborted fetus. In addition to these rather localized anomalies, more severe generalized abnormalities commonly occur, manifested by marked growth retardation and gross malformations with few recognizable anatomic details.

Chromosome studies in abortuses likewise demonstrate a much higher prevalence of chromosomal anomalies with an overall frequency of about 50% in fetuses aborted by 20 weeks' gestation. The most common single chromosome abnormality is 45,XO, occurring in 18% of the chromosomally abnormal fetuses. This is followed by triploidy in 17% of those with an abnormal karyotypes. Both XO and triploidy are much more common in abortuses than in newborns.

As a group, the trisomies account for 50% of all chromosome anomalies among aborted fetuses. The most frequent, accounting for almost one third of the trisomies, is trisomy 16, which does not occur in newborns. Trisomy 21, the most common trisomy in newborns, occurs in less than 10% of all trisomic fetuses.

Unbalanced products of translocations account for 2% to 4% of all chromosomally abnormal fetuses and are three to six times more frequent than in newborns. In stillborn infants the frequency of chromosomal anomalies is much lower, about 5%.

The total prevalence of chromosomal abnormalities in aborted fetuses, like the overall frequency of malformations, is much increased over that in newborns. In addition, specific anomalies in each category markedly diminish the chance of fetal survival to term.

Minor malformations and phenotypic variants

Major malformations often are not difficult to identify. Minor anomalies, however, by their nature are more subtle and may not be appreciated unless specifically looked for. They are nevertheless significant for several reasons. First of all, they may be important as part of a characteristic pattern of malformations and thus may provide the basis for a diagnosis. Second, they are more likely associated with a remarkable pregnancy outcome such as low birth weight, postmaturity, and stillbirths.

Table 38-4. Common phenotypic variants

Phenotypic variant	Percent of newborns
Craniofacial	
Flat nasal bridge	7.3
Ear	
Folding-over of upper helix	43.0
Darwinian tubercle	11.0
Skin	
Capillary hemangioma on face and/or posterior aspect of neck	14.3
Mongolian spots in blacks and Orientals	45.8
Hand	
Hyperextensibility of thumbs	12.3
Foot	
Mild calcaneovalgus	4.7
Genital	
Hydrocele	4.4

Data from Marden, P.M., Smith, D.W., and McDonald, M.J.: J. Pediatr. **64**:357, 1964.

Third, their occurrence may be an indication of the presence of a more serious anomaly. Table 37-1 shows the frequencies of the more common minor malformations. Approximately 12% of newborns will have a single minor anomaly. Multiple minor anomalies, however, are uncommon. About 0.8% of newborns will have two minor malformations; three or more occur in only 0.5%. In those infants with three or more minor anomalies, however, the probability of at least one major malformation is 90%. A single minor anomaly, on the other hand, is associated with a major malformation in only 1.4% of cases.

Minor malformations are most frequent in areas of complex and variable features, such as the face and distal extremities. Among the most common are a lack of a helical fold of the pinna and complete or incomplete simian crease patterns. Typical simian creases occur in almost 3% of normal newborns, as indicated in Table 37-1. There is a natural overlap between minor anomalies and

Table 38-5. Frequency of common congenital malformations in various racial groups (per 1,000)

Malformation	U.S. whites*	U.S. blacks*	Chinese†
Anencephaly-myelo-meningocele-encephalocoele	2.4	0.9	1.5
Cleft lip and palate	1.1	0.6	1.3
Cleft palate	.6	.4	
Clubfoot (talipes equinovarus)	3.9	2.3	0.1
Polydactyly	1.2	11.0	1.5
Hypospadias	2.4	1.2	0.6

*Data from Erickson, J.D.: Ann. Hum. Genet. **39**:315, 1976.
†Data from Emanuel, I., and others: Teratology **5**:159, 1972.

Table 38-6. Racial differences in the frequencies of some minor malformations (per 100)

Malformation	White	Black
Third sagittal fontanel	3.8	11.7
Metopic suture open to bregma	0.7	2.4
Brushfield spots	9.4	0.3
Flat nasal bridge	0.8	5.4
Prominent nasal bridge	2.4	0.4
Preauricular sinus	0.3	2.9
Accessory nipple	0.2	1.6
Umbilical hernia	0.9	6.9
Sacral dimple	4.9	0.4
Scrotum up on penis	4.4	1.0
Prominent heel	3.7	8.8

Data from Holmes, L.B.: N. Engl. J. Med. **195**:204, 1976.

normal variants, and the latter are arbitrarily distinguished by a prevalence greater than 4%. As shown in Table 38-4, capillary hemangioma on the face or posterior aspect of the neck are common, occurring in 14% of newborns. In other locations, however, they are present in only 1% and constitute a minor anomaly. Among the most frequent phenotypic variants are a folded-over helix of the pinna and mongolian spots in blacks and Orientals. Before attributing medical significance to an apparent minor anomaly or phenotypic variation, it is useful to determine whether it is present in other family members or whether it is common in that particular racial or ethnic group. It is particularly not unusual for isolated minor anomalies to be familial.

Racial differences in the prevalence of congenital malformation

The prevalence of congenital malformations varies significantly between racial groups. This may be partly the consequence of differing genetic predispositions as well as variable environmental factors operating in diverse areas. Table 38-5 shows the prevalence of common major congenital malformations in American whites and blacks and in Chinese. It is of interest that certain anomalies are especially common in a particular race, such as polydactyly in blacks and hypospadias and clubfoot in whites. Minor malformations may show an equally striking racial predisposition, as shown in Table 38-6. Brushfield spots are common in whites but rare in blacks. Umbilical hernias, on the other hand, are common in black infants but relatively infrequent in whites. The widely varying frequencies of various traits in different races demonstrate that whether any given characteristic is considered a minor malformation or a phenotypic variant may be strongly dependent on the race of the patient being studied. One of the best examples is mongolian spots, which occur in almost 50% of black or Oriental infants but in only 0.2% of white infants.

EVALUATION OF THE INFANT WITH CONGENITAL MALFORMATIONS
History

Every infant with a congenital malformation deserves a thorough diagnostic evaluation, which always begins with a detailed history. The important goal is to attempt to identify a possible etiology in terms of genetic predisposition and environmental factors. It is useful to begin with the pregnancy and document complications, illnesses, maternal use of any medications, or possible exposure to teratogens (Chapter 12). The extent of smoking and alcohol consumption should be determined. A careful family history charted in a concise manner, using squares for males and circles for females, should be drawn up. Horizontal lines are used to indicate genetic union and vertical lines for genetic descent. All abortions and stillbirths must be noted. A question should always be specifically asked in regard to possible consanguinity. A simple way to inquire is to ask if the families of the parents are related. If so, then the charting should indicate the exact relationship. The presence of other relatives with congenital anomalies of any type should be recorded along with other pertinent information, such as the maternal and paternal ages and the nature of the anomaly. Family photographs are often very useful in clarifying questions of possible unusual phenotypic features. The pedigree should, at a minimum, include all siblings and parents of the proband as well as aunts, uncles, cousins, and grandparents. In the case of dominant or X-linked disorders a more extensive pedigree may be needed if many relatives are affected.

Physical examination

The goal of the examination of an infant with congenital anomalies is to detect a recognizable pattern of malformations so that a specific etiologic diagnosis can be made. The usual physical examination forms the foundation for this assessment (p. 254). In addition, careful attention must be directed not only to an exact description of the major malformation but also to apparent minor anomalies or variations. For the most part this involves detailed inspection and measurement of various features of external anatomy wherever appropriate. In this section an outline of this external examination will be presented by region or structure and certain helpful points, as well as aspects of the differential diagnosis, will be discussed. Greater detail in regard to examination and abnormalities of various organ systems is given in other relevant chapters in this book.

Skin

The normal infant skin, particularly when exposed to cold, shows a marbling pattern termed cutis marmorata or livido reticularis. In rare instances this may be unusually prominent and familial, inherited as an autosomal dominant trait. A similar prominent pattern may occur in the Cornelia de Lange syndrome, hypothyroidism, trisomy 21, and homocystinuria.

A variety of lesions with altered pigmentation may provide useful clues to a diagnosis. Cafe au lait spots are characteristic of neurofibromatosis but also occur in the McCune-Albright syndrome, Bloom's syndrome, and the Russell-Silver syndrome. Hypopigmented macules may be the earliest manifestation of tuberous sclerosis in the young infant. Multiple irregular pigmented lesions arranged in whorls is very suggestive of incontinentia pigmenti. An angiomatous patch over one side of the face may be an isolated anomaly or part of the Sturge-Weber or Klippel-Weber-Trenaunay syndrome.

Hair

The relative sparseness or prominence of body hair should be noted. Sparse hair is characteristic of an ectodermal dysplasia but occurs in other syndromes, such as cartilage hair hypoplasia and oculodentodigital syndrome. Hirsutism is typical of Cornelia de Lange syndrome and the fetal hydantoin and alcohol syndromes but may occur in trisomy 18. It also may be a racial or familial characteristic.

Abnormal scalp hair patterns may reflect underlying brain abnormalities. In microcephaly there may be a lack of the normal parietal whorl, or it may be displaced more centrally or posteriorly. In addition, the frontal hair may show a prominent upsweep. A low posterior hairline occurs with a short neck or webbed neck, as in Noonan's syndrome. Punched-out scalp lesions in the parietal occipital area are typical of trisomy 13 (Fig. 38-1).

Head

The size of the head, measured by the maximum head circumference, and the sizes of the anterior and other fontanels should be compared with appropriate standards (p. 375). Head size will vary with age, sex, and

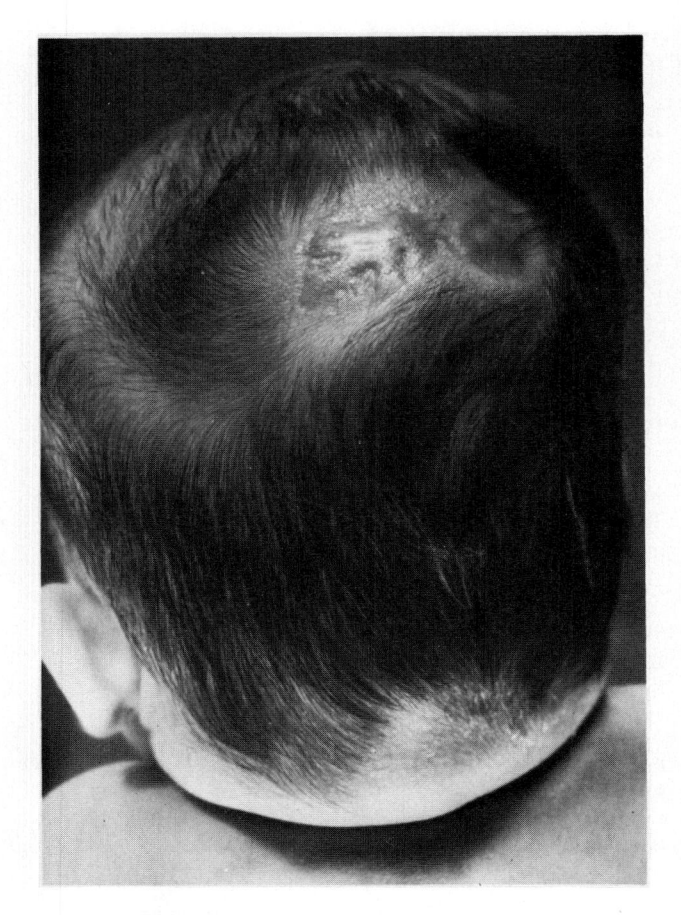

Fig. 38-1. Scalp lesions in trisomy 13.

racial group and has a general correlation with body size. Macrocephaly as an isolated anomaly is often familial and inherited in an autosomal dominant fashion. Determining the head circumferences of the parents may be diagnostic. Macrocephaly, however, also may be a manifestation of a number of disorders, including hydrocephalus and various diseases affecting bones and/or growth, such as achondroplasia. Microcephaly also can be familial, either autosomal dominant or recessive, but is more commonly a manifestation of many syndromes that result in mental retardation. Large fontanels occur in hypothyroidism, trisomies 21, 18, and 13, and many bone disorders, such as hypophosphatasia and cleidocranial dysostosis. A small anterior fontanel may be a sign of failure of normal brain growth.

The normal shape of the head may vary from long-headedness, or dolicocephaly, to short-headedness, or brachycephaly. These terms are precisely defined by the cephalic index (CI), which is the maximum breadth over the maximum length times 100. A CI less than 76 indicates dolichocephaly, and brachycephaly is present when the CI is greater than 80. Intermediate values of CI

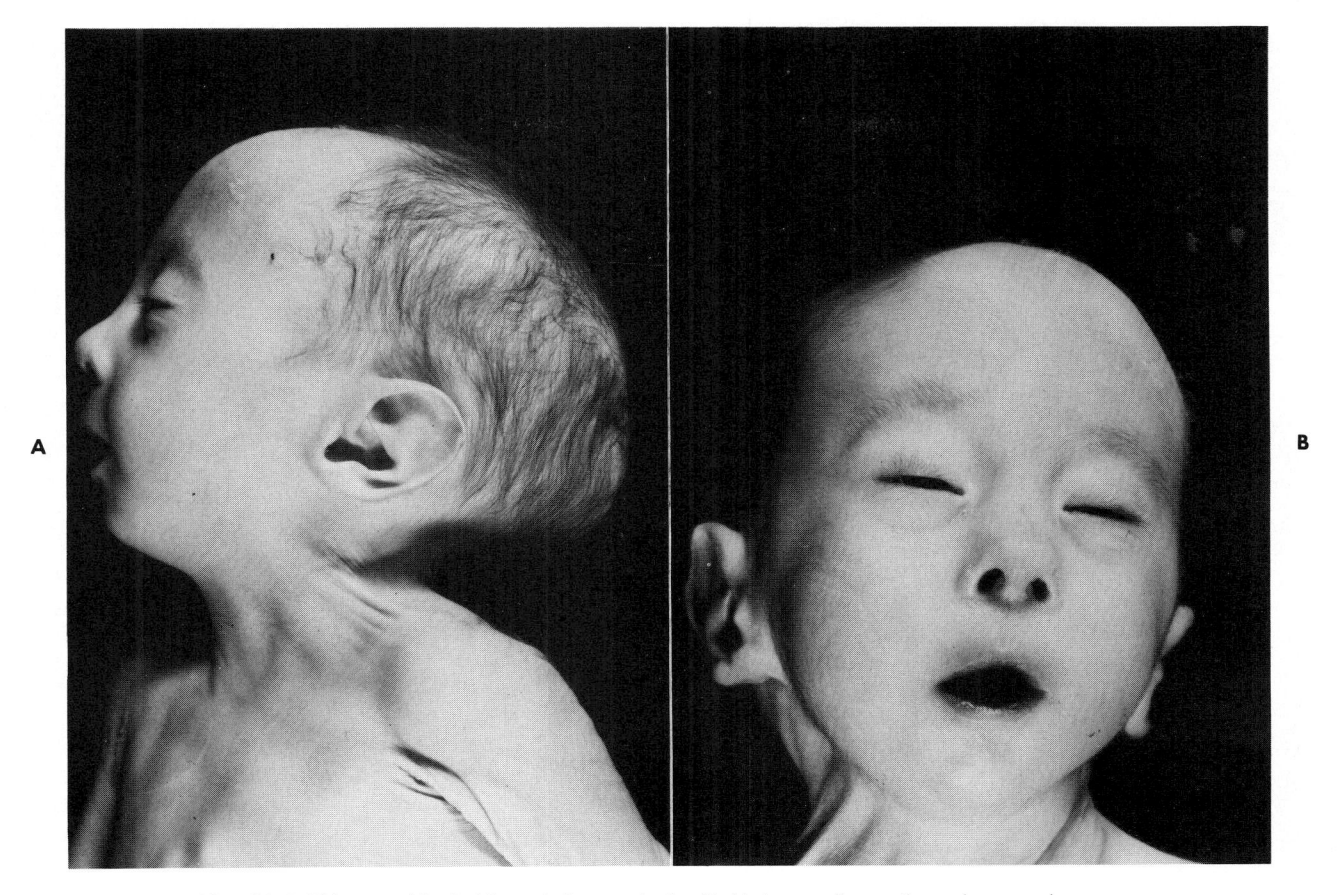

Fig. 38-2. Trisomy 18. **A,** Note dolicocephaly. **B,** Note small mouth and anomalous ears.

denote mesocephaly. Premature infants and those with trisomy 18 characteristically have dolicocephaly (Fig. 38-2), but either type of head shape may be familial or racial. Many Oriental infants, for example, have striking brachycephalic heads.

Premature fusion of cranial sutures results in an abnormal alteration in head shape. Various types occur depending on the sutures involved and are discussed further on p. 382.

A common anomaly in head shape is frontal bossing, which is frequent in many syndromes involving the skeletal system, including achondroplasia, osteopetrosis, I cell disease, and GM_1 gangliosidosis.

Face

The face is composed of a series of structures, each of which demonstrates considerable normal variation and which in toto provide a distinctive and particularly unique appearance to every human being. Since examination of the face is both complex and important, a systematic approach is necessary. It is never sufficient to merely describe the face as "funny looking" or unusual. Specific abnormalities must be analyzed, even though an overall gestalt impression may suggest a diagnosis in some cases. Before considering individual features of the face in detail, it is helpful to review some aspects of facial embryology.

The face has basically a dual embryologic origin, and its development is illustrated in Fig. 38-3. Upper and medial facial structures arise from the frontonasal process. Lateral facial structures develop from the branchial arches. In the embryo of 4 weeks the primitive face consists of an upper frontal prominence, a mouth or stomodeum bordered laterally by maxillary processes, and the mandibular and hyoid arches. Subsequently nasal placodes, which are thickenings of the ectoderm, develop above the stomodeum to either side of the frontal prominence. During the fifth week ridges appear on each side of the nasal placode—the nasolateral and nasomedial processes. The lateral processes eventually form the nasal alae, and the medial processes result in the formation of the middle portion of the nose, the philtrum or middle portion of the upper lip, and that part of the maxilla in which the incisor teeth develop. The nasomedial

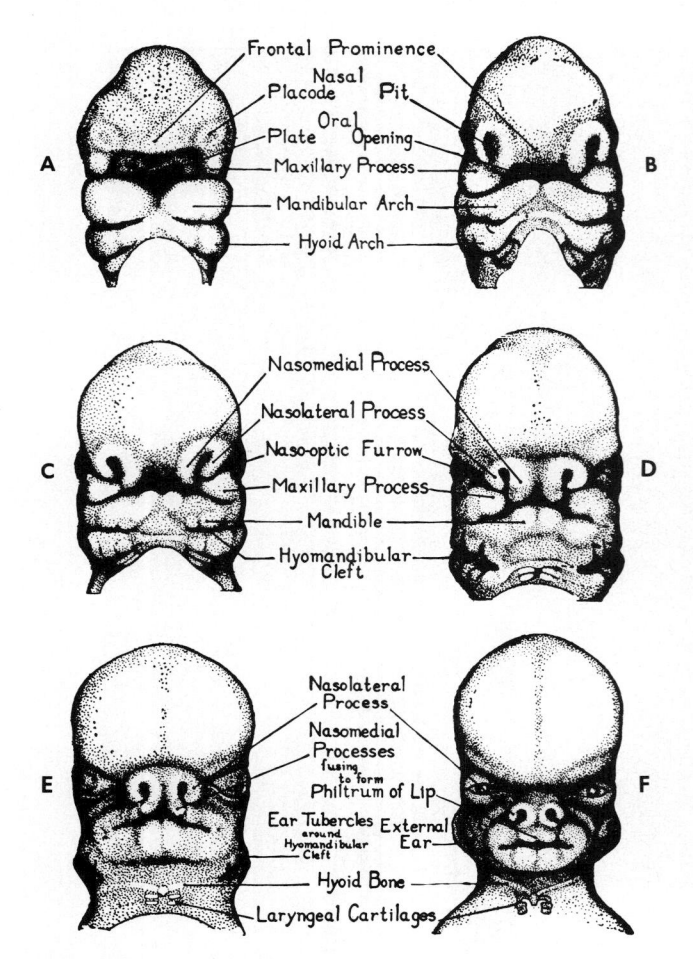

Fig. 38-3. Development of the face. **A,** Four weeks (3.5 mm). **B,** Five weeks (6.5 mm). **C,** Five and a half weeks (9 mm). **D,** Six weeks (12 mm). **E,** Seven weeks (19 mm). **E,** Eight weeks (28 mm). (From Patten, B.M.: Human embryology, New York, 1953, McGraw-Hill Book Co., Inc. Copyright © 1953 by McGraw-Hill Book Co. Used with permission of McGraw-Hill Book Co.)

Table 38-7. Natural developmental junctions of the face along which clefts and other anomalies occur

Junction	Cleft or anomaly
Nasomedial processes with each other	Median notch or cleft of upper lip
Nasomedial process with maxillary process	Common lateral cleft lip
Nasolateral process with maxillary process along line of nasooptic furrow	Oblique facial cleft
Maxillary and mandibular processes	Horizontal cleft/macrostomia
Mandibular and hyoid arch	Pits, sinus tracts, clefts, and ear anomalies
Maxillary process and frontonasal prominence at lateral aspect of lower eyelid	Colobomas of lower eyelid
Mandibular processes with each other	Clefts or pits of lower lip and median cleft mandible

processes fuse during the seventh week, and failure of this fusion leads to a midline cleft. Each nasomedial process also fuses laterally with the corresponding maxillary process, and failure of this fusion results in the common lateral cleft lip. In addition, the maxillary process fuses with the nasolateral process, eventually forming the nasolacrimal duct. An oblique facial cleft results from failure of this fusion. The nasolateral maxillary processes form the medial orbital regions. The maxillary processes, which are derived from the first branchial arch, ultimately give rise to the maxilla, the lateral aspects of the upper lip and gum, and the upper cheek regions. The mandibular processes of the first branchial arch eventuate in the lower lip and gum, the chin, and the lower cheek region. The junction between the mandibular process of the first branchial arch and the hyoid arch derived from the second branchial arch results in the hyoid-mandibular cleft, around which the external ear eventually forms. Defects in this developmental field result in abnormalities of the mandible and ear. As the mandible develops and grows, the relative position of the ears ascends to the level of the eyes. During the tenth week the palatal shelves from the maxillary process fuse with each other and the nasal septum, and a cleft palate results from failure of this fusion. The final adult facial structures and their origins follow:

A. Frontonasal prominence
 1. Frontal bones
 2. Crista galli
 3. Ethmoid bone
 4. Nasal bone
 5. Vomer bone and cartilaginous septum
 6. Premaxillary bone
 7. Anterior palatine triangle
B. Branchial arches
 1. Temporal bone in part and ossicles
 2. Zygomatic arch
 3. Maxillary bone
 4. Mandible
 5. Hard palate

The consequences of various failures of fusion are given in Table 38-7.

Eyes (see also Chapter 35)

The orbits originate partly from the frontonasal prominence, and thus their development is intimately related to the formation of midline structures such as the nose and interorbital region. Hypotelorism occurs when the eyes are unusually close together; when they are too far apart there is hypertelorism. Clinically, hypotelorism and hypertelorism are defined by the interpupillary dis-

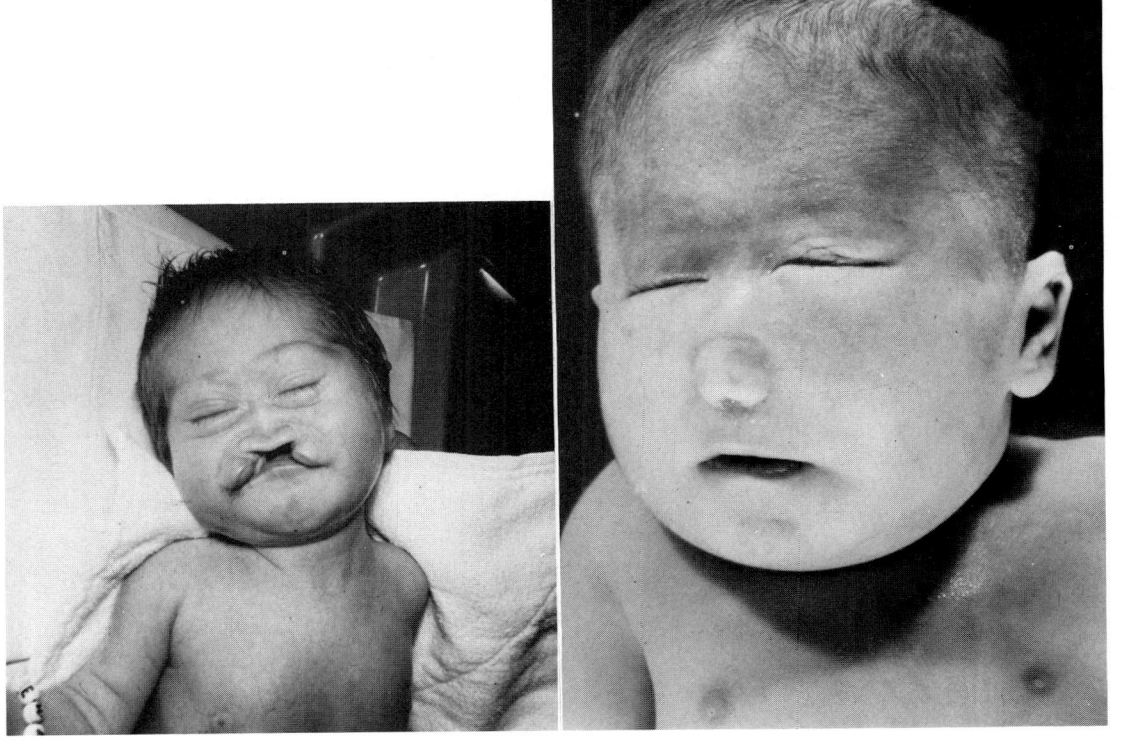

Fig. 38-4. A, Trisomy 13; note anomalous midline facial development with hypotelorism, a midline cleft lip, and lack of a nose. **B,** Trisomy 13; note hypotelorism and an abnormal nose.

tance, which may be estimated in a relaxed patient by approximating a tape measure between the midpoints of the pupils. Two other relevant measures that are useful and relatively easier to obtain are the inner canthal distance and the outer canthal distance. Telecanthus is an increase in the inner canthal distance and may occur in the absence of hypertelorism, such as in Waardenburg's syndrome (p. 977). Other factors that also can cause an illusion of hypertelorism follow:

1. Blepharophimosis
2. Cryptophthalmos
3. Epicanthal folds
4. Exotropia
5. Flat nasal bridge
6. Microphthalmos
7. Small face with normally spaced eyes
8. Small nose
9. Symblepharon
10. Telecanthus
11. Widely spaced eyebrows

For this reason a subjective impression always should be confirmed by measurement of all three distances. From a prognostic and diagnostic point of view it is important to identify hypotelorism, since it is often associated with holoprosencephaly, as in trisomy 13. Examples are shown in Fig. 38-4. Hypertelorism, on the other hand, occurs in a number of syndromes, such as frontonasal dysplasia, and even if it is severe it is less likely to be related to an underlying brain malformation. Figs. 38-5 and 38-6 illustrate hypertelorism with midline facial anomalies.

Epicanthal folds are a feature of normal fetal development but after birth are prominent in less than 1% of normal infants. They are characteristic in trisomy 21 (Fig. 38-7, *A* and *B*) but occur in many other malformation syndromes.

Normally an imaginary line through the inner and outer canthi should be perpendicular to the sagittal plane of the face. When the line slopes upward laterally, there is a mongoloid or upward slant (Fig. 37-7, *B*), and an antimongoloid or downward slant occurs when the line deviates downward laterally in a patient with mandibulofacial dysostosis (Fig. 38-7, *C*). As the term implies, a mongoloid slant is common in trisomy 21, but either type of slant is present in a number of syndromes.

Palpebral fissure length is measured from the inner to the outer canthus. A short palpebral fissure may occur in association with other ocular anomalies, such as micro-

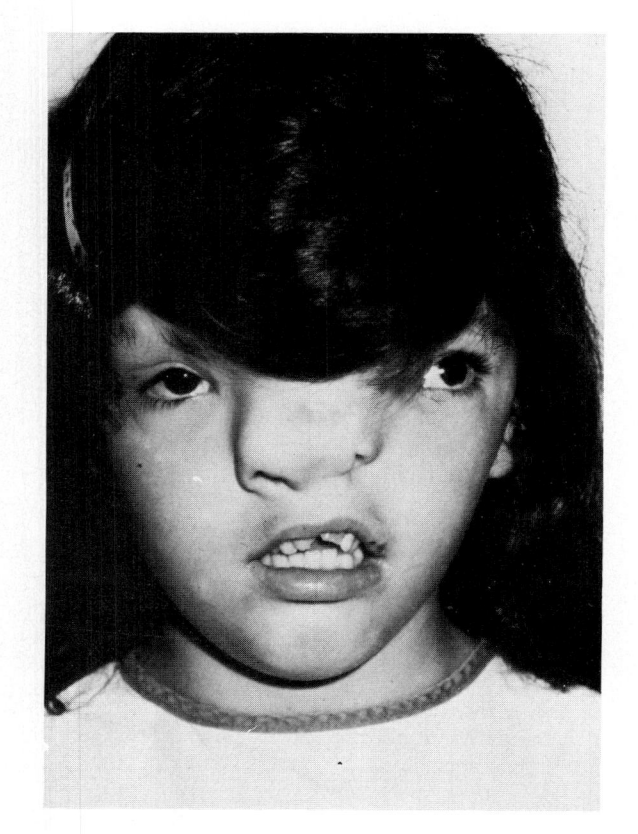

Fig. 38-5. Frontonasal dysplasia with hypertelorism and bifid nose.

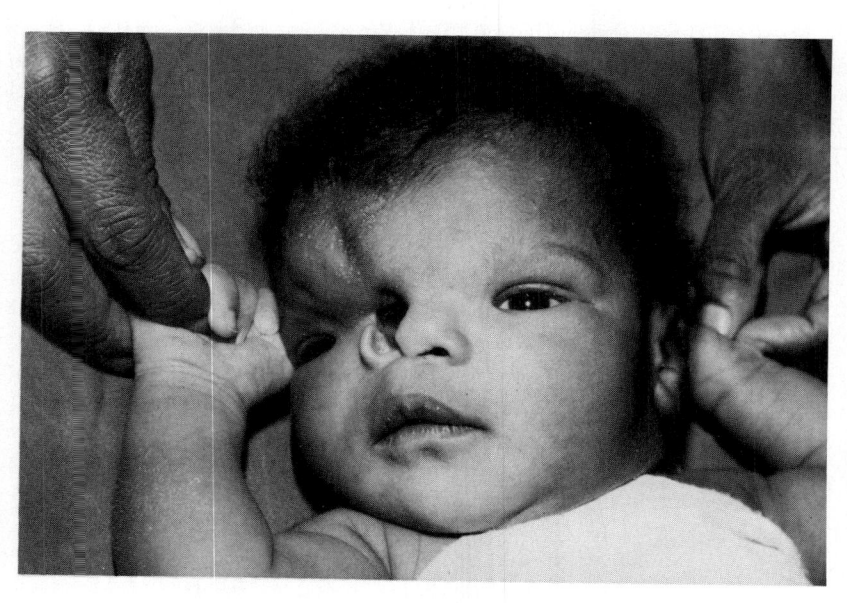

Fig. 38-6. Frontonasal dysplasia with a nasal cleft.

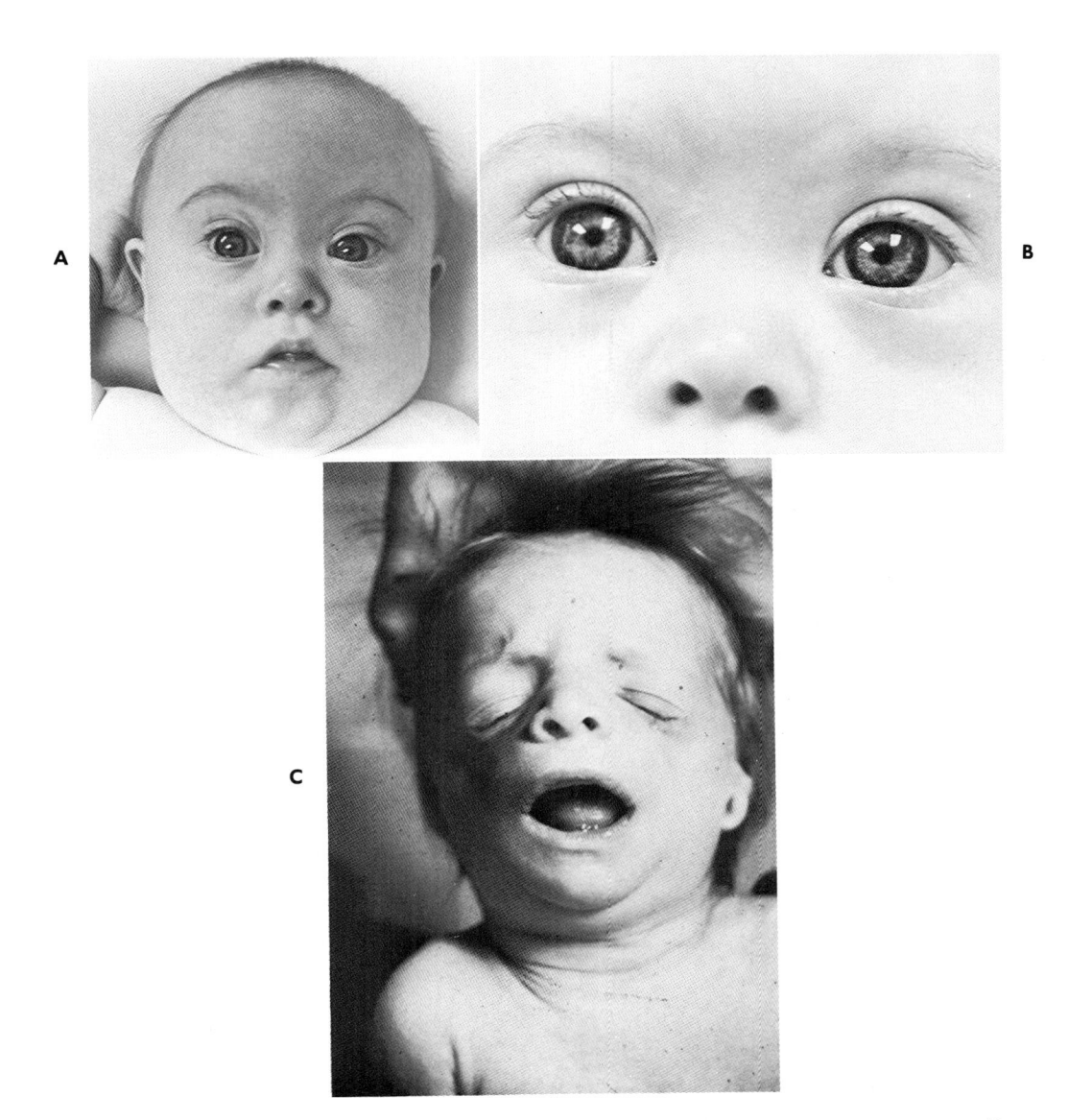

Fig. 38-7. A, Trisomy 21; note epicanthal folds and a mongoloid slant of the eyes. **B,** Enlargement of the eyes of the patient in **A.** Note the Brushfield spots in the irrides. **C,** Mandibulofacial dysostosis (Treacher Collins syndrome) with an antimongoloid slant of the eyes. Note the coloboma, or notch, in the left lower eyelid.

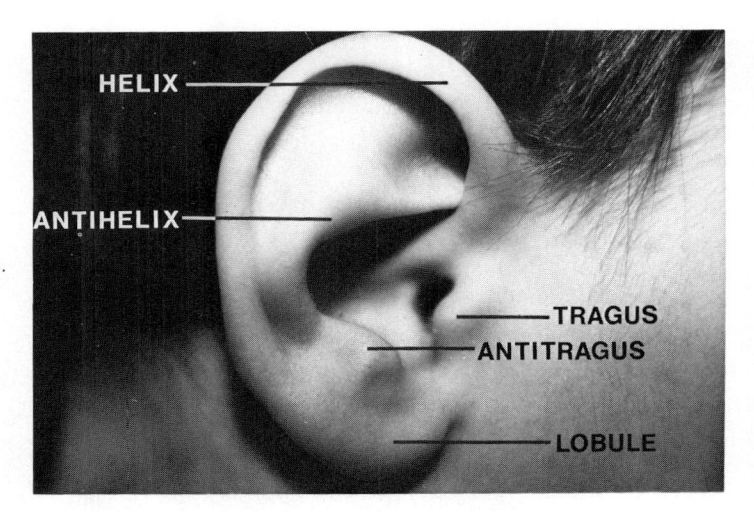

Fig. 38-8. Normal pinna and its landmarks.

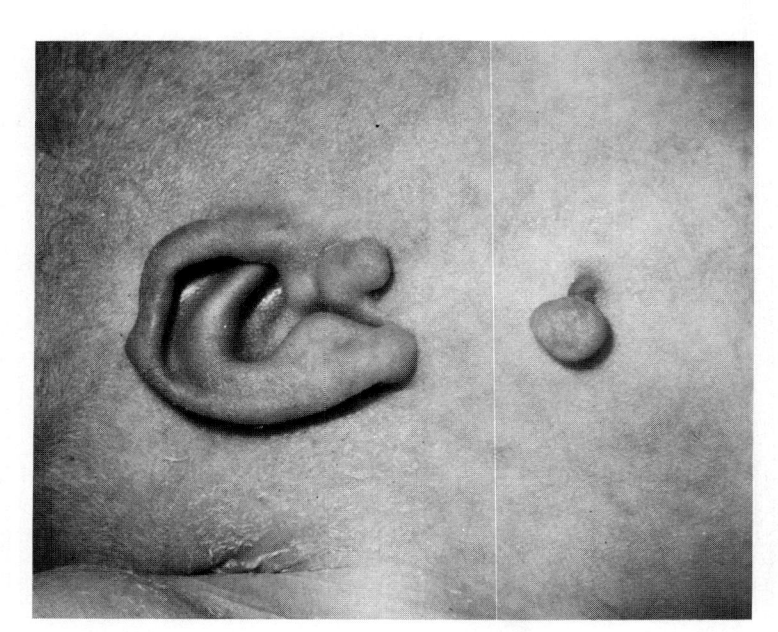

Fig. 38-9. Preauricular tags with a malformed pinna.

Fig. 38-10. Normal pinna and its orientation with respect to the eyes.

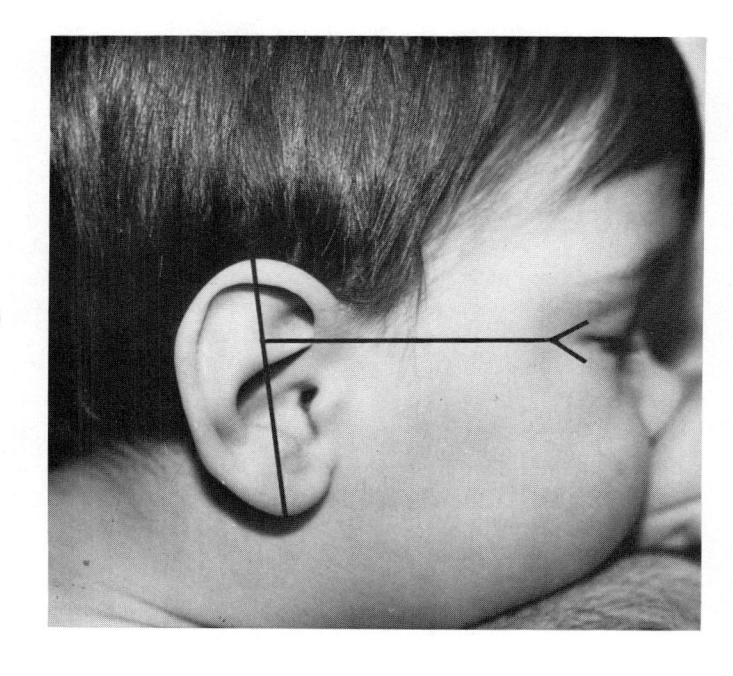

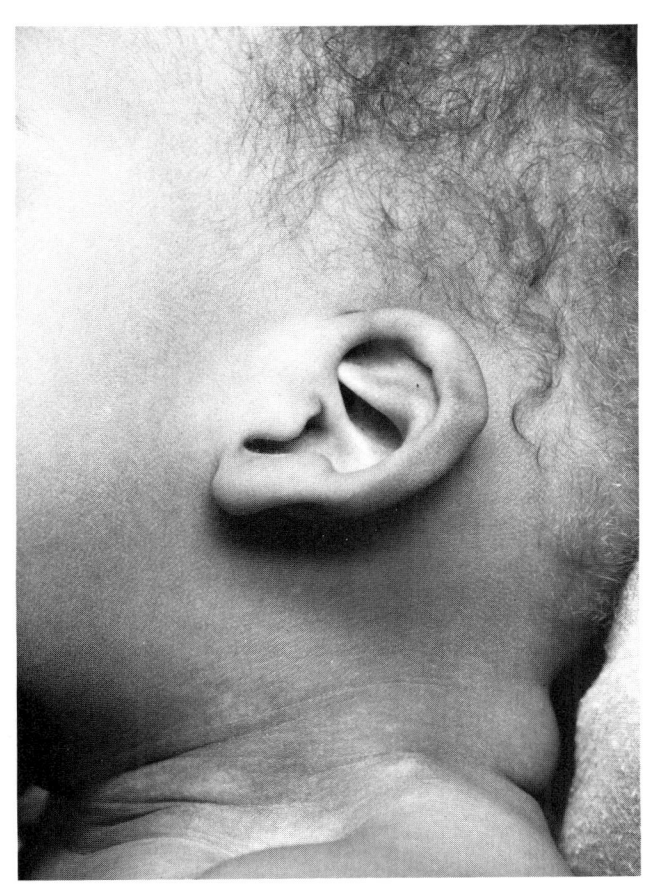

Fig. 38-11. Abnormal pinna that is low set and posteriorly rotated in a patient with the Smith-Lemli-Opitz syndrome.

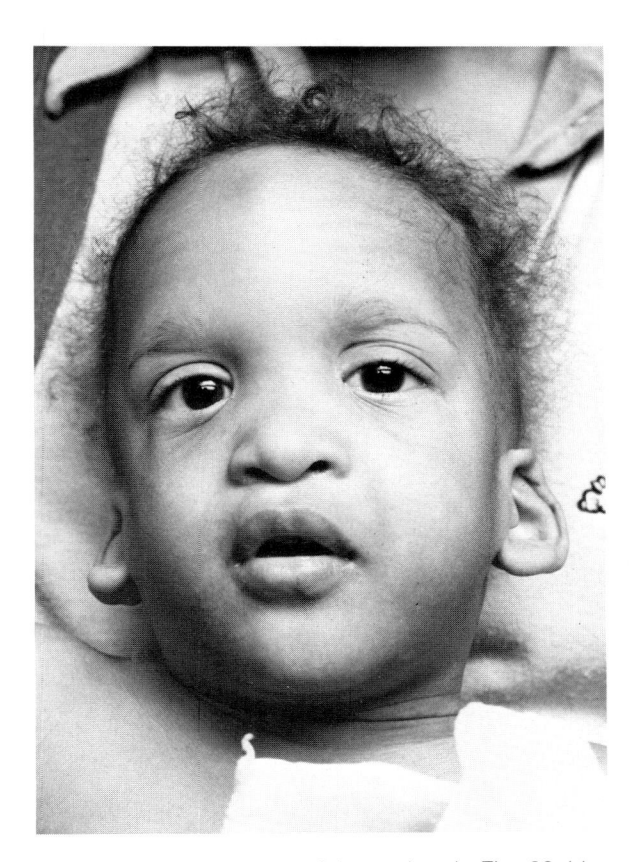

Fig. 38-12. Facial view of the patient in Fig. 38-11.

ophthalmia, and is characteristic of syndromes such as fetal alcohol and trisomy 18 (Fig. 38-2, *B*).

Colobomas are developmental defects in the normal continuity of a structure and may occur in the eyelid border resulting in a notch or angulation of the eyelid margin. Such defects are characteristic in the Goldenhar and Treacher Collins syndromes (see Fig. 38-7, *C*).

Synophrys, or fusion of the eyebrows in the midline, is common in hirsute infants and usually occurs in the Cornelia de Lange syndrome.

Other types of anomalies involving the internal structure of the eyes are discussed in Chapter 35.

Ear

The external ear, or pinna, commonly shows great variation, but a number of anatomic landmarks can be identified and should be evaluated in the anomalous ear. These include the helix, antihelix, tragus, antitragus, external meatus, and lobule (Figs. 38-8 and 38-10). Microtia or macrotia should be determined by measuring the maximum length of the pinna from the lobule to the superior margin of the helix. Preauricular tags or pits may be isolated or associated with other abnormalities of the pinna (Fig. 38-9).

Low-set ears are designated when the helix joins the head below a horizontal plane passing through the outer canthi perpendicular to the vertical axis of the head. It is critical that this be assessed with the head in vertical alignment with the body, since any posterior rotation of the head can easily create an illusion of low-set ears.

When the vertical axis of the ear deviates more than 10 degrees from the vertical axis of the head, the ears are posteriorly rotated. This anomaly is often associated with low-set ears and represents a lag in the normal ascent of the ear during development (Figs. 38-11 and 38-12).

It is important to note that any abnormality of the external ear may be an indication of additional anomalies of the middle or inner ear and associated hearing loss. Therefore an early hearing assessment may be needed in such cases (Chapter 22). Fig. 38-13 illustrates a patient with hemifacial microsomia, a severely malformed pinna, and absent external auditory meatus.

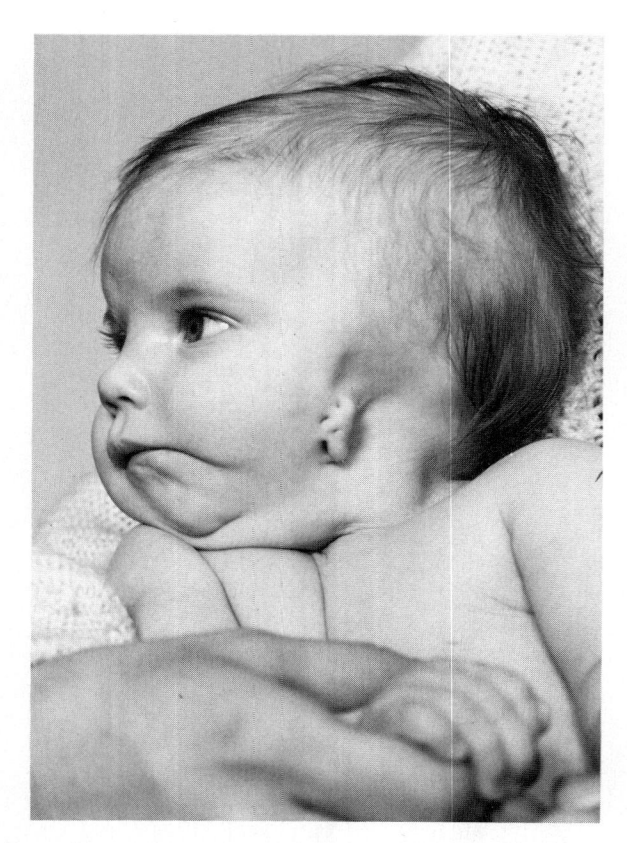

Fig. 38-13. Hemifacial microsomia showing mandibular hypoplasia and a severely malformed pinna and absent ear canal.

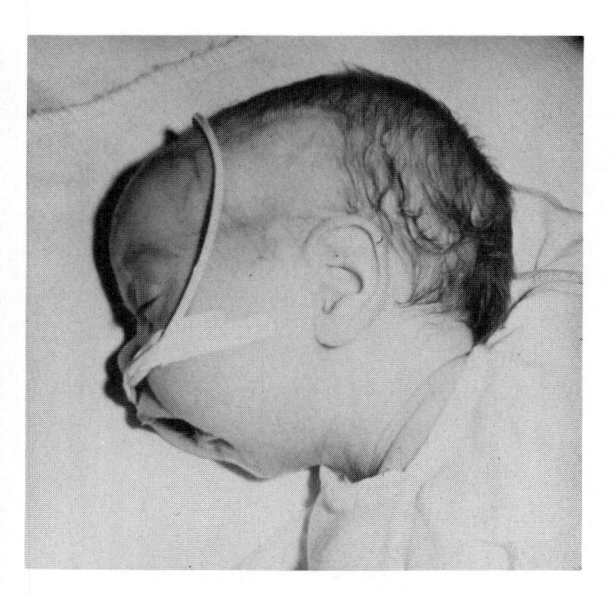

Fig. 38-14. Micrognathia in the Pierre Robin malformation complex.

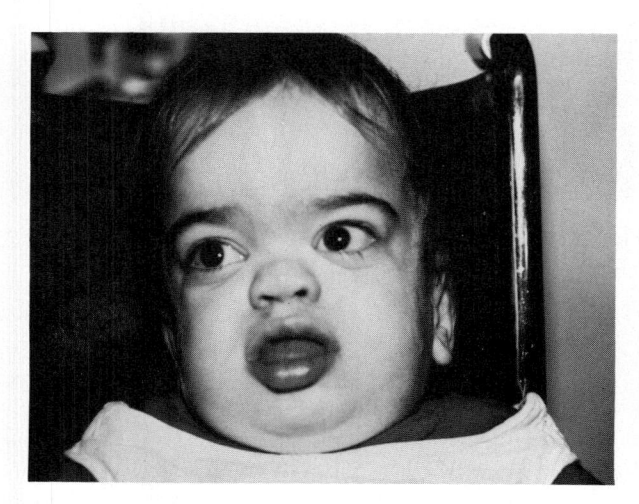

Fig. 38-15. Hurler's disease; note coarse facies, prominent lips, and large tongue.

Nose

The nose, like the external ear, shows great individual variation, but certain alterations in shape are frequent in malformation syndromes involving the face. The nose may be unusually thin with hypoplastic alae nasi, as in Hallerman-Streiff syndrome; or it may be unusually broad, as in the cranial metaphyseal dysplasias and frontonasal dysplasia, or prominent, as in the trichorhinophalangeal syndrome. A depressed nasal bridge with an upturned nose occurs in many skeletal dysplasias, such as achondroplasia. When the depression is severe, the nostrils may appear anteverted and the nose shortened with a high philtrum.

Mouth

The mouth is a complex structure with component parts, each requiring separate evaluation. The lower portion of the mouth is formed by the mandible, which in young infants is relatively small. An excessively small mandible is termed *micrognathia*, which is a feature of many syndromes. It is characteristic in the Pierre Robin malformation complex, which consists of the triad of micrognathia, glossoptosis, and a U-shaped cleft palate, as opposed to the common V-shaped cleft. A typical patient is shown in Fig. 38-14. The Pierre Robin complex may be part of a syndrome, and thus other anomalies must be searched for. In other syndromes the maxilla likewise may be hypoplastic, decreasing the prominence of the upper cheeks.

The size and shape of the mouth may be altered; a small mouth, or *microstomia*, occurs in trisomy 18; severe macrostomia may result in association with a lateral facial cleft. The common cupid's bow configuration of the lips may be exaggerated, leading to a highly tented upper lip, a characteristic of myotonic dystrophy. The corners of the mouth may be downturned, as in the Russell-Silver syndrome. An asymmetric face during crying occurs with congenital deficiency in the depressor anguli oris muscle on one side, and this may be associated with congenital heart defects and other abnormalities.

Prominent full lips occur in various syndromes characterized by coarse facies, such as Hurler's disease (Fig. 38-15). A cleft upper lip is commonly median, as in trisomy 13, or lateral, as in the common multifactorial cleft lip and/or palate anomaly. The presence of pits in the lower lip associated with a cleft lip or palate, however, is suggestive of a different malformation syndrome inherited in an autosomal dominant manner. In fact, there are diverse syndromes with cleft lip and/or palate that are important to identify, since they may have relatively high genetic risks of recurrence. Following is an outline of the common cleft lip and/or palate syndromes.

A. Autosomal dominant
  1. Lip pits
  2. Filiform fusion of eyelids
  3. Ectrodactyly–ectodermal dysplasia (EEC)
  4. Popliteal pterygium
  5. Rapp-Hodgkin ectodermal dysplasia
  6. Acrocephalosyndactyly
  7. Arthroophthalmopathy (Stickler's syndrome)
  8. Mandibulofacial dysostosis
  9. Spondyloepiphiseal dysplasia congenita
  10. Brachial plexus neuritis
  11. Lateral synechial CKSP
  12. Metatropic dysplasia (Kniest's syndrome)
  13. Ectrodactyly
  14. Micrognathia, dysplastic ears, ectrosyndactyly
  15. Joint dislocations, unusual facies (Larsen's syndrome)
  16. Microcephaly, large ears, short stature, proximal thumbs, hypoplastic distal phalanges
B. Autosomal recessive
  1. Encephalocele, polydactyly, polycystic kidneys (Meckel's syndrome)
  2. Ablepharon
  3. Tetraphocomelia (Roberts' syndrome)
  4. Hypertelorism, microtia, ectopic kidney, congenital heart disease, growth deficiency
  5. Orocraniodigital
  6. Diastrophic dwarfism
  7. Multiple pterygium
  8. Stapes fixation and oligodontia
  9. Cerebrocostomandibular
  10. Branchioskeletogenital
  11. Craniostenosis, microcephaly, arthrogryposis, adducted thumbs
  12. Short stature, mental retardation
  13. Joint dislocations, unusual facies (Larsen's syndrome)
  14. Truncus arteriosus, abnormal right pulmonary artery
  15. Micromelic dwarfism
  16. Microcephaly, mental retardation, bulbous nasal tip, clinodactyly of toes (Palint's syndrome)
  17. Growth retardation, flexion contractures of hands, small fingers, and nails, ureteral stenosis, coarse facies (Rudiger's syndrome)
C. X-linked syndromes
  1. Orofaciodigital
  2. Otopalatodigital
  3. Nephritis, deafness (Alport's syndrome)
  4. Micrognathia, talipes equinovarus, atrial septal defect, and persistence of left superior vena cava
  5. Short stature
  6. Submucous connective tissue dysplasia
D. Multifactorial or unknown etiology
  1. Median cleft face
  2. Thoracopagus
  3. Anencephaly
  4. Congenital oral teratoma
  5. Clefting ectropian
  6. Premaxillary agenesis
  7. Short rib, polydactyly (Majewski's syndrome)
  8. Coarse facies, hirsutism, absent fifth finger and toenails (Coffin-Sires syndrome)
  9. Aglossia-adactyly (Hanhart's syndrome)
  10. Buccopharyngeal membrane
  11. Oral duplication
E. Chromosome defects
  1. 1q+
  2. 3p+
  3. 3p−, q+
  4. 4p−
  5. Trisomy 13
  6. 14q+
  7. Trisomy 18
  8. 18q−
  9. Trisomy 22
  10. 49,XXXXY
  11. Triploidy
  12. Many translocations

Isolated cleft palate has a different genetic predisposition than that associated with cleft lip. Mild forms of cleft palate are represented by submucosal clefts, pharyngeal incompetence with nasal speech, and bifid uvula. Occasionally a palatine torus is noted as a midline swelling of the hard palate. It has no particular medical significance but is more common in Orientals and was described in *Homo erectus* from China. A high arched palate may occur normally but is also a feature of many syndromes.

Hypertrophied alveolar ridges are apparent in the palate along the inner margin of the teeth and are suggestive of a mucopolysaccharidosis or mucolipidosis, such as I cell disease. They are also present in the Smith-Lemli-Opitz syndrome (Fig. 38-16).

Macroglossia may be relative, as in the Pierre Robin malformation complex, where the primary abnormality is mandibular hypoplasia. In other cases, such as cretinism, the mucopolysaccharidoses, or a mucolipidosis such as

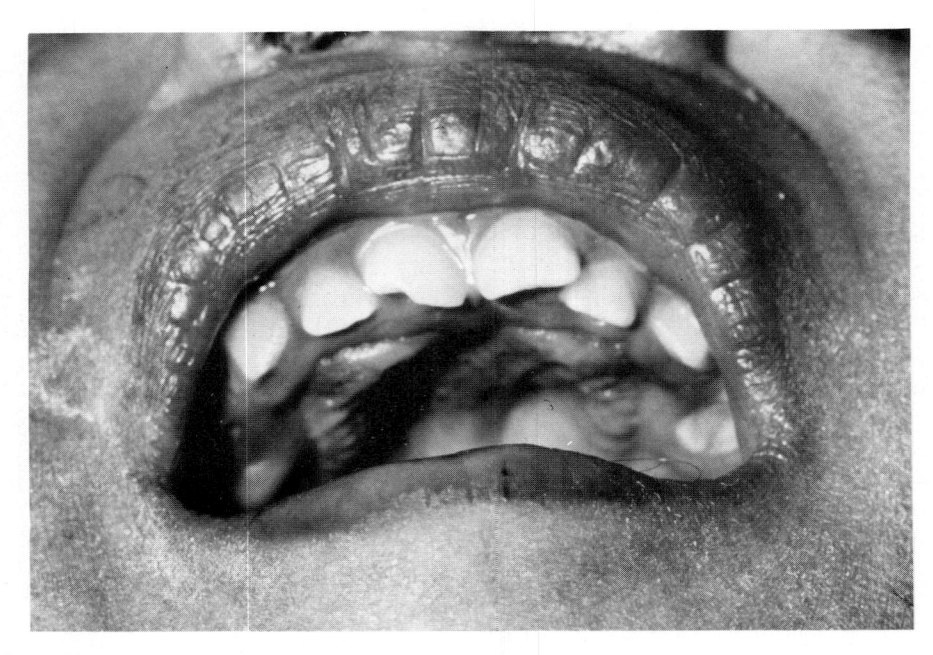

Fig. 38-16. Prominent alveolar ridges in a patient with the Smith-Lemli-Opitz syndrome.

GM₁ gangliosidosis, the tongue appears protruding and enlarged. A cleft or irregular tongue or oral frenula occur in various syndromes such as the orofaciodigital syndrome.

Neck

The neck may be short with limitation of rotation, as in a Klippel-Feil anomaly, with fusion of cervical vertebrae. Excessive skinfolds are characteristic of Turner's or Noonan's syndrome (Fig. 38-17).

Chest

The thoracic cage may be unusually small as part of a skeletal dysplasia, such as thoracic asphyxiating dystrophy (Fig. 38-18). A relative increase in the anteroposterior diameter occurs in Turner's or Noonan's syndrome, but the apparent increase in internipple distance is illusionary, since it is normal relative to the chest width.

The sternum itself may be unusually short, as is typical in trisomy 18, or it may be altered in shape, as in pectus excavatum or pectus carinatum. The latter anomalies are common with a variety of skeletal dysplasias.

Abdomen

Hypoplasia of the abdominal musculature may occur associated with in utero obstruction and other anomalies of the urogenital system resulting in a characteristic prune belly appearance (p. 798). An omphalocele may be part of the Beckwith-Wiedemann syndrome (p. 858). Anomalies of a more minor nature, such as inguinal or

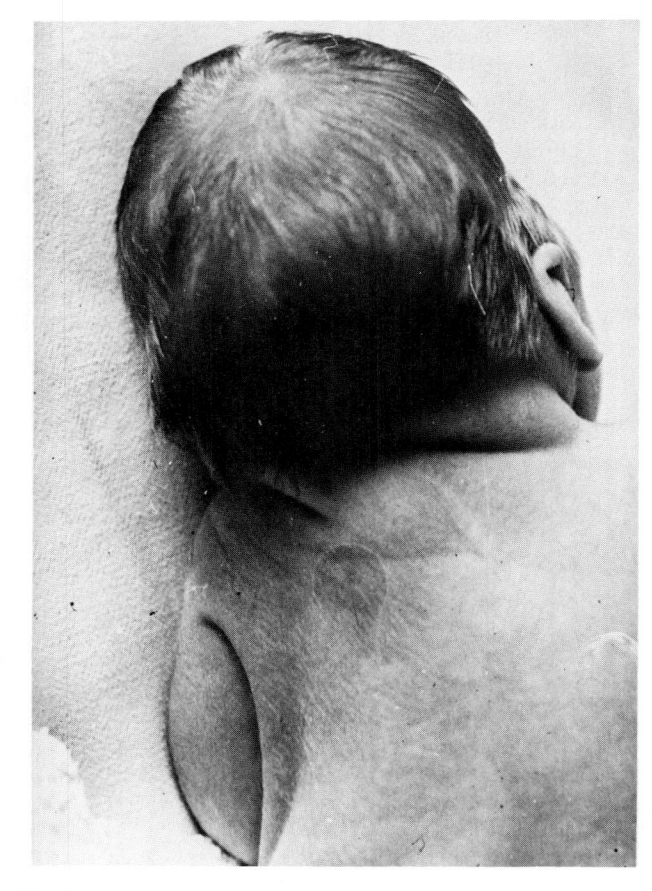

Fig. 38-17. Excess skinfolds of the neck in a patient with Turner's syndrome.

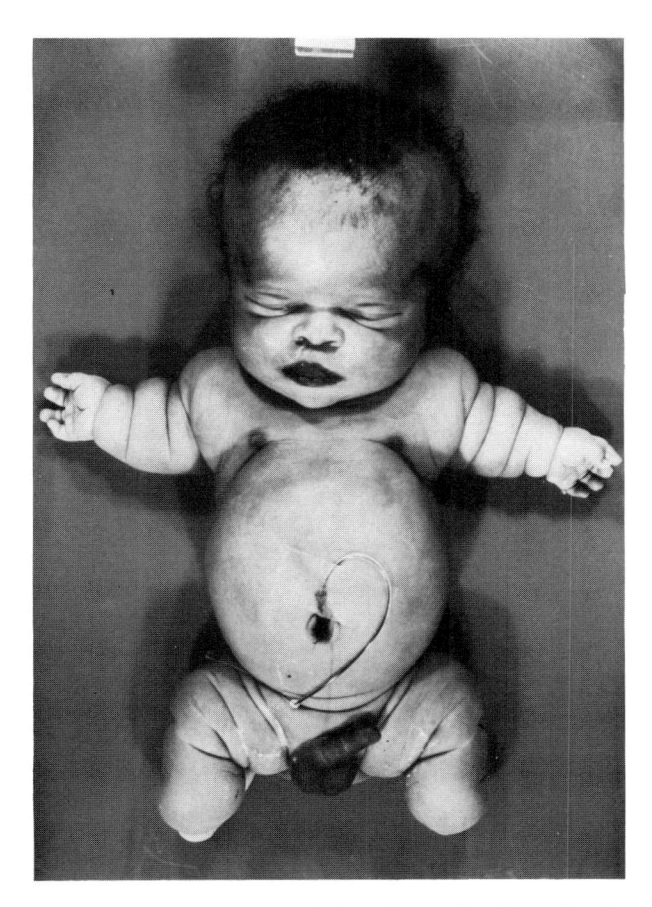

Fig. 38-18. Thoracic asphyxiating dystrophy. Note the short limbs and narrow thoracic cage.

umbilical hernias, occur in normal infants but are more frequent in various syndromes, particularly connective tissue disorders such as the mucopolysaccharidoses.

Anus

Imperforate anus may occur as the mildest expression of a caudal regression malformation complex, which in severe cases has extensive lower-body abnormalities (Chapter 33, part one). It also may be part of a constellation of malformations, such as the VATER association or the VACTERL association, which consists of VATER plus congenital heart and limb anomalies (p. 1035).

Genitalia

Abnormalities in the development of the genitalia and the associated hormonal influences are discussed in Chapter 33, part four.

Spine

Among the most common congenital anomalies are the neural tube defects, which involve abnormalities of the central nervous system along with defects in the associated bony structures. These lesions are discussed in detail on p. 385. Minor external anomalies, particularly of the lower spine, include unusual pigmentary lesions or hair tufts, sacral dimples and sinuses, and pilonidal sinuses. Some of these changes, such as hair tufts, may be an indication of a more significant deeper anomaly, such as diastematomyelia.

Extremities

Abnormalities of length. Extremities may be either relatively long, as occurs in Marfan's syndrome or homocystinuria, or unusually short, as occurs in a diverse number of skeletal dysplasias, the prototype and most common being achondroplasia. A simple guide to evaluating relative extremity length is to determine where the fingertips are in relation to the thighs when the upper extremities are adducted alongside the body. In the normal infant the fingertips fall below the hip joint in the midthigh region. When the upper extremities are short, they align with the hip joint or above (Fig. 38-18), and when they are relatively long, they may reach the knees. A more precise and useful measurement is to determine the upper-to-lower segment ratio. The upper segment is measured from the vertex to the pubic symphysis, and the distance from the pubis to the heel constitutes the lower segment. In normal newborns this ratio is about 1.75 and decreases with age to 0.85 in the adult. A high ratio suggests relative shortening of the extremities, and a low ratio implies either unusually long extremities or a foreshortened trunk, as may occur in spondyloepiphyseal dysplasia.

Paired extremities may be asymmetric in either length or overall size, suggesting either atrophy of one or hypertrophy of the other. The distinction may be difficult to make at times, although it is often evident if an extremity is unusually large or excessively small. Hypertrophy of limbs more often occurs on the right side and may be a manifestation of neurofibromatosis, the Beckwith-Wiedemann syndrome, or the Klippel-Weber-Trenaunay syndrome. There is also an association with Wilms' tumor as well as other tumors of the adrenal glands and liver. Isolated hemiatrophy is more common on the left side and may occur with long-standing corticospinal tract damage as well as in the Russell-Silver syndrome.

Foreshortening of long bones will lead to various limb abnormalities, depending on the segments involved. A number of terms have been used to describe such anomalies. *Amelia* refers to complete absence of a limb. *Peromelia* and *hemimelia* are both used to describe limb defects with shortened or deformed long bones. *Rhizomelia* denotes proximal shortening of the limbs, such as occurs in achondroplasia. *Phocomelia* refers to seal-like limbs in which distal segments such as the hands appear attached to the trunk as a result of marked fore-

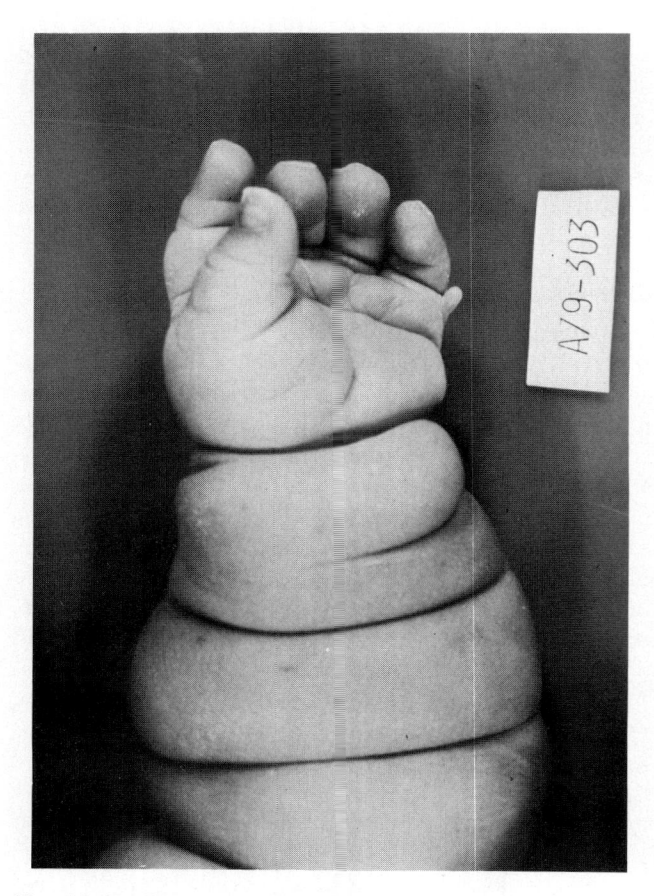

Fig. 38-19. Forearm and hand of the patient in Fig. 38-18. Note the rudimentary postaxial polydactyly.

shortening of the intervening segments. Such defects among other limb anomalies occurred as a consequence of maternal use of thalidomide. A shortened forearm with secondary prominence of skinfolds is shown in Fig. 38-19.

Abnormalities of hands and feet

Dermatoglyphics. The hands and feet have epidermal ridges and creases forming a variety of configurations. These dermatoglyphic patterns may be altered in various malformation syndromes and although the changes are rarely pathognomonic of a particular condition, they provide useful additional diagnostic information. A permanent record may be obtained by using special pads and paper or examination can be done with a magnifying glass. Epidermal ridge patterns and creases are well developed by the fourth month of gestation and are under multifactorial genetic control.

The finger patterns are divided into arches, loops, and whorls (Fig. 38-20). Triradii occur at the juncture of three sets of converging ridges. In the arch pattern, ridges enter from one side and flow to the other in an arch shape. A loop pattern has one triradius and may be open toward either the radial or ulnar side of the hand forming radial or ulnar loops, respectively. Whorls have at least two triradii and may consist of a spiral or ellipse pattern or two interlocking loops in the double whorl. Ridge count is obtained from the total number of ridges crossed by a line from the triradii up to the pattern core. The total finger ridge count averages 145 in males and 127 in females.

Palmar patterns shown in Fig. 38-21 include the distal triradii *a*, *b*, *c*, and *d* found beneath each finger from the index finger to the little finger, respectively. The axial triradius, called *t*, occurs in the axial line of the palm and is usually not more than 10% of the distance from the distal creases of the wrist to the proximal crease of the third finger. It may be displaced distally or to either side in various malformation syndromes. Normally there are two deep transverse palmar creases that do not completely cross the palm. In various conditions, such as trisomy 21, there may instead be a single transverse palmar crease, termed a *simian crease*. Simian creases may be completely transverse across the palm or may be incomplete (Fig. 38-22). They may become more apparent when the palm is slightly flexed. A single phalangeal crease on the fifth finger instead of the normal two also occurs commonly in trisomy 21 (Fig. 38-22).

The foot also has ridge patterns (Fig. 38-21). The great toe may have arches, loops, and whorls, and the hallucal area of the sole usually has a loop or whorl. The absence of the latter pattern, termed an open field, is frequent in trisomy 21 and other disorders. A sandal pattern of furrows is typical of trisomy 8 (Fig. 38-23). Fig. 38-24 illustrates the increased separation of the first and second toes and a prominent interdigital furrow in trisomy 21.

Abnormalities in size and shape. The hands and feet may be enlarged as a result of lymphedema. This can be a generalized process and is characteristic of infants with Turner's or Noonan's syndrome in which the dorsum of the hands and feet may have a puffy appearance (Fig. 38-25). Congenital lymphedema can also be an autosomal dominantly inherited condition with variable expressivity.

Rocker-bottom feet (Fig. 38-26) are manifested by a prominent heel and a loss of the normal concave longitudinal arch of the sole. They are common in trisomy 18 and other syndromes.

Enlargement of the hands and feet may occur as part of a generalized growth disturbance such as cerebral gigantism or the Soto syndrome or may be a manifestation of a partial macrosomia such as in congenital hemihypertrophy, discussed previously.

Significant anomalies of the underlying bony structure will produce alterations in the normal form of the hands and feet. Such abnormalities may be classified into the following categories: absence deformities, polydacty-

Text continued on p. 1058.

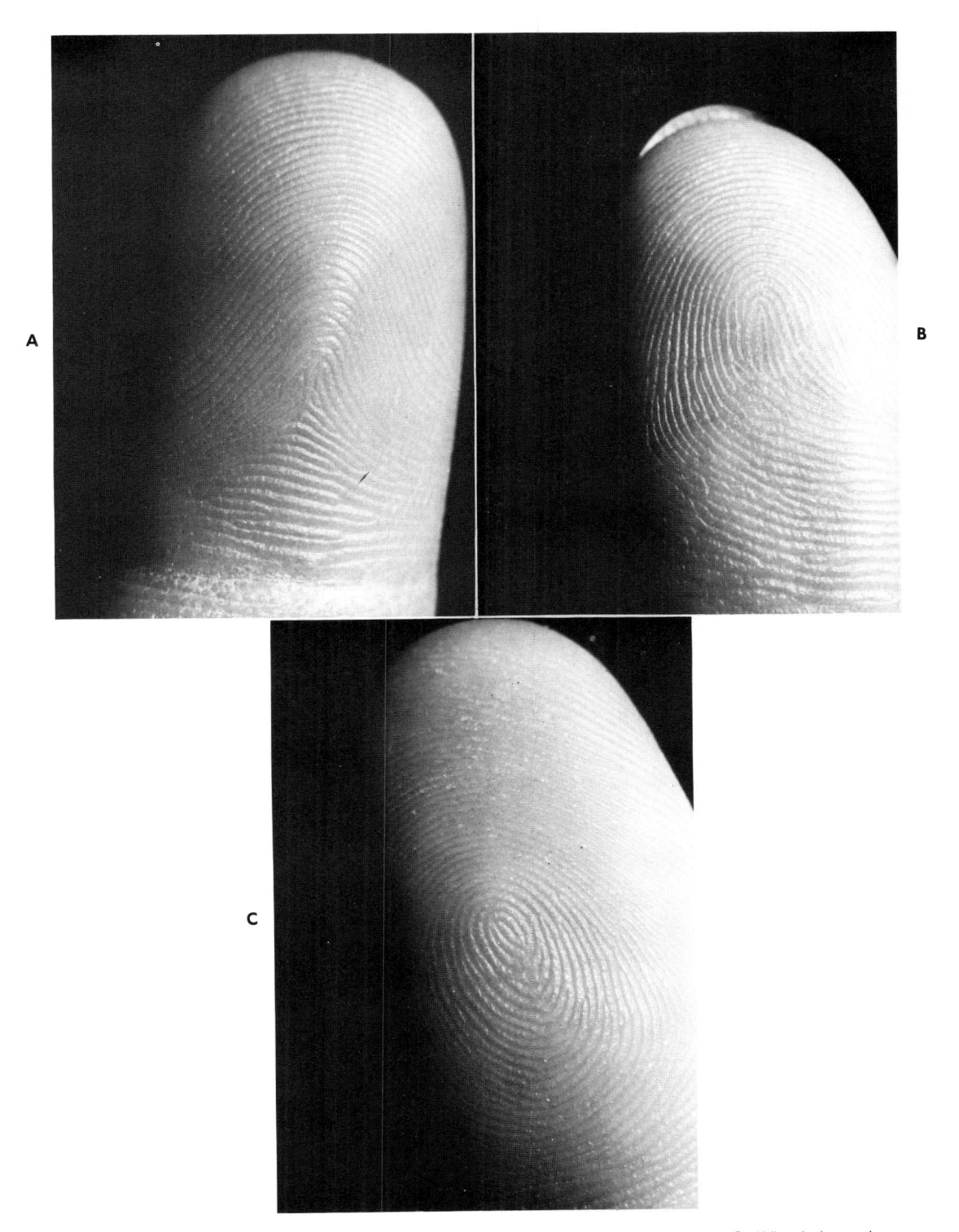

Fig. 38-20. A, Arch dermal ridge pattern. **B,** Loop dermal ridge pattern. **C,** Whorl dermal ridge pattern.

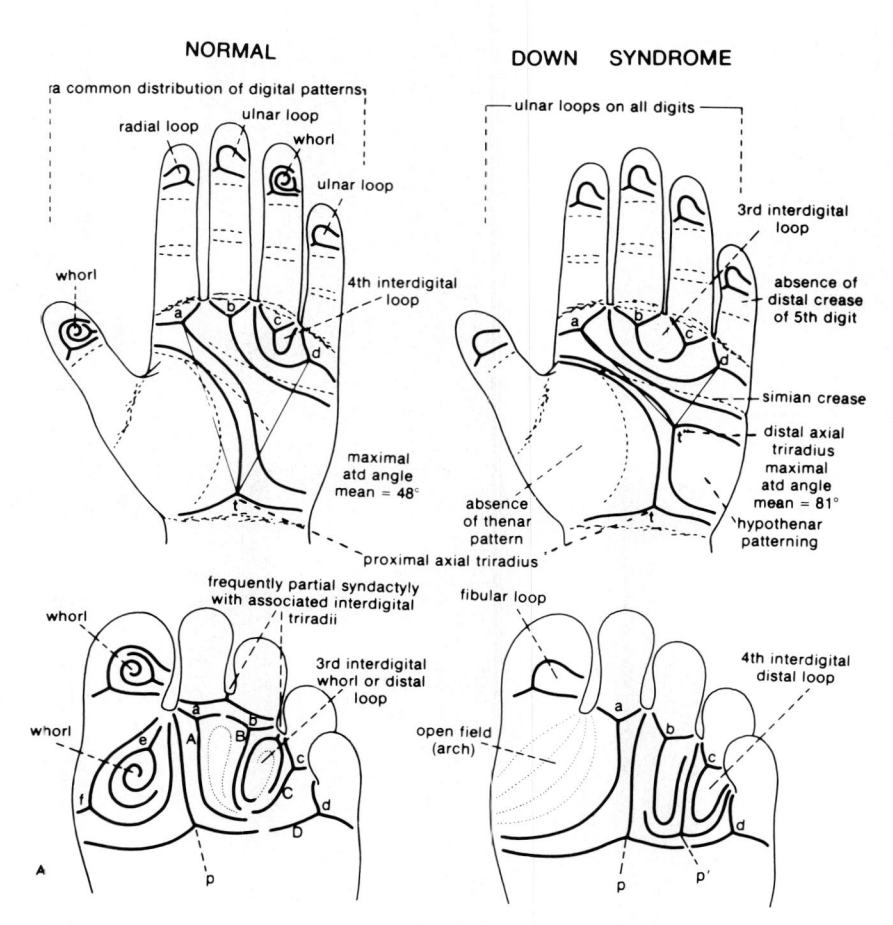

Fig. 38-21. Dermal ridge patterns of the palm and foot: normal and Down's syndrome. (From Smith, D.W.: Recognizable patterns of human malformation, Philadelphia, 1976, W.B. Saunders Co.)

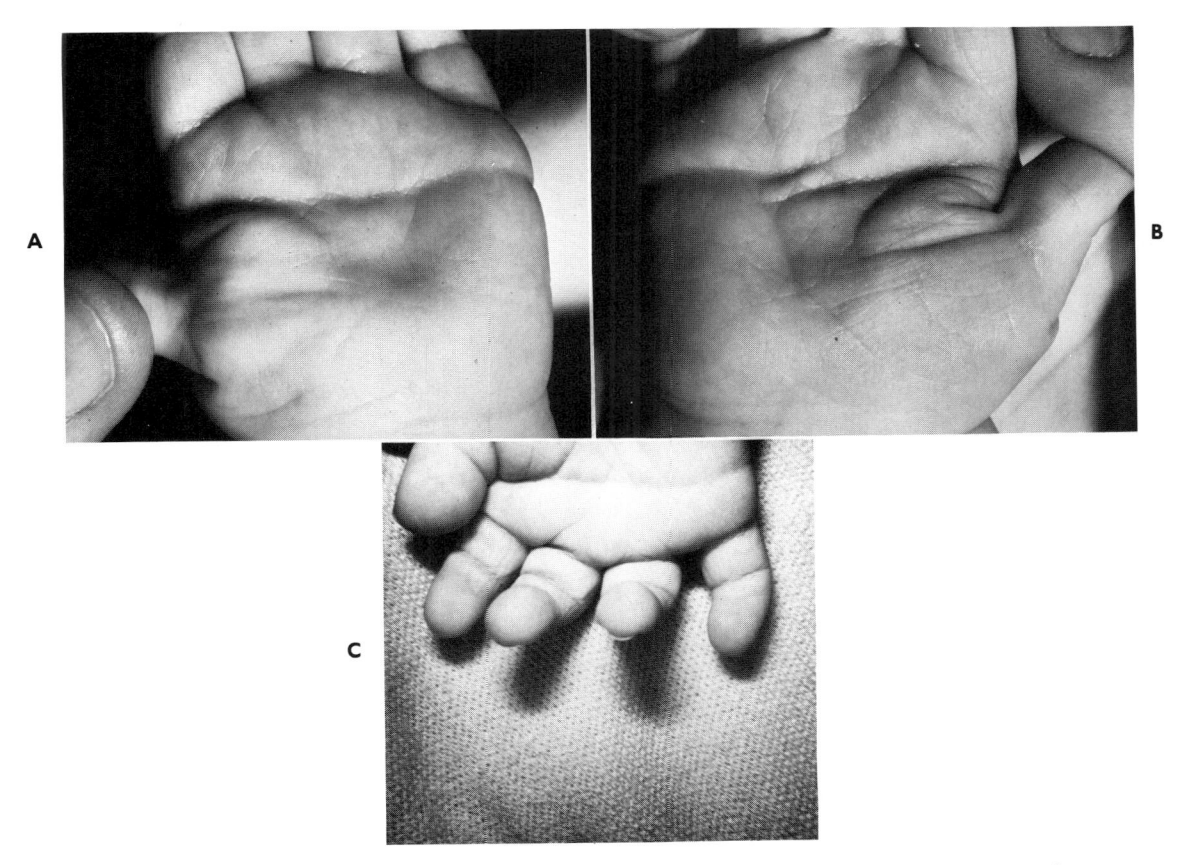

Fig. 38-22. A, Simian crease. **B,** Incomplete bridged simian crease. **C,** The hand of a patient with trisomy 21 showing a simian crease, brachydactyly, and clinodactyly of the fifth finger with a single phalangeal crease.

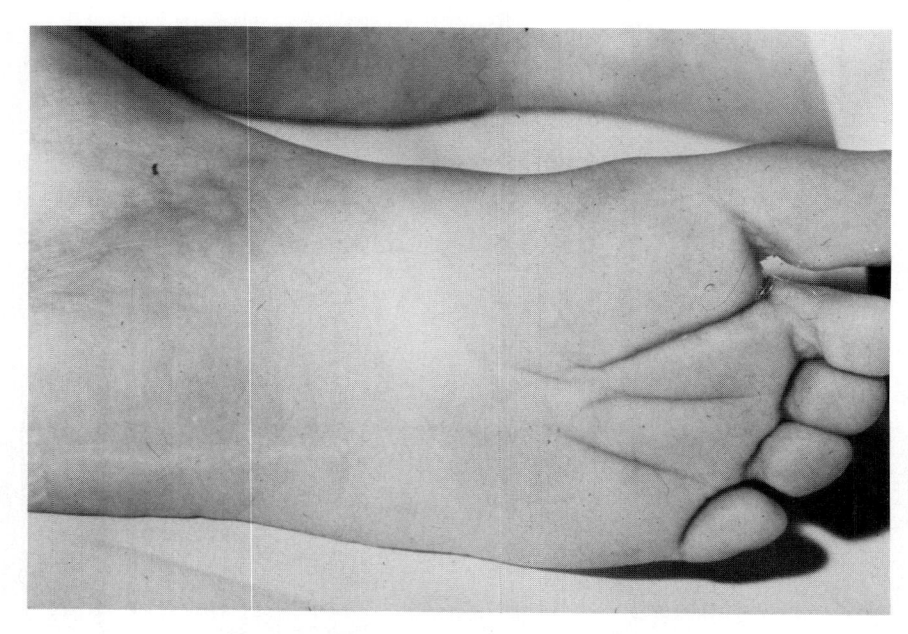

1056 Behrman's neonatal-perinatal medicine: diseases of the fetus and infant

Fig. 38-23. Sandal line furrows in trisomy 8.

Fig. 38-24. Trisomy 21; note increased separation of the first and second toes.

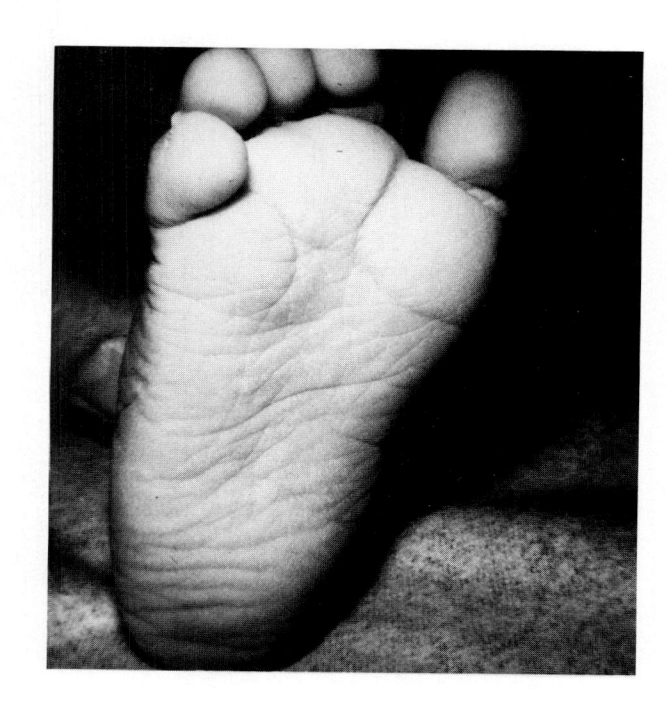

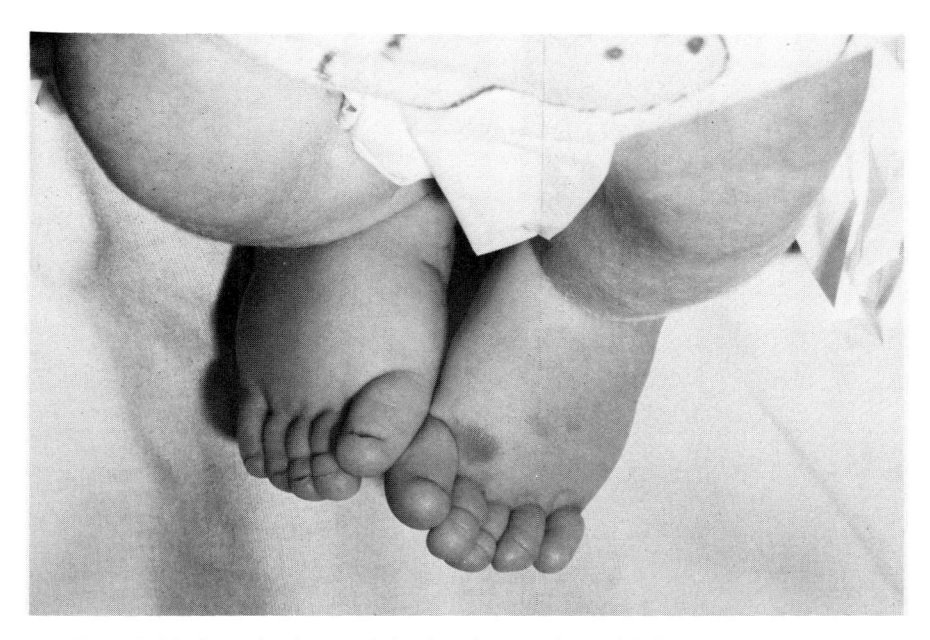

Fig. 38-25. Dorsal edema of the feet in a patient with Turner's syndrome.

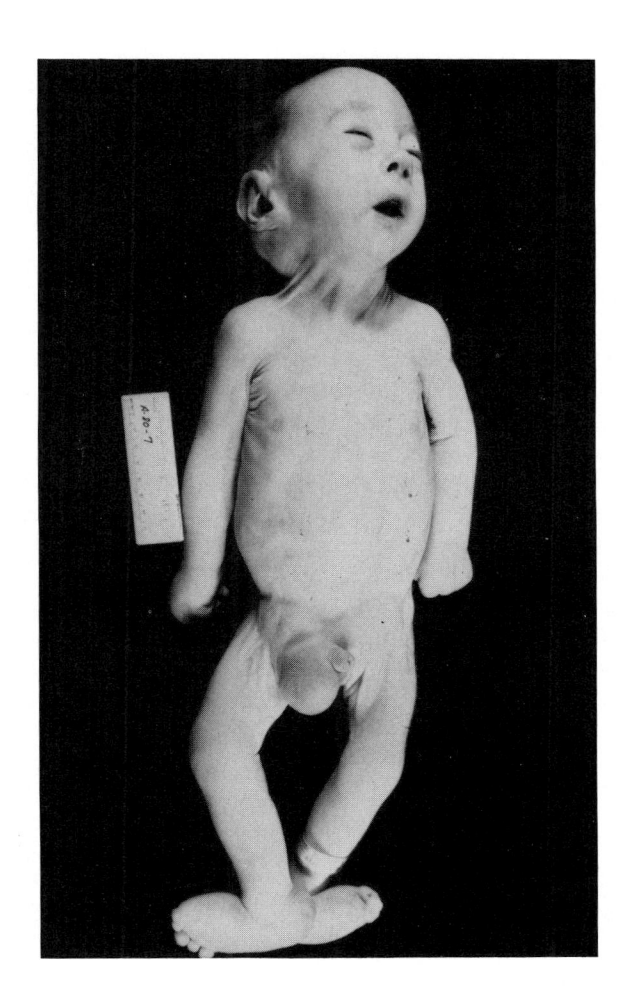

Fig. 38-26. Trisomy 18; note right hydrocele and rocker-bottom feet.

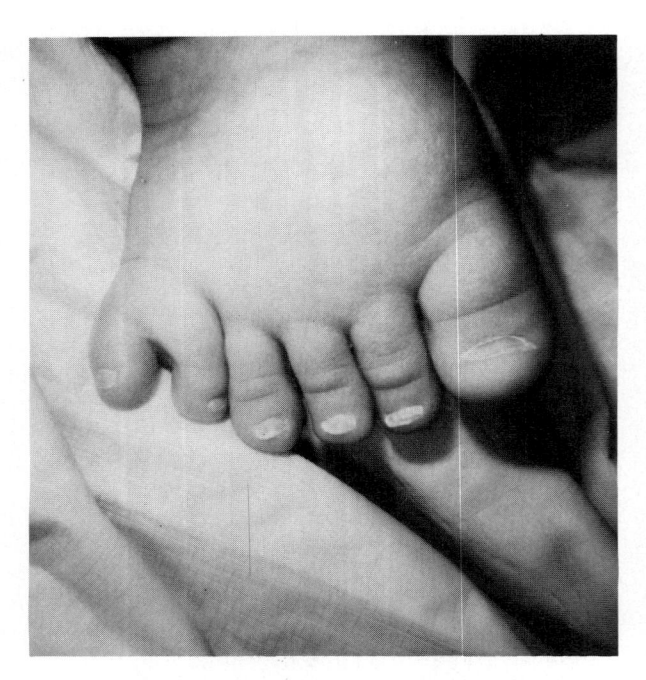

Fig. 38-27. Postaxial polydactyly.

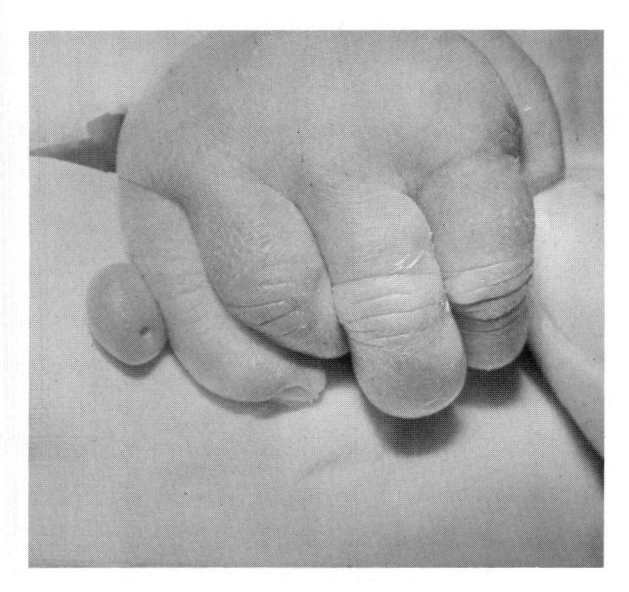

Fig. 38-28. Postaxial polydactyly in trisomy 13.

ly, syndactyly, brachydactyly, arachnodactyly, and contracture deformities. These types of anomalies are briefly discussed (Chapter 36).

The congenital absence of an entire hand is termed *acheria*, whereas absence of both hands and feet is *acheiropody*.

Ectrodactyly refers to a partial or total absence of the distal segments of a hand or foot with the proximal segments of the limbs more or less normal. All such anomalies are examples of terminal transverse defects and may occur sporadically or as part of a syndrome. It is useful to determine whether the defects involve primarily the radial or preaxial side of the limb or the ulnar or postaxial side. For example, blood dyscrasias such as the Fanconi pancytopenia syndrome, the Blackfan-Diamond syndrome, and the thrombocytopenia–absent radius (TAR) syndrome commonly involve radial defects (Chapter 29). Ulnar defects of a limb are frequent in the Cornelia de Lange syndrome.

Polydactyly refers to partial or complete supernumerary digits and is one of the most common hand malformations. Postaxial polydactyly is more frequent than preaxial, particularly in blacks; two types, A and B, can be distinguished. In type A there are fully developed extra digits (Fig. 38-27); in type B there are rudimentary digits. As an isolated anomaly, polydactyly may be inherited as an autosomal dominant trait. It also may be a manifestation of multiple malformations. Postaxial polydactyly may occur in a variety of syndromes, including trisomy 13 (Fig. 38-28), chondroectodermal dysplasia, asphyxiat-

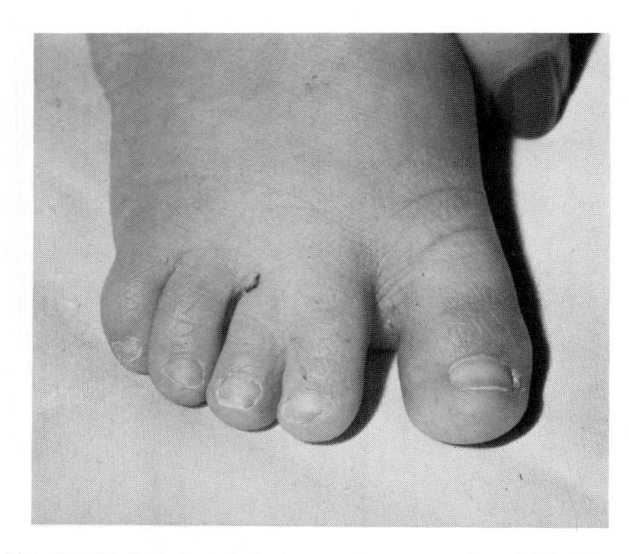

Fig. 38-29. Syndactyly between the second and third toes.

ing thoracic dystrophy (Fig. 38-19), Noonan's syndrome, the Meckel-Gruber syndrome, and the Laurence-Moon-Bardet-Biedl syndrome. Preaxial polydactyly is characteristic of the Carpenter type of acrocephalosyndactyly and the Majewski short rib polydactyly syndrome.

Syndactyly refers to a fusion of digits, which may be solely cutaneous or involve bone as well. It is the most common congenital malformation of the hand and is a normal characteristic in some marsupials, rodents, and

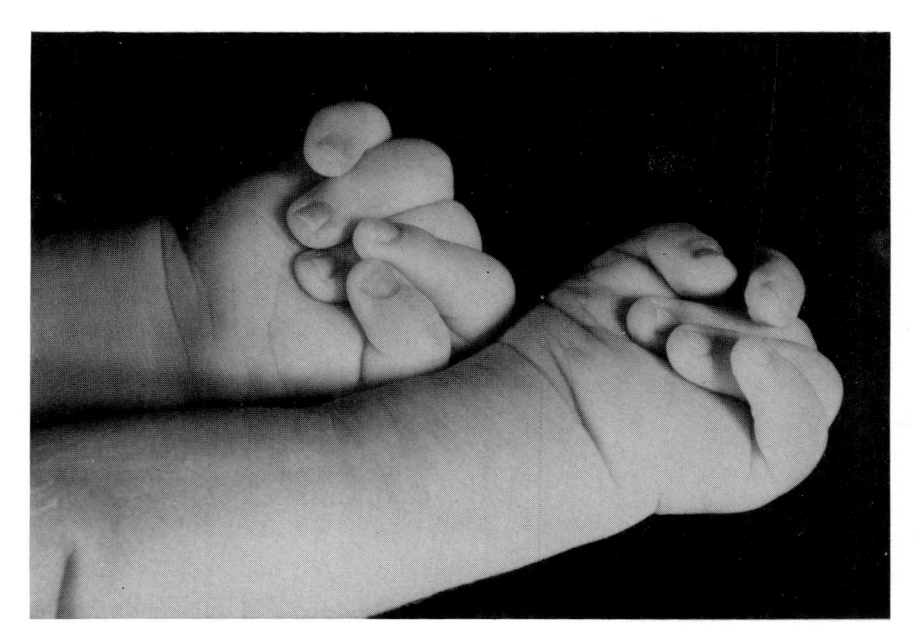

Fig. 38-30. Trisomy 18; note characteristic clinodactyly of the second, fourth, and fifth fingers.

various primates. Minimal syndactyly of the second and third toes is common in normal newborns. An excessive amount is shown in Fig. 38-29. As an isolated anomaly, different clinical types may be distinguished, but each of them is inherited as an autosomal dominant trait with variable expressivity and incomplete penetrance.

Syndactyly also may be part of a syndrome, and typical examples include the various forms of acrocephalosyndactyly, such as the Apert, Saethre-Chotzen, and Pfeiffer syndromes.

Brachydactyly is a shortening of the digits due to anomalous development of any of the phalanges, metacarpals, or metatarsals. Various clinical types may be distinguished, but most isolated forms of brachydactyly are inherited in an autosomal dominant fashion. It is also a component of numerous skeletal dysplasias such as achondroplasia.

Arachnodactyly refers to unusually long, spiderlike digits and is characteristic but not invariable in the Marfan syndrome and homocystinuria. These may be distinguished on various clinical grounds, including the congenital occurrence of ectopia lentis in Marfan's syndrome but not in homocystinuria. Arachnodactyly and associated dolichostenomelia also occur in the Marfanoid hypermobility syndrome, congenital contractural arachnodactyly and the Achard syndrome.

Joint deformities. A variety of congenital joint deformities involving the limbs may occur. *Arthrogryposis* refers to multiple congenital contractures that are most often sporadic and may be associated with oligohydramnios or be the result of some underlying neuromuscular abnormality. Talipes equinovarus or calcaneovalgus deformities of the ankle are common isolated joint contractures (Chapter 36). Limitation of movement of joints or contractures occur in numerous syndromes. Joint hypermobility is frequent in various connective tissue disorders, such as the Marfan and Ehlers-Danlos syndromes.

Cubitus valgus refers to an increase in the angle formed by the arm and forearm with the elbow extended. This angle is more acute in normal females and those with the Turner or Noonan syndrome.

Camptodactyly is a flexion contracture involving the proximaal interphalangeal joints. In the hand it practically always involves the fifth finger but may affect other fingers as well. *Dupuytren's contracture* is a flexion deformity of the digits at their proximal interphalangeal joints due to thickening and shortening of the palmar fascia. Both isolated camptodactyly and Dupuytren's contracture may be inherited as autosomal dominant traits, but they can be distinguished because the latter does not usually appear until middle age. Camptodactyly also may be part of a syndrome such as trisomy 8, trisomy 10q, the cerebrohepatorenal syndrome of Zellweger, and the whistling face syndrome of Freeman-Sheldon.

Camptodactyly should be distinguished from *clinodactyly*, which designates an incurving of a digit, most often the fifth finger. This is common in trisomy 21 and other syndromes. A characteristic clinodactyly involving the fourth and fifth fingers radially and second finger in an ulnar direction occurs in trisomy 18, or less often trisomy 13 (Fig. 38-30).

After the clinical examination

Once the history and clinical findings are noted, various laboratory studies may be indicated to confirm or establish a diagnosis. TORCH titers and chromosome analyses are frequently obtained from blood specimens. Chromosome studies are essential in every case of multiple minor or major malformations of unclear etiology. It must be remembered, however, that multiple malformations also can be the consequence of a single mutant gene. Chromosome studies are therefore only part of the appropriate diagnostic evaluation. They are also indicated in known chromosome syndromes such as Down's syndrome, since the chromosomal aberration may be sporadic or hereditary, and clinical evaluation alone cannot make the distinction. If a structural chromosomal rearrangment is detected, such as an inversion, deletion, or translocation, then additional chromosome studies will usually be necessary in both parents to determine if either is a carrier for an abnormal chromosome. The malformed infant who is stillborn or dies soon after birth also should have a thorough evaluation, including photographs, radiographs, chromosome studies, and complete postmortem examination. A common error is failure to obtain tissue for chromosome studies. Although a blood sample may not be adequate in a dying or dead infant, tissue such as amnion, skin, thymus, lung, or gonad can be obtained sterilely after death for tissue culture and subsequent chromosome analysis. Failure to do so may forever obscure a diagnosis and a significant genetic recurrence risk for the family.

The physician who evaluates infants with congenital anomalies should be familiar with standard references on teratogens and malformation syndromes. These are listed in the bibliography. Puzzling cases may require referral to various specialists, particularly when there are multiple organ system malformations. Ultimately the patient may be seen by a clinical geneticist, who may be involved not only in the initial diagnostic evaluation but also in continued follow-up and treatment as well as providing genetic counseling for the family.

GENETIC COUNSELING (see also p. 1028)

The goals of genetic counseling are to provide information in meaningful fashion to an individual or family in regard to a hereditary or potentially teratogenic condition and to provide emotional support in the adjustment to a serious birth defect. It is equally important to state that a problem is not of genetic origin as it is to explain a specific genetic abnormality. Since many malformations have a relatively low risk of recurrence, a negative family history is common. The family may assume, however, that the absence of affected relatives means that the problem is not a genetic disorder. Furthermore, they may blame themselves or implicate some other unrelated factor as a cause for the condition. It is important to clarify these misconceptions and to relieve the individual and family of any unwarranted guilt for a problem over which they had no control. Malformations that lead to serious disability or death cause a grief reaction in the parents, which may require more extensive supportive counseling.

The basis for an accurate assessment of the risk of recurrence of a birth defect is a specific diagnosis. Abnormalities that are the consequence of a single mutant gene will have a probability of recurrence that depends on the mendelian pattern of inheritance. Thus an autosomal dominant condition will have a 50% recurrence risk for an affected parent. The risk of recurrence for an autosomal recessive trait is 25%, and in this case both parents are usually asymptomatic carriers of the mutant allele. Dominantly inherited conditions may occasionally arise for the first time in a family as a new mutation, and in this situation limited data may make it difficult to differentiate them from an autosomal recessive disorder. The latter is not likely to originate in one individual as a consequence of mutation, since two rare mutational events would be necessary. In X-linked recessive disorders the risk in most cases is confined to male offspring of asymptomatic carrier mothers. For such males the risk is 50%, whereas the female sibs have a 50% chance of being carriers like their mother. In an X-linked recessive disorder, females can be affected only if their mothers are carriers or are affected and their fathers are affected also, an unlikely combination. However, the normal random inactivation of one of the X chromosomes in females can occasionally result in a predominance of cells containing the mutant allele, resulting in some clinical expression in carrier females. X-linked dominant disorders are the least common single gene traits, and in this case male and female offspring have a 50% risk when the mother is affected. When the father is affected, all the daughters will be affected but none of the sons.

Chromosome disorders have variable risks of recurrence depending on the specific abnormality and condition. The common form of trisomy 21 due to nondisjunction has a 1% empirically determined recurrence risk. The general risk also increases particularly with maternal age over 35. Trisomy 21 due to translocation has a risk of recurrence dependent on the nature of the translocation and which parent is the carrier of the abnormal chromosome. It can be as high as 100% in a 21 to 21 translocation.

Many of the common major malformations are inherited in a multifactorial manner, and the risks of recurrence are based on empirical data from large numbers of families. Generally the recurrence risk for a second affected offspring will be approximately 2% to 5%. Unlike mendelian inheritance, the risk increases with the number of affected relatives and decreases with decreasing genetic relationship to the affected proband. Table 37-2 summarizes some empirical risk figures for various common malformations.

In addition to informing the family about recurrence risks, genetic counseling also must consider the possibility of prenatal diagnosis (Chapter 37). Chromosomal and many biochemical disorders are easily diagnosed following amniocentesis and appropriate studies of the amniotic fluid and its cells. The *alpha-fetoprotein* determination in amniotic fluid is very useful in detecting neural tube defects and occasionally other anomalies. Current studies are in progress in the United States to assess the value of maternal serum alpha-fetoprotein for similar purposes.

Advances in ultrasonography (Chapter 8) have made it possible to diagnose various malformations early in pregnancy, and continued developments in the ability to visualize the fetus in utero are likely. This includes fetoscopy, in which the fetus is directly examined with a fiberoptic scope inserted into the uterus. As techniques are improved and newer ones developed, it may eventually be possible to screen all pregnancies for a variety of malformations. Ultimately the prevention of congenital malformations will depend on the elucidation of causal mechanisms as well as advances in prenatal diagnosis.

Thaddeus W. Kurczynski

ACKNOWLEDGMENT

Various photographs of patients were graciously provided by Drs. Haynes B. Robinson, Avroy Fanaroff, and Samuel J. Horwitz.

BIBLIOGRAPHY
General

Beighton, P.: Inherited disorders of the skeleton, New York, 1978, Churchill Livingstone.
Bergsma, D.: Birth defects compendium, New York, 1979, Alan R. Liss.
de Grouchy, J., and Turleau, C.: Clinical atlas of human chromosomes, New York, 1977, John Wiley and sons, Inc.
Dyken, P.R., and Miller, M.D.: Facial features of neurologic syndromes, St. Louis, 1980, The C.V. Mosby Co.
Gellis, S.S., and Feingold, M.: Atlas of mental retardation syndromes, Washington, D.C., 1968, U.S. Government Printing Office.
Goodman, R.M., and Gorlin, R.J.: Atlas of the face in genetic disorders, St. Louis, 1977, The C.V. Mosby Co.
Gorlin, R.J., Cohen, M.M., Jr., and Pindborg, J.J.: Syndromes of the head and neck, New York, 1975, McGraw-Hill Book Co., Inc.
McKusick, V.A.: Mendelian inheritance in man: catalog of autosomal dominant, autosomal recessive, and X-linked phenotypes, Baltimore, 1978, The Johns Hopkins University Press.
Nyhan, W.L., and Sakati, N.O.: Genetic and malformation syndromes in clinical medicine, Chicago, 1976, Year-Book Medical Publishers, Inc.
Patten, B.M.: Human embryology, New York, 1953, McGraw-Hill Book Co., Inc.

Smith, D.W.: Recognizable patterns of human malformation, Philadelphia, 1976, W.B. Saunders co.
Spanger, J.W., Langer, L.O., and Wiedemann, H.R.: Bone dysplasias: an atlas of constitutional disorders of skeletal development, Philadelphia, 1974, W.B. Saunders Co.
Temtamy, S.A., and McKusick, V.A.: The genetics of hand malformations, Birth Defects, vol. 4, no. 3, New York, 1978, Alan R. Liss.
Warkany, J.: Congenital malformations, Chicago, 1971, Year-Book Medical Publishers, Inc.
Wynne-Davies, R.: Heritable disorders in orthopedic practice, Oxford, 1973, Blackwell Scientific Publications.

Terminology

Feingold, N., and Bossert, W.H.: Normal values for selected physical parameters: an aid to syndrome delineation, Birth Defects 10(13): 1, 1974.
Freire-Maia, N.: Congenital skeletal limb deficiencies—a general review, Birth Defects 5(3):7, 1969.
Holmes, L.B.: Inborn errors of morphogenesis: a review of localized hereditary malformations, N. Engl. J. Med. 192:763, 1974.
Holmes, L.B.: Current concepts in genetics: congenital malformations, N. Engl. J. Med. 195:204, 1976.
Montagu, M.F.A.: A handbook of anthropometry, Springfield, Ill., 1960, Charles C Thomas, Publishers.
O'Rahilly, R.: The nomenclature and classification of limb anomalies, Birth Defects 5(3):14, 1969.
Smith, D.W.: Letter to the editor, J. Pediatr. 93:160, 1978.
Spranger, J.: Letter to the editor, J. Pediatr. 93:159, 1978.

Epidemiology and genetics

Carr, D.H., and Gedeon, M.: Population cytogenetics of human abortuses. In Hook, E.B., and Porter, I.H., editors: Population cytogenetics, New York, 1977, Academic Press, Inc.
Emanuel, I., and others: The incidence of congenital malformations in a Chinese population: the Taipei collaborative study, Teratology 5:159, 1972.
Erickson, J.D.: Racial variations in the incidence of congenital malformations, Ann. Hum. Genet. 39:315, 1976.
Holmes, L.B.: Congenital malformations: incidence, racial differences and recognized etiologies. In Biologic and clinical aspects of malformations, Mead Johnson Symposium on Perinatal and Developmental Medicine, no. 7. Evansville, Ind., 1976, Mead Johnson.
Hook, E.B., and others: Some aspects of the epidemiology of human minor birth defects and morphological variants in a completely ascertained newborns population (Madison study), Teratology 13:47, 1976.
Jacobs, D.A., Melville, M., and Ratcliff, S.: A cytogenetic survey of 11,680 newborn infants, Ann. Hum. Genet. 37:359, 1974.
Marden, P.M., Smith, D.W., and McDonald, M.J.: Congenital anomalies in the newborn infant, including minor variations, J. Pediatr. 64:357, 1964.
Nelson, T., Oakley, G.P., Jr., and Shepard, T.H.: Collection of human embryos and fetuses. In Hook, E.B., Javevick, D.T., and Porter, I.A., editors: Monitoring birth defects and environment: the problem of surveillance, New York, 1971, Academic Press, Inc.
Neshemura, H.: Incidence of malformations in abortions. In Fraser, F.C., and McKusick, V.A., editors: Proceedings of the Third International Conference on Birth Defects, New York, 1969, Excerpta Medica.
Warshaw, J.B., and Holmes, L.B.: Congenital malformations—some genetics, embryological and environmental considerations. In Genetics and the perinatal patient, Mead Johnson Symposium on Perinatal and Developmental medicine, no. 1. Evansville, Ind., 1973, Mead Johnson.

Teratogenic states

Clarren, S.K., and Smith, D.W.: The fetal alcohol syndrome, N. Engl. J. Med. 298:1063, 1978.

Clarren, S.K., and others: Brain malformations related to prenatal exposure to ethanol, J. Pediatr. 92:64, 1978.

Committee on Drugs, American Academy of Pediatrics: Anticonvulsants and pregnancy, Pediatrics 63:331, 1979.

Day, R.E., and Insley, J.: Maternal diabetes mellitus and congenital malformation, Arch. Dis. Child. 51:935, 1976.

Dudgeon, J.A.: Infective causes of human malformations, Br. Med. Bull. 32:77, 1976.

Fraser, F.C., Metrakos, J.D., and Zlatkin, M.: Is the epileptic genotype teratogenic? Lancet 1:884 1978.

Hansen, H.: Variability of reproductive casualty in maternal phenylalaninemia, Early Hum. Develop. 2:51, 1978.

Hanshaw, J.B., and Dudgeon, J.A.: Viral diseases of the fetus and newborn, Philadelphia, 1978, W.B. Saunders Co.

Hanson, J.W., Jones, K.L. and Smith, D.W.: Fetal alcohol syndrome, J.A.M.A. 235:1458, 1976.

Hill, R.M.: Fetal malformations and antiepileptic drugs, Am. J. Dis. Child. 130:923, 1976.

Monson, R.R., and others Diphenylhydantoin and selected congenital malformations, N. Engl. J. Med. 289:1049, 1973.

Montouris, G.D., Fenichel, G.M. and McLain, W., Jr.: The pregnant epileptic: a review and recommendations, Arch. Neurol. 36:601, 1979.

Nishimura, H., and Tanimura, T.: Clinical aspects of the teratogenicity of drugs, Amsterdam, 1976, Excerpta Medica, American Elsevier–North Holland.

Passage, E.: Congenital malformations and maternal diabetics, Lancet 1:324, 1965.

Pedersen, L.M., Tygstrup, I., and Pedersen, J.: Congenital malformations in newborn infants of diabetic women, Lancet 1:1124, 1964.

Rowland, T.W., Hubbell, J.P., Jr. and Nadas, A.S.: Congenital heart disease in infants of diabetic mothers, J. Pediatr. 83:815, 1973.

Rutsteins, D.D., and Veech, R.L.: Genetics and addictions to alcohol, N. Engl. J. Med. 298:1140, 1978.

Shephard, T.H.: Catalog of teratogenic agents, Baltimore, 1976, The Johns Hopkins University Press

Simpson, J.L.: Genetics of diabetes mellitus and anomalies in offspring of diabetic mothers. In Merkatz, I.R., and Adam., P.A.J., editors: The diabetic pregnancy: a perinatal perspective, New York, 1979, Grune and Stratton, Inc.

Smith, D.W.: Teratogenicity of anticonvulsive medications, Am. J. Dis. Child. 131:1337, 1977.

Smithells, R.W.: Environmental teratogens of man, Br. Med. Bull 32:27, 1976.

Streissguth, A.P., Herman, C.S., and Smith, D.W.: Intelligence, behavior, and dysmorphogenesis in the fetal alcohol syndrome: a report of 20 patients, J. Pediatr. 92:363, 1978.

Stumpf, D.A., and Frost, M.: Seizures, anticonvulsants, and pregnancy, Am. J. Dis. Child. 132:746, 1978.

Selected malformations

Alexious, D., and others: Frequency of other malformations in congenital hypoplasia of depressor anguli oris muscle syndrome, Arch. Dis. Child. 51:891, 1976.

Banks, H.H.: Birth defects and the orthopedic surgeon, Orthopedic Clinics of North America, vol. 7, no. 2, Philadelphia, 1976, W.B. Saunders Co.

Bergoma, D., and Lenz, W., editors: Morphogenesis and malformations of the limb, Birth Defects, vol. 13, no. 1, 1977.

Collins, E.: The illusion of widely spaced nipples in the Noonan and Turner syndromes, J. Pediatr. 83:557, 1973.

DeMyer, W.: The median cleft face syndrome, Neurology 17:961, 1967.

DeMyer, W.: Median facial malformations and their implications for brain malformations, Birth Defects 11:(7):155, 1975.

Gorlin, R.J., Cervenka, J., and Pruzansky, S.: Facial clefting and its syndromes, Birth Defects 12(7):3, 1971.

Hanson, J.W., and Smith, D.W.: U-shaped palatal defect in the Robin anomalad: developmental and clinical relevance, J. Pediatr. 87:30, 1975.

Hanson, J.W., Smith, D.W., and Cohen, N.N., Jr.: Prominant lateral palatine ridges: developmental and clinical relevance, J. Pediatr. 89:54, 1976.

Heyn, R., Kurczynski, E., and Schmickel, R.: The association of Blackfan-Diamond syndrome, physical abnormalities, and an abnormality of chromosome 1, J. Pediatr. 85:531, 1974.

Jaffe, B.F.: Pinna anomalies associated with congenital conductive hearing loss, Pediatrics 57:332, 1976.

Jones, K.L., Hanson, J.W., and Smith, D.A.: Palpebral fissure size in newborn infants, J. Pediatr. 92:787, 1978.

King, C.R., and Prescott, G.: Pathogenesis of the prune belly anomalad, J. Pediatr. 93:273, 1978.

Noveh, Y., and Friedman, A.: Familial imperforate anus, Am. J. Dis. Child. 130:441, 1976.

Paradice, B.A., and Poland, B.J.: A 94 mm human fetus with the VACTERL association of anomalies, Teratology 13:21, 1976.

Popich, G.A., and Smith, D.W.: The genesis and significance of digital and palmar hand creases: preliminary report, J. Pediatr. 77:1917, 1970.

Quan, L., and Smith, D.W.: The VATER association: vertebral defects, anal atresia, tracheo-esophageal fistula with esophageal atresia, radial dysplasia, Birth Defects 8(2):75, 1972.

Rapin, I., and Ruben, R.J.: Patterns of anomalies in children with malformed ears, Laryngoscope 86:1469, 1976.

Ross, R.B.: Lateral facial dysplasia, Birth Defects 11(7):51, 1975.

Schaumann, B., and Alter, M.: Dermatoglyphics in medical disorders, New York, 1976, Springer-Verlag.

Schnall, B.S., and Smith, D.W.: Normandom laterality of malformations in paired structures, J. Pediatr. 85:509, 1974.

Sedano, H.O., and others: Frontonasal dysplasia, J. Pediatr. 76:906, 1970.

Smith, D.W., and Greely, M.J.: Unruly scalp hair in infancy: its nature and relevance to problems of brain morphogenesis, Pediatrics 61:783, 1978.

Woodard, J.R.: The prune belly syndrome, Urol. Clin. North Am. 5:75, 1978.

Wilkens, L.: The diagnosis and treatment of endocrine disorders in childhood and adolescence, Springfield, Ill., 1966, Charles C Thomas, Publisher.

Wynne-Davis, R., and Lloyd-Roberts, G.C.: Arthrogryposis multiplex congenita, Arch. Dis. Child. 51:618, 1976.

Human genetics and genetic counseling

Bonaiti-Pellie, C., and Smith, C.: Risk tables for genetic counseling in some common congenital malformations, J. Med. Genet. 11:374, 1974.

Fraser, F.C.: Genetic counseling, Am. J. Hum. Genet. 26:636, 1974.

Fraser, F.C.: Current concepts in genetics: genetics as a health-care service, N. Engl. J. Med. 295:486, 1976.

Golbus, M.S., and others: Prenatal diagnosis in 3000 amniocenteses, N. Engl. J. Med. 300:157, 1979.

Hobbins, J.C., and others: Ultrasound in the diagnosis of congenital anomalies, Am. J. Obstet. Gynecol. 134:331, 1979.

Jackson, L.G., and Schimke, R.N.: Clinical genetics: a source book for physicians, New York, 1979, John Wiley & Sons, Inc.

MacIvar, J.: Antenatal detection of fetal abnormality—physical methods, Br. Med. Bull. 32:4, 1976.

Milunsky, A.: Prenatal diagnosis of genetic disorders, N. Engl. J. Med. 295:377, 1976.

The NICHD National Registry for Ammiocentesis Study Group: Midtrimester amniocentesis for prenatal diagnosis, J.A.M.A. 236:1471, 1976.

Nora, J.J., and Fraser, F.C.: Medical genetics: principles and practice, Philadelphia, 1974, Lea & Febiger.

Vogel, F., and Molulsky, A.G.: Human genetics, New York, 1979, Springer-Verlag.

Zellweger, H., and Simpson, J.: Chromosomes of man, Clinics in developmental medicine, nos. 65/66, Philadelphia, 1977, J.B. Lippincott Co.

CHAPTER 39 Diagnostic radiology

In attempting to present a subject as comprehensive as neonatal radiology within the confines of a single chapter, many important aspects of the discipline must be omitted and others mentioned only briefly. It is not our intention to cover the roentgenology of specific disorders that affect the neonate, since these are dealt with elsewhere in this book; rather it is our purpose to discuss the indications and the basic methodology of commonly used roentgenologic examinations. In addition, a roentgenologic approach to diagnosis based on frequently occurring roentgenographic findings is presented.

PATIENT PROTECTION

Prolonged survival of premature infants has resulted in larger numbers of roentgenograms being taken, thus increasing radiation exposure. Consequently, radiologists have become more concerned with the possible long-term effects of low-dosage diagnostic roentgenograms. These effects are extremely difficult to measure, since most data must be obtained from laboratory experiments or following accidental human exposure to high doses of radiation. Investigations such as those showing an apparent increased risk for development of leukemia in children exposed to diagnostic x rays in utero might imply a similar effect on the preterm neonate. A long latent period between low-dose exposure and development of a radiation effect is an additional difficulty in studying current intensive care nursery populations. However, certain practical steps can be taken to prevent unnecessary radiation. These include careful columnation of the x-ray beam to the field of interest, gonadal shielding, avoidance of overexposure and repeat examinations by meticulous attention to technical detail, and a thorough evaluation of the indications for the examination on the part of the attending physician.

ASSESSMENT OF AN ADEQUATE EXAMINATION

A simple check of several technical aspects of the film greatly increases the likelihood of proper interpretation of suspected abnormalities. The following points should be considered:

1. *Exposure.* This is a subjective evaluation and is represented by the degree of blackening of the film. In general, details of the thoracic spine should be visible through the cardiothymic silhouette.
2. *Motion.* This will cause obvious blurring of the images and will result in decreased definition of structures such as the pulmonary vessels and diaphragm.
3. *Positioning.* Rotation will increase magnification of the structures closest to the beam. For example, in the supine position, rotation of the patient to the right will cause magnification of the left ribs and the left hilum. Also, the heart will be projected within the right hemithorax. A simple method of assessing rotation is to compare the relative positions of the anterior ends of a pair of ribs.
4. *Extraneous objects.* A large portion of the chest of a small premature infant can be completely obscured by electrocardiogram electrodes, cutaneous oxygen monitors, and other equipment. When possible, these as well as other opaque densities such as warming mattresses and respirator tubing should be removed prior to roentgenography.
5. *Inspiration.* The roentgenogram should be exposed at the end of inspiration, a difficult task in neonates with rapid respiratory rates. In some the tidal volume is so small that there is little difference in the degree of lung aeration during the respiratory cycle. In others it is difficult to determine whether the resultant increase in lung opacity is due to expiration or a pathologic decrease in lung volume. As a general rule, on a good inspiratory film the right diaphragmatic dome should be projected at about the level of the anterior end of the sixth rib.

CHEST

Chest roentgenograms account for the majority of roentgenographic studies in newborn infants. Most of these are required because of problems of respiratory distress in premature infants. Roentgenographic techniques for the neonate differ from those used in older infants and children because of the small size and rapid respiratory rates of the newborn. Radiologists, neonatologists, and nursery personnel must understand the special requirements for proper roentgenographic examination of these patients.

Methods of examination

Except for special studies, most roentgenography of the chest can be accomplished in the newborn nursery using modern portable roentgenographic equipment. These units employ a single-phase generator capable of exposure times of less than 5 msec at the relatively low kilovoltage required for these infants. In almost every case, blurring due to respiratory motion can be prevented. Recently, further decreases in exposure time (and thus the dose of absorbed radiation) have been achieved by using faster film-intensifying screen combinations. Rare earth screens show promise in this regard, although there is some resultant loss of detail with an increase in graininess or mottle because of increased quantum "noise."

Within the radiology department, most chest roentgenography is done at a distance of 72 inches. This must be reduced to approximately 40 inches when using portable equipment. Although in the larger patient this results in considerable distortion of structures due to magnification, no important degradation of the image occurs with small infants.

Portable roentgenographic examinations of the chest consist of an anteroposterior (AP) view made with a vertical beam and, frequently, a lateral view made with a horizontal beam. Careful positioning, which is often undertaken by the nursery personnel, is of extreme importance in obtaining a high quality roentgenogram. The AP view is made with the patient lying supine, and proper positioning is facilitated by extending the patient's arms above the head and immobilizing the thighs. For the lateral view the x-ray tube can then be moved so that the x-ray beam is directed horizontally. The patient, therefore, need not be turned as would be the case with a vertical beam lateral view. Occasionally a lateral decubitus view is necessary, particularly for evaluation of a pneumothorax. This also is made with a horizontal x-ray beam. The patient is turned so that the unaffected side is dependent.

It is debatable whether a lateral as well as an AP view need be done for each examination. The increased radiation dose and the necessity of further handling of a fragile infant must be weighed against the possibility of significant gain in diagnostic information from the lateral view. In a recent study the addition of a lateral view did not increase the diagnostic accuracy of initial chest roentgenograms made in the nursery. Whether this would hold true for subsequent roentgenographic examinations is not known, but in our nursery we no longer do lateral views routinely.

Other useful roentgenographic techniques in newborn chest disease include magnification radiography, which is done with a small focal spot (0.2 to 0.3 mm) that approximates a point source. The patient is no longer in contact with the film, so divergence of the x-ray beam projects a magnified image onto the film. This usually requires removal of the infant from the incubator. Also, high-kilovoltage films may be made to assess the airways and mediastinal structures. These are done in the radiology department using extra filtration of the x-ray beam. The rationale for this technique is to increase the relative absorption of x rays in bone and soft tissue by using a higher energy beam, thus enhancing the radiolucency of the air-containing structures. This technique also may be combined with magnification roentgenography.

Fluoroscopy, tomography, bronchography, angiography, computed tomography, and radionuclide lung scanning are other roentgenologic techniques that are available for specific diagnostic problems.

Ultrasonography is less useful for chest diagnosis than in the abdomen because of reduced transmission of sound waves in air. However, if an appropriate "window" can be found, it can be very useful in further characterization of intrathoracic masses and fluid collections. This modality is particularly helpful in differentiating cystic from solid masses (Fig. 39-1).

Computed tomography with image acquisition times of 5 seconds or less is capable of producing exquisite anatomic detail of intrathoracic structures even in rapidly breathing newborn infants (Fig. 39-1). The indications for computed tomography in newborn chest diagnosis are usually limited to the evaluation of masses and air- or fluid-containing cysts. An obvious disadvantage of this method of examination is the need to transport the infant to the scanner and to remove the patient from the protective environment during the scan.

Normal chest

The appearance of the normal chest varies throughout the first few days of life. The lungs may be slightly opaque due to retained lung liquid in the early newborn period. The lungs eventually become radiolucent except for well-defined pulmonary vessels branching from the hila. The minor fissure of the right lung is frequently seen as a fine horizontal line in the midportion of the lung field. The cardiophrenic and costophrenic angles

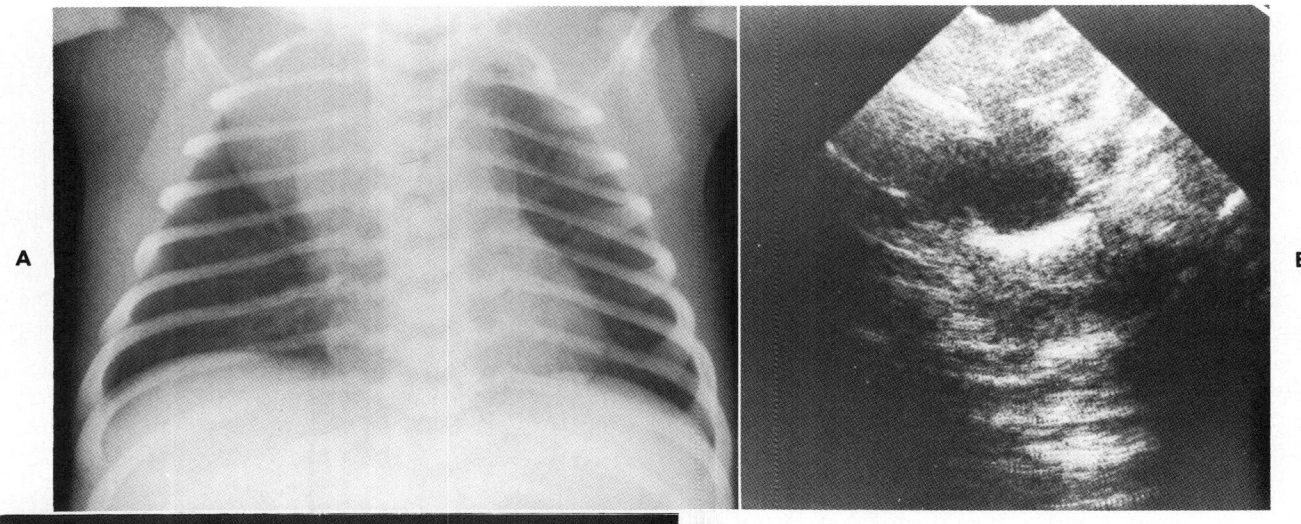

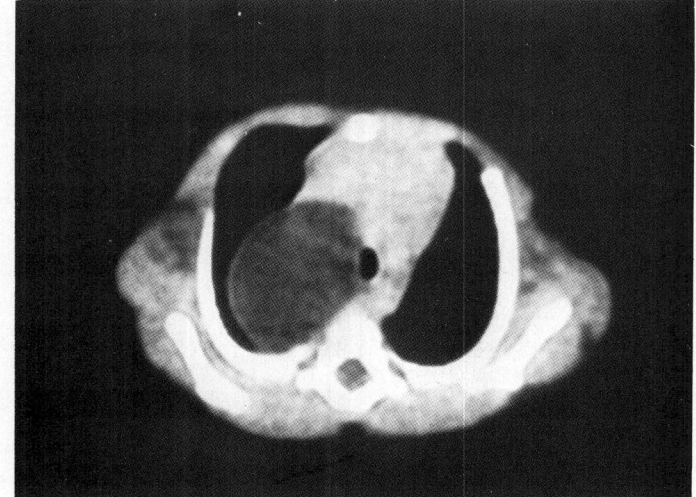

Fig. 39-1. Comparison between conventional radiography, ultrasonography, and computed tomography in a patient with a large right upper mediastinal mass. **A,** The chest radiograph shows a well-defined mediastinal tumor compressing the trachea. There is no indication as to whether the mass is solid (e.g., neurogenic tumor) or cystic. **B,** Ultrasound shows the cystic nature of the lesion. **C,** Computed tomography shows that the cyst has a well-defined, thin wall and contains material of homogeneously decreased attenuation. Note the compression of the right wall of the trachea. The adjacent vertebra is not involved. The lesion was a bronchogenic cyst.

should be clear. The heart borders, except for the portions adjacent to the hila, should be distinct, and the diaphragmatic pleura should be clearly outlined against the lungs except for that portion of the left hemidiaphragm that is contiguous to the heart.

The cardiothoracic ratio should be no greater than 0.60. In the first few days of life a rounded opacity may be seen in the left upper mediastinum due to a normal "ductus bump" associated with the closing ductus arteriosus. The tracheal air shadow should curve gently to the right around the aortic arch. Displacement of the trachea to the left is abnormal and suggests a mediastinal mass or right aortic arch. The descending thoracic aorta is rarely visible in the newborn.

The thymus is frequently prominent in the newborn, and because of its variable configuration, its appearance causes frequent confusion. The thymus overlies the anterior aspect of the pericardium, obscuring much of the cardiac silhouette; thus it may simulate a large heart. It is frequently asymmetric and more prominent on the right, sometimes producing a sail-like appearance. Wavelike undulations of its lateral border may be seen due to pressure of the costal cartilages. Aside from these fairly characteristic normal features, the thymus can generally be identified by its homogenous density, anterior location, lack of associated compression of the trachea, and sharp definition of its edges. A lateral view will often exclude cardiomegaly by demonstrating an absence of posterior enlargement of the heart. The ratio between the transverse diameter of the cardiothymic image and that of the thoracic cage tends to be slightly larger in babies with respiratory distress syndrome (RDS) than in those with normal lungs.

Roentgenologic signs of pulmonary abnormalities

Pulmonary consolidation and pneumonia

The term *consolidation* indicates a process that causes the alveoli to be filled with a substance having the density of water. The most frequent cause is pneumonia, but

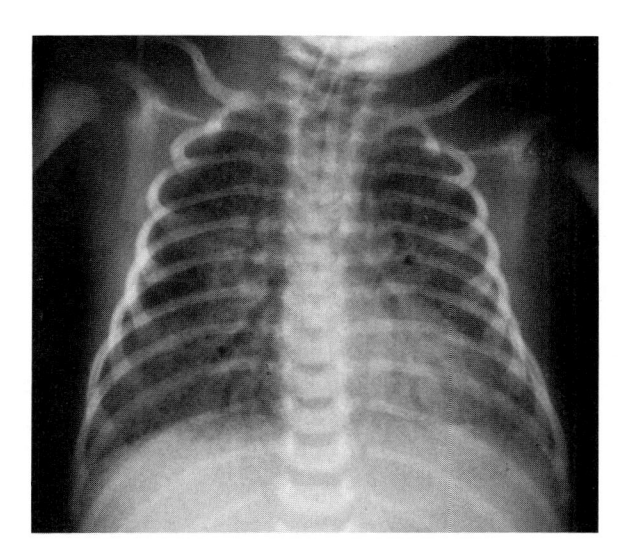

Fig. 39-2. Diffuse bilateral pulmonary consolidation due to pneumococcal pneumonia in the newborn. Note the prominent "air bronchograms" and reticular pattern resembling respiratory distress syndrome. The lungs have increased in volume, an uncommon finding in RDS.

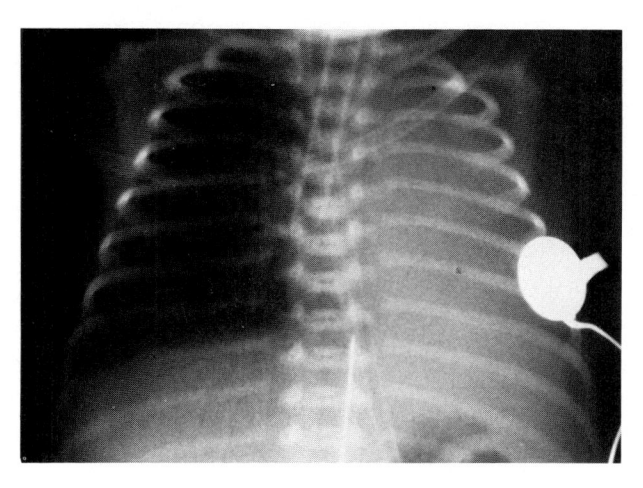

Fig. 39-3. Atelectasis of the entire left lung. The mediastinum has shifted into the left hemithorax. The atelectasis is due to the aberrant position of the endotracheal tube in the right main bronchus.

hemorrhage, pus, and edema also are included under this term. Varying degrees of opacification of the lungs are the result of consolidation. The densities may be localized or diffuse and are frequently "patchy." The edges of the consolidation are indistinct, and there is frequently an "air bronchogram," with visualization of the relatively radiolucent bronchi within the involved area of the lung.

As opposed to a process in which the air spaces are opacified, involvement of the interstitial tissues of the lung may predominate. In this case a diffuse reticular or nodular pattern results. Peribronchial disease results in small ring shadows when the smaller, more peripheral bronchi are seen in cross-sections, but air bronchograms are not seen.

Generalized pulmonary hyperinflation also frequently accompanies diffuse pneumonia and is particularly apparent in meconium aspiration pneumonitis. Completely airless, consolidated lobes and segments of lung tend to be less voluminous than when they are filled with air.

Group B streptococcal pneumonia deserves special mention, since some small premature infants may have a lung pattern which closely resembles that seen in RDS. This pattern, once thought to be specific for RDS, consists of diffuse bilateral reticulogranularity with exaggerated air bronchograms. We have also noted this pattern in neonatal pneumonias of other causes (Fig. 39-2).

Atelectasis

Like consolidation, atelectasis also causes an increase in lung density. Furthermore, until the gas is completely resorbed from the bronchi, an air bronchogram may be present. Lobar atelectasis is primarily manifested as changes in position of the fissures. For example, with lower lobe collapse the major fissure moves posteromedially. In middle lobe collapse the minor fissure is depressed, whereas right upper lobe collapse causes elevation of this fissure.

Atelectasis also results in a shift of the mediastinum toward the side of the collapse (Fig. 39-3). This is most notable in lower lobe atelectasis, but in newborn infants the compliant mediastinal structures will also shift slightly toward the side of an upper lobe collapse. In addition, lower lobe atelectasis results in elevation of the ipsilateral hemidiaphragm. Narrowing of the intercostal spaces is a frequent secondary sign. Compensatory hyperinflation of uninvolved portions of lung or of the opposite lung will also occur and must be differentiated from a primary increase in lung volume, such as that which occurs in congenital lobar emphysema.

In neonates the most frequent site of lobar atelectasis is the right upper lobe. This may be due to occlusion of the right upper lobe bronchus associated with faulty position of an endotracheal tube, but it is also a frequent finding following extubation, probably because of mucus accumulation and decreased ciliary activity.

Diffuse atelectasis occurs in premature infants who

have unstable alveoli due to surfactant deficiency. The roentgenographic hallmark of RDS is a diffuse reticulogranular pattern (Fig. 39-4). This is the result of microatelectases interspersed with dilated air spaces. In more severe RDS a roentgenologic "white-out" may result from generalized atelectasis. A similar appearance may also result from sudden collapse of both lungs in babies who have been breathing high concentrations of oxygen, if they become apneic or develop airway obstruction.

Air leak

Extravasation of alveolar air is a frequent complication of ventilatory assistance for respiratory failure. The extravasated air travels from the alveolus, dissects through the interstitium of the lung, and enters the mediastinum. The air may then perforate the pleural space and result in a pneumothorax. Pneumopericardium and pneumoperitoneum are less common manifestations of extraventilatory air.

Pneumothorax in a newborn infant is usually readily recognizable when the gas in the pleural space clearly outlines the visceral pleura. In addition, there is usually considerable mediastinal shift toward the contralateral side and a varying amount of collapse of both lungs. Occasionally, even fairly large pneumothoraces may not be obvious. This is because the air in the supine neonate's thorax tends to assume a position anterior and

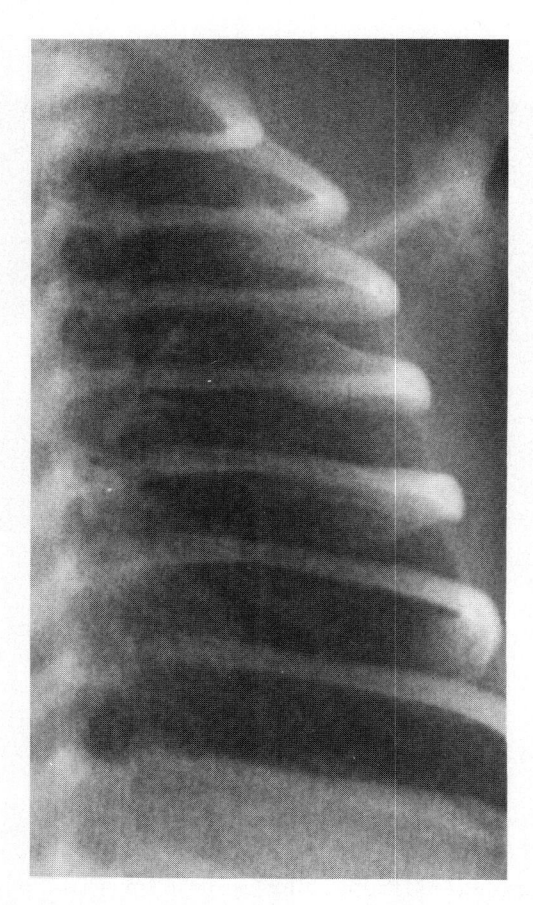

Fig. 39-4. Typical reticulogranular pattern of mild RDS.

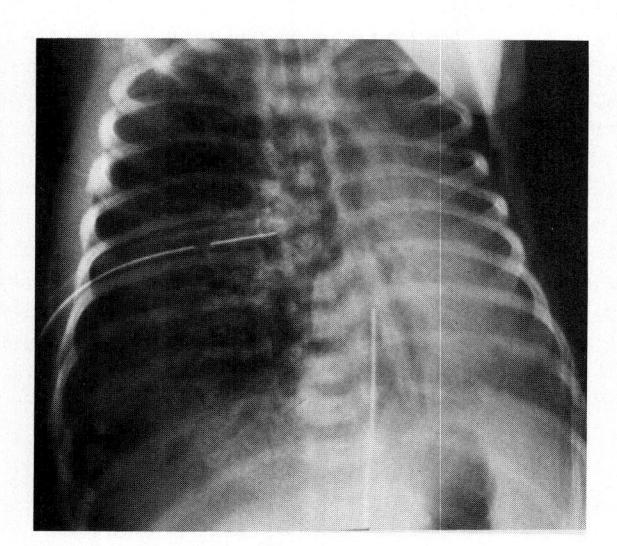

Fig. 39-5. Lateral decubitus film made with the left side down shows a residual right pneumothorax in spite of the presence of a chest tube. Part of the intrapleural gas also is trapped medial to the right lung. The increased right lung volume and streaky lucencies are caused by interstitial emphysema.

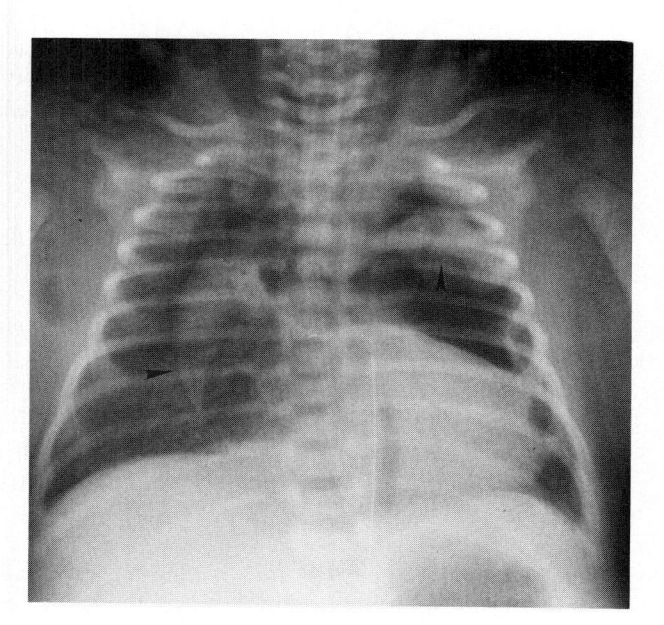

Fig. 39-6. Separation of the thymic lobes (arrowheads) from the pericardial surface due to a large pneumomediastinum. There is also a large amount of air in the neck and soft tissues of the chest wall, which occurs less commonly in the newborn than in the older child.

medial to the lung. The only sign may be enlargement and increased lucency of the affected hemithorax (Figs. 39-5 and 39-26). In this case a lateral decubitus film, made with the normal side dependent, will demonstrate air adjacent to the visceral pleura of the costal surface of the involved lung.

In pneumomediastinum a halo of air may be recognizable on either side of the mediastinum. The hallmark, however, is displacement of the thymus away from the parietal pericardium, the so-called spinnaker sail sign (Fig. 39-6). Air less commonly dissects into the soft tissues of the neck in neonates than it does when pneumomediastinum occurs in older infants and children. Unlike mediastinal emphysema, which is limited inferiorly by the central tendon of the diaphragm, a pneumopericardium completely surrounds the heart and origins of the great vessels.

Interstitial emphysema may be diffuse, bilateral, or localized to a single lung or lobe (Fig. 39-5). The interstitial gas appears as multiple well-defined circular or elongated lucencies contrasted against the collapsed lung parenchyma. In addition, there is a marked increase in volume of the involved portion of lung. Occasionally continued expansion of the interstitial gas collections results in localized pulmonary overdistension resembling congenital lobar emphysema.

Cardiovascular abnormalities
Congestive heart failure

Infants with congestive heart failure exhibit varying degrees of cardiomegaly as demonstrated on AP chest roentgenograms. In a mature infant the heart is considered to be enlarged when the cardiothymic-thoracic ratio is greater than 0.6. In preterm infants the normal ratio is smaller and cardiomegaly often less obvious. Pulmonary venous congestion is manifested by engorgement and increase in size of the pulmonary veins. As pulmonary venous pressure rises, interstitial edema occurs. This is observed as a decrease in the definition of the lung vasculature and by Kerley lines, which are produced by leakage of fluid into the interlobular septa. Kerley B-lines are seen as short horizontal linear densities in the lung extending to the pleural surface. They are typically found above the costophrenic angles but may be seen to better advantage, in infants, in the retrosternal portion of the lungs on lateral views. Kerley A-lines are longer linear densities radiating from the hila. Edema of the subpleural areolar tissue and pleural effusions are more easily seen in small infants than are Kerley lines (Fig. 39-7).

Extravasation of edema fluid into the air spaces results in more diffuse opacification of the lungs, typically involving the perihilar regions. Identical pulmonary

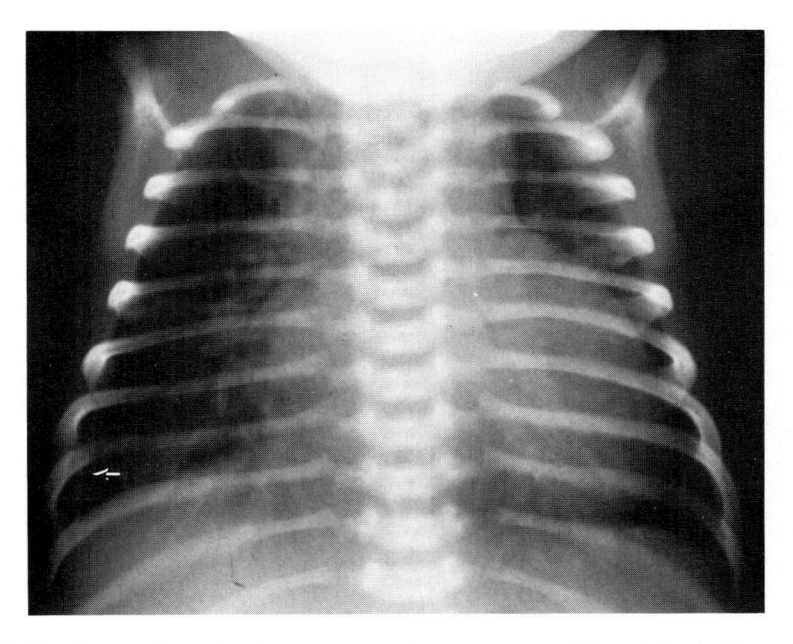

Fig. 39-7. Cardiomegaly and pulmonary vascular engorgement in an infant with coarctation of the aorta and a left-to-right interatrial shunt. Fluid adjacent to or within the minor fissures makes it appear "thickened," and there is a faint vertical density in the right costophrenic angle due to similar involvement of the inferior portion of the major fissure *(arrowhead).*

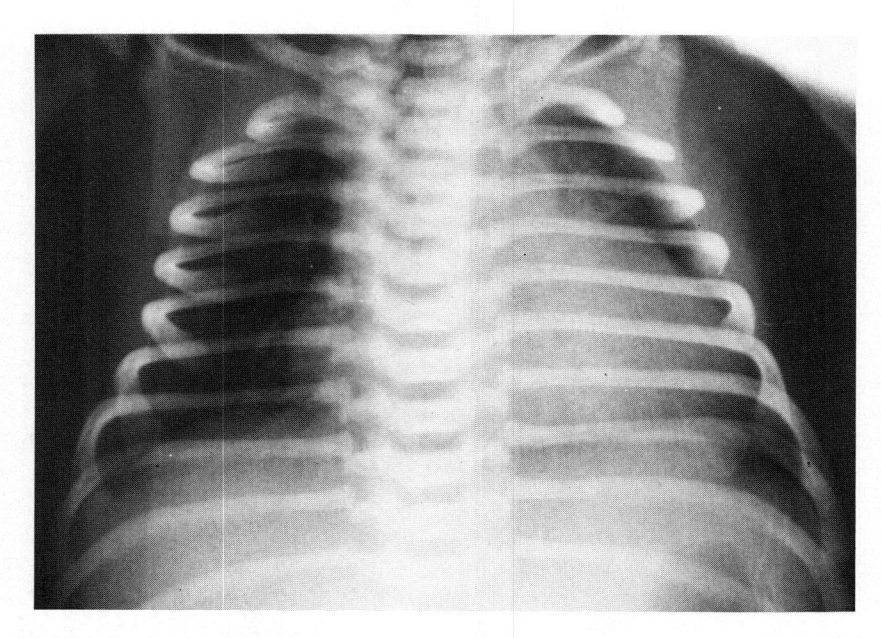

Fig. 39-8. Marked enlargement of the cardiothymic silhouette and diminished caliber of the pulmonary vessels in a patient with the syndrome of persistent fetal circulation, simulating cyanotic congenital heart disease.

changes without cardiomegaly can be observed during resolution of normal alveolar lung liquid.

Left-to-right shunts

An increase in caliber of the pulmonary arteries can be detected when there is a moderate increase in blood flow to the lungs through a left-to-right shunt. The size of the hila as well as the intrapulmonary vessels is increased, and the main pulmonary artery is frequently enlarged. Enlargement of tiny peripheral vessels results in a reticular appearance that superficially resembles interstitial edema. Frank pulmonary edema may then occur due to overload of the pulmonary circulation. This event occurs rapidly in preterm infants with persistent patent ductus arteriosus.

Cyanotic congenital heart disease

The size of the heart may range from relatively normal, as in transposition of the great arteries, to huge, as in Ebstein's anomaly. In most cases the caliber of the pulmonary vessels is reduced. The hila are consequently small and the lungs appear relatively lucent. Also, the thymus tends to be involuted due to stress, and the lungs are often hyperinflated. Pulmonary vascular engorgement, rather than oligemia, accompanies cyanosis in patients with d-transposition of the great arteries due to incomplete mixing of systemic and pulmonary blood. Cyanosis with congestive heart failure and roentgenographic signs of pulmonary edema with a relatively small cardiothymic silhouette suggests the diagnosis of sub-diaphragmatic total anomalous pulmonary venous drainage.

Persistence of the fetal circulation may also, on occasion, mimic cyanotic congenital heart disease on chest roentgenograms, since there may be cardiomegaly and pulmonary oligemia (Fig. 39-8). In other cases congestive heart failure or pulmonary disease may also be present.

GASTROINTESTINAL TRACT

Roentgenologic evaluation of the gastrointestinal tract has become more common, particularly in premature infants, because of the emergence of necrotizing enterocolitis as a serious source of morbidity and mortality. Acute surgical emergencies constitute another major group of disorders that require roentgenologic diagnosis (Figs. 39-9 to 39-13). In addition, roentgenograms taken to localize umbilical catheters have provided incidental experience with the normal plain film appearance of the gut.

Methods of examination

Initial plain film examination usually consists of an AP supine film made with a vertical beam and includes both the chest and the abdomen. As with chest roentgenography, additional lateral and decubitus views are made with a horizontally directed x-ray beam. These films can be made without removing the infant from the incubator and allow visualization of air-fluid levels and permit more precise demonstration of free intraperitoneal air (Fig. 39-

Diagnostic radiology 1071

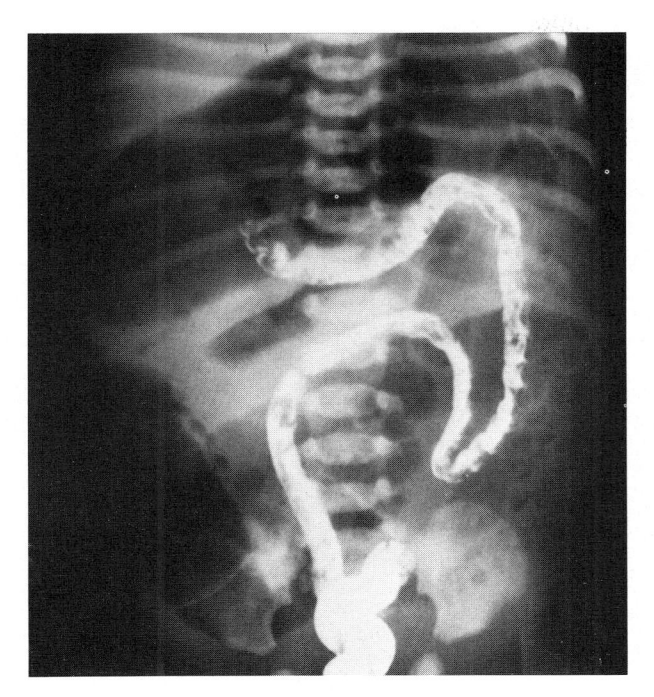

Fig. 39-9. AP recumbent film of the abdomen in an infant with meconium ileus. Note the distended bowel loops of varying sizes, and the bubbly appearance of the intestinal contents, particularly in the left flank (compare with Fig. 39-15). The distal ileal obstruction is reflected by the marked diminution in caliber of the colon (microcolon).

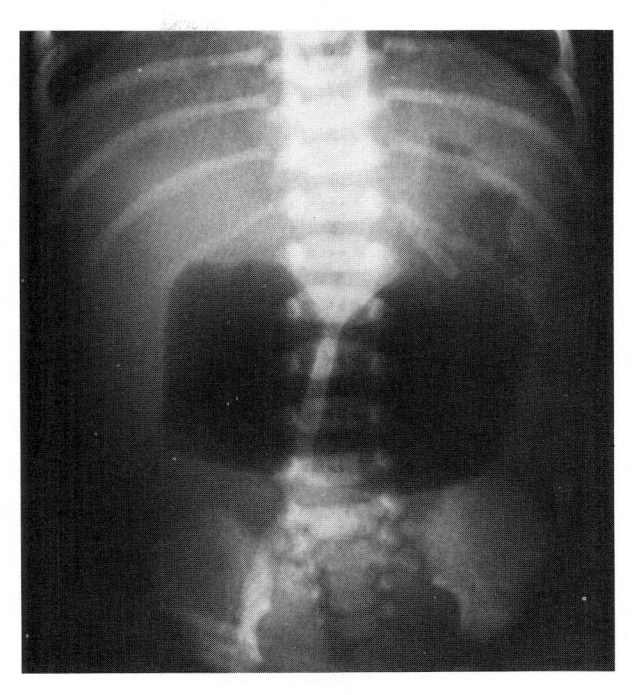

Fig. 39-10. AP recumbent film of the abdomen demonstrating the "double-bubble" due to gaseous distension of the stomach and first portion of the duodenum caused by duodenal atresia. Note the complete absence of gas distal to the duodenum.

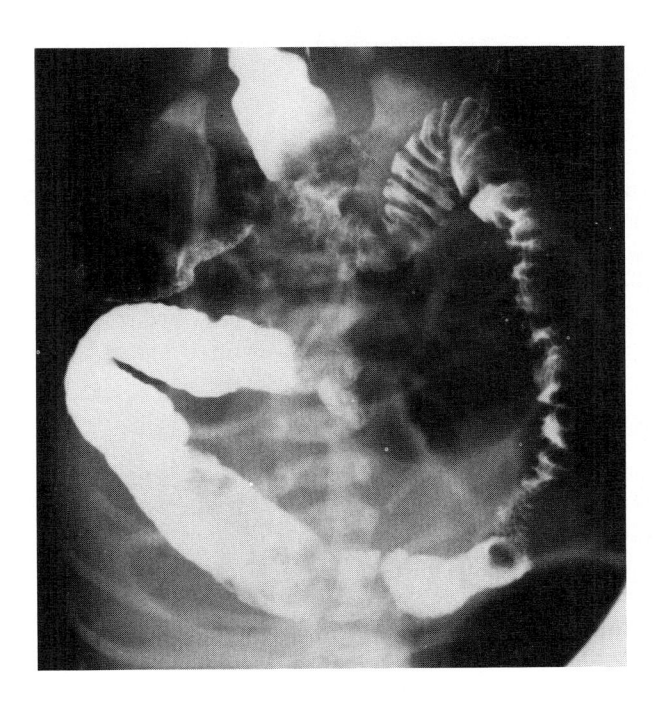

Fig. 39-11. Barium enema demonstrates an abnormally high and medially positioned cecum in a patient with small intestinal obstruction due to malrotation and midgut volvulus.

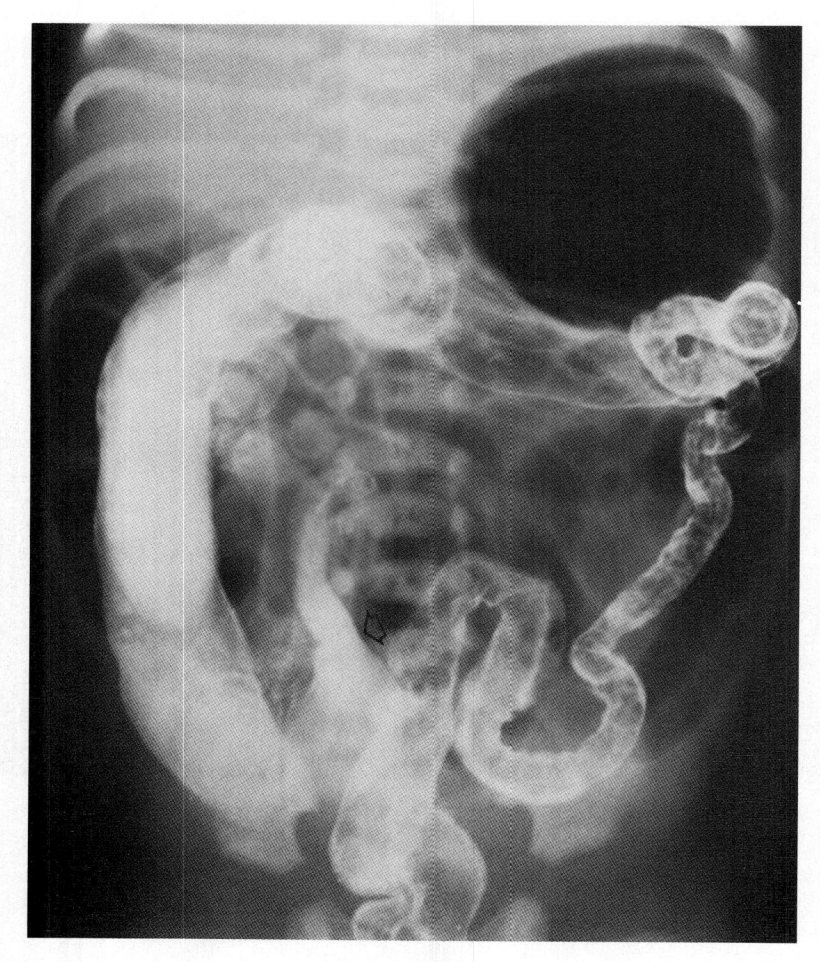

Fig. 39-12. Barium enema demonstrates decreased caliber of the left side of the colon with an apparent transition zone at the splenic flexure. The bowel contains a moderate amount of meconium. Besides Hirschsprung's disease, these findings can occur in infants of diabetic mothers with the neonatal small left colon syndrome and in meconium plug syndrome. Note the large "fetal" appendix.

14). A horizontal beam lateral view of the abdomen with the infant prone is an aid in demonstrating gas in the rectum and sigmoid colon when obstruction is suspected. Roentgenograms made with the infant erect or inverted are not recommended, since they are stressful to the patient and present considerable technical difficulties.

Contrast media

Air is a very satisfactory contrast medium that frequently can be used to demonstrate the site of bowel obstruction. When it is necessary to opacify the stomach or bowel, barium sulfate is usually the medium of choice, since it is relatively inert. On the other hand, water-soluble, iodine-containing contrast media are useful when perforation of the gut is suspected, since they are readily absorbed from the peritoneal surface.

The most frequently used water-soluble contrast medium is Gastrografin, a 76% solution of sodium methyl-glucamine diatrizoate containing 37% bound iodine. The major disadvantage of this product is its high osmolarity (1,900 mOsm/L), which causes a shift of water and electrolytes into the lumen of the bowel. Furthermore, absorption occurs through the bowel wall, enhancing the resultant systemic dehydration. These problems can be avoided by using these substances in isotonic solution (1:5 dilution), at which they remain radiopaque, or by maintaining hydration of the infant by means of intravenous infusions. Nonionic contrast agents are currently being developed that should improve safety. Unfortunately, they are costly and have not yet been approved for general use.

Another problem with water-soluble contrast media is possible mucosal damage of the intact bowel, especially if

Diagnostic radiology **1073**

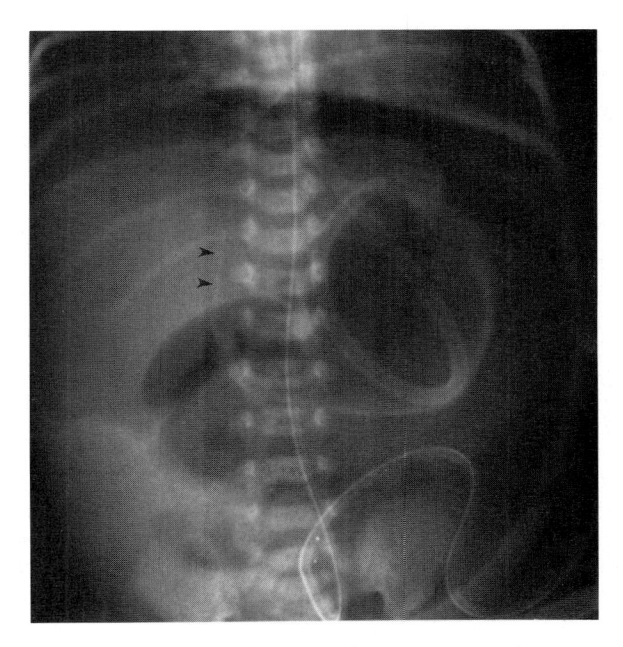

Fig. 39-13. AP recumbent film of the abdomen demonstrates a large pneumoperitoneum, with free air inferior to the diaphragm and outlining the falciform ligament *(arrowheads)*.

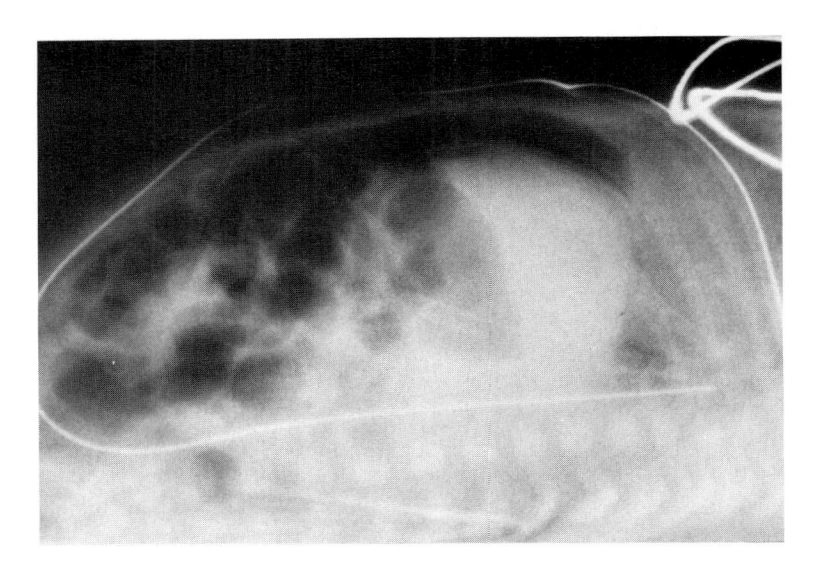

Fig. 39-14. Horizontal-beam lateral view of the abdomen made with the infant supine demonstrates intraperitoneal gas anterior to the liver and adjacent to the anterior abdominal wall. Several examples of the double-wall sign, with the inner wall of the bowel outlined by intraluminal air and the outer wall outlined by intraperitoneal air, also are visible anteriorly. There is no intraperitoneal air fluid level to suggest peritonitis.

the bowel is overdistended with the contrast media. In addition, further compromise of an already tenuous mesenteric vascular supply may occur in the distended loops proximal to a bowel obstruction. Water-soluble media also may produce pulmonary edema if aspirated into the lungs.

Water-soluble contrast media are indicated for therapeutic enemas done to relieve meconium plugs or meconium ileus. For these purposes they are usually used in higher concentrations than for diagnosis. The therapeutic benefits are due to osmosis of water into the lumen of the bowel and resultant softening of the meconium as well as the surface-active properties of Tween 80. This polysorbate wetting agent and emulsifier is contained in Gastrografin in a 0.1% concentration. Other similar substances, such as Hypaque and Renografin also have been used therapeutically, although these do not contain Tween 80.

Contrast enemas must be carried out under fluoroscopic control in the radiology department. Upper gastrointestinal studies also are preferably done fluoroscopically, but if this is contraindicated because of the clinical condition of the infant, the contrast medium can be monitored during its course through the gastrointestinal tract using portable roentgenologic equipment. The opaque media may be fed from a bottle or administered through a nasogastric tube after removal of residual gastric contents.

Opaque enemas in newborn infants are done using a flexible infant feeding tube that is taped in place. Inflation of a balloon catheter in the rectum should be avoided because of the risk of perforation. Preparation of the bowel often is not necessary and is especially contraindicated when there is suspicion of Hirschsprung's disease.

Normal findings

Air is swallowed immediately after birth and reaches the small bowel at about 3 hours of postnatal life. After approximately 6 to 8 hours of age, gas is present throughout the large and small bowel, although rectal gas may not be visible if the bladder is distended. Mild generalized gaseous distension often occurs due to air-swallowing.

Newborn infants present a special diagnostic problem because of the similarity in appearance and caliber of the large and small bowel. However, the colon sometimes can be distinguished by its anatomic position and the presence of haustra. These features are established by 20 weeks of gestation.

The liver often appears prominent in normal infants, and roentgenograms are not an accurate index of hepatomegaly. On roentgenograms taken with the infant supine, the spleen is usually obscured by overlying gas in the stomach and splenic flexure.

Intestinal distension and obstruction

An increase in the amount of intestinal gas does not necessarily indicate obstruction, since it may occur in a variety of conditions, including tracheoesophageal fistula, necrotizing enterolitis, maternal drug therapy, hypothyroidism, septicemia, and hypermagnesemia. In these disorders the gas is distributed throughout the small and large bowel. Obstruction also may be mimicked by excess air-swallowing due to respiratory distress. Furthermore, as in mechanical obstruction, air-fluid levels may be present.

Mechanical bowel obstruction produces gaseous intestinal distension, and air-fluid levels are seen proximal to the site of obstruction. Distal to the obstruction the intraluminal gas may be diminished or absent. A different pattern is often seen, however, in obstruction due to meconium ileus. In this disorder the bowel loops vary in size, are unevenly distributed, and contain few air-fluid levels. The inspissated meconium in the small bowel becomes mixed with air, producing a bubbly appearance (Fig. 39-9).

Duodenal obstruction is usually easily recognizable on plain films because of distension of the stomach and duodenal bulb, which produces the classic "double-bubble" appearance. These structures often contain air-fluid levels, and the amount of gas distal to the obstruction varies with the degree of obstruction. The most common entities that produce this finding are duodenal stenosis or atresia, annular pancreas, and malrotation with peritoneal bands and/or midgut volvulus (Fig. 39-10).

Contrast examinations are often indicated when duodenal obstruction is suspected clinically or is demonstrated on plain films. These studies are particularly urgent because of the importance of recognition and prompt surgical treatment of midgut volvulus with associated mesenteric vascular insufficiency. When the degree of obstruction appears to be incomplete, the volvulus can be diagnosed by introducing barium into the stomach. If there is an associated malrotation of the midgut, the duodenojejunal junction is displaced medially and inferiorly from its normal position in the left upper abdominal quadrant, and the duodenum has a typical corkscrew configuration. When the obstruction is complete, an opaque study of the upper gastrointestinal tract will not add to the information provided by the air within the stomach and duodenum. Under these circumstances, evidence of malrotation can be obtained by a barium enema, which will demonstrate the cecum in an unusually superior or medial position (Fig. 39-11). The cecum may also be abnormally mobile. If there is nonrotation of the bowel, the cecum and entire colon are seen to the left of the midline.

The caliber of the colon is another important observation made on contrast enemas. A ribbonlike microcolon occurs when there is lack of normal distension by intestinal contents due to exclusion of succus entericus from the colon during fetal life (Fig. 39-9). The diminished colonic caliber usually indicates some type of distal ileal obstruction such as meconium ileus or ileal atresia. On the other hand, the caliber of the colon is predicted to be normal in the presence of duodenal or high jejunal obstruction.

Exceptions to this rule may occur, however. If the distal ileal atresia occurs late in fetal life, the caliber of the colon may be normal. On the other hand, the caliber of the colon is decreased in nearly 40% of patients with total colonic aganglionosis, presumably due to functional small intestine obstruction. We have also noted decreased colonic caliber premature infants with duodenal obstruction alone. Localized decrease in caliber of the left colon occurs in Hirschsprung's disease, meconium plug syndrome, and the neonatal small left colon syndrome (Fig. 39-12).

Pneumoperitoneum

Early diagnosis of pneumoperitoneum often depends on its recognition on routine AP supine views. Since the air rises anteriorly, a lucency will be seen overlying the liver adjacent to the inferior surface of the diaphragm. A large collection of air causes generalized abdominal distension, and structures not usually visible, such as the falciform ligament, umbilical vein, or a persistent urachus, may be outlined by the air (Fig. 39-13). Perhaps the most valuable indicator of small amounts of free air is the double-wall sign, in which the mucosal surface of the bowel is outlined by intraluminal air and the serosal surface by intraperitoneal air. The intraperitoneal air is best demonstrated on films made with a horizontal beam in supine or decubitus positions, which show collections of gas adjacent to the anterior abdominal wall or flanks (Fig. 39-14).

Although the most important cause of pneumoperitoneum is perforation of the bowel, the possibility of extension of gas from a pneumomediastinum into the peritoneal cavity must be considered in infants with respiratory distress. An air-fluid level in the peritoneal cavity almost certainly indicates bowel perforation, but absence of an air-fluid level is not a completely reliable sign of an intact gastrointestinal tract. The presence of perforation can be demonstrated by instilling a small amount of water-soluble contrast medium through a nasogastric tube and observing its passage into the peritoneal cavity.

Pneumatosis intestinalis

The most common etiology of pneumatosis intestinalis is necrotizing enterocolitis, although bowel ischemia secondary to intestinal obstruction is also an occasional cause. The intramural gas that collects beneath the serosa or in the submucosa of the intestine may be either localized or diffusely distributed throughout the bowel

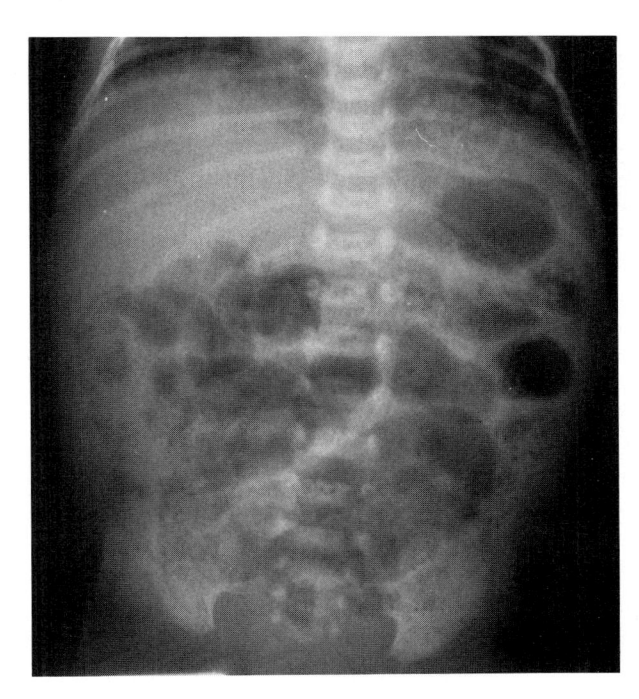

Fig. 39-15. Numerous linear and bubbly lucencies caused by intramural gas associated with necrotizing enterocolitis. The bubbly pattern is difficult to distinguish from the intraluminal bubbles shown in Fig. 39-8.

and appears as small linear or bubbly lucencies (Fig. 39-15). In patients with necrotizing enterocolitis, intestinal distension with air-fluid levels, portal venous gas, inflammatory masses, pneumoperitoneum, or intraperitoneal fluid also may be present.

Intravascular gas

In necrotizing enterocolitis the intramural gas may dissect into the portal venous system and is seen radiating into the liver from the hilus. In the absence of necrotizing enterocolitis, portal vein gas also may be introduced through umbilical venous catheters.

Pulmonary gas embolism is another cause of intravascular gas and is unrelated to gastrointestinal disease. The embolism occurs when alveolar gas ruptures into the pulmonary vascular bed. The gas is then rapidly distributed throughout the systemic vessels, usually resulting in sudden death. The gas is often particularly prominent within the hepatic veins. The roentgenologic findings may be mimicked by postmortem accumulations of gas.

Decreased intraabdominal gas

Since most intestinal gas is produced by ingested air, any mechanism that reduces the infant's ability to swallow causes diminished bowel gas. Thus a reduction in the amount of bowel gas may occur due to central nervous system depression and can indicate deterioration of the infant's condition. Pharyngeal obstruction due to an orotracheal tube has a similar effect. If the swallowed gas contains a high concentration of oxygen, it can be absorbed very rapidly. Curariform drugs are a more recently observed iatrogenic cause of gasless abdomen. Gas also may be expelled by severe vomiting and diarrhea.

Bowel gas is also absent in esophageal atresia without distal tracheoesophageal fistula. In diaphragmatic hernias the intestinal gas is contained within the thorax, and the abdomen is markedly scaphoid.

Ascites

Neonatal ascites is often associated with intrauterine perforation of the bowel. Other causes include obstruction of the portal circulation, urine ascites associated with anomalies of the lower urinary tract, chylous ascites, erythroblastosis, and intrauterine infections such as syphilis. Massive neonatal ascites is accompanied by a relatively gasless abdomen, which is also markedly distended (Fig. 39-16). If any gas-containing loops of bowel are present, they tend to be localized centrally within the abdomen. Separation of the right lateral border of the liver from the adjacent abdominal wall is a helpful sign that can be frequently observed in infants. This has been ascribed to a relatively greater radiodensity of the liver as compared with that of the intraperitoneal fluid. This difference in densities can be enhanced by total body opacification. The presence of even small amounts of intraperitoneal fluid can be well demonstrated by ultrasonography.

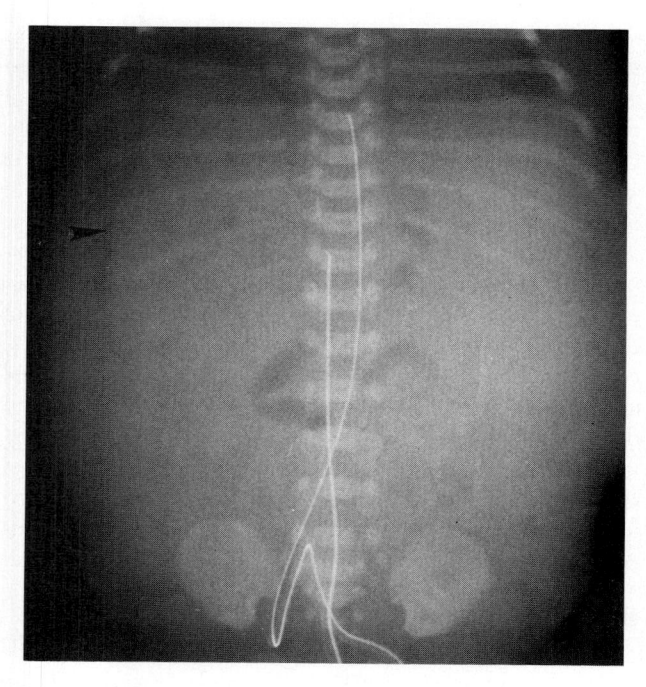

Fig. 39-16. Massive neonatal ascites associated with erythroblastosis. The abdomen is distended and contains little intestinal gas. The lateral liver edge (*arrowhead;* retouched) could be readily seen on the original film because of the difference in radiodensities of the liver and ascitic fluid. An umbilical venous catheter is present. The umbilical arterial catheter is to the left of the midline, extending to the level of T8.

Intraabdominal calcifications

In the fetus and the newborn, intraabdominal calcifications can occur within a few days. Calcifications of the peritoneum, intestinal wall, or even intraluminal contents are occasional but important clues to intestinal disorders.

The most frequently recognized calcifications involve the peritoneum and are caused by sterile meconium peritonitis due to intrauterine bowel perforation associated with meconium ileus or vascular occlusion. The calcifications are usually streaky or plaquelike and often occur over the liver, abdominal surface of the diaphragm, or along the flanks (Fig. 39-17).

Calcifications of intraluminal meconium appear as small rounded densities that follow the course of the small or large bowel. Within the colon they have been seen in association with imperforate anus. Small intestinal calcifications have been documented in cases of ileal stenosis, atresia, and total colonic aganglionosis. Rarely, calcification of the bowel wall may occur in patients with intestinal volvulus or atresia. Neuroblastomas commonly

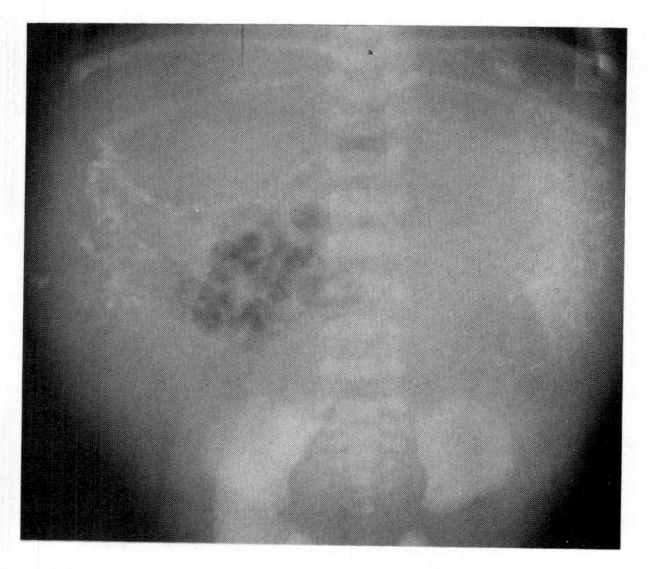

Fig. 39-17. Ascites and peritoneal calcification due to meconium peritonitis.

contain calcium, and intrahepatic calcifications have been observed in the neonate due to transplacental infections and neoplastic lesions.

THE URINARY TRACT

A number of roentgenologic examinations are used to image the urinary tract and retroperitoneum. Selection of the most effective diagnostic modality and the sequence in which it may optimally be employed requires individual consideration of each case and a close dialogue between the referring physician and the radiologist. In this section we outline some of the important indications and diagnostic signs pertaining to the various examinations.

Traditionally the excretory urogram has been the primary mode of examination of the urinary tract. More recently, ultrasound has been recognized as an effective diagnostic tool. Under many circumstances, particularly when anatomic information is required, sonographic examination is now the method of choice. In comparison with sonography, which is noninvasive, computed tomography gives similar but slightly more detailed images, although this is achieved at a higher cost and radiation dosage. The relatively long exposures required, however, make it less practical for use in the neonate. Additional information can be derived from inferior vena cavography. This examination can be carried out prior to urography by injection of contrast medium through a superficial vein in the foot and is particularly useful in the delineation of right-sided abdominal masses. Umbilical aortography is used to delineate the renal arteries as an aid in the diagnosis of absence or hypoplasia of the kidneys. This technique also produces renal parenchymal opacification independent of renal function. Radioisotope renograms are more valuable indicators of renal function than of renal structure. The lower urinary tract and vesicoureteral reflux are best evaluated by means of voiding cystourethrography. Micturating radionuclide studies also are used to identify vesicoureteral reflux.

Excretory urography

The excretory urogram permits assessment of renal function as well as visualization of the morphology of the entire urinary tract and contiguous structures. Thus it provides much more information than is suggested by the commonly used term *intravenous pyelogram*. The urogram must be tailored to individual clinical requirements rather than being done in a routine fashion, particularly with regard to timing of exposures and special views.

There are a number of physiologic differences between the newborn and the older infant that make urography more difficult in the early neonatal period. Because of the relatively large extracellular volume of the newborn, diffusion of contrast medium in plasma is reduced. Plasma flow to the kidneys, glomerular filtration rates, and tubular concentration also are relatively diminished at this age in comparison with later life. As a result, the concentration of contrast medium in the kidney is poor, and maximum opacification is delayed. For these reasons, elective urography should be deferred until after the first month of life. This attitude would particularly affect patients requiring urography because of disorders that are accompanied by a high incidence of minor congenital urinary tract abnormalities.

The contrast media used for excretory urography are 50% to 60% aqueous solutions of sodium or meglumine diatrizoate or meglumine iothalamate containing bound iodine. They have an osmolarity of up to 1,700 mOsm/L. The usual intravenous dosage in the neonate is 2 to 4 ml/kg.

Since reactions to contrast media are rare in newborn infants, contraindications to urography are few. Pulmonary edema, however, has been observed following a bolus injection of relatively high doses of opaque media. In addition, fluids should not be restricted before examination because of the possibility of promoting dehydration due to the high osmolarity of the water-soluble contrast media.

The preliminary abdominal film is an essential part of the examination, and optimum technique is mandatory. The outlines of the kidneys are often poorly visualized on this film because of overlying bowel gas and sparse retroperitoneal fat. Masses or renal enlargement may be indirectly demonstrated by displacement of adjacent gas-filled bowel loops. Absence or malposition of the kidney may sometimes be recognized by medial displacement of the splenic or hepatic flexures into the unoccupied renal fossae. Intraperitoneal fluid due to urinary ascites may increase the roentgenographic density of the abdomen. Calcifications are best seen on films made with relatively low kilovoltages.

A roentgenogram obtained immediately after injection of contrast medium allows observation of opacified abdominal viscera other than the kidneys because of the phenomenon of total body opacification. This technique is very useful in assessing the location and morphology of abdominal masses. Total body opacification occurs when the intravenous contrast material is distributed through the intravascular and extravascular compartments. Abdominal organs become more dense because of their relatively high blood flow, whereas avascular masses, such as cysts, are relatively lucent (Fig. 39-18). For the same reason, central necrosis or hemorrhage within a tumor will appear relatively radiolucent in contrast to its opacified rim. The nephrogram, seen early in the course of the urogram, is produced by contrast that has undergone glomerular filtration and is being concentrated within

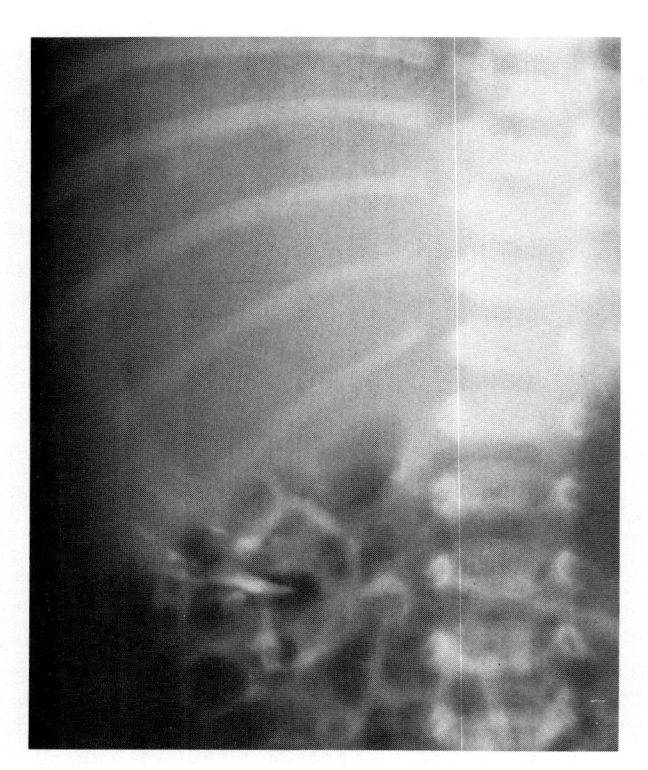

Fig. 39-18. Supine film of the right upper quadrant of the abdomen obtained soon after injection of contrast medium shows a lucent suprarenal mass caused by an adrenal abscess bordered by relatively well-opacified adrenal and liver tissue. Note that the total body opacification phase has persisted into the pyelographic phase of the excretory urogram. The mass is displacing the right kidney inferiorly, but the collecting system is intact and renal function is normal.

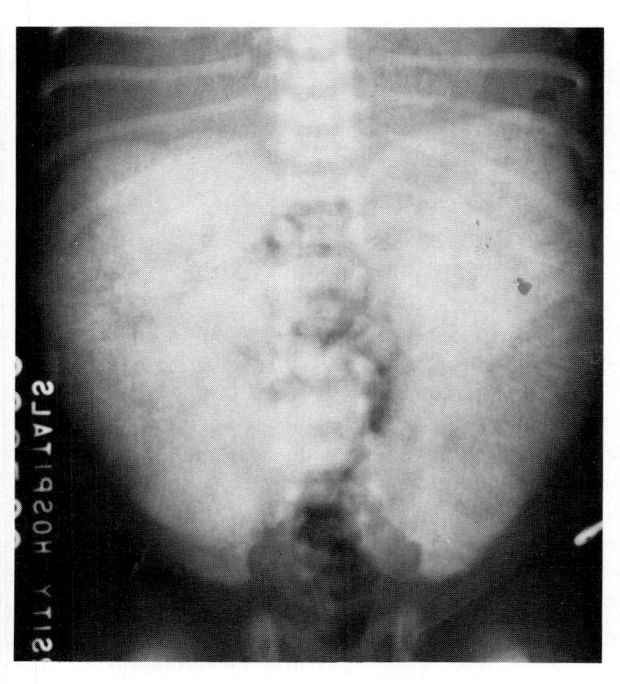

Fig. 39-19. Film of the abdomen 1 hour after contrast administration demonstrates marked bilateral nephromegaly and a prolonged, dense nephrographic phase due to infantile polycystic disease. The mottled streaky appearance is caused by stasis of contrast in dilated collecting tubules.

the renal tubules by tubular reabsorption of water. The pyelographic phase of the urogram frequently occurs while a nephrogram is still present. As a result, a film obtained 5 to 6 minutes after injection often will demonstrate the nephrographic and pyelographic features of the kidneys as well as the ureters and bladder. In normal patients, further filming often is unnecessary, and the examination can be completed in a short time with minimal radiation exposure.

Air-swallowing in an infant often results in abundant intestinal gas that can obscure the renal outlines. When this occurs, a prone film is often helpful. Also, with the patient prone the application of a balloon compression device to the anterior abdominal wall allows better visualization by displacement of the bowel loops. This technique should be avoided when masses are suspected. Routine ureteral compression is not used. Occasionally, oblique or lateral projections also are helpful, and increased distension of the ureters may be obtained and films made after the patient has been held upright for a short time.

Several features are unique to normal neonatal kidneys. The kidneys are more vertically oriented than in the older child and are relatively large. Their length spans approximately 5 vertebral bodies. There may be residual fetal lobulation of the renal margins, and there is a large amount of renal parenchyma with respect to the size of the pelvicalyceal complex.

Poor visualization of one or both kidneys with a delay in appearance of the nephrogram and pyelogram can result from abnormalities of the renal veins, arteries, parenchyma, or collecting system. Roentgenologic visualization of the kidneys may require serial roentgenograms taken over a period of hours or sometimes days. In dehydrated, oliguric infants, bilaterally prolonged dense nephrograms with normal renal collecting systems may be produced by tubular obstruction with Tamm-Horsfall protein. A strikingly dense, prolonged nephrogram occurs in infantile polycystic disease (Fig. 39-19). Typically, both kidneys are markedly enlarged, and the nephrogram has a striated appearance due to stasis of contrast in the dilated tubules. Unilateral delay in

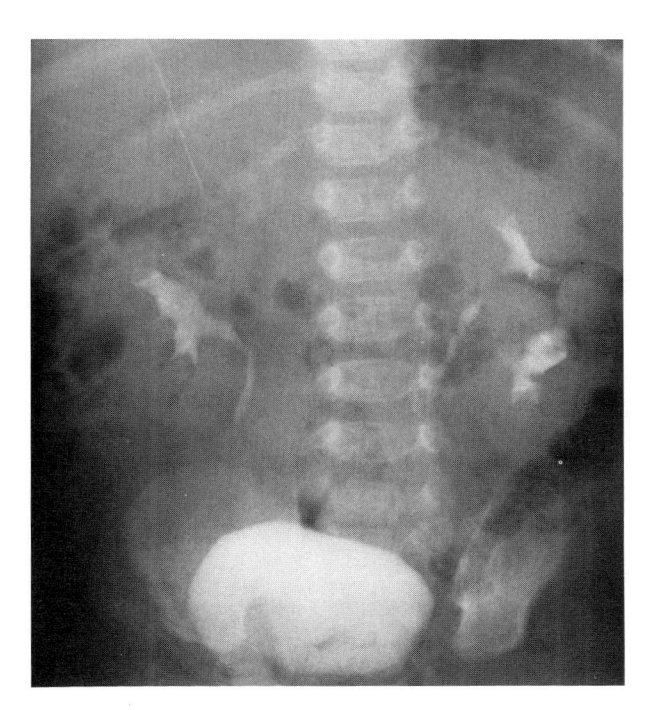

Fig. 39-20. Absence of opacification of the upper portion of the right renal collecting system due to obstruction of the superior moiety of a duplex collecting system associated with an ectopic ureterocele (not visible). The collecting system appears incomplete. Note that the left collecting system also is duplicated without obstruction (compare with Fig. 39-18).

appearance and prolongation of the nephrogram may occur with renal vein thrombosis. In this case the kidney is usually enlarged. Prolongation of the nephrogram also may occur secondary to obstruction of the renal pelvis or the ureter. In these patients the delayed opacification of the collecting system may be preceded by the appearance of calyceal "crescents." These are due to stasis of contrast medium within the collecting tubules that are aligned parallel to the dilated calyces. The crescents are seen in contrast to the relatively radiolucent urine-containing calyces.

As the contrast material slowly filters into the collecting system, there is progressive opacification of the dilated renal calyces, pelvis, and ureter. In obstruction, sufficient opacification eventually may occur to enable identification of its location. Unilateral obstructions occur at the pelviureteric junction or, as with ectopic ureteroceles, at the ureterovesical junction. Bilateral hydronephrosis and hydroureter suggests distal obstruction such as that which occurs in males with posterior urethral valves. Dilatation of the collecting systems or ureters also can occur in the absence of an obstructive lesion due to chronic prenatal or postnatal vesicoureteral reflux. Atrophy of the renal parenchyma may accompany chronic reflux or obstruction.

If the kidney is displaced by an extrarenal mass, alteration of the orientation of the kidney is a guide to the site of origin of the mass, since retroperitoneal lesions displace the kidney according to their vector force. A suprarenal mass will displace the kidney inferiorly and its superior pole laterally, causing a characteristic "drooping lily" appearance (Fig. 39-18). This is not specific and can be seen with adrenal hemorrhage, abscess, and tumor. An obstructed superior moiety of a duplex collecting system may mimic a suprarenal mass. In this case the visualized collecting system of the functioning portion of the kidney appears incomplete (Fig. 39-20). Even intraperitoneal masses, if large enough, may displace the kidney. Renal function is usually normal in the presence of extrinsic masses.

Intrarenal mass lesions cause either focal or diffuse enlargement of the kidney with severe distortion or obstruction of the collecting system. These lesions also may interfere with renal function.

Voiding cystourethrography

In neonates, voiding cystourethrography is useful in the evaluation of vesicoureteral reflux, suspected anatomic abnormalities of the male urethra, ambiguous genitalia, and anorectal malformations.

A small plastic feeding tube serves as an ideal catheter. The water-soluble contrast medium is instilled with a syringe or as a drip infusion. The bladder is filled until the patient voids, during which rapid serial imaging is carried out. A steep oblique position is necessary for visualization of the bladder neck and the entire length of the urethra (Fig. 39-21).

Normally the contour of the bladder is symmetrical and smooth. Slight irregularity appears during voiding. Trabeculation and diverticula suggest outlet obstruction or neurogenic bladder. An ectopic ureterocele may cause a smooth, rounded intraluminal filling defect. This may be missed if the contrast medium is too dense.

Roentgenographic evaluation of the urethra in females is usually unrewarding. During micturition, contrast medium normally may reflux into the vagina. Roentgenographic evaluation of the male urethra, however, is essential to demonstrate anatomic abnormalities such as posterior ureteral valves.

The presence or absence of vesicoureteral reflux is an extremely important observation. Since reflux may be identified only during voiding, careful filming must be carried out during this time. Vesicoureteral reflux also allows morphologic assessment of the ureters and collect-

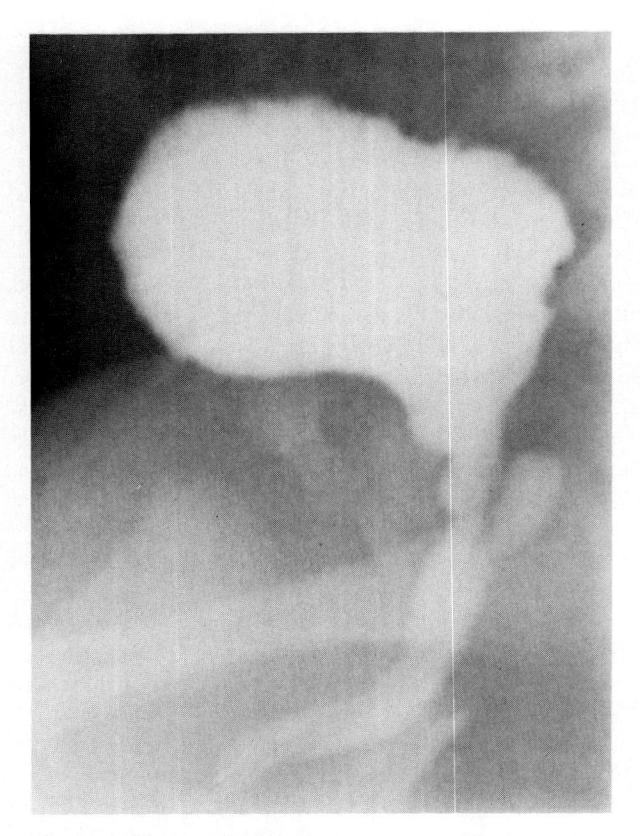

Fig. 39-21. Cystourethrogram done for evaluation of ambiguous genitalia shows a short penile urethra and demonstrates a prostatic utricle, which is prevalent in males with hypospadias. Note the normal irregularity of the dome of the partially emptied bladder.

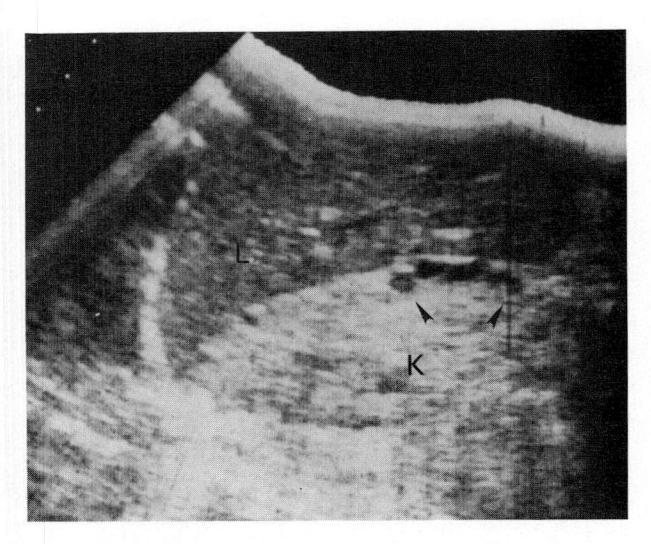

Fig. 39-22. Sagittal supine sonogram in the plane of the right kidney in a patient with typical sonographic findings of infantile polycystic kidney disease. The kidney *(K)* is seen posterior to the liver *(L)* and demonstrates increased echogenicity relative to the liver, multiple cortical cysts *(arrowheads)*, and no demonstrable pelvicalyceal complex.

ing systems in infants with reduced or absent renal function.

Ultrasonography

Ultrasonography is a valuable diagnostic modality for all pediatric patients because of the characteristic interactions of high-frequency sound waves with cystic, solid, and complex tissue (Chapter 8). It is especially useful in neonates, since the majority of abnormalities that occur at this age are cystic in nature. Sonographic demonstration of urinary tract structures also is independent of renal function, and therefore it is an especially useful tool in the evaluation of the genitourinary system in newborn infants (Fig. 39-22). This method of examination is emerging as an important screening procedure because of its versatility, safety, and accuracy. The use of grayscale and high-resolution focused transducers has resulted in greatly improved diagnostic accuracy. Dynamic changes in organs and vascular structures may be assessed using real-time ultrasound equipment.

The technique of sonographic examination and a discussion of physical properties of the equipment that must be adjusted individually to each patient are beyond the scope of this text but are extremely important for accurate diagnosis. It should be emphasized that the sonographic findings must be evaluated in conjunction with all available clinical information and any previous diagnostic study to date.

Ultrasonography is useful in the diagnosis of the majority of suspected retroperitoneal disorders in neonates. Alterations in position and shape of the kidney as well as abnormalities of the parenchyma or collecting systems can be readily evaluated. In addition, a dilated ureter can be followed to its point of obstruction. The exact relationship of juxtarenal masses to the kidney can be determined, and abnormal calcifications can be identified. Important vascular structures, including the inferior vena cava, also can be readily evaluated.

Pelvic anatomy also is easily evaluated using the bladder as a sonographic window. Cystic or solid masses and their relationship to the bladder and adjacent organs can be demonstrated. The internal genitalia also can be evaluated in patients with ambiguous genitalia.

SKELETAL SYSTEM

No attempt is made to describe all of the numerous bone abnormalities that can exist in the neonate. However, important observations can be made from the bones visible on films of the chest and abdomen, which reflect physiologic and pathologic changes.

The bones of a gestationally mature infant are normally

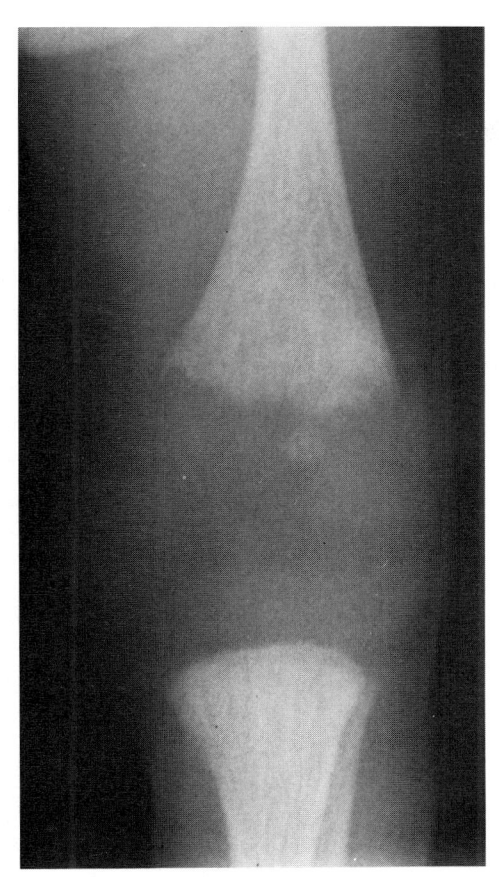

Fig. 39-23. Radiograph of the knee of a full-term infant was prompted by suspicious findings in the proximal humeri on the chest film. There are numerous vertical metaphyseal striations due to intrauterine rubella infection. Note the delayed ossification of the epiphyses.

dense. During the first 4 to 6 weeks of life this density diminishes as bone growth accelerates. By approximately 2 months of age, physiologic periosteal new bone formation may be seen along the shafts of long bones in rapidly growing healthy infants. This usually can be differentiated from abnormal periosteal reaction by its symmetry and lack of underlying osseous lesions. In contrast, the bones of the premature infant appear less well mineralized than normal, and the cortices are relatively thin.

On roentgenograms of the chest and abdomen the proximal metaphyses of the humeri or femurs almost always are visible. Abnormalities of these bony structures may reflect either intrauterine or postnatal disorders.

Antenatal disorders

Intrauterine infections frequently cause metaphyseal abnormalities. In rubella and cytomegalovirus infections the metaphyses typically are rarefied and contain dense, vertical striations that resemble a celery stalk (Fig. 39-23). Syphilis also causes metaphyseal irregularity, proximal to which is a zone of radiolucency. Intrauterine insults, such as meconium peritonitis, produce a horizontal band of increased density in the metaphysis due to growth arrest.

Postnatal disorders

Osteomyelitis in the newborn is usually due to *Staphylococcus*, *Streptococcus*, or *Candida organisms*. These organisms produce focal lucent metaphyseal areas of bone destruction with or without associated septic arthritis. These lesions may be silent and found incidentally on films done for other purposes. Since they are often multifocal, a complete skeletal survey should be done when one lesion is discovered.

Serial films of chronically ill premature infants also should be observed closely for signs of rickets. In this disorder the metaphysis is abnormally lucent, and there is a loss of the zone of provisional calcification, which is the dense line at the metaphyseal end of the bone adjacent to the epiphyseal cartilage plate. This abnormality is accompanied by metaphyseal fraying and cupping. The metaphyses of the knees and wrists are particularly sensitive indicators of rickets as are the anterior rib ends, which may show a rachitic rosary (Fig. 39-24). Rib fractures also are common in these infants.

Spine, pelvis, and hips

These portions of the skeleton also are visible on many routine chest and abdomen films of the neonate. Common anomalies of vertebral segmentation, such as sagittally cleft (butterfly) vertebrae and hemivertebrae, may be incidental roentgenologic findings or accompany other congenital anomalies such as esophageal atresia, imperforate anus, agenesis of the lung, and bronchopulmonary foregut malformations. Spinal dysraphism is manifested on AP views as an increase in the interpediculate distance of the involved portion of the vertebral column, which indicates a widening of the spinal canal (Fig. 39-25). Although this finding is commonly associated with meningomyelocele, lesser degrees of widening of the interpediuate distance may indicate the presence of an occult intraspinal lesion. Varying degrees of caudal regression with agenesis of the lumbosacral spine may be found in infants of diabetic mothers. A thorough evaluation of the genitourinary tract should be performed in all patients with spinal anomalies.

The femoral heads are rarely ossified in the early newborn period. This is unfortunate, since they are important landmarks in the diagnosis of congenital hip dislocation. In the absence of femoral head ossification, this diagnosis is recognized by superolateral displacement of the proximal femoral metaphyses and associated acetab-

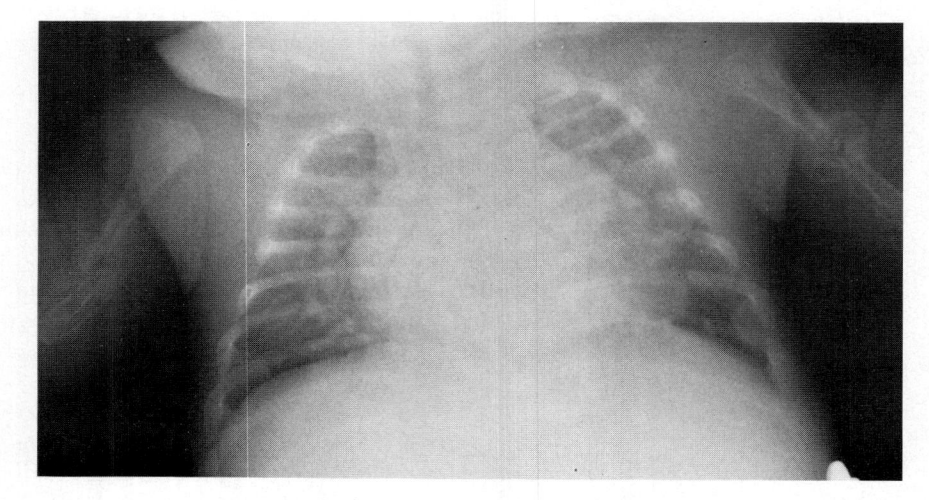

1082 Behrman's neonatal-perinatal medicine: diseases of the fetus and infant

Fig. 39-24. Infant with chronic lung disease has severe osteopenia, flaring and rarefaction of the metaphyses, and expansion of the anterior ends of the lower ribs due to rickets. There also were multiple long bone fractures. An alimentation catheter extends into the superior vena cava.

Fig. 39-25. Supine view of the lumbosacral spine shows widening of the interpediculate distances and dysplasia of the neural arch characteristic of spinal dysraphism. A memingomyelocele has been repaired surgically.

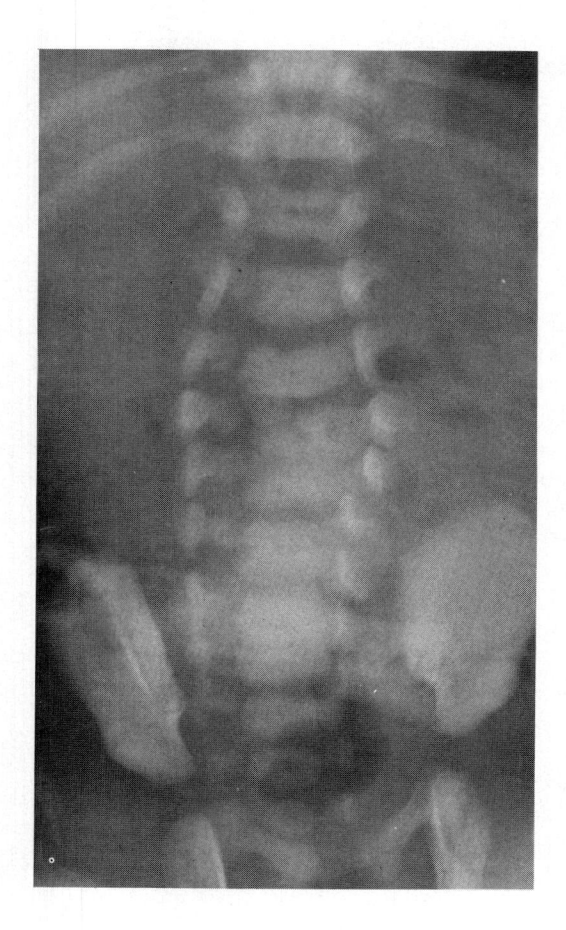

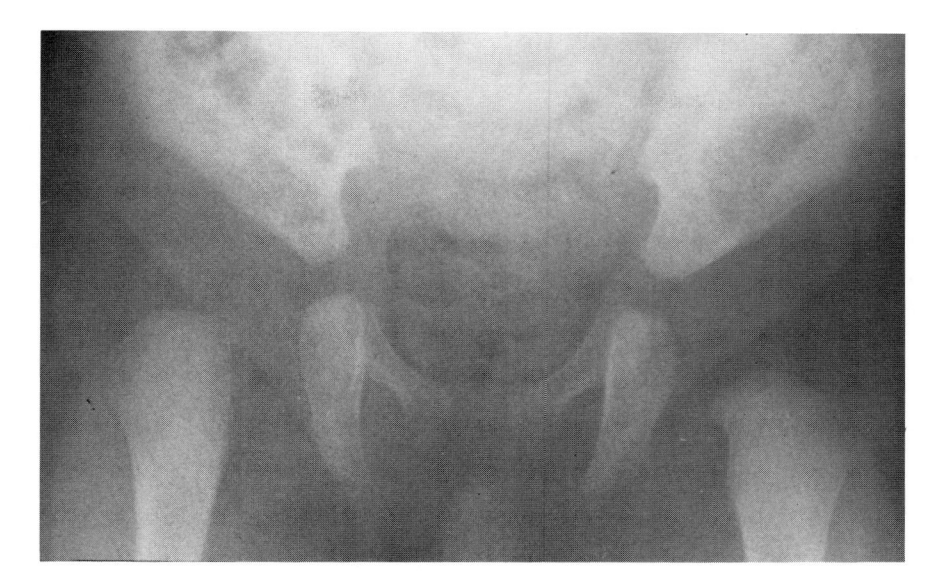

Fig. 39-26. AP view of the hips and pelvis demonstrates superolateral displacement of the right femur in a male with congenital dislocation of the hip. There is an associated dysplasia of the ipsilateral acetabulum manifested by an increased acetabular angle. The left acetabulum is also slightly dysplastic, but there is no subluxation.

Fig. 39-27. Ill-defined streaky lung densities caused by meconium aspiration pneumonia. Note the ossification of the humeral heads and coracoid apophyses *(arrowheads)*. The barely discernible left pneumothorax can be suspected by the increased volume and lucency of the left hemithorax.

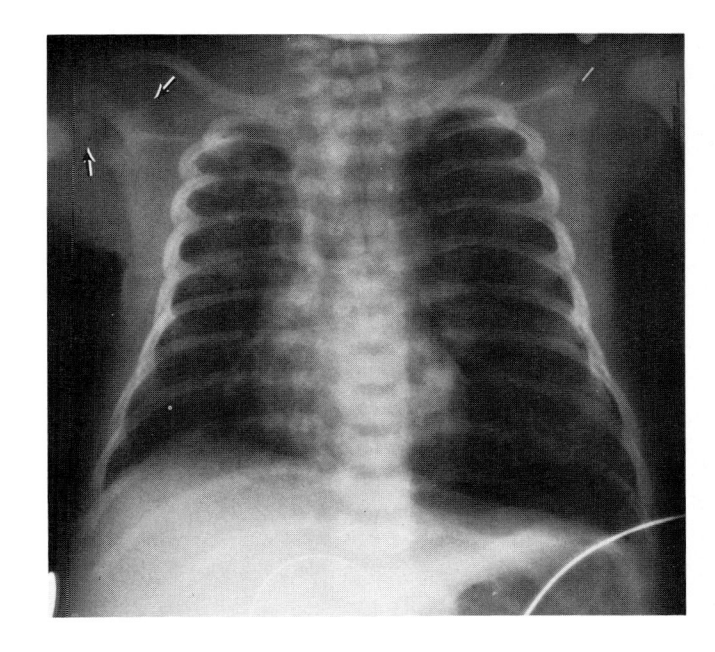

ular dysplasia (Fig. 39-26). Septic arthritis causes rapid subluxation or dislocation of the hips in the absence of acetabular dysplasia.

Estimation of gestational age

Traditionally, ossification of the epiphyseal centers of the knee has been used for roentgenologic assessment of gestational age, although the appearance of these centers is quite variable. In addition, the humeral heads are readily visible on chest roentgenograms. They are rarely ossified before 38 weeks of age and, if visible, indicate gestational maturity. Although their presence is not diagnostic of postmaturity, infants with respiratory distress in whom these centers are ossified have a statistically high chance of having meconium aspiration syndrome (Fig. 39-27).

A delay in ossification of the epiphyses may occur in an SGA fetus. Ossification also may be retarded by severe intrauterine infection such as rubella (Fig. 39-23). However, the lower deciduous molar teeth are more reliable indicators of gestational age and are frequently included on chest roentgenograms. Mineralization of the first deciduous molar indicates at least 33 weeks of gestation, whereas mineralization of the second molar indicates at least 36 weeks.

SKULL AND BRAIN

Although computerized tomography is now established as the primary diagnostic modality for suspected intracranial abnormalities, skull roentgenography is more useful for examination of the calvarium. Other diagnostic modalities, such as nuclear scintigraphy and angiography, have more limited applications in the neonate.

Roentgenographic evaluation of the neonatal skull requires three basic views: frontal, lateral, and Townes. Submental-vertex, tangential, and other views may be obtained for specific indications.

Soft tissues

Soft tissue swelling is common in neonates as a result of caput succedaneum and cephalhematoma. Cephalhematomas are caused by subperiosteal hemorrhage and are confined by the periosteal attachment at the sutural edges. They are most frequent over the parietal bones and eventually ossify and become incorporated into the outer table of the skull. Approximately 5% of cephalhematomas are accompanied by skull fractures.

Calvarium

Considerable experience is required in interpreting skull roentgenograms of infants because of the ongoing changes in craniofacial proportions. Craniofacial proportions are assessed on lateral roentgenograms by comparison of the relative areas of the face and calvarium. At birth the ratio of the cranial area to the facial area is normally about 4:1. A higher ratio indicates macrocrania, which is most often secondary to hydrocephalus. Microcrania reflects micrencephaly (Fig. 39-28).

In the immediate postnatal period the skull may be misshapen due to molding. Later asymmetry and other abnormal skull configurations may indicate underlying abnormalities of the developing brain due to cerebral atrophy and also may be caused by sutural synostoses. Minor degrees of calvarial asymmetry are, however, fairly common in normal infants, and parietooccipital flattening due to prolonged dependency of this portion of the skull is frequent, especially in debilitated infants. Convolutional markings are not usually prominent until the anterior fontanel closes but may be seen posteriorly with parietooccipital flattening or asymmetrically with premature synostosis or cerebral atrophy. They must be differentiated from the rounded dysplastic lucencies seen in craniolacunia and meningomyelocele.

Sutures

There is a wide range of normal suture widths in neonates because of molding, skeletal maturation, and gestational age. The size of the fontanels also is quite variable. During the first few days of life, sutural overriding is usually due to molding, after which the sutures appear relatively wide. The more premature the infant, the smaller the ossification centers of the various membranous bones and the greater the apparent widening of the sutures. With postnatal growth and subsequent ossification the sutures decrease in width. In premature infants the sutures are often difficult to visualize because of lack of mineralization of the adjacent calvarium. Intrasutural (wormian) bones may be normal but also may indicate an alteration of normal membranous ossification due to osteogenesis imperfecta, cleidocranial dysostosis, or hypothyroidism.

Early closure of a suture may be either an isolated primary abnormality or, less commonly, secondary to generalized bone diseases such as hypophosphatasia and rickets, or it may be associated with congenital anomalies, as in Apert's or Crouzon's syndrome. Associated abnormalities of the shape of the cranium due to limitation of directional growth of the brain may precede anatomic closure of the suture. Lack of normal brain growth is an important cause of generalized sutural narrowing (Fig. 39-28).

Calcifications

Artifacts on the scalp, such as bandages, tape, iodoform gauze, electrode paste, blood, and matted hair, may appear as focal areas of increased density suggesting

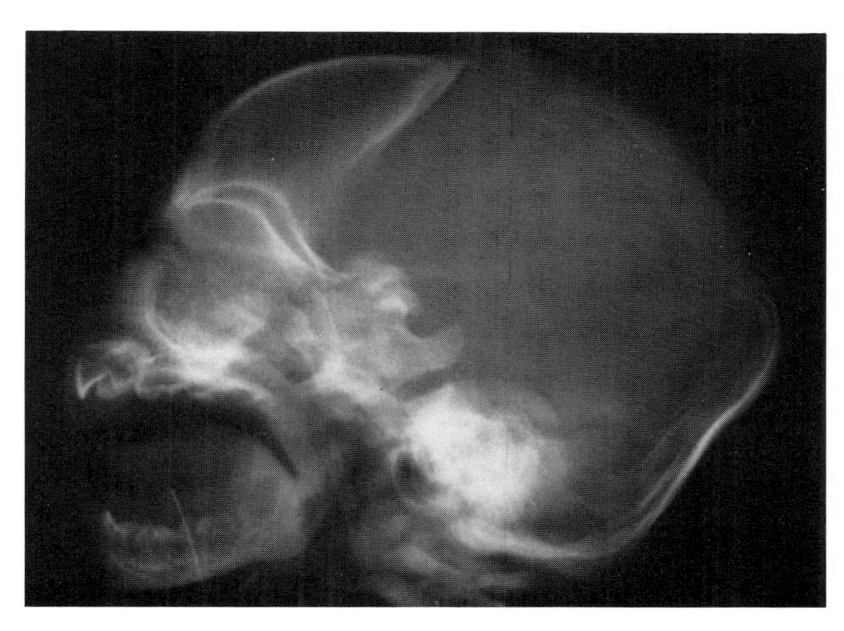

Fig. 39-28. Lateral film of the skull of a micrencephalic infant demonstrates a severely reduced craniofacial proportion of approximately 1.5:1. The sutures are markedly narrowed.

Fig. 39-29. CT scan at the level of the foramen of Monro demonstrates bleeding *(white)* into the lateral and third ventricles with mild ventricular dilatation.

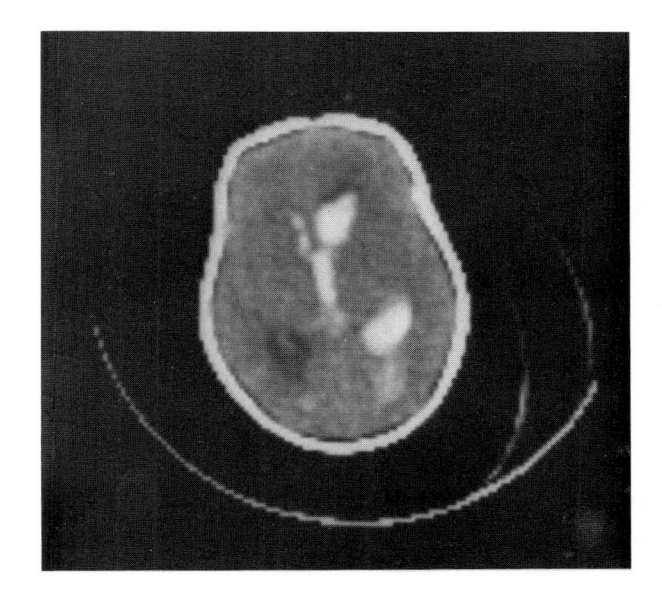

intracranial calcifications. Calcification or ossification of the scalp occurs within soft tissue lesions such as hemangioma or an organizing cephalhematoma. Intracranial calcifications in neonates are usually secondary to intrauterine infections such as herpes, cytomegalovirus, and toxoplasmosis.

Computed tomography (CT)

Discussion of the wide variety of intracranial abnormalities that occur in the neonate and that can be detected by CT scanning is beyond the scope of this text.

However, intracranial hemorrhage is a common and important problem, especially in premature neonates. Posttraumatic hemorrhage is usually subdural or subarachnoid in location. Periventricular hemorrhage associated with prematurity and hypoxia may lead to progressive ventricular dilatation and hydrocephalus (Fig. 39-29). CT is used not only for diagnosis but also for periodic evaluation of the ventricular system. B-mode ultrasonography is now being used for sequential evaluation following the initial diagnostic CT scan (Chapter 22).

MONITORING AND TREATMENT DEVICES

An important aspect of the roentgenologic examination of the newborn infant is the assessment of the position of various devices, such as endotracheal tubes, nasogastric tubes, umbilical catheters, and intravenous alimentation catheters. For obvious reasons these devices must be radiopaque (see Fig. 39-16).

The endotracheal tube is visible on most chest roentgenograms. Its tip should be approximately halfway between the vocal cords and the carina, at approximately the level of the first ribs. In small premature infants, even slight alterations in the degree of flexion of the neck will cause a remarkable difference between the position of the tube as seen on AP and lateral roentgenograms.

The position of the nasogastric tube also should be noted on the chest roentgenogram. Its tip may be displaced inadvertently from the stomach into the lower esophagus. On occasion the tube will be found curled above a previously unsuspected esophageal atresia.

To assess umbilical arterial and venous catheters, a film should done that includes both the chest and the abdomen. The umbilical arterial catheter can be seen in the aorta, to the left of the midline. Proper position of its tip is either in the thoracic aorta between T6 and T10 or in the abdominal aorta just above the aortic bifurcation. The umbilical vein catheter ascends toward the porta hepatis to the right of the midline and bypasses the portal system by entering the ductus venosus, which leads to the inferior vena cava. The optimum position of this catheter tip is in the intrathoracic portion of the inferior vena cava. Intravenous alimentation catheters are usually inserted via the internal or external jugular vein into the superior vena cava so that the tip comes to lie immediately superior to the right atrium.

Barry D. Fletcher
Barry S. Yulish
Gary M. Amundson

BIBLIOGRAPHY
General

Avery, M.E., Fletcher, B.D., and Williams, R.G.: The lung and its disorders in the newborn infant, ed. 4, Philadelphia, 1981, W.B. Saunders Co.

Caffey, J.: Pediatric x-ray diagnosis, ed. 7, Chicago, 1978, Year-Book Medical Publishers, Inc.

Lebowitz, R.L., editor: Pediatric uroradiology, Radiology Clinics of North America, vol. 15, Philadelphia, 1977, W.B. Saunders Co.

Poznanski, A.K.: Practical approaches to pediatric radiology, Chicago, 1976, Year-Book Medical Publishers, Inc.

Reilly, B.J., editor: Neonatal radiology, Radiology Clinics of North America, vol. 13, Philadelphia, 1975, W.B. Saunders Co.

Singleton, E.B., Wagner, M.L., and Dutton, R.V.: Radiology of the alimentary tract in infants and children, ed. 2, Philadelphia, 1977, W.B. Saunders Co.

Methods of examination and contrast media

Colodny, A.H., and Lebowitz, R.L.: The importance of voiding during a cystourethrogram, J. Urol. **111**:838, 1974.

Davis, L.A.: Standard roentgen examination in newborns, infants, and children: techniques, "portable" films, immobilization devices, and fluoroscopy, Progr. Pediatr. Radiol. **1**:3, 1967.

Dunbar, J.S., and Nogrady, B.: Excretory urography in the first year of life, Rad. Clin. North Am. **10**:367, 1972.

Franken, E.W., and others: Initial chest radiography in the neonatal intensive care unit: value of the lateral view, Am. J. Roentgenol. **133**:43, 1979.

Frech, R.S., and others: Meconium ileus relieved by 40 per cent water-soluble contrast enemas, Radiology **94**:341, 1970.

Griscom, N.T.: Total body opacification, Am. J. Roentgenol. **131**:919, 1978.

Haller, J.O., and others: Sonographic evaluation of the chest in infants and children, Am. J. Roentgenol. **134**:1019, 1980.

Harris, P.D., Neuhauser, E.B.D., and Gerth, R.: The osmotic effect of water-soluble contrast media on circulating plasma volume, Am. J. Roentgenol. Radium Ther. Nucl. Med. **91**:694, 1964.

Hope, J.W., and O'Hara, A.E.: Use of air as a contrast medium in the diagnosis of intestinal obstruction of the newborn, Radiology **70**:349, 1958.

Joseph, P.M., and others: Upper airway obstruction in infants and small children: improved radiographic diagnosis by combining filtration, high kilovoltage and magnification, Radiology **121**:143, 1976.

Leonidas, J.C., and others: Possible adverse effect of methylglucamine diatrizoate compounds on the bowel of newborn infants with meconium ileus, Radiology **121**:693, 1976.

Lorenzo, R.L., and Harolds, J.A.: The use of prone films for suspected bowel obstruction in infants and children, Am. J. Roentgenol. **129**:617, 1977.

Lutzger, L.G., and Factor, S.M.: Effects of some water-soluble contrast media on the colonic mucosa, Radiology **118**:545, 1976.

MacEwan, D.W., and others: Pneumothorax in young infants—recognition and evaluation, J. Can. Assoc. Radiol. **22**:264, 1971.

Noblett, H.R.: Treatment of uncomplicated meconium ileus by Gastrografin enema: a preliminary report, J. Pediatr. Surg. **4**:190, 1969.

O'Connor, J.F., and Neuhauser, E.B.D.: Total body opacification in conventional and high dose urography in infancy, Am. J. Roentgenol. Radium Ther. Nucl. Med. **90**:63, 1963.

Shopfner, C.E.: Genitography in intersex problems, Progr. Pediatr. Radiol. **3**:97, 1970.

Standen, J.R., and others: The osmotic effects of methylglucamine diatrizoate (Renografin-60) in intravenous urography in infants, Am. J. Roentgenol. Radium Ther. Nucl. Med. **93**:473, 1965.

Tucker, A.S., and Izant, R.J., Jr.: Inferior venacavagraphy, Progr. Pediatr. Radiol. **3**:82, 1970.

Wagget, J., and others: The nonoperative treatment of meconium ileus by Gastrografin enema, J. Pediatr. **77**:407, 1970.

Wood, B.P., and others: Diatrizoate enemas: facts and fallacies of colonic toxicity, Radiology **126**:441, 1978.

Patient protection

Margulis, A.R.: The lessons of radiobiology for diagnostic radiology, Am. J. Roentgenol. Radium Ther. Nucl. Med. **117**:741, 1973.

Mazzi, E., Herrera, A.J., and Linton, H.: Neonatal intensive care and radiation, Johns Hopkins Med. J. **142**:15, 1978.

Normal findings

Berdon, W.E., Baker, D.H., and James, L.: The ductus bump: a transient physiologic mass in chest roentgenograms of newborn infants, Am. J. Roentgenol. Radium Ther. Nucl. Med. **95**:91, 1965.

Burnard, E.D., and James, L.S.: Radiographic heart size in apparently healthy newborn infants: clinical and biochemical correlations, Pediatrics **27**:726, 1961.

Fletcher, B.D., and others: Thymic response to endogenous and exogenous steroids in premature newborn infants, J. Pediatr. **95:**111, 1979.
Kemp, F.H., Morley, H.M.C., and Emrys-Roberts, E.: A sail-like triangular projection from the mediastinum: a radiographic appearance of the thymus gland, Br. J. Radiol. **21:**618, 1948.
Kleinman, P.K., and others: The neonatal colon: an anatomic approach to plain films, Am. J. Roentgenol. **128:**61, 1977.
Podolsky, M.L., and Jester, A.W.: The distribution of air in the intestinal tract of infants during the first twelve hours as determined by serial roentgenograms, J. Pediatr. **45:**633, 1954.
Shopfner, C.E., and Hutch, J.A.: The normal urethrogram, Rad. Clin. North Am. **6:**165, 1968.
Taybi, H.: Roentgen evaluation of cardiomegaly in the newborn period and early infancy, Pediatr. Clin. North Am. **18:**1031, 1971.

Pulmonary abnormalities

Ablow, R.C., and others: The radiographic features of early onset group B streptococcal neonatal sepsis, Radiology **124:**771, 1977.
Fletcher, B.D., and Avery, M.E.: The effects of airway occlusion after oxygen breathing on the lungs of newborn infants: radiologic demonstration in the experimental animal, Radiology **109:**655, 1973.
Fletcher, B.D., and others: Pulmonary interstitial emphysema in a newborn infant treated by lobectomy, Pediatrics **54:**808, 1974.
Macklin, M.T., and Macklin, C.G.: Malignant interstitial emphysema of the lungs and mediastinum as an important occult complication in many respiratory diseases and other conditions: an interpretation of the clinical literature in the light of laboratory experiment, Medicine **23:**281, 1944.
Moseley, J.E.: Loculated pneumomediastinum in the newborn: a thymic "spinnaker sail" sign, Radiology **75:**788, 1960.
Moskowitz, P.S., and Griscom, N.T.: The medial pneumothorax, Radiology **120:**143, 1976.
Recavarren, S., Benton, C., and Gall, E.A.: The pathology of acute alveolar diseases of the lung, Semin. Roentgenol. **2:**22, 1967.
Wyman, M.L., and Kuhns, L.R.: Lobar opacification of the lung after tracheal extubation in neonates, J. Pediatr. **91:**109, 1977.
Yeh, T.F., Vidyasagar, D., and Pildes, R.S.: Neonatal pneumopericardium, Pediatrics **54:**429, 1974.

Cardiovascular abnormalities

Bauer, C.R., Tsipuras, D., and Fletcher, B.D., Syndrome of persistent pulmonary vascular obstruction of the newborn: roentgen findings, Am. J. Roentgenol. Radium Ther. Nucl. Med. **120:**285, 1974.
Higgins, C.B., and others: Patent ductus arteriosus in preterm infants with idiopathic respiratory distress syndrome: radiographic and echocardiographic evaluation, Radiology **124:**189, 1977.
Kuhn, J.P., Fletcher, B.D., and deLemos, R.A.: Roentgen findings in transient tachypnea of the newborn, Radiology **92:**751, 1969.

Gastrointestinal tract

Berdon, W.E., and others: Necrotizing enterocolitis in the premature infant, Radiology **83:**879, 1964.
Berdon, W.E., and others: Midgut malrotation and volvulus, Radiology **96:**375, 1970.
Burko, H.: Toxic depression of the newborn causing deficient intestinal gas pattern, Am. J. Roentgenol. Radium Ther. Nucl. Med. **88:**575, 1962.
Davis, W.S., and others: Neonatal small left colon syndrome, Am. J. Roentgenol. Radium Ther. Nucl. Med. **120:**322, 1974.
Franken, E.A.: Ascites in infants and children: roentgen diagnosis, Radiology **102:**393, 1972.
Fletcher, B.D., and Yulish, B.S.: Intraluminal calcifications in the small bowel of newborn infants with total colonic aganglionosis, Radiology **126:**451, 1978.
Griscom, N.T., and others: Diagnostic aspects of neonatal ascites: report of 27 cases, Am. J. Roentgenol. **128:**961, 1977.
Kassner, E.G., and others: Gasless abdomen in neonates with orotracheal tubes, Radiology **112:**659, 1974.
Leonidas, J.C., and others: Meconium ileus and its complications, Am. J. Roentgenol. Radium Ther. Nucl. Med. **108:**598, 1970.
Leonidas, J.C., and others: Pneumoperitoneum in ventilated newborns, Am. J. Dis. Child. **128:**677, 1974.
Miller, R.E.: Perforated viscus in infants: a new roentgen sign, Radiology **74:**65, 1960.
Neuhauser, E.B.D.: The roentgen diagnosis of fetal meconium peritonitis, Am. J. Roentgenol. Radium Ther. Nucl. Med. **51:**421, 1944.
Pochaczevsky, R., and Kassner, E.G.: Necrotizing enterocolitis in infancy, Am. J. Roentgenol. Radium Ther. Nucl. Med. **113:**283, 1971.
Pochaczevsky, R., and Leonidas, J.C.: The meconium plug syndrome, Am. J. Roentgenol. Radium Ther. Nucl. Med. **120:**342, 1974.
Robinson, A., Grossman, H., and Brumley, G.: Pneumatosis intestinalis in the neonate, Am. J. Roentgenol. Radium Ther. Nucl. Med. **120:**333, 1974.
Sane, S.M., and Girdany, B.R.: Total aganglionosis coli, Radiology **107:**397, 1973.
Siegle, R.L.: Neonatal gasless abdomen: another cause, Am. J. Roentgenol. **133:**522, 1979.

Urinary tract

Allen, R.P.: The lower urinary tract, Progr. Pediatr. Radiol. **3:**139, 1970.
Alton, D.J., and McDonald, P.: Urinary obstruction in the neonatal infant, Rad. Clin. North Am. **13:**343, 1975.
Berdon, W.E., and others: Tamm-Horsfall proteinuria: its relationship to prolonged nephrogram in infants and children and to renal failure following intravenous urography in adults with multiple myeloma, Radiology **92:**714, 1969.
Dunbar, J.S., and Nogrady, M.B.: The calyceal crescent—a roentgenographic sign of obstructive hydronephrosis, Am. J. Roetgenol. Radium Ther. Nucl. Med. **110:**520, 1970.
Elkin, M.: Renal cystic disease—an overview, Semin. Roentgenol. **10:**99, 1975.
Griscom, N.T.: The roentgenology of neonatal abdominal masses, Am. J. Roentgenol. Radium Ther. Nucl. Med. **93:**447, 1965.

Ultrasonography

Cook, J.H., III, Rosenfield, A.T., and Taylor, K.J.W.: Ultrasonic demonstration of intrarenal anatomy, Am. J. Roentgenol. **129:**831, 1977.
Kangarloo, H., and Sample, W.F.: Ultrasound of the pediatric abdomen and pelvis, Chicago, 1980, Year-Book Medical Publishers, Inc.
Sample, W.F., Gyepes, M.T., and Ehrlich, R.M.: Gray scale ultrasound in pediatric urology, J. Urol. **117:**518, 1977.

Skeletal system

Binstadt, D.H., and L'Heureux, P.R.: Rickets as a complication of intravenous hyperalimentation in infants, Pediatr. Radiol. **7:**211, 1978.
Brill, P.W., and others: Osteomyelitis in a neonatal intensive care unit, Radiology **131:**83, 1979.
Kuhns, L.R., and Poznanski, A.K.: Radiological assessment of maturity and size of the newborn infant, CRC Crit. Rev. Diagn. Imaging **13:**245, 1980.
Lachman, R.S., Yamauchi, T., and Klein, J.: Neonatal systemic candidiasis and arthritis, Radiology **105:**631, 1972.
McCook, T.A., Felman, A.H., and Ayoub, E.: Streptococcal skeletal infections: observations in four infants, Am. J. Roentgenol. **130:**465, 1978.

Merten, D.F., and Gooding, C.A.: Skeletal manifestations of congenital cytomegalic inclusion disease, Radiology **95**:333, 1970.

Singleton, E.B., and others: The roentgenographic manifestations of the rubella syndrome in newborn infants, Am. J. Roentgenol. Radium Ther. Nucl. Med. **97**:82, 1966.

Wolfson, J.J., and Engel, R.R.: Anticipating meconium peritonitis from metaphyseal bands, Radiology **92**:1055, 1969.

Skull and brain

Burstein, J., Papile, L., and Burstein, R.: Subependymal germinal matrix and intraventricular hemorrhage in premature infants: diagnosis by CT, Am. J. Roentgenol. **128**:971, 1977.

Dorst, J.P.: Functional craniology: an aid in interpreting roentgenograms of the skull, Rad. Clin. North Am. **2**:347, 1964.

Haber, K., and others: Ultrasonic evaluation of intracranial pathology in infants: a new technique, Radiology **134**:173, 1980.

Swischuk, L.E.: The normal newborn skull, Semin. Roentgenol. **9**:101, 1974.

Zelson, C., Lee, S.J., and Pearl, M.: The incidence of skull fractures underlying cephalhematomas in newborn infants, J. Pediatr. **85**:371, 1974.

Monitoring and treatment devices

Campbell, R.E.: Roentgenologic features of umbilical vascular catheterization in the newborn, Am. J. Roentgenol. Radium Ther. Nucl. Med. **112**:68, 1971.

Kuhns, L.R., and Poznanski, A.K.: Endotracheal tube position in the infant, J. Pediatr. **78**:991, 1971.

APPENDIX A

Blood specimen collection in the newborn

Blood specimens may be obtained from newborns for diagnostic laboratory tests via skin puncture or venous or arterial sampling. The major considerations are specimen volume and potential for injury to the infant. If the samples are obtained frequently for diagnostic tests or in large volumes, iatrogenic anemia may occur. It is recommended that a daily log be kept in each infant's hospital record showing the amount of blood removed and the time of day each specimen is obtained. If an amount exceeding 10% of the infant's blood volume is removed, the infant will generally require a replacement blood transfusion. The currently available state-of-the-art laboratory analyzers require only microquantities of blood to perform multiple laboratory tests, and with these instruments it is no longer necessary to collect large volumes of blood from infants.

SKIN PUNCTURES

When well-defined guidelines are followed, skin puncture is the least hazardous technique for collecting mass screening blood specimens from newborns. Recent increased interest in screening programs for metabolic defects has resulted in the development of new devices for skin puncture blood collection and has stimulated studies to compare the values of constituents in skin puncture, arterial, and venous blood.

In newborns, skin puncture blood may be obtained from the lateral or medial plantar heel surface. Histologic examination shows that uncomplicated skin puncture wounds heal with minimal scarring and without neuroma formation, although foci of calcification in the heel skin have been reported. To prevent calcaneal puncture and the risk of osteochondritis, heel punctures in the newborn should be done (1) on the most medial or lateral portions of the plantar surface of the heel, (2) no deeper than 2.4 mm, (3) not on the posterior curvature of the heel, and (4) not through previous puncture sites that may become infected. Skin punctures of the finger should not be performed in infants, especially premature ones, since punctures in this site have resulted in local infection and gangrene of the distal phalanx due to the short distance from the skin surface to the underlying bone in newborns.

The skin puncture site must not be swollen, since an accumulation of tissue fluid or blood within the skin will contaminate the blood specimen for diagnostic tests. Before puncture of the skin, the site should be warmed to increase the blood flow to the skin (up to sevenfold). Since the increase is primarily in arterial blood flow, the blood specimen obtained after warming has been called *arterialized skin puncture blood*. This warming step is essential for accurate results when specimens are collected for pH and blood gas determinations, although their use in evaluating arterial Po_2 is extremely limited (Chapter 23, part three). The simplest and least expensive method of warming is to cover the site for 3 minutes with a hot, moist towel at a temperature no higher than 40° C. This warming technique will adequately increase the blood flow but will not burn the skin nor result in a significant change in the values of any chemical constituent routinely measured in a hospital chemistry laboratory.

The chosen skin puncture site should be cleaned with 75% aqueous solution of isopropanol. After cleaning, the skin must be completely dried with a sterile gauze pad before puncture, since any remaining alcohol will cause rapid hemolysis of any blood that contacts it. Betadine should not be used to clean skin puncture sites because blood contaminated with it may have falsely elevated levels of potassium, phosphorus, uric acid, and bilirubin.

The infant's heel should be grasped with a moderately firm grip, and the skin puncture should be at a slight angle to the skin surface. After the puncture, the first drop of blood should be wiped away with a sterile gauze, since it is most likely to contain larger amounts of tissue fluids and not be a representative specimen. The use of heparinized or nonheparinized capillary tubes for collection depends on whether plasma or serum is desired.

After the puncture the blood will form a drop over the site, and when the tip of the capillary tube is placed against the drop, the blood will flow into the tube by capillary action. Blood flow is enhanced if the puncture site is held downward; a gentle continuous pressure (milking) should not be used, since it may increase hemolysis and tissue fluid in the specimen. If an adequate puncture has been performed, 0.5 to 1 ml of blood can be collected from a single puncture site.

After collection of a specimen for pH and blood gas analysis, a small magnetic mixing bar placed in the bore of the tube allows the blood in the tube to be adequately mixed. Specimens obtained for pH and blood gas analysis should be transported in water containing ice chips to prevent a significant change in blood pH.

VENOUS AND ARTERIAL SAMPLING

The increased availability of microtechniques for laboratory tests has reduced the need for obtaining blood from the neonate via venipuncture. Care should always be exercised in drawing venous blood samples from newborns, especially when deep veins are used. Patient hazards include hemorrhage, venous thrombosis, reflex arteriospasm, damage to surrounding tissues, and infection.

Umbilical arterial catheters offer a convenient and ready source of blood for laboratory tests, especially blood gas determinations. The numerous serious hazards of umbilical catheters are described in Chapters 14 and 19. The ability to sample blood accurately for chemical analysis through a catheter being used for administration of peripheral fluids depends on the size of the catheter and the concentration gradient between the chemical constituents in the blood and the parenteral fluid being administered. It has been shown that, when a 10% glucose solution is infused into the umbilical artery through a no. 5F catheter (0.3-ml capacity), a clinically significant glucose contamination occurs in blood specimens drawn through the catheter even after a volume of blood 10 times the catheter capacity has been shunted. It has been recommended that the amount of blood initially shunted from the catheter (and subsequently returned) to obtain accurate chemical measurements should be the following:

1. If using a 3½F catheter: 3 ml for glucose, 1 ml for sodium and potassium, and 0.4 ml for pH.
2. If using a 5F catheter: 4 ml for glucose, 1 ml for sodium or potassium, and 0.4 ml for pH.
3. If using an 8F catheter: 4 ml for sodium, 2 ml for potassium, 1.2 ml for pH, and an amount greater than 6 ml for glucose.

Solutions that contain *benzyl alcohol* or other preservatives should not be used to flush intravascular catheters, since toxicity may occur in the form of metabolic acidosis, CNS depression, respiratory distress (with gasping), hypotension, renal failure, and even seizures and intracranial hemorrhage.

Blood for coagulation studies, activated partial thromboplastin time, and whole blood partial thromboplastin time can be drawn through 5F heparinized umbilical catheters, and accurate results are obtained if 4 ml of blood is shunted before obtaining the sample.

When it is necessary to obtain an arterial blood sample from a newborn, alternative sites to the umbilical artery are the radial and brachial arteries. Scalp and femoral arteries should be avoided because of the risk of cerebral thrombosis and hip damage, respectively.

DIFFERENCES IN VALUES IN SKIN PUNCTURE BLOOD, VENOUS BLOOD, AND ARTERIAL BLOOD IN NEWBORNS

Blood obtained by skin puncture is not specifically blood from capillaries but is a mixture of blood from arterioles, venules, and capillaries and contains interstitial and intracellular fluids. Chemistry values for 12 constituents simultaneously obtained in skin puncture serum, skin puncture plasma, and venous serum have been compared. The effect of warming the skin before the puncture also was studied. No clinically important differences were found in the concentration of the constituents measured in skin puncture serum and plasma with or without warming the skin before puncture. When the concentration of each of the measured constituents was compared between skin puncture blood and venous serum, there were differences in the concentrations of glucose, potassium, total protein, and calcium, which could be clinically significant. Except for those of glucose, the concentrations in venous serum were higher. The degree of hemolysis reflected by plasma (free) hemoglobin concentration was the same in skin puncture serum and plasma, although the total plasma hemoglobin is higher in skin puncture than in venous specimens.

There is poor correlation of Po_2 values in arterialized skin puncture blood and umbilical artery blood in term and preterm infants with a variety of illnesses. Almost uniformly the Po_2 is lower in skin puncture blood, and if these samples are used to determine Po_2, toxic levels of oxygen may be undetected. Therefore arterial or transcutaneous measurements should be used to monitor arterial Po_2. It is also preferable to measure pH and Pco_2 in newborns with cardiopulmonary abnormalities by using arterial blood (or measuring transcutaneous Pco_2).

Thomas A. Blumenfeld

Bibliography
Skin puncture

Blumenfeld, T.A., Hertelendy, W.G., and Ford, S.H.: Simultaneously obtained skin puncture serum, skin puncture plasma, and venous serum compared and effects of warming the skin before puncture, Clin. Chem. 23:1705, 1977.

Blumenfeld, T.A., Turi, G.K., and Blanc, W.A.: Recommended sites and depth of newborn heel skin punctures based on anatomic measurements and histopathology, Lancet 1:230, 1979.

Blumenfeld, T.A., and others: Standard procedures for the collection of diagnostic blood specimens by skin puncture: TSH-4, Villanova, Pa., 1979, National Committee for Clinical Laboratory Standards.

Gambino, S.R.: Blood pH, pCO_2, oxygen saturation, and pO_2, Chicago, 1967, American Society of Clinical Commission on Continuing Education.

Gandy, G., and others: The validity of pH and pCO_2 measurements in capillary samples in sick and healthy newborn infants, Pediatrics 34:192, 1964.

Hicks, J.R., Rowland, G.L., and Buffone, G.J.: Evaluation of a new blood collection device (microtainer) that is suited for pediatric use, Clin. Chem. 22:2034, 1976.

Karna, P., and Poland, R.L.: Monitoring critically ill newborn infants with digital capillary blood samples: an alternative, J. Pediatr. 92:270, 1978.

Lilien, L.D., and others: Neonatal osteomyelitis of the calcaneus: complication of heel puncture, J. Pediatr. 88:478, 1976.

Meites, S., and others: Skin puncture and blood-collecting techniques for infants, Clin. Chem. 25:183, 1979.

Michaelsson, M., and Sjolin, S.: Hemolysis in blood samples from newborn infants, Acta Paediatr. Scand. 54:325, 1965.

Sell, E.J., Hansen, R.C., and Struck-Pierce, S.: Calcified nodules on the heel: a complication of neonatal intensive care. J. Pediatr. 96:473, 1980.

Von Steirteghem, A.C., and Young, D.S.: Povidone-iodine (Betadine) disinfectant as a source of error, Clin. Chem. 23:1512, 1977.

Venipuncture

Blumenfeld, T.A.: Clinical applications of microchemistry. In Werner, M.W., editor: Microtechniques for the clinical laboratory: concept and application, New York, 1976, John Wiley & Sons, Inc.

Differences in values in skin puncture and arterial and venous specimens in newborns

Blumenfeld, T.A., Hertelendy, W.G., and Ford, S.H.: simultaneously obtained skin puncture serum, skin puncture plasma, and venous serum compared and effects of warming the skin before puncture, Clin. Chem. 23:1705, 1977.

Christensen, R.D., and Rothstein, G.: Pitfalls in the interpretation of leukocyte counts of newborn infants, Am. J. Clin. Pathol. 72:608, 1979.

Feusner, J.H., and others: Platelet counts in capillary blood, Am. J. Clin. Pathol. 72:410, 1979.

Gandy, G., and others: The validity of pH and pCO_2 measurements in capillary samples in sick and healthy newborn infants, Pediatric 34:192, 1964.

Langer, P.H., Jr., and Fies, H.L.: Blood sugar values of blood obtained simultaneously from the radial artery, antecubital vein, and the finger, Am. J. Clin. Pathol. 12;559, 1942.

Michaelsson, M., and Sjolin, S.: Hemolysis in blood samples from newborn infants, Acta Paediatr. Scand. 54:325, 1965.

Mountain, K.R., and Campbell, D.G.: Reliability of oxygen tension measurements on arterialized capillary blood in the newborn, Arch. Dis. Child. 45:134, 1970.

Stuart, J., and others: Capillary blood coagulation profile in the newborn, Lancet 2:1467, 1979.

APPENDIX B Therapeutic agents

Agent	Dosage	Comments
ADRENERGICS		
Dobutamine	5-20 µg/kg/min IV	Tolerance may develop with prolonged use (>3 days)
Dopamine	2-5 µg/kg/min IV	"Renal dose" to promote renal blood flow
	5-20 µg/kg/min IV	Inotropic and vasoconstrictive dose
Epinephrine	1:1000 aqueous solution; 0.01 ml/kg/dose SC	Repeat every 2-4 hr as needed
	1:10,000 aqueous solution; 0.1 ml/kg IV, intratracheal, or intracardiac	May repeat after 15 min
	0.05-1.0 µg/kg/min IV in D5W	
Isoproterenol	0.1-4.0 µg/kg/min IV	Continous ECG and blood pressure monitoring essential to prevent hypotension and tachycardia
ANTIBACTERIALS (see also Chapter 27)		
Amikacin	0-7 days: 15 mg/kg/day divided every 12 hr IV, IM	Serum concentrations should be monitored and dosage adjusted to achieve peak concentrations ≤ 40 µg/ml and trough concentrations ≤ 10 µg/ml
	>7 days: 15-22.5 mg/kg/day divided every 8 hr IV	
Ampicillin	0-7 days: 100 mg/kg/day divided every 12 hr IV, IM	Meningitis doses
	50-100 mg/kg/day divided every 12 hr IV, IM	Other indications
	>7 days: 200 mg/kg/day divided every 6-8 hr IV, IM	Meningitis doses
	100 mg/kg/day divided every 6-8 hr IV, IM	Other indications
Carbenicillin	0-7 days: 200-300 mg/kg/day divided every 8 hr IV, IM	Serum sodium and potassium levels should be carefully monitored
	>7 days: 300-400 mg/kg/day divided every 6-8 hr IV, IM	
Cefazolin	0-7 days: 25-50 mg/kg/day divided every 12 hr	
	>7 days: 25-100 mg/kg/day divided every 8 hr	
Ceftriaxone*	50-100 mg/kg/day divided every 12 hr (preliminary recommendation)	Highly potent against group B streptococci, pneumococci, *Staphylococcus aureus, H. influenzae, E. coli, Klebsiella,* and *Serratia;* high CSF penetrance and resistance to degradation by β-lactamases
Chloramphenicol	0-7 days: 25 mg/kg/day divided every 12 hr	Serum concentrations should be monitored; the succinate is not predictably cleaved, and doses should be adjusted to yield peak concentrations ≤25 µg/ml, trough concentrations ≥6 µg/ml
	7-14 days: 25-50 mg/kg/day divided every 8-12 hr	
	>14 days: 25-50 µg/kg/day divided every 8 hr	

*Pending FDA approval.

Agent	Dosage		Comments
Clindamycin	>7 days:	8-20 mg/kg/day divided every 6 hr PO	Not recommended for infants less than 1 month of age
Erythromycin estolate	0-7 days:	20 mg/kg/day divided every 12 hr	
	>7 days:	20 mg/kg/day divided every 6-8 hr PO	
Gentamicin	0-7 days:	5 mg/kg/day divided every 8-12 hr IV, IM	Serum concentrations should be monitored and doses adjusted to achieve peak concentrations ≤10 μg/ml and trough concentrations ≤2 μg/ml
	>7 days:	7.5 mg/kg/day divided every 12 hr IV, IM	
Kanamycin	0-7 days:	15-20 mg/kg/day divided every 12 hr	
	>7 days:	20-30 mg/kg/day divided every 8 hr	
Methicillin	0-7 days:	50-100 mg/kg/day divided every 12 hr IV, IM	
	>7 days:	100-200 mg/kg/day divided every 6-8 hr IV, IM	
Moxalactam*		150-200 mg/kg/day divided every 8 hr IV	Reserved for gram-negative infections and not reliably effective for group B streptococci
Nafcillin	0-7 days:	50-100 mg/kg/day divided every 12 hr IV	
	>7 days:	100-200 mg/kg/day divided every 6-8 hr IV	
Oxacillin	0-7 days:	50-100 mg/kg/day divided every 12 hr IV	
	>7 days:	100-200 mg/kg/day divided every 6-8 hr IV	
Penicillin G	0-7 days:	100,000-150,000 units/kg/day divided every 12 hr IV, IM	Meningitis dose
		50,000-100,000 units/kg/day divided every 12 hr IV, IM	Other indications
	>7 days:	150,000-400,000 units/kg/day divided every 6-8 hr IV, IM	Meningitis dose
		75,000-100,000 units/kg/day divided every 8 hr IV, IM	Other indications
Penicillin G benzathine	0-7 days:	50,000 units/kg single dose IM	For treatment of congenital syphilis when central nervous system is not involved
	>7 days:	50,000 units/kg single dose IM	
Piperacillin*		150-300 mg/kg/day divided every 8-12 hr (preliminary recommendation)	More potent than carboxy-penicillins against gram-negative organisms and provides effective single-drug therapy for Klebsiella, Enterococcus, and Bacteroides
Ticarcillin	0-7 days:	<2,000 gm: 150 mg/kg/day divided every 12 hr	Serum sodium and potassium should be carefully monitored
	0-7 days:	>2,000 gm: 225 mg/kg/day divided every 8 hr	
	>7 days:	225-300 mg/kg/day divided every 6-8 hr	
Tobramycin	0-7 days:	5 mg/kg/day divided every 12 hr IV, IM	Serum concentrations should be monitored and doses adjusted to achieve peak concentrations ≤10 μg/ml and trough concentrations ≤2 μg/ml
	>7 days:	7.5 mg/kg/day divided every 8 hr IV, IM	
Trimethoprim with sulfamethoxazole		5-10 mg trimethoprim and 25-50 mg sulfamethoxazole/kg/day divided every 12 hr IV, PO	Sulfamethoxazole can displace bilirubin; use with caution
		20 mg/kg trimethoprim and 100 mg/kg sulfamethoxazole/kg/day divided every 6 hr IV	Treatment for infections due to Pneumocystis carinii
Vancomycin	0-7 days:	30 mg/kg/day divided every 12 hr IV	Intravenous therapy reserved for Staphylococcus epidermidis or methicillin-resistant Staphylococcus aureus
		10-50 mg/kg/day divided every 12 hr PO	
	>7 days:	45 mg/kg/day divided every 8 hr IV; 10-50 mg/kg/day divided every 8 hr PO	Oral treatment for pseudomembranous enterocolitis

Continued.

Agent	Dosage	Comments
ANTIFUNGALS		
Amphotericin B	0.25-1.0 mg/kg/day IV infusion over 2-4 hr	Patients with *Candida* sepsis generally treated to a total dose of 15-20 mg/kg; serum potassium and creatinine clearance levels should be monitored closely; alternate day therapy may permit better control of electrolyte status
5-Fluorocytosine	50-150 mg/kg/day divided every 6 hr PO; 1,500-4,500 mg/m^2/day divided every 12 hr IV	Should not be employed as a single agent in the treatment of fungal sepsis
Miconazole	20-40 mg/kg/day IV divided every 8 hr	Titrate dose to yield serum concentrations above the MIC for infecting organism; no data available for newborn infants
Nystatin	400,000 units/day divided every 6-8 hr PO	
ANTITUBERCULOUS AGENTS		
Isoniazid	10 mg/kg/day PO	Prophylaxis
	15-30 mg/kg/day as a single dose PO	Therapeutic
	10 mg/kg/day divided every 8-12 hr IM	Therapeutic
Rifampin	10-20 mg/kg/day as a single dose PO	Use with caution in patients with hepatic dysfunction
Streptomycin	20-40 mg/kg/day divided every 12 hr IM	Use higher dose if tuberculous meningitis is present
ANTIVIRAL		
Adenine arabinoside	15 mg/kg/day over 12 hr at a concentration not exceeding 0.45 mg/ml of standard intravenous fluid	Efficacy documented only for herpes simplex virus encephalitis
ANTICOAGULANT		
Heparin	Load with 50 units/kg IV and then maintain with 100 units/kg IV every 4 hr or 20,000 units/m^2/day by continuous IV infusion	These dosing recommendations should serve as a starting point; therapy in each patient should be individualized to give a PTT of 1.5 to 2.5 times the control value
ANTICONVULSANTS		
Carbamazepine	10 mg/kg/day divided twice per day PO for *initial* therapy	Dose will require a gradual increase because of the "autoinduction" phenomenon; titrate to achieve serum concentrations between 4 and 12 µg/ml ($\simeq$20-40 nmol/L); no convenient dosage form available for infants
Paraldehyde	0.1-0.2 ml/kg as a 4% solution by slow IV infusion	Infusion rate should be adjusted to control patient's seizures; rapid infusion may cause cardiopulmonary depression and pulmonary edema
	0.3 ml/kg/dose per rectum every 4-6 hr	
Phenobarbital	Loading dose: 15-20 mg/kg slow IV push (50 mg/kg maximum)	Serum concentrations should be monitored and doses adjusted to maintain concentrations between 15 and 30 µg/ml; the long half-life of the drug suggests that single daily doses will be sufficient; little information available on oral absorption in the first month of life
	Maintenance dose: 4-6 mg/kg/day IV, IM, or PO as a single dose	
Phenytoin	Loading dose: 15-20 mg/kg IV at a rate not to exceed 50 mg/min (30 mg/kg maximum); may be diluted in 0.9% NaCl only to a concentration of 0.1 mg/ml	Loading dose should be administered with continuous ECG monitoring; serum concentrations should be monitored and doses adjusted to maintain concentrations between 10 and 20 µg/ml; oral absorption during the first month of life is negligible; the drug displays dose-dependent kinetics, so great care must be exercised when making a dosage change
	Maintenance dose: 5-8 mg/kg/day IV, PO	
Valproic acid	10-60 mg/kg/day divided every 12 hr PO; initial dose 10-15 mg/kg/day	Little data available for newborns; optimum seizure control in children reported at serum concentrations between 50 and 100 µg/ml

Agent	Dosage	Comments
ANTIDOTES		
Atropine	0.01-0.03 mg/kg IV, SC, or endotracheal	
Methylene blue	1-2 mg/kg/dose IV over 5 min	Treatment for methemoglobinemia
Naloxone	0.01-0.1 mg/kg/dose IV	May be repeated every 10-15 min
Protamine	1 mg for every 100 units of heparin in the previous 3-4 hr by IV drip (50 mg/dose maximum)	
BLOOD DERIVATIVES		
Albumin	1 gm/kg/day IV	May use 5% or 25% if infused over same length of time
Blood, packed cells	5-10 ml/kg IV	
Blood, whole	10-20 ml/kg IV	
Fibrinogen	50 mg/kg IV	Repeat as needed
Plasma, fresh, frozen	10-20 ml/kg IV	
CARDIOVASCULAR DRUGS (see also Chapter 25)		
Diazoxide	3-5 mg/kg IV as a bolus injected within 30 sec; may repeat in 30 min and then every 2-5 hr	Should not be used in treatment of compensatory hypertension such as associated with coarctation of the aorta and arteriovenous shunting
Digoxin	Premature: 0.02-0.04 mg/kg IV 0.01 mg/kg/day divided every 12 hr Full term: 0.04 mg/kg IV 0.01 mg/kg/day divided every 12 hr PO	Total digitalizing dose (load with half) Maintenance dose (may be given once daily) Total digitalizing dose (load with half) Maintenance dose; oral doses (elixir) are 75% as effective as IV doses; based on pharmacokinetics, maintenance dose may be given once daily
Hydralazine	0.2 mg/kg/dose or 1.7-3.5 mg/kg/day divided every 4-6 hr IV, IM 1 mg/kg/day divided every 6 hr to increase as needed up to 7.5 mg/kg/day	
Lidocaine	0.5-1.5 mg/kg/dose by slow intravenous push; may be repeated every 5-10 min as needed 20-50 µg/kg/min continuous IV infusion	Side effects include hypotension, seizures, respiratory arrest, asystole
Nitroprusside	0.5-5 µg/kg/min by continuous IV infusion	Must have continuous intraarterial blood pressure monitoring; may produce profound hypotension, metabolic acidosis, and CNS symptoms; serum thiocyanate concentrations must be monitored
Procainamide	2 mg/kg/dose given over 5 min IV 40-60 mg/kg/day divided every 6 hr PO	
Propranolol	0.01-0.15 mg/kg/dose by slow IV push; then 0.5-1.0 mg/kg/day divided every 6 hr PO Starting dose: 1 mg/kg/day divided every 6 hr PO 0.15-0.25 mg/kg/dose IV	For arrhythmias For hypertension For tetralogy spells
Phenytoin	See anticonvulsant dosage above	Drug of choice for digitalis intoxication
Tolazoline	1-2 mg/kg IV as a test dose; then 1-2 mg/kg/hr by continuous IV infusion	Monitor blood pressure and renal status; may cause gastrointestinal and pulmonary hemorrhages
Verapamil	0.1-0.3 mg/kg by IV infusion over 2 min	Treatment of paroxysmal supraventricular tachyarrhythmias
Neostigmine	2 mg/kg/day divided every 3-4 hr PO	
Pyridostigmine	1-2 mg every 4-12 hr PO 0.05-0.15 mg every 4-8 hr IM	
CHOLINERGIC BLOCKING AGENTS		
Atropine	See antidotes	
Belladonna, tincture	0.1 ml/kg/day divided every 6-8 hr PO	Maximum dose 3.5 ml/day
CHOLINESTERASE INHIBITOR		
Edrophonium	Test dose: 1.0 mg IV for neonates; 0.2 mg/kg/dose IV for infants	Give 20% of test dose initially; if no response in 1 min, give remainder in 1-mg increments; keep atropine available, since drug may precipitate cholinergic crisis

Continued.

Agent	Dosage	Comments
DIURETICS		
Acetazolamide	5 mg/kg/day as a single dose PO, IM	May cause acidosis
Chlorothiazide	20-30 mg/kg/day divided every 12 hr PO	May cause hypokalemia, alkalosis, hyperglycemia
Ethacrynic acid	2-3 mg/kg/day divided every 12 hr PO	Ototoxicity may occur
	0.5-2.0 mg/kg/dose IV	Dosage for infants not well established
Furosemide	1-2 mg/kg/dose every 6-8 hr PO	Ototoxicity may occur in renal disease
	0.5-2.0 mg/kg/dose every 12 hr IM or IV	May cause hypokalemia, alkalosis, and dehydration
Spironolactone	1.7-3.3 mg/kg/day divided every 6-8 hr	May require several days of therapy before effect is seen
ENDOCRINE		
Adrenal		
ACTH	1.6 units/kg/day divided every 6-8 hr IV, IM, SC	
Cortisone	25 mg/m^2/day divided every 8 hr	Physiologic replacement
	12 mg/m^2/day single dose IM	
Desoxycorticosterone	1-3 mg/day IM	
Hydrocortisone	50 mg/kg IV initial dose; then 50-75 mg/kg/day divided every 6 hr	Treatment for gram-negative shock
Prednisone	1-3 mg/kg/day PO	Every other day therapy advisable to minimize growth retardation
Pancreas		
Glucagon	0.025-0.1 mg/kg/dose SC, IV, IM; may repeat every 20-30 min	Treatment for hypoglycemia (1.0 mg maximum dose)
Insulin	0.01-0.1 unit/kg/hour continuous IV infusion	Titrate rate of infusion to achieve desired serum glucose concentration
Pituitary		
Vasopressin	Aqueous: 1-3 ml/day divided every 8 hr SC	
	Tannate in oil: 0.2 ml/dose every 1-3 days IM	
	Nose drops: 1-2 drops at bedtime and every 4-6 hr as needed	
Thyroid		
Desiccated thyroid	Initial: 8-15 mg/day as a single dose PO	Titrate dosage at weekly intervals to normalize serum T$_4$; usual maintenance 50-200 mg/day
Lugol's Solution	One drop 3 times per day PO	
Methimazole	Initial: 0.4 mg/kg/day divided every 8 hr PO	
	Maintenance: 0.2 mg/kg/day divided every 8 hr	
Propylthiouracil	5-10 mg/kg/day divided every 8 hr	Dosage for infants not well established
Triiodothyronine (T$_3$)	Calculate dosage as for desiccated thyroid using the equivalent: 65 mg desiccated thyroid = 25 µg T$_3$	
MINERALS		
Calcium		
Chloride (27% Ca^{++})	250-300 mg/kg/day as a 2% solution divided every 6 hr PO	Do not administer intravenously
Glubionate (90 mg Ca^{++}/gm salt)	500 mg/kg/day divided every 4-8 hr PO	High osmotic load
Gluconate (9.4% Ca^{++})	500 mg/kg/day divided every 4-8 hr PO	
	100-200 mg/kg/dose by slow IV infusion	Monitor heart rate when administering IV
Lactate (13% Ca^{++})	500 mg/kg/day divided every 4-8 hr PO	
Iron		
Ferrous sulfate drops (25 mg Fe/ml)	6 mg elemental iron/kg/day divided in 3 doses PO	Treatment of iron-deficiency anemia
	1-2 mg elemental iron/kg/day divided into 2-3 doses	Prophylaxis
Ferrous gluconate (7 mg Fe/ml)	As above	

Agents	Dosage	Comments
Magnesium		
Sulfate	0.05 ml/kg of a 50% solution every 6 hr IV or IM × 3-4 doses initially; then 12-15 mg/100 ml of maintenance IV fluid	For hypomagnesemia; calcium gluconate should be available as an antidote; monitor serum concentrations
NARCOTICS		
Meperidine	6 mg/kg/day divided every 4-6 hr PO, IV, IM, SC as needed	
Morphine	0.05-0.2 mg/kg/dose repeated every 3-4 hr IV, IM as needed	
SEDATIVES/TRANQUILIZERS		
Chloral hydrate	10-30 mg/kg/day divided every 6-8 hr IV, IM, PO, PR	Sedative dose
	50 mg/kg as a single dose PO or PR	Hypnotic dose
Chlorpromazine	2.0-2.5 mg/kg/day divided every 6 hr PO, IM	
Diazepam	0.1-1.0 mg/kg/day divided every 6-8 hr PO	May displace bilirubin
Promethazine	0.25-1.0 mg/kg/dose divided every 6-8 hr as needed PO, IM	
VITAMINS (daily requirements)		
A	250-750 IU PO	
B_1 (thiamine)	Premature: 200 μg PO	
	Full term: 40 μg PO	
	Treatment: 10 mg given every 6-8 hr	
B_2 (riboflavin)	Premature: 400 μg PO	
	Full term: 60 μg PO	
B_6 (pyridoxine)	Premature: 400 μg PO	Give 50 mg stat for pyridoxine-dependent seizures
	Full term: 35 μg PO	
B_{12} (cyanocobalamin)	Premature: 1.5 μg PO	
	Full term: 0.15 μg PO	
C (ascorbic acid)	Premature: 60 mg PO	
	Full term: 8 mg PO	
D	Premature: 600 IU PO	
	Full term: 40-100 IU PO	
E	Premature: 30 IU PO	
	Full term: 4 IU PO	
K	Premature: 15 μg	
	Full term: 4 μg	Start with 1 mg and adjust to normalize clotting functions
	Treatment: 1-10 mg IM	
MISCELLANEOUS		
Aminophylline	Loading dose: 5-6 mg/kg by slow IV infusion	Serum theophylline concentrations should be monitored and doses adjusted to achieve peak concentrations between 6 and 13 μg/ml
	Maintenance dose: 1-2 mg/kg/dose every 8-12 hr IV or PO	
Caffeine	Loading dose: 10 mg/kg IV or PO	Serum caffeine levels in the range 5-20 μg/ml; caffeine may accumulate in the serum of theophylline-treated infants
	Maintenance dose: 2.5 mg/kg/day as a single dose IV or PO	
Chloroquine	10 mg/kg/day PO	
	5 mg/kg/day IV	
Kayexalate	Calculate dose to desired exchange PO or PR every 6 hr as needed; average is 0.5-1 gm/kg/dose. 1 mEq potassium per 1 gm of resin	
Mannitol	0.5-2.0 gm/kg IV over 1 hr following a 200-mg/kg IV test dose	
Methadone	0.3-0.4 mg/kg/day PO	
Pancuronium bromide (Pavulon)	0.04-0.10 mg/kg/dose repeated as needed IV	Morphine or barbiturate may be considered with Pavulon to ease anxiety
Cimetidine	20-40 mg/kg/day IV, PO divided every 6 hr	

Jeffrey L. Blumer
Thomas A. Blumenfeld

APPENDIX C Tables of normal values

BLOOD PRESSURE

Table 1. Average systolic, diastolic, and mean blood pressures during the first 12 hours of life in normal newborns grouped according to birth weight

Birth weight		1	2	3	4	5	6	7	8	9	10	11	12
1,001 to 2,000 gm	Systolic	49	49	51	52	53	52	52	52	51	51	49	50
	Diastolic	26	27	28	29	31	31	31	31	31	30	29	30
	Mean	35	36	37	39	40	40	39	39	38	37	37	38
2,001 to 3,000 gm	Systolic	59	57	60	60	61	58	64	60	63	61	60	59
	Diastolic	32	32	32	32	33	34	37	34	38	35	35	35
	Mean	43	41	43	43	44	43	45	43	44	44	43	42
Over 3,000 gm	Systolic	70	67	65	65	66	66	67	67	68	70	66	66
	Diastolic	44	41	39	41	40	41	41	41	44	43	41	41
	Mean	53	51	50	50	51	50	50	51	53	54	51	50

(Column group header: Hour)

From Kitterman, J.A., Phibbs, R.H., and Tooley, W.H.: Pediatrics **44**:959, 1969.

URINE AND STOOL

Table 2. Time of first voiding by 500 full-term infants

	Number	Percent	Cumulative percent
Delivery room	85	17.0	17.0
Hours			
12	253	50.6	67.6
12-24	124	24.8	92.4
24-48	35	7.0	99.4
Over 48	3*	0.6	100.0
Totals	500	100.0	

From Sherry, S.N., and Kramer, I.: J. Pediatr. **46**:189, 1955.
*These patients voided at 50, 50, and 51 hours.

Table 3. Time of passage of first urine in 200 premature infants

Time	Number	Percent
Delivery room	45	21.5
Hours		
0-12	86	43.0
12-24	52	26.0
24-48	17	9.5
Over 48		

From Kramer, I., and Sherry, S.N.: J. Pediatr. **51**:374, 1957.

Table 4. Time of passage of first stool by 500 full-term infants

	Number	Percent	Cumulative percent
Delivery room	136	27.2	27.2
Hours			
12	209	41.8	69.0
12-24	125	25.0	94.0
24-48	29	5.8	99.8
Over 48	1*	0.2	100.0
Totals	500	100.0	

From Sherry, S.N., and Kramer, I.: J. Pediatr. **46:**158, 1955.
*Sixty-two hours.

Table 5. Time of passage of first stool in 200 premature infants

Time	Number	Percent
Delivery room	26	13.0
Hours		
0-12	63	31.5
12-24	71	35.5
24-48	28	14.0
Over 48	12	6.0

From Kramer, I., and Sherry, S.N.: J. Pediatr. **51:**373, 1957. From the Department of Pediatrics, Sinai Hospital of Baltimore, Inc.

CEREBROSPINAL FLUID

Table 6. Cerebrospinal fluid in healthy term newborns

	0-24 Hours	1 Day	7 Days	> 7 Days
Color	Clear or xanthochromic	Clear or xanthochromic	Clear or xanthochromic	
Red blood cells/mm^3	9 (0-1,070)	23 (6-630)	3 (0-48)	
Polymorphonuclear leukocytes/mm^3	3 (0-70)	7 (0-26)	2 (0-5)	
Lymphocytes/mm^3	2 (0-20)	5 (0-16)	1 (0-4)	
Proteins (mg/dl)	63 (32-240)	73 (40-148)	47 (27-65)	
Glucose (mg/dl)	51 (32-78)	48 (38-64)	55 (48-62)	
Lactate dehydrogenase (IU/L)	←——— 22-73 ———→ (Birth-7 days)			0-40

Data from Naidoo, B.T.: S. Afr. Med. J. **42:**932, 1968; Neches, W., and Platt, M.: Pediatrics **41:**1097, 1968.

CHEMISTRY

Table 7. Acid-base status of term and premature infants from birth to 3 days of age

Determination	Sample source	Birth	1 Hour	3 Hours	24 Hours	2 Days	3 Days
Vigorous term infants, vaginal delivery							
pH	Umbilical artery	7.26					
	Umbilical vein	7.29					
P_{CO_2} (mm Hg)	Arterial	54.5	38.8	38.3	33.6	34	35
	Venous	42.8					
O_2 sat	Arterial	19.8	93.8	94.7	93.2		
	Venous	47.6					
pH	Left atrial		7.30	7.34	7.41	7.39 (temporal artery)	7.38 (temporal artery)
CO_2 content (mEq/L)			20.6	21.9	21.4		
Premature infants							
	Capillary (skin puncture)						
pH	<1,250 gm				7.36	7.35	7.35
P_{CO_2} (mm Hg)					38	44	37
pH	>1,250 gm				7.39	7.39	7.38
P_{CO_2} (mm Hg)					38	39	38

From Schaffer, A.J.: Diseases of the newborn, ed. 3, Philadelphia, 1971, W.B. Saunders Co. Data from Weisbort and others: J. Pediatr. **52**:395, 1958; Bucci, G., and others: Biol. Neonate **8**:81, 1965.

Table 8. Normal blood chemistry values of term infants

Determination	Sample source	Cord	1-12 Hours	12-24 Hours	24-48 Hours	48-72 Hours
Sodium mEq/L*	Capillary	147 (126-166)	143 (124-156)	145 (132-159)	148 (134-160)	149 (139-162)
Potassium, mEq/L		7.8 (5.6-12)	6.4 (5.3-7.3)	6.3 (5.3-8.9)	6.0 (5.2-7.3)	5.9 (5.0-7.7)
Chloride, mEq/L		103 (98-110)	100.7 (90-111)	103 (87-114)	102 (92-114)	103 (93-112)
Calcium, mg/dl		9.3 (8.2-11.1)	8.4 (7.3-9.2)	7.8 (6.9-9.4)	8.0 (6.1-9.9)	7.9 (5.9-9.7)
Phosphorus, mg/dl		5.6 (3.7-8.1)	6.1 (3.5-8.6)	5.7 (2.9-8.1)	5.9 (3.0-8.7)	5.8 (2.8-7.6)
Blood urea, mg/dl		29 (21-40)	27 (8-34)	33 (9-63)	32 (13-77)	31 (13-68)
Total protein, gm/dl		6.1 (4.8-7.3)	6.6 (5.6-8.5)	6.6 (5.8-8.2)	6.9 (5.9-8.2)	7.2 (6.0-8.5)
Blood sugar, mg/dl		73 (45-96)	63 (40-97)	63 (42-104)	56 (30-91)	59 (40-90)
Lactic acid, mg/dl		19.5 (11-30)	14.6 (11-24)	14.0 (10-23)	14.3 (9-22)	13.5 (7-21)
Lactate, mmol/L†		2.0-3.0	2.0			

From Schaffer, A.J.: Diseases of the newborn, ed. 3, Philadelphia, 1971, W.B. Saunders Co.
*Acharya, P.T., and Payne, W.W.: Arch. Dis. Child. **40**:430, 1965.
†Daniel, S.S., Adamsons, K., Jr., and James, L.S.: Pediatrics **37**:942, 1966.

Table 9. Normal blood and urine chemistry values of newborns

Constituent	Age and value
Ammonia nitrogen[1,2] (plasma)	Newborn, 90-150 µg/dl
α-Fetoprotein[3] (plasma, serum)	Birth, 0-10 mg/dl
Calcium,[4] total (plasma, serum)	Premature, 1 week, 6.0-10.0 mg/dl (1.5-2.5 mmol/L)
	Full-term, 1 week, 7.0-12.0 mg/dl (1.75-3.00 mmol/L)
Cholesterol[1] (plasma, serum)	Premature, cord blood, 47-98 mg/dl (1.2-2.5 mmol/L)
	Full-term, cord blood, 45-98 mg/dl (1.2-2.5 mmol/L)
	Full-term, newborn, 45-167 mg/dl (1.2-4.3 mmol/L)
	3 days-1 year, 69-174 mg/dl (1.8-4.5 mmol/L)
Copper[1] (plasma, serum)	0-6 months, 70 µg/dl
Creatinine[5] (plasma, serum)	Newborn, 0.8-1.4 mg/dl
Free fatty acid[1] (plasma)	Newborn, 905 µEq ± 470 µEq/L
Magnesium[1,2,5] (plasma, serum)	Newborn, 1.52-2.33 mEq/L
Phosphorus[1,2,5] (inorganic plasma, serum)	Premature, at birth, 5.6-8.0 mg/dl (1.81-2.58 mmol/L);
	6-10 days, 6.1-11.7 mg/dl (1.97-3.78 mmol/L)
	20-25 days, 6.6-9.4 mg/dl (2.13-3.04 mmol/L)
	Full-term, at birth, 5.0-7.8 mg/dl (1.62-2.52 mmol/L);
	3 days, 5.8-9.0 mg/dl (1.87-2.91 mmol/L)
	6-12 days, 4.9-8.9 mg/dl (1.58-2.87 mmol/L)
	1 month, 5.9-9.5 mg/dl (1.62-3.07 mmol/L)
Vitamin A[1,5] (retinol) (plasma, serum)	Birth, 20 mg/dl
Creatinine[5] (urine)	Newborn, 8-13 mg/kg/day
Homovanillic acid[6] (HVA) (urine)	1-12 months, 12.9 ± 9.6 (1.2-35) µg/mg creatinine
Vanillylmandelic acid[7] (VMA) (urine)	1 week-1 month, 35-180 µg/kg/day

[1]O'Brien, D., and Rodgerson, D.O.: Interpretation of biochemical values. In Kempe, C.H., Silver, H.K., and O'Brien, D., editors: Current pediatric diagnosis and treatment, ed. 3, Los Altos, Calif., 1974, Lange Medical Publications, pp. 970-994.
[2]O'Brien, D., Ibbot, F.A., and Rodgerson, D.O.: Laboratory manual of pediatric micro-biochemical techniques, ed. 4, New York, 1968, Hoeber.
[3]Karlson, B.W., and others: Acta Paediatr. Scand. **61**:133, 1972.
[4]Meites, S.: C.R.C. Crit. Rev. Clin. Lab. Sci **6**(1):1, 1975.
[5]Meites, S., editor: Pediatric clinical chemistry: a survey of normals, methods and instruments, Washington, D.C., 1977, American Association for Clinical Chemistry.
[6]Gitlow, S.E., and others: J. Lab. Clin. Med. **72**:612, 1968.
[7]Hakolinen, A.: Acta Paediatr. Scand. [Suppl.] 212, 1971.

Table 10. Normal blood chemistry values (average), low birth weight infants, capillary blood, first day

Determination	Birth weight (gm)			
	< 1,000	1,001-1,500	1,501-2,000	2,001-2,500
Sodium, mEq/L	138	133	135	134
Potassium, mEq/L	6.4	6.0	5.4	5.6
Chloride, mEq/L	100	101	105	104
Total CO$_2$, mEq/L	19	20	20	20
Urea, mg/dl	22	21	16	16
Total serum protein, gm/dl	4.8	4.8	5.2	5.3

From Schaffer, A.J.: Diseases of the newborn, ed. 3, Philadelphia, 1971 W.B. Saunders Co. Data from Pincus and others: Pediatrics **18**:939, 1956.

Table 11. Levels of whole blood glucose in normal full-term infants

Group		No.	Maternal	At delivery (umbilical) Vein	At delivery (umbilical) Artery	½	1	1½	2	2½	3	4	6	9	12	24	References
I Blood sugar, mg/dl	Mean	46	108	80	68	60	51	50	52	56	56		56	52	52		Creery and Parkinson (1953)
	SE		4.2	2.6	4.3	2.5	2.4	2.0	1.8	1.8	2.0		1.6	1.4	1.8		
	Range		68	49	40	27	21	19	30	34	30		32-82	30-73	10-75		
			154	126	118	110	87	79	77	90	90			Normal vaginal			
II Blood sugar, mg/dl	Mean	32	Birth		76	77	71		64			63	63	Normal vaginal			Farquhar (1954)
	SE				2.6	3.5	3.7		2.4			2.0	2.0				
	Range				43-105	44-128	39-121		39-102			31-87	38-90				
IIIa True blood sugar, mg/dl		13	Vaginal, no fluid to mother														Cornblath and others (1961)
	Mean		85	66		55	55		48			55	47	Normal			
	SE		4.6	3.5		5.8	5.2		3.5			3.5	3.9				
	Range		63-121	44-84		34-90	35-89		22-73			30-71	27-28				
IIIb		7	Cesarean section, saline IV to mother														
	Mean		85	64		75	76		70			60	57			54	
	SE		11.2	6.0		6.6	11.8		8.5			9.7	5.3			5.0	
	Range		46-131	38-90		58-107	34-136		45-108			47-101	35-76			43-76	
IIIc		23	Cesarean section, glucose IV to mother														
	Mean		149	107		72	67		57			60	53			67	
	SE		17.3	12.6		8.0	8.5		6.1			4.3	3.7			5.7	
	Range		77-354	61-204		31-125	28-117		34-115			27-90	32-77			35-109	
IIId		8	Vaginal, glucose IV to mother														
	Mean		127	89		54	47		41			50	51				
	SE		20.1	12.9		8.4	8.3		5.8			4.8	7.0				
	Range		80-250	54-163		27-98	16-82		19-71			34-80	29-81				

From Cornblath, M., and Schwartz, R.: Diseases of carbohydrate metabolism, Philadelphia, 1966, W.B. Saunders Co.

Table 12. Levels of whole blood glucose in low birth weight infants

Group		Cord blood	Age (hours)									References
			0-3	4-6	12	18	24	30	36	42	48	
I												
True blood sugar, mg/dl	Mean	71		47	45	43	43	44	41	46	50	Ward (1953)
	SE	6.0										
	Range	24-140										
No. determinations		21										
IIa												
Blood glucose, mg/dl	Mean											Somogyi
						15-62	16-60	18-90	25-60	18-78	19-80	
				26-72	18-107	23	14	15	10	14	14	
				20	23							
	Mean		41	47	48				44			Baens and others (1963)
	SE		2.6	2.5	3.1	45			1.7			
	Range		24-72	21-70	25-89	2.5			18-73			
						23-84			49			
No. determinations			20	26	22	37						Glucose oxidase

Group		Age (days)													Conditions and references
		0	1	2	3	4	5	6	7	8	9	10	11	12	13	
III																
True blood sugar, mg/dl	Mean	45	53	55	60	60	58	63	63	66	65	71	65	63	64	Fast, 2-3 hours Norval (1950)
	SE	1.8	1.6	2.0	1.9	2.0	1.4	1.7	1.9	2.1	2.1	2.9	1.7	2.3	2.0	
	Range	←— 15 to 115 mg/100 ml —→														
No. determinations		33							28	25	24	23	23	23	22	Somogyi
IIb		0	1	2	3	4	5	6	7-13	14-20	21-27	28-55				
Blood glucose, mg/dl	Mean	44		39	40	42	43	43	45	56	52	48				Fast, 3½-4 hours Baens and others (1963)
	SE	1.7		1.9	1.9	2.1	2.1	2.2	1.6	2.8	2.9	2.5				
	Range	18-73		15-73	20-64	21-79	18-78	22-83	28-61	23-98	18-77	22-83				
No. determinations		49		45	43	32	33	33	40	33	26	43				Glucose oxidase

From Cornblath, M., and Schwartz, R.: Disorders of carbohydrate metabolism, Philadelphia, 1966, W.B. Saunders Co.

Table 13. Serum iron and iron-binding capacity in the newborn and mother

Serum iron (μg/dl)		Total iron-binding capacity (μg/dl)		References
Infant	Mother	Infant	Mother	
173	98	259	470	Hagberg (1953)
147	80	226	446	Laurell (1947)
193	—	240	—	Sturgeon (1954)
(145-240)		(147-468)		
159	—	—	—	Vahlquist and others (1941)
(106-227)				

From Oski, F.A., and Naiman, J.L.: Hematologic problems in the newborn, ed. 2, Philadelphia, 1972, W.B. Saunders Co.

Table 14. Thyroid function

	Birth	24 Hours	48 Hours	1 Week	2 Weeks	4 Weeks
PBI (μg/dl)	4.3-9.5	7.3-12.9	9.6-16.8	7.3-14.5	4.0-11.0	4.0-11.0
BEI (μg/dl)	5.5	—	—	9.8	7.8	4.8
	(4.5-6.5)			(7.8-12.0)	(7.0-8.2)	(4.0-5.5)
TSH (μU/ml)	8.38	17.1 ± 3	12.8 ± 1.9	—	< 1-10	—
	(3-22)					
Thyroxin (T_4) (μg/dl)	11.2					
	(6.9-16.7)					
		11-23			9-18	
		←—1-3 days—→		←——1 week-1 month——→		

From Meites, S., editor: Pediatric clinical chemistry: a survey of normals, methods, and instruments, Washington, D.C., 1977, American Association for Clinical Chemistry.

Table 15. Serum enzymes in newborns

Enzymes	Age	IU/L
Acid phosphatase*	Birth-1 month	7.4-19.4
Alanine amino transaminase (SGPT)*,§	Birth-10 days	1.3-11
	Birth-1 month	0-54
Aldolase†	Birth-1 month	4-24
Alkaline phosphatase§	Birth-1 month	20-225
	1 month-3 months	73-226
Aspartate amino transaminase (SGOT)*,§	Birth-10 days	6-25
	Birth-1 month	0-67
Creatinine phosphokinase (CPK)‡	Premature	0-210
	Birth-3 weeks	22-267
	3 weeks-3 months	15-134
Gamma glutamyl transpeptidase (GGPT)‡	Premature	56-233
	Birth-3 weeks	0-103
	3 weeks-3 months	4-111
Lactate dehydrogenase (LDH)†	Birth-10 days	150-590
	1 day-1 month	185-404
	1 month-2 years	110-244
Leucine aminopeptidase (LAP)*	Birth-1 month	29-59
	>1 month	15-50

*O'Brien, D., and Rodgerson, D.O.: Interpretation of biochemical values. In Kempe, C.H., Silver, H.K., and O'Brien, D., editors: Current pediatric diagnosis and treatment, ed. 3, Los Altos, Calif., 1974, Lange Medical Publications.
†Meites, S., editor: Pediatric clinical chemistry: a survey of normals, methods and instruments, Washington, D.C., 1977, American Association for Clinical Chemistry.
‡Sitzmann, F.C.: Arch. Kinderheilk. (Suppl.) **57:**1, 1968.
§King, J., and Morris, M.B.: Arch. Dis. Child. **36:**604, 1961.

Table 16. Hormones and steroid metabolites in the healthy newborn

	Age	Male	Female
Plasma and serum			
Follicle-stimulating hormone (FSH)[1]	0-2 years	4-12 IU/L	6-40 IU/L
Luteinizing hormone (LH)[1]	0-2 years	0.6-1.8 IU/L	1.3-3.0 IU/L
Testosterone[1]	0-2 years	4-37 ng/dl	7-18 ng/dl
Human growth hormone (HGH)[2]	Newborn (fasting)	15-40 ng/ml; response to provocation variable	
	After newborn (fasting resting)	0-5 ng/ml; response to natural and artificial provocation (i.e., arginine, insulin, hypoglycemia) > 8 ng/ml	
17-Hydroxyprogesterone[3]	< 4 days	< 15 µg/L	
	> 4 days	< 5 µg/L	
Urine			
17-Hydroxycorticosteroids[4,5]	Birth-14 days	0.05-0.3 mg/day	
	15 days-1 year	0.1-0.5 mg/day	
17-Ketosteroids[6]	Birth-14 days	< 2.5 mg/day	
	15 days-1 year	< 1.0 mg/day	
Pregnanetriol[1]	Birth-14 days	0.0-0.2 mg/day	
	15 days-1 year	0.0-0.1 mg/day	

[1]Meites, S., editor: Pediatric clinical chemistry: a survey of normals, methods and instruments, Washington, D.C., 1977, American Association for Clinical Chemistry.
[2]O'Brien, D., and Rodgerson, D.O.: Interpretation of biochemical values. In Kempe, C.H., Silver, H.K., and O'Brien, D., editors: Current pediatric diagnosis and treatment, ed. 3, Los Altos, Calif., 1974, Lange Medical Publications.
[3]Barnes, N.D., and Atherden, S.M.: Arch. Dis. Child. **47:**62, 1972.
[4]Smith, E.K., Reardon, H.S., and Field, S.H.: J. Pediatr. **64:**652, 1964.
[5]Ulstrom, R.A., and others: J. Clin. Endocrinol. Metab. **20:**1066, 1960.
[6]Mitchell, F.L.: Vitam. Horm. **25:**191, 1967.

Table 17. Serum total protein and electrophoresis fractions in newborns (gm/dl)

Fraction	Cord blood	At birth	1 Week	1-3 Months
Total protein	4.78-8.04	4.6-7.0	4.4-7.6	3.64-7.38
Albumin	2.17-4.04	3.2-4.8	2.9-5.5	2.05-4.46
Alpha-1	0.25-0.66	0.1-0.3	0.09-0.25	0.08-0.43
Alpha-2	0.44-0.94	0.2-0.3	0.30-0.46	0.40-1.13
Beta	0.42-1.56	0.3-0.6	0.16-0.60	0.39-1.14
Gamma	0.81-1.61	0.6-1.2	0.35-1.3	0.25-1.05

Data from Meites, S., editor: Pediatric clinical chemistry: a survey of normals, methods and instruments, Washington, D.C., 1977, American Association for Clinical Chemistry; Ellis, E.F., and Robbins, J.B.: Children are different, Columbus, Ohio, 1970, Ross Laboratories, pp. 72-73.

Table 18. Mean complement levels of sera of newborns of different birth weights and the maternal sera, compared with a normal adult standard serum

	Complement component levels (mean ± 1 SEM)							
	Ratio to standard serum*						mg/dl†	
Group	CH$_{50}$‡	C1q	C2	C3(B$_{1C}$)	C4	C4(B$_{1E}$)	C1q	B$_{1C}$	B$_{1E}$
1. <1,000 gm	0.6 ± 0.1 (7)§	0.5 ± 0.1 (7)	1.2 ± 0.1 (2)	0.6 ± 0.1 (7)	0.5 ± 0.1 (7)	0.6 ± 0.2 (7)	1.1 ± 0.2	89 ± 16	9 ± 3
2. 1,000-1,500 gm	0.7 ± 0.1 (7)	0.4 ± 0.02 (9)	0.4 ± 0.2 (3)	0.7 ± 0.1 (9)	1.4 ± 0.3 (7)	0.8 ± 0.1 (9)	1.1 ± 0.1	94 ± 10	12 ± 2
3. 1,500-2,000 gm	0.7 ± 0.3 (5)	0.7 ± 0.1 (8)	1.2 ± 0.5 (4)	0.9 ± 0.2 (7)	1.0 ± 0.6 (4)	1.0 ± 0.3 (8)	1.6 ± 0.3	141 ± 24	15 ± 4
4. 2,000-2,500 gm	0.9 ± 0.2 (5)	0.8 ± 0.1 (5)	1.0 ± 0.2 (5)	1.0 ± 0.2 (5)	1.2 ± 0.4 (5)	1.4 ± 0.3 (5)	1.9 ± 0.3	151 ± 33	21 ± 5
5. >2,500 gm	0.9 ± 0.1 (8)	0.9 ± 0.5 (11)	1.0 ± 0.2 (6)	1.0 ± 0.1 (11)	1.4 ± 0.2 (7)	1.0 ± 0.1 (11)	2.2 ± 0.1	160 ± 13	16 ± 2
6. Mother	1.5 ± 0.1 (24)	0.9 ± 0.04 (25)	1.2 ± 0.2 (18)	1.8 ± 0.1 (27)	1.9 ± 0.2 (23)	2.3 ± 0.1 (26)	2.3 ± 0.1	254 ± 12	35 ± 2
7. Normal standard	1.0	1.0	1.0	1.0	1.0	1.0	2.5	145.2	15.2

From Sawyer, M.K., and others: Biol. Neonate **19:**148, 1971.
*Determined by titration assay.
†Determined by radial immunodiffusion assay.
‡Total hemolytic complement expressed in 50% hemolytic units.
§Number in parentheses refers to number in group.

Table 19. Serum immunoglobulin levels in newborns (mg/dl)

Age	IgG	IgA	IgM
Newborn	631-1,431	Up to 8	1-21
6 days-4 weeks	400-1,250	4-36	20-80
1-2 months	200-950	5-64	20-142

Data from Stiehm, E.R., and Fudenberg, H.H.: Pediatrics **37**:715, 1966; Allansmith, M., and others: J. Pediatr. **72**:279, 1968; Meites, S., editor: Pediatric clinical chemistry: a survey of normals, methods and instruments, Washington, D.C., 1977, American Association for Clinical Chemistry.

Table 20. Plasma-serum amino acids in premature and term newborns (µmol/L)

Amino acid	Premature, first day	Newborn, before first feeding	16 Days-4 months
Taurine	105-255	101-181	
OH-proline	0-80	0	
Aspartic acid	0-20	4-12	17-21
Threonine	155-275	196-238	141-213
Serine	195-345	129-197	104-158
Asp + Glut	655-1155	623-895	
Proline	155-305	155-305	141-245
Glutamic acid	30-100	27-77	
Glycine	185-735	274-412	178-248
Alanine	325-425	274-384	239-345
Valine	80-180	97-175	123-199
Cystine	55-75	49-75	33-51
Methionine	30-40	21-37	15-21
Isoleucine	20-60	31-47	31-47
Leucine	45-95	55-89	56-98
Tyrosine	20-220	53-85	33-75
Phenylalanine	70-110	64-92	45-65
Ornithine	70-110	66-116	37-61
Lysine	130-250	154-246	117-163
Histidine	30-70	61-93	64-92
Arginine	30-70	37-71	53-71
Tryptophan	15-45	15-45	
Citrulline	8.5-23.7	10.8-21.1	
Ethanolamine	13.4-105	32.7-72	
α-Amino-n-butyric acid	0-29	8.7-20.4	
Methylhistidine			

Data from Dickinson, J.C., Rosenblum, H., and Hamilton, P.B.: Pediatrics **36**:2, 1965; Dickinson, J.C., Rosenblum, H., and Hamilton, P.B.: Pediatrics **45**:606, 1970.

Table 21. Urine amino acids in normal newborns (μmol/day)

Amino acid	μmol/day
Cysteic acid	Tr-3.32
Phosphoethanolamine	Tr-8.86
Taurine	7.59-7.72
OH-proline	0-9.81
Aspartic acid	Tr
Threonine	0.176-7.99
Serine	Tr-20.7
Glutamic acid	0-1.78
Proline	0-5.17
Glycine	0.176-65.3
Alanine	Tr-8.03
α-Aminoadipic acid	
α-Amino-n-butyric acid	0-0.47
Valine	0-7.76
Cystine	0-7.96
Methionine	Tr.0.892
Isoleucine	0-6.11
Tyrosine	0-1.11
Phenylalanine	0-1.66
β-Aminoisobutyric acid	0.264-7.34
Ethanolamine	Tr-79.9
Ornithine	Tr-0.554
Lysine	0.33-9.79
1-Methylhistidine	Tr-8.64
3-Methylhistidine	0.11-3.32
Carnosine	0.044-4.01
β-Aminobutyric acid	
Cystathionine	
Homocitrulline	
Arginine	0.088-0.918
Histidine	Tr-7.04
Sarcosine	
Leucine	Tr-0.918

Adapted from Meites, S., editor: Pediatric clinical chemistry: a survey of normals, methods and instruments, Washington, D.C., 1977, American Association for Clinical Chemistry.

Table 22. Creatinine, urea, and inulin clearance (ml/min/1.73 m^2)

	Premature	Term newborn	1 Month
Creatinine	40-65	40-65	
Urea	3.5-17.3	8.7-33	
Inulin			50 (29-88)

Data from Meites, S., editor: Pediatric clinical chemistry: a survey of normals, methods, and instruments, Washington, D.C., 1977, American Association for Clinical Chemistry; O'Brien, D., Ibbott, F.A., and Rodgerson, D.O.: Laboratory manual of pediatric micro-biochemical techniques, ed. 4, New York, 1968, Hoeber.

Table 23. Haptoglobin levels in low birth weight infants*

Gestation (weeks)	0	5	10	15	21	28
< 32	10 (3)	—	—	—	—	—
32-34	—	18.5 (2)	51.6 (3)	42.6 (3)	12 (1)	12 (1)
34-36	9.8 (9)	14.9 (11)	11.4 (10)	11.6 (9)	7.1 (7)	16.5 (4)
36-38	13.0 (7)	18.3 (3)	16.6 (5)	16.3 (2)	11 (1)	7.5 (1)
38+	9.3 (8)	28.3 (6)	20.9 (4)	10.1 (5)	9.2 (3)	7.0 (1)
Totals	10.5 (27)	19.6 (22)	19.5 (22)	16.1 (19)	8.3 (12)	13.2 (7)

From Philip, A.G.S.: Biol. Neonate **19:**322, 1971.
*Haptoglobin levels are measured as mg/dl MetHb binding capacity. Numbers in parentheses indicate number of samples from which mean values were derived.

Table 24. Haptoglobin levels in full-term infants

	Birth	Fifth day
Haptoglobin (mg/dl Hgb binding capacity)	23.9 (10.6-50.0)	52.3 (14.8-100.0)

Table 25. Serum folic acid (mμg/ml)

Age	Range	Mean ± SD
Normal premature infants		
1-4 days	7.17-52.00	29.54 ± 0.98
2-3 weeks	4.12-15.62	8.61 ± 0.55
1-2 months	2.81-11.25	5.84 ± 0.35
2-3 months	3.56-11.82	6.95 ± 0.50
3-5 months	3.85-16.50	8.92 ± 0.86
5-7 months	6.00-12.25	9.02 ± 0.74
Normal children		
1-6 years	4.12-21.25	11.37 ± 0.82

From Klaus, M.H., and Fanaroff, A.A.: Care of the high risk neonate, Philadelphia, 1973, W.B. Saunders Co. Adapted from Shojania, A., and Gross, S.: J. Pediatr. **64:**323, 1964.

Table 26. Serum vitamin E (mg/dl), mean ± 1 SD

	\multicolumn{10}{c	}{Weeks}
	1	2	3	4	5	6	7	8	9	10
< 1,500 gm, 28-32 weeks	0.40 (0.05)	0.30 (0.04)	0.25 (0.03)	0.25 (0.03)	0.25 (0.03)	0.25 (0.03)	0.25 (0.03)	0.25 (0.03)	0.35 (0.04)	0.45 (0.05)
1,500-2,000 gm, 32-36 weeks	0.45 (0.05)	0.40 (0.05)	0.40 (0.05)	0.45 (0.05)	0.45 (0.05)	0.45 (0.05)	0.50 (0.05)	0.50 (0.05)	0.60 (0.06)	0.70 (0.06)
2,000-2,500 gm, 36-40 weeks	0.50 (0.05)	0.45 (0.05)	0.50 (0.05)	0.60 (0.06)	0.70 (0.06)	0.75 (0.06)	0.75 (0.60)	0.75 (0.60)	0.75 (0.06)	0.80 (0.70)
> 2,500 gm, term	0.55 (0.60)	0.55 (0.60)	0.55 (0.60)	0.60 (0.60)	0.75 (0.70)	0.80 (0.70)	0.85 (0.80)	0.85 (0.80)	0.85 (0.80)	0.85 (0.80)

From Klaus, M.H., and Fanaroff, A.A.: Care of the high risk neonate, Philadelphia, 1973, W.B. Saunders Co.

Table 27. Relationship of age, total blood volume, and body weight of infants*

Age	Body weight (kg) (fiftieth percentile)	Total blood volume (ml)
26 weeks	0.9	104
28 weeks	1.1	127
30 weeks	1.3	150
32 weeks	1.6	185
34 weeks	2.1	242
36 weeks	2.6	299
38 weeks	3.0	345
Birth	3.4	272-340

*Based on total blood volume of: (1) premature infant, 115 ml/kg; (2) newborn, 80-110 ml/kg.

Table 28. Body water (values as percent body weight)

Age	Total body water	Extracellular water	Intracellular water
0-11 days	77.8 (69-84)	42.0 (34-53)	34.6 (28-40)
11 days-6 months	72.4 (63-83)	34.6 (28-57)	38.8 (20-47)

From O'Brien, D., Ibbott, F.A., and Rodgerson, D.O.: Laboratory manual of pediatric micro-biochemical techniques, ed. 4, New York, 1968, Hoeber.

HEMATOLOGY

Table 29. Mean red cell values during gestation

Age (weeks)	Hb (gm/dl)	Hematocrit (%)	RBC (10^6/mm^3)	Mean corpuscle vol (μ^3)	Mean corpuscle Hb ($\gamma\gamma$)	Mean corpuscle Hb conc (%)	Nuc RBC (% of RBCs)	Retic (%)	Diam (μ)
12	8.0-10.0	33	1.5	180	60	34	5.0-8.0	40	10.5
16	10.0	35	2.0	140	45	33	2.0-4.0	10-25	9.5
20	11.0	37	2.5	135	44	33	1.0	10-20	9.0
24	14.0	40	3.5	123	38	31	1.0	5-10	8.8
28	14.5	45	4.0	120	40	31	0.5	5-10	8.7
34	15.0	47	4.4	118	38	32	0.2	3-10	8.5

From Oski, F.A., and Naiman, J.L.: Hematologic problems in the newborn, ed. 2, Philadelphia, 1972, W.B. Saunders Co.

Table 30. Postnatal hematologic values

		1-3 Days	4-7 Days	2 Weeks	4 Weeks	6 Weeks	8 Weeks
< 1,200 gm birth weight	Hgb	15.6	16.4	15.5	11.3	8.5	7.8
	Retic	8.4	3.9	1.9	4.1	5.4	6.1
	Plat	148,000 ±61,000	163,000 ±69,000	162,000	158,000	210,000	212,000
	Leuk	14,800 ±10,200	12,200 ±7,000	15,800	13,200	10,800	9,900
	Seg	46	32	41	28	23	23
	Band	10.7	9.7	8.0	5.9	5.8	4.4
	Juv	2.0	3.9	5.3	3.6	2.6	2.0
	Lymph	32	43	39	55	61	65
	Monos	5	7	5	4	6	3
	Eos	0.4	6.2	1.0	3.7	2.0	3.8
	Nuc/RBC	16.7	1.1	0.1	1.0	2.7	2.0
>1,200-<1,500 gm birth weight	Hgb	20.2	18.0	17.1	12.0	9.1	8.3
	Retic	2.7	1.2	0.9	1.0	2.2	2.7
	Plat	151,000 ±35,000	134,000 ±49,000	153,000	189,000	212,000	244,000
	Leuk	10,800 ±4,000	8,900 ±2,900	14,300	11,000	10,500	9,100
	Seg	47	31	33	26	20	25
	Band	11.9	10.5	5.9	3.0	1.4	2.1
	Juv	5.1	2.4	2.7	1.8	1.7	1.6
	Lymph	34	48	52	59	69	64
	Monos	3	6	3	4	5	5
	Eos	1.3	2.2	2.5	5.1	2.6	2.3
	Nuc/RBC	19.8	0.8	0	0.4	1.4	1.0

From Wolff and Goodfellow: Pediatrics **16**:753, 1955.

Table 31. Normal hematology of the full-term newborn (venous blood)

	Cord blood	Day 1	Day 2	Day 7	Day 20	Day 45	Day 75
Hemoglobin (gm/dl)	16.8	18.4	17.8	17.0	15.9	12.7	11.4
Range	13.7-20.1				11.3-20.5	9.5-15.9	9.6-13.2
	(14.0)*	(14.5)	(14.0)	(14.0)		(10.0)	(10.0)
Hematocrit (%)	53	58	55	54			
	(44)	(48)	(45)	(45)			
Reticulocyte count (%)	3-7	3-7	1-3	0-1	0-1	0-1	0-1
Nucleated RBC/mm³	500	200	0-5	0	0	0	0
(% per 100 WBC)	(10%)	(7%)					
Per 100 RBC	0.1	0.05	0	0			
RBC morphology		Macrocytes					

*Values given in parentheses indicate anemia.

Table 32. White blood cell count and differential count during the first 2 weeks of life

		Neutrophils						
Age	Leukocytes	Total	Seg	Band	Eosinophils	Basophils	Lymphocytes	Monocytes
Birth								
Mean	18,100	11,000	9,400	1,600	400	100	5,500	1,050
Range	9.0-30.0	6.0-26			20-850	0-640	2.0-11.0	0.4-3.1
Mean %	—	61	52	9	2.2	0.6	31	5.8
7 days								
Mean	12,200	5,500	4,700	830	500	50	5,000	1,100
Range	5.0-21.0	1.5-10.0			70-1,100	0-250	2.0-17.0	0.3-2.7
Mean %	—	45	39	6	4.1	0.4	41	9.1
14 days								
Mean	11,400	4,500	3,900	630	350	50	5,500	1,000
Range	5.0-20.0	1.0-9.5			70-1,000	0-230	2.0-17.0	0.2-2.4
Mean %	—	40	34	5.5	3.1	0.4	48	8.8

From Altman, P.L., and Dittmer, D.S.: Blood and other body fluids, Washington, D.C., 1961, Federation of American Societies for Experimental Biology.

Table 33. Venous platelet counts in normal low birth weight infants

Day	No. of infants	Mean mm³	Range 1,000's
0	60	203,000	80-356
3	47	207,000	61-335
5	14	233,000	100-502
7	52	319,000	124-678
10	40	399,000	172-680
14	50	386,000	147-670
21	47	388,000	201-720
28	40	384,000	212-625

From Appleyard, W.J., and Bunton, W.A.: Biol. Neonate **17:**30, 1971.

Table 34. Platelet counts in full-term infants

Day	Mean	Range
Cord	200,000	100,000-280,000
1	192,000	100,000-260,000
3	213,000	80,000-320,000
7	248,000	100,000-300,000
14	252,000	

Table 35. Normal percentile values for micro-ESR in 100 low birth weight infants 3 days of age or less

	ESR (mm/1 hour)	
Percentile	Male*	Female†
10	1.0	1.0
25	1.8	1.8
50	2.5	3.0
75	3.3	4.0
90	4.0	6.0
95	6.0	6.0
99	8.8	8.3

From Evans, H., and others: J. Pediatr. **76:**448, 1970.
*Hematocrit: median 57%, range 43% to 78%.
†Hematocrit: median 54%, range 41% to 77%.

Table 36. Normal percentile values for micro-ESR in 30 low birth weight infants, median age 28 days, range 9 to 56 days

Percentile	ESR (mm/1 hour)*
10	3.0
25	3.8
50	5.5
90	9.5
95	11.0

From Evans, H., and others: J. Pediatr. **76:**450, 1970.
*Hematocrit: median 35%, range 25% to 58%.

Table 37. Bone marrow differential count during the first week of life

	0-24 Hours (%)	7 Days (%)	Adult (%)
Myeloblasts	0-2	0-3	0.3-50
Promyelocytes	0.5-6.0	0.5-7.0	1.0-8.0
Myelocytes	1.0-9.0	1.0-11.0	5.5-22.5
Metamyelocytes	4.5-25.0	7.0-35.0	13.0-32.0
Band forms	10.0-40.0	11.0-45.0	—
Erythroblasts	0-1.0	0-0.5	1.0-8.0
Proerythroblasts	0.5-9.0	0-0.5	2.0-10.0
Normoblasts	18.0-41.0	0-15.0	7.0-32.0
Myeloid:erythroid ratio	1.5:1.0	6.5:1.0	3.5:1.0

From Oski, F.A., and Naiman, J.L.: Hematologic problems in the newborn, ed. 2, Philadelphia, 1972, W.B. Saunders Co. Adapted from Shapiro and Bassen (1941) and Gairdner and others (1952).

Table 38. Coagulation factor and test values in normal pregnant women and newborns*

Category	Fibrinogen (mg/dl)	II (%)	V (%)	VII (%)	VIII (%)	IX (%)	X (%)	XI (%)	XII (%)	XIII (titer)	Euglobulin lysis time (min)	Partial thromboplastin time† (sec)	Prothrombin time (sec)	Thrombin time (sec)
Normal adult or child	190-420	100	100	100	100	100	100	100	100	1/16	90-300	37-50	12-14	8-10
Term pregnancy	483	92	108	170	196	130	130	69	—	1/16	278	44	13	8.0
Premature (1,500-2,500 gm), cord blood	233	25	67	37	80	Dec‡	29	—	—	1/8	214	90	17 (12-21)	14 (11-17)
Term infant, cord blood	216	41	92	56	100	27	55	36	—	1/8	84	71	16 (13-20)	12 (10-16)
Term infant, 48 hours	210	46	105	20	100	Dec	45	39	25	—	105	65	17.5 (12-21)	13 (10-16)

Adapted from Hathaway, W.E.: Pediatr. Clin. North Am. **17**:929, 1970.
NOTE: All levels expressed as means or ranges; if no reference is noted, the value is derived from unpublished data from the author's laboratory.
*Kaolin PTT.
‡Dec, Decreased.

Thomas A. Blumenfeld

Index

A

A type blood, 726
a Wave, 129
  in central venous pressure rise, 540
  seen during umbilical catheterization, 186
Aarskog's syndrome, 63
Abdomen
  congenital malformations of 1050-1051
  inspection of, 255
Abdominal compression, 121
Adbominal diameter, fetal, 84
Abdominal distension
  in gastrointestinal perforation, 485
  in intestinal obstruction, 483
  in jejunoileal obstruction, 502
  in polycystic disease, 796
Abdominal masses, 531-532
  in renal disease, 791
Abdominal wall defects, 529-531
  ultrasonographic detection of, 86
Abdominal wall movement in respiration monitoring, 284-285
Abducens nerve
  examination of, 354-355
  palsy, 222, 224
Abduction contractures, 227
Aberrant fetal growth; *see* Fetal growth, aberrant
Abetalipoproteinemia, 523, 525
ABO incompatibility, 42, 726
  in hereditary spherocytosis, 737
  hyperbilirubinemia in, 759
Abortion
  malformations in, 1037-1038
  spontaneous, due to smoking, 153
Abrasions
  corneal, 976
  of ears, 225
  sustained at birth, 216
Abruptio placentae, 84, 212
  in disseminated intravascular coagulation, 720
  elevated baseline pressure in, 114
  in preeclampsia, 30
  and premature labor, 141
  due to smoking, 153

Abscess
  breast, 670
  scalp
    following FHR monitoring, 190-191, 238, 669
    due to *Neisseria gonorrhoeae*, 673
Absolute neutrophil count, 744
Acanthocytosis, 738
Acantholysis, 946
Acanthosis nigricans, benign congenital, 959
Acardiac fetus, 215
Accelerations in heart rate
  fetal, 99-101
  neonatal, 119
Accountability of perinatal center for population, 5
Acentric fragment, 1017
Acetabular dysplasia, 1009-1012, 1084
Acetabulum, double-notch, 465
Acetaldehyde, 167
Acetaminophen in human milk, 166
Acetazolamide
  dosage for, 1096
  for hydrocephalus, 380
Acetylation
  deficiency of, at birth, 162
  enzymes causing, 158
Acetylcholine decreasing pulmonary artery pressure, 130
Acetylcholinesterase
  in aganglionic tissue, 505
  in amniotic fluid, 1033
N-Acetylglutamate synthetase deficiency, 824
Acetylphenylhydrazine, 735
Acetylsalicylic acid in human milk, 166
Achalasia, 495
Achard syndrome, 1059
Acheria, 1058
Achondrogenesis, 463, 465
Achondroplasia
  differentiation from hydrocephalus, 379
  head shape in, 1041
  homozygous, 463, 465
  nose in, 1048
Acid
  biologic, 320
  gastric, 160
  organic, metabolic disorders of, 824-830

Acid citrate dextrose
  for exchange transfusion, 767
  in hypoglycemia, 863
Acid maltase deficiency, 838
Acid phosphatase values, 1104
Acid reflux test, 494
Acid-base equilibrium
  disturbances of, 322-327
    and callium homeostasis, 871
    due to digitalis toxicity, 62
    fetal, in variable deceleration, 102
    hypocalcemic, 876
  net acid balance, 321-322
  physicochemical mechanisms of, 320
  physiologic mechanisms of, 320-321
Acid-base profile
  fetal, 115
  normal newborn, 1100
Acid-base therapy, 433
Acid-fast organisms, 678
Acidosis, 72-73
  and bilirubin binding, 765
  due to diaphragmatic hernia, 488
  dilution, 324
  first breath caused by, 179
  increased at night in neonatal ICU, 18
  increasing pulmonary artery pressure, 130
  maternal, 117
  in meconium aspiration syndrome, 444
  renal factors in, 786
  renal tubular, 801, 803-804
Acinar region, 407-408
Acne neonatorum, 944
Acoustic nerve examination, 355
Acoustics in hospital units, 293
Acrocephalosyndactyly, 384; see also Apert's syndrome
  eyes in, 976
Acrocephaly, 384
Acrocyanosis, 429
Acrodermatitis enteropathica, 523, 527, 950
ACTH; see Adrenocorticotropic hormone
Actin, 746
  in bilirubin transport, 771
Actinomycin D, 747
Active awake state, 329-331
Active sleep
  apnea during, 458
  in preterm infants, 333-334
  respirations during, 122
  in term infant, 329-331
Acuity, visual, 338
Adaptive problems, perinatal, 70
Addiction
  maternal, effects on neonate, 933-937
  from narcotics in human milk, 167
Addis count, 788
Adenine arabinoside, 1094
Adenomatous lung cysts, 455
  delivery room diagnosis of, 193
  preventing lung expansion, 184
Adenosine deaminase deficiency, 647
Adenosine triphosphate
  embryonic activity of, 479-480
  generation of, 736
  hemoglobin combined with, 710, 711

Adenovirus, 683
Adenyl cyclase activation, 663
Adipose tissue in SGA infants, 66
Adrenal glands
  abscess of, 670
  absent, in hepatoblastoma, 748
  calcified, 233, 234
  drugs for disorders of, 1096
  fetal
    hypoplasia of, 140
    ultrasonic detection of, 86
  growth of, in SGA infant, 66
  hemorrhage of, 233-235, 715
  neuroblastoma on, 748
Adrenal hyperplasia, congenital, 915-922
  malabsorption due to, 525
β-Adrenergics
  antagonists, effect on ventilation, 412
  blocking agents, and FHR variability, 97
  dosages for, 1092
  fetal activity of, 85
  receptor population, 143
  stimulators, 573
Adrenocorticotropic hormone
  dosage for, 1096
  in hypoglycemia, 861
  to test adrenal function, 235
  unresponsiveness, 861-862
Adrenogenital syndrome, 1024
  examination for, 256
  maldigestion due to, 523
Adriamycin; see Doxorubicin
Adult polycystic disease, 796-797
Aerobacter, 805
Aerobic metabolism, fetal, 1151
Aeromonas hydrophila, 683
Afferent inputs to neonatal respiratory center, 456
After-birth period, care of parents during, 243-247
AGA infant; see Appropriate for gestational age infant
Agammaglobulinemia
  B lymphocytes in, 644
  X-linked infantile, 645-646, 961
Aganglionosis, 505
  colonic, 1075
Agar to reduce enteric bilirubin absorption, 770
Age
  and diagnosis of disease, 1024
  as factor in drug absorption, 160
Agranulocytosis, 745
Air
  as contrast medium, 1072
  in rectum, diagnostic, 509
Air bronchogram
  absence of, 470
  in pulmonary consolidation, 1067
  in respiratory distress syndrome, 429
  in tachypnea, 448
Air embolism, 130
Air flow measurement, 424
Air leak, 437
  diagnostic radiology for, 1068-1069
  predisposing to bronchopulmonary dysplasia, 472
  syndromes, 448-451
Air mattress, 123, 124

Air temperature
  in incubator, 261-265, 296-297
  in nursery, 264-265, 296
Air trapping, 448
Air-fluid levels
  bowel patency indicated by, 1075
  plain film visualization of, 1070
Air-swallowing, 1074
  effect on radiologic appearance, 1078
Airway
  development and growth of, 407-408
  gas flow detection in, 284
  oral, for nasal fractures, 223
Airway collapse, 454
Airway obstruction
  mechanical, 180
  and respiratory distress, 462-463
Airway pressure system, 123
Alacrima, 984
Alagille syndrome, 775
Alanine elevation in SGA infant, 73
Alanine amino transaminase
  in fructose intolerance, 833
  in hyperbilirubinemia, 766
  values for, 1104
Alarm system
  in cardiac monitor, 280
  in respiration monitor, 285
Alarm timer in delivery room, 183
Albers-Schönberg disease, 723
Albinism
  complete, 954
  eyes in, 1000
  oculocutaneous, 747
  partial, 954
Albright's syndrome, 952
Albumin
  bililrubin binding of, 754
    reduction of
      in kernicterus, 765
      in Rh hemolytic disease, 759
  ^{51}Cr-labeled, 526
  dosage for, 1095
  in meconium, 518
  in nephrotic syndrome, 800
  salt-poor, 767
  serum
    in bronchopulmonary dysplasia, 474
    displacement of bilirubin from, 165-166
  for systemic hypertension, 567
Albumin-reacting antibodies, 35
Albustix, 788
Alcaptonuria, 820
Alcohol; see also Ethanol
  addiction to, 936
  associated with congenital malformations, 153
Aldactone; see Spironolactone
Aldolase, 1104
Aldosterone effect, 499
Aldosterone hypersecretion, 791
Aleukemic reticulosis, 987
Alexander's disease, 379
Alginic acid, 495
Alimentary tract as origin of abdominal masses, 532
Alimentation, metabolism during, 54

Alkali, delivery room administration of, 185-188
Alkaline phosphatase
  as determinant of fetal growth, 66
  embryonic activity of, 479-480
  values for, 1104
Alkaline picrate method to measure creatinine, 137
Alkalosis
  contraction, 324
  metabolic; see Metabolic alkalosis
  respiratory; see Respiratory alkalosis
Alkylating agents, 154
Allergy
  to antiprostaglandins, 143
  cow's milk, colitis due to, 487
  cow's milk–protein, 526
  soy protein, 526
    colitis due to, 487
Allogeneic cells, 639
Alloisoleucine, 825
Alpha-fetoprotein
  amniotic fluid test for, 1061
  blood values for, 1101
  as determinant of fetal growth, 66
  in hepatoblastoma, 748
  in maternal serum, 1033
  neural tube defect diagnosis with, 1032-1033
Alphaprodine
  for labor, 174
  sinusoidal FHR due to, 106
Alternative pathway of complement system, 633-634
Aluminum silicate, 137
Alveolar dead space, 425
Alveolar overdistension, 423
Alveolar phase of lung development, 407
Alveolar rhabdomyosarcoma, 748
Alveolar ridges, hypertrophied, 1049
Alveoli
  in bronchopulmonary dysplasia, 470-471
  development of, 406, 407, 408
Amaurosis, Leber's congenital, 1000
Amblyopia
  due to congenital esotropia, 989
    accompanying leukoma, 225
  due to lid hemangioma, 980
Amelanosis, 954
Amelia, 1051
American Indians, physiologic jaundice in, 758
Amikacin, 660
  dosage for, 1092
  for sepsis, 655, 656
Amino acid storage disease, 838
Amino acids
  blood values for, 1107
  crystalline, in total parenteral nutrition, 310
  essential for premature infant, 304
  fetal intestinal transport of, 480
  in intravenous nutrient administration, 312
  malabsorption of, 523
  metabolism of
    diagnostic tests for, 1031
    disorders of, 817-822
    inborn errors of, 1036
  placental transport of, 50
  supplementation feedings with, 309
  urine values for, 1108

Aminoaciduria, 802
  hyperdibasic, 802
  microcephaly due to, 381
Aminoglycosides
  eliminated via glomerular filtration, 164
  in human milk, 166
  for meningitis, 658
  for pneumonia, 447
  potentiating noise-induced hearing loss, 273
Aminopeptidase, embryonic activity of, 479-480
Aminophylline
  dosage for, 1097
  neonatal tachycardia due to, 121
  for premature labor, 142
  in weaning from ventilator, 437
Aminopterin, 58, 1026
Amish, incidence of PK deficiency in, 736
Ammonia nitrogen, plasma values for, 1101
Amniocentesis
  in area of fetal small parts, 37
  to detect erythroblastosis fetalis, 35
  to determine fetal lung development 25, 69
  fetal injury during, 1029
  incidence of Down's syndrome and chromosomal abnormalities by, 1030
  for prenatal genetic diagnosis, 1028-1033
  ultrasonic guidance for, 85
  to view placenta, 211
Amniography, 40, 41, 44, 1028
Amnion
  anatomy of, 206
  tears of, 207
Amnion nodosum, 47-48
  pathogenesis of, 207
  in renal agenesis, 793
Amniorrhea, 207
Amniotic bands, 207
Amniotic fluid
  bilirubin in, 757-758
    values for, 39, 40
  biochemical fetal assessment of, 110
  contaminated, 650
  diminished; see Oligohydramnios
  excess; see Polyhydramnios
  Liley's graph of specimen of, 38
  meconium staining of, 443
  in nephrotic syndrome, 800
  optical density of, 136-137
  phospholipids of, 417
  pigments of, 36
  polymorphonuclear leukocytes in, 653
  purulent, 445
  in Rh incompatibility, 727-728
  supernatant, 1029
  viscosity of, 136
  volume of
    in intrauterine growth retardation, 92
    normal, 45
Amniotic fluid analysis
  nonsurfactant tests, 137-138
  surfactant tests, 134-137
Amphetamines
  in human milk, 166
  and intrauterine growth retardation, 58
Amphojel, 792

Amphotericin B
  for candidiasis
    cutaneous, 950
    oral, 684
  for coccidioidomycosis, 685
  dosage for, 1094
Ampicillin, 660
  diarrhea due to, 524
  dosage for, 1092
  estriol secretion affected by, 111
  plasma half-life of, 164
  for sepsis, 655, 656
  for *Streptococcus agalactiae*, 673
Amputations, fetal, 1008
Amyl nitrite, 142
Amylase
  embryonic activity of, 480
  pancreatic, in low birth weight infant, 305
  salivary, 521
α-Amylase, activities of, 516
Amyotonia congenita, 231
Anacrotic notch, 126
Anaerobic infection, 670-671
Anal agenesis, 509
Anal atresia
  delivery room diagnosis of, 194
  ultrasonic detection of, 86
Anal fissure, 510
Anal stenosis, 509
Analeptics, 188
Analgesics
  in human milk, 166
  for normal labor and delivery, 174-175
  teratogenicity of, 155
Anaphase lag, 1016
Anastomosis
  of bile ducts, 779-780
  for cystic fibrosis, 521
  for esophageal atresia, 498
  of facial nerve, 223
  for jejunoileal obstruction, 504
  placental, 215
  in preductal coarctation of aorta, 591
Anatomic dead space, 425
Androgen insensitivity syndromes, 914-915
Androgen-dependent target cells, 913-915
Androgenic hormonal stimulation of fetus, 63
Androgens
  effect on sweat glands, 941
  in genital development, 902
  maternally derived, 922-923
  for pancytopenia, 723
Androstenedione
  blood levels of, in pseudohermaphroditism, 918
  conversion to testosterone, 913
Anemia
  congenital hypoplastic, 721-723
  due to cortical & medullary necrosis, 808
  delayed manifestation of, 730
  due to ecchymoses, 217
  of endocrine insufficiency, 723
  due to erythrocyte underproduction
    acquired, 723-725
    congenital, 721-723
  fetal, 106

Anemia—cont'd
  heart failure due to, 569
    treatment of, 571
  hemolytic, 34
    due to hemorrhage, 712-715
    due to hemorrhagic disorders, 715-721
  maternal
    effect on fetal growth, 58
    fetal asphyxia due to, 180
  neonatal tachycardia due to, 121
  due to red cell destruction, 725-730
Anencephaly
  associated with diminished birth weight, 63
  associated with hydramnios, 193
  associated with prolonged pregnancy, 44
  role of growth hormone in, 55
  ultrasonic detection of, 89, 91
Anesthesia
  conduction, and prolonged FHR decelerations, 104
  for labor and delivery
    normal, 174-175
    in special circumstances, 175-178
Aneuploidy, 1015-1017
Aneurysms
  aortic, 63
  umbilical vessel, 714
Angiocardiography
  in d-transposition, 586-587, 588
  indications for, 622-623
Angiography
  in lobar emphysema, 454
  renal, 788
Angioma
  capillary, 956, 977
  cavernous, 956
  choroidal, 977
  cutaneous, 955-958
  within umbilical cord, 209
Angiotensin in preeclampsia, 28
Anhidrosis, 224
Aniline, methemoglobinemia precipitated by, 733
Animal studies
  on administration of alkali, 185
  on asphyxia, 361
  on cellular proliferation, 478-479
  on drug effects, 158
  on effect of corticosteroids on fetal lung, 417
  on lung development, 412, 414
  on physiologic jaundice, 756-757
Anion, undetermined, 321-322
Aniridia, 991
Anisocoria, 224
Anisometropia, 984
Ankylosis of mandible, 223
Annular constriction bands, 1008
Annular pancreas, 194
  with congenital duodenal obstruction, 501
Anocutaneous fistula, 509
Anodontia, 963
Anomalad sequence, definition of, 1035
Anomalies, congenital; see Congenital malformations
Anomaly, definition of, 1035
Anophthalmia, 982
Anorchia, congenital, 911
Anorectal anomalies, 508-510

Anorectal anomalies—cont'd
  abscess and fistula, 510
  voiding cystourethrography for, 1079
Anorectal fissures, 487
Anovestibular fistula, 509
Anovulvar fistula, 509
Antacids
  bezoars due to, 501
  for hiatal hernia, 495
Antenatal care in intrauterine growth retardation, 66-70
Anterior chamber
  bleeding into, 975
  inspection of, 970
Anterior horn cell disease, 394-395, 461
Anterior perianal anus, 509
Anterior vascular capsule of lens, 257, 259
Anthropomorphic measurements, 49
Antibacterials, 1092-1093
Antibiotic prophylaxis, 688
Antibiotics
  maldigestion due to, 523, 524
  for meconium aspiration syndrome, 445
  for necrotizing enterocolitis, 513
  for respiratory distress syndrome, 433
  for sepsis, 655
  vitamin K deficiency due to, 718
Antibodies
  causing erythroblastosis fetalis, 42-43
  maternal transfer of, in hyperbilirubinemia, 759
  naturally occurring, 726
  19S, 726, 727
  to poliovirus, 680
  relationship of type to placental transfer, 640
  screening for, 34
  7S 726, 727
  in syphilis, 675
Antibody titers, antiacetylcholine receptor, 396
Anti-(C) antibody, 42
Anticoagulants
  dosages for, 1094
  in human milk, 166
  teratogenicity of, 156
Anticonvulsants
  dosages for, 392, 1094
  inducing congenital malformations, 153
  teratogenicity of, 154
Anti-D immune globulin, 727
Antidiuretic hormone, syndrome of inappropriate secretion of, 391
Antidotes, 1095
Anti-(E) antibody, 42
Antierythrogenic toxin, 640
Antifungals, 1094
Anti-Fy[a] antibody, 42
Antigenemia, hepatitis B, 696, 702
Antigenic differences, maternal-fetal, 63
Antigens
  in B cell differentiation, 638
  hepatitis B, 695, 696
  neonatal function of, 638-639
  red cell, 726
  Rh, 35, 726, 727
Antihistamines, 155
Antiinflammatory drugs in human milk, 166
Anti-Kell antibody, 42
Anti-Kell hemolytic disease, 728

Antimetabolites, 154
Antimicrobials
　associated with congenital malformations, 153
　in human milk, 166
　plasma half-lives of, 159
　teratogenicity of, 154
Antimongoloid slant, 1043
　chromosomal abnormalities characterized by, 978
Antinauseants, 155
Antineoplastics
　associated with congenital malformations, 153
　teratogenicity of, 154
Antiperistaltic waves, 481
Antiprostaglandins, 143
Antiproteinase, 472
Anti-Rh₀(D) antibody, 35
　for erythroblastosis fetalis, 758
Antistaphylococcal antibody, 640
Antistreptolysin, 640
Antithrombin III, 716
Antitoxin, tetanus, 677
α-1-Antitrypsin deficiency, 782
Antituberculous agents, 1094
Antiviral agents, 1094
Anus
　congenital malformations of, 1051
　covered, 509
　imperforate, 509, 510, 511, 1051
Aorta
　dimension of, 552
　echocardiographic measurement of, 548, 551
　hypoplasia of, 588
Aortic arch
　double, 615
　interrupted, 591
Aortic compression, 109
Aortic pulse wave analysis, 126
Aortic stenosis
　aortic pressure in, 126
　congenital, 589-590
Aortic thrombi due to umbilical catheterization, 188
Aortic valve, 548
　atresia of, 588
　opening and closing of, 552, 555
　in transposition of great arteries, 583, 584, 587
Aortography, 592
　for abdominal masses, 788
　in heart failure, 569
　umbilical, 1077
Apert's syndrome, 383, 384
　choanal atresia in, 463
　facies in, 976
　suture closure in, 1084
　syndactyly in, 1059
Apgar score, 181-183
　acidosis, and asphyxia, relationship between, 116
　in analysis of mortality, 10
　five-minute, 183
　in hypoxic ischemic encephalopathy, 359-360
　limitations of, 183
　order of disappearance of signs, 182
　person to assign, 183
　time to assign, 183
　value of scoring, 182-183

Aplastic anemia
　in hemolytic disease, 724
　idiopathic acquired, 724
Apnea
　fetal, 110
　idiopathic, 459-460
　neonatal, 122, 126
　obstructive, inability to detect, 286
　patterns in, 125
　of prematurity, 456-460
　primary and secondary, 180, 181
　recurrent, 202
　　incidence of, 203
　during seizures, 389
Apnea monitors, 285, 294
Apocrine glands, 941
Apoproteins, surfactant, 414
Appendicitis, 533
Appropriate for gestational age infant, percentiles for, 197, 198
Apresoline; *see* Hydralazine
Apt test, 486-487
Aqueductal stenosis, 376
Arachidonic acid, 304
　role in onset of labor, 140
Arachnodactyly, 1059
Arachnoid cysts, 379
Arch ridge patterns, 1052, 1054
Arching of back in hiatal hernia, 493
Areolas, 942
　hyperpigmentation of, 943
Arginase deficiency, 824
Arginine, 304
Arginine hydrochloride, 326
Argininosuccinicaciduria, 824
Arm anthropometry, 474
Arnold-Chiari malformation, 375-377
Arousal response criterion in hearing screening, 355
Arousal states
　in preterm infant, 332
　in term infant, 328-331
Arrector pili muscles, 942
Arrhinencephaly, 382
Arrhythmias
　benign, 576
　due to digitalis toxicity, 620
　drug therapy for, 575-576
　due to exchange transfusion, 730
　intermittent, 541-542
　mechanisms of, 575
　pathologic, 576-579
　sinus, 547
　ventricular tachycardia, 579-582
Arterial obstruction, renal, 806
Arterial oxygen saturation
　in cyanosis, 560, 561
　in d-transposition, 586, 588
　in mixed venous and arterial blood, 601
Arterial pulse
　bounding, 541
　in neonatal heart disease, 539, 540
Arterial unsaturation
　in cyanosis, 560, 564
　mechanisms for, 559
Arterial wall pressure, 284
Arteriohepatic dysplasia, 596

1120 Index

Arteriovenous fistula
    intracranial, 608
    pulmonary, 456
        echocardiography in, 557
    systemic, 608-609
Arteriovenous shunts in twin placenta, 215
Arteritis, umbilical, 665
Artery(ies)
    cutaneous, 941
    single umbilical, 61, 62, 209-211
Arthritis, septic, 236, 667-668, 1084
Arthrocentesis, 236
Arthrography, hip, 236
Arthrogryposis, 1008, 1059
    in myotonic dystrophy, 396
Arthrogryposis multiplex congenita, 398
Artifact
    in cardiac monitoring, 280
    in pressure monitoring system, 281
    in respiration monitoring, 285
    in skull radiology, 1084
Artificial bacterial colonization, 688
Ascites, 532-534
    diagnostic radiology for, 1076
    fetal, 92
    and heart failure, 541, 568
    preventing lung expansion, 180
    renal causes of, 791
Ascorbate, 158
Ascorbic acid for methemoglobinemia, 560, 734
Ashkenazi Jews, Tay-Sachs disease in, 1014
Asian influenza, 681
Ask-Upmark kidney, 799
Aspartate amino transaminase
    in fructose intolerance, 833
    in hyperbilirubinemia, 766
    in myotonic dystrophy, 396
    values for, 1104
Aspartate transcarbamylase, 479
Aspergillus niger, 839
Asphyxia
    acute total, 361
    in disseminated intravascular coagulation, 720
    and drug depression, differentiation of, 188-189
    effect on quiet awakeness, 338
    fetal, 2
    intrapartum, 175, 357-358
        brain sites involved in, 358
        and cardiogenic shock, 574
        hypocalcemia in, 875
        urinary retention due to, 789
    neonatal
        antenatal detection of, 66
        effect on other organs, 192
        pathologic features of, 191-192
    partial prolonged, 361-363
    seizures due to, 389
    of SGA infant, 72-73
Asphyxia pallida, 255
Asphyxiating thoracic dystrophy, 1058
Aspiration
    diagnostic, 220
    recurrent, 467
Aspiration syndromes, 445-446
    delivery room treatment of, 184

Aspirin
    persistence of fetal circulation due to, 556
    for premature labor, 143
Asplenia, congenital, 747
Association of malformations, 1035
Asthma due to ectodermal dysplasia, 964
Astrup method of acid-base determination, 325
Asymmetrical crying facies, 374
Atarax; *see* Hydroxyzine
Ataxia-telangiectasia, 961
Atelectasis
    arterial carbon dioxide tension in, 423
    compression, from assisted ventilation, 451
    diagnostic radiology for, 1067-1068
    after extubation, 439
    in phrenic nerve paralysis, 228
    recurrent, 469
    in respiratory distress, 134
Atlas occipitalization, 230
Atrial fibrillation, 578
Atrial flutter, 578
Atrial hypertrophy, 546
Atrial rate, 578
Atrial septal gradient, 603
Atrial septectomy, 587
Atrioventricular block, 580-582
    in atrial flutter, 578
    maternal systemic lupus erythematosus causing, 537
    PR interval in, 547
Atrioventricular canal, common, 607-608
Atrioventricular node arrhythmias, 575
Atrioventricular valve abnormalities, 558
    a waves in, 129
Atrium, single, 601
Atropine
    effect on surfactant, 413
    for cardiac resuscitation, 582
    for cardiovascular disease, 626
    dosage for, 1095
    fetal baroreceptor response altered by, 102
    neonatal tachycardia due to, 121
    rises in FHR due to, 95, 101
Attachment behaviors, 240
Attention and perception in neonate, 337
Atypical familial nephrotic syndrome, 801
Auditory attention, 339-340
Auerbach's plexus, 481
    ganglion cell degeneration in, 495
    in Hirschsprung's disease, 505
Auscultation
    in delivery room, 255
    for neonatal arterial blood pressure, 126
    problems of, 283
Automaticity, disorders of, 575
Autonomic nervous system disorders affecting heart rate, 121
Autoregulation in preterm infant, 370
Autosomal inheritance patterns, 1023-1024
Avascular villi, 61
Awake state
    in preterm infant, 334
    in term infant, 329-331
Axillary temperature measurement, 263
Axis of ear, vertical, 1047
Azotemia, 313
Azygos vein, 603

B

B lymphocytes
  in breast milk, 642
  development of, 637-638
  differentiation of, 639
B type blood, 726
Bacillus subtilis, 651
Background noise in ICU, 16
Bacteria
  phagocytic action on, 632-633
  transplacental acquisition of, 650-651
Bacterial endocarditis, 622
Bacteriuria, 804-806
  during pregnancy, 651
  and premature labor, 141
Bacteroides, 651, 671
Baffle procedure for cardiac surgery, 587, 588
Bagging, oxygen concentration during, 437
Balanced reciprocal translocations, 1017
Balanoposthitis, 790
Ball valve phenomenon in meconium staining, 443-444
Ballard scoring system to assess gestational age, 257, 258
Balloon septostomy, 587, 599, 603
Band neutrophils, 653, 654
Barbiturates
  in human milk, 166
  for hypoxic ischemic encephalopathy, 367
  malformations due to, 1037
  septic shock due to, 128
  in tetanus, 677
Barium enema
  for aganglionosis, 505-506
  in meconium plug syndrome, 507
Barium sulfate, 1072
Barium swallow
  in duodenal malrotation, 502
  in esophageal fistula, 194
  examination after, 483
  in hiatal hernia, 494
  for vascular rings, 496
  for ventricular septal defect, 606
Barlow's test, 1010-1011
Barotrauma, 437
  bronchopulmonary dysplasia due to, 473
Barr body, 1024, 1029
Barrier nursing technique, 687-688
Basal ganglia
  effect of poliovirus on, 680
  status marmorata of, 191
Base deficit, delivery room reduction of, 185
Base substitution, 157
Baseline fetal heart rate, 95-99
Baseline preprogram measurements, 14
Bases, conjugate, 320
Basilar artery, ultrasonic detection of, 83
Bassinets, 294
Battering, and early neonatal separation, 241
Bayley Scales of Infant Development, 18
BCG vaccine, 678, 679
Beak sign, 499
Beckwith's syndrome, 256
  components of, 530
  role of insulin in, 55

Beckwith-Wiedemann syndrome
  capillary hemangiomas in, 956
  hypoglycemia in, 858-859
  limb hypertrophy in, 1051
  omphalocele in, 1050
  polycythemia in, 741
  renal tumors in, 809
Bed rest for premature labor, 142
Beds, open radiantly heated, 270
Behavior
  infant
    with heart disease, 539
    in response to mother, 244
  parenting, 242
  social, in preterm infant, 334-335
Behavioral characteristics
  common among poor women, 59
  of SGA infant, 72
Behavioral teratogens, 152
Belladonna, 1095
Benefit of fetal monitoring, 106
Benign congenital hypotonia, 397
Benzalkonium chloride, 670
Benzoin tincture, 232
Bergmeister's papilla, 998, 1001
Best's vitelliform degeneration, 1000
Betamethasone, 145
  to hasten lung maturity, 427
Bicarbonate
  as blood buffer, 320
  for metabolic acidosis, 326
  renal threshold for, 786
    decreased, 803
Bicarbonate ion concentration, fetal, 116
Bicycling movement, 389
Bifidus factor, 640
Bilateral pudendal block, 175
Bile in vomitus, 483
Bile acids, fetal absorption of, 480
Bile ascites, 533
Bile pigments and neonatal bradycardia, 121
Bile plug syndrome, 781
Bile salts
  absorption of, after ileal resection, 528
  in low birth weight infant, 305
Biliary atresia
  congenital hyperbilirubinemia in, 774-781
  interpretation of liver biopsy for, 777-778
Bilirubin
  amniotic fluid values of, 39, 40
  conjugation of, 754-755
    deficient, 760-764
  enteric absorption of, 756
  excretion of, 756
  hepatic uptake of, 754
  increased production of, 758-760
  serum concentration of, 756, 765
  staining brain, 726
  staining placenta and cord, 208
  synthesis of, 754
  toxicity, 764-766
  transport of
    fetal, 757-758
    in plasma, 754
  unconjugated, photoisomerization of, 768

"Bilirubin hump," spectrophotometric scan of, 38
Biliverdin, 754
Biochemical fetal assessment
  amniotic fluid, 110
  fetoplacental steroid hormones, 110-112
  placental proteins and enzymes, 110
Biopotential electrodes, skin, 277-278, 285
Biopsy
  liver, 777-778
  needle, 788
  of nevocellular nevi, 953
  punch, 964
Biotin therapy, 827, 828
Biot-like breathing, 122
Biotransformation of drugs, 161
Biparietal diameter
  absolute measurement and rate of change of, 67
  cephalometry to obtain, 134
  as determinant of fetal growth, 66
  in twin gestations, 92
  ultrasonography to obtain, 82-84
Birth
  complications in, facilities for, 6-7
  evaluation at, 181-183
  physiologic changes at, 179-181
  premature; see Prematurity
Birth injury
  asphyxia, 357-358
  brachial plexus palsy, 374
  cerebellar hemorrhage, 373
  epidural bleeding, 373
  to extremities, 235-237
  facial nerve palsy, 374
  to genitalia, 237
  to head, 218-226
  hypoxic ischemic encephalopathy, 358-367
  to intraabdominal organs, 232-235
  intracranial hemorrhage, 373
  to neck and shoulder girdle, 226-230
  ocular, 975
  related to intrapartum fetal monitoring, 237-238
  to soft tissues, 216-218
  to spine and spinal cord, 230-232, 373-374
Birth order, effect on fetal size, 62
Birth weight
  classification by, 196
  and gestational age
    classification by, 196-198
    relationships, 56
  mean values of, 50
  and neonatal risk, 196-205
  and placental weight, correlation of, 61
  specific risks of, 199-203
Biscoumacetate in breast milk, 166
Bishydroxycoumarin in breast milk, 166
Black population
  abnormal G6PD enzymes in, 735
  ABO incompatibility in, 726
  congenital malformations in, 1039
  DNA mutation in, 1032
  α-genes in, 732
  infection in, 651
  lactase activity in, 480
  polydactyly in, 1058
  Rh incompatibility in, 727

Black population—cont'd
  rarity of hip dislocation in, 1009
  thanatophoric dwarfism in, 465
Blackfan-Diamond syndrome, 1058
Bladder
  distension of, during ultrasonography, 82
  malfunction of, in spinal injury, 232
  in prune-belly syndrome, 799
  radiologic appearance of, 1079
  trabeculated, 798
  ultrasonic detection of, 86
Blade breakage during fetal blood sampling, 117
  removal technique after, 238
Blalock and Potts shunt, 594
Blastema, nodular, 809
Blastogenic factor, 637
Bleeding; see also Hemorrhage
  in early pregnancy, 133
  epidural, 373
  in newborn, evaluation of, 721
  subarachnoid, 390
  vaginal, 366
Bleeding time, 721
Blennorrhea, inclusion, 983
Blepharophimosis, 980, 1043
Blepharospasm, 983
Blindness, 975
Blistering diseases, 946-947
  hereditary, 947-950
Blood
  citrated, 190
  diagnostic tests for, 1031
  for erythroblastosis, 190
  heparinized, 190
  in 21-hydroxylase deficiency, 918-919
  in hypocalcemia, 877
  in hypoglycemia, 850
  maternal passage of exogenous compounds from, to milk, 165
  in necrotizing enterocolitis, 513
  occult, 487
  pH of, 320
  replacement of, after cardiac surgery, 625
  sequestered, 759
  skin supply of, 941-942
  for systemic hypertension, 567
  venous and arterial mixing of, 601-602
  viscosity of, in polycythemia, 741
  whole
    dosage for, 1095
    glucose, levels of, 1102-1103
    for transfusion, 742
Blood buffers, 325
  distribution of, 320
Blood cells
  red; see Red blood cells
  white; see White blood cells
Blood chemistry values, 1100, 1101
Blood component replacement therapy, 742-743
Blood derivatives, 1095
Blood flow
  cerebral, effects of mechanical ventilation on, 440
  in d-transposition, 586
  in intervillous space, 109
  in mammary glands, 165
  in maternal breast, on hearing infant cry, 244

Blood flow—cont'd
  in pulmonary atresia, 594
Blood gases, 421-424
  in aortic stenosis, 590
  arterial
    in bronchopulmonary dysplasia, 474
    in neonatal heart disease, 558-559
    in transient tachypnea, 448
  in hypoplastic left-heart syndrome, 589
  in pulmonary atresia, 593
  in persistent truncus arteriosus, 601
  postoperative monitoring of, 624
  in preductal coarctation of aorta, 591
  in respiratory distress syndrome, 430-432
  in tricuspid atresia, 597, 599
Blood loss
  after cardiac surgery, 625
  events leading to, 742
  in utero, from twin to twin, 714
Blood pressure
  average, 1098
  labile, 495
  maintenance of, in hypoxic ischemic encephalopathy, 366-367
  neonatal arterial, 281
    aortic pulse wave analysis of, 126
    methods of measurement, 126
    pitfalls in measurement and interpretation of, 127-128
  in neonatal heart disease, 539
  normal, 619
  in preeclampsia-eclampsia, 27-28
  recorders, 294
  systolic
    blood loss indicated by, 742
    newborn values for, 618
  in uremia, 793
  venous, 281
Blood pressure cuff use, 126
Blood sampling
  fetal; see Fetal blood sampling
  venous and arterial, 1090
Blood specimen collection, 1089-1090
Blood types, 726
  in exchange transfusion, 730
Blood urea nitrogen
  effect of amino acid mixtures on, 311
  in renal artery obstruction, 806
Blood-brain barrier
  alteration in, 765
  to bilirubin, 726
Bloom's syndrome, 63
  skin in, 1040
Blue diaper syndrome, 523
Blue nevus, 954
Blue rubber bleb nevus syndrome, 958
Blueberry-muffin rash, 72, 748
B-mode ultrasonography, 84, 368
  following CT scan, 1085
Body composition, fetal, 49-54
Body mass, contributions of organs to, 53
Body plethysmography, 123
Body weight, neonatal
  correlation with arterial blood pressure, 127
  and insensible water loss in incubator, 270
  percentages in, 315
Boerhave's syndrome, 496

Bombesin-like peptides, 522
Bonding with infant, 240
Bone marrow
  allografting, 748
  differential count, 1112
  dysfunction of, and pancreatic insufficiency, 518, 745
  neonatal, 711
  rate of production of, 744
  release of erythrocytes and myeloid precursors from 725-726
  suppression of, 720
  transplantation of, 646, 648
    in aplastic anemia, 724
    in congenital hypoplastic anemia, 723
Bones
  in cretinism, 894
  density of, 1080-1081
  effect of rubella on, 701
  in pancytopenia, 723
Bony spur, 385, 387
Bordetella pertussis, 640
Bossing, frontal, 1041
  in ectodermal dysplasia, 963
Botryoid rhabdomyosarcoma, 748
Bowel
  cavernous hemangiomas of, 958
  obstruction, ultrasonic detection of, 86
Bowel sounds
  in intestinal obstruction, 483
  in meconium plug syndrome, 507
Boyden chamber chemotaxis analysis, 643
Brachial palsy, 226-228, 374
Brachial plexus injury, 224, 226-227
  associated with humeral fractures, 235
Brachial pulse, 539
Brachiocephalic arteries in coarctation of aorta, 591
Brachycephaly, 1040-1041
Brachydactyly, 1059
Bradycardia
  fetal, 97
  heart rate in, 547
  neonatal, 119
  sinus, 576
Bradykinin, in hypoxia, 192
Brain
  abscess of, 620
  bilirubin staining of, 764
  diagnostic radiology for, 1084-1085
  fetal
    blood flow in, 2
    ultrasonic visualization of, 83
  growth of
    abnormal, 1084
    relative sparing of, in SGA infants, 66
  swelling of, in asphyxia, 191, 362-363
  temperature of, in active sleep, 334
  water distribution in, in asphyxia, 363-364
Brain damage
  in bilirubin encephalopathy, 765
  conditions leading to, 357-358
  in Rh hemolytic disease, 759
Brainstem Evoked Response, 355
Branchial arches, 1042
Brazelton Neonatal Behavioral Assessment Scale, 342-343
Breast milk banking, 642
Breast milk jaundice, 762-763

Breast tissue, newborn, 942
Breast-feeding; see also Milk, human
  after early mother-infant contact, 244
  gastrointestinal bleeding due to, 487
  jaundice related to, 762-763
  protein absorption increased by, 480
Breath detector, 285, 286
Breath hydrogen analysis, 481
Breath sounds
  in diphragmatic hernia, 488
  in esophageal atresia, 496
  in pulmonary agenesis, 454
  in respiratory distress syndrome, 429
Breathing; see also Respiration
  chemical and reflex control of, 456-457
  onset of
    blood gas volumes at, 423-424
    functions of, 425
    and physiologic changes, 179-181
  work of, 426
Breech delivery
  anesthesia for, 176-177
  ecchymoses due to, 217
  petechiae due to, 216
  rupture of liver due to, 232-233
Brethine; see Terbutaline
Bricanyl; see Terbutaline
Brock procedure for infundibular obstruction, 596
Bromides, 58
Bronchi, structure of, 406
Bronchial obstruction, 454, 462
Bronchial tree development, 407-408
Bronchiolitis, 476
Bronchodilators, 475
Bronchogenic carcinoma, 747
Bronchomalacia, 462
Bronchopneumonia, 659
Bronchopulmonary dysplasia, 467
  clinical and radiologic features of, 469-470
  as complication of respiratory distress syndrome, 427
  with diffuse pulmonary interstitial emphysema, 451
  etiology of, 471-473
  management of, 473-475
  outcome after, 475-476
  oxygen toxicity and, 441
  patent ductus arteriosus causing, 438
  pathophysiology of, 470-471
  radiographic recognition of, 430
  reduced risk of
    by continuous distending pressure, 435
    by fluid restriction, 432
Bronchoscopy
  in candidiasis, 684
  fiberoptic, 439, 470
  in lobar emphysema, 454
Bronchospasm, 475
Bronchostenosis, 462
Brønsted-Lowry definition, 321
Bronze baby syndrome, 769
Brown bowel syndrome, 518
Brushfield spots, 978
  racial predilection of, 1039
Bryant's traction, 235
B-scanners, 82
Bubble stability test, 135

Bubbly radiographic pattern, 469
Buffy coat smears, 713
Bullous congenital icthyosiform erythroderma, 945-946
Bullous diseases, 950
Bumetanide, 158
Buphthalmos, 988
Bupivacaine, 175
Burns, orbital, 976
Bursa of Fabricius, 637
Busulfan, 58
Butterfly vertebrae, 1081
β-OH-Butyrate, 846
Byler's disease, 782

C

C antigens, 727
c Wave, 186
Cafe au lait spots, 950-952, 1040
Caffeine
  for apnea, 158, 161, 460
  dosage for, 1097
  effect on respiration, 156
  in human milk, 167
Calcaneovalgus deformities, 1059
Calcification
  cortical, 808
  intraocular, 994-995
  intraabdominal, 484
    diagnostic radiology for, 1076
  skull, diagnostic radiology for, 1084-1085
  in subcutaneous fat necrosis, 962
  tramline, 956
Calcitonin, activity of, 873-874
Calcium
  infusion, bradycardia due to, 121
  physiology of, 870-874
  low birth weight infant requirement of, 305-306
  serum, changes in, 547
Calcium antagonists, 142
Calcium chloride
  for cardiovascular disease, 627
  dosages for, 1096
  for heart failure, 572, 582
Calcium glubionate, 1096
Calcium gluconate
  for cardiovascular disease, 627
  in chronic renal insufficiency, 792
  for heart failure, 572
  infusion, during exchange transfusion, 730
  for magnesium overdosage, 33
Calcium lactate, 1096
Calcium/phosphorus ratio, fetal, 50
Calciuria, 474
Callus formation after humeral fracture, 235
Calories
  added, and enhanced fetal weight, 57
  requirements for
    low birth weight infant, 303
    in respiratory distress syndrome, 432
  SGA infant intake of, 75
Calvarium, diagnostic radiology for, 1084
Calyceal crescents, 1079
cAMP; see Cyclic adensosine monophosphate
CAMP test, 672
Camptodactyly, 1008, 1059

Campylobacter, gastroenteritis due to, 662
Campylobacter fetus, 651
Canalicular phase of lung development, 407, 408
Canaliculus, bile, 772
Canavan's disease, 379
Candida
  infection caused by, 683-684
    pulmonary, 467
  skin reactions to, 639, 644
  superinfection with, in mechanical ventilation, 438
Candida albicans
  in amniotic sac, 209
  gastroenteritis due to, 662
  on skin, 947
Candida parapsilosis, 209
Candidiasis
  cutaneous, 950
  oral, 683-684
Canthal distance, 1043
Capacitance pneumography, 123
Capacitive mattress, 123, 124
Capillaries
  brain
    in cytotoxic edema, 363-364
    development of, 347
  cutaneous, 941
Capnograph, 123
Caput succedaneum, 218
  hemorrhage associated with, 715
  soft tissue swelling in, 1084
Carbamazepine
  dosage for, 1094
  elimination of, 161
Carbamylphosphate synthetase deficiency, 823
Carbenicillin, 660
  dosage for, 1092
  for sepsis, 655
Carbidopa, 819
Carbimazole in human milk, 166
Carbohydrate
  absorption of, in developing gastrointestinal tract, 481
  intestinal breakdown of, 521-522
  intolerance for, 22
  low birth weight infant requirement of, 305
  malabsorption of, 524
  metabolism of
    in diabetes, 23
      diagnostic tests for, 1031
      disorders of, 845-867
Carbohydrate oxidation, 54
Carbohydrate tolerance tests, 524
Carbon dioxide
  impaired elimination of, 186
  mechanism of, in acid-base regulation, 320-321
  ventilatory response to, 456-457
Carbon dioxide snow, 980
Carbon dioxide tension, 321
  arterial, 423-424
    after alkali administration, 186
    in causes of cyanosis, 563, 565
    in d-transposition, 586
    ventilator effects on, 436
    ventilatory response affected by, 456-457
  fetal, during variable deceleration, 102
  intrapartum, 179

Carbon dioxide tension—cont'd
  transcutaneous measurement of, 431-432
Carbon monoxide, 58, 59
  in bilirubin synthesis, 754
  production rate of, heme degradation assessed by, 759
Carbonic acid, 320
Carbonic anhydrase activity, 711
Carcinogenesis
  chemical, 157
  transplacental, due to drugs, 152
Carcinoma, squamous cell, 954
Cardiac anomaly causing flat FHR, 106
Cardiac arrest, 582-583
Cardiac ejection, 126
Cardiac function after surgery, 624
Cardiac massage, 582
  in delivery room, 184, 185
Cardiac monitoring; *see also* Fetal heart rate monitoring; Neonatal heart rate monitoring
  equipment for, 296
  neonatal, 277-280
Cardiac pacing, 583
  disordered, 547-548
Cardiac silhouette in bronchopulmonary dysplasia, 469
Cardiac tamponade, 621-622
  after cardiac surgery, 625
  and rise in central venous pressure, 129
Cardioaccelerator components, 120, 121
Cardiofacial syndrome, 374
Cardiogenic shock, 573-575
Cardioinhibitor components, 120, 121
Cardiomegaly
  in congestive heart failure, 1069-1070
  in meconium aspiration syndrome, 444
  in respiratory distress syndrome, 429
  as sign of heart failure, 568
Cardiopulmonary monitoring, neonatal
  arterial blood pressure, 126-128
  central venous pressure, 128-130
  heart rate, 119-122
  pulmonary artery pressure, 130-131
  respiration, 122-126
Cardiopulmonary resuscitation, 185
Cardiopulmonary status determination, 255
Cardioregulatory centers, suppression of, 122
Cardiotachometry, 279-280
  fetal, 25
  neonatal, 119
Cardiothoracic ratio, 1066
Cardiovascular disorders, 615-622
  benefit of electrophysiologic monitoring for, 113
  due to Coxsackie virus, 679, 680
  diagnostic radiology for, 1069-1070
  drug therapy for, 626-628
  from lithium in human milk, 166
  physical examination for, 539-551
  serious results of, 583-615
  signs of, 538-539
Cardiovascular drugs
  in human milk, 166
  teratogenicity of, 156
Cardiovascular reactivity, in preeclampsia, 28-30
Cardiovascular stimulants, 188
Cardioversion, 577
Care goals in outreach education, 13

Care needs for different groups, 6
Care practices, measurement of changes in, 15
Carnitine deficiency, 610
Carotid compression, 121
Carpenter acrocephalosyndactyly, 1058
Carpenter's syndrome, 538
Carrier-mediated drug transport, 160
Cartilage, metaplastic, 794
Cartilage-hair hypoplasia, 981, 1040
Casein, role in late metabolic acidosis, 325
CAT scanning; *see* Computed axial tomography
Catalase
  in chronic granulomatous disease, 746-747
  in neonatal erythrocytes, 735
Cataracts, 72, 993-994
  genetically determined, 993
Catecholamines
  inappropriate sweating due to, 568
  local accumulation of, 955
  release of, in SGA infant, 74
  urinary, in neuroblastoma, 235, 748
  uterine blood flow altered by, 140
Catheter
  balloon, for pleural pressure, 425-426
  balloon flotation, 131
  candidiasis due to, 684
  cardiac, 583
  for central venous pressure, 129, 574
  for direct arterial pressure, 127
  indwelling
    risks of, 129-130
    in spinal injury, 232
  for intrauterine pressure, 114
  for nasojejunal feedings, 309
  polyvinyl, 309
  for pressure monitoring, 281
    problems with, 283
  pulmonary artery, 131
  radiologic monitoring of, 1086
  Silastic, 300, 309
  for suspected anal atresia, 194
  for total parenteral nutrition, 311
  tracheal stimulation with, 457
  umbilical
    for arterial sampling, 430
    end-hole, 566
Catheterization
  arterial, risks of, 296-297
  bladder, 804
  cardiac, 600
    care of neonate after, 623
    indications for, 570, 622-623
    risks of, 622-623
    for ventricular septal defect, 588
  Dudrick's method, 299
  for esophageal atresia diagnosis, 496-497
  retrograde arterial, 605
  for tracheoesphageal fistula, 193-194
  umbilical, 186
    complications from, 187-188
    Dunn standards for, 299
    hepatic ischemic necrosis associated with, 782
Cat's eye reflex, 992
Caudal epidural block, 174
Caudal regression, 1081

Cecum, arrest of, 502
Cefazolin, 1092
Ceftriaxone, 1092
Cell(s)
  allogeneic, 639
  dermal, 941
  effect of rubella on, 63
  epithelial lung, 406-408
  gastrointestinal, proliferation of, 478-479
  giant
    hepatocytes transformed into, 774
    due to subcutaneous fat necrosis, 218
  growth of, 50
    effect of drugs on, 58
  in human milk, 640-642
  intestinal, migration of, and enzyme activity, 480
  mast, disease of, 961-962
  oxygen toxic effects on, 472
  pluripotent hematopoietic stem, 637
  pluripotential, development of, 347
  production of, folic acid for, 306-307
  pyloric ganglion, decrease of, 499
  spur, 738
  type I alveolar, injury to, 472
  type II, 406, 408, 427
  X, 211
β-Cell nesidioblastosis-adenoma spectrum, 859-860
Cellulitis, facial, 673
Central core disease, 397
Central nervous system
  altered states of, in hypoxic ischemic encephalopathy, 359
  bleeding in, 718
  depression of
    at birth, 180
    from ethanol in human milk, 167
  development of, 347
  disorders of, 357-400
    cyanotic spells and, 619-620
    flat FHR caused by, 106
    heart failure and, 569
    from lithium in human milk, 166
    and respiratory distress, 460-461
    due to rubella, 701
    due to toxoplasmosis, 702-703
    ultrasonic detection of, 89
  drugs affecting
    associated with congenital malformations, 153
    in human milk, 166
  insult to, in neonatal asphyxia, 73
  irritability of, in preeclampsia, 30
  nutritive effects on, 302
Central venous and esophageal pressure system, 123
Central venous pressure
  blood loss indicated by, 742
  after cardiac surgery, 624
  in cardiogenic shock, 574
  neonatal, 128-130
    method of measurement, 129
    pressure wave analysis, 129
    risk of monitoring, 129-130
Centralization of regional perinatal center, 9
Centrifugation of amniotic fluid, 135
Centronuclear (myotubular) myopathy, 397
Cephalhematoma
  differentiation from caput succedaneum, 218

Cephalhematoma—cont'd
 infection following, 652
 soft tissue swelling in, 1084
 sustained at birth, 218-220
 from vacuum extraction, 176
Cephalhematoma deformans of Schüller, 220
Cephalic index, 1040
Cephalometry, 82-84
 ultrasonic, 134
Cephalopelvic disproportion, 114
Cephalosporins, 660
 in human milk, 166
Cephalothin, 655
Cerebellar hemorrhage, 373
Cerebral arteries, ultrasonic detection of, 83
Cerebral blood flow in intrapartum asphyxia, 363
Cerebral depression, 72-73
Cerebral hemorrhage in preeclampsia, 31
Cerebral morbidity in SGA infants, 76
Cerebral necrosis
 due to asphyxia, 191
 in hypoxic ischemic encephalopathy, 360
Cerebral palsy
 chorioathetoid, 764
 incidence of, 358
 in SGA infants, 77
 associated with spinal injury, 231
Cerebral peduncles, ultrasonic detection of, 82
Cerebrohepatorenal syndrome, 538
 hyperbilirubinemia in, 782
Cerebrospinal fluid
 in cryptococcosis, 685
 draining from ears or nose, 221
 enterovirus isolated from, 704
 in histoplasmosis, 686
 in meningitis, 657-658
 obstructed flow of, 375-376
 overproduction of, 375
 production of, 375
 values for, 1099
Cervical dilatation, 176-177
 and FHR accelerations, 101
Cervix, incompetent, 141
Cesarean section
 anesthesia for, 177-178
 in erythroblastosis fetalis, 42
 incidence of, and electronic fetal monitoring, 106
Chagas' disease, 213
Chalasia, 495-496
Charcoal, activated, to reduce enteric bilirubin absorption, 770
Chart recorder for cardiac monitor, 279
Charting, 300
 in heart failure, 570
Chédiak-Higashi syndrome, 747
 skin in, 954-955
Chemoreceptors
 aortic, and respiratory drive, 179
 carotid, and respiratory drive, 179
 ventilatory response affected by, 456-457
Chemotactic factor, 637
Chemotaxis, phagocytic, 745
Cherry-red macula, 1001
Chest
 congenital malformations of, 1050
 diagnostic radiology for, 1065-1070

Chest—cont'd
 examination of, 256
Chest drainage after cardiac surgery, 625
Chest leads, QRS patterns in, 543-544
Chest physiotherapy
 in bronchopulmonary dysplasia, 474
 in respiratory distress syndrome, 437
Chest tubes
 in chylothorax, 455
 for pneumothorax with lung disease, 451
Chest wall
 movement of, 458
  paradoxical, 458
  in respiration monitoring, 284-285
 retractions of, 420
Chest x-ray examination
 after cardiac surgery, 625
 in causes of cyanosis, 563, 565
Cheyne-Stokes breathing, 122
 in adult, relationship to neonatal periodic breathing, 458
Chimerism, 908
Chlamydia, pulmonary infection caused by, 467
Chlamydia trachomatis
 conjunctivitis due to, 666
 infection by, 662, 676
 pneumonia caused by, 446
Chloracne, 168
Chloral hydrate, 1097
Chloramphenicol, 660
 dosage for, 1092
 in human milk, 166
 inhibiting glucuronyl transferase, 764
 for sepsis, 655
Chloramphenicol gray baby syndrome, 161
Chlorcyclizine, 157
Chlordiazepoxide in human milk, 166
Chloride; *see also* Electrolytes
 fetal concentration of, 50
 low birth weight infant requirement for, 305
 serum levels of, in heart disease, 559-560
Chloridorrhea, 525
 maldigestion due to, 523
Chloroquine
 dosage for, 1089
 for malaria, 687
Chlorothiazide
 for cardiovascular disease, 627
 dosage for, 1096
 for hypertension, 619
Chlorpromazine
 decreasing pulmonary artery pressure, 130
 dosage for, 1097
Chlorpropamide, hypoglycemia due to, 860
Chlorthalidone in human milk, 166
Chonanal atresia, 462
 delivery room diagnosis of, 193
 examination for, 255
 preventing lung expansion, 180
 and respiratory distress, 463
Cholangiopathy, infantile obstructive, 775
Cholangitis, 781
Cholecalciferol; *see* Vitamin D$_3$
Cholecystokinin-pancreozymin, 516
 pancreatic function after tests with, 517
 properties of, 522

Choledochal cysts, 775
　abdominal masses due to, 532
Choledochus, 772
Cholestasis, 771
　familial recurrent, 782
　intracanalicular, 772
　intracellular, 772
　due to total parenteral nutrition, 312
Cholesterol
　blood values for, 1101
　in skin, 942
Cholesterol side-chain cleavage enzyme deficiency, 921-922
Cholestyramine, 837
Choline phosphorylation, 414, 415
Cholinekinase, 416
Cholinephosphate cytidyltransferase, 416
Cholinephosphotransferase, 416
Cholinergic blocking agents, 1095
Cholinergic mediation of pulmonary surfactant, 413
Chondroectodermal dysplasia, 1058
Chondroitin sulfate B, 941
Chordae tendineae, 614
Chordee, 923
Chorioamnionitis, 209
　due to amniocentesis, 1029
　fetal tachycardia due to, 95
　sepsis associated with, 653
Chorioangioma, 61, 62, 209, 211
　in disseminated intravascular coagulation, 720
Chorion laeve, 206
Chorionic sac, 206
Chorionic surface area, 59
Chorioretinitis, 72, 1000
　due to toxoplasmosis, 702
Choroid plexus
　functions of, 375
　papillomas of, 375
Christmas disease, 717
Chromatography
　in acute metabolic disease, 398
　column, 765, 821
Chromosomal abnormalities, 1013-1033
　in abortuses, 1038
　clinical features of, 1018-1020
　congenital heart disease due to, 537-538
　incidence at birth, by amniocentesis, 1030
　laboratory tests for, 1020-1021
　malformations due to, 1036
　numeric, 1015-1017
　in pancytopenia, 723
　parental counseling in, 1021-1023
　risk of, 1060
Chromosomal deletions, 1036
　ocular findings in, 978-979
Chromosomal determination of fetal growth, 63
Chromosome banding, 1016, 1020, 1036
Chromosome 4p- syndrome, 978
Chromosome 5p- syndrome, 978
Chromosome 18p- syndrome, 978-979
Chromosome 13q- syndrome, 978
Chromosome 18q- syndrome, 978-979
Chronic disease, maternal, 57-58
Chronic granulomatous disease, 645, 746-747
　tests for, 643
Chronic pulmonary insufficiency of prematurity, 467

Chylothorax, 455
Chylous ascites, 533
Chymodenin, 516
　properties of, 522
Cigarette ingredients in human milk, 167
Cimetidine
　dosage for, 1097
　in human milk, 167
Cineesophogram, 494
Cineradiography
　for esophageal fistula, 194
　for hiatal hernia, 493
Circulating blood volume, restoration of, 487
Circulation
　cerebral, in active sleep, 334
　enterohepatic, 754
　transition from fetal to neonatal, 130
　during umbilical catheterization, 186
Circulatory collapse following liver injury, 233
Circumvallate placenta, 61
Cirrhosis
　due to biliary atresia, 781
　Indian childhood, 782
Citrate phosphate dextrose
　for exchange transfusion, 767
　in hypoglycemia, 863
Citric acid cycle, 828
Citrobacter, 651
Citrullinemia, 824
^{14}C-labeled antipyrine, 361, 363
^{14}C-labeled deoxyglucose, 361
Classic pathway of complement system, 633-634
Classification by birth weight and gestational age, 196-198, 203-204
Claw deformity, 228
Cleft lip, 1049
Cleft lip and palate
　in abortuses, 1037
　syndromes of, 1049
Cleft palate, 256
　delivery room diagnosis of, 194
　associated with hydramnios, 193
　isolated, genetic predisposition of, 1049-1050
　in Pierre Robin syndrome, 463
　shapes of, 1048
Cleidocranial dysostosis
　fontanel size in, 1040
　wormian bones in, 1084
Click
　cardiac, 542
　on hip reduction, 1010
Clindamycin, 660
　dosage for, 1093
　for sepsis, 655
Clinics, 6
Clinodactyly, 1059
Clitoromegaly, 922, 923
Cloacal exstrophy, 509
　in abortuses, 1038
Cloquet's canal, 998
Clostridium, 671
　necrotizing enterocolitis due to, 513
Clostridium difficile, 664
Clostridium perfringens, 653
Clotting factors, 716-721
　in Kasabach-Merritt syndrome, 957

Clotting factors—cont'd
　　test values for, 1113
Clubfoot, 1012
　　in arthrogryposis, 398
　　racial predilection of, 1039
Clubhand, 1004
Clutton's joints, 676
Coagulation, congenital disorders of, 717-718
Coagulopathy, gastrointestinal hemorrhage due to, 487
Coarctation of aorta, 127
　　postductal, 591-592
　　preductal, 590-591
　　pulses in, 539
Coccidioides immitis, 684
Coccidioidomycosis, 684-685
Codeine for bile salt malabsorption, 528
Coeur en sabot shape, 594
Cofactor-related phenylketonuria, 819
Cognitive knowledge change, 15
Cognitive program in outreach education, 13-14
Cold acetone precipitation, 134
Cold stress, 121
　　alerting of infant to, 260
　　panniculitis due to, 962
　　subcutaneous fat necrosis due to, 218
Colistimethate, 655
Colistin elimination rate, 164
Colitis
　　bloody diarrhea due to, 487
　　milk-induced, 529
Collagen
　　in clotting cascade, 716
　　in dermal tissue, 941
Collagen disease
　　and benefits of electrophysiologic monitoring, 113
　　associated with placental insufficiency, 108
Collarette of scale, 943-944
Collecting tubules, dilatation of, 796
Collodion baby, 945
Colobomas, 1047
　　of eyelids, 979
　　iris, 991
　　optic disc, 1001-1002
Colon
　　disorders of, 504-512
　　radiologic diagnosis for, 1074-1075
Colonic atresia, 504
Colonic stenosis, 504
Colony-stimulating factor, 744
Color of infant, 255
　　Apgar scoring by, 182
　　at birth, 942
　　in cardiogenic shock, 573
　　in cyanosis, 560, 561
　　harlequin change, 943
　　in heart disease, 559
　　in hyperbilirubinemia, 757
　　in methemoglobinemia, 560
　　phototherapy affecting, 769
　　in septicemia, 653
Colostomy
　　for aganglionosis, 507
　　for colonic atresia, 504
Colostral phase, drug secretion in, 165

Colostrum
　　agglutinins in, 652
　　antibodies in, 640-642
Columella, dislocation of cartilage from, 223
Coma, 349
Comedones, 944
Commitment of parties in outreach education, 13
Community base of outreach education, 12
Community hospitals, 6
Compensation in acid-base disturbances, 322
Complement cascade, 633-634
Complement components
　　deficiencies of, infection due to, 652
　　in isoimmune hemolytic disease, 726
　　Leiner's disease causing defect in, 960
　　phagocyte interactions with, 744
　　serum levels of, 1106
　　tests for, 643
Complement fixation tests
　　in coccidioidomycosis, 685
　　in myxovirus infection, 682
　　in syphilis, 675
Complement system, 633-634
　　neonatal function of, 644
Compressed air, availability of, in hospital units, 293
Computed axial tomography, 356-357, 1085
　　for chest diagnosis, 1065
　　in subependymal germinal matrix hemorrhage, 368
Concanavalin A, 639, 645
Conductive heat losses, 264-265
Condyloma, perianal, 674
Congenital heart disease; *see* Heart disease, congenital
Congenital malformations
　　associated with diabetes, 25-26
　　diagnosis of, 192-194
　　drugs associated with, 153
　　epidemiology and genetics, 1035-1039
　　evaluation of infant with, 1039-1060
　　family care in, 250-251
　　incidence of, by gestation quartiles, 200
　　major nonrenal, from oligohydramnios, 47
　　associated with polyhydramnios, 46
　　possible multifactorial control of, 157
　　related to birth weight and gestational age, 200
　　terminology, 1035
Congestive heart failure, 121
　　with bronchopulmonary dysplasia, 469
　　diagnostic radiology for, 1069-1070
　　ischemic, 73
　　pulmonary hemorrhage associated with, 447
Conjugate eye movements, 354
　　examination for, 968
Conjugate gaze, 972
Conjunctival irritation, 984
Conjunctivitis, 665
　　chemical, 982-983
　　chlamydial, 676
　　gonorrheal, 983
　　nongonococcal bacterial, 983
Connective tissue disorders, 537
Conradi syndrome, 156
Consanguinity
　　dystrophic epidermolysis bullosa in, 949
　　effects of, 1014
　　inquiries about, 1039

Consciousness, level of
　assessment of, 349
　in hypoxic ischemic encephalopathy, 359
Conservation of pulmonary surfactant, 412
Consolidation, pulmonary, 1066-1067
Constant regions of immunoglobulin molecules, 635
Constipation, neonatal, 512
Constriction band syndrome, 1008
Continuous distending airway pressure, 434
　in meconium aspiration syndrome, 445
　pseudocysts caused by, 453
Continuous negative pressure, 436
Continuous positive airway pressure, 412
　for idiopathic apnea, 460
　in phrenic nerve paralysis, 228
　pneumothorax incidence with, 448
　in respiratory distress syndrome, 434-435
Continuous transcutaneous monitoring, 118, 297
Contraction alkalosis, 324
Contraction stress test; see Oxytocin challenge test
Contractions; see also Labor
　abnormal patterns, 114-115
　fetal asphyxia due to, 180
　fetus unable to tolerate, 69
　tetanic, 104, 114, 115
Contralateral collapse, 438
Contrast echocardiography, 555
Contrast media for gastrointestinal tract examination, 1072-1074
Contrast roentgenography, 438
Conus, 1001
Convective heat, 259
　forced, 296
　losses, 264-265
　thermoneutrality and, 269-270
Convulsions
　neonatal bradycardia due to, 121
　in preeclampsia, 32
Cooley's anemia, 733
Coombs' test, 190
　in ABO incompatibility, 42, 726
　in fetal-maternal transfusion, 712
　for hyperbilirubinemia, 766
　in isoimmune hemolytic disease, 728
Copper
　blood values for, 1101
　human milk content of, 306
　intrauterine accumulation of, 306
Coproantibodies, 526
Cor pulmonale, 469
Cor triatriatum, 614
Cord blood
　bilirubin concentration in, 759
　screening, for globin chain abnormalities, 733
Cord clamping, 709
Cord compression
　and FHR acceleration, 101
　and FHR variable deceleration, 102
Cord insertion patterns, abnormal, 62
Cord occlusion
　causing first breath, 179
　stimulating gasping, 181
Cori classification, 834
Cornea
　birth injuries to, 225
　cloudy, 72, 990

Cornea—cont'd
　examination of, 969-970
　necrosis of, 666
Corneal abrasions, 976
Corneal diameter, 988
Corneal reflection techniques, 338
Corneal transplantation, 990
Cornelia de Lange syndrome, 63, 538
　facies in, 976
　hirsutism in, 1040
　hypertrichosis in, 981
　skin in, 1040
　synophrys in, 1047
　ulnar defects in, 1058
Coronal synostosis, 383
Coronary artery, left, anomalous origin of, 611-613
Coronavirus, 698
Corpus callosum
　absence of, 378
　ultrasonic detection of, 83
Cortical and medullary necrosis, 807-808
Cortical thumb, 349-351
Corticosteroids
　for congenital hypoplastic anemia, 722
　to delay delivery, 141
　effect on estriol levels, 111
　effect on fetus, 59
　for lid hemangiomas, 980
　role in phosphatidylcholine synthesis, 417
　stimulation of lung function by, 417-418
　for strawberry nevus, 957
Cortisol
　deficiency of, 861-862
　fetal production of, 140, 847
Cortisone, 1096
Cotazyme, 521
Cough at first breath, 179
Cough and cold medicines, 156
Coumadin, vitamin K supplementation needed with, 718
Countercurrent immunoelectrophoresis, 654, 673
Countershock for arrhythmias, 577
Covermark, 956
Coxsackie B encephalitis, 390
Coxsackie viruses, 679-680
　endocardial fibroelastosis due to, 610
　frequency of infection by, 697
C-peptide, 857
Cracked-pot percussion note, 383
Cradle cap, 960
Cranial metaphyseal dysplasias, 1048
Cranial nerves; see specific nerves
Cranial sutures in SGA infant, 70
Craniofacial dysostosis, 384, 976; see also Crouzon's disease
Craniolacunia, 1084
Craniomeningocele, 388
Craniosynostosis, 382-385
　fontanel condition in, 194
Craniotabes, 194
Cranium bifidum, 388
　position of, 219
C-reactive protein, 633-634
Creatine kinase, 574
Creatine phosphokinase in myotonic dystrophy, 396
Creatinine
　amniotic fluid concentration of, 137-138

Creatinine—cont'd
  blood values for, 1101
  plasma concentration of, 788-789
  serum levels of, in preeclampsia, 30
  urine values for, 1101
Creatinine clearance, 789, 1108
Creatinine phosphokinase, 1104
Credé prophylaxis, 982
Crescent, congenital, 1001
Cresyl violet stain, 735
Cretinism, 890-897
  facies in, 976
  tongue in, 1049-1050
Cri du chat syndrome, 538
  chromosomal deletion in, 1017
  eyes in, 978
Crib-O-Gram, 355
Cricoid pressure during labor, 177, 178
Crigler-Najjar syndrome, 760-761
Crista galli, 1042
Crossovers, chromosome, 1017
Crouzon's disease, 383, 384
  facies in, 976
  suture closure in, 1084
Crown-rump length
  relationship to gastrointestinal tract development, 478, 479
  ultrasonic measurement of, 82
Cry
  in airway obstruction, 463
  at first breath, 179
  of preterm infant, 335
  reflex, 182
  in vocal cord paralysis, 226
Crying
  asymmetric face during, 1049
  blood pressure rise during, 539
  effect on arterial saturation, 564
  due to left atrial pressure drop, 180
  as state of arousal, 329
Cryoprecipitate, 717
Cryotherapy
  for retinoblastoma, 995
  transscleral, 997
Cryptococcosis, 685
Cryptophthalmos, 982, 1043
Cryptorchidism, 925
Cryptothyroid, 890
Crypts of Lieberkühn, 478
Crystals used in ultrasonography, 82
Cubitus valgus, 908, 1059
Curettage of placenta, 212
Current leakage pathways, 287-288
Cushing's syndrome, 617
Cutdown technique for pulmonary artery catheter, 131
Cutis hyperelastica, 963
Cutis laxa, 596, 962-963
Cutis marmorata, 1040
Cyanide, 59
Cyanide-nitroprusside test, 821
Cyanocobalamin; see Vitamin B_{12}
Cyanosis, 255
  assessment of, 421
  central, 561-565
  generalized, 565-566
  due to methemoglobinemia, 734

Cyanosis—cont'd
  neonatal, 130
  oxygen therapy for, 296
  peripheral, 561
  in phrenic nerve paralysis, 228
  recognition of, 560-564
  in respiratory distress syndrome, 429
Cyanotic spells, 619-620
Cyclic adenosine monophosphate, 142
  intrathyroidal, 885
  phosphatidylcholine synthesis and, 417
  in respiratory drive, 460
Cyclic guanosine monophosphate, 747
Cyclophosphamide
  combined with phenobarbital, 157
  for neuroblastoma, 748
  postnatal effects of, 152
  for retinoblastoma, 995
  teratogenicity of, 157
Cyproheptadine, 962
Cystathionine synthetase, 820
Cysteine
  as antiteratogen, 158
  in human milk protein, 304
Cystic fibrosis, 467, 518-521, 1032
  liver injury due to, 782
  and risk for intestinal obstruction, 483
Cystic hygroma, 958
Cystinosis, 802
Cystinuria, 802
Cystourethrography, 509
  in ascites, 533
  voiding, 788, 1079
Cytidine diphosphocholine pathway, 414
Cytochrome P_{450}
  increasing teratogenicity of cyclophosphamide, 157
  multiple forms of, 162
Cytochromes in bilirubin synthesis, 754
Cytodifferentiation of respiratory epithelium, 408-409
Cytolysis from placental infection, 63
Cytomegalic inclusion disease, 781
Cytomegalovirus infection
  congenital, 700
  in donated milk, 307
  effect on fetal growth, 63
  frequency of, 695
  manifestations of, 698
  metaphyseal abnormalities due to, 1081
  microcephaly due to, 381
  nephrotic syndrome due to, 801
  structural malformations and, 1014
  treatment and prevention of, 705
Cytoplasmic receptors in fetal lung, 417
Cytotoxic edema, 363-364

D

D antigens, 727
Dacron graft
  for coarctation of aorta, 591
  for persistent truncus arteriosus, 602
Dacryocystitis, 983
Dandy-Walker syndrome, 375
Dane particles, 696
Daraprim; see Pyrimethamine
Darvon; see Propoxyphene

DDT in human milk, 167-168
De novo structural rearrangement, 1018
Decelerations in heart rate
    fetal, 69
        early, 101
        late, 103-104
        prolonged, 104
        variable, 101-103
    neonatal, 119
Decerebrate posturing, 389, 390
Decidua capsularis, 206
Decompression
    bowel, 484
    intraabdominal, 486
    nasogastric, 489
    nerve, 223
    for osteomyelitis, 668
    in pneumomediastinum, 451
    in pneumothorax, 449
Decorticate posturing, 389
Decubitus ulcer, 232
Deep tendon reflexes, 353
Defecation causing neonatal bradycardia, 121
Deflation stability of lung, 410, 411
Dehydration, renal thrombosis due to, 806
Dehydroepiandrosterone, 111
Dehydroepiandrosterone-sulfate loading test, 111-112
Dehydroisoandrosterone clearance studies, 57
Delivery
    anesthesia for, 174-178
    of asymmetrically growth-retarded fetus, 70
    in erythroblastosis fetalis, 35-36, 110
    of fetus with rises in FHR, 97
    indications for, after oxytocin challenge test, 69
    infection acquired during, 651
    modes of, after positive oxytocin challenge test, 69-70
Delivery room
    keeping baby warm in, 266
    physical examination in, 255-256
Demerol; see Meperidine
Denitrogenation, 177
Densitometry, 134
Depression
    delayed, due to analgesia, 188-189
    neonatal
        from chordiazepoxide in human milk, 166
        delivery room treatment of, 183-184
        from drugs, distinguishing from asphyxia, 188-189
        from meperidine used during labor, 174
    neurologic, in meconium aspiration syndrome, 444
    respiratory, in meconium aspiration syndrome, 444
    due to spinal cord injury, 461
Depressor anguli oris muscle, 1049
Dermal sinuses, 388
    in spina bifida, 386
Dermatan sulfate, 941
Dermatitis, eczematous contact, 960
Dermatoglyphics, 1014-1015, 1052
Dermatome patterns, 353, 354
Dermatoses, 961-962
Dermis, structure of, 941
Dermographism, 962
Dermoids, 388
    of eyelid, 980
    orbital, 985-986

Dermoids—cont'd
    in spina bifida, 386
Descemet's membrane, rupture of, 225, 975
Desferrioxamine, 722
Desiccated thyroid, 896
    dosage for, 1096
Desiccytes, 736
17,20-Desmolase, 913
Desoxycorticosterone, 1096
Desoxycorticosterone acetate, 919
Desquamation, physiologic, 944
de Toni–Fanconi syndrome, 838
Developmental abnormalities, 385-388
    pulmonary, 453-456
Developmental outcome of SGA infants, 76-77
Devil's eye configuration, 384
Dexamethasone, 145
    to hasten lung maturity, 427
    prior to extubation, 439
Dextroamphetamine, 536
Dextrocardia with situs inversus, 614-615
Dextrose, 574
Dextrostix, 74, 559
    in cardiogenic shock, 574
    in causes of cyanosis, 563, 565
Dextrotransposition; see Transposition of great arteries
Diabetes mellitus, 830-831
    anesthesia for labor and delivery in, 175
    and benefit of electrophysiologic monitoring, 113
    delaying fetal pulmonary maturation, 135
    hyperbilirubinemia due to, 764
    intrapartum complications due to, 23-26
    juvenile-onset, 22
    associated with polyhydramnios, 46
    postpartum care in, 26
    transient neonatal, 55
    ultrasonic diagnosis of, 92-94
Diamine oxidase, 66
Diamnionic monochorionic twinning, 61
Diamond-Blackfan anemia, 721
Diamox; see Acetazolamide
Diaper dermatitis, 960-961
    candidal, 950
Diaphorase, NADH-dependent, 733, 734
Diaphragm
    disorders of, 465
    eventration of, 489-490
    fibrous, 504
    role in breathing, 420
    surgery on, 229
Diaphragmatic hernia, 121
    bronchopulmonary dysplasia with, 469
    clinical manifestations of, 488-489
    delivery room diagnosis of, 193
    differentiation from lung cysts, 455
    preventing lung expansion, 184
    prognosis in, 489
    pulmonary hypoplasia associated with, 453
    treatment for, 489
Diarrhea
    due to *Escherichia coli*, 663
    hypoglycemia associated with, 863-864
    infectious, 523-524
    intractable, 528-529
    malabsorption and, 521-529

Diarrhea—cont'd
 parenteral, 526
 from penicillins in human milk, 166
 due to physical and chemical agents, 524
 water loss in, 319
Diastematomyelia, 388, 1051
Diastole
 arterial pressure during, 126
 Doppler method to detect, 284
 echocardiographic measurement during, 549-550
 uterine, 115
Diathermy for retinoblastoma, 995
Diatrizoate, 787
Diazepam
 for cardiovascular disease, 627
 dosage for, 1097
 in human milk, 166
 multicompartmental model of elimination, 165
 for seizures, 392, 658, 677
Diazoxide
 for cardiovascular disease, 627
 dosage for, 1095
 for hypertension, 619
 for hyperglycemia, 865
 for premature labor, 142
Dichorionic placentation, 214
Dieldrin, 168
Diet
 in fructose intolerance, 833
 influence on drug effects, 152
 in phenylketonuria, 818-819
 for preeclamptic patient, 32
 for pregnant diabetic, 23-24
Diethylstilbestrol
 genital anomalies due to, 922-923
 teratogenicity of, 157
 transplacental carcinogenesis due to, 152
Diffuse neonatal hemangiomatosis, 957-958
DiGeorge phenotype, 390
DiGeorge syndrome, 646-647
Digital pulse, 539
Digitalis
 for heart failure, 570
 neonatal bradycardia due to, 121
 septic shock due to, 128
 toxicity, 570, 620-621
Digitalization
 in bronchopulmonary dysplasia, 475
 for cardioversion, 577
 maternal, 97
 neonatal, 571
Diglucuronide, bilirubin, 755
Digoxin
 for arrhythmias, 577
 for cardiovascular disease, 626
 dosage for, 1095
 in human milk, 166
 multicompartmental model of elimination, 165
 steady-state plasma concentrations of, 164
Dihydrobiopterin reductase, 817
Dihydroorotase, 479
Dihydrotachysterol, 793
Dihydrotestosterone, 902, 903
 fetal excretion of, 905
1,25-Dihydroxycholecalciferol, 793

1α, 25-Dihydroxycholecalciferol, 873
Diiodotyrosine, 884
Dilantin; see Phenytoin
Dilution acidosis, 324
Dimethyl-triazenoimidazole-carboxamide, 748
Dimple
 anal, 509
 sacral, 1051
 in spina bifida, 386, 388
2,4-Dinitrophenylhydrazine test, 822, 825
Dioctyl sodium sulfosuccinate, 510
Dipalmitoyl lecithin, 134
Dipalmitoyl-phosphatidylcholine, 413
Dipeptidases, 480
Diphenoxylate, 528
Diphosphoglycerate, 422
2,3-Diphosphoglycerate
 buildup of, 736
 combined with hemoglobin, 711
 Hb F interaction with, 731
2,3-Diphosphoglycerate mutase deficiency, 760
Diphtheria antitoxin, 640
Diploic bone, 220
Direct measurement of arterial blood pressure, 126, 127
Director of obstetric and neonatal services, 7-8
Direct-reacting bilirubin, 776
Direct-Yellow-7, 765
Disaccharidases, 479-480
Disaccharide malabsorption, 523, 524
Dishabituation to stimulus, 337, 339
Disinfection, 295
Dislocations
 congenital, 1009-1011
 of extremities, 236
 facial bone, 223-224
Dispermy, 1017
Display and recording section of monitor, 277, 278-279
Disseminated intravascular coagulation, 720
 associated with cord vessel thrombosis, 211
 gastrointestinal hemorrhage due to, 487
 platelet count in, 216
Distal femoral epiphysis, fetal, 134
Distributive phase of plasma concentration of drug, 164
Districhiasis, 969, 981
Diuresis
 avoiding forced, 792
 in preeclampsia, 32
 in respiratory distress syndrome, 432
Diuretics
 and amniotic fluid creatinine levels, 137
 dosage for, 1096
 for heart failure, 571
 in human milk, 166
 septic shock due to, 128
 teratogenicity of, 156
 for uremic hypertension, 793
Diuril; see Chlorothiazide
Diverticula
 bladder, 1079
 urethral, 798
DNA
 complementary, 1032
 defective repair mechanism of, 723
 effect of seizures on, 388
 loss of, syndromes resulting from, 978

1134 Index

DNA—cont'd
   reactions with active metabolites, 157
   recombinant, 1032
   restriction endonuclease examination of, 731-732
   role in phosphatidylcholine synthesis, 416
   synthesis
      in breast T cells, 640, 642
         measurement of, 645
   ultraviolet light–damaged, 953
   viruses, 682, 683
Dobutamine
   for cardiovascular disease, 627
   dosage for, 1092
Dobutrex; *see* Dobutamine
Dolichocephaly, 1040-1041
   biparietal diameter changes due to, 92
Doll's eye movement, 354-355, 972, 973
L-Dopa, 819
Dopamine
   altering arterial blood pressure, 127
   for cardiovascular disease, 628
   dosage for, 1092
   for heart failure, 572, 573
   increasing pulmonary artery pressure, 130
   for systemic hypertension, 567
Doppler method
   for blood pressure, 294
   for cerebral blood flow velocity, 357
   with sphygmomanometer, 283
Doppler shift, 283, 284
Doppler ultrasound
   for arterial blood pressure, 126
   to detect fetal breathing, 109
   for fetal heart rate, 95
Dorsalis pedis pulse, 539
Dosage guidelines, neonatal, 164-165
"Double-bubble" sign, 483, 1074
Double-outlet right ventricle, 602
Double-track sign, 499
Double-wall sign, 1075
Doula, 243
Down's syndrome, 63, 400; *see also* Trisomy 21
   congenital heart disease in, 537
   duodenal obstruction in, 501
   eyes in, 978
   Hirschsprung's disease with, 504
   incidence at birth by amniocentesis, 1030
   intestinal obstruction in, 483
   maternal age and, 1016
   polycythemia in, 741
   prevalence of, 1036
Doxorubicin, 747
DPT-Schick test, 643, 644
Dressing around phlebotomy site, 311
Drooping lily appearance, 1079
   in urinary tract obstruction, 798
Drowsiness, 329-331, 334
Drug administration
   during labor and delivery, 174-175
   routes of, 158, 169
Drug antagonists in resuscitation, 138
Drug interactions, 157
Drug toxicity
   antibiotics, 660-661
   fetal mechanisms of, 157-158

Drug toxicity—cont'd
   septic shock due to, 128
Drugs
   absorption of, in newborn, 158-160
   for arrhythmias, 575-578
   biotransformation of, 161
   cardioactive, postoperative use of, 625
   cardiovascular, 626-628
      dosages for, 1095
   effect on fetus, 150-158
   effect on neonate, 158-164
   effect on quiet awakeness, 338
   elimination from body, 161
   hyperbilirubinemia due to, 764
   neonatal asphyxia due to, 180
   for neonatal heart failure, 572
   for neonatal hypertension, 619
   plasma half-lives of, 159, 161, 162
   for premature labor, 142-146
   protein binding of, 160-161
   renal excretion of, 163-164
   taken by mother
      effects on fetal growth, 58-59
      hyperglycemia induced by, 860
   therapeutic, table of, 1092-1097
   for unconjugated hyperbilirubinemia, 769-770
Dubowitz scoring system, 257, 351
Dubowitz syndrome, 63
Duchenne muscular dystrophy, 396
Duchenne-Erb paralysis, 226
Duct ligation for heart failure, 569
Ductal phase of bile excretion, 772
Ductal shunting, 424
Ductus arteriosus
   flow in, at birth, 179, 180
   patent; *see* Patent ductus arteriosus
Dudrick's method of catheterization, 299
Duffy blood group, 728
Duhamel procedure, 507
Dunn standards for umbilical catheterization, 299
Duodenal atresia, 194
   duodenal obstruction due to, 501
   ultrasonic detection of, 86
Duodenal obstruction
   congenital, 501-502
   hyperbilirubinemia associated with, 763
Duodenostomy, 502
Duodenum
   intubation of, 761
   radiologic diagnosis for, 1074
Duplication
   of collecting system, 797-798
   of digits, 1008
   in regional care system, 9
Duplicitas supercilia, 981
Dupuytren's contracture, 1059
Dural tear, 222
Duration of pregnancy, definition of, 133
Dwarfism, 63
   differentiation from hydrocephalus, 380
   short-limbed, 465
   thanatophoric, 465
Dye-binding methods, 765
Dynamic placentation, 85
Dysautonomia, familial, 63, 495-496, 984

Dysconjugate eye movements, 355
Dysphagia due to vascular rings, 496
Dysraphism, spinal, 1081
Dystocia
  due to cystic kidneys, 795
  secondary to cephalopelvic disproportion, 216

E

E form of bilirubin, 729
Ear oximeter, 564
Ears
  agenesis of, 193
  birth injuries to, 225
  congenital malformations of, 1047
  in renal anomalies, 194
Ebstein's anomaly, 599-601
Eccrine glands, 941
  absence of, 964
  innervation of, 942
Ecchymoses
  of ears, 225
  sustained at birth, 217
ECHO virus infection, 680, 693, 694
Echocardiography
  diagnostic applications of, 548-560
  in d-transposition, 587
  fetal, 1028
  in heart failure, 568
  in left-to-right shunting, 438
  in persistent pulmonary hypertension, 130-131
  in respiratory distress syndrome, 430
  two-dimensional, 557-558
Ecthyma gangrenosum, 669
Ectodermal dysplasia, 981
  anhidrotic, 963-964
  hair in, 1040
Ectopia lentis, 999
  in homocystinuria, 820
Ectopic beats, 580
Ectopic pacemaker tissue, 575
Ectrodactyly, 1058
Ectropion, 945
Eczema, 960-961
Edema
  interstitial, in renal disease, 790-791
  nerve root, 465
  due to neuromuscular blockade, 437
  peripheral
    in neonatal heart disease, 541
    as sign of heart failure, 568
  in preeclampsia, 28
  pulmonary, 130, 467
    with bronchopulmonary dysplasia, 475
    hemorrhagic, 447
    due to left-to-right shunts, 1070
    due to opaque contrast media, 1077
Edema foam, 410
Edrophonium, 462
  for cardiovascular disease, 626
  dosage for, 1095
  to increase vagal tone, 576
  for myasthenia gravis, 396
EDTA to lower serum calcium, 621
Education, implications of perinatal health services for, 10
EEC syndrome, 964

Egg-on-side appearance of heart, 585
Ehlers-Danlos syndrome, 596, 963
  cardiac defects in, 537
  joint deformities in, 1059
Ehrlich diazo reaction, 753
Eisenmenger's complex, 58
Ejection click, 542
  in aortic stenosis, 589
Elastic components of breathing, 419, 420
Elastic tissue
  in cutis laxa, 963
  embryogenesis of, 941
  inadequate development of, 471
Elastolysis, generalized, 962-963
Electrical axes of newborn heart, 545-546
Electrical diaphragmatic pacing, 229
Electrical stimulation of phrenic nerve, 228, 229, 230
Electricity in hospital units, 293
Electrocardiographic abnormalities, 547-548
Electrocardiography
  diagnostic applications of, 543-548
  display of, 279-280
  fetal
    abdominal, 95
    transabdominal, 108
  in heart failure, 568
Electrodes
  Clark, 430
  oxygen, for arterial sampling, 430
Electrodesiccation, 959
Electroencephalography
  for nevus flammeus, 956
  for seizures, 392
  in states of arousal, 332, 333, 334
Electrolyte gel, 278
Electrolytes
  electrocardiography to detect disturbances of, 546-547
  provision of, 314-319
    adequate, determination of, 316-318
    in heart failure, 571-573
    modifiers of, 318-319
  requirements for
    after cardiac surgery, 624
    low birth weight infant, 305
  serum, in neonatal heart disease, 559-560
  in total parenteral nutrition, 310
Electromyogram, 280
Electrophilic metabolites, 157
Electrophoresis, 211
Electrophoresis fractions, 1105
Electroretinography, 972, 975
Elimination phase of plasma concentration of drug, 164
Elliptocytosis, hereditary, 737
Ellis–van Creveld syndrome, 63, 538
  respiratory distress in, 463, 465
Embolism, pulmonary gas, 1075
Embryo, period of, drug effects during, 152
Embryogenesis
  critical periods in, 152
  facial, 1041-1042
  genital, 901-904
  esophageal, 491
  gastrointestinal, 477-478
  hematopoietic, 708
  lung, 407

Embryogenesis—cont'd
  lymphocytic, 637
  neurologic, 347
  ocular, 974
  pancreatic, 516
  radiation effects on, 1026-1027
  respiratory, 407-408
  retinal, 996
  of stomach, 498
  thyroid, 883
  toxic effects during, 1026
Embryonal rhabdomyosarcoma, 748
Emergencies
  in delivery room, 179-195
  gastrointestinal, 483-490
Emissivity of skin, 265
Emphysema
  in bronchopulmonary dysplasia, 471
  congenital lobar, 454-455
  cystic, 469
  interstitial
    radiologic examination for, 1069
    pulmonary, 451-453, 467
Encephalocele, 388
  orbital, 987
Encephalofacial angiomatosis, 956
Encephalomeningocele, 388
Encephalomyocarditis, 679
Encephalooculofacial angiomatosis, 977
Encephalopathy
  bilirubin, 764-766
  with fatty degeneration of viscera, 823
End diastole, 551
End systole, 551
Endocardial fibroelastosis, 590, 610-611
Endocarditis, infective, 557
Endocrine system
  disorders of
    anemia due to, 723
    cataracts associated with, 993
    drugs for, 1096
    in hypoglycemia in SGA infants, 74
    polycythemia associated with, 741
    in sexual differentiation, 901-930
    thyroid, 883-899
  drugs affecting, in human milk, 166-167
  fetal gonadal function, 903-904
Endocrinopathy, cutaneous candidiasis associated with, 950
Endogenous smiling, 335
Endometrial disease, congenital tuberculosis due to, 677
Endonuclease deficiency, 953
Endoplasmic reticulum, 754
Endoscopy, 116-117
  for gastrointestinal hemorrhage, 487
Endothelium
  blood vessel, 716
  swelling of, in subcutaneous fat necrosis, 218
Endotoxin-coated Oil Red O particle ingestion, 643
Endotracheal intubation
  alternatives to, in respiratory distress syndrome, 434-435
  during breech delivery, 177
  complications with, 438-439
  plastic, 181
    positive pressure through, 183-184
  radiologic monitoring of, 1086

Endotracheal intubation—cont'd
  role in bronchopulmonary dysplasia, 473
  size requirements for, 437
Enema
  barium, 505-507
  opaque, 1074
Energy expenditure
  of low birth weight infant, 303
  of neonatal growth, 154
Enflurane, 174
Enolase, 734
Enophthalmos, 224
Enteric cysts, 504
Enteric somatic antibodies, 640
Enterobacter, 662
Enterocolitis, 505
Enterokinase
  activities of, 516
    embryonic, 480
  deficiency of, 517
Enterostomy, 521
Enterovirus
  diarrhea due to, 523
  manifestations of, 699
Entropion, 969
Enucleation in retinoblastoma, 995
Environment
  effect on arousal state, 330-331
  effect on development of SGA infant, 77
  nursery, control of, 295
  physical; *see* Physical environment
  temperature of, 264-266
Environmental chemicals, 156-157
Environmental disorders, 1026-1028
Enzymes
  converting, effect of hypoxia on, 192
  defects of, in Ehlers-Danlos syndrome, 963
  in developing gastrointestinal tract, 479-480
  fetal, 847
  pancreatic
    for cystic fibrosis, 521
    in developing gastrointestinal tract, 480
    embryonic activity of, 516
  for phosphatidylcholine synthesis, 416
  proteolytic, 472
  replacement of, 648
  serum, 1104
  testosterone, 912-913
Eosinophilia, 676
  in incontinentia pigmenti, 950
Eosinophilic membrane in lungs, 427
Ephedrine, 104
Epicanthal folds, 1043
Epicanthus, 980
Epicanthus inversus, 980
Epidemiology
  to delineate drug effects, 158
  of erythroblastosis fetalis, 34
  of preeclampsia, 28
  of viral infection, 694-695
Epidermal growth factor, 55
Epidermal nevus syndrome, 959
Epidermis, structure of, 939
Epidermolysis bullosa, 947-949
Epidural bleeding, 373

Epiglottis, floppy, 462
Epilepsy, risk of, 1037
Epinephrine, 744
　altering arterial blood pressure, 127
　for cardiac resuscitation, 582
　for cardiovascular disease, 628
　dosage for, 1092
　for heart failure, 572
　for hypoglycemia, 865
　neonatal tachycardia due to, 121
　increasing pulmonary artery pressure, 130
　for uterine relaxation, 142
Epinephrine-isoxsuprine inhalations, 439
Epiphora, 983
Epiphyses
　ossification of, in SGA infant, 70
　overgrowth of, 235
　radiographic visualization of, 134
　separation of, 236
Epiphysiolysis, 236
Epispadias, 799
Epistaxis due to decreased platelets, 718
Epithelial cells in amniotic fluid, 138
Epithelium, gastrointestinal, 477
Epstein-Barr virus, 682-683
Erb's palsy, 374
E600-resistant acid esterase, 839
Ergot in human milk, 167
Erythema
　in eczema, 960
　sustained at birth, 216
Erythema toxicum, 943
Erythroblastopenia of childhood, transient, 723-724
Erythroblastosis, 726
Erythroblastosis fetalis
　ABO incompatibility, 42
　clinical applications for, 40-42
　clinical manifestations of, 35-36
　color of placenta in, 211
　delivery room procedures for, 190
　diagnosis, 34-35
　in disseminated intravascular coagulation, 720
　epidemiology of, 34
　history in, 34
　hypoglycemia in, 858
　management of, 35, 36-39
　other antibodies causing, 42-43
　polyhydramnios associated with, 46
　prevention of, 43
　Rh, 34-42
Erythrocytes; *see also* Red blood cells
　in cerebrospinal fluid, 372
　circulating
　　destruction of, hyperbilirubinemia due to, 758
　　mass of, in SGA infants, 75
　destruction of, 759
　fetal, 721-722
　of newborn, 710
　underproduction of, anemia due to, 721-725
Erythrogenesis imperfecta, 721
Erythroid hypoplasia, congenital, 723, 724
Erythromycin, 660
　for chlamydial pneumonia, 447
　dosage for, 1093
　in human milk, 166

Erythropoiesis, ineffective, 733
Erythropoietic porphyria, congenital, 760
　phototherapy contraindicated in, 769
Erythropoietin, 711
　in congenital hypoplastic anemia, 722
　SGA infant synthesis of, 75
Escape rhythms, 575
Escherichia coli
　bacteriuria due to, 805
　colitis due to, 487
　diarrhea due to, 523
　hyperbilirubinemia due to, 760
　in icteric infants, 653
　in mechanical ventilation, 438
　meningitis due to, 657
　necrotizing enterocolitis due to, 513
　pneumatoceles due to, 471
　pneumonia due to, 446
　in septic shock, 128
　subdivisions of, 662-663
Esophageal atresia
　in polyhydramnios, 44
　with tracheoesophageal fistula, 496-498
　ultrasonic detection of, 86
Esophageal duplications and cysts, 491
Esophageal dysmotility, 491-492
　in familial dysautonomia, 495
Esophageal hiatus, herniation through, 489
Esophageal motility in preterm infant, 481
Esophageal pressure determinations, 425-426
Esophageal rupture, 496
Esophageal varices, 487
Esophageal vestibule, 491-492
Esophagitis, 495
Esophagoscopy 487
Esophagus, disorders of, 491-501
Esotropia, 980, 989
Estetrol, 110
Estradiol
　plasma levels of, in premature labor, 140
　synthesis of, 904
　to test fetal well-being, 110
Estriol
　levels of
　　in erythroblastosis fetalis, 36
　　in preeclampsia, 30
　plasma
　　to determine fetal well-being, 69, 111-112
　　diurnal variations in, 111
　urinary
　　determinations of, 66
　　to determine fetal well-being, 25, 69
　　diurnal variations in, 111
　　maternal excretion of, 111
Estriol-16-glucuronide, 111
Estriol-3-sulfate-16-glucuronate, 111
Estrogens
　effect on sweat glands, 941
　fetal production of, 140
　levels of, in pregnancy, 23
　placental, 111
　role in phosphatidylcholine synthesis, 417
Ethacrynic acid
　dosage for, 1096
　potentiating noise-induced hearing loss, 273

Ethambutol, 678
Ethanol, 58; *see also* Alcohol
　in human milk, 167
　malformations due to, 1037
　for premature labor, 143
　saturation kinetics of, 165
Ethanolamine phosphorylation, 414
Ethchlorvynol, 391
Ethical issues in neonatal-perinatal medicine, 3
Ethical problems in ICU, 16
Ethmoid bone, 1042
Ethmoiditis, 673
Ethnic background
　and genetic disorders, 1014
　and physiologic jaundice, 758
Ethosuximide in human milk, 166
Ethyl ether, 142
Euglobulin lysis time, 721
　in anemia, 716
　test values for, 1113
Euglycemia, 26
Eustachian tube, 664
Euthanasia, 387
Evaporative heat losses, 265-266
Eventration of diaphragm, 489-490
Eversion of eyelids, 969
Evoked potentials
　auditory, 339, 355
　visual, 338
Examination
　behavioral, 342-343
　general pediatric, 348-349
　microscopic renal, 788
　neurologic
　　Brazelton Neonatal Behavioral Assessment Scale, 343
　　cranial nerves, 353-355
　　interpretation of, 355-356
　　level of consciousness, 349
　　motor system, 349-353
　　　in meningomyelocele, 386
　　sensory system, 353
　radiologic, assessment of, 1064
　vaginal, causing prolonged FHR decelerations, 104
Excretory urography, 1077-1079
Exenteration for orbital teratoma, 986
Exercises in brachial palsy, 227-228
Exfoliation, 947
Exodeviation, 984
Exogenous compound passage from maternal blood to milk, 165-166
Exogenous smiling, 335
Exophthalmos
　hyperthyroid, 986
　due to tumors, 986
Exotropia, 989, 1043
Exposure of radiologic film, 1064
Exstrophy, bladder, 799
Extracellular fluid ionization, 278
Extrahepatic bile ducts, 772-774
Extramembranous gestation, 207
Extravasation during parenteral therapy, 299
Extremities
　birth injury to, 235-237
　congenital malformations of, 1051-1052

Extubation
　accidental, 438
　atelectasis after, 439
Eye
　abnormalities of, due to infection, 1037
　birth injury to, 224-225
　closed, 982
　congenital malformations of, 1042-1047
　development of, in preterm infant, 338
　dry, 984
　effect of phototherapy on, 767
　examination of, 967-971
　　in multiple malformations, 1014-1015
　injury to, 975-976
　internal, diseases of, 991-1002
　large, 987-989
　purulent, 982-983
　red, 984
　small, 987
　watery, 983-984
Eye drops, adverse effects of, 338
Eye movement in term infant, 337
Eyebrows
　fusion of, 1047
　sparse, 981
　widely spaced, 1043
Eyelashes, sparse, 981
Eyelids
　abnormal, 979-980
　injuries to, 224
　penetration of, by spiral scalp electrode, 238
　separation of 969
　tumors of, 980-981

F

Face
　abnormal, 976-979
　birth injuries to, 222-224
　congenital malformations of, 1041-1042
　development of, 1041-1042
　developmental junctions of, 1042
　in DiGeorge syndrome, 647
　in idiopathic infantile hypercalcemia, 537
　in sclerema neonatorum, 962
　in trisomies, 1018-1020
Face masks
　deleterious effects of, 440
　for respiratory distress syndrome, 434
Facial clefts, 976-977
Facial expression of preterm infant, 334-335
Facial nerve examination, 355
Facial nerve paralysis, 374
　sustained at birth, 222-223
Failure to breathe at birth, 180
Failure of differentiation of parts, 1004, 1008
Failure of formation of parts, 1004
Failure to thrive, 240, 241
　due to hiatal hernia, 493
False alarms in cardiac monitoring, 280
False labor, 141-142
False lumen perforation during umbilical catheterization, 187
Family planning for diabetic woman, 26
Fanconi's anemia, 722, 723
Fanconi's pancytopenia, 63

Fanconi's syndrome
    radial defects in, 1058
    urine excretion in, 802
Farber's disease, 840
Fasting states, metabolism during, 54
Fat
    absorption of, in developing gastrointestinal tract, 480-481
    fetal, 50
    intestinal breakdown of, 521
    in intravenous nutrient administration, 313
    low birth weight infant requirement for, 304-305
Father
    age of, as factor in Down's syndrome, 1016
    care of, throughout pregnancy, 240-251
    drug ingestion by, effect on fetus, 151-152
Fatty acids
    and breast milk jaundice, 763
    free; *see* Free fatty acids
    for phosphatidylcholine synthesis, 416
    polyunsaturated
        effect of vitamin E on, 306
        requirements for, 304
Favism, 735
Fecal nutrient loss, 303
Fecal retention in spinal injury, 232
Fecal water losses, 317, 319
Feeding
    in chylothorax, 455
    constipation due to changes in, 512
    difficulties in, as sign of heart failure, 568
    in heart failure, 571
    hyperosmolar, 513
    for low birth weight infant, 308-313
    in necrotizing enterocolitis, 513, 516
    parenteral fluids, 298-300
    after pyloromyotomy, 500
    in respiratory distress syndrome, 433
Feet
    congenital malformations of, 1052-1059
    epidermal ridge patterns of, 1052, 1054
Femoral pulse, 590, 592
Femur
    fetal, ultrasonic measurement of, 84
    fracture of, 235-236
    hypoplasia of, 1004
    radiologic appearance of, 1081-1084
Fenoterol, 145, 146
Ferric chloride tests, 822
Ferrous gluconate, 1096
Ferrous sulfate, 1096
Fetal activity monitoring, 40
Fetal alcohol syndrome, 58, 936
    anomalies of, 153
    hair in, 1040
    pattern of malformations in, 1037
    renal hypoplasia in, 794
Fetal anatomy, seen with ultrasonography, 86
Fetal asphyxia, 2
Fetal assessment
    antepartum
        biochemical, 110-112
        clinical applications of, 112
        electrophysiologic monitoring, 107-108
        fetal breathing, 109-110
        fetal movement, 108

Fetal assessment—cont'd
    antepartum—cont'd
        "movements alarm signal," 108
        nonstress monitoring, 108
        oxytocin challenge test, 108-109
    intrapartum
        blood sampling technique, 116-118
        electrophysiologic monitoring, 112-115
        future outlook, 118
        of pH, 115-116
Fetal blood sampling, 1033
    complications of, 190-191
    injuries related to, 104
    during late deceleration, 104
    precautions concerning, 117
    technique of, 116-118
Fetal breathing assessment, 109-110
Fetal circulation
    as factor in placental transfer of drugs, 151
    persistent, 73; *see also* Persistence of fetal circulation
Fetal death, ultrasonic diagnosis of, 92
Fetal growth
    aberrant; *see also* Intrauterine growth retardation
        maternal contributions to, 55-59
        in SGA infant, 64-66
    and body composition, 49-54
    cessation of, management of, 70
    genetic determinants of, 62
    population norms for, 64
    rate of, assessing, 196-197
    variation in, 197
Fetal heart heard with stethoscope, as index of maturity, 134
Fetal heart rate; *see* Heart rate, fetal
Fetal heart rate monitoring
    baseline FHR, 95-99
    benefit of, 106
    injuries related to, 238
    ominous patterns in, 104-106
    periodic FHR changes, 99-104
Fetal hydantoin syndrome, 1037
    hair in, 1040
Fetal maturity, estimation of, 133-138
Fetal metabolism, 54-55
Fetal monitoring, 2
    intrapartum, injuries related to, 237-238
Fetal movement
    associated with FHR accelerations, 99
    maternal perception of, 108
    monitoring of, 108
Fetal organ blood flow, 2
Fetal period, environmental effects during, 1026
Fetal/placental ratio, 211
Fetal repiratory responses, 180-181
Fetal urine, 47
Fetal weight, 51
    following eclampsia, 58
Fetal-maternal hemorrhage, 742-743
Fetal-to-adult hemoglobin switch, 731
Fetoplacental steroid hormones, 110-112
Fetoscopy, 1028, 1033
Fetus
    aborted, malformations in, 1037-1038
    adverse drug effects in, 150-158
    auditory responses of, 339
    body composition of, 53

Fetus—cont'd
  determinants of growth of, 62-63
  harlequin, 945
  perception of, by parents, 241-242
  period of, 152
  sucking reflex in, 336-337
Fever
  control of, 272
  in ectodermal dysplasia, 964
  maternal, causing fetal tachycardia, 95
  neonatal tachycardia due to, 121
Fibrin split products, 720
Fibrinogen, 716
  dosage for, 1095
  levels of, 721
    in preeclampsia, 30
  test values for, 1113
Fibrinosis, diffuse, 61
Fibrin-stabilizing factor deficiency, 717
Fibroblast growth factor, 55
Fibroma, sternocleidomastoid, 230
Fibrosis
  idiopathic pulmonary, 467
  ventricular, 377
Fibrous cords, 775
Fibula, absent, 1004
Filtration process of drug transport, 160
Financial considerations for perinatal health services, 10
Fingerprint body myopathy, 397
Fingers, epidermal ridge patterns of, 1052, 1053, 1054
FIO_2, in respiratory distress syndrome, 435
FIO_2, maternal, during cesarean section, 178
First breath; see Breathing, onset of
First-order kinetics, 164-165
Fish mouth deformity, 945
Fixation, visual, 337-338, 354, 974
  examination for, 968
Flaccid paralysis in facial nerve palsy, 222
Flavobacterium meningosepticum, 651, 657
Flocculation tests, 675
Flow dynamics before labor, 113
9α-Fludrocortisone acetate, 920
Fluid
  body
    in late edema, 791
    shift in distribution of, 709
    volume and composition of, 315-316
  in fetal lung, 180
  providing adequate, 317-319
  requirement for, 318
Fluid and electrolytes
  in preeclampsia, 30
  in renal insufficiency, 792-793
Fluid management in chronic pulmonary disease, 474-475
Fluid replacement, central venous pressure to aid, 128, 129
Fluid restriction
  in bronchopulmonary dysplasia, 474
  after cardiac surgery, 624
  in chest tube use, 451
Fluid space distribution, 52
Fluid therapy, 316-317
  for chronic pulmonary disease, 473
  in heart failure, 571-573
  for respiratory distress syndrome, 432-433
Fluorescein angiography, 977

Fluorescent polarization technique, 136
Fluorescent treponema antibody absorption test, 675
5-Fluorocytosine
  for cutaneous candidiasis, 950
  dosage for, 1094
Fluoroscopy
  in airway obstruction, 463
  for catheter placement, 131
  in cystourethrography, 788
  in phrenic nerve palsy, 228
Fluothane, 142
Flush technique for arterial blood pressure, 126
Focal dermal hypoplasia, 962
Folate
  deficiency of, 724
  serum concentration of, 307, 724, 725
Folic acid
  deficiency of, 724-725
  malabsorption of, 523
  requirement for, 306-307
  serum values for, 1109
  for unstable hemoglobin, 734
Folinic acid, 705-706
Follicle-stimulating hormone
  blood values for, 1105
  estradiol synthesis by, 904
Following, visual, 337-338, 354, 974
  examination for, 968
Follow-up of SGA infants, 76-78
Fontan conduit procedure
  for single ventricle, 602
  for tricuspid atresia, 599
Fontanel
  anterior
    in craniosynostosis, 384
    fullness of, 191, 368
    palpation of, 194
    as site for intracranial pressure monitoring, 357
    vulnerabilitry to external pressure, 101
  interparietal, mistaken for fracture, 221
  large, 1040
  posterior, 194
Foramen of Bochdalek, 488
Foramen ovale, 179
  catheterization through, 586, 587, 591
  shunting across, 599
Forceps
  cephalhematoma due to, 218
  for delivery, 176
  erythema and abrasions due to, 216
  skull fractures due to, 220
  for umbilical catheterization, 186
Forebrain cleavage anomalies, 378
Formalin, 964
Formaminoglutamic acid, 724
Formula feedings
  high-calorie, 474
    lactobezoars due to, 501
  and protein requirements, 304
Fovea, 974
Fractional shortening, 551
  reduced left ventricular function indicated by, 555
Fracture
  of clavicle, 226
  facial bone, 223-224

Fracture—cont'd
  of femur, 235-236
  greenstick, 226, 235
  of humerus, 235
  rib, due to rickets, 1081
  skull, 220-222
    associated with cephalhematoma, 219
    elevation of, 221
Fragmentary clonic movement, 389
Fragments, complement, 633-634
Frame shift mutations, 157
Franceschetti syndrome, 977
Freckles, 943
  axillary, 952
Free fatty acids
  bilirubin binding diminished by, 765
  during maternal fasting, 54
  plasma values for, 1101
  in SGA infants, 73
  in skin, 942
Freeman-Sheldon whistling face syndrome, 1059
Frejka pillow, 1011
Frequency
  of mechanical ventilators, 436-437
  sound, neonatal response to, 339
  of tremors, 353
  ultrasonographic, 81-82, 548
Friederich's ataxia, 538
Frog breathing, 179
Frontonasal dysplasia, 1043, 1048
Frontonasal prominence, 1042
Fructose
  for glucose-galactose malabsorption, 524
  intolerance to 833, 863
  metabolic disorders of, 833-834
Fructose-1,6-diphosphate deficiency, 833-834
Fructosuria, 833
Functional residual capacity, 411
  in chronic pulmonary insufficiency, 467
  establishment of, 425
  grunting to maintain, 421
Fundal height recording, 66
Fundus, ocular
  abnormal, 999-1000
  examination of, 971, 989
Fundus albipunctatus, 999-1000
Funduscopy, 354
Funisitis, 213
Funnel deformity, 226
Furosemide
  calciuria due to, 474
  for cardiovascular disease, 627
  for congestive heart failure, 571, 572
  dosage for, 1096
  for hypertension, 619
  potentiating noise-induced hearing loss, 273
  for respiratory distress syndrome, 432

G

Galactokinase deficiency, 831
Galactose
  -free diet, 994
  metabolic disorders of, 831
Galactosemia, 63, 831-832, 862
  cataracts due to, 994

Galactosemia—cont'd
  liver injury due to, 782
Galactose-1-phosphate uridyltransferase, 831
  deficiency of, 994
GALANT, 353
Galeazzi's sign, 1011
Gallbladder, bile collection from, 761
Gallop rhythm, 568
  in hyperplastic left-heart syndrome, 588
Gallstones, 736
Gametogenesis, toxic effects on, 1026
Gamma camera scanning, 777
Gamma-aminobutyric acid, absence of, 391
Gammaglobulin
  for hepatitis, 706
  for myxovirus infection, 682
  for Rh incompatibility, 727
Gamma-glutamyl transpeptidase
  test for, during total parenteral nutrition, 312
  values for, 1104
Ganglioneuroma, diarrhea due to, 525
Ganglioside storage disease, 840-842
Gangliosidosis, 63, 841-842
Gangrene
  in gastroschisis, 529
  intrauterine, 1008
Gantrisin; see Sulfisoxazole
Garment nevus, 953
Gas dilution studies, 424
Gas exchange
  in bronchopulmonary dysplasia, 470-471
  in developing lung, 408-409
  fetal, compromised, 70
Gasless abdomen
  due to neuromuscular blockade, 437
  radiologic diagnosis of, 1075-1076
Gas-liquid chromatography, 671
Gasoline inhalation, 156-157
Gasping, 122
  aspiration of amniotic fluid during, 446
  pattern of, 109, 125
  reinitiation of, 181
  rhythmic, 180-181
Gastric air bubble, medial displacement of, 233
Gastric aspirate in intestinal obstruction, 483
Gastric emptying time
  delayed, 309
  effect on drug absorption, 160
  in preterm infant, 481
Gastric hypersecretion, 527
Gastric inhibitory peptide, 522
Gastric lavage, 620
Gastrin, 522
Gastroenteritis, 662-664
Gastroenteropathy, allergic, 526
Gastroesophageal reflux, 467, 491-492
Gastrografin, 507, 521, 1072
Gastrointestinal tract
  assimilation of fat in, by low birth weight infant, 305
  cellular proliferation in, 478-479
  development of, 477-482
  diagnostic radiology for, 1070-1077
  disorders of
    abdomen, 529-532
    colon, 504-512

Gastrointestinal tract—cont'd
　disorders of—cont'd
　　delivery room diagnosis of, 194
　　esophagus, 491-498
　　pancreas, 516-521
　　stomach, 498-501
　　sucking and swallowing, 490-491
　　total parenteral nutrition for, 311
　　ultrasonic detection of, 86-89
　drug absorption through, 158, 160
　duplications in, 504
　enzymatic development in, 479-480
　hemorrhage in, 486-487
　perforation of, 73, 485-486
Gastropexy
　for hiatal hernia, 495
　for volvulus of stomach, 499
Gastroschisis, 89
Gastroscopy, 487
Gastrostomy, 300
　for continuous intestinal decompression, 489
　for esophageal atresia, 497-498
　for gastrointestinal perforation, 486
Gaucher's disease, 63
　chronic nonneuropathic form, 840
　hyperbilirubinemia associated with, 782
　malignant form, 840
Gavage feeding, 299-300
　in heart failure, 571
　neonatal bradycardia due to, 121
Gel filtration in pulmonary hemorrhage, 447
Genetic counseling
　in cardiovascular disease, 623
　in congenital malformations, 1060-1061
　in multiple malformations, 1015
Genetic determinants
　in congenital heart disease, 538
　of fetal growth, 62
　of fetal response to drugs, 157
　for globin chain synthesis, 731, 732
　in 21-hydroxylase deficiency, 921
　in physiologic jaundice, 758
Genetic diagnosis, prenatal, 1028-1033
Genetic disease, 1013-1033
Genital duct development, 901-902
Genitalia
　ambiguous, 925-930
　　voiding cystourethrography for, 1079
　birth trauma to, 237
　congenital malformations of, 1051
　differentiation of, control of, 905-907
　examination of, 256
　external, development of, 902-903
　female, of SGA infant, 72
　internal, in renal agenesis, 794
Genitourinary system
　anomalies of
　　delivery room diagnosis of, 194
　　ultrasonographic detection of, 86
　bacteria in, 651
Genotype
　effect on birth weight, 62-63
　effect on fetal response to drugs, 157
Genotypic studies, 1028
Gentamicin, 660

Gentamicin—cont'd
　dosage for, 1093
　effect on gastrointestinal activity, 516
　multicompartmental model of elimination, 164-165
　for sepsis, 655, 656
Genu recurvatum, 1011
Gestational age
　classification by, 196
　estimation of, 133
　　in nursery, 256-259
　　radiologic, 1084
　　ultrasonographic, 82-84
　as factor in infection outcome, 694
　and neonatal risk, 196-205
　specific risks by, 199-203
Gestational diabetes; see Diabetes, in pregnancy
Gestational sac visualization, 82
Giant hairy nevus, 953-954
Giemsa stain, 666, 676, 686
Gigantism, cerebral, 1052
Gingival cysts, 462
Glabella, lesions in, 943
Glandular stage of lung development, 407
Glaucoma, 72, 983-984, 988
　in microphthalmia, 987
Glioma, 987
Globin chain synthesis, disorders of, 731-741
α_2-Globulin in preeclampsia, 28
Glomerular filtration rate
　decrease in, 790
　neonatal, 163, 785
　substance clearance and, 789
Glomeruli, variability of, 786
Glomeruloendotheliosis, 28
　differentiation from preeclampsia, 27
Glomerulonephritis
　acute, 799
　chronic, 799-800
Glomerulosclerosis, 787
　differentiation from chronic glomerulonephritis, 800
Glossopharyngeal nerve examination, 355
Glossoptitis, 256, 1048
Glucagon
　congenital deficiency of, 862
　dosage for, 1096
　for hypoglycemia, 866
　intravenous, causing neonatal tachycardia, 121
　levels of, in SGA infant, 74
Glucagon tolerance test, 864
Glucagon-like gut immunoreactants, 522
Glucocorticoids
　deficiency of, 862
　fetal production of, and surfactant production, 135
　in human milk, 166
　prepartum, to hasten lung maturity, 427
Gluconeogenic amino acid precursors, 73
Glucose
　and bilirubin conjugation, 755
　blood levels of
　　in malabsorption, 524
　　in pregnant diabetic, 23
　　range of, 202
　　in SGA infant, 74
　fetal intestinal transport of, 481
　fetal metabolism of, 846-847

Glucose—cont'd
　hepatic, 848
　intravenous, 864-865
　　for nutrient administration, 312
　　for respiratory distress syndrome, 185
　low birth weight infant requirement for, 305
　during maternal fasting, 54
　maternal storage of, 57
　neonatal metabolism of, 847-849
　oxidation of, in neutrophils, 745
　for phosphatidylcholine synthesis, 415-416
　renal reabsorption of, 802
　supplementation of feedings with, 309
　in total parenteral nutrition, 310
　whole blood levels of, 1102-1103
Glucose homeostasis disturbances, 202, 835-836
Glucose phosphate isomerase, 734
Glucose-galactose malabsorption, 524-525
Glucose-6-phosphate dehydrogenase deficiency, 735
　geographic influences on, 758
　hyperbilirubinemia in, 759-760
α-Glucosidases, embryonic activity of, 480, 611
Glucosuria, 801-802
Glucuronic acid
　bilirubin conjugated with, 754
　conjugated with estriol, 111
β-Glucuronidase
　deficiency of, 839
　enteric bilirubin absorption with, 756
Glucuronidation
　absence of, in fetal liver, 162
　enzymes causing, 158
Glucuronyl transferase
　decreased activity of, 499
　deficiency of, 761-762
　hepatic activity of, 761
　inhibitors of, in serum, 763
Glutaric aciduria, 830
Glutathione, detoxifying electrophilic metabolites, 157
Glutathione peroxidase
　function with tocopherol, 739
　in neonatal erythrocytes, 735
Gluten-sensitive enteropathy, 961
Glutethimide, 153
Glyceraldehyde-3-phosphate, 734
D-Glyceric aciduria, 830
Glycogen
　epidermal, 942
　hepatic, in SGA infants, 73
　myocardial, 73
Glycogen storage disease, 611, 862-863
　heart disease due to, 537-538
Glycogenolysis, 73
Glycogenoses, 834-836
Glycolysis
　anaerobic, 185
　during cold stress, 260
Glycolytic red blood cell enzymes, 711
Glycopyrrolate, 177
GM_1 gangliosidosis
　cherry-red macula in, 1001
　head shape in, 1041
　tongue in, 1050
　causing trophoblastic vacuolization, 213
Goiters, 897

Goiters—cont'd
　airway obstruction due to, 462
　endemic, 891
Gold salts, neutropenia induced by, 744
Goldberg's syndrome, 1001
Goldenhar's syndrome
　eyes in, 1047
　facies in, 977
Goltz's syndrome, 962
Gonadal dysgenesis, 908-910
Gonadotropin, 912
Gonads
　developmental disorders of, 907-912
　fetal, endocrine function in, 903-904
　streak, 904-905
　in Turner's syndrome, 908-909
Gonococcal disease, 673-674
Gonorrhea, 673
Goretex shunt, 594
Gorham's disease, 958
Gower hemoglobins, 731
Gowning procedures in nursery, 295
Graft-versus-host reaction, 647, 648
　after exchange transfusion, 730
Granulocytes
　fetal, 708
　transfusion with, 743
Granulomas
　in cryptococcosis, 685
　endometrial, 678
　immunologic aspects of, 636
Graves' disease, 986
Gray matter
　effect of poliovirus on, 680
　as site of asphyxia, 358
Gray-scale instrumentation, 81
Gray-wire sign, 500
Greek population, G6PD deficiency in, 758
Greenhouse effect in incubator, 265
Greig's hypertelorism, 977
Grimacing
　during seizures, 389
　testing for, 355
Ground glass sign, 543
　corneal, 990
Grounding in electronic monitor use, 287-288
Group A β-hemolytic streptococci, 667, 669
Group B β-hemolytic streptococci, 672-673
Group B Ia plasma factor, 652
Group B streptococci
　endocarditis due to, 557
　pneumonia due to, 446
Growth
　catch-up, after intrauterine growth retardation, 76
　energy requirement for, 303
　factors in, 55
　fetal; see Fetal growth
　postnatal, as percent increment of body weight, 52
　retardation of, intrauterine; see Intrauterine growth retardation
Grunting, 335
　assessment of, 420-421
　effect on arterial oxygen tension, 434
　to improve oxygenation, 412
Guarnieri's bodies, 683
Guillain-Barré syndrome, 681

Gut, effect of hypoxia on, 192
Gynecomastia, 167

H

Habituation to stimulus, 337, 339
Haemophilus influenzae, 640, 651, 654
  antibodies to, 638
  otitis media due to, 664
Hair
  congenital malformations of, 1040
  growth of, 940
  patch of, in spina bifida, 385, 386, 388
Hallerman-Streiff syndrome
  facies in, 977
  nose in, 1048
Halogenated aromatic hydrocarbons, 157
Halothane, 177
Hamartomas, 211
  renal, 808
Hamman-Rich syndrome, 467
Handicaps due to stage IV bronchopulmonary dysplasia, 476
Hands, congenital malformations of, 1052-1059
Hand-washing techniques
  infections due to inadequate, 651
  in nursery, 295, 300
Haptoglobin
  low birth weight levels, 1108
  normal levels, 1109
Harlequin fetus, 945
Harlequin infant, 561
Hartnup disease, 523, 527
Haustra, 1074
Hb Bart's, 732
HB$_c$Ag
  in hepatitis, 696
  in oriental population, 695
HB$_s$Ag
  in hepatitis, 696
  liver injury associated with, 781
  in oriental population, 695, 696
^{3}H-choline, 408
Head
  birth injuries to, 218-226
  circumference, in hydrocephalus, 378
  congenital malformations of, 1040-1041
  examination of, 256
Head/abdomen circumference ratio, 68
Head/body ratio, fetal, 92
Head box, pressurized, 434
Head compression, 121
Head growth, normal, 379
Head hoods, 270
Head shape
  abnormalities of, 382-385
  values for, 1040-1041
Head size
  abnormal
    enlarging, 375-381; *see also* Hydrocephalus
    small, 381-382; *see also* Microcephaly
  ECHO virus affecting, 680
Head's reflex, 457
Health services
  perinatal, 4-11
  public, 8

Hearing disorders
  external ear abnormalities indicating, 1047
  due to rubella, 701
Hearing screening, 355
Heart
  areas of, echocardiographic transection of, 548-549
  examination of, 256
  fetal blood flow in, 2
Heart disease
  congenital, 613-615
    etiology of, 536-538
    hyperoxia-hyperventilation test to determine, 424
    hypoglycemia in, 863
    incidence of, 200, 536
    due to rubella, 701
  cyanotic
    diagnostic radiology for, 1070
    echocardiography for, 556-557
  differentiation from lung disease, 566-567
Heart failure
  advanced, near-terminal, 569
  management of, 570-573
  recognition of, 567-570
  without structural heart disease, 569-570
Heart rate
  Apgar scoring of, 182
  fetal
    decelerations in, 69, 156
    delivery room monitoring of, 181
    and fetal hemorrhage, 36
    flat, 104-105
    in meconium aspiration syndrome, 445
    ominous patterns of, 104-106
    periodic changes in, 99-104
    sinusoidal, 106
    variability of, 97
  neonatal
    alterations in, causes of, 121
    baseline changes in, 119-121
    ECG time intervals in, 544-545
    normal, 119, 541-542
    resting, 544
    variability in, 121-122
Heart shape, evaluation of, 543
Heart size
  consideration of, in heart disease evaluation, 542-543
  in persistent truncus arteriosus, 601
Heart sounds
  during cardiac resuscitation, 582
  diagnosis of, 542
  in Ebstein's anomaly, 599-600
  in persistent truncus arteriosus, 601
  in pulmonary atresia, 594
Heat exchange, physics of, 262
Heat loss, 264-266; *see also* Temperature regulation
  at birth, 179
Heat stress, 121
Heel prick
  in causes of cyanosis, 563, 565
  in methemoglobinemia, 560
  in heart disease, 558
Heinz bodies
  in dextrocardia, 615
  in G6PD deficiency, 735
  removal of, by spleen, 746

Heinz bodies—cont'd
  suggesting splenic disorders, 541
  and unstable hemoglobins, 734
Helium dilution, 468
Helix of ear, 1047
Hemangioma
  airway obstruction due to, 462
  capillary, 980, 1038, 1039
  cavernous, 985
  eyelid, 980
  giant, of liver, 608-609
  macular, 943
  orbital, 985
  in spina bifida, 385, 386, 388
Hematemesis, 487
Hematocele, 237
Hematochezia, 486, 487, 663
Hematocrit
  after acute hemorrhage, 189
  blood replacement corroborated by, 742
  in causes of cyanosis, 563, 565
  elevated
    heart failure indicated by, 569
    in SGA infant, 75
  normal newborn values, 708-711
  in polycythemia, 741
  in preeclampsia, 30
  in pulmonary hemorrhage, 447
  in respiratory distress syndrome, 433
  in subependymal germinal matrix hemorrhage, 368
Hematogenous dissemination, 685
Hematoidin, 208
Hematologic evaluation in gastrointestinal bleeding, 487
Hematologic values
  normal full-term, 1111
  postnatal, 1110
Hematomas
  of ear, 225
  orbital, 985
  retroplacental
    pathogenesis of, 212
    recognition of, 206
  in sternocleidomastoid injury, 230
Hematopoietic system
  changes in, 711-712
  cortical and medullary necrosis affecting, 808
  cytomegalovirus affecting, 700
  fetal, 708
  normal newborn, 708-711
Hematotympanum, 222
Hematuria, 790
Heme
  bilirubin derived from, 754
  degradation of
    carbon monoxide assessment of, 759
    increased, 758
Heme oxygenase, 754
Hemiclonic movement, 389
Hemifacial atrophy of Romberg, 977
Hemihypertrophy with hepatoblastoma, 748
Hemimelia, 1051
Hemoconcentration in preeclampsia, 30
Hemodialysis, 793
Hemodynamics
  in aortic stenosis, 590

Hemodynamics—cont'd
  in coarctation of aorta, 591, 592
  in d-transposition, 586-587, 588
  in Ebstein's anomaly, 600
  in left-to-right shunt, 605, 606, 608
  in myocardial disorders, 610, 613
  in pulmonary arterial stenosis, 597
  in pulmonary atresia, 592, 594
  in total anomalous venous return, 602-604
  in tricuspid atresia, 599
Hemoglobin
  A_{1c}, in maternal diabetes, 26
  absolute concentration of, 560
  as blood buffer, 320
  conversion to bilirubin, 754
  disorders of, 731-734
  fetal, 711
    hereditary persistence of, 733
  fetal-to-adult ratio, 561
  normal newborn values, 708-711
  oxygen binding of, 422
  oxygen-carrying capacity of, 185
  structure of, 731
  unstable, 734
  values
    after acute hemorrhage, 189
    blood replacement corroborated by, 742
Hemoglobin C disease, 733
Hemoglobin F, 722, 731
Hemolysis
  due to ABO incompatibility, 726
  drug-induced, 735
  in preeclampsia, 31
  severe, and risk of kernicterus, 759
Hemolytic complement assay, 634
Hemolytic disease
  amniotic fluid bilirubin in, 757-758
  isoimmune, 726, 728-730
Hemoperitoneum, 233, 715
Hemophilia, 717-718
Hemorrhage
  acute neonatal, 189
  adrenal, 233-235
  anemia due to, 712-715
  cerebellar, 373
  cerebral, 31
  after fetal blood sampling, 191
  gastrointestinal, 486-487
  internal, and hepatic ischemic necrosis, 782
  intracranial, 372-373
    due to cephalhematoma, 219
  intraocular, 225, 354
  intraventricular, with pneumothorax, 449
  lid, 975
  obstetric, 714-715
  orbital, 224
  postnatal, 715
  pulmonary, 447
  retinal, 975
  retrobulbar, 975
  due to skull fractures, 221
  subconjunctival, 224, 975
Hemorrhagic disorders
  anemia due to, 715-721
  petechiae from, 216

Hemosiderin, 208
Hemosiderosis, 722
Hemostasis
 development of, 715-717
 after fetal blood sampling, 117
 laboratory assessment of, 721
Henderson-Hasselbalch equation, 320
Heparin
 in breast milk, 166
 chromosomal diagnosis with, 1020
 dosage for, 1094
 to reduce risk of arterial thrombi, 430
Heparinization, 720
Hepatic cysts, 532
Hepatic enzymatic assay, 761
Hepatic fibrosis, congenital, 782
Hepatic glycogen content, 73
Hepatic neoplasms, 532
Hepatic uptake of bilirubin, 754
 deficiency of, 760
Hepatitis
 conjugated hyperbilirubinemia in, 774-781
 idiopathic neonatal, 774
 infection causing, 781
 interpretation of liver biopsy for, 778
 syphilitic, 674
Hepatitis B, 702
 frequency of infection, 696-697
 treatment and prevention of, 706
Hepatitis B immune globulin, 706
Hepatoblastoma, 748-749
 conjugated hyperbilirubinemia due to, 782
Hepatocellular phase of bile excretion, 771
Hepatocytes, 754
Hepatomegaly
 fetal, 92
 causing rupture of liver, 232
Hepatosplenomegaly, 72
 in β-thalassemia, 733
Hereditary persistence of fetal hemoglobin, 733
Hering-Breuer reflex, 434, 457
Hering's canal, 772
Hermaphroditism, true, 907-908
Hernia
 in connective tissue disorders, 1050-1051
 in cutis laxa, 963
 examination for, 194
 sites of, 489
Heroin
 addiction to, 934-935
 in human milk, 167
 and intrauterine growth retardation, 58
 withdrawal from, 934-935
  maldigestion due to, 523
Herpes simplex
 frequency of infection by, 697
 manifestations of, 699
 microcephaly due to, 381
 neonatal, 703
 treatment and prevention of, 705
Herpes zoster–immune globulin, 683
Herpesvirus, seizures from, 390
Herpesvirus hominis, 669
Herxheimer's reactions, 676
Heterochromia, 971, 992

Heterochromia—cont'd
 ptosis associated with, 981
Heterophile antibody, 640
Hexachlorophene
 dilute, 300
 routine bathing in, 688
Hexanoic/butanoic aciduria, 830
Hexoprenaline, 146
Hexosaminidase A, 840
Hiatal hernia, 492-495
High-risk patients
 Apgar score to determine, 183
 according to birth weight and gestational age, 196-205
 with central nervous system disorders, 398-400
 diabetics as, 22-23
 facilities for, 290-291
 follow-up of, 10
 frequency of problems of, 8
 need for recognition of, 1
 small for gestational age determining, 49
Hip
 diagnostic radiology for, 1081-1084
 dislocation of, 236
  congenital, 1009-1011
 septic arthritis in, 1084
 subluxatable, 1011
Hippus, 969
Hirschberg test, 989
Hirschsprung's disease, 504-507
 colon caliber in, 1075
 with intestinal obstruction, 483, 484
 iris bicolor in, 992
Hirsutism, 1040
His-Purkinje system, 575, 580
Histamine
 intradermal injection of, 496
 liberation of, 636
  in mastocytosis, 962
Histidine, 304
Histidinemia, 822
Histiocytosis, 987
 eczema in, 961
Histoplasma capsulatum, 686
Histoplasmosis, 686
History
 in congenital malformations, 1039
 indicating intrauterine growth retardation risk, 66
 of infection, 703-704
 neurologic, 348
 ocular, 968
HLA identical, mixed leukocyte culture nonreactive donor, 723
HLA typing, 648
Hodgkin's disease, 747
 following Chédiak-Higashi syndrome, 955
Holoprosencephaly, 1043
Holt-Oram syndrome, 538, 1035
Homeostasis
 disorders of
  due to hypomagnesemia, 880
  in preeclampsia, 28, 29
 glucose, disturbances in, 202
Homeothermy, 260-262
Homocystinuria, 820-821
 arachnodactyly in, 1059
 ectopia lentis in, 999

Homocystinuria—cont'd
  extremity length in, 1051
Homogentisic acid, 820
Homograft
  aortic, 602
  for pulmonary atresia, 594
Homovanillic acid, 1101
Hormones
  abnormalities of, diarrhea and malabsorption due to, 525-526
  epithelial changes due to, 942
  fetal, 846-847
  gastrointestinal, 522, 874
  newborn values for, 1105
  for phosphatidylcholine synthesis, 417
  placental transport of, 846
  teratogenicity of, 155
  thyroid, 883-890
Horner's syndrome, 224
  in brachial palsy, 227, 374
  heterochromia in, 992
  miosis in, 968
  pupillary size in, 981
Hospital facilities, measurement of changes in, 15
Host defense mechanisms
  antibody-mediated immunity, 634-636
  cell-mediated immunity, 636
  complement system, 633-634
  disorders of, 645-648
  neonatal
    evaluation of function in, 642-645
    specific, 638-639
  phagocytic, 632-633
  T and B lymphocytes, 637-638
Howell-Jolly bodies
  in dextrocardia, 615
  removal of, by spleen, 746
HpaI enzyme, 1032
Hubner's artery, 370
Human chorionic gonadotropin, 903-904
Human chorionic somatomammotropin
  effects on maternal metabolism, 110
  levels of, in pregnant diabetic, 23
  during maternal fasting, 54
Human growth hormone, 55
  blood values for, 1105
  fetal, 847
  for hypoglycemia, 866
  for hypoglycemia with hypopituitarism, 861
Human pancreatic polypeptide, 522
Human placental lactogen; see Human chorionic somatomammotropin
Human tetanus–immune globulin, 677
Humerus
  fracture of, 235
  radiologic appearance of, 1084
Humidification
  in eczema, 961
  of inspired gases, 474
Humidity
  distinction from vapor pressure, 265
  in incubators, 259, 296
  in oxygen therapy, 298
Huntington's chorea, 1024
Hurler's syndrome, 538
  facies in, 1049

Hurler's syndrome—cont'd
  mucopolysaccharide accumulation in, 990
Hürthle cell tumor, 897
Hutchinson's teeth, 676
H-Y antigen, 904, 909, 910
Hyaline membrane disease; see also Respiratory distress syndrome
  derivation of term, 427
Hyaloid artery, persistence of, 1001
Hyaluronic acid, 941
Hydantoin, 58
  embryogenetic effects of, 1026
  vitamin K supplementation with, 718
Hydatidiform change, 61
Hydralazine
  for cardiovascular disease, 627
  dosage for, 1095
  for hypertension, 32, 619
Hydranencephaly, 379
Hydration, enzymes causing, 158
Hydrocephalus, 375-381
  ex vacuo, 375
  and hydramnios, 46, 193
  neonatal bradycardia due to, 121
  due to subependymal hemorrhage, 192, 370-371
  ultrasonic detection of, 89, 90
    appearance of ventricles in, 83
Hydrochloric acid
  fetal production of, 498
  in metabolic acidosis, 326
  spillage of, after perforation, 486
Hydrochlorothiazide
  for cardiovascular disease, 627
  for heart failure, 571, 572
Hydrocolpos, 532
Hydrocortisone, 145
  defective biosynthesis of, 943
  dosage for, 1096
  for eczema, 961
  for hypoglycemia, 865
Hydrocortisone sodium succinate
  for cardiogenic shock, 574
  for hypotension, 656
Hydrodiuril; see Hydrochlorothiazide
Hydrogen, excretion of, 524
Hydrogen peroxide
  possible role in tissue damage, 472
  production of, in neutrophils, 745
Hydrometra, 532
Hydronephrosis, 531
  following breech delivery, 237
  ultrasonic detection of, 86, 88
  in urinary tract obstruction, 797
Hydropneumothorax, 496
Hydrops fetalis
  and delay in pulmonary maturation, 135
  gene deletion causing, 732
  "nonimmune," 541
  in Rh incompatibility, 727
  stigmata of, 34
  due to syphilis, 674
Hydrothorax, 180
Hydroxyapatite synthesis, 322
2-(4-Hydroxybenzeneazo) benzoic acid, 765
25-Hydroxycholecalciferol, 872-873

17-Hydroxycorticosteroids
 urinary excretion of, 235
 urine values for, 1105
16-Hydroxy-dehydroepiandrosterone, 111
Hydroxyl radical, 472
11β-Hydroxylase deficiency, 920-921
17α-Hydroxylase deficiency, 922
21-Hydroxylase deficiency, 916-920
17-Hydroxyprogesterone
 blood values for, 1105
  in female pseudohermaphroditism, 918
 elevations of, 913
17-α-Hydroxyprogesterone caproate, 139
3β-Hydroxysteroid dehydrogenase deficiency, 921
17β-Hydroxysteroid oxidoreductase, 913
5-Hydroxytryptophan, 181, 819
Hydroxyzine
 during labor, 174
 and neonatal seizures, 391
Hygroma, cystic, 462
Hyoid arch, 1042
Hyperaldosteronism, 617
Hyperalert state, 349
Hyperalimentation in bronchopulmonary dysplasia, 474
Hyperammonemia, 121, 398
 idiopathic, self-limited neonatal, 822-823
 sex-linked, 824
Hyperbilirubinemia
 due to cephalhematoma, 219
 conjugated
  defined, 753
  diseases that may be seen as, 774
  pathophysiology of, 771-774
  specific disorders of, 774-782
 displacing drug from albumin-binding site, 160
 due to ecchymoses, 217
 in G6PD deficiency, 735
 indirect, 499
 in isoimmune hemolytic disease, 728
 mixed, 753
 in pyruvate kinase deficiency, 736
 transient familial neonatal, 763
 unconjugated
  defined, 753
  management of, 766-770
  pathologic states of, 758-764
  physiology of, 754-756
Hypercalcemia
 causing craniosynostosis, 382
 heart disease due to, 537
 iatrogenic, 879
 idiopathic, 878-879
Hypercapnia, 121
Hypercarbia, 428
Hyperglycemia, 866-867
 and fetal macrosomia, 24
 and gestational age, 202
 associated with intravenous supplementation feedings, 313
 nonketotic, 821-822
 due to total parenteral nutrition, 311
Hyperinflation of lung, 1067
 ipsilateral, 438
 in meconium aspiration syndrome, 444
 in stage IV bronchopulmonary dysplasia, 469
Hyperinsulinemia, fetal, 24

Hyperkalemia
 ECG changes due to, 547
 neonatal bradycardia due to, 121
Hyperkeratosis, 945
Hyperlipidemia, 837
Hyperlipoproteinemia, 836-837
Hyperlysinemia, 999
Hypermagnesemia, 880-881
Hypermethioninemia, 819-820
Hypermetropia, 987
Hypernatremia, 185-186
Hyperoxia, 130
Hyperoxia-hyperventilation test, 424
Hyperparathyroidism, 878
Hyperphenylalaninemia, 819
Hyperphosphatemia, 792
Hyperpigmentation
 diffuse, 950
 localized, 950-954
 postinflammatory, 953
Hyperplastic phase of cell growth, 50
Hyperplastic visceromegaly syndrome, 741, 858-859
Hyperpnea
 primary, 180
 during seizures, 389
Hyperstat; see Diazoxide
Hypertelorism, 1042-1043
 in craniosynostosis, 383
 syndromes associated with, 985
Hypertension
 chronic, 27, 28
 chronic maternal, effect on fetal growth, 57
 endocrine, 127
 fetal, 102
 neurogenic, 127
 pulmonary
  after diaphragmatic hernia surgery, 489
  ECG systolic time intervals in, 554
  heart failure due to, 569
  in meconium aspiration syndrome, 444
 renal, 127
 systemic, 617-618
  in coarctation of aorta, 592
 systolic, 127-128
 transient, differentiation from preeclampsia, 27
 due to uremia, 793
Hyperthermia, fetal, 74
Hyperthyroidism
 maternal, 95
 causing neonatal tachycardia, 121
Hypertonia, 191
Hypertrichosis, 981
 disorders with, 940
Hypertrichosis lanuginosa, 981
Hypertrophic phase of cell growth, 50
Hyperventilation, 121
 cerebral, 448
 for persistent fetal circulation, 445
Hyperviscosity, 863
Hyperviscosity-polycythemia syndrome, 75
Hypervolemia
 postinfusion, prevention of, 487
 pulmonary hemorrhage due to, 447
Hyphema, 976, 984
 sustained at birth, 225

Hypoadrenalism, 723
Hypocalcemia
　due to calcium/phosphorus ratio in formulas, 305-306
　early, 874-875
　late, 875-877
　from neonatal asphyxia, 73
　seizures due to, 390
Hypochromia, 712
Hypocortisolemia, 918
Hypodermoclysis, 298
Hypodontia, 963
Hypofibrinogenemia, 720
　associated with preeclampsia, 30-31
Hypogammaglobulinemia, 646
Hypoglossal nerve examination, 355
Hypoglycemia
　asymptomatic transient, 851
　clinical problems of, 849-864
　due to cold stress, 260
　diagnostic evaluation of, 864
　and gestational age, 202
　iatrogenic causes of, 863
　with infection, 654
　leucine-induced, 860
　in neonatal heart disease, 559
　and pituitary deficiency, 860-861
　and ponderal index relationships, 75
　seizures due to, 390
　in SGA infants, 73-74
　symptomatic transient, 851-854
　treatment of, 864-867
Hypoglycemic drugs, teratogenicity of, 155
Hypomagnesemia, 879-880
　with hypocalcemia, 876
　maldigestion due to, 523
　seizures due to, 390
Hypomelanosis of Ito, 955
Hyponatremia, 315-316
　associated with human milk feedings, 305
　with infection, 654
　due to respiratory distress therapy, 432-433
　seizures due to, 390-391
Hypoparathyroidism
　due to hypocalcemia, 877
　maternal, 871
Hypoperfusion, 366
Hypophosphatasia, 63
　causing craniosynostosis, 382
　fontanels in, 1040
　respiratory distress due to, 463
　suture closure in, 1084
Hypopigmentation, 954-955
Hypopituitarism
　anemia due to, 723
　hypoglycemia and, 860-861
Hypoplasia
　limb, 1004
　pulmonary, 453-454
　unilateral mandibular, 223
Hypoplastic left-heart syndrome, 588-589
　echocardiography in, 556
　hepatic ischemic necrosis in, 782
Hypopyon, 994
Hypospadias, 256, 923-924
　racial predilection of, 1039

Hypotelorism, 1042, 1043
　syndromes associated with, 984
Hypotension
　diastolic, 128
　effect on gut drug absorption, 160
　maternal, causing fetal asphyxia, 180
　postural, 495
　systemic, 567
　systolic, 128
　transient fetal, 99-101
Hypothalamic-pituitary-adrenal axis, 111
Hypothalamic-pituitary-thyroid axis, 885
Hypothalamus, thyroid hormone secretion and, 885
Hypothermia due to hypoglycemia, 863
Hypothyroidism
　congenital, 890-897
　hyperbilirubinemia in, 764
　microcephaly due to, 381
　neonatal bradycardia due to, 121
　neonatal screening for, 892-897
　wormian bones in, 1084
Hypotonia
　due to asphyxia, 191
　cerebral, 231
　determination of, 351-352
Hypotrichosis, 981
　disorders with, 940
　in ectodermal dysplasia, 963, 964
Hypovolemia, 126
Hypoxemia
　fetal, 103-104
　maternal, effect on fetal growth, 58
　renal function affected by, 164
　in respiratory distress syndrome, 428
Hypoxia
　during abnormal contractions, 114
　fetal
　　characterized by FHR variability, 97
　　causing fetal tachycardia, 95-97
　causing first breath, 179
　increasing pulmonary artery pressure, 130
　kernicterus and, 764-765
　neonatal, 72-73
　pulmonary hemorrhage associated with, 447
Hypoxic ischemic encephalopathy, 358-367
Hysteresis, 410

I

i antigen 722, 723
I cell disease, 63, 842
　head shape in, 1041
　palate in, 1049
Ichthyosis, 944-945
Idiopathic thrombocytopenic purpura, 639, 718
　as contraindication to fetal blood sampling, 118
I/E ratio, 436
IgA antibody
　in breast milk, 642
　cord blood elevations of, 639
　secretory, 635
　　response, 481-482
　structure and properties of, 635-636
IgD antibody, 635, 636
IgE antibody, 635, 636

IgG antibody
  antinuclear, 537
  in erythroblastosis fetalis, 34, 35
  in isoimmune hemolytic disease, 726
  in malaria, 686
  in neonatal immune thrombocytopenia, 718
  in nephrotic syndrome, 800
  placental transport of, 639
  structure and properties of, 635
  against TORCH agents, 704
IgM antibody
  cord blood
    in congenital infection, 72, 705
    elevations of, 639
    in pneumonia, 447
  against cytomegalovirus, 695
  in erythroblastosis fetalis, 35
  in pre-B cells, 637
  rubella-specific, 696
  serum concentration of, 653-654
  structure and properties of, 635, 636
  test of, in syphilis, 675
  in variola, 683
^{131}I-labeled rose bengal for ascites diagnosis, 533
Ileal atresia, 86, 88
Ileocecal valve, 527
Ileostomy, 507
  for cystic fibrosis, 521
Ileum, in necrotizing enterocolitis, 514
Imidazolepyruvic acid, excretion of, 822
Iminoglycinuria, 802
Immune response, fetal, 481
Immune serum globulin, 646
Immunity
  antibody-mediated, 634-636, 644
  cell-mediated, 636, 644-645
  passive, 639
  specific, in neonate, 638-639
  tests for, 643
Immunization
  maternal, in erythroblastosis fetalis, 34
  Rh, 34
  tetanus, 677
Immunodeficiency, 467
  developmental, 648
  malnutrition associated with, 648
  severe combined, 647-648
Immunoglobulins
  cord blood, in pneumonia, 447
  in glomerulonephritis, 799
  infection due to deficiency of, 652
  normal values for, 636
  phagocyte interactions with, 744
  serum levels of, 1107
  structure of, 634-636
Immunologic function
  disorders of, diarrhea due to, 525
  human milk increasing, 307
  intestinal, development of, 481-482
  in mother-child relationship, 639-642
  in SGA infants, 75
Immunoperoxidase technique, 782
Immunotherapy for neuroblastoma, 748
Impedance pneumography, 123, 124, 294
Imperforate anus, 509, 510, 511, 1051

Imperforate anus—cont'd
  associated with hydramnios, 193
Impetigo, bullous, 946-947
In utero constraining factor, 78
Inandione drug group, 166
Inborn errors of metabolism
  amino acid, 817-822
  amniotic fluid diagnosis of, 1030-1032
  cataracts associated with, 993
  fructose, 833-834
  galactose, 831-832
  glycogenoses, 834-836
  lipid, 836-837
  lysosomal function, 837-842
  monosaccharide, 830-831
  organic acid, 824-830
  screening tests for, 816-817
  urea cycle, 822-824
Inclusion blennorrhea, 983
Incontinentia pigmenti, 949-950, 954, 1040
Incubator
  air temperature in
    by age, 297
    by birth weight, 297
  chambers of, 267
  computer-controlled, 260
  convectively heated, 266-269
  in heart failure management, 570
  maintenance of, 294
  specifications for, 294
  survival incidence with, 259
Inderal; see Propranolol
Indian childhood cirrhosis, 782
Indomethacin
  for closure of ductus arteriosus, 1581
  contraindications to use of, 605
  to inhibit prostaglandin synthesis, 605
  for nephrogenic diabetes insipidus, 803
  persistence of fetal circulation due to, 566
  for premature labor, 143
Inducer T cells, 636, 637
Industrial by-products in human milk, 168
Infantile polycystic disease, 532, 796-797
  radiologic appearance of, 1078
Infants; see Neonates
  low birth weight; see Low birth weight infants
  SGA; see Small for gestational age infants
Infants of diabetic mothers, 854-858
  echocardiography for, 551-552
  hypocalcemia in, 875
  malformation incidence in, 1036, 1037
Infarcts
  placental, 212
  retroplacental, 62
Infection
  anaerobic, 670-671
  bacterial and yeast, of skin, 946-947
  in bronchopulmonary dysplasia, 471
  in chronic granulomatous disease, 645, 746-747
  control of, in chronic pulmonary disease, 475
  in disseminated intravascular coagulation, 720
  effect on fetal growth, 63, 64
  due to exchange transfusion, 730
  focal, due to cephalhematoma, 220
  frequency of, 694-698

Infection—cont'd
  genital, as contraindication to fetal blood sampling, 118
  gram-negative, granulocyte transfusion for, 743
  hepatitis due to, 781
  hypoglycemia with, 863
  local, after blood sampling, 117-118
  nosocomial, prevention of, 295
  ocular, 982-983
    intrauterine, 1000
  of organ systems, 656-670
  pathogenesis of, 692-694
  postnatally acquired, 650-688
  prevention of, in neonatal unit, 687-689
  respiratory tract
    after bronchopulmonary dysplasia, 475-476
    in ectodermal dysplasia, 964
  due to severe combined immunodeficiency disease, 647
  thrombocytopenia due to, 720
  TORCH, 72
  following umbilical catheterization, 187-188
  urinary tract, 782
    in secondary chalasia, 495
  viral and protozoal, 692-706
Inflammation
  perivascular, 218
  of placental membranes, 208-209
Inflammatory bowel disease, 111
Influenza, 681-682, 693
Infusate
  for intravenous nutrient administration, 312
  for total parenteral nutrition, 310
Inguinal hernias, 483
Inheritance patterns, malformations due to, 1036
Initial contact in outreach education, 13
Innominate veins, 603
Insensible water loss, 316, 318, 432
Inspiration, radiologic examination during, 1064
Inspissated bile syndrome, 730, 782
Inspissated milk syndrome, 508
Insulin
  dosage for, 1096
  fetal, 846-847
    as growth-enhancing hormone, 24, 54-55
  in lipodystrophy, 837
  during maternal fasting, 54
Insulin growth factors, 55
"Insulin resistance" of pregnancy, 23
Insulin therapy during pregnancy, 24
Intellectual function in SGA infants, 76
Intensities of ultrasound instruments, 81
Intensive care unit, 6-8
  nursery, 291-292
  and reduction of neurologic sequelae, 5, 8
  stimuli in, 343
  stress of staff in, 15-20
Interdigital furrow, 1052
Interface in monitoring equipment, 277
Interferon, 636, 637
Interhemispheric fissure, 83
Intermittent mandatory ventilation, 436-437
  for bronchopulmonary dysplasia, 474
Intermittent negative pressure ventilation, 435-436
Intermittent positive pressure ventilation, 129
  in bronchopulmonary dysplasia, 469
  in respiratory distress syndrome, 435-436

Internal podalic version, 177
Interpupillary distance, 1042-1043
Intersex problems, 925-930
Interventricular septum, 551
  abnormal thickness of, 552
  motion of, 555
Intestinal atresia, 483
Intestinal distension, diagnostic radiology for, 1074-1075
Intestinal duplications
  abdominal masses due to, 532
  rectal bleeding due to, 487
Intestinal motility and drug absorption, 160
Intestinal obstruction, 483-485
  diagnostic radiology for, 1074-1075
  hyperbilirubinemia associated with, 763
Intestine
  aganglionic, 505
  bilirubin reabsorption in, 754
  carbohydrate absorption in, 481
  development of, 480-482
  fat absorption in, 480-481
  immunologic function in, 481-482
  motility of, 481
  protein absorption in, 480
Intraabdominal gas, decreased, 1075-1076
Intraabdominal organs, birth injury to, 232-233
Intracellular volume, 315-316
Intracranial hemorrhage, 121, 372-373
  and alkali administration, 185-186
  as complication of respiratory distress syndrome, 440
  computed tomography for, 1085
  seizures due to, 390
  due to vacuum extraction, 176
Intracranial pressure monitoring, 282, 357
Intragastric infusion, continuous, 309-310
Intrahepatic bile ducts, 774
Intramyometrial injection, 142
Intraocular hemorrhage, 225
Intrapulmonary malformations, 455-456
Intrauterine growth retardation
  antenatal care for, 66-70
  asymmetrical, mode of delivery in, 70
  due to drug exposure, 152
  fetal determinants of, 62-63
  fetal growth and body composition in, 49-54
  fetal metabolism in, 54-55
  follow-up for, 76-78
  low profile and late flattening patterns of, 64
  malformations accompanying, 1014
  maternal contributions to, 55-59
  neonatal problems due to, 72-75
  placental determinants of, 59-62
  associated with preeclampsia, 30
Intrauterine transfusion; see Transfusion, intrauterine
Intrauterine volume measurements, 92
Intravascular clotting cascade, 716
Intravascular gas, diagnostic radiology for, 1075
Intravenous nutrients for low birth weight infant, 312-313
Intravenous pyelogram, 1077
  in abdominal masses, 532
Intropin; see Dopamine
Intubation
  of immature infant, 190
  for localized pulmonary interstitial emphysema, 452
  of moderately depressed infants, 183

Intussusception, 508
  rectal bleeding due to, 487
Inulin clearance, 789, 1108
Inventory process in outreach education, 13
Inversions of chromosomes, 1036
Iodide
  in human milk, 166
  pump, 884
  trapping, defective, 891
Iodine
  compounds containing, in nursery, 295
  associated with congenital malformations, 153
  in contrast media, 1072
  human milk content of, 306
  kinetics of, 889
  protein-bound, 885
  thyroid hormones and, 884
  time in pregnancy to administer, 1027
Iodotyrosines, 891
Ionization of drugs
  influencing concentration in milk, 165
  influencing placental transfer, 151
Ionizing radiation, 538
Iophenoxic acid, 886
IQ
  after cytomegalovirus infection, 700
  effect of protein intake on, 304
  after hydrocephalus, 380, 381
  in microcephaly, 381
Iridodonesis, 999
Iris
  colobomas of, 991
  examination of, 970-971
  pigmentation of, 970-971, 992
Iron
  intrauterine accumulation of, 306
  in methemoglobinemia, 733-734
  neonatal levels and requirements for, 712
  serum values for, 1104
  storage of, 730
  supplementation, 740-741
  teratogenicity of, 156
  trivalent, 738
Iron chelation therapy
  for congenital hypoplastic anemia, 722
  for pancytopenia, 723
Irradiation
  of blood for transfusion, 742, 743
  genetic defects due to, 1026-1027
  whole-body, 748
Irregular breathing patterns, 122
Irritability
  from ergot extracts in human milk, 167
  due to hiatal hernia, 493
  reflex, Apgar scoring of, 182
Irritating eczema, 960
Ischemia
  local, causing subcutaneous fat necrosis, 218
  gastrointestinal, 485
  necrotizing enterocolitis due to, 513
  uterine, 57
Ischemic villous necrosis, 61
Ischemic-hypoxic encephalopathy, 73
Islets of Langerhans, congenital absence of, 55

Isoagglutinins
  in hypogammaglobulinemia, 646
  titer, 643
Isochromosome, 1017
Isoflurane, 174
Isolation
  in impetigo, 946
  of pathogen, 704
Isolation circuits in monitors, 288
Isoleucine, 825
Isomaltase, embryonic activity of, 480
Isomerization of bilirubin, 768
Isoniazid
  dosage for, 1094
  in human milk, 166
  for tuberculosis, 678
Isoproterenol
  altering arterial blood pressure, 128
  for cardiac resuscitation, 582
  for cardiovascular disease, 628
  dosage for, 1092
  for heart failure, 572, 573
  neonatal bradycardia due to, 121
  in premature labor, 144
  pulmonary artery pressure decreased by, 130
Isotopes, use during lactation, 167
Isovaleric acidemia, 829
Isoxsuprine
  for premature labor, 144
  stimulating phospholipid, 412
Isuprel; *see* Isoproterenol
IUD for diabetic woman, 26
Ivemark's syndrome, 747

J

Jaundice, 72
  breast milk, 762-763
  classification of, 753
  effect on quiet awakeness, 338
  exaggerated neonatal, 764
  physiologic, 756-758
  after postnatal hemorrhage, 715
  in Rh incompatibility, 727
Jaw, airway obstruction due to conditions of, 462
Jaw-winking syndrome, 968
Jejunal atresia, 194
Jejunal obstruction, 763
Jejunoileal obstruction, 502-504
Jendrassik and Grof technique, 753
Jet ventilation, high-frequency, 436
Jetane's procedure for cardiac surgery, 587, 588
Jeune's syndrome, 463
  cortical dysplasia in, 796
Jitteriness
  from amphetamines in human milk, 166
  from caffeine in human milk, 167
  characteristics of, 353
Job's syndrome, 632
Jobst garments, 956
Joints
  abnormalities of, 1059
  in sclerema neonatorum, 962
Juxtaductal coarctation, 539, 540

K

K₁ capsular antigen, 642
K1 strain of *Escherichia coli*, 654, 657, 658
Kahn test, 675
Kanamycin, 661
  dosage for, 1093
  for sepsis, 655, 656
  for tuberculosis, 678
Karyotypes
  hermaphroditic, 907
  in robertsonian translocation, 1018
  in testicular disorders, 910-912
  trypsin G-banded, 1020, 1021
Kasabach-Merritt syndrome, 957
Kasai procedure, 775, 781
Kayexalate; *see* Polystyrene sodium sulfonate
Kell blood group, 728
Keloids, 949
Kent's bundle, 578
Keratectasia, 667
Keratinocytes, 939
Keratoconjunctivitis palmoplantaris, 819
Keratopathy, 990
Kerley lines, 1069
Kernicterus, 764-766
  in isoimmune hemolytic disease, 729
Ketoacidosis, 398
  maternal, 24-25
α-Ketoadipic aciduria, 830
α-Ketoisocaproic acid, 825
Ketone bodies during maternal fasting, 54
Ketonuria, 827
17-Ketosteroids, urine values for, 1105
  in female pseudohermaphroditism, 919
β-Ketothiolase deficiency, 827
Kidd blood group, 728
Kidney
  aplastic, 794-795
  bilateral dysplastic, 453
  disease of; *see* Renal disease
  drugs excreted by, plasma half-lives of, 159
  effect of hypoxia on, 192
  end-stage, 787
  fetal blood flow in, 2
  function of, 785-786
  hemorrhage involving, 715
  horseshoe, 810
  immature, reaction to injury, 786-787
  maldevelopment of, 793-797
  microcystic, 800
  multicystic, 794-796
  orientation of, 1078
  radiologic visualization of, 1077
  role in regulation of amniotic fluid, 47
  solitary, 810
  tumors of, 808-810
  ultrasonic identification of, 86
  unilateral multicystic, 531
  vascular disorders of, 806-808
Kinetoarteriography, ultrasound, 283-284
Klebsiella
  bacteriuria due to, 805
  diarrhea due to, 523
  gastroenteritis due to, 662

Klebsiella—cont'd
  in mechanical ventilation, 438
  necrotizing enterocolitis due to, 513
  pneumatoceles due to, 471
  pneumonia due to, 446
  in septic shock, 128
Kleihauer-Betke slide elution technique, 36, 712-713
  to detect Hb F cells, 731
Klein-Waardenburg syndrome, 955
Klinefelter's syndrome, 911-912
  prevalence of, 1036
Klippel-Feil syndrome
  differentiation from sternocleidomastoid injury, 230
  neck appearance in, 1050
Klippel-Weber-Trenaunay syndrome
  limb hypertrophy in, 1051
  skin in, 956, 1040
Klumpke's paralysis, 226, 374
Knee dislocation, 236
  congenital, 1011
Koch-Weeks bacillus, 666
Kolmer test, 675
Koplik's spots, 681
Korotkoff sounds, 126, 283
Kostmann's syndrome, 745
Kupffer cells, 778
Kyphoscoliosis, 959
  in muscle diseases, 397

L

Labia majora
  birth injury to, 237
  hypertrophy of, 922
Labor; *see also* Contractions
  anesthesia for, 174-178
  care of parents during, 242-243
  FHR accelerations during, 99
  FHR decelerations during, 101
  induction of, 25
    contraindications for, 109, 141
    in erythroblastosis fetalis, 42
  position for, after positive oxytocin challenge test, 69
  premature
    clinical evaluation and management of, 141-142
    drug therapy for, 142-146
    effects of, 139
    mechanisms of, 139-141
    pathogenesis of, 141
  stimulating fetal lung development, 417
  variable deceleration prolonged during, 102-103
  who should be monitored during, 113-114
Laboratory tests
  for acid-base disturbances, 325-326
  availability of, 294-295
  for chromosomal abnormalities, 1020-1021
  for congenital malformations, 1060
  for conjugated hyperbilirubinemia, 776
  for cryptococcosis, 685
  for cyanosis, 562-565
  to differentiate heart disease and lung disease, 567
  for intractable diarrhea, 528-529
  for intrauterine growth retardation, 66
  for meningitis, 657-658
  for metabolic disorders, 815-817
  for septicemia, 653-654

Laboratory tests—cont'd
  for unconjugated hyperbilirubinemia, 766
Lacerations
  of ears, 225
  of lid or globe, 975, 976
  sustained at birth, 218
Lacrimal duct blockage, 983
Lacrimal secretion, congenital absence of, 984
Lactase, 479-480
Lactate, in SGA infant, 73
Lactate dehydrogenase, 1104
Lactation
  in diabetic woman, 26
  drug administration during, 168
  drugs affecting, 165-168
Lactic acid, fetal
  anaerobic metabolic production of, 102
  rise in concentration of, 116
Lactic acid dehydrogenase, aqueous humor levels of, 995
Lactic acidosis, 828-829
Lactobacillus, 305
Lactobezoars, 501
Lactoferrin, 642
Lactoperoxidase, 640
Lactose
  in infant formulas, 305
  malabsorption of, 481
    diarrhea due to, 524
Lacy densities in bronchopulmonary dysplasia, 469
Ladd's bands, 502, 503
Lagophthalmos, 224
Lambdoid stenosis, 383
Lamellar bodies in pneumonocytes, 408
  after vagotomy, 413
Lamellar icthyosis, 954
Laminar air flow, 293
Laminectomy
  for dermal sinuses, 388
  exploratory, 232
Langhans chorionic layer, 674
Lanoxin; *see* Digoxin
Lanugo, 939-940
Laparotomy
  for biliary atresia, 779
  for gastrointestinal bleeding, 487
  for intraabdominal trauma, 233
Laplace's law, 409, 410
Large for gestational age infants
  diabetes causing, 854
  percentiles for, 197, 198
  phrenic nerve injury in, 465
Larson's dwarf, 55
Laryngeal obstruction, 462
Laryngeal stenosis, 193
Laryngeal web, 462
  preventing lung expansion, 180
Laryngoscopy, 181, 183
  in cleft palate, 194
  in stridor, 226
Laryngospasm, 462
Lasix; *see* Furosemide
Latex agglutination test, 685
LATS; *see* Long-acting thyroid stimulator
Laurence-Moon-Biedl-Bordet syndrome, 538
  polydactyly in, 1058

Lazy leukocyte syndrome, 746
Lead in human milk, 167
Leber's congenital amaurosis, 1000
Lecithin
  disaturated, 135
  reduced synthesis of, 185
Lecithin: cholesterol acyltransferase, 738
Lecithin/sphingomyelin ratio
  to determine late gestation, 25
  to estimate fetal maturity, 134-136
  patterns of, 135
  to predict respiratory distress syndrome, 110
  in preeclampsia, 31
  in supraventricular tachycardia, 576
Left atrial dimension, 551
Left atrial hypertrophy, 548
Left atrium
  ECG measurements of, 548, 551
  enlargement of, 555
  pressure in, at birth, 179-180
  size of, 552-553
Left axis deviation, 548
Left ventricle
  enlargement of, 555
  hypoplasia of, 588, 589
  in Pompe's disease, 538
  wall thickening of, 555
Left ventricular diastolic dimension, 551
Left ventricular failure, 568
Left ventricular function, 555
Left ventricular hypertrophy, 548
  due to bronchopulmonary dysplasia, 475
Left ventricular pressure, 587
Left-sided heart failure, 130
  in pulmonary hemorrhage, 447
Left-sided heart obstruction, 588-592
Left-to-right shunt
  aortic diastolic pressure drops in, 126
  diagnostic radiology for, 1070
  echocardiography for, 552-553
  in patent ductus arteriosus, 438
  specific types of, 604-609
  after surfactant therapy, 434
Legal issues in neonatal-perinatal medicine, 3
Legs, spastic paresis of, 371
Leiner's syndrome, 644, 960
Leiomyoma, 809
Lens
  dislocated, 999
  in prematurity, 974
Lentigines, 943
Leprechaunism, 63
  role of insulin in, 55
Leptomeningeal cyst, 222
Leptomeningeal melanocytosis, 954
Leroy's syndrome; *see* I cell disease
Lesions
  bone, 701
  bullous, 669
  candidal, 684
  cutaneous
    flat, 950-953
    raised, 953-954
  ephemeral, 942-944
  extraneural, in bilirubin toxicity, 764

Lesions—cont'd
  intestinal obstruction due to, 483
  metabolic, in spherocytosis, 737
  paronychial, 950
  syphilitic, 674
  varicella-zoster, 682
  variola, 683
  venous and arterial blood mixing produced by, 601-604
  viral, 947
Lethargy
  characteristics of, 349
  from diazepam in human milk, 164
Letterer-Siwe disease, 987
Leucine, in maple syrup urine disease, 825
Leucine aminopeptidase, 1104
Leukemia
  myeloid, 745
  postirradiation risk for, 1064
Leukemic transformation, 723
Leukocyte-inhibiting factor, 637
Leukocytes; *see also* White blood cells
  count at birth, 711
  defects in response of, 652
  fetal, 708
Leukocytosis, 653
  in thrombocytopenia, 719
Leukocyturia, 788
  values for, 805
Leukoma, 225
Leukopenia, 653
Levator palpebrae superioris muscle, 981
Levels I, II, and III facilities
  medical policy and administration of, 290-292
  services provided by, 7, 289-292
Levocardia with situs inversus, 614-615
Levocardiogram, 592
Levotransposition; *see* Transposition of great arteries
Lewis blood group, 728
Leydig cells, 901
LGA infant; *see* Large for gestational age infant
Lichenification, 960
Lid retractors, 969, 970
Lidocaine
  for arrhythmias, 576
  for cardiac resuscitation, 582
  for cardiovascular disease, 626
  dosage for, 1095
  during labor, 174
  for ventricular tachycardia, 579
Ligandin
  binding bilirubin, 754
  developmental deficiency of, 757
Lighting
  in hospital units, 292
  in nurseries, 273
Liley's graph of prognostic zones for erythroblastosis fetalis, 36, 38
Limb blanching during umbilical catheterization, 187
Limb defects
  longitudinal, 1004
  prevalence of, 1036
  transverse, 1004
Limb epidermis, 939-941
Linea alba, 942
Linear array scanner, 82
Linoleic acid requirement, 304-305

Linolenic acid, 304
Lipase
  activities of, 516
    embryonic, 480
  deficiency of, 518
  pancreatic, in low birth weight infant, 305
Lipid
  elevated, 315-316
  metabolism of
    diagnostic tests for, 1031
    disorders of, 836-837
  skin surface, 942
Lipid extraction and concentration, 134
Lipid peroxidation, 157
Lipid solubility of drugs
  as factor in placental transfer, 151
  increasing absorption, 160
  influencing concentration in milk, 165
Lipidoses
  complex, 840
  neutral, 839
Lipodystrophy, 63, 837
Lipogranulomatosis, 218
Lipoid adrenal hyperplasia, 921-922
Lipolysis due to cold stress, 260
Lipomas, 388
  in spina bifida, 385, 386, 388
Lipoprotein
  blood, absence of, 525
  matrix of, defects of, 955
  X, 776
Lips, abnormalities of, 1048-1949
Listeria
  hepatitis due to, 781
  pneumonia due to, 446
  seizures due to, 390
  in septic shock, 128
Listeria monocytogenes, 671-672
  meningitis due to, 657
  transplacentally acquired, 650
Listeriosis, 213, 671
Lithium in human milk, 166
Lithium carbonate, 537
Livedo reticularis, 942, 1040
Liver
  biopsy of, 777-778
  central venous pressure and, 540
  conjugation of estriol in, 111
  in cytomegalovirus, 700
  disorders of
    clotting factor decrease due to, 721
    hypocalcemia in, 876
    malabsorption due to, 525
  fatty, 782
  giant hemangioma of, 608-609
  growth of, in SGA infants, 66
  hemorrhagic necrosis of, 188
  in hepatitis, 697
  in hypoxia, 192
  injury to
    in metabolic disorders, 782
    associated with parenteral nutrition, 782
  neuroblastoma metastasized to, 748
  in rubella, 701
  rupture of, 232-233, 715

Liver—cont'd
  size of, in neonatal heart disease, 540, 568
  transplantation of, 781
Liver enzymes, 30
Lloyd's reagent, 137
Loading dose to achieve plasma concentration, 165
Lobectomy
  in lobar emphysema, 454-455
  in localized pulmonary interstitial emphysema, 452-453
Lobes of lung
  in congenital lobar emphysema, 454
  malformation of, 455-456
Local anesthetics
  causing loss of FHR variability, 97
  causing neonatal bradycardia, 121
  toxicity from, 188
Local infiltration analgesia, 175
Local participation in outreach education, 12
Localized malformations
  in abortuses, 1038
  incidence of, 1036
Log of fetal activity, 69
Long-acting thyroid stimulator
  fetal tachycardia due to, 95
  placental transport of, 890
  in thyrotoxicosis, 526, 897-898
Long-term heart rate variability, 121
Loop ridge patterns, 1052, 1054
Loopogram, 509
Loupe, ocular, 969
Low birth weight infant
  apnea in, 456-460
  calorie requirements for, 303
  carbohydrate requirements for, 305
  electrolyte requirements for, 305
  human milk for, 307
  incidence of, 1, 8
  and later disability, risk of, 1
  mineral requirements for, 305-306
  patent ductus arteriosus in, 438
  prognosis for, 398-400
  protein requirements for, 303-304
  and retrolental fibroplasia, 997
  vitamin requirements for, 306-307
Low forceps deliveries, anesthesia for, 176
Lowe's syndrome, 802-803
LSD, 1026
Lugol's solution, 1096
Lumbar epidural block, 174
Lumbar puncture
  in ECHO virus infection, 680
  for tuberculosis, 678
Lung compliance
  dynamic, 426
  retractions indicating, 420
  values for, 426
Lung cysts, 455
Lung expansion
  in heart disease evaluation, 542
  initial, 179
Lung function tests, 448
Lung immaturity, 180
Lung profile, 135-136
Lung volumes
  measurements of, 424-425

Lung volumes—cont'd
  stretch receptors affecting, 457
  in Werdnig-Hoffmann disease, 461
Lungs
  appearance of, in respiratory distress syndrome, 427
  developmental biology of, 404-418
  disorders of, differentiation from heart disease, 566-567
  examination of, 256
  fetal blood flow in, 2
  hypoplastic, 180
  in hypoxia, 192
  liquid- and air-filled, pressure volume characteristics of, 409-410
  perforation of, from chest tubes, 451
  in rubella, 701
Luteinizing hormone
  blood values for, 1105
  fetal pituitary, deficiency of, 912
  testosterone secretion by, 903-904
Lymph, skin supply of, 941-942
Lymph nodes, periductal, enlarged, 782
Lymphangiectasia
  intestinal, 536
  pulmonary, 467
    congenital, 456
Lymphangioma
  cavernous, 958
  cutaneous, 958
  eyelid, 980
Lymphangioma circumscriptum, 958
Lymphatic obstruction, 533
Lymphedema
  hands and feet in, 1052
  primary, 791
  in pulmonary lymphangiectasia, 456
Lymphocytes
  defects of, in reticular dysgenesis, 745
  deficiency of, in SGA infants, 75
  engraftment, 728
  fetal, 708
Lymphocytosis, 679
Lymphokines, 637
Lymphoma, orbital, 987
Lymphopenia, 646
Lymphopoiesis, fetal, 481
Lymphosarcoma, 747
Lymphotoxin, 637
Lyon hypothesis, 735, 1024
Lysine intolerance, 824
Lysis of peritoneal bands, 502
Lysosomal function disorders, 837-842
Lysosomal phospholipase A_2, 140
Lysozyme, 642

M

M hemoglobins, 734
Maceration of skin, 945
Macrocephaly, 1040
Macrocrania, 1084
Macrocytosis
  in congenital hypoplastic anemia, 722
  in isoimmune hemolytic disease, 728
Macroglossia, 462, 1049-1050
  examination for, 256
Macromolecular composition patterns, fetal, 50
Macrophage inhibitory factor, 636, 637

Macrophages
  activated, 636
  alveolar, 472
    fat globules in, 313
  breast milk, 642
  lipid-laden, 841
  splenic, 746
Macrosomia
  and adrenal hemorrhage, 233
  due to diabetes, 94
  risk for, 22
Macrostomia, 1048-1049
Macrotia, 1047
Macula
  abnormal, 1000-1001
  effect of retinal hemorrhage on, 225
  function of, 974
  hypoplasia of, 987
  pigmentation of, 971
Maffucci's syndrome, 958
Magnesium
  deficiency of, 306
  deposition in fetal bone, 50
  intrauterine accumulation of, 306
  physiology of, 879
Magnesium sulfate
  for cardiovascular disease, 627
  dosage for, 1097
  for preeclampsia, 31, 32-33
  for premature labor, 142
Magnet mattress/pad, 123, 124
Magnetometer, 285
Maintenance dosage adjustments, 165
Majewski short rib polydactyly syndrome, 1058
Malabsorption syndromes, 524-525
Malar flush, 821
Malaria, 63, 686-687
  congenital, 703
  frequency of, 697-698
  treatment and prevention of, 706
Male sex, and enhanced birth weight, 62
Malformation complex, definition of, 1035
Malnutrition
  effect on head growth, 379
  immunodeficiency associated with, 648
Malrotation
  of gastrointestinal tract, 502
  of gut, 194
  radiologic diagnosis of, 1074
Maltase, 480
Mammary tissue, drug uptake by, 165
Mandelamine, 111
Mandibular hypoplasia, 462, 1049
Mandibular process, 1042
Mandibulofacial dysostosis, 977
Manipulation of fetus causing subcutaneous fat necrosis, 218
Mannitol
  for cardiovascular disease, 627
  dosage for, 1097
Mannosidosis, 842
Manometry, anorectal, 505, 506
Manual remodeling of nasal fracture, 223
Maple syrup urine disease, 825-827
  maldigestion due to, 523, 527
  and neonatal seizures, 391

Marasmus-kwashiorkor, 75
Marcaine; see Bupivacaine
Marcus Gunn syndrome, 968
  ptosis in, 982
Marfanoid hypermobility syndrome, 1059
Marfan's syndrome
  arachnodactyly in, 1059
  cardiac defects in, 537
  extremity length in, 1051
  inheritance pattern of, 1023
Maroteaux-Lamy syndrome, 990
Masculinization, 915-923
Mastitis, 670
Mastocytosis, 954, 961-962
Maternal contributions to aberrant fetal growth, 55-59
Maternal deprivation, 240
Maternal mortality committees, 4
Maternal plasma determinations, 25
Maternal sensitive period, 243
Mattress to detect body movement, 285
Mauriceau maneuver, 177
  causing facial bone fractures, 223
Maxillary processes, 1042
McCoy cells, 676
McCune-Albright syndrome, 1040
Mean airway pressure, 473
Mean blood pressure, 126
Mean corpuscular hemoglobin concentration, 710-711
Measles, 681, 693
Measurement of program effectiveness, 14-15
Mechanical resonance in pressure monitoring system, 281
Mechanical ventilation
  increasing pulmonary artery pressure, 130
  long-term, 474
  for respiratory distress syndrome, 435-437
Meckel-Gruber syndrome, 63
  polydactyly in, 1058
Meckel's diverticulum, 487
  with diaphragmatic hernia, 488
  with hepatoblastoma, 748
  in intussusception, 508
Meckel's syndrome, 795-796
Meconium
  in amniotic fluid, 70
    effect on L/S ratio, 135
  bilirubin in, 757
  calcifications due to, 1076
  delayed passage of, 483
  monitoring fetuses who pass, 113-114
  suctioning of, in delivery room, 184
Meconium aspiration syndrome, 73, 443-445, 467
  arterial carbon dioxide pressure in, 423
Meconium ileus, 483
  due to cystic fibrosis, 518
  perforation due to, 485
  radiologic appearance of, 1074
  ultrasonic detection of, 86
Meconium peritonitis, 533
Meconium plug syndrome, 507-508, 1075
  seen in contrast study, 484
Mediastinal masses, 455
  airway obstruction due to, 462
Mediastinal shift
  in air leak syndromes, 450
  in atelectasis after extubation, 439

Mediastinal shift—cont'd
  in diaphragmatic hernia, 488
Medical policy and administration in nurseries, 290, 291, 292
Mediterranean background predisposition to β-thalassemia, 733
Medroxyprogesterone, 139
Medullary ductal ectasia, 797
Medullated nerve fibers, 1001
Megacolon, congenital aganglionic, 504-507
Megakaryocytes, hypoplasia of, 719
Megalencephaly, 379
Megalocornea, 988
Megalophthalmos, 988
Megavitamin therapy, 816
Meglucamine diatrizoate, 507, 508, 521
Meiosis, disorders of, 1016-1018
Meissner's plexus, 481
  in Hirschsprung's disease, 505
Meissner's tactile organs, 942
Melanin, 939
Melanocytes, 939
Melanocytosis, leptomeningeal, 954
Melanosis, transient neonatal pustular, 943-944
Melanosomes, giant, 952
Melena, 663
  due to decreased platelets, 718
Membrane pressure, 282
Mendelian inheritance
  disorders of, 1023-1025
  malformations of, 1036
Mendosal structures mistaken for fractures, 221
Meningitis
  associated with cephalhematoma, 220
  neonatal bacterial, 656-658
  seizures due to, 390
Meningocele, 385
  cranial, 219
  orbital, 987
Meningoencephalitis, 670
Meningoencephalocele, 89
Meningomyelocele, 385, 386-388
  ultrasonic detection of, 89
Menke's syndrome, 63
Menstrual history, 133
Mental retardation due to phenylketonuria, 1037
Menthol for glucuronide conjugation testing, 762
Meperidine
  dosage for, 1097
  during labor, 174
Mepivacaine, 391
Meprobamate in human milk, 166
Mercurochrome, to promote epithelialization, 530
Mercury in human milk, 167
Merkel-Ranvier corpuscles, 942
Mesangial sclerosis, 800
  in nephrotic syndrome, 800
Mesenteric cysts, 532
Metabisulfite test for sickling, 733
Metabolic acidosis, 322
  fetal
    during late deceleration, 104
    during variable deceleration, 102
  late, 324-325
  after massive bowel resection, 528
  neonatal
    due to prolonged exposure, 181

Metabolic acidosis—cont'd
  neonatal—cont'd
    due to prolonged heat production, 260
    associated with protein intake, 304
    and respiratory distress syndrome, 433
    treatment of, 326
Metabolic alkalosis, 322-323
  due to hypertrophic pyloric stenosis, 499
  treatment of, 326
Metabolic disorders, 73-74
  acute, 398
  calcium, 870-879
  carbohydrate, 845-867
  associated with diminished birth weight, 63
  in infants of addicted mothers, 933-937
  liver injury in, 782
  magnesium, 879-881
  prenatal diagnosis of, 1031
  due to total parenteral nutrition, 311, 312
Metabolic rate, monitoring of, 269
Metabolism
  aerobic, 115
  amino acid, errors of, 1036
  drug, in newborn, 161-163
  fetal, 54-55
  inborn errors of; see Inborn errors of metabolism
  intrapartum, unstable, 23-24
  maternal, adjustments in, 54
  oxidative
    in Chédiak-Higashi syndrome, 747
    in neutrophils, 745
  placental, alteration of, 61
Metabolites, active, 157
Metaphyseal abnormalities, 1081
Metaphyseal dysostosis, 518
Metatarsus varus, 1012
Methadone
  addiction to, 935-936
  dosage for, 1097
  in human milk, 167
  and intrauterine growth retardation, 58
  and neonatal seizures, 391
  withdrawal from, 935-936
    maldigestion due to, 523
Methemoglobin reductase, NADH-dependent, 711
Methemoglobinemia, 733-734
  diagnostic tests for, 560
  maternal, causing fetal asphyxia, 180
Methenamine silver stains, 687
Methicillin, 661
  dosage for, 1093
  for sepsis, 655, 656
Methimazole
  dosage for, 1096
  in human milk, 166
  neutropenia induced by, 744
Methionine, 304
Methisazone, 683
Methotrexate, 58
Methoxamine, 626
β-Methyl crotonylglycinuria, 829-830
Methylation pathway, 414, 415
  caffeine produced via, 163
Methylcellulose
  for alacrima, 984

Methylcellulose—cont'd
  for facial nerve palsy, 223
Methyldopa
  for cardiovascular disease, 626
  for hypertension, 32, 619
Methylene blue
  dosage for, 1095
  esophageal introduction of, 498
  for methemoglobinemia, 560, 734
3-OH,3-Methylglutaric aciduria, 830
Methylmalonic acid, 827
Methylmalonic acidemia
  and neonatal seizures, 391
Methylmercury
  embryogenetic effects of, 1026
  in human milk, 167
  poisoning from, 156
Methylxanthines, 163
Metopic suture, 383
Metronidazole in human milk, 166
Miconazole
  for cutaneous candidiasis, 950
  dosage for, 1094
Micrencephaly, 1084
Micro–blood gas analysis, 114
Micro-blood sampling, 116
Microcephaly, 63, 76, 381-382, 1040
  due to cytomegalovirus, 700
  hair pattern in, 1040
  associated with hydramnios, 193
  ultrasonic detection of, 89
Microcolon, 483-484, 503, 504
  radiologic appearance of, 1074-1075
Microcytosis, 712
MicroESR, normal percentile values for, 1112
Micrognathia, 256, 1048
  in Pierre Robin syndrome, 463
Micromelia, 465
Micropenis, 924-925
Microphthalmia, 987, 1043
  colobomatous, 987
  complicated, 987
  simulating true anophthalmia, 982
Micropolygyria, 377
Microspherocytes, 728, 729
Microstomia, 1048
Microtia, 1047
Microviscometry, 136
Micturition
  disorders of, 789-790, 798
  neonatal bradycardia stimulating, 121
Midbrain, ultrasonic detection of, 82
Midforceps deliveries, anesthesia for, 176
Midwives, 4, 242-243
Mikulicz enterostomy, 504
Mild preeclampsia, 27
Milia, 942
Miliaria, 944
Miliary disease, 677, 678
Miliary hemangiomatosis, 957-958
Milk
  allergy to, 526
  comparison of kinds of, and protein requirements, 304
  cow's
    fat in, 305

Milk—cont'd
  cow's—cont'd
    hypocalcemia due to, 875-876
    protein content of, 304
  daily intake of, 165
  donor, 307
  glutathione peroxidase levels in, 739
  human
    bacteriostatic effect of, 652
    compounds in, 166-167
    environmental pollutants in, 167-168
    immunologic properties of, 640-642
    jaundice due to, 762-763
    for low birth weight infant, 307
    mineral content of, 306
    for necrotizing enterocolitis, 516
    nontherapeutic agents in, 167
    passage of exogenous compounds from maternal blood to, 165
    protein content of, 304, 307
  in hypocalcemia, 871
  net acid in, 321
Milroy's disease, 791
Mima polymorpha, 651
β-Mimetic drugs, 143-146
Minamata disease, 156, 167
Mineral oil, 510, 512
Mineralocorticoid replacement therapy, 920
Minerals, low birth weight infant requirement for, 305-306
Minimal brain dysfunction, 765
"Mini-residency," 11
Minute volume, 456
  in bronchopulmonary dysplasia, 471
Miosis, 968
  in Horner's syndrome, 224
Mirror bands, 1008
Mitogenic factor, 637
Mitosis, disorders of, 1016
Mitral valve
  atresia of, 588
  ECG examination of, 549-550, 551
  motion of, 555
Mittendorf dot, 998
Mixed gonadal dysgenesis, 910
M-mode echocardiography, 548
Mobitz block, 580
Möbius syndrome, 63, 222, 374
  airway obstruction in, 462
  eyes in, 977
Molars, mineralization of, 1084
Molecular sieving, 447
Molecular weight of drugs
  and absorption, 160
  and concentration in milk, 165
  and placental transfer, 151
Mongolian spots, 942-943
  racial predilection of, 1039
Mongolism; see Down's syndrome; Trisomy 21
Mongoloid slant, 1043
  chromosomal abnormalities characterized by, 978
Moniliasis, oral, 669, 684
Monitoring
  after cardiac surgery, 624-625
  chemical, during total parenteral nutrition, 311
  electrophysiologic fetal
    antepartum, 107-108

Monitoring—cont'd
  electrophysiologic fetal—cont'd
    intrapartum, 112-115
  in heart failure, 571
  of incubators, 268-269
  nonstress fetal, 108
  therapeutic, in neonatal drug therapy, 164-165
Monochorionic placentation, 214
Monochorionic twins, 46
Monocytes, 744
Monoglucuronide, bilirubin, 755
Monoiodotyrosine, 884
Mononucleosis, infectious, 682
Monosaccharides
  malabsorption of, 523, 524
    transient, 525
  metabolic disorders of, 830-831
Monosomy, 1015-1016
Monotropy, 247
Monozygosity, 213-214
Morbidity
  differences according to geographic area, 5
  neonatal, patterns of, 199
Morgagni's foramen
  herniation through, 489
  infection in, 510
Moro reflex, 353
  asymmetric, 256
  after fracture of clavicle, 226
  in humeral fractures, 235
  in lower extremity dislocations, 236
Morphine
  for cardiovascular disease, 627
  dosage for, 1097
  for heart failure, 572, 573
  in human milk, 167
Morquio's syndrome, 990
Mortality
  fetal
    division of, by weight groups, 9-10
    due to maternal ketoacidosis, 24
  maternal
    analysis of, 10
    in preeclampsia, 30
  neonatal, 198-199
    division of, by weight groups, 9-10
    as indication of regional conditions, 10
    from prematurity, 139, 260
    due to septicemia, 650
    statistics for, in United States, 8, 398
  perinatal
    for baseline preprogram measurements, 14
    in breech presentations, 176
    factors associated with, 5
    in preeclampsia, 30
    reduction in, 8-9
  viral and parasitic agents associated with, 693
Mosaicism, 1016
  fetal diagnosis of, 1030
  in trisomies, 1020
  in Turner's syndrome, 909
Mosquito clamps, 451
Mother
  care of
    after birth, 243-247

Mother—cont'd
  care of—cont'd
    during labor, 242-243
    practical considerations in, 247-249
    before pregnancy, 241
    during pregnancy, 241-242
  drug consumption by, effect on fetus, 150
  of premature or sick neonate, 249-251
Mother-infant contact, 245-247
Motilin, 522
Motion in radiologic examination, 1064
Motor behavior
  fetal, 340
  in preterm infant, 341-342
Motor system, assessment of, 349-353
Mouth
  airway obstruction due to conditions of, 462
  congenital malformations of, 1048-1050
Movement
  assessment of, 353
  conjugate eye, 354
  ocular, 972
"Movements alarm signal," 108
Moxalactam, 661
  dosage for, 1093
  for meningitis, 658
  for sepsis, 655
Mucociliary function, in bronchopulmonary dysplasia, 472-473
Mucolipidoses, 841, 842
  palate and tongue in, 1049-1050
Mucopolysaccharidoses, 839
  corneal effects of, 990
  diagnostic tests for, 1031
  hernias associated with, 1050-1051
  palate and tongue in, 1049-1050
Mucosal biopsy, 484
"Mucosal choke," 492
Mucous membranes
  in ectodermal dysplasia, 964
  infections of, 669-670
  verroucous nevi in, 959
Mucus
  in cystic fibrosis, 518
  in intestine, 507
Mulberry molars, 676
Müllerian ducts
  aplasia of, 925
  development of, 901-902
  persistent, 912
Müllerian-inhibiting factor, 903
Multicore myopathy, 397
Multidisciplinary orientation of outreach education, 12
Multifactorial defects, 1025-1026
Multifactorial inheritance, 1036
Multifocal tissue ischemia, 364
Multiple gestation; see also Twins
  effect on fetal growth, 56
  identifying placentas in, 85
  and placental disorders, 61-62, 213-215
  associated with polyhydramnios, 46
Multiple malformations
  evaluation of neonate with, 1014-1015
  incidence of, 1036
Multiple sutures, 383
Multiplication-stimulating action factor, 55

Mumps, 681-682, 693
  endocardial fibroelastosis due to, 610
Mural thrombosis, 209
Murmurs, cardiac
  diagnosis of, 542
  in d-transposition, 584
  parasystolic, 588
  in respiratory distress syndrome, 429
  systolic, 589, 590, 592, 604, 605
Murphy drip, 300
Murphy-Pattee test, 886
Muscle biopsy, 398
Muscle fiber, congenital disproportion of, 397
Muscle fibrillation potentials, 223
Muscle tone
  Apgar scoring of, 182
  examination of, 351
  in preterm infant, 341
Muscles
  abdominal, absence of, 798-799
  depressor, of mouth, 222
  diseases of, 396-398
  external ocular, injuries to, 224
  involved in brachial palsy, 227
  percent of fetal weight, 50
  sternocleidomastoid, 230
Muscular dystrophies, 396-397
Musculoskeletal malformations, 1004-1008
Mustard procedure for cardiac surgery, 587, 588
Myasthenia gravis, 395-396
  congenital, 180
  respiratory distress caused by, 461-462
Mycobacterium tuberculosis, 677
Mycocel agar, 950
Mycocel slants, 685
Mycoplasma fermentans, 651
Mycoplasma hominis, 651
Myelination, 347
Myelitis, transverse, 231
Myelodysplasia
  cervical, 230
  differentiation from spinal injury, 231
Myelography, 373
Myelomeningocele, 400
Myeloperoxidase, 633
Myelopoiesis, 744
Myeloschisis, 385, 386-388
Myocardial disorders, 609-613
Myocardial glycogen reserves, 73
Myocardial infarction, 548
Myocarditis, 609-610
  in cardiogenic shock, 574
  gallop rhythm in, 568
Myoclonic movement, 389
Myositis, 230
Myotonic dystrophy, 396
  respiratory distress caused by, 462
Myringotomy, 665
Myxovirus infections, 681-682

N

NADH-reductase, 734
Nafcillin, 661
  dosage for, 1093
  for sepsis, 655, 656

Nails
  defects of, syndromes associated with, 940-941
  verroucous nevi affecting, 959
Nalline; *see* Nalorphine
Nalorphine, 627
Naloxone
  dosage for, 1095
  for resuscitation, 188
Naphthalene, 759
Naproxen, 143
Narcotics
  dosages for, 1097
  effect on primary hyperpnea and apnea, 181
  in human milk, 167
  during labor, 175
  loss of FHR variability due to, 97
Nasal bridge, 1043
Nasal placodes, 1041
Nasal prongs for continuous positive airway pressure, 434-435
Nasogastric infusion, 309
  radiologic monitoring of, 1086
Nasojejunal feeding, 300-309
Nasolabial fold, 222
Nasolacrimal duct, 1042
Nasopharyngeal intubation, 435
Navajo Indians, persistence of NADH-dependent diaphorase deficiency in, 733
Nebulizers, 298
Neck
  birth injuries to, 226-230
  congenital malformations of, 1050
  examination of, 256
Necropsy, after umbilical catheterization, 188
Necrotizing enterocolitis, 512-516, 664
  in disseminated intravascular coagulation, 720
  associated with high rate of fluid administration, 318
  neutropenia associated with, 744
  pneumatosis intestinalis due to, 1075
  related to birth weight and gestational age, 202-203
  in respiratory distress syndrome, 432
Needle biopsy for kidney, 788
Neisseria catarrhalis, 664
Neisseria gonorrhoeae, 673-674
  conjunctivitis due to, 983
Neisseria meningitidis, 651, 654
Nemaline myopathy, 397
Neomycin, 661
  for sepsis, 655
Neonatal heart rate; *see* Heart rate, neonatal
Neonatal heart rate monitoring, 119-122
Neonatal monitoring
  biochemical engineering aspects of
    cardiac, 277-280
    future of, 288
    pressure, 280-284
    respiratory, 284-286
    safety considerations, 286-288
  equipment for, 294
Neonatal period, 1
Neonatal problems
  asphyxia, 72-73
  hyperviscosity-polycythemia syndrome, 75
  of metabolism, 73-74
  temperature regulation, 74-75

Neonatal-perinatal medicine
  concepts of, 1-3
  ethical and legal issues in, 3
Neonates
  of addicted mothers, 933-937
  care of
    along with mother and father, 246-251
    charting, 300
    feeding, 298-300
    in hospital units, 292-298
    in intensive care unit, 292
    in maternal gonococcal infection, 674
    at night, compared with during day, 18
    in normal newborn nursery, 289-290
    skin, 300
    in transitional care nursery, 290-291
    in transport unit, 292
  classification of, by birth weight and gestational age, 196-198
  drug use, disposition, and metabolism in, 158-164
  floppy, 393
    with hypotonia and weakness, 394-396
    with muscle disease, 396-398
  immature, delivery room procedures for, 190
  with multiple malformations, 1014-1015
  too hot, 271-272
Neostigmine
  to diagnose myasthenia gravis, 462
  dosage for, 1095
  to increase vagal tone, 576
Neo-Synephrine; see Phenylephrine
Neovascularization, retinal, 996
Nephrectomy
  for hypertension, 619
  for renal artery thrombosis, 807
  for tumors, 810
Nephritis, 799-800
  maternal, 57
Nephroblastomatosis, 809
Nephrocalcinosis, 804
Nephrogenic diabetes insipidus, 803
Nephrogram, 1077-1078
Nephrolithiasis, 647
Nephroma, congenital mesoblastic, 747, 808
Nephrons
  urine concentration by, 785
  variability of, 786
Nephrosialidosis, 842
Nephrotic syndrome, 800-801
Nerve; see also specific nerves
  cutaneous, 942
  laryngeal, 226
  root, avulsion of, 228
Nerve fibers, medullated, 1001
Nerve growth factor, 55
Nesidioblastosis, 55
Neural crest tumors, 523, 525
Neural tube defects, 1051
  in abortuses, 1037
  alpha-fetoprotein diagnosis of, 1033
Neuraminidase deficiency, 1001
Neuraxis, defects in closure of, 385-388
Neuroblastoma, 618, 747-748
  abdominal masses due to, 532
  as calcification, 1076-1077
  conjugated hyperbilirubinemia due to, 782

Neuroblastoma—cont'd
  differentiation from adrenal hemorrhage, 235
  orbital, 986
Neurocirculatory control, 119
Neurodevelopment in SGA infants, 76, 77
Neurofibromatosis
  eyelid involvement in, 980-981
  limb hypertrophy in, 1051
  orbital defects due to, 987
Neurogenic bladder, 799
Neurohumoral regulation of surfactant secretion, 412-413
Neurologic assessment
  of gestational age, 257-288
  neonatal, 347-356
  of SGA infant, 72
Neurologic impairment due to maternal alcohol ingestion, 153
Neurologic sequelae, reduction of, 5, 8
Neuroma, plexiform, 987
Neuromuscular blockade
  during mechanical ventilation, 437
  placental transmission of, causing myasthenia gravis, 461
Neuromuscular disease and respiratory distress, 461-462
Neuronal necrosis, in bilirubin encephalopathy, 764
Neurons, seizure activity of, 389
Neuropathy, peripheral, 395
Neuroplasty, 223
Neuropraxis lesion, 228
Neurosyphilis, 676
Neutral thermal environment, 262
Neutropenia, 645, 744-745
  cyclic, 745
  after multiple exchange transfusions, 730
  in Schwachman's syndrome, 518
  tests for, 643
Neutrophils, kinetics of, 744
Nevocellular nevi, 952-953
Nevus
  blue, 954
  compound, 954
  giant hairy, 953-954
  intraabdominal, 954
  nevocellular, 952
  strawberry, 956-957
Nevus achromicus, 955
Nevus anemicus, 955
Nevus flammeus, 956, 977
Nevus unius lateris, 958
Nezelof syndrome, 648
Nicotinamide, 158
Nicotinamide adenosine dinucleotide phosphate oxidase, 633
Nicotine in human milk, 167
Niemann-Pick disease, 841
  cherry-red macula in, 1001
  hyperbilirubinemia associated with, 782
Nipple sign, 499
Nisentil; see Alphaprodine
Nissen fundiplication, 495
Nitrates, maldigestion due to, 523, 524
Nitrites, methemoglobinemia precipitated by, 733
Nitroblue tetrazolium dye reduction test, 643
Nitrofurantoin, 661
Nitrogen
  balance
    in preeclampsia, 30
    after total parenteral nutrition, 310

Nitrogen—cont'd
  intrauterine accumulation of, 306
Nitrogen washout technique, 471
Nitroprusside, 1095
Nitrous oxide–oxygen inhalation analgesia, 174
No reflow phenomenon, 364
Noise
  in incubators, 272-273
  in nursery, 293
Nonbreathing periods, 126
Nonbullous congenital icthyosiform erythroderma, 945
Nondisjunction, 1015-1017
Noninvasive diagnostic tools, 356-357
Nonketotic hyperglycinemia, 391
Nonlipid solubility of drug, 160
Nonreactive nonstress test, 108
Non-REM sleep, 122; see also Quiet sleep
Nonscarring dermal lesions, 948-949
Nonstress fetal monitoring, 108
Nonstress testing
  to determine acceleration of fetal heart rate, 69
  fetal reactivity measured by, 99
Nonsurfactant tests, 137-138
Nonvertex presentation, 113
Noonan's syndrome
  congenital heart disease in, 537
  hairline in, 1040
  hands and feet in, 1052
  neck and chest in, 1050
  polydactyly in, 1058
Norepinephrine
  increasing pulmonary artery pressure, 130
  release of, due to cold stress, 260
Norrie's disease, 998
Northern Europeans
  PK deficiency in, 736
  spherocytosis in, 737
Nose
  airway obstruction due to conditions of, 462
  congenital malformations of, 1048
  fracture of, 223
Nova Scotia Fetal Risk Project, 8
Novobiocin, 764
Novocain; see Procaine
Nuclear agenesis, 222
Nuclear aplasia, 977
5'-Nucleotidase test, 312
Numeric chromosomal abnormalities, 1015-1017
Nursery
  intensive care, 291-292
    keeping baby warm in, 266-271
  normal newborn, 289-290
  physical examination in, 256-259
  transitional care, 290-291
Nursery services, 4-20
Nurses
  effects of stress on, in ICU, 16
  on nursery staff, 289, 290, 291
Nursing services, perinatal, 8
Nutramigen, 832
Nutrient delivery for low birth weight infant
  continuous transpyloric or intragastric infusions, 309-310
  intravenous
    by peripheral vein, 312-313
    supplementing oral feedings, 313

Nutrient delivery for low birth weight infant—cont'd
  total parenteral nutrition, 310-312
Nutrient flow
  monitoring of, 113
  reduction in, metabolic acidosis due to, 115-116
Nutrients
  and intestinal adaptation, 527
  intrauterine accumulation of, 306
  placental transport of, 846
  recommended intake of, for low birth weight infant, 303
Nutrition
  in chronic pulmonary disease, 474
  in chronic renal insufficiency, 792-793
  effect on central nervous system, 302
  for low birth weight infant, 302-307
  methods of delivery for, 308-313
  maternal, 54, 56-57
  in respiratory distress syndrome, 432-433
Nutritionist as part of health care team, 24
Nystagmus
  fundal rhythm in, 971
  jerky, 389
  opticokinetic, 354, 974, 975
  pendular, 994
  rotational, 973, 974
Nystatin
  for cutaneous candidiasis, 950
  dosage for, 1094
  for moniliasis, 684
  for sepsis, 655

O

O type blood, 726
Oasthouse urine disease, 523, 527
Obesity, maternal, 56
Oblique discs, 1002
Obstetric trauma causing subcutaneous fat necrosis, 218
Obstipation, 512
  in inspissated milk syndrome, 508
Occipital meningocele, 90
Occiput posterior position, 114
Ochoa syndrome, 799
OCT; see Oxytocin challenge test
Ocular compression, 121
Ocular examination sequence, 967
Ocular findings, normal, 972-975
Ocular injuries, 975-976
Ocular measurements, 972
Ocular movement during seizures, 389
Oculoauricular dysplasia, 977
Oculocerebrorenal dystrophy, 802-803
Oculodentodigital syndrome, 1040
Oculoencephalography, 975
Oculomandibulofacial dyscephaly, 977
Oculomotor nerve
  examination of, 354-355
  palsy, 224
Oculovestibular response, 191
Oil retention enema, 512
Olfactory nerve examination, 353
Oligohematuria, 806
Oligohydramnios, 47-48
  pulmonary hypoplasia associated with, 453-454
Oligonephronic hypoplasia, 794-795
Oliguria, 789-790

Oliguria—cont'd
  in cortical and medullary necrosis, 808
  in preeclampsia, 28
Olive (pyloric mass), 499
Omphalitis, 665
Omphalocele, 1050
  bronchopulmonary dysplasia developing after repair of, 469
  and gastroschisis, comparison of, 530
  ultrasonic detection of, 88, 89
Opacification
  of left side of heart, 603
  left ventricular, 607
  renal parenchymal, 1077
  total body, 1077
  in urography, 787
Opacity
  corneal, 945
  of lens, 992, 993
  retinal, 997
  in vitreous, 994
Open field sole pattern, 1052
Ophthalmic consultation, 975
Ophthalmitis, 665-667
  due to *Neisseria gonorrhoeae*, 673
Ophthalmoscopy, 971
  for white pupil 992
Opisthotonos, 390
  in tetanus, 677
Opsonization, 634, 635
  of group B streptococci, 672
Optic atrophy, 225
  congenital, 1002
  in craniosynostosis, 383
Optic disc
  abnormalities of, 1001-1002
  blue-white, 225
  pallor of, 354
Optic nerve
  birth injuries to, 224-225
  examination of, 353-354, 971
  hypoplasia of, 1002
Optic pit, 1002
Optical density
  of amniotic fluid, 136-137
  change in, in erythroblastosis fetalis, 110
Optical density technique, 758
Optimum use of facilities and personnel, 6
Optokinetics, 972
Oral contraceptives
  problems with, in diabetes, 26
  use during lactation, 166-167
Oral movements, 336-337
Orbits
  abnormal, 984-985
  examination of, 969
  injury to, 224
  tumors of, 985-987
Orchiopexy, 925
Orciprenaline, 146
Organ culture techniques, 158
Organ maturity in SGA infant, 72
Organ weights, deviation of, following intrauterine growth retardation, 65
Organization of perinatal health services, 4-11
Orgasm, correlation with premature labor, 141

Oriental population
  abnormal G6PD enzymes in, 735
  congenital malformation frequency in, 1039
  HB_sAg and HB_eAg carriage in, 695
  head shape in, 1041
  palatine torus in, 1049
  physiologic jaundice in, 758
  Rh incompatibility in, 727
  thalassemia in, 732
Ornithine carbamyltransferase deficiency, 824
Orofaciodigital syndrome, 1050
Oropharyngeal airway, plastic, 181
Oropharyngeal suctioning, 70
Orthopedic problems, 1004-1012
Ortolani's maneuver, 1010
Oscillation, high-frequency, 436
Oscillatory breathing, 122
Oscillometry, 126
Oscilloscope
  for cardiac monitor, 279
  for combined functions, 285
Osmiophilic lamellar bodies, 408
Osmotic fragility, 737
Ossification, delay in, 1084
Osteochondritis, 674
Osteogenesis imperfecta, 63, 194, 463, 465
  renal artery rupture in, 537
  scleral color in, 991
  wormian bones in, 1084
Osteomyelitis, 667-668
  radiologic diagnosis of, 1081
Osteopetrosis
  anemia due to, 723
  head shape in, 1041
O'Sullivan-Mahan criteria for diabetes in pregnancy, 23
Otitis media, 664-665
  tuberculous, 678
Otorrhea, cerebrospinal fluid, 221
Ouabain, 620
Outreach education, perinatal
  classic approaches, 11-12
  comprehensive program components of, 13-14
  evaluation of, 14-15
  principles of, 12-13
  rationale of, 11
  responsibility of regional center for, 7, 8
Ovarian cysts, 532
Ovaries, differentiation of, 900
Overdrive pacing, 578
Overshoot in pressure monitoring, 281
Ovotestis, 907-908
Ovum, blighted, 82
Oxacillin, 661
  dosage for, 1093
  for sepsis, 655, 656
Oxidase, membrane-bound, 746
Oxidation, bilirubin reactions of, 768
Oxidation-reduction reaction in electrodes, 278
Oxidizable substrates in ovine fetus, 54
Oximeter, fiberoptic, 430
Oxycephaly, 976
Oxygen
  availability of, in hospital units, 293
  100% breathing of, in causes of cyanosis, 562, 564
  humidification of, 298

Oxygen—cont'd
  ventilatory response to, 457
Oxygen consumption
  and caloric intake, relationship of, 75
  change in, in incubator, 269-270
  fetal, 54
  in quiet sleep state, 330
  in SGA infants, 75
Oxygen delivery, reduced, 539
Oxygen dissociation curve, 422, 561
  fetal, 711
Oxygen radical, 472
Oxygen saturation
  arterial, at birth, 179
  environmental, effect on fetal growth, 58
Oxygen tension
  arterial, 422-423
    constricting ductus arteriosus at birth, 180
    in d-transposition, 586
    during grunting, 420
    in meconium aspiration syndrome, 445
    and retrolental fibroplasia, 997
    sampling for, 430
    sleep state comparison of, 458-459
    ventilator effects on, 436
    ventilatory response affected by, 456-457
  fetal
    decline in, during variable deceleration, 102
    in hypoxia, 108
  and hepatic oxidation, 164
  skin electrodes to measure, 430
  transcutaneous measurement of, 118, 297, 430-432
Oxygen therapy
  in heart failure, 571
  in nursery, 296-298
  retrolental fibroplasia due to, 995-996
Oxygen toxicity
  etiology of, 472-473
  due to respiratory distress syndrome, 440-441
Oxygen transport
  Hb F affecting, 731
  reduced, during deceleration, 103-104
Oxygenation
  extracorporeal membrane, 437
  for diaphragmatic hernia, 489
Oxygen-carrying capacity after treatment of anemia, 571
Oxyhemoglobin, 320
Oxymetholone, 723
Oxytocin
  elevating baseline intrauterine pressure, 114
  fetal, 140
  maternal, 140
  secretion of, from nipple stimulation, 244
  to simulate stress of labor, 107
  stimulating fetal lung development, 417
Oxytocin challenge test
  in antepartum fetal assessment, 108-109
  to detect erythroblastosis fetalis, 36
  to predict fetal demise, 69
Oxytocin induction in preeclampsia, 32
Oxytocinase, 66

P

P wave
  axis of, 546

P wave—cont'd
  in heart failure, 568
  in supraventricular tachycardia, 577
  in ventricular septal defect, 606
Pacemaker
  for atrioventricular block, 581-582
  for sinoatrial node disorders, 580
Pacing
  overdrive, 578, 621
  transvenous, 574
PaCO$_2$; *see* Carbon dioxide tension, arterial
Pain
  decreased sensation to, 495
  effect on sleep states, 334
  testing response to, 353
Paired contractions, 114-115
Palate, examination of, 256
Palatine triangle, anterior, 1042
Palmar grasp, 353
Palmar patterns, 1052
Palmar pulse, 539
Palpation
  abdominal, 791
  for neonatal arterial blood pressure, 126
Palpebral fissures, 1043-1047
Pancreas
  agenesis of, 63
  aplasia of, 55
  disorders of, 516-521
    malabsorption due to, 525
    drugs for, 1096
Pancreatectomy, 866
Pancreatic α-cells, 847
Pancreatic insufficiency and bone marrow dysfunction, 518
Pancreatin, 521
Pancrepilase, 521
Pancuronium bromide
  altering arterial blood pressure, 127
  for cardiovascular disease, 627
  dosage for, 1097
  neonatal tachycardia due to, 121
Pancytopenia, constitutional, 723
Panhypopituitary fetus, 55
Panniculitis
  cold, 962
  nodular nonsuppurative, 218
PaO$_2$; *see* Oxygen tension, arterial
Papanicolaou smear, 704
Papillary muscle infarction, 574
Para-aminohippurate clearance, 163
Para-aminohippuric acid, 44
Para-aminosalicylic acid, 678
Paracentesis
  for ascites, 533
  for intraabdominal trauma, 233
Paracentric inversion, 1017
Paracervical block, 174
  prolonging FHR decelerations, 104
Paradoxical breathing, 122
Paraldehyde
  dosage for, 1094
  for seizures, 392
Paralysis
  orbicular muscle, 222
  phrenic nerve, 228-230

Paralysis—cont'd
  in poliomyelitis, 681
  vocal cord, 225-226
Paramedics in nurseries, 289, 291, 292
Paraneoplastic syndrome, 879
Paraplegia following spinal injury, 231
Paraplegia-in-flexion, 231, 232
Parasitemia, 686
Parasympathetic control of heart rate, 121
Parasympathetic drugs, 97
Parathyroid hormone, 871-872
Paregoric, 538
Parenchyma
  pulmonary
    agenesis of, 453
    disease of, 130
    opacification of, 469
    proline in development of, 454
  renal
    disease of, 787
    hypoplasia of, 794
Parents
  genetic counseling for, 1015, 1021-1023, 1024-1025, 1027-1028, 1033
  of infant with cardiovascular disease, 623
  of infant with chronic pulmonary disease, 475
  of infant in intensive care, 300-301
Parietal foramina mistaken for fractures, 221
Paronychia, 669
  lesions of, 950
Parotitis, 670
Partial thromboplastin time, 721
  in anemia, 716
  in disseminated intravascular coagulation, 720
  test values for, 1113
Parvoviruses, 698
Pasteurella multocida, 651
Patau's syndrome, 978
Patch angioplasty, 592
Patella, congenital dislocation of, 1011
Patent ductus arteriosus, 121, 604-605
  in high rate of fluid administration, 318
  persistent, incidence of, 201
  postductal coarctation of aorta with, 591-592
  related to birth weight and gestational age, 200
  relationship between fluid therapy, bronchopulmonary dysplasia, and, 473
  with respiratory distress syndrome, 432, 438
  right atrial pressure in, 129
  thrill in, 541
  with ventricular septal defect, 607
Pathologic conditions, effect on arousal state, 331
Patient movement, minimal, 5-6
Patient outcome, measurement of change in, 15
Patient protection in radiology, 1064
Pavulon; *see* Pancuronium bromide
P_{CO_2}; *see* Carbon dioxide tension
Peak inspiratory pressure, 436
  bronchopulmonary dysplasia due to, 473
Pectus carinatum, 256
  sternum in, 1050
Pectus excavatum, 256
  sternum in, 1050
Pedigree
  formation of, 1039

Pedigree—cont'd
  in multiple malformations, 1014
Pelvis, diagnostic radiology for, 1081-1084
Pendred's syndrome, 891
Penicillin
  for anaerobic infection, 671
  in human milk, 166
  for neonatal pneumonia, 433, 447
  neutropenia induced by, 746
  requiring tubular excretion, 164
  for sepsis, 655, 656
  for staphylococcal scalded skin syndrome, 947
Penicillin G, 661
  aqueous, 673, 676
  benzathine, 676
  dosage for, 1093
  for meningitis, 658
  for ophthalmitis, 666
  for *Streptococcus agalactiae*, 673
Pentamidine isethionate, 687
Pentazocine, 391
Pepsin, fetal, 498
Peptic ulcer disease, 500-501
  due to antiprostaglandins, 143
Peptococcus, 671
Peptostreptococcus, 671
Perception, measurement of, 337
Pericardial effusion, 621-622
  echocardiography in, 555-556
  heart failure due to, 541
Pericardiocentesis, 622
Pericentric inversions, 1017
Perichondritis, postoperative, 225
Peridontosis, 963
Perihilar streaking, 448
Perinatal health services, 5-10
Perinatal nursing services, 8
Perinatal outreach education; *see* Outreach education, perinatal
Perinatal period, 1
Perineal analgesia, 175
Periodic acid–Schiff reagent, 687
  for α-1-antitrypsin deficiency, 782
Periodic breathing, 122, 125, 126, 457-458
Periostitis, 674
Peripheral nerve injuries, 236-237
Perisinusoidal space of Disse, 772
Peristaltic waves, 481
  esophageal, 490
  in hypertrophic pyloric stenosis, 499
Peritoneal dialysis
  preoperative, 798
  for renal insufficiency, 792, 793
Peritonitis, 485-486
  calcifications due to, 1076
  infectious, 533
  meconium, 533
Periventricular leukomalacia, 371
  site of lesions in, 358
Peromelia, 1051
Persistence of fetal circulation
  echocardiographic systolic time intervals in, 554
  hyperoxia-hyperventilation test to determine, 424
  in meconium aspiration syndrome, 444
  in pulmonary agenesis, 454
  radiologic mimicking of congestive heart failure, 1070

Personnel performance, effect of stress on, 17-19
Pesticides in human milk, 167-168
Petechiae
  due to decreased platelets, 718
  lid, 975
  sustained at birth, 216-217
Peutz-Jeghers syndrome, 953
Peyer's patches, 481
Pfeiffer syndrome, 1059
pH
  arterial, 563, 565
  of blood, 320
  esophageal, 494
  as factor in drug absorption, 160
  fetal
    fall in, during variable deceleration, 102
    intrapartum assessment of, 115-116
    scalp, 116
  of milk, 321
  in neonatal heart disease, 558-559
  tissue, continuous measurement of, 432
  urinary, 789
Phagocytic mechanisms, 632-633
  neonatal, 643-644
Phagocytosis, 743-747
  tests for, 643
Pharmacokinetics, neonatal, 164-165
Pharmacology, developmental
  in fetus, 150-158
  during lactation, 165-168
  in newborn, 158-165
Pharyngeal incompetence, 1049
Pharyngeal stimulation, 121
Phase-contrast microscopy, 718, 736
Phenacetin, 733
Phencyclidine, 58
Phenergan; see Promethazine
Phenobarbital
  addiction to, 937
  congenital heart disease due to, 537
  dosage for, 1094
  for glucuronyltransferase deficiency, 757, 762
  hepatic effects of, 769-770
  potentiating teratogenicity of cyclophosphamide, 157
  postnatal elimination of, 162
  in preeclampsia, 32
  for seizures, 392, 658
Phenobarbitone, 437
Phenolic disinfectants, 295
Phenothiazines
  in human milk, 166
  intoxication by, 677
  septic shock due to, 128
Phenotypic mapping, 1020, 1028
Phenotypic variants of malformations, 1038-1039
Phenylalanine, 304
  metabolic disorders, 817-822
  altering arterial blood pressure, 127
Phenylephrine
  for cardiovascular disease, 626
  for cyanotic spells, 620
Phenylketonuria, 817-819
  cofactor-related, 819
  eczema in, 961
  maldigestion due to, 523, 527

Phenylketonuria—cont'd
  malformations due to, 1037
  maternal, 63
  skin in, 954
Phenytoin
  for arrhythmias, 576
  for cardiovascular disease, 626
  congenital heart disease due to, 537
  dosage for, 1094, 1095
  in human milk, 166
  malformations due to, 1037
  postnatal elimination of, 162
  protein binding of, 160
  for seizures, 392
  teratogenicity of, 157
Pheochromocytoma, 121, 127, 617
Philtrum, 1041, 1048
Phimosis, 790
Phlebitis
  associated with intravenous nutrient administration, 313
  umbilical, 665
Phlebotomy, 311
Phocomelia, 719, 1051-1052
Phonocardiography, 108, 560
  for fetal heart rate monitoring, 95
Phonopneumograph, 123, 124
Phosphate
  as blood buffer, 320
  in hypocalcemia, 870-871
Phosphate loading, 876
Phosphatidic acid phosphatase, 416
Phosphatidyl inositol, 135
Phosphatidylcholine
  deficiency of, 134
  in fetal lung, 414-415
  mechanisms for production of, 414
  in pulmonary surfactant, 413-414
  synthesis, regulation of, 415-417
Phosphatidylcholine-lysophosphatidylcholine cycle, 414, 415
Phosphatidyl-N,N-dimethylethanolamine, 414
Phosphatidylethanolamine, 738
Phosphatidylglycerol, 136
  in amniotic fluid, 25
  to predict respiratory distress syndrome, 110
  in surfactant, 413-414
Phosphaturia, 801
Phosphodiesterase, 460
Phosphofructokinase, 734
6-Phosphogluconic dehydrogenase deficiency, 760
Phosphoglycerate kinase, 734
Phospholipids
  artificial aerosolized, 433
  protein-free, 434
  pulmonary surfactant, 134, 413-414
    synthesis of, 408
  low birth weight infant requirement for, 305-306
Photobilirubin, 768
Photocoagulation, 995
Photoelectric pneumograph, 123
Photometry, reflectance, 766
Photophobia
  in Chédiak-Higashi syndrome, 954
  in congenital glaucoma, 983
Photosensitivity, cutaneous, 954

Phototherapy
    for cephalhematoma causing jaundice, 219
    for Crigler-Najjar syndrome, 761
    for ecchymoses, 217
    guidelines for, 768
    for isoimmune hemolytic disease, 729
    ocular effects of, 769
    for unconjugated hyperbilirubinemia, 768-769
Phrenic nerve paralysis, 228-230
    and respiratory distress, 465
O-Phthalaldehyde in xylene, 964
Phthisis bulbi, 998
Physical criteria to assess gestational age, 256-257, 258
Physical environment
    effect on cardiac embryogenesis, 538
    to manage stress, 19
    of mother, effects on fetal growth, 55-56
    nonthermal sensory, 272-273
    pollution in, 273
    thermal, 259-272
Physical examination
    in congenital malformations, 1039-1059
    in delivery room, 255-256
    maternal, for infection, 703-704
    in multiple malformations, 1014-1015
    in nursery, 256-259
    in transition period, 254-255
Physicians' offices for health services, 6
Physiologic central cyanosis, 561, 564
Physiologic dead space, 425
Physiologic functions, influence of arousal state on, 330, 331
Phytohemagglutinin, 639, 645
    in chromosomal diagnosis, 1020
    response of SGA infants to, 75
Picornaviruses, 679, 680, 693
Piebaldism, 954
Pierre Robin syndrome, 256
    airway obstruction in, 462
    facies in, 977
    mouth in, 1048
    and respiratory distress, 463
    tongue in, 1049-1050
Piezoelectric property, 81
Piezoelectric transducers, 109
Pigmentation
    abnormalities of, 950-955
    congenital grouped, 1000
    embryonic activity of, 939
    iris, 224, 227
    lesions of, 942-943
Pilonidal sinuses, 1051
Pinna
    anatomy of, 1047
    anomalies of, 1038, 1039
Pinocytosis, 160
    for fetal lipid absorption, 480
Piper forceps, 177
Piperacillin, 1093
Piston mobility, 1011
Pituitary gland, drugs for disorders of, 1096
pK′, in acid-base disorders, 325
pK_a of drug, 168
Pl^{a1} antigen, 718
Placenta
    calcification of, 84, 92, 206

Placenta—cont'd
    circumvallate, 207, 211
    color of, 207-208, 211
    cystic, 211
    examination of, 206
    fetal blood flow in, 2
    growth rate of, 59
    growth-promoting roles of, 59
    increased thickness of
        in diabetes, 94
        in Rh incompatibility, 92
    large anterior, ultrasound scan of, 36, 37
    lobes of, abnormal, 211
    localization of, ultrasonic, 84-85
    low-lying, 85
    membranes of, 206-209
    migration of, 84-85
    multilobular, 714
    in nephrotic syndrome, 800
    nutrient support of, 55
    pathologic conditions of, 206-215
    in preeclampsia, 28
    viral passage across, 692-694
    weight of, and gestational age, relationship of, 60
Placenta previa
    mechanism of blood loss in, 189
    and premature labor, 141
    due to smoking, 153
    ultrasonic detection of, 84-85
Placental bed biopsy, 212
Placental blood flow, effects of ritodrine on, 145
Placental determinants of fetal growth, 59-62
Placental function and reserve, estimation of
    by antepartum fetal assessment, 107-112
    by fetal heart rate monitoring, 95-106
    by intrapartum fetal assessment, 112-118
Placental insufficiency, 61
    chronic, 108-109
    polycythemia associated with, 741
Placental proteins and enzymes, biochemical assessment of, 110
Placental separation, 135
Placental transport
    of drugs, 151
    of IgG antibodies, 639
    of nutrients and hormones, 846
Placidyl; see Ethchlorvynol
Placing response, 353
Plain films, 1070
Planarity of membrane, 283
Plantar grasp, 353
Plasma
    bilirubin transport in, 754
    contrast medium flow in, 1077
    creatinine concentration in, 788-789
    fetal, 151
    fresh frozen, 717, 720
        dosage for, 1095
    half-lives of drugs in, 159, 161
    lactescence of, 836
    maternal
        concentrations of drugs in, 151
        determination of, 25
    osmolality of, 315
    urea concentration in, 788-789
Plasma aminograms, abnormal, 311-312

Plasma aminograms—cont'd
    associated with intravenous supplementation feedings, 313
Plasma estriol; *see* Estriol, plasma
Plasma lipids, 315-316
    acanthocytosis due to abnormalities of, 738
Plasma volume in SGA infants, 75
Plasmacellular response in placental membranes, 209
Plasmodium, 686
Plasticizers, 513
Platelet count, 721
    at birth, 711
    in infection, 653
    venous, 1112
Platelet factor 3, 716
    to stimulate clotting, 718
    disorders of, 718-720
    for disseminated intravascular coagulation, 720
    fetal, 708
    release of, in hemostasis, 716
    transfusion with, 743
Pleiotropy, 1024
Pleocytosis, 670
    in syphilis, 674
Pleomorphic rhabdomyosarcoma, 748
Plethysmography, body, 424
Pleural effusion
    in chylothorax, 955
    heart failure due to, 541
Pleurodynia, 703
Plication of diaphragm, 490
PM 60-40, 792
Pneumatoceles, 455
    due to *Staphylococcus aureus*, 659
Pneumatosis, 513
Pneumatosis intestinalis, 487
    diagnostic radiology for, 1075
Pneumococcus, antibodies to, 638
Pneumocystis carinii, 687
Pneumomediastinum
    delivery room procedures for, 189-190
    in meconium aspiration syndrome, 444
    with pneumothorax, 449
    radiologic appearance of, 1069
Pneumonia, 658-662
    bacterial, 446-447
    chlamydial, 447
    diagnostic radiology for, 1066-1067
    intrauterine, 184
    neonatal, 446-447
        antibodies for, 433
        inability to differentiate respiratory distress from, 429-430
        due to phrenic nerve injury, 465
        following spinal injury, 231
        viral, 446, 467
Pneumonitis
    due to neonatal asphyxia, 73
    recurrent, 467
Pneumonocytes
    development of, 408
    hormones in, 417
    after vagotomy, 413
Pneumopericardium
    neonatal bradycardia due to, 121
    with pneumomediastinum, 449

Pneumoperitoneum
    in air leak syndromes, 449
    diagnostic radiology for, 1075
Pneumotachograph, 123
Pneumotachometer, 424
Pneumothorax, 448-457
    decreased incidence of, with appropriate ventilation, 436
    delivery room procedures for, 189-190
    in meconium aspiration syndrome, 444
    due to neonatal asphyxia, 73
    neonatal bradycardia due to, 121
    radiologic examination for, 1068
        position for, 1065
    tension
        in esophageal rupture, 496
        and rise in central venous pressure, 129
Po$_2$; *see* Oxygen tension
Poikilocytosis, 735
Polarity of drugs, 160
Polarization in cardiac monitoring electrodes, 278, 280
Polio vaccine, oral, 75
Poliomyelitis, 680-681
Poliovirus, 693
Pollicization, 1004
Pollution, 273
Polybrominated biphenyls, 168
Polychlorinated biphenyls, 58, 168
Polychromatophilia, 712
Polycyclic aromatic hydrocarbons, 157
Polycystic disease, 796
Polycythemia, 741-742
    increasing pulmonary artery pressure, 130
    in nephrotic syndrome, 800
    in SGA infants, 75
    in twin, 714
Polydactyly, 1058
    in thoracic dystrophy, 465
Polygraph to measure sleep states, 330, 332-333
Polyhydramnios
    associated conditions, 46
    clinical manifestations, 44
    delivery room diagnosis of, 193
    dilution of bilirubin value in, 39
    with esophageal atresia, 496
    intestinal obstruction due to, 483
    laboratory evaluation of, 44
    malformations accompanying, 1014
    prognosis in, 46-47
    in thanatophoric dwarfism, 465
    treatment of, 46
Polymorphonuclear leukocytes
    actions of, 632-633
    in amniotic cavity, 208-209
    in impetigo, 946
    oxygen toxicity and, 472
Polymyxin B, 661
    for sepsis, 655
Polyploidy, 1017
    in amniotic cells, 1030
Polyposis, small bowel, 953
Polyps, gastrointestinal, 487
Polysaccharide storage disease, 838-839
Polysaccharides activating classic pathway, 633-634
Polysplenia-heterotaxia syndrome, 775

Polystyrene sodium sulfonate
  dosage for, 1097
  for oliguria, 792
Polysystole, 114, 115
Polyuria, 790
Pompe's disease, 256, 611, 838-839
  cardiac disorders in, 537-538
Ponderal index and neonatal hypoglycemia, relationship of, 75
Population means to classify birth weight, 64
Porencephaly, 378
  differentiation from hydrocephalus, 379
Pores of Kohn, 449
Portland hemoglobin, 731
  in α-thalassemia, 732
Portocholecystostomy, 781
Portoenterostomy, 781
Port-wine stain, 956, 977
Poseiro effect, 109
Position
  infant
    in hiatal hernia treatment, 495
    immediately after delivery, 181
    to limit heat loss, 260
    for nasojejunal feeding, 309
    in phrenic nerve paralysis, 228
    in radiologic examination, 1064
    in sternocleidomastoid injury, 230
    during transcutaneous monitoring, 431
  maternal, in fetal blood sampling, 116
Positive end expiratory pressure, 436
  to improve gas exchange, 412
  pneumothorax incidence with, 448
Postductal gases, obtaining, 424
Posterior tibial pulse, 539
Postmaturity
  echocardiography in, 546
  in meconium aspiration syndrome, 444
  physiologic jaundice due to, 757
Postmeiotic chromosomal nondisjunction, 215
Postpartum care for diabetics, 26
Postrenal failure, 792
Posture
  examination of, 349-351
  in heart failure management, 571
  in hiatal hernia, 493
  in preterm infant, 341
Potassium; see also Electrolytes
  requirement for
    in heart failure, 573
    low birth weight infant, 305
  restriction of, in renal insufficiency, 792
  serum levels, in heart disease, 559-560
Potter's facies, in renal agenesis, 793
Potter's syndrome, 48, 63
  with pneumothorax, 449
  with pulmonary hypoplasia, 454
PR interval, 544-545
  in atrioventricular block, 580
  in hypokalemia and hyperkalemia, 547
  prolongation of, 547, 600
  shortening of, 547
  variation of, 547-548
Preauricular tags and pits, 1047
Precocious puberty, 1024
Precordial impulse, 541

Precordial leads, 544
Prediction of risk, 203
Prednisolone in human milk, 166
Prednisone
  for congenital hypoplastic anemia, 722
  dosage for, 1096
  in human milk, 166
  for hypoglycemia, 865
Preductal coarctation, 539, 540
Preductal gases, obtaining, 424
Preeclampsia-eclampsia
  amniotic fluid creatinine levels in, 137
  clinical manifestations of, 30-31
  complicated by placental insufficiency, 61
  diagnosis of, 27-28
  in disseminated intravascular coagulation, 720
  effect on fetal growth, 57
  epidemiology of, 28
  etiology of, 28
  pathogenesis of, 28-30
  prevention of, 31
  treatment of, 31-33
Preejection period, 553-555
Preejection period/ejection time ratio, 130
Preexcitation syndrome, 578-579
Pregnancy
  acceptance of, 241
  bilirubin activity during, 762
  care of parents during, 241-251
  dating of, 133
  diabetic, 22-26
    urinary estriol levels in, 111
  early, 82-84
  fears in, 241-242
  high-risk, 92-94
  immunized, against erythroblastosis fetalis, 34, 35
  metabolic adjustments during, 845-846
  termination of
    due to drug exposure, 152
    factors concerning, 133
Pregnancy-induced hypertension; see Preeclampsia-eclampsia
Pregnanediol, 110
Pregnane-3α,20 β-diol, 763
Pregnanetriol, urine values for, 1105
  in female pseudohermaphroditism, 919
Pregnenolone, 139
Preleukemic conditions, 724
Prematurity
  apnea of, 456-460
  associated with diabetes, 25
  electrocardiography in, 546
  family care in, 249-250
  heart disease in, 536
  hemoglobin concentration in, 708-709
  hyperglycemia in, 866
  hypocalcemia in, 874-875
  in nephrotic syndrome, 800
  obstetric management of
    amniotic fluid analysis, 134-138
    clinical evaluation, 141-142
    clinical manifestations, 133-134
    drug therapy, 142-146
    effects of, 139
    mechanisms of labor, 139-141
    radiography and ultrasound, 134

Prematurity—cont'd
　ocular disorders due to, 974-975
　physiologic desquamation in, 944
　physiologic jaundice in, 757
　and retrolental fibroplasia, 996
　due to smoking, 153
　systolic time intervals in, 554
Prenatal diagnosis, 2
Preovulatory interval, 133
Prepyloric gastric antral webs, 500
Prerenal failure, 792
Pressure
　capillary, in pulmonary hemorrhage, 447
　continuous distending, 434
　continuous negative, 434
　esophageal, 434
　　during swallowing, 492
　intraocular, 990
　intrathoracic, 179
　neonatal monitoring of, 280-284
　physics of, 280, 282
　pleural, 425-426
Pressure curves, 436
Pressure gradient in d-transposition, 587
Pressure pulse, 126
Pressure transducer
　for fetal monitoring, 114
　for neonatal monitoring, 280-281
Pressure transducer mattress, 123, 124
Pressure wave analysis, 129
Pressure-cycled ventilators, 435, 436
Pressure-volume characteristics, 410
Primary care units, 6
Primidone, 166
Primigravida, eclampsia in, 31
Priscoline; see Tolazoline
Procainamide
　for arrhythmias, 576, 577
　for cardiovascular disease, 626
　dosage for, 1095
Procaine, 186
Procaine penicillin, 676
Processor component in monitoring equipment, 277, 278
Professional growth as means of managing stress, 19
Progesterone
　levels of, in pregnancy, 23
　production of, in preeclampsia, 28
　role in onset of labor, 139
　synthesis of, in placenta, 110
Progestogens, 537
Prognostic stratification, 204
Program use, assessment of, 15
Proinsulin, 846
Prolactin
　role in anencephaly, 55
　secretion of, 244
Prolapsed cord causing prolonged FHR decelerations, 104
Proline, 454
Promethazine
　dosage for, 1097
　during labor, 174
Pronestyl; see Procainamide
Properdin system, 633-634
Propionate pathway, 827
Propionic acidemia, 827

Propoxyphene, 391
Propranolol
　for arrhythmias, 577
　for cardiomyopathy, 552
　for cardiovascular disease, 626
　associated with congenital malformations, 153
　dosage for, 1095
　effect on fetus, 59
　effect on increased ventilation, 412
　in human milk, 166
　for hypertension, 619
　and intrauterine growth retardation, 58
　neonatal bradycardia due to, 121
Proptosis
　in Apert's syndrome, 976
　congenital malformations producing, 987
　tumors causing, 985
Propylthiouracil
　associated with congenital malformations, 153
　dosage for, 1096
Prosobee, 832
Prostaglandin D_2, 567
Prostaglandin E_1
　after cardiac surgery, 625
　in coarctation of aorta, 591
　for d-transposition, 587
　for pulmonary atresia, 593-594
Prostaglandins
　constricting ductus arteriosus, 180
　to decrease pulmonary vascular resistance, 489
　in onset of labor, 140
　regulating surfactant turnover, 413
Prostatic utricle, 923
Protamine, 1095
Protective ptosis, 982
Protein
　absorption of, in developing gastrointestinal tract, 480
　cross β-fibrous, 945
　α-fibrous, 945
　intestinal breakdown of, 521
　intracellular intestinal, 480
　nonhemoglobin heme, 754
　plasma, as blood buffer, 320
　reactions with active metabolites, 157
　renal excretion of, 790
　requirements for
　　in diabetic pregnancy, 24
　　low birth weight infant, 303-304
　role in late metabolic acidosis, 324
　serum total, values for, 1105
　supplementation of, and fetal neurodevelopment, 57
　synthesis of
　　in active sleep, 334
　　fetal, 50
　　　calorie expenditure necessary for, 54
　urinary, 788
Protein binding of drugs
　in newborn, 160-161
　in placental transfer, 151
Protein hydrolysate, 310
Protein hydrolysis, incomplete, 480
Protein kinase, 737
Protein-bound iodine test, 885
Proteinuria, 790
　in preeclampsia, 27, 28, 30

Index

Proteus, 651
  bacteriuria due to, 805
  exaggerated unconjugated hyperbilirubinemia due to, 760
Prothrombin, 716
Prothrombin time, 721
  in anemia, 716, 717
  determination of, before liver biopsy, 777
  in disseminated intravascular coagulation, 720
  test values for, 1113
Protozoal infections, 692-706
Proximal tibial epiphysis, fetal, 134
Prune-belly syndrome, 63, 1050
  in urethral obstruction, 798
Pruritus, 962
Pseudarthrosis, 1011-1012
Pseudocysts, 453
Pseudodislocation, 236
Pseudoesotropia, 980
Pseudohermaphroditism
  female, 915-923
  male, 910-911
Pseudohyperaldosteronism, 803
Pseudohypoparathyroidism, 876
Pseudomonas
  bacteriuria due to, 805
  diarrhea due to, 523
  gastroenteritis due to, 662
  in mechanical ventilation, 438
  pneumatoceles due to, 471
  pneumonia due to, 446
  in septic shock, 128
Pseudomonas aeruginosa, 651, 653
Pseudooptic atrophy, 354
Pseudostrabismus, 990
Pseudotruncus arteriosus, 594, 601
Pseudotumor cerebri, 831
Psychomotor retardation, 76-77
Psychoprophylaxis during labor, 175
Psychotropic agents, 154-155
Pterins, quantitation of, 818
Ptosis, 981-982
  due to birth injury, 224
  in facial nerve palsy, 374
  in oculomotor palsy, 224
Public health services offered by regional care system, 8
Puborectalis sling, 508
Pulmonary agenesis, 453
Pulmonary artery
  banding of, 588, 601, 602
  in d-transposition, 587
Pulmonary artery pressure
  after cardiac surgery, 624
  neonatal, 130-131
Pulmonary atresia
  with intact ventricular septum, 592-594
  with open ventricular septum and tetralogy of Fallot, 594-596
Pulmonary disorders
  diagnostic radiology for, 1066-1069
  residual, after respiratory distress syndrome, 439-440
Pulmonary function
  blood gases, 421-424
  in bronchopulmonary dysplasia, 471
  after cardiac surgery, 624
  clinical observations in, 419-421
  after esophageal reanastomosis, 498

Pulmonary function—cont'd
  physiologic measurement of, 424-426
Pulmonary hemorrhage, 447
Pulmonary hypoplasia, 453-454
  due to diaphragmatic hernia, 488
Pulmonary maturation
  bronchopulmonary dysplasia affecting, 471
  pharmacologic acceleration of, 427
Pulmonary rupture, 449
Pulmonary stenosis, multiple peripheral arterial, 596-597
Pulmonary surfactant
  biochemistry of, 413-418
  neonatal deficiency of, 411-412
  oxygen altering, 472
  physiology of, 409-413
  understanding of, chronology of advances in, 405
Pulmonary valve
  isolated absence of, 613-614
  opening and closing of, 552-555
  pinhole orifice in, 592
Pulmonary valvotomy, 594
Pulmonary vascular bed, decreased cross-sectional area of, 130
Pulmonary vascular obliterative disease, 588
Pulmonary water loss, 318
Pulmonic stenosis
  thrill in, 541
  in Turner's syndrome, 537
Pulse
  alteration in, during umbilical catheterization, 187
  blood loss indicated by, 742
  examination of, 256
Pulsus alternans, 568
Punch biopsy, 964
Puncta, lacrimal, 969
  obstruction of, 983
  occlusion of, 984
Pupil
  dilated
    in cardiac arrest, 582
    in oculomotor palsy, 224
  examination of, 968-969
  Marcus Gunn, 969
  white, 992-998
Pupillary light reflex, 989
Pupillary membranes, persistent, 991
Pupillary response, abnormal, 191
Pure red cell aplasia, 721
Purpura, 234
Pyelocalyceal occlusion, 795
Pyelonephritis, 805
  and premature labor, 141
  vesicoureteral reflux and, 799
Pyknocytosis, infantile, 760
Pyloric stenosis
  congenital hypertrophic, 499-500
  associated with hydramnios, 193
  hyperbilirubinemia in, 763-764
Pyloromyotomy, 500
Pylorospasm
  in hiatal hernia, 494
  intravenous glucagon for, 499
Pyoderma, 944
Pyridostigmine, 1095
Pyridoxine; *see* Vitamin B_6
Pyridoxine dependency, and neonatal seizures, 391

Pyrimethamine
 for chorioretinitis, 1000
 for toxoplasmosis, 705
Pyrimidine synthesis, 479
Pyruvate kinase
 deficiency of, 732, 735-736
 erythrocyte, deficiency of, 760
Pyuria, 790

Q

Q wave, 590
Q-banding, 1016, 1030
QRS complex, 543-544
 axis of, 546
 in hyperkalemia, 547
 in supraventricular tachycardia, 577
 wide, 548
QT interval, 545
 in hypocalcemia and hypercalcemia, 547, 877
QT_c interval, 548
Quality standard of perinatal care, 5
Quickening, 108; *see also* Fetal measurement
 normal occurrence of, 133
Quiet alert state, 349
Quiet awake state in term infant, 329-331
Quiet sleep
 fetal analogue of, 108
 in preterm infants, 333-334
 respirations during, 122
 in term infant, 329-331
Quinacrine fluorescence, 1016
Quinidine
 for arrhythmias, 576, 577
 for cardiovascular disease, 626
 in human milk, 166

R

R wave, 543
Racemic epinephrine aerosols, 437
Rachitic rosary, 1081
Racial differences in congenital malformation prevalence, 1039
Radial aplasia, 63
Radial diffusion, 643, 644
Radial palsy, 236
Radial pulse, 539
Radiant heat, 259
 losses, 265
 thermoneutrality and, 270
Radiography
 for adrenal hemorrhage, 234
 for air leak syndromes, 449-451
 for anorectal abnormalities, 509
 for bronchopulmonary dysplasia
  differential diagnostic, 469-471
  stages of, 469
 for cardiogenic shock, 574
 for cephalhematoma, 219
 chest, 542-543
 for chronic pulmonary diseases, 469-470
 for craniosynostosis, 384
 for cystic fibrosis, 519-521
 to detect tube displacement, 438
 to estimate fetal maturity, 134
 for hypertrophic pyloric stenosis, 499
 for intestinal obstruction, 483

Radiography—cont'd
 for lobar emphysema, 454
 for multiple malformations, 1015
 for nevus flammeus, 956
 for phrenic nerve paralysis, 228
 for pneumonia, 446, 659-662
 for prenatal genetic diagnosis, 1028
 for pulmonary hypoplasia, 454
 for respiratory distress syndrome, 429-430
 for seizures, 392
 for skull fractures, 221
 for syphilis, 674-675
 for umbilical catheterization, 186
Radioimmunoassay
 IgE, 643
 thyroid-stimulating hormone determination by, 887
 thyroxine determination by, 886
 triiodothyronine determination by, 887
Radioisotopic renal diagnosis, 787, 789, 1077
Radionuclide accumulation method, 145
Radionuclide effects on fetus, 1027
Radiotherapy
 for Kasabach-Merritt syndrome, 957
 for neuroblastoma, 748
Radius
 absent, 1004
 congenital dislocation of, 1011
Rales
 in cardiogenic shock, 573
 in esophageal atresia, 496
 in meconium aspiration syndrome, 444
 as sign of heart failure, 568
Rapid eye movement; *see* REM sleep
Rapid maturation, 135
Rapid surfactant test, 135
Rare earth screens, 1065
Rastelli procedure for persistent truncus arteriosus, 602
Rate meter on cardiac monitor, 280
RDS; *see* Respiratory distress syndrome
Reactive nonstress test, 108
Reactive period of neonate, 254
Reactivity, fetal, 99
Reagins, 675
Real-time scanning, 81, 82, 109
 in neurologic examinations, 356
Rectal bleeding
 due to anal fissure, 510
 causes of, 487
Rectal dilatation, 505
Rectal temperature, 262-263
 monitoring of, 271
Rectosphincteric reflex in preterm infants, 481
Red blood cells; *see also* Erythrocytes
 destruction of, 725-730
 enzymes of
  deficiencies of, 734-736
  jaundice due to, 760
 in erythroblastosis fetalis, 34
 gestational values for, 1110
 glycerolized irradiated, 648
 in malaria, 686
 membrane disorders of, 737-741
 transfusion with, 742-743
 in urine, 788
Red reflex, 992

Reduced penetrance of genes, 1024
Reducing body myopathy, 397
5α-Reductase deficiency, 913-914
Reflexes
 absence of, in brachial palsy, 227
 assessment of, 353
 Head, 457
 Hering-Breuer, 434, 457
 ocular, 972
 pulmonary irritant, 457
 sucking, 335-337
 total body, fetal, 340
Regional anesthesia, 176
Regional center workshop, 13
"Regional Services in Reproductive Medicine," 5
Regionalization of health services, 7-8
Regular breathing pattern, 122, 125, 126
Regurgitation, 492
 mitral, 568
  in l-transposition, 584, 588
 tricuspid, 593
Reid's law of lung development, 408
Reilly bodies, 841
REM sleep, 122, 329; see also Active sleep
 changes in, according to age, 333
 in preterm infants, 334
 smiling during, 335
Renal acidifying mechanism, 789
Renal agenesis
 bilateral, 793-794
 associated with oligohydramnios, 44, 47, 48
 pulmonary hypoplasia with, 453
Renal clearance, 788-789
Renal disease
 and benefit of electrophysiologic monitoring, 113
 differentiation from preeclampsia, 27
 investigation of, 787-789
 signs and symptoms of, 789-791
Renal dysplasia, 794-797
 ultrasonography for, 86, 88
Renal excretion of drugs, 163-164
Renal failure, 791-793
 after cardiac surgery, 625
Renal hypoplasia, 794-795
Renal insufficiency, 791-793
Renal malformations, 793-799
 with pneumothorax, 449
Renal shutdown from umbilical catheterization, 188
Renal tubules
 in acid-base regulation, 321
 anomalies of, 801-804
Renal vein thrombosis, 532
Renin
 plasma, 806
 in preeclampsia, 28
Renogram, 787
Reovirus type 3, 775
Research on stress in ICU, 20
Resection, bowel, 502
Reserpine, 462
Resistive components of breathing, 419, 420
Respiration
 control of, 456-460
 fetal, 109-110, 180-181

Respiration—cont'd
 neonatal
  monitoring of, 123, 284-286
  patterns of, 122-126
  role of surfactant in, 409-410
  support of, 474
Respiratory acidosis, 323
 fetal, 102
 in respiratory distress syndrome, 433
 treatment of, 326
Respiratory alkalosis, 323-324
 in transient tachypnea, 448
 treatment of, 326-327
Respiratory distress
 extrapulmonary causes of, 460-465
 in phrenic nerve paralysis, 228
 in polycythemia, 741
 in vocal cord paralysis, 226
Respiratory distress syndrome
 associated with birth weight and gestational age, 200-201
 blood gases in, 430-432
 clinical features of, 428-429
 complications of, 437-441
 follow-up evaluation of, 441
 heart failure due to, 569
 heart rate variability decrease in, 122
 incidence of, 427
 lecithin/sphingomyelin ratio in, 135
 pathophysiology of, 427-428
 in preterm infants, 334
 radiologic findings in, 429-430, 1066, 1068
 surfactant activity in, 134
 treatment for, 432-437
 type II, 447
 understanding, chronology of advances in, 405
Respiratory effort, Apgar scoring of, 182
Respiratory epithelium, 408-409
Respiratory monitoring methods, 124
Respiratory movement
 fetal, 456
  decreased, 453
 paradoxical, 465
Respiratory patterns, 457-458
 in causes of cyanosis, 562, 564
 in heart disease, 539
Respiratory quotient, 75
Respiratory rate
 assessment of, 419-420
 average median, 125
 in d-transposition, 584
 stimulation of, 457
Respiratory system, 404-476
 architecture of, 405-407
 development of, 407-408
Rest-activity cycles, fetal, 332
Resuscitation
 cardiac, 582-583
 decision to initiate, 195
 delivery room preparation for, 181
 delivery room procedure for, 184-188
 in heart failure, 573
Resuscitation equipment, infection through, 651
 prevention of, 688-689
Retardation, intrauterine; see Intrauterine growth retardation
Reticular dysgenesis, 745

Reticulocytes
    in cord blood, 709
    glycolysis in, 736
Reticulocytopenia
    in aplastic crises, 724
    in hypoplastic anemia, 721
Reticulocytosis, fetal, 798
Reticuloendothelial system
    actions of, 632-633
    and bilirubin synthesis, 754
Reticulogranular pattern, 429
Retina
    diseases of, producing white pupil, 994-998
    examination of, 971
    function of, at birth, 972
    hemorrhage of, 225
    oxygen toxicity affecting, 440
Retinal dysplasia, 998
Retinal folds, 1000
Retinitis, due to rubella, 701
Retinitis pigmentosa, 1000
Retinoblastoma, 994-995
Retinol; see Vitamin A
Retinopathy, 57
Retinoschisis, 999
Retractions, respiratory, 420
Retrobulbar neuritis, 678
Retrolental fibroplasia, 296, 995-998
    examination for, 975
Retroplacental hematoma; see Abruptio placentae
Reverse transport of neonates, 9
Review and update in outreach education, 14
Rewarming cold infant, 271
Reye's syndrome, 823
Rh antigen, 34, 35
Rh immune globulin, 34
Rh incompatibility, 726-728
    anemia due to, 569
    ultrasonic diagnosis of, 92, 93
Rh sensitization, 727
    amniotic fluid creatinine level in, 137
    and hyperbilirubinemia, 758-759
    sinusoidal FHR due to, 106
Rhabdomyosarcoma, 748
    orbital, 986
Rh$_o$(D)-immune globulin, 43
Rhinitis
    allergic, 964
    syphilitic, 674
Rhinorrhea, 664
    cerebrospinal fluid, 221
Rhizomelia, 1051
Rhonchi
    in esophageal atresia, 496
    as sign of heart failure, 568
Rhythm
    in aganglionic colon, 506
    fundal, suggesting nystagmus, 971
    between mother and infant, 244, 246
    sucking, 336
Rib cage abnormalities, and respiratory distress, 463-465
Rib-gap syndrome, 463
Riboflavin; see Vitamin B$_2$
Richner-Hanhart syndrome, 819

Rickets
    with bronchopulmonary dysplasia, 474
    causing craniosynostosis, 382
    in hepatitis, 779
    serial films for, 1081
    vitamin D–dependent, 876
Rifampin
    dosage for, 1094
    for tuberculosis, 678
Right atrial hypertrophy, 548
Right axis deviation, 548
Right ventricle
    double-outlet, 601, 602
    in d-transposition, 587
    failure of
        central venous pressure in, 129
        hyperdynamic quality at cardiac apex indicating, 541
    hypertrophy of, 548
Right-sided heart failure, 567-568
Right-sided heart obstruction, 592-601
Right-to-left shunt, 130
    at birth, 179-180
    blood "contamination" due to, 559
    in cyanosis, 566
    after diaphragmatic hernia surgery, 489
    in meconium aspiration syndrome, 444
    in pneumothorax, 449
    in preductal coarctation of aorta, 590
    ventilation/perfusion ratio in, 422
Riley-Day syndrome, 495
    eyes in, 984
Riley-Smith syndrome, 958
Ring chromosomes, 1017, 1036
Ritodrine
    for premature labor, 145-146
    causing rises in FHR, 95
Ritter's disease, 669, 947
Robert's syndrome, 63
Robertsonian translocations, 1017-1018
Rocker-bottom feet, 1052
Rod-body myopathy, 397
Roentgenography; see Radiography
Role confusion in ICU, 16
Rose bengal I 131 excretion test, 776-777
Rotating tourniquets, 573
Rotavirus, 662, 698
Roviralta's syndrome, 494
Rowing movement, 389
RPR test, 675
RR interval, 121, 122
    in supraventricular tachycardia, 577
Rubella
    congenital, 700-702
    effect on fetal growth, 63
    frequency of, 695-696
    heart disease due to, 537
    manifestations of, 698
    metaphyseal abnormalities due to, 1081
    microcephaly due to, 381
    pulmonary arterial stenosis due to, 596
    structural malformations due to, 1014
    treatment and prevention of, 705
Rubella embryopathy syndrome, 993
Rubella keratopathy syndrome, 990
Rubenstein-Taybi syndrome, 956

Rubeola, 681-682
Rumination syndrome, 494
Russell-Silver dwarf, 63
Russell-Silver syndrome
  limb hypertrophy in, 1051
  mouth in, 1049
  skin in, 1040

S

S wave, 543
Saber shins, 676
Sabouraud's medium, 685, 950
Sacrococcygeal teratomas, 749
Saddle block, 174
Saethre-Chotzen syndrome, 1059
Safety considerations in neonatal monitoring, 286-288
Sagittal synostosis, 382-383
Salbutamol, 146
Salicylamide, 762
Salicylazosulfapyridine, 166
Salicylic acid, 959
Saline
  in contrast echocardiography, 555
  contrast peripheral vein injection, 558
  pulmonary artery injection with, 557
Saline-glucose infiltration, 298
Saline-reacting antibodies, 35
Saliva, drug concentrations obtained from, 161
Salivation, excessive, 495
Salk killed polio vaccine, 644
Salmon patches, 943
Salmonella, 651
  diarrhea due to, 523
  gastroenteritis due to, 662
Salmonella flagella, 640
Salt-losing adrenal crisis, 919-920
Sandal pattern, 1052
Sandifer's syndrome, 493-494
Sarcoma, radiation-induced, 995
Sarcoplasmic protein concentration, 50
Sarcotubular myopathy, 397
Scaling, eczematous, 960
Scalp edema, 41
Scalp electrodes, 95
Scaly baby, 944-947
Scaphocephaly, 382
Scaphoid abdomen
  in diaphragmatic hernia, 488
  in esophageal atresia, 496
Scarring, 949
Scheie's syndrome, 990
Schwachman-Diamond syndrome, 745
Schwachman's syndrome, 518
  thrombocytopenia due to, 720
Schwann cells in neurofibromatosis, 981
Sciatic palsy, 236
Scimitar sign, 543
Scintiscan, 494
Sclera, 990-991
Sclerema neonatorum, 962
  differentiation from subcutaneous fat necrosis, 218
Scoliosis, 230
Scotoma, 1002

Scrotum
  birth injury to, 237
  pigmentation of, 942
  shawl, 923
Sebaceous glands, 941
  verrucous nevi in, 958
Seborrheic eczema, 960
Seckel's syndrome, 63
Secretagogues, 516, 517
Secretin
  activities of, 516
  properties of, 522
Secretin-pancreozymin, 480
Secretory granules, 413
Sector scanner, 82
Sedatives
  dosages for, 1097
  loss of FHR variability due to, 97
  teratogenic potential of, 153
Segmental lumbar epidural block, 174
Seizures, 388-393
  due to drug withdrawal, 391
  forms of, 352
  in hypoxic ischemic encephalopathy, 359, 360
  in leptomeningeal melanocytosis, 954
  phenobarbital concentrations during, 163
Selenium
  in glutathione peroxidase synthesis, 340, 739
  to resist oxygen toxicity, 472
Self-administered nontherapeutic agents, 153-156
"Selfish mother" hypothesis, 57
Semen, drugs in, 151-152
Semicircular canals, 354
Semilunar valve
  in d-transposition, 555
  opening and closing of, 553
Seminiferous tubule dysgenesis, 911-912
Sensation, cutaneous, 942
Sensorimotor development
  Brazelton Neonatal Behavioral Assessment Scale for, 342-343
  attention and perception, 337
  auditory attention, 339-340
  facial expression and social behaviors, 334-335
  motor behavior, 340-342
  states of arousal, 328-334
  sucking, 335-337
  visual attention, 337-339
Sensory stimuli in incubators, 273
Sensory system examination, 353
Sephadex G-25, 765
Sephardic Jews, abnormal G6PD enzymes in, 735
Sepsis
  bacterial, manifestations of, 699
  factors causing, 651-653
  hyperbilirubinemia due to, 782
  neonatal tachycardia due to, 121
  low incidence of, in breast-fed infants, 305
  reducing homeothermy, 271
  seizures due to, 390
  during total parenteral nutrition, 311
Septal dislocation, 223
Septal dropout, 608
Septicemia
  in cephalhematoma, 219
  heart failure due to, 569-570

Septicemia—cont'd
    neonatal, 650-656
      neutropenia associated with, 744
Septum pellucidum, 83
Sequestered lung lobes, 455-456
Serial antibody titers, 35
Serial Apgar score, 183
Serologic studies in infection, 704-705
Serotonin, ^{14}C-labeled, 718
Serotypes
    group B streptococcal, 672
    Listeria, 671
Serratia marcascens, 651
Sertoli cells, 901
Serum
    bilirubin concentration in, 756-757, 765
    chemoattractant factors of, 632
    enzymes, 1104
    folic acid levels in, 1109
    glucuronyl transferase inhibitor in, 763
    half-life of phenytoin, 163
    hyperimmune, 781
    lecithin/sphingomyelin ratio in, 135
    maternal, alpha-fetoprotein in, 1033
    osmolality of, 315
    thyroid hormone values for, 888
    vitamin E levels in, 1109
Serum glutamic oxaloacetic transaminase; *see* Aspartate amino transaminase
Serum glutamic pyruvic transaminase; *see* Alanine amino transaminase
Serum human placental lactogen concentration, 66
Servo system for pressure monitoring, 283
Servocontrol of incubator, 267, 268, 271, 296
Setting sun sign, 377
Severe preeclampsia, 28
Sex
    determination of fetal, 1029, 1030
    and limited expression of disorders, 1024
Sex predilection
    in congenital heart disease, 536
    in congenital hip dislocation, 1009
    in cystic fibrosis, 518
    for hair growth, 940
    in incontinentia pigmenti, 949
    in infection, 652
    in renal agenesis, 793
    in strawberry nevus, 957
    in transposition of great arteries, 583
    in urinary tract obstruction, 797, 798
    in X-linked ichthyosis, 945
Sex of rearing
    in ambiguous genitalia, 928-929
    in 21-hydroxylase deficiency, 920
Sex-related differences in growth rate, 197
Sexual differentiation
    abnormalities of, 900-930
    control of, 904-907
    embryology and endocrinology of, 900-904
SGA infant; *see* Small for gestational age infant
SGOT; *see* Aspartate amino transaminase
SGPT; *see* Alanine amino transaminase
Shake test, 135, 136
Shampoos for eczematous scalp, 961
Sheep erythrocyte rosette technique, 643, 644, 647

Shetland pony breeding experiments, 56
Shigella, 651
    diarrhea due to, 523
    gastroenteritis due to, 662
Shigella flexneri, 640
Shire horse breeding experiments, 56
Shock, 121
    in air leak syndromes, 449
    cardiogenic, 128, 573-575
    central venous pressure measurement in, 128
    in disseminated intravascular coagulation, 720
    due to ecchymoses, 217
    electrical, hazard of, 287
    hypovolemic, 128
    neurogenic, 128
    renal causes of, 808
    septic, 128, 656
Short bowel syndrome, 502
Short stature, 722
Short-gut syndrome, 527
Short-term heart rate variability, 121
Shoulder
    congenital dislocation of, 1011
    girdle, birth injuries to, 226-230
"Shoulders" acceleration, 102
Shunt
    arteriovenous, 956
    Blalock and Potts, 594
    causal placental, 215
    Goretex, 594
    left-to-right; *see* Left-to-right shunt
    right-to-left; *see* Right-to-left shunt
    ventriculocardiac, 379
    Waterston, 588
Shunting
    in d-transposition, 586
    ductal, 424
    for hydrocephalus, 380
    intrapulmonary, 422-423
Sialic acid, 672
Sialidoses, 841-842
Sibling visitation, 300
Sibship, recurrence risk in, for congenital malformations, 1026
Sick sinus syndrome, 580
Sickle cell anemia, 58
Sickle cell disease, 724, 733
Sickle cell hemoglobinopathy, 984
Sickle cell trait, 730
Sickledex, 733
Sighing, 122
Signal processing in cardiac monitor, 278-279
Silent carrier, 732
Silicone gel in fetal blood sampling, 116
Silver nitrate, 158
    to cauterize anal fissure, 510
    causing corneal haziness, 225
    ophthalmia neonatorum due to, 982
    withholding application of, 248
Silver–silver chloride electrodes, 278, 280
Simian creases, 1038, 1052
Similac, 571
Simple diffusion of drug molecules, 160
Single ventricle, 602
Single-gene defects, effect on fetal growth, 63
Singlet excited oxygen, 472

Sinoatrial node
  arrhythmias in, 575
  disorders of, 580
Sinoatrial node pacemaker, 121
Sirenomelia, 1035
  in renal agenesis, 794
Situs inversus, 584
Size-dates discrepancy, 66
Skeletal anomalies
  delivery room diagnosis of, 194
  diagnostic radiology for, 1080-1084
  in Goltz's syndrome, 962
  milk composition and, 306
  ultrasonic detection of, 89-92
Skewed contractions, 114, 115
Skill acquisition in outreach education, 14
Skin
  biology of, 939-942
  blood and lymph supply to, 931-942
  blotching of, 495
  care of, 300
  congenital diseases of, 962-963, 1040
  diagnostic techniques for, 964
  infections of, 669-670, 946-947
  innervation of, 942
  lesions of, 942-944
  normal newborn, 942
  principles of therapy for, 964-965
  of SGA infant, 70, 72
  temperature measurement of, 263-264
Skin biopsy, 945
Skin blanching response, 939
Skin flare, abnormal, 496
Skin punctures, 1089-1090
Skin reactive factor, 637
Skin webs, 1008
Skinfold thickness, 65
  neck, excessive, 1050
  thigh, asymmetry of, 1011
Skin-sensitizing antibody, 640
Skull
  birth injury to, 218-222
  diagnostic radiology for, 1084-1085
  fractures of, 220-222
  lacunar, 221
Sleep states
  development of, 332-334
  and interpretation of heart rate, 119
  respiration during, 126, 458-459
  in term infant, 329-331
Slit-lamp examination, 990
  for white pupil, 992
Slow-reacting substance of anaphylaxis, 636
SMA, 792
Small for gestational age infant
  aberrant fetal growth patterns of, 64-66
  approach to, 70-72
  follow-up of, 76-78
  hypoglycemia in, 852-853
  IgG levels in, 639
  due to maternal consumption of alcohol, 153
  neonatal heart rate in, 119
  percentiles for, 197, 198
  physical appearance of, 70, 72
  synonyms for, 49

Small intestine
  disorders of, 501-504
  massive resection of, 526-528
Small left colon syndrome, neonatal, 507-508
Smallpox, 683
Smiling, in preterm infant, 334-335
Smith-Lemli-Opitz syndrome, 63
  palate in, 1049
Smoking during pregnancy, 651
  effect on fetus, 153, 156
  and intrauterine growth retardation, 58-59
  and premature labor, 141
"Snowstorm" appearance on radiograph, 444, 543
  differentiation from pneumonia, 446
Snuffles, 674
Soave procedure, 507
Socialization, 240
  in preterm infant, 334-335
Socioeconomic status
  fetal growth influenced by, 59
  prematurity influenced by, 141
  sepsis development influenced by, 651
  viral infection influenced by, 695
Sodium; see also Electrolytes
  fetal concentration of, 50
  membrane permeability to, 737
  requirement for
    in heart failure, 573
    low birth weight infant, 305
  retention of, in preeclampsia, 30
  serum levels, in heart disease, 559-560
Sodium benzoate, 765
Sodium bicarbonate
  to adjust pH, 559
  delivery room administration of, 185
  for heart failure, 572
  for respiratory distress syndrome with severe
    acidosis, 433
Sodium citrate for renal tubular acidosis, 803
Sodium nitroprusside, 619
Sodium sulfacetamide, 983
Sodium-L-thyroxine, 896
Soft tissues
  birth injuries to, 216-218
  radiology for, 1084
Solu-Cortef; see Hydrocortisone sodium succinate
Somatomedins, 55
Somatostatin
  for hypoglycemia, 866
  properties of, 522
Sonocardiogram, 108
Sonograms, serial, 92
Soto syndrome, 1052
Sound stimulation in nonstress testing, 108
Sound velocity in tissue, 81
Southern Europeans, abnormal glucose-6-phosphate dehydrogenase
    enzymes in, 735
Spastic paralysis, 222
Spectrophotometric scan
  of amniotic fluid, 36
  to measure bilirubin pigments, 35
  in Rh incompatibility, 727-728
  salicylate displacement, 765
Spectroscopy, 560
Speech therapy after tracheostomy, 475

Spherocytes, 726
Spherocytosis, hereditary, 737
 exaggerated jaundice due to, 760
 transient red cell hypoplasia with, 724
Sphingomyelinase, 841
Sphygmomanometry, 283-284
Spina bifida, 385-386
 aperta, 385
 associated with hydramnios, 193
 occulta, 194, 385-386
 ultrasonic detection of, 89, 91
Spinal accessory nerve examination, 355
Spinal block, low, 174
Spinal cord
 injury to
  intrapartum, 230-232, 373-374
  and respiratory distress, 461
 transection of, 373
Spinal fluid
 analysis of, 391-392
 block, 232
Spine
 birth injury to, 230-232
 congenital malformations of, 1051
 diagnostic radiology for, 1081-1084
 ultrasonic examination of, 89
Spinnaker sail configuration, 451
Spiral arteriolar pressure, 114
Spirochetemia, 674
Spirometer, 123
Spironolactone
 for cardiovascular disease, 627
 dosage for, 1096
 for heart failure, 571, 572
 in human milk, 166
Spitz-Holter valve, 569
Splanchnic vascular circulation required for drug absorption, 160
Splanchnopleure, 477
Spleen
 growth of, in SGA infants, 66
 host defense roles of, 745-746
 in neonatal heart disease, 540-541
 rupture of, 233, 715
Splenectomy, 233
 in congenital hypoplastic anemia, 722
 Heinz body and hemoglobin increase after, 734
 for red cell membrane disorders, 737
Splenic cysts, 532
Splinting
 for brachial palsy, 227
 of humeral fractures, 235
Splitting of heart sounds, 542
Spondyloepiphyseal dysplasia, 1051
Spondylothoracic dysplasia, 463
Spongiosis, 946
 in eczema, 960
Sporangia, 684
Sprengel's deformity, 230
Spur cells, 738
Squames in fetal lung, 443
Squamous debris in amniotic fluid, 445
Squamous metaplasia, 297
Staccato cough, 659, 676
Staff
 for delivery room resuscitation, 184

Staff—cont'd
 education of, 11-12
 in intensive care unit, 291-292
  stress of, 15-20
 interaction of, 19-20
 necessary for regional perinatal center, 9
 in normal newborn nursery, 289
 operating room, 150
 in transitional care nursery, 290-291
Staphylococcal scalded skin syndrome, 947
Staphylococcus
 pneumatoceles due to, 471
 pneumonia due to, 446
 in septic shock, 128
Staphylococcus aureus
 osteomyelitis due to, 667
 skin infection due to, 669, 946, 947
 superinfection with, in mechanical ventilation, 438
Staphylococcus epidermidis, 651, 946
Staphylococcus pneumoniae, 664
Staphyloma, 990
Stationary dystrophy, congenital hereditary, 990
Status marmoratus
 due to asphyxia, 191
 in hypoxic ischemic encephalopathy, 361
Steady-state flow during labor, 113
Steatorrhea
 in abetalipoproteinemia, 525
 in pancreatic insufficiency, 516
Stensen's duct, 670
Stepping response, 353
Stercobilins, 754
Sterility necessary during resuscitation, 184
Sterilization, gas, 295
Sternocleidomastoid muscle
 injury to, 230
 visualization of, 355
Sternum, abnormalities of, 1050
Steroids
 associated with congenital malformations, 153
 effect on embryonic enzyme activity, 480
 for hypoglycemia, 865
 and intrauterine growth retardation, 58
 for spinal cord trauma, 373
Stertorous breathing, 389
Sticky eye, 982
Stiff skin syndrome, 842
Stillbirth
 associated with diabetes, 25
 in polyhydramnios, 46
 due to renal agenesis, 794
Stimulation
 in apnea, 459-460
 in chronic pulmonary disease, 475
Stimulus-response testing of fetal heart rate, 108
Stoichiometric relationships, 322
Stomach
 digestive process in, 521
 fluid in, 194
 lactobezoars in, 501
 volvulus of, 498-499
Stomatocytosis, hereditary, 737
Stomodeum, 1041
Stools
 acholic, 775, 779

Stools—cont'd
    bilirubin excretion in, 756
    color of, in choledochal cysts, 779
    effect of phototherapy on, 769
    enterovirus isolated from, 704
    examination of, 487
    in gastroenteritis, 663
    loose, 523
    in necrotizing enterocolitis, 513
    softening of, 510
    time of passage of first, 1099
Storage in hospital units, 293
Strabismus, 989-990
    in craniosynostosis, 383
    accompanying leukoma, 225
    associated with protein intake, 304
    in retinoblastoma, 994
Strain gauge
    for central venous pressure measurement, 129
    for direct measurement of arterial blood pressure, 126
    mercury-in-rubber, 123
    in respiration monitoring, 284-285
Stratum corneum, permeability of, 939
Strawberry nevus, 956-957
Strength assessment, 351-353
Streptococcus in septic shock, 128
Streptococcus agalactiae, 651, 672-673
Streptococcus faecalis, 650
Streptococcus pneumoniae, 654
Streptomycin, 661
    dosage for, 1094
    inhibiting glucuronyl transferase, 764
    for tuberculosis, 678
Stress
    in intensive care staff, 15-20
    intrauterine, 130
Stretch receptors, pulmonary, 457
Stridor
    due to airway obstruction, 462-463
    in vocal cord paralysis, 226
String sign, 499
Stromal fibroblasts, 990
Structural malformations, 152
Strychnine, 822
Stupor, 349
Sturge-Weber syndrome
    nevi in, 956
    skin in, 1040
Subarachnoid block, 175
Subarachnoid hemorrhage, 372
Subcapsular splenic hematoma, 532
Subclavian artery
    anomalous, 496
    for patch angioplasty, 592
Subconjunctival hemorrhage, 224
Subcutaneous fat necrosis, 217-218, 962
    hypercalcemia due to, 878-879
Subdural hematoma
    differentiation from hydrocephalus, 378
    due to hydrocephalus, 381
Subdural hemorrhage, 372-373
Subependymal germinal matrix hemorrhage/intraventricular hemorrhage, 367-371
    due to asphyxia, 191-192

Subependymal—cont'd
    site of lesions in, 358, 369
Subglottic stenosis
    due to intubation, 439, 474
    respiratory rate in, 420
Submucosal clefts, 1049
Substrates for phosphatidylcholine, 415-416
Succenturiate placental lobes, 207
Succinyl CoA: 3-keto acid CoA-transferase deficiency, 830
Succinylcholine
    for cardiovascular disease, 627
    during labor, 177
Succus entericus, exclusion of, 1075
Sucking
    disorders of, 490-491
        transpyloric infusions for, 309
    pattern of, 490
    in response to visual stimuli, 338
    during seizures, 389
Sucking reflex, 335-337, 353
Sucrase, 480
Sucrose, 305
Sucrose-isomaltose malabsorption, 524
Suction apparatus, 181
Suction biopsy, 506
Suctioning
    at birth, 181-182, 183
    with chest tubes, 451
    continuous intercostal, 489
    of meconium, 184
    nasogastric, 502
    neonatal bradycardia due to, 121
    in respiratory distress syndrome, 437
    tracheal, 445
Sudden infant death syndrome, 580
Sulfadiazine, 705
Sulfates
    bilirubin conjugation with, 755
    maldigestion due to, 523, 524
Sulfide oxidase deficiency, 999
Sulfisoxazole, 232
Sulfobromophthalein, 754
Sulfonamides, 661
    bilirubin binding diminished by, 765
    in human milk, 166
    neutropenia induced by, 744
Sulfuric acid, 325
Superinfection, pulmonary, 475
Superoxide dismutase, 472
Superoxide radical, 746
Suppressor T cells, 636, 637
Suprapubic aspiration, 804
Supraventricular tachycardia, 97
Surface balance experiments, 410
Surface tension
    laboratory assessment of, 410
    surfactant for, 411
Surface-active material; *see* Pulmonary surfactant
Surfactant, pulmonary; *see* Pulmonary surfactant
Surfactant tests for amniotic fluid analysis, 134-137
Surfactant therapy, 433-434
Surgery
    for adrenal hemorrhage, 235
    cardiac
        altering arterial blood pressure, 127

Surgery—cont'd
  care of neonate after, 623-625
  treatment of complications after, 625
 for craniosynostosis, 384
 for diaphragmatic hernia, 489
 to elevate skull fractures, 222
 for esophageal atresia, 497-498
 for gastrointestinal perforation, 486
 for intestinal obstruction, 484
 for late FHR deceleration, 104
 for lung cysts, 455
 for meningomyelocele, 386
 nasal, 223
 for necrotizing enterocolitis, 513
 for neuroblastoma, 748
 open-heart, 603-604
 for patent ductus arteriosus, 438
 for phrenic nerve paralysis, 229
 for preductal coarctation of aorta, 591
 for sternocleidomastoid injury, 230
 for supraventricular tachycardia, 578
Sutures
 abnormalities of, 383
 closure of, in craniosynostosis, 382
 diagnostic radiology for, 1084
 premature fusion of, 1041
 separation of, in hydrocephalus, 377
Suturing of lacerations, 218, 225
Swaddling to prevent heat loss, 266
Swallowing
 disorders of, 490-491
  aspiration syndromes and, 446
  in cyanosis, 565
  transpyloric infusions for, 309
 fetal, 47, 48, 481
 in myotonic dystrophy, 462
 pattern of, 490
Sweat losses, 317
Sweat test, 519
Sweating
 absence of, 963, 964
 onset of, 941
 as sign of heart failure, 568
Sweaty feet syndrome, 829, 830
"Sweet spirits of nitre," 733
Swenson procedure, 507
Symblepharon, 1043
Sympathetic blastoma, 986
Sympathetic control of heart rate, 121
Sympathetic nervous system, birth injuries to, 224
Sympathomimetic amines
 constricting ductus arteriosus, 180
 response of cardiovascular muscle to, 185
Synchondroses, innominate, 221
Syncytial knots, 61
Syncytial trophoblast layer of placenta, 61
Syndactyly, 1058-1059
 associated with craniosynostosis, 384
 treatment for, 1004, 1008
Syndrome, definition of, 1035
Syndrome complexes in cardiovascular disease, 621, 622
Syndromes associated with diminished birth weight, 63; *see also* specific syndromes
Synophrys, 976, 981, 1047

Synostosis, 1004
Syphilis, 63, 674-676
 acute glomerulonephritis due to, 799
 airway obstruction due to, 462
 chronic villitis due to, 213
 metaphyseal abnormalities due to, 1081
 nephrotic syndrome due to, 801
Syringocystadenoma papilliferum, 959
Systemic lupus erythematosus, 639
 congenital atrioventricular block due to, 537
 thrombocytopenia due to, 718
Systemic vascular disease, maternal, causing fetal asphyxia, 180
Systemic-pulmonary collateral arteries, 596
Systole
 Doppler method to detect, 284
 echocardiographic measurement during, 549-550
 pressure pulse during, 126
 time intervals of, 553-555
 uterine, 115

T

T cells, 964
T lymphocytes
 in breast milk, 642
 in cell-mediated immunity, 636
 development of, 637-638
T vector, 544
T wave
 in aortic stenosis, 590
 axis of, 546
 in hyperkalemia and hypokalemia, 547
 inversion, 597, 598
T_3; *see* Triiodothyronine
T_4; *see* Thyroxine
Tachycardia
 fetal, 95-97
 heart rate in, 547
 maternal, 142
 due to methemoglobinemia, 734
 neonatal, 119
 paroxysmal, 580
 as sign of heart failure, 568
 sinus, 576
 supraventricular, 576-577
 ventricular, 579-582
Tachypnea
 due to methemoglobinemia, 734
 as sign of heart failure, 568
 transient, 447-448
  arterial carbon dioxide tension in, 423
  cyanosis due to, 565
Tachysystole, 114, 115
Tactile discrimination, 942
Takayasu's disease, 596
Talipes calcaneovalgus, 1012
Talipes equinovarus, 1012, 1059
 in myotonic dystrophy, 396
Talipes varus, 1012
Talwin; *see* Pentazocine
Tamm-Horsfall protein, 1078
Tamponade
 for adrenal hemorrhage, 235
 for liver trauma, 233
Tarsorrhaphy, 984
Taste, increased sensation of, 495

Taurine, 755
Tay-Sachs disease, 840-841, 1014
　cherry-red macula in, 1001
　megalencephaly in, 379
Team service in perinatal care, 6
Tearing
　excessive, 983
　lack of, 984
　reflex, 972
Technetium sulfur colloid, 494
Teeth
　in ectodermal dysplasia, 963
　in thoracic dystrophy, 465
Telangiectasia, 957
Telecanthus, 1043
　measurement of, 972
Telescoping sign, 1011
Temperature
　environmental, 264-266
　internal, 262-263
　normal body, 262
　skin, 263-264
Temperature regulation, 259-272
　after cardiac surgery, 624
　central nervous system control of, 941-942
　during exchange transfusion, 730
　in hospital units, 293
　in nursery, 296
　for respiratory distress syndrome, 432
　of SGA infants, 74-75
　of skin electrodes, 431
Tenotomy, 228
Tensilon; see Edrophonium
Teratogenicity of drugs, 150-157
Teratoma, 749
　abdominal masses due to, 532
　airway obstruction due to, 462
　orbital, 986
Terbutaline
　for premature labor, 144-145
　stimulating increase in phospholipid, 412
Terminal sac period of lung development, 407
Testes
　developmental disorders of, 910-912
　differentiation of, 900
　dysgenetic, 910-911
　functional disorders of, 912-913
　injury to, 237
　rudimentary or small, 911
Testicular feminization, 914-915
Testicular regression syndromes, 911
Testosterone
　biosynthetic defects of, 912-913
　blood values for, 1105
　　in female pseudohermaphroditism, 918-919
　enzymes of, 912-913
　fetal excretion of, 905
　in gonadal development, 903
Tetanic contractions, 114, 115
　causing prolonged FHR decelerations, 104
Tetanolysin, 676
Tetanospasmin, 676
Tetanus antitoxin, 640
Tetanus infection, 676-677
Tetany, postacidotic, 876

Tetracaine, 174
2,3,7,8,-Tetrachlorodibenzo-p-dioxin, 168
Tetracycline, 661
　diarrhea due to, 534
　in human milk, 166
Tetrahydrobiopterin, 817-818
Tetralogy of Fallot
　bronchopulmonary dysplasia developing after repair of, 469
　echocardiography for, 557
　associated with maternal hypoxemia, 58
　with pulmonary atresia, 594-596
Tetraploidy, 1017
Thalamus, ultrasonic detection of, 83
Thalassemias, 732-733
　color of placenta in, 211
Thalidomide
　congenital heart disease due to, 536
　limb defects due to, 1052
　teratogenicity of, 150
　　metabolic activation requirement of, 157
Thanatophoric dwarfism, 463, 465
　ultrasonic appearance of, 91
Thayer-Martin media, 673
Theobromine, 167
Theophylline
　for apnea, 158, 161, 460
　bronchial effects of, 475
　in human milk, 167
　producing caffeine via methylation pathways, 163
　role in phosphatidylcholine synthesis, 417
Thermal environment
　at birth, 179
　effect on quiet sleep, 334
Thermal transfer coefficient, 262
Thermistor, 123, 124, 263
　nasal, 424
　in respiration monitoring, 284
Thermocouples, 263
Thermoneutrality
　convective heating and, 269-270
　radiant heating and, 270
Thiamine; see Vitamin B_1
Thiazides, 475
Thigh
　asymmetric skinfolds of, 1011
　swelling of, after femoral fracture, 235
Thin-layer chromatography, 134
　two-dimensional, 136
Thiobarbiturates, 171
Thiocyanate in human milk, 167
Thiopental sodium, 177
Third ventricle, ultrasonic identification of, 83
Thoracentesis
　in chylothorax, 455
　in esophageal rupture, 496
Thoracic cage, abnormal size of, 1050
Thoracic dystrophy, asphyxiating, 465
Thoracic gas volume, 448
Thoracotomy, extrapleural, 498
Thrills, cardiac, 541
Thrombin time
　in anemia, 716
　in disseminated intravascular coagulation, 720
　test values for, 1113
Thromboatheroma, 430

Thrombocytopenia, 718-720
  due to antiprostaglandins, 143
  differentiation from other disorders, 216
  hemangioma associated with, 957
  platelet transfusion for, 743
Thrombocytopenia–absent radius syndrome, 719-720, 1058
Thrombocytopenic purpura, 701
Thromboembolism, renal vascular, 806
Thrombosis
  arterial, 430, 567
  cerebral, 620
  after exchange transfusion, 730
  renal vein, 807
    nephrotic syndrome due to, 801
Thrush, 683-684
Thumb, absent, 1004
Thymic dysplasia, 525
Thymic hypoplasia, 646-647
Thymic silhouette in respiratory distress syndrome, 430
Thymidine kinase, 479
Thymocytes, 637
Thymosin, 648
Thymus
  growth of, in SGA infants, 66
  radiologic appearance of, 1066
Thyroglobulin, 884
  defective synthesis of, 891
Thyroglossal cysts, 462
Thyroid
  chemical function tests for, 885-887
  in DiGeorge syndrome, 646-647
  disorders of, 883-899
    drugs for, 1096
  embryogenesis of, 883
  fetal-maternal relationships affecting, 887-890
  function, values for, 1104
  lingual, 893
  regulation of, 885
  suppression of, 166
Thyroid hormones
  in hypoglycemia, 860-861
  physiologic action of, 883-884
  release of, due to cold stress, 260
  role in birth weight, 55
  role in phosphatidylcholine synthesis, 417
  synthesis of, 884-885
Thyroid-stimulating hormone
  functions of, 885
  radioimmunoassay to test, 887
Thyrotoxicosis, 128, 897-899
  maldigestion due to, 523, 526
Thyroxine
  actions of, 883-884
  determination of
    by competitive protein binding, 886
    by radioimmunoassay, 886
  effect on embryonic enzyme activity, 480
  free, 886-887
  in human milk, 166
  synthesis of, 884-885
    errors of, 890
Thyroxine-binding globulin, 885
  familial abnormalities of, 899
  test for, 887
Thyroxine-binding prealbumin, 885

Thyroxine-binding protein saturation, assessment of, 887
Thyroxine-column test, 885-886
Tibia, pseudarthrosis in, 1011-1012
Ticarcillin, 1093
Tidal volume; see also Lung volume
  in bronchopulmonary dysplasia, 471
  control of, through ventilators, 436
Tight junction of bile canaliculus, 772
Time intervals
  electrocardiographic, 544-545
  systolic, echocardiographic measurement of, 553-554
Tissue biopsy, 1021
Tissue density, 81
Tissue necrosis, 365
Tissue perfusion
  adequate, in gastrointestinal bleeding, 487
  in cardiogenic shock, 574
T-mycoplasmas, 651
Tobramycin, 661
  dosage for, 1093
  for sepsis, 655, 656
Tocodynamometer, 108, 109
  to measure uterine activity, 95
α-Tocopherol; see Vitamin E
Tolazoline
  for cardiovascular disease, 627
  decreasing pulmonary artery pressure, 130
  dosage for, 1095
  for Ebstein's anomaly, 601
  after hernia surgery, 489
  neonatal bradycardia due to, 121
  for persistent fetal circulation, 566
Tolbutamide, 860
Tongue
  abnormalities of
    airway obstruction due to, 462
    in Pierre Robin syndrome, 463
  circumvallate papillae of, absent, 496
  examination of, 256
    in cyanosis, 561, 564
  fasciculation of, 461
  forward suturing of, 463
Tonic movement, 389
Tonic neck reflex, 353
Tonic-clonic movements, 353, 389
Tonometry, 281-282
TORCH infections, 72
  causing chronic villitis, 213
  malformations due to, 1037
  screening for, 381, 382, 704-705
  seizures due to, 390
  thrombocytopenia due to, 721
Torsion spasms, 493
Torticollis, 230
Tortuosity
  of retinal veins, 997
  ureteral, 798
Torulopsis, 651
Torus, palatine, 1049
Total hemolytic complement assay, 643, 644
Total parenteral nutrition
  in chylothorax, 455
  for low birth weight infant, 310-312
  after massive bowel resection, 527
Total pulmonary resistance, 426

"Toward Improving the Outcome of Pregnancy," 5
Toxemia; *see also* Preeclampsia-eclampsia
    anesthesia for labor and delivery in, 175-176
    and premature labor, 141
Toxin
    in gastroenteritis, 664
    tetanus, 676
Toxoplasma gondii, 693
    hepatitis due to, 781
    microcephaly due to, 381
    myocarditis due to, 609
Toxoplasmosis, 63
    congenital, 702-703
    differentiation from syphilis, 801
    frequency of, 697
    manifestations of, 698
    treatment and prevention of, 705-706
Trabeculation, bladder, 1079
Tracheal cyst, 462
Tracheal fluid, composition of, at birth, 180
Tracheal lesions, 438, 439
Tracheal secretions, 475
Tracheal stenosis, 462
Tracheal stimulation, 121
Tracheoesophageal fistula
    airway obstruction due to, 462
    delivery room diagnosis of, 193-194
    with esophageal atresia, 496-498
    without esophageal atresia, 498
    H-type, 467
    associated with hydramnios, 193
Tracheomalacia, 462
Tracheostomy
    for laryngeal stenosis, 193
    for laryngeal web, 183
    in Pierre Robin syndrome, 463
    after prolonged intubation, 474
    for subglottic stenosis, 439
    in vocal cord paralysis, 226
Traction-suspension, 235
Transaminase, 702
Transcephalic impedance determination, 368
Transcutaneous measurement of oxygen tension, 297, 430-432
    continuous, 118
    in cyanotic heart disease, 559
    fall in, and pneumothorax, 449
    in retrolental fibroplasia, 997
Transcutaneous monitoring
    of fetal scalp pH, 118
    in meconium aspiration syndrome, 445
Transducer
    to measure skin temperature, 264
    motion-sensing, 355
Transendonasal perforation for choanal atresia, 463
Transfer factor, 637
Transfusion
    for anemia, 571, 722
    in DiGeorge syndrome, 647
    exchange, 433
        complications of, 767
        for Crigler-Najjar syndrome, 761
        with heparinized blood, 720
        for isoimmune hemolytic disease, 729-730
        partial, in polycythemia, 741
        in thrombocytopenia, 718

Transfusion—cont'd
    exchange—cont'd
        for unconjugated hyperbilirubinemia, 766-767
    fetal-maternal, 712-714
    in gastrointestinal hemorrhage, 486
    granulocyte, 743
    for intraabdominal trauma, 233
    intrauterine
        for erythroblastosis fetalis, 39, 759
        for Rh incompatibility, 728
    neutrophil, 744
    of placental blood, 709
    platelet, 743
        for Kasabach-Merritt syndrome, 957
        for thrombocytopenia, 718
    red cell, 742-743
    in respiratory distress syndrome, 433
    twin-twin, 714, 741
Transfusion syndrome, 211
Transient renal impairment, 792
Transillumination
    cranial, 368
    in hydrocephalus, 378
    for pneumothorax, 449
Transition period, 254-255
Transitional sleep, 333-334
Translocation of chromosomes, 1017-1018, 1036
    in abortuses, 1038
Transplantation
    allogeneic, 723
    bone marrow, 646, 648, 723, 724
    corneal, 990
    kidney, 801
    liver, 781
    thymus, 647
Transport unit, care in, 292
Transportation in regional care system, 9
Transport-referral conference, 14
Transposition of great arteries, 557
    d-, 584-588
        echocardiographic systolic time intervals in, 555
    incidence of, 583
    l-, 588
    pathology of, 583-584
    tricuspid atresia with, 599
Transpulmonary pressure, 121
Transpyloric infusions, continuous, 309-310
Transthoracic electrical impedance, 285
Trauma, cataracts associated with, 993
Treacher Collins syndrome
    choanal atresia in, 463
    eyes in, 977, 1047
Tremors, 353
Treponema pallidum, 674
    hepatitis due to, 781
    transplacentally acquired, 650
Treponema pallidum immobilization test, 675
Treponemal antigen tests, 675
Trichiasis, 969
Trichloracetic acid, 788
Trichorhinophalangeal syndrome, 1048
Tricuspid atresia, 597-599
    echocardiography for, 557
Tricuspid insufficiency, isolated congenital, 614
Tricyclic antidepressants in human milk, 166

Trident iliac bones, 465
Tridione; *see* Trimethadione
Triethylenemelamine, 995
Trigeminal nerve
 examination of, 355
 irritation of, 983
Trigger digits, 1008
Triglycerides
 fetal synthesis of, 54
 in infant formulas, 305
 in SGA infants, 73
 in skin, 942
Triiodothyronine, 1096
 actions of, 883-884
 determination of, by radioimmunoassay, 887
 synthesis of, 884-885
Triiodothyronine-resin uptake test, 887
Trimethadione, 58
 embryogenetic effects of, 1026
Trimethoprim-sulfamethoxazole, 687
 dosage for, 1093
Triphalangeal thumbs, 722
Triple dye for cord, 158
Triploidy, 1017
 in abortuses, 1038
Triradii, 1052
Tris(hydroxymethyl)aminomethane, 185
 for respiratory acidosis, 326
Trismus, 677
Trisomies
 in abortuses, 1038
 autosomal, 63, 1016
 fontanel size in, 1040
 joint deformities in, 1059
 ocular findings in, 978
 placental pathology in, 213
 prevalence of, 1036
 sclerotic glomeruli in, 787
 thrombocytopenia due to, 720
Trisomy 8, 1052
Trisomy 13
 capillary hemangiomas in, 956
 characteristics of, 978
 cleft lip in, 1049
 congenital heart disease in, 537
 eyes in, 1043
 polydactyly in, 1058
 scalp lesions in, 1040
Trisomy 18
 biliary atresia in, 775
 characteristics of, 978
 with double-outlet right ventricle, 602
 eyes in, 1047
 feet in, 1052
 hair in, 1040
 hepatitis associated with, 775
 mouth in, 1048
 sternum in, 1050
Trisomy 21; *see also* Down's syndrome
 characteristics of, 978
 eyes in, 1043
 palmar patterns in, 1052
 risk for, 1060
Tristichiasis, 981

Trochlear nerve
 examination of, 354-355
 palsy, 224
Tromethamine, 326
Tromethamine buffer, 572
Trophoblasts on chorionic sac, 206
Truncal incurvation reflex, 353
Truncometry, 66, 69
Truncus arteriosus
 echocardiography for, 556
 persistent, 601-602
 type IV, 594
Trypsin
 activities of, 516
 embryonic, 480
Trypsin G-banding, 1021
Trypsinogen
 deficiency of, 517
 inactivation of, 517
Tryptophan, 817-818
Tuberculin sensitivity, 636
Tuberculin test, 678
Tuberculosis, 677-679
Tuberous sclerosis
 macules indicating, 1040
 white spots in, 955
d-Tubocurarine, 177
Tubular necrosis, 73
Tumor cells, inhibition of attachment of, 158
Tumors
 of eyelids, 980-981
 intracardiac, 557
 renal, 808-810
 solid, 747-749
 spinal cord, 231
 uterine, 222
Tungstate, 137
Tunica vaginalis, hematocele in, 237
Tunica vasculosa lentis, 998
Turner's syndrome, 63, 908-910
 anaphase lag in, 1016
 congenital heart disease in, 537
 eyes in, 978
 hands and feet in, 1052
 neck and chest in, 1050
 prevalence of, 1036
Tuttle and Grossman test, 494
Tween 80 stabilized material, 678
 properties of, 1074
Twins; *see also* Multiple gestations
 biparietal diameter of, 92
 blood loss in utero from one to other, 714
 delivery of, 177
 monochorionic, 46
 placentas of, 214-215
 polycythemia in, 741, 742
 and placental disorders, 61
Tympanocentesis, 665
Tyrosinase deficiency, 954
Tyrosine, 304
 metabolic disorders of, 817-822
Tyrosinemia, 819-820
 ethnic predilection for, 1014
 liver injury due to, 782
Tyrosinosis, 819-820

Tzanck test, 947

U

U wave, in hyperkalemia, 547
Ulcerative colitis, 487
Ulcers
 in gastroenteritis, 663
 peptic, 500-501
 due to strawberry nevus, 957
Ulegyria
 due to asphyxia, 191
 in hypoxic ischemic encephalopathy, 361
Ultrasonic cephalometry, 134
Ultrasonography
 for abdominal masses, 532
 for adrenal hemorrhage, 234
 for central nervous system disturbances, 356
 for chest diagnosis, 1065
 to detect fetal movement, 340
 to detect polyhydramnios, 44
 to diagnose early pregnancy, 82-84
 to diagnose fetal anomalies, 85-92
 to estimate fetal growth, 66
 to estimate fetal maturity, 134
 to estimate gestational age, 82-84
 for high-risk pregnancy, 92-94
 indications for, 85
 for placental localization, 36, 84-85
 for prenatal genetic diagnosis, 1028
 principles of, 81-82
 renal, 787
 for urinary tract, 1080
Ultraviolet light, hypersensitivity to, 953
Umbilical artery, absent, 794
Umbilical cord
 length of, 209
 parenteral therapy through, 299
 pathologic conditions of, 209-211
 velamentous, 206, 211
Umbilicus
 care of, 688
 as portal of entry for *Clostridium tetani*, 677
Umbrella sign, 499
Undernutrition, maternal, effect on fetal growth, 61
Unresponsive period of neonate, 254
Upper-to-lower segment ratio, 1051
Upright suspension of infant, 351
Urea
 diffusion of, across cell membrane, 316
 nephrotic, 785
 permeability in ovine placenta, 60
 plasma concentration of, 788-789
Urea clearance, 789, 1108
Urea cycle, disorders of, 822-824
Ureter, nonpatency of, 795
Ureteral atresia, 795
Ureteral reflux, 798
Ureterocele, ectopic, 797, 1079
Ureteropelvic junction, obstruction at, 798
Urethra
 male, voiding cystourethrography for, 1079
 valvular obstruction of, 798
Uridine diphosphogalactose 4-epimerase deficiency, 832
Uridine diphosphoglucose dehydrogenase, 755
Uridine diphosphoglucuronic acid, 755, 757

Uridine diphosphoglucuronyl transferase, 755
Uridine kinase, 479
Urinary estriol; *see* Estriol, urinary
Urinary osmolality, 317
 in oliguria, 789
Urinary output
 decreased, 270
 values for, 792
Urinary retention following spinal injury, 231
Urinary tract
 diagnostic radiology for, 1077-1080
 infection of, 668-669, 804-806
  hyperbilirubinemia associated with, 782
 obstruction of, 789, 797-799
  ascites due to, 532-533
Urine
 color of, in erythropoietic porphyria, 760
 drug-screening methods for, 937
 fetal, 47
 in 21-hydroxylase deficiency, 919
 specimen, 788
  collection of, 804
 time of passage of, 1098
 water losses in, 316-317, 318
Urine chemistry values, 1101
Urobilinogens, 754
Urobilinoids, 756
Urogastrone, 522
Urography
 excretory, 787-788, 796, 1077-1079
 high-dose, 795
 intravenous, 788
Urticaria pigmentosa, 954
Uterine blood flow, alterations in, 140-141
Uterine capacity, 56
Uterine ischemia, 57
Uterine size, 133-134
Uvula, bifid, 1049

V

V Wave, 129
 seen during umbilical catheterization, 186
Vaccines, 694, 695
Vaccinia, 683, 693
Vaccinia-immune globulin, 683
VACTERL syndrome, 63
 imperforate anus in, 1051
Vacuoles in lens, 994
Vacuolization, trophoblastic, 213
Vacuum extraction, anesthesia for, 176
Vagal mediation of FHR deceleration, 102
Vagal stimulation of fetal heart rate, 101
Vaginal agenesis, 925
Vaginal compression, lung function effects of, 448
Vaginal epithelium, infant, effects of oral contraceptives on, 167
Vaginitis, gonococcal, 673
Vagotomy, 413
Vagus nerve
 examination of, 355
 injury of, 225-226
 role in heart rate variability, 121
Valine, 825
Valium; *see* Diazepam
Valproic acid, 1094
Valsalva maneuver, during labor, 176

Valsalva phase of breathing, 420
Valvuloplasty, tricuspid, 601
van den Berg reaction, 753
Vancomycin, 1093
Vanillylmandelic acid
   in neuroblastoma, 235
   in systemic hypertension, 618
   urine values for, 1101
Vanishing testes syndrome, 911
Vapor pressure, 265-266
Variability of baseline fetal heart rate, 97
Variable expressivity, 1024
Varicella-zoster, 63, 682-683, 693, 694
Varices of umbilical vessels, 714
Variola, 683, 693
Vasa previa, 211
Vascular accidents, intrauterine
   intestinal cysts due to, 504
   jejunoileal obstruction due to, 502
Vascular disease and hypercalcemia, heart disease due to, 537
Vascular insufficiency, effect on fetal growth, 57
Vascular resistance, pulmonary
   after first breath, 179
   and pH, 185
   in pulmonary hypoplasia, 453
   systolic time intervals associated with, 554
   during transition from fetal to neonatal circulation, 130
Vascular rings, 462, 463, 496, 615-617
Vascularization, retinal, to ora serrata, 997
Vasculature
   aberrant, airway obstruction due to, 462
   ocular, examination of, 971
   pulmonary, 406-407
      in bronchopulmonary dysplasia, 471
      consideration of, in heart disease evaluation, 543
      development and growth of, 407-408
      in pulmonary atresia, 593
      in pulmonary hypoplasia, 453
   retinal, in retrolental fibroplasia, 996
Vasculitis, 657
Vasoactive intestinal peptide, 522
Vasoconstriction
   pulmonary, in cardiogenic shock, 574
   to reduce heat loss, 260
Vasodilan; see Isoxsuprine
Vasodilatation in cyanosis diagnosis, 561
Vasodilators, 128
Vasogenic edema, 365
Vasomotor tone, cutaneous, 941-942
Vasopressin
   dosage for, 1096
   renal tubule insensitivity to, 803
Vasospasm in preeclampsia, 28-30
Vasoxyl; see Methoxamine
VATER syndrome, 63, 538, 1035
   imperforate anus in, 1051
Vater-Pacini bodies, 942
VDRL antibodies, 640
   in syphilis, 675
Vectorcardiography, 560
Vectors, cardiac, 543
Veillonella, 671
Vein of Galen
   arteriovenous fistula in, 608
   malformations of, 377

Velpeau bandage, 235
Vena caval compression
   from contracting uterus, 109
   fetal asphyxia due to, 180
Vena caval syndrome, 175
Venacavogram, 788
Venous pressure
   in neonatal heart disease, 539-540
   systemic, 568
Venous return
   changes in, 129
   pulmonary
      obstruction of, 130
      total anomalous, 467, 602-604
         echocardiography for, 556
Ventilation
   alveolar
      in air leak syndromes, 448
      in persistent fetal circulation, 566
      in pulmonary atresia, 593
   assisted
      for chronic pulmonary disease, 473
      complications of, 437-438
      for diaphragmatic hernia, 489
      in meconium aspiration syndrome, 445
      in severe depression, 184
   for cyanotic spells, 619
   effect on pulmonary surfactant, 412
   maldistribution of, 471
   in nursery, 293
   pulmonary, 184
   in tetanus, 677
Ventilation equipment, infection through, 651
   prevention of, 688-689
Ventilation/perfusion ratio, 422
Ventilator-incubator, 435
Ventilatory response, 456-457
   sleep state comparisons in, 459
Ventral silon pouch, 489
Ventral suspension of infant, 351
Ventricle
   common, 584
   echocardiographic measurement of, 549-551
   preejection period in, 554
   single, 602
Ventricular asystole, 582
Ventricular ejection time, 553-555
Ventricular fibrillation, 582
Ventricular hypertrophy, 546
Ventricular inversion, 584
Ventricular opacification, 592
Ventricular rate in supraventricular tachycardia, 576-577
Ventricular septal defect, 605-607
   combined with patent ductus arteriosus, 607
   with d-transposition, 587-588
   with l-transposition, 584, 588
   thrill in, 541
   tricuspid atresia with, 597-599
Ventricular septum
   intact
      d-transposition with, 584-587
      pulmonary atresia with, 591-592
   open
      d-transposition with, 587-588
      pulmonary atresia with, 594-596

Ventriculitis, 657
Verapamil
  for arrhythmias, 577
  for cardiovascular disease, 626
  dosage for, 1095
Vernix caseosa, 942
  in SGA infants, 72
Verrucous nevi, 958-959
Version and extraction, anesthesia for, 177
Vertebrae
  butterfly, 1081
  fusion of, 1050
Verumontanum, cysts of, 798
Vesicobullous eruptions, 946
Vesicoureteral reflux, 799
  radiologic identification of, 1077
  voiding cystourethrography for, 1079
Vessel thrombosis, fetal, 61
Vestibular anus, 509
Vestibular portion of acoustic nerve, 354, 355
Vestibuloocular reflex, 973-974
Vidarabine, 705
Video recording of fetal chest wall movements, 109
Villi, embryonic intestinal, 478
Villitis, 61, 63
  chronic, 212-213
  due to syphilis, 674
Villous area of placenta, 61
Vincristine, 747
Viokase, 521
Viral infections, 692-706
  biliary atresia due to, 775
  cataracts associated with, 993
  hepatitis due to, 775
  lesions due to, 947
  maternal, congenital heart disease due to, 537
  pneumonia due to, 446
Viremia, effect on fetal growth, 63
Viscosity of amniotic fluid, 136
Vision testing, 353-354
Vistaril; see Hydroxyzine
Visual acuity at birth, 974
Visual attention
  in preterm infant, 338-339
  in term infant, 337-338
Vitamin A
  blood values for, 1101
  dosage for, 1097
Vitamin B$_1$, 1097
Vitamin B$_2$, 1097
Vitamin B$_6$, 1097
Vitamin B$_{12}$
  deficiency of, 724-725
  dosage for, 1097
  malabsorption of, 523, 527
Vitamin C
  as chelation enhancer, 722
  dosage for, 1097
Vitamin D
  for chronic renal insufficiency, 792-793
  deficiency of
    in bronchopulmonary dysplasia, 474
    dietary, 876
  dosage for, 1097
  in human milk, 306

Vitamin D—cont'd
  metabolism of, 872-873
    disorders of, 876-877, 878-879
  for neonatal hepatitis, 779
Vitamin D$_3$, 872
Vitamin E
  deficiency of, 306
    anemia due to, 738-741
    in cystic fibrosis, 518
  dosage for, 1097
  to reduce risk of retrolental fibroplasia, 997
  role in resisting oxygen toxicity, 472
  serum values for, 1109
Vitamin K
  administered at birth, 158
  deficiency of, 717-718
  dosage for, 1097
  for gastrointestinal bleeding, 487
  high-dose synthetic, 759
  malabsorption of, 518
  for neonatal hepatitis, 779
Vitamins
  as antiteratogens, 158
  low birth weight infant requirement for, 306-307
  teratogenicity of, 156
  in total parenteral nutrition, 310
Vitiligo, 954
Vitreous
  diseases of, 994-998
  hemorrhage of, 225
  persistent hyperplastic primary, 998
Vivonex, 863
Vocal cords
  during breathing, 420
  effects of intubation on, 439
  paralysis of, 225-226, 462
Voiding cystourethrography, 1079
Volume-cycled ventilators, 435, 436
Volvulus
  in duodenal malrotation, 502
  associated with hydramnios, 193
  intestinal, 485
  midgut, radiology for, 1074
  of stomach, 498-499
Vomer bone, 1042
Vomerine groove, dislocation of cartilage from, 223
Vomiting
  bilious, 502
  due to gastrointestinal hemorrhage, 486
  due to hiatal hernia, 493
  in hypertrophic pyloric stenosis, 499
  in intestinal obstruction, 483
  neonatal bradycardia due to, 121
  in severe uremia, 793
Von Gierke's disease, 862-863
von Recklinghausen's disease; see Neurofibromatosis
Vulvovaginitis, 790

W

Waardenburg's syndrome
  facies in, 977-978
  heterochromia in, 992
  telecanthus in, 1043
Walls in hospital units, 292-293
Warfarin, 58

Warfarin—cont'd
  associated with congenital malformations, 153
    incidence of, 1036
  undetectable in human milk, 166
Wash basins in hospital units, 293
Wasserman antibody, 640
Wasserman test, 675
Water
  allowances of, in fluid therapy, 317, 318-319
  body, as percent of body weight, 1110
  oxidants in, methemoglobinemia due to, 733, 734
  provision of, 314-319
    adequate, determination of, 316-318
    modifiers of, 318-319
Water bed for sensory stimulation, 460
Water loss during phototherapy, 769
Water retention, and weight gain, 303
Water-soluble contrast media, 1073-1074
Waterston shunt, 588, 594, 599
Wax esters, 942
Weakness disorders, 394-398
Weaning from ventilator, 437, 474
Weeping skin, 960
  treatment for, 961
Wegner's sign, 675
Weight, as factor in renal excretion of drugs, 164
Weight gain
  effect of metabolic acidosis on, 325
  fetal, 49-50
    composition of, 53
  from human milk feeding, 303
  during intravenous nutrient administration, 312
  during pregnancy, 56-57
  during total parenteral nutrition, 311
  after transpyloric infusions, 309
Weight loss
  from diazepam in human milk, 166
  insensible, measurement of, 265
Weill-Marchesani syndrome, 999
Werdnig-Hoffmann disease, 395
  with cyanosis, 565
  differentiation from spinal cord transection, 373
  respiratory distress in, 461
Western equine encephalitis virus, 693
Wet lung, 447
White blood cells; see also Leukocytes
  in cryptococcosis, 685
  in histoplasmosis, 686
  normal counts for, 1111
  in pneumonia, 446
  in urine, 788
White classification of pregnant diabetics, 23
White matter
  as site of asphyxia, 358
  thinning of, in hydrocephalus, 377
White population
  cystic fibrosis in, 518
  malformation frequency in, 1039
White-out, radiologic, 1068
Whorl ridge patterns, 1052, 1054
William's syndrome, 63
Wilms' tumor, 532, 707, 808-810
  aniridia with, 991
  differentiation from adrenal hemorrhage, 235
  limb hypertrophy with, 1051

Wilson-Mikity syndrome, 467, 469
Wimberger's sign, 674
Wisconsin Perinatal Care Program, 8
Wiskott-Aldrich syndrome, 646
  eczema in, 961
  maldigestion in, 523, 525
  thrombocytopenia due to, 720
Withdrawal symptoms
  heroin, 934-935
  methadone, 935-936
  from narcotics in human milk, 167
  phenobarbital, 937
Wolffian ducts, development of, 901-902
Wolff-Parkinson-White syndrome, 578-579
  electrocardiographic findings in, 547, 548
Wolman's disease, 839
  maldigestion in, 523, 527
Wood's lamp examination, 955
Workshop in Gestational Diabetes (1979), 22-23
Wormian bones, 1084
Wright's stain, 686
Wrist-drop due to peripheral nerve injuries, 236

X

X cells, 211
X chromosome
  deletion of, 909
  disorders carried on, 1024
  G6PD gene on, 735
  monosomy, 1016
  in ovarian development, 904-905
Xanthochromia, 372
  in hydrocephalus, 375
Xanthogranuloma, juvenile, 961
Xanthoma, cutaneous, 776
Xanthomatosis, 836
Xenobiotic compounds, need to eliminate, 163
Xeroderma pigmentosum, 953
X-irradiation for retinoblastoma, 995
X-linked ichthyosis, 945
X-linked inheritance patterns, 1023-1024
45,XO anomaly, 1036, 1038
XX gonadal dysgenesis, 909
47,XXX anomaly, 1036
XXXXX syndrome, 538
XXXXY syndrome, 538
47,XXY syndrome, 911-912, 1036
XY gonadal agenesis, 911
XY gonadal dysgenesis, 910
Xylocaine; see Lidocaine
Xylose, 755
47,XYY anomaly, 1036

Y

Y chromosome
  abnormal, 908-909
  extra, in renal agenesis, 793
  gonadal differentiation controlled by, 904
Y protein, 755
Yeast phagocytosis, 643
Yeast phase antigen, 686
Yersinia, 662
Y-fluorescent bodies, 1029
Yolk sac, 206
Yusho disease, 168

Yutopar; *see* Ritodrine

Z

Z form of bilirubin, 729
Z protein, 754
Zellweger's syndrome
    cortical dysplasia in, 796
    joint deformities in, 1059
Zeroing of pressure transducers, 114
Zinc
    human milk content of, 306
Zinc—cont'd
    intrauterine accumulation of, 306
    metabolic defects of, 950
Zinc oxide, 961
Zinc sulfate, 950
Zygomatic arch, 1042
    absence of, 977
Zygote, period of, adverse drug effects during, 152
Zymogen, embryonic activity of, 480
Z-plasty for constriction bands, 1008